Handbook of
SMALL
ANIMAL
PRACTICE

SECTION EDITORS

Section II: *Cardiovascular System*
Matthew W. Miller, D.V.M., M.S.

Section III: *Respiratory System*
Brendan C. McKiernan, D.V.M.

Section IV: *Neurologic System*
Karen Dyer Inzana, D.V.M., Ph.D.

Section V: *Digestive System*
Albert E. Jergens, D.V.M., M.S.

Section VI: *Endocrine and Metabolic System*
C. B. Chastain, D.V.M., M.S.

Section VII: *Urinary System*
Gregory F. Grauer, D.V.M., M.S.

Section VIII: *Reproductive System*
Janice L. Cain, D.V.M.

Section IX: *Hemolymphatic System*
Karen M. Young, V.M.D., Ph.D.

Section X: *Immune System*
Kevin T. Schultz, D.V.M., Ph.D.

Section XI: *Musculoskeletal System*
Joseph Harari, D.V.M., M.S.

Section XII: *Dermatologic System*
Diane E. Bevier, D.V.M.

Section XIII: *Diseases of the Eye*
Cynthia S. Cook, D.V.M., Ph.D.

Section XV: *Infectious Diseases*
Johnny D. Hoskins, D.V.M., Ph.D.

RHEA V. MORGAN, D.V.M.

Diplomate
American College of Veterinary Internal Medicine and
American College of Veterinary Ophthalmologists
Chief of Staff
Rowley Memorial Animal Hospital
Springfield, Massachusetts

Handbook of
SMALL
ANIMAL
PRACTICE

3rd Edition

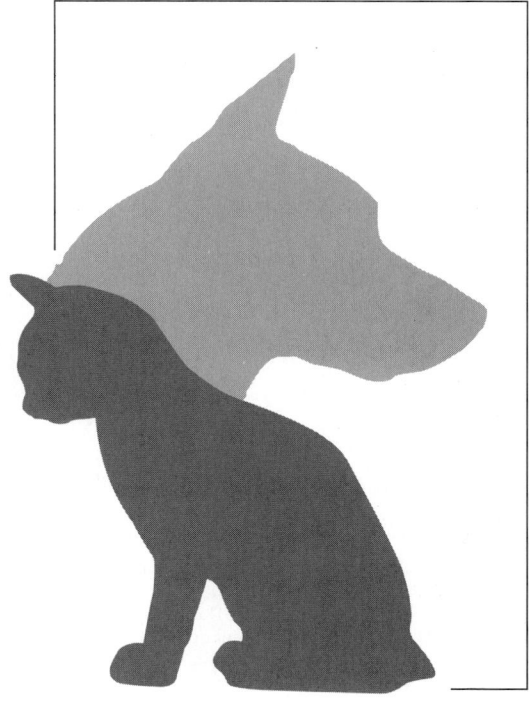

W.B. SAUNDERS COMPANY
A Division of Harcourt Brace & Company
Philadelphia London Toronto Montreal Sydney Tokyo

W.B. SAUNDERS COMPANY
A Division of Harcourt Brace & Company

The Curtis Center
Independence Square West
Philadelphia, Pennsylvania 19106

Library of Congress Cataloging-in-Publication Data

Handbook of small animal practice / [edited by] Rhea V. Morgan—3rd ed.

p.   cm.

ISBN 0–7216–3329–3

1. Dogs—Diseases—Outlines, syllabi, etc.   2. Cats—Diseases—Outlines,
syllabi, etc. 3. Dogs—Physiology—Outlines, syllabi, etc.
4. Cats—Physiology—Outlines, syllabi, etc.   5. Pet medicine—Outlines,
syllabi, etc.   I. Morgan, Rhea Volk.

SF991.H228 1997

636.7′089—dc20   96-45945

HANDBOOK OF SMALL ANIMAL PRACTICE, 3rd edition   ISBN 0–7216–3329–3

Printed in the United States of America.

Last digit is the print number: 9   8   7   6   5   4   3   2

The third edition of the
Handbook of Small Animal Practice
is dedicated to my parents:

Louis and Joyce Volk

*They rose from humble beginnings and survived difficult
times to raise a large, close-knit family. They taught us the
importance of education, hard work, and dedication to the
task at hand. They gave us simple and good rules to live by:
be honest, forthright, kind, compassionate. They encouraged
us to explore the world and travel to far-off places, but
also reminded us to never forget family, church, and our
local community. They trained us to be independent and to
think for ourselves, and always supported us in whatever
endeavor we chose to attempt. For all the 56 years of their
married life, their love and devotion to us have been
unwavering. For that, and for all they have given us, I will
be eternally grateful.*

With love,
Rhea

Contributors

William H. Abbott, D.V.M., M.S.
Resident in Dermatology, Animal Allergy and Dermatology, Virginia Beach, VA
Idiopathic Dermatoses

Lowell J. Ackerman, D.V.M.
Diplomate, American College of Veterinary Dermatology; Dermatology Consultant, Scottsdale, AZ
Immune-Mediated Skin Diseases

Richard K. Anderson, D.V.M.
Diplomate, American College of Veterinary Dermatology; Staff Dermatologist, Angell Memorial Animal Hospital, Boston, MA
Nutritional Disorders of the Skin

Jeanne A. Barsanti, D.V.M., M.S.
Diplomate, American College of Veterinary Internal Medicine; Professor, Department of Small Animal Medicine, College of Veterinary Medicine, University of Georgia, Athens, GA
Diseases of the Prostate Gland

Claudia L. Barton, D.V.M.
Diplomate, American College of Veterinary Internal Medicine; Professor, Department of Small Animal Medicine and Surgery, College of Veterinary Medicine, Texas A&M University, College Station, TX
Diseases of the Uterus

Ann D. Beebe, D.V.M.
Resident in Animal Behavior, Department of Clinical Studies, School of Veterinary Medicine, University of Pennsylvania, Philadelphia, PA
Feline Behavioral Disorders

Philip J. Bergman, D.V.M., M.S.
American Cancer Society PRTA Fellow, Department of Cell Biology, M.D. Anderson Cancer Center; Medical Oncologist, Gulf Coast Veterinary Oncology and Specialists, Houston, TX
Paraneoplastic Syndromes

Kristen A. Bernard, D.V.M., Ph.D.
Postdoctoral Fellow, Department of Microbiology and Immunology, University of North Carolina–Chapel Hill, Chapel Hill, NC
Immune-Mediated Diseases

Diane E. Bevier, D.V.M.
Diplomate, American College of Veterinary Dermatology; Medical and Technical Consultation, Heska Corporation, Fort Collins, CO
Introduction (Dermatologic System); Degenerative Skin Diseases

Julia T. Blue, D.V.M., Ph.D.
Associate Professor of Clinical Pathology, Department of Pathology, College of Veterinary Medicine, Cornell University, Ithaca, NY
Disorders of the Spleen

John D. Bonagura, D.V.M., M.S.
Diplomate, American College of Veterinary Internal Medicine; Gilbreath-McLorn Professor of Veterinary Cardiology, College of Veterinary Medicine, University of Missouri, Columbia, MO
Congenital Diseases

Mary K. Boudreaux, D.V.M., Ph.D.
Associate Professor, Department of Pathobiology, College of Veterinary Medicine, Auburn University, Auburn, AL
Platelet and Coagulation Disorders

Ronald M. Bright, D.V.M., M.S.
Diplomate, American College of Veterinary Surgeons; Alumni Distinguished Service Professor and Professor of Surgery, Department of Small Animal Clinical Sciences, College of Veterinary Medicine, University of Tennessee, Knoxville, TN
Diseases of the Salivary Glands

Michele M. Brignac, D.V.M.
Staff Dermatologist, Emerald Coast Veterinary Specialists, Fort Walton Beach, FL
Degenerative Skin Diseases

Scott A. Brown, V.M.D., Ph.D.
Associate Professor, Department of Physiology and Pharmacology and Department of Small Animal Medicine, College of Veterinary Medicine, University of Georgia, Athens, GA
Diseases of the Kidney

Douglas E. Brum, D.V.M.
Staff Veterinarian, Director of Wellness Service, Angell Memorial Animal Hospital, Boston, MA
Selected Diagnostic and Therapeutic Procedures

Robert G. Buerger, D.V.M.
Diplomate, American College of Veterinary Dermatology; Veterinary Dermatology Center, Baltimore, MD
Congenital/Developmental Dermatoses

Susan E. Bunch, D.V.M., Ph.D.
Diplomate, American College of Veterinary Internal Medicine; Professor of Medicine, Department of Companion Animal and Special Species Medicine, College of Veterinary Medicine, North Carolina State University, Raleigh, NC
Diseases of the Large Intestine

Janice L. Cain, D.V.M.
Diplomate, American College of Veterinary Internal Medicine; Staff Internist, Norris Canyon Veterinary Medical Center, San Ramon, CA
Introduction (Reproductive System); Diseases of the Ovaries; Diseases of the Uterus; Disorders of Canine Reproduction; Disorders of Feline Reproduction

Karen L. Campbell, D.V.M., M.S.
Diplomate, American College of Veterinary Dermatology and American College of Veterinary Internal Medicine; Associate Professor, Department of Veterinary Clinical Medicine, College of Veterinary Medicine, University of Illinois, Urbana, IL
Infectious Skin Diseases

Thomas L. Carson, D.V.M., M.S., Ph.D.
Diplomate, American Board of Veterinary Toxicology; Professor of Veterinary Pathology, Veterinary Diagnostic Laboratory, College of Veterinary Medicine, Iowa State University, Ames, IA
Introduction (Toxicology); Rodenticides; Insecticides and Mulluscacides; Herbicides; Bacterial and Mold Toxins; Household and Metal Toxicants; Household Drugs; Toxic Plants and Zootoxins; Adverse Drug Reactions

C. B. Chastain, D.V.M., M.S.
Diplomate, American College of Veterinary Internal Medicine; Associate Dean for Academic Affairs, College of Veterinary Medicine, University of Missouri, Columbia, MO
Introduction (Endocrine and Metabolic System)

Cynthia S. Cook, D.V.M., Ph.D.
Diplomate, American College of Veterinary Ophthalmologists; Research Assistant Professor, Department of Growth and Development, University of California, San Francisco, CA; Ophthalmologist, Veterinary Vision, San Mateo, CA
Introduction (Diseases of the Eye); Diseases of the Orbit

Autumn P. Davidson, D.V.M.
Diplomate, American College of Veterinary Internal Medicine; Associate Professor, University of California, Davis, CA; Staff Internist, Encina Veterinary Hospital, Walnut Creek, CA
Disorders of Canine Reproduction

Jacqueline R. Davidson, D.V.M., M.S.
Diplomate, American College of Veterinary Surgeons; Assistant Professor of Companion Animal Surgery, Department of Veterinary Clinical Science, School of Veterinary Medicine, Louisiana State University, Baton Rouge, LA
Diseases of Muscles and Tendons

Michael G. Davidson, D.V.M.
Diplomate, American College of Veterinary Ophthalmologists; Associate Professor of Ophthalmology, Department of Companion Animal and Special Species Medicine, College of Veterinary Medicine, North Carolina State University, Raleigh, NC
Diseases of the Anterior Uveal Tract

Linda J. DeBowes, D.V.M., M.S.
Diplomate, American College of Veterinary Internal Medicine and American Veterinary Dental College; Associate Professor, Department of Clinical Sciences, College of Veterinary Medicine, Kansas State University, Manhattan, KS
Diseases of the Oral Cavity and Pharynx

Robert C. DeNovo, Jr., D.V.M., M.S.
Diplomate, American College of Veterinary Internal Medicine; Associate Professor of Medicine, Department of Small Animal Clinical Sciences, College of Veterinary Medicine, University of Tennessee, Knoxville, TN
Diseases of the Stomach

Nishi Dhupa, B.V.M.
Diplomate, American College of Veterinary Internal Medicine and American College of Veterinary Emergency and Critical Care; Assistant Clinical Professor, Department of Medicine, Tufts University School of Veterinary Medicine North Grafton, MA
Burns; Hypothermia and Frostbite

David A. Dzanis, D.V.M., Ph.D.
Diplomate, American College of Veterinary Nutrition; Veterinary Nutritionist, U.S. Food & Drug Administration, Center for Veterinary Medicine, Rockville, MD
Introduction (Nutritional Disorders); Nutrition Through the Life Cycle; Disorders of Nutritional Deficiency; Disorders of Nutritional Excess

Robert V. English, D.V.M., Ph.D.
Diplomate, American College of Veterinary Ophthalmologists; Visiting Assistant Professor, Department of Companion Animals and Special Species, College of Veterinary Medicine, North Carolina State University, Raleigh, NC
Diseases of the Lens and Vitreous

Alicia M. Faggella, D.V.M.
Diplomate, American College of Veterinary Emergency and Critical Care; Director, Intensive Care Unit, Angell Memorial Animal Hospital, Boston, MA
Introduction to Critical Care; Electric Cord and Smoke Inhalation Injuries

Peter J. Felsburg, V.M.D., Ph.D.
Trustee Professor of Clinical Immunology, Chairman, Department of Clinical Studies, School of Veterinary Medicine, University of Pennsylvania, Philadelphia, PA
Immunodeficiency Disorders

David J. Fisher, D.V.M.
Diplomate, American College of Veterinary Pathologists; Veterinary Clinical Pathologist, CVD/IDEXX Veterinary Services, Inc., West Sacramento, CA
Disorders of Red Blood Cells

Carol S. Foil, D.V.M., M.S.
Diplomate, American College of Veterinary Dermatology; Professor, Department of Veterinary Clinical Sciences, School of Veterinary Medicine, Louisiana State University, Baton Rouge, LA
Infectious Skin Diseases

Theresa W. Fossum, D.V.M., M.S., Ph.D.
Diplomate, American College of Veterinary Surgeons; Associate Professor, Department of Small Animal Medicine and Surgery, College of Veterinary Medicine, Texas A&M University, College Station, TX
Pleural Cavity Diseases

Joni L. Freshman, D.V.M., M.S.
Diplomate, American College of Veterinary Internal Medicine; East Springs Animal Hospital, Colorado Springs, CO
Diseases of the Testes and Epididymides

Angela E. Frimberger, V.M.D.
Diplomate, American College of Veterinary Internal Medicine; Postdoctoral Research Fellow, Cancer Center, University of Massachusetts, Worcester, MA
Principles of Oncology

Urs Giger, Dr.Med.Vet., M.S.
Diplomate, American College of Veterinary Internal Medicine; Professor of Medicine and Medical Genetics, Chief, Section of Medical Genetics, School of Veterinary Medicine, University of Pennsylvania, Philadelphia, PA
Transfusion Medicine; Immunodeficiency Disorders

Michael H. Goldschmidt, M.Sc., B.V.M.S., M.R.C.V.S.
Diplomate, American College of Veterinary Pathologists; Professor, Veterinary Pathology, and Chief, Surgical Pathology, School of Veterinary Medicine, University of Pennsylvania, Philadelphia, PA
Cutaneous Neoplasia

Melissa F. Goodman, D.V.M.
Veterinary Referral Center, Frazer, PA
Disorders of Canine Reproduction

W. Dunbar Gram, D.V.M.
Diplomate, American College of Veterinary Dermatology; Clinical Dermatologist, Animal Allergy and Dermatology, Virginia Beach, VA
Idiopathic Dermatoses

Gregory F. Grauer, D.V.M., M.S.
Diplomate, American College of Veterinary Internal Medicine; Professor, Department of Clinical Sciences, Section Chief, Small Animal Medicine, College of Veterinary Medicine and Biomedical Sciences, Colorado State University, Fort Collins, CO
Introduction (Urinary System); Diseases of the Kidney

Jean A. Hall, D.V.M., Ph.D.
Diplomate, American College of Veterinary Internal Medicine; Assistant Professor, Veterinary Teaching Hospital, College of Veterinary Medicine, Oregon State University, Corvallis, OR
Diseases of the Exocrine Pancreas

Terrance A. Hamilton, D.V.M.
Diplomate, American College of Veterinary Internal Medicine; Veterinary Oncologist, Veterinary Referral Clinic, Cleveland, OH
Pulmonary Parenchymal Disorders

Joseph Harari, D.V.M., M.S.
Diplomate, American College of Veterinary Surgeons; Director of Surgery, Rowley Memorial Animal Hospital, Springfield, MA
Introduction (Musculoskeletal System); Diseases of Bone

Lori Ellen Hartzband, D.V.M.
Diplomate, American College of Veterinary Radiology; Staff Radiologist, Angell Memorial Animal Hospital, Boston, MA
Contrast Radiography

Jean-Pierre Held, Dr.Med.Vet.
Diplomate, American College of Theriogenologists; Associate Professor, Department of Large Animal Clinical Sciences, College of Veterinary Medicine, University of Tennessee, Knoxville, TN
Diseases of the External Genitalia

Stuart C. Helfand, D.V.M.
Diplomate, American College of Veterinary Internal Medicine, Associate Professor, Department of Medical Sciences, School of Veterinary Medicine, University of Wisconsin, Madison, WI
Immunoproliferative Diseases; Diseases of the Thymus

Mark E. Hitt, D.V.M., M.S.
Diplomate, American College of Veterinary Internal Medicine and American Board of Veterinary Practitioners; Chief of Medicine, Atlantic Veterinary Internal Medicine at Chesapeake Veterinary Referral Center, Annapolis, MD
Diseases of the Oral Cavity and Pharynx; Miscellaneous Endocrine and Metabolic Disorders

Giselle Hosgood, B.V.Sc., M.S.
Diplomate, American College of Veterinary Surgeons; Associate Professor of Companion Animal Surgery, Department of Veterinary Clinical Sciences, School of Veterinary Medicine, Louisiana State University, Baton Rouge, LA
Diseases of Muscles and Tendons

Johnny D. Hoskins, D.V.M., Ph.D.
Diplomate, American College of Veterinary Internal Medicine; Professor Emeritus, Department of Veterinary Clinical Sciences, Louisiana State University School of Veterinary Medicine, Baton Rouge, LA
Introduction (Infectious Diseases); Viral Infections; Bacterial Infections; Mixed Infections; Rickettsial Infections

Thomas N. Hribernik, D.V.M.
Diplomate, American College of Veterinary Internal Medicine; Staff Internist, Friendship Veterinary Clinic, Inc., Ft. Walton, FL
Rickettsial Infections

Karen Dyer Inzana, D.V.M., Ph.D.
Diplomate, American College of Veterinary Internal Medicine; Associate Professor, Department of Small Animal Clinical Sciences, Virginia–Maryland Regional College of Veterinary Medicine, Virginia Polytechnic Institute, Blacksburg, VA
Introduction (Neurologic System); Disorders of Peripheral Nerves

John D. Jacobson, D.V.M., M.S.
Diplomate, American College of Veterinary Anesthesiologists; Associate Professor, Department of Small Animal Clinical Sciences, Virginia–Maryland Regional College of Veterinary Medicine, Virginia Polytechnic Institute, Blacksburg, VA
Cardiopulmonary Resuscitation

Christine C. Jenkins, D.V.M.
Diplomate, American College of Veterinary Internal Medicine; Adjunct Associate Professor of Medicine, Department of Small Animal Clinical Sciences, College of Veterinary Medicine, University of Tennessee, Knoxville, TN
Diseases of the Stomach

Albert E. Jergens, D.V.M., M.S.
Diplomate, American College of Veterinary Internal Medicine; Associate Professor, Department of Veterinary Clinical Sciences, College of Veterinary Medicine, Iowa State University, Ames, IA
Introduction (Digestive System); Diseases of the Esophagus; Miscellaneous Endocrine and Metabolic Disorders

Lynelle Johnson, D.V.M., M.S.
Diplomate, American College of Veterinary Internal Medicine; Ph.D. Candidate, Department of Veterinary Biomedical Sciences, University of Missouri, Columbia, MO
Diseases of the Trachea

Thomas J. Kern, D.V.M.
Diplomate, American College of Veterinary Ophthalmologists; Associate Professor of Ophthalmology, Department of Clinical Sciences, College of Veterinary Medicine, Cornell University, Ithaca, NY
Disorders of the Lacrimal and Nasolacrimal System

Richard D. Kienle, D.V.M.
Diplomate, American College of Veterinary Internal Medicine; Staff Cardiologist, Mission Valley Veterinary Cardiology, Gilroy, CA
Pericardial Diseases

Rebecca Kirby, D.V.M.
Diplomate, American College of Veterinary Internal Medicine and American College of Veterinary Emergency and Critical Care; Adjunct Assistant Professor, Department of Small Animal Surgery, School of Veterinary Medicine, University of Wisconsin, Madison, WI; Chief of Medicine, Animal Emergency Center, Milwaukee, WI
Acute Abdomen Syndrome

Susan E. Kirschner, D.V.M.
Diplomate, American College of Veterinary Ophthalmologists; Ophthalmologist, Oregon Veterinary Referral Center, Portland, OR
Diseases of the Cornea and Sclera

Barbara E. Kitchell, D.V.M., Ph.D.
Diplomate, American College of Veterinary Internal Medicine; Assistant Professor of Medicine, Department of Veterinary Clinical Medicine, College of Veterinary Medicine, University of Illinois, Urbana, IL
Diseases of the Mammary Glands

Joyce S. Knoll, V.M.D., Ph.D.
Diplomate, American College of Veterinary Pathologists; Assistant Professor, Department of Pathology, Section Head in Clinical Pathology, Tufts Veterinary Diagnostic Laboratory, Tufts University School of Veterinary Medicine; North Grafton, MA
Disorders of White Blood Cells

Kim Knowles, D.V.M., M.S.
Diplomate, American College of Veterinary Internal Medicine; Assistant Professor of Medicine, Department of Medicine, Tufts University School of Veterinary Medicine, North Grafton, MA
Diseases of the Middle and Inner Ear; Deafness

D. J. Krahwinkel, Jr., D.V.M., M.S.
Diplomate, American College of Veterinary Surgeons and American College of Veterinary Anesthesiologists; Professor of Surgery, Head, Department of Small Animal Clinical Sciences, College of Veterinary Medicine, University of Tennessee, Knoxville, TN
Diseases of the Anus and Perineum

India F. Lane, D.V.M., M.S.
Diplomate, American College of Veterinary Internal Medicine; Assistant Professor and Medicine Service Chief, Department of Companion Animals, Atlantic Veterinary College, University of Prince Edward Island; Charlottetown, Prince Edward Island, Canada
Disorders of Micturition

Michael R. Lappin, D.V.M., Ph.D.
Diplomate, American College of Veterinary Internal Medicine; Associate Professor, Department of Clinical Sciences, College of Veterinary Medicine and Biomedical Sciences, Colorado State University, Fort Collins, CO
Protozoal Infections

Linda B. Lehmkuhl, D.V.M., M.S.
Diplomate, American College of Veterinary Internal Medicine; Assistant Professor, Department of Veterinary Clinical Sciences, College of Veterinary Medicine, Ohio State University, Columbus, OH
Congenital Diseases

Cynthia R. Leveille-Webster, D.V.M.
Diplomate, American College of Veterinary Internal Medicine; Assistant Professor, Department of Medicine, Tufts University School of Veterinary Medicine, North Grafton, MA
Diseases of the Hepatobiliary System

Denise M. Lindley, D.V.M., M.S.
Diplomate, American College of Veterinary Ophthalmologists; President, Animal Eye Consultants, Crestwood, IL
Diseases of the Eyelids

Andrew S. Loar, D.V.M.
Diplomate, American College of Veterinary Internal Medicine
Diseases of the Mammary Glands

Cheryl A. London, D.V.M.
Diplomate, American College of Veterinary Internal Medicine; Postdoctoral Research Fellow, Immunology Research Division, Department of Pathology, Harvard Medical School and Brigham and Women's Hospital, Boston, MA
Principles of Oncology

Jody P. Lulich, D.V.M., Ph.D.
Diplomate, American College of Veterinary Internal Medicine; Associate Professor, Department of Small Animal Clinical Sciences, College of Veterinary Medicine, University of Minnesota, St. Paul, MN
Diseases of the Ureter; Diseases of the Urinary Bladder

Ann Marie Manning, D.V.M.
Resident in Emergency and Critical Care Medicine, Department of Medicine, Tufts University School of Veterinary Medicine, North Grafton, MA
Heat Prostration

Christiane Massicotte, D.V.M.
Resident in Neurology, Department of Small Animal Clinical Sciences, Virginia–Maryland Regional College of Veterinary Medicine, Virginia Polytechnic Institute, Blacksburg, VA
Disorders of Peripheral Nerves

Michael E. Matz, D.V.M.
Diplomate, American College of Veterinary Internal Medi-

cine; Staff Internist, Southwest Veterinary Specialty Center, Tucson, AZ
Acute Gastric Dilatation-Volvulus

Dianne Mawby, D.V.M., M.V.Sc.
Diplomate, American College of Veterinary Internal Medicine; Clinical Instructor, Department of Small Animal Clinical Sciences, College of Veterinary Medicine, University of Tennessee, Knoxville, TN
General Physical Examination of the Dog and Cat

Paul E. McCarthy, D.V.M.
Diplomate, American College of Veterinary Surgeons; Assistant Professor of Surgery, College of Veterinary Medicine, Mississippi State University, Starkville, MS
Diseases of the External Ear and Pinna

Robert K. McDonald, D.V.M.
Diplomate, American College of Veterinary Internal Medicine; Internal Medicine Dermatology Clinic, Starkville, MS
Diseases of the Pituitary Gland

Brendan C. McKiernan, D.V.M.
Diplomate, American College of Veterinary Internal Medicine; Professor of Medicine, Department of Veterinary Clinical Medicine, College of Veterinary Medicine, University of Illinois, Urbana, IL
Introduction (Respiratory System); Diseases of the Nasal and Nasopharyngeal Cavities and Paranasal Sinuses

Linda Medleau, D.V.M., M.S.
Diplomate, American College of Veterinary Dermatology; Professor of Dermatology, Department of Small Animal Medicine, College of Veterinary Medicine, University of Georgia, Athens, GA
Parasitic Skin Diseases

Sandra R. Merchant, D.V.M.
Diplomate, American College of Veterinary Dermatology; Associate Professor of Dermatology, Department of Veterinary Clinical Sciences, School of Veterinary Medicine, Louisiana State University, Baton Rouge, LA
Introduction (Diseases of the Ear); Diseases of the External Ear and Pinna

Kathryn M. Meurs, D.V.M.
Assistant Professor, Department of Veterinary Clinical Sciences, College of Veterinary Medicine, Ohio State University, Columbus, OH
Myocardial Disease

Matthew W. Miller, D.V.M., M.S.
Diplomate, American College of Veterinary Internal Medicine; Associate Professor of Cardiology, Department of Small Animal Medicine and Surgery, College of Veterinary Medicine, Texas A&M University, College Station, TX
Introduction (Cardiovascular System); Heartworm Disease

Jaime F. Modiano, V.M.D., Ph.D.
Assistant Professor, Department of Veterinary Pathobiology, College of Veterinary Medicine, Texas A&M University, College Station, TX
Immunoproliferative Diseases; Diseases of the Thymus

William E. Monroe, D.V.M., M.S.
Diplomate, American College of Veterinary Internal Medicine; Associate Professor, Department of Small Animal Clinical Sciences, Virginia–Maryland Regional College of Veterinary Medicine, Virginia Polytechnic Institute, Blacksburg, VA
Diseases of the Parathyroid Glands

Cecil P. Moore, D.V.M., M.S.
Diplomate, American College of Veterinary Ophthalmologists; Associate Professor and Ophthalmology Section Chief, Department of Veterinary Medicine and Surgery, College of Veterinary Medicine, University of Missouri, Columbia, MO
Disorders of the Conjunctiva and Third Eyelid

Frances M. Moore, D.V.M.
Diplomate, American College of Veterinary Pathologists; Section Head, Veterinary Division, Marshfield Laboratories, Marshfield, WI
Diseases of the Peritoneum

Rhea V. Morgan, D.V.M.
Diplomate, American College of Veterinary Internal Medicine and American College of Veterinary Ophthalmologists; Chief of Staff, Rowley Memorial Animal Hospital, Springfield, MA
Collection and Interpretation of Laboratory Data; Selected Diagnostic and Therapeutic Procedures

Karen A. Moriello, D.V.M.
Diplomate, American College of Veterinary Dermatology; Clinical Associate Professor of Dermatology, Department of Medical Science, School of Veterinary Medicine, University of Wisconsin, Madison, WI
Inflammatory Skin Diseases

Karen R. Muñana, D.V.M., M.S.
Diplomate, American College of Veterinary Internal Medicine; Assistant Professor, Department of Companion Animal and Special Species Medicine, College of Veterinary Medicine, North Carolina State University, Raleigh, NC
Disorders of the Brain

Robert J. Murtaugh, D.V.M., M.S.
Diplomate, American College of Veterinary Internal Medical and American College of Veterinary Emergency and Critical Care; Professor, Department of Medicine, Tufts University School of Veterinary Medicine, North Grafton, MA
Heat Prostration

Rhett Nichols, D.V.M.
Diplomate, American College of Veterinary Internal Medicine; Eastern Regional Director of Consulting Services, Antech Diagnostics, Farmingdale, NY
Diseases of the Pituitary Gland; Diseases of the Adrenal Gland

Carl A. Osborne, D.V.M., Ph.D.
Diplomate, American College of Veterinary Internal Medicine; Professor, Department of Small Animal Clinical Sciences, College of Veterinary Medicine, University of Minnesota, St. Paul, MN
Diseases of the Ureter; Diseases of the Urinary Bladder

Gary D. Osweiler, D.V.M., M.S., Ph.D.
Diplomate, American Board of Veterinary Toxicology; Professor of Veterinary Toxicology; Director, Iowa State University Veterinary Diagnostic Laboratory, College of Veterinary Medicine, Iowa State University, Ames, IA
Introduction (Toxicology); Rodenticides; Insecticides and Molluscacides; Herbicides; Bacterial and Mold Toxins; Household and Metal Toxicants; Household Drugs; Toxic Plants and Zootoxins; Adverse Drug Reactions

Karen L. Overall, V.M.D., Ph.D.
Diplomate, American College of Veterinary Behaviorists; Consultant, Animal Behavior, Department of Clinical Studies, School of Veterinary Medicine, University of Pennsylvania, Philadelphia, PA
Introduction (Behavioral Disorders); Canine Behavioral Disorders; Feline Behavioral Disorders

Mark A. Oyama, D.V.M.
Resident in Cardiology, Department of Medicine, School of Veterinary Medicine, University of California, Davis, CA
Pericardial Diseases

Philip Padrid, D.V.M.
Assistant Professor of Medicine and Immunology, Section of Pulmonary and Critical Care Medicine, Chief of Academic Programs, Department of Comparative Medicine and Pathology, University of Chicago, Chicago, IL
Diseases of the Lower Airway

David L. Panciera, D.V.M., M.S.
Diplomate, American College of Veterinary Internal Medicine; Staff Internist, Alameda East Veterinary Hospital, Denver, CO
Diseases of the Thyroid Glands

Michael M. Pavletic, D.V.M.
Diplomate, American College of Veterinary Surgeons; Professor of Surgery, Department of Surgery, Tufts University School of Veterinary Medicine, North Grafton, MA
Burns

Robert L. Peiffer, Jr., D.V.M., Ph.D.
Diplomate, American College of Veterinary Ophthalmologists; Professor and Director of Laboratories, Departments of Ophthalmology and Pathology, School of Medicine, University of North Carolina, Chapel Hill, NC; Staff Ophthalmologist, Animal Ophthalmology of North Carolina and Virginia, Durham NC
Glaucoma

Mark E. Peterson, D.V.M.
Diplomate, American College of Veterinary Internal Medicine; Head, Division of Endocrinology, Department of Medicine, Associate Director, Caspary Research Institute, Animal Medical Center, New York, NY
Diseases of the Adrenal Gland

Michael Podell, M.Sc., D.V.M.
Diplomate, American College of Veterinary Internal Medicine; Assistant Professor, Director, Comparative Neurology Service, Department of Veterinary Clinical Sciences, College of Veterinary Medicine, Ohio State University, Columbus, OH
Seizures and Sleep Disorders

Philip E. Prater, D.V.M.
Diplomate, American College of Theriogenologists; Bedford Hill Veterinary Hospital, Paris, KY
Diseases of the External Genitalia

James C. Prueter, D.V.M.
Diplomate, American College of Veterinary Internal Medicine; Director of Operations, Veterinary Referral Clinic, Cleveland, OH
Pulmonary Parenchymal Disorders

Steven M. Roberts, D.V.M., M.S.
Diplomate, American College of Veterinary Ophthalmologists; Associate Professor of Ophthalmology, Department of Clinical Sciences, College of Veterinary Medicine and Biomedical Sciences, Colorado State University, Fort Collins, CO
Neuro-ophthalmology

Kenita S. Rogers, D.V.M., M.S.
Diplomate, American College of Veterinary Internal Medicine; Associate Professor, Department of Small Animal Medicine and Surgery, College of Veterinary Medicine, Texas A&M University, College Station, TX
Diseases of the Mediastinum

Rodney A. W. Rosychuk, D.V.M.
Diplomate, American College of Veterinary Internal Medicine; Assistant Professor, Department of Clinical Sciences, College of Veterinary Medicine and Biomedical Sciences, Colorado State University, Fort Collins, CO
Endocrine/Metabolic Skin Diseases

James K. Roush, D.V.M., M.S.
Diplomate, American College of Veterinary Surgeons; Associate Professor, Department of Clinical Sciences, College of Veterinary Medicine, Kansas State University, Manhattan, KS
Diseases of Joints and Ligaments

Michael Schaer, D.V.M.
Diplomate, American College of Veterinary Internal Medicine and American College of Veterinary Emergency and Critical Care; Professor and Associate Department Chair, Department of Small Animal Clinical Sciences, College of Veterinary Medicine, University of Florida, Gainesville, FL
Diseases of the Endocrine Pancreas (Islet Cells)

Kevin T. Schultz, D.V.M., Ph.D.
Executive Director, Worldwide Animal Science Research and Development, Merck & Company, Rahway, NJ
Introduction (Immune System)

Howard B. Seim, III, D.V.M.
Diplomate, American College of Veterinary Surgeons; Associate Professor, Chief, Small Animal Surgery, Department of Clinical Sciences, College of Veterinary Medicine and Biomedical Sciences, Colorado State University, Fort Collins, CO
Diseases of the Urethra

Frances S. Shofer, Ph.D.
Adjunct Assistant Professor of Epidemiology and Biostatistics, School of Veterinary Medicine, University of Pennsylvania, Philadelphia, PA
Cutaneous Neoplasia

Susan F. Soderberg, D.V.M.
Diplomate, American College of Veterinary Internal Medicine; East Detroit Animal Hospital, Eastpointe, MI
Disorders of the Canine Vagina

Rebecca L. Stepien, D.V.M., M.S.
Diplomate, American College of Veterinary Internal Medicine; Clinical Assistant Professor, Department of Medical Sciences, School of Veterinary Medicine, University of Wisconsin, Madison, WI
Dysrhythmias

Steven J. Susaneck, D.V.M., M.S.
Diplomate, American College of Veterinary Internal Medicine; Greater Houston Veterinary Specialists, Houston, TX
Diseases of the Ovaries

James F. Swanson, D.V.M., M.S.
Diplomate, American College of Veterinary Ophthalmologists; Veterinary Ophthalmologist, Gulf Coast Animal Eye Clinic, P.C., Houston, TX
Ocular Manifestations of Systemic Disease

Margaret S. Swartout, D.V.M.
Diplomate, American College of Veterinary Internal Medicine; Veterinary Specialty Consultation Service, Inc., Knoxville, TN
Endocrine/Metabolic Skin Diseases

Joseph Taboada, D.V.M.
Diplomate, American College of Veterinary Internal Medicine; Associate Professor, Department of Veterinary Clinical Sciences, Interim Director of Professional Instruction and Curriculum, School of Veterinary Medicine, Louisiana State University, Baton Rouge, LA
Systemic Mycoses

William B. Thomas, D.V.M., M.S.
Diplomate, American College of Veterinary Internal Medicine; Assistant Professor of Neurology/Neurosurgery, Department of Small Animal Clinical Sciences, College of

Veterinary Medicine, University of Tennessee, Knoxville, TN
Disorders of the Spinal Cord

Leland Thompson, D.V.M.
Research Scientist, Department of Clinical Development, Pfizer Animal Health Group, Lee's Summit, MO
Diseases of the Pituitary Gland; Diseases of the Adrenal Gland

David M. Vail, D.V.M., M.S.
Diplomate, American College of Veterinary Internal Medicine; Associate Professor of Oncology, Department of Medical Sciences, School of Veterinary Medicine, University of Wisconsin, Madison, WI
Diseases of the Thyroid Glands; Diseases of Lymph Nodes and Lymphatics

Anjop J. Venker-van Haagen, D.V.M., Ph.D.
Diplomate, European College of Veterinary Surgeons; Associated Professor, Department of Clinical Sciences of Companion Animals, Faculty of Veterinary Medicine, University of Utrecht, Utrecht, The Netherlands
Diseases of the Larynx

Melissa S. Wallace, D.V.M.
Diplomate, American College of Veterinary Internal Medicine; Staff Internist, Department of Medicine, Animal Medical Center, New York, NY
Disorders of Canine Reproduction

Wendy A. Ware, D.V.M., M.S.
Diplomate, American College of Veterinary Internal Medicine; Associate Professor, Departments of Veterinary Clinical Sciences and Veterinary Physiology and Pharmacology,

College of Veterinary Medicine, Iowa State University, Ames, IA
Acquired Valvular Diseases

Cynthia A. Wheeler, D.V.M.
Diplomate, American College of Veterinary Ophthalmologists; Ophthalmologist, Animal Eye Care of Michigan, Laingsburg, MI
Disorders of the Posterior Segment

David A. Williams, Vet.M.B., Ph.D., M.R.C.V.S.
Diplomate, American College of Veterinary Internal Medicine; Professor and Chief, Small Animal Medicine, Department of Small Animal Clinical Sciences, Purdue University, School of Veterinary Medicine, West Lafayette, IN
Diseases of the Small Intestines

Peggy M. Wykes, D.V.M., M.S.
Diplomate, American College of Veterinary Surgeons; Staff Surgeon, Reference Surgical Veterinary Practice, Englewood, CO
Disorders of the Canine Vagina

Karen M. Young, V.M.D., Ph.D.
Clinical Associate Professor of Clinical Pathology, Department of Pathobiological Sciences, School of Veterinary Medicine, University of Wisconsin, Madison, WI
Introduction (Hemolymphatic System); Myeloproliferative Disorders

Debra L. Zoran, D.V.M.
Diplomate, American College of Veterinary Internal Medicine; Lecturer, Small Animal Medicine, Department of Small Animal Medicine and Surgery, College of Veterinary Medicine, Texas A&M University, College Station, TX
Diseases of the Oral Cavity and Pharynx

Preface to the Third Edition

The third edition of the *Handbook of Small Animal Practice* represents a continued effort on the part of all its authors to provide the most current information on practical veterinary medicine in a concise and easy-to-use format. Once again half of the authors have returned to revise their material from the second edition, and one half of the authors have composed new text, thereby bringing a new perspective to many diseases and disorders.

The outline format and chronology of the book remain the same, so subjects should be easy for readers to find, and pertinent information easy to retrieve. In some instances chapter titles have changed, mainly as a reflection of the different emphasis brought by authors new to this edition. The four appendices at the end of the book contain similar information to those of the second edition; however, the drug appendix has been expanded to include many of the new drugs and new applications that have been developed in the last 5 years.

Production of the third edition of the *Handbook* would not have been possible without the hard work and dedication of numerous people. I am particularly grateful for the participation of the thirteen section editors. Their expertise was essential in preparing the manuscripts for the book. I would also like to thank all the contributors for their hard work and dedication to the project. Without them, there would be no *Handbook*. A special thank you is due Ms. Elizabeth Hatter at W.B. Saunders for supervising production of the book. Beth is the most efficient and organized editor I have worked with, and she made my job much easier. Thanks are also due Ms. Marlene D'Amato and Ms. Beverly Boudreau for their help in processing the manuscripts and proofs.

Publication of the third edition of this text finds me back in Massachusetts and once again employed at an MSPCA hospital. Working at a busy, high-volume practice has reminded me of the daily challenges of practicing clinical medicine. It is my hope, and the goal of all the contributors, that the material presented in this edition of the *Handbook* will continue to help veterinarians meet those daily challenges.

Rhea V. Morgan, D.V.M.

Preface to the Second Edition

Welcome to the second edition of the *Handbook of Small Animal Practice*. In keeping with the *Handbook's* unusual style and format, this edition is a unique combination of state-of-the-art material from the first edition and new information from the latest developments in clinical veterinary medicine.

Readers familiar with the first edition will notice that the basic chronology of the text is largely unchanged. Two new sections pertaining to Dermatology and Ophthalmology have been added, but the order of other sections and chapters, as well as the sequence of subjects within each chapter, remains the same. Each subject is again described in a concise outline format, under the headings of definition, causes, pathophysiology, diagnosis, differential diagnosis, treatment, and patient monitoring. For those already accustomed to the first edition, it should not take long to feel comfortable with this revision.

Approximately one half of the original authors and section editors have returned to revise their initial material. New contributors have chosen to either recreate chapters or build upon existing chapters, making alterations and additions where indicated. Credit must be given to *all* the authors of the first edition, who provided the scaffolding upon which the second edition has been built.

Production of a text this size is an enormous undertaking.

I would like to thank the thirteen section editors, who worked diligently and expertly to ensure the accuracy and quality of each specialty section. I am deeply grateful to all the contributors, who worked so carefully to provide concise, practical, and applicable material for each subject. I also appreciate their efforts in mastering the outline style, and their patience with and tolerance of my editing. A special thank you must be extended to Ms. Karen Darcy and Ms. Myrna Snyder for their invaluable help in preparing the final manuscripts, and to Dr. Mary Dulisch for providing many new illustrations.

On a personal note, publication of the second edition of the *Handbook* marks an important milestone in my career. For fourteen years I was privileged to be a member of the staff of Angell Memorial Animal Hospital, Boston, Massachusetts. Composed of truly dedicated and selfless people, the AMAH staff played a major role in my professional education and development. I will forever be indebted to the wealth of knowledge they shared, the encouragement they lent, and the camaraderie they provided me. It was at Angell that I learned to be a clinician and practitioner. It is my sincere hope that this second edition of the *Handbook of Small Animal Practice* adequately addresses the changing needs of clinicians and practitioners everywhere.

Rhea V. Morgan, D.V.M.

Preface to the First Edition

With the recent plethora of veterinary publications, including new journals and new texts, as well as recent revisions of old texts, one might ask why another book would be worthwhile. The answer lies in a major difference between this book and many other texts: the presentation of its material. The *Handbook of Small Animal Practice* is written entirely in an outline format. Every effort has been made to keep standardized prose to a minimum. The book is exciting not only for its simplicity, but also for its ability to present to the busy practitioner the latest, most applicable information on a subject in a concise and easily retrievable manner.

Each subject is explored under a variety of headings, including definition, cause, pathophysiology, clinical signs, diagnosis, differential diagnoses, treatment, and patient monitoring. The information presented emphasizes practical and applicable methods of diagnosis, treatment, and follow-up care.

This book is not intended to provide an in-depth, detailed discussion of selected diseases. Instead it is designed as a reference text, one that contains concise descriptions of most of the medical disorders affecting dogs and cats. Its ultimate goal is to provide the veterinary practitioner with material that is instantly applicable as well as easily retrievable. A bibliography at the end of each chapter lists references available for further reading.

The *Handbook* consists of seventeen sections, beginning with patient evaluation. It continues with sections on each of the eleven body systems, and closes with sections on infectious diseases, behavioral and nutritional disorders, toxicology, and environmental injuries. Wherever appropriate, each section is subdivided into chapters based on the anatomic components of that body system. In turn, each chapter is organized in a chronological fashion beginning with congenital and developmental disorders and followed by degenerative, infectious, inflammatory, idiopathic, parasitic, metabolic/toxic, immune-mediated, vascular, nutritional, neoplastic, and traumatic diseases. This chronology is maintained wherever possible so that the reader can predict and find the location of a given subject within each chapter.

To complete a task of this magnitude requires the participation and commitment of many people. I am deeply grateful to the ninety contributors who expended so much effort in writing this book. I am indebted to their diligence in writing each chapter, to their punctuality in completing the manuscripts, and to their acceptance and tolerance of my editing. I would like to thank Dr. Mary Dulisch for providing many of the illustrations, and Ms. Colleen Tully, Mrs. Geraldine Rennie, and Ms. Betty Stevens for their help in preparing the final mansucripts. Thanks are also due to my family, friends, and colleagues for their unfailing support and enthusiasm.

The people at Churchill Livingstone have believed in this project from the beginning and have demonstrated great faith in allowing me to supervise its completion. I very much appreciate their support, and the opportunity to participate in the project. It has been an exciting and educational experience.

It is the hope of all the contributors and myself that the *Handbook of Small Animal Practice* will become a valuable and time-proven tool for the veterinarian. We hope it is a book that the practitioner will use often.

Rhea V. Morgan, D.V.M.

Contents

Patient Evaluation

General Physical Examination of the Dog and Cat

Dianne Mawby

GENERAL EXAMINATION

I. The basic equipment required for a complete physical examination includes stethoscope, thermometer, sterile lubrication and rubber gloves, otoscope, and ophthalmoscope or indirect lens and penlight.
  A. The examiner must use all of the senses during the examination, including seeing, hearing, smelling, and feeling.
  B. More is missed by not looking than by not knowing.
II. There are two phases of the physical examination.
  A. General observational examination, including assessment of alertness, responsiveness, body condition, posture, gait, and hair coat
  B. Hands-on examination
III. The observational examination continues while the palpation examination and auscultation are occurring.
IV. Certain procedures of the physical examination require extra time.
  A. Thoracic auscultation of heart and lungs
  B. Abdominal palpation
V. Each animal must be assessed for signs of aggression or fear biting by body posture and behavior. If there is any indication that the animal may be dangerous, a muzzle is applied to protect the examiner and holder.
VI. The examination should cover every aspect of the animal, "from nose to toes to tail." The hands-on examination usually begins at the head and moves toward the tail.

HEAD AND NECK

I. Skull
  A. While the examiner is holding the head, the shape and symmetry of the skull can be assessed.
  B. The skull can also be checked for open fontanelles.
II. Eyes
  A. Each eye is examined separately from anterior to posterior.
  B. Examination should include assessment of the following:
    1. Evidence of ocular discharge or blepharospasm
    2. Eye position and movement with normal head movements
    3. Vision and lid movement by eliciting menace reflex
    4. Eyelids and eyelashes
    5. Conjunctivae and third eyelids
    6. Corneal edema, defects, and vascularization
    7. Depth and clarity of the anterior chamber
    8. Color, integrity, and pupillary response to light of the iris and pupil
    9. Lens position and clarity
    10. Fundus, with either an indirect lens or direct ophthalmoscope
III. Ears
  A. The external pinnae should move in response to sound and to a light touch on the interior side.
  B. Ear canals are examined grossly initially, followed by an otoscopic examination of the entire canal and the tympanic membrane.
IV. Nose
  A. The bridge of the external nose is examined for shape and symmetry.
  B. The planum nasale is examined for color and erosions.
  C. The nares are examined for discharge and patency.
    1. Patency can be tested by placing a microscope slide in front of, but not touching, the nose.

2. Condensation on the slide from each nostril occurs with respiration (exhalation).

D. The interior of the nasal cavity cannot be examined without heavy sedation or general anesthesia.

V. Mouth

A. The mouth can be opened by grasping the maxillae with one hand and the mandible with the other. Resistance to opening can indicate pain at the temporomandibular joint or may reflect only the animal's behavior.

B. The lips and mucocutaneous junctions are examined for erosive lesions.

C. The mucous membranes are examined for color and for dryness. The capillary refill time can be assessed by gently pushing on the gums to blanch the capillaries and then observing for refill time.

D. The gums, hard palate, and soft palate are checked for color and integrity. These are especially important to assess in pediatric patients.

E. The teeth are visualized and can be palpated for pain or looseness. The cheeks are retracted from the teeth, and the vestibular surface of the teeth and the cheek pouch are examined.

F. The tongue is examined for color and movement.

1. The underside of the tongue is checked for masses, a string foreign body, or laceration of the frenulum as a result of a string.

2. This procedure can be done using a cotton tipped swab to deviate the tongue dorsally or by pushing up with the thumb/finger in the intermandibular space.

G. The tonsils and edge of the soft palate can be visualized by depressing the base of the tongue.

H. Swallowing and the gag reflex can be assessed by placing an index finger at the base of the tongue.

I. The odor of the breath can be indicative of disease.

1. Uremia
2. Poisons such as strychnine
3. Dental tartar and gingival disease
4. Ketonemia

VI. Salivary glands

A. Parotid glands are located at the junction of the head and neck at the base of the ear.

B. The mandibular gland lies caudal to the angle of the jaw.

C. The sublingual gland is closely related to the anterior end of the mandibular gland.

VII. Lymph nodes

A. Lymph nodes are differentiated from salivary glands because they are usually more mobile than the glands (Fig. 1–1).

B. Parotid lymph nodes are palpated at the rostral base of the ear.

C. Mandibular lymph nodes are located ventral to the angle of the jaw.

VIII. Neck

A. The neck is flexed, extended, and turned to each side to check for pain.

1. The eye position is monitored for normal nystagmus during this procedure.

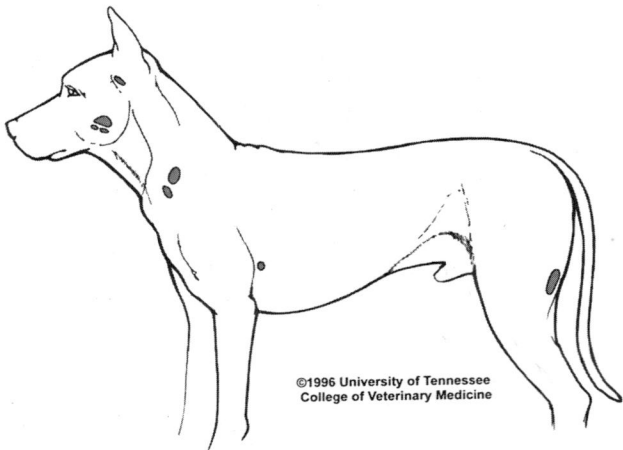

Figure 1–1. Palpable peripheral lymph nodes in the dog. (Courtesy of University of Tennessee College of Veterinary Medicine.)

2. Pressure exerted over the cervical vertebrae by slight pinching can also detect pain.

B. The larynx is palpated, and the trachea then is palpated from the larynx to the thoracic inlet. Slight squeezing of the trachea may elicit a cough.

C. The thyroid gland lies adjacent to the trachea.

1. Enlargement of the gland can be detected by using the thumb and forefinger in a steady movement to trace the tracheal margins from the larynx to the thoracic inlet. The head should be extended while the examiner is performing this manipulation.

2. In cats, an enlarged gland is palpated as it slips through the fingers (Fig. 1–2).

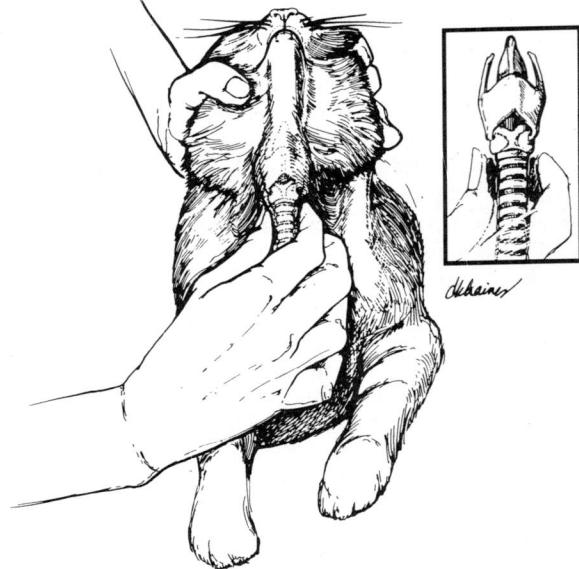

©1996 University of Tennessee
College of Veterinary Medicine

Figure 1–2. Palpation of the feline thyroid glands. (Courtesy of University of Tennessee College of Veterinary Medicine.)

D. The esophagus is not readily palpable in the cervical region. If there is an abnormal enlargement, the esophagus may be seen to be ballooning out at the thoracic inlet.

E. The jugular veins can be visualized by occlusion at the thoracic inlet. A jugular pulse may be seen prior to occlusion in instances of heart disease.

INTEGUMENT

I. The general appearance of the hair coat is seen on initial observational examination.
   A. The coat is observed for cleanliness and hair thickness.
   B. Areas of alopecia are noted as local or symmetrical, and the underlying skin is examined for pathologic conditions.
II. The body surface can be quickly palpated by running both hands over the entire body.
   A. This is especially important in long-haired animals in which the skin cannot be visualized.
   B. This quick overview can detect cutaneous and subcutaneous masses.
   C. The skin texture is described as normal, greasy, or dry. Dander is also noted.
III. Look for external parasites. Evidence of fleas can be found by examining around the tail head for flea dirt and self-abrasions.
   A. Pruritus may be observed on examination.
   B. The ear scratch test is done by scratching the edges of the pinnae to elicit a scratch response. This can be suggestive of sarcoptic mange or other chronic pruritic diseases.
IV. The skin of the abdomen is examined for thickness and for pathology such as pustules and papules.
V. The nails, nail beds, and footpads are examined on each foot for color, symmetry, and masses.
   A. Check between the toes of all four feet for masses or foreign bodies.
   B. Check for discoloration of the fur on the feet, which can indicate excessive licking.
VI. Each mammary gland is thoroughly palpated along the entire chain to check for masses. Each nipple is visually examined for masses or discharge.

FORELIMBS/AXILLAE

I. The animal is usually observed at presentation for signs of lameness. The origin of any lameness should be localized to a limb and area on that limb by palpation and flexion/extension.
II. Each forelimb is examined from the scapula to the toes. The axillary region is palpated to detect any abnormalities between the scapula and limb.
III. The prescapular (or superficial cervical) lymph nodes are palpated to evaluate size and shape. The axillary lymph node may be palpated on the thorax, just caudal to the shoulder joint.
IV. Each limb is examined by flexing and extending each

joint. The joints are also palpated to detect any joint effusions, pain, or heat.

V. A cursory neurologic exam can be done by observing whether the toenails have been worn on the dorsal surface from dragging.
   A. The foot can be placed in flexed position with the dorsum of the paw on the table.
   B. The animal should immediately right the foot, indicating conscious proprioception.

THORAX

I. The thoracic cage is observed and palpated to evaluate the integrity of the ribs. Pressure can be placed over the vertebrae to detect back pain.
II. The thoracic cage is compressible in the normal cat.
   A. This can be checked by holding the thorax with the sternum in the palm of the hand and gently squeezing the sides of the chest between the fingers and thumb.
   B. Abnormal resistance can indicate space-occupying problems in the feline thoracic cavity.
III. The respiratory system is evaluated next.
   A. The breathing pattern and rate are evaluated prior to auscultation. The pattern is a description of the relationship between inspiration and expiration plus the depth of respiration (Table 1–1).
      1. The animal's posture and attitude can reflect respiratory distress.
      2. Orthopnea, open mouth breathing, and extension of the head and neck indicate severe forms of respiratory distress.
   B. Auscultation of the lungs is done separately from that of the heart.
      1. Upper airway sounds can be reflected to the lower airway.
      2. The animal should not be panting or purring during the exam.
      3. The mouth of a panting dog can be gently held closed during the time of auscultation.
      4. Purring may be stopped by carrying the cat toward a tap with running water or by placing alcohol on the tip of the nose.
   C. The lung fields are auscultated in a systematic method. Adventitious lung sounds are described as continuous (wheezes) or discontinuous (crackles).

Table 1–1. Normal Physiologic Parameters

	Dog	Cat
Heart rate (beats/min)	60–160 in adults Up to 180 in toy breeds Up to 220 in puppies	160–240 maximum Mean, 197
Respiratory rate (breaths/min)	24	26
Temperature	100.2–103.8°F 37.9–39.9°C	100.5–102.5°F 38.1–39.2°C

Data from Lunney and Ettinger, 1995; Swenson, 1984.

1. The exact location of the abnormal lung sounds is recorded.
2. The absence of lung sounds may indicate pleural space disease (pneumothorax, pleural effusion, or masses) or lung lobe consolidation.

D. A cough may be elicited by gently squeezing the trachea in the cervical region.

E. Percussion of the chest wall can aid in identifying areas of fluid or air or solid regions in the thoracic cavity. If pleural effusion is present, a fluid line may be identified by using percussion to differentiate the fluid–air interface (Fig. 1–3).

IV. Cardiac examination involves the following:

A. Auscultation of the heart utilizes both the diaphragm and the bell of the stethoscope. The diaphragm is used for high- and medium-frequency sounds, and the bell is used for low-frequency sounds.

B. The heart rate is taken and the pulses are palpated simultaneously to check for pulse deficits. The femoral pulse is the easiest pulse to feel while auscultating the chest (see Table 1–1).

C. The rhythm of the heart is assessed as being regular, regular-irregular (as in sinus arrhythmia), or irregular-irregular (as in atrial fibrillation).

1. Arrhythmias can result from abnormalities in the atria or ventricles.
2. An electrocardiogram is usually necessary to diagnose the exact arrhythmia.

D. The heart sounds are ausculted over the area of the valves. The pulmonic, aortic, and mitral valves are assessed on the left side, and the tricuspid valve is assessed on the right side.

E. The location of each valve is as follows (Fig. 1–4):

1. Pulmonic valve: third left intercostal space, ventral
2. Aortic valve: fourth left intercostal space

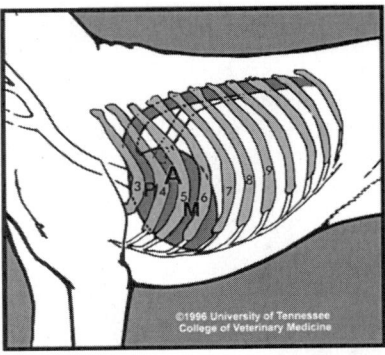

Figure 1–4. Cardiac valve positions and their relationship to the thoracic ribs. P = pulmonic valve; A = aortic valve; M = mitral valve. (Courtesy of University of Tennessee College of Veterinary Medicine.)

3. Mitral valve: fifth left intercostal space above the middle of the lower third of the thorax
4. Tricuspid valve: fourth right intercostal space at the level of the costochondral junction

F. The heart sounds are produced by the closing of the valves, the flow of blood, and the contraction of the heart muscle.

1. The first heart sound (S1) occurs during ventricular contraction and the closure of the atrioventricular valves. This is the normal "lub" in the "lub dub" of the heart.
2. The second heart sound (S2) is produced by the closure of the aortic and pulmonic valves. This is the "dub" in the normal "lub dub" of the heart.
3. The third heart sound (S3) is produced by the sudden cessation of the rapid ventricular filling with vibration of the walls and muscles. This sound is not normally heard in the dog and cat and may indicate dilated cardiomyopathy or decompensated mitral or tricuspid insufficiency (Gompf, 1995).
4. The fourth heart sound (S4) is the result of atrial contraction ejecting blood into the ventricles. This sound is not normally heard in dogs and cats and may indicate atrial dilatation (Gompf, 1995).

G. Any murmurs should be described in relation to the heart sound, position or site, intensity, duration, and radiation.

1. Intensity can be graded on a 6-point scale, with 6 being the loudest (Gompf, 1995).
   a) Grade 1/6 is very soft and can be heard only by listening for a long period of time.
   b) Grade 2/6 is very soft.
   c) Grade 3/6 is of low to moderate intensity.
   d) Grade 4/6 is very loud, but there is no "thrill" palpated on the thorax.
   e) Grade 5/6 is very loud, and a "thrill" can be palpated on the thorax.
   f) Grade 6/6 is very loud and can be heard with the stethoscope held slightly off the thorax or without the use of a stethoscope.
2. The quality of the murmur is subjective, but

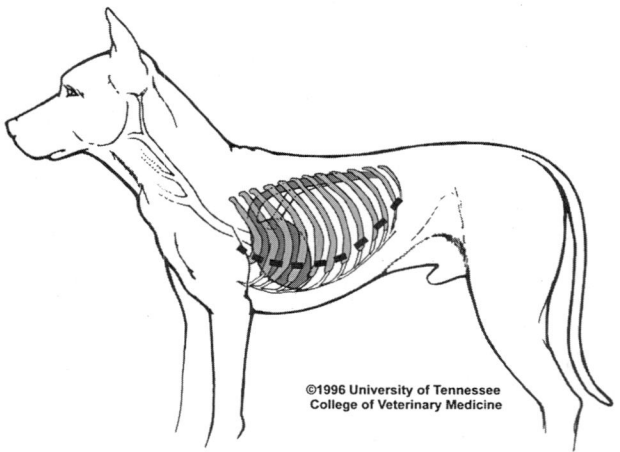

Figure 1–3. Depiction of a pleural fluid line and its relationship to the ribs and heart. (Courtesy of University of Tennessee College of Veterinary Medicine.)

it can be described as regurgitant, ejection, machinery, or blowing.

3. Feline hearts are much smaller, and therefore it may be difficult to assess the exact location of a murmur accurately.

ABDOMEN

I. When palpating the abdominal cavity, a light but forceful touch is required. Some animals tense the abdominal muscles in response to the procedure. It must be determined whether the cause is from pain or from anxiety.

II. When palpating the abdomen, a systematic approach ensures completeness.
   A. Moving cranial to caudal and dorsal to ventral in the abdomen ensures that nothing is overlooked.
   B. When palpating, the tips of the fingers are sensitive to the size and shape of the organs or any masses felt (Fig. 1–5).

III. The animal may arch its back when the abdomen is palpated.
   A. If the primary problem is back pain, the examiner may mistakenly interpret this as abdominal pain.
   B. It is useful to check for back pain prior to abdominal palpation.
   C. This is done by exerting pressure over each lumbar vertebra in a serial manner.

IV. The muscles of the abdominal wall should be palpated to check for masses and for any hernias in the body wall. It is important to check for umbilical hernias in pediatric patients.

V. The liver is the most cranial organ and cannot be entirely palpated.
   A. The edges of the liver may be felt at or just cranial to the costal margins.
      1. On the left, the caudal edges of the left lateral hepatic lobe may be felt.
      2. On the right, the medial lobe of the right hepatic lobe and the caudate process may be palpated.
   B. With diffuse enlargement, the liver can be palpated extending caudally past the costal margins. The edges may seem sharp or rounded.
   C. With solitary masses, only those extending caudally can be discretely palpated.

VI. If the stomach is enlarged, it may be palpated in the cranial left quadrant of the abdomen. A grossly distended stomach extends beyond the costal margins and is palpable as a taut air-, food-, or fluid-filled vesicle.

VII. The pancreas is not usually palpable; however, if inflammation is occurring, a local peritonitis may result in pain in the right cranial quadrant of the abdomen.

VIII. The kidneys lie in the dorsal, cranial abdomen.
   A. Canine kidneys are fixed in the retroperitoneal space. The right kidney is more anterior than the left, and therefore only the caudal end may be felt. The left kidney is more posterior and can be readily palpated.
   B. Feline kidneys are more mobile than those of the canine. Each kidney can be gently grasped and inspected entirely.
   C. Each kidney is evaluated for size, shape, symmetry, location, pain, consistency, and smoothness.
   D. The kidney surface is smooth, and the medial surface is indented by the hilus.
   E. Kidney size varies with size of the dog, with the average being 6–9 cm in length, 4–5 cm in width, and 3–4 cm in thickness (Evans and Christiansen, 1974).
   F. The size of the normal feline kidney is 4–4.5 cm in length and 3–3.5 cm in width (Thrall, 1994).

IX. The spleen lies on the left side of the abdomen, and the tail can be felt lying on the ventral abdominal floor.
   A. The spleen should be palpated for increase in size and for nodules or large masses.
   B. If the tip of the spleen is folded over, it may be mistaken for a mass.

X. The intestines are palpable throughout the abdominal cavity.
   A. Initially, using two hands in large dogs and one hand in small dogs and cats, the fingers are brought together dorsally and gently moved ventrally. The loops of bowel can be felt as they slide through the fingers.
   B. Individual sections of small intestine are difficult to distinguish on palpation. The cecum can sometimes be isolated and identified.
   C. The bowel is evaluated for thickness, rigidity, and irregular masses. Feces can be contained in the bowel and mistaken for a mass. The feces are usually compressible with gentle pressure.
   D. The colon and rectum can be palpated dorsally in the abdomen and may be filled with feces.

XI. The size of the bladder is variable.
   A. Filled bladders can be easily palpated in the caudal abdomen. Partially filled or empty bladders may require extra palpation.

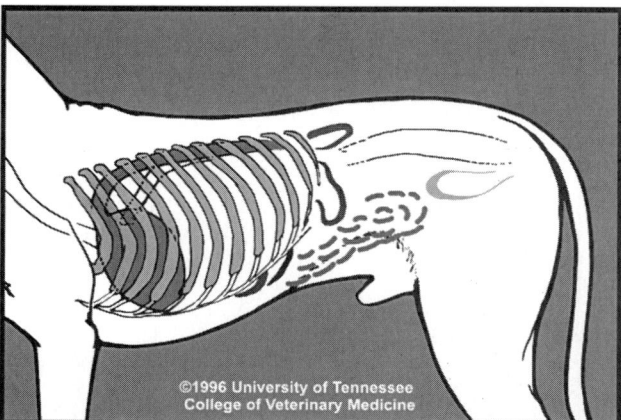

©1996 University of Tennessee
College of Veterinary Medicine

Figure 1–5. Diagram of the approximate location of the palpable abdominal organs, including bladder, small and large intestines, kidneys, liver, and spleen. (Courtesy of University of Tennessee College of Veterinary Medicine.)

B. The bladder can be located by gently laterally compressing the caudal abdomen and moving cranial to caudal. The bladder feels like a fluid-filled vesicle.

XII. Urogenital examination is also performed.
A. The uterus in an intact, non-pregnant, normal female is not palpable. If there is a pregnancy or pyometra, the uterus can be palpated as an enlarged organ dorsal to the bladder.
B. The prostate of an intact, normal dog is not usually palpable. If there is prostatic enlargement, the cranial portion of the prostate may be felt by deep palpation into the caudal abdomen.

XIII. Lymph nodes may also be detected.
A. The cranial mesenteric lymph nodes may be palpated if abnormally large.
B. These lymph nodes are present along the vessels of the great mesentery.

REAR LIMBS/PELVIS/TAIL

I. As with the forelimbs, any sign of lameness should be detected prior to the general examination.
II. Each limb is palpated and examined in a manner similar to that used for the front limbs.
III. The popliteal lymph nodes are palpated to evaluate size and shape. The superficial inguinal lymph nodes may be palpated between the abdominal wall and the medial surface of the thigh.
IV. The position and movement of the tail are evaluated initially.
A. The tail is examined for any abnormal masses or hair loss.
B. Applying gentle pressure to the tail by pulling in a rostral direction can detect lumbosacral pain.
V. Early signs of generalized weakness can be detected in the rear limbs. This may be seen as ataxia or as weakness, especially when applying pressure over the hips.
VI. Conscious proprioception is also evaluated in the rear limbs in a manner similar to that used for the forelimbs.

EXTERNAL UROGENITAL AND PERINEAL AREA

I. Female vulva
A. The external vulva is examined for discharge or swelling.
B. The mucous membranes of the vulva may be used to assess mucous membrane color, especially if the mucous membranes of the mouth are pigmented.
II. Male
A. The prepuce is examined for discharge around the external orifice.
B. The prepuce is retracted to allow examination of the penis.

C. The scrotum is palpated to examine the testicles. Both testicles should be descended and symmetrical. The epididymis can normally be palpated on each testicle.
III. The anus and perineum
A. This area is examined when the rectal temperature is taken (see Table 1–1).
B. The area is examined for masses, especially in male dogs.

RECTAL EXAMINATION

I. A gloved and well-lubricated finger is gently inserted into the rectum.
II. Many structures can be evaluated during this examination, such as rectal wall thickness, anal glands, contours of the pelvis and sacrum, pelvic urethra, pelvic arteries, prostate in the male and vaginal tract in the female, and the obturator foramen and the anterior brim of the pelvis.
III. The gloved finger can also apply pressure dorsally to the sacrum to evaluate for pain.
IV. The prostate gland may be enlarged and protruding cranially over the pelvic brim. To assist in rectal palpation, the other hand of the examiner can be used to gently push the prostate into more dorsal caudal position via abdominal palpation.
V. The feces are examined for color and consistency.

NEUROLOGIC EXAMINATION

I. The neurologic examination begins with the initial evaluation of the animal's demeanor and behavior.
II. As the physical examination continues, the neurologic system is assessed with each step.
A. The cranial nerves and neck pain are evaluated when the head is examined.
B. Back pain is assessed while the thorax and abdomen are examined.
C. Proprioception is assessed with examination of the limbs.
D. Neurologic evaluation of the reflexes is performed with a complete neurologic examination.

Bibliography

Evans HE, Christiansen GC: Miller's Anatomy of the Dog. 2nd Ed. WB Saunders, Philadelphia, 1974

Gompf RE: History taking and physical examination of the cardiovascular system. p. 1. In Miller MS, Tilley LP (eds): Manual of Canine and Feline Cardiology. 2nd Ed. WB Saunders, Philadelphia, 1995

Lunney J, Ettinger SJ: Cardiac arrthymias. p. 959. In Ettinger SJ, Feldman EC (eds): Textbook of Veterinary Internal Medicine: Diseases of the Dog and Cat. 4th Ed. WB Saunders, Philadelphia, 1995

Swenson MJ: Duke's Physiology of Domestic Animals. 10th Ed. Comstock Publishing Associates, Ithaca, New York, 1984

Thrall DE: Textbook of Veterinary Diagnostic Radiology. 2nd Ed. WB Saunders, Philadelphia, 1994

2

Collection and Interpretation of Laboratory Data

Rhea V. Morgan

This chapter presents the techniques and procedures for collecting samples for certain laboratory tests (Tables 2–1 to 2–5). Normal values and interpretative guidelines are included. (For normal physiologic values, see Appendix I.)

ANION AND OSMOLAL GAPS

Anion Gap

Definition

I. By the law of electroneutrality, the concentration of circulating anions equals that of circulating cations.
II. Cations and anions are classified as measured or unmeasured.
  A. Measured
    1. Anions: Cl, HCO_3
    2. Cations: Na, K
  B. Unmeasured
    1. Anions (UA): albumin, alpha and beta globulins, PO_4, SO_4, organic acids, certain toxins and drugs
    2. Cations (UC): gamma globulins, Ca, Mg, certain drugs
  C. $Na + K + UC = Cl + HCO_3 + UA$
III. Anion gap is the difference between measured cation and anion concentrations.
  A. Denotes an alteration in some unmeasured component of the equation
  B. Anion gap = $(Na + K) - (Cl + HCO_3)$
    1. Normal: 12 mEq/L; range: 8–16 mEq/L
    2. May be increased by either a decrease in UC or an increase in UA
    3. Is decreased by either an increase in UC or a decrease in UA
    4. Potassium sometimes deleted from equation because of its low, constant concentration

Causes

I. Causes of increased anion gap
  A. Increase in unmeasured anions
  B. Increase in serum lactate, ketoacids, uremia
  C. Certain medications: carbenicillin, penicillin
  D. Dehydration: concentrated normal anions
  E. Alkalemia
  F. Decrease in unmeasured cation concentrations: Ca, Mg
  G. Increase in serum albumin
  H. Toxins: ethylene glycol, methanol, salicylate, paraldehyde
II. Causes of decreased anion gap
  A. Increase in normal cations, especially Ca, Mg, globulins
  B. Retention of abnormal cations (e.g., multiple myeloma)
  C. Loss of unmeasured anions: hypoalbuminemia

Clinical Significance

I. Increases index of suspicion that unexpected (or unmeasured) cations or anions are present in serum
II. Allows further definition and classification of metabolic acidotic states
  A. Metabolic acidosis with normal or decreased anion gap is usually caused by renal or intestinal loss of bicarbonate (hyperchloremic acidosis).
  B. Metabolic acidosis associated with an increased anion gap may have various causes.
    1. Diabetic ketoacidosis
    2. Lactic acidosis
    3. Ethylene glycol or paraldehyde intoxication
    4. Acute renal failure

Text continued on page 15

Table 2–1. *Endocrine Assays*

Test	Protocol	Sample Required	Normal Values	Interpretation of Abnormal Values
Basal T_3, T_4 assay		Serum	Dog: T_3 = 80–200 ng/dl = 0.8–2 ng/ml = 1.2–3.1 nmol/L; T_4 = 1.3–4 µg/dl = 13–40 ng/ml = 20–52 nmol/L; Cat: T_3 = 60–150 ng/dl = 0.6–1.5 ng/ml = 0.6–1.9 nmol/L; T_4 = 1–4.5 µg/dl = 10–45 ng/ml = 15–55 nmol/L	Suggestive of hypothyroidism—dog: T_3 < 30 ng/dl, T_4 < 1 µg/dl, < 19 nmol/L. Hyperthyroidism Cat: T_3 >200 ng/dl, T_4 > 5 µg/dl, Dog: T_3 > 290 ng/dl, T_4 > 4 µg/dl
Free T_4 by dialysis		Serum	Dog: FT_4 = 16–30 pmol/L; Cat: FT_4 = 15–48 pmol/L	Dog: FT_4 <16 pmol/L suggestive of hypothyroidism, but may accompany other diseases. Cat: FT_4 > 48 pmol/L indicative of hyperthyroidism
Thyroid-stimulating hormone (TSH) response test	Dog: 0.1 IU TSH/kg IV (Thytropar)	Measure serum T_4 at 0 and 4 or 6 h after TSH.	Post-TSH T_4 ≥ 2 × basal T_4 or > 35 nmol/L	Post-TSH T_4 < 2 × basal T_4 or < 35 nmol/L = diagnostic of hypothyroidism
Canine TSH		Serum	Dog: 2–30 µU/L 2.7–7.9 ng/ml	Primary hypothyroidism: T_4 decreased, TSH increased (20–30 ng/ml)
TRH stimulation test	Dog: 0.2 mg TRH (Thypinone) IV	Measure serum T_4 before and 2–4 h after TRH	Dog: Post-T_4 > 2 µg/dl or > basal T_4 + 0.5 µg/dl	Hypothyroidism: Post-T_4 < 0.5 µg/dl
T_3 suppression test	Cat: give 25 µg T_3 PO TID × 7 doses.	Measure T_4 at 0 and 4 h after last dose of T_3.	T_4 ≤ 15 ng/mL ≤ 20 nmol/L	Hyperthyroid cats: T_4 does not suppress.
Adrenocorticotropic hormone (ACTH) response test	A. Synthetic ACTH (Cortrosyn) 0.25 mg IM or IV. B. ACTH gel (Cortigel) 2.2 U/kg IM	A. Measure plasma cortisol at 0 and 1 h after ACTH. B. Measure plasma cortisol at 0 and 2 h after ACTH.	Dog: Pre-ACTH 1.1–8 µg/dl, 25–125 nmol/L, Post-ACTH 6.2–16.8 µg/dl, 200–500 nmol/L; Cat: Pre-ACTH 0.33–2.6 µg/dl, 15–150 nmol/L, Post-ACTH 4.8–7.6 µg/dl, 130–450 nmol/L	Hyperadrenocorticism Pre-ACTH 4–10.8 µg/dl, Post-ACTH 11.7–50 µg/dl. Primary hypoadrenocorticism Pre- and post-ACTH ≤ 1 µg/dl, 30 nmol/L
ACTH assay	Draw sample into chilled syringe and insert into chilled EDTA tube. Transfer sample to plastic tube and cool for 20 min in ice water. Centrifuge sample for short time, retrieve plasma into another plastic tube, add Trasylol. Freeze sample immediately and transport on dry ice.		Dog: 20–100 pg/ml (avg. 45); Cat: 2–15 pmol/L, 20–61 pg/ml, 1–20 pmol/L	Pituitary-dependent hyperadrenocorticism: ACTH ≥ 40–500 pg/ml, > 88 pmol/L. Functional adrenal tumor: ACTH ≤ 20 pg/ml, ≤ 4.4 pmol/L
Low-dose dexamethasone suppression test	0.01 mg/kg dexamethasone sodium phosphate IV	Measure plasma cortisol at 0, 4, and 8 h after dexamethasone.	Dog: Pre = 1.1–8 µg/dl Post = < 1 µg/dl (Normal dogs suppress)	Hyperadrenocorticism: no suppression 4 h post: 30% of pituitary hyperadrenocorticism suppresses. 8 h post: > 1 µg/dl or 30 nmol/L

Test	Dose/Protocol	Sample	Values	Interpretation
High-dose dexamethasone suppression test	0.1 mg/kg dexamethasone sodium phosphate IV	Measure plasma cortisol at 0 and 4 h after dexamethasone.	Pre values reflect hyperadrenocorticism: 4–10.8 μg/dl.	Pituitary hyperadrenocorticism 1. 75% have post values < 50% of pre value. 2. 25% fail to suppress. Adrenal tumor: 100% do not suppress, post = >1.5 μg/dl or 40 nmol/L.
Urine cortisol:creatinine ratio		Fresh urine sample	Urine cortisol (nmol/L): urine creatinine (mmol/L) ≤ 35 (dog), < 28 (cat)	Ratio > normal is suggestive of hyperadrenocorticism.
Insulin assay		Measure serum insulin after 24-h fast or during episodes of hypoglycemia.	6–22 μU/ml	Values < normal preclude diagnosis of insulinoma. Values > normal should be checked against the amended insulin:glucose ratio.
Growth hormone (GH) assay		Serum	Dog: 0–10 ng/ml (usually 2–3 ng/ml) Cat: 0–8.5 ng/ml (mean = 1.21 ± 1.0 ng/ml)	Values >90 ng/ml have been associated with neoplasia causing diencephalic syndrome in the dog and acromegaly in the cat. Low values are difficult to assess; stimulation tests should be performed.
Clonidine stimulation test	10 μg clonidine kg IV (Catapresan)	Measure plasma GH at 0, 15, 30, 45, 60, and 120 min after clonidine. Keep samples frozen until assayed.	Normal dogs show increase in GH between 15 and 45 min with a peak of 25–40 ng/ml.	Clonidine is a GH stimulant. Pituitary dwarfs demonstrate either no or little response to clonidine.
Xylazine stimulation test	100 μg/kg IV (Rompun)	Measure plasma GH at 0, 15, 30, 45, 60, and 120 min after xylazine. Keep samples frozen until assayed.	Normal dogs show increase in GH between 15 and 45 min with a peak of 25–40 ng/ml.	Pituitary dwarfs show no response to xylazine.
Gastrin assay		Plasma after 12-h fast	Dog: 45–125 pg/ml Cat: 28–135 pg/ml	Plasma gastrin levels are increased with primary gastrointestinal tract disease (e.g., functional gastrinomas) or secondary to other systemic diseases, especially chronic renal failure.
Antidiuretic hormone (ADH) response test	Perform water deprivation test first. Give desmopressin acetate 2–4 drops conjunctivally or 2–5 μg/dog SQ	Empty bladder. Collect urine at 60, 120, 180, and 240 min.	Normal: sp. gr. >1.025	Central diabetes insipidus: sp. gr. >1.015 Nephrogenic diabetes insipidus or medullary washout: sp. gr. <1.015
Parathormone (PTH) assay		Serum	Dog: 2–13 pmol/L 16–136 pg/ml Cat: 3.3–22.5 pg/ml	Hypoparathyroidism: PTH = low or undetectable Parathyroid adenoma: PTH as high as 45 pmol/L Secondary hyperparathyroidism (renal failure): PTH grossly elevated
Calcitonin assay		Plasma	Dog: ≤ 25 pg-Eq/ml	Values of plasma calcitonin are difficult to interpret at this time. Extreme elevations may be caused by calcitonin-producing thyroid tumors.
Erythropoietin		Serum	Dog: 5–15 mU/ml Cat: 5–22 mU/ml	Low: primary polycythemia, chronic renal failure Normal or high: Secondary polycythemia Very elevated: asplastic anemia, certain renal tumors
Ionized calcium		Serum	1.12–1.42 nmol/L	Primary hyperparathyroidism: increased values Malignant hypercalcemia: increased values Renal failure: Normal or increased values Hypoparathyroidism: decreased values

Table 2–2. Gastrointestinal Studies

Test	Protocol	Sample Required	Normal Values	Interpretation
Bile acid assays	1. Fast animal 12 h. 2. Feed a routine meal.	Serum samples are collected after 12-h fast and 2 h after a meal.	Dog: Fasting $\leq$ 5 μmol/L Postprandial $\leq$ 15.5 μmol/L Cat: Fasting $\leq$ 2 μmol/L Postprandial $\leq$ 10 μmol/L	Elevations indicate dysfunction of normal hepatobiliary physiology, with the degree of elevation providing quantitative information.
Ammonium tolerance test	Give 100 mg/kg NH_4Cl PO (max. dose 3 g).	1. Draw blood sample into EDTA before and 30 min after NH_4Cl. 2. Cool blood on ice immediately.	Fasting $\leq$ 120–150 μg/dl Post-NH_4Cl $\leq$ 200–250 μg/dl	Elevation of blood ammonia indicates either hepatic dysfunction of shunting of portal blood away from the liver (i.e., portocaval shunt).
Glucagon tolerance test	1. Fast animal 2 h. 2. Give glucagon 0.03 mg/kg IV.	Measure serum glucose at 0, 15, 30, 60, and 90 min after glucagon administration.	Serum glucose rises in response to glucagon, with peak at 15 min, and returns to normal by 90 min.	Glucose curve remains flat with severe hepatic insufficiency, portocaval shunt, glycogen storage disease, and prolonged anorexia or starvation.
BT-PABA test (*N*-benzoyl-L-tyrosyl-*p*-aminobenzoic acid)	1. Fast animal 18 h. 2. Give 5 ml 1% BT-PABA/kg PO followed by 25–100 ml water. 3. Stomach tubing is preferred. 4. Avoid concurrent use of chloramphenicol, sulfonamides, diuretics, and pancreatic extracts for 5 days before test.	Heparinized plasma is obtained for measuring plasma PABA at 0, 30, 60, 90, and 120 min.	Dog: > 5μg/ml Cat: >7.5 μg/ml (at 90 min)	Indirectly measures chymotrypsin activity. Values < 1.25 μg/ml are compatible with pancreatic exocrine insufficiency. Also reflects small intestinal absorption capabilities. Values of 1.25–4 μg/ml are compatible with malabsorption.
Trypsin immunoreactivity	Fast animal 12 h.	Serum	Dog: 5–35 μg/L Cat: 17–49 μg/L	Maldigestion: < 2 μg/L (dog), < 8 μg/L (cat) Malabsorption: > 5 μg/L (dog) Pancreatitis: > 35 μg/L (dog) >60 μg/L (cat)
Fecal proteolytic activity	Collect at least 3 fresh specimens.	Feces	Cat: 29–207 ACU/g Dog: 19–200 ACU/g Dog: 6–24 mm radial enzyme diffusion	Maldigestion: <29 ACU/g (cat) < 19 ACU/g (dog)
Folate levels	Fast animal 12 h.	Serum	Dog: 6.7–17.4 μg/L Cat: 13.4–38 μg/L	Increased with GI bacterial overgrowth Low with small intestine malabsorption
Cobalamin levels	Fast animal 12 h.	Serum	Dog: 225–660 ng/L Cat: 200–1680 ng/L	Low with cobalamin malabsorption or pancreatic exocrine insufficiency

Table 2–3. Renal Function Tests

Test	Protocol	Sample Required	Normal Values	Interpretation
Phenolsulfonphthalein (PSP) excretion in urine	A. 1. Empty bladder via catheterization 2. Give 6 mg PSP IV. B. Give 1 mg PSP/kg IV.	A. Catheterize bladder 20 min later and collect all urine. B. Collect 4 ml heparinized plasma before and 60 min after PSP administration.	A. Normal: >30% excretion of PSP B. Normal: 80 µg/dl Suspicious: 80–120 µg/dl Abnormal: ≥ 120 µg/dl	A. Assesses renal blood flow B. Assesses renal tubular function; abnormal retention occurs with renal insufficiency.
Sodium sulfanilate (SS) clearance	Give 0.2 ml of 10% solution/kg IV after a 12-h fast.	Obtain heparinized blood at 30, 60, and 90 min.	Results are expressed as the time needed to clear 50% of dye from the blood ($t_{1/2}$). Normal $t_{1/2}$ = 32–84 min	SS retention in plasma above normal reflects diminished glomerular filtration rate (GFR). SS clearance is usually reduced before the development of either azotemia or urine concentration defects.
Endogenous creatinine clearance	1. Acclimate animal to metabolism cage. 2. Catheterize and empty bladder. 3. Allow access to free choice water. 4. Collect all urine for 24 h; emtpy bladder again at end of test. 5. Avoid contamination of urine with feces. 6. Store urine in closed, refrigerated container until test is concluded. 7. Record total volume of urine.	1. Submit serum sample obtained midway through test for creatinine assay (SC). 2. Submit urine sample from the pooled collection for creatinine measurement (UC). 3. Use equation to calculate clearance: $$GFR = \frac{UC\ (mg/dl) \times urine\ volume\ (ml)}{SC\ (mg/dl) \times 1440\ min \times weight\ (kg)}$$	Normal, dogs: 2–5 ml/min/kg Normal, cats: 1.6–4 ml/min/kg	Decreased GFR occurs with decreased renal blood flow (prerenal), obstruction of urine outflow (postrenal), and renal parenchymal disease. Decreased GFR in an otherwise normal dog indicates renal insufficiency.
Urine protein quantitation	Follow protocol outlined above for endogenous creatinine clearance. Most common assay is trichloroacetic acid–ponceau S method.	1. Submit pooled urine sample. 2. Protein excretion/24 h = urine protein (mg/dl) × urine volume (dl) 3. Protein excretion/kg = total protein (mg)/weight (kg)	1. Protein/kg/day ≤ 30 mg/kg/ day 2. Total protein: 333 ± 309 mg/ day	Significant proteinuria occurs with glomerular disease. Other causes include Bence Jones proteinuria, myoglobinuria, and severe urinary tract trauma.
Urine protein:creatinine ratio (UP/C ratio)	Random sample	Dog: urine	Normal ≤ 1.0	Significant proteinuria: UP/C > 1.0 Results are affected by both pyuria and gross blood contamination.

Table 2-4. Interpretation of Serologic Tests

Disease/Disorder	Test	Interpretation
Brucellosis	A. Rapid slide agglutination test (RSAT)	A. Good screening test False-positives occur, so perform further serologic assay to confirm the diagnosis. Becomes positive within 2 wk, but false-negative can occur up to 8 wk.
	B. Tube agglutination tests 1. TAT	B. 1. Becomes positive by 3–6 wk Titer results: 1:50—early or recovering infection 1:50—1:100—suspicious $\geq$ 1:200—active infection
	2. 2-Mercaptoethane TAT (ME-TAT)	2. Fewer false-positives Becomes positive 1–2 wk after TAT $\geq$ 1:100—active infection
	C. Agar-gel immunodiffusion (AGID)	C. Becomes positive in 5–10 wk Very specific; used to confirm diagnosis Both somatic and cytoplasmic tests available Results reported as positive, suspicious, or negative Repeat in 4–6 wk if first results are suspicious.
	D. ELISA	D. Very specific, but less sensitive than TAT tests; not recommended
Leptospirosis	A. Microscopic agglutination test (MAT)	A. Titers <1:300 may be postvaccinal. Titers >1:3200 usually indicate infection. Paired samples 2–4 wk apart are tested; a fourfold increase in titer is diagnostic.
	B. ELISA	B. IgM–titer: Develops after 1 wk IgG–titer: Develops in 2–3 wk Vaccinates: High IgG titer with low or negative IgM titer
Feline infectious peritonitis (FIP)	IFA, ELISA	Titer >1:1600 or fourfold increase over 2–4 wk is compatible with a positive diagnosis. Titer <1:240 is inconclusive. *Note:* This titer cross-reacts with other feline coronaviruses, so is not specific for FIP.
Canine parvovirus (CPV)	Latex agglutination, ELISA	Positive diagnosis: Single high IgM titer Fourfold rise in IgG titer over 2–4 wk
Ehrlichiosis	A. Indirect immunofluorescence B. Western immunoblotting assay C. PCR assay	A. Titer >1:20 is considered positive in endemic areas. Any measurable titer (>1:10) is significant in nonendemic areas. Submit a second sample 2 wk later if suspicious case is negative on first sample.
Rocky Mountain spotted fever (RMSF)	A. Indirect microimmunofluorescence test (micro-IF) for IgG	A. Submit acute and convalescent titers 2–3 wk apart. Titer $\leq$ 1:64—normal Titer $\geq$1:1024 in East, $\geq$1:25 in West = infected Fourfold increase in titers is diagnostic. Titers stay elevated for 6–10 mo.
	B. Micro-IF for IgM	B. Single high titer indicates active infection.
Borreliosis (Lyme disease)	IFA, ELISA, immunoblot techniques	Titers are difficult to interpret. Symptomatic dogs usually have titers >1:1024. Fourfold increase in paired samples submitted 2–4 wk apart is supportive.
Toxoplasmosis	A. Antibody assay IgM: IFA, ELISA IgG: IFA	A. IgM titers: Develop within 2 wk Usually nondetectable after 16 wk Positive: titer > 1:256 IgG titers: Develop in 3–4 wk and may persist for life Increasing titer over 4 wk may indicate active or recent infection.
	B. Antigen assay C. PCR assay	B. Can test serum, CSF, or aqueous humor Antigenemia may be intermittent. C. Can test aqueous humor

Table 2–4. **Interpretation of Serologic Tests** (Continued)

Disease/Disorder	Test	Interpretation
Blastomycosis	A. AGID	A. If positive, animal has 91% chance of having active disease but may be negative in acute stages. If negative, sensitivity is 90–98%.
	B. ELISA	B. More sensitive than AGID test
Cryptococcosis	Latex agglutination test	Dog: Positive results, even as low as 1:16, confirm the diagnosis. False-negative can occur; test cross-reacts with toxoplasmosis. Titers tend to correlate well with extent and course of disease. May be assayed in blood, urine, CSF Cat: Titer >1:10 indicative of active infection.
Coccidioidomycosis	A. Tube precipitin test	A. Becomes positive in 2–6 wk. Detects IgM; is a qualitative test and fades quickly
	B. Complement fixation (CF) titer	B. Detects IgG; therefore appears in 8–10 wk. Titer ≤1:4—negative. Titer ≥1:16 suspicious, chronic or localized disease. Titer ≥1:32—active disease. Rise or drop in titer corresponds well with clinical course.
Histoplasmosis	A. CF titer B. Skin histoplasmin test	Neither test is considered reliable in dogs and cats for definitive diagnosis.
Aspergillosis	Immunodiffusion gel precipitin test	Positive results correlate well with active infection. Cross-reacts with *Penicillium* spp.

CSF = cerebrospinal fluid; ELISA = enzyme-linked immunosorbent assay; IFA = indirect fluorescent antibody test; PCR = polymerase chain reaction.

Osmolal Gap

Definition

I. Osmolal gap is the difference between measured serum osmolality and calculated osmolality
II. Serum osmolality can be measured with an osmometer.
   A. The major osmotically active solutes are Na, K, glucose, and urea.
   B. Normal osmolality is 285–300 mOsm/kg.
III. Calculated serum osmolality is derived from the following equation.

$$2(Na + K) + \frac{Glucose}{18} + \frac{BUN}{3}$$

IV. A difference >10 mOsm between the measured and calculated values is significant.

Causes

I. If the calculated value exceeds the measured value, a mathematical or laboratory error exists.
II. If the measured value is normal but the calculated value is low, a decrease in serum water is the usual cause.
III. When both values are elevated and a significant gap exists, an unmeasured osmole should be suspected.
   A. Mannitol, glycerin
   B. Sorbitol, acetone
   C. Ethylene glycol, alcohol
   D. Myeloma protein, hyperlipidemia
   E. Infused hyperosmotic solutions

Clinical Significance

I. Directs attention to laboratory errors
II. Detects presence of unmeasured osmoles (e.g., ethylene glycol)
III. Can be used to confirm hyperproteinemia and hyperlipidemia

Table 2–5. **Precautions for Collection and Handling of Blood Samples for Clotting Tests**

1. Obtain all blood samples with plastic syringes by *careful* venipuncture.
2. To avoid activation of clotting during collection, the best method for obtaining samples of animal blood is to put the desired amount of anticoagulant into the syringe beforehand.
3. Trisodium citrate is the anticoagulant of choice for coagulation and platelet work (i.e., 1 part 3.8% citrate to 9 parts whole blood).
4. Keep all samples in plastic or silicone-coated glass test tubes.
5. Plasma samples prepared from fresh blood are kept cool and tested immediately or frozen for testing later. Frozen samples can be stored at −40°C or lower temperatures for several months.
6. Platelet tests must be performed on fresh samples within 2–4 h of collection. Polycarbonate is an ideal plastic surface for platelet preparations. Samples are kept at room temperature because platelet shape is altered by heat or cold.
7. Normal control samples from the *same* species and prepared the same way should be measured along with test samples for comparison and to check reagents.

Courtesy of Dr. W. Jean Dodds.

Bibliography

Aguilera-Tejero E, Mayer-Valor R, Gomez-Cardenas G: Quantification of plasma bile acids in the dog with a direct spectrophotometric method. J Small Anim Pract 29:705, 1988

Bagley RS, Center SA, Lewis RM et al: The effect of experimental cystitis and iatrogenic blood contamination on the urine protein/creatinine ratio. J Vet Intern Med 5:66, 1991

Center SA, Baldwin BH, Erb HN, Tennant BC: Bile acid concentrations in the diagnosis of hepatobiliary disease in the dog. J Am Vet Med Assoc 187:935, 1985

Crawford MA, Kittleson MD, Fink GD: Hypernatremia and adipsia in a dog. J Am Vet Med Assoc 184:818, 1984

Eigenmann JE: Diagnosis and treatment of dwarfism in a German shepherd dog. J Am Anim Hosp Assoc 17:798, 1981

Feldman BF, Rosenberg DP: Clinical use of anion and osmolal gaps in veterinary medicine. J Am Vet Med Assoc 178:396, 1981

Feldman EC: Comparison of ACTH response and dexamethasone suppression as screening tests in canine hyperadrenocorticism. J Am Vet Med Assoc 182:506, 1983

Feldman EC: Distinguishing dogs with functioning adrenocortical tumors from dogs with pituitary-dependent hyperadrenocorticism. J Am Vet Med Assoc 183:195, 1983

Feldman EC, Krutzik S: Case reports of parathyroid levels in spontaneous canine parathyroid disorders. J Am Anim Hosp Assoc 17:393, 1981

Feldman EC, Nelson RW: Canine and Feline Endocrinology and Reproduction. 2nd Ed. WB Saunders, Philadelphia, 1996

Giger U: Erythropoietin and its clinical use. Compend Contin Educ Pract Vet 14:25, 1992

Grauer GF, Grauer RM: Veterinary clinical osmometry. Compend Contin Educ Pract Vet 5:539, 1983

Greene CE (ed): Infectious Diseases of the Dog and Cat. WB Saunders, Philadelphia, 1990

Greene CE, Burgdorfer W, Cavagnolo R et al: Rocky Mountain spotted fever in dogs and its differentiation from canine ehrlichiosis. J Am Vet Med Assoc 186:465, 1985

Greene RT, Levine JF, Breitschwerdt EB et al: Clinical and serologic evaluations of induced Borrelia burgdorferi infection in dogs. Am J Vet Res 49:752, 1988

Hasler AH, Popkave CG, Shafer FS et al: Serum erythropoietin in polycythemic cats. J Vet Intern Med 9:187, 1995

Henry CJ, Clark TP, Young DW, Spano JS: Urine cortisol:creatinine ratio in healthy and sick cats. J Vet Intern Med 10:123, 1996

Kaufman CF, Kirk RW: The 60-minute plasma phenolsulfonphthalein concentration as a test of renal function in the dog. J Am Anim Hosp Assoc 9:66, 1973

Kemppainen RJ, Mansfield PD, Sartin JL: Endocrine responses of normal cats to TSH and synthetic ACTH administration. J Am Anim Hosp Assoc 20:737, 1984

Kuehn NF, Gaunt SD: Clinical and hematologic findings in canine ehrlichiosis. J Am Vet Med Assoc 186:355, 1985

Lappin MR, Greene CE, Prestwood AK et al: Diagnosis of recent Toxoplasma gondii infection in cats by use of an enzyme-linked immunosorbent assay for immunoglobulin. Am J Vet Res 50:1580, 1989a

Lappin MR, Greene CE, Prestwood AK et al: Enzyme-linked immunosorbent assay for the detection of circulating antigens of Toxoplasma gondii in the serum of cats. Am J Vet Res 50:1586, 1989b

Leib MS, Wingfield WE, Twedt DC, Bottoms GD: Plasma gastrin immunoreactivity in dogs with acute gastric dilatation-volvulus. J Am Vet Med Assoc 185:205, 1984

Mack RE, Feldman EC: Comparison of two low-dose dexamethasone suppression protocols as screening and discrimination tests in dogs with hyperadrenocorticism. J Am Vet Med Assoc 197:1603, 1990

Maddison JE, Pascoe PJ, Jansen BS: Clinical evaluation of sodium sulfanilate clearance for the diagnosis of renal disease in dogs. J Am Vet Med Assoc 185:961, 1984

Medleau L, Marks MA, Brown J, Borges WL: Clinical evaluation of a cryptococcal antigen latex agglutination test for diagnosis of cryptococcosis in cats. J Am Vet Med Assoc 196:1470, 1990

Middleton DJ: Duodenal ulceration associated with gastrin-secreting pancreatic tumor in a cat. J Am Vet Med Assoc 183:461, 1983

Nelson RW, Ihle SL, Feldman EC, Bottoms GD: Serum free thyroxine concentration in healthy dogs, dogs with hypothyroidism, and euthyroid dogs with concurrent illness. J Am Vet Med 198:1401, 1991

Nicoletti P, Chase A: An evaluation of methods to diagnose Brucella canis infection in dogs. Compend Contin Educ Pract Vet 9:1071, 1987

Panciera DL: Hypothyroidism in dogs: 66 cases (1987–1992). J Am Vet Med Assoc 204:761, 1994

Polzin DJ, Stevens JB, Osborne CA: Clinical application of the anion gap in evaluation of acid-base disorders in dogs. Compend Contin Educ Pract Vet 4:1021, 1982

Refsal KR, Nachreiner RF, Stein BE et al: Use of the triiodothyronine suppression test for diagnosis of hyperthyroidism in ill cats that have serum concentration of iodothyronines within normal range. J Am Vet Med Assoc 199:1594, 1991

Reusch CE, Feldman EC: Canine hyperadrenocorticism due to adrenocortical neoplasia. J Vet Intern Med 5:3, 1991

Schaer M, Chen CL: A clinical survey of 48 dogs with adrenocortical hypofunction. J Am Anim Hosp Assoc 19:443, 1983

Smiley LE, Peterson ME: Evaluation of a urine cortisol:creatinine ratio as a screening test for hyperadrenocorticism in dogs. J Vet Intern Med 7:163, 1993

Smith MC, Feldman EC: Plasma endogenous ACTH concentrations and plasma cortisol responses to synthetic ACTH and dexamethasone sodium phosphate in healthy cats. Am J Vet Res 48:1719, 1987

Strombeck DR: Evaluation of 60-minute blood p-aminobenzoic acid concentration in pancreatic function testing of dogs. J Am Vet Med Assoc 180:419, 1982

Vail DM, Panciera DL, Ogilvie GK: Thyroid hormone concentrations in dogs with chronic weight loss, with special reference to cancer cachexia. J Vet Intern Med 8:122, 1994

White JV, Olivier NB, Reimann K, Johnson C: Use of protein-to-creatinine ratio in a single urine specimen for quantitative estimation of canine proteinuria. J Am Vet Med Assoc 185:882, 1984

Williams DA, Scott-Moncrieff C, Bruner J: Validation of an immunoassay for canine thyroid-stimulating hormone and changes in serum concentration following induction of hypothyroidism in dogs. J Am Vet Med Assoc 209:1730, 1996

3

Selected Diagnostic and Therapeutic Procedures

Douglas E. Brum
Rhea V. Morgan

CENTRAL VENOUS PRESSURE MEASUREMENT

Definition

Central venous pressure (CVP) is the measurement of fluid pressure in the anterior vena cava or right atrium. It is a dynamic function of both cardiac output and venous return to the heart.

Indications

I. Assess IV fluid therapy
II. Monitor circulating hemodynamics during shock
III. Diagnostic aid in cases of heart failure and pericardial effusion with tamponade

Restraint

I. The animal may be placed in either sternal or lateral recumbency.
II. Sedation is not indicated or desirable.

Technique

I. Insert an indwelling IV catheter into the external jugular vein, bringing the tip of the catheter to rest in the right atrium.
II. Connect catheter to male end of three-way stopcock via extension tubing.
III. Attach a manometer calibrated in centimeters to stopcock, perpendicular to the catheter line (Table 3–1).
IV. Attach IV infusion solution to third portal of stopcock.
V. Fill tubing and manometer with heparinized saline or IV solution.
VI. Hold manometer so the zero mark is level with the right atrium.

A. Sternal recumbency: 4th intercostal space, 2–3 in. above sternum
B. Lateral recumbency: parallel to sternum near 4th sternebra
VII. Turn stopcock so that infusion set is off and the manometer to the catheter is free-flowing.
VIII. Allow liquid in manometer to equilibrate.
IX. Note pressure at point where meniscus stops descending.
X. If the meniscus falls below zero, refill the manometer and lower it so that the zero point is now at the 5-cm mark, with values between 0 and 5 cm denoting negative measurements.

Sources of Error

I. Incorrect positioning of manometer
II. Rapid or labored breathing
III. Kinking of catheter or extension tubing
IV. Clots within the catheter
V. Malfunctioning of stopcock

Interpretation

I. CVP is an insensitive test. The sensitivity can be increased by using minimal lengths of connective tubing and removing all extraneous catheter adapters.
II. The trends that develop with sequential CVP recordings are more significant than isolated or individual measurements.
III. See Appendix I for normal CVP values.

PERICARDIOCENTESIS

Definition

Pericardiocentesis is the transthoracic insertion of a needle or cannula into the pericardial space for the collection of fluid for diagnostic or therapeutic purposes.

17

Table 3–1. **Diagnostic and Therapeutic Instruments**

Manometer: Pharmaseal Manometer Tray—Baxter Healthcare Corp., Pharmaseal Division, Valencia, CA 91355

Blood pressure monitors

Dinamap oscillometric veterinary blood pressure monitor Model 8300—Critikon, Inc., Tampa, FL 33634

Parks ultrasonic Doppler flow detector model 811-B—Parks Medical Electronics, Inc., Aloha, OR 97007

Indwelling chest tube: Argyle trochar catheter with Sentinel Eye—Argyle Division of Sherwood Medical, St. Louis, MO 63103

One-way air valve: Heimlich Chest Drain Valve—Becton, Dickinson and Co, Franklin Lakes, NJ 07417

Continuous evacuation pump

Pleur-Evac—Deknatel, Division of Howmedica, Queens Village, NY 11429

Closed chest suction—Argyle Division of Sherwood Medical Products, St. Louis, MO 63103

Nasal oxygen tubes and nasal feeding tubes

Kaofeed II polyurethane feeding tube—Ivac Corp., San Diego, CA 92121-1579

Sterile single-use feeding tube and urethral catheter—Monoject, Division of Sherwood Medical, St. Louis, MO 63103

Argyle nasogastric feeding tube—Argyle Division of Sherwood Medical, St. Louis, MO 63103

Nasal oxygen humidification: Hudson Humidifier—Oxygen Therapy Sales Company, Wadsworth, OH 44281

Tracheostomy tube: Portex—Portex, Wilmington, MA 01887

Transtracheal fluid trap: Lukens Specimen Container—Sherwood Medical Products, St. Louis, MO 63103

Percutaneous gastrostomy tubes

Medicut intravenous cannula—Sherwood Medical Industries, Inc., St. Louis, MO 63103

Bard urologic catheter—Bard Urologic Division of C.R. Bard, Covington, GA 30209

Silicone percutaneous endoscopic gastrostomy kit—Mill-Rose Laboratories, Inc., Mentor, OH 44060

Bone marrow biopsy needles

Osgood bone marrow needle—Becton, Dickenson and Co., Franklin Lakes, NJ 07417

Rosenthal bone marrow needle—Becton, Dickenson and Co., Franklin Lakes, NJ 07417

Jamshidi bone marrow needle—Kor Med, Inc., Minneapolis, MN 55420

Bone biopsy instrument: Michel trephine biopsy instrument—Miltex Instrument Co., Lake Success, NY 11042

Indications

I. Pericardial effusion
   A. Collection of fluid for gross, cytologic, and bacterial analysis
   B. Therapeutic removal of pericardial fluid when diastolic filling or pulmonary function is compromised by the presence of that fluid

II. Cardiac tamponade
   Removal of fluid that can cause right-sided heart failure because of restriction of diastolic filling of the ventricles

III. Radiographic contrast studies
   Intrapericardial administration of positive or negative contrast media to enhance radiographic visualization of intrapericardial structures

Restraint

I. Physical restraint in lateral or sternal recumbency or in standing position

II. Mild chemical sedation [diazepam (Valium), 0.2–0.6 mg/kg IV] sometimes beneficial, depending on the temperament and physical status of the patient

Technique

I. A rectangular area of the right lateral thoracic skin is clipped and prepared aseptically from the sternum to the midthorax and from the 2nd to the 8th intercostal spaces.

II. Ideally, thoracic ultrasound should be used for needle placement.

III. If ultrasound is unavailable, the site for needle insertion is selected based on review of the dorsoventral and lateral thoracic radiograph to assess the location of the pericardial silhouette.
   A. Usually the 4th, 5th, or 6th intercostal space is best.
   B. The right side is preferable, owing to the absence of pulmonary tissue in the region of the cardiac notch (approximately the 4th intercostal space).
   C. A point one-fourth the distance from the sternabrae to the costochondral junction is selected. The ventral location reduces the risk of coronary artery laceration by the needle.
   D. The skin and subcutaneous and intercostal tissues may be infiltrated with a local anesthetic before needle insertion.
   E. A through-the-needle intravenous catheter is selected (19-gauge needle). The needle is passed through the skin, subcutis, and intercostal muscles until it is in the pericardial space.
      1. The catheter is advanced, and the needle is withdrawn from the chest wall.
      2. The stylet is removed, and a three-way stopcock and sterile syringe (12 or 20 ml) are attached.
   F. Fluid is aspirated. If no fluid is obtained, the catheter is slowly withdrawn while applying intermittent suction. After completion of fluid collection, the catheter is withdrawn.
   G. The fluid is transferred to EDTA tubes for cytologic study and to transport medium for bacteriologic analysis.

Complications

I. Cardiac arrhythmias can be induced by the needle contacting or penetrating the myocardium. Electrocardiographic (ECG) monitoring during the procedure is advised.

II. Laceration of a coronary artery can lead to hemorrhage and tamponade.
   A. Collection of bloody fluid that clots soon after collection may indicate coronary artery laceration.
   B. Insertion of the needle in a ventral location (near cardiac apex) or under guidance with fluoroscopy or ultrasonography reduces the likelihood of this complication.

THORACENTESIS

Definition

Thoracentesis is the surgical puncturing of the chest wall for drainage of fluid or air from the pleural cavity.

Indications

I. Alleviation of pneumothorax
II. Obtaining fluid samples for analysis
III. Removal of fluid to relieve dyspnea

Restraint

I. Sternal recumbency is preferred so that gravity causes intrathoracic fluid to be positioned ventrally in the chest and air to be trapped dorsally.
II. Compromised patients are restrained manually.
III. Fractious or anxious animals may be mildly tranquilized.
   A. Cat: 0.1 ml ketamine HCl IV
   B. Dog: 0.05–0.15 ml acepromazine IV
   C. Butorphanol
      1. Dose: 0.2–0.4 mg/kg IV
      2. May be combined with diazepam 0.2 mg/kg IV or midazolam 0.1–0.2 mg/kg IV for added sedation

Technique

I. Shave hair and with sterile technique prepare the skin at the site of puncture.
   A. Air: aspirate dorsally at 7th to 9th intercostal spaces.
   B. Fluid: aspirate ventrally at the 7th or 8th intercostal space. Avoid the apex beat of the heart.
II. Aspirate either air or fluid using appropriate equipment.
   A. Air: 20- or 22-gauge 1.5-in. needle, three-way stopcock, and 12- to 20-ml syringe
   B. Fluid: 17- or 19-gauge through-the-needle IV catheter, three-way stopcock, and 12- to 20-ml syringe
III. Pass the needle through the skin, intercostal muscles, and parietal pleura into the pleural cavity.
IV. If an IV catheter is used, thread the catheter into the chest for several inches and withdraw the needle.
V. Apply negative pressure to the syringe with the three-way stopcock in the open position.

Complications

I. Accidental puncture of the internal thoracic artery, intercostal or coronary vessels, and myocardium
II. Accidental pneumothorax if the three-way stopcock is left open or connections in the aspiration line become loose

CHEST TUBE PLACEMENT

Definition

Chest tube placement refers to insertion of an indwelling chest tube for therapy of pleural cavity disease.

Indications

I. Provide access to the pleural space for repeated intermittent aspiration of free pleural fluid
II. Provide continuous evacuation of air in cases of severe and/or tension pneumothorax
III. Provide a means for installation and subsequent drainage of intrathoracic antibiotics and lavage solutions

Restraint

I. For insertion of the chest tube, the animal is placed in lateral recumbency. Manual restraint is preferred, but light sedation may be considered.
II. Once the chest tube is inserted and positioned, actual aspiration of the chest may be attempted in any position that facilitates removal of the fluid or air.

Technique

I. The hair is shaved and the skin prepared with sterile technique.
II. If time allows, the skin and musculature are infiltrated with a local anesthetic one to two ribs caudal to the insertion site.
III. The sites chosen for insertion are similar to those for thoracentesis.
   A. Air: dorsal 7th or 8th intercostal spaces
   B. Fluid: ventral 6th to 8th intercostal spaces
   C. One or more tubes inserted uni- or bilaterally
IV. A stab incision is made through the skin with a scalpel blade over the infiltrated site.
V. The chest tube with trocar is inserted through the incision and advanced cranially under the skin to the desired site. With a quick, forceful movement the tube is pushed through the intercostal muscles and into the thorax (Fig. 3–1).
VI. As the trocar is removed, the tube is cross-clamped, and the free end is attached to a three-way stopcock, one-way valve, or continuous evacuation pump (see Table 3–1).
VII. The clamp is released, the patency of the tube ensured, and a pursestring suture placed in the skin where the tube exits. A non–water-soluble ointment is applied at the exit site.
VIII. The tube is fixed to the chest by placing stay sutures through a tape butterfly surrounding the free end of the tube. A light chest wrap is then applied to protect the tube from dislodgement.

Complications

I. Inadvertent laceration of intercostal, internal thoracic, or cardiac vessels

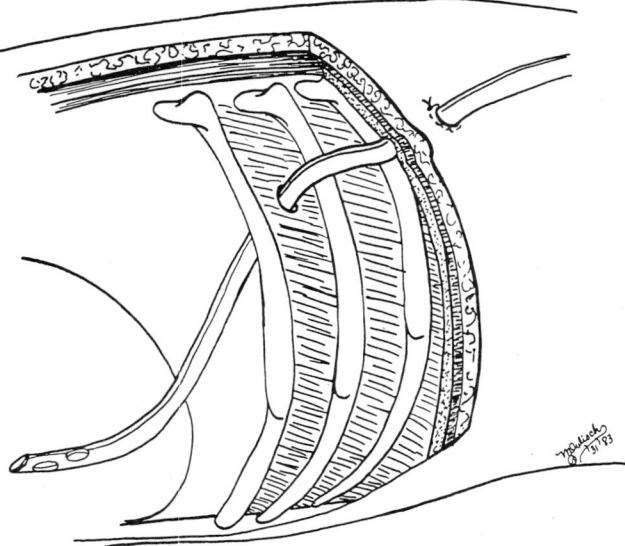

Figure 3–1. Technique for inserting an indwelling chest tube. (From Morgan RV: *Manual of Small Animal Emergencies*. Churchill Livingstone, New York, 1985, with permission.)

II. Accidental pneumothorax during removal of the trocar
III. In the days after insertion of the chest tube, close monitoring is necessary to ensure the following:
   A. The chest tube remains patent, and all moving parts remain free of viscous discharges.
   B. The position of the tube is correct within the chest, and it does not back out.
   C. All connections are tight, with no leakage of air into the chest.
   D. All portals are protected from bacterial contamination.

NASAL OXYGEN ADMINISTRATION

Definition

Nasal cannulation allows the administration of oxygen from a tube placed through the nares into the ventral nasal meatus to provide for increased arterial blood oxygen concentration in the compromised patient.

Indications

I. Any cause of hypoxia
   A. Cardiopulmonary disease
   B. Hematologic abnormalities
   C. Metabolic disease
   D. Shock
II. Useful in the animal too mobile for an oxygen mask or too large for an oxygen cage

Restraint and Technique

I. Topical anesthesia is usually all that is required.

   A. With the head extended, 0.1–0.5 ml of 2% lidocaine is dripped into the nares.
   B. Lidocaine gel is also applied to the junction of the skin and the nares laterally, allowing several minutes for the region to become anesthetized.
II. A fenestrated polyurethane catheter of appropriate size (usually a 4, 6, or 8 French) is selected.
III. The tube is measured from the nares to approximately the level of the fourth premolar tooth and marked.
IV. The tube is then passed through the nares into the ventral nasal meatus until the predetermined mark is reached.
V. It is sutured to the skin lateral to the nares using 3-0 or 2-0 nylon.
   A. It is important to place this first suture as close to the nasal mucosa as possible to ensure good tube stability.
   B. Once the first knot is placed, the suture material is passed several times around the tube in a "boot-lace" pattern.
VI. A second suture is placed on the midline of the forehead, fixing the skin to an adhesive tape butterfly placed around the tube.
VII. Humidified oxygen is delivered to the animal.
   A. Commercially available humidifiers may be used (see Table 3–1).
   B. A homemade humidifier can be made (Fitzpatrick and Crowe, 1985).
     1. An IV extension tube is attached to the nasal oxygen tube (see Table 3–1) and into the administration port of a half-full bottle of warm saline.
     2. The tube carrying the oxygen source is attached to the vent hole of the bottle, and the oxygen is bubbled through the water.
   C. The oxygen flow rate is set at 50–150 ml/min/kg body weight initially and then adjusted as needed.

Complications

I. If the oxygen flow rate is too high, nasal mucosal erosions ("jet lesions") and nasal irritation may occur.
II. Gastric dilation can occur if the tube is placed too far caudally toward the pharynx or if the oxygen flow rate is too high.
III. Unhumidified oxygen causes dryness of the respiratory passages.
IV. Traumatic tube placement may result in mild epistaxis.

TRACHEOSTOMY TUBE INSERTION

Definition

A tracheostomy is the surgical creation of an opening into the trachea for insertion of a tracheostomy tube.

Indications

I. Provide a means for delivering air or oxygen past an upper airway obstruction
II. Allow a means to evacuate secretions from the airway
III. Facilitate passage of air or oxygen to the lungs under positive pressure

Restraint

I. General anesthesia is preferred.
II. In an emergency, physical restraint, with or without local anesthesia, may be all that is required.

Technique

I. Shave the hair and by sterile technique prepare the skin from the angular process of the jaw to the thoracic inlet while the animal is in dorsal recumbency.
II. Make an incision over the trachea immediately caudal to the larynx or caudal to the obstruction.
III. Separate the two sternohyoid muscles with blunt dissection (Fig. 3–2A).
IV. Incise the trachea between the cartilaginous rings. For high obstructions, make the incision between rings 2 and 3 or 3 and 4.
V. Enlarge the incision with a scalpel blade, being careful not to lacerate the endotracheal tube (Fig. 3–2B).

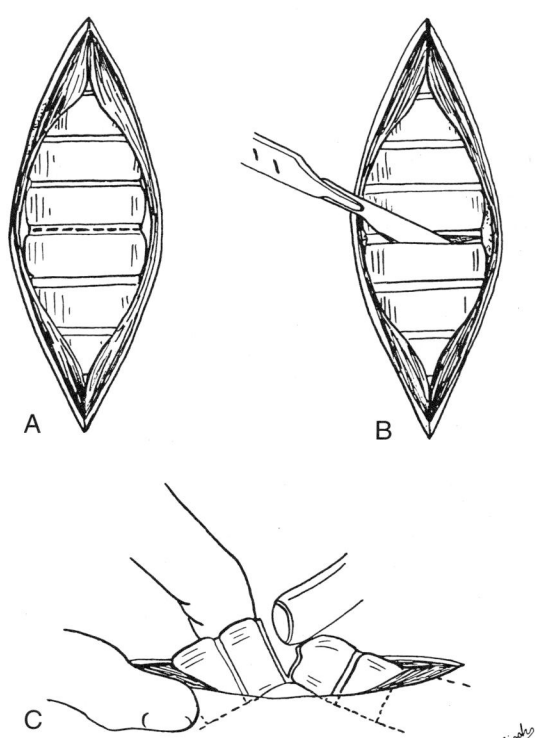

Figure 3–2. Technique for insertion of a tracheostomy tube. (From Morgan RV: Manual of Small Animal Emergencies. Churchill Livingstone, New York, 1985, with permission.)

VI. Withdraw the endotracheal tube and insert a tracheostomy tube (Fig. 3–2C and Table 3–1).
VII. If the tracheostomy tube is supplied with an obturator, remove it.
VIII. Tie the tracheostomy tube in place with umbilical tape, and/or suture it to the skin of the neck.
IX. Sterile endotracheal tubes may be used in giant-breed or thick-necked dogs in which ordinary tubes cannot be adequately secured.

Complications

I. Patency of the airway may be compromised during the tracheostomy procedure by blood and secretions. Suction the airway immediately after inserting the tube.
II. The normal warming and humidification of air by the nasal passages is bypassed with a tracheostomy tube. Thick, dry mucus may accumulate as a result and diminish the tube's patency. Measures can be taken to prevent it.
   A. Suction the tube every 2 or 4 hours using aseptic technique.
   B. Liquefy secretions.
      1. Nebulize with saline or diluted acetylcysteine every 4–8 hours.
      2. Instill 1 ml saline into tracheal tube every 2–8 hours.
   C. Maintain normal body hydration with SQ or IV fluids.
III. When the tracheostomy tube is removed, the site is left open to heal by second intention.
   A. The open site is cleaned several times daily.
   B. Surgical closure of the tracheostomy site may result in subcutaneous emphysema or pneumomediastinum.

TRANSTRACHEAL ASPIRATION

Definition

Transtracheal aspiration (TTA) is the placement of a cannula from the rostral trachea into the lower respiratory tract for the collection of uncontaminated bronchial secretions.

Indications

I. To determine the cause of inflammatory conditions of the respiratory tract
   A. Bacterial
   B. Viral
   C. Fungal
   D. Allergic
   E. Parasitic
   F. Neoplastic
Note: Although neoplastic cells from bronchial or pulmonary tumors may be identified microscopically in TTA specimens, there is a high incidence of false-negative results with pulmonary tumors.

II. Prognostic aid after smoke inhalation or exposure to fire and toxic fumes

Restraint

I. Dogs

Mild sedation (butorphanol 0.2–0.4 mg/kg IV, and diazepam 0.2 mg/kg IV) may be indicated depending on the temperament and physical status of the patient.

II. Cats
  A. Intravenous induction of general anesthesia with an untrashort-acting thiobarbiturate
  B. Heavy sedation with ketamine 2–4 mg/kg IV and diazepam 0.1–0.2 mg/kg IV
  C. Sternal or lateral recumbency

Technique

I. Dogs
  A. The ventral cervical skin is clipped and prepared aseptically.
  B. The site for catheter insertion is palpated. Either the cricothyroid membrane or the space between any of the first three tracheal rings may be used.
  C. The skin and subcutaneous tissues are infused with a local anesthetic.
  D. A 16-, 17-, or 18-gauge IV catheter is advanced through the skin and subcutis and into the tracheal lumen at the selected site (Fig. 3–3).
  E. Once the needle is within the tracheal lumen, it is directed downward toward the carina, and the catheter is advanced. A transient cough reflex usually occurs during this step.

F. The needle is retracted from the site and the stylet removed.
G. A sterile syringe containing a multiple-electrolyte solution (1 ml/5 lb body weight) is attached. Aspiration on the syringe yields air if the catheter is placed correctly.
H. If central suction is available, the entire calculated dose of fluid is injected. The syringe is disconnected from the catheter, and a Lukens specimen container, 14 French with 20-ml trap and male adapter plug, is attached to the catheter (see Table 3–1).
  1. Central suction is applied to the trap, and fluid is collected.
  2. When a sufficient specimen has been collected, suction is turned off and the catheter is withdrawn.
I. If central suction is not available, the fluid is injected at 2-ml increments with intermittent aspiration until fluid, not air, is retrieved. The volume of fluid necessary may vary from 2–25 ml. The actual specimen collected is usually 0.5–2 ml.

II. Cats
  A. The technique is basically the same as for the dog except that it is performed under sedation through a sterile endotracheal tube.
  1. Immediately on sedation by intravenous injection, a sterilized endotracheal tube is carefully placed in the trachea by intubation.
  2. The catheter is advanced through the endotracheal tube, and fluid is administered and collected in the same manner as described for the dog.

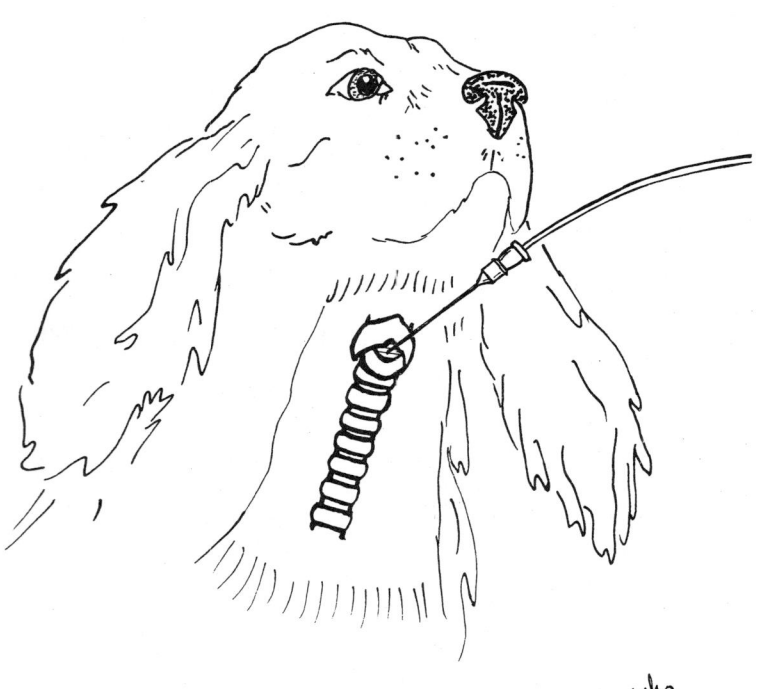

Figure 3–3. Transtracheal aspiration is accomplished by inserting an intravenous catheter through the criocothyroid membrane of the larynx into the trachea. The catheter is then advanced into the lower airway.

B. An alternative method is to perform the technique outlined for the dog.

III. Specimen handling
 A. A portion of the fluid is placed in transport medium for microbiologic analysis.
 B. The remainder of the fluid is spun in a centrifuge, and the cellular fraction is examined microscopically. If immediate cytologic analysis is not possible, several drops of 10% formalin solution are added, and centrifugation is performed just before microscopic examination.

Complications

I. Most complications are mild and transient in nature.
 A. Coughing
 B. Subcutaneous or mediastinal emphysema
 C. Hemoptysis
 D. Subcutaneous hematoma

II. Inadvertent collection of pharyngeal or upper tracheal secretions may yield inappropriate results.

III. The use of collection fluids containing bacteriostatic agents may cause false-negative culture results.

CEREBROSPINAL FLUID COLLECTION

Definition

A cerebrospinal fluid (CSF) tap is used to collect CSF by percutaneous needle aspiration of the subarachnoid space.

Indications

I. Retrieval of CSF for analysis when organic dysfunction of the central nervous system (CNS) is suspected
 A. Recent history of neurologic symptoms
 B. Neurologic deficits present on examination

II. Insertion of contrast medium into the subarachnoid space as an aid to localizing spinal cord lesions

Restraint

I. General anesthesia is always indicated for CSF tap in dogs and cats.

II. Proper positioning is critical to accomplish accurate needle placement.
 A. Cisternal tap
  The animal is placed in lateral recumbency with the head flexed ventrally to open the atlanto-occipital interspace. The ears are pulled forward to tense the skin. A towel or sandbag may be positioned under the head to maintain the entire spine a consistent distance from the table surface.
 B. Lumbar tap
  The animal is placed in sternal recumbency with an assistant pulling the hind legs in a cranial and dorsal direction to open the interarcual space between the caudal lumbar vertebrae. The entire spine must be kept straight.

Technique

I. Cisternal tap
 A. The hair is clipped, and the skin is aseptically prepared on the dorsal cervical region from 2 cm rostral to the occipital protuberance to the level of the 3rd cervical vertebra.
 B. With the left hand, the operator digitally palpates the external occipital protuberance and the rostral wings of the atlas. The index finger can be used to palpate a depression between these three structures. This depression marks the site for needle placement (Fig. 3–4).
 C. A spinal needle with stylet is slowly inserted through the skin, subcutaneous tissues, and muscles.
  1. Large dogs: 20-gauge 3.5-in. needle
  2. Small dogs, cats: 22-gauge 1.5- or 3.5-in. needle
 D. The combined dura mater and arachnoid membranes are penetrated.
  1. The stylet is withdrawn with each advancement of the needle through the membranes to check for the presence of fluid.
  2. Always replace the stylet before advancing the needle. (The stylet is not used in small animals so there can be constant observation for fluid.)
 E. Immediately on the appearance of fluid through the needle, a spinal manometer with three-way stopcock is attached.
  1. The manometer is held perpendicular to the long axis of the needle, and the stopcock is turned so that CSF flows into the manometer.
  2. A reading (in centimeters) is taken when the

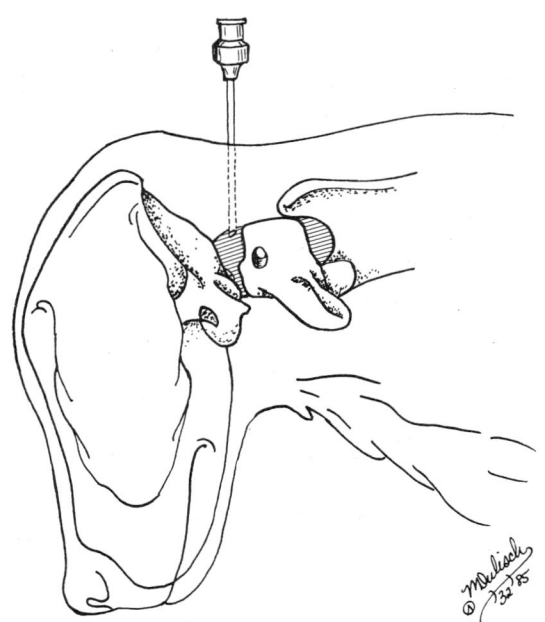

Figure 3–4. Cisternal puncture for spinal fluid collection and/or insertion of contrast medium for myelographic study.

fluid level has stabilized within the manometer.

3. It is important that no external pressure is exerted on any part of the body during pressure measurement, and the jugular veins must be free of compression.

F. A 3-ml syringe is attached to the female end of the three-way stopcock, and CSF is collected by careful, gentle aspiration.
   1. It is important not to move the needle during pressure measurement and fluid collection.
   2. Fluid from the manometer may be aspirated into the syringe to increase the volume of the specimen.
   3. In small animals (<7 kg), the small volume of CSF present prohibits the measurement of pressure. Instead, a syringe is attached directly to the needle, or CSF is allowed to drip into a sterile collection tube.
   4. The quantity of fluid saved varies.
      a) Large dogs: 1.0–3.5 ml
      b) Small dogs, cats: 0.5–1.5 ml

G. If indicated, contrast material may be administered for myelography.

H. The needle is carefully and smoothly withdrawn.

I. Fluid is placed in a sterile tube for microscopic, chemical, and microbiologic analysis.

II. Lumbar tap

A. The skin over the dorsal lumbar spine is clipped and aseptically prepared.

B. The dorsal spinous processes of the lumbar vertebrae are palpated. Optimal sites for the collection of CSF are at the L4–L5 or L5–L6 interspace (Fig. 3–5).

C. A 20- or 22-gauge 3.5-in. spinal needle is inserted immediately cranial to the dorsal spinous process of the vertebra at the caudal aspect of the planned puncture site.
   1. The needle is advanced toward the spinal canal until it contacts a dorsal laminar surface.

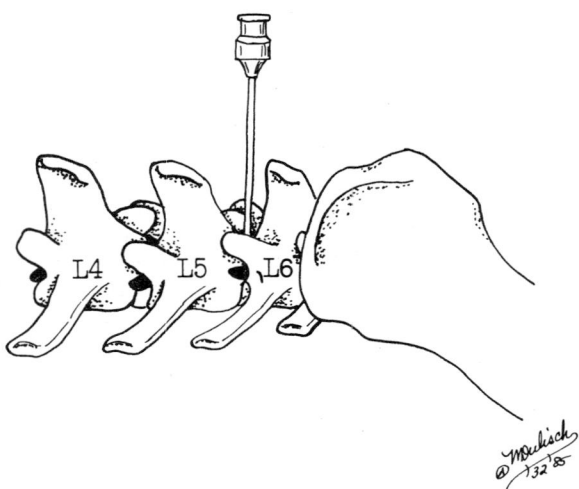

Figure 3–5. A lumbar spinal tap is demonstrated at the interarcual space between lumbar vertebrae 5 and 6.

The needle must be maintained parallel to the dorsal spinous processes.

2. The needle is "walked" cranially or caudally along the laminar surface until it drops into the interarcual space. A twitch in the rear legs or tail may indicate proper needle placement (see Fig. 3–5).

D. The stylet is withdrawn, a syringe is attached to the needle, and gentle aspiration is applied until fluid is recovered.
   1. The depth of needle insertion may be adjusted slightly during aspiration.
   2. The subarachnoid space is small in the region of the lumbar cord, and only a small quantity of fluid may be recovered (0.5–2.5 ml).

E. At this point, contrast medium can be injected if myelographic study is indicated.

F. The needle is removed and fluid placed into a sterile tube for microscopic, chemical, and microbiologic analysis.

Complications

I. Direct needle trauma to the parenchyma of the brain or spinal cord can occur if careful, controlled advancement of the needle is not practiced.

II. Iatrogenic hemorrhage may make interpretation of laboratory results difficult. If contamination with blood occurs, consider the following correction factors.
   A. One white blood cell (WBC) is expected for every 500 red blood cells (RBCs).
   B. One thousand RBCs will increase CSF protein by approximately 1 mg/dl.

NASAL FEEDING TUBE PLACEMENT

Definition

I. A nasal feeding tube is a tube placed from the external nares into the stomach (nasogastric) or distal esophagus (nasoesophageal) for administration of fluids and nutrients or to achieve decompression of the dilated stomach.

II. If the esophagus is functional, a nasoesophageal tube should be placed; if the esophagus is nonfunctional (e.g., megaesophagus or esophageal stricture), a nasogastric tube should be placed.

Indications

I. To provide nutritional support to patients unwilling or unable to eat for various reasons
   A. Facial, maxillary, and mandibular fractures
   B. Oral and esophageal disease
   C. Prolonged anorexia from a systemic disorder (e.g., hepatic lipidosis)

II. For temporary decompression of the stomach before or after corrective surgery for gastric dilatation volvulus

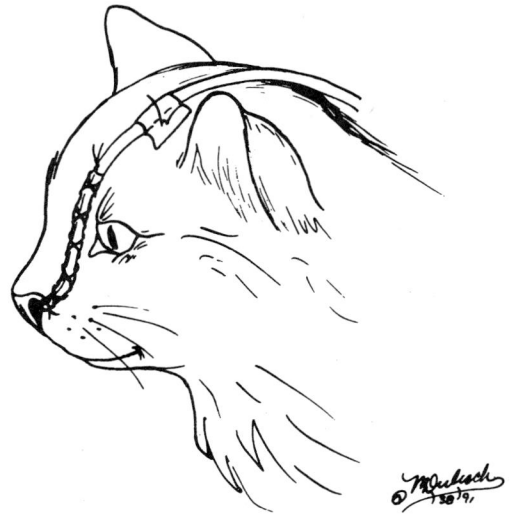

Figure 3–6. Correct placement of a nasal feeding tube.

Restraint

I. Usually local anesthesia is all that is required.
II. Occasionally mild sedation is useful.
   A. Dog: butorphanol 0.2–0.4 mg/kg IV
   B. Cat: diazepam 0.1–0.5 mg/kg IV with or without ketamine 0.2 mg/kg IV

Technique

I. Based on the patient's size, a 3.5–8 French polyurethane or polyvinylchloride tube is selected (see Table 3–1).
II. The distance from the tip of the nares to the last rib is measured and the tube marked accordingly.
III. Instill 2% lidocaine down the nostril (several drops for cats; 0.5–1 ml for dogs). Keep the head slightly elevated for 1–2 minutes as the lidocaine takes effect.
IV. The tube, nares, and skin where the sutures are to be applied are lubricated with 2% lidocaine jelly (Fig. 3–6).
V. The tube is then advanced through the nostril and into the ventral nasal meatus.
   A. In dogs, the tube is inserted dorsomedially for the first centimeter to avoid the alar fold and nasal vestibule, and then advanced ventrally. Alternatively, the external naris is pushed dorsally as the tube is advanced in a caudoventral, medial direction (Abood and Buffington, 1991).
   B. In cats, the tube may initially be directed ventromedially because of the lack of a well-developed alar fold.
VI. As the tube enters the pharynx, the animal is encouraged to swallow, allowing for easy passage into the esophagus.
   A. When placing a nasoesophageal tube, advance the tube until the tip is in the distal esophagus. The previously placed mark on the tube should be exposed for 2–4 cm.
   B. In placing a nasogastric tube, the tube is advanced until the premarked spot reaches the tip of the nares.
VII. Inject a small quantity of air and then saline into the tube to check for correct placement.
   A. Abdominal auscultation indicates air bubbling in the stomach.
   B. The injection should be well tolerated by the patient without struggling or coughing.
   C. A lateral caudal thoracic radiograph is taken if there is any uncertainty of the final location of the tube.
VIII. The tube is secured in place using 3-0 nonabsorbable sutures.
   A. The first suture is placed in the skin as close to the lateral margin of the external nares as possible, to ensure tube stability.
   B. Once the first ligature is made, the suture is passed around the tube several times in a "bootlace" pattern and then tied in place.
   C. The second suture is passed through an adhesive butterfly tape around the tube and into the skin along the dorsal midline of the head.
IX. An IV extension tube is attached to the exposed end of the nasal tube to allow for appropriate connections and free movement of the animal.
X. An Elizabethan collar is usually required to prevent tube removal by the animal.
XI. The tube may be left open to allow constant decompression of gas, or it may be opened intermittently for infusion of nutrients. A variety of canine and feline liquid diets are available (Table 3–2).

Table 3–2. **Liquid Diets for Use in Tube Feeding**

Brand	Manufacturer	Indications
CliniCare	CliniCare Products Pet-Ag, Inc. Elgin, IL 60120	Specifically formulated to meet protein caloric requirements of dogs and cats but requires functional gastrointestinal integrity
CliniCare Renal	CliniCare Products Pet-Ag, Inc. Elgin, IL 60120	Specifically formulated for dogs and cats with renal or liver disease
Travasorb MCT	Baxter Healthcare Corp. Deerfield, IL 60015	Recommended for use in animals with gastrointestinal disease because very digestible Comes in a powder and needs to be well blended so tubes do not clog May cause diarrhea at higher concentrations
Osmolite HN	Ross Labs Columbus, OH 43216	High in both protein content and quality but difficult to balance both protein and caloric requirements
Peptamen	Clintec Nutrition Co. Deerfield, IL 60015	Complete elemental diet for use in animals with impaired gastrointestinal function

XII. The tube is flushed periodically to maintain lumen patency.

Complications

I. Mild discomfort and rhinitis can occur, although patient compliance is usually quite good.

II. Nasogastric tubes may produce gastric irritation causing vomition. This can be decreased by placing the tube in the distal esophagus.

III. Vomiting or regurgitation from other causes including gastroesophageal reflux can alter tube location. Consider the use of pharmacologic agents that reduce gastric fluid acidity (e.g., cimetidine) or decrease gastric emptying time (e.g., metoclopramide) to minimize vomiting and regurgitation.

IV. If the liquid diet is too thick, the tube may become plugged.

V. If hyperosmolar solutions are used, diarrhea may occur. This can be minimized by diluting the formulation to an osmolarity between 200 and 300 mOsm/kg.

PERCUTANEOUS TUBE GASTROSTOMY

Definition

This procedure involves the placement of a feeding tube directly through the skin and into the gastric lumen with the use of an endoscope.

Indications

I. To provide nutritional support to animals unwilling or unable to eat for various reasons
   A. Facial and head trauma
   B. Oral and esophageal disease or after surgery
   C. Anorexia secondary to a systemic disorder

II. The larger diameter of the gastrotomy tube allows for more routine feeding (e.g., a mixture of blended canned food and water).

III. Nutrition is easily administered while the animal is cared for at home.

Restraint

I. General anesthesia with either injectable or inhalation anesthetics is required.

II. The animal is placed in right lateral recumbency, and a mouth gag is used to facilitate the passage of the endoscope.

Technique

I. The skin of the left paracostal region is clipped and aseptically prepared.

II. The endoscope is advanced through the mouth and esophagus into the gastric lumen. The stomach is insufflated with air until the gastric wall is under tension and in contact with the abdominal wall.

III. A gastrostomy tube and cannula are selected.
   A. Silicone percutaneous endoscopic gastrostomy kit (see Table 3–1)
   B. A sized 14–20 French mushroom tipped catheter with a 16-gauge medicut intravenous cannula and stylet (see Table 3–1)

IV. A small 3–4 mm skin incision is made caudal to the last rib and over the insufflated stomach.

V. The cannula (with stylet in place) is advanced through the skin incision, abdominal wall, and gastric wall and into the gastric lumen.

VI. The stylet is removed and a No. 1 or 2 nonabsorbable suture is placed through the catheter into the stomach.

VII. The suture is grasped in the stomach by a snare from the endoscope, and together they are pulled cranially toward the oral cavity.

VIII. The cannula is removed from the abdominal wall and passed tapered end first over the suture exiting the mouth.

IX. The funneled end of the gastrostomy tube is cut to fit inside the catheter, and the two are sutured together using 3-0 nylon on a straight needle that passes transversely through the catheter sheath and tube.

X. A water-soluble lubricant is applied to the cannula and tube, and they are passed through the oral cavity and esophagus and into the stomach, using gentle traction from the transabdominal suture.

XI. Correct positioning of the gastrostomy tube is checked with the endoscope.

XII. Using the transabdominal suture exiting the abdomen, the cannula and gastrostomy tube are pulled through the gastric and abdominal walls until the mushroom end of the tube comes to rest in the gastric lumen.

XIII. The gastrostomy tube is then secured to the skin using traction sutures. It is important to mark the tube at the skin margin and monitor it for any signs of migration.

XIV. An adapter and three-way stopcock are placed at the end of the tube to allow for intermittent feedings, and a light abdominal bandage is applied over the tube.

XV. The tube should remain in place for a minimum of 5 days to 2 weeks to decrease the incidence of peritonitis after tube removal.

XVI. To remove the tube, the sutures are cut and one of two methods is used.
   A. Steady outward traction is applied to the tube until the mushroom tip collapses and the tube can be pulled out through the abdominal wall.
   B. Pull the tube up against the body wall and then cut it flush at the skin, allowing the mushroom tip to fall back into the stomach and pass out the gastrointestinal tract (medium to large dog) or be retrieved endoscopically (small dogs and cats).

Complications

I. Wound infection, peritonitis

II. Migration of mushroom catheter tip into the pyloric antrum, causing vomiting

III. Splenic or intestinal laceration if either organ slips between the stomach and body wall during cannulation

IV. Pneumoperitoneum

CYSTOCENTESIS

Definition

Cystocentesis is the transabdominal needle puncture of the urinary bladder for collection of urine without contamination by cells, debris, or bacteria from the lower urinary or genital tract.

Indications

I. To obtain urine for gross, microscopic, chemical, physical, and microbiologic analysis in suspected cases of urinary tract infection
   A. To identify and classify cellular, crystalline, and bacterial contents of urine as a guide to selection of specific therapeutic measures
   B. To aid in the differentiation of infection of the vagina, prostate, or urethra from infections of the kidneys or urinary bladder

II. To aid in identification of the site of origin of hematuria (e.g., prostatic versus renal hemorrhage)

III. Therapeutic uses
   A. Temporary removal of urine from the animal with lower urinary tract obstruction
   B. Before hydropropulsive techniques for the dislodgement of urethral calculi
      1. Collection of specimen before contamination by urethral flush fluids
      2. Relief of intraluminal pressure before the addition of more fluid volume by hydropropulsive technique

Restraint

I. Usually no chemical restraint is needed.

II. Lateral recumbency with the hindlimbs extended in a caudal direction is the preferred position for cats and small dogs.

III. For larger animals, the animal is placed in dorsal recumbency with the hindlimbs extended in a caudal direction.

IV. The standing position may also be used.

Technique

I. The first step is manual palpation of the urinary bladder, assessing it for size and location. If the bladder is empty or near empty, the technique is not performed.

II. With manual location of the bladder, an appropriate area of skin is selected, clipped, and prepared aseptically.
   A. If the lateral recumbent position is used, the ventral paralumbar region is appropriate.
   B. The ventral caudal abdominal midline is appropriate if the standing or dorsal recumbent position is used.

III. While the bladder is immobilized (usually against the abdominal wall) with one hand, the operator slowly inserts a 22-gauge 1.5- or 2.5-in. needle through the muscles at a right angle. The optimal placement of the needle through the bladder wall is at a 45°–90° angle in its ventral or ventrolateral aspect.

IV. Aspiration on the syringe should result in recovery of urine. If no urine is obtained, the needle is carefully redirected while the bladder is positively identified by palpation.

Complications

I. Transient hematuria may occur.

II. In the microscopic analysis of a specimen collected by cystocentesis, variable amounts of red blood cells may be present because of the technique, resulting from hemorrhage of the bladder mucosa at the site of needle puncture.

III. Leakage of urine through the needle puncture site into the peritoneal cavity, resulting in peritonitis, is rare and more likely in the obstructed patient in which the bladder wall may be experiencing vascular compromise or necrosis.

IV. Inadvertent aspiration of an enlarged prostate or prostate cyst or abscess may yield confusing results.

BLOOD PRESSURE MEASUREMENT

Definition

I. Direct methods of measuring blood pressure involve inserting a saline-filled catheter into an artery and using a pressure transducer. These methods are the most accurate, yet are impractical in an average clinical setting.

II. Indirect methods of measuring blood pressure involve using an inflatable cuff and measuring arterial wall motion or blood flow after arterial occlusion. These methods are clinically most practical, and further discussion is limited to indirect measurements.

Indications

I. Surgical monitoring of critical patients
II. Shock assessment
III. Detection of hypertensive states
   Hypertension has been associated with cardiovascular disease, renal disease, endocrine disorders, neurologic disease, ocular disease, hypercalcemia, anemia, polycythemia, obesity, and aging.

Restraint

I. Animals should be relaxed, minimally restrained, and placed in lateral recumbency.

II. Measurements on larger dogs may be made while they are standing.

III. Chemical restraint should not be used, since blood pressure may be affected.

Technique

I. Oscillometric
   A. An inflatable cuff is placed between the elbow and carpus on the foreleg or just below the hock on the hind leg.
   B. The width of the cuff should be approximately 40% of limb circumference.
   C. The cuff is automatically inflated and deflated at a predetermined rate.
   D. The machine automatically displays pulse rate and systolic, diastolic, and mean arterial blood pressure.
   E. Several readings are taken for accuracy.
   F. This method is most accurate in animals over 15 pounds.
II. Doppler
   A. An inflatable cuff is placed in one of the following locations.
      1. Mid foreleg
      2. Just distal to the hock
      3. Around the tail base
      4. Below the stifle (cats)
   B. The width of the cuff should be approximately 40% of limb circumference.
   C. A patch of hair is clipped distal to the cuff over the palpable artery on the palmar or plantar surface.
   D. The ultrasound transducer with coupling gel is placed over the clipped skin and positioned so that arterial flow is audible. The transducer is taped in place.
   E. The cuff is inflated by a sphygmomanometer until arterial flow ceases and audible flow has disappeared.
   F. Cuff pressure is slowly reduced until flow is reestablished and flow sounds can be heard. Systolic blood pressure is read at this point from the sphygmomanometer.
   G. Continued reduction of cuff pressure results in a change in sound quality that corresponds to diastolic pressure.
   H. Several readings are taken for accuracy.
   I. Diastolic blood pressure measurements may not be accurate or obtainable in many animals.

Complications

I. Stress may cause a falsely elevated blood pressure.
II. Inappropriate cuff size or placement may give erroneous results.
III. Doppler readings are somewhat subjective in relying on auditory signals for measurements.
IV. Oscillometric measurements may be difficult to determine in low flow states.

BONE MARROW BIOPSY

Definition

Bone marrow samples may be obtained by aspiration through a bone marrow needle or by punch biopsy through a trephine instrument (core biopsy).

Indications

I. Aspirate or core biopsy
   A. Nonregenerative anemias
   B. Suspected bone marrow disease (e.g., myeloid or erythroid suppression or neoplasia)
   C. Certain clotting disorders, especially involving platelets
II. Core biopsy
   A. To study the structural architecture of the bone marrow
   B. When aspiration biopsies have been unsuccessful
   C. When searching for metastatic or occult neoplasia
   D. Certain metabolic disorders of bone

Restraint

I. Most bone marrow biopsies may be performed using local anesthesia with or without mild sedation.
II. The position of restraint is determined by the site to be biopsied.
   A. Wing of ilium (Fig. 3–7)
      1. Large dog: standing or sternal recumbency
      2. Small dog or cat: sternal recumbency with hind legs drawn up alongside the abdomen
   B. Proximal femur: lateral recumbency (Fig. 3–8)
   C. Rib: sternal or lateral recumbency (Fig. 3–9)
   D. Proximal humerus: lateral recumbency (Fig. 3–10)
   E. Other less commonly used sites: ischial tuberosity and sternum

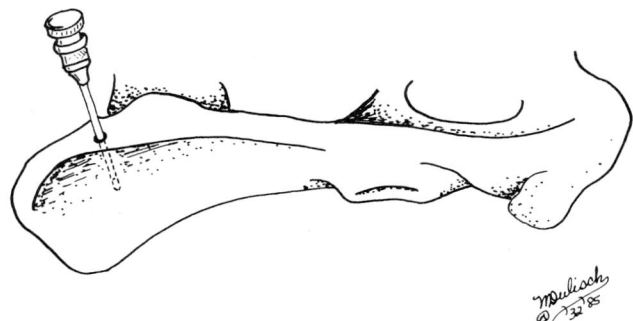

Figure 3–7. Insertion of bone marrow needle through the dorsal iliac spine into the marrow cavity of the wing of the ilium. The medial and lateral aspects of the spine are localized with the thumb and forefinger of one hand. With the other hand the needle is directed ventrally and slightly laterally into the central portion of the wing of the ilium.

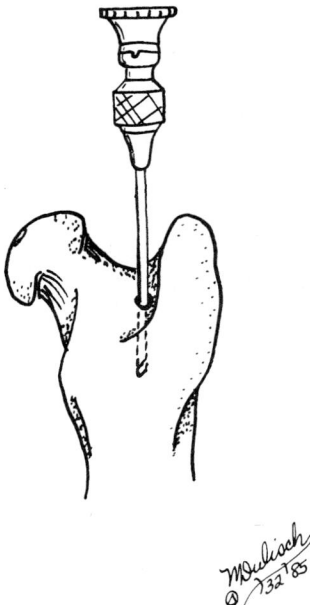

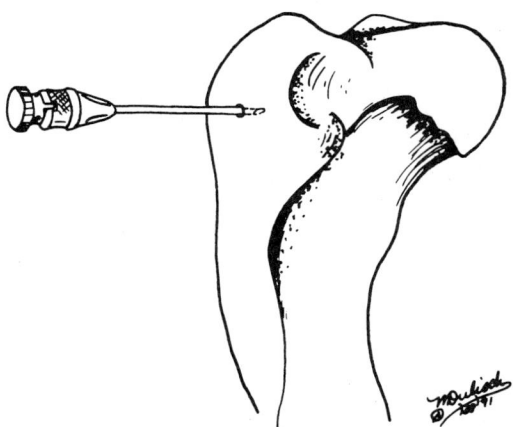

Figure 3–10. Bone marrow from the humerus is obtained by palpating the bony prominence of the greater tubercle lateral to the biceps tendon. The needle is inserted at a spot perpendicular to the long axis of the bone.

Figure 3–8. To retrieve a sample from the marrow cavity of the proximal femur, a bone marrow needle is advanced through the trochanteric fossa caudal and medial to the greater trochanter and directed laterally in a line parallel to the shaft of the femur.

Technique

  I. The hair over the biopsy site is shaved, and the site is prepared with sterile technique and infiltrated with a local anesthetic.

  II. A small stab incision is made in the skin with a scalpel blade.

  III. Bone marrow is aspirated.

    A. A 16- or 18-gauge 1.5-in. Osgood or Rosenthal (see Table 3–1) biopsy needle is chosen. With the stylet in place, the needle is advanced through the soft tissues until it meets resistance at bone.

    B. The needle is pushed through the bone by applying pressure with a simultaneous rotating motion. Decreased resistance indicates that the needle has passed through the cortex into the marrow cavity.

    C. After advancing the needle into the marrow, the stylet is removed, a 12-ml syringe is attached, and negative pressure is exerted on the syringe. Evidence of pain with aspiration usually indicates that the needle is located within the marrow cavity.

    D. When marrow appears in the syringe, aspiration is halted and the syringe disconnected.

    E. Overzealous aspiration may lead to contamination of the sample with peripheral blood. Smears are quickly made on glass slides, and any clot is saved in formalin for histologic examination. A sample may also be submitted for culture.

    F. If adequate marrow is retrieved, the needle is withdrawn. The skin incision may be sutured or left to heal by second intention.

  IV. Core biopsy

    A. A core biopsy instrument (e.g., Jamshidi bone marrow needle) is chosen. The needle, with the stylet in place, is advanced through the soft tissues and then into bone with steady pressure and a back-and-forth rotating motion.

    B. Once through the cortex, the stylet is removed

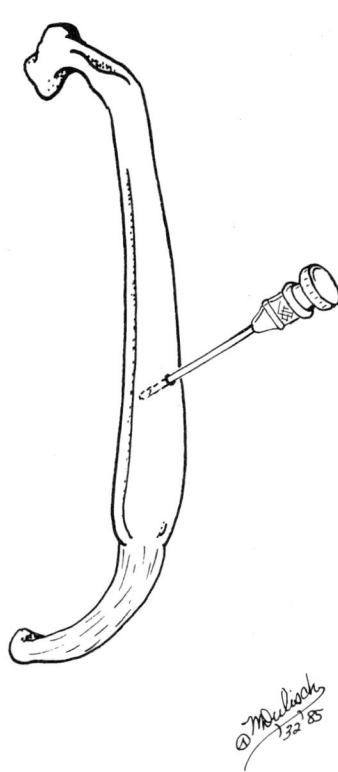

Figure 3–9. Bone marrow aspiration from a rib. Usually the 7th, 8th, or 9th rib is chosen. The biopsy needle is inserted at a slightly ventral angle at a point midway from the neck of the rib to the costal cartilage.

and the trephine instrument is pushed into the marrow. It is advanced for 1–2 cm and then rotated around its long axis several times.
  C. The needle is removed. The core sample is retrieved using the extending probe and is placed in formalin.

Complications

  I. Complications are rare.
 II. Damage to adjacent structures may occur.
   A. Poor positioning of the needle in the trochanteric fossa may damage the sciatic nerve.
   B. Accidental pneumothorax or laceration of intercostal vessels may accompany rib biopsies.
III. Infiltration of the trochanteric fossa with local anesthetic may result in transient paresis of the sciatic nerve.

ARTHROCENTESIS

Definition

Arthrocentesis is the percutaneous placement of a needle into a synovial cavity for the collection of synovial fluid for laboratory analysis.

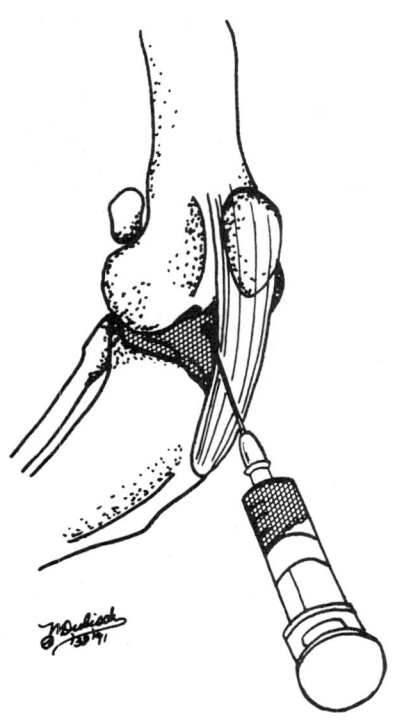

Figure 3–11. With the stifle joint partially flexed, the distal edge of the patella and proximal edge of the tibial tuberosity are palpated. The joint is entered at a spot approximately one third of the way between these two structures. Insert the needle into the joint just lateral to the straight patellar ligament and direct it slightly medially into the area between the two femoral condyles.

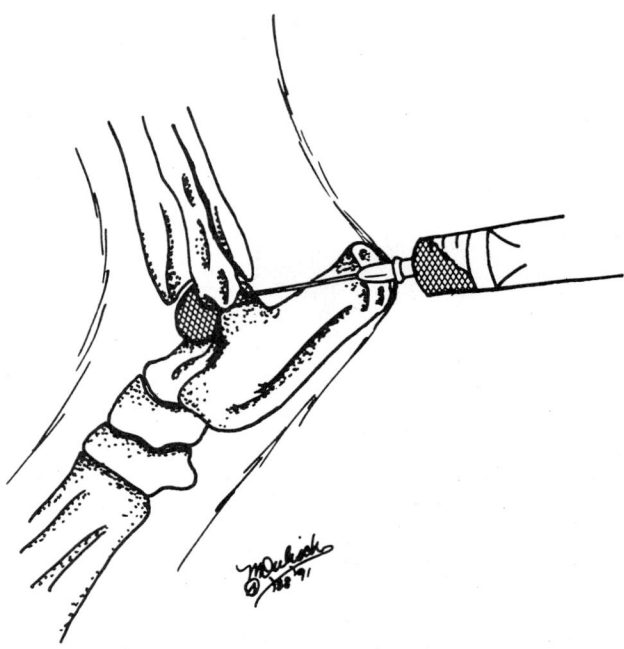

Figure 3–12. With the hock partially flexed, the tibiotarsal joint is entered laterally by inserting the needle under the malleolus from the plantar side. Care is taken to avoid the caudal branch of the lateral saphenous vein.

Indications

  I. As a diagnostic aid in suspected cases of inflammatory joint disease
     Analysis of synovial fluid may be beneficial in differentiating among septic or infectious arthritis, immune-mediated arthritis, hemarthrosis, and traumatic synovial effusion.
 II. Insertion of contrast medium for radiographic evaluation (see Chap. 4)
III. Administration of therapeutic agents intrasynovially

Restraint

  I. Local anesthesia and mild chemical sedation may be necessary depending on the temperament of the patient.
 II. Lateral recumbency is used for centesis of the stifle, hock, elbow, and shoulder joints.
III. Centesis of the carpal joint may be performed in either lateral or sternal recumbency.

Technique

  I. The skin over the affected joint is clipped and prepared aseptically.
 II. Palpation of the distended joint capsule or the joint space must be precise before placing the needle. A thorough knowledge of the joint and periarticular anatomy is essential for accurate needle placement (Figs. 3–11 to 3–13).
III. A 22-gauge needle attached to a 3- or 6-ml syringe is advanced slowly through the skin, subcutaneous,

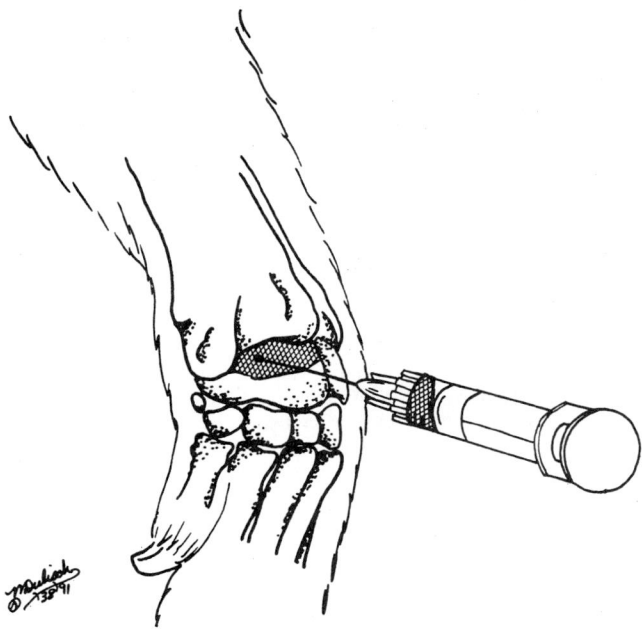

Figure 3–13. With the carpus partially flexed, the carpal joint is aspirated by inserting a needle into the medial radiocarpal space or between any of the palpable intercarpal spaces.

periarticular, and synovial tissues to enter the synovial cavity.

IV. Aspiration of the syringe should result in collection of synovial fluid.

V. Suction is released, and the needle is withdrawn when sufficient fluid (0.1–0.5 ml) has been collected.

VI. The fluid is placed in EDTA tubes for cytologic study and in transport medium or thioglycolate broth for microbiologic analysis. Thin smears are prepared and air-dried. It is useful to evaluate the viscosity of the fluid while preparing slides.

VII. In suspected cases of polyarthritis, multiple joints are aspirated.

Complications

I. Inadequate preparation of the skin may result in bacterial inoculation of the joint or contamination of the specimen.

II. Intrasynovial trauma from the needle may result in hemarthrosis or abrasion of the articular cartilage if technique is suboptimal.

III. Direct needle-induced damage to the periarticular blood vessels or nerves may occur if anatomic considerations are overlooked.

IV. Contamination of the sample with iatrogenic hemorrhage may necessitate centesis of another joint or repeated centesis of the same joint 48 hours later.

BONE BIOPSY

Definition

A trephine bone biopsy is the collection of a full-thickness specimen of bone for histopathologic and microbiologic analysis.

Indications

I. Obtain a specimen for histologic examination after radiographic evaluation of a lesion involving bone in certain suspected cases
   A. Primary or secondary neoplasia of bone
   B. Bacterial, mycotic, or parasitic infection of bone
   C. Developmental (idiopathic) or degenerative diseases of bone, including panosteitis, hypertrophic osteodystrophy, and hypertrophic pulmonary osteoarthropathy
II. Obtain material for culture

Restraint

General anesthesia is required.

Technique

I. A wide area of skin around the affected site is clipped and prepared for aseptic surgery.

II. Radiographs are used to select an appropriate site to insert and direct the biopsy instrument.

III. A 1-cm incision is made over the selected site. The subcutaneous, muscle, tendon, and deep fascial tissues are retracted to gain access to the periosteal surface.

IV. Using an appropriately sized Michel trephine biopsy instrument without stylet (see Table 3–1), an oscillating twisting motion guides advancement of the instrument through the cortical bone, across the medullary cavity, and through the opposite cortex. Palpation of the trephine in the subcutaneous tissues indicates complete full-thickness biopsy.

V. The trephine is withdrawn, and the stylet is inserted to eject the core into bacteriologic transport medium or 10% formalin solution for microbiologic and histopathologic examination, respectively.

VI. Bleeding from the biopsy site is controlled with direct pressure and closure of the deep tissues.

VII. Additional specimens may be collected until the surgeon is comfortable that a diagnostic sample has been obtained.

Complications

I. False-negative results may be obtained if inadequate or inappropriate tissues have been collected. Careful radiographic analysis and collection of multiple samples minimize this occurrence.

II. Pathologic fractures may result from weakening of the bone.
   A. Such problems may be avoided by selecting smaller trephines and limiting the number of samples taken.
   B. External coaptation is used postoperatively if a secondary pathologic fracture is feared.

Bibliography

Abood SK, Buffington CA: Improved nasogastric intubation technique for administration of nutritional support in dogs. J Am Vet Med Assoc 199:577, 1991

Armstrong JA, Hardie EM: Percutaneous endoscopic gastrostomy: a retrospective study of 54 clinical cases in dogs and cats. J Vet Intern Med 4:202, 1990

Bailey CS: Lumbar puncture for collection of cerebrospinal fluid. Proc Am Anim Hosp Assoc 40:289, 1973

Bright RM, Burrows CF: Percutaneous endoscopic tube gastrostomy in dogs. Am J Vet Res 49:629, 1988

Bright RM, Okrasinski EB: Percutaneous tube gastrostomy for enteral alimentation in small animals. Compend Contin Ed Pract Vet 13:15, 1991

Conner GH, Gupta BN, Krehbiel JD: A technique for bone marrow biopsy in the cat. J Am Vet Med Assoc 158:1702, 1971

Creighton SR, Wilkins RJ: Transtracheal aspiration biopsy: technique and cytologic evaluation. J Am Anim Hosp Assoc 10:219, 1974

Crowe DT: Clinical use of a indwelling nasogastric tube for enteral nutrition and fluid therapy in the dog and cat. J Am Anim Hosp Assoc 22:675, 1986

Crowe DT: Use of a nasogastric tube for gastric and esophageal decompression in the dog and cat. J Am Vet Med Assoc 188:1178, 1986

Crowe DT: Nutrition in critical patients: administering the support therapies. Vet Med 84(2):152, 1989

Deeley TJ: The drill biopsy of bone lesions. Clin Radiol 23:536, 1972

Dukes J: Hypertension: a review of the mechanisms, manifestations and management. J Small Anim Pract 33:119, 1992

Fitzpatrick RK, Crowe DT: Nasal oxygen administration in dogs and cats: experimental and clinical investigations. J Am Anim Hosp Assoc 22:293, 1985

Grandy JL, Dunlop CI, Hodges DS et al: Evaluation of the doppler ultrasonic method of measuring systolic arterial blood pressure in cats. Am J Vet Res 53:1166, 1992

Harvey CE, O'Brien JA: Management of respiratory emergencies in small animals. Vet Clin North Am 2:243, 1972

Hunter JS Jr, McGrath CJ, Thatcher CD et al: Adaptation of human oscillometric blood pressure monitors for use in dogs. Am J Vet Res 51:1439, 1990

Jamshidi K, Swaim WR: Bone marrow biopsy with unaltered architecture: a new biopsy device. J Lab Clin Med 77:335, 1971

Krahwinkel DJ: Thoracic trauma. p. 268. In Kirk RW (ed): Current Veterinary Therapy VII. WB Saunders, Philadelphia, 1980

Mathews SA, Binnington AG: Percutaneous incisionless placement of a gastrostomy tube using a gastroscope: preliminary observations. J Am Anim Hosp Assoc 22:601, 1986

McCartney RD, McMurty RJ: Complications of transtracheal aspiration. N Engl J Med 289:1094, 1973

Morgan RV: Manual of Small Animal Emergencies. Churchill Livingstone, New York, 1985

Osborne CA, Schenk MP: Technique of urine collection. Proc Am Anim Hosp Assoc 44:431, 1977

Spano JS, Hoerlein BF: Laboratory examinations. p. 136. In Hoerlein BF (ed): Canine Neurology. WB Saunders, Philadelphia, 1978

Contrast Radiography

Lori Ellen Hartzband

GENERAL CONSIDERATIONS

Purpose

I. To enhance radiographic visibility of a particular anatomic structure or system
II. To give functional information about an organ or system

Contrast Materials

I. Classification
   A. Positive contrast media are more opaque than soft tissue because of high atomic number and include agents such as barium sulfate and iodinated contrast media.
   B. Negative contrast media are more lucent than soft tissue because of low density. Examples include gases such as air, carbon dioxide, and nitrous oxide.
   C. Double-contrast procedures use a combination of these two types of contrast media to coat surfaces with a positive contrast medium and highlight them with a negative contrast medium.
II. Barium sulfate
   A. Insoluble, inert metallic compound that is not absorbed or digested but passes through the gastrointestinal tract (GIT) unchanged, coating mucosal surfaces and enhancing their visibility
   B. Not recommended in cases of suspected esophageal or gastrointestinal perforation because may cause granulomatous reactions when it leaks extraluminally
   C. Available products (Table 4–1)
      1. Barium sulfate powder
         a) Requires mixing with water before use
         b) Tends to flocculate in the GIT
         c) Inexpensive
      2. Barium sulfate colloidal liquid suspension
         a) Most desirable form for imaging the GIT
         b) Used 100% w/v or diluted depending on the procedure
      3. Barium sulfate paste: used for imaging of the esophagus where longer-lasting mucosal coating is desirable

III. Organic iodide compounds
   A. Tri- or hexa-iodinated organic compounds
      1. Most compounds have low protein binding and are excreted through the kidneys by glomerular filtration.
      2. Higher protein binding allows for increased excretion through the biliary system (e.g., ioxaglate).
      3. Increased biliary and intestinal excretion occur when there is poor renal function (vicarious excretion).
   B. Available products (see Table 4–1)
      1. Commonly used iodine concentrations vary from 140–400 mg I/ml.
      2. Single or multiple dose vials are available for oral, intravenous, intrathecal, and other uses.
   C. Classification of water-soluble iodinated media
      1. High osmolar ionic contrast media (HOCM)
         a) Include diatrizoate, iothalamate, and metrizoate
         b) Associated with a higher incidence of local and systemic contrast reactions than low osmolar and nonionic media
         c) Can be administered by all routes except intrathecal and are inexpensive
         d) Are combined with sodium or methylglucamine (meglumine) as salts
         e) Sodium salts: more toxic and irritating than meglumine salts; meglumine salts: more viscous and therefore more difficult to inject as a rapid bolus
      2. Low osmolar ionic contrast media (LOCM/ ionic)
         a) Include ioxaglate, a hexa-iodinated dimer
         b) Associated with fewer contrast reactions than HOCM because of lower osmolality
         c) Not for intrathecal use (ionic)
         d) More expensive than HOCM
      3. Low osmolar nonionic contrast media (LOCM/nonionic)
         a) Include metrizamide, iopamidol, iohexol, ioversol, iopromide (tri-iodinated monomer), iodixanol, and iotrolan (hexa-iodinated dimer)

Table 4–1. **Media for Contrast Procedures**

Procedures	Brand Name	Class	Generic Name	Concentration	Manufacturer
Nonselective angiocardiography, pleurography, peritoneography, intravenous urography	Renografin-60	HOCM	Diatrizoate Meg & Na	292 mg I/ml	Squibb
	Renografin-76		Diatrizoate Meg & Na	370 mg I/ml	Squibb
	Hypaque 50%		Diatrizoate Na	300 mg I/ml	Winthrop
	Hypaque 60%		Diatrizoate Meg	282 mg I/ml	Winthrop
	Conray		Iothalamate Meg	282 mg I/ml	Mallinckrodt
	Conray 400		Iothalamate Na	400 mg I/ml	Mallinckrodt
	Conray 325		Iothalamate Na	325 mg I/ml	Mallinckrodt
	Omnipaque-240	LOCM	Iohexol	240 mg I/ml	Winthrop
	Omnipaque-300	Nonionic	Iohexol	300 mg I/ml	Winthrop
	Omnipaque-350		Iohexol	350 mg I/ml	Winthrop
	Isovue-300		Iopamidol	300 mg I/ml	Squibb
	Isovue-370		Iopamidol	370 mg I/ml	Squibb
Myelography	Amipaque	LOCM	Metrizamide	170 mg I/ml	Winthrop
	Isovue-200	Nonionic	Iopamidol	200 mg I/ml	Squibb
	Omnipaque-180		Iohexol	180 mg I/ml	Winthrop
	Omnipaque-240		Iohexol	240 mg I/ml	Winthrop
Cystourethrography	Cysto-Conray	HOCM	Iothalamate Meg	202 mg I/ml	Mallinckrodt
Arthrography	Hypaque 25%		Diatrizoate Na	150 mg I/ml	Winthrop
	Omnipaque-140	LOCM Nonionic	Iohexol	140 mg I/ml	Winthrop
Esophagram	Esophotrast	—	Barium paste	100% w/v BaSO₄	Armour Pharmaceutical
Esophagram, upper gastrointestinal study, barium enema	Liquid Polibar	—	Barium sulfate susp.	100% w/v	E-Z-EM
	Novopaque	—	Barium sulfate susp.	60% w/v	Picker
	Gastrografin	HOCM	Diatrizoate Meg & Na	367 mg I/ml	Squibb
	Hypaque Oral	HOCM	Diatrizoate Na	249 mg I/ml	Winthrop
	Omnipaque-240	LOCM Nonionic	Iohexol	240 mg I/ml	Winthrop

Na = sodium; Meg = meglumine.

b) Associated with the fewest systemic and local reactions
c) Safe for intrathecal use (nonionic) and all other routes
d) More expensive than HOCM

IV. Negative contrast media
   A. Carbon dioxide and nitrous oxide are considered safer than room air because these gases are more soluble in blood should they accidentally enter the vascular system (air embolization).
   B. Air embolization is an infrequent occurrence that can result in acute death of the animal.
   C. Left lateral recumbency is the safest body position to maintain because any air will be trapped in the right ventricle, where it is less likely to enter the pulmonary artery segment and cause an obstruction to blood flow.

Contrast Reactions

I. Barium sulfate
   A. Although generally soothing to the GIT, it may cause mild constipation.
   B. Granulomatous reactions occur if barium leaks extraluminally into the mediastinal, pleural, or peritoneal spaces.
   C. If aspirated into the tracheobronchial tree, it is usually rapidly cleared by coughing and mucociliary mechanisms.
   D. If aspirated into the lung tissue, barium may remain there. Small amounts are considered innocuous, but larger amounts can be associated with respiratory compromise, pneumonitis, and granuloma formation.

II. Iodinated contrast media
   A. Oral agents are unpalatable and may stimulate drooling and/or emesis.
   B. Because HOCM are hyperosmolar, oral preparations can cause osmotic diarrhea and dehydration; this does not occur with LOCM.
   C. If aspirated into the lungs, HOCM cause severe, osmotically induced pulmonary edema; this is less likely with LOCM.
   D. HOCM and ionic LOCM are severely neurotoxic and should never be used intrathecally.
   E. Nonionic LOCM are the media of choice for intrathecal use, but mild leptomeningitis, mild exacerbation of clinical neurologic signs, radicular pain, or seizures may occur after use.
   F. Intra-articular injection of HOCM causes mild synovial effusion and inflammation; a less severe reaction occurs when LOCM are used.
   G. Types of systemic reactions and treatment

1. Osmotic diuresis
   a) Very common reaction after intravenous (IV) administration of contrast media, particularly HOCM
   b) Usually self-limiting
2. Idiosyncratic/anaphylactoid reactions
   a) Skin erythema, urticaria, pruritus, facial and laryngeal edema
   b) Altered mentation, seizures
   c) Circulatory collapse characterized by hypotension, tachycardia, arrhythmia
   d) Symptomatically treated with IV fluids, epinephrine, corticosteroids, dopamine, antihistamines, and anticonvulsants
3. Nonidiosyncratic reactions
   a) Local pain, nausea, vomiting
   b) Cerebral and pulmonary edema
   c) Cardiovascular collapse characterized by hypotension, bradycardia (vasovagal response), and arrhythmias
   d) Symptomatically treated with IV fluids, atropine, and corticosteroids
4. Contrast medium–induced renal failure
   a) Variable severity, lasting 4–14 days in people
   b) Usually reversible with symptomatic therapy (IV fluids)
   c) Found to be dose-related in the face of preexisting renal disease but idiosyncratic (non–dose-related) in patients without renal disease
   d) Known risk factors: dehydration, renal disease, diabetes mellitus, multiple myeloma
H. Incidence of systemic contrast reactions
   1. Reactions are rare, particularly serious/life-threatening ones.
   2. Most systemic reactions occur within 5–30 minutes of administration of the contrast agent.
I. Risk factors for increased systemic reactions
   1. High-dose procedures
      a) Angiocardiography, intravenous urography, computed tomography
      b) When the total dose/procedure exceeds 20 g iodine (in people)
   2. Dehydration, azotemia
   3. Renal, cardiovascular disease
   4. Diabetes mellitus, multiple myeloma, sickle cell anemia (in people)
   5. Very old or very young patients
   6. History of previous contrast reaction
      a) This is controversial.
      b) Pretreatment of these patients with corticosteroids and use of LOCM may decrease risk of recurrence.

NONSELECTIVE ANGIOGRAPHY

Definition

I. Bolus intravenous injection of aqueous iodinated contrast agent through a large peripheral vein while taking multiple sequential exposures

II. Allows evaluation of the major vessels of the systemic and pulmonary circulatory systems and the chambers of the heart

Indications

I. Evaluate the size and shape of the heart chambers when the cardiac silhouette is enlarged radiographically
II. Differentiate between major categories of feline cardiomyopathy
III. Differentiate heart enlargement from pericardial effusion or mass
IV. Evaluate the heart valves for stenosis or insufficiency
V. Detect right to left cardiac shunts and abnormalities of the major systemic and pulmonary vasculature, both congenital and acquired
VI. Identify filling defects in the heart such as thrombus and tumor

Contraindications

I. Congestive heart failure, cardiovascular or respiratory infection, severe arrhythmias
II. Least helpful in big dogs in which a rapid bolus injection of a large volume of contrast material is difficult to achieve; best results with cats and small dogs (<15 kg)

Alternative Procedures

I. Selective angiocardiography
II. Echocardiography with or without Doppler examination

Materials and Methods

I. Avoid patient anxiety and motion during the study.
   A. Examples of appropriate tranquilizers
      1. Ketamine (dogs: 6–10 mg/kg, cats: 4 mg/kg) and diazepam 0.2 mg/kg IV
      2. Butorphanol 0.2–0.4 mg/kg followed by diazepam 0.2 mg/kg IV (do not mix together in syringe)
      3. Propofol (Diprivan) or ultrashort-acting barbiturate given to effect
   B. Use atropine only if severe bradycardia is detected.
   C. Provide adequate restraint with sandbags, tape, and other positioning devices.
II. A wide, short intravenous catheter (18–20 gauge for cats, 14–20 gauge for dogs, 1.5–2.0 in.) is placed in a large peripheral vein (jugular, cephalic, saphenous).
III. The catheter is flushed with heparinized saline.
IV. Plain radiographs are obtained before injection.
V. Inject 1–2 ml/kg of HOCM or LOCM (250–400 mg I/ml) rapidly by hand or with a power injector.
   A. If using an IV extension set, prime this with contrast medium before injecting.
   B. Warming the contrast agent before injection decreases viscosity and increases ease of injection.
VI. Perform the study with the patient in lateral recum-

bency and then repeat the study while in dorsal recumbency.
- A. Increase exposure techniques by approximately 5–10 kVp from the survey study.
- B. Obtain multiple sequential exposures using a rapid film changer or a cassette tunnel.
- C. Begin exposures when 50–80% of the calculated volume of contrast agent has been injected.
- D. The exposure sequence will vary with the equipment used, the animal's heart rate, and the underlying cardiovascular disease.
  1. Cassette tunnel: one to two exposures per second for 4–5 seconds and then two to three more exposures over the next 4–5 seconds
  2. Rapid film changer: four to six exposures per second for 5 seconds and then one to two per second for 5–10 seconds

Interpretation

- I. Normal sequence of filling is right atrium, right ventricle, pulmonary arteries, lung, pulmonary veins, left atrium, left ventricle, aorta. Typical transit times are listed in Table 4–2.
- II. Abnormal transit times
  - A. Decreased transit time (rapid flow): hypertrophic cardiomyopathy (variable), right-to-left shunts such as reverse patent ductus arteriosus and tetralogy of Fallot
  - B. Increased transit time (slow flow): congestive heart failure, dilated cardiomyopathy, valvular insufficiency
- III. Altered chamber/vessel size and wall thickness
  - A. Hypertrophic cardiomyopathy: large left atrium, thick left ventricle with small lumen and enlarged papillary muscles
  - B. Dilated cardiomyopathy: thin-walled and enlarged left ventricle, poorly opacified aorta caused by poor cardiac output
  - C. Heartworm disease: enlarged right ventricle and pulmonary artery segment, enlarged or tortuous or pruned pulmonary arteries

Table 4–2. Positive Contrast Transit Times Through the Heart

Animal or Condition	Transit Time (sec)
Normal transit times for contrast bolus[a]	
Cat	6–8
Small dog	6–8
Medium dog	7–9
Large dog	7–10
Transit times with some cardiac diseases	
Hypertrophic cardiomyopathy (cat)	3–4
Dilated cardiomyopathy	10–20
Patent ductus arteriosus (right-to-left shunt)	3–4
Ventricular septal defect (right-to-left shunt)	3–4

[a]Time from arrival of bolus at right atrium until bolus has reached the aortic arch.

- IV. Filling defects: thrombi, tumors, enlarged papillary muscles, heartworms
- V. Pericardial effusion or mass
  - A. The heart occupies a smaller percentage of the cardiac silhouette.
  - B. The heart may have an eccentric location within the pericardium if a mass exists.

Complications

- I. Peripheral vasculitis or thrombosis
- II. Systemic contrast reactions
  - A. Arrhythmias, hypotension, renal failure
  - B. Air, clot, or catheter embolus
  - C. Sepsis

PLEUROGRAPHY/ PERITONEOGRAPHY

Definition

Injection of positive or negative contrast medium into the pleural or peritoneal space to better visualize the parietal and visceral surfaces

Indications

- I. Better visualize fissures between lung lobes, aiding in localization of pulmonary lesions
- II. Evaluate the contour and integrity of the parietal pleural or peritoneal surfaces
- III. Evaluate the diaphragm for masses, rupture, and congenital defects
- IV. Increase the ability to define visceral peritoneal surfaces

Contraindications

- I. Unstable cardiovascular status
- II. Pleural or peritoneal effusion
  - A. This is a relative contraindication.
  - B. The effusion will dilute the contrast medium and must be removed before the study.

Alternative Procedures

- I. Ultrasonography
- II. Computed tomography

Materials and Methods

- I. Negative contrast media are rarely used because of potential cardiovascular compromise with induced pneumothorax or air embolism.
- II. Sterile HOCM or LOCM (250–400 mg I/ml) are used at a dose of 0.5–1 ml/kg body weight (pleural) and 1–2 ml/kg (peritoneal).
  - A. To reduce discomfort, contrast medium can be mixed with 2% lidocaine (0.5 ml lidocaine/10 ml contrast medium) before injection (not for use in cats).

B. Warming the contrast agent decreases discomfort and reduces viscosity.

C. Local skin blocks or sedation may be needed.

III. Pleural injections are made using a short 18–22-gauge IV catheter, placed aseptically in the 7th to 9th intercostal space at the widest point of the thorax.

    A. Avoid the intercostal vessels caudal to each rib.

    B. Connect to a stopcock and short IV extension set to reduce movement of the catheter and chance of iatrogenic pneumothorax while attaching the syringe.

    C. Aspirate before injecting to avoid intrapulmonary administration and to remove pleural fluid or air.

IV. Peritoneal injections are made using a short 18–22-gauge IV catheter or winged infusion set, slightly to the right of midline, approximately at the level of the umbilicus.

    A. This location prevents gastric, splenic, and falciform fat injections.

    B. Remove peritoneal effusion before injecting.

V. Roll the animal to distribute the contrast material.

    A. Do so cautiously if diaphragmatic rupture is suspected.

    B. Four views are recommended, including both laterals, dorsoventral, and ventrodorsal.

    C. Increase exposure techniques approximately 5–10 kVp from precontrast studies.

Interpretation

I. Normal findings

    Pleural and peritoneal surfaces should be evenly coated, demonstrating smooth parietal and visceral surfaces.

II. Abnormal findings

    A. Passage of contrast agent from one body cavity across the body wall or diaphragm indicates a hernia or rupture.

    B. The contrast agent may coat pleural or abdominal masses, increasing their visibility.

Complications

I. Laceration of thoracic or abdominal viscera or vasculature during needle placement can result in pneumothorax and pleural, pericardial, or peritoneal hemorrhage.

II. Iatrogenic infection is usually avoided with sterile preparation of the injection site.

III. Accidental intrapulmonary or pericardial injection may cause pulmonary edema or cardiac tamponade.

IV. In the presence of a diaphragmatic rupture, iatrogenic pneumothorax can occur during peritoneography if a closed injection system is not employed.

MYELOGRAPHY

Definition

Introduction of contrast medium into the subarachnoid space (SAS) to outline the spinal cord and delineate the SAS

Indications

I. Clinical signs of spinal cord or spinal canal disease, but negative or ambiguous findings on survey radiographs

II. Better localize (lateralize) known spinal cord or canal lesions before surgery

Contraindications

I. Increased intracranial pressure

II. Premedication with phenothiazine derivatives or neuroleptic agents because of increased risk of seizures

III. May see increased toxicity of contrast material if meningitis or dehydration is present

Alternative Procedures

I. Computed tomography

II. Magnetic resonance imaging

III. Electromyography and nerve conduction studies

Materials and Methods

I. Place animal under general anesthesia.

II. Obtain good quality lateral and ventrodorsal survey radiographs.

III. Use *only* nonionic LOCM such as iohexol (180–240 mg I/ml) or iopamidol (200 mg I/ml).

    A. Avoid metrizamide because of high incidence of seizures.

    B. Iohexol may be least epileptogenic (Dennis and Herrtage, 1989).

    C. Dose is 0.25–0.45 ml/kg.

        1. Use the lower dosage for large or obese animals or if injecting close to the suspected lesion (e.g., lumbar injection for lumbar lesion).

        2. Use the higher dosage if the injection is made far from the suspected lesion.

        3. Inject close to the lesion to decrease dosage, potentially diminishing toxic effects.

        4. Warm contrast medium to body temperature before injection.

IV. Perform the cerebrospinal fluid tap (see Chap. 3).

    A. Save fluid for analysis.

    B. If fluid is grossly turbid or bloody, wait for analysis before injection of contrast medium.

V. Inject the contrast agent slowly over 2–5 minutes.

    A. Tilt the animal to encourage flow in the direction needed.

    B. If fluoroscopy is available, stop injecting when satisfactory filling is achieved.

VI. Obtain lateral and ventrodorsal views within 30 minutes, increasing exposure factors by 5–10 kVp.

    A. Collimate to reduce scatter.

    B. Elevate head between exposures and after study to reduce intracranial accumulation of contrast medium.

VII. Additional radiographic views may be needed.

    A. Cervical disk disease: right and left ventrodorsal oblique

B. Cervical vertebral instability: lateral with neck in flexion or extension, lateral with cranial traction
   1. Flexion and extension may exacerbate the degree of spinal cord compression, therefore perform with caution.
   2. Traction views are obtained by making an exposure while pulling the head cranially, widening the disk spaces, and relieving some ligamentous compressive lesions.
C. Lumbosacral disease: flexion and extension of the lumbosacral junction

Interpretation

I. Normal findings
   A. The SAS should be seen in all areas of the spinal cord as a thin, opaque line with the ventral column often thinner than the dorsal column.
   B. The dorsal column is widest within C1 and C2 and also broadens at the cervicothoracic junction.
   C. There is normally a slight dorsal lifting of the ventral column over the C2–3 disk space without narrowing of the dorsal space.
   D. The ventral SAS may not fill well in the mid to caudal thoracic region because both the cord and SAS appear most narrow at this level.
   E. The contrast columns are slightly narrowed within C6 and C7, L4 and L5 because of the thoracic and lumbar intumescences.
   F. The spinal cord tapers at L5, and so lesions caudal to this point may not be well demonstrated.
   G. A normal myelogram can be seen in degenerative myelopathy, fibrocartilaginous embolism, and meningitis.
II. Abnormal findings (Fig. 4–1)
   A. Extradural lesions
      1. Examples include disk protrusion or extrusion, ligamentous hypertrophy, vertebral malformation, hematoma, abscess or granuloma, and neoplasia.
      2. The SAS is narrowed and deviated away from the wall of the vertebral canal focally.
      3. Projected at 90°, the cord may appear widened and the SAS tapered.
   B. Intradural-extramedullary lesions
      1. These include neoplasia, granulomas, and cysts.
      2. The spinal cord may deviate away from the lesion.
         a) The SAS may end abruptly, showing the mass as a lucent filling defect.
         b) A "golf tee" sign (column forked) may be present at each end of the mass.
      3. Projected at 90°, the cord may appear widened and the SAS tapered.
   C. Intramedullary lesions
      1. Neoplasia, spinal cord edema, malformations such as syringomyelia, and occasionally infarction can produce an intramedullary pattern.
      2. The spinal cord is usually not deviated.

   3. The cord appears focally widened on both views with the SAS tapering at the point of swelling.
D. Other myelographic changes
   1. Streaking or pooling of the contrast medium usually indicates cord malacia, a grave sign.
   2. A small, well-defined focal area of contrast agent within the cord at the injection site indicates intraparenchymal injection, which can have variable consequences, from none to malacia.
   3. A thin line of contrast agent centrally within the cord over a variable distance indicates central canal filling.
      a) If very fine, this is of no great significance.
      b) If wide, it may indicate prior dilation of the canal (congenital or acquired) or excessive injection pressure and can be associated with increased neurotoxicity.
   4. Pooling of the contrast agent in soft tissues dorsal or lateral to the spine indicates unsuccessful SAS injection, and a repeat injection is needed.
   5. Scalloping of the ventral column (lifting over each intervertebral foramen) and outlining of the nerve roots indicate epidural injection of contrast medium.
      a) Wait 15–20 minutes for epidural contrast agent to fade.
      b) Reinject if not enough contrast medium is seen in SAS on repeat lateral exposure.

Complications

I. Respiratory arrest or altered anesthetic plane can occur during or shortly after intrathecal injection.
II. Intraparenchymal injection or trauma to the spinal cord during needle placement can result in neurologic deficit or death depending on the location and severity of the damage.
III. Postmyelographic seizures are minimized by use of LOCM, prolonging anesthesia for 30–60 minutes after injection, and by elevating the head.
IV. Contrast medium–induced hemorrhagic leptomeningitis manifests as hyperesthesia, hyperreflexia, radicular pain, or worsening of neurologic deficits.

EPIDUROGRAM

Definition and Indications

I. Injection of iodinated contrast medium into the epidural space (ES)
II. Evaluates for compressive or mass lesions caudal to L5 (cauda equina syndrome) that are not apparent on survey radiographs

Contraindications

I. The animal must be able to undergo general anesthesia.

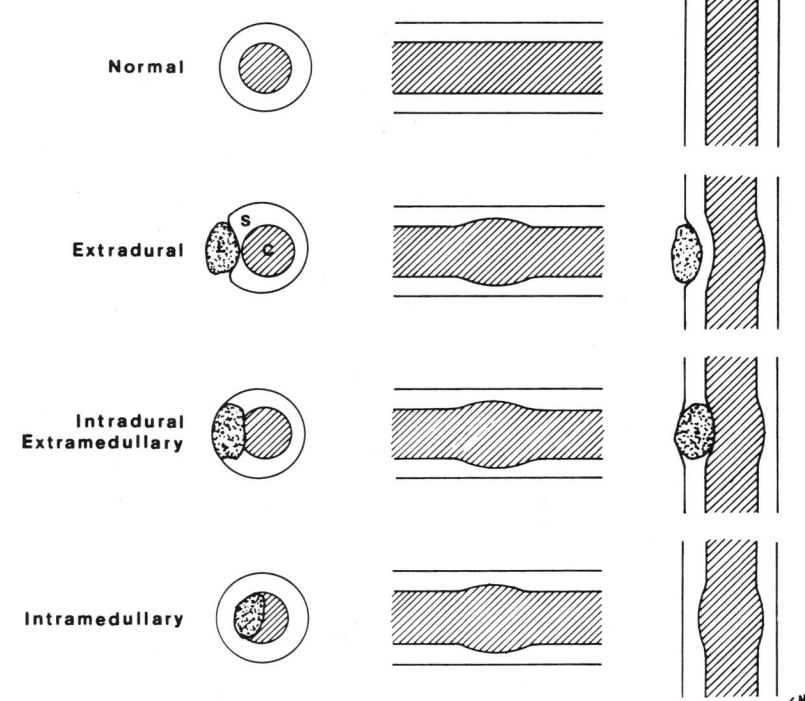

Figure 4–1. Schematic of spinal cord (C) and subarachnoid space (S) with and without the presence of a mass lesion (L). Presented in cross section and two orthogonal (at 90°) myelographic views.

II. The soft tissue and bone of the tail base should not be contaminated or infected, so that the needle can be placed aseptically in the epidural space.

Alternative Procedures

I. Computed tomography
II. Magnetic resonance imaging
III. Flexion and extension myelography of lumbosacral spine
IV. Vertebral sinus venography
V. Diskography

Materials and Methods

I. Use needles and contrast agent as described for myelography.
II. Inject on the dorsal midline in one of several locations.
  A. Sacrococcygeal junction
  B. One of first few coccygeal interspaces
  C. Lumbosacral junction
III. Inject 0.15 ml/kg initially, adding 0.1 ml/kg as needed to fill ES using a short IV extension set so that additional contrast agent can be added without manipulating the needle.
IV. Best results are obtained if injection is performed under fluoroscopic guidance.

Interpretation

I. Normal findings
  A. Contrast medium fills the epidural space and leaks out the intervertebral foramina around the nerve roots.
  B. The appearance can be quite varied because of the presence of epidural fat.
II. Abnormal findings
  A. Filling defects can be produced by disk extrusion or prolapse, ligamentous hypertrophy, neoplasia, and granuloma.
  B. Narrowing of the ES occurs with bony stenosis of the vertebral canal.

Complications

I. Trauma to the nerve roots or epidural hemorrhage during needle placement
II. Iatrogenically induced infections (rare)

ESOPHAGRAM

Definition

Administration of oral positive contrast medium for morphologic evaluation of the lumen of the pharynx and esophagus as well as functional assessment of the oral, pharyngeal, cricopharyngeal, and esophageal phases of swallowing

Indications

I. Clinical signs of pharyngeal and esophageal disease
  A. Gagging, retching, dysphagia, regurgitation
  B. Cough or emesis immediately after eating
II. Recurrent, unexplained aspiration pneumonia

III. Assess swallowing function
  A. Before laryngeal or pharyngeal surgery
  B. Evaluate residual function in known esophageal motility disease (megaesophagus)
IV. Demonstrate pharyngeal and esophageal foreign bodies and strictures suspected from survey views
  A. Focal retention of gas, fluid, or food
  B. Focal or regional dilation
V. Determine the degree of esophageal involvement in cervical and thoracic disorders (e.g., trauma, inflammation, neoplasia)
VI. Evaluate the cranial and caudal esophageal sphincters and esophageal hiatus

Contraindications

I. Uncooperative patient
  A. Tranquilization is undesirable.
  B. Use of a muzzle is not practical.
II. Esophageal perforation (relative contraindication)
  A. Iodinated contrast medium is used initially rather than barium to avoid granulomatous reactions.
  B. Very small perforations may go undetected with iodinated media, requiring the use of barium.
III. Esophageal-respiratory fistula
  A. When fistula is suspected, procedure is performed under fluoroscopic guidance to minimize the amount of contrast medium entering the respiratory tract.
  B. Small amounts of iodinated contrast agent or barium will be cleared from the upper airways spontaneously, but these substances are undesirable in the lungs.

Alternative Procedures

I. Endoscopy
II. Radioisotope esophagram

Materials and Methods

I. Food should be withheld for 6–24 hours so that the animal will eat voluntarily.
II. Tranquilize only if absolutely necessary because sedation may alter motor function. Use acetylpromazine 0.025–0.05 mg/kg IV (max = 1.5 mg), IM, or SQ (max = 3 mg).
III. Obtain survey radiographs of the neck and thorax, including lateral, ventrodorsal, and ventrodorsal obliques (as needed).
IV. Administer barium sulfate.
  A. Paste (100% w/v)
    1. The medium of choice for esophagus
    2. Excellent, persistent mucosal coating
  B. Liquid suspension (100% w/v)
    1. Inferior mucosal coating, short-lasting
    2. Useful for fluoroscopic evaluation to simulate normal drinking
    3. May demonstrate small tears better than paste
  C. Barium meatballs
    1. Paste or liquid mixed with canned pet food or marshmallows
    2. Simulates normal eating
    3. Better dilation of esophageal walls to demonstrate strictures
V. Iodinated contrast medium is less desirable except in cases of perforation.
  A. Unpalatable: emesis, drooling
  B. Can cause osmotic diarrhea, dehydration
  C. Inferior to barium for mucosal coating
  D. LOCM minimize side effects and are safer than HOCM if aspirated into respiratory tract.
VI. Administer 5–15 ml contrast agent per os.
  A. If possible, perform with patient in lateral recumbency so radiographs can be obtained quickly before contrast medium clears.
    1. Obtain lateral, ventrodorsal, and oblique views as needed.
    2. Administer additional contrast medium if more than 2 minutes elapse.
    3. Iodinated medium fades faster than barium.
  B. If fluoroscopy is available, follow the bolus from mouth to stomach.
    1. Repeat the study using liquid, paste, and then meatballs.
    2. Record on videotape or cine film to allow review.

Interpretation

I. Normal findings
  A. The pharynx is lightly coated without significant accumulation of contrast medium in the valleculae or piriform recesses.
  B. No contrast agent enters the nasopharynx or passes through the larynx.
  C. The esophagus is lightly coated.
    1. Six to 12 linear parallel streaks are seen in the dog.
    2. The cat esophagram shows a vertically striated "herringbone" pattern in the caudal third of the esophagus.
    3. Accumulation of small amounts of contrast agent in the caudal cervical and cranial thoracic esophagus may occur but clears quickly with the next swallowed bolus.
  D. Gastroesophageal reflux occurs infrequently.
    1. Contrast material should clear quickly from the distal esophagus.
    2. Tranquilization may increase the frequency of reflux.
  E. Some redundancy of the esophagus is normal at the thoracic inlet in brachycephalic breeds.
    1. Contrast material should not accumulate here.
    2. Extending the neck eliminates the redundancy and differentiates it from a true diverticulum.
II. Abnormal findings
  A. Foreign body
    1. May absorb contrast medium or be coated by it
    2. Typical locations: pharynx, heart base, and caudal esophagus
  B. Mucosal disease: neoplasia, granuloma, ulcer, esophagitis

C. Mural disease
  1. Smooth filling defect
  2. Circumferential narrowing
  3. Neoplasia, abscess, granuloma, stricture
D. Megaesophagus: focal vs. generalized
E. Distal esophageal sphincter
  1. Hiatal hernia
  2. Gastroesophageal intussusception
  3. Gastric reflux with esophagitis
F. Extravasation of contrast medium: perforation, fistula
G. Stricture
  1. Vascular ring anomaly
  2. Previous injury
  3. Neoplasia
H. Esophageal displacement
  1. Tracheobronchial lymph nodes
  2. Intrathoracic neoplasia
  3. Diaphragmatic rupture

Complications

I. Aspiration of contrast medium
  A. Usually indicates pharyngeal, cricopharyngeal, or laryngeal dysfunction
  B. Possible esophageal-respiratory fistula
  C. If cough or dyspnea occurs during the study
    1. Obtain lateral thoracic exposure.
    2. Discontinue administration of contrast medium if aspiration has occurred.
II. False impression of motility disorder possible with tranquilization

UPPER GASTROINTESTINAL STUDY

Definition

Administration of liquid positive contrast medium into the stomach, monitoring its passage through the stomach and small intestine by performing sequential exposures

Indications

I. Evaluate GIT mucosal characteristics, luminal patency, and motility
  A. Chronic vomiting, diarrhea, or weight loss
  B. Suspect ulcer or bleeding mass (melena)
  C. Suspect obstruction, but survey study is inconclusive
  D. Suspect foreign body, but none seen on survey study
II. Confirm abnormal location of GIT
  A. Diaphragmatic rupture
  B. Body wall hernia
III. Assess effect of intra-abdominal mass on GIT
  A. Displacement
  B. Altered motility

Contraindications

I. Inadequate gastrointestinal preparation (except in emergency situations)
II. Recent sedation, which may alter GIT motility
III. Confirmed surgical disease such as obstruction or perforation
IV. Abnormal electrolyte status with altered motility
V. Pharynx, esophagus, or stomach unable to withstand passage of orogastric tube or volume of contrast medium to be administered

Alternative Procedures

I. Endoscopy
II. Ultrasonography
III. Nuclear scintigraphy
  A. Motility study
  B. Ulcer labeling (labeled sucralfate)
  C. Localization of GIT bleeding
IV. Surgical exploratory laparotomy

Materials and Methods

I. Perform standard gastrointestinal preparation except in cases of acute obstruction or other emergencies.
  A. Withhold food for 12–24 hours.
  B. Administer cathartics, laxatives, and enemas as needed to clear colon of feces.
II. Obtain right lateral and ventrodorsal survey radiographs.
III. Sedate only if absolutely necessary.
  A. Chemical restraint may alter motility of GIT.
  B. Use drugs that alter motility the least.
    1. Dog: acetylpromazine 0.025–0.05 mg/kg IV, SQ, IM; max = 1.5 mg IV or 3 mg SQ, IM
    2. Cat: ketamine 4–6 mg/kg IV with diazepam 0.2 mg/kg IV (do not mix in same syringe)
IV. Pass lubricated orogastric tube through an oral speculum.
  A. Pick an appropriate-sized orogastric tube.
    1. Use 14 French, 24 in. for cats and small dogs.
    2. Use 24–40 French, 36 in. for medium to large dogs.
    3. Mark the tube at a point approximating the distance from the tip of the nose to the costal arch.
  B. Pass the tube into the stomach and verify gastric location.
    1. On initial passage of tube, some characteristic-smelling gas may escape through the tube.
    2. Aspirate the tube to remove any remaining fluid in the stomach, which could interfere with interpretation by diluting the contrast agent or giving a false impression of mural thickening.
    3. Blow into the tube and auscult over the stomach.
    4. Palpate the animal's neck for the presence of the tube being distinct from the trachea.
V. Administer positive contrast medium through the tube.
  A. Barium
    1. 30–50% w/v liquid barium suspension
    2. Dose: 12 ml/kg
  B. Iodinated contrast medium, LOCM

1. 240 mg I/ml
2. Dose: dilute 1:2 or 1:3 with water, use 10 ml/kg after dilution
3. Safer than barium if perforation suspected
4. Good quality study compared with barium except inferior mucosal coating
5. Similar transit times compared with barium study

C. Iodinated contrast medium, HOCM
1. 250–370 mg I/ml
2. Dose: 2–4 ml/kg
3. Advised only if suspect perforation and LOCM unavailable
   a) May cause emesis, diarrhea, dehydration
   b) Dilutes itself rapidly because of high osmolality, therefore not effective for imaging beyond the stomach and proximal small bowel
   c) Rapid transit when compared with barium and LOCM

D. Contrast medium administered per os if necessary
1. Increased risk of aspiration in some patients
2. Palatability problems (drooling, emesis) especially with iodinated media

VI. Obtain right lateral and ventrodorsal views.
A. Immediate, 0.5, 1, 3, 5, and 24 hours
B. If stomach is of major interest
1. Obtain right and left lateral, dorsoventral, and ventrodorsal views at 0.5 and 1 hour.
2. For improved gastric mucosal evaluation, it may be desirable to perform a double-contrast gastrogram (Evans and Laufer, 1981).
   a) Administer 1.5–3 ml/kg liquid barium suspension (100% w/v) by stomach tube and then distend stomach with air (approximately 12–20 ml/kg).
   b) Obtain right and left lateral, dorsoventral, and ventrodorsal views.
   c) For optimal evaluation of mucosa, consider use of glucagon to induce temporary hypomotility.
     (1) Dose is 0.1–0.35 mg glucagon IV, with additional doses of 0.1 mg IV as needed (up to a maximum of 1 mg total).
     (2) Do not use glucagon if patient has unregulated diabetes mellitus or a pheochromocytoma.
     (3) Glucagon interferes with a motility study.

Interpretation

I. Normal findings
A. For normal transit times see Table 4–3.
B. The stomach should distend smoothly, more so in the fundus and least in the pylorus.
1. Rugae are more parallel in the body than the fundus.
2. The pylorus has the least folds.

Table 4–3. Normal Transit Times During Upper Gastrointestinal Study

Event Evaluated	Dog	Cat
Times when barium or LOCM are used		
Stomach empty within	2–3 h	1–2 h
Duodenum fills in	10–15 min	5–10 min
Jejunum and ileum fill in	1–2 h	30–60 min
Reaches colon	1.5–2 h	30–60 min
Most of barium in colon	3–5 h	2–3 h
Times when iodinated HOCM are used		
Passes through small intestine	30–60 min	30 min

3. Approximately six contractions per minute are seen with fluoroscopy.
C. The small intestine has a mucosal pattern that is either smooth or finely fimbriated.
1. The intestine moves freely on its mesentery, changing position and diameter frequently.
2. The duodenum has a distinct appearance.
   a) Dog: lymphoid follicles in the antimesenteric border present as multiple square, shallow depressions called "pseudoulcers."
   b) Cat: multiple peristaltic contractions result in a beaded appearance called the "string of pearls" sign.

II. Abnormal findings
A. Rapid transit: rarely specific, common in enteritis
B. Delayed gastric emptying
1. Pyloric outflow disease: foreign body, muscular or mucosal hypertrophy, or pylorospasm from pain or parvovirus infection
2. Diminished gastric motility
3. Delayed onset of emptying
   a) This is common in stressed animals, especially cats.
   b) Once emptying starts, transit times should normalize.
C. Delayed intestinal transit
1. Disordered or diminished motility
2. Mechanical obstruction
   a) Luminal mass: neoplasia, polyp, foreign body, intussusception
   b) Stricture: scar, circumferential tumor ("apple core")
3. Functional obstruction
   a) Infiltrative mural disease
   b) Electrolyte disturbances
   c) Vascular compromise (infarction)
   d) Iatrogenic (drugs)
D. Filling defects: foreign body, ascarids, neoplasia, granuloma
E. Mucosal disease: inflammation, ulcer, infiltrative neoplasia
F. Displacement of GIT caused by adhesion, abdominal mass, or hernia
G. Plication caused by linear foreign body

   H. Diverticulum
   I. Extravasation of contrast medium caused by perforation

Complications

   I. Trauma to mouth, pharynx, esophagus, or stomach from stomach tube
   II. Administration of contrast agent into respiratory tract from improper orogastric tube placement or aspiration during oral administration
   III. Gastric rupture caused by overfilling of a diseased stomach
   IV. Leakage of barium into peritoneal cavity as a result of GIT perforation
   V. Osmotic diarrhea and dehydration caused by iodinated contrast agent (HOCM)

BARIUM ENEMA/ PNEUMOCOLONOGRAPHY

Definition

   I. These procedures use positive contrast medium (barium enema), negative contrast medium (pneumocolonography), or both (double-contrast barium enema) to evaluate the large intestinal lumen and mucosa.
   II. Pneumocolonography is most useful to identify the colonic lumen and demonstrate large filling defects.
   III. Barium enema gives improved luminal contrast and mucosal detail.
   IV. Double-contrast barium enema is best for subtle mucosal disease.

Indications

   I. Signs of large bowel disease, to evaluate mucosa for disease
   II. Identify colon when not well seen on survey radiographs
   III. Demonstrate intraluminal masses such as intussusception and neoplasia
   IV. Detect perforation or fistulation

Contraindications

   I. Inadequate patient preparation
   II. Perforation or recent colonic biopsy (avoid use of barium)
   III. Fluid or electrolyte imbalance
      A. Cleansing enemas and cathartics may exacerbate these.
      B. Postpone study until problem is corrected.
   IV. Unable to undergo sedation or anesthesia

Alternative Procedure

Endoscopy

Materials and Methods

   I. The colon should be free of fecal material.
      A. Feed low-residue diet for 24 hours, followed by 24-hour fast.
      B. Administer cathartics, laxatives, and enemas as needed until colon is empty.
         1. Soapy enemas prevent good coating of mucosa with barium.
         2. Warm water or saline enemas are preferred.
      C. A less stringent preparation is needed if identification of the colonic lumen is the only goal of the study.
   II. Obtain survey radiographs to determine whether colonic preparation is adequate.
   III. Sedation may be adequate for pneumocolonography.
      A. Dog
         1. Butorphanol 0.2–0.4 mg/kg followed by diazepam 0.2 mg/kg IV (do not mix)
         2. Butorphanol 0.2–0.4 mg/kg and acetylpromazine 0.025–0.05 mg/kg IV
      B. Cat: ketamine 4–6 mg/kg and diazepam 0.2 mg/kg IV
   IV. General anesthesia is preferred for positive contrast procedures.
   V. Prepare the needed materials.
      A. Bardex or Foley catheter 18–30 gauge for dog, smaller Foley catheter for small dog or cat
      B. Lubricating jelly, stopcock, syringes, or enema bag
   VI. Place catheter in rectum and inflate bulb.
   VII. Fill colon with contrast medium (7–14 ml/kg) and clamp off tube to prevent leakage.
      A. For barium enema use 15–20% w/v barium sulfate suspension.
      B. Iodinated contrast medium is substituted if perforation is suspected or endoscopy is to follow. Dose is 7–14 ml/kg of HOCM or LOCM with 150–200 mg I/ml.
      C. For pneumocolonography use air, carbon dioxide, or nitrous oxide.
      D. A double-contrast study can be performed by draining the contrast medium after a barium enema and administering negative contrast medium.
      E. Do not overfill the colon.
         1. Monitor the filling with fluoroscopy or take test exposures.
         2. Goal is to smoothly fill the colon and cecum without reflux into the ileum.
   VIII. Obtain right and left lateral, ventrodorsal, and oblique views as needed.
      A. Decrease technique by 5 kVp for pneumocolonography.
      B. Increase technique by 5–10 kVp for barium enema.

Interpretation

   I. Normal findings
      A. The colon is smooth and nonsacculated.
      B. The ascending, transverse, and descending colon and the cecum should fill with contrast material.
         1. The canine cecum is coiled.
         2. The feline cecum is small and pointed, blending with the colon.
   II. Abnormal findings

A. Filling defects: intussusception, neoplasia, polyp, foreign body, pseudomass caused by fecal material
B. Perforation: ulcer, trauma, iatrogenic
C. Abnormal position: mass, adhesion
D. Mucosal irregularity: ulceration, colitis, typhlitis, neoplasia
E. Stricture: annular neoplasia, scar

Complications

I. Barium peritonitis from perforation
II. Necrosis at site of catheter bulb from excessive or prolonged inflation

INTRAVENOUS UROGRAPHY

Definition

I. This study is performed by injecting aqueous iodinated contrast material into a peripheral vein, with subsequent clearing of the contrast agent through the urinary tract.
II. Sequential radiographs show contrast medium enhancement of the renal vasculature, parenchyma, and collecting system, followed by the ureters and bladder.
III. Intravenous urography (IVU) provides morphologic information and a crude assessment of renal and ureteral function.

Indications

I. Evaluate the size, shape, and position of the kidneys, ureters, and bladder
II. Detect renal pelvic abnormalities such as hydronephrosis, mass, or calculus
III. Investigate the source of hematuria, pyuria, or incontinence
IV. Determine the effect of intra-abdominal and retroperitoneal masses or abdominal trauma on the structure and function of the urinary tract
V. Crude assessment of renal and ureteral function before and after surgical intervention

Contraindications

I. Except in rare emergencies, delay IVU until the results of renal diagnostics such as blood urea nitrogen (BUN), creatinine, and urinalysis are obtained.
II. Screen the patient for high-risk factors associated with serious systemic contrast medium reactions.
A. Patients must not be dehydrated!
B. Renal disease is a relative contraindication.
1. A poor study may result with significantly reduced renal function (BUN >75 mg/dl).
2. A higher dose of contrast agent will be needed in an attempt to obtain a diagnostic study.
3. Increased risk of contrast medium–induced renal failure and other systemic reactions exists with increased dose and decreased renal function.
4. Despite increased dose, renal opacification is

unlikely with BUN >150 mg/dl and/or creatinine >3.5 mg/dl.
III. Except in emergency situations, this study is not performed on animals without proper preparation.
A. Withhold food from animals for 12–24 hours.
B. Use cathartics, laxatives, and enemas as needed to empty colon of fecal material.

Alternative Procedures

I. Ultrasonography
II. Renal angiography
III. Computed tomography
IV. Magnetic resonance imaging
V. Radioisotope urogram

Materials and Methods

I. A standard, 24-hour gastrointestinal preparation is completed before the study.
II. Obtain lateral and ventrodorsal survey radiographs.
III. Sedate only if needed.
A. Sedate nervous, uncooperative animals.
B. Evaluation for ectopic ureter may require the patient to be under chemical restraint for placement of a urethral catheter to perform a pneumocystogram or a retrograde urethrogram.
IV. A wide, short intravenous catheter (18–20 gauge for cats, 14–20 gauge for dogs, 1.5–2 in.) is placed in a large peripheral vein (jugular, cephalic, saphenous).
V. Use HOCM or LOCM containing 250–400 mg I/ml.
A. Dosage is 800 mg I/kg (range 600–1000 mg I/kg), or approximately 2–3 ml/kg.
B. Impaired renal function may necessitate use of 1600 mg I/kg to obtain a diagnostic study.
VI. With the patient in dorsal recumbency, make a rapid bolus intravenous injection of the contrast medium and perform the following sequence of exposures.
A. Ventrodorsal exposure within 20 seconds
B. Right lateral and ventrodorsal exposures at 5, 20, 40, and 60 minutes
C. The use of abdominal compression to transiently distend the renal pelvis and diverticula is controversial and a matter of personal preference (Feeney et al., 1982b).
D. Obtain ventrodorsal oblique views of the caudal abdomen while performing a pneumocystogram when evaluating for the presence of ectopic ureters.

Interpretation

I. Normal findings
A. The vascular phase (opacified renal artery and vein) persists only a few seconds and may not be seen.
1. Multiple renal arteries (two to three per kidney) may be seen as an anatomic variant.
2. If the renal blood supply is of major interest, consider renal angiography.
B. The nephrogram (opacified renal parenchyma) should be relatively uniform and most opaque at 5 minutes, fading gradually over 1–2 hours.

1. Kidneys are bean-shaped to oval with smooth borders.
2. Both kidneys should be the same size.
    a) Dogs: 2.5–3.5 × length of second lumbar vertebra (ventrodorsal view)
    b) Cats: 2.4–3 × length of second lumbar vertebra (ventrodorsal view)
        (1) Females tend to have small kidneys.
        (2) Intact males have larger kidneys.
3. The nephrogram can appear normal despite significant renal disease.

C. The pyelogram (opacified collecting system) is seen by 3 minutes; the pelvis and diverticula are best seen at 20 and 40 minutes.
    1. The pelvis is crescent-shaped and 1 mm wide.
    2. The diverticula (three to five pairs per kidney) are fine, finger-like projections from the pelvis.
    3. The proximal ureter is <2.5 mm in diameter in the dog and typically 1 mm in the cat.
    4. Distal ureters are 0.5–2 mm and are seen incompletely on any single exposure because of peristalsis.

II. Abnormal findings
    A. Nonvisualization of both kidneys
        1. Inadequate dosage
        2. Bilateral poor renal function
    B. Nonvisualization of one kidney
        1. Renal agenesis
        2. Lack of blood supply: avulsion, thrombosis
        3. Unilateral poor renal function
        4. Prior nephrectomy
    C. Abnormal renal shape or size
        1. Large smooth kidneys
            a) Infiltrative neoplasia
            b) Inflammation
            c) Acute infection
            d) Hydronephrosis
        2. Large irregular kidneys
            a) Neoplasia
            b) Granulomas
            c) Polycystic disease
        3. Small, pitted kidneys
            a) Chronic, end-stage renal disease
            b) Renal dysplasia
    D. Persistent nephrogram
        1. Contrast medium–induced renal failure
        2. Severe hypotension
        3. Renal vein thrombosis
        4. Obstruction (renal tubular or ureteral)
    E. Abnormal collecting system
        1. Pelvis and diverticula
            a) Dilation is seen with hydronephrosis, pyelonephritis, and renal calculus.
            b) Blunted, misshapen diverticula are seen in chronic pyelonephritis and renal dysplasia.
            c) Deviation or compression of diverticula or pelvis occurs with renal mass lesions such as cyst, abscess, or neoplasia.
        2. Ureters
            a) Neoplasia, granuloma, calculus
            b) Ectopic ureter
            c) Hydroureter
                (1) Functional obstruction: inflammation, trauma
                (2) Mechanical obstruction: calculus, neoplasia, stricture
    F. Extravasation of contrast material into the retroperitoneal or peritoneal spaces
        1. Trauma
        2. Erosion by inflammation or neoplasia
        3. Best seen at 20 or 40 minutes after injection

Complications

I. Systemic contrast medium reactions
II. Aspiration of vomitus while in dorsal recumbency
    A. Emesis is common within minutes of contrast medium administration.
    B. Do not leave muzzled animals unattended.

CYSTOURETHROGRAM

Definition

Examination of the bladder and urethra using negative contrast medium (pneumocystogram), iodinated contrast medium (positive contrast examination), or both (double-contrast)

Indications

I. Suspected lower urinary tract disease
    A. Signs of dysuria, pollakiuria, hematuria, pyuria, incontinence
    B. Recurrent lower urinary tract infections
    C. Prostatomegaly, other caudal abdominal masses
    D. Abnormal bladder shape, opacity, or position
II. Type of study
    A. Positive contrast cystogram
        1. To locate a bladder not seen on survey study
        2. Demonstrate bladder patency
    B. Pneumocystogram
        1. Evaluate bladder wall thickness
        2. Improve visualization of luminal structures such as stones and masses
        3. Aid in evaluation for ectopic ureters during excretory urography
    C. Double-contrast cystogram
        1. To obtain superior mucosal detail
        2. Provides best evaluation of intraluminal and mural lesions such as masses and stones
    D. Retrograde urethrogram
        1. Evaluate causes of dysuria, incontinence, hematuria
        2. To detect calculi, masses, strictures, rupture, ectopic ureter

Contraindications

I. Known bladder rupture
II. Inadequate gastrointestinal preparation (except in emergency)

III. Inability to undergo anesthesia or heavy sedation

Alternative Procedures

I. Ultrasonography
II. Urethrocystoscopy
III. Magnetic resonance imaging

Materials and Methods

I. Use standard gastrointestinal preparation.
  A. No food for 12–24 hours
  B. Cathartics, laxatives, and enemas as needed to remove feces from the colon
II. General anesthesia is preferable to sedation.
  A. Reduces straining against a full bladder
  B. Increases ease of urethral catheterization, particularly in female dogs, all cats, and animals in pain.
III. Obtain survey radiographs before catheterization.
IV. Insert a lubricated, sterile urethral catheter.
  A. For dogs use a 6–12 French urinary catheter.
    1. Foley catheter for female
    2. Urethral or ureteral catheter for male
  B. For cats use a 3–5 French tom cat catheter.
  C. Wash the prepuce or vulva with surgical scrub before catheterization.
  D. Empty the bladder completely before administration of contrast medium.
    1. Save a urine sample in a sterile container for urinalysis and culture.
    2. If the bladder is incompletely emptied, positive contrast medium becomes diluted with urine. When performing a pneumocystogram, residual urine leads to a false impression of bladder wall thickening.
    3. Flush bladder with saline to remove clots if significant hematuria is present.
V. For positive contrast cystogram use HOCM or LOCM with 150–200 mg I/ml.
  A. Instill 4–10 ml/kg until the bladder is evenly distended. Smaller amounts may be adequate to identify the bladder and determine its patency.
    1. Palpate the bladder through the body wall to monitor distention or take an exposure to confirm size during the filling.
    2. Do not rely on syringe back pressure alone or the bladder may be overfilled, risking iatrogenic rupture.
  B. Obtain lateral and ventrodorsal views, increasing radiographic technique by 5–10 kVp.
VI. For a pneumocystogram use air, carbon dioxide, or nitrous oxide.
  A. Carbon dioxide and nitrous oxide are preferred because of decreased risk of air embolism, and left lateral recumbency is recommended while filling the bladder.
  B. Infuse 4–10 ml/kg of gas until bladder is smoothly distended but not overfilled.
    1. Overdistention can mask small mucosal defects.
    2. Diseased bladders are more susceptible to iatrogenic rupture.

  C. Obtain lateral and ventrodorsal views, decreasing radiographic technique by 5 kVp.
VII. Double-contrast cystogram combines both techniques.
  A. Use HOCM or LOCM 150–200 mg I/ml.
  B. After performing a pneumocystogram, add 0.25–0.50 ml/kg of positive contrast agent to the gas-filled bladder.
    1. Roll the animal to coat the mucosal surfaces with positive contrast medium.
    2. The contrast agent will form a central puddle surrounded by the lucent gas.
    3. Obtain right and left ventrodorsal oblique and lateral views.
VIII. To perform a retrograde urethrogram use HOCM or LOCM with 150–200 mg I/ml.
  A. Before the urethral study, the bladder should be moderately full or inadequate distention of the proximal urethra will result.
  B. The following urethral studies are advised.
    1. Male dogs
      a) Make an exposure while injecting caudal to the prostate and again caudal to the base of the os penis.
      b) If contrast medium leaks around the catheter, a Foley or other balloon catheter can be used.
    2. Female dogs
      a) Place Foley bulb as far caudal in the urethra as possible and expose while injecting.
      b) For full evaluation of the urethra, perform an additional injection with the Foley bulb in the caudal vagina (vaginogram).
    3. Cats: single injection with catheter tip in the distal urethra
  C. Inject a 3–20 ml (depends on size of animal) bolus of contrast medium through the catheter and make an exposure near the end of the injection.
    1. Obtain lateral and oblique views as needed, repeating the injection.
    2. Increase radiographic technique by 5–10 kVp from the cystogram technique.

Interpretation

I. Normal findings in the dog
  A. The bladder is pear-shaped with a smoothly tapering trigone.
    1. When filled, the bladder is predominantly abdominal.
    2. The bladder has a more pelvic location when empty.
    3. Some breeds such as the greyhound and the Doberman pinscher have a ''pelvic bladder,'' which has occasionally been associated with incontinence.
  B. The bladder wall should be smooth and uniformly thin (1 mm) when distended.
  C. The female urethra has a relatively uniform diameter and smooth walls.

D. The male urethra consists of prostatic, membranous, and penile portions.
  1. Normal sites of widening are the prostatic urethra, membranous urethra, and proximal penile urethra.
  2. Normal sites of narrowing are just distal to the prostate, at the ischial arch, and within the os penis.
II. Normal findings in the cat
  A. The bladder is round or oval.
    1. Abdominal location
    2. Smooth, thin wall (0.5–1 mm)
  B. The urethra is long.
    1. The female urethra is of uniform diameter.
    2. The male urethra tapers gradually from the trigone distally.
III. Abnormal bladder findings
  A. Wall thickening
    1. Inflammation (diffuse or in apex)
    2. Neoplasia (often trigonal)
    3. Hematoma (variable)
  B. Mucosal irregularity or staining: inflammation, neoplasia
  C. Nondistensible, small capacity
    1. Fibrosis
    2. Severe inflammation or edema
    3. Neoplastic infiltrate
    4. Ectopic ureter
  D. Filling defects
    1. Calculi (usually central)
    2. Neoplasia (variable, often trigonal)
    3. Inflammatory polyp (often in apex)
    4. Blood clots (irregular)
    5. Ureterocele (trigonal, rounded)
    6. Air bubbles (round, peripheral)
  E. Altered shape
    1. Urachal remnant (apex)
    2. Mucosal hernia (usually apex)
    3. Old trauma (variable)
  F. Altered position
    1. Displacement by mass or adhesions
    2. Hernia: body wall, perineal, inguinal
    3. Pelvic bladder
  G. Extravasation of contrast medium
  H. Vesicoureteral reflux
    1. It occurs when valvular function is lost because of inflammatory or neoplastic disease.
    2. It also occurs in healthy adult animals under general anesthesia and in young animals.
IV. Abnormal urethral findings
  A. Filling defects
    1. Calculi (variable appearance)
    2. Neoplasia (variable appearance)
    3. Blood clots (irregular)
    4. Scar or inflammatory tissue (mural, variable)
    5. Air bubbles (round, peripheral)
  B. Mucosal irregularity or staining
    1. Urethritis: trauma, infection
    2. Neoplasia
  C. Extravasation of contrast agent
    1. Rupture caused by trauma or infection

2. Communication with prostatic ducts and cysts allowing filling of these during urethrogram
  a) Chronic prostatitis or abscess
  b) Cystic hyperplasia
  c) Neoplasia
  d) Normal in small amounts
    (1) Should not coalesce
    (2) Extends less than the width of the prostatic urethra into the prostate tissue (Feeney and Johnston, 1986)
D. Retrograde filling of ectopic ureter
E. Urethral stricture

Complications

I. Iatrogenic infection
II. Iatrogenic rupture of bladder or urethra
  A. Direct trauma from catheter
  B. Overdistention
III. Catheter complications
  A. Knotting within bladder
  B. Iatrogenic foreign body caused by breakage
IV. Air embolism (rare)

ARTHROGRAPHY

Definition

Intra-articular injection of positive or negative contrast material to better demonstrate articular joint surfaces, joint capsule, and bursal extensions

Indications

I. Enhance visualization of cartilaginous defects or joint capsule disease not seen on plain radiographs
II. Better localize bone fragments and foreign bodies to intra- or extra-articular locations

Contraindications

Animal must be able to undergo anesthesia or heavy sedation.

Alternative Procedures

I. Ultrasonography
II. Computed tomography
III. Magnetic resonance imaging
IV. Arthroscopy

Materials and Methods

I. Materials needed are needles (20–22 gauge), syringes (6–12 ml), sterile fluid collection tubes, and culture medium (see Chap. 3).
  A. Use HOCM or LOCM containing 100–150 mg I/ml, diluting contrast agent with saline or sterile water to achieve this iodine concentration.
  B. Negative contrast agent can be substituted.
  C. Inject approximately 2–6 ml per joint.

II. The patient is anesthetized or sedated heavily.
   A. Preinjection high-detail radiographs (two views) are obtained.
   B. After sterile preparation of the injection site, the needle is placed in the joint and synovial fluid aspirated to confirm needle placement, to minimize dilution of contrast material, and to obtain a sample for analysis.
   C. Contrast agent is then injected and the needle withdrawn.
   D. The joint is flexed and extended to distribute the contrast medium.
   E. At least two views are obtained, increasing radiographic techniques by 5 kVp over the survey study.

Interpretation

I. Normal articular surfaces are smooth and well defined.
   A. Joint capsule size and contour vary with the joint examined.
   B. Consult references for typical appearance (Suter and Carb, 1969; Ticer, 1984; Muhumuza et al., 1988; van Bree, 1990).
II. A filling defect in the contrast medium can be caused by a blood clot, cartilage flap, joint mouse, villonodular mass, or neoplasm.
III. Leakage of contrast agent beyond the normal confines of the joint capsule occurs with capsular rupture, synovial hernia (contrast agent remains confined in a hernial sac), or synovial fistula (contrast medium is seen within a communicating structure such as a tendon sheath).

Complications

I. Iatrogenic laceration of cartilage, joint hemorrhage, and infection occur rarely.
II. Transient, mild synovitis is common after HOCM arthrography; LOCM are less irritating.

Bibliography

Ackerman N, Wingfield WE, Corley EA: Fatal air embolism associated with pneumourethrography and pneumocystography in a dog. J Am Vet Med Assoc 160:1616, 1972

Adams WM: Myelography. Vet Clin North Am 12:295, 1982

Agut A, Sanchez-Valverde MA, Lasaosa JM et al: Use of iohexol as a gastrointestinal contrast medium in the dog. Vet Radiol Ultrasound 34:171, 1993

Bettman MA: Angiographic contrast agents: conventional and new media compared. AJR 139:787, 1982

Bonagura JD, Myer CW, Pensinger RR: Angiocardiography. Vet Clin North Am 12:239, 1982

Cohan RH, Dunnick NR, Bashore TM: Treatment of reactions to radiographic contrast material. AJR 151:263, 1988

Cox FH, Jakovljevic S: The use of iopamidol for myelography in dogs: a study of 27 cases. J Small Anim Pract 27:159, 1986

Debatin JF, Cohan RH, Leder RA et al: Selective use of low osmolar contrast media. Invest Radiol 26:17, 1991

Dennis R, Herrtage ME: Low-osmolar contrast media: a review. Vet Radiol 30:2, 1989

Evans SM, Biery DN: Double contrast gastrography in the cat. Vet Radiol 24:3, 1983

Evans SM, Laufer I: Double contrast gastrography in the normal dog. Vet Radiol 22:2, 1981

Feeney DA, Barber DL, Johnston GR: The functional aspects of the nephrogram in excretory urography: a review. Vet Radiol 23:42, 1982a

Feeney DA, Barber DL, Johnston GR, Osborne CA: The excretory urogram: part I. Compend Contin Educ Pract Vet 4:233, 1982b

Feeney DA, Barber DL, Johnston GR, Osborne CA: The excretory urogram: part II. Compend Contin Educ Pract Vet 4:321, 1982c

Feeney DA, Johnston GR: Urogenital imaging: a practical update. Semin Vet Med Surg 1:144, 1986

Feeney DA, Wise M: Epidurography in the normal dog: technique and radiographic findings. Vet Radiol 22:35, 1981

Fischer HW: Catalog of intravascular contrast media. Radiol 159:561, 1986

Fox PR, Bond RB: Nonselective and selective angiocardiography. Vet Clin North Am 13:259, 1983

Hall FM, Rosenthal DI, Goldberg RP, Wyshak G: Morbidity from shoulder arthrography: etiology, incidence, and prevention. AJR 136:59, 1981

Herrtage ME, Dennis R: Contrast media and their use in small animal radiology. J Small Anim Pract 28:1105, 1987

Hogan PM, Aronson E: Effect of sedation on transit time of feline gastrointestinal contrast studies. Vet Radiol 29:85, 1988

Lamb JT: Iohexol vs iopamidol for myelography. Invest Radiol 20:S37, 1985

Lang J: Flexion–extension myelography of the canine cauda equina. Vet Radiol 29:242, 1988

McClennan B: Low-osmolality contrast media: premises and promises. Radiology 162:1, 1987

Muhumuza L, Morgan JP, Miyabayashi T et al: Positive contrast arthrography: a study of the humeral joints in normal beagle dogs. Vet Radiol 29:157, 1988

Puglisi TA, Green RW, Hall CL et al: Comparison of metrizamide and iohexol for cisternal myelographic examination of dogs. Am J Vet Res 47:1863, 1986

Simon JH, Ekholm SE, Kido DK et al: High dose iohexol myelography. Radiology 163:455, 1987

Spencer CP, Chrisman CL, Mayhew IG, Kaude JV: Neurotoxic effects of the nonionic contrast agent iopamidol on the leptomeninges of the dog. Am J Vet Res 43:1958, 1982

Suter PF: Thoracic Radiography: A Text Atlas of Thoracic Diseases of the Dog and Cat. PF Suter, Wettswil, Switzerland, 1984

Suter PF, Carb AV: Shoulder arthrography in dogs—radiographic anatomy and clinical application. J Small Anim Pract 10:407, 1969

Ticer JW: Radiographic Technique in Veterinary Practice. 2nd Ed. WB Saunders, Philadelphia, 1984

van Bree H: Evaluation of the prognostic value of positive-contrast shoulder arthrography for bilateral osteochondrosis lesions in dogs. J Am Vet Med Assoc 51:1121, 1990

van Sonnenberg E, Neff CC, Pfister RC: Life threatening hypotensive reactions to contrast media: comparison of pharmacologic and fluid therapy. Radiology 162:15, 1987

Wheeler SJ, Davies JV: Iohexol myelography in the dog and cat: a series of 100 cases and a comparison with metrizamide and iopamidol. J Small Anim Pract 26:247, 1985

Widmer WR: Iohexol and iopamidol: new contrast media for veterinary myelography. J Am Vet Med Assoc 194:1714, 1989

Williams J, Biller D, Miyabayashi T, Leveille R: Evaluation of iohexol as a gastrointestinal contrast medium in normal cats. Vet Radiol Ultrasound 34:310, 1993

Wood AKW: Iohexol and iopamidol: new nonionic contrast media for myelography in dogs. Compend Contin Educ Pract Vet 10:32, 1988

Cardiovascular System

5

Introduction

Matthew W. Miller

BASIC FUNCTIONS

I. Oxygen and nutrient transport
II. Transport of carbon dioxide and other metabolic waste to excretory organs
III. Distribution of hormones, enzymes, and related substances throughout the body
IV. Thermoregulation
V. Urine formation

PREREQUISITES FOR NORMAL FUNCTION

I. Adaptable coronary circulation
   A. Ability to meet demands of the heart under a variety of circumstances
   B. Provides adequate supply of oxygen and other essential nutrients
II. Adaptable myocardium
   A. Alterations in contractility represent a mechanism by which cardiac performance can be acutely modified.
   B. Myocardial hypertrophy (eccentric and concentric) represents an adaptive response to chronic workload.
III. Competent cardiac valves
   A. Optimize forward flow
   B. Prevent excessive regurgitation
IV. Adaptable heart rate and normal cardiac rhythm
   A. Alterations in heart rate represent a mechanism by which acute changes in cardiac output can be made.
   B. Organized depolarization and subsequent contraction of the myocardium are necessary for optimal performance.
V. Adaptable vasculature
   A. Alterations in arterial tone are required for regulation of blood pressure and perfusion.
   B. Alterations in venous tone influence cardiac filling and cardiac output.

PATHOPHYSIOLOGY OF DYSFUNCTION

I. Reduced coronary blood flow
   A. Systemic hypotension shock
   B. Abbreviation of diastole (tachyarrhythmias)
   C. Anatomic obstruction (very uncommon)
   D. Rarely a primary problem in small animals
II. Valvular dysfunction
   A. Stenosis: narrowing of valve orifice
     1. Impedes forward flow
     2. Increased pressure in chamber proximal to affected valve
   B. Incompetence or insufficiency
     1. Regurgitation during systole or diastole
     2. Decreases forward flow and therefore cardiac output
     3. Imposes a volume load on the cardiac chambers on either side of the valve
III. Decreased myocardial systolic performance (contractility)
   A. Primary: idiopathic dilated cardiomyopathy
   B. Secondary
     1. Myocarditis: viral, protozoal agents
     2. Hypoxemia, electrolyte disturbances, acid–base imbalance
     3. Anesthetics, sedatives
     4. Nutritional disorders
       a) Carnitine deficiency
       b) Taurine deficiency
IV. Reduction in cardiac filling
   A. Elevated filling pressures
     1. Congestive heart failure (CHF)
     2. Pericardial diseases
     3. Intraluminal masses
     4. Hypertrophic cardiomyopathy
   B. Reduced venous return
     1. Volume depletion
     2. Shock
V. Chronic superimposed workload
   A. Increased volume (preload)
     1. Intracardiac shunts: ventricular septal defect

2. Extracardiac shunts: arteriovenous fistula, patent ductus arteriosus
3. Valvular regurgitation
4. Hyperthyroidism, anemia

B. Increased pressure (afterload)
1. Fixed or dynamic obstruction to ventricular ejection
2. Semilunar valve stenosis, e.g., subvalvular, supravalvular
3. Systemic and pulmonary arterial hypertension

VI. Abnormal cardiac rhythm
A. Tachyarrhythmias
1. Decrease time for cardiac filling
2. Decrease time for coronary perfusion
3. Increase myocardial oxygen demand

B. Bradyarrhythmias: decreased cardiac output as a result of decreased rate

E. Arterial pulse palpation
F. Thoracic auscultation

IV. Cardiac rhythm
A. Electrocardiography
B. Holter monitoring

V. Cardiac anatomy and performance
A. Thoracic radiography
B. Echocardiography
C. Doppler echocardiography
D. Cardiac catheterization
E. Nuclear cardiology
F. Computed tomography
G. Magnetic resonance imaging

VI. Peripheral circulation
A. Palpation: temperature, pulse
B. Central venous pressure
C. Blood pressure: direct, indirect
D. Angiography, venography

CLINICAL ASSESSMENT

I. Signalment
There are important breed, age, and sex predilections for many of the common congenital and acquired diseases (see Chaps. 6, 9, 10, and 11).

II. Complete and accurate history
A. Exercise history
B. Respiratory pattern
C. Medications

III. Complete cardiovascular physical examination
A. Mucous membranes
B. Capillary refill time
C. Jugular venous evaluation
D. Precordial palpation

TREATMENT

I. There continue to be important developments in both the diagnosis and management of cardiovascular disease in companion animals.

II. Veterinarians need to be familiar with new and innovative approaches to medical and surgical management of cardiovascular disease.

III. Improved quality and, hopefully, duration of life for the animals we treat is our primary goal.

IV. In the chapters that follow, the current standards for the diagnosis and therapy of the more common acquired and congenital cardiac disorders are addressed.

6

Congenital Diseases

Linda B. Lehmkuhl
John D. Bonagura

VALVULAR LESIONS

Ventricular Outflow Tract Obstructions

Aortic Stenosis

Definition

I. Aortic stenosis is an obstruction to left ventricular outflow.
II. Left ventricular outflow obstruction is common in the dog but rare in the cat.
III. In dogs, it is usually caused by abnormal tissue located below the aortic valve (subaortic stenosis [SAS]) (Pyle et al., 1976).
IV. Dynamic subvalvular obstruction associated with malformations of the mitral valve apparatus may also occur in dogs (Sisson, 1992; Buoscio et al., 1994).

Causes

I. SAS is inherited in dogs.
II. The pattern of transmission is most compatible with an autosomal dominant single gene trait with variable expression (Patterson, 1991).

Pathophysiology

I. Obstruction generates a pressure overload on the left ventricle.
   A. The left ventricle generates an increased systolic pressure to eject blood across the stenosis.
   B. The resultant pressure gradient (higher ventricular than aortic systolic pressure) generally correlates with disease severity.
      1. Pressure gradient (awake or lightly sedated Doppler gradient) <50 mmHg: mild
      2. Pressure gradient of 50–100 mmHg: moderate
      3. Pressure gradient >100 mmHg: severe
   C. Left ventricular hypertrophy (LVH) develops to minimize ventricular wall stress.
II. Myocardial ischemia often occurs.
   A. Increased myocardial oxygen demand and decreased myocardial perfusion are present.
   B. It leads to ventricular arrhythmias.
III. Mitral regurgitation and aortic regurgitation may develop.
IV. Left-sided congestive heart failure (CHF) or low cardiac output failure may occur.
V. The lesion often progresses in severity (Pyle et al., 1976; Nakayama et al., 1996).
VI. Dogs are predisposed to aortic valve endocarditis regardless of SAS severity (Muna et al., 1978).

Clinical Signs

I. Mildly affected animals are usually asymptomatic.
II. Moderate to severely affected dogs may be asymptomatic or develop the following (Kienle et al., 1994).
   A. Exercise intolerance, rear limb weakness
   B. Syncope
   C. Sudden death, probably due to ventricular arrhythmias
   D. Left-sided CHF: cough, shortness of breath
III. Endocarditis (fever, lethargy, anorexia, CHF) may develop.

Diagnosis

I. Signalment: usually large-breed dogs (Buchanan, 1992)
   A. Newfoundland
   B. Golden retriever
   C. Rottweiler
   D. Boxer
   E. German shepherd dog
II. Physical examination
   A. Mild disease
      1. Systolic murmur generated by high velocity, turbulent flow crossing the stenosis
         a) Heard best just caudoventral to the aortic valve (left base)
         b) Crescendo-decrescendo ejection murmur
         c) Soft to moderately intense: grade 1–3/6
         d) Soft radiation of murmur to the right
      2. Normal femoral arterial pulses
   B. Moderate to severe disease

1. Systolic murmur: all dogs
   a) Heard best at the left and right cardiac base
   b) Crescendo-decrescendo ejection murmur
   c) Moderately intense to loud: grade 4–6/6
   d) Radiates widely: craniodorsally, apically, to the right, and even to the head
2. Holosystolic murmur of mitral regurgitation over the left apex: some dogs
3. Diastolic murmur of aortic regurgitation heard best over the left or right cardiac base: small percentage of dogs
4. Weak and late rising arterial pulses

III. Thoracic radiography
   A. Abnormalities are detected only in moderately to severely affected animals.
      1. Left ventricular enlargement
      2. Loss of the cranial waist on the lateral view from post-stenotic dilation of the ascending aorta
      3. Left atrial enlargement, especially if concurrent mitral regurgitation
   B. Left-sided CHF occasionally develops.
      1. Perihilar edema
      2. Pulmonary venous congestion

IV. Electrocardiography (ECG)
   A. Abnormal only in moderately to severely affected animals
   B. Evidence of left ventricular enlargement
      1. R waves in lead II >3 mV (dog), >0.9 (cat)
      2. Left axis deviation
   C. ST-segment depression from LVH or myocardial ischemia
   D. Ventricular tachyarrhythmias

V. Echocardiography
   A. Mildly affected animals
      1. May have no detectable structural lesions
      2. Increased left ventricular outflow tract velocity (>2.2 m/sec)
   B. Moderate to severely affected animals (Wingfield et al., 1983)
      1. Subvalvular obstructive lesion
      2. LVH
      3. Post-stenotic dilation of the aorta
      4. Hyperechoic segments of the left ventricular myocardium indicating subendocardial fibrosis
      5. Increased left ventricular to aortic systolic pressure gradient as measured by Doppler (Lehmkuhl et al., 1995)
         a) Estimated from the peak left ventricular outflow velocity using the modified Bernoulli equation
         b) Pressure gradient = (velocity in meters/sec)^2 × 4

Differential Diagnosis

I. "Functional" murmurs
   A. Mild SAS can be difficult (or impossible) to differentiate from a functional murmur.
   B. This distinction is important for genetic counseling.

C. Functional murmurs are generally heard best craniodorsal to the pulmonic or aortic valve.
D. A Doppler velocity exceeding 2.2 m/sec in the left ventricular outflow tract is suggestive of SAS as opposed to a functional murmur.

II. Pulmonic stenosis (PS)
   A. Similar murmur but best heard more cranioventral and radiates more dorsal on the left chest wall
   B. Different breed predispositions
   C. Produces right-sided enlargement on ECG, radiography, and echocardiography

Treatment

I. Do not breed affected animals.
II. Institute prophylaxis for bacterial endocarditis as needed.
III. In moderate to severe disease, therapeutic options are frustratingly limited and unproven.
   A. Surgery
      1. Limited successes employing dilation, resection, or bypassing obstruction (Orton and Monnet, 1994)
      2. High costs, high mortality rates, and limited availability
   B. Balloon catheter dilation (DeLellis et al., 1993; Lehmkuhl and Bonagura, 1995)
      1. A 50% decrease in the gradient at the time of the procedure is typical.
      2. In some dogs, this benefit is maintained; but in others, it attentuates over time.
   C. Medical therapy
      1. Restricted exercise
      2. Beta-adrenergic blocking drugs
         a) For history of syncope (without CHF), Doppler gradient > 100 mmHg, significant ST-T changes, or ventricular arrhythmias
         b) Atenolol 12.5–50 mg PO BID
         c) May decrease myocardial oxygen demands and protect against ventricular arrhythmias
      3. CHF (see Chap. 9)
         a) Furosemide, digoxin, sodium restriction
         b) Cautious use of angiotensin-converting enzyme inhibitors
      4. Endocarditis (see Chap. 9)

Patient Monitoring

I. Monitor for clinical signs of endocarditis, such as fever or lameness.
II. Mildly affected animals are likely to be near-normal pets.
III. Moderate to severely affected animals may develop mitral regurgitation, aortic regurgitation, and atrial fibrillation leading to clinical deterioration.
   A. Perform physical examination, ECG (or 24-hour Holter monitor), and echocardiogram every 6–12 months.
   B. Institute ventricular antiarrhythmics as necessary.

Pulmonic Stenosis

Definition
I. Pulmonic stenosis is an obstruction to right ventricular outflow.
II. It is common in the dog but is rarely diagnosed as an isolated lesion in the cat.
III. Dysplasia of the pulmonary valve is the most common anatomic form in dogs and is characterized by valve leaflet thickening, fusion, and hypoplasia (Patterson et al., 1981).
IV. Infundibular, subvalvular, and supravalvular obstruction also occur (Fingland et al., 1986; Thomas, 1995).

Causes
I. Valve dysplasia is inherited in beagle dogs (and possibly other breeds) as a polygenetic trait (Patterson et al., 1981; Patterson, 1991).
II. Abnormal development of the coronary arteries may also be present (Buchanan, 1990).
   A. English bulldogs and boxers are most often affected.
   B. Anomalous left main coronary artery originates from a single right coronary artery.
   C. Anomalous vessel encircles the stenotic right ventricular outlet and likely contributes to the embryogenesis of the subvalvular obstruction.
   D. Inheritance of this defect is undefined (Patterson, 1991).

Pathophysiology
I. Obstruction creates a pressure overload on the right ventricle.
   A. The right ventricle generates an increased systolic pressure to eject blood to the lungs.
   B. The resultant pressure gradient generally correlates with disease severity (Thomas, 1995).
      1. Pressure gradient (awake or lightly sedated Doppler gradient) <50 mmHg: mild
      2. Pressure gradient of 50–80 mmHg: moderate
      3. Pressure gradient >80 mmHg: severe
   C. Right ventricular hypertrophy (RVH) develops.
II. Tricuspid regurgitation may develop.
   A. Concurrent tricuspid valve dysplasia
   B. Secondary changes in valve apparatus related to ventricular hypertrophy and valve thickening
III. Right-sided CHF or low output failure may occur.
IV. Hypoxemia may arise from right-to-left shunting through a concurrent atrioventricular septal defect or patent foramen ovale (Lombard et al., 1989).

Clinical Signs
I. Many animals are asymptomatic.
II. Clinical signs are more likely in dogs >1 year of age.
   A. Syncope, exercise intolerance from low cardiac output
   B. Ascites, exercise intolerance from right-sided CHF
   C. Sudden death
   D. Gasping, cyanosis from right-to-left shunt (Lombard et al., 1989)

Diagnosis
I. Signalment (Buchanan, 1992)
   A. Beagle
   B. Chihuahua
   C. English bulldog: males > females
   D. Keeshond
   E. Samoyed
   F. Mastiff
   G. Bullmastiffs: males > females (Malik et al., 1993)
   H. Newfoundland
   I. Boxer
   J. Other terriers and spaniels
II. Physical examination
   A. Systolic murmur: all dogs
      1. Heard best at the left base
      2. Crescendo-decrescendo ejection murmur
      3. Radiating to the left craniodorsal cardiac base and to the right hemithorax
   B. Holosystolic murmur of tricuspid regurgitation heard over the right hemithorax: some dogs
   C. Abnormal jugular pulsation or distention
   D. Palpable right-sided thoracic heave
III. Thoracic radiography (Fingland et al., 1986)
   A. Right ventricular enlargement
   B. Post-stenotic dilation of the main pulmonary artery
   C. Pulmonary underperfusion
IV. Electrocardiography (Thomas, 1995)
   A. Evidence of right ventricular enlargement
      1. Right axis deviation
      2. S waves in leads I, II, III, and AVF
      3. Increased amplitude S waves in left chest leads (V3 and V6)
   B. Right atrial enlargement if concurrent tricuspid regurgitation
V. Echocardiography
   A. Obstructive lesion: often a deformity and narrowing in pulmonic valve area
   B. RVH
   C. Secondary muscular narrowing of the right ventricular outflow tract
   D. Post-stenotic dilation of the main pulmonary artery
   E. Visualization of anomalous coronary artery or asymmetrical aortic valve sinuses
   F. Increased right ventricular to pulmonary artery systolic pressure gradient with Doppler study (see earlier discussion of SAS)
VI. Cardiac catheterization
   A. Unnecessary as a diagnostic aid in many cases
   B. Important in detecting anomalous left coronary artery

Differential Diagnosis
I. Subaortic stenosis (see earlier)
II. Atrioventricular septal defects
   A. Atrial septal defect (ASD)
      1. "Relative" PS murmur of ASD similar to anatomic PS murmur
      2. Right ventricular enlargement with both PS and ASD

3. May have split second heart sound with ASD
4. Pulmonary overcirculation with ASD

B. Ventricular septal defect (VSD)
1. "Relative" PS murmur of VSD similar to anatomic PS murmur
2. VSD shunting murmur similar to tricuspid regurgitation associated with PS
3. Pulmonary overcirculation with VSD
4. Often LVH on ECG, radiography, or echocardiography with VSD

Treatment
I. Do not breed affected animals.
II. Invasive intervention may be considered.
   A. Indications
      1. Animals with clinical signs
      2. Asymptomatic animals with significant radiographic, ECG, and echocardiographic changes (Thomas, 1995)
         a) Severe disease (>80 mmHg): intervention recommended
         b) Moderate disease (50–80 mmHg): consider activity level of dog, evidence of progressive cardiomegaly or increasing gradient, presence or absence of tricuspid regurgitation, client expectations, and whether the gradient is closer to 50 or 80
         c) Mild disease (<50 mmHg): no intervention
   B. Contraindications: subvalvular PS and a single right coronary artery
      1. Most surgical procedures (Buchanan, 1990) and balloon dilation (Kittleson et al., 1992) may result in severing or rupture of the anomalous left coronary artery.
      2. The best option in these animals is conduit implantation.
   C. Surgery
      1. Numerous procedures including valve dilation, open valvulotomy, patch-graft valvuloplasty and conduits are possible (Orton and Monnet, 1994).
      2. Best procedure for an individual animal depends on the following.
         a) Anatomy of obstruction
         b) Severity of subvalvular muscular hypertrophy
         c) Concurrent defects
         d) Surgeon's capabilities, experience, and facilities
         e) Presence or absence of an anomalous coronary artery
      3. High costs, high mortality, and limited availability remain problematic.
   D. Balloon catheter dilation (Brownlie et al., 1991)
      1. It is most effective when the valves are thin and fused and the annulus is not hypoplastic.
      2. A decrease in the pressure gradient by 50% or more occurs in most dogs (Thomas, 1995).
III. Medical therapy may be tried for moderate to severely affected dogs.
   A. Restricted exercise

B. CHF (see Chap. 9)
1. Digitalis, furosemide, dietary sodium restriction, and rest are instituted.
2. After initial stabilization, balloon dilation or surgery may be considered.

Patient Monitoring
I. Dogs with mild and even moderate PS usually have normal lifespans.
II. Moderate to severely affected animals require more monitoring.
   A. Tricuspid regurgitation and development of arrhythmias (especially atrial fibrillation) may lead to clinical deterioration.
   B. Perform physical examination, ECG, and echocardiogram every year.

Dysplasia of the Atrioventricular Valves

Tricuspid and Mitral Valve Dysplasia

Definition
I. Malformation of the atrioventricular valves is characterized by a wide spectrum of morphologic changes in the valve leaflets, chordae tendineae, and papillary muscles (Liu and Tilley, 1975, 1976).
II. These defects are common in both dogs and cats.
III. Ebstein's malformation, a downward displacement of the tricuspid valve's basal attachment, may occur with tricuspid dysplasia (TD) in some dogs (Eyster et al., 1977a; Moise, 1995).

Causes
I. The cause of atrioventricular valve dysplasias in dogs and cats is unknown.
II. Breed predilections in dogs suggests a genetic etiology (Liu and Tilley, 1975; Moise, 1995).

Pathophysiology
I. Atrioventricular valve dysplasia results in regurgitation of blood from the ventricle into the atrium on the affected side.
   A. Volume overload of ipsilateral cardiac chambers
   B. Possibly limited cardiac output
II. Rarely, some dysplastic valves are also stenotic and obstruct ventricular filling (Fox et al., 1992).
III. Right-sided (TD) or left-sided (mitral dysplasia) CHF or low output failure may develop.
IV. There is a predisposition to atrial arrhythmias owing to atrial enlargement.
V. In TD, right-to-left shunting through a patent foramen ovale or an ASD may occur.

Clinical Signs
I. Mildly affected animals are usually asymptomatic.
II. Moderate to severely affected dogs may develop the following.
   A. CHF
      1. Right-sided CHF: ascites, jugular vein pulsation, hepatomegaly, weakness

2. Left-sided CHF: cough, tachypnea, pulmonary crackles
B. Exercise intolerance
C. Rarely, syncope or sudden death

Diagnosis
I. Signalment
   A. Tricuspid dysplasia is most common in large-breed male dogs, especially the Labrador retriever (Buchanan, 1992).
   B. Mitral dysplasia (MD) is very common in cats and Great Danes, German shepherd dogs, bull terriers, golden retrievers, and Newfoundlands (Liu and Tilley, 1975; Bonagura and Darke, 1995).
II. Physical examination
   A. A holosystolic regurgitant murmur is heard best over the left apex (MD) or right hemithorax (TD) in dogs.
   B. In cats, a holosystolic murmur is heard just to the left (MD) or right (TD) of the sternum.
   C. Rarely, a soft diastolic rumble is ausculted over the inflow tract of the affected ventricle, suggesting concurrent valvular stenosis.
   D. Signs of CHF may be evident if the dysplasia is severe.
III. Thoracic radiography
   A. Enlargement of the affected side of the heart, especially the atrium
   B. ± Evidence of CHF
      1. TD: enlarged caudal vena cava
      2. MD: pulmonary edema, pulmonary venous congestion
IV. Electrocardiography
   A. Atrial and ventricular enlargement patterns of the affected side may be present.
   B. Intraventricular conduction disturbances are common in dogs with TD (Bonagura and Darke, 1995; Moise, 1995).
   C. Atrial tachyarrhythmias are common, especially atrial fibrillation.
V. Echocardiography
   A. It documents abnormal shape, location, motion, or attachment of the valve.
   B. Enlargement of the ipsilateral atrium (often huge) and ventricle is often present.
   C. Doppler studies demonstrate a regurgitant jet, valvular stenosis, or both.

Differential Diagnosis
I. Main differential for TD is a VSD.
   A. Both TD and VSD generate holosystolic right-sided murmurs, but usually a VSD murmur is slightly more ventral.
   B. Pulmonary overcirculation occurs with VSD.
   C. Often LVH is demonstrated by ECG, radiography, or echocardiography with a VSD.
II. The main differential considerations for MD are acquired causes of mitral regurgitation such as hypertrophic cardiomyopathy in the cat or dilated cardiomyopathy in the dog.

Treatment
I. Medical management of CHF and arrhythmias is instituted as described for chronic valvular disease (see Chap. 9).
II. Surgical management of these lesions is difficult and rarely done.

Patient Monitoring
I. Atrioventricular valve dysplasia is often tolerated for many years; however, signs of CHF and death may occur in very young patients with severe disease.
II. Progressive cardiomegaly on radiography suggests a guarded prognosis.
III. Development of atrial arrhythmias on ECG warrants concern.

LESIONS CAUSING SYSTEMIC TO PULMONARY SHUNTING

Patent Ductus Arteriosus

Definition and Cause
I. Patent ductus arteriosus (PDA) is a persistent communication between the descending aorta and pulmonary artery that fails to close after birth.
II. It is the most common congenital heart defect in the dog but occurs infrequently in cats (Buchanan, 1992).
III. PDA is an inherited defect transmitted as a polygenic trait in dogs (Patterson et al., 1971; Patterson, 1991).

Pathophysiology
I. PDA allows continuous shunting of blood from the descending aorta to the main pulmonary artery (left-to-right) because the aortic pressure exceeds that of the pulmonary artery throughout the cardiac cycle.
II. Increased pulmonary flow and increased venous return to the left atrium and left ventricle result in volume overload of the left side of the heart.
III. Left-sided CHF may develop from volume overload.
IV. Mitral regurgitation may occur secondary to left ventricular dilation or concurrent MD.

Clinical Signs
I. May be asymptomatic
II. Left-sided CHF: cough, shortness of breath

Diagnosis
I. Signalment
   A. Females > males (Buchanan, 1992)
   B. Breeds at greatest risk: collie, Maltese, poodle, Pomeranian, English springer spaniel, keeshond, bichon frisé, Yorkshire terrier, and Shetland sheepdog (Buchanan, 1992)
II. Physical examination
   A. Continuous (machinery) murmur
      1. Heard best at the craniodorsal left cardiac base
      2. Radiates cranial to the manubrium and to the right base
   B. Holosystolic left apical murmur of mitral regurgitation often present

C. Hyperkinetic arterial pulses due to the increased pulse pressure

D. Tachypnea and pulmonary crackles if left-sided CHF

III. Thoracic radiography
   A. Left-sided cardiomegaly
   B. Pulmonary overcirculation
   C. Main pulmonary artery dilation
   D. Dilation of the descending aorta (''ductus bump'')

IV. Electrocardiography
   A. Left atrial enlargement: wide P waves
   B. Left ventricular dilation: increased voltage Q and R waves in leads II, III, and AVF

V. Echocardiography
   A. Indications
      1. To verify diagnosis in animals lacking classic noninvasive findings
      2. To rule out concurrent defects, especially in predisposed breeds
      3. To assess myocardial function
      4. Not necessary in most patients
   B. Findings
      1. Enlarged left atrium and ventricle
      2. Dilation of the aorta and pulmonary artery
      3. Ventricular shortening fraction decreased in some dogs, probably from chronic severe volume overload
      4. ± Imaging of ductus
      5. Doppler study
         a) Continuous flow through ductus can be imaged in some animals.
         b) Continuous and abnormal retrograde flow may be seen in the pulmonary artery.
         c) Mild increases in aortic velocity (generally <2.5 m/sec) may be detected.
         d) It may demonstrate mitral and pulmonic valve insufficiency.

Differential Diagnosis
I. VSD with aortic regurgitation (AR)
   A. Right sternal border murmur of VSD is not typical for PDA.
   B. Combined VSD and AR murmur is not loudest at the second heart sound and does not have machinery characteristic of PDA murmur.
   C. No ductus bulge is seen on radiography.

II. SAS with AR
   A. PDA has pulmonary overcirculation and ductus ''bump'' on radiography.
   B. PDA murmur is loudest at second heart sound and has machinery characteristic.

III. Aorticopulmonary window: very rare

Treatment
I. Do not breed affected animals.
II. Surgical ligation is recommended in all cases of left-to-right shunting PDA diagnosed in animals <2 years of age.
   A. Prognosis with surgery is excellent unless advanced CHF or atrial fibrillation is present (Eyster et al., 1976b; Birchard et al., 1990; Bonagura and Darke, 1995).

B. The decision to perform surgery in an older pet can be difficult and is best made in concert with a cardiologist.

III. Coil embolization via transcatheter delivery of a Gianturco coil may also be performed.
   A. It is a recently reported technique to occlude PDA without thoracic surgery (Snaps et al., 1995; Grifka et al., 1996).
   B. Pulmonary embolism of the coil is the most common complication.

Patient Monitoring
I. More than half of affected dogs die within 1 year of diagnosis without surgery (Eyster et al., 1976).
II. Most dogs undergoing surgery lead normal lives.
   A. Secondary murmurs (mitral regurgitation) resolve by the time of suture removal.
   B. Radiographically, overall heart size may normalize, but the heart and great vessels continue to be misshapen.
   C. Echocardiography is used to follow up those animals with reduced myocardial function.
   D. Doppler echocardiography may detect trivial residual shunting; in the absence of a murmur or infection, this is ignored.

Ventricular Septal Defect

Definition
I. It is an abnormal communication between the ventricles allowing blood to shunt from left to right.
II. This defect is common in both dogs and cats.
III. Typical defect is located dorsally or ''high'' on the ventricular septum.
   A. Left-sided location of the defect is below the aortic valve.
   B. Right ventricular location is just below the tricuspid valve septal leaflet.
IV. Some lesions result in prolapse of the aortic valve into the defect in dogs (Sisson et al., 1991).

Causes
I. The cause of most ventricular septal defects is unknown.
II. A genetic basis is suspected in some dog breeds (English springer spaniel) and documented in Keeshonds with malformations of the conotruncal septum (Patterson et al., 1993).

Pathophysiology
I. Magnitude and direction of shunting depend on the size of the orifice and the relative resistances in the systemic and pulmonary circulations (Friedman, 1992).
II. Typically, blood shunts from the systemic to the pulmonary vessels (left-to-right).
III. Left ventricle does most of the additional volume work as much of the shunted flow is pumped across the defect and immediately into the pulmonary artery.
IV. As pulmonary flow increases, there is increased venous return and enlargement of the left atrium and left ventricle.

V. Left-sided CHF may develop when the shunt is large.

Clinical Signs
  I. Most animals are asymptomatic.
  II. Left-sided CHF (cough, shortness of breath) and exercise intolerance are possible.

Diagnosis
  I. Signalment: many breeds, especially English bulldog and English springer spaniel
  II. Physical examination
    A. Holosystolic murmur is heard best along the cranial right sternal border.
    B. Systolic ejection murmur of relative pulmonic stenosis may be heard at the left base.
    C. Rarely, a diastolic murmur of aortic regurgitation is present.
  III. Radiographic findings in dogs with VSDs are quite variable.
    A. Left-sided enlargement
    B. Pulmonary overcirculation
    C. Dilated main pulmonary artery
    D. Variable degrees of right ventricular enlargement
  IV. Electrocardiographic findings are also variable.
    A. Left atrial enlargement
    B. Left ventricular dilation
    C. Possible right ventricular enlargement
    D. Abnormal early ventricular septal activation characterized by a Q wave that is wide or contains high-frequency notching
  V. Echocardiography confirms the diagnosis.
    A. Delineates the defect and secondary volume loading of the left atrium and left ventricle
    B. Favorable prognostic findings
      1. Maximal defect diameter is <40% that of the aorta.
      2. Doppler studies identify a high velocity jet (>4.5 m/sec) typical of a small or "restrictive" defect.
      3. Doppler-estimated right ventricular systolic pressure is <45 mmHg.
      4. Significant aortic regurgitation is not evident.

Differential Diagnosis
  I. Tricuspid dysplasia
  II. Pulmonic stenosis
  III. For VSD with AR: PDA

Treatment
  I. Most animals >6 months without clinical signs tolerate the defect and do not require therapy.
  II. Surgery is rarely performed.
    A. Definitive repair requires cardiopulmonary bypass.
    B. Pulmonary artery banding creates supravalvular pulmonary stenosis and decreases the magnitude of left-to-right shunting (Eyster, 1977).
  III. Medical therapy for CHF is started as needed.
    A. Digoxin and furosemide
    B. Arterial vasodilators
      1. Enalapril, hydralazine

      2. May be especially beneficial because decreasing systemic vascular resistance decreases left-to-right shunting
  IV. Prophylactic use of antibiotics to prevent endocarditis may be prudent (Brown, 1995).

Patient Monitoring
  I. Dogs with small defects usually have a normal life span.
  II. Dogs with large defects are monitored at least yearly by physical examination, ECG, and thoracic radiography for development of left-sided CHF or arrhythmias.

LESIONS CAUSING PULMONARY TO SYSTEMIC SHUNTING

Tetralogy of Fallot
Definition and Cause
  I. Tetralogy of Fallot is composed of the following.
    A. Subaortic VSD
    B. Right ventricular outflow tract obstruction, i.e., pulmonic stenosis (PS)
    C. Dextropositioned or overriding aorta
    D. Right ventricular hypertrophy secondary to PS
  II. It is the most common cause of cyanotic heart disease in small animals.
  III. In the keeshond, tetralogy of Fallot is a severe manifestation of conotruncal hypoplasia, which is transmitted as an autosomal recessive trait with variable expression (Patterson et al., 1993).

Pathophysiology
  I. PS results in elevated right ventricular systolic pressure.
  II. Desaturated blood shunts from the right ventricle through the VSD into the left ventricle (right-to-left shunt).
  III. Hypoxemia, decreased hemoglobin oxygen saturation, cyanosis, and secondary polycythemia develop.
  IV. Left atrium and left ventricle are small from decreased pulmonary flow.

Clinical Signs
  I. Poor growth (Ringwald and Bonagura, 1988)
  II. Shortness of breath, gasping with excitement
  III. Cyanosis
  IV. Exercise intolerance, weakness
  V. Seizures or syncope
  VI. Sudden death

Diagnosis
  I. Signalment: common in the keeshond and English bulldog (Buchanan, 1992)
  II. Physical examination
    A. PS murmur is present unless pulmonary atresia and/or severe polycythemia occur.
    B. Right hemithorax murmur is not uncommon.

1. Radiation from PS
2. From VSD
C. Most dogs are cyanotic. Exercise or excitement may induce cyanosis by increasing right-to-left shunting.
III. Thoracic radiography
A. Mild right ventricular enlargement
B. Pulmonary undercirculation
IV. Electrocardiography: right ventricular enlargement
V. Echocardiography
A. Right ventricular hypertrophy
B. Large subaortic VSD: right-to-left shunting on Doppler or contrast echo
C. Right ventricular outflow obstruction
D. Overriding aorta
E. Small left atrium and left ventricle
VI. Laboratory evaluation
A. Decreased arterial P_{O_2} and P_{CO_2}
B. Commonly polycythemic (Ringwald and Bonagura, 1988)

Differential Diagnosis
I. Isolated PS
II. Other right-to-left shunts
A. ASD, VSD, or PDA with pulmonary hypertension
B. ASD, VSD with PS
C. ASD with tricuspid stenosis

Treatment
I. Surgery
A. Definitive repair to close the VSD and remove or bypass PS is rarely done.
B. Creation of a systemic to pulmonary shunt improves clinical signs in some animals and increases the contribution of oxygenated blood to the systemic circulation by increasing pulmonary venous return (Eyster et al., 1977b).
II. Medical therapy
A. Exercise restriction
B. Beta-blocking agents (Eyster et al., 1976a)
1. Decrease dynamic right ventricular muscular obstruction
2. May improve clinical signs in some animals
C. Phlebotomy to maintain the PCV at 62–68%
1. To control signs of hyperviscosity
2. Replace removed blood volume with crystalloid fluids

Patient Monitoring
I. Many dogs tolerate tetralogy of Fallot for years (Ringwald and Bonagura, 1988).
II. Monitor for polycythemia, cardiac arrhythmias, and hypoxemia every 4–6 months.

VASCULAR RING ANOMALIES

Persistent Right Aortic Arch

Definition and Cause
I. Persistent right aortic arch (PRAA) is the retention of the embryonic right, as opposed to left, fourth aortic arch.

II. A vascular ring around the esophagus results, with the following components.
A. Right: aorta
B. Left: pulmonary artery
C. Ventral: heart base
D. Dorsal: ligamentum arteriosum (may be PDA)
III. This defect occurs commonly in dogs but only rarely in cats.
IV. PRAA is most likely genetic and transmitted by a complex inheritance pattern (Patterson, 1991).

Pathophysiology
I. Esophageal obstruction causes food retention cranial to the vascular ring with regurgitation.
II. Secondary aspiration pneumonia is common.

Clinical Signs
I. Regurgitation: begins during weaning to solid foods
II. Weight loss despite good appetite
III. Evidence of pneumonia: fever, tachypnea, cough

Diagnosis
I. Signalment: usually large-breed dogs
A. German shepherd dog
B. Great Dane
C. Irish setter
II. Thoracic radiography
A. Survey radiographs reveal distention of esophagus cranial to the heart base.
B. Barium swallow shows distention of esophagus cranial to constriction at the cardiac base.

Differential Diagnosis
I. Other vascular rings (VanGundy, 1989)
A. Double aortic arch
B. Aberrant subclavian artery
II. Primary esophageal diseases
A. Megasophagus: dilation extends past the cardiac base
B. Stricture: endoscopy may be necessary to differentiate

Treatment and Patient Monitoring
I. Surgery
A. Divide the ligamentum arteriosum.
B. Free the esophagus from surrounding adhesions.
C. Persistent left cranial vena cava may be an incidental finding at surgery.
D. Persistent esophageal dysfunction often causes clinical signs to persist postoperatively (Shires and Liu, 1981).
II. Feed frequent small meals with head elevated for 8 weeks postoperatively.
III. Modified feeding regimens may be required for life.
IV. Antibiotic therapy is instituted for pneumonia when present.

Bibliography

Birchard SJ, Bonagura JD, Fingland RD: Results of ligation of patent ductus arteriosus in dogs: 201 cases (1969–1988). J Am Vet Med Assoc 12:2011, 1990

Bonagura JD, Darke PGG: Congenital heart disease. p. 892. In Ettinger SJ, Feldman EC (eds): Textbook of Veterinary Internal Medicine. 4th Ed. WB Saunders, Philadelphia, 1995

Brown WA: Ventricular septal defects in the English springer spaniel. p. 827. In Bonagura JD (ed): Kirk's Current Veterinary Therapy XII. WB Saunders, Philadelphia, 1995

Brownlie SE, Cobb MA, Chambers J et al: Percutaneous balloon valvuloplasty in four dogs with pulmonic stenosis. J Small Anim Pract 32:165, 1991

Buchanan JW: Pulmonic stenosis caused by single coronary artery in dogs: four cases (1965–1984). J Am Vet Med Assoc 196:115, 1990

Buchanan JW: Causes and prevalence of cardiovascular disease. p. 648. In Kirk RW, Bonagura JD (eds): Current Veterinary Therapy XI: Small Animal Practice. WB Saunders, Philadelphia, 1992

Buoscio DA, Sisson DD, Zachary JF et al: Clinical and pathological characterization of an unusual form of subvalvular aortic stenosis in four golden retriever puppies. J Am Anim Hosp Assoc 30:100, 1994

DeLellis LA, Thomas WP, Pion PD: Balloon dilation of congenital subaortic stenosis in the dog. J Vet Intern Med 7:153, 1993

Eyster GE: Pulmonary artery banding for ventricular septal defect in dogs and cats. J Am Vet Med Assoc 170:434, 1977

Eyster GE, Anderson LA, Sawyer DC et al: Beta adrenergic blockade for management of tetralogy of fallot in a dog. J Am Vet Med Assoc 169:637, 1976a

Eyster GE, Eyster JT, Cords GB et al: Patent ductus arteriosus in the dog: characteristics of occurrence and results of surgery in one hundred consecutive cases. J Am Vet Med Assoc 168:435, 1976b

Eyster GE, Anderson LA, Evans AT et al: Ebsteins's anomaly: a report of 3 cases in the dog. J Am Vet Med Assoc 170:709, 1977a

Eyster GE, Braden TD, Appleford M et al: Surgical management of tetralogy of Fallot. J Small Anim Pract 18:387, 1977b

Fingland RB, Bonagura JD, Myers CW: Pulmonic stenosis in the dog: 29 cases 1975–1984. J Am Vet Med Assoc 189:218, 1986

Fox PR, Miller MW, Liu S: Clinical, echocardiographic, and Doppler imaging characteristics of mitral valve stenosis in two dogs. J Am Vet Med Assoc 201:1575, 1992

Friedman W: Congenital heart disease in infancy and childhood. p. 887. In Braunwald E (ed): Heart Disease: A Textbook of Cardiovascular Medicine. WB Saunders, Philadelphia, 1992

Grifka RG, Miller MW, Frischmeyer KJ et al: Transcatheter occlusion of a patent ductus arteriosus in a Newfoundland puppy using the Gianturco-Grifka vascular occlusion device. J Vet Intern Med 10:42, 1996

Kienle RD, Thomas WP, Pion PD: The natural history of canine congenital subaortic stenosis. J Vet Intern Med 8:423, 1994

Kittleson MD, Thomas W, Loyer C et al: Letter to the editor. J Vet Intern Med 6:250, 1992

Lehmkuhl LB, Bonagura JD: Subaortic stenosis in the dog. p. 822. In Bonagura JD (ed): Kirk's Current Veterinary Therapy XII. WB Saunders, Philadelphia, 1995

Lehmkuhl LB, Bonagura JD, Jones DE et al: Comparison of catheterization and Doppler derived pressure gradients in subaortic stenosis. J Am Soc Echocardiogr 8:611, 1995

Liu S, Tilley LP: Malformation of the canine mitral valve complex. J Am Vet Med Assoc 167:465, 1975

Liu S, Tilley LP: Dysplasia of the tricuspid valve in the dog and cat. J Am Vet Med Assoc 169:623, 1976

Lombard CW, Ackerman N, Berry CR et al: Pulmonic stenosis and right-to-left atrial shunt in three dogs. J Am Vet Med Assoc 194:71, 1989

Malik R, Church DB, Hunt GB: Valvular pulmonic stenosis in bullmastiffs. J Small Anim Pract 34:288, 1993

Moise NS: Tricuspid valve dysplasia in the dog. p. 813. In Bonagura JD (ed): Current Veterinary Therapy XII. WB Saunders, Philadelphia, 1995

Muna WF, Ferrans VJ, Pierce J et al: Discrete subaortic stenosis in Newfoundland dogs: association of infective endocarditis. Am J Cardiol 41:746, 1978

Nakayama T, Wakao Y, Ishikawa R et al: Progression of subaortic stenosis detected by continuous wave doppler echocardiography in a dog. J Vet Intern Med 10:97, 1996

Orton C, Monnet E: Pulmonic stenosis and subvalvular aortic stenosis: surgical options. Semin Vet Med Surg (Small Anim) 9:221, 1994

Patterson DF: Genes and the heart: congenital heart disease. Acad Vet Cardiol Proc 13, 1991

Patterson DF, Pyle R, Buchanan JW et al: Hereditary patent ductus arteriosus and its sequelae in the dog. Circ Res 29:1, 1971

Patterson DF, Haskins ME, Schnarr WR: Hereditary dysplasia of the pulmonary valve in beagle dogs. Am J Cardiol 47:631, 1981

Patterson DF, Pexieder T, Schnarr WR et al: A single major-gene defect underlying cardiac conotruncal malformations interferes with myocardial growth during embryonic development. Am J Hum Genet 52:388, 1993

Pyle RL, Patterson DF, Chacko S: The genetics and pathology of discrete subaortic stenosis in the Newfoundland dog. Am Heart J 92:324, 1976

Ringwald RJ, Bonagura JD: Tetralogy of fallot in the dog: clinical findings in 13 cases. J Am Anim Hosp Assoc 24:33, 1988

Shires PK, Liu W: Persistent right aortic arch in dogs: a long term follow-up after surgical correction. J Am Anim Hosp Assoc 17:773, 1981

Sisson D, Luethy M, Thomas WP: Ventricular septal defect accompanied by aortic regurgitation in five dogs. J Am Anim Hosp Assoc 27:441, 1991

Sisson DD: Fixed and dynamic subvalvular aortic stenosis in dogs. p. 760. In Kirk RW, Bonagura JD (eds): Current Veterinary Therapy XI: Small Animal Practice. WB Saunders, Philadelphia, 1992

Snaps FR, McEntee K, Saunders JH et al: Treatment of patent ductus arteriosus by placement of intravascular coils in a pup. J Am Vet Med Assoc 207:724, 1995

Thomas WP: Therapy of congenital pulmonic stenosis. p. 817. In Bonagura JD (ed): Kirk's Current Veterinary Therapy XII. WB Saunders, Philadelphia, 1995

VanGundy T: Vascular ring anomalies. Compend Contin Educ Pract Vet 11:35, 1989

Wingfield WE, Boon JA, Miller CW: Echocardiographic assessment of congenital subaortic stenosis in dogs. J Am Vet Med Assoc 183:673, 1983

7

Dysrhythmias

Rebecca L. Stepien

GENERAL CONSIDERATIONS

Cardiac Dysrhythmias

Definition and Causes

I. Dysrhythmias can be defined as variations in the normal rhythm of the heart, including disturbances in the rate, rhythm, or sequence of conduction of the atria and ventricles.

II. Cardiac dysrhythmias may result from direct damage to the heart (through congenital or acquired disease) or be a consequence of systemic abnormalities (Table 7–1).

Pathophysiology

I. Several mechanisms for development of cardiac dysrhythmias have been documented (abnormal automaticity, triggered activity, re-entry), but the underlying mechanism of any given dysrhythmia is often unknown.

II. Abnormalities causing dysrhythmias include changes in resting membrane potential or threshold potential, changes in control of transmembrane ion flux, or changes in conductivity.

III. These abnormalities are induced by myocardial stretch, necrosis, trauma, hypoxia, electrolyte, or acid-base abnormalities or toxicity.

Clinical Signs

I. Lack of substrate delivery from inadequate cardiac output
   A. Exercise intolerance
   B. Weakness, syncopal episodes
   C. Chest pain/angina: difficult to document in animals

II. Electrical instability
   A. Syncope

Table 7–1. *Potential Causes of Cardiac Dysrhythmias*

Intrinsic Cardiovascular Disease	Hypoxia	Infection	Metabolic Disease	Autonomic Nervous System Disorders
Myocardial disease	Systemic	Sepsis	Acid–base disorders	Vagal disorders
Cardiomyopathies	Pulmonary disease	Septic shock	(especially acidosis)	Situational
Infiltrative diseases	Anesthesia	Pyrexia	Electrolyte disorders	Pathologic
Inflammatory disease	Anemia		Potassium	Sympathetic nervous
Pericardial disease	Others		Calcium	system stimulation
Pericardial effusion	Local		Magnesium	Stress
Pericarditis	Myocardial infarction		Neurologic disease	Drugs
Neoplasia			Elevated intracranial	Pain
Ischemia (infarction)			pressure	
Hypo- or hypertension			Brain stem disorders	
Sinoatrial dysfunction			Organ failure (many)	
Conduction disorders			Acute renal failure	
Congenital heart disease			Hepatic failure	
Acquired valvular diseases			Endocrine disorders	
Trauma			Thyrotoxicosis	
Congestive heart failure			Hypothyroidism	
			Others	

Multiple causes may contribute to generation of dysrhythmias in an individual animal; examples of most common etiologies are given.

Table 7–2. *Normal Lead II ECG Findings in Cats and Dogs*

ECG Parameter	Cat	Dog
Resting heart rate	120–200 beats/min*	60–70 to 120–140 beats/min*
Rhythm	Sinus rhythm	Sinus rhythm
		Sinus arrhythmia (respiratory)
P wave duration (sec)	max: 0.04	max: 0.04
P wave amplitude (mV)	max: 0.2	max: 0.4
P-Q interval (sec)	0.05–0.09	0.06–0.13
QRS duration (sec)	max: 0.04	max: 0.05–0.06
R wave amplitude (mV)	max: 0.9	max: 2.5–3.0
Q-T interval (sec)	0.12–0.18	0.15–0.25
T wave amplitude (mV)	max: 0.3	max: $\leq\frac{1}{4}$ of R amplitude
Mean electrical axis (°)	0–160 (highly variable)	40–100

max = maximum; sec = seconds; mV = millivolts.
*Heart rate ranges noted are for adult, awake, resting animals. Animals with normal cardiovascular systems may exhibit heart rates outside of these ranges when hypothermic, hyperthermic, sleeping, systemically ill, immature, or excited. Deflection measurements are as recommended by Tilley (1992).

B. Sudden death
III. Refractory or worsening heart failure
    A. Sudden development of dysrhythmia (e.g., atrial fibrillation) may lead to decompensation of previous stable congestive signs.
    B. Signs of dysrhythmia (e.g., lethargy, weakness) may be confused with signs of heart failure.
IV. Clinical findings of end-organ damage
    A. Azotemia may be prerenal or renal in nature.
    B. Elevated alanine aminotransferase (ALT) levels may result from decreased hepatic blood flow.

Diagnosis

I. Cardiac dysrhythmias may be suggested by physical examination, but an electrocardiographic (ECG) diagnosis is mandatory prior to therapy.
    A. Disorders of rate
        1. Normal rates: see Table 7–2
        2. Bradydysrhythmias: rate of normal or abnormal depolarization is below accepted normal range
        3. Tachydysrhythmias: rate of normal or abnormal depolarization is above accepted normal range
    B. Disorders of rhythm
        1. Identify normal complex and conduction pattern (Fig. 7–1).
        2. Identify ectopic depolarizations.
          a) Ectopic depolarizations differ in appearance or timing.
          b) Ectopic depolarizations may be early (''premature'') or late (''escape'').
        3. Identify frequency and pattern of ectopy.
    C. Disorders of conduction
        1. Disturbance in atrioventricular (AV) nodal transmission may result in any of the following.
          a) Prolonged P-Q interval (first degree AV block)
          b) Intermittent transmission failure (second degree AV block)
          c) Complete transmission failure and development of an escape rhythm (third degree AV block)
        2. Intraventricular conduction disturbances result in changes in the QRS morphology but do not affect cardiac rhythm (Fig. 7–2).
II. Certain cardiac disorders are associated with a high probability of dysrhythmia (e.g., canine dilated cardiomyopathy).

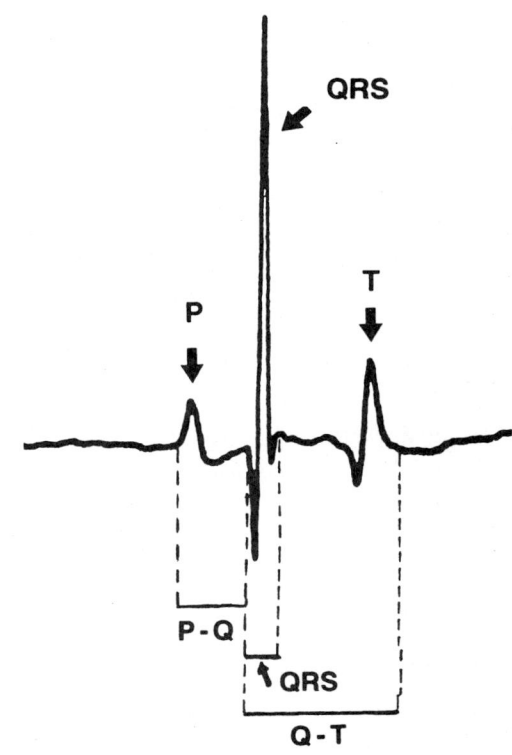

Figure 7–1. Normal lead II ECG complex. P wave, QRS complex, and T wave are identified. Each marked interval represents electrical activity in a specific anatomic location. P wave: atrial depolarization; P-Q interval: atrioventricular transmission of impulse; QRS width: ventricular depolarization; Q-T interval: ventricular repolarization. Atrial repolarization is usually not identifiable on the surface lead II ECG.

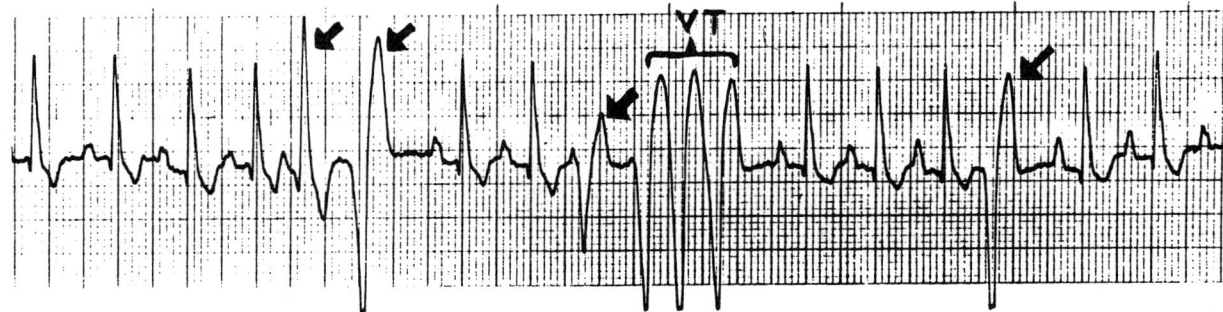

Figure 7–2. Lead II rhythm strip (25 mm/sec, 1 cm = 1 mV) recorded from a dog. An underlying sinus rhythm is present and is conducted with an intraventricular conduction defect. The sinus rhythm is interrupted by multiform single VPCs (arrows) and paroxysmal ventricular tachycardia (VT) showing "R-on-T" morphology (see text for details).

III. Diagnosis of intermittent abnormalities may require prolonged ECG monitoring.
  A. Multiple lengthy "rhythm strips"
  B. Portable 24-hour monitoring devices with "off-line" analysis (Holter monitors)
IV. The presence of any of the following abnormal physical findings in conjunction with an irregular heart rhythm suggests pathologic rhythm abnormalities.
  A. Pulse deficits
    1. Definition: lack of a palpable peripheral pulse to accompany a thoracic auscultable or palpable "beat"
    2. Usually accompany true premature contractions
  B. Irregular jugular pulses
    1. Cannon a waves occur when the atrium contracts against a closed AV valve and generated pressure is transmitted retrograde to the jugular veins.
    2. Intermittent occurrence of cannon a waves (i.e., not every beat) is consistent with the presence of dysrhythmia.
V. Some non-cardiac diseases or clinical conditions are associated with dysrhythmias, e.g., splenic or gastric torsion (Muir and Bonagura, 1984).

Differential Diagnosis

I. In dogs, cardiac dysrhythmias may be mistaken on physical examination for respiratory sinus arrhythmia (RSA).
II. Occasionally, extra heart sounds (S3 or S4 gallops) may be confused with premature contractions during auscultation.
III. In all cases, a properly recorded ECG establishes a diagnosis.

Treatment

I. Specific therapy with antidysrhythmic medications (Table 7–3)
  A. Decision to treat is based on many clinical considerations.
    1. Frequency of ectopy

      a) More than 20–30 ectopic beats/min are usually associated with hemodynamic compromise.
      b) Infrequent ectopic beats are not usually treated.
    2. Repetitiveness of the event
      a) Paroxysmal or sustained tachycardias >160 beats/min (dogs) or 240 beats/min (cats) are usually treated directly.
      b) Single ectopic complexes may not be treated if they are relatively infrequent (<20–30/min), especially if there are no clinical signs.

Table 7–3. **Options for Therapy of Dysrhythmias**

I. Improvement of animal's external and internal environment
  A. Supply oxygen.
    1. Oxygen-enriched environment
    2. Blood transfusion, if needed
  B. Rectify electrolyte and acid–base abnormalities via fluid and electrolyte therapy.
  C. Institute therapy of underlying disorder.
    1. Antibiotics for sepsis or bacterial endocarditis
    2. Definitive therapy of metabolic disorders
    3. Discontinuance or decreased dosage of suspected toxic medications
  D. Institute treatment for pain.
II. Direct medical antidysrhythmic therapy
  A. Vagolytics
  B. Vagomimetics, e.g., digoxin
  C. Sympathomimetics
  D. Antidysrhythmic medications*
    1. Class I: inhibit fast sodium currents
    2. Class II: β-antagonists (β-blockers)
    3. Class III: prolong action potential duration
    4. Class IV: calcium channel antagonists (calcium channel blockers)
III. Synchronous or asynchronous defibrillation
IV. Surgical intervention
  A. Pacemaker implantation
  B. Surgical or radiofrequency catheter ablation of abnormal conduction pathways

*Individual animals may require combinations of medications or combinations of medications and supportive therapy.

3. Relationship to clinical signs
    a) Dysrhythmias that are associated with clinical signs (e.g., syncope) are treated directly.
    b) Innocuous-appearing dysrhythmias that are documented in animals with typical clinical signs (e.g., weakness, exercise intolerance, syncope) may be treated on a trial basis or be investigated further with 24-hour monitoring.
4. Risk of sudden death
    a) Direct antidysrhythmic therapy is recommended for specific dysrhythmias accompanying certain breed-related cardiac diseases, especially those associated with sudden death (Harpster, 1983; Rush and Keene, 1989).
    b) Some animals have atypical reasons for their clinical signs; severe dysrhythmias should be documented prior to empiric therapy, even in typically affected breeds (Calvert et al., 1996).
5. Concurrent heart failure
    a) Uncontrolled dysrhythmias may decrease cardiac output and worsen signs of heart failure.
    b) Prolonged hypoxia due to congestive heart failure may worsen dysrhythmias.
6. Availability and efficacy of medication for specific dysrhythmias
    a) Few antidysrhythmic medications have been studied in dogs and cats with naturally occurring disease.
    b) Formulations may not be appropriate for small animals.
7. Side effects
    a) Side effects may be local (prodysrhythmia) or distant (systemic) in nature.
    b) Side effects may occur at serum drug concentrations known to be toxic or be unrelated to serum drug concentrations.
    c) Side effects may be idiosyncratic and unpredictable.
  B. Antidysrhythmic therapy is not warranted for all dysrhythmias.
II. Systemic therapy to rectify any underlying/concurrent abnormalities (see Tables 7–1 and 7–3)

Patient Monitoring

  I. Follow-up ECG monitoring
    A. Antidysrhythmic drug must be allowed to reach effective plasma concentration.
    B. Dysrhythmia may be abolished, decreased in frequency or repetitiveness, or converted to another abnormal rhythm.
 II. Clinical progress of animal
III. Therapeutic drug monitoring
    A. Indications
      1. To provide evidence of drug toxicity
      2. To ensure adequate dosing/compliance
    B. Drug pharmacokinetics and sampling time

1. Peak concentrations ensure effective dosage.
2. Trough concentrations may reflect toxicity.

SPECIFIC DYSRHYTHMIAS

Respiratory Sinus Arrhythmia

Definition

  I. Respiratory sinus arrhythmia (RSA) is an irregular rhythm that originates in the sinoatrial (SA) node.
 II. The rate of SA nodal discharge increases and decreases with variations in vagal tone that accompany respiration.
III. Respiratory sinus arrhythmia is considered to be a normal variation in dogs, but is not seen in normal cats.

Causes

  I. Respiratory sinus arrhythmia may be normal (dogs) or associated with accentuated vagal activity (dogs and cats).
 II. Accentuated vagal tone is usually caused by some respiratory disease or abnormality, gastrointestinal disease, or drug effects (e.g., digoxin).

Clinical Signs

  I. Dogs: usually normal or may show signs of underlying respiratory disease
 II. Cats: usually associated with signs of respiratory disease

Diagnosis

  I. Physical examination
    A. Slow to normal heart rate
    B. Heart rhythm irregular, varies with respiratory cycle
    C. Normal pulse strength with *no* pulse deficits
 II. ECG (Fig. 7–3)
    A. PQRST complexes are normal in appearance.
    B. P wave may vary in appearance cyclically (wandering pacemaker).
    C. Heart rate increases with inspiration and decreases with expiration in a repeating pattern.

Differential Diagnosis

  I. Atrial fibrillation
    A. P waves are present with RSA.
    B. Heart rate is within normal range with RSA.
 II. Atrial premature depolarizations
    A. P waves are uniform or undergo gradual changes in appearance with RSA.
    B. Depolarizations are predictable in timing with RSA (depolarization rate speeds and slows gradually).

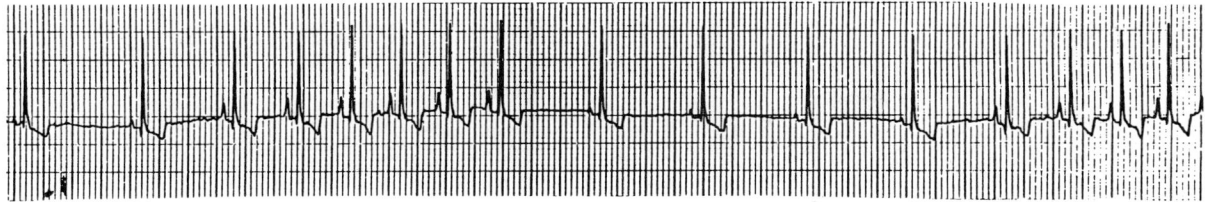

Figure 7–3. Lead AVF rhythm strip (25 mm/sec, 1 cm = 1 mV) recorded from a dog with respiratory sinus arrhythmia and a wandering pacemaker. Notice the gradual change in P wave morphology associated with changes in heart rate.

Treatment

I. No direct therapy required.
II. Treat underlying disease, if present.

BRADYDYSRHYTHMIAS

Sinus Bradycardia

Definition

I. Sinus bradycardia is a sinus rhythm in which the rate of depolarization is below normal.
II. Sinus arrest is temporary cessation of SA nodal discharge.
III. In both cases, the origin of the rhythm is the SA node.

Causes

I. Increased vagal tone
  A. Resting, sleeping, or athletic animals
  B. Secondary to gastrointestinal or respiratory disease
  C. Secondary to ocular or carotid manipulation
II. Systemic abnormalities
  A. Environmental: hypothermia
  B. Metabolic
    1. Hyperkalemia
    2. Hypothyroidism
    3. End-stage renal or hepatic failure (impending cardiac arrest)
  C. Neurologic lesions
    1. Brain stem lesions
    2. Elevated intracranial pressure
  D. Drugs or drug toxicity
    1. Antidysrhythmic drugs
    2. Anesthetics, analgesics, and tranquilizers

Pathophysiology

I. Low heart rates limit cardiac output if stroke volume is unchanged.
II. If bradycardia is chronic, it may result in cardiac changes consistent with volume overload.

Clinical Signs

I. Often no clinical signs, other than signs of underlying disease

II. Signs of decreased cardiac output
  A. Lethargy, weakness
  B. Exercise intolerance
  C. Syncope

Diagnosis

I. Physical examination
  A. May be normal, other than slow heart rate
  B. May show concurrent signs of heart disease or heart failure
    1. Heart murmur
    2. Pulmonary crackles, dyspnea (if left-sided heart failure)
    3. Distended jugular veins, ascites, pleural effusion (if right-sided heart failure)
    4. Pale mucous membranes with prolonged capillary refill time
  C. Pulses strong if no concurrent systolic dysfunction
II. ECG (Fig. 7–4)
  A. Sinus rhythm: upright P waves in lead II, variable in morphology if "wandering pacemaker" is present
  B. Sinus depolarization rate below normal range
  C. May be irregular with periods of sinus arrest (temporary cessation of SA nodal discharge) and escape beats originating from any non-sinus physiologic pacemaker
  D. Normal ECG complexes unless concurrent conduction disease present

Treatment

I. Rectify causal situation or treat underlying disease.
II. Vagolytic drugs may be effective acutely or for short periods of time (Table 7–4).
  A. Injectable atropine, glycopyrrolate: acutely increase SA discharge rate
  B. Oral propantheline bromide: tolerance may develop with chronic use
III. β-Agonists can be used for heart rate support in emergency situations.
  A. Dobutamine IV
  B. Isoproterenol IV
IV. Pacemaker implantation is necessary for permanent resolution of symptomatic bradycardia.
  A. Permanent pacemaker implantation is recommended when the animal is symptomatic and the underlying cause cannot be found and rectified.

Table 7-4. **Summary of Antidysrhythmic Medications**

Drug	Mode of Action	Indications	Contraindications	Dose	Side Effects	Comments
Atenolol [Class II]	Selective (β-1) β-receptor antagonism	D: supraventricular tachycardias, some ventricular tachycardias; C: supraventricular tachycardias, ventricular tachycardias, thyrotoxicosis	Sinus bradycardia, AV block, hypotension, CHF, concurrent use of calcium channel blockers	D: 6.25-12.5 mg/dog PO BID; C: 6.25-12.5 mg/cat PO SID-BID	Bradycardia, AV block, worsening of CHF	May be used with digitalis to slow ventricular response rate in AF
Atropine sulfate	Parasympatholytic	Sinus bradycardia, first or second degree AV block, bradycardias related to anesthesia, atropine response test	Tachydysrhythmias, Gastrointestinal disease (relative)	D, C: 0.01-0.04 mg/kg SQ, IM, IV*	Gastrointestinal stasis, sinus tachycardia, dry mouth	Bradycardias related to anesthesia may respond to decreases in anesthetic depth
Digoxin	Increased vagal tone, Na^+,K^+-ATPase pump inhibitor	Supraventricular tachycardias, especially if heart failure is present	Digitalis toxicity, Ventricular dysrhythmias; Relative: Hypokalemia, Concurrent quinidine, Renal dysfunction	D: 0.005-0.01 mg/kg PO BID; C: 2-3 kg cat: 0.0321 mg PO QOD; 4-5 kg cat: 0.0312 mg PO SID; >6 kg cat: 0.0312 mg PO BID	Bradycardia, AV block, junctional and ventricular tachycardias, nausea, vomiting, diarrhea	Presence of relative contraindications may require reductions in digoxin dosage
Digoxin immune Fab (ovine)	Binds digoxin in blood stream	Acute digoxin toxicity		D: for acute ingestion: 40 mg per mg ingested		May need to repeat dose
Diltiazem [Class IV]	Calcium channel antagonism	Supraventricular tachycardias	Sinus bradycardia, AV block, concurrent β-blockade	D: 0.5-1.5 mg/kg PO TID; C: 1.75-2.4 mg/kg PO BID-TID	Sinus bradycardia, AV block, worsening of CHF	May be used with digitalis to slow ventricular response rate in AF
Esmolol [Class II]	Selective (β-1) β-receptor antagonism	Acute therapy of supraventricular tachycardias, occasionally ventricular tachycardias	Sinus bradycardia, AV block, hypotension, CHF, concurrent use of calcium channel blockers	D, C: 250-500 µg/kg slow IV bolus; CRI: 50-200 µg/kg/min	Hypotension, bradycardia, AV block	Ultra-short acting (effects last about 20 minutes)
Glycopyrrolate	Anticholinergic	Acute therapy of sinus bradycardia, first or second degree AV block, bradycardias related to anesthesia	Tachydysrhythmias, Gastrointestinal disease (relative)	D, C: 0.005-0.01 mg/kg IM, IV or 0.01-0.02 mg/kg SQ	Gastrointestinal stasis, sinus tachycardia, dry mouth	Bradycardias related to anesthesia may respond to decreases in anesthetic depth
Isoproterenol	β-Receptor antagonism	Emergency therapy of bradycardias	Tachydysrhythmias	D: 0.2-0.5 mg in 250 ml dextrose in water (D5W), 0.01 µg/kg/minute IV, increase to effect	Hypotension, tachydysrhythmias	
Lidocaine [Class IB]	Membrane stabilization	Emergency therapy of ventricular tachydysrhythmias	Presence of escape rhythms; Relative: concurrent use of cimetidine or β-blockade	D: 2-4 mg/kg IV (to a maximum of 8 mg/kg over a 10-minute period); CRI: 25-75 µg/kg/min; C: 0.25-0.75 mg/kg slow IV bolus	Vomiting, tremors, nystagmus, seizures	Side effects common in cats; Presence of relative contraindications may require reduction in dosage

Drug [Class]	Mechanism	Indication	Contraindication	Dosage	Adverse Effects	Comments
Mexiletine [Class IB]	Membrane stabilization	D: chronic therapy of ventricular arrhythmias	Presence of escape rhythms	D: 5–8 mg/kg PO BID–TID	Vomiting, neurotoxicity	May be combined with class I or II drugs to treat VT
Procainamide [Class IA]	Prolongation of effective refractory period	D: ventricular tachycardias C: refractory ventricular tachycardias	Sick sinus syndrome, presence of escape rhythms	D: 10–20 mg/kg IM, PO QID; 8–20 mg/kg IV bolus CRI: 25–50 μg/kg/min C: 3–8 mg/kg PO TID–QID; 1–2 mg/kg IV bolus† CRI: 10–20 μg/kg/min* IV	Hypotension (after rapid IV administration), gastrointestinal signs, prodysrhythmia	
Propantheline	Anticholinergic	Chronic therapy of bradydysrhythmias	Gastrointestinal disease (relative)	0.25–0.5 mg/kg PO BID–TID		In animals that respond initially, condition may become refractory
Propranolol [Class II]	Nonselective (β-1 and β-2) β-receptor antagonism	D: supraventricular, some ventricular tachycardias C: supraventricular, ventricular tachycardias, thyrotoxicosis	Sinus bradycardia, AV block, hypotension, CHF, concurrent use of calcium channel blockers	D, C: 0.02–0.06 mg/kg IV over 5–10 minutes D: 0.2–1.0 mg/kg PO TID C: 2.5–5.0 mg PO BID–TID	Hypotension, bradycardia, AV block, worsening of CHF, bronchospasm	May be used with digitalis to slow ventricular response rate in AF, may be combined with class I agents to treat VT
Quinidine gluconate [Class IA]	Prolongation of effective refractory period, changes in autonomic tone	D: supraventricular, ventricular tachycardias, termination of acute AF C: refractory ventricular dysrhythmias	Sick sinus syndrome, bradycardia, presence of escape rhythms Relative: concurrent digoxin therapy	D: 6–20 mg/kg IM QID of base (324 mg = 202 mg quinidine) 6–20 mg/kg PO TID–QID of base	Hypotension, ventricular dysrhythmias, worsening of CHF, AV block, gastrointestinal signs, many others	Differing formulations have differing "base-equivalent" levels of quinidine, may need to decrease dose of digoxin if used with quinidine to avoid digoxin toxicity
Tocainide [Class IB]	Membrane stabilization	D: chronic therapy of ventricular dysrhythmias		D: 10–20 mg/kg PO TID	Anorexia, vomiting, neurotoxicity	
Verapamil [Class IV]	Calcium channel antagonism	Acute therapy of supraventricular tachycardias	Sinus bradycardia, AV block, CHF, profound hypotension	D, C: 0.05 mg/kg IV over 5 minutes, administered every 10–30 minutes to effect *Total dose not to exceed 0.2 mg/kg*	Bradycardia, AV block, hypotension, worsening of CHF	Inject slowly to avoid acute hypotension

Roman numerals in brackets indicate anti-arrhythmic classification. Doses are approximate and may need to be modified for individual animals according to clinical circumstances.
D = dog; C = cat; AF = atrial fibrillation; CHF = congestive heart failure; CRI: = continuous rate infusion; VT = ventricular tachycardia.
*0.04 mg/kg IM for atropine response test.
†Harpster, 1992.

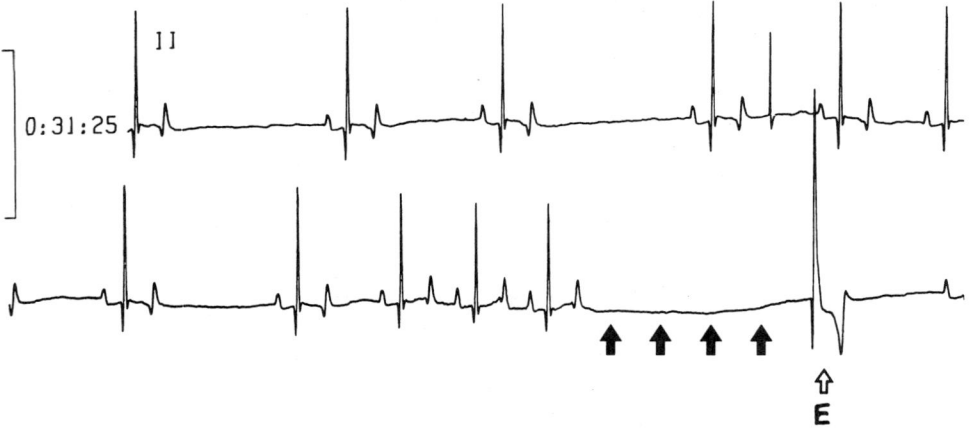

Figure 7–4. Lead II rhythm strip (25 mm/sec, 1 cm = 1 mV) recorded from a dog with sinus bradycardia (heart rate = 60 beats/min). There is a period of sinus arrest (arrows) with an escape beat of ventricular morphology (E).

B. A temporary pacemaker may be used to check clinical response prior to permanent implantation.

Patient Monitoring

I. Continuous ECG or frequent rhythm strips are needed to monitor response to emergency therapy.

II. Repeat ECG after several days of propantheline therapy to ensure response, then monitor clinical response and repeat rhythm strips to monitor for development of drug tolerance.

III. Most animals show noticeable improvement in clinical status immediately after successful pacemaker implantation.

IV. Permanent pacemakers are monitored for position and performance.
   A. Thoracic radiographs are checked immediately after implantation to ensure proper lead and pulse generator placement, and yearly thereafter.
   B. ECG recordings during and after pacemaker implantation ensure adequate "capture" of the heart rhythm.
   C. ECG rhythm strips are monitored frequently initially, then every 6 months to 1 year.

V. Complications may arise.
   A. Early pacemaker malfunction usually is a result of inadequate lead placement or improper pacemaker programming.
      1. Lead placement problems are diagnosed via analysis of radiographs and the ECG.
      2. Improper pacemaker programming is diagnosed and rectified using ECG analysis and commercial pacemaker interrogation units.
   B. Pacemakers have variable battery lifespans depending on age of the battery and previous use at the time of implantation.
      1. New batteries may last up to 5–7 years.
      2. Battery failure is usually signalled by change in pacemaker output to an asynchronous discharge at a preset, low rate.
      3. Pacemaker generators can be replaced without dislodging the lead wire from the heart.
   C. Surgical site complications may occur at the site of the implant.

1. Seromas may be treated with hot packing and external bandages. Avoid surgical drainage to prevent contamination of the implant site.
2. Surgical site infection is treated with appropriate antibiotics (based on culture and sensitivity results) for prolonged periods (3–6 months).
3. In rare instances, replacement of the pacemaker may be required to resolve wound infection.
   D. Ectopic depolarizations may interrupt the paced rhythm.
      1. Postoperative ventricular dysrhythmias may be self-limiting, and no therapy is required.
      2. Persistent or severe ventricular dysrhythmias may require permanent antidysrhythmic therapy.
VI. Prognosis is as follows.
   A. Most pacemakers function well for the life of the battery.
   B. Chronic volume load-related ventricular dilation may result in myocardial failure after prolonged ventricular pacing (usually years).

Sick Sinus Syndrome (Bradycardia/Tachycardia)

Definition

I. The term "sick sinus syndrome" describes a clinical syndrome involving irregular discharge of the SA node.

II. In some animals, sinus bradydysrhythmias are accompanied by periods of sinus node arrest and development of escape rhythms, whereas other animals develop alternating periods of sinus bradydysrhythmias and atrial tachydysrhythmias.

III. Sick sinus syndrome occurs primarily in small-breed dogs, particularly miniature schnauzers, but may be seen in any breed.

IV. Sick sinus syndrome appears to be rare in cats.

Causes

I. Sick sinus syndrome has been associated with fibrous replacement or degeneration of the SA nodal tissue.

II. The initiating cause of this degeneration is unknown but may be genetic, ischemic, or inflammatory.

Clinical Signs

I. Periods of sinus arrest without development of an escape rhythm for >3–5 seconds lead to neurologic signs.
  A. Animal may suddenly appear "dizzy," i.e., have a dazed facial expression or stagger.
  B. Sinus arrest or failure of escape rhythm for longer periods may lead to syncope.
II. Recovery from episodes is quick and complete (within minutes).
III. Sinus arrest seldom leads to sudden death, but frequency of events may severely affect quality of life.

Diagnosis

I. Physical examination
  A. Usually normal, other than markedly irregular heart rate
  B. Not associated with heart failure unless other cardiac disease is present
  C. Variable pulse quality
    1. Pulses following long pauses are strong.
    2. Pulses during tachydysrhythmias may be weak with pulse deficits.
II. ECG
  A. Sinus bradycardia with long pauses in which P waves are absent
  B. May or may not develop appropriate escape rhythm
  C. Periods of bradycardia interrupted by paroxysms of supraventricular tachycardia (Fig. 7–5)
  D. Sinus P waves and QRS complexes relatively normal during bradycardic periods unless concurrent conduction disease present

Treatment

I. Response to vagolytic medications is unpredictable and usually not sustained.

II. Permanent pacemaker implantation is the definitive therapy.
III. Supraventricular antidysrhythmic therapy may be needed to control concurrent tachydysrhythmias.
  A. Consistent pacing may allow resolution of tachydysrhythmia without more specific therapy.
  B. Antidysrhythmic therapy for supraventricular dysrhythmias should *not* be initiated until successful pacemaker implantation is completed.

Patient Monitoring

I. Monitoring of pacemaker implantation is similar to that recommended for sinus bradycardia.
II. Prognosis for control of clinical signs is good; most animals respond well to pacing with or without supraventricular antidysrhythmic medication.

Atrial Standstill (Atrial Asystole)

Definition

I. Atrial standstill is defined as the lack of electrocardiographic evidence of atrial depolarization.
II. Failure of atrial transmission of the SA nodal discharge leads to development of an escape rhythm, which may be conducted normally or associated with AV nodal or ventricular conduction disturbances (bundle branch blocks).

Causes

I. Physiologic: hyperkalemia secondary to urinary obstruction or hypoadrenocorticism
II. Pathologic
  A. Severe atrial muscle pathology associated with chronic heart disease
  B. Replacement of atrial tissue
    1. Neoplasia
    2. Neuromuscular disease associated with cardiomyopathy (e.g., fascioscapulohumeral or scapulohumeral muscular dystrophy)

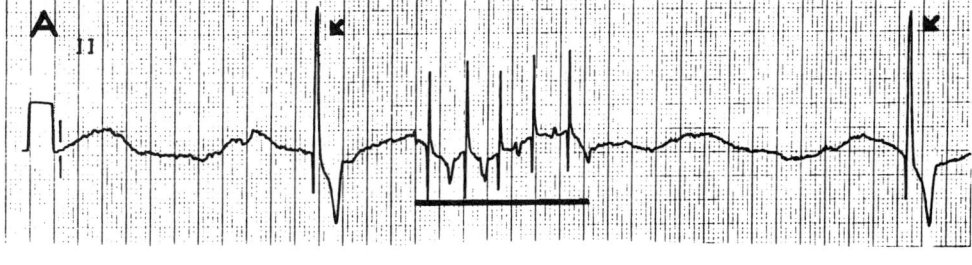
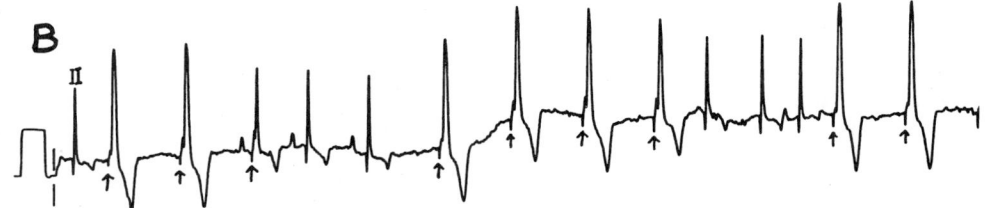

Figure 7–5. A. Lead II rhythm strip (25 mm/sec, 1 cm = 1 mV) recorded from a dog with sick sinus syndrome. Arrows mark ventricular escape beats following periods of sinus arrest. A paroxysm of supraventricular tachycardia (black bar) is present. B. Lead II rhythm strip recorded from the same dog after pacemaker implantation. Arrows indicate pacing spikes.

a) Springer spaniels (Miller et al., 1992)
b) Sporadic occurrence in other breeds (Tilley and Liu, 1983)
III. Toxic: severe digitalis glycoside toxicity

Clinical Signs

I. Hyperkalemia
  A. Signs typical of associated condition (e.g., urinary obstruction)
  B. Weakness, collapse
  C. Sudden death due to ventricular asystole
II. Atrial muscle pathology or replacement
  A. Weakness of affected peripheral muscles
  B. Weakness, collapse
  C. Clinical signs of left- or right-sided congestive heart failure (CHF)

Diagnosis

I. Physical examination
  A. Signs consistent with underlying disease
  B. Slow, irregular heart rate
  C. Weak pulses, poor perfusion
  D. Signs of CHF
    1. Distended jugular veins, ascites, pleural effusion (right-sided CHF)
    2. Dyspnea, cough, pulmonary crackles (left-sided CHF)
  E. Signs of neuromuscular disease, e.g., scapulohumeral atrophy
II. ECG
  A. Bradydysrhythmia with no P waves in any lead
  B. QRS morphology normal if ventricular conduction normal
  C. QRS morphology wide and bizarre if ventricular conduction abnormality present
  D. Other changes associated with hyperkalemia (inconsistent)
    1. Tall, tented T waves
    2. First degree AV block
    3. Wide and distorted QRS morphology
    4. "Sine wave" appearance of QRS complexes possible at high plasma potassium concentrations
III. Elevated serum digoxin concentrations (canine therapeutic range: 0.8–2 ng/dl)

Treatment

I. Emergency therapy for hyperkalemia
  A. 0.9% saline infusion
  B. Sodium bicarbonate administration: 1–2 mEq/kg IV slowly
  C. Calcium gluconate: 10% solution, 0.5–1 ml/kg IV slowly
  D. Therapy for underlying cause of hyperkalemia
II. Atrial pathology
  A. Specific therapy of CHF, if present
  B. Permanent pacemaker implantation
III. Digoxin toxicity

A. Acute toxicity: digoxin immune Fab (ovine) therapy (Senior et al., 1991)
  1. Fab fragment of ovine anti-digoxin antibodies acutely binds digoxin.
  2. Dose is based on amount of digoxin ingested (40 mg IV per mg of digoxin ingested).
B. Chronic toxicity
  1. Discontinue digoxin administration.
  2. Provide supportive care.

Patient Monitoring

I. Follow-up
  A. Hyperkalemia-related atrial standstill
    1. ECG changes respond quickly to acute therapy for hyperkalemia.
    2. Resolution of underlying disease prevents recurrence.
  B. Atrial pathology–related atrial standstill
    1. Monitoring of pacemaker implantation is similar to that recommended for sinus bradycardia.
    2. CHF signs are controlled with typical medications (diuretics, vasodilators).
II. Prognosis
  A. Prognosis is good for hyperkalemia-related atrial standstill if underlying disease is adequately controlled.
  B. Progressive nature of most atrial muscular dystrophies leads to a guarded prognosis for affected dogs.
  C. Dogs with non-progressive atrial muscle replacement who respond to permanent pacemaker implantation may survive months to years with adequate CHF control.

Atrioventricular Blocks

Definition

I. Atrioventricular block is a temporary or permanent failure of conduction between the atria and the ventricles.
II. The condition usually involves the atrioventricular (AV) node, but it may be impossible to distinguish the exact location of the abnormality.
III. Atrioventricular block is subdivided into three types, based on the severity of the block.
  A. First degree AV block: All atrial depolarizations are conducted to the ventricles, but AV conduction time is prolonged.
  B. Second degree AV block: Occasionally or frequently, atrial depolarizations are not conducted to the ventricles.
    1. Named according to the ratio of atrial to ventricular depolarizations, e.g., 3:2 AV block
    2. Higher ratios deemed "high grade" second degree block
    3. May occur concurrently with first degree AV block
  C. Third degree AV block: There is complete disruption of AV conduction.

Causes

I. Congenital: rare, e.g., large ventricular septal defect obliterates nodal tissue
II. Physiologic: first and second degree block
   A. Enhanced vagal tone
   B. Electrolyte disturbances, e.g., hyperkalemia
III. Atrioventricular nodal pathology
   A. Infection, usually associated with aortic valve vegetative endocarditis lesions
   B. Fibrosis
   C. Neoplastic
   D. Breed-related abnormalities in pugs, Doberman pinschers, cocker spaniels
IV. Toxic: digitalis glycosides, β-blockers, calcium channel blockers

Pathophysiology

I. Atrioventricular block from pathologic changes in the AV node may be progressive, i.e., may advance from mild, incomplete, clinically silent first degree AV block through second degree AV block to complete and irreversible third degree AV block.
II. When complete (third degree) AV block occurs, failure to transmit atrial depolarizations to the ventricle necessitates development of a ventricular escape rhythm at heart rates of 25–40 beats/min (dogs) and 80–100 beats/min (cats).
III. Prolonged bradycardia and abnormal depolarization and contraction sequences lead to decreased cardiac output and volume overload.

Clinical Signs

I. First degree AV block
   A. Usually clinically silent
   B. Signs of underlying condition, e.g., respiratory disease
II. Second degree AV block
   A. May be clinically silent, especially in cats
   B. May be associated with exercise intolerance, weakness, or syncope
III. Third degree AV block
   A. May be clinically silent, especially in cats
   B. Decrease in exercise capacity (possibly mistaken by owner for "normal aging change" in older animals)
   C. Exercise intolerance, weakness, syncope
   D. Signs of right-sided heart failure in some animals

Diagnosis

I. Physical examination
   A. First degree AV block
      1. Usually normal
      2. May be associated with sinus bradycardia or second degree AV block
   B. Second degree AV block
      1. Normal heart rate or bradycardia
      2. Irregular rhythm with audible pauses, no pulse deficits

3. Irregular jugular pulses (cannon a waves)
      4. Not associated with cardiac murmurs or heart failure unless other cardiac abnormalities present
   C. Third degree AV block
      1. Regular or irregular bradycardia on auscultation
      2. Irregular jugular pulses (cannon a waves) in some animals
      3. May be associated with soft systolic AV valve murmurs caused by dilation and asynchronous AV contraction.
II. ECG (Fig. 7–6)
   A. First degree AV block
      1. Prolonged P-Q interval, may vary slightly from beat to beat (see Table 7–2)
      2. Normal QRS complexes unless intraventricular conduction disease present
      3. May be associated with sinus bradycardia
   B. Second degree AV block
      1. Mobitz type I
         a) Gradual lengthening of P-Q interval until P waves occur without QRS complexes
         b) One or more P waves unconducted to ventricles
         c) Conduction resumes without development of escape rhythm
         d) May be physiologic, associated with enhanced vagal tone
      2. Mobitz type II
         a) Constant P-Q interval with occasional blocked P waves
         b) Usually associated with pathology of the AV node
   C. Third degree AV block
      1. P waves and QRS complexes have no repeatable relationship to each other.
      2. Escape rhythm is usually ventricular in origin.
         a) Wide and bizarre complexes
         b) Escape rate usually 25–40 beats/min (dog), 80–100 beats/min (cat)

Treatment

I. Investigating vagal contributions to AV block
   A. First and second degree AV block may be due to enhanced vagal tone.
   B. Third degree AV block is never due only to enhanced vagal tone.
   C. Atropine response test is helpful.
      1. Atropine is administered to animals with first or second degree AV block to rule out enhanced vagal tone as a cause for the abnormality.
      2. If normal response to atropine is documented, therapy is directed at the cause of the enhanced vagal tone, and AV block usually resolves without direct therapy.
      3. Record baseline lead II ECG rhythm strip.
      4. Administer 0.04 mg/kg atropine IM (IV administration may lead to acute and temporary worsening of AV block).

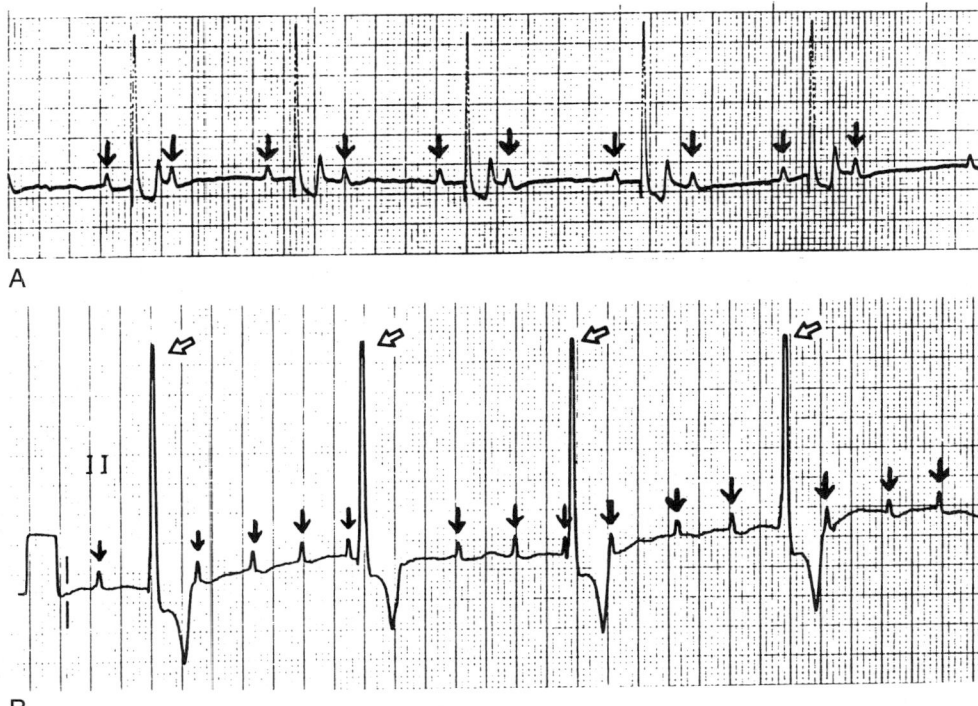

Figure 7–6. A. Lead II rhythm strip (25 mm/sec, 1 cm = 1 mV) recorded from a dog with first and 2:1 second degree heart block. P waves are marked by arrows. B. Lead II rhythm strip (25 mm/sec, 1 cm = 1 mV) recorded from a dog with third degree heart block. P waves (solid arrows) are not related to QRS complexes (open arrows).

5. Repeat lead II rhythm strip 30 minutes after atropine administration.
6. A ≥50% increase in heart rate with normal sinus rhythm and normal conduction pattern is considered a positive (normal) response.

II. No or submaximal response to atropine
  A. First degree AV block
    1. No direct therapy is indicated.
    2. Rule out underlying disease, e.g., bacterial endocarditis, neoplasia.
    3. Monitor for progression of block or development of clinical signs.
  B. Second degree AV block
    1. Rule out underlying disease.
    2. If ventricular rate is within normal range and no clinical signs are present, monitor for progression.
    3. If bradycardia or clinical signs are present, permanent pacemaker implantation is recommended.
  C. Third degree AV block
    1. Rule out underlying intracardiac disease.
    2. In dogs, permanent pacemaker implantation is recommended.
    3. In cats, therapy varies.
      a) Definitive therapy is permanent pacemaker implantation.
      b) Many cats do well without a pacemaker if escape rate is at least 100 beats/min but should be monitored for development of clinical signs.

Patient Monitoring

I. Therapy and follow-up for any underlying disease are based on disease severity.
II. Periodic ECGs are used to monitor progression of non–atropine-responsive heart block that was not treated with pacemaker implantation.
III. Monitoring of implanted pacemaker is similar to that recommended for sinus bradycardia.

TACHYDYSRHYTHMIAS

Sinus Tachycardia

Definition

I. Sinus tachycardia is a rhythm originating in the SA node in which depolarization occurs at a rate higher than the normal sinus range for a given animal.
II. Sinus tachycardias are usually conducted normally and are secondary dysrhythmias, reflecting the cardiac response to systemic disturbances relating to body temperature, blood pressure, exercise, anxiety, or other abnormalities.

Causes

I. Rarely a primary rhythm disorder
II. Occurs secondary to systemic changes
  A. Temperature increase (hyperthermia)
  B. Decreased blood pressure

1. Cardiac disease or cardiac failure
2. Dehydration, hypovolemia
3. Shock
  C. Increased metabolic demands
1. Pyrexia
2. Metabolic disease, e.g., thyrotoxicosis
3. Anemia
  D. Psychologic factors, e.g., pain, fear
  E. Exercise

Clinical Signs

   I. Usually no obvious outward signs
  II. May detect signs of underlying disease
 III. If associated with CHF, signs of heart disease or heart failure
    A. Heart murmur
    B. Pulmonary crackles, dyspnea (if left-sided heart failure)
    C. Distended jugular veins, ascites, pleural effusion (if right-sided heart failure)
    D. Pale mucous membranes with prolonged capillary refill time, poor pulse strength

Diagnosis

   I. Physical examination
    A. Findings typical of underlying condition
    B. Rapid, regular heart rate with *no* pulse deficits
  II. ECG
    A. Heart rate elevated above normal range
1. Sinus tachycardia range (dog): 140–260 beats/min
2. Sinus tachycardia range (cat): 200–300 beats/min
    B. Upright (positive) P waves in lead II
    C. Normal conduction sequence

Differential Diagnosis

   I. Sinus tachycardia may be confused with atrial tachycardia (Table 7–5).
  II. Atrial tachycardias are usually treated with antidys-rhythmic drugs or physiologic manipulations (see later).

Treatment and Monitoring

   I. Diagnose and treat underlying cause of tachycardia.
  II. No direct antidysrhythmia therapy is recommended for sinus tachycardia.
 III. If presumed sinus tachycardia is not responsive to therapy of underlying causes, the ECG should be reevaluated to confirm correct diagnosis.
    A. ECG consultation, i.e., second opinion
    B. Vagal maneuver (see Table 7–5)
    C. Response to acute administration of supraventricular antidysrhythmic drugs
  IV. Persistent sinus tachycardia in an animal with heart disease but no evidence of CHF may be treated with digoxin, β-blockers, or calcium channel blockers.

Atrial Premature Depolarizations

Definition and Causes

   I. Atrial premature depolarizations (APDs) are supraventricular depolarizations that originate somewhere other than the SA node.
  II. The "native" discharge rate of these foci is usually higher than the normal rate of SA nodal discharge, but sinus tachycardia may suppress some ectopic atrial depolarizations.
 III. Although APDs may occur secondary to many systemic abnormalities (see Table 7–1), they are often associated with atrial muscle stretch (from congenital or acquired cardiac disease) or atrial muscle pathology (e.g., fibrosis secondary to chronic heart disease, neoplastic infiltration).

Pathophysiology

   I. Single APDs are associated with an instantaneous decrease in stroke volume, because the prematurity of the ectopically stimulated contraction does not allow for adequate ventricular filling.
  II. A solitary APD is not hemodynamically significant,

*Table 7–5. **Differentiation of Sinus Tachycardia from Atrial Tachycardia***

	Sinus Tachycardia	Atrial Tachycardia
Depolarization rate*	• ≤260 beats/min (dog) • ≤300 beats/min (cat)	• >260 beats/min (dog) • >300 beats/min (cat)
Conduction sequence	• AV conduction usually 1:1	• May be conducted with second degree AV block
P wave morphology	• Positive in lead II	• May be positive or negative in lead II • Often "buried" in previous T wave
Response to vagal maneuver	• Gradual slowing of rate	• Abrupt change in rate and/or rhythm
Response to IV β-blocker or calcium channel blocker	• Induction of AV block or gradual slowing of sinus rate	• Acute termination of rhythm with or without AV block, followed by resumption of normal sinus rhythm

IV = intravenous.
*Rates given are *approximate* ranges; individual animals may vary.

but frequent or repetitive occurrence of APD (atrial tachycardia) leads to physiologically significant decreases in cardiac output and blood pressure.

Clinical Signs

  I. Single APD: clinical signs rare
 II. May see signs of associated cardiac abnormalities or heart failure
III. Frequent or repetitive APD, especially in association with structural heart disease
   A. Refractory or recurrent signs of heart failure
   B. Lethargy, weakness, exercise intolerance
   C. If atrial tachycardia: episodic weakness, syncope

Diagnosis

  I. Physical examination
   A. Auscultation
     1. May hear prematurely occurring contraction of decreased intensity followed by a short pause ("compensatory pause")
     2. May hear pause only ("dropped beat")
   B. Peripheral pulse
     1. Premature contraction is accompanied by a pulse deficit.
     2. Pulse following the pause is increased in strength.
   C. Findings typical of associated heart disease or heart failure
 II. ECG
   A. "Early" depolarization: occurs prior to the next expected sinus depolarization
   B. Abnormal P wave morphology (usually differs from sinus P wave)
   C. Conduction sequence
     1. Conduction sequence is normal unless concurrent conduction disease is present, e.g., bundle branch block.
     2. Ectopic P wave may be "blocked" if very premature (Fig. 7–7).

Treatment

  I. Rectify underlying disease and/or heart failure, if possible.
 II. Therapy is based on frequency of occurrence of APD, clinical signs, and presence of documentable cardiac disease.
   A. "Lone" atrial ectopy: single APDs without documentable cardiac disease

     1. Usually no clinical signs
     2. If ≥20–30 per minute or occurring in pairs
       a) β-blockers (see Table 7–4)
       b) Calcium channel blockers
   B. If associated with structural heart disease/heart failure
     1. Digoxin (see Table 7–4)
     2. If uncontrolled with therapeutic serum digoxin concentrations
       a) Add β-blockers (contraindicated if CHF is present).
       b) Add calcium channel blockers.
       c) Concurrent use of β-blockers and calcium channel blockers is *not* recommended.

Patient Monitoring

  I. Repeat ECG monitoring after stable serum drug concentrations are established.
   A. Digoxin: stable drug concentrations in 10–14 days (dog)
   B. β-Blockers and calcium channel blockers: should see improvement in 1–2 days
 II. Monitor for drug complications and side effects (see Table 7–4).

Atrial Tachycardia/Atrial Flutter

Definition

  I. Atrial tachycardia is the rapid ectopic depolarization of a non-sinus atrial pacemaker.
 II. The rapid supraventricular depolarization is often conducted 1:1 to the ventricle, resulting in extremely rapid ventricular depolarization (>250 beats/min in dogs, Fig. 7–8).
III. Atrial flutter is a rapid depolarization of the atria that results in a "sawtooth" pattern of P waves, characterized by P waves occurring so rapidly that no isoelectric baseline is evident between P waves.
 IV. Both atrial tachycardia and atrial flutter may be conducted with second degree AV block, resulting in an irregular ventricular response.

Causes

  I. The causes are the same as those for atrial premature depolarizations.
 II. Atrial and re-entry tachydysrhythmias may occur in animals with no other discernible cardiac or systemic abnormalities.

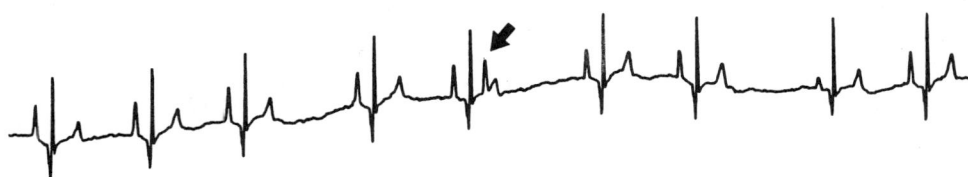

Figure 7–7. Lead II rhythm strip (25 mm/sec, 1 cm = 1 mV) recorded from a dog. The arrow identifies a premature atrial depolarization that is not conducted to the ventricle as a result of physiologic second degree heart block (see text).

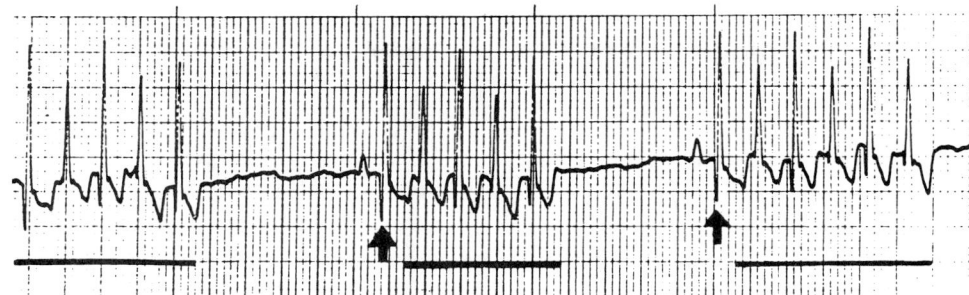

Figure 7–8. Lead II rhythm strip (25 mm/sec, 1 cm = 1 mV) recorded from a dog with paroxysmal supraventricular tachycardia. Brief pauses in the sinus rhythm are terminated by single beats of sinus origin (arrows), followed by short bursts of tachycardia. The tachycardia is characterized by tall and narrow QRS complexes, consistent with a supraventricular origin. Ectopic P waves are not repeatably observed in this strip.

III. Abnormal re-entrant pathways in the atrium or AV junction may lead to re-entry supraventricular tachy-dysrhythmias indistinguishable from atrial tachycardia.

Pathophysiology

I. Extremely rapid ventricular contractions result in marked shortening of diastole.
  A. Decreased stroke volume
   1. Decreased ventricular filling time
   2. Loss of synchronized atrial contraction contribution during physiologic second degree AV block
  B. Promotion of myocardial ischemia
   1. Increased myocardial oxygen consumption due to increased rate of contraction
   2. Inadequate myocardial perfusion due to shortened diastole
II. Decreased cardiac output leads to clinical signs.
III. Myocardial ischemia leads to worsening of any underlying cardiac pathology.

Clinical Signs

I. General signs
  A. Lethargy, inappetence, general malaise
  B. Occasionally no clinical signs
II. Cardiovascular signs
  A. Exercise intolerance, episodic weakness, syncope
  B. Sudden occurrence or acute decompensation of previously stable CHF

Diagnosis

I. Physical examination
  A. Rapid, irregular cardiac rhythm
  B. Weak, variable pulses with pulse deficits
  C. Signs of underlying cardiac disease or CHF
II. ECG
  A. Rate of atrial depolarization is extremely rapid.
   1. Atrial tachycardia
    a) P waves usually differ from sinus P waves in polarity or contour.
    b) P waves may be conducted 1:1 to ventricle, or variable second degree AV block may be present.
   2. Atrial flutter
    a) Baseline exhibits "sawtooth" appearance because of the rapidity of P wave occurrence.
    b) Irregular conduction to the ventricles (because of second degree block) is more common than 1:1 conduction.
  B. QRS complexes are normal in appearance (positive and narrow in lead II) unless concurrent ventricular conduction abnormality is present.
  C. Paroxysms of tachycardia begin and end abruptly.

Differential Diagnosis

I. When atrial flutter is conducted 1:1 to the ventricle, it is impossible to distinguish it from atrial tachycardia.
II. A vagal maneuver (e.g., ocular pressure, carotid massage) may induce second degree AV block and allow examination of the typical "sawtooth" baseline associated with atrial flutter.
III. The two rhythms are treated in a similar manner (see later).

Treatment

I. Acute therapy
  A. Vagal maneuver
   1. Sudden increases in vagal tone may abruptly convert atrial tachycardia or atrial flutter to sinus rhythm by slowing ectopic pacemaker discharge or causing second degree AV block.
   2. Ocular pressure and/or carotid massage (ventral to ear, caudal to the angle of the jaw) are the most frequently used techniques.
   3. Conversion is usually not permanent.
  B. Chemical intervention (IV administration recommended)
   1. Esmolol (see Table 7–4)
    a) Rapid-acting β-blocker (effects last ~ 20 minutes)

b) Slows sinus rate and causes AV block
c) Used with caution if CHF present because of negative inotropic effects

2. Diltiazem
   a) Calcium channel blocker
   b) Oral or IV preparations (IV recommended for acute use)
   c) Slows sinus rate and causes AV block
   d) Preferable to esmolol if CHF present, but proceed with caution because of negative inotropic effects

3. Adenosine
   a) Causes acute and transient (3–5 seconds) AV block
   b) Little information published regarding clinical use in dogs and cats

II. Chronic therapy
   A. β-blockers: propranolol, atenolol, metoprolol
   B. Calcium channel blockers: diltiazem
   C. Digoxin
      1. Digoxin is recommended if tachydysrhythmia is accompanied by CHF or structural heart disease.
      2. Digoxin toxicity may cause supraventricular tachydysrhythmias, especially if hypokalemia is present.
   D. Ancillary therapy for CHF: diuretics, vasodilators

III. Recurrent re-entry tachycardia pathways: disrupted surgically or via radiofrequency catheter ablation (Kuck & Schluter, 1993; Scherlag et al., 1993)

Patient Monitoring

I. Heart rate may be monitored by owners to ensure that heart rate is consistently in normal range, with decreased or no episodes of tachydysrhythmia.

II. Repeated ECGs or continuous 24-hour ECG monitoring is recommended if clinical signs recur.

III. If significant heart disease or heart failure is present, a routine ECG is recorded at each reevaluation examination.

IV. Animals with no discernible underlying heart disease are re-examined every 6 months to 1 year as long as there are no clinical signs apparent.

Atrial Fibrillation

Definition

I. Atrial fibrillation (AF) is a rapid supraventricular rhythm in which no organized atrial depolarization is present on the ECG recording.

II. The rapid, chaotic atrial rhythm is transmitted with varying degrees of AV block to the ventricles and results in rapid and irregular ventricular depolarization.

Causes

I. As for atrial premature depolarizations

II. Usually occurs in the presence of significant atrial muscle pathology (stretch or fibrosis)

III. Commonly associated with dilated cardiomyopathy in large-breed dogs

IV. Occasionally documented in giant-breed dogs with otherwise normal cardiac examinations, e.g., Irish wolfhounds, St. Bernards
   A. Ventricular response rate usually within normal range of heart rate for dogs
   B. May be early sign of dilated cardiomyopathy

Pathophysiology

I. Atrial muscle pathology (usually due to severe and long-standing disease of myocardium or valves) disrupts normal depolarization propagation pathways through the atrial tissue.

II. The mechanism by which AF occurs is incompletely understood but is thought to involve microscopic re-entry pathways.

III. Cardiac output is compromised by high rate of ventricular contraction and by loss of the atrial contribution to ventricular filling (approximately 15–20%).

Clinical Signs

I. Typical clinical signs associated with AF include weakness, exercise intolerance, and signs related to the underlying heart disease or CHF.

II. Acute AF may be associated with sudden decompensation of previously stable CHF.

Diagnosis

I. Physical examination
   A. Rapid, irregular heart rate
   B. Dramatic variations in pitch and intensity of ausculted heart sounds
   C. Findings associated with underlying disease (heart murmurs, gallop rhythms) or CHF (pulmonary crackles, ascites)
   D. Pulses variable in intensity with marked pulse deficits

II. ECG (Fig. 7–9)
   A. Irregularly irregular tachycardia (no repeatable pattern to the irregularity; R to R intervals highly variable)
   B. No P waves present; small, rapid fibrillation waves (f waves) possibly present
   C. QRS complexes supraventricular in appearance (tall and narrow in lead II)

III. Atypical ECG findings
   A. Ventricular response rate normal and/or regular
      1. Concurrent medical intervention or drug toxicity, e.g., digoxin therapy
      2. Concurrent AV block
   B. QRS complexes wide and bizarre
      1. Concurrent bundle branch block (if rate is normal or increased)
      2. Concurrent third degree AV block with ventricular escape rhythm (if rate is below normal range)

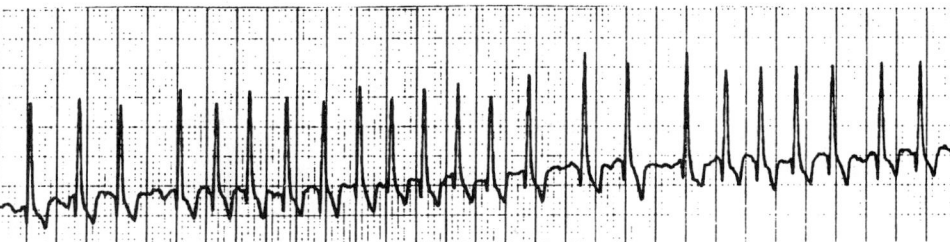

Figure 7–9. Lead II rhythm strip (25 mm/sec, 1 cm = 1 mV) recorded from a dog with atrial fibrillation. The rate of ventricular response is rapid (220–240 beats/min), and the rhythm is irregularly irregular. No P waves are present, and the QRS complexes are supraventricular in appearance.

Treatment

I. Acute therapy
   A. Acute therapy is recommended if AF is of recent onset (<24–48 hours).
   B. No further therapy may be needed if no underlying cardiac pathology is present.
   C. "Converted" AF frequently recurs if structural heart disease is present.
   D. Medical therapy (see Table 7–4) with diltiazem (IV or PO) or quinidine gluconate (IM) may be instituted.
   E. Synchronized cardioversion has been performed but is seldom used clinically in animals.
II. Chronic therapy
   A. Goal is to control ventricular response rate.
      1. Dogs: approximately 140–180 beats/min
      2. Cats: approximately 180–200 beats/min
   B. Institute medical therapy with digoxin if CHF or structural heart disease is present.
   C. β-Blockers *or* calcium channel blockers may be added if digoxin alone does not control heart rate once CHF is resolved.

Patient Monitoring

I. Monitor the heart rate (rate of ventricular response).
   A. Daily heart rates taken by owners allow assessment of drug efficacy in achieving target heart rates without adverse effects.
      1. Increases in the rate of ventricular response in a previously stable medicated animal may result from changes in systemic status (e.g., dehydration, pyrexia), decompensation of CHF, or progression of cardiac disease.
      2. Decreases in ventricular response rate below the recommended level may indicate drug toxicity or result in signs of low cardiac output or worsening of CHF.
   B. Repeat ECG whenever there is a change in clinical status or heart rate as noted by the owners or veterinarian.
II. Atrial fibrillation in giant-breed dogs with no other signs of cardiac disease may be clinically silent for several years before discernible cardiac changes occur.
III. Atrial fibrillation concurrent with significant structural heart disease worsens signs of heart failure, complicates therapy, and may shorten survival.

Junctional Tachydysrhythmias

Definition

I. Junctional or "nodal" tachydysrhythmias are rhythms that originate in or near the AV node and are usually transmitted both retrograde (toward the atria) and antegrade (to the ventricles).
II. In order for junctional ectopic depolarizations to become apparent on the ECG, their rate of discharge must exceed all other pacemakers in the heart, including the SA node.
III. Junctional rhythms usually discharge at a rate slightly less than that of the SA node (normal junctional depolarization rate, approximately 60–80 beats/min in dogs).
IV. Junctional tachycardias occur when the junctional rate is accelerated concurrent with slowing of the SA rate of discharge.

Causes

I. More frequently related to systemic illness than primary cardiac disease (see Table 7–1)
II. May indicate "mismatch" of vagal and sympathetic tone related to systemic or neurologic disease
III. Occasionally the result of AV nodal abnormality
IV. May indicate digitalis toxicity

Pathophysiology

I. Junctional tachycardias are usually hemodynamically stable.
II. The typical rate of discharge of junctional tachycardia is within the normal range, and the ventricles depolarize normally, leading to correct contraction sequence and reasonable cardiac output.

Clinical Signs

I. Often no clinical signs
II. Signs consistent with underlying disease/condition, e.g., digoxin toxicity

Diagnosis

I. Physical examination
   A. Mild irregularity in heart rhythm may be detected.
   B. There are usually *no* pulse deficits present.
II. ECG

A. Premature depolarizations and tachycardia are characterized by tall and narrow QRS complexes in lead II.
B. P waves typically are negative and follow the QRS complex (may be "buried" in the S-T segment).
C. P waves may not be visible.

Differential Diagnosis

When P waves are not visible, junctional tachycardia can be differentiated from AF in an unmedicated animal by the regularity of the junctional discharge rate and the relatively normal heart rate.

Treatment

I. Digoxin toxicity
   A. Confirm with serum digoxin concentration.
   B. Discontinue digoxin temporarily; may need to adjust dose chronically.
   C. Consider digoxin immune Fab (ovine) therapy if toxicity is acute and severe (see Table 7–4).
II. Systemic disease
   A. Rectify underlying problem.
   B. No direct antidysrhythmic therapy may be needed.
III. Persistent dysrhythmia despite resolution of underlying problem
   A. No therapy is needed if heart rate is within normal range and blood pressure is stable.
   B. Consider β-blocker or calcium channel blocker therapy.

Patient Monitoring

I. Digoxin toxicity
   A. Confirm resolution of dysrhythmia after digoxin toxicity is adequately treated.
   B. Reestablish therapeutic serum digoxin levels after 10–14 days of new dosage level.
II. Confirm normal ECG after resolution of systemic abnormalities that caused junctional dysrhythmia.
III. Repeat ECGs every 3–6 months while on medical therapy.

Ventricular Premature Depolarizations/Ventricular Tachycardia

Definition and Causes

I. Ventricular premature depolarizations (VPDs) are ectopic depolarizations that originate from any location in the ventricle.
II. VPDs usually result in ventricular, but not atrial, contraction.
III. The occurrence of three or more VPDs sequentially is termed "ventricular tachycardia" (VT).
IV. Ventricular dysrhythmias are often associated with severe cardiac or systemic disease (see Table 7–1).

Pathophysiology

I. Incomplete ventricular filling and an abnormal sequence of contraction associated with VPD result in decreased stroke volume for that contraction.
II. Ventricular tachycardia occurring at high heart rates (>300 beats/min in dogs) tends to become electrically unstable as the premature depolarization encroaches on the "vulnerable period" of the ventricle, i.e., depolarization occurs when the ventricle is not yet fully repolarized.
III. On an ECG, this phenomenon appears as the QRS complex of the premature depolarization occurring during the T wave of the previous depolarization (see Fig. 7–2).
IV. Sustained VT results in significant decreases in arterial blood pressure (Fig. 7–10).

Clinical Signs

I. May have no clinical signs
II. Clinical signs associated with underlying disease if VPD secondary to systemic illness
III. Refractory or recurrent CHF
IV. Signs of low cardiac output: lethargy, exercise intolerance
V. Episodic weakness, syncope
VI. Sudden death

Diagnosis

I. Physical examination
   A. Irregular cardiac rhythm
   B. Variable pulse strength with pulse deficits
   C. Findings typical of underlying heart disease and/or heart failure
   D. Signs of underlying systemic disease
II. ECG
   A. Tachycardia
   B. Wide and bizarre QRS complexes with no associated P wave
      1. Unconducted P waves may be visible in ECG baseline (Fig. 7–11).
      2. P waves may not be visible if rate of VT is rapid.
   C. Morphology of complex indicative of origin
      1. R wave positive in lead II: probable right ventricular origin
      2. R wave negative in lead II: probable left ventricular origin
   D. Ectopic depolarizations or VT: uniform (all ectopic complexes of similar morphology) or multiform (ectopic complexes of varying morphology, see Fig. 7–2)

Differential Diagnosis

Accelerated idioventricular rhythms may be mistaken for true ventricular tachycardia (see Accelerated Idioventricular Rhythms, later).

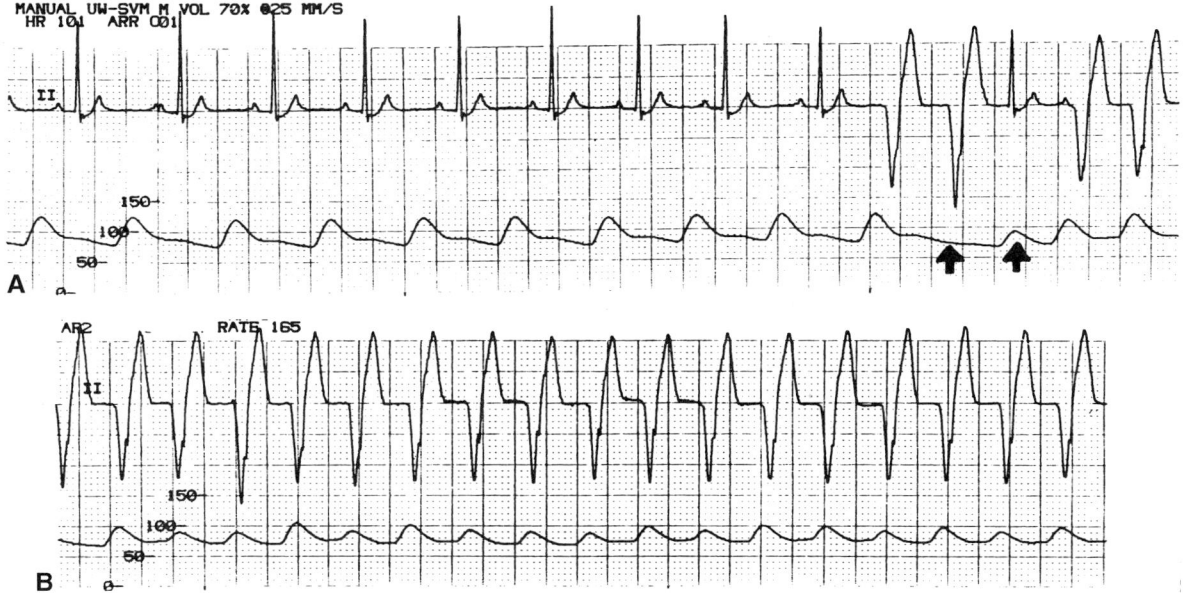

Figure 7–10. A. Lead II rhythm strip (25 mm/sec, 1 cm = 1 mV) recorded with simultaneous invasive arterial blood pressure tracing (blood pressure calibration at left end of strip). During sinus rhythm, systolic blood pressure = 120 mmHg, diastolic = 80 mmHg, and mean arterial pressure = 100 mmHg. Pressure pulses are markedly attenuated during ectopic depolarizations (arrows). B. Sustained ventricular tachycardia in the same dog results in disproportionate decreases in systolic blood pressure (95 mmHg), diastolic pressure (70 mmHg), and mean arterial pressure (78 mmHg).

Treatment

I. Emergency therapy (IV recommended, see Table 7–4)
  A. Lidocaine (IV only)
  B. Procainamide (IV, IM, or PO)
  C. DC cardioversion (synchronous defibrillation)
    1. Animal must be heavily sedated, e.g., opioid and benzodiazepine.
    2. Electrical discharge must be synchronized by cardioversion unit to occur on the R wave of the QRS complex to avoid ventricular fibrillation.
    3. Administer 1 joule/kg discharge.
    4. Ventricular fibrillation may occur; immediate defibrillation is necessary to return to sinus rhythm.
II. Elimination of underlying/associated problems
  A. Discontinue or decrease offending medications.
  B. Rectify electrolyte and acid–base disorders.
  C. Provide definitive therapy for underlying disease.
  D. Begin ancillary therapy for CHF, if present.
III. Chronic antidysrhythmic therapy
  A. Class I antidysrhythmics: procainamide, mexiletine, tocainide
  B. Class II antidysrhythmics: propranolol, atenolol, sotalol
  C. Class III antidysrhythmics: sotalol, amiodarone
  D. Combined antidysrhythmic therapy (class I + class II)
IV. No therapy for single or infrequent VPDs (<20/min)

Patient Monitoring

I. Emergency monitoring
  A. Continuous ECG monitoring recommended until conversion of VT to sinus rhythm
  B. Continuous or repeat monitoring to ensure continuing sinus rhythm

Figure 7–11. Lead II rhythm strip (25 mm/sec, 1 cm = 1 mV) recorded from a dog with paroxysmal ventricular tachycardia. Arrows indicate P waves "buried" within the ectopic rhythm. Ectopic deflections are predominantly positive in lead II, indicating probable right ventricular origin (see text).

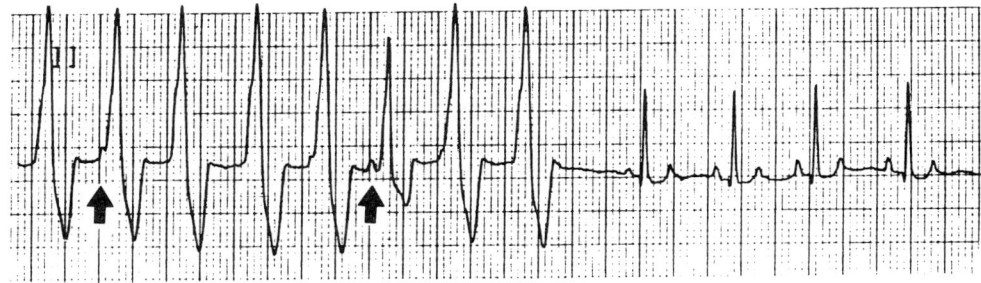

C. Invasive arterial pressure measurement to monitor for hypotension secondary to dysrhythmias

II. Chronic monitoring
   A. Therapeutic drug monitoring is performed to ensure plasma drug concentration (e.g., procainamide) is within therapeutic range.
   B. Repeat ECGs at 3-month intervals in stable animals, or obtain an ECG whenever a change in clinical condition occurs.
   C. Holter (24 hour) ECG recordings may be helpful to ensure efficacy of antidysrhythmic therapy.

Accelerated Idioventricular Rhythms

Definition and Causes

I. Accelerated idioventricular rhythm (AIR; alternative terms: fast idioventricular rhythm, slow ventricular tachycardia, or idioventricular tachycardia) is a ventricular rhythm initiated after a pause in sinus rhythm in which the rate of discharge is no more than 5–10 beats/min faster than the prevailing sinus rhythm.

II. AIR is most frequently diagnosed in dogs.

III. AIR usually arises in association with thoracic or myocardial trauma, neurologic disease, or severe systemic illness.

Pathophysiology

I. Basis for dysrhythmia
   A. Disturbances in autonomic balance
      1. Enhanced vagal tone to sinus node (respiratory sinus arrhythmia often present)
      2. Increased sympathetic stimulation to AV node or ventricular tissue
   B. Possibly result of ischemia/reperfusion

II. Physiologic response
   A. Heart rate and blood pressure relatively stable
   B. Occasionally associated with clinically significant hypotension

Clinical Signs

I. Often no clinical signs
II. Outward signs related to underlying problem

Diagnosis

I. Physical examination
   A. Usually no abnormalities other than those related to causative condition
   B. May have signs of low cardiac output
      1. Pale mucous membranes, slow capillary refill time
      2. Weak pulses or variable pulse strength
      3. Weakness, lethargy

II. ECG (Fig. 7–12)
   A. Wide and bizarre QRS complexes occur with no consistent relationship to P waves.
   B. Onset of ectopic rhythm is late in diastole, often closely following a normally timed P wave.
   C. "Run" of ventricular depolarizations often begins and ends with a fusion complex.
   D. Ectopic rhythm emerges on the ECG during the slow phases of respiratory sinus arrhythmia.
   E. Discharge rate of ectopic rhythm is 5–10 beats faster than sinus rhythm.

Differential Diagnosis

I. Ventricular tachycardia
   A. VT rates are usually >160 beats/min.
   B. VT is usually associated with hypotension.
   C. VT is often associated with evidence of heart disease and/or heart failure.

II. Ventricular escape rhythm
   A. First beat of escape rhythm usually follows a long (>1–3 seconds) pause in the sinus rhythm.
   B. Discharge rate of ventricular escape rhythms is usually 25–40 beats/min.

Treatment

I. Diagnose and treat the underlying problem.
   A. Supply oxygen and respiratory assistance, as needed.
   B. Acutely manage electrolyte and acid–base abnormalities with corrective fluid therapy.
   C. Provide specific therapy for underlying disorder, e.g., antibiotics if infection is present.
   D. Institute pain management.

II. No direct antidysrhythmic therapy is indicated if *all* of the following criteria apply.

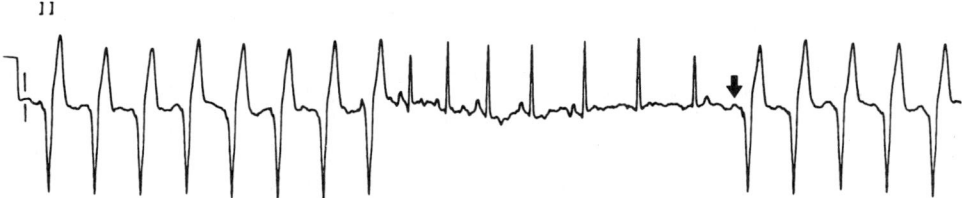

Figure 7–12. Lead II rhythm strip (25 mm/sec, 1 cm = 1 mV) recorded from a dog with an accelerated idioventricular rhythm. The underlying rhythm is a sinus arrhythmia with rates of depolarization that vary from 120–150 beats/min. The ectopic ventricular rhythm (approximately 135 beats/min) is manifest when the sinus rate slows. The arrow identifies a non-conducted P wave (see text).

A. If heart rate and blood pressure are within normal ranges and stable
B. If no clinical signs are apparent
C. If no other ventricular ectopic depolarizations interrupt "stable" AIR

III. Direct antidysrhythmic therapy may be indicated if *any* of the following occur.
A. Heart rate >130–160 beats/min
B. Hypotension or unstable blood pressure
C. If premature ventricular ectopic depolarizations initiate or interrupt "stable" AIR, or if R wave of ectopic depolarization occurs on the T waves of the previous depolarization ("R-on-T")
D. Clinical signs of poor cardiac output

IV. For specific medical therapy, see Ventricular Tachycardia, earlier.

Patient Monitoring

I. Repeated or continuous ECG
II. Invasive blood pressure measurement
A. If no antidysrhythmic therapy is being employed, occurrence of hypotension signals the need to directly treat the dysrhythmia.
B. If direct antidysrhythmic therapy is employed, blood pressure monitoring ensures efficacy.

Ventricular Fibrillation

Definition

I. Ventricular fibrillation (VF) is an irregular and chaotic rhythm initiated in the ventricles.
II. VF is usually a terminal rhythm in animals.

Causes and Pathophysiology

I. Ventricular fibrillation often signals the deterioration of a rapid ventricular tachycardia, which may result from any of the causes previously listed for ventricular tachycardia.
II. VF may result from a single premature depolarization occurring during ventricular repolarization, resulting in generation of multiple "wavelets" of depolarization and chaotic contraction.
III. Ventricular fibrillation results in weak and asynchronous contraction of multiple areas of the ventricular myocardium.
IV. Stroke volume decreases drastically, resulting in severely decreased cardiac output and hypotension.

Clinical Signs

I. Acute collapse with unconsciousness and cyanosis
II. Sudden death

Diagnosis

I. Physical examination
A. Lack of audible heart beat
B. Pulselessness
C. Pale/cyanotic mucous membranes, slow or absent capillary refill time

D. If collapse observed acutely, mucous membranes and capillary refill time still normal

II. ECG
A. No discernible P, QRS, or T deflections
B. Fibrillation waves may be large ("coarse fibrillation") or small ("fine fibrillation")

Differential Diagnosis

I. Artifacts
A. One or more lead wires dislodged from the animal
B. Purring or shivering artifact
C. Baseline electrical interference (60-cycle interference)

II. Ventricular tachycardia
A. Extremely rapid ventricular tachycardia may be mistaken for coarse VF.
B. Rapid VT usually responds to medical intervention, e.g., lidocaine.

Treatment

I. Initiate cardiopulmonary resuscitation procedures (see Chap. 8).
A. Electrical defibrillation
B. Drug therapy
C. Chemical defibrillation

II. Prognosis for recovery is best if VF is caused by trauma in a healthy animal.
III. Successful defibrillation may need to be followed by weeks of intensive medical management in order to return the animal to functional status.

MISCELLANEOUS CONDITIONS

Ventricular Pre-excitation

Definition

I. Ventricular pre-excitation refers to premature ventricular depolarization occurring in response to SA nodal discharge.
II. The ventricle depolarizes prematurely as a result of rapid conduction of supraventricular impulses through fast-conducting accessory pathways, bypassing the AV node and resulting in a shortened P-Q interval on the ECG.
III. Although generally uncommon in the veterinary population, ventricular pre-excitation has been clinically documented in both dogs and cats (Hill and Tilley, 1985; Miller et al., 1988).

Causes and Pathophysiology

I. Abnormal pathways bypassing the AV node may be congenital or develop subsequent to myocardial trauma, inflammation, or infarction.
II. Ventricular pre-excitation is hemodynamically benign but predisposes the heart to development of reciprocating or re-entrant tachycardias.

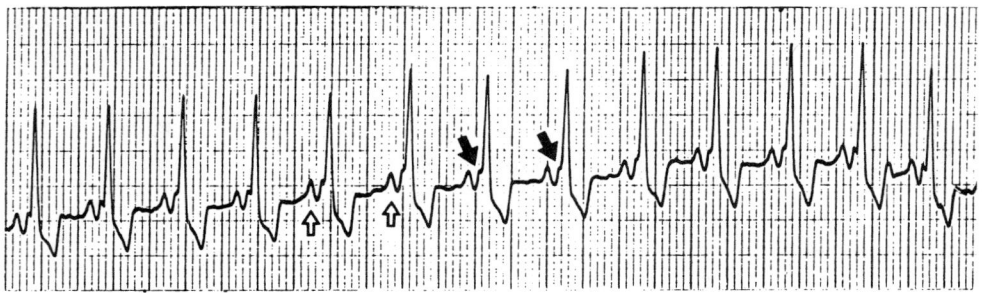

Figure 7–13. Lead II rhythm strip (25 mm/sec, 1 cm = 1 mV) recorded from a dog with ventricular pre-excitation. The P waves (open arrows) are of normal morphology; but the P-Q interval is short, and delta waves (solid arrows) are present.

III. Re-entrant tachycardias are supraventricular in appearance and may result in hypotension and clinical signs of low cardiac output.

Clinical Signs

I. No clinical signs occur during sinus rhythm.
II. Supraventricular tachycardia (SVT) may result in hypotension with episodic weakness or syncope.

Diagnosis

I. Physical examination: unremarkable unless SVT present
II. ECG (Fig. 7–13)
  A. Sinus discharge rate within normal range
  B. Shortened P-Q interval with normal P wave morphology
  C. QRS normal or have slurred upstroke (delta wave)
  D. Paroxysmal SVT associated with ventricular pre-excitation usually conducted 1:1 to ventricle

Differential Diagnosis

I. Other supraventricular tachycardias: ventricular pre-excitation includes short P-Q interval during sinus rhythm, and the abnormal upstroke of QRS during sinus rhythm usually "normalizes" during SVT.
II. Ventricular dysrhythmias: short P-Q interval seen in ventricular pre-excitation may be confused with wide and bizarre QRS contour of ventricular ectopic depolarizations.

Treatment and Monitoring

I. Ventricular pre-excitation without SVT requires no therapy.
II. If SVT is present, consider the following.
  A. Vagal maneuvers (ocular or carotid sinus pressure) may be used to acutely terminate SVT.
  B. β-Blockers, calcium channel blockers, or Class I antidysrhythmics may be used chronically to control recurrent SVT.
III. Survival of animals with ventricular pre-excitation has not been studied extensively.

IV. Control of SVT episodes usually eliminates clinical signs.
V. Ventricular pre-excitation is permanent but does not appear to be progressive.
VI. Most affected animals require lifelong therapy.

Bibliography

Bonagura JD, Muir WW: Antiarrhythmic therapy. p. 320. In Tilley LP (ed): Essentials of Canine and Feline Electrocardiography. 3rd Ed. Lea & Febiger, Philadelphia, 1992

Calvert CA, Jacobs GJ, Pickus CW: Bradycardia-associated episodic weakness, syncope, and aborted sudden death in cardiomyopathic Doberman pinschers. J Vet Intern Med 10:88, 1996

Harpster NK: Boxer cardiomyopathy. p. 329. In Kirk RW (ed): Current Veterinary Therapy VIII: Small Animal Practice. WB Saunders, Philadelphia, 1983

Harpster NK: Feline arrhythmias: diagnosis and management. p. 744. In Kirk RW, Bonagura JD (eds): Current Veterinary Therapy XI: Small Animal Practice. WB Saunders, Philadelphia, 1992

Hill BL, Tilley LP: Ventricular preexcitation in seven dogs and nine cats. J Am Vet Med Assoc 187:1026, 1985

Kuck KH, Schluter M: Junctional tachycardia and the role of catheter ablation. Lancet 341:1386, 1993

Miller MS, Tilley LP, Atkins CE: Persistent atrial standstill (atrioventricular muscular dystrophy). p. 786. In Kirk RW, Bonagura JD (eds): Current Veterinary Therapy XI: Small Animal Practice. WB Saunders, Philadelphia, 1992

Miller MW, Bonagura JD, DiBartola SP: ECG of the month. J Am Vet Med Assoc 192:336, 1988

Muir WW, Bonagura JD: Treatment of cardiac arrhythmias in dogs with gastric distention-volvulus. J Am Vet Med Assoc 185:1366, 1984

Rush JE, Keene BW: ECG of the month. J Am Vet Med Assoc 194:52, 1989

Scherlag BJ, Wang X, Nakagawa H et al: Radiofrequency ablation of a concealed accessory pathway as treatment for incessant supraventricular tachycardia in a dog. J Am Vet Med Assoc 203:1147, 1993

Senior DF, Feist EH, Stuart LB, Lombard CW: Treatment of acute digoxin toxicosis with digoxin immune Fab (ovine). J Vet Intern Med 5:302, 1991

Tilley LP: Analysis of canine P-QRS-T deflections. p. 60. In Tilley LP (ed): Essentials of Canine and Feline Electrocardiography. 3rd Ed. Lea & Febiger, Philadelphia, 1992a

Tilley LP: Analysis of feline P-QRS-T deflections. p. 100. In Tilley LP (ed): Essentials of Canine and Feline Electrocardiography. 3rd Ed. Lea & Febiger, Philadelphia, 1992b

Tilley LP, Liu SK: Persistent atrial standstill in the dog and cat. Proc Am Coll Vet Intern Med 3:43, 1983

8

Cardiopulmonary Resuscitation

John D. Jacobson

CARDIOPULMONARY ARREST

Definitions

I. Cardiopulmonary arrest (CPA): loss of effective spontaneous circulation and effective spontaneous ventilation
II. Cardiopulmonary resuscitation (CPR): actions taken for the treatment of CPA

Causes

I. Hypoxia
II. Acid-base, fluid, and electrolyte imbalance
III. Autonomic nervous system imbalance
IV. Excessive or inappropriate drugs
V. Cardiac disease or arrhythmias

Clinical Signs

I. Absence of auscultable heart beat or palpable pulse
II. Absence of breathing (agonal attempts to breathe may be present)
III. Other clinical signs
    A. Dilated pupils
    B. Gray or purple mucous membranes
    C. Delayed capillary refill time
    D. Absence of bleeding at the surgical site

Diagnosis

I. If there is no pulse and the animal is not breathing, other signs are not necessary to make the diagnosis of CPA.
II. A search for additional supporting evidence may result in an unnecessary and possibly detrimental delay in treatment.

Treatment Considerations

I. Treatment of CPA requires a minimum of three participants.

    A. Someone to provide breaths
    B. Someone to perform compressions
    C. Someone to administer drugs and evaluate therapy
II. If a crash cart is not used, the animal is taken to a predetermined location where CPR is performed and emergency supplies and drugs are located.
III. Based on previous studies, the survival rate in animals requiring CPR is very low, although it may be somewhat higher in closely monitored anesthetized patients. CPR recommendations change with great frequency based on results of new studies.
IV. Guidelines for discontinuing or not performing CPR are as follows.
    A. If an untreatable terminal illness is present
    B. If there has been inadequate blood flow for more than about 15 minutes
    C. If the owner requests that CPR not be performed

Treatment (ABCs)

I. Airway (Fig. 8–1)
    A. Provide a patent airway. Use an endotracheal tube of appropriate diameter and length.
    B. Secure the endotracheal tube. The endotracheal tube is easily dislodged if not secured.
    C. Evaluate thoracic compliance (by administering positive pressure ventilation while no one is compressing the chest). If it is very difficult for the animal to breathe, there may be an airway obstruction, tension pneumothorax, or severe pleural effusion.
    D. Tracheostomy is performed if orotracheal intubation is not possible.
II. Breathing
    A. Use breathing rates of 20 breaths/min.
    B. Administer 100% oxygen and discontinue anesthetics.

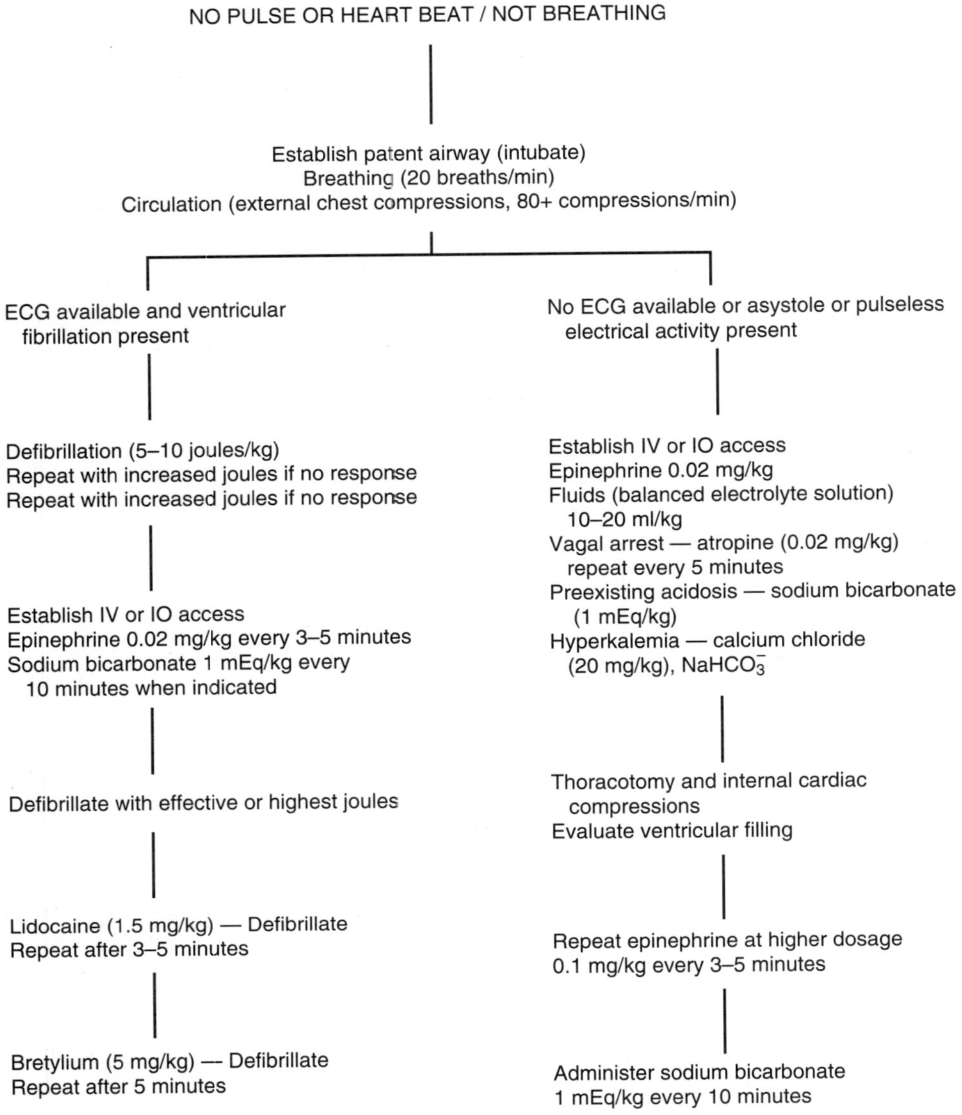

NO PULSE OR HEART BEAT / NOT BREATHING

Establish patent airway (intubate)
Breathing (20 breaths/min)
Circulation (external chest compressions, 80+ compressions/min)

ECG available and ventricular
fibrillation present

No ECG available or asystole or pulseless
electrical activity present

Defibrillation (5–10 joules/kg)
Repeat with increased joules if no response
Repeat with increased joules if no response

Establish IV or IO access
Epinephrine 0.02 mg/kg
Fluids (balanced electrolyte solution)
   10–20 ml/kg
Vagal arrest — atropine (0.02 mg/kg)
   repeat every 5 minutes
Preexisting acidosis — sodium bicarbonate
   (1 mEq/kg)
Hyperkalemia — calcium chloride
   (20 mg/kg), $NaHCO_3^-$

Establish IV or IO access
Epinephrine 0.02 mg/kg every 3–5 minutes
Sodium bicarbonate 1 mEq/kg every
   10 minutes when indicated

Defibrillate with effective or highest joules

Thoracotomy and internal cardiac
   compressions
Evaluate ventricular filling

Lidocaine (1.5 mg/kg) — Defibrillate
Repeat after 3–5 minutes

Repeat epinephrine at higher dosage
0.1 mg/kg every 3–5 minutes

Bretylium (5 mg/kg) — Defibrillate
Repeat after 5 minutes

Administer sodium bicarbonate
1 mEq/kg every 10 minutes

Figure 8–1. Management of cardiopulmonary arrest.

III. Circulation
   A. External chest compressions (ECC)
      1. Institute a minimum of 80 compressions/ min; rates of 100–120 compressions/min are considered in smaller patients.
      2. A faster compression rate should not be achieved at the expense of compression quality.
      3. Compressions may be performed with the animal in lateral or dorsal recumbency. The optimal position has not been determined and may vary with the patient chest conformation.
      4. Hand placement varies with the size of the animal; the heel of the hand is usually used to perform compressions.
      5. About a 1:1 compression to relaxation ratio is used.
      6. Relaxation between compressions must be complete (allow the chest to return to its normal position before beginning the next compression).
      7. Depth of compressions is $1/4$–$1/3$ of the width of the chest.
      8. Compressions should be *uninterrupted*! Do not stop compressions to make frequent attempts to determine whether spontaneous contractions have begun.
      9. The goal of compressions is to produce effective blood flow through the heart and brain until spontaneous activity can be achieved.
     10. Effectiveness of compressions is evaluated by palpating a pulse with each compression.
     11. Methods that may be used to enhance the effectiveness of ECC include the following.
      a) Simultaneous compression and ventilation (SCV) is breathing for the animal at the same time the chest is compressed.
         (1) During ECC, blood flow may be

caused by increased intrathoracic pressure rather than actual compression of the heart; SCV further increases intrathoracic pressure, thus improving blood flow. Increased survival rates using SCV have not been demonstrated.

    (2) The value of SCV may be uncertain; however, positive pressure ventilation between compressions decreases blood return to the heart.

    (3) Breaths are administered immediately before, during, or after compressions, and do not dominate the time in between compressions because of the negative effect on venous return.

  b) Abdominal binding (e.g., using a towel) may help shunt blood flow toward heart and brain. However, this technique may increase injury to abdominal organs.

  c) Interposed abdominal compressions (pressing the abdomen cranially in between chest compression) may be preferred to abdominal binding because abdominal organs are less likely to be injured during chest compressions. This technique can be performed when extra people are available, but there is no proof that it improves survival.

B. Internal chest compressions (ICC)
1. Current literature does not heartily endorse the practice of ICC; however, application of ICC early in the course of CPA has not been studied in clinical settings.
2. Some authors recommend that ICC begin as early as 2 minutes following onset of CPA and no later than 5 minutes after onset of CPA.
3. There are a few situations in which ECC should not be attempted, but ICC immediately employed.
  a) Thoracotomy has already been performed
  b) Significant chest trauma
  c) Pleural effusion
  d) Pneumothorax
  e) Pericardial tamponade
  f) Diaphragmatic hernia
4. If spontaneous cardiac activity does not begin following initial drug therapy (see Drugs) while using ECC, ICC should be strongly considered.
5. Advantages of ICC vs. ECC are as follows.
  a) Allows assessment of gross mechanical activity of the heart
  b) Allows assessment of ventricular filling
  c) Higher cardiac output attained
  d) Potentially less traumatic
  e) Thoracotomy possibly diagnostic of underlying cause
6. Clipping the hair and preparing the skin are

too time consuming and are not performed prior to thoracotomy, but sterile gloves are worn (skin preparation can be performed before closure if resuscitation is successful).
  a) Lateral thoracotomy is performed at the 4th to 6th intercostal space.
    (1) A scalpel is used for the skin and muscle, or a scalpel for the skin and Mayo scissors for muscle, with entrance into the thoracic cavity coordinated with ventilation.
    (2) Avoid the internal thoracic artery (ventrally) and avoid the vertebral artery (dorsally) by extending the incision dorsally and ventrally with the fingers.
    (3) Intercostal arteries are avoided by making the incision in the center of the intercostal space.
    (4) Self-retaining retractors are helpful to increase exposure.
  b) Incision of the pericardium is not essential for compressions, but it does allow the heart to be grasped easier. The pericardium is incised before closing the thoracotomy to prevent pericardial effusion from accumulating.
    (1) Avoid the phrenic nerve.
    (2) Avoid incising the auricles.
7. Use the palmar surfaces of your fingers and/or hand to compress the heart.
8. Compress from apex to base.
9. Ventricular filling can be evaluated with each compression; this will help determine compression rate and the need for additional epinephrine and fluid therapy.
10. Intermittent aortic compression or cross-clamping has been advocated to improve cerebral and coronary blood flow (Beardow and Dhupa, 1995). Exposure of the descending aorta is made with a left lateral thoracotomy.

IV. Drugs
A. Fluids
1. Balanced electrolyte solution (lactated Ringer's solution)
  a) Standard recommendation is 90 ml/kg/h IV, but if severe hemorrhage has not occurred, excessive fluid administration is likely.
  b) In the absence of significant hypovolemia, fluids serve an important role in flushing medications toward the heart when peripheral catheters are used.
  c) Administer 10–40 ml/kg IV as rapidly as possible, then reevaluate; this volume can be administered with a syringe in small animals.
  d) Use a large bore catheter, preferably not in the caudal half of the body.
2. Fluid alternatives
  a) If severe hemorrhage (blood loss >20–

30 ml/kg) has contributed to CPA, packed red blood cells or whole blood are necessary.

b) Hypertonic saline (7.5% NaCl) 3–5 ml/kg IV (up to 10 ml/kg), alone or in combination with a colloid, may prove to be a superior resuscitative fluid.

c) Colloids (e.g., dextran 70, hetastarch), by themselves or in combination with hypertonic saline, may prove to be superior resuscitative fluids. Smaller volumes are used, e.g., 5–10 ml/kg IV (up to 20 ml/kg).

B. Epinephrine
  1. Route of administration
    a) First choice: intravenous (IV), ideally a central (jugular vein) catheter
    b) Second choice: intraosseous (IO), if IV access is unavailable or not readily obtainable
    c) Third choice: intratracheally, with dosages 2–5 × IV dose
    d) Last choice: intracardiac
      (1) Compressions must be interrupted.
      (2) Pericardial tamponade may occur if blood seeps from the injection site or from lacerated coronary vessels into the pericardial sac, where it cannot escape.
      (3) Accidental intraventricular injections in the cardiac muscle lead to intractable ventricular fibrillation.
  2. Dosage
    a) Initial dosage is 0.01–0.02 mg/kg (0.5–1 ml of 1:10,000/10 lb) IV or IO. Dilute 1:1000 solution (1 mg/ml) with sterile saline (1 ml epinephrine with 9 ml saline) to create a 1:10,000 solution.
    b) If initial epinephrine administration is not successful, higher dosages are recommended at 0.1–0.2 mg/kg (0.5–1 ml of 1:1000/10 lb) IV or IO every 3–5 minutes.
  3. Purpose of using epinephrine
    a) Causes peripheral vasoconstriction and enhances venous return
    b) Used in virtually all cases of CPA except ventricular tachycardia
    c) May convert fine ventricular fibrillation (VF) to coarse fibrillation

C. Corticosteroids
  1. Dexamethasone sodium phosphate (Azium-SP) 4–8 mg/kg IV (0.5–1 ml/lb)
  2. Prednisolone sodium succinate (Solu-Delta-Cortef) 10–30 mg/kg IV
  3. Causes vasodilation and hypotension when administered rapidly
  4. Controversial; possibly not beneficial to cardiovascular or cerebral resuscitation

D. Anticholinergics
  1. Atropine (rather than glycopyrrolate) is used most frequently because its response is more reliable.
  2. The primary indication is a vagally induced arrest. However, one could argue that vagal tone is always high during the first few minutes of arrest or that almost any situation could involve a vagal component.
  3. Atropine is currently recommended for treatment of asystole and slow pulseless electrical activity, but administration of epinephrine is preferred initially.
  4. Dosage is 0.02–0.04 mg/kg IV or about 1 ml/40 lb (0.5 mg/ml) every 5 minutes.

E. Calcium salts
  1. Previously indicated for treatment of pulseless electrical activity, but this recommendation has been discontinued because calcium may contribute to a poor neurologic outcome.
  2. Indications for calcium salt administration include the following.
    a) Hypocalcemia: caused by massive transfusions of citrated blood products, hypoparathyroidism, renal failure, pancreatitis, long-term use of loop diuretics, excessive hyperventilation, or following the use of alkalinizing agents
    b) Hyperkalemia: calcium antagonizes potassium's effect on the myocardium
    c) Calcium channel blocker toxicity
  3. Dosage of calcium chloride is 10–20 mg/kg IV (0.2 ml/kg of 10% calcium chloride).
  4. Dosage of calcium gluconate is 2–5 times higher.

F. Sodium bicarbonate
  1. Previously administered as a first line drug; however, it has been shown that significant metabolic acidosis may not occur until 5–10 minutes after the onset of CPA.
  2. Potential problems associated with indiscriminate administration include metabolic alkalosis, paradoxical central nervous system acidosis, hyperosmolality, hypernatremia, and shifts of the oxyhemoglobin curve to the left.
  3. Recommendation is to administer immediately if moderate to severe metabolic acidosis preexisted; otherwise, administer 0.5–1 mEq/kg IV 5–10 minutes after the onset of CPA and every 5–10 minutes thereafter.
  4. When available, bicarbonate administration can be based on blood gas analysis.
    a) Venous blood gas analysis, reflecting tissue pH, may be more useful than arterial blood gases.
    b) Arterial pH usually reflects the result of hyperventilation.

G. Lidocaine
  1. Indications include ventricular tachycardia and ventricular ectopy.
  2. It may be prudent to administer lidocaine prior to epinephrine administration in situations in which a defibrillator is not available,

but the value of this practice has not been determined.
3. Dosage is 0.5–2 mg/kg IV with a maximum dose of 8 mg/kg every 10 minutes. *Caution*: Lidocaine may cause asystole!
4. Procainamide may be used if lidocaine is not effective at 2–4 mg/kg IV over 5 minutes.

Patient Monitoring

I. Evaluation of the effectiveness of internal or external cardiac compressions
   A. Pulse quality: usually femoral or lingual artery
   B. Doppler ultrasonic flow detector: crystal placed over or under the eyelid or over peripheral artery (extremely helpful to detect when spontaneous activity begins)
   C. Direct arterial blood pressure: diastolic blood pressure ideally maintained >40 mmHg
   D. End-tidal carbon dioxide using capnometry: values <10 mmHg associated with poor outcomes
II. Electrocardiogram (ECG)
   Note: Initiation of CPR should not be delayed because an ECG is not immediately available.
   A. Asystole (flat line)
      1. Eliminate the possibility that fine ventricular fibrillation is present by confirming asystole in more than one lead.
      2. Institute ABCs, oxygen, epinephrine, and IV or IO fluids; then atropine.
      3. Rule out common causes such as hypoxia, hyperkalemia, hypokalemia, preexisting acidosis, and hypothermia.
   B. Pulseless electrical activity
      1. It is a normal ECG in the presence of cardiovascular collapse due to absence of mechanical contractions or contractions too weak to produce a pulse; previously referred to as electromechanical dissociation and includes idioventricular rhythms and ventricular escape rhythms.
      2. Institute ABCs, oxygen, epinephrine, and IV or IO fluids (and atropine, if bradycardia is present).
      3. Rule out common causes such as hypovolemia, hypoxia, cardiac tamponade, tension pneumothorax, hypothermia, hyperkalemia, and acidosis.
   C. Ventricular fibrillation (squiggly ECG)
      1. Precordial thump is not a currently recommended technique.
      2. Defibrillation is performed immediately.
         a) External defibrillation: 5–10 joules/kg
         b) Internal defibrillation: 0.5–2 joules/kg
         c) Defibrillation initially effective, but the rhythm converts back to ventricular fibrillation: repeat the effective dose
         d) First attempt at defibrillation not effective initially: increase joules about 25–50%
         e) Second attempt not successful: increase joules an additional 25%

f) These three attempts administered one after the other without delay
3. Refractory ventricular fibrillation
   a) Continue ABCs.
   b) Administer epinephrine (if not administered already, or if 3–5 minutes have elapsed since last administration); repeat every 3–5 minutes.
   c) Defibrillate using highest recommended joules.
   d) Give lidocaine 1–2 mg/kg IV; repeat in 3–5 minutes.
   e) Consider bretylium 5 mg/kg IV; repeat in 5 minutes.
   f) Consider procainamide 40 μg/kg/min IV infusion.
   g) Alternate administration of these medications in the order listed here, and repeat defibrillation using the highest recommended joules within 30–60 seconds after administration of each medication.
4. Chemical defibrillation
   a) It is rarely effective and involves the use of acetylcholine to convert the rhythm to asystole.
   b) Acetylcholine is not a commonly used drug and has a short shelf life.
   D. Ventricular ectopy: lidocaine
   E. Bradycardia: atropine
III. Post-CPR management
   The amount of post-resuscitation care is usually related to the animal's pre-CPA condition and the difficulty encountered during resuscitation.
   A. Central nervous system monitoring
      1. Parenteral atropine does not alter pupil size.
      2. Treat or prevent cerebral edema.
         a) Keep head elevated.
         b) Give dexamethasone 2 mg/kg IV every 6–8 hours if deteriorating, or 0.2–0.4 mg/kg if stable or improving.
         c) Give mannitol 0.25–0.5 g/kg over 10–15 minutes, but do not overload with fluids.
         d) Give furosemide 0.7–1 mg/kg IV 15 minutes following mannitol; repeat mannitol and furosemide 1–2 times at 3–4 hour intervals (Fenner, 1995).
      3. Provide padded bedding and turn frequently.
      4. Provide analgesia and/or sedation as needed with morphine 0.1 mg/kg IV, oxymorphone 0.05 mg/kg IV, or diazepam 0.2 mg/kg IV.
   B. Cardiovascular system monitoring
      1. Continuous ECG monitoring until arrhythmias are absent for several hours
      2. Pulse oximetry monitoring until oxygenation is normal when the animal is breathing room air
      3. Blood pressure (peripheral pulse quality): maintain mean blood pressure >60–70 mmHg
      4. Acid-base and electrolyte status evaluated daily or more frequently if severe abnormalities exist

5. Central venous pressure (CVP) monitored to avoid fluid overload
6. Therapy for hypotension
    a) Dobutamine 5–15 μg/kg/min IV infusion
    b) Dopamine 1–7 μg/kg/min IV infusion
C. Respiratory system monitoring
    1. Provide oxygen via nasal tube or an oxygen cage until the animal can breathe room air without becoming hypoxemic.
    2. Ventilation is supported as necessary to prevent hypercapnia.
    3. Monitor oxygenation and ventilation using pulse oximetry, capnometry, and/or arterial blood gas analysis.
    4. Evaluate for the presence of pulmonary edema, pulmonary contusions, and/or pleural effusion with thoracic radiographs and frequent auscultation if patient is tachypneic.
D. Renal monitoring
    1. Urine output: minimum of 1–2 ml/kg/h
    2. Treatment of oliguria/anuria
        a) Administer IV fluids, but avoid fluid overload by monitoring CVP and urine output.
        b) Administer dopamine 0.5–3 μg/kg/minute IV infusion.
        c) Consider furosemide 1 mg/kg IV or 1 mg/kg/h IV infusion.
        d) Consider mannitol 0.25–0.5 g/kg IV or

dextrose 50% 1.6 ml/kg IV, followed by 5–10% dextrose maintenance solution to maintain diuresis.
E. Gastrointestinal monitoring
    Provide supportive therapy for hemorrhagic diarrhea, septic shock, and impaired hepatic function.
F. Disseminated intravascular coagulation
    1. Always a possible sequela of prolonged low circulatory states
    2. See Chap. 66.

Bibliography

American Heart Association: Guidelines for cardiopulmonary resuscitation and emergency cardiac care. JAMA 268:2171, 1992

Beardow AW, Dhupa N: Cardiopulmonary arrest and resuscitation. p. 425. In Miller MS, Tilley LP (eds): Manual of Canine and Feline Cardiology. WB Saunders, Philadelphia, 1995

Fenner WR: Diseases of the brain. p. 578. In Ettinger SJ, Feldman EC (eds): Textbook of Veterinary Internal Medicine. WB Saunders, Philadelphia, 1995

Montgomery WH: Mechanisms and methods of cardiopulmonary resuscitation. Anesthesiology Clin North Am 13:767, 1995

Otto CW: Vasopressor therapy for advanced cardiac life support. Anesthesiology Clin North Am 13:835, 1995

Schleien CL, Gelman B, Kuluz JW: Pediatric cardiopulmonary resuscitation. Anesthesiology Clin North Am 13:943, 1995

Wass CT, Lanier WL: Improving neurologic outcome following cardiac arrest. Anesthesiology Clin North Am 13:869, 1995

Acquired Valvular Diseases

Wendy A. Ware

DEGENERATIVE DISORDERS

Chronic Atrioventricular Valve Disease

Definition

I. Chronic, degenerative atrioventricular (AV) valve disease results in mitral and sometimes tricuspid valve insufficiency.
   A. It is the most common cause of mitral regurgitation (MR) and congestive heart failure in dogs (Buchanan, 1992).
   B. Tricuspid regurgitation (TR) is less common than, but frequently coexists with, degenerative mitral valve disease.
   C. A minority of dogs have degenerative TR without MR.
II. Other names include endocardiosis, mucoid or myxomatous valvular degeneration, and chronic valvular fibrosis.
III. Clinically recognized degenerative valve disease is rare in cats (Buchanan, 1992).

Causes

I. The underlying etiology is unknown.
   A. Affected dogs are usually small to mid-size.
      1. Greater prevalence in poodles, miniature schnauzers, Chihuahuas, fox terriers, cocker spaniels, Boston terriers (Buchanan, 1992)
      2. Especially high incidence (54–59% of dogs >4 years) and early onset in cavalier King Charles spaniels (Haggstrom et al., 1992; Beardow and Buchanan, 1993; Darke, 1995)
   B. Genetic factors involving collagen degeneration are suspected (Buchanan, 1992).
II. The disease prevalence increases with age (Sisson, 1987; Buchanan, 1992).

A. Over 30% of small breed dogs >10 years are affected.
B. Males are affected more often than females.

Pathophysiology

I. Progressive anatomic changes in the valve complex occur with age.
   A. Small nodules initially form along the free edges of the valve leaflets, then gradually enlarge and begin to merge with each other.
   B. The affected valves become thickened as larger plaque-like lesions form.
      1. The chordae tendineae also become thickened near their valvular attachment site.
      2. The valve gradually begins to leak.
   C. As the disease advances, the valve leaflets become grossly deformed, thick, and shrunken.
      1. Diseased chordae tendineae are weakened and may rupture.
      2. The valve may appear to bulge (prolapse) toward the atrium like a parachute or balloon.
      3. Valvular insufficiency is usually clinically evident at this stage.
II. Mitral valve insufficiency leads to other cardiac changes.
   A. The left atrium, mitral valve annulus, and left ventricle dilate, and varying degrees of endocardial fibrosis may occur.
   B. Jet lesions may develop from the impact of the regurgitant blood.
   C. Partial- or full-thickness tears can occur in the left atrial wall in advanced cases, especially in male miniature poodles, cocker spaniels, and dachshunds.
III. The pathophysiology of MR relates to left ventricular and atrial volume overload.
   A. Regurgitation gradually worsens as the mitral valve becomes more deformed.
   B. Compensatory changes in atrial and ventricular size and blood volume allow most dogs to remain

asymptomatic for a prolonged time. Some cases never show signs of heart failure.

C. If left atrial pressure increases sufficiently, pulmonary venous congestion and edema develop.
  1. Gradual increases in atrial and pulmonary capillary hydrostatic pressure allow compensatory increases in pulmonary lymphatic flow.
  2. Overt pulmonary edema develops when the capacity of the pulmonary lymphatic system is exceeded.

D. Left atrial enlargement allows a slowly increasing regurgitant volume to be accommodated at low filling pressures because of increased atrial compliance (Kihara et al., 1988).
  1. Massive atrial enlargement may develop before any signs of heart failure appear. Left mainstem bronchus compression and coughing can result.
  2. Chordal rupture may acutely increase MR and left atrial pressure, leading to pulmonary edema regardless of atrial size.
  3. Full-thickness tears cause bleeding into the pericardial space and, potentially, fatal cardiac tamponade.

E. The left ventricle dilates and undergoes eccentric hypertrophy over time as an increasing regurgitant volume must be pumped in addition to the normal forward output. Ventricular dilation stretches the mitral annulus, which further exacerbates the regurgitation.
  1. Compensatory hypertrophy allows for normalized myocardial wall tension at a larger volume (Braunwald, 1992a).
  2. Ventricular contractility is maintained fairly well until late in the disease (Kittleson et al., 1984).
    a) Severe congestive failure can result from MR in spite of normal contractility.
    b) Reduced contractility eventually results from chronic volume overload when dilation exceeds the heart's ability to adequately hypertrophy (Braunwald, 1992a).
    c) Reduced contractility exacerbates ventricular dilation and MR and therefore may worsen congestive failure.
    d) Reduced ventricular contractility and compliance tend to increase left atrial pressure and congestion.
  3. Assessment of myocardial contractility is difficult because loading conditions are altered with MR.
    a) Ejection phase indices (e.g., echocardiographic fractional shortening) overestimate contractility (Braunwald, 1992b).
    b) The end-systolic volume index and end-systolic stress or pressure–end-systolic volume indices are better, although not ideal (Braunwald, 1992c; Davila-Roman et al., 1993).

IV. Chronic TR leads to right heart dilation and other changes analogous to those occurring in the left heart from MR.

A. TR causes volume overload of the right atrium and ventricle.
  1. Increased pulmonary vascular resistance due to concurrent left heart failure promotes right ventricular dilation and exacerbates TR.
  2. Congestive heart failure develops when low right atrial pressures (e.g., <10–12 mmHg) cannot be maintained.

B. Compensatory circulatory mechanisms increase blood volume and enhance vasoconstriction (Braunwald, 1992a; Ware, 1994).
  1. Increased sympathetic neural tone and attenuated vagal activity occur.
  2. Increased angiotensin II formation results from enhanced renal renin release.
  3. Antidiuretic hormone (vasopressin) and other vasoconstrictor peptides have also been identified in heart failure.
  4. Changes begin early and intensify with worsening heart failure.
  5. Intrarenal circulatory adjustments contribute to volume retention.

C. Complicating factors frequently develop.
  1. Tachyarrhythmias may occur intermittently and without clinical signs, or may be severe enough to cause decompensated congestive failure and/or syncope.
  2. Rupture of chordae tendineae may cause fulminant, refractory pulmonary edema within hours.
    a) This may occur in previously asymptomatic dogs or those with chronic MR.
    b) The acute decrease in forward volume may cause weakness and other signs of low cardiac output.
    c) Ruptured chordae may be an incidental finding (on echocardiogram or necropsy), especially if 2nd or 3rd order chordae are involved.
  3. A full-thickness (usually left) atrial tear allows bleeding into the pericardial space; signs of cardiac tamponade quickly develop.
  4. Diminished myocardial contractility contributes to clinical decompensation.

Clinical Signs

I. Many dogs with degenerative AV valve disease show no clinical signs.

II. Signs of MR usually relate to decreased exercise tolerance and pulmonary congestion and edema.
A. Mild signs include diminished exercise capacity and cough or tachypnea with exertion.
B. As pulmonary congestion and interstitial edema worsen, the resting respiratory rate also increases.
C. Cough may occur at night and early morning as well as with activity.
D. Severe edema produces obvious respiratory distress and often a moist cough, with anxiety and reluctance to lie down (orthopnea).

E. Signs of severe pulmonary edema can develop gradually or acutely.

F. Decreased interest in food is typical as heart failure worsens; total anorexia is common with severe edema.

G. Many dogs have intermittent episodes of symptomatic pulmonary edema between times of compensated heart failure over a period of months to years.

H. Episodes of transient weakness or acute collapse may occur secondary to arrhythmias, coughing, or atrial tear.

III. Clinical signs of TR usually relate to systemic venous congestion, ascites, pleural effusion, and rarely, peripheral tissue edema.

A. Gastrointestinal signs may result from splanchnic congestion.

B. Tachyarrhythmias can exacerbate congestion and cause transient weakness or syncope, as with MR.

1. Atrial premature complexes are common.

2. Paroxysmal atrial tachycardia and atrial fibrillation are more likely to precipitate worsened clinical signs by their adverse hemodynamic effects (Sisson et al., 1995).

3. Ventricular premature complexes and tachycardia are less common than atrial tachyarrhythmias.

C. Cardiac tamponade from an atrial tear can also cause pleural effusion or ascites.

Diagnosis

I. Physical examination

A. Chronic MR is accompanied by a holosystolic murmur best heard in the area of the left apex (left 4th to 6th intercostal space).

1. The murmur may radiate in any direction.

2. A murmur heard only in early systole (protosystolic) may accompany mild MR.

3. Loud MR murmurs have been associated with more advanced diseases (Buchanan, 1979; Haggstrom et al., 1995).

4. Nevertheless, the murmur may be soft or inaudible with massive regurgitation and severe heart failure.

5. Some dogs have an audible mid- to late systolic click, with or without a murmur.

6. Occasionally the murmur sounds like a musical tone or whoop.

7. An S3 gallop is sometimes noted at the left apex with advanced MR. This diastolic sound is of lower pitch (frequency) than the first and second heart sounds.

B. TR causes a holosystolic murmur similar to MR but best heard at the right apex. Radiation of a MR murmur to the right chest wall may mimic TR or mask a TR murmur.

C. Lung sounds may be normal or abnormal.

1. Normal breath sounds are heard in the absence of congestive failure or with mild pulmonary edema.

2. Accentuated, harsh breath sounds and end-inspiratory crackles (especially in ventral lung fields) develop as edema worsens.

3. Widespread inspiratory as well as expiratory crackles and wheezes can be heard with fulminant pulmonary edema.

4. Some dogs with chronic MR have abnormal lung sounds associated with underlying pulmonary or airway disease rather than heart failure.

5. Pleural effusion associated with TR causes diminished pulmonary sounds ventrally.

D. Other physical parameters may be non-contributory.

1. Peripheral capillary perfusion and arterial pulse strength are usually good.

2. Pulse deficits may occur with tachyarrhythmias.

3. A palpable precordial thrill accompanies loud (grade 5–6/6) murmurs.

4. Jugular vein distention or pulsations are not expected with MR, unless there is concurrent TR.

5. With TR, jugular pulsations occur during ventricular systole.

   a) These may be more evident after exercise or with excitement.

   b) Jugular vein distention results from elevated right heart filling pressures.

   c) Jugular pulsations and distention are more evident with cranial abdominal compression (positive hepatojugular reflux).

6. Abdominal signs of right heart failure (e.g., hepatomegaly, ascites) may occur with TR.

II. Radiography typically shows some degree of left atrial and ventricular enlargement that worsens over months to years with MR.

A. Left atrial enlargement is seen on the lateral view as bulging of the dorsocaudal heart border.

1. Elevation of the left and sometimes right mainstem bronchi, with compression of the left mainstem bronchus, occurs when enlargement is severe.

2. Left auricular enlargement produces a bulge in the 2 to 3 o'clock position on dorsoventral (DV) or ventrodorsal (VD) views.

B. Left ventricular enlargement causes lengthening of the heart shadow on the lateral projection with elevation of the carina and caudal vena cava.

1. The caudal heart border becomes more rounded.

2. Rounding and enlargement in approximately the 2 to 5 o'clock position is seen on DV or VD views.

C. Use of the vertebral heart score (VHS) has been suggested as a means to quantify the presence and degree of cardiomegaly (Buchanan and Bücheler, 1995).

1. Cardiac long axis and the perpendicular short axis are measured in number of vertebrae (to the nearest 0.1) beginning with T4.

2. Both measurements are added to yield the VHS.
3. VHS ≤10.5 vertebrae is considered normal for most breeds.

D. The earliest radiographic sign of left heart failure is pulmonary venous congestion.
   1. Lobar veins appear wider and denser than the accompanying artery.
   2. This is most easily seen in the cranial lobar veins on lateral view.

E. Pulmonary edema initially accumulates around vessels and in the interstitial tissue, blurring vascular markings.
   1. Peribronchial cuffing appears.
   2. Advanced pulmonary edema fills alveolar spaces, causing fluffy, indistinct opacities and "air bronchograms."
   3. The classic distribution of cardiogenic pulmonary edema in dogs is hilar, dorsocaudal, and bilaterally symmetrical.
   4. The presence and severity of pulmonary edema are not necessarily correlated with the degree of cardiomegaly.
      a) Acute, severe MR can cause cardiogenic edema with minimal left atrial enlargement.
      b) Slowly developing MR can produce massive left atrial enlargement with no evidence of congestive failure.

III. Radiographically, some degree of right heart enlargement is evident with chronic TR.
   A. This may be masked by left heart and pulmonary changes secondary to concurrent mitral disease.
   B. Progressive rounding of the right heart border and widening of the cardiac shadow are typical.
   C. Caudal vena cava distention, pleural fissure lines, and hepatomegaly are early signs of right heart failure.
   D. Overt pleural effusion and ascites occur with advanced failure.

IV. The electrocardiogram (ECG) is often normal but may suggest chamber enlargement or document an arrhythmia.
   A. Wide P waves (>0.04 second) suggest left atrial enlargement but are not a very sensitive indicator.
   B. Tall P waves (>0.4 mV) suggest right atrial enlargement, but this change is often absent with TR.
   C. Tall R waves in lead II or AVF (>3 mV) suggest left ventricular enlargement, although this ECG finding is also not always present.
   D. QRS prolongation (>0.05–0.06 second) has also been used as an indicator of left ventricular enlargement.
   E. An S wave in lead I, right axis deviation, or other criteria for right ventricular enlargement are occasionally seen with severe TR.
   F. Atrial tachyarrhythmias are common with advanced disease; ventricular tachyarrhythmias are less frequent.

V. Echocardiography is useful for assessing cardiac structural and functional changes (Bonagura, 1994; Jacobs et al., 1995).
   A. With chronic mitral valve degeneration the following may be noted.
      1. The mitral valve appears thickened and "knobby."
         a) Balloon-like systolic prolapse of one or both leaflets may be observed.
         b) Valve leaflet tips and attached chordal remnants flail into the atrium in systole when major chordae tendineae rupture.
         c) Mitral valve motion appears exaggerated on M-mode exam.
         d) It is usually not possible to differentiate bacterial endocarditis lesions from degenerative valve thickening with certainty.
      2. Severity of left atrial and left ventricular enlargement can be evaluated on two-dimensional and M-mode.
      3. Pericardial fluid is evident with a left atrial tear.
      4. Left ventricular function can be estimated.
         a) Left ventricular wall and septal motion appears exuberant with severe regurgitation and good myocardial function.
         b) High normal to increased fractional shortening is expected in the presence of significant mitral regurgitation when contractility is normal.
         c) The end-systolic volume index can be derived, although assumptions about volume calculation may cause significant inaccuracy (Kittleson et al., 1984).
         d) There is little to no mitral "E" point-septal separation on M-mode except when contractility is decreased.
   B. With chronic tricuspid valve degeneration, look for the following.
      1. Right ventricular and atrial enlargement are seen with significant TR.
      2. Severe volume overload of the right ventricle may cause paradoxical septal motion.

VI. Doppler echocardiography identifies regurgitant flow.
   A. Systolic pressure gradients between affected atrium and ventricle can be estimated from the maximum regurgitant jet velocity with spectral Doppler echocardiography.
   B. Color flow Doppler echocardiography can demonstrate the orientation of the regurgitant jet.
      1. A rough estimate of severity can be based on the extent of turbulent retrograde flow (Feigenbaum, 1994).
      2. Other techniques (e.g., proximal flow convergence) allow more accurate quantitation (Feigenbaum, 1994).

Differential Diagnosis

I. Other causes of left-sided systolic murmurs must be differentiated; echocardiography is most helpful.
   A. Mitral regurgitation may be secondary to another disease.

1. Bacterial endocarditis (see later)
2. Dilated cardiomyopathy causing MR from mitral annulus dilation and papillary muscle dysfunction (see Chap. 10)
   a) This is less common in small breed dogs, except the cocker spaniel.
   b) Echocardiography shows poor ventricular motion as well as dilation.
3. Congenital malformation (dysplasia) of the mitral valve (see Chap. 6)
   a) The murmur is present since birth.
   b) Malformations of the valve apparatus as well as changes from chronic MR are seen on echocardiography.
B. The murmur of ventricular outflow obstruction could be confused with MR, although these ''ejection'' type murmurs are usually heard best at the left heart base.
   1. Congenital subaortic stenosis is usually heard best low at the left base; the murmur should have been present since the dog was a puppy or young adult.
   2. Congenital pulmonic stenosis is heard best at the cranial left base rather than the left apex, with the murmur present since puppyhood.
   3. Ventricular outflow obstruction in dogs occasionally develops from an intracardiac tumor or hypertrophic cardiomyopathy.
C. Innocent or physiologic flow murmurs (e.g., secondary to anemia) are usually best heard at the left base.
II. Rule out other causes of cough or respiratory distress.
   A. Determine whether congestive heart failure has resulted, or whether the respiratory signs are caused by another disease, e.g., chronic bronchitis, collapsing trachea, pneumonia, pulmonary neoplasia, pulmonary fibrosis, non-cardiogenic pulmonary edema, or pleural space disease.
   B. Heartworm disease must be considered in endemic areas.
   C. Mechanically stimulated cough (from left main bronchus compression) may occur with or without congestive failure.
III. Differential considerations for degenerative TR include other causes of right-sided systolic murmurs.
   A. TR occurs with dilated cardiomyopathy, congenital tricuspid dysplasia, or rarely, bacterial endocarditis.
   B. Congenital ventricular septal defect murmurs are usually heard near the right sternal border rather than right apex.
   C. Subaortic stenosis murmurs may be loud at the cranial right base.
IV. Other causes of pleural effusion or ascites must be differentiated from right heart failure with TR (see Chap. 19).

Treatment

I. Treatment of congestive heart failure centers on enhancing forward flow, reducing regurgitant volume, controlling pulmonary edema, and perhaps most importantly, modulating the neurohumoral compensatory mechanisms.
   A. Surgical valve replacement is still not a practical option.
   B. Drugs that decrease left ventricular size (e.g., diuretics, vasodilators, and positive inotropic drugs) may reduce regurgitant volume by decreasing mitral annulus size.
   C. Arteriolar vasodilation also enhances forward cardiac output and reduces regurgitant volume by decreasing systemic arteriolar resistance.
II. Asymptomatic dogs with degenerative MR are usually not treated.
   A. Whether the benefits of angiotensin-converting enzyme inhibitor (ACEI) therapy outweigh the expense in asymptomatic dogs with significant left atrial enlargement is unclear at present.
   B. The possibility that ACEI therapy delays the onset of clinical signs and/or increases survival time in dogs with MR needs further exploration (Hamlin et al., 1996).
   C. A diet moderately restricted in sodium may be helpful because compensatory neurohumoral mechanisms interfere with normal renal excretion of sodium. Avoid high salt food or ''treats.''
III. Dogs with clinical signs during exercise or activity are treated with several modalities (Table 9–1).
   A. The severity of heart failure and the presence of complicating factors influence the choice of drugs and aggressiveness of therapy.
   B. Moderate dietary sodium restriction (e.g., diets formulated for dogs with kidney disease or geriatric dogs) is recommended.
      1. Diets formulated for dogs with heart failure provide further sodium restriction and can be

Table 9–1. **Drugs for Heart Failure (Dogs)**

Angiotensin-Converting Enzyme Inhibitors (ACEI)
Enalapril	0.5 mg/kg PO SID-BID
Captopril	0.5–2 mg/kg PO BID-TID
Lisinopril	0.5 mg/kg PO SID
Benazepril	0.25–0.5 mg/kg PO SID-BID

Other Vasodilators
Hydralazine	0.5–2 mg/kg PO BID (start low, especially if concurrent with ACEI)
Nitroglycerin ointment	¼–1 in. q 4–6 h, cutaneously
Nitroprusside	1 µg/kg/min IV (initial), titrate upwards based on blood pressure

Diuretics
Furosemide	1–4 mg/kg PO SID-TID chronically PO; or 2–4 mg/kg IV, IM, SQ q 2–6 h
Spironolactone	2 mg/kg PO SID
Hydrochlorothiazide	2–4 mg/kg PO SID-BID

Digoxin 0.005–0.01 mg/kg PO BID

Antiarrhythmic Agents
Atenolol	0.2–3 mg/kg PO SID-BID (start low, titrate to effect)
Propranolol	0.2–2 mg/kg PO BID-TID (start low, titrate to effect)
Diltiazem	0.5–1.5 mg/kg PO TID

used initially or reserved for dogs with more advanced failure.

   2. A reducing diet is recommended for overweight dogs.

C. An ACEI is generally prescribed for dogs with signs of failure (COVE Study Group, 1995; IMPROVE Study Group, 1995; King et al., 1995).

   1. Although ACEIs are not pure arteriolar vasodilating agents, their overall effects in modulating the neurohumoral response to heart failure make them more advantageous for chronic use.

   2. Hydralazine is a non-ACEI, pure arteriolar vasodilator that is less expensive, but it does not antagonize and may exacerbate neurohumoral compensatory mechanisms.

D. Dogs with radiographic evidence of pulmonary edema and/or more severe clinical signs are also treated with furosemide.

   1. If it is unclear whether respiratory signs are caused by heart failure or non-cardiac causes, an initial trial course of the diuretic furosemide is indicated.

   2. Once signs of failure are controlled, the dose and frequency of drug are reduced to the lowest effective levels.

   3. The use of furosemide alone (e.g., without an ACEI or digoxin) for heart failure is not recommended.

E. Digoxin therapy is regaining favor in the treatment of MR.

   1. Its benefit may come from its sensitizing effects on baroreceptors and resulting inhibition of sympathetic activation in heart failure (Ferguson, 1992).

   2. Digoxin is often added after an ACEI and furosemide have been initiated, especially if marked left ventricular enlargement is present.

   3. Other indications include frequent atrial premature beats or tachycardia, atrial fibrillation, or recurrent episodes of pulmonary edema despite use of furosemide and ACEI.

   4. Caution is required to avoid toxicity.

     a) Azotemia, hypokalemia, and some drugs (e.g., quinidine) predispose to toxicity.

     b) Serum drug concentrations are measured after 7–10 days of initiating or changing therapy; samples are drawn 8–10 hours after a dose.

     c) Therapeutic serum concentrations range from 0.8–2 ng/ml.

F. Exercise is restricted until signs of failure are well controlled, then mild to moderate activity as tolerated is encouraged.

IV. Dogs with shortness of breath at rest and evidence of severe pulmonary edema are treated aggressively.

A. Maximal restriction of activity, preferably cage rest, is enforced.

B. Oxygen supplementation is provided via cage, nasal tube, etc.

C. Furosemide 2–4 mg/kg IV is repeated every 1–4 hours as needed.

D. Vasodilator therapy with hydralazine 1–2 mg/kg PO BID may be considered.

   1. Hydralazine is used for acute therapy because of its direct and rapid vasodilating effect on arterioles.

   2. The neurohormonal activation of heart failure can be exacerbated by hydralazine, especially if hypotension is induced.

E. Alternatively, an ACEI can be used but has slower onset and less pronounced initial effect (see Table 9–1).

F. Topical nitroglycerin ¼–1 in. q 4–6 h can be used to reduce pulmonary venous pressure by direct venodilation, although its effectiveness is unclear.

G. Nitroprusside 1 μg/kg/min IV can be used instead of other vasodilators and provides arteriolar dilation and venodilation, but blood pressure must be closely monitored to avoid hypotension.

H. Stress is minimized by avoiding repeated handling and oral medication when possible.

I. Mild sedation with morphine 0.1–0.2 mg/kg SQ can be useful to reduce anxiety.

J. Bronchodilator therapy (e.g., aminophylline 6–10 mg/kg IM, SQ, PO TID) has been used to counteract possible bronchospasm with severe pulmonary edema. Effectiveness is unclear, although methylxanthines help support respiratory muscle function.

K. Digoxin treatment is started (or continued) (see Table 9–1) when paroxysmal atrial tachycardia or atrial fibrillation is present.

   1. Several days are needed to achieve therapeutic blood concentration at oral maintenance doses; intravenous digitalization is generally avoided unless the arrhythmia appears to be life threatening.

   2. Diltiazem or atenolol can be used instead of or in addition to digoxin for supraventricular tachyarrhythmias (see Chap. 7).

   3. If the animal with acute dyspnea has not previously received digoxin, maintenance therapy is initiated when the dyspnea has subsided.

L. When the animal is stabilized, medications are adjusted over several days to weeks to determine the best level for chronic treatment.

   1. Furosemide is titrated to the lowest dose (and longest dosing interval) that controls the signs.

   2. If hydralazine or nitroprusside was used initially, switching to an ACEI for chronic therapy is recommended.

V. Additional therapy may be needed for dogs with TR and right-sided congestive signs.

A. Pleural effusion characterized as more than "mild" is aspirated to improve pulmonary function.

B. Ascites severe enough to impede respiration or cause discomfort is drained.

VI. Emergency intervention may be needed for a left atrial tear.
  A. Acute cardiac tamponade can cause sudden death (see also Chap. 11).
  B. Immediate pericardiocentesis is indicated.
    1. Cautious fluid therapy or blood transfusion may help support cardiac output.
    2. Continued bleeding requires repeated pericardiocentesis or surgical attempt to close the atrial tear.

Patient Monitoring

I. Owners of asymptomatic dogs are educated as to the disease process and early signs of congestive heart failure.
  A. Instruct the owners to periodically check and record the pet's resting respiratory rate.
    1. An increase of over 15–20% that persists for several days may indicate early pulmonary edema.
    2. Accumulation of pleural effusion from TR tends to increase respiratory effort rather than respiratory rate.
  B. Resting heart rates can also be counted.
  C. Reevaluation of the animal's status is recommended at least once per year.
    1. A routine preventive health program is continued or implemented.
    2. Regular hematologic and biochemical testing is useful to screen for potentially complicating concurrent illness.
II. The reevaluation schedule for dogs receiving heart failure medications depends on the stability of the animal.
  A. Dogs with recently diagnosed or decompensated heart failure are checked more frequently (every several days to a week) until stable.
  B. Dogs with chronic congestive heart failure that appears well controlled are reevaluated several times per year.
  C. Reevaluation includes a general physical exam as well as a careful cardiovascular exam.
    1. An ECG is advisable if an arrhythmia or unexpectedly low or high heart rate is ausculted.
    2. If abnormal pulmonary sounds are ausculted, if the owner reports coughing or other respiratory signs, or if an increased resting respiratory rate is detected, chest radiographs are warranted.
    3. Measure at least serum electrolytes and renal function.
    4. Measure serum digoxin concentration 7–10 days after initiation or dosage change.
III. Reevaluate the animal with any recurrence of cough or respiratory distress to determine whether congestive heart failure has decompensated or another problem has developed.
  A. Abnormal pulmonary sounds or an arrhythmia as well as other abnormalities may be detected on physical exam.

B. Chest radiographs are indicated to identify the presence of pulmonary edema or patterns suggestive of other respiratory disease.
C. When an arrhythmia is suspected but not documented on routine ECG, 24-hour Holter monitoring may be helpful.
D. Echocardiography may show evidence of chordal rupture, progressive cardiomegaly, or worsened myocardial function.
E. Blood and urine tests may reveal abnormalities in other body systems.
F. Other causes of cough are considered if neither pulmonary edema nor venous congestion is seen radiographically and if resting respiratory rate has not increased.
  1. Compression of the left main bronchus by the enlarged left atrium can stimulate cough.
  2. Cough suppressants are used after other causes of cough are ruled out.
G. If decompensated congestive heart failure is present, therapy is intensified or modified as needed for the individual (see earlier discussion).
  1. Some dogs respond to an increased furosemide dose and rest for a few days and then can return to their previous medication levels.
  2. Increasing ACEI (e.g., enalapril) administration from SID to BID can be effective.
  3. If ACEI and furosemide doses are already maximized, low-dose hydralazine therapy could be added.
    a) Blood pressure is monitored carefully until the animal is stabilized.
    b) The ACEI dose may need to be reduced.
  4. The addition of another diuretic with a different mechanism of action (e.g., spironolactone 2 mg/kg BID) may reduce chronic refractory pulmonary edema.
  5. Continued monitoring, especially of renal function and serum electrolytes, is important.
IV. Episodes of transient weakness or syncope may be caused by intermittent tachyarrhythmias, atrial bleeding, cough-induced syncope, or other causes of reduced cardiac output.

INFECTIOUS DISEASES

Infectious Endocarditis

Definition

Invasion of any cardiac valve or endocardial surface by an infectious agent

Causes

I. Bacteria are the most common agents.
  A. *Streptococcus* spp., *Staphylococcus* spp., *Escherichia coli*, *Pasteurella* spp., *Corynebacterium* spp., *Pseudomonas aeruginosa,* and *Erysipelothrix rhusiopathiae* have been reported most often (Sisson, 1994).

1. Other bacterial and (rarely) fungal infections may occur.
2. *E. rhusiopathiae* isolates from dogs with endocarditis have also been identified as *Erysipelothrix tonsillarum* (Takahashi et al., 1993; Sisson, 1994).
   B. Bacteremia, either persistent or transient, is necessary for endocardial infection.
   1. Recurrent bacteremia can result from infections of the skin, mouth, urinary tract, prostate, lungs, and other organs.
   2. Dental procedures are known to cause transient bacteremia (Black et al., 1980).
   3. Other procedures presumed to cause transient bacteremia are endoscopy, urethral catheterization, and anal surgery.
II. Bacterial cultures are frequently negative.
   A. Some cases may be caused by fastidious organisms such as *Bartonella* spp. (Breitschwerdt et al., 1995).
   B. Negative blood cultures may occur with intermittent bacteremia.
   C. Sterile vegetations, consisting mainly of platelets and fibrin, may form at areas of endothelial damage.
   1. This is termed nonbacterial thrombotic endocarditis.
   2. Nonseptic emboli may break off from such vegetations and cause infarctions elsewhere.
   3. Bacteremia can also cause secondary infective endocarditis at these sites.
III. Physical damage to a valve or endothelial surface predisposes to infection if bacteremia occurs.
   A. Damage and/or hemodynamic factors resulting from turbulent blood flow cause lesions to be located downstream to disturbed flow (Korzeniowski and Kaye, 1992).
   B. Common sites include the ventricular side of the aortic valve with subaortic stenosis, the right ventricular side of a ventricular septal defect, and the atrial surface of the mitral valve with MR.
   C. Subaortic stenosis is associated with an increased incidence of aortic valve endocarditis (Muna et al., 1978; Sisson and Thomas, 1984).
IV. The incidence of bacterial endocarditis is relatively low in dogs and cats (Calvert et al., 1985; Elwood et al., 1993; Sisson, 1994).
   A. The prevalence of endocarditis increases with age.
   B. Male dogs are affected more commonly than females.
   C. Immunocompromised animals are thought to be at greater risk.
   D. Highly virulent organisms or a heavy bacterial load increases the chance of cardiac infection.

Pathophysiology

I. The mitral and aortic valves are most commonly infected in small animals (Sisson, 1994).
II. Vegetative lesions typically form on the infected valve surface.

   A. Vegetations consist of platelets, fibrin, red and white blood cells, and bacteria.
   B. Valve dysfunction occurs as a result of perforations and/or tearing of the leaflet(s).
   C. Valve stenosis caused by large vegetations is uncommon.
III. Infection can extend into adjacent structures (e.g., the valve annulus, myocardium, or pericardium) (Sisson, 1994).
   A. Rupture of infected chordae tendineae can lead to acute pulmonary edema.
   B. Aortic valve endocarditis may extend into the AV node to cause partial or complete AV block.
   C. Atrial or ventricular tachyarrhythmias may result from myocarditis or myocardial infarction.
IV. Embolization of other body sites with fragments of vegetative lesions causes diverse signs from infarction and/or metastatic infection.
   A. Emboli may be septic or bland (sterile).
   B. Septic arthritis, diskospondylitis, urinary tract infections, and renal and splenic infarctions may occur.
   C. Myocardial infarction occasionally occurs secondary to coronary embolization.
   D. Hypertrophic osteopathy has also been associated with bacterial endocarditis (Vulgamott and Clark, 1980; Sisson and Thomas, 1984).
V. Circulating immune complexes contribute to the disease syndrome.
   A. Sterile polyarthritis, glomerulonephritis, and other immune-mediated organ damage may result (Bennett and Taylor, 1988; Sisson, 1994).
   B. Results of rheumatoid factor and antinuclear antibody tests may be positive.
VI. Hemodynamic changes relate to acute or chronic valve insufficiency and resulting volume overload.
   A. Because left heart valves are usually affected, pulmonary congestion and edema from left-sided heart failure is most common.
   B. In the rare instance that valve stenosis might result from a large, obstructive vegetation, a pressure overload to the upstream chamber and murmur of valve obstruction would be expected.

Clinical Signs

I. Clinical signs are quite variable; so a high index of suspicion for this disease is important.
   A. Nonspecific signs of lethargy, weight loss, inappetence, and weakness may predominate.
   B. A clear history of predisposing factors is frequently absent.
II. Although cardiac signs (e.g., resulting from left-sided congestion or arrhythmias) may be the cause for presentation, they may also be overshadowed by dysfunction or infection of other organs.
III. Systemic signs result from infarction, infection, and immune-mediated damage.
   A. Recurrent fever is a suggestive sign but may be absent.
   B. Urinary signs are related to infection and hema-

turia, infarction and azotemia, or glomerulonephritis.

   C. Lameness can result from immune-mediated polyarthritis, septic arthritis, and diskospondylitis.
   D. Other signs can include gastrointestinal upsets, neurologic abnormalities, and signs of peripheral vasculitis.

Diagnosis

   I. Physical examination findings are variable.
      A. Auscultation of a cardiac murmur in a patient with no previously noted murmur may indicate infective valve damage; however, other causes of murmurs must be considered as well.
         1. The onset of a diastolic murmur at the left heart base is suspicious for aortic valve endocarditis, especially when fever or other signs are present.
         2. Endocarditis can also develop in an animal with a known murmur from other cardiac disease.
      B. Labored or rapid respirations, cough, and abnormal pulmonary sounds accompany left heart failure.
      C. Cardiac arrhythmias may be noted.
      D. Diverse signs of disease in any organ caused by septic or sterile emboli, primary infection, or immune phenomena make endocarditis "the great imitator" of other diseases.
   II. Radiographs may be unremarkable or show evidence of left heart failure.
      A. Cardiomegaly is absent or minimal early in the disease.
      B. Valve dysfunction and insufficiency cause cardiomegaly over time.
      C. Radiographic abnormalities may reflect other organ involvement (e.g., diskospondylitis).
   III. Electrocardiography may document premature beats, tachycardias, conduction disturbances, or evidence of myocardial ischemia.
   IV. Echocardiography is used to identify suspected vegetative lesions and abnormal valve motion.
      A. False-positive and false-negative "lesions" can mistakenly be identified, so cautious interpretation is important.
      B. Differentiation of mitral vegetations from degenerative thickening may be impossible.
      C. Poor or marginal quality images or use of lower frequency transducers may cause some vegetations to be missed because of suboptimal resolution.
      D. Measurement of chamber size and estimation of regurgitant volume and ventricular function are also done.
   V. Laboratory findings vary depending on the extent and distribution of disease.
      A. Blood cultures are submitted (Table 9–2).
         1. Submit at least three samples of ≥10 ml blood collected aseptically over a 24-hour period.

Table 9–2. *Criteria for Diagnosing Bacterial Endocarditis*

Possible Bacterial Endocarditis

Persistently positive (≥2) blood cultures plus one of the following:
- Preexisting valvular or predisposing congenital heart disease
- Clinical evidence of embolic phenomenon
- Fever (on presentation or documented historically)

Negative or intermittently positive blood cultures plus all of the following:
- Preexisting valvular or predisposing congenital heart disease
- Evidence of embolic phenomenon
- Fever (on presentation or documented historically)

Probable Bacterial Endocarditis

Persistently positive (≥2) blood cultures plus one of the following:
- Visible valve vegetation or leaflet destruction (echocardiography)
- Preexisting valvular or predisposing congenital heart disease, fever, and evidence of embolic phenomenon
- New regurgitant murmur (no murmur on prior recent examination)

Negative or intermittently positive blood cultures plus any of the following:
- Visible valve vegetation or leaflet destruction (echocardiography)
- Diastolic murmur, bounding pulses, and fever
- New systolic regurgitant murmur, fever, and evidence of embolic phenomenon

Definite Bacterial Endocarditis

Histologic confirmation of infective endocarditis
Bacteriology of vegetation or peripheral embolus

Modified from Sisson D: Bacterial endocarditis, p 84. In Proceedings of the 18th Annual WALTHAM/OSU Symposium for the Treatment of Small Animal Diseases. Cardiology, October 1994. Vernon, CA, 1994. Used with permission.

         2. Time between samples should be >1 hour.
         3. Both aerobic and anaerobic cultures are done.
         4. Prolonged incubation (3 weeks) is recommended because some bacteria are slow growing.
      B. Blood cultures are positive in approximately 75% of canine cases (Sisson, 1994).
         1. A negative culture does not rule out infective endocarditis.
         2. Chronic endocarditis, recent antibiotic therapy, fastidious or slow growing organisms, and noninfective endocarditis are some causes of negative cultures.
      C. Hematologic abnormalities often reflect acute or chronic inflammation.
         1. Neutrophilia with a left shift is typical with acute endocarditis.
         2. Mature neutrophilia with or without monocytosis tends to develop with chronicity.
         3. Non-regenerative anemia has been associated with about 50% of canine cases (Calvert et al., 1985).
      D. Other laboratory abnormalities are variable.
         1. Elevations in serum creatinine and urea nitro-

Table 9–3. *Miscellaneous Causes of Acquired Valvular Dysfunction*

Pulmonic Regurgitation
    Heartworm disease
    Other causes of pulmonary hypertension
Tricuspid Regurgitation
    Pulmonic stenosis
    Other causes of chronic RV outflow obstruction
    Dilated cardiomyopathy
    Traumatic papillary muscle avulsion
Mitral Regurgitation
    Chronic LV outflow obstruction
    Chronic LV volume overload (e.g., PDA)
    Dilated cardiomyopathy
    Traumatic papillary muscle avulsion

RV = right ventricular; LV = left ventricular; PDA = patent ductus arteriosus.

gen levels may occur with renal involvement, with or without heart failure.
  2. Urinalysis may show evidence of urinary tract infection or glomerulonephritis.

Differential Diagnoses

I. Cardiac considerations are related to the valve(s) involved (Table 9–3).
  A. Other causes of AV valve insufficiency include degenerative valve disease, congenital malformation (dysplasia), and dilated cardiomyopathy (in larger breeds).
  B. A diastolic murmur at the left heart base is usually caused by aortic insufficiency.
    1. Although endocarditis is the most common cause, congenital malformations of the left ventricular outflow tract can cause aortic regurgitation as well as a systolic murmur.
    2. Degenerative disease rarely causes audible aortic regurgitation in small animals.
    3. Pulmonic regurgitation is occasionally audible, especially with pulmonary hypertension.
II. Differential lists for systemic signs are extensive and include causes of local as well as disseminated infections, primary immune-mediated diseases, and other causes of fever.

Treatment

I. Aggressive therapy with bactericidal antibiotics capable of penetrating fibrin is indicated.
II. The choice of drug is ideally guided by positive culture results.
  A. Broad spectrum combination therapy is usually begun immediately after blood samples have been obtained for culture.
  B. Therapy can be changed if necessary when culture results are available.
  C. Patients with negative cultures are continued on the broad spectrum regimen.
III. An initial combination of a cephalosporin (e.g., cefa-

zolin 25 mg/kg QID) or penicillin 20–40 $\times 10^3$ U/kg QID with an aminoglycoside (e.g., gentamicin 2–4 mg/kg TID or amikacin 5–10 mg/kg TID) is commonly employed.
IV. Antimicrobial administration is IV or IM for at least the first week in order to obtain higher and more predictable blood concentrations.
V. Duration of antimicrobial therapy is at least 2–4 weeks to increase the likelihood that all bacteria have sufficient exposure to the drug. Therapy for 6–8 weeks is often recommended.

Patient Monitoring

I. Close monitoring is important to detect and treat complications as soon as possible.
  A. Adverse drug effects can occur (e.g., renal toxicity, GI disturbances).
  B. Cardiovascular decompensation can develop.
    1. Congestive heart failure is treated as described previously.
    2. Tachyarrhythmias and conduction abnormalities are monitored and treated appropriately (see Chap. 7).
  C. Complications related to the primary source of infection, embolic events, or immune reaction must be addressed.
II. The prognosis tends to be guarded to poor for the long term (O'Grady, 1995).
  A. Death is usually related to congestive heart failure, sepsis, embolic events, or renal failure.
  B. Aortic valve involvement and gram-negative organisms independently appear to worsen the prognosis.
III. The use of prophylactic antimicrobial drugs in animals at risk is controversial.
  A. If the experience in people is applicable to dogs and cats, most cases of infective endocarditis are not preventable (Korzeniowski and Kaye, 1992).
  B. In view of the increased incidence of this disease with subaortic stenosis, antimicrobial prophylaxis is recommended for these animals prior to dental or other "dirty" procedures (e.g., involving the intestinal or urogenital systems).
  C. Antimicrobial prophylaxis may also be considered in immunocompromised animals.

Bibliography

Beardow AW, Buchanan JW: Chronic mitral valve disease in cavalier King Charles spaniels: 95 cases (1987–1991). J Am Vet Med Assoc 203:1023, 1993

Bennett D, Taylor DJ: Bacterial endocarditis and inflammatory joint disease in the dog. J Small Anim Pract 29:347, 1988

Black AP, Crichlow AM, Saunders JR: Bacteremia during ultrasonic teeth cleaning and extraction in the dog. J Am Anim Hosp Assoc 16:611, 1980

Bonagura JD: Echocardiography. J Am Vet Med Assoc 204:516, 1994

Braunwald E: Pathophysiology of heart failure. p. 393. In Braunwald E (ed): Heart Disease: A Textbook of Cardiovascular Medicine. 4th Ed. WB Saunders, Philadelphia, 1992a

Braunwald E: Assessment of cardiac function. p. 419. In Braunwald E (ed): Heart Disease: A Textbook of Cardiovascular Medicine. 4th Ed. WB Saunders, Philadelphia, 1992b

Braunwald E: Valvular heart disease. p. 1007. In Braunwald E (ed): Heart Disease: A Textbook of Cardiovascular Medicine. 4th Ed. WB Saunders, Philadelphia, 1992c

Breitschwerdt EB, Kordick DL, Malarkey DE et al: Endocarditis in a dog due to infection with a novel *Bartonella* subspecies. J Clin Microbiol 33:154, 1995

Buchanan JW: Chronic valvular disease (endocardiosis) in dogs. Adv Vet Sci Comp Med 21:75, 1979

Buchanan JW: Causes and prevalence of cardiovascular disease. p. 647. In Kirk RW, Bonagura JD (eds): Current Veterinary Therapy XI: Small Animal Practice. WB Saunders, Philadelphia, 1992

Buchanan JW, Bücheler J: Vertebral scale system to measure canine heart size in radiographs. J Am Vet Med Assoc 206:194, 1995

Calvert CA, Greene CE, Hardie EM: Cardiovascular infections in dogs: epizootiology, clinical manifestations and prognosis. J Am Vet Med Assoc 187:612, 1985

COVE Study Group: Controlled clinical evaluation of enalapril in dogs with heart failure: results of the cooperative veterinary study group. J Vet Intern Med 9:243, 1995

Darke PGG: Mitral valve disease in cavalier King Charles spaniels. p. 837. In Bonagura JD (ed): Kirk's Current Veterinary Therapy XII. WB Saunders, Philadelphia, 1995

Davila-Roman VG, Creswell LL, Rosenbloom M et al: Myocardial contractile state in dogs with chronic mitral regurgitation: echocardiographic approach to the peak systolic pressure/end systolic area relationship. Am Heart J 126:155, 1993

Donoghue S, Kronfeld DS: Home-made diets. p. 445. In Wills JM, Simpson K (eds): The Waltham Book of Clinical Nutrition of the Dog and Cat. Pergamon/Elsevier Science Inc, Tarrytown, New York, 1994

Elwood CM, Cobb MA, Stepien RL: Clinical and echocardiographic findings in 10 dogs with vegetative bacterial endocarditis. J Small Anim Practice 34:420, 1993

Feigenbaum H: Acquired valvular heart disease. p. 239. In Feigenbaum H: Echocardiography. 5th Ed. Lea & Febiger, Philadelphia, 1994

Ferguson DW: Digitalis and neurohormonal abnormalities in heart failure and implications for therapy. Am J Cardiol 69:24G, 1992

Haggstrom J, Hansson K, Karlberg BE et al: Plasma concentration of atrial natriuretic peptide in relation to severity of mitral regurgitation in cavalier King Charles spaniels. Am J Vet Res 55:698, 1994

Haggstrom J, Hansson K, Kvart C et al: Chronic valvular disease in the cavalier King Charles spaniel in Sweden. Vet Rec 131:549, 1992

Haggstrom J, Kvart C, Hansson K: Heart sounds and murmurs: changes related to severity of chronic valvular disease in the cavalier King Charles spaniel. J Vet Intern Med 9:75, 1995

Hamlin RL, Benitz AM, Ericsson GF et al: Effects of enalapril on exercise tolerance and longevity in dogs with heart failure produced by iatrogenic mitral regurgitation. J Vet Intern Med 10:85, 1996

IMPROVE Study Group: Acute and short-term hemodynamic, echocardiographic, and clinical effects of enalapril maleate in dogs with naturally acquired heart failure: results of the invasive multicenter prospective veterinary evaluation of enalapril study. J Vet Intern Med 9:234, 1995

Jacobs GJ, Calvert CA, Mahaffey MB et al: Echocardiographic detection of flail left atrioventricular valve cusp from ruptured chordae tendineae in 4 dogs. J Vet Intern Med 9:341, 1995

Kaplan PM, Fox PR, Garvey MS et al: Acute mitral regurgitation with papillary muscle rupture in a dog. J Am Vet Med Assoc 191:1436, 1987

Kihara Y, Sasayama S, Miyazaki S et al: Role of the left atrium in adaptation of the heart to chronic mitral regurgitation in conscious dogs. Circ Res 62:543, 1988

King JN, Mauron C, Kaiser G: Pharmacokinetics of the active metabolite of benazepril, benazeprilat, and inhibition of plasma angiotensin-converting enzyme activity after single and repeated administration to dogs. Am J Vet Res 56:1620, 1995

Kittleson MD, Eyster GE, Knowlen GG et al: Myocardial function in small dogs with chronic mitral regurgitation and severe congestive heart failure. J Am Vet Med Assoc 184:455, 1984

Korzeniowski OM, Kaye D: Infective endocarditis. p. 1078. In Braunwald E (ed): Heart Disease: A Textbook of Cardiovascular Medicine. 4th Ed. WB Saunders, Philadelphia, 1992

Lewis LD, Morris ML, Hand MS: Small Animal Clinical Nutrition III. Mark Morris Associates, Topeka, Kansas, 1987

Malik R, Hunt GB, Porges WL et al: Traumatic tricuspid insufficiency in a dog. J Am Anim Hosp Assoc 27:467, 1991

Muna WFT, Ferrans VJ, Pierce JE et al: Discrete subaortic stenosis in Newfoundland dogs: association of infective endocarditis. Am J Cardiol 41:746, 1978

O'Grady MR: Acquired valvular heart disease. p. 944. In Ettinger SJ, Feldman EC (eds): Textbook of Veterinary Internal Medicine. 4th Ed. WB Saunders, Philadelphia, 1995

Pedersen HD, Kock J, Poulsen K et al: Activation of the renin-angiotensin system in dogs with asymptomatic and mildly symptomatic mitral valvular insufficiency. J Vet Intern Med 9:328, 1995

Sisson D: Acquired valvular heart disease in dogs and cats. p. 59. In Bonagura JD (ed): Contemporary Issues in Small Animal Practice—Cardiology. Churchill Livingstone, New York, 1987

Sisson D: Bacterial endocarditis. Proc Annual Watham/OSU Symposium on Cardiology 18:79, 1994

Sisson D, Thomas WP: Endocarditis of the aortic valve. J Am Vet Med Assoc 184:570, 1984

Sisson D, Brown W, Riepe R: Hemodynamic effects of atrial fibrillation in dogs with experimentally induced mitral regurgitation. Proc Am Coll Vet Intern Med 13:1015, 1995

Takahashi T, Tamura Y, Yoshimura H et al: *Erysipelothrix tonsillarum* isolated from dogs with endocarditis in Belgium. Res Vet Sci 54:264, 1993

Vulgamott JC, Clark RG: Arterial hypertension and hypertrophic pulmonary osteopathy associated with aortic valvular endocarditis in a dog. J Am Vet Med Assoc 177:243, 1980

Ware WA: Congestive heart failure: pathophysiology and therapeutic implications. Proc Annual Watham/OSU Symposium on Cardiology 18:15, 1994

10

Myocardial Disease

Kathryn M. Meurs

CANINE DILATED CARDIOMYOPATHY

Definition

I. It is a functional abnormality of the myocardium causing systolic dysfunction.
II. Boxer cardiomyopathy is a primary myocardial disorder characterized by unique histologic changes of the myocardium.
   A. Dilation of the atria and ventricle is typically mild.
   B. Ventricular arrhythmias are common.
III. Dilated cardiomyopathy also occurs in the cocker spaniel, Doberman pinscher, and other large- and giant-breed dogs, including the Great Dane, Irish wolfhound, and Newfoundland.
IV. Breed and species differences exist.

Causes

I. Cause is usually unknown.
II. Carnitine deficiency has been reported in one family of boxers (Keene et al., 1991).
III. American cocker spaniels may have dilated cardiomyopathy associated with decreased serum taurine and/or carnitine levels, although a cause and effect relationship has not been established.

Pathophysiology

I. Decreased left ventricular systolic function is the primary abnormality; diastolic dysfunction also occurs.
II. Left atrial and left ventricular dilation may occur before obvious functional changes develop.
III. Dilation of the ventricle and mitral valve annulus may cause mitral regurgitation.
IV. Pulmonary edema may develop secondary to elevated ventricular filling pressures.
V. Arrhythmias may contribute to clinical signs.

Clinical Signs

I. The average age of affected boxers is 8 years (6 months to 15 years).
   A. Three clinical classifications are reported (Harpster, 1983).
   B. Class I dogs are asymptomatic but have an arrhythmia detected by physical examination.
   C. Class II dogs have a history of syncope or episodic weakness.
   D. Class III dogs may present with congestive heart failure and arrhythmias.
II. Affected cocker spaniels are between 2 and 9 years of age. Clinical signs include cough, acute dyspnea, exercise intolerance, and ascites.
III. The average age of affected Doberman pinschers is 6.5 years (1–14.5 years). Incidence of disease increases with age.
   A. Males may present more frequently than females.
   B. Clinical signs may include cough, respiratory distress, exercise intolerance, and weight loss.
   C. Sudden death is reported frequently.
IV. Giant- and large-breed dogs have similar presentations.
   A. Males appear to be affected more frequently than females.
   B. Clinical signs include exercise intolerance, dyspnea, coughing, and ascites.

Diagnosis

I. Physical examination
   A. Boxers
      1. A systolic murmur and/or gallop (S3) may be ausculted at the left apex.
      2. Arrhythmias are common.
      3. Signs of right heart failure (ascites and jugular venous distention) may be observed.
   B. Cocker spaniels
      1. A systolic murmur and/or gallop rhythm (S3) at the left apex or an arrhythmia may be ausculted.

2. Ascites and jugular venous distention may be observed.

C. Doberman pinschers
1. A systolic murmur and/or gallop rhythm (S3) is frequently ausculted at the left apex.
2. An arrhythmia may be noted.
3. Biventricular failure occasionally occurs; clinical signs may include ascites and jugular venous distention.

D. Large and giant breeds
1. A systolic murmur, gallop rhythm (S3), or arrhythmia may be ausculted.
2. Jugular venous distention and ascites may be noted when right ventricular failure occurs.

II. Electrocardiography
A. Boxers
1. Ventricular premature complexes (VPCs) may be present singly, in pairs, and in runs of paroxysmal ventricular tachycardia. VPCs typically have a wide, upright QRS in leads I, II, III, and AVF.
2. Supraventricular premature complexes are occasionally seen.

B. Cocker spaniels
1. Increased R wave amplitude (>3 mV in lead II) is suggestive of left ventricular enlargement.
2. Supraventricular or ventricular arrhythmias may occur.

C. Doberman pinschers
1. Left ventricular enlargement (R >3.5 mV in lead II) or left bundle branch block (QRS >0.08 second) may be noted.
2. Ventricular arrhythmias are common.
3. Atrial fibrillation is reported in at least 20% of cases.

D. Large and giant breeds
1. Atrial fibrillation is the most common arrhythmia observed.
2. Increased R wave amplitude (3.5 mV in lead II) is suggestive of left ventricular enlargement.
3. Ventricular premature complexes may occur.

III. Radiography
A. Boxers
1. Thoracic radiographs may be normal.
2. Generalized cardiomegaly with pulmonary edema and/or pleural effusion may be noted.

B. Cocker spaniels
1. Left atrial and ventricular enlargement or generalized cardiomegaly may be seen.
2. Pulmonary venous distention and pulmonary edema may be noted.

C. Doberman pinschers
1. Left atrial and ventricular enlargement is common.
2. Pulmonary venous distention with a patchy distribution of pulmonary edema denotes left-sided congestive heart failure.

D. Large and giant breeds
1. Generalized cardiomegaly may be seen.

2. Pulmonary edema and, less commonly, pleural effusion may be observed.

IV. Echocardiography
A. Boxers
1. Ventricular dimensions may be normal to increased.
2. Contractility may be normal or decreased.

B. Cocker spaniels
1. Left ventricular and left atrial dilation are common.
2. Decreased systolic function is seen in the majority of cases.

C. Doberman pinschers
1. Left ventricular and left atrial dilation are frequently seen.
2. Occult disease is suspected if left ventricular diastolic dimension is >46 mm and left ventricular systolic dimension is >38 mm (O'Grady, 1995).
3. Systolic dysfunction is frequently severe.

D. Large and giant breeds
1. Left atrial and ventricular dilation with decreased systolic function may be seen.
2. Right ventricular dilation may also be noted.

V. Clinical pathology
A. Baseline chemistry panel and electrolytes are evaluated before starting therapy.
B. American cocker spaniels require further testing.
1. Decreased plasma taurine levels have been reported in some American cocker spaniels with dilated cardiomyopathy.
2. Plasma taurine levels (normal range; 44–224 nmol/ml) may be evaluated to help guide therapeutic interventions.

Differential Diagnosis

I. Primary valvular disease: see Chap. 9
II. Congenital cardiac disease: see Chap. 6
III. Pleural disease: see Chap. 19
IV. Thoracic or mediastinal neoplasia: see Chap. 20

Treatment

I. Treatment is individualized based on breed, clinical signs, presence of arrhythmias, and/or congestive heart failure.
II. If pleural effusion is present, thoracocentesis is performed and as much fluid is removed as possible. Fluid is then submitted for analysis.
III. If thoracic radiographs document pulmonary edema, furosemide is given.
A. If the dog is dyspneic, furosemide may be given IV, IM, or SQ at 2–4 mg/kg BID-TID.
B. Once the dog's condition is stabilized, the dosage is decreased to 1–2 mg/kg PO SID-BID.
IV. Digoxin is given for its positive inotropic effects at a dose of 0.22 mg/m² PO BID.
V. Angiotensin-converting enzyme inhibitors are given for their vasodilation and favorable neurohormonal effects. Enalapril may be given at 0.25–0.5 mg/kg PO SID-BID.

VI. Antiarrhythmic therapy is initiated as needed for specific arrhythmias (see Chap. 7).

VII. Taurine supplementation can be tried, especially in American cocker spaniels, at a dose of 500 mg PO TID.

Patient Monitoring

I. Serum electrolytes, blood urea nitrogen (BUN), and creatinine are measured before starting therapy, 7 days after starting therapy, and then every 4–6 weeks.

II. Serum digoxin level is evaluated 10–14 days after starting therapy and should be between 1–2 ng/ml 8 hours after the pill is administered. Serum digoxin levels are also reevaluated if signs of digoxin toxicity (vomiting, nausea, loss of appetite, or arrhythmias) occur.

III. Thoracic radiographs are repeated as needed for evaluation of any tachypnea and dyspnea that may occur as the disease progresses.

IV. Electrocardiography is repeated if syncope has developed, heart rate has increased, or a new arrhythmia has been ausculted.

V. Echocardiography is reevaluated if there is a sudden decrease in the animal's condition or the animal does not appear to respond to appropriate therapy.

VI. Prognosis varies among breeds.
   A. Boxers
      1. Class I dogs have a fairly good prognosis (>1 year) but are still at a risk of sudden death.
      2. Class II dogs have a variable prognosis and are at risk of sudden death.
      3. Class III dogs have the worst prognosis (possibly <6 months).
   B. Cocker spaniels: accurate prognostication difficult
   C. Doberman pinschers
      1. They have the worst prognosis.
      2. Once clinical signs have developed, death usually occurs as a result of heart failure or sudden death within 6 months.

FELINE DILATED CARDIOMYOPATHY

Definition and Causes

I. It is a functional abnormality of the myocardium causing systolic dysfunction.

II. Taurine deficiency is the most common cause.

III. A small percentage of cats have dilated cardiomyopathy and normal plasma taurine levels; the cause in these cases is unknown.

Pathophysiology

I. Decreased left ventricular systolic function is the primary abnormality; diastolic dysfunction also occurs.

II. Left atrial and left ventricular dilation may occur before obvious functional changes develop.

III. Dilation of the ventricle and mitral valve annulus may cause mitral regurgitation.

IV. Pulmonary edema may develop secondary to elevated ventricular filling pressures.

V. Arrhythmias may contribute to clinical signs.

VI. Thrombi may develop in the dilated atria.

Clinical Signs

I. Middle-aged or older cats are typically affected.

II. Dyspnea and respiratory distress are frequent presenting complaints.

III. Acute hindlimb paralysis suggests distal aortic embolization.

Diagnosis

I. Physical examination
   A. An auscultable murmur and/or gallop rhythm (S3) is commonly detected.
   B. Arrhythmias less commonly occur.
   C. Retinal changes may be noted with taurine deficiency.
   D. Distal aortic embolization may cause stiffened hindlimbs, absent or weak femoral pulses, and pale, cold footpads. These findings may be bilateral or unilateral (see also Chap. 25).

II. Electrocardiography
   A. Increased QRS amplitude (>1.0 mV R in lead II) suggests left ventricular enlargement.
   B. Ventricular tachyarrhythmias are occasionally noted.
   C. Conduction disturbances can occur.

III. Radiography
   A. Left atrial and ventricular enlargement or generalized cardiomegaly may be observed.
   B. Pulmonary venous distention, patchy pulmonary edema, and pleural effusion denote congestive heart failure.

IV. Echocardiography
   A. Left atrial and ventricular dilation with decreased left ventricular systolic function is observed.
   B. Left atrial thrombi may be seen.
   C. Right atrial and ventricular enlargement can occur secondary to chronic pulmonary edema and pulmonary hypertension.

V. Laboratory evaluation
   A. Baseline chemistry panel and electrolyte levels are evaluated before starting therapy.
   B. Plasma taurine levels are measured (normal mean is 90 nmol/ml; range, 40–140 nmol/ml). Taurine levels are typically low (<30 nmol/ml) with taurine deficiency.
   C. Pleural effusion is most commonly a modified transudate, but chylous effusions also occur.

Differential Diagnosis

I. Primary valvular disease: see Chap. 9

II. Congenital cardiac disease: see Chap. 6

III. Pleural disease: see Chap. 19
IV. Thoracic or mediastinal neoplasia: see Chap. 20

Treatment

I. Treatment is individualized based on clinical signs, presence of arrhythmias, and/or congestive heart failure.
II. If pleural effusion is present, thoracocentesis is performed to remove as much fluid as possible. Fluid is then submitted for analysis.
III. If thoracic radiographs document pulmonary edema, furosemide is given.
   A. If the cat is dyspneic, furosemide is given IV, IM, or SQ at 1–3 mg/kg BID-TID.
   B. Once the cat's condition is stabilized, the dose is decreased to 1–2 mg/kg PO SID-BID.
IV. Digoxin is given for its positive inotropic effects at 0.0312 mg/cat PO QOD-SID.
V. Taurine supplementation is given until taurine deficiency is ruled out at a dose of 250–500 mg PO BID.
VI. Angiotensin-converting enzyme inhibitors may be given for their vasodilation and favorable neurohormonal effects. Enalapril is used at 0.25–0.5 mg/kg PO SID-QOD.
VII. Antiarrhythmic therapy is initiated as needed for specific arrhythmias (see Chap. 7).
VIII. If thromboembolism has occurred, acepromazine (0.1–0.2 mg/kg SQ TID) is given for sedation and mild vasodilation. Heparin may be given at 100 IU/kg SQ TID to prevent additional clot formation (Harpster and Baty, 1995).
IX. Prevention of thromboembolism may be attempted with aspirin or coumadin; however, thromboembolism may still occur.
   A. Aspirin: 25 mg/kg PO q 72 h
   B. Warfarin (Coumadin): dosage based on frequent monitoring; spontaneous hemorrhage a potential complication

Patient Monitoring

I. Serum electrolytes, BUN, and creatinine are measured before starting therapy, 7 days after starting therapy, and every 4–6 weeks during therapy.
II. Serum digoxin level is evaluated 10–14 days after starting therapy and should be between 1 and 2 ng/ml 8 hours after administration.
III. Radiographs are repeated as necessary for any tachypnea and dyspnea that may occur as the disease progresses.
IV. Echocardiography is repeated after starting taurine therapy. Cats with taurine deficiency often show echocardiographic improvement in 4–6 weeks.
V. If taurine deficiency exists and is diagnosed before severe congestive heart failure occurs, the prognosis is good.
VI. If dilated cardiomyopathy is not caused by taurine deficiency, the prognosis is usually poor.
VII. If thromboembolism has occurred, perfusion of the hindlegs is provided by collateral circulation and some muscle function may return. However, a second embolic episode may occur, and this is usually associated with a poor prognosis.

CANINE HYPERTROPHIC CARDIOMYOPATHY

Definition and Cause

I. Left ventricular concentric hypertrophy and increased ventricular muscle mass in absence of causative systemic or cardiac disease
II. Etiology unknown

Pathophysiology

I. Hypertrophy of the left ventricular free wall and/or interventricular septum causes diastolic dysfunction. Increased myocardial stiffness and decreased lumen size due to hypertrophy are contributing factors.
II. Mitral regurgitation frequently develops from distortion of the mitral valve apparatus.
III. Increased left atrial pressure develops to fill the stiffened left ventricle. Elevated pulmonary venous pressure and pulmonary edema may develop.

Clinical Signs

I. The disease is rare, and clinical information is sparse.
II. Clinical presentation can vary from asymptomatic to congestive heart failure.
III. Syncope can occur.

Diagnosis

I. Physical examination
   A. Systolic murmur or a gallop rhythm (S4) may be auscultated.
   B. Weak femoral pulses may be present.
II. Electrocardiogram
   A. Conduction abnormalities, including left anterior fascicular block, are common.
   B. The electrocardiogram may be normal.
III. Echocardiography
   A. Left ventricular free wall and/or septal hypertrophy may be observed.
   B. Dynamic obstruction of the left ventricle may be observed.

Differential Diagnosis

I. Subaortic stenosis
II. Infiltrative myocardial disease
III. Systemic hypertension

Treatment

I. If pleural effusion is present, thoracocentesis is performed and as much fluid as possible is removed. Fluid is then submitted for analysis.
II. If thoracic radiographs document pulmonary edema, furosemide is given.

A. If the animal is dyspneic, furosemide is given IV, IM, or SQ at 2–4 mg/kg TID.

B. Once the animal is stabilized, the dose is decreased to 1–2 mg/kg PO SID-BID.

III. If the animal is symptomatic or tachycardiac, consider beta blocker or calcium channel blocker therapy.

A. Beta blockers are preferred with dynamic outflow obstruction or persistent tachycardia. Atenolol, a selective β_1 blocker, may be given at 6.25–25 mg/dog PO BID.

B. Calcium channel blockers are sometimes preferred. Diltiazem may be given at 0.5–1.5 mg/kg PO TID.

IV. If refractory heart failure exists, consider adding enalapril at a dose of 0.25–0.5 mg/kg PO SID-BID.

Patient Monitoring

I. Electrolytes, especially potassium, BUN, and serum creatine are monitored before starting therapy, 7 days after starting therapy, and then every 4–6 weeks.

II. Owners can monitor respiratory rate and watch for signs of dyspnea at home.

III. Radiographs are taken to evaluate for pulmonary edema if dyspnea or tachypnea develops.

IV. An electrocardiogram is evaluated 2 weeks after starting therapy and then every 8–12 weeks.

V. Echocardiography is reevaluated every 16–20 weeks, or if the animal's condition suddenly deteriorates.

FELINE HYPERTROPHIC CARDIOMYOPATHY

Definition and Cause

I. Left ventricular concentric hypertrophy and increased ventricular muscle mass in the absence of causative systemic or cardiac disease

II. Etiology unknown

III. Familial hypertrophic cardiomyopathy in Maine coon cats

Pathophysiology

I. Hypertrophy of the left ventricular free wall and/or interventricular septum causes diastolic dysfunction. Increased myocardial stiffness and decreased lumen size due to hypertrophy are contributing factors.

II. Mitral regurgitation and systolic anterior motion of the mitral valve frequently develop from distortion of the mitral valve apparatus.

III. Increased left atrial pressure develops to fill the stiffened left ventricle. Elevated pulmonary venous pressure and pulmonary edema may develop.

IV. Pulmonary hypertension and right ventricular enlargement may occur.

V. Thrombi may develop in the dilated atria.

Clinical Signs

I. Affected cats may be asymptomatic.

II. Cough, dyspnea, and shortness of breath may be presenting complaints.

III. Acute hindlimb paralysis suggests distal aortic embolization.

IV. Sudden death can occur.

Diagnosis

I. Hyperthyroidism and systemic hypertension can cause concentric hypertrophy and a similar clinical presentation. A diagnosis of hypertrophic cardiomyopathy should not be made until these have been excluded (see Chaps. 41 and 47).

II. Physical examination

A. A systolic murmur and/or gallop rhythm are common.

B. Distal aortic embolism may cause stiffened hindlimbs, absent or weak femoral pulse, and pale, cold footpads. These findings may be bilateral or unilateral (see also Chap. 25).

III. Electrocardiography

A. Increased R wave amplitude (1 mV R in lead II) suggests left ventricular enlargement.

B. Increased P wave width (0.04 second) suggests left atrial enlargement.

C. Conduction disturbances and arrhythmias (ventricular and supraventricular) may be noted.

IV. Thoracic radiography

A. Generalized cardiomegaly with biatrial enlargement and pleural effusion is seen most frequently.

B. Pulmonary venous distention and patchy pulmonary edema are less common.

V. Echocardiography

A. Left ventricular free wall and/or interventricular septal hypertrophy (>6 mm at end-diastole) are typical.

B. Left atrial or biatrial dilation may be noted.

C. Systolic anterior motion of the mitral valve with mitral regurgitation may be observed.

D. Thrombi may be observed in the left atria.

Differential Diagnosis

I. Hyperthyroidism

II. Aortic stenosis

III. Infiltrative myocardial disease

IV. Systemic hypertension

Treatment

I. If pleural effusion is present, thoracocentesis is performed and as much fluid is removed as possible. Fluid is then submitted for analysis.

II. If thoracic radiographs document pulmonary edema, furosemide is given.

A. If the animal is dyspneic, furosemide is given IV, IM, or SQ at 1–3 mg/kg TID.

B. Once the animal is stabilized, the dose is decreased to 1–2 mg/kg PO SID-BID.

III. If the animal is symptomatic or tachycardiac, consider beta blocker or calcium channel blocker therapy.
   A. Beta blockers are preferred in cats with dynamic outflow obstruction or persistent tachycardia. Atenolol, a selective β_1 blocker, may be given at 6.25–12.5 mg/cat PO SID-BID.
   B. Calcium channel blockers are sometimes preferred. Diltiazem may be given at 1.5–2.4 mg/kg PO BID-TID.
   C. If refractory heart failure exists, consider adding enalapril at a dose of 0.25–0.5 mg/kg SID-QOD.
   D. Prevention of thromboembolism may be attempted with aspirin or Coumadin; however, thromboembolism may still occur (Harpster and Baty, 1995).
      1. Aspirin: 25 mg/kg PO q 72 h
      2. Warfarin (Coumadin): requires frequent monitoring; spontaneous hemorrhage a potential complication

Patient Monitoring

I. Electrolytes, especially potassium, BUN, and serum creatine are monitored before starting therapy, 7 days after starting therapy, and then every 4–6 weeks.
II. Owner should monitor respiratory rate and watch for signs of dyspnea at home. Radiographs are taken to evaluate for pulmonary edema or pleural effusion if dyspnea or tachypnea develops.
III. Heart rate is evaluated 2 weeks after starting therapy.
   A. Optimal heart rate after starting therapy is between 140 and 160 beats/min.
   B. Heart rate is then reevaluated every 4–6 weeks.
IV. Echocardiography is reevaluated every 4–6 months and if the animal's condition suddenly deteriorates.
V. Prognosis is as follows.
   A. If the cat is asymptomatic at the time of diagnosis, with mild hypertrophy and normal atrial size, the prognosis may be good for an extended period of time.
   B. If the cat is asymptomatic with significant hypertrophy but normal left atrial size, the prognosis is fair. If the left atrium is enlarged, there is an increased risk of thromboembolism, and prognosis is poorer.
   C. Prognosis for cats that have suffered an embolic episode is poor. Although cats may regain some motor function of the hindlegs, there is a risk of a second embolic episode, and progression of significant heart disease may also occur.

FELINE RESTRICTIVE CARDIOMYOPATHY

Definition and Cause

I. It is a myocardial disorder characterized by a thickened, fibrotic endocardium, variable wall thickness, stiffened ventricular wall, and impaired ventricular filling.

II. Systolic function may be normal or decreased.
III. Etiology is unknown.

Pathophysiology

I. Increased left atrial pressure develops to fill the stiffened left ventricle. Elevated pulmonary venous pressure and pulmonary edema may then occur.
II. Pulmonary hypertension and right ventricular enlargement may occur.
III. Thrombi commonly develop in the markedly dilated atria.

Clinical Signs

I. Middle-aged or older cats are affected most commonly.
II. Historical complaints may include decreased activity, tachypnea, and respiratory distress.
III. Physical examination may reveal the following.
   A. A gallop rhythm (S3 or S4), systolic murmur, or arrhythmia may be ausculted.
   B. If there is concurrent right ventricular involvement, jugular venous distention can occur.
IV. The risk of thromboembolism appears to be higher than that of dilated or hypertrophic cardiomyopathy and may be suspected if physical examination reveals the following.
   A. Stiffened hindlimbs with absent or weak femoral pulses (bilateral or unilateral)
   B. Pale, cold footpads (bilateral or unilateral)

Diagnosis

I. Suspicious history and physical examination findings
II. Electrocardiography
   A. A widened QRS complex (>0.05 second) or tall R wave amplitude (>1 mV in lead II) suggests left ventricular enlargement.
   B. Left bundle branch block and other conduction disturbances may occur.
   C. Ventricular and atrial arrhythmias are occasionally seen.
III. Radiography
   A. Marked left atrial enlargement is common.
   B. Left ventricular enlargement or generalized cardiomegaly may be noted.
   C. Pulmonary venous distention and pulmonary edema associated with left heart failure may be observed.
   D. Pleural effusion and right atrial and right ventricular enlargement may be seen secondary to pulmonary hypertension.
IV. Clinical pathology
   A. Baseline chemistry panel and electrolytes are evaluated before starting therapy and are typically within normal limits.
   B. Fluid analysis of pleural fluid may be consistent with transudate, modified transudate, or chyle.
V. Echocardiography
   A. Left atrial or biatrial enlargement is usually marked.

B. Left ventricular dilation is usually mild.

C. Fractional shortening and other contractile parameters may be decreased.

D. Focal or diffuse subendocardial hyperechogenicity (fibrosis) may be found, with a thickened hyperechoic fibrous tissue bridging the septum and free wall.

E. Atrial or ventricular thrombi may be observed.

Differential Diagnosis

I. Primary thoracic or pulmonary disorders (neoplasia, lung lobe torsion) that result in pleural effusion

II. Infiltrative cardiac disease: neoplasia, amyloidosis

Treatment

I. If the cat is symptomatic, consider the following.
   A. If the animal is dyspneic, furosemide 1–3 mg/kg IV, IM, or SQ TID
   B. Enalapril 0.25–0.5 mg/kg PO SID-QOD
   C. Aspirin 25 mg/kg PO every third day for prevention of thromboembolism

II. If the cat is in respiratory distress, treat as previously described for dilated cardiomyopathy.
   A. Enalapril, furosemide, and aspirin as recommended above
   B. Digoxin for myocardial systolic dysfunction at a dose of 0.031 mg PO QOD-SID

Patient Monitoring

I. Monitor electrolytes, BUN, and creatinine before starting therapy, 7 days after starting therapy, and then every 4–6 weeks.

II. Monitor digoxin serum level 10–12 days after starting therapy. Digoxin level is maintained at 1–2 ng/ml.

III. Prognosis is guarded but variable. Some cats may be controlled medically for up to 2 years after diagnosis.

IV. If thromboembolism has occurred, prognosis is poor.

VIRAL MYOCARDITIS

Definition and Cause

I. It is a focal or diffuse inflammation and necrosis of the myocardium caused by direct invasion by a viral organism.

II. Primary cause is parvovirus in the dog.

Pathophysiology

I. Extensive inflammation of the myocardium occurs with infiltration of lymphocytes and plasma cells, myocardial cell fragmentation, and lysis.

II. Arrhythmias and congestive heart failure may develop.

Clinical Signs

I. There are two classic presentations of parvovirus myocarditis.

A. Sudden onset of severe dyspnea and pulmonary edema at 6–9 weeks of age (typically without concurrent enteritis) is the most common presentation.

B. Congestive heart failure with systolic dysfunction at 6–9 months of age also occurs.

II. Physical examination often reveals the following.
   A. Auscultable arrhythmias, systolic murmur, and/or gallop rhythm (S3)
   B. Tachypnea and dyspnea

Diagnosis

I. High degree of suspicion based on signalment and clinical presentation

II. Electrocardiogram: tachycardia and arrhythmias

III. Radiography
   A. Pulmonary venous distention and diffuse pulmonary edema
   B. Generalized cardiomegaly

IV. Echocardiography: left ventricular dilation with decreased systolic function

V. Histopathology
   A. Large basophilic intranuclear inclusion bodies may be seen.
   B. Histopathology may provide a definitive diagnosis.

Treatment

I. Oxygen therapy (nasal oxygen, oxygen cage, oxygen mask) is given for respiratory distress.

II. Furosemide is given if pulmonary edema is present.
   A. If the animal is very dyspneic, give furosemide at a dose of 2–4 mg/kg IV, IM, or SQ BID-TID.
   B. Once the animal is stabilized, the dose may be decreased to 1–2 mg/kg PO BID-TID.

III. Congestive heart failure at 6–9 weeks of age is poorly responsive to therapy.

IV. Older animals (6–9 months) that develop systolic dysfunction and heart failure may be more responsive to therapy.
   A. Digoxin may be given for its positive inotropic effects at a dose of 0.22 mg/m² PO BID.
   B. Enalapril may be given for vasodilation and positive neurohormonal effects at a dose of 0.25–0.5 mg/kg PO SID-BID.

Patient Monitoring

I. Puppies that develop clinical signs of heart failure at 6–9 weeks of age have a very poor prognosis.

II. Dogs that develop systolic dysfunction and heart failure at 6–9 months of age may be controlled on medical therapy for a longer period of time; however, reversal of cardiac dysfunction will not occur.

PARASITIC MYOCARDITIS

Definition and Cause

One of the most common causes of parasitic myocarditis is a protozoan parasite, *Trypanosoma cruzi* (Chagas' disease).

Pathophysiology

I. Direct damage to the myocardium occurs as the parasite ruptures myocytes.
II. Myocardial inflammation develops secondary to parasitic invasion of the myocardium.

Clinical Signs

I. Chagas' disease has been diagnosed only in the dog.
II. Sudden death is frequent.
III. Congestive heart failure with predominantly right ventricular dysfunction is typical.
   A. Arrhythmias may be ausculted.
   B. Jugular venous distention with ascites may be noted.

Diagnosis

I. Suggestive history
   Increased suspicion for the disease exists if the dog has lived or traveled in the southern United States or Central or South America.
II. Electrocardiogram
   A. Right bundle branch block is the most frequent conduction disturbance reported.
   B. Ventricular premature complexes and ventricular tachycardia frequently exist.
III. Echocardiography
   A. It may be normal.
   B. Right atrial and ventricular dilation may be seen.
   C. Progressive left ventricular dysfunction can develop.
IV. Radiography
   A. Thoracic radiographs may be within normal limits.
   B. Right ventricular enlargement (mild) may be observed.
V. Clinical pathology
   A. Complete blood count and biochemistry profile are nonspecific.
   B. A serum indirect fluorescent antibody test may be performed for antemortem diagnosis.
   C. Endomyocardial biopsy may provide a definitive diagnosis.

Treatment

I. Ventricular arrhythmias are frequently poorly responsive or refractory to antiarrhythmic therapy (see Chap. 7).
II. Diuretics, digoxin, and vasodilators are used as described for dilated cardiomyopathy to control signs of congestive heart failure.

Patient Monitoring

I. Animals that show clinical signs at a younger age (average 4.5 years) seem to have a poorer prognosis than dogs that develop clinical signs at an older age.
II. Death may be sudden secondary to a malignant arrhythmia or progressive right-sided congestive heart failure.

DOXORUBICIN CARDIOMYOPATHY

Definition and Cause

I. It is a progressive myocardial degeneration secondary to the toxic effects of doxorubicin, an antineoplastic agent.
II. The mechanism by which doxorubicin results in cardiotoxicity is poorly understood, but free radical generation and lipid membrane peroxidation have been suggested.

Pathophysiology

I. Myocyte degeneration and fibrosis occur with toxicity.
II. Toxicity can be manifested by the development of arrhythmias, conduction disturbances, and/or congestive heart failure.
   A. The likelihood of drug-induced congestive heart failure increases with the cumulative dose.
   B. Arrhythmias and conduction disturbances are not directly associated with congestive heart failure.
III. Breeds with increased risk of cardiomyopathy (boxer, Doberman pinscher, giant breeds) or animals with preexisting cardiac abnormalities may be at an increased risk of cardiotoxicity.

Clinical Signs

I. Congestive heart failure can be a delayed development even after the doxorubicin treatment is completed.
II. Electrocardiographic changes (arrhythmias, conduction disturbances) can occur with or without heart failure.

Diagnosis and Treatment

I. Radionuclide angiography is the most sensitive indicator of early onset cardiotoxicity but is not clinically practical.
II. Although electrocardiography and echocardiography are not as sensitive indicators of cardiotoxicity as radionuclide angiography, they are much more practical.
   A. Before starting treatment, electrocardiography and echocardiography are performed to screen for preexisting cardiac abnormalities.
   B. Animals are reevaluated with an electrocardiogram and echocardiogram at the 4th, 5th, and 6th treatments, or earlier if an arrhythmia, gallop rhythm, or new murmur develops.
   C. If myocardial contractility is decreased slightly in comparison with pretreatment, or if an occasional ventricular or supraventricular premature complex exists, treatment is delayed by 2 weeks followed by reevaluation.
   D. If significant alterations in cardiac function, arrhythmias, or conduction disturbances have de-

veloped, treatment with doxorubicin is discontinued.

III. Treatment is individualized based on clinical signs, presence of arrhythmias, and/or congestive heart failure.
   A. Antiarrhythmic therapy is based on the type of arrhythmia present (see Chap. 7).
   B. If systolic dysfunction exists, digoxin may be used at 0.22 mg/m² PO BID.
   C. If congestive heart failure develops, treatment and monitoring as given for dilated cardiomyopathy is recommended.

Patient Monitoring

I. If doxorubicin treatment is discontinued after the development of mild cardiotoxicity (mild function alterations), the prognosis is good.

II. If cardiotoxicity is severe and significant cardiac dysfunction or congestive heart failure has occurred, prognosis is guarded.

TRAUMATIC MYOCARDITIS

Definition and Causes

I. Myocardial contusions and ischemia occur secondary to blunt trauma to the chest.

II. It is most commonly seen after automobile accidents; however, other types of blunt trauma are also important.

Pathophysiology

I. Blunt trauma may result in myocardial inflammation and necrosis.

II. Ischemia, hypoxemia, and electrolyte and acid-base imbalances frequently observed with acute trauma and shock contribute to the significance of the arrhythmias and cardiac dysfunction.

Clinical Signs

I. Arrhythmias develop 24–72 hours after trauma.

II. Pulse deficits or decreased pulse quality may be palpated.

Diagnosis

I. History of recent trauma

II. Electrocardiography
   A. Idioventricular tachycardia (see Chap. 7)
      1. This is a ventricular rhythm that is initiated after a brief pause in rhythm.
      2. Typically the heart rate is only 5–10 bpm faster than the underlying sinus rate.
   B. Ventricular premature complexes or ventricular tachycardia

III. Radiography
   A. Pulmonary contusions may be noted.
   B. Cardiac silhouette is frequently normal.
   C. Rib fractures, diaphragmatic hernia, and pleural effusion may be observed.

IV. Echocardiography
   A. Usually within normal limits.
   B. Focal areas of abnormal wall motion may be observed.
   C. Asynchronous wall motion may be noted during arrhythmia.

Differential Diagnosis

I. Other systemic trauma causing ventricular arrhythmias

II. Splenic trauma or disease as a cause of ventricular arrhythmias

III. Previously undiagnosed cardiovascular disease

Treatment

I. Idioventricular rhythm may not need specific therapy as long as the heart rate is regular, the heart rate is within 10 bpm of the normal rate, and peripheral perfusion remains normal.

II. If ventricular tachycardia occurs, it is treated as follows.
   A. Nasal or cage oxygen is administered.
   B. Fluid and electrolyte balance is carefully evaluated, and any abnormalities are corrected.
   C. Lidocaine may be given at 2 mg/kg IV bolus up to a total dose of 8 mg/kg. If this effectively establishes conversion to normal sinus rhythm, an infusion at 40–80 µg/kg/min IV may be considered.
   D. If there is no response to lidocaine, consider procainamide at 8–20 mg/kg IV slowly over 5 minutes or as a continuous rate infusion at 25–50 µg/kg/min IV (or to effect).

Patient Monitoring

I. Continuously monitor the electrocardiogram for the first 24–72 hours after trauma to evaluate for arrhythmias.

II. Monitor electrolyte and fluid balance every 24 hours.

III. Arrhythmias typically begin to resolve in 72–96 hours.

Bibliography

Abbott JA: Traumatic myocarditis. p. 846. In Bonagura JD (ed): Kirk's Current Veterinary Therapy XII. WB Saunders, Philadelphia, 1995

Atkins CE, Gallo AM, Kurzman ID et al: Risk factors, clinical signs and survival in cats with a clinical diagnosis of idiopathic hypertrophic cardiomyopathy: 74 cases (1985–1989). J Am Vet Med Assoc 201:613, 1992

Atkins CE, Snyder PS, Keene BW et al: Efficacy of digoxin for treatment of cats with dilated cardiomyopathy. J Am Vet Med Assoc 196:1463, 1990

Bonagura JD, Fox PR: Restrictive cardiomyopathy. p. 863. In Bonagura JD (ed): Kirk's Current Veterinary Therapy XII. WB Saunders, Philadelphia, 1995

Bright JM, Golden AL, Gompf RE et al: Evaluation of the

calcium channel blocking agents diltiazem and verapamil for treatment of feline hypertrophic cardiomyopathy. J Vet Intern Med 5:272, 1991

Fox PR: Canine myocardial disease. p. 467. In Fox PR (ed): Canine and Feline Cardiology. Churchill Livingstone, New York, 1988

Fox PR: Feline myocardial disease. p. 435. In Fox PR (ed): Canine and Feline Cardiology. Churchill Livingstone, New York, 1988

Fox PR, Liu SK, Maron BJ: Echocardiographic assessment of spontaneously occurring feline hypertrophic cardiomyopathy: an animal model of human disease. Circulation 92:2645, 1995

Harpster NK: Boxer cardiomyopathy. p. 329. In Kirk RW (ed): Current Veterinary Therapy X. WB Saunders, Philadelphia, 1983

Harpster NK: Boxer cardiomyopathy: a review of the long-term benefits of antiarrhythmic therapy. Vet Clin North Am [Small Anim Pract] 21:989, 1991

Harpster NK, Baty C: Warfarin therapy of the cat at risk of thromboembolism. p. 868. In Bonagura JD (ed): Kirk's Current Veterinary Therapy XII. WB Saunders, Philadelphia, 1995

Keene BW, Panciera DP, Atkins CE: Myocardial L-carnitine deficiency in a family of dogs with dilated cardiomyopathy. J Am Vet Med Assoc 198:647, 1991

Kittleson MD: CVT update: feline hypertrophic cardiomyopathy. p. 854. In Bonagura JD (ed): Kirk's Current Veterinary Therapy XII. WB Saunders, Philadelphia, 1995

Kittleson MD, Pion PD, Youstry M: Hypertrophic cardiomyopathy in a group of highly interrelated Maine coon cats. Proc Am Coll Vet Intern Med 11:930, 1993

Laste NJ, Harpster NK: A retrospective study of 100 cases of feline distal aortic thromboembolism: 1977–1993. J Am Anim Hosp Assoc 31:492, 1995

Liu SK, Keene BW, Fox PR: Myocarditis in the dog and cat. p. 842. In Bonagura JD (ed): Kirk's Current Veterinary Therapy XII. WB Saunders, Philadelphia, 1995

Kramer GA, Kittleson MD, Fox PR, et al: Plasma taurine concentrations in normal dogs and in dogs with heart disease. J Vet Intern Med 9:253, 1995

Meurs KM, Miller MW, Helman RG: Canine chagas myocarditis. p. 850. In Bonagura JD (ed): Kirk's Current Veterinary Therapy XII. WB Saunders, Philadelphia, 1995

O'Grady M: Occult dilated cardiomyopathy in the Doberman pinscher. Proc Am Coll Vet Intern Med 13:298, 1995

Page RL, Keene BW: Doxorubicin cardiomyopathy. p. 783. In Bonagura JD (ed): Kirk's Current Veterinary Therapy XII. WB Saunders, Philadelphia, 1995

Sisson DD, Knight DH, Helinski C et al: Plasma taurine concentrations and M-mode echocardiographic measures in healthy cats and in cats with dilated cardiomyopathy. J Vet Intern Med 5:232, 1991

11

Pericardial Diseases

Richard D. Kienle
Mark A. Oyama

GENERAL INFORMATION

Pericardial Anatomy

I. The normal pericardium consists of a fibrous outer layer and an inner serosal layer.
  A. Visceral pericardium (epicardium): portion of the serosal layer attached to the myocardium
  B. Parietal pericardium: the outer fibrous layer (collagen fibers interlaced with wavy elastic fibers) lined by a portion of the inner serosal layer
II. The cone-shaped pericardial sac is formed by reflection of the serous layer from the inner surface of parietal pericardium over the surface of the heart to form the epicardium. The pericardial space lies between these serosal layers.
  A. It contains 1–15 ml of clear serous fluid that is an ultrafiltrate of plasma.
  B. The fibrous tissue of the pericardium blends with the adventitial layer of the great vessels and forms ligamentous attachments to the sternum and diaphragm.
III. The pericardium is innervated by the vagus and left recurrent laryngeal nerves. The phrenic nerves are embedded in the right and left dorsal aspects of the parietal pericardium as they course to the diaphragm.

Pericardial Function

I. Pericardium: not an essential structure, true physiologic role controversial (Lorell and Braunwald, 1992)
II. Ligamentous function: stabilizes the heart in an optimal functional position and prevents excessive motion during changes in body position
III. Barrier function: provides a physical barrier to infection and malignancy
IV. Membranous function: lubricates the heart and reduces external friction
V. Restraint function: limits acute distention of the heart
VI. Hemodynamic function: equalizes surface forces on the heart, balances transmural pressure of left and right ventricles and helps balance right and left ventricular output

CONGENITAL PERICARDIAL DISEASES

Pericardial Defects

Definition

I. Pericardial defects are small communications between the pericardial cavity and the pleural space.
II. A portion of the heart may be herniated or incarcerated into the defect.
III. Complete absence of the pericardium has been reported (Thomas, 1989).

Causes

I. Pericardial defects are thought to be developmental anomalies.
II. In middle-aged to older animals, trauma is a potential cause of acquired pericardial defects.

Pathophysiology

I. They occur as round or oval openings usually on the left side (Thomas, 1989).
II. Most are clinically insignificant and identified as incidental findings at necropsy.
III. If there is any clinical consequence, it is generally related to the area and degree of cardiac herniation and strangulation.

Clinical Signs

I. Most animals are asymptomatic.
II. Clinical signs may include sudden death, weakness and collapse, dyspnea, and/or signs of right congestive heart failure.

Diagnosis

I. Radiography
   A. Herniated portions of the heart may be seen as unusual protuberances from the cardiac silhouette.
      1. These changes may be dynamic in nature, appearing on some studies and not others, depending on the phase of cardiac cycle.
      2. Fluoroscopy can be used to document these dynamic herniations.
   B. Angiographic studies may identify the chamber or vessel protruding through the defect.
II. Ultrasonography may demonstrate dilated or strangulated cardiac chambers or vessels that underlie the defect.

Differential Diagnosis

I. Primary (congenital) heart disease
II. Pericardial cyst
III. Peritoneopericardial diaphragmatic hernia (PPDH)

Treatment and Monitoring

I. Defects causing clinical signs are treated by surgical closure of the defect or subtotal pericardectomy (Miller and Sisson, 1995).
II. Recovery is usually complete, and prognosis after a successful surgery is excellent (Miller and Sisson, 1995).

Pericardial Cysts

Definition and Causes

I. Pericardial cysts are fluid-filled mass lesions that occur within the pericardial space.
II. They have primarily been reported in young dogs, suggesting a developmental or congenital etiology.
III. Those reported in dogs do not meet the gross pathologic or histologic criteria of congenital cysts in humans, but rather appear to resemble acquired cystic hematomas (Sisson et al., 1993).

Pathophysiology

I. Pericardial cysts may arise from herniated omental or falciform fat in dogs with small PPDH or umbilical hernias or may arise from abnormal development of thoracic mesenchymal tissue.
II. They are commonly located in the right or left costrophrenic angle and usually have a pedicular attachment to the apex of the parietal pericardium.

Clinical Signs

I. Signs are similar to those of cardiac tamponade (see later).
II. Presenting complaints include exertional fatigue, abdominal distention, and dyspnea.
III. Muffled heart sounds may be heard on auscultation.

IV. If cardiac tamponade is present, jugular venous distention, hepatomegaly, and ascites may be detectable (Sisson et al., 1993).

Diagnosis

I. Electrocardiography may demonstrate small amplitude R waves (<1 mV), without electrical alternans, in all leads (Sisson et al., 1993).
II. Cardiomegaly is common on thoracic radiographs. The heart may assume a spherical shape, or the contour of the cardiac silhouette may be interrupted by an abnormal protrusion.
III. Pneumopericardiography or echocardiography is necessary for definitive diagnosis.
IV. Other imaging techniques such as computed tomography or magnetic resonance imaging may also establish the diagnosis (Sisson et al., 1993).

Differential Diagnosis

I. Pericardial effusion
II. Peritoneopericardial diaphragmatic hernia
III. Primary (congenital) heart disease

Treatment and Monitoring

I. Treatment is necessary when clinical signs are present.
II. The treatment of asymptomatic animals is controversial. Generally, they are reevaluated at regular intervals.
III. Surgical removal of the cyst and its pedicle, followed by subtotal pericardectomy, appears to result in resolution of clinical signs (Thomas, 1989).

Peritoneopericardial Diaphragmatic Hernia

Definition

I. Peritoneopericardial diaphragmatic hernia (PPDH) is a persistent communication between the pericardial and peritoneal cavities that may allow abdominal contents to enter the pericardial cavity.
II. PPDH is the most frequent congenital pericardial anomaly reported in dogs and cats (Evans and Biery, 1980; Hay et al., 1989).

Causes

I. Although a genetic cause is suspected for PPDH, none has been proved.
II. All PPDHs are considered to be congenital.

Pathophysiology

I. Abnormal fusion of the septum transversus with the pleuroperitoneal folds during embryonal development leads to incomplete development of the ventral diaphragm. This allows a communication between the peritoneal and pericardial cavities.

II. There is often an accompanying defect in the ventral abdominal wall or caudal sternebrae.

III. The size of the defect may vary from clinically silent, small communications involving herniation of the omentum to very large defects with herniation of other abdominal organs (Thomas, 1989).

IV. The liver and gallbladder tend to herniate most frequently, followed by the small intestines, spleen, and stomach (Evans and Biery, 1980).

Clinical Signs

I. Animals with a PPDH have a variable presentation depending on presence of organ entrapment, cardiac compression, and compromise of the pleural cavity by an enlarged pericardium (Hay et al., 1989).

II. In many instances, the PPDH is identified as an incidental finding while evaluating other problems or at necropsy.

III. The age at onset of clinical signs ranges from 4 weeks to 15 years, with most diagnoses being made within the first year of life (Evans and Biery, 1980; Hay et al., 1989).

IV. Clinical signs are primarily related to the gastrointestinal system and the respiratory tract and include vomiting, diarrhea, weight loss, exertional fatigue, dyspnea/tachypnea, and cough.

V. Cardiac signs include muffled heart sounds, signs of cardiac tamponade, and rarely a systolic heart murmur.

Diagnosis

I. Physical findings may be normal with smaller defects.

II. With larger defects, findings may include diminished or displaced heart sounds, umbilical or abdominal hernias, caudal sternal deformities, inability to palpate abdominal organs, and rarely, signs of cardiac tamponade and right-sided congestive heart failure.

III. Electrocardiography may demonstrate reduced amplitudes as a result of the addition of abdominal contents in the pericardial sac, and the mean electrical axis may be shifted because of cardiac displacement.

IV. Survey thoracic radiography may show generalized cardiomegaly and silhouetting of the caudal heart border and the diaphragm. The cardiac silhouette may have a heterogeneous density (soft tissue, gas, and/or fat) from the varied contents of the pericardial cavity.

V. Abdominal radiography may reveal the peritoneal cavity to be devoid of organs, and gastrointestinal gas patterns may be seen extending from the peritoneal cavity into the pericardial cavity.

VI. Two-dimensional echocardiography often allows direct visualization of an extracardiac, intrapericardial mass that displaces the heart, with or without a small amount of pericardial effusion (Kienle and Thomas, 1995). Occasionally, the discontinuity in the diaphragm can be seen, and herniated tissue appears to be continuous with abdominal contents.

VII. Fluoroscopy, nonselective angiocardiography, upper gastrointestinal barium studies, and/or pneumopericardiography may also help establish the diagnosis (Thomas, 1989).

Differential Diagnosis

I. Pericardial effusion
II. Primary cardiac disease
III. Traumatic diaphragmatic hernia

Treatment and Monitoring

I. Surgical correction via laparotomy and/or thoracotomy is the recommended treatment.

II. In asymptomatic adult animals or animals with small hernias, treatment may not be indicated.

III. Postoperative prognosis for most animals is excellent.

PERICARDIAL EFFUSION AND CARDIAC TAMPONADE

Definition

I. Pericardial effusion is an abnormal accumulation of fluid within the pericardial space.

II. Cardiac tamponade is an increase in intrapericardial pressure, secondary to pericardial effusion, that results in elevation of intracardiac pressures, impairment of diastolic ventricular filling, and a decrease in stroke volume and cardiac output (Lorell and Braunwald, 1992).

Causes

I. Reported causes of pericardial effusion in the dog include neoplasia, infectious disease, pericardial cysts, PPDH, left atrial tears, trauma, coagulopathies, uremia, idiopathic disease, and pericardial foreign bodies (Thomas, 1989; Berg and Wingfield, 1984).

II. Pericardial effusion in the cat has been associated with infectious disease (e.g., feline infectious peritonitis, bacterial infections, cytauxzoonosis), neoplasia, cardiomyopathies, uremia, trauma, left atrial tears, idiopathic disease, and PPDH (Rush et al., 1990).

Pathophysiology

I. The development of increased pericardial pressure secondary to pericardial effusion is dependent on the volume of effusate, the rate of fluid accumulation, and the physical nature of the pericardium.

A. The normal pericardium is able to accommodate small volumes of pericardial fluid with little rise in intrapericardial pressures. As the amount of effusion increases, the elastic limit of the pericardium is met and intrapericardial pressures rise dramatically (Fig. 11–1).

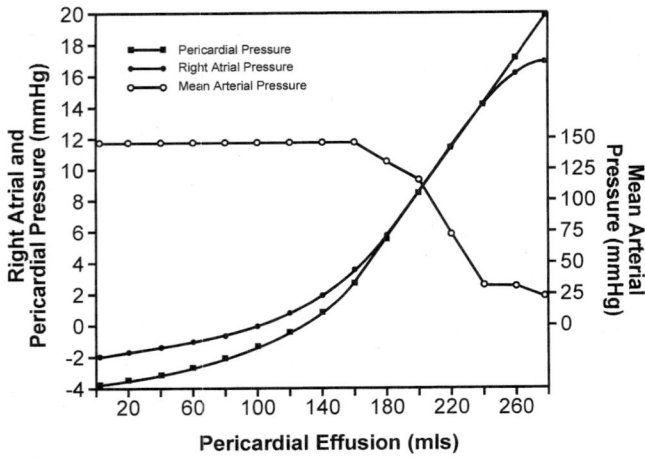

Figure 11–1. Graphic representation of the hemodynamic consequences of cardiac tamponade in a dog with acute pericardial effusion. Once the elastic limit of pericardium is reached (shown here at approximately 160 ml), small increases in the volume of the effusion result in large increases in right atrial and pericardial pressures as well as a decline in systemic arterial pressure.

  B. If fluid accumulation is rapid, the pericardium does not hypertrophy and cardiac tamponade occurs at relatively low volumes (100–200 ml in dogs).
  C. If fluid accumulation is slow, the pericardium hypertrophies and stretches and can accommodate much larger volumes (up to 1800 ml in large dogs) with little increase in pericardial pressure.
  D. When pericardial compliance is reduced, smaller effusions produce cardiac tamponade.
    1. Older animals have a less compliant pericardium as a result of age-related changes in the pericardial elastic fibers.
    2. Pericardial fibrosis also causes the pericardium to become less compliant.
II. Cardiac tamponade is characterized by an elevation of intracardiac diastolic pressures, progressive limitation of ventricular filling, and a reduction of cardiac stroke volume.
  A. Once the ventricular transmural distending pressure (difference between the intracardiac and pericardial pressures) reaches zero, the diastolic pressure of all chambers of the heart equilibrate with intrapericardial pressure, and diastolic filling is compromised.
  B. The resulting decrease in stroke volume and cardiac output and the increase in filling pressures cause signs of heart failure, either congestive, low output, or both.
  C. The right ventricle is more susceptible to compression by pericardial effusion, and congestive right-sided heart failure is a common finding (Thomas, 1989).
  D. Ventricular systolic function is usually normal.
III. Increased sympathetic tone leads to an increase in heart rate, increased contractility, and systemic vasoconstriction, which initially help maintain forward cardiac output.

Clinical Signs

  I. Clinical signs are variable and influenced by the rate of effusion and degree of cardiac compression. Mild effusions may not cause clinically apparent disease.
  II. Moderate volume and/or slowly accumulating effusions generally cause signs of right-sided heart failure.
    A. Lethargy, anorexia, weakness
    B. Dyspnea, tachypnea, cough from pleural effusion and/or severe ascites
    C. Abdominal distention from ascites and hepatomegaly
    D. Syncope, usually upon exertion
  III. Large volume or rapid accumulations of fluid generally lead to signs of low cardiac output.
    A. Marked weakness or collapse
    B. Dyspnea and tachypnea
    C. Sudden death

Diagnosis

  I. The classic physical finding of pericardial tamponade is Beck's triad—systemic venous hypertension, reduced stroke output, and muffled heart sounds.
    A. Systemic venous hypertension is recognized by jugular venous distention and pulsation.
    B. Decreased stroke work causes a weak arterial pulse and in some cases pulsus paradoxus (an exaggerated decrease in arterial pulse pressure during inspiration).
    C. Diminished or muffled heart sounds and a reduced precordial impulse are suggestive of cardiac compression by fluid.
    D. Other findings include pale mucous membranes, tachycardia, hepatosplenomegaly, ascites, peripheral edema (rare), pleural effusion with diminished lung sounds, and arrhythmias.
  II. Electrocardiography may reveal the following.
    A. Diminished QRS amplitudes (<1 mV in dogs) in all leads (Berg and Wingfield, 1984; Miller and Sisson, 1995)
    B. Electrical alternans (beat-to-beat variation in QRS amplitudes) as the heart swings within the pericardial fluid (Fig. 11–2), in approximately 50–60% of canine cases (Berg and Wingfield, 1984)
    C. Nonspecific ST segment deviation
    D. Commonly sinus tachycardia (80%)
    E. Other ventricular or supraventricular arrhythmias occasionally (Berg and Wingfield, 1984)
  III. Thoracic radiography often reveals generalized cardiomegaly.
    A. Small effusions may not alter the cardiac silhouette or may cause only mild cardiomegaly. A normal chest radiograph does not exclude the possibility of a hemodynamically important effusion.
    B. Large amounts of effusion cause severe generalized cardiomegaly.
    C. The shape of the cardiac silhouette is usually round or globoid in both views, with loss of the

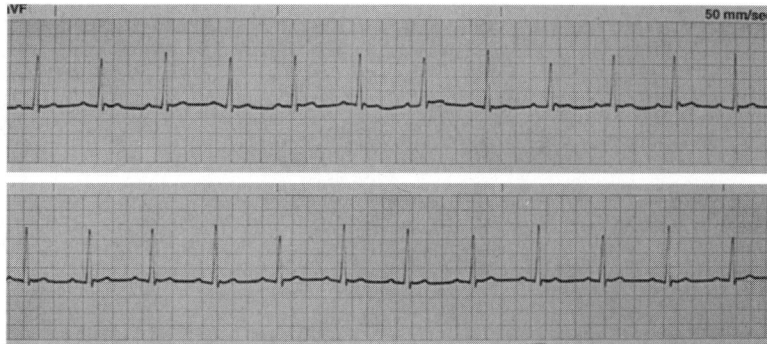

Figure 11–2. Electrical alternans in a dog with pericardial effusion. Note the mild beat-to-beat variation in R wave amplitude (lead aVF, 50 mm/sec).

normal cardiac shape. In the lateral projection, the cranial cardiac waist is lost, but the caudal cardiac waist is usually maintained.

D. Other radiographic findings may include pleural effusion, enlargement of the caudal vena cava, pulmonary metastatic disease, mass lesions producing tracheal deviation, or abnormal protuberances of the cardiac silhouette.

E. Special radiographic studies such as pneumopericardiography, angiocardiography, and fluoroscopy may help identify the underlying cause; however, these studies have largely been supplanted by echocardiography.

IV. Echocardiography is highly sensitive for detecting pericardial effusion and is the diagnostic test of choice for confirming the diagnosis and attempting to determine the underlying cause. It can detect as little as 15 ml of pericardial fluid (Bonagura and Pipers, 1981; Kienle and Thomas, 1995).

A. M-mode echocardiography (Bonagura and Pipers, 1981)
   1. Pericardial fluid is identified as an echo-free space between the posterior pericardial and epicardial surfaces (Fig. 11–3A).
   2. Paradoxical septal wall motion can occur secondary to the swinging of the heart within the pericardial sac.

B. Two-dimensional echocardiography
   1. An echo-free pericardial fluid space surrounds the heart (Fig. 11–3B).
   2. The heart is often seen to swing (usually from left to right) within the fluid.
   3. Diastolic collapse of the right atrium and ventricle is often identified and is highly suggestive of cardiac tamponade (Kienle and Thomas, 1995).
   4. It identifies and localizes pericardial and cardiac masses in about 90% of cases with neo-

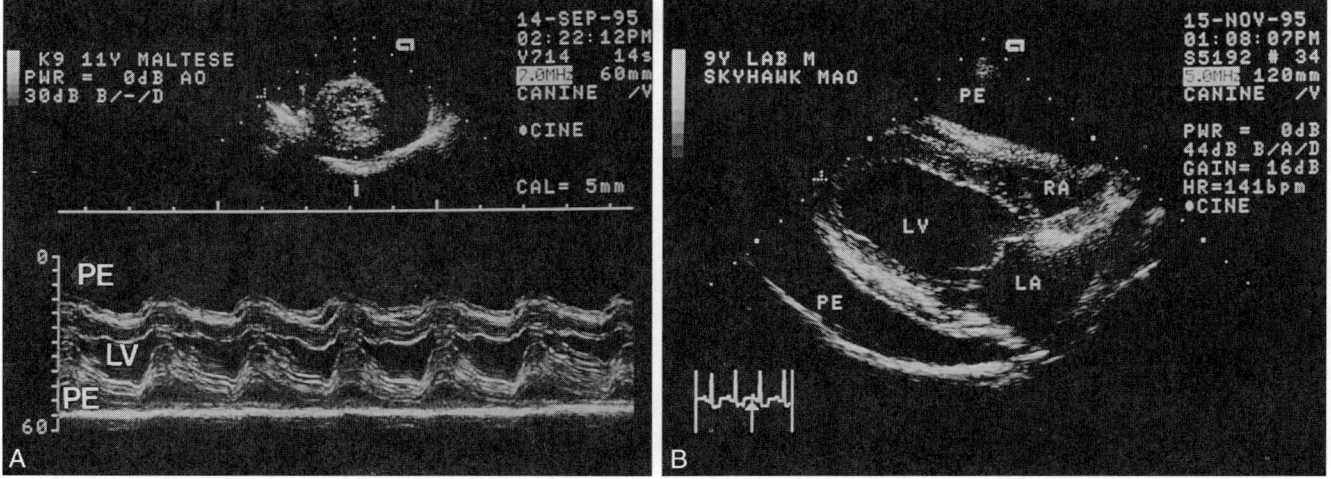

Figure 11–3. A. M-mode echocardiogram from a dog with pericardial effusion. The effusion appears as a hypoechoic rim of fluid posterior to the left ventricular free wall and a large hypoechoic area anterior (toward the top of the scan) to the right ventricular free wall. Note the paradoxical septal wall motion during systole (the septum moves toward the right ventricle in systole). B. Two-dimensional echocardiogram from a dog with pericardial effusion (right parasternal long axis view). There is a hypoechoic fluid space surrounding the heart. This image was taken during diastole (arrow on the electrocardiogram indicates timing). Note the diastolic collapse of the right atrium (RA), suggesting cardiac tamponade. PE = pericardial effusion; LV = left ventricle; LA = left atrium.

plastic effusions; however, failure to identify a mass does not exclude the diagnosis of a diffuse neoplastic process such as mesothelioma.

C. Doppler echocardiography

It may reveal the variations in diastolic mitral and tricuspid inflows and systolic aortic and pulmonary artery outflows that occur with pulsus paradoxus (Chandraratna, 1991).

V. Cardiac catheterization can be used to document characteristic hemodynamic changes seen with cardiac tamponade, such as the elevation and equilibration of diastolic pressure in all four cardiac chambers.

VI. Pericardial fluid analysis and cytology have limited clinical value in identifying the cause of a pericardial effusion (Sisson et al., 1984).

A. Most effusions in dogs are serosanguineous with high red blood cell counts, moderate protein levels (1–6 g/dl), and variable nucleated cell counts.

1. Purulent and chylous effusions are usually easily distinguished; however, neoplastic and inflammatory effusions are not.

2. Cytologic exam is unreliable and confounded by reactive mesothelial cells leading to a high incidence of both false-negative (75%) and false-positive (13%) diagnoses of cardiac neoplasia (Sisson et al., 1984).

B. Determining the pH of the pericardial fluid has been proposed as a way to differentiate neoplastic from non-neoplastic (inflammatory) effusions. In a study of 51 dogs with pericardial effusion, dogs with neoplastic disorders tended to have a more alkaline effusion (pH 7.0–7.5) than those with inflammatory diseases (pH 6.5–7.0) (Edwards, 1996).

C. Bacterial culture and sensitivity are indicated if the effusion contains high numbers of neutrophils that appear degenerative or if actual microbes are identified on cytology.

VII. Other laboratory findings are usually mild and reflect the underlying cause of the effusion or the hemodynamic consequences.

A. Mild elevation in blood urea nitrogen and creatinine (prerenal azotemia)

B. Mild elevation of hepatic enzymes secondary to passive congestion

C. Anemia and/or presence of nucleated red blood cells with hemangiosarcoma

D. Leukocytosis with a left shift from infectious pericarditis

Differential Diagnosis

I. Other causes of congestive right-sided heart failure

A. Dilated cardiomyopathy, tricuspid insufficiency (congenital and acquired), constrictive pericarditis, and cor pulmonale/pulmonary hypertension

B. Distinguished from pericardial effusion based on physical examination, thoracic radiography, and echocardiography

II. Other disorders that lead to abdominal distention

A. Abdominal neoplasia or other abdominal masses

B. Other causes of abdominal effusion (e.g., trauma, peritonitis, hypoproteinemia)

III. Other causes of muffled heart sounds and characteristic electrocardiographic changes

A. Any cause of pleural effusion

B. Obesity

C. Pneumothorax

D. Thoracic masses

E. Diaphragmatic hernia

Treatment

I. An algorithm for the treatment of pericardial effusion is shown in Figure 11–4.

II. Pericardiocentesis is indicated in virtually all effusions of clinical significance.

III. Subsequent treatment depends on the cause.

A. Idiopathic (benign) hemorrhagic pericardial effusion

1. Pericardiocentesis is curative in approximately 50% of cases (Thomas, 1989). Repeated pericardiocentesis can be performed if the effusion recurs.

2. In refractory cases (cases that have recurred >3 times), surgical subtotal pericardectomy is considered because repeated pericardiocentesis may result in pericardial fibrosis and ultimately pericardial constriction. Prognosis

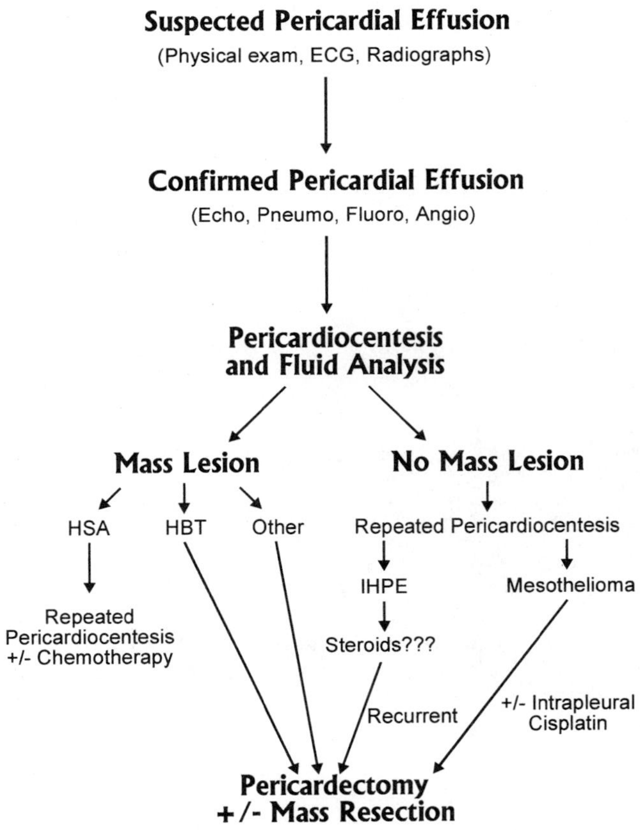

Suspected Pericardial Effusion
(Physical exam, ECG, Radiographs)

Confirmed Pericardial Effusion
(Echo, Pneumo, Fluoro, Angio)

Pericardiocentesis and Fluid Analysis

Mass Lesion — **No Mass Lesion**

HSA · HBT · Other — Repeated Pericardiocentesis

Repeated Pericardiocentesis +/- Chemotherapy

IHPE

Steroids???

Mesothelioma

Recurrent

+/- Intrapleural Cisplatin

Pericardectomy +/- Mass Resection

Figure 11–4. Algorithm for the diagnosis and treatment of serosanguineous pericardial effusion in the dog. HSA = hemangiosarcoma; HBT = heart base tumor; IHPE = idiopathic hemorrhagic pericardial effusion.

is good following pericardectomy (Berg et al., 1984; Matthiesen and Lammerding, 1985).
3. Oral corticosteroid therapy has been proposed as a treatment for idiopathic effusions, although its efficacy is unknown (Miller and Sisson, 1995).

B. Heart base tumor
1. Conservative management consists of repeated pericardiocentesis.
2. Pericardectomy is considered in cases of recurrent effusions as a palliative measure.
   a) Heart base tumors are usually slow growing, and pericardectomy provides relief from recurrent pericardial tamponade.
   b) Survival after pericardectomy is variable (months to years) (Miller and Sisson, 1995).
3. Surgical reduction or resection of the tumor may be attempted if the tumor is surgically accessible.

C. Hemangiosarcoma
1. Conservative therapy by repeated pericardiocentesis is usually recommended.
2. Hemangiosarcomas are usually very aggressive, and surgery (pericardectomy and/or resection) does not appear to provide increased survival or improved quality of life (Aronsohn, 1985).
3. Surgical resection may be considered for small tumors that are easily accessible. However, the prognosis appears to remain unchanged.
4. Chemotherapy may also be tried (see Neoplasia, later).

D. Infectious pericarditis
   It requires surgical drainage and long-term antibiotics.

E. Other causes
   Most other types of pericardial effusion require subtotal pericardectomy (Thomas, 1989).

Patient Monitoring

I. Continuous electrocardiographic monitoring to help detect ventricular arrhythmias is recommended during pericardiocentesis and subtotal pericardectomy.
II. Following pericardiocentesis or surgery, animals are observed for blood loss, arrhythmias, and dyspnea.
III. A chest tube is placed for a variable amount of time following pericardectomy.
IV. Follow-up examination after the initial diagnosis is within the first 2 weeks.
V. Subsequent rechecks are determined by the cause and severity of the underlying disorder.

CONSTRICTIVE AND CONSTRICTIVE-EFFUSIVE PERICARDITIS

Definition

I. Constrictive pericarditis occurs when cardiac compression and restriction result from a thickened, fibrotic, and non-compliant pericardium without effusion.
II. Constrictive-effusive pericarditis is similar, except for the presence of a small amount of pericardial fluid (usually not enough to cause cardiac tamponade alone).

Causes

I. Most cases of constrictive pericarditis are idiopathic.
II. Any chronic pericardial effusion may result in constriction if the pericardium becomes fibrotic.
III. Known causes in dogs include recurrent idiopathic hemorrhagic pericardial effusion, intrapericardial foreign bodies, chronic septic pericarditis, intrapericardial neoplasia, and traumatic pericardial hemorrhage (Thomas et al., 1984).
IV. Constrictive pericardial disease in cats is extremely rare but has been associated with dilated cardiomyopathy and congestive heart failure (Bunch, 1981).

Pathophysiology

I. Pericardial constriction occurs when the parietal and/or visceral (epicardium) pericardium are histologically altered by a disease process that interferes with their normal mechanical properties.
II. The normal pressure-volume relationship is altered so that minimal increases in total pericardial volume (i.e., normal ventricular filling) cause dramatic increases in pericardial pressure.
III. In some cases, the pericardial space is obliterated by complete fusion of the parietal and visceral layers; in others, a small fluid space remains (constrictive-effusive pericarditis).
IV. The pathophysiology is similar to cardiac tamponade in that the main consequences are limitation of diastolic ventricular volume, elevation and equilibration of diastolic pressures throughout the heart, and ultimately the development of right-sided congestive heart failure and/or cardiogenic shock.
V. Constrictive pericardial disease differs from pericardial effusion in that diastolic filling is not impeded throughout the entire diastolic period. Most of ventricular filling occurs in early diastole, followed by an abrupt cessation in mid-diastole as the elastic limit of the pericardium is reached.

Clinical Signs

I. Presenting complaints and physical findings are similar to those of cardiac tamponade, of which abdominal enlargement (ascites) is the most common.
II. Jugular distention is a common finding but usually without pulsation.
III. Less common complaints include dyspnea, tachypnea, fatigue, weakness, syncope, and weight loss.
IV. Weak peripheral pulses are common, but pulsus paradoxus is rarely observed (Hancock, 1980).
V. Pericardial knocks and gallop sounds are reported in humans (Blake, 1983) but occur infrequently in dogs (Thomas et al., 1984).

Diagnosis

I. The definitive diagnosis of constrictive pericarditis is difficult and often requires cardiac catheterization. It is often an exclusionary diagnosis in dogs and is arrived at with signs of right-sided heart failure that cannot be explained by other causes.

II. Electrocardiographic findings include small R waves in all leads (<1 mV), increased P wave duration (>45 msec in lead II), and right axis shift. Supraventricular arrhythmias are common, especially during anesthesia (Thomas, 1989).

III. Radiographic findings are often subtle and inconsistent (Thomas, 1989).
   A. Mild cardiomegaly with or without rounding of the heart shadow
   B. Enlargement of the caudal vena cava
   C. Pleural effusion
   D. Left or right atrial enlargement

IV. Echocardiography may reveal the following.
   A. Decreased left ventricular end-diastolic dimension, rapid premature closure of the mitral valve, and changes in Doppler blood flow velocities are suggestive of constrictive disease but are not reliable findings, especially in the dog (Oh et al., 1994).
   B. Dogs more commonly have constrictive-effusive pericarditis. The presence of only a small effusion on echocardiography in a dog with signs of right-sided heart failure or cardiogenic shock is highly suggestive of constrictive-effusive pericarditis.
   C. If pleural effusion and pericardial effusion are present, the pericardium is seen between the two fluid spaces, and abnormal thickening of the parietal pericardium may be noted.

V. Cardiac catheterization demonstrates elevated diastolic filling pressures and venous wave forms indicative of rapid early diastolic filling with abrupt cessation (characteristic of pericardial constriction).

Differential Diagnosis

See Pericardial Effusion and Cardiac Tamponade.

Treatment and Monitoring

I. The treatment of pericardial constriction requires subtotal pericardectomy.

II. In cases in which the epicardium is significantly involved in the constrictive process, pericardectomy may only partially alleviate the clinical signs. Unfortunately, epicardial involvement can be determined only by exploratory thoracotomy.

III. Postoperative pulmonary thrombosis has been reported in dogs (Thomas et al., 1984).

IV. Monitoring is similar to that required for pericardial effusion and cardiac tamponade.

PERICARDIAL NEOPLASIA AND OTHER MASS LESIONS

Definition and Causes

I. Pericardial mass lesions are space-occupying lesions within the pericardial space, arising from the pericardium, surrounding vessels, or myocardium.

II. Neoplastic masses account for 40–60% of all cases of pericardial effusion (Berg, 1994).
   A. Common intrapericardial tumors in the dog include chemodectoma, hemangiosarcoma, mesothelioma, and thyroid adenocarcinoma.
      1. Hemangiosarcomas represent approximately 60% of all cardiac neoplasia in dogs (Berg and Wingfield, 1984). They usually originate from the right atrium or auricle, are invasive and aggressive, and have often metastasized by the time of diagnosis (Fruchter et al., 1992).
      2. Chemodectomas (nonchromaffin paragangliomas) arise from chemoreceptor tissue associated with the aortic and carotid bodies (Patnaik et al., 1975). They usually originate at the heart base, are slow growing, and infrequently metastasize.
      3. Mesothelioma is a diffuse tumor of the serous lining of the pericardium, pleural cavity, and/or peritoneum.
         a) Pericardial mesothelioma usually produces large amounts of effusion that is refractory to repeated pericardiocentesis (McDonough et al., 1992).
         b) Puncture of the pericardium during pericardiocentesis or pericardectomy may hasten the spread of the tumor to the pleural cavity with resulting pleural effusion.
      4. Thyroid adenocarcinomas arise from ectopic thyroid tissue around the heart base and are usually non-functional.
   B. Other reported intrapericardial tumors in the dog include rhabdomyosarcoma, myxoma, fibrosarcoma, and lymphoma.
   C. Reported intrapericardial tumors in the cat include lymphosarcoma, malignant melanoma, chemodectoma, hemangiosarcoma, and a variety of carcinomas (Rush et al., 1990).

III. Other non-neoplastic mass lesions seen in dogs include fungal granulomas, bacterial abscesses, pericardial cysts, and abdominal viscera (peritoneopericardial hernias).

Pathophysiology

I. Mass lesions usually produce pericardial effusion and cardiac tamponade (see earlier).

II. Mass lesions may cause infiltration, displacement, and/or compression of cardiac chambers or great vessels.

III. Signs of illness may also reflect paraneoplastic syndromes or primary involvement in other organs.

Clinical Signs

I. Clinical signs are variable and are dependent on the type, size, and location of mass; they are often associated with pericardial effusion or fibrosis. Systemic involvement may also influence clinical signs.
II. Nonspecific signs include lethargy, weakness, anorexia, dyspnea, and cough.
III. Signs of right-sided heart failure are related to pericardial effusion or constriction.
IV. Head and neck swelling develop from obstruction of the cranial vena cava.
V. Signs of low cardiac output occur with obstruction of ventricular outflow.

Diagnosis

I. Physical, electrocardiographic, and radiographic findings are usually consistent with pericardial effusion (see earlier).
II. Occasionally thoracic radiography demonstrates abnormal protuberances or densities within the cardiac silhouette suggesting the presence of a mass.
III. Pneumopericardiography or angiography may outline the external or intracardiac margins of the mass.
IV. Echocardiography is the most specific diagnostic technique (Cobb and Brownlie, 1992).
   A. Two-dimensional echocardiography often accurately identifies and localizes masses in all pericardial regions when adequate pericardial effusion is present.
   B. In the absence of pericardial effusion, some smaller masses may be overlooked and/or the total extent of the mass may be underestimated.
   C. A negative echocardiographic exam for mass lesions does not rule out the presence of small masses (<0.5 cm) or mesothelioma.
V. Fine needle aspiration of pericardial masses is generally non-diagnostic and may be contraindicated because of the high risk of complications.
VI. Determination of the pH of pericardial effusion may be of value in distinguishing neoplastic effusions from non-neoplastic effusions (see Pericardial Effusion).
VII. Additional laboratory and radiographic evaluations are indicated to determine the systemic effects and metastatic nature of any mass.
VIII. Definitive characterization of the mass may require surgical biopsy with histopathology.

Differential Diagnosis

See Pericardial Effusion and Cardiac Tamponade.

Treatment

I. Treatment for most pericardial neoplasia is symptomatic and is targeted at relieving pericardial effusion

via repeated pericardiocentesis or pericardectomy (see Fig. 11–4).
II. Subtotal pericardectomy in cases of slow-growing tumors may be of benefit, as the effusate is more readily reabsorbed by the pleural than by the pericardial surface. The potential spread of tumor to the pleural cavity must be considered (i.e., mesothelioma).
III. Surgical resection is generally unrewarding because of the vascular nature of most tumors (chemodectoma, hemangiosarcoma) and presence of metastatic disease (hemangiosarcoma) at the time of surgery.
IV. Pericardectomy and/or right atrial resection for hemangiosarcoma are controversial, and their effect on survival time appears minimal (Miller and Sisson, 1995).
V. Chemotherapy agents have been rarely used, and their efficacy and safety are largely undetermined.
   A. Intracavitary cisplatin has been used for pleural and pericardial mesothelioma with limited success. The accumulation of effusion may be slowed, but the effect on survival is minimal (Moore, 1991).
   B. Combination therapy with doxorubicin, cyclophosphamide, and vincristine has been used in isolated right atrial hemangiosarcoma (deMadron et al., 1987). Although reduction in tumor size has been documented, survival is only increased by a few weeks in most cases.

Patient Monitoring

I. Serious postoperative complications (hemorrhage, disseminated intravascular coagulation, arrhythmias) are frequent (Aronsohn, 1985).
II. In most cases treatment is considered palliative, and the overall effect on long-term survival is minimal.
   A. Especially with the more aggressive tumors (hemangiosarcoma and mesothelioma), survival is only a few months.
   B. Animals with heart-based tumors (chemodectoma or thyroid adenocarcinoma) may survive several months to years following pericardectomy.

Bibliography

Aronsohn M: Cardiac hemangiosarcoma in the dog: a review of 38 cases. J Am Vet Med Assoc 187:922, 1985
Berg J: Pericardial disease and cardiac neoplasia. Semin Vet Med Surg 9:185, 1994
Berg RJ, Wingfield W: Pericardial effusion in the dog: a review of 42 cases. J Am Anim Hosp Assoc 30:721, 1984
Berg RJ, Wingfield WE, Hoopes PJ: Idiopathic hemorrhagic pericardial effusion in eight dogs. J Am Vet Med Assoc 185:988, 1984
Blake S: The clinical diagnosis of constrictive pericarditis. Am Heart J 106:432, 1983
Bonagura JD, Pipers FS: Echocardiographic features of pericardial effusion in dogs. J Am Vet Med Assoc 179:49, 1981
Bunch S: Pericardial effusion with restrictive pericarditis associated with congestive cardiomyopathy in a cat. J Am Anim Hosp 17:739, 1981

Chandraratna PA: Echocardiography and Doppler ultrasound in the evaluation of pericardial disease. Circulation 84(Suppl 1):1–303, 1991

Cobb MA, Brownlie SE: Intrapericardial neoplasia in 14 dogs. J Small Anim Pract 33:309, 1992

deMadron E, Helfand SC, Stebbins KE: Use of the chemotherapy for treatment of cardiac hemangiosarcoma in a dog. J Am Vet Med Assoc 190:887, 1987

Edwards NJ: The diagnostic value of pericardial fluid pH determination. J Am Anim Hosp Assoc 32:63, 1996

Evans SM, Biery DN: Congenital peritoneopericardial diaphragmatic hernia in the dog and cat: a literature review and 17 additional case histories. Vet Radiol 21:108, 1980

Fruchter AM, Miller CW, O'Grady MR: Echocardiographic results and clinical considerations in dogs with right atrial/auricular masses. Can Vet J 33:171, 1992

Hancock EW: On the elastic and rigid forms of constrictive pericarditis. Am Heart J 100:917, 1980

Hay WH, Woodfield JA, Moon MA: Clinical, echocardiographic and radiographic findings of peritoneopericardial diaphragmatic hernia in two dogs and a cat. J Am Vet Med Assoc 195:1245, 1989

Kienle RD, Thomas WP: Echocardiography. p. 198. In Nyland TG, Mattoon JS (eds): Veterinary Diagnostic Ultrasound. WB Saunders, Philadelphia, 1995

Lorell BH, Braunwald E: Pericardial disease. p. 1465. In Braunwald E (ed): Heart Disease. WB Saunders, Philadelphia, 1992

Matthiesen DT, Lammerding A: Partial pericardiectomy for idiopathic hemorrhagic pericardial effusion in the dog. J Am Anim Hosp Assoc 21:41, 1985

McDonough SP, MacLachlan NJ, Tobias AJ: Canine pericardial mesothelioma. Vet Pathol 29:256, 1992

Miller MW, Sisson DD: Pericardial disorders. p. 1032. In Ettinger SD (ed): Textbook of Veterinary Internal Medicine. 4th Ed. WB Saunders, Philadelphia, 1995

Moore AS: Intracavitary cisplatin. J Vet Intern Med 5:227, 1991

Oh JK, Hatle LK, Seward JB et al: Diagnostic role of Doppler echocardiography in constrictive pericarditis. J Am Coll Cardiol 23:154, 1994

Patnaik AK, Liu SK, Hurvitz AI et al: Canine chemodectoma (extra-adrenal paragangliomas): a comparative study. J Small Anim Pract 16:785, 1975

Rush JE, Keene BW, Fox PR: Pericardial disease in the cat: a retrospective evaluation of 66 cases. J Am Anim Hosp Assoc 26:39, 1990

Sisson DD, Thomas WP, Ruehl WW et al: Diagnostic value of pericardial fluid analysis in the dog. J Am Vet Med Assoc 184:51, 1984

Sisson D, Thomas WP, Reed J et al: Intrapericardial cysts in the dog. J Vet Intern Med 7:364, 1993

Thomas WP: Pericardial disorders. p. 1132. In Ettinger SD (ed): Textbook of Veterinary Internal Medicine. 3rd Ed. WB Saunders, Philadelphia, 1989

Thomas WP, Reed JR, Bauer TG et al: Constrictive pericardial disease in the dog. J Am Vet Med Assoc 184:546, 1984

12

Heartworm Disease

Matthew W. Miller

CANINE HEARTWORM DISEASE

Definition

I. Heartworm disease (HWD): obstructive pulmonary vascular disorder
II. Distribution
   A. Suitable mosquito vectors exist worldwide in temperate and tropical climates.
   B. A serious endemic problem exists in many parts of the world including southern Canada, Mexico, the Caribbean, South America, Australia, Asia and the Pacific, Japan, western and southern Africa, and southern Europe, especially northern Italy.
   C. In the United States, canine HWD has been detected in every state, and feline HWD has been reported in 30 states (Soll and Knight, 1996).
III. Primary hosts and principal reservoirs of infection
   A. Domestic canines
   B. Wild canines, particularly coyotes in northern California
IV. Other susceptible hosts
   A. Domestic and captive non-domesticated (African lion) cats
   B. Ferret
   C. California sea lion
V. Aberrant hosts
   Most other mammals, including humans, may be infected but do not become microfilaremic, so do not serve as reservoirs of infection.

Cause

I. Caused by the mosquito-borne filarial parasite *Dirofilaria immitis*
II. Life cycle of *D. immitis* (Katoni and Powers, 1982)
   A. Microfilaria/embryo stage (L1)
      1. Microfilariae (MF) may circulate in the blood of an infected host for more than 2 years after being released by a gravid female.
      2. MF must be ingested by a suitable mosquito vector before development can continue.
   B. Third stage (L3)
      1. MF molt twice (L1→L2, L2→L3) in the mosquito to reach the infective third stage (L3).
      2. MF migrate to the proboscis of the infected mosquito within 12–40 days depending on ambient temperature (Otto, 1983).
      3. They are deposited on the skin and enter the definitive host through a mosquito bite wound.
   C. Tissue migratory stages (L4, L5)
      1. Infective larvae promptly molt (2 weeks) to the precardiac fourth stage (L4).
      2. Maturation to the fifth larval stage (juvenile adult, L5) occurs about 50–70 days after infection.
   D. Adult stage
      1. Fifth stage larvae reach the circulation by penetrating systemic veins between 70 and 110 days.
      2. After embolizing the pulmonary arteries, they mature and release MF usually by 5–6.5 months after infection.
      3. Adult worms may survive up to 8 years.
III. Pathogenic life cycle stages
   A. The adult heartworm is directly responsible for nearly all primary pathologic changes.
   B. Some pulmonary parenchymal and renal glomerular changes have been attributed to deposition and immunologic destruction of MF.

Pathophysiology

I. Pulmonary vascular disease (Knight, 1983, 1987a)
   A. Endothelial injury by adult heartworms and release of growth factor by adhering platelets are proposed as the cause of myointimal proliferation (Schaub et al., 1983).
   B. Factors causing increased pulmonary vascular resistance include the following.
      1. Myointimal proliferation in occupied pulmonary arteries
      2. Obstructive fibrosis in end arteries
      3. Live heartworms, worm emboli, and associated thrombosis

C. Severity of pulmonary hypertension depends on several factors.
  1. Severity of infection (number of parasites)
  2. Number of parasitized arteries
  3. Degree of luminal narrowing
  4. Daily level of physical activity (Soll and Knight, 1996)
II. Cardiac disease
  A. Sequelae of pulmonary hypertension
    1. Right ventricular hypertrophy
    2. Right-sided congestive heart failure (R-CHF)
  B. Tricuspid valve regurgitation
    1. Dilatation of tricuspid annulus from right ventricular enlargement
    2. Mechanical interference by heartworms (caval syndrome, see later)
III. Pulmonary parenchymal disease
  A. Diffuse interstitial infiltration by eosinophils
  B. Pulmonary granulomas around areas of thrombosis
IV. Caval syndrome
  A. Associated with heavy adult worm infections and pulmonary hypertension
  B. Displacement of worms to the right atrium, caudal vena cava, and hepatic veins
  C. Presence of the worms within the tricuspid valve annulus preventing closure of tricuspid valve
V. Glomerulonephritis
  A. Deposition of immune complexes containing worm antigen in the glomerular basement membrane
  B. Physical damage to glomerulus by viable MF
  C. May lead to proteinuria and eventually renal failure

Clinical Signs

I. Clinical pattern
  A. Although heartworm infection can cause devastating disease, lightly infected animals often remain asymptomatic indefinitely.
  B. Because of the parasite's long life cycle, clinical signs seldom occur before a year after infection and ordinarily do not become evident for several years.
  C. Heightened surveillance and widespread use of chemoprophylaxis have reduced the incidence of symptomatic clinical cases.
II. Signs associated with chronic cardiopulmonary disease
  A. Nonproductive cough
  B. Variable degree of respiratory distress
  C. Exertional fatigue and lethargy
  D. Syncope triggered by sudden exercise or excitement
  E. Weight loss and loss of lean muscle mass (cardiac cachexia)
  F. Ascites (sometimes accompanied by pleural effusion)
  G. Hemoptysis (uncommon)
III. Acute signs associated with caval syndrome
  A. Anorexia, depression, lethargy, weakness

B. Hemolytic crisis: icterus, hemoglobinuria, bilirubinuria, pale mucous membranes
C. Tachycardia, bounding pulses
D. Occasionally also signs of severe cardiopulmonary disease, as listed previously

Diagnosis

I. Systemic evidence of HWD
  A. Physical findings
    1. Heart murmurs (inconsistently present)
      a) Systolic murmur of tricuspid regurgitation may develop secondary to right ventricular dilatation or from worms interfering with closure of the tricuspid valve in cases of caval syndrome.
      b) A murmur of tricuspid regurgitation is detected in >90% of all animals with caval syndrome.
      c) Diastolic murmur of pulmonary regurgitation may arise secondary to pulmonary hypertension and dilatation of the main pulmonary artery annulus (uncommon).
      d) Splitting of the second heart sound is occasionally heard in association with pulmonary hypertension.
    2. Lung sounds
      Fine to coarse inspiratory crackling is heard sometimes and is associated with eosinophilic pneumonitis.
    3. General physical findings related to R-CHF
      a) Jugular venous pulsation/distention
      b) Hepatomegaly and ascites
      c) Pleural effusion (muffled heart and lung sounds)
      d) Chronic weight loss
      e) Gallop rhythm (accentuated third heart sound)
  B. Thoracic radiography
    1. Pulmonary radiographic features are recognizable first in the caudal lung lobes and best appreciated in the dorsoventral projection.
    2. The earliest radiographic changes include indistinct expansion and linear opacification of peripheral pulmonary arteries.
    3. Moderate disease is characterized by increased interstitial pulmonary radiodensity and tortuosity, loss of uniform tapering, and truncation of peripheral pulmonary arteries and lobar branches.
    4. In addition to worsening of these, advanced disease is characterized by enlargement of the main pulmonary artery and right side of the heart.
    5. A dense interstitial lung pattern radiating from the hilum, and obscuring the vascular features, is typical of eosinophilic pneumonitis.
    6. Blotchy pulmonary parenchymal densities are indicative of focal granulomas and major arterial thrombosis.
    7. Eosinophilic granulomas are more distinct tis-

sue densities with clearly defined borders that may reach several centimeters in diameter.

C. Electrocardiography (ECG)
   1. ECG evidence of right ventricular hypertrophy (RVH) occurs only in the presence of chronic, severe pulmonary hypertension.
   2. Hemodynamically significant arrhythmias are quite uncommon, even with severe disease, but may include atrial fibrillation and paroxysmal or sustained ventricular tachycardia (see Chap. 7).

D. Echocardiography
   1. Enlargement of the right atrium and ventricle
   2. Hypertrophy of the papillary muscles of the tricuspid valve and right ventricular free wall
   3. Paradoxical motion of the interventricular septum in some cases of pulmonary hypertension and CHF
   4. Indicated in dogs with evidence of CHF or those suspected of having caval syndrome

E. Clinical laboratory findings
   1. Findings typically nonspecific
   2. Hematology: eosinophilia, basophilia, normocytic hypochromic anemia
   3. Serum biochemical profile
      a) Hypergammaglobulinemia ± hypoalbuminemia
      b) Elevation of enzymes reflecting hepatic necrosis and congestion
      c) Elevated levels of serum creatinine, urea nitrogen (BUN)
   4. Urinalysis
      a) Albuminuria
      b) Hemoglobinuria, hyperbilirubinuria

II. Definitive diagnosis
   A. Species identification of circulating MF
      1. Microfilariae of *D. immitis* should be identified and treated for the following reasons.
         a) Reservoirs of infection can then be eliminated.
         b) Some microfilaremic dogs do not have detectable amounts of circulating heartworm antigen and are missed with serologic testing.
         c) Diethylcarbamazine is hazardous to MF-positive dogs.
      2. Concentration techniques (Knott test and filter method) are superior to fresh blood smears as screening tests.
      3. False-negative results can occur with the use of nonconcentrating techniques and with occult infections.
      4. False-positive results can occur with contaminated filter holders or with persistent MF after death of adult heartworms.
   B. Serologic testing
      1. Approximately 20–75% of infected dogs do not have circulating MF for one of the following reasons.
         a) Prepatent infection
         b) Host hypersensitivity to MF (immune occult)

         c) Unisex infection
         d) Microfilaricide (chemoprophylaxis) suppression of MF
         e) Infertile heartworms
      2. Methodology
         a) Detection of circulating *D. immitis* antigen by monoclonal antibody enzyme-linked immunosorbent assay (ELISA), bifunctional antibody hemagglutination, and immunochromatography has replaced indirect fluorescent antibody (IFA) and ELISA methods that detect host antibody to HW antigen.
         b) Commercially available HW antigen detection kits are applicable, without modification, for all host species, with the exception of the bifunctional antibody/hemagglutination test (VetRED).
         c) The target antigen is produced primarily by mature females.
         d) Cross-reactivity with other filarial parasites is not a problem.
         e) False-negative results are caused by low antigenemia.
            (1) Prepatent (immature) infections
            (2) Light infections with <5 worms
            (3) Unisex (male) infections
         f) False-positive results are uncommon.
            (1) Technical errors: most related to inadequate wash cycles
            (2) Nonspecific binding to sample debris
      3. Interpretation of results
         a) When screening in areas where prevalence of infection is low, the predictive value of a positive test result depends more on the specificity of a test than its sensitivity.
         b) A positive HW antigen test is indicative of current or recently terminated (within 12–20 weeks) infection with adult heartworms.
         c) The strength of the test reaction (not applicable for the hemagglutination test) is proportional to the number of mature adults and is a measure of infection but not severity of disease.
         d) Unexpected positive (faint) results should be verified by repeating the test using meticulous technique.
         e) When results are ambiguous in animals with no objective evidence of infection, defer adulticide administration and retest after several months.
      4. Microfilarial and antigen detection tests are complementary and, when combined, yield a slightly higher rate of positive diagnoses.
   C. Direct visualization of adult heartworms via two-dimensional echocardiography
      1. The right cardiac chambers, the main pulmonary artery and the right branch, and the caudal vena cava can be adequately imaged to identify adult heartworms.

2. Findings are usually negative except in heavily infected cases.
3. Failure to visualize heartworms does not rule out the disease.
4. A cluster of worms surging back and forth through the tricuspid valve is a classic feature of caval syndrome.

Differential Diagnosis

I. Pulmonary thrombosis
   A. Hyperadrenocorticism
   B. Renal amyloidosis
   C. Idiopathic pulmonary thrombosis
II. Pulmonary neoplasia
III. Primary chronic respiratory disease
   A. Chronic bronchitis
   B. Pneumonia
   C. Tracheal collapse
IV. Heart failure
   A. Dilated cardiomyopathy
   B. Pericardial disease
   C. Valvular heart disease
V. Microfilaremia
   A. Filarial species other than *D. immitis* and *Dipetalonema reconditum* rarely found in the United States
   B. Irish *Dipetalonema* spp.: Ireland, Great Britain, Florida
   C. Miscellaneous unnamed *Dirofilaria* spp.: Florida

Treatment

I. Pretreatment patient evaluation
   A. Thorough physical examination
   B. Thoracic radiographs
      1. Assess degrees of cardiac and pulmonary arterial changes
      2. Indispensable for classifying disease and determining prognosis
   C. Selective laboratory tests
      1. Complete blood count
      2. Serum biochemical profile
      3. Urinalysis
      4. Semi-quantitative HW antigen assessment
   D. Additional special studies depending on clinical circumstances
      1. ECG
      2. Echocardiography
      3. Angiography (seldom necessary)
II. Patient classification
   Note: Animals need not display all characteristics of a given classification to be assigned that class of disease.
   A. Class 1: subclinical disease
      1. Weakly positive HW antigen test
      2. No clinical signs
      3. Normal physical examination
      4. Thoracic radiographs normal or mild evidence of pulmonary arterial or parenchymal changes (see earlier)
      5. Laboratory data within normal limits

   B. Class 2: moderate disease
      1. Moderately positive HW antigen test
      2. Moderate exercise intolerance and/or an occasional cough
      3. Good to fair general condition
      4. Moderate right ventricular and/or main pulmonary artery enlargement, moderate enlargement of the pulmonary arteries with truncation, diffuse perivascular pulmonary parenchymal infiltrates on radiography
      5. ± Mild anemia, circulating eosinophilia, moderate proteinuria
   C. Class 3: severe disease
      1. Strongly positive HW antigen test
      2. Obvious clinical signs: significant exercise intolerance, respiratory distress, persistent cough, ascites, anorexia, weight loss
      3. Poor to fair general condition, increased respiratory sounds, easily elicited cough, jugular venous distention, ascites, prolonged capillary refill time, pale mucous membranes
      4. Right ventricular and atrial enlargement; enlarged pulmonary arteries with pruning, truncation, and loss of arterial arborization; diffuse pulmonary parenchymal infiltrates with evidence of pulmonary thromboembolism
      5. Marked anemia and proteinuria; decreased plasma protein; elevated levels of BUN, creatinine, and hepatic enzymes
   D. Special considerations
      1. Dogs older than 9 years of age and/or weighing <7.5 kg are typically assigned a disease classification one class greater than diagnostic tests would suggest.
      2. Surgical extraction of heartworms, via jugular venotomy, from dogs with caval syndrome should be performed without delay (Jackson et al., 1977).
III. Elimination of adult heartworms
   A. Melarsomine HCl (Immiticide)
      1. Give dogs with class 1 and class 2 disease two injections at 2.5 mg/kg IM 24 hours apart.
      2. Give dogs with class 3 disease one injection at 2.5 mg/kg IM, wait 30 days and then give two injections at 2.5 mg/kg IM 24 hours apart (split-dosing regimen).
      3. Meticulous attention to injection technique minimizes local inflammation (medication must be given by deep lumbar intramuscular injection).
      4. Efficacy against adult females surpasses that of thiacetarsamide, and incidence of acute hepatic and renal toxicity is much less.
      5. Minimize exercise for 4–6 weeks after treatment or 8–10 weeks if using the split-dosing regimen.
      6. Most common complications are local inflammation and thromboembolic disease.
   B. Thiacetarsamide sodium (Caparsolate)
      1. Give dogs 2.2 mg/kg (0.22 ml/kg) IV BID at 6- to 8-hour intervals for 2 days, with the overnight interval not exceeding 16 hours.

2. Underdosing is totally ineffective.
3. Survival of some adult female worms (usually immature females) is common (>25%).
4. If the injection series is interrupted, repeat all four doses.
5. Minimize exercise for 4–6 weeks after treatment.
6. Most common complications are acute hepatic or renal toxicity, and local cellulitis secondary to perivascular injection and thromboembolism.

C. Surgical extraction of adult heartworms
1. Straight alligator forceps or endoscopic basket retrieval device (Jackson et al., 1977)
2. Indicated only in caval syndrome in which heartworms in the right atrium and venae cavae can be reached via jugular venotomy
3. Performed under local anesthesia
4. Timing of further adulticide therapy (if indicated) based on clinical response

IV. Elimination of MF
A. Ivermectin
1. Dose in dogs is 50 μg/kg PO, repeated in 10 days if MF persist. The cattle parasiticide may be diluted 1:9 with propylene glycol; the dose is 0.5 ml/10 kg PO.
2. Dosage in collies must be precise.
3. Microfilaricidal reactions may occur within 8 hours in dogs with high MF counts, so hospitalization and monitoring are prudent.
4. Administration of prednisone at a dose of 1 mg/kg PO 1 hour before and 6 hours after administration prevents most adverse reactions seen with high circulating MF counts.
5. Prophylactic dose is also microfilaricidal, often resulting in elimination of circulating MF within 6–12 months.

B. Milbemycin oxime
1. Prophylactic dose (500 μg/kg PO) is also microfilaricidal.
2. Microfilaricidal reactions may occur within 8 hours in dogs with high MF counts, so hospitalization and monitoring are prudent.
3. Administration of prednisone at a dose of 1 mg/kg PO 1 hour before and 6 hours after administration of milbemycin prevents most adverse reactions seen with high circulating MF counts.

V. Methods of chemoprophylaxis
A. Ivermectin
1. Dosage is 6–12 μg/kg PO once monthly.
2. Protection is provided for exposure period of at least 45 days preceding administration.
3. It may provide up to 4 months "reach-back" protection if given for 12 consecutive months (Soll and Knight, 1996).
4. Long-term administration to dogs with prepatent or patent infections results in suppression of MF.
5. It is safe in all breeds of dogs.

B. Milbemycin oxime
1. Dosage is 500 μg/kg PO once monthly.

2. It also controls roundworm, hookworm, and whipworm infection.
3. It may provide up to 3 months "reach-back" protection if given for 12 consecutive months (Soll and Knight, 1996)
4. Long-term administration to dogs with prepatent or patent infections results in suppression of MF.
5. It is safe in all breeds of dogs.

C. Diethylcarbamazine citrate (DEC)
1. Dosage is 6.6 mg/kg PO SID preceding infection and for 60 days following last exposure to mosquitos.
2. It is contraindicated if MF are present.
3. It may be continued in dogs that subsequently become microfilaremic as long as daily administration is not interrupted.
4. It may be used immediately in occult (MF-negative) infections.

VI. Retreatment with adulticide
A. Justifications
1. Interrupted treatment
2. Evidence of persistent infection and disease

B. Considerations
1. Adult heartworms become more susceptible with age, but a second treatment with thiacetarsamide may be no more successful than the first.
2. Additional doses of melarsamine are typically associated with a higher likelihood of seroconversion (Soll and Knight, 1996).
3. Re-treat dogs with persistent microfilaremia.
4. Nonworking, asymptomatic MF-negative dogs with presumed light infections that are receiving prophylaxis face little risk if their infection is not completely eradicated (disease vs. infection).

VII. Ancillary treatments
A. Prednisolone
1. Dosage is 1–2 mg/kg PO divided BID in diminishing doses over 7–14 days.
2. It effectively decreases pulmonary parenchymal inflammation caused by the following.
a) MF hypersensitivity–induced allergic pneumonitis
b) Heartworm thromboembolic pulmonary granulomas
3. It may help control mild hemoptysis.
4. Results of recent studies suggest that routine postadulticide administration (1 mg/kg PO QOD) may be beneficial despite the tendency to promote pulmonary thrombosis (Otto, 1983; Soll and Knight, 1996).

B. Aspirin
1. The regression of pulmonary endovascular lesions and reduction in pulmonary thromboembolism originally attributed to low-dose aspirin therapy in dogs have not been substantiated (Otto, 1989).
2. The American Heartworm Society no longer advocates the use of aspirin in the manage-

ment of heartworm disease (Soll and Knight, 1996).

C. Arterial vasodilators

1. The use of arterial vasodilators such as hydralazine may reduce the severity of pulmonary hypertension in some animals but also may be associated with adverse effects including systemic hypotension and reflex tachycardia.

2. Supplemental oxygen administration remains the safest and most effective means by which to induce pulmonary vasodilation in these animals.

D. R-CHF therapy

1. Strict exercise limitation
2. Digoxin
3. Diuretics in modest doses
4. Dietary sodium restriction
5. Supplemental oxygen

Patient Monitoring

I. Complications of therapy

A. Adulticide (thiacetarsamide)

1. Perivasculitis at the venipuncture site

a) Do not inject if venipuncture is anything less than perfect.

b) Stop injection immediately if a bleb occurs or needle must be repositioned.

c) Painful, edematous swelling may be evident within 1 hour.

d) At first indication of injection accident, clip area and apply topical dimethyl sulfoxide (DMSO) every 4–6 hours until pain subsides. Hot compresses and astringents may have value.

e) Monitor severe cases for skin slough after several days.

2. Systemic toxicosis

a) Anorexia, vomiting, and icterus may become evident during the injection series (first 2 days).

b) Proceed cautiously if only anorexia develops.

c) Discontinue treatment with the appearance of icterus, depression, fever, or vomiting.

d) There are no laboratory tests that are helpful in predicting which animals are likely to become toxic.

e) No specific antidotes are available; most animals recover with supportive treatment.

f) Adulticide treatment can be repeated 4–6 weeks later and is usually completed without further complications.

3. Pulmonary thromboembolism

a) Fever, tachypnea, cough, and sometimes hemoptysis are evident.

b) Clinical signs usually manifest as the worms die, 5–10 days after treatment.

c) Disseminated intravascular coagulation may develop in seriously ill animals.

d) Prednisolone is useful (see earlier).

e) Antibiotics are reserved for severe cases with extensive parenchymal damage.

f) Exercise restriction is essential until clinical signs have disappeared for at least 2 weeks.

B. Microfilaricides

1. Ivermectin

a) Miscalculated, off-label use as a microfilaricide may produce dose-dependent side effects.

(1) Minor signs (within 10–12 hours) include salivation, vomiting, mydriasis, tachypnea, disorientation, stupor, mild ataxia, and tremors.

(2) Severe signs that may begin within 4–6 hours are marked ataxia, tremors, seizures, recumbency, coma, and death.

(3) Therapy for toxicosis involves supportive care with fluid therapy.

(4) Most dogs, even if comatose, usually recover in a few days.

b) Side effects from a rapid reduction in MF may be confused with toxicosis.

(1) Onset within 6–8 hours: listlessness, fever, anorexia, vomiting, diarrhea, cough, shock

(2) Therapy: supportive care with fluid therapy and corticosteroids

2. Milbemycin oxime

a) No adverse reactions attributed to a direct toxic effect have been reported to date.

b) Side effects from a rapid reduction in MF have been reported.

(1) Onset within 6–8 hours: listlessness, fever, anorexia, vomiting, diarrhea, cough, shock

(2) Therapy: supportive care with fluid therapy and corticosteroids

C. Chemoprophylaxis

1. Ivermectin

a) No confirmed reports of adverse reaction at prophylactic dose

b) Safe in all breeds at this dose

2. Milbemycin oxime

a) No confirmed adverse reactions to date

b) Has potential side effects in dogs with high MF numbers related to its microfilaricidal activity

3. DEC reactions

a) Systemic type I hypersensitivity (anaphylactic shock) may develop in D. immitis MF–positive dogs within 20 minutes of receiving DEC.

(1) Emesis, diarrhea, salivation

(2) Depression, lethargy, incoordination, prostration

(3) Hypovolemic shock

(4) Disseminated intravascular coagulation

b) Reaction peaks within 1–2 hours, with recovery in most cases by 6 hours. Fatalities do occur.

c) Supportive therapy consists primarily of fluid replacement and administration of dexamethasone.

II. Assessing efficiency of adulticide treatment
 A. Clinical signs of efficacy
  1. Development or worsening of respiratory signs 5–10 days after treatment
  2. Eventual improvement in respiratory signs
 B. Heartworm antigenemia
  1. Persistence beyond 12–20 weeks after treatment is indicative of a residual infection.
  2. Disappearance within 12–20 weeks indicates complete eradication or survival of very few worms.
 C. Microfilaremia
   Disappearance of MF does not guarantee all adults have been killed, as residual unisex infections are common.
III. Assessing efficacy of microfilaricides
 A. Timing of re-examinations
   Ivermectin should eliminate MF within 2 weeks (usually within 72 hours).
 B. Persistent MF
  1. Occasionally there is a postadulticide inability to achieve MF-negative status.
   a) Persistent dual sex infection
   b) Inadequate dose of microfilaricide
   c) Noncompliance with microfilaricide administration
  2. There may be postadulticide return of MF within weeks of an initially successful microfilaricide treatment.
   a) Persistent dual sex infection
   b) Female unisex infection continuing to release MF
  3. There may be a postadulticide return of MF 6 months or more after successful microfilaricide treatment because of reinfection with a new generation of heartworms.
   a) Inadequate dose or duration of chemoprophylactic agent.
   b) Noncompliance with chemoprophylactic administration.

FELINE HEARTWORM DISEASE

Definition

I. Heartworm disease (HWD): obstructive pulmonary vascular disorder
II. Distribution
 A. Suitable mosquito vectors exist worldwide in temperate and tropical climates.
 B. A serious endemic problem exists in many parts of the world.

C. In the United States, feline HWD has been reported in 30 states (Soll and Knight, 1996).

Cause

I. Caused by the mosquito-borne filarial parasite *D. immitis*
II. Life cycle of *D. immitis* (Katoni and Powers, 1982)
 A. L1 to L4 stages similar to that in the dog (see earlier)
 B. Tissue migratory stages (L4, L5)
  1. Infective larvae promptly molt (2 weeks) to the precardiac fourth stage (L4).
  2. Maturation to the fifth larval stage (juvenile adult, L5) occurs about 50–70 days after infection.
 C. Adult stage (L5)
  1. Fifth stage larvae reach the circulation by penetrating systemic veins between 70 and 110 days.
  2. After embolizing the pulmonary arteries, they mature and release MF usually by 6.5–8 months after infection.
  3. Adult worms usually survive only 1–3 years.

Clinical Signs

I. Clinical signs are not as stereotyped as in dogs and do not correlate as well with the presence of heartworms.
II. Signs can include the following.
 A. Coughing
 B. Intermittent dyspnea
 C. Sporadic vomiting sometimes associated with eating and not usually in association with respiratory signs
 D. Lethargy, weight loss
 E. Hemoptysis (uncommon)
 F. Nonspecific neurologic signs (aberrant migration/location)
 G. Sudden death

Diagnosis

I. Systemic evidence of HWD
 A. Physical findings
  1. Heart murmurs: exceptionally uncommon (Atkins et al., in press)
  2. Lung sounds
   a) Fine to coarse inspiratory crackling is sometimes heard.
   b) Increased bronchovesicular sounds are common.
  3. General physical findings related to R-CHF
   a) Jugular venous pulsation/distention
   b) Pleural effusion (muffled heart and lung sounds)
   c) Chronic weight loss
   d) Gallop rhythm (accentuated third heart sound)
 B. Thoracic radiography
  1. Pulmonary radiographic features are recogniz-

able first in the caudal lung lobes and best appreciated in the dorsoventral (DV) projection.
2. The earliest radiographic changes include indistinct expansion and linear opacification of peripheral pulmonary arteries.
3. Moderate disease is characterized by increased interstitial pulmonary radiodensity, and tortuosity, loss of uniform tapering, and truncation of peripheral pulmonary arteries and lobar branches.
4. The radiographic finding that correlates best with a diagnosis of feline HWD is enlargement of the caudal pulmonary arteries (ratio >1.6:1) when compared with the 9th rib in the DV or ventrodorsal projection (Schafer and Berry, 1995).
5. Pleural effusion (chylous) has been documented in both experimental and spontaneous cases of feline HWD.

C. Electrocardiography (ECG)
1. ECG evidence of right ventricular hypertrophy (RVH) in HWD may occur in the presence of chronic, severe pulmonary hypertension.
2. Hemodynamically significant arrhythmias are quite uncommon.

D. Echocardiography
1. Enlargement of the right atrium and ventricle
2. Dilation of the main pulmonary artery with visualization of adults

E. Clinical laboratory findings
1. Findings are typically nonspecific.
2. See previous laboratory findings in the dog.

II. Definitive diagnosis of infection
A. Serologic testing
1. More than 80% of cats with HWD do not have circulating MF for one of the following reasons.
   a) Prepatent infection
   b) Host hypersensitivity to MF (immune occult)
   c) Unisex infection
2. Methodology
   a) Commercially available heartworm antigen (HW-Ag) detection kits are applicable, without modification, for all host species, with the exception of the bifunctional antibody/hemagglutination test (VetRED).
   b) False-negative results are caused by low antigenemia.
      (1) Prepatent (immature) infections
      (2) Light infections with <5 worms
      (3) Unisex (male) infections
   c) False-positive results are uncommon.
      (1) Technical errors: most related to inadequate wash cycles
      (2) Nonspecific binding to sample debris
   d) A commercially available heartworm antibody (HW-Ab) test has recently been

shown to be both sensitive and specific (Soll and Knight, 1996).
3. Interpretation of results
   a) A positive HW-Ag test is indicative of current or recently terminated (within 12–20 weeks) infection with adult heartworms.
   b) The strength of the test reaction is proportional to the number of mature adults and is a measure of infection but not severity of disease.
   c) A negative HW-Ag test does not eliminate the diagnosis.
   d) A negative HW-Ab test essentially eliminates HWD as a differential diagnosis.
   e) A positive HW-Ab test simply documents exposure; it does not establish a diagnosis of an adult worm infestation.

B. Direct visualization of adult heartworms with two-dimensional echocardiography
1. The right cardiac chambers, the main pulmonary artery and the right branch, and the caudal vena cava can be adequately imaged to identify adult heartworms.
2. Findings may be positive even when all other tests are negative.
3. Failure to visualize heartworms does not rule out the disease but makes it quite unlikely.
4. A cluster of worms surging back and forth through the tricuspid valve is a classic feature of caval syndrome.

Differential Diagnosis

I. Other causes of pulmonary thrombosis
II. Pulmonary neoplasia
III. Primary chronic respiratory disease
   A. Chronic bronchitis (asthma)
   B. Pneumonia
   C. Lungworms
IV. Heart failure
   A. Cardiomyopathy
   B. Pericardial disease
   C. Valvular heart disease

Treatment

I. Because of the severity of post-adulticide complications encountered in cats, a significant controversy exists as to whether or not cats should receive any form of adulticide therapy.
II. Pretreatment patient evaluation involves the following.
   A. Thorough physical examination
   B. Thoracic radiography
      1. Assess degrees of cardiac and pulmonary arterial and parenchymal changes
      2. May help differentiate feline HWD from other differential diagnoses
   C. Selective laboratory tests
      1. Complete blood count

2. Serum biochemical profile
3. Urinalysis
4. Semi-quantitative HW-Ag assessment
5. HW-Ab assessment
   D. Additional special studies depending on clinical circumstances
   1. ECG (seldom indicated)
   2. Echocardiography
      a) Sensitivity is much greater in cats than in dogs.
      b) It is imperative that the bifurcation of the pulmonary artery be imaged.
      c) Worms appear as hyperechoic parallel lines.
   3. Non-selective pulmonary angiography
      a) Allows for critical evaluation of pulmonary vascular size and tortuosity, even in the presence of pulmonary parenchymal infiltrate
      b) May detect intraluminal filling defects
      c) May help rule out important differential diagnoses
III. Most investigators recommend *against* the use of adulticide therapy for elimination of adult heartworms in cats. Instead, supportive therapy with corticosteroids and bronchodilators is preferred.
   A. Melarsomine HCl (Immiticide)
   1. Minimal information is available regarding safety or efficacy in cats.
   2. One recent study suggested that a single dose of 2.5 mg/kg IM resulted in a 35% worm kill with no significant adverse effects (Goodman, 1996). This degree of adulticide efficacy was not significantly different from placebo.
   B. Thiacetarsamide sodium (Caparsolate)
   1. Give cats 0.22 ml/kg IV BID at 8-hour intervals for 2 days, with the overnight interval not exceeding 16 hours.
   2. Minimize exercise for 4–6 weeks after treatment.
   3. Most common complications are acute hepatic or renal toxicity, local cellulitis secondary to perivascular injection, and thromboembolism.
   4. A fatal idiosyncratic pulmonary reaction resulting in pulmonary edema has been reported.
   C. Surgical extraction of adult heartworms
   1. Horse hair brush or endoscopic basket retrieval device (Glaus et al., 1995)
   2. Indicated only in caval syndrome in which heartworms in the right atrium and venae cavae can be reached via jugular venotomy
   3. Performed using heavy sedation and local anesthesia
IV. Elimination of MF is almost never needed in cats because of the exceptionally high number (>80%) of MF-negative cases.
   A. Ivermectin
      The prophylactic dose (24 μg/kg PO) is also microfilaricidal, often resulting in elimination of circulating MF within 6–12 months.

   B. Milbemycin oxime
   1. Prophylactic dose (500 μg/kg) is also microfilaricidal.
   2. Microfilaricidal reactions may occur within 8 hours in cats with high MF counts (very uncommon).
V. Methods of chemoprophylaxis are as follows.
   A. Ivermectin
   1. Dosage is 24 μg/kg PO once monthly (4 times the canine dose).
   2. Protection is provided for an exposure period of at least 45 days preceding administration.
   3. Long-term administration to cats with prepatent infections may suppress microfilaremia.
   B. Milbemycin oxime
   1. Dosage is 500 μg/kg PO once monthly (same as the canine dose).
   2. It provides protection for prior 30 days, if administered at 60 and 90 days after exposure.
VI. Ancillary treatments may be used.
   A. Prednisolone
   1. Dosage is 1–2 mg/kg PO divided twice daily in diminishing doses over 7–14 days.
   2. It effectively decreases pulmonary parenchymal inflammation caused by the following.
      a) MF hypersensitivity–induced allergic pneumonitis
      b) Heartworm thromboembolic pulmonary granulomas
   3. It may help control mild hemoptysis.
   B. Bronchodilators
   1. Used to control bronchoconstriction associated with eosinophilic parenchymal inflammation
   2. Preferred: Theo-Dur 25 mg/kg PO SID in the evening
   C. R-CHF therapy
   1. Strict exercise limitation
   2. Digoxin
   3. Diuretics in modest doses
   4. Dietary sodium restriction
   5. Supplemental oxygen

Patient Monitoring

I. Complications of therapy
   A. Adulticide (thiacetarsamide)
   1. Similar to those seen in the dog (see earlier discussion)
   2. Perivasculitis at the venipuncture site
   3. Systemic toxicosis
   4. Pulmonary thromboembolism
      a) Fever, tachypnea, cough, and sometimes hemoptysis are evident.
      b) Clinical signs usually manifest as the worms die, 5–10 days after treatment.
      c) Disseminated intravascular coagulation may develop in seriously ill animals.
      d) Prednisolone is useful, as for dogs (see earlier).
      e) Antibiotics are reserved for severe cases with extensive parenchymal damage.

f) Exercise restriction is essential until clinical signs have disappeared for at least 2 weeks.

g) It is usually more severe than in dogs.

B. Microfilaricides

Complications associated with the use of microfilaricides are uncommon, as they are infrequently used in cats, but when encountered are similar to those seen in dogs (see earlier).

C. Chemoprophylaxis

1. Ivermectin
   a) No confirmed reports of adverse reaction at prophylactic dose
   b) Safe in all breeds at this dose
2. Milbemycin oxime
   a) No confirmed adverse reactions to date
   b) Has potential side effects in cats with high MF numbers related to its microfilaricidal activity

II. Assessing efficiency of adulticide treatment

A. Clinical signs of efficacy

1. Development or worsening of respiratory signs 5–10 days after treatment
2. Eventual improvement in respiratory signs

B. Heartworm antigenemia

1. Persistence beyond 12–20 weeks after treatment is indicative of a residual infection.
2. Disappearance within 12–20 weeks indicates complete eradication or survival of very few worms.
3. It is not as useful as in the dog, because some cats are heartworm antigen negative prior to therapy and have the diagnosis made on echocardiography or angiography.
4. It has been estimated that there is a 30% mortality associated with adulticide therapy in cats (Atkins et al., in press).

Bibliography

Ackerman N: Radiographic aspects of heartworm disease. Semin Vet Med Surg 2:15, 1987

Atkins C, DeFrancesco TR, Miller MW et al: Prevalence of heartworm infection in cats with cardiorespiratory abnormalities. J Am Vet Med Assoc (in press)

Castleman WL, Wong MM: Light and electron microscopic pulmonary lesions associated with retained microfilariae in canine occult dirofilariasis. Vet Pathol 19:355, 1982.

Chalifoux L, Hunt RD: Histochemical differentiation of *Dirofilaria immitis* and *Dipetalonema reconditum*. J Am Vet Med Assoc 158:601, 1971

Courtney CH, Zeng Qi-Yun: Immunodiagnosis of occult heartworm infection. Cal Vet Jan:12, 1989

Glaus TM, Jacobs GJ, Rawlings CA et al: Surgical removal of heartworms from a cat caval syndrome. J Am Vet Med Assoc 206:663, 1995

Goodman JG: Safety and efficacy of melarsomine dihydrochloride in cats with experimentally induced dirofilariasis [abstract 88]. Proc Am Assoc Vet Parasitol, 1996

Ishihara K, Kitagawa H, Okima M et al: Clinicopathological studies in canine dirofilarial hemoglobinuria. Jpn J Vet Sci 40:525, 1978

Ishihara K, Sasaki Y, Kitagawa H: Development of a flexible alligator forceps: a new instrument for removal of heartworms in the pulmonary arteries of dogs. Jpn J Vet Sci 48:989, 1986

Jackson RF, von Lichtenberg F, Otto GF: Occurrence of adult heartworm in the venae cavae of dogs. J Am Vet Med Assoc 141:117, 1962

Jackson RF, Seymour WG, Growney PJ et al: Surgical treatment of the caval syndrome of canine heartworm disease. J Am Vet Med Assoc 171:1965, 1977

Katoni T, Powers KG: Developmental stages of *Dirofilaria immitis* in the dog. Am J Vet Res 43:2199, 1982

Knight DH: Heartworm disease. p. 1097. In Ettinger SJ (ed): Textbook of Veterinary Internal Medicine. 2nd Ed. WB Saunders, Philadelphia, 1983

Knight DH: Heartworm infection. Vet Clin North Am [Small Anim Pract] 17:1463, 1987a

Knight DH: Thiacetarsamide treatment of heartworm infection in dogs. Semin Vet Med Surg 2:36, 1987b

Knight DH: Multifaceted hypothesis for the pathogenesis of caval syndrome. Proc Am Coll Vet Intern Med 8:875, 1990

Otto GF (ed): Proceedings of the Heartworm Symposium 1977. Veterinary Medical Publishing, Bonner Springs, Kansas, 1978

Otto GF (ed): Proceedings of the Heartworm Symposium 1980. Veterinary Medical Publishing, Edwardsville, Kansas, 1981

Otto GF (ed): Proceedings of the Heartworm Symposium 1983. Veterinary Medical Publishing, Edwardsville, Kansas, 1983

Otto GF (ed): Proceedings of the Heartworm Symposium 1986. American Heartworm Society, Washington, DC, 1986

Otto GF (ed): Proceedings of the Heartworm Symposium 1989. American Heartworm Society, Washington, DC, 1989

Rawlings CA: Pulmonary arteriography and hemodynamics during feline heartworm disease: effects of aspirin. J Vet Intern Med 4:285, 1990

Schafer M, Berry CR: Cardiac and pulmonary artery mensuration in feline heartworm disease. Vet Radiol Ultrasound 36:499, 1995

Schaub RC, Keigh JC, Rawlings CA: The effect of acetylsalicylic acid on vascular damage and myointimal proliferation in canine pulmonary arteries subjected to chronic injury by *Dirofilaria immitis*. Am J Vet Res 44:449, 1983

Soll MD, Knight DH (eds): Proceedings of the Heartworm Symposium 1995. American Heartworm Society, Batavia, IL, 1996

Respiratory System

13

Introduction

Brendan C. McKiernan

PULMONARY DEFENSE MECHANISMS

I. Defense mechanisms must exist to protect the airways and enable the respiratory system to maintain normal function.

II. Nonspecific mechanisms include natural defenses.
   A. Convoluted, branching air passageways created by nasal turbinates and lower airway bifurcations help keep debris from penetrating deep into the lungs.
      1. Inertial impaction causes particles ≥ 10 μm diameter to settle out in the upper airways (nose, pharynx, larynx, and trachea).
      2. Particles in the 0.5–2 μm range are affected by sedimentation (gravity) but are capable of reaching the distal airways.
      3. Particles ≤ 0.5 μm diameter may reach the alveoli and remain suspended unless diffusion (brownian motion) causes them to impact the surface.
   B. A mucociliary blanket traps particulate material and soluble vapors for clearance; inhaled gases are warmed and humidified.
      1. Mucus is produced by goblet cells and the submucosal glands.
      2. Cilia beat to move mucus and trapped material toward the pharynx at rates up to 20 mm/min in the trachea.
      3. Mucus contains substances that assist in pulmonary defenses: immunoglobulins, lysozyme, lactoferrin, interferon, and protease inhibitors.
   C. Normal protective reflexes serve to clear foreign material from the surface of the larger airways and prevent particulate material from deeply penetrating into the lungs.
      1. Upper airway reflexes include sneezing, reverse sneezing, and laryngospasm.
      2. Lower airway reflexes include coughing and bronchospasm.
   D. Intraepithelial lymphocytes and plasma cells are found in the airway walls. Aggregates of lymphocytes, submucosal lymphocytic nodules, and lymph nodes are important processing centers of inhaled antigens and actively participate in both local and systemic immune responses.
   E. The function of phagocytes (macrophages [MO] and neutrophils) is to assist in clearance of debris from the respiratory system through attachment, ingestion, phagolysosome formation, and particle killing.

III. Specific mechanisms are immunologically mediated defenses that develop after natural exposure to foreign antigens or after vaccination.
   A. Antigen specific antibody (humoral immunity) is secreted by B lymphocytes in response to presentation of antigen by pulmonary macrophages; the latter are responsible for the induction of the immune response.
      1. Different classes of immunoglobulins predominate in the mucosal secretions of the upper and lower airways.
      2. IgG is the most common immunoglobulin in lavage fluid from the lower airways/alveoli, appearing as the result of both diffusion from serum and local production.
      3. IgA is the predominant immunoglobulin in fluid recovered from the upper airways; IgA assists in agglutination and virus neutralization and prevents adherence among other functions.
   B. Cellular immunity involves T lymphocytes.
      1. Function in delayed hypersensitivity and cytotoxic responses
      2. Are stimulated to replicate after interaction with antigen processing MO
      3. Modulate MO function through the release of various lymphokines

RESPIRATORY PHYSIOLOGY

I. Ventilation: It is the process of moving air into and out of the lungs in sufficient quantity to meet the metabolic demands of the tissues.
   A. Inspiration is an active process; the muscles of

135

inspiration must expend energy to overcome three forces.
1. Frictional resistance to air flow
    a) Lung resistance (RL), or the amount of pressure required per unit of air flow, is measured as the change in pressure (ΔP)/change in air flow (ΔV).

$$RL = \Delta P/\Delta V, \text{ with units of cm } H_2O/ml/sec$$

    b) Approximately 50–70% of the total pulmonary resistance is in the upper airways, predominantly in the large central airways.
    c) Because of their very large cross-sectional area, diffuse small airway disease must exist before overall pulmonary resistance is increased or clinical signs are noted.
    d) RL is *increased* in such common clinical conditions as laryngeal paralysis, hilar lymphadenopathy, and chronic bronchitis.
2. Lung and chest wall elasticity
    a) Lung compliance (C), or how easily the lungs are distended, is measured as the change in tidal volume (ΔVT)/the change in pressure.

$$C = \Delta VT/\Delta P, \text{ with units of ml/cm } H_2O$$

    b) Diseases that cause pulmonary fluid or cellular infiltrates result in the lung becoming less compliant (stiffer) and more difficult to inflate.
    c) C is *decreased* in such common clinical conditions as pulmonary edema, fibrosis, severe obesity, pleural effusion, and pneumonia.
3. Inertia of tissue and gases within the airways
    a) Is minimal
    b) Is not normally measured
B. Expiration during quiet (resting or nonexertional) breathing is always a passive process.
    1. It occurs as the result of elastic fiber recoil in the lungs and also the recoil of the chest wall to normal position (functional residual capacity) after expansion (enlargement) of the rib cage during inspiration.
    2. Any active expiratory effort (abdominal muscular contraction) that occurs while resting is indicative of diffuse, obstructive intrathoracic (typically small) airway disease.
II. Distribution: Inhaled gases must be evenly distributed to all exchange units in the lungs to allow for O_2 uptake and CO_2 elimination.
    A. Regional differences in RL and C influence distribution.
    B. Clinical hypoxemia occurs because of this maldistribution of gases.
    C. Maldistribution (hypoxemia) is accentuated when respiratory rate increases, e.g., when metabolic demand increases with exercise.

III. Diffusion: Once in the alveolus, inhaled gas must equilibrate with pulmonary capillary blood across the alveolar capillary membrane.
    A. Factors that affect the diffusion of gas across the alveolar capillary membrane include the following.
        1. Surface area available for diffusion: decreased in true emphysema cases
        2. Wall thickness: increased with pulmonary edema and some infiltrative diseases
        3. Difference in partial pressure of the gas between alveolus and pulmonary capillary blood
        4. Solubility of the gas: CO_2 20-fold more soluble than O_2
        5. Time the blood flow is exposed to the membrane: pulmonary capillary blood transit time decreases as blood flow increases with exercise
    B. A major clinical factor in gas diffusion is driving pressure; this is why O_2 therapy works to increase PaO_2 levels.
IV. Perfusion: The amount of blood flow should match the amount of inhaled gas delivered to all gas exchange units.
    A. The normal ventilation/perfusion (V/Q) ratio is approximately 1.
    B. Pulmonary artery obstructive diseases (e.g., heartworms and pulmonary emboli) are common clinical examples of V/Q mismatching in dogs and cats.

LOCALIZING THE PROBLEM

I. History
    A. Excessive work of breathing, or *dyspnea*, is thought of as the interpretative description of any respiratory pattern (rate and/or effort) that is disproportionate to the level of the animal's recent activity.
    B. Excessively frequent reflexes are common presenting complaints and are associated with disorders affecting different anatomic sites.
        1. Sneezing/reverse sneezing: nasal/nasopharyngeal disease
        2. Coughing: characteristic sound; may be suggestive of a specific cause
        3. Wheezing heard by owners: airway narrowing
II. Physical examination
    A. Observation of the pattern and work of breathing
        1. Obstructive diseases are associated with increased RL, which classically lead to a slower respiratory rate and deeper tidal volume compared with normal.
            a) Increased inspiratory effort and/or inspiratory time are usually found with upper airway (extrathoracic) obstructive diseases (e.g., laryngeal paralysis, nasopharyngeal obstruction).
            b) Increased expiratory effort and/or expiratory time are usually noted with lower airway (intrathoracic) obstructive diseases (e.g., chronic bronchitis).

c) Fixed (when both inspiration and expiration are affected) and non-fixed (when only one is affected) airway obstructions may occur.

2. Restrictive diseases are associated with decreases in C and classically lead to a faster respiratory rate and a decreased tidal volume compared with normal.

3. Diseases associated with diffusion and/or perfusion abnormalities are not associated with a specific breathing pattern.

B. Auscultation

1. Normal lung sounds: note presence, location, and intensity
   a) Expiratory sound is louder and longer than inspiratory sound when heard over the trachea (bronchial lung sounds) but is normally quieter over the lung periphery.
   b) Vesicular sounds are normally very quiet (depending on tidal volume) and are best heard in the lung periphery.

2. Localization of adventitious or abnormal lung sounds
   a) When heard outside their normal location, bronchial sounds are abnormal and usually indicate lung consolidation.
   b) Crackles are associated with airways snapping open on inspiration and are commonly heard with bronchitis, edema, and pneumonia.
   c) Wheezes are associated with airway narrowing, are more noticeable on expiration, and are commonly heard with laryngospasm, bronchospasm, and airway obstruction.
      (1) Stridor: an inspiratory wheeze/noise that localizes to upper airway or larynx, most common with laryngeal diseases
      (2) Laryngeal brake: an expiratory wheeze that localizes to the larynx (sounds like whining); commonly due to diffuse lower airway disease

3. Type of cough
   a) Dry cough: tracheobronchial disease
   b) Moist cough: pneumonia or exudative process
   c) Snap or click with coughing: tracheobronchial collapse

C. Palpation of symmetry of chest wall motion, nasal airflow, abdominal muscle effort on expiration, degree of tracheal sensitivity

Bibliography

Bienenstock J: Immunology of the Lung and Upper Respiratory Tract. McGraw-Hill, New York, 1984

Murray JF: The Normal Lung. 2nd Ed. WB Saunders, Philadelphia, 1986

Murray JF, Nadel JA: Textbook of Respiratory Medicine. 2nd Ed. WB Saunders, Philadelphia, 1994

Robinson NE: Airway physiology. Vet Clin North Am [Small Anim Pract] 22:1043, 1992

14

Diseases of the Nasal and Nasopharyngeal Cavities and Paranasal Sinuses

Brendan C. McKiernan

DEVELOPMENTAL DISORDERS

Brachycephalic Syndrome

Definition and Causes

  I. It is a series of anatomic disorders in brachycephalic animals that, singly or in combination, result in varying degrees of upper airway obstruction.
 II. The syndrome consists of one or more of the following.
   A. Stenotic nares
   B. Elongated (often edematous) soft palate
   C. Laryngeal mucosal edema
   D. Collapse of the laryngeal cartilage(s)
   E. Everted or edematous lateral (laryngeal) saccules
   F. Tracheal hypoplasia
III. Commonly seen in the English bulldog, Boston bulldog, Pekingese, pug, Lhasa apso, and Shih Tzu. Less commonly encountered in brachycephalic cats.
 IV. No genetic studies on the syndrome have been published.
   A. It is assumed that the conformational selection process for these breeds perpetuates the clinical problem.
   B. Severely affected animals are not recommended for breeding.
  V. Factors that increase the risk of acute upper respiratory obstruction include the following.
   A. Hot, humid, ambient temperature with increased panting
   B. Recovery from anesthesia or sedation
   C. Obesity

Pathophysiology

  I. Abductor muscles function to dilate the non-rigid portions of the upper airways (nares, pharynx, larynx).
   A. Most dogs maintain respiration without any major effort of these muscles while at rest.
   B. English bulldogs require continuous muscle activity to maintain airway patency; relaxation during sleep routinely leads to hemoglobin desaturation and hypoxemia (Hendricks, 1992).
   C. Sedation and/or general anesthesia relax the dilating effect of these muscles.
    1. As a result, an animal may encounter some degree of airway obstruction.
    2. Brachycephalic animals are constantly at risk for developing upper airway obstruction and hypoxemia.
 II. The airway narrowing that occurs in brachycephalic breeds results in increased (primarily inspiratory) work of breathing, alveolar hypoventilation, and hypoxemia.
III. Over an extended period of time, increased negative airway pressures lead to further obstruction from the development of mucosal edema, saccular eversion, and eventually laryngeal collapse (Robinson, 1992; Hobson, 1995).

Clinical Signs

  I. History
   A. Exercise intolerance, excessive airway sounds (snoring, gurgling), and coughing are commonly reported by owners.
   B. Sounds often worse when the animal is sleeping.

II. Physical examination
   A. Careful handling is required to avoid undue stress in these animals.
   B. Hyperthermia and hypoxemia may occur following exercise, exertion, or stress.

Diagnosis

I. Signalment alone is enough to suspect this syndrome.
II. Confirmation of stenotic nares is based on the lack of a visible opening into the nares, with dynamic collapse of the alar fold during inspiration.
III. Laryngoscopy is required (under anesthesia) to fully assess the airway.
   A. Elongated soft palate: should just touch the tip of the epiglottis
   B. Laryngeal edema: mucosa is glistening or gelatinous in appearance
   C. Collapse of the laryngeal cartilage(s): typically collapsed at rest and is worse with increasing inspiratory effort
   D. Everted or edematous lateral (laryngeal) saccules: seen ventrally in the glottic lumen; may dynamically evert during forced breathing and return to a normal position quickly
IV. Tracheal hypoplasia is a radiographic diagnosis (see Chap. 16) and should be considered in any brachycephalic dog.

Differential Diagnosis

I. Nasopharyngeal obstruction
   A. Tumor or polyp, especially in the cat
   B. Pharyngeal mucocele
   C. Foreign body
II. Laryngeal paralysis (see Chap. 15)
III. Tracheal obstruction
   A. Chondroma or other mass
   B. Stenosis

Treatment

I. A temporary tracheostomy may be necessary.
   A. To relieve airway obstruction in severely affected animals
   B. To ensure a patent airway for the first 24–48 hours postoperatively
II. Medical treatment is usually indicated.
   A. Mucosal edema and swelling of the soft palate, the larynx, and/or the laryngeal saccules commonly occur.
   B. Short-term corticosteroids are indicated to reduce mucosal swelling and edema and may be repeated 1–2 times.
      1. Dexamethasone sodium phosphate 0.2–2.2 mg/kg IV
      2. Prednisolone 1–2 mg/kg SQ, IM
III. Various surgical procedures are available for the relief of upper airway obstructions in brachycephalics (Aron and Crowe, 1985; Hobson, 1995).
   A. Stenotic nares are corrected as early in life as

possible via removal of a small wedge-shaped portion of the alar fold.
   B. An elongated soft palate is surgically shortened.
   C. Collapse of the laryngeal cartilage(s) is more serious and requires either laryngeal prosthesis ("tie back") surgery or permanent tracheostomy.
   D. Everted saccules are removed if they cause significant laryngeal obstruction.
   E. Tracheal hypoplasia is not surgically correctable (see Chap. 16).

Patient Monitoring

I. Brachycephalic animals are at risk for developing upper airway obstruction during recovery from anesthesia.
II. Mucosal edema and postoperative swelling worsen airway obstruction.
III. Prognosis is good, especially if surgical correction is performed early in life.

INFECTIOUS/INFLAMMATORY DISEASES

Rhinitis/Sinusitis

Definition

Inflammation of the mucosa of the nasal cavity or sinuses without regard to etiology (cause) or duration (acute vs. chronic)

Causes

I. Primary nasal causes: conditions arising within the nose
   A. Viral infections
      1. Many different viruses are capable of infecting the upper respiratory tract.
         a) Dog: distemper, parainfluenza, herpesvirus, adenovirus
         b) Cat: calicivirus and rhinotracheitis virus
      2. Clinical signs often become more apparent with development of a secondary bacterial infection.
   B. Bacterial infections
      1. Primary infections are rare (Harvey, 1984). *Bordetella bronchiseptica* and *Pasteurella multocida* may be associated with primary bacterial rhinitis in the dog (Bedford, 1995).
      2. Secondary infections are common.
         a) Miscellaneous causes: any primary nasal disease
         b) Dental disease: one of the most common causes of secondary rhinitis in the middle-aged dog and cat (Manfra, 1992; McKiernan, 1995)
         c) Intranasal foreign bodies: plant material, metallic objects, stones, and teeth
         d) IgA deficiency: incriminated as a cause of rhinitis in dogs (Shofer et al., 1990; Felsburg, 1994)

e) Ciliary dyskinesia: ineffective mucociliary clearance, secretion retention, recurrent respiratory tract infections (Van Pelt and McKiernan, 1992)

C. Fungal infections (Wolf, 1992)
   1. Dogs (in order of frequency): *Aspergillus*, *Cryptococcus*, *Penicillium*, *Rhinosporidium* spp.
   2. Cats (in order of frequency): *Cryptococcus*, *Sporothrix*, *Aspergillus*, *Histoplasma* spp.
   3. Rare: *Alternaria*, *Exophiala*, *Prototheca*

D. Parasitic infections
   1. Nasal mite (*Pneumonyssoides caninum*) infections have been reported in dogs (Mundell and Ihrke, 1990).
   2. Capillariasis (*Capillaria* sp.) has been diagnosed in the nasal cavity of dogs and one cat but is more commonly found in the lower respiratory tract (King et al., 1990).
   3. Gapeworm (*Syngamus ierei*) infection has been reported in 33% of stray cats surveyed from Puerto Rico (Cuadrado et al., 1980).
   4. Miscellaneous parasites include grubs (*Cuterebra* spp.) and tongue worms (*Linguatula serrata*).

E. Neoplasia
   1. Adenocarcinoma (most common) and other types of tumors occur in both dogs and cats.
   2. Secondary bacterial infections are common (Ogilvie and LaRue, 1992).

F. Idiopathic rhinitis
   1. No definitive cause can be determined, yet a thick nasal discharge persists.
   2. Examples include the following.
      a) Chronic rhinosinusitis of cats (Cape, 1992)
      b) Irish wolfhound rhinitis (Wilkinson, 1969)
      c) Chronic hyperplastic rhinitis in whippets and dachshunds (Sullivan, 1991)

G. Other causes
   1. Allergy
      a) Eosinophils on cytology, but no parasite identified
      b) Reported in small-breed dogs, especially dachshunds (van Oosterhout et al., 1989)
   2. Lymphoplasmacytic rhinitis
      a) Lymphocytes and plasma cells on biopsy or cytology
      b) Turbinate destruction common (Burgener et al., 1987)
      c) Probably related to chronic (undetermined) antigenic stimulation
   3. Cleft palate with secondary irritation of the nasal cavity
   4. Trauma

II. Extranasal causes: primary process outside the nasal cavity (McKiernan, 1995)
   A. Pneumonia
   B. Chronic vomiting or regurgitating
      1. Cricopharyngeal disorders
      2. Megaesophagus
      3. Primary and secondary causes of vomiting

Pathophysiology

I. Stimulation of subepithelial receptors initiates protective reflexes that function to facilitate removal of irritants and particulate matter from the mucosal surfaces of the nasal cavity.
   A. Sneezing is a forceful expiration associated with nasal cavity irritation.
   B. Reverse sneezing is a forceful inspiration associated with irritation of the dorsal nasopharyngeal mucosa.

II. These reflexes may diminish or disappear with chronic diseases.

III. Irritation also leads to glandular stimulation and an increase in serous secretions. The character of the secretions may change with time if secondary infection ensues.

Clinical Signs

I. Signalment
   A. Nasal tumors are more common in older animals.
   B. Dental-related rhinitis is common in middle-aged to older animals.
   C. Aspergillosis is more common in younger, large-breed dogs.

II. History
   A. Sneezing
      1. Acute onset of paroxysmal sneezing is suggestive of intranasal foreign body, and the owner may indicate that the animal has access to fields and brushy areas.
      2. The sneeze reflex often decreases in frequency with chronic disease.
   B. Nasal discharge
      1. Onset: may be difficult to determine because animals tend to lick secretions from their nares
      2. Duration
      3. Character: serous, mucoid, purulent, blood-tinged; epistaxis
      4. Initial side of involvement, any progression to bilateral involvement
         a) Typical unilateral diseases: foreign body, dental disease, aspergillosis, neoplasia
         b) Typical bilateral diseases: infectious agents, cilial dyskinesia, IgA deficiency
      5. Response to previous medical therapy
         A transient response to antibiotics is common with a foreign body, tooth abscess, or chronic rhinosinusitis in the cat.

III. Miscellaneous signs
   A. Pawing at the face is characteristic of intranasal foreign body.
   B. Teeth chattering is common with chronic dental disease.

Diagnosis

I. Physical examination
   A. Facial asymmetry may be found.

1. Nasal tumors may result in gross facial distortion (typically involving the nasal, maxillary, or frontal bones).
2. Focal swelling and drainage may be associated with a tooth abscess.
3. Examine the hard and soft palates carefully.
    a) Nasopharyngeal masses (e.g., polyps in cats) often cause a ventral bulge in the soft palate or can be felt through the soft palate.
    b) Hard palate involvement is often present as nasal tumors grow and invade adjacent structures.
B. Pain may arise from periosteal involvement by a tumor or infection (most often *Aspergillus* spp.).
C. The primary process may result in tonsillar or submandibular, retropharyngeal, or prescapular lymph node enlargement.
D. Compare air flow at both nostrils to determine whether flow is symmetrical or decreased on one side.
    1. A healthy animal should be able to breathe comfortably at rest while one nostril is being held closed.
    2. Feel air flow against your skin.
    3. Listen for the sound of air flowing through the nose; partial obstruction results in increased air turbulence and louder sound.
    4. Observe any discomfort (or effort) an animal experiences breathing through a partially obstructed nasal cavity.
    5. Measure the area of condensation when the animal exhales onto a cool surface (glass slides, stainless steel exam table).
E. Miscellaneous signs may be noted.
    1. Ulceration or loss of pigmentation on the nasal planum or alar fold is frequently encountered with canine aspergillosis (Wolf, 1992).
    2. Halitosis may be noted with dental disease, intranasal foreign body, or lower airway infection (pneumonia).
    3. Cats may be anorexic if they cannot smell their food.
    4. Fever, lethargy, and depression are present only with long-standing or severe disease.
    5. Ocular discharge may occur with infectious agents (conjunctivitis) or if there is nasolacrimal duct involvement/obstruction.

II. Clinical pathology
A. A routine blood count, urinalysis, and serum chemistry panel do not reveal a specific cause for rhinitis or sinusitis.
B. If nasal bleeding (blood-tinged discharge or frank epistaxis) is present, perform a platelet count and coagulation profile and rule out systemic hypertension.

III. Nasal cytology (French, 1987; Rebar et al., 1992)
A. Nonspecific rhinitis (predominantly neutrophils) is the most common cytologic finding.
B. Cytologic findings that are indicative of a specific disease are as follows.

1. Mycotic elements: *Aspergillus* spp., *Cryptococcus* spp.
2. Parasitic rhinitis: eggs or larvae
3. Neoplasia (see later)

IV. Microbiology
A. Results of nasal bacteriology or mycology must be interpreted with caution because of the high prevalence of airway colonization by microbial agents.
B. Bacterial cultures of the nasal cavity and/or secretions are of questionable value (Ford, 1989).
C. Results of fungal cultures are felt to be indicative of active infection only if the results are compatible with the other clinical findings (e.g., radiography, rhinoscopy) (Harvey, 1984).

V. Fungal serology
A. Various serologic tests (e.g., agar gel immunodiffusion, counterimmunoelectrophoresis, and enzyme-linked immunosorbent assay [ELISA]) can be used in the diagnosis of nasal aspergillosis in dogs (Wolf, 1992).
    1. Negative serology does not exclude the diagnosis.
    2. Positive results support the diagnosis but do not confirm the diagnosis because there is the potential for false-positive reactions.
    3. Serology results must be correlated with other clinical findings.
B. The latex cryptococcal antigen test (LCAT) is felt to be an accurate diagnostic test.
    1. Titers may also be used to monitor the response to therapy (Wolf, 1992).
    2. LCAT titers of $\geq 1:1$ are considered positive (Van Pelt and Lappin, 1992).
C. Although histoplasmosis and blastomycosis have occasionally been reported in the nasal cavity, serologic testing is not considered a definitive diagnostic test for either.

VI. Diagnostic imaging
A. Radiography is one of the main diagnostic tests for nasal diseases.
    1. Changes typically seen include the following.
        a) Increased density compatible with the accumulation of exudate, hemorrhage, and soft tissue (tumor, polyp, granuloma)
        b) Decreased density most often seen with turbinate loss (destructive rhinitis) or following chronic nasal inflammation (aspergillosis, chronic bacterial infection)
        c) Loss of turbinates
    2. The recommended radiographic views are the lateral, open mouth or intraoral ventrodorsal, and rostrocaudal (frontal sinus) views (McKiernan, 1995).
B. Computed tomography (CT) and magnetic resonance imaging (MRI) help distinguish between the different causes of chronic nasal disease (Codner et al., 1993) and can often detect changes not visible on routine radiography (Park et al., 1992).

VII. Rhinoscopy
A. Rhinoscopy is recognized as a very important

diagnostic procedure for nasal and nasopharyngeal diseases (van Oosterhout et al, 1989; McCarthy and McDermaid, 1990; Lent and Hawkins, 1992).
  B. The limiting factor in selecting equipment is patient size. Flexible endoscopes are recommended because of their overall versatility (Ford, 1990).
     1. Small (3–5 mm diameter), flexible endoscopes allow for both anterior and posterior (retroflexed) rhinoscopy, depending on the size of the patient.
     2. Although visual examination of the nasopharynx may be done using a dental mirror and spay hook, flexible endoscopes provide a better view during posterior rhinoscopy.
  C. Rhinoscopy procedure/techniques are described elsewhere (McCarthy and McDermaid, 1990).
  D. Sinoscopy is recommended if sinus involvement is apparent on radiography and normal nasal structures prevent access via routine anterior rhinoscopy (McCarthy and McDermaid, 1990).
VIII. Nasal biopsy
  A. Blind biopsy is performed if the lesion is not visualized during the biopsy procedure.
     1. Tumor location is based on radiographic assessment or gross findings.
     2. Care must be taken not to penetrate beyond the medial canthus of the eye (location of the cribriform plate).
     3. Bleeding is common but manageable in most cases (Withrow et al., 1985).
        a) Punch (Tru-Cut needle) biopsy (diagnostic accuracy of 86%)
        b) Aspiration (coring) biopsy
           (1) Performed with a stiff 3–7 mm diameter plastic tube or catheter connected to a syringe
           (2) Diagnostic accuracy of 97% with confirmed neoplasias
  B. A nasal flush technique uses an angled, rigid plastic catheter aggressively inserted into the nasal cavity (Withrow, 1977).
     1. The procedure dislodges and flushes tissue fragments from the nasal cavity.
     2. A 10% povidone-iodine solution is used to decrease the bacterial numbers in the nasal cavity.
  C. Rhinoscopy-assisted biopsy allows direct visualization of the lesion, as well as gross evaluation of changes within the nasal cavity, and has an 83% diagnostic success rate with all types of rhinitis (Lent and Hawkins, 1992).
  D. Surgical biopsy (e.g., rhinotomy) may be required for definitive diagnosis if other less invasive techniques fail to provide adequate tissue.
IX. Dental examination
  A. Probing the periodontal sulcus of all maxillary teeth is indicated for all rhinitis cases, regardless of the radiographic and rhinoscopic findings.
  B. Intraoral dental radiographs may also be helpful (see Chap. 27).

Differential Diagnosis

  I. Other causes of chronic licking, nasal discharge, and excoriation of the nasal planum: discoid lupus erythematosus, pemphigus erythematosus
  II. Other causes of nasal discharge: pneumonia, megaesophagus, chronic vomiting
  III. Other causes of epistaxis: coagulopathies

Treatment

  I. Symptomatic therapy
    A. Nursing care is important in animals with chronic nasal diseases.
       1. Secretions are cleaned from the nares as needed.
       2. Systemic hydration and body temperature are maintained.
    B. Broad-spectrum antibiotics are recommended if nasal secretions are purulent.
       1. Amoxicillin 11–20 mg/kg PO, IV TID
       2. Clindamycin 12.5 mg/kg PO BID
    C. Decongestants are of unknown efficacy and are used only short term (Boothe and McKiernan, 1992).
       1. Phenylephrine (1.25%) applied as nose drops BID-TID
       2. Pseudoephedrine
          a) Dogs: 15–50 mg total (to maximum of 4 mg/kg) PO BID-TID
          b) Cats: 2–4 mg/kg PO BID-TID
       3. Diphenhydramine 2–4 mg/kg PO TID
  II. Dental-related rhinitis
    A. The affected tooth is removed.
    B. Mucosal flaps are used to cover any oronasal fistula.
    C. Broad-spectrum antibiotics (e.g., amoxicillin 11–20 mg/kg PO, IV TID) are indicated for 7–10 days.
  III. Intranasal foreign body
    A. Endoscopic removal is frequently possible.
       1. Biopsy, grasping, or snare forceps may be used to retrieve the foreign body.
       2. Plant material—frequently fragments and multiple pieces—must be recovered.
       3. Some nasal foreign bodies may be retropulsed out of the nose and into the nasopharynx using a large saline-filled syringe and vigorous flushing while the nostrils are held closed.
    B. Vigorous anterior-to-posterior saline retropulsion may be used to dislodge foreign material from the nasal cavity.
    C. Surgical rhinotomy and turbinectomy may be required when the foreign body cannot be dislodged by the previously stated methods.
    D. Broad-spectrum antibiotics (e.g., amoxicillin 11–20 mg/kg PO, IV BID) are indicated for 7–10 days.
  IV. Fungal diseases
    A. *Aspergillus* and *Penicillium*
       1. Oral ketoconazole at 5 mg/kg PO BID has been approximately 50% successful; higher

doses are associated with anorexia and liver enzyme elevations.
2. Oral fluconazole at 1.25–2.5 mg/kg PO BID was shown to be approximately 60% successful in a group of 10 dogs with nasal fungal disease (Sharp et al., 1991).
3. Oral itraconazole at 5 mg/kg PO BID for 2–3 months is approximately 70% successful and induces less side effects than ketoconazole.
4. Topical clotrimazole with a 1 hour contact time has been used to successfully treat a number of cases using surgically implanted tubes (Davidson and Pappagianis, 1995).
5. Topical enilconazole has been the most effective treatment (~90% success rate) for treating canine nasal/sinus aspergillosis, but the medical grade solution (Imaverol, Pitman Moore) is not available in the United States at this time.
   a) The recommended dose is 10 mg/kg BID in approximately 10 ml of solution divided between both nasal cavities and delivered via surgically (sinus and nasal) implanted tubes for 10–14 days.
   b) An enilconazole-containing fungicide (Clinifarm EC, Sterwin Labs) is available and has been used by the author to successfully treat six dogs with nasal aspergillosis via endoscopically placed nasal and frontal sinus tubes.
6. Surgery is not recommended as the sole treatment for nasal aspergillosis.
B. *Cryptococcus*
1. For cats, fluconazole at 50 mg PO BID for 2–6 months is recommended.
   a) It is preferred in cats with concurrent liver disease.
   b) Drug resistance may develop.
2. Itraconazole is given for at least 2 months after clinical resolution and is preferred in animals with impaired renal function.
   a) Dogs: 5–10 mg/kg PO BID
   b) Cats ≤3.2 kg: 50 mg PO SID (Medleau et al., 1995)
   c) Cats ≥3.2 kg: 100 mg PO SID (Medleau et al., 1995)
C. *Sporothrix*
1. Give itraconazole at 5 mg/kg PO BID for at least 1 month after clinical resolution.
2. Check feline leukemia and feline immunodeficiency viral status, as they are potential immunosuppressants that may allow *Sporothrix* to develop.
D. Rhinosporidiosis: rhinotomy and surgical excision of the nasal granulomas
V. Parasitic diseases
A. *Pneumonyssoides caninum:* ivermectin 300 μg/kg PO weekly for 2–3 treatments
B. *Capillaria* spp.: single dose of ivermectin 300 μg/kg PO
C. *Cuterebra* spp.: surgical removal

D. *Syngamus ierei, Linguatula serrata:* no known treatments
VI. Lymphoplasmacytic and allergic rhinitis
A. Begin prednisolone 2 mg/kg/day PO for 14 days.
B. Doses will vary and are based on clinical response.
VII. Neoplasia: see later

Patient Monitoring

I. Sneezing and nasal discharge should decrease in frequency with effective treatment.
II. Failure to respond (or relapses) may warrant further diagnostic testing.
III. Owners should be warned that, when destructive rhinitis is present, some nasal discharge and occasional sneezing persist.
IV. Evaluate liver chemistries every 1–2 months in animals receiving itraconazole or ketoconazole therapy.

Nasopharyngeal Stenosis

Definition and Cause

I. It is a membrane or web of tissue formed dorsal to the soft palate and coursing transversely across the nasopharynx with a very small hole remaining in the center through which the animal breathes (Mitten, 1992).
II. It is presumed to represent a cicatricial membrane following prior severe, chronic upper respiratory inflammation.
III. Histopathology reveals chronic inflammation and submucosal fibrosis with inflammatory cell infiltrates.

Clinical Signs

I. There is a long history of marked inspiratory effort and wheezing.
II. A history of exercise intolerance is common.
III. Nasal discharge and sneezing are usually minimal.

Diagnosis

I. Suspect the condition in cats with inspiratory airflow obstruction, especially if the following are evident.
A. Stridor is ausculted and localizes over the larynx/pharynx.
B. Cat is able to breathe normally through the mouth.
C. No ventral deviation of the soft palate (e.g., polyp) is noted.
II. General anesthesia is required for a definitive workup and diagnosis.
A. Skull radiographs rarely show any abnormality.
B. The nasopharynx is examined; a small catheter is passed posteriorly from the nares and used to detect an obstruction in the nasopharynx.
C. Posterior rhinoscopy is performed using either a dental mirror and spay hook or a small flexible endoscope.

1. A small (1–3 mm diameter) opening is found in a transverse web of tissue across the nasopharynx.
2. Other obstructive nasopharyngeal diseases (e.g., foreign body, tumor, polyp) are excluded.

Differential Diagnosis

I. Chronic upper respiratory tract infection (viral, bacterial, fungal)
II. Nasopharyngeal polyp or tumor
III. Laryngeal disorders (see Chap. 15)

Treatment

I. Sharp surgical resection of the tissue is performed after splitting the soft palate.
II. Broad-spectrum antibiotics (e.g., amoxicillin at 11–20 mg/kg PO BID) are recommended postoperatively for 5–7 days.

Patient Monitoring

I. Potential complications following surgery include breakdown of the soft palate incision and recurrence of the stenosis.
II. Owners should monitor for return of stertor or the original breathing pattern that accompanied the obstruction.
III. Repeat rhinoscopy is indicated to assess the nasopharyngeal patency 4–6 weeks postoperatively or sooner if signs recur.

NEOPLASIA

Nasal and Nasopharyngeal Polyps

Definition

I. Small, benign masses that cause obstruction of the nasal cavity and nasopharynx in dogs and cats
II. Solid tissue or fluid-filled masses

Pathophysiology and Causes

I. These small mass lesions are associated with foci of inflammation and result in varying degrees of upper airway obstruction.
II. Actual etiology in cats is unknown.
A. Polyps are typically solid.
B. Proposed causes include the following (Kapatkin et al., 1990; Pope, 1995).
1. Chronic otitis media or otitis externa
2. Calicivirus infection
3. Development from branchial arch remnants
III. They occur less commonly in dogs than in cats, and the etiology is also uncertain.
A. Polyps are typically cystic and fluid filled.
B. Proposed causes in dogs are as follows.
1. In one young dog, the polyp was felt to be developmental in origin (Pook and Meric, 1990).
2. They may be sequelae to significant loss of nasal turbinates (as a result of chronic destructive rhinitis, surgical turbinectomy, or post–radiation therapy).

Clinical Signs

I. There is a gradual onset of nasal airway obstruction that is progressive in nature.
A. Inspiratory noise when breathing: stertor, wheezing
B. Nasal discharge and sneezing
II. Otitis externa is commonly reported in cats.
III. Horner's syndrome is a common, but typically transient (≤1 month), complication in cats (Pope, 1995).

Diagnosis

I. Physical examination of upper (nasopharyngeal) airway
A. Sneezing, nasal discharge, gagging, and coughing may be noted.
B. In cats, a nasopharyngeal location is common.
1. Most cats are able to breathe through their mouth without difficulty or with increased airway sounds (stertor).
2. Soft palate may be depressed ventrally by the mass.
3. Otitis externa may be present, and the polyp may extend into the ear canal.
C. In dogs, polyps can be located either in the nasal cavity or in the nasopharynx.
D. Palpation through the soft palate may detect a mass lesion.
E. The polyp may be visualized by pulling the soft palate forward.
II. Skull radiography
A. Lateral radiograph may reveal a soft tissue density in the nasopharynx.
B. Intraoral radiograph may reveal increased soft tissue density on the affected side.
C. Radiographs of the bullae often demonstrate middle ear involvement.
III. Rhinoscopy (anterior/posterior): allows visualization of the mass
IV. Surgical exploration: allows definitive diagnosis

Differential Diagnosis

I. Nasopharyngeal or soft palate tumor or foreign body
II. Laryngeal tumor
III. Feline upper respiratory disease complex

Treatment

I. Gentle traction placed on the polyp, with forceps attached as close to the base of the stalk as possible, removes the polyp from its attachment.
II. Ventral bulla osteotomy is recommended when there

is radiographic evidence of bullae involvement (Pope, 1995).

III. Bulla osteotomy is considered on the side of the origin of the polyp regardless of whether there is radiographic evidence of bullae involvement or not, in order to minimize the chance for recurrence (Kapatkin et al., 1990).

Patient Monitoring

I. Medical therapy may help with secondary signs.
   A. Prednisolone (1–2 mg/kg PO BID) or dexamethasone (0.25–1 mg/kg IV) is given if signs of pharyngeal mucosal edema develop postoperatively.
   B. Antibiotics are not routinely indicated.

II. Recurrence is common (30–40%) within 1–12 months if bulla osteotomy is not performed, but rare (3%) when bulla osteotomy is performed (Kapatkin et al., 1990).

III. Recurrence is suggested by return of upper airway obstructive signs.

Malignant Tumors

Definition

I. Nasal tumors account for up to 2.4% of all tumors in dogs and up to 4.2% of all tumors in cats (Ogilvie and LaRue, 1992).

II. In the older dog, malignant nasal tumors are the most common cause of nasal discharge (Bedford, 1995).

Causes

I. Dogs
   A. Epithelial origin
      1. Adenocarcinoma
      2. Squamous cell carcinoma
   B. Nonepithelial origin
      1. Chondrosarcoma
      2. Osteosarcoma
      3. Lymphosarcoma
      4. Fibrosarcoma
      5. Miscellaneous: neuroblastoma, neuroendocrine tumor, melanoma, transmissible venereal tumor

II. Cats
   A. Epithelial origin
      1. Adenocarcinoma
      2. Squamous cell carcinoma
   B. Nonepithelial origin
      1. Lymphosarcoma
      2. Fibrosarcoma
      3. Chondrosarcoma
      4. Miscellaneous: neuroblastoma

Pathophysiology

I. Growth of neoplastic tissue results in airflow obstruction and invasion of adjacent structures (bones of the nose, face, and oral cavity).

II. Approximately 41% of the tumors metastasize to regional lymph nodes or to more distant structures.

III. Rates of metastasis appear to vary with tumor type.

Clinical Signs

I. They vary widely depending on the site and extent of tumor.

II. Typically the signs have been present for months prior to diagnosis.

III. They typically start unilaterally and progress to bilateral involvement.

IV. Nasal discharge may be bloody, mucoid, or purulent.

V. Airflow obstruction and respiratory distress are often noted.

VI. Facial deformity is common.

VII. Miscellaneous signs include sneezing, epiphora, coughing, and ocular or neurologic signs.

Diagnosis

I. Signalment (Hayes et al., 1982; Ogilvie and LaRue, 1992)
   A. Mean age at diagnosis of most nasal tumors is as follows.
      1. Dogs: 9 years
      2. Cats: 8–10 years
   B. Dolichocephalic dog breeds have a 2.5-fold increased risk; brachycephalic dogs have a lower risk.
   C. Male dogs have a 1.3-fold increased risk compared with female dogs; male cats also are more commonly affected than female cats.

II. History and physical findings
   A. Nasal obstruction: decreased airflow through one or both nostrils, stertor on auscultation
   B. Chronic sneezing and nasal discharge: mucoid, mucopurulent to bloody discharge
   C. Deformation of facial bones: the frontal, maxillary, or nasal bones and/or the hard palate

III. Nasal cytology
   A. In the epithelial tumors, cells typically are found in clusters, and secondary inflammation and hemorrhage are common.
      1. The most common type is adenocarcinoma.
      2. Other types include squamous cell carcinoma and undifferentiated carcinoma.
   B. In mesenchymal tumors, cells exfoliate poorly.
      1. Typically, single cells are found and secondary inflammation and hemorrhage are also common.
      2. Examples include fibrosarcoma, chondrosarcoma, and osteosarcoma.
   C. Round cell tumors exfoliate readily and have distinctive cytologic morphology.
      1. Lymphosarcoma vs. lymphoid hyperplasia
      2. Mast cell tumor
      3. Transmissible venereal tumor

IV. Diagnostic imaging
   A. Skull radiography is very helpful (Sullivan et al., 1987; O'Brien et al., 1996).
      1. The dorsoventral, intraoral view is the best

radiographic view for the detection of nasal neoplasia.

2. Increased radiodensity has been reported in more than 70% of the radiographs from dogs with nasal tumors (Sullivan et al., 1987).
3. Turbinate destruction is common.
4. Unilateral bone lysis, turbinate destruction, and loss of teeth are commonly reported in cats.

B. Thoracic radiographs, including both left and right lateral views, are taken to check for metastases.

C. CT and MRI better define the extent of nasal tumors as compared with conventional skull radiography.

1. Extension of nasal neoplasia into the brain (through the cribriform plate) can often be appreciated.
2. Both techniques are useful for planning radiation therapy.

V. Rhinoscopy and nasal biopsy

A. It is valuable for obtaining biopsy samples for histopathologic confirmation of the tumor and ruling out other causes of nasal discharge (see earlier).

B. Nasal biopsy may be performed via blind biopsy, nasal flushing, rhinoscopic-assisted nasal biopsy, or open rhinotomy.

Differential Diagnosis

I. Nasal fungal infection
   A. Aspergillosis
   B. Cryptococcosis
II. Chronic dental disease
III. Coagulopathy
IV. Nasal foreign body

Treatment

I. As a result of secondary bacterial involvement, a transient response to antibiotic therapy may be reported.

II. Because of local tissue invasion, surgical treatment alone is not recommended.

III. Radiation therapy is the recommended treatment for most nasal tumors.

A. Radiation therapy is relatively effective in treating nasal tumors in dogs and cats (median survival time: 23 and 20 months, respectively) (Ogilvie and LaRue, 1992).

B. Orthovoltage therapy is reported to be slightly better than megavoltage therapy but requires surgical debulking because of the relatively poor penetration of this form of radiotherapy (Ogilvie and LaRue, 1992).

C. Megavoltage therapy (cobalt, linear accelerator) can be used without prior surgical debulking.

D. Animals with facial deformity are not excluded from receiving radiotherapy, as they do as well as those without facial deformity (Evans et al., 1989).

IV. Chemotherapy is indicated for selected tumors of the nasal cavity and nasopharynx.

A. Lymphosarcoma (see Chaps. 67 and 70)
B. Transmissible venereal tumor (see Chaps. 58 and 70)
C. Mast cell tumor (see Chaps. 64 and 70)
D. May be used concurrently with radiation therapy

Patient Monitoring

I. Survival times for dogs who receive cryotherapy, immunotherapy, or surgery alone, or for those who are not treated average 3–5 months (Ogilvie and LaRue, 1992).

II. Metastases are rare early, but often develop late in the course of the disease.

III. Complications of radiation treatments are variable.

A. Early side effects (within 1 month) are very common and include oral mucositis, rhinitis, keratoconjunctivitis sicca, and moist dermatitis over the radiation portal (Ogilvie and LaRue, 1992).

B. Late side effects (6 months or more after therapy) occur in less than 5% of patients and include retinal damage, cataracts, and bone or brain necrosis (Ogilvie and LaRue, 1992).

Bibliography

Abramson AL, Isenberg HD, McDermott LM: Microbiology of the canine nasal cavities. Rhinology 18:143, 1980

Aron DN, Crowe DT: Upper airway obstruction. Vet Clin North Am [Small Anim Pract] 15:891, 1985

Bedford PGC: Diseases of the nose. p. 551. In Ettinger SJ, Feldman EC (eds): Textbook of Veterinary Internal Medicine. 4th Ed. WB Saunders, Philadelphia, 1995

Boothe DM, McKiernan BC: Respiratory therapeutics. Vet Clin North Am [Small Anim Pract] 22:1231, 1992

Burgener DC, Slocombe RF, Zerbe CA: Lymphoplasmacytic rhinitis in five dogs. J Am Anim Hosp Assoc 23:55, 1987

Cape L: Feline idiopathic chronic rhinosinusitis: a retrospective study of 30 cases. J Am Anim Hosp Assoc 28:149, 1992

Codner EC, Lurus AG, Miller JB et al: Comparison of computed tomography with radiography as a noninvasive diagnostic technique for chronic nasal disease in dogs. J Am Vet Med Assoc 202:1106, 1993

Cuadrado R, Maldonado-Moll JF, Segarra J: Gapeworm infection of domestic cats in Puerto Rico. J Am Vet Med Assoc 176:996, 1980

Davidson AP, Pappagianis D: Treatment of nasal aspergillosis with topical clotrimazole. p. 899. In Bonagura JD (ed): Kirk's Current Veterinary Therapy XII. WB Saunders, Philadelphia, 1995

Evans SM, Goldschmidt M, McKee LJ et al: Prognostic factors and survival after radiotherapy for intranasal neoplasms in dogs: 70 cases (1974–1985). J Am Vet Med Assoc 194:1460, 1989

Felsburg PJ: Overview of the immune system and immunodeficiency diseases. Vet Clin North Am [Small Anim Pract] 24:629, 1994

Ford RB: Noninfectious diseases of the upper respiratory tract. p. 755. In Sherding RD (ed): The Cat. Churchill Livingstone, New York, 1989

Ford RB: Endoscopy of the upper respiratory tract of the dog and cat. p. 297. In Tams TR (ed): Small Animal Endoscopy. CV Mosby, St. Louis, 1990

French TW: The use of cytology in the diagnosis of chronic nasal disorders. Compend Contin Educ Pract Vet 9:115, 1987

Harvey CE: Therapeutic strategies involving antimicrobial treatment of the upper respiratory tract in small animals. J Am Vet Med Assoc 185:1159, 1984

Hawkins JB: Periodontal disease. Vet Clin North Am [Small Anim Pract] 16:835, 1985

Hayes HM, Wilson GP, Fraumeni JF: Carcinoma of the nasal cavity and paranasal sinuses in dogs: descriptive epidemiology. Cornell Vet 72:168, 1982

Hendricks JC: Brachycephalic airway syndrome. Vet Clin North Am [Small Anim Pract] 22:1145, 1992

Hobson HP: Brachycephalic syndrome. Semin Vet Med Surg (Small Anim) 10:109, 1995

Kapatkin AS, Matthiesen DT, Noone KE et al: Results of surgery and long-term follow-up in 31 cats with nasopharyngeal polyps. J Am Anim Hosp Assoc 26:387, 1990

King RR, Greiner EC, Ackerman N et al: Nasal capillariasis in a dog. J Am Anim Hosp Assoc 26:381, 1990

Legendre AM: Antimycotic drug therapy. p. 327. In Bonagura JD (ed): Kirk's Current Veterinary Therapy XII. WB Saunders, Philadelphia, 1995

Lent SEF, Hawkins EC: Evaluation of rhinoscopy and rhinoscopy-assisted mucosal biopsy in diagnosis of nasal disease (1985–1989). J Am Vet Med Assoc 201:1425, 1992

Manfra SM: Chronic rhinitis and dental disease. Vet Clin North Am [Small Anim Pract] 22:1101, 1992

McCarthy TC, McDermaid SL: Rhinoscopy. Vet Clin North Am [Small Anim Pract] 20:1265, 1990

McKiernan BC: Sneezing and nasal discharge. p. 79. In Ettinger SJ, Feldman EC (eds): Textbook of Veterinary Internal Medicine. 4th Ed. WB Saunders, Philadelphia, 1995

Medleau L, Jacobs GJ, Marks MA: Itraconazole for treatment of *Cryptococcus* in cats. J Vet Intern Med 9:39, 1995

Mitten RW: Acquired nasopharyngeal stenosis in cats. p. 801. In Kirk RW, Bonagura JD (eds): Current Veterinary Therapy XI: Small Animal Practice. WB Saunders, Philadelphia, 1992

Miyabayashi T, Biller DS, Haider PR et al: Radiographic appearances of the nasal conchae in dogs using different screen-film systems: a postmortem study. J Am Anim Hosp Assoc 30:382, 1994

Mundell AC, Ihrke PJ: Ivermectin in the treatment of *Pneumonyssoides caninum:* a case report. J Anim Hosp Assoc 26:393, 1990

O'Brien RT, Evans SM, Wortman JA et al: Radiographic findings in cats with intranasal neoplasia or chronic rhinitis: 29 cases (1982–1988). J Am Vet Med Assoc 208:385, 1996

Ogilvie GK, LaRue SM: Canine and feline nasal and paranasal sinus tumors. Vet Clin North Am [Small Anim Pract] 22:1133, 1992

Orsini P, Hennet P: Anatomy of the mouth and teeth of the cat. Vet Clin North Am [Small Anim Pract] 22:1265, 1992

Park RD, Beck ER, LeCouteur RA: Comparison of computed tomography and radiography for detecting changes induced by malignant nasal neoplasia in dogs. J Am Vet Med Assoc 201:1720, 1992

Pook HA, Meric SM: Caudal nasal cyst in a dog: retrograde rhinoscopic management. J Anim Hosp Assoc 26:169, 1990

Pope ER: Feline inflammatory polyps. Semin Vet Med Surg (Small Anim) 10:87, 1995

Rebar AH, Hawkins EC, DeNicola DB: Cytologic evaluation of the respiratory tract. Vet Clin North Am [Small Anim Pract] 22:1065, 1992

Robinson NE: Airway physiology. Vet Clin North Am [Small Anim Pract] 22:1043, 1992

Sharp N: Nasal aspergillosis. p. 1106. In Kirk RW (ed): Current Veterinary Therapy X: Small Animal Practice. WB Saunders, Philadelphia, 1989

Sharp NJH, Harvey CE, O'Brien JA: Treatment of canine nasal aspergillosis/penicilliosis with fluconazole (UK-49,858). J Small Anim Pract 32:513, 1991

Shofer FS, Glickman LT, Payton AJ et al: Influence of parental serum immunoglobulins on morbidity and mortality of beagles and their offspring. Am J Vet Res 51:239, 1990

Sullivan M: Differential diagnosis of chronic nasal disease. p. 37. In Boden E (ed): Canine Practice. Bailliere Tindall, London, 1991

Sullivan M, Lee R, Skae CA: The radiological features of sixty cases of intra-nasal neoplasia in the dog. J Small Anim Pract 28:575, 1987

van Oosterhout CAM, Meij BP, Venker-van Haagen AJ: Rhinoscopy in small animal clinics: an analysis of the results of 223 rhinoscopies and 97 bacterial cultures from nasal swabs. Tijdschr Diergeneesk 114:94S, 1989

Van Pelt DR, Lappin MR: Pathogenesis and treatment of feline rhinitis. Vet Clin North Am [Small Anim Pract] 22:807, 1992

Van Pelt DR, McKiernan BC: Pathogenesis and treatment of canine rhinitis. Vet Clin North Am [Small Anim Pract] 22:789, 1992

Widdecombe JG: Reflexes from the upper respiratory tract. p. 372. In Fishman AP, Cherniack NS, Widdicombe JG (eds): Handbook of Physiology. The Respiratory System. American Physiological Society, Bethesda, Maryland; 1986

Wilkinson GT: Some observations on the Irish wolfhound rhinitis syndrome. J Small Anim Pract 10:5, 1969

Withrow SJ: Diagnostic and therapeutic nasal flush in small animals. J Am Anim Hosp Assoc 13:704, 1977

Withrow SJ, Susaneck SJ, Macy DW et al: Aspiration and punch biopsy techniques for nasal tumors. J Am Anim Hosp Assoc 21:551, 1985

Wolf AM: Fungal diseases of the nasal cavity of the dog and cat. Vet Clin North Am [Small Anim Pract] 22:1119, 1992

Wolf AM, Troy GC: Deep mycotic diseases. p. 439. In Ettinger SJ, Feldman EC (eds): Textbook of Veterinary Internal Medicine. 4th Ed. WB Saunders, Philadelphia, 1995

15

Diseases of the Larynx

Anjop J. Venker-van Haagen

CONGENITAL DISEASES

Familial Laryngeal Hypoplasia

Definition and Causes

I. This disorder consists of hypoplasia of the laryngeal cartilaginous structures.
II. This disorder is familial, but the mode of inheritance is not known.

Pathophysiology

I. The cartilaginous structures (thyroid, arytenoid, and cricoid cartilages) and the laryngeal opening are too small for more than basic ventilation.
II. The cartilaginous structures are not firm and thus give inadequate support for laryngeal abduction.
III. The hypoplastic arytenoid and epiglottic cartilages tend to fold together and obstruct the laryngeal opening.
IV. Edema and hyperplasia of the laryngeal mucosa develop as a consequence of forced ventilation through the narrow passage.
V. Eversion of the lateral laryngeal ventricles results from forced ventilation.

Clinical Signs

I. Signalment
   A. Brachycephalic breeds: English bulldog, French bulldog, Pekingese
   B. No sex predilection
   C. Onset of clinical signs in the first months of life, with severity increasing over the years
II. Physical examination
   A. Moderate to severe respiratory distress may be found.
   B. Panting and inspiratory/expiratory laryngeal stridor (sound of sawing wood with a hand saw) are common.
      1. Palpation of laryngeal area changes the sound of the stridor.

2. During an episode of respiratory distress and panting, the following may be noted.
   a) Auscultation of the thorax reveals only the predominant laryngeal stridor.
   b) The body temperature may rise to 40°C or higher.
C. The mucous membranes may be red or pale pink. Cyanosis or an ashen color indicates a critical condition.

Diagnosis

I. A presumptive diagnosis can be made from the signalment and the clinical signs.
II. Laryngoscopy is used to make the definitive diagnosis.
   A. Light anesthesia is required to minimize the loss of laryngeal function caused by anesthesia.
   B. Findings at laryngoscopy include the following.
      1. The larynx is small for the dog's size and is more round than oval in shape.
      2. Abduction of the vocal folds opens the laryngeal inlet only moderately.
      3. The laryngeal inlet may be obstructed by the aryepiglottic folds.
      4. Observation of the vocal folds may be hindered by the everted lateral ventricles.
      5. Hyperplasia and edema of the laryngeal mucosa are often observed.
      6. Hyperemia or inflammation of the laryngeal mucosa is often evident after prolonged panting.
III. Radiography does not give conclusive information about the laryngeal structures.

Differential Diagnosis

I. Stenotic nares: nasal stridor
II. Narrow pharyngeal cavities: pharyngeal stridor
III. Hyperplasia of the base of the tongue
IV. Tracheal hypoplasia
V. Lung disease: no stridor
VI. Heart failure: no stridor

Treatment

I. There is no definitive treatment for this congenital defect.
  A. Surgery of the larynx in an attempt to widen the laryngeal inlet usually does not result in clinical improvement.
  B. Surgery may actually lead to further narrowing.
II. Care of the critical animal involves these measures.
  A. Cool the dog if hyperthermic.
  B. Restore respiration.
    1. Emergency intubation
    2. Temporary tracheostomy for severe laryngeal edema
    3. Corticosteroid therapy of questionable benefit
  C. After further physical examination, restore circulation.
  D. Radiograph the lungs to detect pulmonary edema.

Patient Monitoring

I. Warn the owner to prohibit excessive exercise.
II. Advise the owner that keeping the dog cool may be life saving.
III. Consider surgery of stenotic nares or an elongated soft palate to reduce overall respiratory distress.

Anomaly of the Larynx

Definition and Causes

I. It is a congenital malformation of the laryngeal structures (Venker-van Haagen et al., 1981b).
II. It is the result of abnormal development during the embryonal stage.

Pathophysiology

I. Idiopathic disturbance of the normal development of the cartilaginous and muscular parts of the larynx
II. Not known to be a hereditary trait

Clinical Signs

I. Signalment and onset of clinical signs
  A. Dogs and cats of all breeds
  B. No sex predilection
  C. Variable onset of clinical signs: usually diagnosed in the first 6 months of life
II. Physical examination revealing signs of airway obstruction
  A. Abnormal vocalization, abnormal purring
  B. Inspiratory effort, respiratory distress: moderate or severe
  C. Laryngeal stridor
III. No concurrent abnormalities elsewhere

Diagnosis

I. Radiographic examination of the pharyngeal, laryngeal, and tracheal structures may indicate the extent of the anomaly.
II. Laryngoscopy performed under light anesthesia may reveal the following defects.

A. Abnormal development of the vestibular area: The epiglottis, arytenoid cartilages, and aryepiglottic folds may be abnormal.
  B. Abnormal development of the glottic area: The vocal folds and the arytenoid cartilages may be abnormal.
  C. Abnormal development of the infraglottic area: The cricoid cartilage may be abnormal.
III. Bronchoscopy under general anesthesia may reveal concurrent tracheal and bronchial abnormalities that are masked by the predominance of laryngeal signs.

Differential Diagnosis

I. Pharyngeal malformations: polyps causing obstruction of the glottis
II. Tracheal malformations: dysplasia of the first few cervical tracheal rings
III. Laryngeal lesions caused by trauma

Treatment

I. There is no treatment for this congenital defect.
II. Surgical restoration of vocalization or purring is usually impossible.
III. Corrective surgery may improve air flow through the larynx or reduce the respiratory distress.
  A. In animals younger than 6 months of age, laryngeal surgery has a guarded prognosis because it may adversely influence further cartilaginous development.
  B. Aspiration of pharyngeal contents into the airway with secondary pneumonia is a potential risk after surgical dilatation of the malformed laryngeal opening.
IV. Refrain from surgery under these conditions.
  A. The animal's life is not threatened by the condition.
  B. The risk of asphyxia remains high; permanent tracheostomy or euthanasia should be discussed with the owner in these cases.

Patient Monitoring

I. In obstructive laryngeal disease, the owner is advised to prohibit strenuous exercise.
II. Exercise in high environmental temperatures is also avoided.
III. When aspiration occurs intermittently, antibiotic treatment is indicated.

Brachycephalic Syndrome
See Chap. 14.

LARYNGITIS

Acute Laryngitis
Definition

Acute inflammation of the laryngeal mucosa

Causes

I. Infectious diseases
  A. In dogs, kennel cough (a viral/bacterial disease

in which canine parainfluenza virus, canine adenovirus-2, and *Bordetella bronchiseptica* are involved) is a major cause (Swango, 1995).

   B. In cats, feline calicivirus and rhinotracheitis virus are major causes (Barr et al., 1995).

  II. Local mucosal irritation
    A. Dog: continuous barking, panting
    B. Dog and cat: after long-standing intratracheal intubation
    C. Dog and cat: inhalation of caustic gases or other irritants

Pathophysiology

  I. In infectious diseases, viruses and bacteria are mainly transmitted by aerosols (sputum particles and respiratory secretions) from dog to dog and from cat to cat.
    A. Stress may compromise immunoresistance.
    B. Concurrent disease may suppress immunoresistance.
  II. Mechanical irritation of the laryngeal mucosa causes hypervascularization, edema, and stimulation of the laryngeal cough receptors.
  III. Changes in the laryngeal mucosa, especially edema, may cause impairment of vocal and respiratory functions.

Clinical Signs

  I. Signalment and history
    A. No definite sex and breed predilection
    B. Stress such as that evoked by change of environment
    C. Kennel or cattery housing
    D. Recent surgery
  II. Physical examination
    A. Soft palpation of the laryngeal area elicits a cough.
    B. Cough may evoke gagging.
    C. Severe edema causes a laryngeal stridor.
    D. Body temperature is normal in uncomplicated laryngitis.
  III. Acute onset of frequent loud dry coughing
  IV. Hoarse voice or normal voice
  V. Cough upon vocalization
  VI. Possibly complicated by signs of tracheitis, bronchitis, and interstitial pneumonia

Diagnosis

  I. A presumptive diagnosis can be made from the history, the clinical signs, and the physical examination findings.
  II. Laryngoscopy reveals hypervascularization of the laryngeal mucosa and edema. In cats, laryngeal edema is prominent.
  III. Hematology and serum chemistries are unremarkable.
  IV. Electromyography reveals that there is no muscular involvement.

Differential Diagnosis

  I. Dogs
    A. Tracheobronchitis (also from kennel cough)
    B. Noninfectious tracheitis
    C. Chronic laryngitis
  II. Cats
    A. Laryngeal neoplasia
    B. Laryngeal edema of other origins

Treatment

  I. Acute laryngitis is self-limiting and lasts no more than 14–21 days.
  II. Symptomatic therapy for coughing in dogs is as follows.
    A. Advise owner to prevent barking, straining on the leash, and panting.
    B. Give extra water orally during episodes of coughing, 1 ml/kg, and repeat when necessary.
    C. For coughing during the night, phenobarbital may be given at 2 mg/kg PO SID 2 hours before bedtime.
    D. Refractory coughing in dogs may be controlled with butorphanol at 0.05–0.1 mg/kg PO BID-TID or hydrocodone bitartrate at 0.22 mg/kg PO SID-TID.
  III. Laryngeal edema in cats is treated as follows.
    A. Amoxicillin/clavulanate 12.5 mg/kg SQ, PO TID for 10 days
    B. For severe obstruction: tracheostomy for 5–10 days
  IV. Air conditioning with 70% humidity is also helpful.

Patient Monitoring

  I. Advise owner to prohibit all activity while the dog is symptomatic.
  II. Reevaluate when symptoms indicate complications.
  III. Advise owners to keep affected cats inside while symptomatic.
  IV. In animals with a tracheostomy, the laryngeal function (laryngoscopy) is evaluated before removing the cannula.

Chronic Laryngitis

Definition

  I. In dogs, this is a continuous state of inflammation with thickening of the laryngeal mucosa and incidental mucosal atrophy.
  II. It is not known to occur in cats.

Causes

  I. Not always apparent
  II. Habits of frequent panting, frequent barking, and straining against the collar
  III. Frequent coughing as in tracheal collapse
  IV. Insufficient laryngeal opening

Pathophysiology

Continuous mechanical irritation of the larynx occurs.

Clinical Signs

  I. Signalment
     A. Usually dogs >5 years old
     B. No definite sex or breed predilection
  II. Physical examination
     A. Palpation of the laryngeal area elicits cough.
     B. Coughing may evoke gagging.
     C. There are no signs of general illness.
  III. Gradual onset
  IV. Recurrent periods of coughing
  V. Hoarse voice or normal voice
  VI. Cough evoked upon vocalization

Diagnosis

  I. A presumptive diagnosis can be made from the history, the clinical signs, and the physical examination findings.
  II. Laryngoscopy reveals reddened and thickened laryngeal mucosa.
  III. The vocal folds are voluminous and red.
  IV. Sometimes the laryngeal mucosa is thin and the cartilages of the corniculate processes are clearly visible through the transparant mucosa.
  V. Electromyography sometimes reveals complex repetitive discharges in the thyroarytenoid muscles, indicating muscle involvement of the vocal folds.

Differential Diagnosis

  I. Chronic tracheitis
  II. Chronic tracheobronchitis

Treatment

  I. Symptomatic treatment is aimed at reducing mechanical irritation.
     A. Change the contributing habits of the dog.
     B. Use a harness instead of a collar.
  II. Cough suppressants are usually not helpful.
  III. In severe cases or periods of severe signs, alternate-day treatment with predisone (1–2 mg/kg PO SID) may suppress the signs, but no definite cure is to be expected from medication.

Patient Monitoring

  I. Repeated counseling and encouragement of the owner is often necessary.
  II. Reevaluate when symptoms indicate possible complications, such as pneumonia.

Chronic Epiglottitis

Definition and Cause

  I. Deformation of the cartilage of the epiglottis together with inflammation of the mucosa

  II. Cause unknown

Clinical Signs

  I. Dogs >5 years
  II. Gagging
  III. Repeated swallowing actions independent of food or water intake
  IV. Sometimes stridorous breathing and respiratory distress

Diagnosis

  I. Laryngoscopy reveals the epiglottis is stiff and sometimes ossified, and often the tip is curled upward or downward and is fixed in this position.
  II. Radiography shows the ossification and often other deformations of the epiglottis as well.

Differential Diagnosis

  I. Pharyngitis
  II. Foreign body in the caudal pharyngeal cavity

Treatment

  I. Symptomatic treatment is similar to that for chronic pharyngitis.
     A. Feed small portions of blended food, 3–4 times daily.
     B. Give 0.5–1 tbsp syrup or honey 20 minutes before the meal.
  II. No cure is to be expected from medication.
  III. There are no reports of the results of surgical removal of the epiglottis.

Patient Monitoring

  I. Advise the owner to continue the feeding regimen, even when the signs are diminished. The epiglottis will not become fully normal again.
  II. Restrict exercise when respiratory distress is prominent.
  III. Progression of the deformation of the epiglottis may lead to dysphagia.

LARYNGEAL PARALYSIS

Definition and Causes

  I. It is a complete or partial loss of function of the larynx caused by neurogenic, muscular, neuromuscular, or ankylotic (cricoarytenoid articulation) disease (Venker-van Haagen, 1992, 1995).
  II. There are two possible causes of neurogenic laryngeal paralysis.
     A. Primary or secondary trauma to the recurrent laryngeal nerve(s)
        1. Primary laceration or rupture during a surgical procedure
        2. Direct injury during trauma as in bite wounds

3. Secondary trauma during scar tissue formation after surgery or other trauma
4. Tumor infiltration of the thyroid gland
5. Abscesses in the neck region
B. Neurogenic degenerative disease affecting the recurrent laryngeal nerves and the motoneurons (nucleus ambiguus) (Venker-van Haagen, 1995)

Pathophysiology

I. Primary or secondary trauma to the recurrent laryngeal nerves may be unilateral or bilateral.
A. The recurrent laryngeal nerves pass adjacent to the cervical trachea in a dorsolateral position. In severe tracheal trauma, the nerve(s) may be injured.
B. Trauma to the recurrent laryngeal nerve may occur during thyroidectomy or removal of a thyroid tumor.
C. During surgical repair of tracheal lacerations, the recurrent laryngeal nerves may damaged.
D. More often, scar tissue formation causes laryngeal nerve damage after trauma in the area around the trachea.
E. Foreign body penetration may cause abscesses in the neck region. The trauma to the recurrent laryngeal nerves may be primary or secondary.
II. Neurogenic degenerative diseases result in bilateral laryngeal paralysis involving both the abductor and adductor muscles. Each muscle is partly denervated, and progression of the disease (increased number of affected motoneurons) results in increasing dysfunction of each muscle.
A. A hereditary trait is proved (Venker-van Haagen et al., 1981a) or suggested in familial laryngeal paralysis (O'Brien and Hendriks, 1986).
B. In all cases—hereditary, familial, or nonfamilial—the primary defect is not yet known.
C. In most cases the disease affects only the recurrent laryngeal nerves, but concurrent peroneal nerve paralysis can occur (Venker-van Haagen, 1980).
III. Laryngeal paralysis may also result from polymyositis or myasthenia gravis.
IV. Laryngeal paralysis may be caused by fixation of the cricoarytenoid articulations.
V. Laryngeal paralysis has been associated with hypothyroidism.

Clinical Signs

I. Signalment
A. Trauma to the recurrent laryngeal nerves can occur in dogs and cats of all ages.
B. Laryngeal paralysis caused by neurogenic degenerative disease has been described only in dogs.
1. It occurs in both sexes.
2. Age of onset varies from 5–8 months of age for the Bouvier (Venker-van Haagen et al., 1978) to 3 years and older in other breeds (White, 1989).

3. It usually develops in large dogs (>20 kg), but can occur in small and medium-size dogs.
C. Polymyositis can occur in all dogs of all ages (Kornegay, 1995).
D. Acquired myasthenia gravis has been observed in adult dogs of all sizes, but particularly in German shepherd dogs (Braund, 1995).
E. Cricoarytenoid ankylosis occurs in dogs >10 years.
II. Physical examination
A. With trauma, there is evidence or signs of trauma in the lateral and ventral area of the neck.
1. In unilateral laryngeal paralysis, there is no stridor or respiratory distress at rest.
2. In bilateral laryngeal paralysis, the stridor and respiratory distress are determined by the degree of paralysis and level of exertion.
3. In traumatic bilateral laryngeal paralysis, the stridor is severe and the respiratory distress is life-threatening.
4. Usually no systemic illness exists except for other traumatic injuries.
B. In neurodegenerative disease, there is a history of progressive stridor and respiratory distress. No systemic illness accompanies it.
C. In polymyositis, general clinical features of skeletal muscle disease are present (Kornegay, 1995).
D. In myasthenia gravis, skeletal muscle weakness occurs during exercise (Braund, 1995).
E. In cricoarytenoid articulation ankylosis, no systemic illness is observed.
F. Other signs of hypothyroidism may be evident.

Diagnosis

I. A presumptive diagnosis is made on the basis of laryngeal stridor, respiratory distress, and the history.
II. Thoracic radiographs are normal.
III. Laryngoscopy under light anesthesia reveals insufficient or no abduction on the paralyzed side(s) of the larynx.
IV. Electromyography of the intrinsic laryngeal muscles reveals several abnormalities.
A. After trauma to the laryngeal nerves, fibrillation potentials occur in all muscles on the side of the affected recurrent laryngeal nerve(s).
B. In neurodegenerative disease, there are normal action potentials, fibrillation potentials, and complex repetitive discharges in most or all intrinsic laryngeal muscles (Venker-van Haagen et al., 1978).
C. In polymyositis, there are predominantly complex repetitive discharges and myotonic discharges.
D. In myasthenia gravis, there are specific electromyographic findings in the skeletal muscles (Braund, 1995), but these are not known to occur in the laryngeal muscles.
E. In ankylosis, electromyograms are normal.

Differential Diagnosis

   I. Laryngeal tumor
  II. Laryngeal stenosis
 III. Stenosis in the first few cervical tracheal rings
 IV. Laryngeal edema

Treatment

   I. Unilateral laryngeal paralysis: no treatment necessary
  II. Neurogenic bilateral laryngeal paralysis and respiratory distress: temporary tracheostomy followed by lateral fixation of one vocal fold (Harvey and Venker-van Haagen, 1975; White, 1989)
 III. Polymyositis: sometimes temporary tracheostomy and treatment of polymyositis (see Chap. 80)
 IV. Myasthenia gravis: treatment of the disease (see Chap. 25)
  V. Ankylosis: temporary tracheostomy followed by lateral fixation of one vocal fold
 VI. Hypothyroidism: thyroid supplementation (see Chap. 41)

Patient Monitoring

   I. In unilateral laryngeal paralysis, no monitoring is needed.
  II. After lateral fixation of one vocal fold, do the following.
    A. Use a harness in place of a collar.
    B. Restrict exercise, especially in temperatures above 20°C.
    C. Aspiration of food is rare but may occur and cause aspiration pneumonia.

LARYNGEAL NEOPLASIA

Definition and Causes

   I. Tumors can arise from all structures in the larynx (Saik et al, 1986; Venker-van Haagen, 1992).
  II. Examples in dogs include the following.
    A. Leiomyoma
    B. Rhabdomyosarcoma
    C. Squamous cell carcinoma
    D. Oncocytoma
    E. Mast cell tumor
    F. Chondrosarcoma
 III. Examples in cats are as follows.
    A. Lymphosarcoma
    B. Squamous cell carcinoma

Clinical Signs

   I. Signalment: dogs and cats of both sexes and all ages
  II. Physical examination
    A. Loss of voice
    B. Laryngeal stridor and respiratory distress
    C. In cats: a palpable enlargement of the laryngeal structures

Diagnosis

   I. Suspicious clinical signs
    A. Gradually progressive clinical signs
    B. Abrupt loss of voice
  II. Laryngoscopy revealing the tumor and the laryngeal structures involved
 III. Needle aspirate for cytology or excisional biopsy for histopathology

Differential Diagnosis

   I. Dogs: laryngeal polyps, pharyngeal mucocele
  II. Cats: laryngeal edema, laryngitis

Treatment

   I. Dogs
    A. Noninvasive tumors may be resected.
    B. No curative treatment currently exists for more extensive tumors.
    C. Symptomatic therapy involves either a temporary or permanent tracheostomy.
  II. Cats
    A. Lymphoma may be temporarily suppressed with prednisolone 2 mg/kg PO SID, alone or in conjunction with other chemotherapeutic agents (see Chap. 67).
    B. No curative treatment currently exists for invasive tumors such as squamous cell carcinoma, although several modalities are being investigated (see Chap. 70).

Patient Monitoring

   I. After resection or prednisolone therapy, monitor for recurrent dyspnea.
  II. Animals with a tracheal cannula/temporary tracheostomy usually remain in the hospital for continuous care.
 III. A permanent tracheostomy requires constant observation and frequent cleaning.
    A. Clean environment
    B. No swimming
 IV. The prognosis for noninvasive tumors is good when total resection is accomplished. For invasive tumors, the prognosis is poor.

LARYNGEAL TRAUMA

Definition and Causes

   I. Blunt or sharp trauma causing laceration of the laryngeal structures
  II. Usually bite wounds

Clinical Signs

   I. Signalment: dogs more often affected than cats
  II. Physical examination
    A. Stridorous breathing, respiratory distress

B. Usually multiple bite wounds in the area
C. Subcutaneous emphysema in the neck region
D. Shock, hemorrhage, and other signs caused by trauma

Diagnosis

I. The clinical signs and the history lead to the presumptive diagnosis.
II. Radiography reveals subcutaneous emphysema in the area of the larynx.
III. In progressive emphysema, diagnostic surgical exploration (followed by reconstruction) is indicated.

Differential Diagnosis

I. Tracheal laceration or rupture
II. Pharyngeal laceration or trauma

Treatment

I. Restore the general function if compromised.
II. Perform an intratracheal intubation followed by a tracheostomy.
III. If emphysema increases, surgical reconstruction of the larynx is indicated.
IV. Administer amoxicillin/clavulanate 12.5 mg/kg SQ, PO TID for at least 10 days.

Patient Monitoring

I. Hospitalize for as long as the tracheostomy is needed (often 10 or more days).
II. General malaise can be expected, so physical examinations must be repeated daily.
III. Wound infection often occurs.
IV. Permanent laryngeal stenosis may result.

Bibliography

Barr CM, Olsen CW, Scott FW: Feline viral diseases. p. 425. In Ettinger SJ, Feldman EC (eds): Textbook of Veterinary Internal Medicine. 4th Ed. WB Saunders, Philadelphia, 1995
Braund KG: Peripheral nerve disorders. p. 712. In Ettinger SJ, Feldman EC (eds): Textbook of Veterinary Internal Medicine. 4th Ed. WB Saunders, Philadelphia, 1995
Harvey CE, Venker-van Haagen AJ: Surgical management of pharyngeal and laryngeal airway obstruction in the dog. Vet Clin North Am 5:515, 1975
Kornegay JN: Disorders of skeletal muscles. p. 730. In Ettinger SJ, Feldman EC (eds): Textbook of Veterinary Internal Medicine. 4th Ed. WB Saunders, Philadelphia, 1995
O'Brien JA, Hendriks J: Inherited laryngeal paralysis. Analysis in the husky cross. Vet Q 8:301, 1986
Saik JE, Toll SL, Diters RW et al: Canine and feline laryngeal neoplasia: a 10-year survey. J Am Anim Hosp Assoc 22:359, 1986
Swango LJ: Canine viral diseases. p. 404. In Ettinger SJ, Feldman EC (eds): Textbook of Veterinary Internal Medicine. 4th Ed. WB Saunders, Philadelphia, 1995
Venker-van Haagen AJ: Investigations on the pathogenesis of laryngeal paralysis in the Bouvier [thesis]. p. 70. University of Utrecht, Utrecht, The Netherlands, 1980
Venker-van Haagen AJ: Diseases of the larynx. Vet Clin North Am [Small Anim Pract] 22:1155, 1992
Venker-van Haagen AJ: Diseases of the throat. p. 572. In Ettinger SJ, Feldman EC (eds): Textbook of Veterinary Internal Medicine. 4th Ed. WB Saunders, Philadelphia, 1995
Venker-van Haagen AJ, Bouw J, Hartman W: Hereditary transmission of laryngeal paralysis in Bouviers. J Am Anim Hosp Assoc 17:75, 1981a
Venker-van Haagen AJ, Engelse EJJ, van den Ingh TSGAM: Congenital subglottic stenosis in a dog. J Am Anim Hosp Assoc 17:223, 1981b
Venker-van Haagen AJ, Hartman W, Goedegebuure SA: Spontaneous laryngeal paralysis in young Bouviers. J Am Anim Hosp Assoc 14:714, 1978
White RAS: Unilateral arytenoid lateralization: an assessment of technique and longterm results in 62 dogs with laryngeal paralysis. J Small Anim Pract 30:543, 1989

16

Diseases of the Trachea

Lynelle Johnson

CONGENITAL DISORDERS

Hypoplastic Trachea

Definition

I. Tracheal hypoplasia is caused by a congenital malformation that results in a fixed and narrowed tracheal lumen. It may be segmental or involve the entire tracheal length.

II. The ends of the tracheal rings meet or overlap rather than being C-shaped, and the dorsal tracheal membrane is typically short or absent.

Causes

I. A congenital or inherited lesion is purported.

II. An increased incidence has been reported in the bulldog, Boston terrier, and boxer (Coyne, 1992).

III. The disorder has also been reported in the Labrador retriever, German shepherd dog, Weimaraner, basset hound, and a litter of husky mix dogs (Van Pelt, 1988).

IV. The incidence is reportedly greater in males than in females (2:1) (Coyne, 1992).

Pathophysiology

I. Narrowing of the tracheal lumen results in primarily inspiratory dyspnea and a failure to clear respiratory secretions, which could potentially predispose to recurrent respiratory infections, although this has not been documented in retrospective studies.

II. Hypoplastic trachea is associated with an increased incidence of other congenital anomalies, such as elongated soft palate, stenotic nares, cardiac defects (pulmonic or aortic stenosis), and megaesophagus.

Clinical Signs

I. Dyspnea
II. Stridor
III. Coughing or gagging
IV. Exercise intolerance
V. Syncope
VI. Signs worse with excitement

Diagnosis

I. History, signalment, and the presence of typical clinical signs in a breed commonly affected by tracheal hypoplasia are suggestive.

II. Physical examination may reveal increased tracheal sensitivity.
   A. The trachea may feel narrow on palpation.
   B. Inspiratory wheezes or musical sounds may be auscultated over the trachea owing to turbulent air flow through the narrowed lumen.
   C. A thorough physical examination is recommended to detect concurrent congenital anomalies.

III. Radiographs of the chest establish the diagnosis.
   A. The cardinal finding is decreased tracheal diameter.
   B. Two methods may be used to evaluate tracheal diameter.
      1. A ratio can be constructed of the tracheal lumen diameter at the thoracic inlet (TD) to the diameter of the thoracic inlet (TI).
         a) Tracheal hypoplasia is present if TD:TI is less than the standard value.
         b) The normal value for the bulldog is 0.127, for non-bulldog brachycephalic dogs it is 0.160, and for non-brachycephalic dogs it is 0.204.
      2. A ratio can be constructed of the tracheal lumen diameter halfway between the thoracic inlet and the carina (TT) to the width of the 3rd rib (3R). Normal is >3.0, and tracheal hypoplasia is present if TT:3R is <3.0.

Differential Diagnosis

I. Tracheal collapse
II. Brachycephalic upper airway syndrome
III. Tracheal obstruction
IV. Primary ciliary dyskinesia

Treatment

I. The severity of clinical signs is related to the presence of other disorders and is *not* related to the degree of reduction in tracheal diameter.

II. Concurrent respiratory or cardiac abnormalities associated with tracheal hypoplasia must be identified and managed.
  A. Upper airway abnormalities that can be surgically corrected, such as elongated soft palate and everted laryngeal saccules, are managed early in the course of disease, thereby substantially alleviating clinical signs.
  B. Respiratory infection must be controlled early in the course of disease.
  C. Management of obesity is strongly recommended.
  D. Judicious use of diuretics and vasodilators is indicated for treatment of congestive heart failure.

Patient Monitoring

I. Most dogs with tracheal hypoplasia enjoy a good quality of life and can be maintained relatively free of clinical signs or respiratory distress.
II. Affected dogs benefit from avoidance of hot and humid conditions.
III. Rechecks are advised at least yearly for early detection of complicating diseases.

TRACHEAL COLLAPSE

Definition

I. Tracheal collapse is characterized by dynamic reduction in the luminal diameter of the cervical and/or intrathoracic trachea.
II. Flattening of the tracheal rings normally occurs in a dorsoventral orientation, which results in lengthening of the dorsal tracheal membrane.
III. A component of the dynamic collapse is associated with prolapse of the dorsal membrane into the tracheal lumen.

Causes

I. The etiology is unknown, but abnormal chondrocyte function leading to cartilage defects has been documented in some affected dogs.
II. An increased incidence of disease is seen in small dogs such as the poodle, Yorkshire terrier, Pomeranian, and Chihuahua.
  A. Because signs are often seen at an early age, some authors believe that the disorder may be congenital.
  B. Poor nutrition or metabolic influences may also lead to a failure of chondrogenesis and the development of abnormal cartilage metabolism in these breeds.
III. Originally, tracheal collapse was thought to result from deficient innervation of the dorsal tracheal membrane, but this has not been proved.

Pathophysiology

I. In normal animals, the trachea is a rigid but flexible structure that exhibits only slight changes in intra-luminal diameter in response to pressure changes during respiration.
  A. On inspiration, a pressure drop occurs with progression from the glottis toward the bronchioles, and this is responsible for the flow of air into the lung.
  B. On expiration, rising intrapleural pressures result in air flowing down the pressure gradient toward an equal pressure point near the thoracic inlet.
  C. Throughout expiration, the cartilage within airway walls prevents airway collapse.
II. Some affected dogs lack chondroitin sulfate and glycosaminoglycan in the cartilage ring structure of the trachea, which results in decreased water binding within the cartilage matrix and weakening of the tracheal cartilage.
  A. Malacic changes in the tracheal cartilage allow flattening of the cervical (extrathoracic) trachea in response to the drop in pressure that occurs on inspiration.
  B. The intrathoracic airways may also be weakened, so when intrapleural pressure rises (e.g., on expiration or during a cough) and transmural pressure overcomes airway rigidity, the intrathoracic trachea collapses.
  C. When smaller airways are affected, a diffuse form of airway collapse (bronchomalacia) can lead to severe obstructive lung disease.
III. Chronic intermittent airway obstruction results in dyspnea and cough, which perpetuate laryngeal, tracheal, and bronchial irritation.
  A. Affected animals may suffer frequent episodes of respiratory distress or cough before veterinary attention is sought.
  B. The presence of concurrent disorders such as upper airway obstruction, chronic bronchitis, or cardiac failure may produce serious clinical signs in a previously asymptomatic patient.
  C. Other trigger events have been suggested, such as endotracheal intubation and respiratory infections.
  D. Obesity results in poor thoracic compliance and decreased diaphragmatic excursion, which reduce the ability of the lung to expand on inspiration, leading to relative pulmonary atelectasis, abnormal pressure gradients in the lung, and increased tendency toward airway collapse.
IV. Two sites of tracheal collapse may be distinguished.
  A. Cervical (extrathoracic) tracheal collapse is characterized by signs of cough or airway obstruction on inspiration, when a rapid drop in intraluminal pressure occurs. Upper airway obstruction as a result of laryngeal paralysis, everted laryngeal saccules, or elongated soft palate accentuates the pressure drop across the upper airway and potentiates collapse.
  B. Intrathoracic tracheal collapse causes clinical signs on expiration when intrapleural pressure exceeds the ability of the airway walls to remain open.
    1. Signs are generally more severe during a

forced expiration or cough and are therefore enhanced by bronchitis or heart failure.
  2. Collapse of the mainstem bronchi may be seen with or without tracheal collapse.
  C. Cervical and intrathoracic tracheal collapse may occur alone or together in any given animal.

Clinical Signs

  I. Dogs generally have a long history of respiratory abnormalities.
   A. Cervical tracheal collapse results in inspiratory difficulty.
   B. Intrathoracic tracheal collapse or collapse of the mainstem bronchi is associated with worsened clinical signs on expiration.
  II. Paroxysms of coughing, classically described as a ''goose honk'' cough, are common.
  III. Signs are often elicited by excitement, by pressure exerted on the trachea, by environmental conditions such as high heat or humidity, and by eating or drinking.
  IV. The cough is often followed by retching in an attempt to clear accumulated secretions from the upper airway.
  V. Dyspnea, exercise intolerance, cyanosis, and collapse may also be reported.

Diagnosis

  I. Signalment and clinical signs are often very suggestive of the diagnosis of tracheal collapse.
  II. Upon physical examination, the following may be noted.
   A. Affected dogs are often obese, and hepatomegaly of undetermined etiology may be present.
   B. The animal may appear normal at rest, but excitement often induces a honking cough, airway obstruction, or respiratory distress.
   C. Marked tracheal sensitivity is typical, and even gentle palpation can precipitate a crisis.
   D. The cervical trachea may be flattened to the extent that the free edges of the cartilage rings can be palpated at the most lateral aspect.
   E. Tracheal auscultation reveals musical inspiratory noises in animals with cervical collapse.
    1. Pay specific attention to laryngeal auscultation.
    2. The presence of stridor is suggestive of concurrent laryngeal paralysis, which has been reported in 14–30% of affected dogs.
   F. Intrathoracic tracheal collapse is characterized by respiratory difficulties on expiration. An end-expiratory snap may be heard over the thoracic cage as the intrathoracic trachea and/or mainstem bronchi collapse.
   G. Wheezes or harsh crackles suggest the presence of concurrent bronchitis.
   H. Cardiac auscultation often reveals the presence of coexisting mitral valve insufficiency, with or without congestive heart failure. The presence of a right-sided heart murmur or gallop or a split

second heart sound indicates that pulmonary hypertension may be a complicating disorder.
  III. Radiographs of the chest are an essential component of the diagnosis.
   A. Lateral chest radiographs are taken on both full inspiration and expiration to detect the dynamic nature of cervical and intrathoracic tracheal collapse.
   B. Normal static films do *not* rule out the diagnosis of tracheal collapse.
    1. The cervical trachea may be seen to collapse on inspiration or ''balloon'' open on expiration.
    2. The intrathoracic trachea collapses on expiration and may ''balloon'' open at the carina on inspiration.
   C. Fluoroscopy is useful in suspected cases that have normal chest radiographs, but when it is unavailable, obtaining radiographs during a cough can aid in the detection of collapsing airways.
   D. Both lateral and ventrodorsal chest radiographs are closely evaluated to identify concurrent pulmonary disease or cardiac failure.
   E. Obesity can confuse interpretation of pulmonary infiltrates and lead to artifactual enlargement of the cardiac silhouette.
   F. The degree of obesity in an animal can be determined by measuring the thickness of the fat pad between the ribs and the skin on the ventrodorsal radiograph.
  IV. Confirmation of tracheal collapse is best achieved through bronchoscopy.
   A. Bronchoscopy can be used to obtain respiratory samples and to visualize dynamic airway changes. The grade, extent, and severity of tracheobronchial collapse can be definitively documented.
   B. Airway sampling is recommended to identify underlying pulmonary infection or inflammation.
    1. If a tracheal wash is performed, oral intubation is used, rather than a transtracheal approach, to diminish tracheal trauma, and a small diameter endotracheal tube is used to reduce tracheal irritation.
    2. Cytologic analysis and cultures for bacteria and *Mycoplasma* are performed on airway samples.
     a) Because the trachea is not a sterile environment, positive cultures must be interpreted in light of cytologic findings.
     b) Oropharyngeal contamination is indicated by the presence of squamous cells or *Simonsiella* bacteria.
     c) True infection is accompanied by septic, suppurative inflammation on cytology.
  V. When either a tracheal wash or bronchoscopy is performed, upper airway function is always evaluated at the beginning of the procedure to rule out laryngeal paresis or paralysis. The presence of this disorder complicates management of tracheal collapse.

Differential Diagnosis

I. Infectious tracheobronchitis
II. Tracheal obstruction
III. Chronic bronchitis
IV. Congestive heart failure
V. Pneumonia

Treatment

I. Treatment of coexisting problems is essential.
II. Dogs that have upper airway abnormalities such as laryngeal paralysis or everted laryngeal saccules may become less symptomatic for tracheal collapse when these obstructive disorders are corrected surgically and pressure fluctuations within the airway are reduced.
III. Dogs with bronchitis or small airway disease complicating intrathoracic tracheal collapse also require treatment of their primary airway disease (see Chap. 17).
IV. Corticosteroids may be required to treat chronic bronchial disease. These drugs also decrease tracheal inflammation but have the disadvantage of promoting weight gain and increasing panting, both of which place added stress on the respiratory system.
V. Bronchodilators can provide relief by dilating small airways and reducing the pressure gradient within intrathoracic airways, thereby decreasing the likelihood that collapse will occur on expiration.
   A. Theophylline (Theo-Dur) 20 mg/kg PO BID, or theophylline (Slo-bid Gyrocaps) 25 mg/kg PO BID
   B. Terbutaline 1.25–2.5 mg/dog PO BID-TID
   C. Albuterol 50 μg/kg PO BID
VI. Antibiotic use is warranted when infection is documented by cytology and culture results.
VII. Cough suppressants are used to reduce mechanical irritation of the tracheal epithelium only when infectious processes have been ruled out.
   A. Often the severity of cough in these patients requires the use of narcotic agents.
   B. Examples include butorphanol 0.5–1 mg/kg PO BID-QID or hydrocodone 0.22 mg/kg PO every 4–8 hours as needed.
VIII. Cardiac failure due to valvular insufficiency is treated as described in Chap. 9.
   A. Dogs with mitral regurgitation and malacic airways may develop obstruction of the left mainstem bronchus as a result of compression by an enlarged left atrium.
   B. Therapy that reduces the regurgitant fraction may decrease bronchial compression and alleviate clinical signs.
IX. Obese animals are started on a gradual weight-loss program of regular exercise combined with a high-fiber, low-fat diet.
X. During leash walking, the use of a harness is encouraged to avoid mechanical irritation of the trachea.
XI. Dogs with tracheal collapse are very susceptible to exacerbation of clinical signs when exposed to environmental stressors such as heat and humidity, and efforts should be made to avoid exposure to these elements.
XII. Excessive excitement and stress must also be avoided, as these may precipitate clinical signs. Judicious use of tranquilizers should be considered.
XIII. Surgical placement of ring prostheses may be tried in animals with cervical tracheal collapse that fail to respond to medical management.
   A. Placement of tracheal ring prostheses is technically demanding.
   B. Laryngeal paralysis can occur postoperatively (19%), necessitating a permanent tracheostomy (Buback et al., 1996).
   C. Although a relatively high rate of both immediate and long-term complications such as cough and dyspnea may occur after surgery, these conditions are usually manageable and acceptable to owners.
   D. The majority of animals that have undergone surgical intervention have an improved quality of life and reduction in clinical signs.

Patient Monitoring

I. Dogs with tracheal collapse remain variably symptomatic throughout their entire life span, and owners must understand that some coughing will always be present.
II. Owners should be counseled regarding risk factors that exacerbate disease and should understand the need for follow-up examinations.
III. Concurrent diseases and/or obesity require separate and rigorous monitoring.

TRACHEITIS

Infectious Tracheobronchitis

Definition

Tracheitis is characterized by inflammation of the epithelial lining of the trachea and is typically associated with erosion of the mucosal surface, goblet cell hyperplasia, mucus accumulation, and disruption of the mucociliary clearance apparatus.

Causes and Pathophysiology

I. Exposure to viral infections such as parainfluenza virus, canine adenovirus, or canine distemper virus results in infection of respiratory epithelial cells.
II. Viral damage to the epithelium predisposes to secondary infection with bacteria (primarily *Bordetella* and/or *Mycoplasma*). (See also Chap. 112.)
III. The highly contagious nature of the disease leads to rapid spread among susceptible patients, with clinical signs seen 2–10 days after exposure in an infected animal.
IV. Neonates and immune-compromised animals are susceptible to the development of *Bordetella* or *Mycoplasma* pneumonia.

Clinical Signs

I. Signs often follow exposure to an animal from a shelter or kennel.

II. A characteristic finding is the sudden development of a dry, paroxysmal, "seal bark" cough in the absence of systemic signs of illness.

III. Coughing is easily elicited by tracheal manipulation.

Diagnosis

I. Diagnosis is often based on a history of exposure to a potential carrier of the infection and on finding typical clinical signs in an otherwise healthy animal.

II. The primary physical examination finding is markedly increased tracheal sensitivity.
   A. Lung sounds are normal in uncomplicated cases.
   B. Fever, anorexia, lethargy, and naso-ocular discharge are indicators of systemic disease.

III. A complete diagnostic work-up is reserved for animals with systemic illness.

IV. A complete blood count is typically performed in ill animals.
   A. Lymphopenia suggests a viral etiology but is present only in the early course of disease.
   B. Neutrophilia can indicate the presence of concurrent bacterial infection, especially bronchopneumonia.

V. Chest radiographs are often normal because only tracheal inflammation is present.
   A. A generalized interstitial pattern is compatible with viral pneumonia.
   B. The presence of an alveolar infiltrate suggests that secondary bacterial pneumonia is present.

VI. In complicated cases, a transtracheal wash for cytologic analysis and bacterial and *Mycoplasma* cultures are performed. Antibiotic sensitivity testing is recommended to provide optimal therapy.

Differential Diagnosis

I. Tracheal collapse

II. Tracheal obstruction

III. Pneumonia

IV. Acute bronchitis

V. Parasitic bronchitis or pneumonia

Treatment

I. Generalized supportive care measures such as maintaining a warm, draft-free environment, ensuring adequate systemic hydration, and providing good nutritional support are implemented.

II. Antibiotics are indicated for treatment of secondary infection.
   A. Antibiotics with efficacy against *Bordetella* and *Mycoplasma* are chosen and administered for 7–10 days.
   B. Reasonable choices include chloramphenicol 50 mg/kg PO TID (beware of drug-induced fever or bone marrow suppression), enrofloxacin 2.5 mg/kg PO BID (beware of cartilage deformation in young animals), and doxycycline 5 mg/kg PO BID (beware of staining of the teeth in young animals).
   C. Intratracheal gentamicin or gentamicin nebulization by face mask may be helpful in treating resistant or recurrent cases of infectious tracheobronchitis.

III. Judicious use of antitussives is indicated after infection is cleared to decrease tracheal irritation. If used too early in the course of disease, however, antitussives may encourage the development of pneumonia by trapping bacteria in the lower airways.

IV. Owners are instructed to avoid using a collar to reduce direct tracheal irritation.

Patient Monitoring

I. Infectious tracheobronchitis is generally a self-limited disease, with signs resolving within 7–10 days. Longer duration of illness or the presence of constitutional signs suggests pulmonary involvement.

II. Contact with other dogs must be discouraged, given the highly infectious nature of the disease.

III. Bleach can be used to disinfect the area contaminated by an infected dog.

IV. Use of an intranasal vaccine against *Bordetella bronchiseptica* may reduce the incidence or severity of infection in susceptible animals.

Parasitic Tracheitis

Definition and Causes

I. *Oslerus osleri* is a nematode parasite that infects the carina and major bronchi in dogs.

II. This parasite has a worldwide distribution, is responsible for disease in both wild and domestic canids, and more commonly infects younger animals.

Pathophysiology

I. Transmission from bitch to offspring is believed to occur primarily through grooming activity or possibly regurgitant feeding.

II. Direct, horizontal transmission has been shown experimentally but is unlikely to occur in the natural setting.

III. Infection occurs through ingestion of first-stage larvae that migrate from the intestine to the right heart and then to the tracheal wall during a 10- to 21-week prepatent period.

IV. Adult parasites live in nodules within the larger airways, causing cough due to tracheal irritation and dyspnea associated with physical obstruction of the airway.

V. Eggs and infective L1 larval stages are coughed up, swallowed, and shed intermittently in the feces.

Clinical Signs

I. Dogs often present with a chronic, dry cough that is nonresponsive to antibiotic therapy.

II. Severely parasitized animals develop dyspnea, anorexia, and exercise intolerance.

Diagnosis

I. Physical examination findings are often nonspecific.
  A. Increased tracheal sensitivity is virtually always present.
  B. Severely affected animals show a restrictive breathing pattern and are often debilitated and cachectic.
II. Fecal examination via Baermann technique or zinc sulfate flotation is done to detect first-stage larvae, but samples are often falsely negative because of intermittent shedding.
III. Tracheal nodules associated with *O. osleri* are occasionally visible on radiographs.
IV. Bronchoscopy permits easy visualization of nodules at the carina, and these can be biopsied for definitive diagnosis of parasitic tracheitis.
V. Transtracheal wash or bronchoalveolar lavage cytology or tracheal swabs may reveal larvae or eggs.
VI. Eosinophilia is variably present on evaluation of a complete blood count or on cytology of airway washes.

Differential Diagnosis

I. Chronic bronchitis
II. Parasitic pneumonia or lung worm infection
III. Infectious or irritant tracheobronchitis
IV. Tracheal collapse

Treatment

I. No single therapy has proved universally efficacious for eradicating *O. osleri,* and combinations of drugs may be required for resolution of disease.
  A. Ivermectin 200–300 μg/kg in a single dose PO or SQ
  B. Fenbendazole 50 mg/kg/day PO for 10–30 days
  C. Thiabendazole 32–140 mg/kg/day PO for 10–23 days
  D. Levamisole 7.5 mg/kg/day PO for 10–30 days
  E. Benzimidazoles or levamisole may cause vomiting.
II. Horizontal transmission in a kennel situation is unlikely, but routine cleaning and maintenance of a kennel in which *Oslerus* has been identified are recommended.
III. Removal of infected bitches from a breeding colony reduces the incidence of disease in the offspring.

Patient Monitoring

I. Resolution of clinical signs may be a reliable way to determine efficacy of treatment.
II. Fecal examinations are unreliable, given the intermittent shedding of larvae.
III. Radiographs may be used to follow resolution of tracheal nodules if they were visualized initially.

IV. Bronchoscopy can be used to follow regression of intraluminal nodules after therapy.

Irritant Tracheitis

Definition and Causes

Tracheal irritation may result from blunt trauma, inhalation of noxious fumes, use of an overly large endotracheal tube, overdistention of an endotracheal tube cuff, or as a chronic sequela to bronchial or pulmonary disease.

Pathophysiology

Chronic cough results in a cycle of epithelial erosion and desquamation, increased mucus production, and trapping of secretions, which perpetuates tracheal inflammation.

Clinical Signs

I. Classic signs include the presence of a chronic, nonproductive cough and increased tracheal sensitivity on physical examination.
II. Signs related to the inciting event, such as facial burns associated with smoke inhalation or cervical swelling related to choke-chain trauma, may also be detected.

Diagnosis

I. Historical features such as smoke inhalation, recent endotracheal intubation, or recent pulmonary infection should heighten the suspicion of this disorder.
II. Other causes of cough should be ruled out.
III. Bronchoscopic evaluation of the airway shows irritation, erythema, increased mucus, and hemorrhage in the trachea.

Differential Diagnosis

I. Infectious tracheobronchitis
II. Tracheal collapse
III. Parasitic tracheobronchitis

Treatment

I. Environmental features such as excessive smoke or noxious fumes should be eliminated during the recovery period (see also Chap. 132).
II. Antitussives may be used to decrease chronic irritation associated with coughing. Infectious diseases must be ruled out prior to using antitussives, as decreased clearance of secretions worsens the course of disease caused by infection.
III. A short course (2–5 days) of prednisone or prednisolone at anti-inflammatory dosages (0.5 mg/kg/day PO) can help alleviate tracheitis.

Patient Monitoring

I. Use of a harness may facilitate resolution of clinical signs by decreasing pressure on the trachea.

II. Animals with severe inflammation are monitored with repeat bronchoscopy, as indicated clinically.

III. Severely affected animals are at risk for developing tracheal stenosis, or tracheal necrosis may occur, resulting in air leakage into the subcutaneous space.

OBSTRUCTION

Definition and Causes

I. Tracheal obstruction is narrowing of the tracheal lumen by internal obstruction, stenosis, or external compression.

II. Foreign bodies causing obstruction include grass awns, tree needles, teeth, and dental tartar.

III. Intratracheal mass lesions may be caused by neoplasia, abscess formation, and parasitic or fungal granulomas.

IV. Tracheal stenosis can result from a congenital deformation or, more commonly, is secondary to trauma (e.g., endotracheal intubation, an automobile accident, tracheostomy, or penetrating injury).

V. Extraluminal obstruction of the trachea may result from an esophageal mass or diverticulum; megaesophagus; thyroid cyst; lymphadenopathy; or a mediastinal mass, abscess, or hemorrhage.

Pathophysiology

Tracheal narrowing results in increased resistance to airflow, mechanical irritation of the trachea, stimulation of cough receptors, and increased susceptibility to airway infection.

Clinical Signs

I. Chronic cough, with or without hemoptysis
II. Acute or progressive dyspnea, panting, or respiratory distress
III. Anxiety, pawing at the face
IV. Dysphagia, halitosis
V. Exercise intolerance

Diagnosis

I. Historical features, such as aspiration, intubation, or trauma, are helpful in raising the suspicion of a tracheal foreign body or obstruction.

II. Physical examination often reveals increased tracheal sensitivity.
  A. High-pitched, musical sounds can be heard over the trachea when the lumen is narrowed by an obstruction or increased secretions.
  B. Stridor may be detected in animals with high cervical tracheal obstruction.
  C. A cervical mass or esophageal enlargement may result in a palpable thickening of the neck region.

III. Radiographs may reveal a radiodense foreign body within the tracheal lumen; a focal narrowing of the tracheal air column, suggesting a stenotic lesion; or an external mass compromising the tracheal lumen.

IV. Bronchoscopy can be used to confirm the diagnosis of an intraluminal mass or foreign body, stenotic lesion, or extraluminal obstruction.

Differential Diagnosis

I. Tracheal collapse
II. Infectious tracheobronchitis
III. Tracheal hypoplasia
IV. Parasitic tracheitis
V. Feline bronchial disease

Treatment

I. Tracheal foreign bodies are best removed via bronchoscopy. Aerobic and anaerobic bacterial cultures are performed, because infection with *Actinomyces* or *Nocardia* is often found in association with foreign bodies.

II. Bougienage or, preferably, balloon dilatation may be attempted for resolution of tracheal stenosis.
  A. The inflammatory response generated by the procedure generally leads to rapid re-formation of the stricture.
  B. The risk of tracheal laceration with resultant pneumomediastinum or subcutaneous emphysema must also be considered.

III. Tracheal stenosis usually requires surgical resection and anastomosis. Only lesions involving fewer than 8–10 tracheal rings can be resected without risking excessive stress on the incision line and breakdown of the anastomotic site.

IV. Extraluminal compressive lesions require surgical exploration.

Patient Monitoring

I. Recurrent hemoptysis or pneumonia and chronic cough can be indications that foreign bodies remain within the airway or that infection persists.

II. Postoperatively, cough suppressants are indicated to reduce irritation of the tracheal mucosa, and harness-style restraints can be used to restrict neck motion that places excessive tension on the anastomotic site.

NEOPLASIA

Definition and Causes

I. Neoplasia results from uncontrolled overgrowth of abnormal epithelial or mesenchymal cells within the lower airways.

II. Adenocarcinoma, lymphosarcoma, squamous cell carcinoma, melanoma, and chondrosarcoma have been reported in the dog and cat.

III. Osteochondroma is the most common tracheal tumor, and it is often found in young dogs (Carlisle et al., 1991).

Pathophysiology

Mass lesions within the trachea cause upper airway obstruction or respiratory distress owing to narrowing of the tracheal lumen and increased resistance to airflow.

Clinical Signs

   I. Dyspnea, panting
   II. Exercise intolerance
   III. Coughing
   IV. Increased inspiratory noises
   V. Cyanosis, syncope
   VI. Systemic signs often absent

Diagnosis

   I. Physical examination may reveal abnormal respiratory sounds.
     A. Musical or wheezing noises can be heard over the trachea.
     B. Increased tracheal sensitivity may also be present.
   II. Plain chest radiographs may show an intraluminal mass lesion.
   III. Bronchoscopy often allows visualization and biopsy of the mass.

Differential Diagnosis

   I. Tracheal collapse
   II. Tracheal obstruction: foreign body, granuloma, *O. osleri*
   III. Laryngeal paralysis
   IV. Congestive heart failure
   V. Chronic bronchitis
   VI. Pulmonary hypertension

Treatment

   I. Prepare for an emergency tracheotomy in any case in which neoplasia of the cervical trachea is suspected.
   II. Mass removal via bronchoscopy may be possible in cases in which the mass is attached to the mucosa by a pedunculated stalk.
   III. Tracheal resection and anastomosis can be curative in animals with local disease only. Involvement of greater than 8–10 tracheal rings may prohibit surgical treatment owing to the risk of excessive tension on the suture line after anastomosis.
   IV. Aggressive neoplasms may require subsequent chemotherapy or radiation therapy.
     A. Lymphoma of the trachea often responds to standard chemotherapy regimens.
     B. Palliation of clinical signs may be achieved through use of a permanent tracheostomy distal to the tumor, with radiation therapy or chemotherapy used to slow neoplastic growth.

Patient Monitoring

   I. Animals are closely monitored for clinical signs of systemic spread and for local recurrence of neoplasia through bimonthly radiographs.

   II. Osteochondromas are associated with an excellent prognosis when the tumor can be fully resected.
   III. Response to therapy is variable for malignant neoplasms affecting the trachea.

TRAUMA

Definition and Causes

   I. Tracheal trauma usually results from penetrating neck injuries, bite wounds, gunshot wounds, or automobile accidents.
   II. Iatrogenic tracheal trauma can occur with use of excessive force or styleted tubes during endotracheal intubation or when high intrapulmonary pressures are obtained during anesthesia or ventilator therapy.
   III. Breakdown of a tracheotomy or tracheostomy site results in traumatic wounds to the trachea.

Pathophysiology

   I. Damage to the tracheal cartilage or annular ligament allows leakage of air into the fascial planes of the cervical region with each inspiration.
   II. Excessive air accumulation within the neck region may compress the trachea and lead to respiratory embarrassment. Decreased flow of oxygen into the lung results in alveolar hypoventilation.

Clinical Signs

   I. Clinical signs may not become evident for days to weeks after a traumatic episode owing to delayed tracheal necrosis or stenosis.
   II. Subcutaneous emphysema is commonly encountered.
   III. Inspiratory dyspnea, tachypnea, and occasionally cyanosis may be noted.

Diagnosis

   I. History of a predisposing event is highly suggestive, even if the onset of signs is delayed.
   II. Physical examination may reveal the following.
     A. Subcutaneous emphysema usually originates in the neck region but may extend across the entire body.
     B. Bite wounds, lacerations, or other evidence of trauma may be found in the cervical region.
   III. Radiographs may show subcutaneous air accumulation in the cervical region, pneumomediastinum, or potentially pneumothorax.
   IV. Tracheoscopy is generally unrewarding in locating tracheal lacerations but may be worthwhile in cases with very large rents, hemorrhage, or bruising in the damaged area.

Differential Diagnosis

   I. Infection with gas-producing bacteria
   II. Other causes of tracheal stenosis and obstruction

Treatment

I. Conservative management is usually successful when signs are mild, such as in cases of blunt trauma without tracheal or airway penetration.
   A. The wound is securely bandaged to prevent additional air leakage without restricting respiratory effort or venous return, and an oxygen-enriched environment is provided to reduce respiratory distress and alleviate hypoxemia.
   B. Forced cage rest is encouraged.
II. If respiratory distress is significant because of subcutaneous accumulation of air, 18- to 20-gauge needles can be placed under the skin and air expelled from the subcutaneous space to relieve external compression of the airway.
III. Emergency surgical treatment is required in severe cases to prevent further leakage of air into the subcutaneous space and to stabilize respirations.
   A. Surgical débridement and meticulous closure of tracheal rents are indicated in cases refractory to conservative therapy.
   B. Tracheal resection and anastomosis may be required in patients with substantial tracheal damage.

Patient Monitoring

I. Uncomplicated cases of tracheal injury show resolution of subcutaneous air accumulation within 7–10 days.
II. The animal is closely monitored for complications related to laryngeal damage or paralysis and esophageal injury.
III. Tracheal stenosis or stricture can occur weeks to months after tracheal trauma as a late sequela to injury.

Bibliography

Bauer MS, Currie J: Generalized subcutaneous emphysema in a dog. Can Vet J 29:836, 1988

Buback JL, Boothe HW, Hobson HP: Surgical treatment of tracheal collapse in dogs: 90 cases (1983–1993). J Am Vet Med Assoc 208:380, 1996

Carlisle CH, Biery DN, Thrall DE: Tracheal and laryngeal tumors in the dog and cat: literature review and 13 additional patients. Vet Radiol 32:229, 1991

Corcoran BM: Post-traumatic tracheal stenosis in a cat. Vet Rec 124:342, 1989

Coyne B: Hypoplasia of the trachea in dogs: 103 cases (1974–1990). J Am Vet Med Assoc 201:768, 1992

Dallman MA, McClure RC, Brown EM: Histochemical study of normal and collapsed tracheas in dogs. Am J Vet Res 49:2117, 1988

Done SH, Drew RA: Observations on the pathology of tracheal collapse in dogs. J Small Anim Pract 17:783, 1976

Ford RB: Infectious tracheobronchitis. p. 905. In Bonagura JD (ed): Current Veterinary Therapy XII. WB Saunders, Philadelphia, 1995

Harvey CE: Inherited and congenital airway conditions. J Small Anim Pract 30:184, 1989

Lappin MR, Prestwood AK: *Oslerus osleri*: clinical case, attempted transmission, and epidemiology. J Am Anim Hosp Assoc 24:153, 1988

Lotti U, Niebauer GW: Tracheobronchial foreign bodies of plant origin in 153 hunting dogs. Compend Contin Educ Pract Vet 14:900, 1992

McKiernan BC, Smith AR: Bacterial isolates from the lower trachea of clinically healthy dogs. J Am Anim Hosp Assoc 20:139, 1982

Randolph JF, Rendano VT: Treatment of *Filaroides osleri* infestation in a dog with thiabendazole and levamisole. J Am Anim Hosp Assoc 20:795, 1984

Smith MM, Gourley IM, Amis TC: Management of tracheal stenosis in a dog. J Am Vet Med Assoc 196:931, 1990

Tangner CH, Hedlund CS: Tracheal surgery in the dog—part I. Compend Contin Educ Pract Vet 5:599, 1983a

Tangner CH, Hedlund CS: Tracheal surgery in the dog—part II. Compend Contin Educ Pract Vet 5:738, 1983b

Tangner CH, Hobson HP: A retrospective of 20 surgically managed cases of collapsed trachea. Vet Surg 11:146, 1982

Van Pelt RW: Confirming tracheal hypoplasia in husky-mix pups. Vet Med 83:266, 1988

White RAS, Williams JM: Tracheal collapse in the dog—is there a role for surgery? A survey of 100 cases. J Small Anim Pract 35:191, 1994

Wong WT, Brocke KA: Tracheal laceration from endotracheal intubation in a cat. Vet Rec 134:622, 1994

17

Diseases of the Lower Airway

Philip Padrid

CONGENITAL DISORDERS

Primary Ciliary Dyskinesia

Definition

I. Primary ciliary dyskinesia is an ultrastructural or metabolic abnormality of cilia leading to dysfunction of ciliated cells throughout the body (respiratory tract, middle ear, sperm). It has been reported only in dogs.
II. Primary ciliary dyskinesia is also referred to as immotile cilia syndrome.

Causes and Pathophysiology

I. The most common abnormality involves abnormal function of ciliary microtubules owing to the absence of one or both of the inner and outer dynein arms (Dungworth, 1993).
II. The absence of dynein arms from the peripheral doublets of ciliary microtubules causes ciliary immobility.
III. The normal function of the "mucociliary escalator" to transport mucus orad is impaired, leading to retention of tracheobronchial secretions.
IV. This predisposes the airways and lung parenchyma to recurrent bacterial/viral infection.

Clinical Signs

I. Signalment (Morrison et al., 1987; Hoover et al., 1989)
   A. Dogs are usually younger than 18 months of age.
   B. It is reported most frequently in purebred sporting and working breed dogs such as English pointers, English springer spaniels, golden retrievers, and rottweilers.
   C. It has also been diagnosed in the Old English sheepdog, dalmatian, chow chow, Doberman pinscher, Shar pei, elkhound, and Border collie.

II. Mucopurulent nasal discharge
III. Chronic productive cough
IV. Bronchopneumonia ± fever, general debilitation

Diagnosis

I. A definitive diagnosis can be obtained only from electron microscopic examination of ciliary structure. Common biopsy sites include nasal and tracheal mucosa. Spermatozoa may also be examined for motility and defects in flagella structure.
II. Chronic upper and lower respiratory infections (including rhinitis, sinusitis, otitis, bronchitis, and pneumonia) in young large-breed dogs suggest the possibility of primary ciliary dyskinesia.
III. Radiography may be helpful.
   A. Thoracic radiographs commonly reveal evidence of bronchitis, bronchiectasis, or pneumonia.
   B. Evidence of situs inversus, including dextrocardia in young dogs (Kartagener's syndrome), with chronic respiratory infections and/or infertility is extremely suggestive.
IV. Tracheobronchial culture of specimens obtained by transtracheal aspiration (TTA, see Chap. 3), bronchial wash (BW), or bronchoalveolar lavage (BAL) may be positive for bacteria and commonly contain large numbers of *Staphylococcus* and *Pasteurella* spp.

Differential Diagnosis

I. Other causes of mucopurulent nasal discharge
II. Other causes of bronchitis and bronchiectasis
III. Other causes of bronchopneumonia

Treatment

There is no primary treatment for this congenital defect. The goal of therapy is to sterilize and remove the tracheobronchial mucus to minimize the frequency and severity of infections.

I. Antibiotics: based on culture and sensitivity data
II. Nebulization (see Acute Bronchitis)
III. Chest physical therapy (see Bronchiectasis)

Patient Monitoring

I. Some dogs with primary ciliary dyskinesia have been maintained with antibiotic therapy for as long as 5 years.
II. Most dogs with this disease succumb to the chronic infections relatively early in life, so prognosis is guarded (Hawkins et al., 1989).
III. Early, aggressive antibiotic therapy is indicated at the first signs of infection anywhere within the respiratory system.
IV. If there is a lack of response to antibiotics, obtain more tracheobronchial secretions for repeat culture and sensitivity.

INFLAMMATORY DISEASES

Acute Bronchitis

Definition

Bronchitis is literally inflammation of the bronchi.

Causes

I. Viral infections
   A. Dog: parainfluenza, adenovirus-2, herpesvirus, reovirus
   B. Cat: calicivirus, herpesvirus
II. Bacterial infections
   A. Dog: *Bordetella bronchiseptica,* other predominantly gram-negative organisms, *Mycoplasma* spp.
   B. Cat: *Pasteurella* spp., alpha-hemolytic *Streptococcus* spp., *Mycoplasma* spp.
III. Inhalation of irritants: pollen, smoke, dust, etc.

Pathophysiology

I. Infection occurs via inhalation, aspiration, or direct inoculation (endotracheal intubation).
II. Pathogenic organisms may infect airways for a variety of reasons.
   A. Normal airway flora altered by administration of antibiotics
   B. Concurrent disease/debilitation
   C. Disturbance of normal mucociliary clearance (*Bordetella* infection)
   D. Disruption of epithelial integrity by production of oxygen radicals (*Mycoplasma* infection)
III. Stimulation of irritant (cough) receptors occurs, resulting in cough and production of increased tracheobronchial mucus.

Clinical Signs

I. Signalment
   A. Almost always dogs <2 years of age; usually young cats

B. No definite sex or breed predilection, although large/hunting breed dogs may have an increased incidence
   C. Recent exposure to other animals, often with similar signs
II. Physical examination
   A. Inspection, including assessment of breathing pattern is generally unremarkable.
   B. Palpation of trachea frequently elicits a paroxysm of coughing.
   C. Chest percussion is unremarkable.
   D. Occasional crackles may be heard on auscultation.
III. Acute onset of dry, hacking, paroxysmal cough
   A. May be high-pitched or ''honking''
   B. May terminate in gagging or retching
IV. Usually not systemically ill except for occasional and intermittent low-grade fever
V. May also have upper respiratory tract involvement with conjunctivitis or rhinitis (especially cats)

Diagnosis

I. A presumptive diagnosis can often be made from the history, physical examination findings, and presenting clinical signs.
II. Thoracic radiography is usually normal; peribronchial infiltrates (more common in cats) are occasionally seen.
III. Hematology and serum chemistries are generally unremarkable.
IV. Bronchoscopy may show marked erythema of tracheobronchial mucosa.
   A. Structural integrity of airway walls unaffected
   B. Mild increase in observable tracheobronchial mucus (small amount of mucus is often observed in healthy cat airways)
V. Tracheobronchial cytology may show relative increased numbers of neutrophils in TTA, BW, or BAL.
VI. Tracheobronchial culture may be positive for aerobic bacteria or *Mycoplasma* spp.

Differential Diagnosis

I. Tracheobronchial foreign body: plant material, string, rocks, plastic
II. Tracheobronchial trauma
III. Collapsing trachea

Treatment

I. Acute bronchitis is generally a self-limited syndrome of 10–14 days duration. If signs persist or are distressing to either the animal or the owner, therapy may be considered.
II. Antibiotics with proven in vitro efficacy to organisms commonly recovered from airway include the following.
   A. Cats
      1. Amoxicillin 10 mg/kg PO BID–TID for 7–10 days

2. Tetracycline 10 mg/kg PO TID for 10–14 days (as tolerated)
3. Chloramphenicol 25 mg/kg PO BID (if tolerated) for 10–14 days for mycoplasmosis
B. Dogs
   1. Chloramphenicol 50 mg/kg PO TID for 10–14 days
   2. Enrofloxacin 2.5 mg/kg PO BID for 10–14 days
III. Antitussives are indicated only for persistent paroxysmal coughing and are to be avoided with concurrent bacterial infections.
   A. Dog: hydrocodone bitartrate 0.22 mg/kg PO SID–TID (do not exceed 20 mg daily)
   B. Butorphanol 0.05–0.1 mg/kg PO, SQ SID–TID
IV. Humidification and nebulization are often helpful.
   A. Humidified saline will reach the extrathoracic structures and may help decrease the incidence of cough associated with upper airway mucosal irritation.
   B. Nebulized saline will reach the intrathoracic structures and may decrease irritation of the airway mucosa and subsequently the frequency of coughing and susceptibility to infection. It may also help to liquefy tracheobronchial secretions and facilitate their removal.

Patient Monitoring

I. Advise the owner to discourage excessive exercise or play while the animal is symptomatic.
II. If the animal is not significantly better within 10–14 days, consider the following.
   A. Chest radiographs to look for signs of increased peribronchial inflammation or an additional alveolar component, which would indicate the need to reevaluate the diagnosis of acute bronchitis
   B. TTA, BW, or BAL with culture to reevaluate infectious bacterial etiology or efficacy of antibiotic therapy
   C. Reevaluation of the initial diagnosis

Chronic Bronchitis

Definition

In the dog, chronic bronchitis is defined as a condition of recurrent or persistent coughing with excessive mucus production, occurring on most days for at least 2 months (Wheeldon et al., 1974).

Causes

I. Environmental pollutants: ozone, sulfur dioxide, passive tobacco smoke inhalation, and/or dusts
II. "Allergic" hypersensitivity
III. Mycoplasmal infections (cat)
IV. Parasites (Georgi, 1987)
   A. Dog: *Oslerus osleri, Capillaria aerophila, Crenosoma vulpis*
   B. Cat: *Mammomonogamus* spp.
V. Usually unknown

Pathophysiology

I. An undetermined agent(s) elicits a chronic, active inflammatory response in the airway epithelium mucosa and submucosa, resulting in the following.
   A. Epithelial desquamation, hyperplasia
   B. Goblet cell hypertrophy and hyperplasia
   C. Submucosal glandular hypertrophy, hyperplasia, hypersecretion
   D. Edema and cellular infiltration into mucosa, submucosa
   E. Smooth muscle hypertrophy (rare)
   F. Submucosal fibrosis (occasional)
II. Submucosal nodules may form in distal trachea and mainstem bronchi with *Oslerus* infestation.
III. Stimulation of irritant (cough) receptors results in a cough and secretion of abnormal amounts of unusually viscous tracheobronchial mucus.
IV. Airway obstruction occurs from mucus within the lumen, edema and cellular infiltration of the airway wall, and occasional reversible smooth muscle contraction.
V. Intrathoracic airway collapse occurs on expiration, especially during exercise, excitement, or during and after coughing.

Clinical Signs

I. Signalment (Moise et al., 1989; Padrid, 1995)
   A. Usually dog or cat ≥ 8 years
   B. No definite sex or breed predilection
      1. Siamese cats may be at increased risk.
      2. Toy/small-breed dogs (poodle, sheltie, Pomeranian) appear to have an increased incidence.
II. Physical examination (Padrid et al., 1990)
   A. Prolonged expiratory phase of breathing is usually noted.
   B. Wheezes are commonly ausculted over all lung fields.
III. Hacking cough
   A. May be dry or seemingly productive (gags at end of cough)
   B. May be paroxysmal or insidious in onset
IV. Exercise intolerance: common, but variable
V. Excess mucus production: animal gags/swallows at end of cough episode
VI. Mild expiratory dyspnea or increased expiratory effort

Diagnosis

I. Presence of chronic, daily cough for which other known causes such as chronic heart failure, heartworm disease, or pneumonia have been ruled out is required for diagnosis.
II. Chest radiography usually demonstrates mild to moderate peribronchial infiltrates.
   A. A normal thoracic radiograph does not rule out the diagnosis of chronic bronchitis.
   B. Right middle lobe atelectasis may be found in cats.
III. Bronchoscopy reveals several characteristic findings (Padrid et al., 1990).

A. Mucosa is erythematous, and abundant mucus may partially or totally occlude the smaller airways.
B. The airway wall has an irregular contour.
C. Airways from mainstem to tertiary bronchi may partially or totally collapse during passive expiration.
D. Tracheobronchial nodules may be seen with *Oslerus*.
E. Biopsy findings include epithelial hypertrophy and desquamation, submucosal gland hypertrophy, goblet cell hyperplasia, mixed mucosal/submucosal cellular infiltrates, and (occasionally) submucosal fibrosis.

IV. Cytology via TTA may reveal primarily a neutrophilic infiltrate; however, the alveolar macrophage is usually the predominant cell type recovered on BAL.
A. Eosinophils are more common in cats.
B. Use of a cytology brush results in a higher percentage of epithelial cells recovered and is not recommended.

V. Culture of secretions obtained by TTA are more often positive for aerobic bacteria than are secretions obtained via endoscopy.
A. A pure culture of any bacterial species that does not require subculture in enrichment media for identification may indicate a true pathogenic infection (Padrid et al., 1991).
B. Antibiotic therapy is based on sensitivity data.
C. Anaerobes are more often recovered from BAL than from TTA, but the significance of this finding is unknown.

VI. Abnormal hemograms and serum chemistries usually reflect unrelated disease processes.

VII. Other tests to consider include the following (Padrid et al., 1990).
A. Arterial blood gases
1. Hypoxemia (PaO_2 <80 mmHg) occurs 30–50% of the time.
2. Hypercapnia ($PaCO_2$ >40 mmHg) is rare.
B. Tidal breathing flow volume loop
1. The ratio of expiratory time/inspiratory time is often increased, e.g., ≥1.31.
2. Airflow at 25% of tidal volume is often reduced as the airway narrows or collapses at the end of expiration.
3. It can be used to document efficacy of bronchodilation treatment.
C. Ventilation scans: often display nonhomogeneous distribution of airflow, suggesting ventilation/perfusion inequality

Differential Diagnosis

Rule out any other cause of cough.
I. Heart failure
II. Heartworm disease
III. Pneumonia
IV. Bronchopulmonary neoplasia
V. Bronchial asthma (cat)
VI. Extrathoracic tracheal collapse (dog)
VII. Chronic foreign body

Treatment

I. Corticosteroids are the mainstay of therapy.
A. Prednisone is given initially at 1 mg/kg PO BID for 10–14 days.
B. Maintenance dose is 0.1–0.25 mg/kg PO BID every other day or at the lowest effective dose to control coughing.
C. Corticosteroid therapy is tapered to maintenance dose slowly, over a 2- to 3-month period.

II. Antibiotics are indicated when there is evidence of superimposed infection as implied by culture. Avoid prophylactic or long-term antibiotic therapy.
A. There is no objective evidence that bacterial infection plays a significant role in the cause or perturbation of canine or feline chronic bronchitis.
B. Antibiotic therapy is indicated only as determined by culture, with the initial choice of antibiotic being the same as for acute bronchitis.

III. Antitussives are indicated only when the animal is syncopal following cough or cannot sleep because of cough, or the owners cannot sleep because of the animal's cough. They are avoided in cats.
A. Butorphanol 0.05–0.1 mg/kg PO, SQ SID–TID
B. Hydrocodone bitartrate 0.22 mg/kg PO SID–TID

IV. Bronchodilators are indicated on a trial basis when the animal's ability to exercise is limited by the respiratory disorder, or when wheezes are ausculted.
A. Dog
1. Albuterol (Proventil, Ventolin) 0.02 mg/kg PO SID–TID for 3–5 days, then 0.05 mg/kg PO SID–TID (side effects include transient musculoskeletal tremors and hyperactivity)
2. Long-acting theophylline (Theo-Dur *tablets*) 20 mg/kg PO BID
B. Cat
1. Terbutaline 0.625 mg/cat PO BID
2. Long-acting theophylline (Theo-Dur *tablets*) 25 mg/kg PO SID at night

V. Humidification and nebulization may be helpful as outlined earlier in Acute Bronchitis.

VI. Remove any underlying cause(s).
A. Parasites (see Chap. 16)
B. Inhaled irritants: tobacco smoke

Patient Monitoring

I. Chronic bronchitis is a progressive syndrome that is rarely cured; therefore, client education is critical so that expectations are realistic.
A. The cough frequency can be reduced, but rarely does the cough completely disappear for any extended period of time.
B. Exercise tolerance can often be increased, the degree to which may be predicted by the amount of intrathoracic airway collapse seen during bronchoscopy.

II. Weight reduction in obese animals often significantly reduces exercise intolerance and improves PaO_2.

III. Reevaluate the animal's physical status and drug therapy every 3–6 months if clinical signs are stable.

IV. Reevaluate the animal immediately if the cough increases in severity or frequency, if there is decreased exercise tolerance, or if the animal becomes systemically ill.

Bronchiectasis

Definition

I. Bronchiectasis means irreversible dilation of the bronchi as a result of inflammatory destruction of the airway wall.
II. Bronchiectasis, either congenital or acquired, is a rare disorder of cats.

Causes

I. Primary bronchial infections: viral, bacterial, fungal (Swartz, 1988)
II. Secondary infections: as seen with primary ciliary dyskinesia
III. Obstruction of airways
  A. Neoplasia
  B. Foreign body
  C. Inspissated mucus: chronic bronchitis, purulent pneumonia
IV. Following chronic inflammation
  A. Aspiration of noxious substances
  B. Accompanying chronic bronchopulmonary disease
V. Congenital bronchiectasis: reported in the dog, with other congenital abnormalities such as Kartagener's syndrome

Pathophysiology

I. Bronchiectasis is a common finding in dogs with severe chronic bronchitis and is rarely diagnosed ante mortem in cats.
II. It is assumed to result from a combination of airway luminal obstruction and primary or secondary infection leading to bronchial wall destruction (Swartz, 1988; Spencer, 1985).
III. Airway lumen obstruction leads to several sequelae.
  A. Resorption atelectasis or parenchymal fibrosis
    1. Compensatory stretching or dilation of unobstructed air passages
    2. Bronchial dilation
    3. Mucus accumulation with superimposed infection
    4. Bronchial wall inflammation with loss of structural (cartilaginous) support
  B. An increase in the size and number of bronchial artery anastomoses

Clinical Signs

I. Clinical signs usually reflect other coexisting respiratory disorders such as chronic bronchitis (Hawkins et al., 1989).
II. Chronic cough is usually present.
  A. Productive: often purulent

B. Commonly temporary remission after antibiotics are administered
C. Hemoptysis
III. Note the following on physical examination.
  A. Auscultation: crackles, occasional wheezes
  B. Systemic signs: fever, anorexia, halitosis, general debilitation

Diagnosis

I. Clinical signs and physical findings are rarely definitive.
II. The presence of frankly purulent bronchial secretions is uncommon in simple chronic bronchitis and may indicate underlying bronchiectasis.
III. Thoracic radiography often suggests the diagnosis (Meyer and Burt, 1973; Kneller, 1986).
  A. Plain radiographs do not suggest the presence of bronchiectasis until the disease is advanced.
    1. Increased size of bronchial lumen
    2. Changes consistent with severe chronic bronchitis, i.e., severe diffuse peribronchial infiltrates
    3. Focal atelectasis and consolidation
  B. Contrast bronchography is the definitive method of diagnosis (O'Brien et al., 1966; Cantwell and Blevins, 1981).
    1. Selective bronchography is preferred.
    2. Bilateral bronchography should be avoided, to minimize airflow obstruction and inflammation secondary to the contrast agent.
    3. Bronchography is not indicated unless surgical resection of the bronchiectatic segment or lung lobe is contemplated.
IV. Bronchoscopy can confirm the diagnosis in most cases.
V. Culture of tracheobronchial secretions facilitates the choice of appropriate antibiotic therapy.

Differential Diagnosis

I. Chronic bronchitis without bronchiectasis
II. Occult pneumonia with purulent productive cough
III. Bronchopulmonary tumor with secondary infection

Treatment

I. The goal of therapy is to sterilize retained secretions and facilitate their removal by the cough reflex.
II. Antibiotics are indicated.
  A. The choice of antibiotics is based on culture and sensitivity data of tracheobronchial secretions.
  B. Prolonged therapy (14–21 days minimum) is required and is repeated at the first signs of exacerbation of symptoms.
III. Bronchodilators may be partially effective in controlling symptoms of airflow obstruction associated with coexisting chronic bronchitis or bronchial asthma. (See treatment of Chronic Bronchitis, earlier.)
IV. Chest physical therapy assists in drainage of inspissated, infected bronchopulmonary secretions (Haskins, 1986).

A. Postural drainage: Position the animal in left, right, sternal, and dorsal recumbency and rotate at 30-minute intervals.
B. Percussion: It involves a rapid series of thumps applied to the chest wall by cupped hands to generate vibrational energy, mechanically dislodge secretions, and stimulate coughing.
V. Surgery (partial lobectomy) is indicated in those animals with severe symptoms when attributable to a localized area or single lobe.

Patient Monitoring

I. Generalized bronchiectasis is an incurable condition. Response to therapy is usually temporary, and relapses are common. Long-term prognosis for good quality of life is unfavorable.
II. Early recognition of any exacerbation of symptoms is important in minimizing extension of the disease.
A. Obtain a tracheobronchial wash every 3–6 months.
B. Repeat radiography every 3–6 months.
C. Immediately reevaluate the animal if signs worsen.

Emphysema

Definition

Emphysema is alteration of lung parenchyma characterized by abnormal enlargement of the air spaces distal to the terminal bronchiole, accompanied by destruction of the alveolar walls without obvious fibrosis.

Causes

I. The pathogenesis of emphysema in dogs and cats is unknown.
II. It may develop as an extension of the pathophysiology underlying chronic bronchitis (dogs) and bronchial asthma (cats).
A. Alveolar macrophages and other inflammatory cells release enzymes capable of digesting elastic and collagenous components of the alveolar wall.
B. Chronic bronchiolar obstruction results in air trapping and overdistention of alveoli, with eventual disruption of alveolar wall integrity (Spencer, 1985).

Pathophysiology

I. Mild emphysema confined to the periphery of lung lobes is a frequent finding on necropsy examination of pulmonary tissue obtained from dogs and cats with the clinical diagnosis and histologic evidence of chronic bronchitis or bronchial asthma.
II. Destruction of interstitial parenchyma and capillary beds results in the following.
A. Hypoxemia, pulmonary hypertension, and potentially cor pulmonale
B. Loss of radial traction and reduction in airway diameter

C. Loss of inherent elasticity and lung recoil leading to increased lung compliance, functional residual capacity, residual volume, and total lung capacity
III. The final result is airflow resistance primarily during expiration.

Clinical Signs and Diagnosis

I. Emphysema rarely occurs in the absence of airway disease, so clinical signs reflect the underlying bronchial disease.
II. Histologic analysis of lung tissue is required for the definitive diagnosis of emphysema.
III. Thoracic radiography may demonstrate the following.
A. Hyperinflation of lung fields
1. Flattened diaphragm (may occur with airway pathology in absence of emphysema)
2. Attenuation of pulmonary vascular pattern, especially in the peripheral lung fields
3. Posterior extension of costophrenic portions of the lungs
B. Bullous cysts, rarely pneumothorax (Kramer et al., 1985)
C. Evidence of chronic bronchial disease
IV. Other tests may be considered.
A. The primary noninvasive test used to diagnose emphysema in human medicine measures the efficiency of alveolar capillary gas exchange, as reflected by the diffusing capacity of carbon monoxide.
B. In experimentally induced emphysema in dogs, the diffusing capacity is reduced to 40% of its normal value (Pushpakom, 1970).

Differential Diagnosis

I. Chronic bronchitis, bronchial asthma, bronchiectasis
II. Pulmonary vascular disease: heartworm infestation, pulmonary hypertension
III. Any cause of airway obstruction
IV. Radiographic artifacts

Treatment

I. The goal of therapy is to treat the underlying disease processes, including impaired oxygenation, expiratory airflow resistance, and secondary right heart failure.
II. Theoretically, emphysema may be helped by use of the following.
A. Bronchodilators (see treatment of Chronic Bronchitis, earlier)
B. Oxygen
1. Oxygen minimizes pulmonary vasoconstriction and exercise intolerance owing to hypoxemia.
2. Administer oxygen (28–40%) continuously during hospitalization for exacerbation of clinical signs.
3. Observe for 2–4 hours off oxygen for increasing dyspnea before discharging from hospital.

Patient Monitoring

I. Emphysema is a clinically important finding only insofar as it is a component of other chronic airway diseases such as chronic bronchitis or bronchial asthma.

II. Pulmonary emphysema is an irreversible disorder that can be expected to progress.

III. Evaluation and monitoring are directed toward better definition and interruption of the primary underlying disorder.

IMMUNOLOGIC DISORDERS

Bronchial Asthma/Allergic Bronchitis

Definition

I. Bronchial asthma is a condition of lower airway obstruction that may reverse spontaneously or in response to therapy.
   A. It is associated with chronic airway inflammation and airway hyper-reactivity, i.e., increased smooth muscle contraction following exposure to stimuli that do not cause a similar amount of smooth muscle contraction in nonasthmatics.
   B. It is a feline disease. Naturally occurring, clinically significant *spontaneous* bronchoconstriction is exceedingly rare in the dog.
   C. A clear distinction between extrinsic (type I hypersensitivity) and intrinsic (nonallergic) asthma in cats has not been demonstrated.

II. Allergic bronchitis is a poorly defined syndrome.
   A. Its distinction from chronic bronchitis is arbitrary and is usually based on the finding of large numbers of eosinophils in tracheobronchial secretions in dogs, combined with a rapid response to corticosteroid therapy.
   B. Allergic bronchitis is distinct from asthma in that acute bronchoconstriction is not a feature of bronchitis.

Causes

I. In the vast majority of cases the etiology is unproved. It is assumed that many different inhaled environmental agents may be responsible.

II. Commonly implicated potential allergens and/or irritants include the following.
   A. Pollen
   B. Aerosolized litter dust
   C. Cigarette and cigar smoke
   D. Perfume, scented litter
   E. Carpet cleaning solutions
   F. Household dust and molds
   G. Human dander
   H. Migrating parasite larvae

Pathophysiology

I. The bronchial smooth muscle hypercontracts in response to multiple stimuli that cause a lesser degree of bronchoconstriction in nonaffected individuals. Hypersecretion of mucus and submucosal edema may contribute to generalized small airway obstruction.

II. IgE antigen links bivalently with antibody fixed to previously exposed airway mast cells. Release of preformed (histamine, serotonin) and secreted (platelet activating factor, thromboxane A_2, leukotrienes, oxygen radicals) mediators causes direct bronchoconstriction.

III. Release of mediators from mast cells and basophils stimulates sensory fibers, in turn causing increased efferent neural discharge and reflex bronchoconstriction.

IV. Chronic inflammation of the mucosal epithelium increases airway muscle contraction to a variety of potential agonists.
   A. Eosinophils are implicated as primary effector cells in causing epithelial damage by the release of preformed toxic proteins, including major basic protein and eosinophilic cationic protein.
   B. Eosinophils are stimulated to leave the vascular space and enter airways by cytokines and chemokines secreted by activated T lymphocytes and airway epithelium.
   C. This is consistent with the finding of eosinophils and other inflammatory cells in the airways of cats with bronchial asthma and helps explain the development of hyper-reactive airways.

Clinical Signs

I. Signalment
   A. Cats are generally middle-aged, although cats of all ages have been treated for signs of bronchial disease. Younger dogs (<5 years of age) may be seen with greater frequency (Moise et al., 1989; Padrid, 1995, 1996a, 1996b).
   B. The Siamese breed seems predisposed to the syndrome. There is no apparent sex predilection in dogs or cats (Moise et al., 1989; Padrid, 1995, 1996a; Dye and McKiernan, 1996).
   C. Malamutes and huskies may have an increased incidence.

II. Physical examination
   A. Physical examination findings in dogs with allergic bronchitis are similar to those in dogs with chronic bronchitis. In general, dogs with allergic bronchitis do not present in acute respiratory distress.
   B. Physical examination of cats with asymptomatic asthma may be completely normal.
   C. Close inspection may reveal excessive expiratory effort with abdominal lifting.
   D. Percussion of dogs may reveal hyper-resonance consistent with increased total lung volume and air trapping. This finding is difficult to appreciate in cats.
   E. Auscultation may demonstrate diffuse wheezes and/or crackles.
      1. If the disease is advanced, airflow may be so limited that these sounds are not heard.

2. This is a grave finding in a symptomatic cat.
III. Chronic paroxysmal cough, often terminating in gagging or retching
IV. Paroxysmal dyspnea
    A. This occurs primarily during expiration unless the disease is advanced, then open-mouth breathing or panting is seen in cats.
    B. Resting tachypnea may occur between episodes of dyspnea.
V. Systemically well between clinically significant episodes

Diagnosis

I. The formal diagnosis of asthma requires the demonstration of hyperactive airways, which has been documented in cats by pulmonary function testing (Dye and McKiernan, 1996).
II. A presumptive diagnosis of asthma may be made in a cat with sudden onset of expiratory effort and wheezing.
III. Thoracic radiography is often helpful (Padrid and Koblik, 1990).
    A. Air trapping may be best appreciated from end-expiratory films, with the finding of hyperlucency of lung fields, flattening of the diaphragm, and an appearance similar to end-inspiratory films.
    B. Peribronchial cuffing is frequently found and can be distinguished from interstitial nodules by use of a magnifying glass to identify airway lumina.
    C. The changes accompanying allergic bronchitis are similar to but more dramatic than those associated with chronic bronchitis.
IV. Hematology may demonstrate a peripheral eosinophilia, but this is a nonspecific finding, as many nonrespiratory conditions cause peripheral eosinophilia in the cat (Center et al., 1990).
V. Serum chemistries are unremarkable.
VI. Arterial blood gases may show hypoxemia, severe hypercarbia, and acute respiratory acidosis (Moise and Spaulding, 1981).
VII. Bronchoscopy is a useful tool to rule out foreign body as a cause of cough or acute tachypnea and to evaluate the extent of airway pathology for prognosis.
    A. Profound mucosal erythema and edema
    B. Copious mucus production
    C. Intact structural integrity of airway walls (common in cats, variable in dogs)
    D. Significant circumferential reduction in airway lumen
VIII. Tracheobronchial cytology commonly reveals profound eosinophilia.
    A. Tracheobronchial eosinophilia in normal cats limits the interpretation of this finding (Padrid et al., 1991).
    B. A small number of cats with bronchial asthma have relatively large numbers of neutrophils in their airway washings.
    C. The presence of many alveolar macrophages with foamy cytoplasm and other features of "activation" is a normal finding in cats and does not assist in the diagnosis of asthma.
IX. Tracheobronchial culture may be positive for many bacterial species, including *Staphylococcus, Streptococcus,* or *Pasteurella* spp.
    A. These organisms exist commensally in the airways and may not contribute to the disease process (Padrid, 1995; Dye and McKiernan, 1996).
    B. The presence of *Mycoplasma* may contribute to the pathophysiology of bronchial asthma in cats (see Chronic Bronchitis).
X. Immunologic testing may be undertaken.
    A. Radioallergosorbent testing (RAST) to measure serum IgE in dogs is available, but its clinical utility has not been confirmed.
    B. Skin testing in dogs may aid in the identification of factors that contribute to clinical signs.
    C. IgE has not been clearly identified in cats, therefore RAST is inappropriate.
    D. Skin testing may be used in an attempt to identify some causes of bronchial asthma in cats.
XI. Terbutaline 0.01 mg/kg IM or SQ may be given to cats with signs of asthma and difficulty breathing or wheezes.
    A. If the respiratory rate decreases, respiratory effort is lessened, or wheezes diminish within 30 minutes, a presumptive diagnosis of reversible bronchospasm (consistent with asthma) can be made.
    B. Measurement of lung resistance and dynamic compliance before and after terbutaline challenge documents the degree of reversible airway disease (Dye and McKiernan, 1996).

Differential Diagnosis

I. Any nonrespiratory cause of panting: fear, excitement, hyperthermia, fever, profound anemia
II. Congestive heart failure
III. Pneumonia
IV. Diseases of the pleural space: pneumothorax, pleural effusion, diaphragmatic hernia

Treatment

I. Handle the acutely dyspneic dog or cat with minimal restraint (Padrid, 1996b).
    A. Bronchodilators: terbutaline 0.01 mg/kg IM, SQ
    B. Oxygen 100%: cage, mask, nasal cannula
    C. Corticosteroids given IV
        1. Seem to produce a rapid decrease in symptoms even though their onset of action theoretically is 3–6 hours
        2. Prednisolone sodium succinate 0.5–1 mg/kg IV, repeat in 4–6 hours as needed
II. An animal that shows signs of imminent respiratory arrest may be anesthetized with 0.1 mg/kg ketamine IV and intubated. Administer 100% oxygen and 0.5% halothane until bronchodilator, oxygen, and corticosteroid therapy reverse the acute symptoms.

III. Maintenance therapy for the patient with chronic intermittent symptoms must be individualized.
   A. Attempt to identify and avoid situations or substances that provoke an attack.
   B. Corticosteroids are the mainstay of therapy and are used consistently and chronically rather than episodically.
      1. Give prednisone 1–2 mg/kg PO BID initially.
      2. Taper slowly over 2–3 months to lowest effective alternate-day schedule if possible.
   C. Bronchodilators may be used in conjunction with corticosteroids on a chronic basis for animals that do not respond optimally to corticosteroids alone.
      1. Terbutaline given orally
         a) Dog: 0.05–0.1 mg/kg PO BID–TID PRN
         b) Cat: 0.625 mg/cat PO BID
      2. Terbutaline given parenterally
         a) 0.01 mg/kg IM or SQ
         b) May be given by the owner at home for acute dyspnea in cats
      3. Long-acting theophylline (Theo-Dur *tablets*)
         a) Dog: 20 mg/kg PO BID
         b) Cat: 25 mg/kg PO SID at night
   D. Antibiotics are reserved for cases in which cultures of tracheobronchial secretions are positive for *Mycoplasma* or suggest true infection (see Chronic Bronchitis).

Patient Monitoring

I. Instruct clients to report early symptoms such as increased cough or subtle wheezing immediately and encourage them to return the animal for examination if such signs persist.
II. Adjustment of medications is based on a detailed knowledge of the animal's history and may occasionally be done by phone conversation.
III. If symptoms are becoming more frequent or more severe, repeat chest radiographs to rule out other pulmonary conditions such as pneumonia or pneumothorax.

Bibliography

Boothe DM, McKiernan BC: Respiratory therapeutics. Vet Clin North Am [Small Anim Pract] 22:1231, 1992

Cantwell HD, Blevins WE: Metrizamide insufflation bronchography: a new diagnostic approach. Vet Rad 22:184, 1981

Center SA, Randolph JF, Erb HN, Reiter S: Eosinophilia in the cat: a retrospective study of 312 cases (1975–1986). J Am Anim Hosp Assoc 26:349, 1990

Dungworth DL: The respiratory system. p. 575. In Jubb KVF, Kennedy PC, Palmer N (eds): Pathology of Domestic Animals. 4th Ed. Academic Press, San Diego, 1993

Dye JA, McKiernan BC: Bronchopulmonary disease in the cat—historical, physical, radiographic, clinicopathologic and pulmonary functional evaluation of 24 diseased and 15 healthy cats. J Vet Intern Med 10:385, 1996

Georgi JR: Parasites of the respiratory tract. Vet Clin North Am 17:1421, 1987

Haskins SC: Physical therapeutics for respiratory disease. Semin Vet Med Surg 1:276, 1986

Hawkins EC, Ettinger SJ, Suter PF: Diseases of the lower respiratory tract and pulmonary edema. p. 816. In Ettinger SJ (ed): Textbook of Veterinary Internal Medicine. 3rd Ed. WB Saunders, Philadelphia, 1989

Hoover JP, Howard-Martin MO, Bahr RJ: Chronic bronchitis, bronchiectasis, bronchiolitis, bronchiolitis obliterans and bronchopneumonia in a rottweiler with primary ciliary dyskinesia. J Am Anim Hosp Assoc 25:297, 1989

Kneller SK: Thoracic radiography. p. 250. In Kirk RW (ed): Current Veterinary Therapy: Small Animal Practice. WB Saunders, Philadelphia, 1986

Kramer BA, Caywood DD, O'Brien TD: Bullous emphysema and recurrent pneumothorax in the dog. J Am Vet Med Assoc 186:971, 1985

McKiernan BC, Dye JA, Powell EA et al: Terbutaline pharmacokinetics in cats. J Vet Intern Med 5:122, 1991

Meyer W, Burt JK: Bronchiectasis in the dog: its radiographic appearance. J Am Vet Med Assoc 14:3, 1973

Moise NS, Spaulding GL: Feline bronchial asthma: pathogenesis, pathophysiology, diagnostics and therapeutic consideration. Compend Contin Educ Pract Vet 3:1091, 1981

Moise NS, Wiedenkeller D, Yeager AE et al: Clinical, radiographic and bronchial cytologic features of cats with bronchial disease: 65 cases (1980–1986). J Am Vet Med Assoc 194:1467, 1989

Morrison WB, Wilsman NJ, Fox LE et al: Primary ciliary dyskinesia in the dog. J Vet Intern Med 1:67, 1987

O'Brien J, Reik J, Schryver H: Clinico-pathologic conference. J Am Vet Med Assoc 149:1317, 1966

Padrid PA: Diagnosis and management of canine chronic bronchitis. p. 908. In Bonagura JD (ed): Kirk's Current Veterinary Therapy XII. WB Saunders, Philadelphia, 1995

Padrid PA: New treatment strategies for cats with exacerbations of asthma. Proc Compar Resp Soc p. 49, 1996

Padrid PA: Asthma and bronchitis in cats. p. 370. In Tilley LP, Smith F (eds): The Five Minute Veterinary Consult. WB Saunders, Philadelphia, 1997

Padrid PA, Feldman BF, Funk K et al: Feline bronchoalveolar lavage. Results of cytological, microbiological and biochemical analysis from 24 clinically healthy cats. Am J Vet Res 52:1300, 1991

Padrid PA, Hornof WJ, Kurpershoek CJ, Cross CE: Canine chronic bronchitis. A pathophysiologic evaluation of 18 cases. J Vet Intern Med 4:172, 1990

Padrid PA, Koblik PD: The techniques used to diagnose feline respiratory disorders. Vet Med 9:956, 1990

Pushpakom R: Experimental papain induced emphysema in dogs. Am Rev Respir Dis 102:778, 1970

Spencer H: Diseases of the bronchial tree. p. 131. In Spencer H (ed): Pathology of the Lung. 4th Ed. Pergamon Press, Oxford, 1985

Swartz MN: Bronchiectasis. p. 1553. In Fishman AP (ed): Pulmonary Diseases and Disorders. 2nd Ed. McGraw-Hill, New York, 1988

Wheeldon EB, Pirie HM, Fisher EW et al: Chronic bronchitis in the dog. Vet Rec 94:466, 1974

18

Pulmonary Parenchymal Disorders

James C. Prueter
Terrance A. Hamilton

DISORDERS OF PULMONARY EDEMA

Pulmonary Edema

Definition

I. There is an abnormal accumulation of pulmonary water and solutes in the alveoli, interstitium, or both. It is the result of a disease process rather than a disease itself.

II. Edema usually develops first within the interstitium and progresses to involve the alveoli.

Causes and Classification

I. Increased pulmonary capillary pressure
  A. Cardiac disease: mitral valve disease, left ventricular failure
  B. Excessive fluid therapy

II. Decreased plasma oncotic pressure: hypoproteinemia
  A. Liver insufficiency
  B. Malnutrition, malabsorption
  C. Protein-losing enteropathy, nephropathy
  D. Chronic blood loss
  E. Burns

III. Increased negative interstitial pressure
  A. Following pericardiocentesis
  B. Rapid correction of pneumothorax or pleural effusion

IV. Lymphatic insufficiency: infiltrative neoplasms

V. Altered alveolar-capillary membrane permeability
  A. Pneumonia: infectious, aspiration
  B. Inhaled toxins or smoke
  C. Exogenous toxins: snake venom, paraquat, alpha-naphthylthiourea (ANTU)
  D. Endogenous vasoactive substances or toxins: acute pancreatitis, uremia
  E. Disseminated intravascular coagulopathy
  F. Acute respiratory distress syndrome
  G. Electric shock
  H. Oxygen toxicity

VI. Edema of unknown mechanisms
  A. High-altitude
  B. Neurogenic, postictal
  C. Drug-induced
  D. Associated with eclampsia
  E. Following anesthesia or cardioversion

Pathophysiology

I. Certain factors provide for normal clearance of pulmonary water and solutes.
  A. Starling's forces, i.e., balance between hydrostatic and oncotic pressures
  B. Integrity of capillary wall ultrastructure
  C. Normal lymphatic function

II. Movement of water and solutes from pulmonary capillary beds into the pulmonary interstitium is normally continuous.
  A. Rapid removal of both fluid and proteins takes place through perivascular and peribronchial lymphatics.
  B. Lymphatic drainage occurs via hilar nodes and terminates at the thoracic duct.

III. Pulmonary edema results from aberrations of one or more factors.
  A. Increased pulmonary capillary hydrostatic pressure
  B. Decreased plasma oncotic pressure
  C. Increased negative interstitial pressure
  D. Altered capillary permeability
  E. Pulmonary lymphatic insufficiency

IV. Inhibition or inactivation of surfactant further contributes to the development of edema.

V. In some instances, the pathogenesis of the edema remains to be defined.

Clinical Signs

I. May be slow or acute onset
II. Respiratory distress, orthopnea, tachypnea
    A. The magnitude is directly related to the cause and severity of the edema.
    B. Usually both inspiratory and expiratory respiratory distress occur.
III. Cough: productive, blood-tinged, and frothy with severe edema
IV. Anxiety: often proportional to level of respiratory distress
V. Cyanosis, exercise intolerance
VI. Widespread crackles on inspiration and expiration with auscultation
    A. May be absent with consolidation
    B. May be obscured by sounds referred from the upper airway
VII. Abnormal heart sounds
    A. Murmurs, arrhythmias
    B. Presence of a third heart sound with myocardial dysfunction
    C. Splitting of the second heart sound with pulmonary hypertension

Diagnosis

I. Cardiogenic edema
    A. Abnormal heart sounds: murmurs, gallops, arrhythmias
    B. Abnormal echocardiographic findings (see Chaps. 8 and 9)
    C. Abnormal electrocardiographic (ECG) findings (see Chaps. 7 and 9)
    D. Elevated pulmonary wedge pressure
    E. Thoracic radiography
        1. Cardiomegaly ± abnormal contours to cardiac silhouette
        2. Dog: hilar, mixed alveolar densities
        3. Cat: diffuse, peripheral, alveolar, or mixed pattern, especially in diaphragmatic lobes
        4. ± Pleural effusion
II. Noncardiogenic edema
    A. History and clinical signs may be helpful.
        1. Many predisposing causes are evident on presentation, e.g., near drowning, smoke inhalation, trauma, burns.
        2. There may be a history of recent fluid therapy, drug administration, or previous illnesses.
        3. Note the presence of ventral dependent edema, ascites, and hydrothorax.
    B. Thoracic radiographs are compatible with pulmonary edema (Table 18–1).
    C. Obtain a database of a hemogram, biochemical profile, and urinalysis.

Differential Diagnosis

I. Pneumonia
II. Pulmonary contusion

Table 18–1. **Radiographic Changes with Parenchynmal Diseases**

Disease	Radiographic Signs
Pneumonia	
Bronchopneumonia	Alveolar or mixed alveolar-bronchial pattern; air bronchograms present; changes present in multiple lobes and throughout the lobes
Aspiration	Most commonly affects ventral portions of middle lobes; may be uni- or bilateral; mixed alveolar-interstitial pattern; air bronchograms present unless consolidated
Inhalation	Early changes confined to interstitial pattern with peribronchial infiltrates; late changes show mixed alveolar-interstitial pattern with air bronchograms present; early changes are widespread and diffuse; later changes may affect dependent portions of lungs, mimicking aspiration.
Pulmonary contusion	Irregular, patchy areas of mixed alveolar-interstitial patterns or consolidation; often contain air bronchograms; may be associated with rib fractures, pneumothorax, or atelectasis
Pulmonary edema	
Cardiogenic	
Dog	Hilar, mixed alveolar-interstitial densities
Cat	Diffuse, peripheral alveolar or mixed pattern
Electric shock, snakebite, inhalation	Generalized, severe mixed pattern; often most pronounced in diaphragmatic lobes; bilateral, symmetrical; air bronchograms present
Hypoproteinemia	Mixed pattern with air bronchograms late; often accompanied by hydrothorax
Feline asthma	Increased interstitial densities and peribronchial markings; increased thoracic size; straightening of diaphragm; hyperlucency of lungs; ± aerophagia; emphysematous bullae with chronic asthma

From Morgan RV: Manual of Small Animal Emergencies. Churchill Livingstone, New York, 1985, with permission.

III. Diffuse parenchymal neoplasia

Treatment

I. Treatment objectives are as follows.
   A. Improve oxygenation
   B. Combat the edema
   C. Reverse or remove the cause
II. Ensure a patent airway.
   A. Handle gently; minimize stress.
   B. Administer oxygen via mask, nasal cannula, or cage (see Chap. 3).
   C. Intubate and begin positive pressure ventilation if oxygenation cannot be accomplished by other methods.
III. Institute diuretic therapy with furosemide 2 mg/kg SQ, IM, IV q 4–12 h.
IV. Institute specific therapies for each cause.
   A. Hypoproteinemia: see Chap. 69
   B. Heart diseases: see Chaps. 7, 9, and 10
   C. Smoke inhalation: see Chap. 132

Patient Monitoring

I. Evaluate oxygen delivery.
   A. Color of mucous membranes
   B. Arterial and venous blood gas analysis (see Appendix I)
   C. Oximetry devices
II. Monitor respiratory rate and effort.
III. Monitor ECG.
   A. Check heart rate and rhythm.
   B. ST segment changes may reflect poor oxygenation, i.e., ischemia.
IV. Repeat thoracic radiography.
   A. Abnormalities should clear and correspond to clinical improvement.
   B. Watch for secondary pulmonary complications such as pneumonia.
V. Other monitoring tools include packed cell volume (PCV), total solids, urine output, central venous pressure (CVP), arterial blood and pulmonary wedge pressures, and daily body weight.

Near Drowning

Definition

I. Near drowning is associated with submersion in water.
   A. Cessation of respiration occurs, which creates an elevation in carbon dioxide concentration in the blood stream, which in turn stimulates breathing efforts.
   B. Aspiration of water results in pulmonary damage.
II. Laryngospasm occurs in approximately 10% of cases and prevents aspiration of water, thereby minimizing pulmonary injury.

Causes and Pathophysiology

I. Damage to pulmonary parenchyma occurs through various mechanisms.

A. Fresh water dilutes surfactant, resulting in alveolar collapse and decreased compliance.
   B. Salt water causes the diffusion of water from the interstitial tissues into the alveoli, creating more pulmonary edema (secondary drowning).
   C. Bacteria in water may cause complicating infections.
   D. Aspiration of vomitus, debris, and chemicals may predispose the animal to pneumonia.
II. Hemodynamic abnormalities such as circulatory collapse, hypothermia, severe arrhythmias, or cardiac arrest may further complicate any pulmonary changes.

Clinical Signs

I. Loss of consciousness
II. Respiratory distress or arrest
III. Hypothermia
IV. Hypoxemia, acidosis, shock, cardiac arrest
V. ± Evidence of external trauma
   A. Boat propeller injury
   B. Overzealous rescue or resuscitation efforts

Diagnosis

I. Diagnosis is obvious at the time of rescue.
II. The extent of pulmonary involvement is evaluated by the following tests.
   A. Thoracic radiography is useful.
      1. Perform immediately if stable.
      2. Obtain serial exposures to detect secondary pneumonia, consolidation, or abscessation.
   B. Consider transtracheal wash for culture and sensitivity following aspiration.
   C. Measurement of arterial blood gases often reveals hypoxemia and acidosis.
III. Submit samples for hemograms, biochemistry profile, and urinalysis.

Treatment

I. Clear/remove any debris or obstruction from airway.
II. Provide oxygen supplementation via mouth to muzzle, nasal cannula, cage, or positive pressure ventilation (intubation).
III. Institute bronchodilator therapy with aminophylline 11 mg/kg PO QID (dog).
IV. Begin fluid therapy for shock, and consider bicarbonate supplementation for acidosis (see Chap. 131).
V. Correct electrolyte and serum protein abnormalities with the appropriate fluids and plasma transfusions.
VI. Institute antiarrhythmic therapy as needed.
VII. Consider diuretic therapy for evidence of persistent pulmonary edema (see earlier).
VIII. The use of corticosteroids for near drowning (other than for shock) is controversial.

Patient Monitoring

I. To evaluate the hemodynamic status of the animal and response to therapy, monitor the following.
   A. PCV, total solids

B. CVP
C. Arterial and/or venous blood gases
D. Urine output
E. Body temperature
F. Serial thoracic radiographs
II. The prognosis for survival is dependent on several factors, such as type and temperature of the water, amount of fluid aspirated, duration of immersion, and predisposing physical illnesses.
   A. Exposure to cold water has a better prognosis than exposure to warm water.
   B. Immersion in salt water is inherently more serious than in fresh water.

INFECTIOUS/INFLAMMATORY DISORDERS

Bacterial Pneumonia

Definition

I. Bronchopneumonia is pneumonia beginning in the terminal bronchioles after inhalation of an infective organism.
II. Lobar pneumonia is pneumonia confined to a given lung lobe.
III. Interstitial pneumonia is an infection or inflammation of the interstitium.

Causes

I. Pathogens vary in prevalence for several reasons.
   A. Geographic differences
   B. Community vs. hospital or institution (kennel, pound) microbiologic populations
II. Both aerobic and anaerobic bacteria may be involved.
   A. Aerobic
      1. *Streptococcus, Staphylococcus* spp.
      2. *Escherichia coli, Proteus* spp., *Pasteurella multocida*
      3. *Bordetella bronchiseptica*
      4. *Pseudomonas* spp.
   B. Anaerobic
      1. *Actinomyces, Nocardia* spp.
      2. *Bacteroides, Fusobacterium* spp.
      3. *Clostridium* spp., others

Pathophysiology

I. Routes of transmission
   A. Infection by inhalation: most common
      1. Extension from upper respiratory infection
      2. Secondary or superseding infection following viral disease, aspiration, antibiotics, or immunosuppressive therapy
   B. Hematogenous spread
      1. Less common
      2. May occur in immunosuppressed animals
   C. Direct extension
      1. Penetrating wound

2. Migrating foreign bodies
3. Perforating esophageal lesions
4. Iatrogenic: diagnostic or surgical procedures
II. Modes of intrapulmonary spread
   A. Air space to air space via direct communication or via pores of Kohn
   B. Inflammatory debris entering air space through small airways
   C. Interstitial spread: more common with viral and mycoplasmal pneumonia
III. Predisposing factors
   A. Alterations in immune status
      1. Poor maternal antibody levels or passage
      2. Inadequate vaccination status
      3. Neoplasia
      4. Concurrent use of immunosuppressive drugs
      5. Poor nutrition
      6. Other illnesses: heart disease, burns, chronic bronchial disease
   B. Inactivity, prolonged recumbency
      1. Effects of hypostatic congestion
      2. Effects of atelectasis
      3. Examples: spinal disorders, following surgery
   C. Trauma and other environmental insults

Clinical Signs

I. The onset of pneumonia may be overshadowed by symptoms of preexisting diseases.
II. Acute signs may be noted in sudden, acquired infections.
   A. Fever, malaise
   B. Anorexia, lethargy
   C. Restlessness, tachypnea
III. Signs of upper respiratory infection may precede pulmonary involvement.
IV. Once pneumonia is established, the following signs are common.
   A. Fever
   B. Depression, often profound
   C. Anorexia
   D. Cough, often productive
   E. Dyspnea, polypnea
   F. Exercise intolerance
   G. Nasal discharge

Diagnosis

I. Symptoms are usually compatible with a respiratory infection but may not localize the problem to pulmonary parenchyma.
II. Some physical examination findings are suggestive.
   A. Auscultation is variable.
      1. Increased bronchovesicular sounds
      2. Crackles
      3. Diminished breath sounds over areas of consolidation or atelectasis
   B. Percussion may produce dull tones.
III. Signalment and history may help delineate the etiology.
   A. Note age, vaccination status.

B. Determine housing conditions and exposure to other animals.
C. Determine animal's geographic area of origin or travel pattern.
D. Note any concurrent administration of drugs.
E. Note any prior or concurrent illnesses.
IV. Laboratory tests usually reflect inflammation.
  A. Hemogram may indicate an underlying disease or reveal leukocytosis with a left shift.
  B. Biochemical organ profile is usually normal or reflects an underlying disease.
V. Thoracic radiography is required to characterize the pulmonary changes.
  A. Bronchopneumonia often has a cranioventral distribution (see Table 18–1).
    1. Air bronchograms are present.
    2. Peripheral involvement spreads toward the hilum.
    3. Both mixed air space (alveolar) and interstitial involvement may be present.
  B. Lobar pneumonia is characterized by a regional alveolar pattern with air bronchograms. Focal consolidation may be seen.
  C. Interstitial pneumonia has a diffuse reticular pattern that is difficult to differentiate from early pulmonary edema and inhalation pneumonia.
VI. Respiratory secretions are obtained for cytology and culture.
  A. Sources include transtracheal aspiration, bronchoalveolar lavage, fine-needle aspiration, or specimens obtained at surgery.
  B. Bacterial pneumonia is associated with the following (Bauer, 1988).
    1. Packed white blood cells (WBCs) except in some immunosuppressed patients
    2. Fewer than 10 epithelial cells per high power field (hpf)
    3. More than 25 WBCs/hpf
    4. Intracellular bacteria usually present
  C. Isolation of a bacterial agent is essential to support the diagnosis.
    1. Request both aerobic and anaerobic cultures.
    2. Interpret results in light of the source, collection method, and health status of the animal.
VII. Histopathologic examination is advised for any pulmonary biopsy specimen retrieved.

Differential Diagnosis

I. Other forms of infectious pneumonia: viral, protozoal, mycoplasmal, mycotic
II. Aspiration and inhalation pneumonia
III. Pulmonary edema
IV. Pulmonary contusion
V. Parasitic and eosinophilic parenchymal disease
VI. Infiltrative neoplasia

Treatment

I. Antibiotics are the primary therapy.
  A. Antibiotic of choice depends on culture and sensitivity testing.

  B. Animals should be maintained on a selected antibiotic for a minimum of 2 weeks after all clinical and radiographic changes have resolved.
II. Nebulization/humidification may increase clearance of secretions.
  A. Nebulize via mask, closed cage, or intubation.
  B. Humidify an enclosed area, e.g., bathroom or other small room.
III. Therapeutic percussion (coupage) and mild exercise help stimulate coughing and secretion clearance.
IV. Bronchodilators may be helpful for small airway obstruction.
V. Expectorants are of uncertain or unlikely benefit.
VI. Oxygen is indicated if cyanosis or hypoxemia is present.
VII. Maintaining hydration with SQ or IV fluid therapy is of dramatic importance.
VIII. Thoracotomy for lobectomy is required in cases of consolidated lung lobes that are not responsive to medical therapy.

Patient Monitoring

I. Monitor respiratory rate, lung sounds, amount and type of coughing, body temperature, and WBC count.
II. Obtain serial thoracic radiographs.
  A. Radiographic improvement frequently lags days behind improvement in systemic signs or physical findings, hence the reason for maintaining antibiotics until x-ray results are normal.
  B. Repeat every 7–10 days until resolution is observed.
III. In the animal that fails to respond favorably to initial therapy, consider the following.
  A. Inappropriate antibiotic choice, dosage, or frequency
  B. Poor client compliance with antibiotic administration
  C. Complication of primary infection, i.e., bacteremia, abscessation, or consolidation
  D. Superinfection with resistant agents
  E. Incorrect diagnosis

Mycobacterial Disease

Definition

I. Mycobacterial infections may involve the regional lymph nodes only or may disseminate throughout the body.
II. Cats typically have involvement of the intestinal tract, whereas dogs usually demonstrate pulmonary involvement.

Causes

I. *Mycobacterium tuberculosis*
II. *M. bovis* (true tuberculosis)
III. *M. avium*
IV. Saprophytic, "atypical" mycobacteria
V. *M. fortuitum*

Pathophysiology

See Chap. 111.

Clinical Signs

I. Symptoms depend on the area affected, and rarely are pulmonary signs the primary complaint.
II. Prior lack of response to antibiotics may be reported.
III. Basset hounds may be predisposed to *M. avium* infections (Carpenter et al., 1988).

Diagnosis

I. Radiology
   A. Pulmonary involvement usually shows hilar lymphopathy and a nodular interstitial pattern.
   B. Granuloma formation, mineralization of pulmonary masses, pleural effusion, or pericardial effusion may be present.
   C. Hypertrophic pulmonary osteopathy may also be noted.
II. Cytology: tracheal wash, bronchoalveolar lavage
   A. Intracellular organisms may be demonstrated, but more often a nonspecific mixed inflammation is noted.
   B. Acid fast staining enhances the appearance of organisms.
III. Culture
   A. Specimens are cultured in order to differentiate saprophytic and nonsaprophytic agents; however, remember that mycobacteria are slow growing and treatment should not be delayed.
   B. When respiratory tract cultures are negative, consider culturing urine, a lymph node aspirate, joint fluid, or feces.
IV. Histopathology
   Definitive diagnosis may not be achieved until there is histopathologic identification of organisms on biopsy or post mortem.

Differential Diagnosis

I. Neoplasia
II. Severe nontuberculous bacterial pneumonia
III. Mycotic pulmonary disease

Treatment

I. Active "true" tuberculosis is usually not treated because of potential human innoculation, and euthanasia is recommended.
II. Long-term treatment (6–9 months) is paramount, may not be successful, and is potentially toxic (hepatotoxicity).
III. A variety of drugs may be tried for pathogenic or true tuberculosis.
   A. Isoniazid (Laniazid) 10–20 mg/kg PO SID
   B. Rifampin (Rifadin) 10–20 mg/kg PO SID
   C. Isoniazid combined with rifampin (Rifamate)
   D. Streptomycin 10 mg/kg IM BID
   E. Ethambutol (Myambutol) 15 mg/kg PO SID

IV. For a saprophytic mycobacterium, consider the following antibacterials.
   A. Kanamycin 10 mg/kg SQ BID-TID
   B. Amikacin 10 mg/kg IM, IV TID
   C. Minocycline 5–12.5 mg/kg PO BID
   D. Doxycycline 5–10 mg/kg PO SID
   E. Trimethoprim/sulfadiazine 15 mg/kg PO BID
   F. Amoxicillin/clavulanate 10–20 mg/kg SQ, PO BID-TID
V. Large granulomas or consolidated lung lobes may require surgical excision.

Patient Monitoring

I. Pathogenic or true tuberculosis warrants a grave prognosis.
II. Prognosis with saprophytic forms is guarded.
III. There is a potential of zoonotic transmission, although there are no reported incidents.

Mycotic Lung Disease

Definition

I. It is a pulmonary infection with one of the fungal or fungus-like organisms.
II. Lung involvement in disseminated disease is commonplace.

Causes

I. *Coccidioides immitis*
II. *Blastomyces dermatitidis*
III. *Histoplasma capsulatum*
IV. *Cryptococcus neoformans*
   A. Primary involvement is in the nasal cavity, nasal sinuses, eyes, skin, or brain of cats and central nervous system (CNS) in dogs.
   B. Pulmonary lesions are reported in 50% of feline cases.
V. *Aspergillus flavus*
   A. Predominant involvement is in the nasal cavity and sinuses of the dog.
   B. Pulmonary involvement is typical only with severe infections and immunosuppression from steroid administration or other concomitant diseases.

Pathophysiology

See Chap. 109.

Clinical Signs

I. Signs depend on the route of entry, localization, or dissemination.
   A. Silent infection; asymptomatic
   B. Acute signs with localized disease
   C. Chronic signs that remain localized to the chest
   D. Disseminated disease with multiple organ system signs
II. With aspergillosis and cryptococcosis, nasal signs may predominate.

III. Pulmonary findings are similar to other forms of pneumonia.
  A. Respiratory distress, polypnea
  B. Cough, often unproductive
  C. Wheezing with airway obstruction
  D. Localized crackles
  E. Loss of breath sounds with consolidation or pleural effusions

Diagnosis

I. Culture may be unrewarding, as these agents can be difficult to retrieve and reproduce.
II. Serology may be diagnostic (see Chap. 109).
III. Histopathology or cytopathology of tissues from clinically affected areas is usually diagnostic.
IV. With thoracic radiography, certain changes are highly characteristic.
  A. Miliary dissemination
  B. Numerous nodular lesions
  C. Lobar air space involvement
  D. Hilar lymphadenopathy
  E. ± Cavitary lesions

Differential Diagnosis

I. Pulmonary neoplasia, primary or metastatic
II. Bacterial and parasitic pneumonia
III. Eosinophilic lung disease
IV. Chronic bronchitis

Treatment and Monitoring

I. See Chap. 109 for treatment advice.
II. Frequent reexamination is necessary to evaluate resolution of pulmonary disease and monitor for side effects of drug therapy.
III. Thoracic radiography is repeated every 2–3 weeks until resolution, and then periodically to detect early exacerbations and recurrences.

Viral Lung Disease

See Chaps. 110 and 112.

Protozoal Lung Disease

Toxoplasma Pneumonia

Definition and Cause

I. *Toxoplasma gondii* can occur in the dog or cat; however, the cat is the definitive host.
II. Immune deficiency disease or concurrent problems, such as feline leukemia virus and canine distemper, predispose animals to clinical toxoplasmosis.
III. Pulmonary disease is more common in acute toxoplasmosis than in chronic toxoplasmosis.

Pathophysiology

See Chap. 114.

Clinical Signs

I. The history and physical findings are typical of any severe lower respiratory disease.
II. Generalized lymph node enlargement may also occur.
III. Fundic examination may reveal a chorioretinitis.

Diagnosis

I. Radiography reveals fluffy interstitial and alveolar densities throughout the lung fields. Nodular consolidation can also occur.
II. Tracheal or bronchial washings for cytology may reveal organisms, but more often only a nonspecific mixed inflammation is found.
III. Histopathology may be required for definitive identification of organisms.
IV. Utilization of serum titers is described in Chap. 114.

Treatment and Monitoring

I. For specific therapeutic advice, see Chap. 114.
II. Acute, fulminant toxoplasmal pneumonia is often fatal, but some cats may survive with long-term therapy.

Pneumocystis Pneumonia

See Chap. 114.

Aspiration Pneumonia

Definition

I. Inhalation of any foreign substance
II. May be acute and fulminant or represent chronic aspiration of small amounts of material

Causes

I. Ingesta
  A. Pharyngeal abnormalities, following laryngectomy
  B. Esophageal disorders with regurgitation
  C. Vomiting
  D. Recumbency or unconsciousness with reflux of gastric contents
II. Foreign debris or discharges
  A. Aerosolization of particulate material, e.g., asbestos, lime dust, chemicals, noxious gases
  B. Contamination of airway with oral secretions caused by dental disease, abscesses, necrotic infections, tumors
III. Iatrogenic
  A. Mistaken intubation of the airway, e.g., barium, mineral oil, gruels, foodstuffs
  B. Lack of animal cooperation during administration of oral medications

Pathophysiology

I. The severity of injury is related to various factors.
   A. Volume of aspirate
   B. pH of aspirate: ≤2.5 most severe
   C. Inherent toxicity of any particulate matter
II. Aspiration produces several abnormalities.
   A. Immediate alveolar wall injury
   B. Hemorrhage and edema
   C. Necrosis of airway epithelial cells
   D. Influx of inflammatory cells
   E. Obstruction and collapse of alveoli
III. Infection is not inevitable, but is a frequent sequela.
   A. Pathogens aspirated at the time of initial injury
   B. Secondary to chemical or structural injury

Clinical Signs

I. Acute aspiration
   A. Most commonly recognized episode
      1. Respiratory distress
      2. Tachycardia
      3. Hypotension
      4. Wheezing, coughing, gagging
   B. Rapidly progressive: fever, malaise, cyanosis, orthopnea
II. Subacute or chronic aspiration
   A. History of vomiting or potential aspiration several days prior to onset of respiratory signs
   B. Gradual onset of systemic and respiratory signs
      1. Cough, usually productive
      2. Polypnea, respiratory distress, ± cyanosis
      3. Localized crackles
      4. Depression, anorexia, exercise intolerance
      5. Fever, malaise

Diagnosis

I. Clinical signs and history usually allow a presumptive diagnosis.
II. Laboratory findings are compatible with inflammation.
   A. Hemogram: often dramatic leukocytosis with a left shift
   B. Organ profile: often normal unless prerenal azotemia is present
III. Thoracic radiography may reveal a characteristic pattern (see Table 18–1).
   A. Distribution tends to be patchy or focal.
   B. Ventral (dependent) areas of apical and middle lobes are classically involved.
   C. Alveolar infiltrates with air bronchograms are seen peripherally.
   D. Pleural effusion may be noted.
   E. Other thoracic abnormalities may be discovered, e.g., megaesophagus.
IV. Examination of respiratory secretions is indicated to differentiate the type of pneumonia present.
   A. Cytology
      1. Degenerative epithelial cells, toxic neutrophils, ± bacteria
      2. Particulate debris free or within neutrophils

B. Culture results
   1. Aspiration pneumonia may be sterile depending on the cause and circumstances of sampling.
   2. Culture may yield primary pathogens or opportunists.

Differential Diagnosis

I. Hematogenous pneumonia
   It tends to produce a more diffuse pattern on radiography, affecting multiple lobes and all portions of the lobes.
II. Lobar bronchopneumonia
III. Acute respiratory distress syndrome
IV. Pulmonary edema

Treatment

I. Prevent further aspiration.
   A. Intubate if animal remains in a state of depressed consciousness, in order to prevent further aspiration.
   B. Reposition nasogastric or other feeding tubes.
II. Administer oxygen.
   A. Nasal cannula or oxygen cage is required.
   B. For acute hypoxemia, intubate and mechanically ventilate with positive pressure.
III. Institute antibiotics based on culture results.
   A. No evidence exists to support the prophylactic use of antibiotics.
   B. Aspiration during hospitalization often yields bacteria with unusual and multiple resistance patterns.
IV. Bronchodilator therapy is often helpful.
V. Because cellular injury occurs within seconds, there is no known benefit to the use of corticosteroids after aspiration, and protracted use of corticosteroids may enhance the development of secondary infection.
VI. For other supportive therapy, see Bacterial Pneumonia, earlier, and Smoke Inhalation in Chap. 132.

Patient Monitoring

I. With known aspiration, monitor closely for development of pneumonia and infection.
   A. Perform frequent auscultation.
   B. Monitor body temperature.
   C. Repeat thoracic radiographs 24–72 hours after the episode or as clinical symptoms change.
   D. Repeat hemogram 24–72 hours after the episode.
II. Treat underlying disorder if possible.

Solitary Lung Lesions

Definition

I. All of these conditions radiographically represent localized changes in radiodensity.
II. Cavitation refers to a primary radiodense focus that becomes radiolucent centrally by drainage via bronchial communication.

Causes

I. Bronchogenic cysts (Ball and Girard, 1942)
  A. Usually considered developmental aberrations
  B. Assumed to represent maturation defects of the most distal bronchioles
II. Bullae and blebs (Frazer and Pare, 1977)
  A. Represent large-scale destruction of alveolar walls
  B. Result in "compartmentalization" of large numbers of alveolar exchange units
    1. Cause usually unknown
    2. Can include any of the causes of emphysema (see Chap. 17)
III. Cavitary lesions
  A. Abscesses
    1. Focal pneumonia
    2. Migration of foreign body or direct puncture of pulmonary parenchyma
    3. Complication of chronic bronchitis or bronchiectasis
    4. Primary mycotic or parasitic infection
  B. Neoplasia: primary or metastatic (see later)
  C. Parasitic lesions
    1. Dirofilariasis
    2. Rarely, *Aeleurostrongylus*
    3. Paragonimiasis
      a) Flukes reach lower lobes via diaphragmatic migration.
      b) Lesions are initially cystic and communicate with a bronchus, but they may become lined with epithelial cells late.
  D. Eosinophilic lung diseases
    1. Chronic eosinophilic pneumonia in cats
    2. Granulomatous disease in dogs
    3. Focal pneumonia, especially from ischemia or trauma

Pathophysiology

I. Pleural disease, pneumothorax
  A. Lesion may rupture, producing spontaneous pneumothorax and/or hemothorax.
  B. Cysts, bullae, and blebs are most commonly involved.
  C. Abscesses may rupture, causing empyema.
II. Infection
  A. Lung may become secondarily infected.
  B. Infection may spread to adjacent lobes via bronchial communication.
III. Loss of substantial amounts of functional parenchyma
  A. Pneumatoceles may occupy the major portion or all of a lobe.
  B. Multiple lesions have a cumulative effect.
IV. Airway obstruction can develop from extraluminal compression by solid lesions.

Clinical Signs

I. May be absent and the lesion recognized only on routine thoracic radiographs
II. Respiratory distress from pneumothorax, adjacent pneumonia, or loss of functioning lung volume (capacity)
III. Cough: often associated with airway compression
  A. Productive with draining infection
  B. Hemoptysis
IV. Fever from infection or necrosis
V. Systemic signs: lethargy, malaise, anorexia, exercise intolerance
VI. Hypertrophic pulmonary osteoarthropathy (see Chap. 79)

Diagnosis/Differential Diagnosis

I. Thoracic radiographs (oblique, lateral, or standing views) are useful for defining the type of lesion but do not often determine the cause (Suter and Lord, 1984).
  A. Thick-walled lesions with gas and fluid densities with abnormal adjacent parenchyma
    1. Abscesses
    2. Cavitation of a neoplasm
    3. Infarcts (rare)
  B. Thin-walled structures with usually normal adjacent parenchyma
    1. Blebs
    2. Cysts
    3. Pneumatoceles
  C. No distinct wall and no fluid density
    1. Bullae
    2. Loculated pneumothorax
II. Analysis of airway secretions is often useful, as most lesions communicate with a bronchus.
  A. If done via bronchoscopy, distal brushings may be obtained.
  B. Cytology may aid in the diagnosis of the primary cause if infection or neoplasia is present.
III. Ultrasonography may be helpful in evaluating solid, peripheral lesions and in allowing a guided transthoracic biopsy.
IV. Exploratory thoracotomy may be necessary to characterize the lesion, define the cause, and provide definitive treatment.

Treatment

I. Cysts, bullae, and blebs may require no immediate treatment, but should be monitored, as they may predispose the animal to spontaneous pneumothorax.
II. Medical therapy with antimicrobial or antifungal agents is instituted as indicated by culture, cytology, or histopathology.
  A. *Paragonimus* infections should be treated by praziquantel (Droncit) 5 mg/kg PO TID for 3 days or albendazole 25 mg/kg PO BID for 10 days.
  B. Tube thoracostomy and water seal drainage are applied for pneumothorax (see Chap. 3).
III. Surgical therapy is indicated for the following.
  A. Most solid lung lesions, persistent localized infection, or a suspected abscess
  B. Neoplasia

C. Persistent pneumothorax
   1. Confirmed bullous lesion (see Chap. 19)
   2. Suspected or confirmed foreign body

Patient Monitoring

I. Thoracic radiography is performed.
   A. Repeat in 1 month if animal is asymptomatic.
   B. Six-month follow-up is also advisable.
II. Collect airway secretions if radiographic changes are present on subsequent evaluation.
III. Monitor postoperative animals for development of new lesions with repeat radiographs 1–3 months after surgery.

IDIOPATHIC DISORDERS

Acute Respiratory Distress Syndrome

Definition

I. Syndrome of delayed respiratory failure associated with a known underlying illness or traumatic event
II. Characterized by widespread pulmonary air space infiltrates on thoracic radiography
III. Synonym: ''shock lung syndrome''

Causes

I. Shock
II. Infection
III. Trauma: thoracic or nonthoracic
IV. Aspiration syndromes
V. Inhaled gases: smoke, chemicals, 100% oxygen
VI. Multiple transfusions
VII. Disseminated intravascular coagulopathy
VIII. Pancreatitis
IX. Burns
X. Postcardiac arrest and resuscitation
XI. Following major surgical procedures

Pathophysiology

I. Diffuse, widespread pulmonary injury occurs and is characterized by alveolar membrane alterations and noncardiogenic pulmonary edema.
   A. Edema results from multiple factors.
      1. Altered capillary permeability
      2. Decreased lymphatic flow
      3. Shifts in oncotic pressure
      4. Loss of surfactant
   B. Functioning lung capacity is reduced.
   C. Pulmonary compliance is reduced.
   D. Severe hypoxemia results from arteriovenous shunting and ventilation/perfusion irregularities.
   E. Increased pulmonary vascular resistance occurs from vasoconstriction, microembolization, and capillary obstruction.
II. Histologic findings are nonspecific and may not indicate an underlying cause.

III. Although the events that occur during acute respiratory distress syndrome are well described, it is not known why or how the syndrome develops.

Clinical Signs

I. Respiratory distress, hyperventilation: unresponsive to oxygen
II. May not be cyanotic
III. Tachycardia
IV. Anxiety, restlessness, agitation
V. Crackles and wheezes (initially)

Diagnosis

I. Onset of acute clinical signs follows precipitating event by a few hours to several days.
II. Radiography is compatible with noncardiogenic pulmonary edema.
III. Arterial blood gases are abnormal.
   A. Hypoxemia: progressive and usually profound
   B. Hypocapnia: respiratory alkalosis a classic finding
IV. Cardiogenic pulmonary edema is ruled out by a normal or low pulmonary wedge pressure.

Differential Diagnosis

I. Other causes of pulmonary edema, including congestive heart failure (CHF)
II. Pulmonary contusions
III. Acute pneumonia
IV. Aspiration without respiratory distress syndrome

Treatment

I. Treat underlying cause if possible.
II. Promote tissue oxygenation.
   A. Supplemental oxygen via nasal cannula or cage
   B. Intubation
      1. Mechanical ventilation
      2. Positive end-expiratory pressure (PEEP)
III. Establish euvolemia with cautious fluid therapy.
   A. Administer smallest volume that maintains cardiac output and blood pressure.
   B. Pulmonary artery catheter is used to measure cardiac output and pulmonary wedge pressure.
   C. Alternatively, insert a CVP catheter.
IV. Steroids are of unconfirmed benefit.
V. No specific therapy exists at this time.

Patient Monitoring

I. Repeat routine chest radiographs SID-BID.
II. Measure arterial blood gases SID-QID.
III. Monitor urinary output continuously.
IV. Despite aggressive medical care, this disorder continues to have a grave prognosis and a high mortality rate.

Lung Lobe Torsion

Definition and Causes

I. Lung lobe torsion is rotation of a lung lobe along its long axis, with strangulation of the bronchus and its vascular pedicle.
II. The exact mechanism that induces or precipitates lung rotation is unknown.
 A. Spontaneous, idiopathic
 B. Thoracic surgery
 C. Trauma
 D. Secondary to pleural effusion

Pathophysiology

I. Rotation causes obstruction of venous drainage and ventilation.
 A. Artery remains partially patent.
 B. Progressive lobar engorgement with blood occurs.
 C. Lobe becomes an expansile mass.
II. Copious bloody pleural effusion accumulates, which further decreases tidal volume.
III. Infarction and necrosis of parenchyma may occur.
IV. With chronicity, the lobe may shrink in size, with the normal anatomy being replaced by fibrous connective tissue.

Clinical Signs

I. It occurs most frequently in dogs, especially large deep-chested breeds such as the Afghan hound.
II. It is occasionally observed in cats.
III. Preexisting pleural or pulmonary disease may mask signs initially.
IV. Signs caused by the torsion are often acute and rapidly progressive.
 A. Respiratory distress, ± cyanosis
 B. Cough, ± hemoptysis
 C. Hypotension and collapse
 D. Systemic signs: fever, depression, weakness

Diagnosis

I. Physical examination findings are compatible with pleural effusion (see Chap. 19).
II. Plain radiographic changes vary with progression of the disease.
 A. Pleural effusion usually obscures parenchymal detail; remove the effusion via thoracentesis and repeat the films.
 B. Lobar consolidation is seen.
 C. Air bronchograms occur early, but air is reabsorbed late with atelectasis.
 D. Rounding of lung edges is seen as the lung becomes expansile.
 E. Bronchus may lie in the wrong anatomic plane.
III. Contrast pleurography and bronchography or induced pneumothorax may help enhance the radiographic detail.
IV. For an interpretation of pleural fluid analysis, see Chap. 19.

V. Bronchoscopy may delineate rotation of the bronchus but is rarely indicated.
VI. Surgical exploration may be necessary to confirm the diagnosis and should be considered in the presence of the previously listed radiographic signs, especially when accompanied by a bloody pleural effusion.

Differential Diagnosis

I. Other causes of bloody pleural effusion (see Chap. 19)
II. Pulmonary parenchymal or pleural mass
III. Diaphragmatic hernia
IV. Pneumonia
V. Pulmonary contusion

Treatment

I. Improve oxygenation and stabilize the animal.
 A. Supplemental oxygen
 B. IV fluid therapy to maintain hydration and blood pressure
 C. Thoracentesis with removal of free pleural fluid
 D. Indwelling chest tube as needed (see Chaps. 3 and 19)
II. Surgical resection of the affected lobe is the only effective therapy.
 A. Determine side affected, and approach that side with the animal in lateral recumbency.
 B. Monitor anesthesia carefully; there is a higher than expected incidence of respiratory arrest on induction.

Patient Monitoring

I. Postoperative maintenance of an indwelling chest tube is usually required for 12–48 hours.
II. Monitor the respiratory rate and effort, mucous membrane color, and function of the chest tube carefully.
III. Surgical resection is usually curative; occurrence in another lobe is rare.

HYPERSENSITIVITY AND IMMUNE DISORDERS

Hypersensitivity (Eosinophilic) Diseases

Definition

I. It encompasses a large group of disorders characterized by pulmonary eosinophilic infiltrates.
 A. These diseases may be classified as primarily bronchial or parenchymal.
 B. Bronchial diseases include feline and canine allergic bronchitis and bronchial parasite infections (see Chap. 17).
II. Parenchymal diseases are best known as pulmonary infiltrates with eosinophilia (PIE). Although the syndrome is seen in dogs and cats, it is not as well defined as in people.

III. Peripheral eosinophilia may be present intermittently or absent, depending on the specific disorder.

Causes

I. Most cases are idiopathic and may include intrinsic or extrinsic allergens that affect the lungs.
II. Some cases are characterized by widespread infiltration of other organs with eosinophils (hypereosinophilic syndrome).
III. Eosinophilic infiltrates may also be associated with larva migrans or specific parasites that affect the lung (see later).
IV. Neoplasia such as pulmonary lymphosarcoma and mast cell tumors may be associated with pulmonary eosinophilia.
V. Immune-mediated polyarthritis (rheumatoid arthritis) may occasionally be associated with pulmonary eosinophilia.
VI. Fungal diseases can cause pulmonary eosinophilia.

Pathophysiology

I. Although these disorders differ in their anatomic distribution and severity, certain pathologic responses may be shared.
II. A single common denominator is the presence of eosinophils in the pulmonary parenchyma and the airways.
   A. The use of the term PIE has led to some confusion.
   B. The term implies the consistent presence of eosinophils in the peripheral blood, which is not always seen in animals.
III. The pathogenesis of these disorders appears to be predominantly immunologic (Lord et al., 1975).
   A. The immunologic aspects are not fully elucidated.
   B. Antigen-antibody interactions in the animal's serum may form immune complexes that activate complement.
   C. Complement activation probably accounts for many of the acute features of these disorders.
   D. Cell-mediated (delayed) hypersensitivity may play a significant role in the disorder's chronicity.

Clinical Signs

I. Clinical signs are extremely variable.
II. Coughing is the primary sign and is unresponsive to antibiotic therapy.
III. Weight loss, lethargy, anorexia, and fever may be noted.

Diagnosis

I. Hemogram may denote peripheral eosinophilia.
II. Thoracic radiographs show an increased interstitial pattern, alveolar densities, or even large masses.
   A. Hilar lymphadenopathy is occasionally found.

B. Dilated tortuous pulmonary arteries may be present as a result of prolonged hypertension.
III. Cytology is usually diagnostic.
   A. Predominance of eosinophils may be found by tracheal wash, bronchial lavage, thoracic aspiration, or lung biopsy.
   B. Mast cells may also be noted.
IV. Further evaluation should be pursued to determine specific causes.
   A. Thorough physical examination, including funduscopy
   B. Fecal flotation for parasites
   C. Screening for microfilariae
   D. Serology for systemic mycoses

Differential Diagnosis

I. Chronic allergic bronchitis
II. Primary parasitic lung disease
III. Bronchopneumonia: bacterial, mycotic
IV. Diffuse infiltrative neoplasia
V. Mononuclear granulomatous diseases
   A. These diseases are described in the human literature as pulmonary parenchymal diseases with mononuclear inflammatory cell infiltration.
   B. They include Wegener's granulomatosis, lymphomatoid granulomatosis, Goodpasture's syndrome, and systemic lupus erythematosus (SLE).
   C. Wegener's granulomatosis and lymphomatoid granulomatosis are characterized by necrotizing vasculitis and granulomatosis inflammation.
   D. Goodpasture's syndrome is a result of anti–basement membrane antibodies, which attach to the basement membranes of pulmonary alveoli and capillaries.
   E. SLE is a multisystemic autoimmune disease, and lung vasculature may be occasionally involved.
   F. Causes are rarely identified.
   G. They may represent immune-mediated or preneoplastic conditions.
   H. Some infectious agents such as feline infectious peritonitis virus, rickettsia, atypical bacteria, protozoa, fungi, parasites, and bacteria secondary to foreign bodies may cause similar parenchymal reactions.

Treatment

I. Corticosteroids are the primary therapy.
   A. Begin prednisolone 0.5–1 mg/kg/day PO BID.
   B. Responsiveness to corticosteroids varies.
II. Consider the use of other immunosuppressive agents such as azathioprine 2 mg/kg PO for 10–30 days, then every other day for unresponsive cases.
III. Antibiotics are indicated only if infection is confirmed by cultures obtained on initial work-up.
IV. Bronchodilators may be useful, especially when tapering the daily dosage of corticosteroids.
V. Also institute treatment of any specific diseases identified.

Patient Monitoring

I. Measure total peripheral eosinophil counts.
   A. Performed monthly if eosinophilia is noted initially
   B. May be useful to monitor efficacy of steroid therapy
II. Repeat diagnostic tests if cough or tachypnea returns.
III. Monitor thoracic radiographs.
   A. Useful in evaluating steroid therapy if mild signs return
   B. To assess progression to granulomatous disease
IV. Monitor hemogram if using azathioprine, because of its bone marrow suppressant effects.
V. As clinical and radiographic signs resolve, taper prednisone to alternate-day therapy to avoid iatrogenic hyperadrenocorticism.
VI. Lifetime therapy may be necessary for idiopathic cases.

PARASITIC LUNG DISEASE

Definition

I. It is a parasitic infestation of the bronchi and pulmonary parenchyma.
II. It may represent aberrant migration or a normal phase of parasite development in the canine or feline host.
III. *Paragonimus kellicotti* often causes solitary lung lesions (see earlier).
IV. Parasites that may affect bronchopulmonary functions, but are not discussed here, include *Crenosoma vulpis, Angiostrongylus vasorum, Ancylostoma caninum, Toxocara canis, Toxocara cati,* and *Dirofilaria immitis* (see also Chaps. 12 and 17).

Causes

I. Dog
   A. *Oslerus* spp.
   B. *Capillaria aerophila*
II. Cat
   A. *Aeleurostrongylus abstrusus*
   B. *Capillaria aerophila*

Pathophysiology

I. Transmission is as follows.
   A. *Oslerus* spp.
      1. Ingestion of contaminated fecal material
      2. Ingestion of organisms from environmental surfaces
   B. *Aeleurostrongylus abstrusus* (Scott, 1973)
      1. Expectoration and ingestion of first stage larvae occur.
      2. Fecal spread of larvae to intermediate hosts (slugs, snails) and secondary spread to transport hosts (lizards, birds) occur.
      3. Ingestion of infected intermediate and transport hosts leads to infection of previously noninfected cats.

   C. *Capillaria aerophila:* directly, by ingestion of eggs
II. Anatomic distribution of lesions in the bronchopulmonary tree is variable.
   A. *Oslerus* spp.
      1. *O. hirthi* and *O. milksi* infections are characterized by granuloma formation in the pulmonary parenchyma with a predilection for the caudal lobe.
      2. *O. osleri* may affect the parenchyma, but intraluminal airway lesions predominate.
   B. *Aeleurostrongylus abstrusus*
      1. Interstitial involvement with granuloma formation is a common finding.
      2. Widespread airway involvement can also occur.
      3. Rarely widespread alveolar involvement may develop.
   C. *Capillaria aerophila*
      1. Airway involvement is most common.
      2. Infrequently, air space involvement leads to consolidation.
III. These parasites induce antibody production in animals, but antibody levels do not necessarily correlate with the severity of infection or reflect protection.
IV. Hypersensitivity to parasitic antigens appears to be clinically important, producing the following changes.
   A. Eosinophilia: systemic, airway, parenchymal
   B. Bronchospasm
   C. Granuloma formation
   D. Hypertrophy of bronchial smooth muscle and alveolar ducts
   E. Airway exudates and consolidation of air space

Clinical Signs

I. Respiratory symptoms are variable and nonspecific.
   A. Cough, usually nonproductive
   B. Respiratory distress, may be marked
      1. Bronchospasms with wheezing
      2. Auscultable crackles
II. Systemic signs occur infrequently.
   A. Fever
      1. May abruptly rise with specific therapy directed toward the parasite
      2. May denote concurrent bacterial infection
   B. Weight loss

Diagnosis

I. Clinical signs and physical findings are nonspecific.
II. Peripheral eosinophilia is common.
III. Thoracic radiography shows the following.
   A. Predominantly, parenchymal changes
      1. Air space infiltrates
      2. Interstitial densities
      3. Nodular densities: vary in size
      4. Accentuations of bronchial pattern: mild to marked
   B. Miliary lesions
   C. Localized cystic or cavitated lesions

IV. Examination of respiratory secretions is imperative.
  A. Larvae may be present.
  B. Eosinophils in airway secretions are a classic finding.
V. Other tests may be needed to confirm the diagnosis.
  A. Fecal examination: direct, flotation, sedimentation, Baermann's techniques
  B. Bronchoscopy
    1. Allows visualization of intraluminal granulomas
    2. Useful for obtaining biopsies
    3. Permits collection of airway secretions

Differential Diagnosis

I. Chronic bronchitis, especially allergic
II. Pneumonia: bacterial, viral, fungal, protozoal
III. Eosinophilic lung disease that is nonparasitic in origin
IV. Neoplasia, especially diffuse forms
V. Nonparasitic bronchogenic cysts and granulomas

Treatment

I. Institute antiparasitic (anthelmintic) drugs.
  A. Tetramisole 2 mg/kg SQ QOD × 2–4 doses for *Oslerus* spp.
  B. Thiabendazole 70 mg/kg PO BID × 2 days, then 35 mg/kg PO BID × 20 days for *Oslerus* spp.
  C. Levamisole (Ripercol) 7.5 mg/kg BID or 25 mg/kg QOD PO × 10 days
    1. Good activity against *Aeleurostrongylus, Oslerus*
    2. Poorly tolerated by cats
  D. Ivermectin: dog and cat, 400 µg/kg PO once
    1. Good activity against *Capillaria* spp.
    2. Reports of successful treatment against *Aeleurostrongylus* and *Oslerus*
    3. Not yet licensed for these disorders, although the most effective agent with the least side effects
II. Manual removal of *Oslerus* larvae via bronchoscopy has been attempted, but with limited success.
III. Prevent secondary sequelae.
  A. Monitor for secondary bacterial infections, and institute antibiotics when indicated.
  B. Clinical signs may worsen initially as the death of parasites results in liberation of increased amounts of antigen and/or greater antigen-antibody interaction.
  C. Corticosteroids are used concurrently in anti-inflammatory dosages, e.g., prednisone 0.5–1 mg/kg PO BID.

Patient Monitoring

I. Respiratory signs can be associated with pulmonary parasites.
  A. Should respond dramatically to therapy
  B. Factors responsible for lack of response
    1. Concurrent bacterial infection
    2. Overwhelming parasitic population

3. Irreversible chronic lesions
4. Airway obstruction of another cause
II. Resolution of radiographic lesions occurs as the disease resolves.
  A. Air space infiltrates usually resolve early, often within 10–21 days.
  B. Some lesions may persist, such as cysts and bronchial thickening.
  C. Repeat radiographs in 2–3 weeks.
III. Resolution of respiratory and peripheral eosinophilia correlates well with correction of the disease process.
IV. Prevent reexposure to the parasite.

VASCULAR DISORDERS

James C. Prueter

Pulmonary Thromboembolism

Definition

I. Occlusion of the pulmonary vasculature by clot material
II. Usually originate at a distant site
III. Generally enter the pulmonary arterial circulation as multiple and peripheral clot fragments
IV. Can be central and single

Causes

I. Cardiac disease
  A. Heartworm disease
  B. Dilatative cardiomyopathy
  C. Chronic mitral valvular insufficiency, endocarditis
II. Neoplasia
  A. Lymphosarcoma
  B. Bronchoalveolar carcinoma
  C. Pancreatic carcinoma
III. Disseminated intravascular coagulation
IV. Sepsis
V. Hyperadrenocorticism
VI. Renal disease
  A. Amyloidosis
  B. Glomerulonephritis
VII. Pancreatitis
VIII. Eosinophilic lung disease
IX. Hair emboli
X. Immune-mediated diseases: autoimmune hemolytic anemia
XI. Iatrogenic: indwelling vascular catheters, transfusions
XII. Idiopathic causes

Pathophysiology

I. Thromboembolic phenomena
  A. Venous stasis
    1. Clearance of activated clotting factors by the liver is inhibited.
    2. Fibrinolysis is blocked.
  B. Vascular epithelial injury

1. Promotes platelet plug formation and fibrin thrombus formation
2. Can be secondary to surgery, trauma, or inflammation

II. Pulmonary response
  A. Abnormal ventilation/perfusion relationships
    1. Hypoxemia and hypocapnia
    2. Occasionally, hypercapnia in severe cases
  B. Pulmonary hypertension
    1. Massive obstruction
    2. Reflex vasoconstriction
    3. Can cause cor pulmonale
  C. Increased airway resistance
    1. Regional bronchial constriction
    2. Secondary to vagal reflexes or vasoactive substances associated with the thrombus

III. Other potential complications
  A. Decreased cardiac blood flow
  B. Pleural effusion

Clinical Signs

I. Respiratory distress and tachypnea
II. Coughing and occasionally hemoptysis
III. Auscultation
  A. Crackles are rarely present.
  B. Bronchial sounds may be increased.
  C. Split second heart sounds may develop secondary to pulmonary hypertension.

Diagnosis

I. Vague history and nonspecific clinical signs
II. Thoracic radiography
  A. Normal
  B. Diminution or loss of peripheral vessels
  C. Increased size of central pulmonary artery
  D. Mild enlargement of the right side of the heart
  E. ± Mild pleural effusion
III. Arterial blood gas analysis
  A. Hypoxemia
  B. Hypocapnia; hypercapnia with severe disease
  C. Metabolic acidosis
IV. Electrocardiography
  A. Dependent on the presence or absence of cardiac disease
  B. ST segment abnormalities from hypoxia
  C. Sinus bradycardia secondary to pulmonary hypertension
  D. Discordant T waves occasionally seen
V. Pulmonary angiography
  A. Allows definitive antemortem diagnosis
  B. Most sensitive and specific test
  C. Positive study: filling defects or sudden termination of blood flow
  D. Vessel dilation and rapid contrast transit in unaffected areas
VI. Nuclear perfusion scintigraphy
  A. Safe and sensitive procedure
  B. Nonspecific test

Differential Diagnosis

I. Airway obstruction
II. Other forms of parenchymal disease
III. Pulmonary hypertension

Treatment

I. Supportive care
  A. Supplemental oxygen
  B. Strict cage confinement
  C. Careful use of parenteral fluid therapy
II. Shock therapy: prednisolone sodium succinate 10–30 mg/kg IV once
III. Anticoagulant therapy
  A. Prevents further clot formation
  B. Allows fibrinolysis
  C. Warfarin or coumarin derivatives (Coumadin)
    1. Provides long-term interference with coagulation; monitor coagulation times
    2. Dosage: 0.1 mg/kg PO SID
  D. Heparin
    1. It provides rapid onset, short-term effects.
    2. Begin with 200 U/kg IV, followed by 50–100 U/kg SQ TID-QID.
  E. Aspirin
    1. Decreases platelet function
    2. Dog dosage: 5–10 mg/kg PO BID
    3. Cat dosage: 6 mg/kg PO q 48–72 h
      a) Glucocorticoids may be a better choice in cats with heartworm disease.
      b) Consider prednisone 1–2 mg/kg PO SID.
IV. Fibrinolytic therapy
  A. Agents include streptokinase, urokinase, and tissue plasminogen activator.
  B. Tissue plasminogen activator has been effective in a feline model of pulmonary embolism (Pion and Kittleson, 1989).
  C. They lack selectivity and are expensive.
V. Embolectomy
  A. Risk of mortality extremely high
  B. Should be considered only for central pulmonary artery obstruction
VI. Treatment of the underlying cause: most important part of therapy

Patient Monitoring

I. Partial thromboplastin time (PTT) and prothrombin time (PT) are measured before initiating anticoagulant therapy.
  A. Goal of heparin therapy is to increase PTT 1.5–2 times above the baseline value.
  B. Goal of coumarin therapy is to increase PT 1.5–2 times above the baseline value.
II. Arterial partial pressure of oxygen (PaO_2) increases with resolution of the clot.
III. Recurrences are possible, especially if the primary cause is not resolved.
IV. Large central pulmonary artery obstruction and recurrent episodes of the thromboembolism have a guarded prognosis.

NEOPLASIA

Terrance A. Hamilton

Definition

I. Primary pulmonary neoplasms are uncommon, representing approximately 1.2 and 0.5% of all tumors in the dog and cat, respectively.
II. Older animals (>10 years) are affected most often, except for dogs with lymphomatoid granulomatosis, which occurs in young dogs (1–6 years).
III. Most studies do not recognize a breed or sex predilection for dogs. Female cats are more commonly affected than male cats.
IV. Metastatic lung tumors are more common than primary pulmonary neoplasms.

Causes

I. Primary pulmonary neoplasms
  A. Dog
    1. Carcinomas are the most common histologic type of primary lung tumors.
      a) Bronchoalveolar (>70%)
      b) Squamous cell (epidermoid)
      c) Bronchogenic or bronchial gland
      d) Alveolar: anaplastic–small cell, large cell, and adenomatous
    2. Sarcomas are uncommon.
      a) Lymphosarcoma
      b) Fibrosarcoma
      c) Hemangiosarcoma
      d) Osteosarcoma
    3. Others include lymphomatoid granulomatosis and malignant histiocytosis in Bernese mountain dogs.
  B. Cat
    1. Benign tumors are rarely reported.
    2. Malignant tumors are more common.
      a) Adenocarcinoma: papillary, bronchioloalveolar
      b) Squamous cell carcinoma
      c) Bronchial gland carcinoma
      d) Rare sarcomas: hemangiosarcoma, spindle cell sarcoma, reticulum cell sarcoma
II. Metastatic pulmonary neoplasms
  A. Mammary carcinoma
  B. Osteosarcoma
  C. Thyroid carcinoma
  D. Transitional cell carcinoma
  E. Melanoma
  F. Hemangiosarcoma
  G. Squamous cell carcinoma
  H. Renal carcinoma
  I. Carcinoma of unknown primary origin
  J. Any other malignant tumor

Pathophysiology

I. Primary lung tumors may metastasize to bronchial lymph nodes, lung, brain, bone, and pleura via lymphatics, airways, blood vessels, and transpleural routes.
II. Paraneoplastic syndromes may be associated with primary pulmonary neoplasia.
  A. Hypertrophic osteopathy
  B. Polyneuropathy
  C. Hypercalcemia
  D. Neutrophilic leukocytosis
  E. Polymyopathy
  F. Fever
  G. Ectopic production of adrenocorticotropic hormone (ACTH)
III. About 50% of undifferentiated carcinomas and 90% of squamous cell carcinomas metastasize.
IV. Metastasis to the lungs occurs by spread of tumor emboli via lymphatic or blood vessels. Because of the capillary network in the lungs, tumor emboli are trapped, and may proliferate and form nodules.
V. Environmental factors such as passive cigarette smoke have been implicated as causes.

Clinical Signs

I. Cough: 52%
II. Respiratory distress: 24%
III. Lethargy: 18%
IV. Weight loss: 12%
V. Tachypnea: 5%
VI. Pyrexia: 6.4%
VII. Lameness: 3.8%

Diagnosis

I. Plain thoracic radiographs are a useful diagnostic aid.
  A. Evaluation of both lateral thoracic views (right and left) increases tumor detection rates.
  B. Approximately 11% of pulmonary neoplasms are missed on survey radiographs.
    1. Small size of lesions (5–10 mm)
    2. Lack of tumor contrast with pulmonary parenchyma
    3. Position of the tumor in a hidden location: subpleural space or paraspinal recesses
    4. Presence of pleural fluid or atelectasis of one or more lung lobes
  C. Five radiographic patterns may be found.
    1. Solitary nodule: most common pattern
    2. Circumscribed multiple nodules
    3. Interstitial disseminated reticulonodular pattern
    4. Mixed disseminated alveolar pattern
    5. Homogeneous lobar consolidation
  D. Calcification and cavitation of masses have been associated with adenocarcinomas.
  E. Other radiographic changes include pleural effusion, pleural thickening, and thoracic lymphadenopathy.
  F. The right side and diaphragmatic lung lobes are the most common locations for primary pulmonary neoplasms in dogs.
  G. The left lung lobes are affected more often in cats.
  H. The most common radiographic pattern seen with

metastatic neoplasms is that of disseminated circumscribed nodules.

II. Percutaneous transthoracic fine-needle aspiration or biopsy for cytologic or histologic evaluation may be diagnostic.

III. Cytologic evaluation of tracheal wash, bronchoalveolar lavage, or pleural fluids may detect neoplastic cells in some cases.

IV. Bronchoscopy may be valuable to evaluate perihilar masses.

V. Exploratory thoracotomy and biopsy may be necessary to provide a definitive diagnosis and aid in staging the tumor.

Differential Diagnosis

I. Non-neoplastic solitary lung lesions
II. Mycotic pneumonia
III. Aspiration pneumonia
IV. Focal parasitic parenchymal disease

Treatment

I. Surgery
   A. Lobectomy is the treatment of choice for solitary lung tumors.
   B. Adjunctive chemotherapy may improve survival in some cases (Withrow, 1989).

II. Chemotherapy
   A. Lymphomatoid granulomatosis may be responsive to combination chemotherapy using prednisone, vincristine, and cyclophosphamide.
   B. Malignant histiocytosis in Bernese mountain dogs may be responsive to doxorubicin, cyclophosphamide, and vincristine.
   C. Complete and partial responses have been reported in the treatment of metastatic neoplasms (hemangiosarcoma, thyroid carcinomas, squamous cell carcinoma, and mammary adenocarcinomas) with doxorubicin, cyclophosphamide, and vincristine.
   D. Cisplatin and vinblastine can help in primary pulmonary carcinoma cases.

Patient Monitoring

I. Factors that decrease survival time include large tumor burden, thoracic lymph node involvement, and other metastases.

II. Small (<5 cm), solitary lesions without metastasis or malignant effusion are associated with prolonged survival (>1 year).

III. Monitor thoracic radiographs after treatment every 1–3 months.

IV. In cats, the prognosis is poor, as >75% are inoperable at the time of diagnosis.

Bibliography

Ball V, Girard H: Congenital air cysts of the lung. Rec Med Vet 118:5, 1942

Barr IF, Gruffydd-Jones TJ, Brown PJ et al: Primary lung tumors in the cat. J Small Anim Pract 28:1115, 1987

Bauer TG: Pulmonary parenchymal disorders. p. 195. In Morgan RV (ed): Handbook of Small Animal Practice. Churchill Livingstone, New York, 1988

Berry CR, Moore PF, Thomas WP et al: Pulmonary lymphomatoid granulomatosis in seven dogs (1976–1987). J Vet Intern Med 4:157, 1993

Carpenter JL, Myers AM, Connor MW et al: Tuberculosis in five basset hounds. J Am Vet Med Assoc 192:1563, 1988

Dorn CR, Taylor DO, Frye FL, Hibbard HH: Survey of animal neoplasms in Alameda and Contra Costa Counties, California. J Natl Cancer Inst 50:295, 1968

Frazer RG, Pare JA: Diagnosis of Diseases of the Chest. 2nd Ed. WB Saunders, Philadelphia, 1977

Lord PF, Schaer M, Tilly L: Pulmonary infiltrates with eosinophilia in the dog. J Am Vet Radiol Soc 16:115, 1975

Mehlhaff CJ, Mooney S: Primary pulmonary neoplasia in the dog and cat. Vet Clin North Am [Small Anim Pract] 15:1061, 1985

Miles KG: A review of primary lung tumors in the dog and cat. Vet Radiol 29:122, 1988

Moore AS, Middleton DJ: Pulmonary adenocarcinoma in three cats with non-respiratory signs only. J Small Anim Pract 23:501, 1982

Moore PF: Systemic histiocytosis in Bernese mountain dogs. Vet Pathol 21:554, 1984

Ogilvie GK, Haschek WM, Withrow SJ et al: Classification of primary lung tumors in dogs: 210 cases (1975–1985). J Am Vet Med Assoc 195:106, 1989

Ogilvie GK, Weigel RM, Haschek WM et al: Prognostic factors for tumor remission and survival in dogs after surgery for primary lung tumor: 76 cases (1975–1985). J Am Vet Med Assoc 195:109, 1989

Pion PD, Kittleson MD: Therapy for feline aortic thromboembolism. p. 295. In Kirk RW (ed): Current Veterinary Therapy X: Small Animal Practice. WB Saunders, Philadelphia, 1989

Postorino NC, Wheeler SL, Park RD et al: A syndrome resembling lymphomatoid granulomatosis in the dog. J Vet Intern Med 3:15, 1989

Reif JS, Dunn K, Ogilvie GK, Harris CK: Passive smoking and canine lung cancer risk. Am J Epidemiol 135:234, 1992

Rosin A, Moore P, Dubielzig R: Malignant histiocytosis in Bernese mountain dogs. J Am Vet Med Assoc 188:1041, 1986

Scott DW: Current knowledge of aeleurostrongylosis in the cat. Cornell Vet 63:483, 1973

Suter PF, Lord PF: Thoracic Radiography. A Text Atlas of Thoracic Diseases of the Dog and Cat. P. F. Suter, Wettswil, Switzerland, 1984

Withrow SJ: Tumors of the respiratory system. p. 215. In Withrow SJ, MacEwen EG (eds): Clinical Veterinary Oncology. JB Lippincott, Philadelphia, 1989

19

Pleural Cavity Diseases

Theresa W. Fossum

PNEUMOTHORAX

Definition

I. Pneumothorax is an accumulation of air or gas in the pleural space. It may occur spontaneously, as a result of an underlying pulmonary pathologic process, in association with trauma, or it may be iatrogenic.

II. Pneumothorax may be classified as follows.
  A. Open or pleurocutaneous: There is direct communication between the external atmosphere and the pleural space.
  B. Closed: Free air is present within the pleural space, but there is no communication with external atmospheric air. The source of the air may be the trachea, bronchi, or lungs (pleuropulmonary) or the esophagus (pleuroesophageal).
  C. Tension: Usually occurs when there is a tear in the pleura that acts as a one-way valve so that air accumulates in the pleural space during inspiration but is not expelled during expiration. This condition is rapidly fatal (as a result of hypoxemia and shock) if appropriate therapy is not instituted.

III. With subcutaneous emphysema the air may gain entry to the subcutaneous space from an external skin defect, from the pleural space, or from the mediastinum, cervical trachea, or esophagus.

Causes

I. Traumatic
  A. The source of the air may be pleuropulmonary, pleurocutaneous, or pleuroesophageal.
  B. It generally occurs as a result of vehicular trauma, bite wounds, puncture wounds, or gunshot wounds.

II. Spontaneous
  A. This is pneumothorax that occurs in the absence of a history or evidence of trauma.
  B. It may be either primary (unassociated with clinical or radiographic evidence of significant pulmonary disease) or secondary (pulmonary disease is present).

1. The primary form is usually associated with rupture of an air-containing space.
  a) Bulla: lined partly by a thickened fibrotic pleura, partly by fibrous tissue within the lung itself, and partly by emphysematous lung
  b) Bleb: air accumulation entirely within the pleura
  c) Etiology: not well understood, but probably multifactorial

2. The secondary form is associated with underlying pulmonary disease, including neoplasia, abscesses, granulomatous lesions, pneumonia, fungal infections, and parasites (e.g., *Paragonimus kellicotti, Aelurostrongylus* spp., and dirofilariasis).

III. Iatrogenic
  A. During or following diagnostic or therapeutic procedures
  B. Following intrathoracic surgery or surgery near the diaphragm (e.g., circumcostal gastropexy) or ribs (e.g., en bloc resections)
  C. Result of thoracentesis or pericardiocentesis, chest tube placement, lung aspiration or biopsy, tracheal intubation, or generation of excessive pressures during intermittent positive pressure ventilation

Pathophysiology

I. The effect on pulmonary function depends largely on its severity, although reductions in lung volumes and flow rates may also occur as a response to concurrent pleural or thoracic pain.

II. Alterations are predominantly associated with inadequate ventilation, unless there is significant underlying or associated pulmonary disease.
  A. Hypoventilation occurs with reductions in tidal volume and functional residual capacity, causing hypoxemia and respiratory acidosis.
  B. Ventilation-perfusion mismatching also contributes to the hypoxemia.
  C. Cardiac output may be compromised, leading

to reduced pulmonary perfusion and physiologic shunting.

III. Tension pneumothorax collapses the lungs and great veins, resulting in inadequate ventilation and reduction in cardiac output.

Clinical Signs

I. The severity of clinical signs depends on the amount of air present in the pleural space, rate of accumulation, and severity of any associated parenchymal disease.

II. Mild pneumothorax is associated with an increased respiratory rate and possibly exercise intolerance.

III. Severe pneumothorax usually results in rapid, shallow respirations, with or without cyanosis.
  A. Respiratory distress at rest, standing with the elbows abducted and the neck and head elevated (orthopneic position)
  B. Unable to rise, cyanotic, in shock, with poor capillary refill and weak peripheral pulses

Diagnosis

I. History
  A. Question the owner to determine whether there was any observed or any possible unobserved trauma.
  B. Coughing may precede pneumothorax secondary to pneumonia or abscessation associated with a foreign body (e.g., grass awn, stick or splinter, or other plant material).
  C. Ascertain any previous diagnostic and therapeutic procedures (prior anesthesia, thoracentesis) and any concurrent diseases or abnormalities.
  D. Determine the onset, duration, and progressive nature of the respiratory abnormality.

II. Physical examination
  A. Note: tachypnea, dyspnea, cyanosis, shock, fever, chest wall trauma (fractured ribs, lacerations), other signs of trauma such as fractures, and subcutaneous emphysema
  B. Auscultation: muffled lung and heart sounds, tachycardia, arrhythmias
  C. Percussion: increased resonance, particularly dorsally
  D. Usually bilateral in small animals

III. Needle thoracentesis
  A. Perform prior to radiography in animals that are severely distressed, because removal of even small amounts of air substantially improves ventilation and decreases the risk associated with manipulation for radiographs.
  B. Use a 19- to 23-gauge butterfly needle attached to a three-way stopcock and syringe, or an over-the-needle catheter attached to extension tubing, three-way stopcock, and syringe.
  C. Select the appropriate site based on physical examination findings or, if available, radiographic findings.
    1. Aspiration of either side usually drains the contralateral hemithorax.

  2. Common sites include the 7th, 8th, or 9th intercostal spaces, in the dorsal third of the chest wall.
  D. Consider using a local anesthetic block (optional) with minimal restraint and the animal in sternal recumbency.
  E. Provide oxygen by face mask if the animal will tolerate it.
  F. Aseptically prepare the skin and introduce the needle into the middle of the selected intercostal space, taking care to avoid the large vessels associated with the caudal rib margins.
    1. The needle is advanced into the pleural space until the pleura has been punctured.
    2. Aspirating while the needle is being advanced allows prompt recognition of the appropriate needle placement.
    3. During aspiration, the needle is positioned against the body wall with the bevel of the needle facing inward.

IV. Thoracic radiography
  A. Radiographic diagnosis of pneumothorax depends on the demonstration of free pleural air.
    1. Retraction of the lungs from the parietal pleura with the intervening space appearing more radiolucent than the pulmonary tissue
    2. Absence of pulmonary vasculature in the peripheral pleural space
    3. Improved visualization of the contrast between free pleural air and the collapsed lung
  B. In a recumbent lateral view the heart may shift so that it appears to be elevated from the sternum.
  C. Evaluation of the costophrenic angles may reveal small accumulations of air.
  D. Bullae or blebs are often not evident radiographically.
    1. Making the distinction between spontaneous and traumatic pneumothorax is difficult in cases in which the possibility of trauma exists but cannot be documented.
    2. Closely examine all radiographs for underlying parenchymal disease (pneumonia, abscesses, pulmonary contusions), the presence of rib fractures, diaphragmatic hernias, and other signs of trauma.
  E. The presence of concurrent pleural effusion produces a distinct fluid line on a standing lateral radiograph.

V. Additional tests
  A. Check the patient for parasites with direct smears, fecal sedimentation, and flotation.
  B. Positive contrast bronchography or pleurography is occasionally used to help identify affected lung lobes in animals with unresponsive or recurrent pneumothorax, often of an undetermined origin.
  C. Exploratory thoracotomy is often indicated in patients with spontaneous pneumothorax or traumatic pneumothorax that has not responded to appropriate conservative therapy. If there is no obvious pulmonary abnormality, a median sternotomy allows exploration of both hemithoraces.

Differential Diagnosis

I. Pleural effusion
II. Diaphragmatic hernia
III. Pulmonary contusion and thromboembolism
IV. Pneumonia
V. Asthma

Treatment

I. Traumatic
   A. Most animals with traumatic pneumothorax can be managed conservatively, without surgery.
      1. Often with mild distress, cage rest suffices until resorption of pleural air occurs.
      2. However, monitor the animal closely for evidence of shock or increasing dyspnea.
   B. Perform needle thoracentesis in animals with moderate distress, and closely monitor them for increasing respiratory rate.
   C. In animals with severe distress, needle thoracentesis is first performed; then if air continues to accumulate and requires frequent or repeated thoracentesis, a chest tube is placed (see Chap. 3).
      1. Oxygen and cage rest are generally needed.
      2. Air accumulation may be so great as to necessitate continuous suction with a water trap.
      3. Alternatively, a Heimlich valve (Bard-Parker, Rutherford, NJ) may be used; however, it should be used with caution in small patients (excessive pressures are required to overcome atmospheric pressure) and those with concurrent pleural effusion (fibrin may cause the valve to stick and malfunction).
   D. Treatment of animals with open pneumothorax is directed at re-establishing negative intrathoracic pressures by placing an occlusive bandage over the wound.
      1. Thoracentesis is then performed once the wound has been covered.
      2. Primary closure of the wound is delayed until the animal is stable.
   E. Chest tubes are generally removed when air production has become negligible (1–2 ml/kg on aspiration) for >12–24 hours and no further accumulation of air is detected on thoracic radiographs.
   F. If air leakage continues for >5–6 days, surgical exploration should be considered.
   G. Any evidence of esophageal perforation requires immediate surgical intervention.
II. Spontaneous
   A. Spontaneous pneumothorax usually requires surgical intervention (Holtsinger et al., 1993).
      1. Although the pneumothorax may initially resolve with chest tube drainage, recurrence rates in animals with primary spontaneous pneumothorax are high unless surgery is performed.
      2. With secondary pneumothorax, the underlying disease itself may necessitate prompt surgery (e.g., lung abscess).

   B. A median sternotomy is the approach of choice because it allows exploration of both sides of the thoracic cavity.
   C. Use of an automatic stapling device (US Surgical Corp., Norwalk, CT) facilitates partial lobectomies.
   D. Pleurodesis may be tried to decrease recurrence and is accomplished by gently abrading the visceral and parietal pleura with a dry gauze sponge. For pleurodesis to occur, the lungs must be in contact with body wall; therefore, if pneumothorax persists postoperatively, use continuous suction drainage until the pneumothorax resolves (generally 3–5 days).

Patient Monitoring

I. Monitor respiratory rate, lung sounds, cardiac rate and rhythm, capillary refill time, and mucous membrane color every 1–2 hours.
II. Air production should be monitored and recorded for each thoracentesis. Sudden increases in volumes of air indicate a problem with the chest tube (malposition, loose connection, damage) or further damage to the pulmonary parenchyma.
III. If commercial chest tubes with radiopaque lines are used, correct placement of drainage holes can be verified each time radiographs are performed.
IV. The major complication associated with the use of chest tubes is leakage of air into the chest from biting or scratching the tube or loosening of the tube connections or adaptors.
   A. The risk of these complications can be minimized by placing a hemostat or C-clamp close to the exit site of the tube, by securing the tube to the adaptors, and by proper bandaging of the chest and tube.
   B. Constant surveillance of animals with chest tubes is recommended.
V. A rough estimate of the volume of air production can be determined with sequential radiographs taken every 2–3 days. Resolution of pneumothorax and normal re-expansion of pulmonary tissue should be verified radiographically prior to the animal's release from the hospital.

PLEURAL EFFUSION

Definition

I. Pleural effusion is the accumulation of fluid within the pleural space.
II. The pleura is a serosal surface consisting of a single layer of flattened mesothelial cells with an underlying connective-tissue layer containing blood vessels and lymphatics.
III. The pleural space is the potential space between the visceral and parietal pleura.
   A. Visceral pleura: covers the serosal surface of the lungs, receiving its blood supply from the pulmonary circulation

B. Parietal pleura: lines the thoracic walls, mediastinum, and diaphragm, receiving its blood supply from the systemic circulation

C. Normal pleural space: 2–3 ml of fluid serve as a lubricant for the lungs during normal respiratory movements

Causes and Classification

I. Classification
   A. Pleural effusions are generally classified as transudates, modified transudates, or exudates on the basis of the protein content (TP = total protein or solids) and cellularity (TNCC = total nucleated cell count).
   B. They may also be classified based on their general cytologic features as hemorrhagic, inflammatory, obstructive, chylous, neoplastic, septic, or pyogranulomatous effusions.

II. Transudates
   A. Occur when the mechanical factors influencing the formation or reabsorption of pleural fluid are altered, such as decreased plasma osmotic pressure or elevated systemic or pulmonary hydrostatic pressures
   B. Are fluids that have a low protein content (<1.5 g/dl) and low cellularity (<1000/μl)
   C. Result from hypoalbuminemia ($\leq$1.5 g/dl) associated with decreased protein production (e.g., chronic liver disease), protein-losing nephropathy or enteropathy, intestinal malabsorption and maldigestion, malnutrition, chronic blood loss, and burns
   D. Also occur from increased hydrostatic pressure in blood vessels or lymphatics draining the pleural cavity, from congestive heart failure (CHF)
      1. In dogs, this occurs as a result of either right-sided heart failure or a combination of left- and right-sided failure.
      2. In cats, cardiomyopathy is the most common cause.
      3. With chronicity these effusions become modified transudates.

III. Modified transudates
   A. Are long-standing transudates in which protein and cellularity are increased secondary to localized inflammation in the pleura; have intermediate characteristics between transudates and exudates
   B. TP between 1.5 and 3.0 g/dl, TNCC between 1000 and 5000/μl

IV. Exudates
   A. Result from inflammation or other diseases of the pleural surface, such as occurs in pneumonia, pyothorax, immune-mediated disease, chylothorax, neoplasia, and feline infectious peritonitis (FIP)
   B. TP >3.0 g/dl, TNCC >5000/μl
   C. May also be classified as exudates if the ratio of pleural fluid TP to serum TP is >0.5

Pathophysiology

I. Fluid movement through the pleural space is a result of a balance between filtration and reabsorption forces. Normally, pleural fluid moves through capillaries of the parietal pleura into the pleural space, where it is absorbed by capillaries of the visceral pleura and by lymphatics.

II. The movement of pleural fluid is in accordance with Starling's forces.
   A. A net force of 9 cm H_2O favors movement of fluid from the parietal pleura into the pleural space (Forrester et al., 1988).
      1. The forces promoting fluid transudation into the pleural space are the capillary hydrostatic pressure, a negative intrapleural pressure, and the pleural fluid colloid osmotic pressure.
      2. The only opposing force is the systemic colloid osmotic pressure in the capillaries of the parietal pleura.
   B. Absorption of fluid by the visceral pleura is facilitated by the colloid osmotic pressure of the visceral capillary network.
      1. The forces opposing resorption of pleural fluid include the negative intrapleural pressure, the pleural fluid colloid osmotic pressure, and the pulmonary capillary hydrostatic pressure.
      2. The resulting gradient is 10 cm H_2O, a net of 1 cm H_2O, favoring resorption.

III. Fluid not absorbed by the pleural capillaries returns to the circulation via lymphatics.
   A. The lymphatics are the only route by which high-protein fluid can be reabsorbed.
   B. Lymphatic absorption in animals occurs primarily in the lower mediastinal pleura and in the costal parietal pleura (Forrester et al., 1988).

IV. Anything that results in increased hydrostatic pressure, such as CHF (cardiomyopathy, pericardial effusion, cardiac tamponade, heartworm disease), diaphragmatic hernias, lung lobe torsion, neoplasia, or protein-losing conditions, causes increased formation or decreased resorption of pleural fluid.

V. Diseases causing decreased oncotic pressure (hypoalbuminemia and neoplasia) result in increased formation of pleural fluid.

VI. Diseases producing increased vascular or lymphatic permeability or obstruction, such as immune-mediated diseases (systemic lupus erythematosus and rheumatoid arthritis), inflammatory or infectious conditions (bacterial, viral, or rickettsial pneumonia, fungal infections, parasitic disease), uremia, pancreatitis, trauma, and neoplasia (lymphosarcoma, metastatic mammary neoplasia, and mesothelioma), result in increased formation or decreased resorption of pleural fluid.

VII. Decreased intrapleural pressure from severe upper airway obstruction can also promote formation of pleural fluid.

Clinical Signs

I. Signs vary depending on the underlying etiology, rapidity of fluid accumulation, and volume of fluid.

II. Most animals do not exhibit clinical signs until there is significant impairment of ventilation.

III. Acute signs include tachypnea, cyanosis, open mouth breathing, orthopnea, and coughing.

IV. With chronic pleural disease, weight loss, coughing, anorexia, and lethargy may be present.

Diagnosis/Differential Diagnosis

I. Physical examination
  A. Thoracic percussion
    1. Hyporesonance is present ventrally with moderate or severe amounts of pleural fluid.
    2. With the animal standing or in sternal recumbency, a line of normal resonance may be percussed dorsal to an area of decreased resonance (see Chap. 1).
  B. Chest compression
    A noticeable decrease in the ability to compress the anterior chest is present in many cats with cranial mediastinal masses and pleural effusion.
  C. Auscultation
    1. Muffling of heart and ventral lung sounds
    2. Murmurs or arrhythmias
    3. Increased bronchovesicular sounds, particularly in the dorsal lung field
  D. Additional findings
    1. Nonspecific findings include fever, depression, anorexia/weight loss, pale mucous membranes, and ascites.
    2. Jugular pulses may be present in animals with right-sided heart failure.

II. Thoracentesis
  A. Place 5 ml of fluid in an EDTA tube for analysis of cellularity and an additional 5 ml of fluid in a clot tube for measurement of biochemical parameters.
  B. Make 6–8 direct smears for cytologic evaluation.
  C. Smears are also made by centrifuging the pleural fluid and smearing the pellet of cells in the bottom of the tube on a slide. If substantial blood contamination is present, a buffy coat smear is best.
  D. Submit the remaining fluid for aerobic and anaerobic culture.

III. Thoracic radiography
  A. Perform a thoracentesis first if the animal is extremely dyspneic.
  B. Evidence of pleural effusion includes blurring of the cardiac silhouette, interlobar fissure lines, rounding of the lung margins at costophrenic angles, scalloping of the lung margins at the sternal border, widening of the mediastinum, increased density of the pleural space, and separation of the lung borders from the thoracic wall.
  C. Small quantities of fluid are best seen on expiratory radiographic views and result in widening of the interlobar fissure lines. In a ventrodorsal position (dorsal recumbency), small amounts of fluid may be detected as ''blunting'' or ''rounding'' of the costophrenic angles (Myer, 1978).

D. Fluid may be classified as free or encapsulated.
    1. Free fluid moves easily to both sides of the pleural space, and its distribution is affected by gravity.
    2. Encapsulated fluid is confined by fibrinous adhesions, its distribution is not affected by gravity, and it is commonly associated with chylothorax and pyothorax.

IV. Ultrasonography
  A. Ultrasonography is best performed prior to the removal of pleural fluid because the pleural fluid acts as an ''acoustic'' window, enhancing visualization of structures of the thoracic cavity.
  B. It is used to evaluate cardiac function and anatomy and to detect pericardial effusion or mediastinal masses.

V. Fluid analysis (Table 19–1)
  A. Color and clarity
    1. Clear and colorless: generally transudates
    2. Clear, amber to red-tinged: transudates or modified transudates
    3. Mildly turbid and amber to red-tinged: usually modified transudates
    4. Moderately to markedly turbid, amber to red-tinged: typically exudates
    5. Yellow, tan, white, and opaque: chylothorax, pyothorax
    6. Red, opaque: hemorrhagic or hemothorax
  B. Viscosity
    1. Viscous fluid may be associated with FIP or highly cellular fluids with a large number of ruptured cells.
    2. Viscous fluids are identified by their ''stringy'' or ''rope-like'' appearance when placed between fingers that are slowly pulled apart.
  C. Cytology
    1. Care must be taken to differentiate reactive mesothelial cells from neoplastic cells, as the cytologic characteristics of the two may be confused.
    2. The predominant cell type is used to help characterize the effusion.
      a) Mesothelial cells and macrophages: transudate or modified transudate
      b) Neutrophils and macrophages: modified transudate or exudate (pyothorax, chylothorax, fungal disease, immune-mediated disease, and neoplasia)
      c) Mature lymphocytes: chylothorax
      d) Lymphoblasts: lymphosarcoma
      e) Eosinophils >10% of the cell population: eosinophilic pleural effusion, possibly associated with pneumothorax, parasites, neoplasia, infections, or idiopathic causes
    3. Except for lymphosarcoma, many primary and metastatic neoplasms do not exfoliate into pleural fluid.
    4. Rarely, pleural effusion may be the only clinical manifestation of immune-mediated disease.
      a) The presence of rheumatoid cells or lupus

Table 19–1. *Specific Pleural Effusions Associated with Pleural Cavity Diseases*

Type of Effusion	Causes	Color	Diagnostic Features	Predominant Cell Types
Chylothorax	Mediastinal masses: neoplasia (particularly lymphosarcoma), fungal granuloma Cardiovascular disease: cardiomyopathy, heartworm infestation, venous thrombi, pericardial disease, congenital heart disease (particularly endocardial cushion defects) Trauma Idiopathic	White or pink, opaque	Remains opaque following centrifugation Contains chylomicrons Compare pleural fluid and serum triglyceride concentrations to confirm Ether clearance test has been used to diagnose chylous effusions; however, it is not quantitative or easily interpreted	Neutrophils or lymphocytes Neutrophils often predominate in chylous effusions or in animals receiving multiple thoracenteses
Pyothorax	Foreign body, bite wound, etc. Etiology often not apparent	White-gray, pink, or red	Confirm by presence of bacteria in pleural fluid cytology To differentiate from contamination—look for phagocytosis of bacteria, presence of numerous neutrophils and degenerative neutrophils Occasionally foul-smelling, especially when anaerobes are present Perform microbial cultures; anaerobes may not grow	Neutrophils: often degenerative and toxic appearing
Hemothorax	Trauma Coagulopathies Neoplasia	Red	Blood in the pleural space rapidly becomes defibrinated; therefore, true hemothorax produces a hemorrhagic-appearing sample that does not clot (as opposed to inadvertent aspiration of a vessel or heart) Hematocrit similar to peripheral blood	Red cells White cells in quantities similar to peripheral blood
Feline infectious peritonitis	Vasculitis	Straw-colored, yellow, or tan	Appears thick and stringy owing to high protein content (>6.0 g/dl)	Acute: neutrophils (nondegenerative) Chronic: macrophages and mesothelial cells
Malignant effusions	Associated with thoracic neoplasia: Pleural mesothelioma Lymphosarcoma Metastatic tumors (e.g., mammary tumors) Pulmonary tumors	Red or pink, occasionally white or straw-colored	Difficult to differentiate between malignant cells and reactive mesothelial cells Diagnostics under evaluation for sensitivity and specificity are flow cytometry, pleural fluid cytogenetics, immunohistochemistry, analysis of biochemical parameters (e.g., carcinoembryonic antigen) Mesotheliomas (rare in dogs) are associated with a serosanguineous fluid, which may quickly accumulate in large quantities and inhibit respiration; diagnose with open biopsy	Neoplastic cells may not be present Neoplastic cells and reactive mesothelial cells may be difficult to differentiate

erythematosus (LE) cells is suggestive; however, these cells may also be induced by certain drugs, such as procainamide.

    b) In humans, a pleural fluid antinuclear antibody (ANA) titer has been helpful in diagnosing immune-mediated pleural effusions.

D. Culture

    1. Positive cultures are not obtained in all animals with pyothorax, particularly if anaerobic organisms are present.

    2. The most common etiologic agents of pyothorax in dogs are *Actinomyces, Bacteroides, Fusobacterium,* and *Nocardia.* In cats, *Bacteroides, Pasteurella, Fusobacterium, Actinomyces,* and *Clostridium* are common (Sherding, 1979; Dow et al., 1986).

E. Protein electrophoresis

    1. In effusions other than FIP, albumin is >48% of the total protein, gamma globulin is <32% of total protein, and the albumin/globulin ratio is ≥0.82 (Shelly et al., 1988).

    2. With FIP, gamma globulin is >32% of TP and the albumin/globulin ratio is <0.81.

F. Cholesterol and triglyceride analysis

    1. True chylous effusions

      a) The pleural fluid triglyceride is greater than the serum triglyceride (Fossum et al., 1986b).

      b) These may occur with cardiomyopathy, mediastinal masses, heartworm disease, fungal granulomas, venous thrombi, and pericardial effusion.

    2. Pseudochylous effusions

      a) Pleural fluid cholesterol is greater than the serum cholesterol, and pleural fluid triglyceride is less than or equal to the serum triglyceride (Fossum et al., 1986b).

      b) It is "rare" but may be associated with tuberculosis.

      c) Note: Cholesterol content of the pleural fluid must be greater than the serum cholesterol to be a true pseudochylous effusion.

    3. Sampling method

      a) Because appearance and triglyceride content of the fluid are affected by dietary fat intake, chylous effusions in anorexic animals may not appear white and may have lower than expected triglyceride concentrations.

      b) Pleural fluid samples should be submitted following a feeding in such animals.

G. Pleural fluid pH

    1. Pleural fluid pH has been reported to help differentiate pyothorax from malignant effusion in cats (Stewart et al., 1990).

    2. Suspect pyothorax if the pH is <6.9; malignancy if pH is >7.2.

H. Pleural fluid amylase and glucose

    1. Although increased amylase levels in humans are associated with pancreatitis, esophageal rupture, and malignancies, they have not been reported in dogs and cats.

    2. Low glucose values (<10 g/dl) have been observed in cats with pyothorax (Stewart et al., 1990).

Treatment

I. General considerations

A. The treatment of pleural effusion varies, depending on the underlying etiology.

B. Sometimes treatment of the underlying condition can render specific treatment of the effusion unnecessary.

II. Chylothorax

A. Determine and treat the underlying etiology, if possible. In most animals with chylothorax, the underlying etiology is not apparent (idiopathic) (Fossum et al., 1986a).

B. If no underlying disease is detected, consider medical management.

    1. Repeated thoracentesis can be tried. Chest tube placement is seldom indicated or beneficial and is expensive.

    2. Low-fat diets are instituted.

      a) Hill's r/d

      b) Homemade diet consisting of boiled rice or potato, oatmeal, or pasta (1 cup), 1 cup low-fat (2%) cottage cheese, 1 vitamin/mineral tablet, ½ tsp calcium carbonate (e.g., Tums), and 15 ml of MCT oil per 12–15 lb

      c) Skinned, boiled chicken breast or water-packed tuna substituted for cottage cheese

    3. Supplementation with MCT oil (Mead Johnson) given at 1–2 ml/kg/day orally may be considered; however, MCT is not palatable, particularly to cats.

    4. Medical therapy is generally successful in animals with chylothorax secondary to trauma, but trauma is a relatively rare cause.

    5. Effusion should resolve in 2 weeks if caused by trauma.

    6. In some animals with idiopathic chylothorax, the effusion spontaneously resolves with several months of medical therapy.

    7. Consider long-term therapy with benzopyrones (e.g., rutin 50 mg/kg PO TID) to improve fluid resorption and decrease fibrosis.

C. Some animals with idiopathic chylothorax do not respond to medical management and require surgical intervention. Surgical options include mesenteric lymphangiography and thoracic duct ligation, passive pleuroperitoneal shunting, active pleuroperitoneal or pleurovenous shunting, and pleurodesis.

    1. Mesenteric lymphangiography and thoracic duct ligation

      a) Procedure (Kagan and Breznock, 1979; Birchard et al., 1982)

        (1) Identification of mesenteric lymphatics: Animals are fed corn oil or cream

3 hours prior to surgery, or methylene blue (American Quinine, Shirley, NY) is injected into a mesenteric lymph node at surgery.

(2) Identification of thoracic duct and branches: Catheter is placed in a mesenteric lymphatic, and thoracic radiographs are taken following injection of a contrast agent.

(3) Ligation of thoracic duct and branches: A thoracotomy or transdiaphragmatic approach is used to locate the caudal thoracic duct (often there are multiple branches), and the thoracic duct is ligated using 2-0 or 3-0 silk suture and hemoclips.

(4) Verification of complete ligation: The lymphangiogram is repeated to verify ligation of all branches.

b) Mechanism: Abdominal lymphaticovenous anastomoses form for transport of chyle to the venous system, thereby bypassing the thoracic duct.

c) It results in complete resolution of pleural effusion approximately 50% of the time in dogs (Birchard et al., 1988). In cats, the success rate is 25–50% (Fossum et al., 1991b; Kerpsack et al., 1994).

d) Advantages: If successful, it results in complete resolution of pleural fluid (as compared with palliative procedures described later).

e) Disadvantages: These include prolonged surgery time, high incidence of continued or recurrent chylous or nonchylous (from pulmonary lymphatics) effusion, and mesenteric lymphangiography may be difficult to perform (particularly in cats).

2. Passive pleuroperitoneal shunting (not recommended by author)

a) Procedure (Peterson et al., 1988)

(1) It may be performed in conjunction with thoracic duct ligation or alone.

(2) Perforated medical-grade Silastic sheeting (Dow Corning Co., Midland, MI) is cut to fit defects created in the diaphragm.

(3) Sheeting is fixed to the edges of the diaphragmatic defect using nonabsorbable suture material (Prolene, Ethicon, Somerville, NJ).

b) Mechanism: chyle absorbed from the abdominal cavity owing to increased surface area, preventing respiratory distress

c) Success rates not reported in a large number of animals, but spontaneous resolution of pleural fluid may occur in some animals (Peterson et al., 1988)

d) Advantages: inexpensive, easy, short duration of surgery

e) Disadvantages: possible development of fibrosing pleuritis if chylothorax continues, and inadequate drainage if holes are covered by fibrin or abdominal organs

f) Not to be used in animals with cardiac disease or portal hypertension, as the effusion may not be reabsorbed from the abdominal cavity

g) Note: has been associated with development of gastric neoplasia, presumably associated with chronic irritation (Fossum, unpublished data)

3. Active pleuroperitoneal or pleurovenous shunting

a) Procedure is as follows (Willauer and Breznock, 1987; Smeak et al., 1987)

(1) One arm of a commercially made shunt catheter (Denver double-valve peritoneal-venous shunt, Denver Biomaterials Inc., Evergreen, CO) is placed into the thorax, and the other arm is placed into either the abdomen or the venous system (jugular or azygous vein or caudal vena cava).

(2) The pump chamber is placed over the rib cage so that it can be effectively compressed.

(3) Fluid is manually pumped into the abdomen or venous system by compressing the pump chamber 200–300 times, 3–4 times a day.

b) Advantages are that it may allow more complete drainage of the thorax than passive peritoneal drainage. Pleurovenous shunting overcomes problems with inadequate peritoneal absorption, which may occur with pleuroperitoneal shunting.

c) Disadvantages are that the shunts are expensive, they may easily occlude with fibrin, some animals do not tolerate compression of the pump chamber, and they require a high degree of owner compliance and dedication. Additionally, thrombosis, venous occlusion, sepsis, and electrolyte abnormalities may occur.

4. Pleurodesis (not recommended by author)

a) Pleurodesis is the formation of generalized adhesions between the visceral and parietal pleura.

b) Adhesions may occur spontaneously in association with pleural effusion or in some species they can be induced following instillation of an irritating substance into the pleural cavity.

c) Procedure is as follows (Birchard and Gallagher, 1988).

(1) Place bilateral chest tubes and completely drain the pleural space.

(2) Instill 15–20 mg/kg of tetracycline hydrochloride diluted in 75 ml of sterile water into the chest cavity.

(3) Instill 200 ml of air to ensure contact of the solution with the pleural surface.

(4) Rotate the patient to distribute the solution and drain the pleural space in 2 hours.

(5) Remove chest tubes when drainage is less than 150 ml over a 24-hour period.

d) It is inexpensive and easily performed (does not require a thoracotomy or general anesthetic other than for chest tube placement).

e) It seldom causes generalized adhesions to form; appropriate dosages, concentrations, and dwell times have not been determined for dogs or cats; and with the exception of one study (Gallagher et al., 1990), experimental studies have not been performed in dogs or cats.

f) For pleurodesis to occur, the lungs must be able to contact the body wall; however, many animals with chronic chylothorax have some thickening of their visceral pleura, which prohibits normal lung expansion (see fibrosing pleuritis, later).

D. Chronic chylothorax is extremely irritating to the pleura and may result in severe fibrosing pleuritis (Glennon et al., 1987; Fossum et al., 1992).

1. Cats appear to be more susceptible than dogs.

2. The recommended treatment for fibrosing pleuritis is pleural decortication.

a) Technically, decortication is the removal of visceral pleura in order to allow the lungs to expand.

b) In some cases, the fibrous sheet does not appear to be firmly attached to the underlying pleura and can be removed without excessive damage to the pleura or lungs.

c) When the pleura is diffusely involved, the prognosis is extremely guarded.

III. Pyothorax

A. Place a chest tube(s) and perform thoracic lavage.

1. Instill 10 ml/kg of warmed lactated Ringer's solution with heparin (1500 U/100 ml of lavage solution) into the thoracic cavity and withdraw after 1 hour.

2. Antibiotics can also be added at half the systemic dose; however, this is of questionable benefit and is not recommended.

3. Repeat the lavage BID–TID until cytologic (the effusion clears and bacteria are not seen in direct smears of pleural fluid) and symptomatic (normal temperature, improved appetite, normal respiration) improvement is evident (4–6 days).

B. Start antibiotics based on results of culture and sensitivity.

1. See Table 19–2 for suggested initial antibiotic therapy while awaiting culture results.

2. Antibiotics are continued for a minimum of 3–4 weeks.

C. Surgery is indicated in animals that have underlying disease (lung abscess, lung lobe torsion, foreign body) and in those that do not respond to medical management.

1. If the lesion is delineated radiographically, an intercostal thoracotomy should be performed on the appropriate side.

2. If the underlying lesion is not identified, a median sternotomy approach should be performed.

3. Abnormal lung tissue is removed and the thoracic cavity lavaged with warmed saline or lactated Ringer's solution.

4. Chest tubes are placed during surgery, and thoracic lavage is continued postoperatively until fluid production decreases to <2 ml/kg and bacteria are no longer visible cytologically.

5. Animals with long-standing pyothorax may develop fibrosing pleuritis and require decortication.

IV. Hemothorax

A. Thoracentesis is performed for diagnostic purposes; large amounts of blood are removed only if the effusion is compromising the animal's respiration, because most red cells are absorbed from the thoracic cavity intact (autotransfusion).

B. Transfusion may be required if the hemorrhage has significantly lowered the hematocrit.

C. Correct any underlying coagulation defects (see Chap. 66).

V. Malignant effusions

A. Treatment is directed at controlling the primary tumor.

1. Primary malignancies (lung, heart) are sometimes surgically resectable.

2. Lymphosarcoma is usually responsive to chemotherapy.

B. When there is no effective systemic treatment, palliative treatment of the effusion may be indicated to prolong the animal's life.

1. In some animals, palliation may be accomplished by repeated thoracentesis.

2. Intracavitary instillation of chemotherapeutic agents or radioactive isotopes has been effective in the treatment of malignant pleural effusions in people and in a dog (Shapiro and Turrel, 1988).

3. Pleurodesis has been reported in the dog, but its effectiveness is unproved.

C. Metastasis of mesotheliomas to intrathoracic organs is common in dogs, and therapy is generally restricted to controlling pleural effusion with repeated thoracentesis and/or chemotherapy. The prognosis in dogs for long-term survival is poor.

Patient Monitoring

I. Vital signs

A. Constantly observe for onset or return of severe respiratory distress.

B. Repeatedly assess mucous membrane color, temperature, respiratory rate, lung sounds, cardiac rate and rhythm, and mental status.

Table 19–2. **Morphologic and Culture Characteristics of Bacteria Commonly Associated with Pyothorax**

Bacteria	Oxygen Requirements	Gram's Stain	Morphology	Antibiotic Sensitivity
Actinomyces	Facultative anaerobe to strict anaerobe	Gram-positive	Small bacilli; may form filaments; often beaded and difficult to discern in clinical specimens; may form sulfur granules	**Penicillin** (includes penicillin G, ampicillin, and amoxicillin), amoxicillin + clavulanic acid, cephalosporin, clindamycin, chloramphenicol, erythromycin
Bacteroides	Obligate anaerobe	Gram-negative	Bacilli pleomorphic and may be beaded or cocci; often stain poorly and are difficult to see	Most bacteroides—**penicillin,** cephalosporin, clindamycin, chloramphenicol, metronidazole *B. fragilis*—**metronidazole, amoxicillin + clavulanic acid,** clindamycin, chloramphenicol
Clostridium	Obligate anaerobe	Gram-positive	Bacilli; large, frequently encapsulated, motile; spores uncommon from clinical specimens	Most clostridia—penicillin, amoxicillin + clavulanic acid, chloramphenicol, metronidazole *C. perfringens*—**penicillin,** amoxicillin + clavulanic acid, cefoxitin, clindamycin, chloramphenicol, metronidazole, erythromycin
Fusobacterium	Obligate anaerobe	Gram-negative	Bacilli; often have a cigar-shaped appearance; may be filamentous	**Penicillin,** amoxicillin + clavulanic acid, clindamycin, chloramphenicol, metronidazole
Klebsiella	Facultative anaerobe	Gram-negative	Bacilli; encapsulated	**Cephalosporin,** gentamicin, tobramycin, ticarcillin
Nocardia	Aerobe	Gram-positive (partially acid-fast)	Small bacilli; may form filaments; often beaded and difficult to discern in clinical specimens; may form sulfur granules	**Trimethoprim-sulfa, amikacin**
Pasteurella	Facultative anaerobe	Gram-negative	Coccobacilli; pleomorphic, bipolar staining from tissues	Penicillin, amoxicillin + clavulanic acid
Pseudomonas	Aerobe	Gram-negative	Bacilli; slender, motile	**Carbenicillin (IV),** gentamicin, tobramycin, amikacin, ticarcillin, cefotaxime, moxalactam

Bold type = drug of choice.

II. Hydration and electrolyte status
   A. Provide fluid therapy as needed.
      1. Fluids should be administered with caution in patients with heart failure.
      2. The volume of fluid removed from the thoracic cavity is quantified, and calculated maintenance fluid volumes are supplemented accordingly.
   B. Animals undergoing frequent thoracentesis may develop severe electrolyte abnormalities.
      1. Hyperkalemia and hyponatremia are most common (Willard et al., 1991).
      2. Monitor electrolytes every 2–3 days in patients undergoing thoracentesis; if electrolyte abnormalities are documented, measure them every 12 hours and treat appropriately.
III. Nutritional status
   A. Animals with pleural effusion may have progressive weight loss and hypoproteinemia.
   B. Chylothorax may result in severe debilitation owing to the loss of fat and protein into the thoracic cavity. Management of these animals with re-
stricted diets also contributes to hypoproteinemia.
   C. Parenteral or enteral hyperalimentation should be considered in animals that have severe malnutrition (see Chaps. 3 and 32).

DIAPHRAGMATIC HERNIA

Definition and Causes

   I. Diaphragmatic hernia is the protrusion of an abdominal organ through an abnormal opening in the diaphragm.
  II. With most congenital diaphragmatic hernias, there is open communication between the pleuroperitoneal membrane and the pericardial sac.
 III. For traumatic hernias, the most common cause is motor vehicle accidents; however, any forceful blow (being kicked by a horse, blunt blows, falls from high elevations) may be a cause.

Pathophysiology

I. Congenital diaphragmatic hernia
  A. May be either pleuroperitoneal or peritoneopericardial
    1. Pleuroperitoneal types are often associated with severe dyspnea, and many affected individuals die in the early neonatal period (Valentine et al., 1988).
    2. Of the two, peritoneopericardial hernias are more common.
  B. The most widely accepted theory regarding the embryogenesis of this defect is that the hernia arises because of faulty development or prenatal injury of the septum transversum.
  C. The combination of congenital cranial abdominal wall, caudal sternal, diaphragmatic, and pericardial defects has been reported in dogs.
    1. Ventricular septal defects or other intracardiac defects may also be found.
    2. The heredity has not been determined, but several littermates with this condition have been reported. Breeds that appear to be predisposed include Weimaraners and cocker spaniels.
II. Traumatic diaphragmatic hernia
  A. The abrupt increase in intra-abdominal pressure that accompanies forceful blows to the abdominal wall causes the lungs to rapidly deflate (if the glottis is open) and results in a large pleuroperitoneal pressure gradient, which causes the diaphragm to tear at its weakest points, the muscular portions.
  B. The location and size of the tear(s) depend on the position of the animal at the time of the impact and the location of the viscera.
  C. There is no breed or sex predisposition; however, a majority of animals are young (1–2 years of age).
  D. The duration may range from a few hours to years because many animals are not diagnosed until long after the traumatic incident.

Clinical Signs

I. Congenital diaphragmatic hernia
  A. These are sometimes not diagnosed until the animal is middle-aged or older, because clinical signs are variable and may be intermittent.
  B. Clinical signs are referable to the gastrointestinal (GI), cardiac, or respiratory systems and include anorexia, depression, vomiting, diarrhea, weight loss, wheezing, respiratory distress, orthopnea, exercise intolerance, and pain following ingestion of food.
  C. Neurologic signs occur if hepatoencephalopathy is present.
II. Traumatic diaphragmatic hernia
  A. Animals are frequently presented in shock, with evidence of pale or cyanotic mucous membranes, tachypnea, tachycardia, and oliguria.

  B. Cardiac arrhythmias are common and are associated with significant morbidity.
  C. Other clinical signs are dependent on which organs herniate and may be attributed to the GI, respiratory, or cardiovascular system.
  D. The liver is the most common organ herniated and often causes hydrothorax owing to entrapment and venous occlusion.

Diagnosis/Differential Diagnosis

I. Physical examination
  A. Congenital hernias: respiratory distress, ascites, muffled heart sounds, murmurs caused by displacement of the heart by visceral organs or by intracardiac defects, and concurrent ventral abdominal wall defects
  B. Traumatic hernias
    1. Gut sounds may be heard on thoracic auscultation.
    2. Other findings include respiratory distress, ascites, muffled heart and lung sounds (often unilaterally), increased bronchovesicular sounds, arrhythmias secondary to traumatic myocarditis, and absence of normally palpable structures in the abdominal cavity.
    3. The animal may appear thin if most of the intestinal loops and stomach are in the thoracic cavity.
II. Radiography
  A. Congenital hernias
    1. Look for enlarged cardiac silhouette, dorsal displacement of the trachea, overlap of the diaphragmatic and caudal heart borders, discontinuity of diaphragmatic silhouette, presence of gas- or barium-filled small intestines or stomach in the pericardium, and concurrent sternal defects.
    2. Contrast studies are undertaken only if a definitive diagnosis cannot be made on plain films or upon ultrasonographic evaluation.
  B. Traumatic hernias
    1. Definitive diagnosis is via radiography or ultrasonography. If significant pleural effusion is present, thoracentesis may be necessary to allow diagnostic radiographs.
    2. Look for loss of the diaphragmatic line, loss of the cardiac silhouette, dorsal or lateral displacement of lung fields, and presence of gas- or barium-filled stomach or intestines in the thoracic cavity.
    3. Occasionally, positive-contrast celiography aids in the diagnosis (Stickle, 1984).
      a) Prewarmed water-soluble contrast agent is injected into the abdominal cavity at a dosage of 1.1 ml/kg (dose is doubled if ascites is present).
      b) The patient is gently rolled from side to side or the pelvis is elevated, and films are taken immediately following the injection and manipulation.
      c) The criteria used in evaluating these films

include the presence of contrast medium in the pleural cavity, the absence of a normal liver lobe outline in the abdomen, and incomplete visualization of the abdominal surface of the diaphragm.

   d) Interpret positive-contrast celiograms with caution, because omental and fibrous adhesions may seal the defect, resulting in false-negative diagnoses.

III. Ultrasonography
   A. Discontinuity of the diaphragm can often be detected.
   B. The liver or gas-filled intestines may also be detected in the thorax.

IV. Thoracoscopy: allows differentiation of lung mass from liver herniation

Treatment

I. Congenital diaphragmatic hernia
   A. Surgical repair is performed as early as possible, generally when the animal is 8–16 weeks of age.
      1. At this age it is unlikely that adhesions will be present, and the pliable nature of the skin, muscles, sternum, and rib cage facilitates closure of large defects.
      2. Early correction prevents acute decompensation and the potential development of acute postoperative pulmonary edema.
   B. Most peritoneopericardial hernias can be corrected via a ventral midline abdominal incision; if increased exposure is needed, the incision can be extended cranially into the sternum.
   C. The diaphragmatic defect is closed with a simple continuous suture using either a nonabsorbable material such as polypropylene or an absorbable material such as polydioxanone.
   D. Air is removed from the pleural cavity following closure of the defect by placing a chest tube or by aspirating air through the closed diaphragm with a catheter attached to an extension tubing and three-way stopcock for easy manipulation.

II. Traumatic diaphragmatic hernia
   A. Studies have shown a significantly higher mortality when surgery is performed <24 hours after the injury; therefore, surgical repair should be delayed until the animal has been stabilized.
   B. With herniation of the stomach, evaluate carefully for gastric distention and perform a herniorrhaphy at the earliest opportunity, once the animal is stable.
   C. The surgical approach is similar to that described for congenital hernias.

Patient Monitoring

I. Take radiographs following surgery if respirations become labored.
   A. Respiratory distress occurs following incomplete removal of air from the thoracic cavity after diaphragmatic closure.
   B. Pulmonary edema may also occur postoperatively.

II. Re-expansion pulmonary edema
   A. This is a potential complication associated with rapid lung re-expansion following surgical repair, especially in cats. Although the origin is unknown and probably multifactorial, it does not appear to be associated with cardiac failure.
   B. Initially following surgery, the animal appears improved, but after a few hours, respiratory distress and tachypnea develop. The distress is progressive and is associated with marked, diffuse pulmonary edema related to decreased lung compliance. Hypoxia develops and persists despite intense oxygen therapy.
   C. The etiology of the edema is unknown but may be associated with decreased mitochondrial superoxide dismutase and cytochrome oxidase (Jackson et al., 1988; Inauen et al., 1989; Stampley and Waldron, 1994). The reoxygenation of chronically collapsed lungs is thought to release superoxide radicals that cannot be effectively scavenged, resulting in increased pulmonary capillary permeability and pulmonary edema.
   D. Prophylaxis and therapy are difficult and poorly understood.
      1. Re-expansion of chronically collapsed lung tissue should be accomplished *slowly,* and high ventilation pressures are avoided in these patients.
      2. Current recommendations include the use of positive end-expiratory pressure (PEEP) ventilation and drugs that stabilize the pulmonary capillary membranes, such as methylprednisolone.
      3. A number of other pharmaceutical agents are currently being investigated, but conclusive evidence of their beneficial effects is not yet available.
   E. Pulmonary hypoplasia may be present with peritoneopericardial hernias, contributing to the development of high intrapleural pressures and re-expansion pulmonary edema; care must be taken to avoid rapid and excessive pulmonary re-expansion in these animals.

FLAIL CHEST

Definition and Causes

I. Flail chest is a paradoxical movement of the chest wall with respiration, owing to multiple rib fractures.
II. Trauma is the usual cause.
III. It occurs when several ribs on both sides of the point of impact are fractured such that the intervening rib segments lose their continuity with the remainder of the thorax.

Pathophysiology/Clinical Signs

I. Paradoxical movement of the chest wall occurs during respiration owing to intrapleural pressure changes; the fractured segment moves inward during inspiration and outward during expiration.

II. Pulmonary abnormalities in patients with flail chest may be severe and lead to decreased vital capacity, reduced functional residual capacity, hypoxemia, decreased compliance, increased airway resistance, and increased work of breathing.

III. The abnormal respiratory parameters were once thought to be caused primarily by the movement of the flail segment, but it is now believed that the underlying lung damage and hypoventilation from chest pain are much more important factors in the development of respiratory insufficiency.

Diagnosis

I. The diagnosis is made from the classic physical findings and confirmed with radiography.

II. Be sure to evaluate the thoracic cavity for evidence of additional trauma (e.g., pulmonary contusions, pneumothorax).

Treatment

I. Initially, the flail segment can be immobilized by positioning the patient with the affected side down. This may not be effective in barrel-chested dogs.

II. If pulmonary contusions are present, mechanical ventilation is the treatment of choice but is often not possible or practical for many veterinary patients.

III. Surgical stabilization is indicated to prevent further damage to intrathoracic structures, improve pulmonary ventilation, and decrease pain associated with movement of fragments.

A. The affected ribs can be stabilized by securing them to a sheet of plastic splinting material (Orthoplast, Pittman-Moore) that has been molded to conform to the thoracic wall.

1. Sutures can usually be placed circumferentially around the affected ribs under local anesthesia.

2. The suture ends are placed through holes drilled in the splint with a small Steinmann pin.

3. Aluminum rods may be substituted for the plastic splinting material.

B. Occasionally, open stabilization is indicated, particularly for intramedullary pinning of the affected ribs (proximally and distally); to repair the defect with a muscle flap transfer, diaphragm, or polypropylene mesh; or to directly suture the flail segment to adjacent ribs.

Patient Monitoring

I. Administer oxygen via nasal intubation, an oxygen cage, high-frequency jet ventilation, or intermittent positive pressure ventilation until signs of respiratory failure abate.

II. Monitor mucous membrane color, capillary refill time, respiratory rate, lung sounds, and heart rate and rhythm closely for the initial 72–96 hours.

III. Take radiographs at 48- to 96-hour intervals to ensure resolution of pulmonary abnormalities.

IV. Analgesics are indicated if the animal appears to be in severe pain, but drugs that may cause respiratory depression are contraindicated.

A. Consider butorphanol tartrate 0.2–0.4 mg/kg IV, IM, or SQ q 2–4 h (as needed).

B. Oxymorphone 0.05–0.1 mg/kg IV, IM, or SQ q 4–6 h (as needed) may also be used.

C. Perform an intercostal nerve block with bupivacaine supplied as 0.5% solution (2 mg/kg maximum dose).

1. This drug can also be injected into the thoracic cavity while the animal is under anesthesia (dilute to 0.25% solution).

2. Animals given bupivacaine intrathoracically are placed with the affected side down for 20 minutes.

Bibliography

Birchard SJ, Cantwell HD, Bright RM: Lymphangiography and ligation of the canine thoracic duct: a study in normal dogs and three dogs with chylothorax. J Am Anim Hosp Assoc 18:769, 1982

Birchard SJ, Gallagher L: Use of pleurodesis in treating selected pleural diseases. Compend Contin Educ Pract Vet 10:826, 1988

Birchard SJ, Smeak DD, Fossum TW: Results of thoracic duct ligation in dogs with chylothorax. J Am Vet Med Assoc 193:68, 1988

Boudrieau RJ, Fossum TW, Birchard SJ: Surgical correction of primary pneumothorax. J Am Vet Med Assoc 186:75, 1985

Dow SW, Jones RL, Adney WS: Anaerobic bacterial infections and response to treatment in dogs and cats: 36 cases (1983–1985). J Am Vet Med Assoc 189:930, 1986

Forrester SD, Troy GC, Fossum TW: Pleural effusions: pathophysiology and diagnostic considerations. Compend Contin Educ Pract Vet 10:121, 1988

Fossum TW, Birchard SJ, Jacobs RM: Chylothorax in 34 dogs. J Am Vet Med Assoc 188:1315, 1986a

Fossum TW, Jacobs RM, Birchard SJ: Evaluation of cholesterol and triglyceride concentrations in differentiating chylous and nonchylous pleural effusions in dogs and cats. J Am Vet Med Assoc 188:49, 1986b

Fossum TW, Forrester SD, Swenson CL et al: Chylothorax in cats: 37 cases (1969–1989). J Am Vet Med Assoc 198:672, 1991

Fossum TW, Evering WN, Miller MW et al: Severe bilateral fibrosing pleuritis associated with chronic chylothorax in dogs and cats. J Am Vet Med Assoc 201:317, 1992

Gallagher LA, Birchard SJ, Weisbrode SE: Effects of tetracycline hydrochloride on pleurae in dogs with induced pleural effusion. Am J Vet Res 51:1682, 1990

Glennon JC, Flanders JA, Rothwell JT, Shelly S: Constrictive pleuritis with chylothorax in a cat: a case report. J Am Anim Hosp Assoc 23:539, 1987

Holtsinger RH, Beale BS, Bellah JR et al: Spontaneous pneumothorax in the dog: a retrospective analysis of 21 cases. J Am Anim Hosp Assoc 29:195, 1993

Inauen W, Suzuki M, Granger DN: Mechanisms of cellular injury: potential sources of oxygen free radicals in ischemia/reperfusion. Microcirc Endothelium Lymphatics 5:143, 1989

Jackson RM, Brannen AL, Curtis FV, Fulmer JD: Superoxide

dismutase and cytochrome oxidase in collapsed lungs: possible role in reexpansion edema. J Appl Physiol 65:235, 1988

Kagan KG, Breznock EM: Variations in the canine thoracic duct system and the effects of surgical occlusion demonstrated by rapid aqueous lymphography, using an intestinal lymphatic trunk. Am J Vet Res 40:948, 1979

Kerpsack SJ, McLoughlin MA, Birchard SJ et al: Evaluation of mesenteric lymphangiography and thoracic duct ligation in cats with chylothorax: 19 cases (1987–1992). J Am Vet Med Assoc 205:711, 1994

Myer W: Radiography review: pleural effusion. J Am Vet Radiol Soc 19:75, 1978

Peterson SL, Pion PD, Breznock EM: Passive pleuroperitoneal drainage for management of chylothorax in two cats. J Am Anim Hosp Assoc 25:569, 1988

Shapiro W, Turrel J: Management of pleural effusion secondary to metastatic adenocarcinoma in a dog. J Am Vet Med Assoc 192:530, 1988

Shelly SM, Scarlett-Kranz J, Blue JT: Protein electrophoresis on effusions from cats as a diagnostic test for feline infectious peritonitis. J Am Anim Hosp Assoc 24:495, 1988

Sherding RG: Pyothorax in the cat. Compend Contin Educ Pract Vet 1:247, 1979

Smeak DD, Gallagher L, Birchard SJ, Fossum TW: Management of intractable pleural effusion in a dog with pleuroperitoneal shunt. Vet Surg 12:212, 1987

Stampley AR, Waldron DR: Reexpansion pulmonary edema after surgery to repair a diaphragmatic hernia in a cat. J Am Vet Med Assoc 203:1699, 1994

Stewart A, Padrid P, Lobingier R: Diagnostic utility of differential cell counts and measurement of LDH, total protein, glucose and pH in the analysis of feline pleural fluid. Proc Am Coll Vet Intern Med 8:1121, 1990

Stickle RL: Positive-contrast celiography (peritoneography) for diagnosis of diaphragmatic hernia in dogs and cats. J Am Vet Med Assoc 185:295, 1984

Valentine BA, Cooper BJ, Dietze AE, Noden DM: Canine congenital diaphragmatic hernia. J Vet Intern Med 2:109, 1988

Willard MW, Fossum TW, Torrance A, Lippert A: Hyponatremia and hyperkalemia associated with spontaneous and experimentally-induced chylothorax in the dog. J Am Vet Med Assoc 199:359, 1991

Willauer CC, Breznock EM: Pleurovenous shunting technique for treatment of chylothorax in three dogs. J Am Vet Med Assoc 191:1106, 1987

20

Diseases of the Mediastinum

Kenita S. Rogers

PNEUMOMEDIASTINUM

Definition

Pneumomediastinum (mediastinal emphysema) is the presence of free gas within the mediastinal space.

Causes

I. Penetrating wounds of the head, neck, and cranial thorax: air dissects into the mediastinum by following fascial planes
II. Airway or alveolar rupture
   A. Iatrogenic injury: bronchoscopy, mechanical ventilation, transtracheal wash, tracheostomy, overinflation of endotracheal tube cuff, traumatic intubation
   B. External trauma
   C. Severe, diffuse parenchymal disease
III. Esophageal rupture
   A. Perforating esophageal foreign body
   B. External trauma
   C. Esophageal ulceration with perforation
   D. Therapeutic procedures (e.g., ballooning or bougienage)
   E. Esophageal neoplasia
IV. Following abdominal surgery or rupture of a gas-filled viscus
V. Secondary to mediastinal infection by gas-producing organisms (rare)

Pathophysiology

I. Pneumomediastinum may be a benign condition with no overt clinical signs, but it can also be associated with subcutaneous emphysema and/or pneumothorax.
   A. A buildup of excessive air in the mediastinal space beyond 20 mmHg can cause rupture of the mediastinal pleura, leading to pneumothorax.
   B. The presence of air within the mediastinum may result in a local inflammatory reaction.

II. Gas within the mediastinum can originate from five sites.
   A. Lung
   B. Mediastinal airway: trachea, proximal mainstem bronchi
   C. Esophageal rupture
   D. Neck trauma or cervical surgical and diagnostic procedures
   E. Abdominal cavity

Clinical Signs

I. Clinical signs depend on the etiology of pneumomediastinum, the volume and pressure of mediastinal air, and the presence or absence of concurrent pneumothorax and infection.
II. Many animals are relatively asymptomatic.
III. Subcutaneous emphysema may be mild to profound.
IV. Respiratory distress and coughing occur with tracheal injury and significant pneumothorax.
V. Esophageal rupture and concurrent mediastinitis lead to thoracic pain, fever, and dysphagia.
VI. When air does not freely escape from the mediastinum into the neck, markedly elevated pressures can occur within the anterior thorax, leading to secondary sequelae.
   A. Ventilatory embarrassment or failure
   B. Diminished venous return from compression of the great veins
      1. Engorged neck veins
      2. Hypotension

Diagnosis

I. Compatible historical information
II. Physical examination findings and clinical signs as described earlier
III. Radiography
   A. Plain films are characterized by an ability to visualize structures not normally identified, e.g.,

cranial vena cava, azygous vein, brachiocephalic trunk, aorta, esophagus, and tracheal wall.
  B. Subcutaneous emphysema may be present, and fascial planes of the neck and front limbs may be recognized.
  C. Concurrent pneumothorax, pneumoretroperitoneum, and hydrothorax may be seen.
  D. Pneumopericardium is rare.
  E. An esophageal foreign body may be visualized.
IV. Endoscopy may help localize the lesion.
  A. Bronchoscopy can help confirm a large airway tear.
  B. Esophagoscopy is used to confirm and remove foreign bodies.

Treatment

  I. Uncomplicated cases are usually self-limiting and require no therapy.
  II. Most patients with significant dyspnea have concurrent pneumothorax that requires either simple thoracentesis or tube thoracostomy with frequent manual evacuation or continuous water seal drainage.
  III. Fresh neck wounds are treated with primary wound closure, and a neck bandage helps limit the spread of subcutaneous air.
  IV. Tracheal injuries require surgical intervention if the site does not seal spontaneously.
  V. Esophageal perforations require immediate surgical intervention.
  VI. If subcutaneous emphysema is extensive, needle aspiration may hasten resolution.

Patient Monitoring

  I. Resolution of the pneumomediastinum may take as long as 7–14 days after the primary disease is cured.
  II. Subcutaneous emphysema usually dissipates within 5–7 days.
  III. Serial radiographs are taken to determine if the condition is resolving or progressing. Progression is indicated by pneumothorax, pneumoretroperitoneum, and expansion of subcutaneous emphysema.

MEDIASTINITIS

Definition

  I. Mediastinitis is an acute, subacute, or chronic process producing inflammation within the mediastinal space.
  II. In animals, mediastinitis is associated primarily with infectious agents, particularly bacterial and fungal.

Causes

  I. Esophageal perforation or rupture
    A. Subsequent to foreign bodies such as bones, fish hooks, sticks, caustic agents
    B. Traumatic injuries
    C. Iatrogenic rupture during endoscopic examination, biopsy, or therapeutic procedures, e.g., bougienage, ballooning

    D. Primary esophageal neoplasm
  II. Tracheal perforation or rupture
    A. Traumatic injuries
    B. Iatrogenic with stylet usage during intubation
    C. Iatrogenic during bronchoscopic examination
  III. Penetrating thoracic trauma
    A. Bite wounds, projectiles
    B. Migrating foreign body, e.g., grass awn, sewing needle
  IV. Direct extension of infection from adjacent tissues such as the head, neck, and axillary region via fascial planes
  V. Direct extension of infection from intrathoracic tissues such as the pericardium, pleura, lymph nodes, and lungs
  VI. Complication of tube thoracostomy
  VII. Complication of thoracic surgery, particularly of mediastinal structures
  VIII. Secondary to bacteremia (rare)

Pathophysiology

  I. Acute mediastinitis is usually caused by bacterial organisms.
    A. The most common are *Streptococcus* spp., *Staphylococcus* spp., and *Escherichia coli* (Aronsohn, 1988).
    B. Anaerobic bacteria are an important component if the infection is caused by esophageal perforation.
    C. The infection can be diffuse or localized to single or multiple abscesses.
  II. Chronic mediastinitis is usually caused by fungal organisms.
    A. The most common are histoplasmosis, coccidioidomycosis, blastomycosis, and cryptococcosis.
    B. Bacteria such as *Actinomyces* spp., *Nocardia* spp., and *Corynebacterium* spp. may also cause chronic mediastinitis.
    C. Chronic mediastinitis occurs more commonly as discrete abscesses or granulomas.

Clinical Signs

  I. Acute mediastinitis: rapid onset, profound clinical signs
  II. Chronic mediastinitis: often insidious, few distinct signs
  III. Respiratory distress, dysphagia
  IV. Thoracic pain
  V. Fever
  VI. Concurrent pneumothorax or hydrothorax
  VII. Edema of the neck, head, and/or forelegs (cranial vena caval syndrome)

Diagnosis

  I. Compatible historical information
  II. Physical examination findings and clinical signs
  III. Radiography
    A. There may be no definitive findings on initial examination.

B. The mediastinum may be widened, with loss of detail and difficulty in visualizing normal structures.
C. With esophageal or tracheal rupture, air may be seen within the mediastinum or soft tissues of the neck.
D. Thoracic films may reveal a concurrent pneumothorax or hydrothorax.
E. Deviation of the trachea or esophagus can occur with abscesses or granulomas.
F. Consider a positive-contrast esophagram to evaluate esophageal integrity (see Chap. 4).
IV. Advanced imaging techniques: computed tomography scanning, magnetic resonance imaging
V. Fine-needle aspiration: culture and sensitivity, cytology
VI. Surgical biopsy via thoracotomy

Differential Diagnosis

I. Mediastinal masses, including neoplasia
II. Mediastinal hemorrhage secondary to trauma, thoracic surgery, coagulopathies, or thymic vascular disruption
III. Mediastinal edema secondary to infections, trauma, heart failure, and lymphangiectasis
IV. Mediastinal fat secondary to obesity
V. Esophageal diverticula

Treatment

I. Specific treatment is based on the etiology and severity of the underlying disease.
II. Medical therapy includes the following.
A. Antibiotics are indicated for suspected bacterial causes.
B. Choice of antibiotic is broad-spectrum, including activity against anaerobes. Therapy is continued for at least 3–6 weeks.
C. Antifungal therapy is started when a fungal disease is diagnosed (see Chap. 109) and is often continued for at least 3–6 months.
III. Surgical therapy may be considered.
A. Indicated in cases of esophageal or tracheal perforation
B. May be necessary to collect culture and biopsy specimens
C. May be required to establish pleural or local drainage, particularly after conservative methods have failed
D. For any large abscess or granuloma causing an obstructive mass
E. May be difficult and require segmental pulmonary resection
F. Postoperative chest tube drainage for several days to treat concurrent pyothorax

Patient Monitoring

I. Monitor clinical condition daily while animal is febrile, painful, or in respiratory distress.
II. Monitor radiographs at weekly intervals for bacterial disease and every 2–3 weeks for fungal disease. After clinical improvement, radiographs are evaluated at 2- to 4-week intervals.
III. Monitor hemograms at weekly intervals until condition stabilizes, then evaluate at 2- to 4-week intervals.
IV. If medical management fails to resolve the clinical signs, consider surgical exploration of the thoracic cavity.
V. Postoperatively, repeat thoracic radiographs at 2- to 4-day intervals. Remove the chest tube after the development of residual thoracic fluid is minimal.
VI. Monitor at periodic intervals for evidence of disease recurrence or incomplete resolution.

MASS LESIONS OF THE MEDIASTINUM

Definition

I. Space-occupying lesions within the mediastinal pleura
II. Includes enlargement of lymph nodes within the mediastinal compartments (particularly sternal, tracheobronchial, and hilar lymph nodes)

Causes and Pathophysiology

I. Abscess or granuloma (bacterial or fungal disease)
A. Local manifestation of a systemic infection
B. Secondary to contamination from a bite wound or esophageal perforation
II. Cysts (uncommon)
A. Usually benign and found in ventral compartment
B. Arise from diffuse cell lines, including pleural, lymphatic, bronchogenic, and thymic
III. Neoplasia
A. Primary and spontaneous from a mediastinal structure: lymph nodes, thymus, trachea, esophagus, or fat
B. Extension from adjacent structures: heart, lung, thoracic inlet, chemoreceptors, paravertebral tissues
C. Component of a multicentric or diffuse tumor: lymphosarcoma, histiocytic disorders
D. From ectopic tissue of the third and fourth branchial pouches: thyroid and parathyroid glands
E. Metastatic disease from a distant site
IV. Mediastinal lymphadenopathy
A. Infectious disorders
1. Bacterial organisms, particularly those associated with a concurrent mediastinitis or pyothorax or higher bacteria such as *Actinomyces* spp. and *Nocardia* spp., have been implicated.
2. The most common fungal infections are coccidioidomycosis, histoplasmosis, blastomycosis, and cryptococcosis.
3. Mycobacteria causing primary tuberculosis in dogs and cats are rare in the United States.

B. Neoplasia
  1. Lymphosarcoma (see Chap. 67)
      a) Multicentric form in the dog
      b) Presence of anterior mediastinal mass in dogs: poor prognosis (Rosenberg et al., 1991)
      c) Anterior mediastinal form in the cat
  2. Lymhomatoid granulomatosis
  3. Metastatic neoplasia
  4. Histiocytic disorders
C. Noninfectious granulomatous disorders with eosinophilia
  1. May or may not have extramediastinal involvement
  2. May also have pulmonary masses, peripheral eosinophilia, and eosinophils in pleural fluid

Clinical Signs

I. Clinical signs: reflect the underlying disease process
II. No clinical signs
  A. Small, slowly growing tumors or lymph nodes
  B. Small or walled-off abscess or granuloma
III. Associated clinical signs or findings
  A. Coughing and respiratory distress caused by tracheal or segmental bronchial compression or pleural effusion
  B. Dysphagia and drooling caused by esophageal compression or megaesophagus
  C. Edema of face, neck, and forelimbs secondary to compression of the vena cava (cranial vena caval syndrome)
  D. Laryngeal paralysis owing to peripheral nerve entrapment with resultant upper airway obstruction, changes in vocalization, and stridor
  E. Horner's syndrome
  F. Myasthenia gravis, hypogammaglobulinemia, hypercalcemia, and aplastic anemia with thymoma

Diagnosis

I. Compatible historical information
II. Physical examination findings and clinical signs
  A. Often nonspecific
  B. May include noncompressible anterior thorax in the cat
III. Thoracic radiography
  A. Abnormal density in any compartment of the mediastinum
  B. Compression or displacement of trachea, heart, or esophagus
  C. Esophagram demonstrating esophageal pathology and extrinsic displacement or compression
IV. Imaging techniques
  A. Ultrasonography may be useful in detecting an abscess, cyst, or neoplasm and pleural and pericardial effusion and in obtaining a biopsy.
  B. Radioisotope studies are useful to diagnose ectopic thyroid tissue.
  C. Advanced imaging techniques can help define involved tissues.

V. Cytology of lung and lymph node aspirates, pleural fluid, or biopsy specimens
VI. Culture and sensitivity of aspiration and biopsy specimens
VII. Serology for infectious diseases
VIII. Bronchoscopy for examination, biopsy, culture, or bronchoalveolar lavage
IX. Biopsy via thoracotomy
  A. Open biopsy may be necessary to make a diagnosis.
  B. Make impression smears if lymphoma is suspected, as chemotherapy (not excision) is the treatment of choice.
  C. Excisional biopsy is attempted for other masses.
  D. Completely explore the thoracic cavity to define the limit of the disease process.

Differential Diagnosis

The primary differential considerations would include any extramediastinal abnormality that causes increased soft tissue density in the area of the mediastinum, including lung masses, cardiac masses, diaphragmatic hernias, or mediastinal widening caused by fat, and esophageal diverticula or masses.

Treatment

I. Abscess or granuloma
  A. Specific antibacterial or antifungal agents
  B. Surgical drainage or removal
II. Cyst
  A. Extrathoracic drainage via needle aspiration
    1. Structure may shrink in size or disappear.
    2. If it recurs, consider surgery.
  B. Surgical removal
III. Neoplasia
  A. Surgical excision is indicated for selected cases of thymoma, chemodectoma, lipoma, teratoma, thyroid and parathyroid tumors.
  B. Chemotherapy is the treatment of choice for lymphosarcoma and some metastatic tumors (see Chap. 67).
  C. Radiation therapy may be indicated as adjunctive therapy for lymphosarcoma and thymoma.

Patient Monitoring

I. Postoperatively, an indwelling chest tube may be indicated for intermittent evacuation of fluid or air or for thoracic lavage.
II. Radiograph thorax 24–72 hours after surgery to check for persistent pneumothorax or effusion.
III. If a mediastinal abscess has been diagnosed, monitor body temperature and perform a complete blood count frequently for evidence of persistent infection.

Bibliography

Aronsohn MG: Diseases of the mediastinum. p. 227. In Morgan RV (ed): Handbook of Small Animal Practice. Churchill Livingstone, New York, 1988

Bauer T, Woodfield JA: Mediastinal, pleural, and extrapleural diseases. p. 812. In Ettinger SJ, Feldman EC (eds): Textbook of Veterinary Internal Medicine. 4th Ed. WB Saunders, Philadelphia, 1995

Fraser RG, Pare JAP, Pare PD et al: Diseases of the mediastinum. p. 2794. In Fraser RG (ed): Diagnosis of Diseases of the Chest. 3rd Ed. WB Saunders, Philadelphia, 1991

Pierson DJ: Disorders of the mediastinum: general principles and diagnostic approach. p. 2235. In Murray JF, Nadel JA (eds): Textbook of Respiratory Medicine. 2nd Ed. WB Saunders, Philadelphia, 1994

Postorino NC, Wheeler SL, Park RD et al: A syndrome resembling lymphomatoid granulomatosis in the dog. J Vet Intern Med 3:15, 1989

Rosenberg MP, Matus RE, Patnaik AK: Prognostic factors in dogs with lymphoma and associated hypercalcemia. J Vet Intern Med 5:268, 1991

Thrall DE: The mediastinum. p. 277. In Thrall DE (ed): Textbook of Veterinary Diagnostic Radiology. 2nd Ed. WB Saunders, Philadelphia, 1994

Neurologic System

21

Introduction

Karen Dyer Inzana

FUNCTIONAL ORGANIZATION

Anatomic Localization

I. Anatomically, the nervous system can be divided into seven different regions that contain one or more functional classes of neuron (Jenkins, 1978; Evans, 1993).

II. Lesions can be localized to each of these seven regions based on the specific upper motor neurons (UMNs), lower motor neurons (LMNs), sensory neurons (SNs), or integrative neurons (INs) affected.

  A. Motor unit disease

    1. The motor unit is defined as a single LMN, neuromuscular junction, and all the muscle fibers innervated by that LMN. Based on proximity, SN may be affected by disorders of the motor unit.

    2. It is difficult to distinguish between injury to each of these structures by clinical signs alone. However, it is common to clinically refer to injury to the motor unit as causing LMN signs.

    3. Clinical signs of injury to the motor unit or LMN signs include the following.

      a) Weakness to paralysis

      b) Diminished or absent spinal reflexes (see Table 21–1)

      c) Muscle atrophy

      d) Loss of sensation if the sensory neuron is also affected

    4. Clinical signs may be confined to one region or may be generalized if multiple motor units are affected.

  B. Spinal cord

    1. Each segment of the spinal cord contains LMNs, central extensions of SNs, and axons of UMNs.

    2. Unilateral injury causes deficits on the same side of the body as the injury. The clinical pattern of signs varies with the region affected.

      a) Spinal cord segments L4-S3

        (1) This region contains the LMNs that provide motor control to the rear limbs, tail, and anal and urinary sphincters.

        (2) Clinical signs of injury to this area cause motor unit or LMN signs to the rear limbs.

      b) Spinal cord segments T2-L4

        (1) This region contains LMNs for intercostal and abaxial skeletal muscle, sensory axons from these regions as well as those from more caudal regions, and axons from UMNs that are controlling the rear limb LMNs.

        (2) Clinical signs of motor unit injury to individual intercostal or abaxial muscles are difficult to detect; loss of UMN control to the LMNs innervating the pelvic limbs are commonly referred to as UMN signs to the rear limbs.

        (3) UMN signs include weakness to paralysis, exaggerated spinal reflexes, more gradual muscle atrophy, and loss of sensation if axons from SN are damaged.

      c) Spinal cord segments C6-T2

        (1) This region contains the LMNs for the thoracic limbs and axons from SNs and UMNs that control the pelvic limbs.

        (2) Clinical signs of injury to this region create LMN signs to the thoracic limbs and UMN signs to the pelvic limbs.

        (3) Preganglionic sympathetic neurons to the head and neck are located in spinal cord segments T1-T2. Injury to this area may cause Horner's syndrome (see Chap. 102).

      d) Spinal cord segments C1-C6

        (1) This region contains LMNs for cervical musculature and axons from SNs and UMNs.

(2) Clinical signs of injury to this region result in UMN signs to all four limbs.

(3) Severe injury results in respiratory compromise and death due to paralysis of both diaphramatic and intercostal muscles.

C. Pontomedullary region of the brain stem
1. The pons and medulla oblongata constitute the caudal regions of the brain stem and contain LMNs for cranial nerve nuclei V-XII, axons from peripheral SNs, and axons from some UMNs as well as some UMN cell bodies. Two integrative systems are also located in the pontomedullary region of the brain stem: the reticular formation and the cerebellum.
2. Clinical signs of injury to the pons and medulla consist of the following.
   a) LMN signs to structures innervated by cranial nerves V-XII (see Table 21-2)
   b) Upper motor neuron signs to all four limbs
   c) Gait and postural reaction deficits on the same side as a unilateral injury
   d) Mental dullness to coma with severe, diffuse injury to the pontomedullary reticular system

D. Cerebellum
1. The cerebellum is an integrative structure that embryologically is a part of the pons.
2. It coordinates voluntary motor activity and contributes to the vestibular system.
3. Clinical signs of cerebellar injury consist of loss of coordinated movement, generalized ataxia, intention tremors, and vestibular dysfunction if the flocculonodular lobes of the cerebellum are affected.

E. Midbrain region of the brain stem
1. The midbrain contains LMNs for cranial nerves III and IV, UMNs, axons from UMNs located in the cerebrum, axons from SN, and the reticular system.
2. Clinical signs of injury to the midbrain consist of LMN signs to structures innervated by cranial nerves III and IV and milder signs of UMN injury to the limbs.
3. Unilateral injury usually causes limb deficits more severe on the side opposite the lesion.
4. Derangements in consciousness and decerebrate body posture characterized by rigid extension of all four limbs and opisthotonos occur with severe injury.

F. Thalamus and hypothalamus
1. The thalamus functions largely as a relay center to the cerebrum for all sensory modalities.
2. Clinical signs are difficult to distinguish from cerebral lesions and consist of seizures, mild gait deficits, and behavioral changes.
3. The hypothalamus contains neurons that regulate autonomic and endocrine functions.
4. Clinical signs of injury to the hypothalamus include alterations in appetite, thirst, temperature regulation, electrolyte balance, behavior, and endocrine function.
5. Because of proximity to the optic chiasm, lesions in this area can also cause blindness and loss of pupillary light reflexes.

G. Cerebrum
1. The cerebrum consists largely of integrative structures as well as a few UMN nuclei.
2. Clinical signs of cerebral injury include mild gait deficits on the opposite side of the body, behavioral changes, and vision loss with normal pupillary light reflexes.
3. Stupor and coma may be seen with diffuse lesions.
4. Seizures are also seen with cerebral lesions.

EXAMINATION PROCEDURES

Physical Examination

I. Objectives of a neurologic examination are to determine the presence or absence of injury to the nervous system and to establish the location and extent of the injury.
II. There are four components to a thorough neurologic examination (Oliver and Lorenz, 1993; Braund, 1986).
   A. Observation at a distance (Fig. 21–1)
      1. Mentation/level of consciousness
         a) Abnormalities range from depression to coma.
         b) Changes are nonspecific but indicate a lesion rostral to the foramen magnum.
      2. Body posture
         a) Pontomedullary lesions cause a marked head tilt with the down ear usually directed to the side of the lesion.
         b) Lesions in the frontal lobe of the cerebrum create an aversive syndrome with the head turned toward the side of the lesion.
         c) Lesions in the thalamus and midbrain are more variable in their effect on body posture but may also cause head deviations, usually toward the side of the lesion.
   B. Gait/postural reactions
      1. Normal coordinated gait requires multiple levels of the nervous system (SN, LMN, UMN, and IN).
      2. Postural reactions include conscious proprioception, hopping, hemiwalking, wheelbarrowing, and extensor postural thrust.
      3. All are designed to put the foot in an abnormal position to bear weight and to test the animal's ability to recognize this incorrect position (SN) and correct it (UMN and LMN).
      4. Because multiple levels are necessary, gait/postural reactions are better at confirming a neurologic condition rather than localizing the level of the lesion.
      5. Gait/postural reaction deficits confined to the

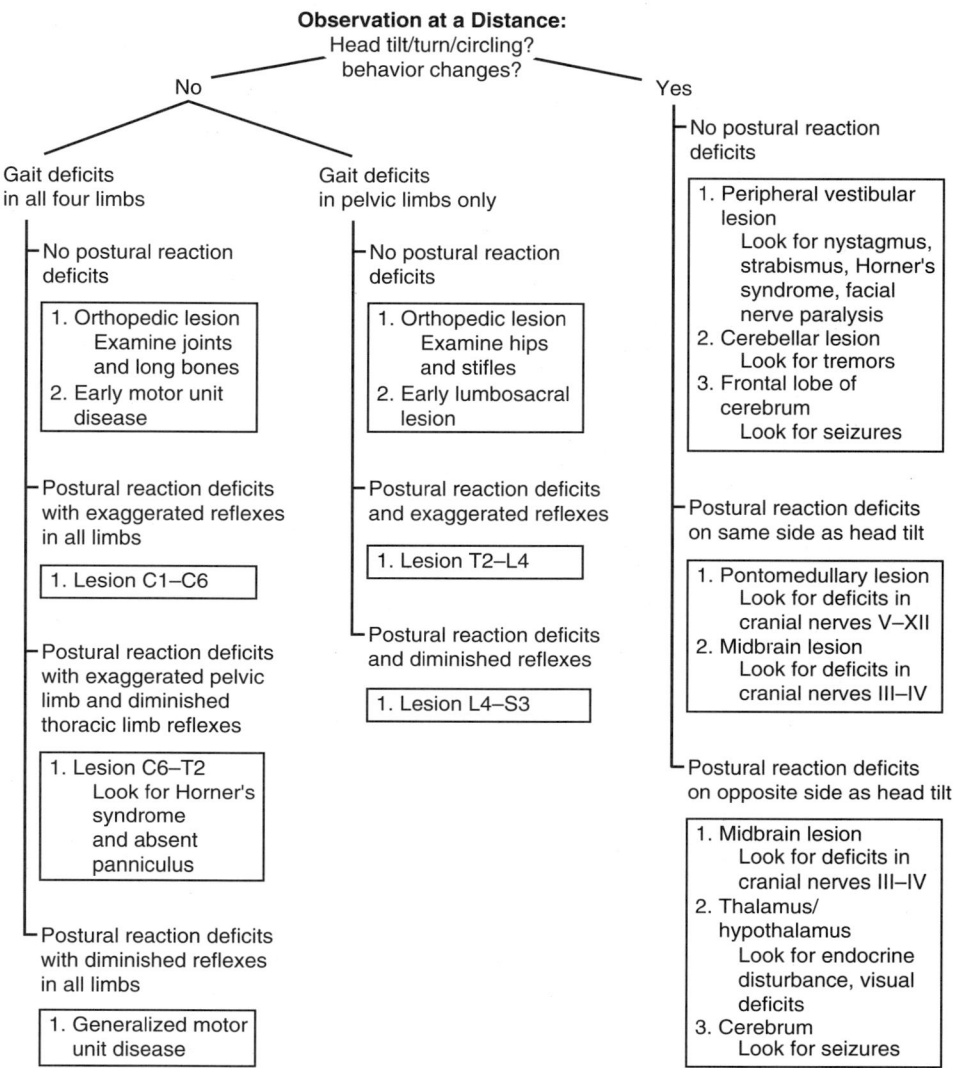

Figure 21–1. Small animal neurologic examination.

rear limbs (paraparesis or paraplegia) indicate a lesion caudal to spinal cord segments T2.

6. Gait/postural reaction deficits in all four limbs (quadriparesis or quadriplegia) indicate a lesion rostral to T2 spinal cord segments or generalized motor unit disorders.

7. Gait/postural reaction deficits on one side of the body (hemiparesis) indicate a unilateral lesion on the same side in the spinal cord or pontomedullary area of the brain stem; but they indicate a lesion on the opposite side if in midbrain, thalamus, or cerebrum.

C. Spinal reflexes
1. Spinal reflexes test the integrity of the motor unit (and associated sensory neurons).
2. Diminished reflexes are a strong indication of motor unit disorders.
3. Exaggerated reflexes indicate that UMNs and INs are no longer effectively modulating the response of LMNs.
4. Specific reflexes and the peripheral nerve and

spinal cord segments evaluated are listed in Table 21–1.

D. Cranial nerve examination
1. Cranial nerve deficits may occur after injury to the brain stem or peripheral course of the nerve.
2. Associated clinical signs help localize the site of injury.
3. Brain stem injury usually produces profound deficits in postural reactions, whereas peripheral nerve injury does not.
4. Specific cranial nerves and their functions are listed in Table 21–2.

Cerebrospinal Fluid Analysis

I. Cerebrospinal fluid (CSF) analysis is indicated to confirm central nervous system involvement in the disease process and to aid in the differentiation between degenerative, inflammatory, or neoplastic diseases (Vandeveld and Spano, 1977; Kornegay, 1981).

Table 21–1. **Spinal Reflexes**

Reflex	Procedure	Response	Peripheral Nerve	Spinal Cord Segments
Patellar reflex	Percuss patellar tendon	Extension of stifle	Femoral nerve	L4-L6
Gastrocnemius reflex	Percuss Achilles tendon	Extension of hock	Tibial branch of sciatic nerve	L6,7-S1
Cranial tibial reflex	Percuss muscle belly directly	Flexion of hock	Peroneal branch of sciatic nerve	L6,7-S1
Flexor reflex—pelvic limb	Noxious stimuli to limb	Flexion of limb	Medial toe: femoral nerve; lateral toe: sciatic nerve	L4-S1
Biceps reflex	Percuss biceps tendon	Flexion of elbow	Musculocutaneous nerve	C6-C8
Triceps reflex	Percuss triceps tendon	Extension of elbow	Radial nerve	C7-T2
Extensor carpi radialis reflex	Percuss muscle belly	Extension of carpus	Radial nerve	C7-T2
Flexor reflex—thoracic limb	Noxious stimuli to limb	Flexion of limb	Dorsal surface: radial nerve; palmar surface: median and ulnar nerves	C7-T2
Perineal reflex	Noxious stimuli to perineum	Constriction of anal sphincter and flexion of tail	Perineal nerve	S2-S3

II. CSF may be collected from the cisterna magna or lumbar cistern (see Chap. 3).

III. Increased intracranial pressure from any cause, including hemorrhage, edema, or mass lesions, increases the risk of displacement of the caudal cerebellar vermis through the foramen magnum or displacement of the temporal cerebral cortex beneath the tentorium cerebelli (Kornegay et al., 1983).

IV. Parameters routinely evaluated in CSF are as follows (see also Appendix I).

Table 21–2. **Cranial Nerves**

Cranial Nerve	Location	Anatomic Course	Function	Evaluation
CN I Olfactory	Cerebrum Pyriform cortex	Enters cribriform plate to olfactory lobe of cerebrum	Smell	Not routinely evaluated
CN II Optic	Thalamus	Enters optic foramen to optic chiasm to optic tracts	Vision, pupillary light reflexes	Menace response, pupillary light reflexes, avoidance of objects, visual placing
CN III Oculomotor	Midbrain	Orbital fissure through basilar sinus to midbrain	Parasympathetic to pupil, motor to medial, dorsal and ventral rectus, ventral oblique extraocular muscles	Pupillary light reflexes, conjugate eye movement, resting lateral strabismus
CN IV Trochlear	Midbrain	Orbital fissure through basilar sinus to midbrain; crosses in roof of 4th ventricle	Motor to dorsal oblique extraocular muscle	Eye movement (not routinely tested in dogs), resting rotational strabismus
CN V Trigeminal	Pons and medulla	Mandibular nerve: oval foramen; maxillary nerve: round foramen; ophthalmic nerve: orbital fissure	Motor to muscles of mastication; sensory to face	Jaw tone, masticatory muscle mass, sensation to face
CN VI Abducens	Pons and medulla	Orbital fissure through basilar sinus to pons and medulla	Motor to lateral rectus and retractor bulbi extraocular muscles	Eye movement, resting medial strabismus
CN VII Facial	Pons and medulla	Stylomastoid foramen, through middle ear to internal acoustic meatus	Motor to muscles of facial expression; parasympathetic to lacrimal gland	Blink, retract lip, move ear, tear production
CN VIII Vestibulocochlear	Pons and medulla	Jugular foramen to lateral surface of pons and medulla	Balance, hearing	Body posture, eye movement, hearing
CN IX Glossopharyngeal	Pons and medulla	Jugular foramen to lateral surface of pons and medulla	Sensory and motor to pharynx	Gag reflex, swallow
CN X Vagus	Pons and medulla	Jugular foramen to lateral surface of pons and medulla	Sensory and motor to pharynx, parasympathetic to viscera	Gag reflex, swallow
CN XI Accessory	Pons and medulla	Jugular foramen to lateral surface of pons and medulla	Motor to trapezius and brachiocephalicus muscles	Shoulder and neck muscle tone and mass
CN XII Hypoglossal	Pons and medulla	Hypoglossal canal to ventral surface of pons and medulla	Motor to tongue muscles	Tongue movement

A. Pressure (Simpson and Reed, 1987)
1. Dog: normally <160–170 mm H$_2$O
2. Cat: normally <100 mm H$_2$O, but not routinely measured

B. Physical appearance
1. CSF is normally clear and colorless.
2. CSF appears cloudy or turbid if there are >500 cells/ml.
3. CSF appears red if there are >6000 RBC/ml, and this indicates recent hemorrhage or contamination by peripheral blood during the procedure.
4. CSF appears yellow or xanthochromic if hemorrhage occurred into the subarachnoid space prior to obtaining the CSF sample. Crenated RBCs or RBCs within macrophages are also reliable signs of previous hemorrhage.

C. Total cell counts
1. Both RBC and WBCs degenerate rapidly in CSF because the protein content is too low to support most cells. Cell counts must be performed within 20–30 minutes of collecting the sample.
2. Normal WBC counts are <8 from the cisterna magna and <12 from the lumbar cistern.
3. The types of WBCs present can be of diagnostic significance (see Chap. 23).

D. Total protein
1. Normal protein concentration for CSF is <25 mg/dl when collected from the cisterna magna and <40 mg/dl when collected from the lumbar cistern.
2. Protein is elevated in any condition that causes necrosis of the CNS or disruption of the blood-brain barrier.

E. Antibody titers
1. Antibody titers to a number of infectious agents can be measured in CSF.
2. Any disruption of the blood-brain barrier results in antibody leakage into the CSF.
3. Techniques exist that establish the amount of peripheral blood contamination in CSF samples by comparing the amount of albumin in CSF and peripheral blood (Bichsel et al., 1984; Sorjonen, 1987; Sorjonen et al., 1989).

F. Culture
1. If CSF cytology indicates marked inflammation, especially if neutrophils are present, both anaerobic and aerobic bacterial cultures or fungal cultures of CSF fluid should be attempted (Dow et al., 1988).
2. False-negative results are common for bacterial infections.

Neuroradiology

I. Survey radiography
A. Nervous tissue is surrounded by bone and is therefore not readily visible on routine radiographs, but the bone is in intimate contact with neural tissue.
B. Changes in vertebral or skull density or position are helpful in diagnosing fractures, osteolytic tumors, or infections of bone or disk spaces.

II. Contrast studies
A. Myelography is the injection of iodinated contrast material into the subarachnoid space around the spinal cord and is the most commonly used technique to critically evaluate spinal cord compression.
B. Second-generation monometric nonionic triiodinated materials (iopamidol or iohexol) are the most commonly used for radiographic contrast materials (see Chap. 4).

III. Radioisotope scanning
A. A radionucleotide-labeled pharmaceutical (e.g., technetium-99m) is injected into a peripheral vein. If the blood-brain barrier has been disrupted, this radiopharmaceutical enters the nervous tissue and creates a focal area of radioactivity.
B. This technique is most commonly used to identify brain tumors.

IV. Computed tomography
A. Computer-assisted reconstruction of x-ray diffraction patterns allows differentiation of nervous tissue from surrounding bone (Fike et al., 1981; Kaufman et al., 1981).
B. Intravenous injection of iodinated contrast material can be used to identify focal areas with altered vascularity.
C. CT is most useful for mass lesions in the brain and allows sensitive assessment of any bony changes in the skull or vertebral column (Kornegay, 1990).

V. Magnetic resonance imaging (MRI)
A. Outer valence protons of molecules are "excited" by a large magnetic field. The energy released as these protons are then exposed to radiowaves produces a signal that can be recorded and reconstructed with computers to create an image similar to a CT scan (Thomson et al., 1993).
B. Paramagnetic material (gadolinium) can be injected intravascularly to better visualize focal areas of altered vascularity such as tumors.
C. MRI is more sensitive than CT at identifying changes in soft tissue structures; however, bone is poorly visualized.

Electrophysiology

I. Electromyography (EMG)
A. EMG measures the electrical activity of muscle fibers (Chrisman et al., 1972; Kimura, 1983).
B. Normal muscle at rest is electrically silent.
C. Voluntary contraction of a muscle causes synchronous contraction of motor units and produces characteristic motor unit potentials.
D. If the muscle is injured by disease or is denervated, it produces a variety of abnormal electrical potentials collectively referred to as spontaneous activity.
E. EMG helps identify motor unit disease but does

not reliably differentiate diseases affecting muscles from diseases affecting motor neurons or their axons.

II. Motor nerve evoked potentials

    A. By stimulating a peripheral nerve in several sites and recording from the same muscle, conduction rates of motor axons can be determined (Kimura, 1983).

        1. The amplitude and duration of the muscle action potential produced by electrical nerve stimulation reflects the synchrony of muscle contraction. Decreased amplitude and prolonged action potentials typically indicate neuropathy.

        2. Slow motor nerve conduction velocity is seen with demyelination of peripheral nerves but may also occur with cooling of the limb and in either young or older animals.

    B. Repetitive stimulation of the motor nerve at rates of 1–3 stimuli per second produces identical muscle action potentials in normal animals. Successively smaller action potentials during repetitive stimulation indicate inhibition of neuromuscular transmission as occurs in myasthenia gravis (Sims and McLean, 1990).

III. Sensory nerve conduction

    A. Sensory nerves may be evaluated by stimulating a peripheral nerve that contains only sensory fibers or stimulating a mixed motor and sensory nerve and recording directly from the spinal cord (Holliday et al., 1977; Holliday, 1992).

    B. Pure sensory neuropathies are rare.

IV. Evoked potentials

    A. Evoked potentials are action potentials recorded from nervous tissue that occur after either electrical or receptor-mediated stimulation.

    B. Evoked potentials evaluate the functional integrity of the nervous system and are useful for identifying both the severity and distribution of injury.

    C. Evoked potentials (EPs) useful in clinical medicine include the following.

        1. Visual EPs are used to evaluate visual receptors and the visual pathways to the occipital cortex following flashes of light (Sims et al., 1989).

        2. Brain stem auditory EPs are used to evaluate auditory receptors and the pathways through the brain stem that are activated following a series of clicking stimuli in the ear (Sims, 1988).

        3. Spinal cord evoked potentials are used to evaluate the sensory tracts in the spinal cord following electrical stimulation of a peripheral nerve (Holliday, 1992).

        4. Cortical evoked potentials are used to evaluate the integrity of sensory pathways through the brain stem to the somatosensory cortex following electrical stimulation of a peripheral nerve (Purinton et al., 1983).

V. Electroencephalography (EEG)

    A. The spontaneous electrical activity of the cerebral cortex and thalamus can be recorded by placing electrodes across the skull (Redding and Knecht, 1984).

    B. The action potentials recorded by this technique represent the summation of electrical activity occurring in the area of the recording electrode.

    C. Normal cortical electrical activity varies with age and level of arousal. It is also strongly influenced by anesthetics.

    D. Many diseases including congenital disorders, encephalitis, toxins, metabolic diseases, trauma, and neoplasia cause abnormal electrical activity in the EEG.

    E. There is considerable overlap in the abnormal EEG pattern produced by different diseases; therefore, abnormal EEG data must be correlated with other information to achieve an accurate diagnosis.

Bibliography

Bailey CS, Higgens RJ: Comparison of total white blood cell count and total protein content of lumbar and cisternal cerebrospinal fluid of healthy dogs. Am J Vet Res 46:1162, 1985

Bichsel P, Vandevelde M, Vandevelde E et al: Immunoelectrophoretic determination of albumin and IgG in serum and cerebrospinal fluid in dogs with neurologic diseases. Res Vet Sci 37:101, 1984

Braund KG: Clinical Syndromes in Veterinary Neurology. Williams & Wilkins, Baltimore, 1986

Chrisman CL, Burt JK, Wood PK, Johnson EW: Electromyography in small animal clinical neurology. J Am Vet Med Assoc 160:311, 1972

Chrisman CL: Problems in Small Animal Neurology. 2nd Ed. Lea & Febiger, Philadelphia, 1991

deLahunta A: Veterinary Neuroanatomy and Clinical Neurology. 2nd Ed. WB Saunders, Philadelphia, 1983

Dow SW, LeCouteur RA, Henik RA et al: Central nervous system infection associated with anaerobic bacteria in two dogs and two cats. J Vet Intern Med 2:171, 1988

Evans HE: Miller's Anatomy of the Dog. 3rd Ed. WB Saunders, Philadelphia, 1993

Fike JR, LeCouteur RA, Cann CE: Anatomy of the canine brain using high resolution computed tomography. Vet Radiol 22:236, 1981

Holliday TA: Electrodiagnostic examination: somatosensory evoked potentials and electromyography. Vet Clin North Am [Small Anim Pract] 22:833, 1992

Holliday TA, Ealand BG, Weldon NE: Sensory nerve conduction velocity: technical requirements and normal values for branches of the radial and ulnar nerves of the dog. Am J Vet Res 38:1543, 1977

Kandel ER, Schwartz JH: Principles of Neural Science. 3rd Ed. Elsevier, New York, 1991

Kaufman HH, Cohen G, Glass TF et al: CT atlas of the dog brain. J Comput Assist Tomogr 5:529, 1981

Kimura J: Electrodiagnosis in Diseases of Nerve and Muscle: Principles and Practice. FA Davis, Philadelphia, 1983

Kornegay JN: Cerebrospinal fluid collection, examination, and interpretation in dogs and cats. Compend Contin Ed Pract Vet 3:85, 1981

Kornegay JN: Imaging brain neoplasms. Computed tomography and magnetic resonance imaging. Vet Med Report 2:372, 1990

Kornegay JN, Oliver JE, Gorgacz EJ: Clinicopathologic features of brain herniation in animals. J Am Vet Med Assoc 182:1111, 1983

Lee AF, Bowen JM: Evaluation of motor nerve conduction velocity in the dog. Am J Vet Res 31:1361, 1970

Oliver JE, Lorenz MD: Handbook of Veterinary Neurology. 2nd Ed. WB Saunders, Philadelphia, 1993

Oliver JE, Horelein BF, Mayhew IG: Veterinary Neurology. WB Saunders, Philadelphia, 1987

Puglisi TA, Green RW, Hall CL et al: Comparison of metrizamide and iohexol for cisternal myelographic examination of dogs. Am J Vet Res 47:1863, 1986

Purinton PT, Oliver JE, Kornegay JN et al: Cortical averaged evoked potentials produced by pudendal nerve stimulation in dogs. Am J Vet Res 44:446, 1983

Redding RW, Knecht CE: Atlas of Electroencephalography in the Dog and Cat. Praeger, New York, 1984

Simpson ST, Reed RB: Manometric values for normal cerebrospinal fluid pressure in dogs. J Am Anim Hosp Assoc 23:629, 1987

Sims MH: Electrodiagnostic evaluation of auditory function. Vet Clin North Am [Small Anim Pract] 18:913, 1988

Sims MH, McLean RA: Use of repetitive nerve stimulation to assess neuromuscular function in dogs. A test protocol for suspected myasthenia gravis. Prog Vet Neurol 1:311, 1990

Sims MH, Laratta LJ, Bubb WJ et al: Waveform analysis and reproducibility of visual-evoked potentials in dogs. Am J Vet Res 50:1823, 1989

Sorjonen DC: Total protein, albumin quota, and electrophoretic patterns in cerebrospinal fluid of dogs with central nervous system disorders. Am J Vet Res 48:301, 1987

Sorjonen DC, Cox NR, Swango LJ: Electrophoretic determination of albumin and gamma globulin concentrations in the cerebrospinal fluid of dogs with encephalomyelitis attributable to canine distemper virus infection: 13 cases (1980–1987). J Am Vet Med Assoc 195:977, 1989

Thomson CE, Kornegay JN, Burn RA et al: Magnetic resonance imaging—a general overview of principles and examples in veterinary neurodiagnosis. Vet Radiol Ultrasound 34:2, 1993

Thomson CE, Kornegay JN, Stevens JB: Analysis of cerebrospinal fluid from the cerebellomedullary and lumbar cisterns of dogs with focal neurologic disease: 145 cases (1985–1987). J Am Vet Med Assoc 196:1841, 1990

van Bree H, Van Rijssen B, Van Ham L: Comparison of nonionic contrast agents iohexol and iotrolan for cisternal myelography in dogs. Am J Vet Res 52:926, 1991

Vandeveld M, Spano JS: Cerebrospinal fluid cytology in canine neurologic disease. Am J Vet Res 38:1827, 1977

Widmer WR, DeNicola DB, Blevins WE et al: Cerebrospinal fluid changes after iopamidol and metrizamide myelography in clinically normal dogs. Am J Vet Res 53:396, 1992

22

Seizures and Sleep Disorders

Michael Podell

SEIZURES

Definition

I. A seizure is defined as a nonspecific, sudden, often catastrophic event.

II. An epileptic seizure is the clinical manifestation of excessive and/or hypersynchronous abnormal neuronal activity in the cerebral cortex.
   A. An epileptic seizure has a specific neural origin, which is not true of all seizures.
   B. Absolute confirmation that a seizure is epileptic may be difficult, as it requires simultaneous visualization of behavioral and electroencephalographic (EEG) changes. As a result, historical information is often used in human and veterinary medicine to diagnose an epileptic seizure.
   C. Characteristics of a seizure include the following.
      1. Aura: the initial manifestation of a seizure
         a) It can last from minutes to hours.
         b) Animals can exhibit stereotypic sensory or motor behavior (pacing, licking), autonomic patterns (salivating, urinating, vomiting), or even unusual psychic events (excessive barking, increased or decreased attention seeking).
      2. Ictus: the actual seizure event manifested by involuntary muscle tone or movement and/or abnormal sensations or behavior, usually lasting from seconds to minutes
      3. Postictus: the period immediately after the ictal event
         a) An animal can exhibit unusual behavior, disorientation, inappropriate bowel or bladder activity, excessive or depressed thirst and appetite, and actual neurologic deficits of weakness, blindness, and sensory and motor disturbances (Todd's paralysis) during this time.
         b) The postictal period can last from minutes to days and rarely longer.

III. Status epilepticus is continuous seizure activity for 30 minutes or longer without a return to normal consciousness during this time.

IV. Epilepsy is a chronic brain disorder characterized by recurrent epileptic seizures.

Causes

I. Recurring or nonrecurring epileptic seizures (EEG evidence of epileptic activity)
   A. Primary epileptic seizures
      1. Cryptogenic: neurophysiologic or neurochemical abnormality of the brain that is undetectable
      2. Idiopathic: undetermined cause
      3. Genetic basis believed to be the common denominator
   B. Secondary epileptic seizures: structural abnormality of the brain present
      1. Developmental anomaly: hydrocephalus, lissencephaly
      2. Inflammatory disorders: canine distemper virus, granulomatous meningoencephalitis
      3. Trauma
      4. Neoplasia
      5. Vascular disorders: stroke, vasculitis
      6. Degenerative diseases: lysosomal storage disorders
   C. Reactive epileptic seizures
      1. Normal brain reacting to an abnormality in systemic metabolism
      2. Examples: hepatic encephalopathy, uremia, hypoglycemia

II. Nonepileptic seizures (no EEG evidence of epileptic activity)
   A. Non-neurologic
      1. Cardiovascular: arrhythmia-induced syncope
      2. Metabolic disorders: Addison's disease
      3. Toxicities: strychnine
   B. Neurologic
      1. Vestibular attacks

2. Myasthenia gravis
3. Narcolepsy

Pathophysiology

I. The pathogenesis of epilepsy is multifactorial.
   A. Genetically determined "seizure susceptibility factors" play a crucial role in the brain's response to triggering or precipitating factors.
   B. Seizures in these individuals may be activated from unrecognized changes in neuronal activity or intrinsic neurochemical transmission or by environmental stimuli that do not cause seizures in the normal brain.
   C. A basic tenet in the mechanism of epilepsy is the presence of an imbalance in excitatory and inhibitory neurotransmission (Fenner and Hass, 1989). A seizure develops when the balance shifts toward excessive excitation.
      1. Glutamate is the principal excitatory neurotransmitter in the brain.
      2. Gamma-aminobutyric acid (GABA) is the principal inhibitory neurotransmitter in the brain.
   D. Conditions leading to excessive excitation or loss of inhibition lead to depolarization of neurons without normal regulatory feedback mechanisms (McNamara, 1992).
      1. The result is a paroxysmal depolarization shift of a neuronal aggregate.
      2. In response to this sudden change in brain activity, local surround inhibitory zones are established to try to prevent the spread of this epileptogenic activity.
      3. If inhibition is unsuccessful, other neuronal aggregates are excited through thalamocortical recruitment, intrahemispheric association pathways, or interhemispheric commissural pathways.
      4. Successful recruitment of a critical number of areas with synchronized depolarization leads to a seizure.

II. Alterations in neurologic function can occur with seizures.
   A. Acute brain damage in the epileptic animal begins at the subcellular level, progresses to the cellular level, and over time results in overt pathologic changes to the brain and eventual permanent changes in brain function.
   B. Mechanisms of neuronal cytotoxicity are multifactorial.
      1. Excitotoxicity from excessive accumulation of glutamate
      2. Uncoupling of cerebral metabolic demand and energy sources
         a) Higher metabolic activity of the brain during seizure events
         b) Reduction in aerobic glycolysis, resulting in less energy for cells
         c) Ischemia, which reduces delivery of glucose and other nutrients to the brain
      3. Cerebral edema from physiologic disruption of the blood-brain barrier, with subsequent increase in intracranial pressure and possible ischemia
      4. Physiologic systemic changes
         a) Hyperthermia
         b) Hypoventilation leading to hypoxia
         c) Systemic arterial hypertension
   C. Clinical manifestations are as follows.
      1. Vision loss
      2. Circling
      3. Paresis
      4. Profound disorientation
      5. Personality changes
   D. The most common chronic change in neurologic function is persistent behavior disturbances.
      Lack of obedience, withdrawal activity, changes in socialization with other animals or people in the household, and unprovoked aggressive behavior can all occur as interictal manifestations of a chronic epileptic condition in the dog.

III. Propagation of further seizures involves the following.
   A. In the initial stages of idiopathic epilepsy, an animal may possess only a single or limited number of epileptic foci.
   B. With recurrent seizure activity, however, the number of cells with an intrinsic pattern of high spontaneous firing activity (pacemaker cells) increases in the epileptic focus, which is highly correlated with increased seizure frequency.
   C. As an animal continues to have seizures, the number of areas of the brain that are randomly and spontaneously able to initiate a seizure increases.
   D. A mirror focus of actively firing epileptogenic neurons may also develop in a homologous region in the opposite hemisphere, and the number of epileptic foci can multiply rapidly.
   E. Prevention of this sequence relies primarily on early identification of the underlying etiology of the seizure disorder, followed by initiation of proper medical therapy.

Clinical Signs

I. Partial seizures are the manifestation of a focal epileptogenic event in the cerebral cortex. The focal nature of this seizure type is associated with a higher incidence of focal intracranial pathology.
   A. Simple partial
      1. Asymmetrical motor or sensory signs occur without a change in consciousness.
      2. Examples include facial focal seizures or excessive pawing or biting of a body part.
   B. Complex partial
      1. Impaired consciousness occurs and is often associated with unusual behaviors.
      2. Examples include "fly-biting" behavior patterns, aggressiveness without provocation, incessant howling or barking, restlessness, or a variety of motor disturbances.

II. Generalized seizures are characterized by impaired consciousness coupled with bilateral motor signs and are not necessarily associated with focal cerebrocortical disease.
   A. Convulsive (grand mal) seizure
      1. The most common type of seizure observed in the dog
      2. Tonic-clonic: alternating rigid extension and rapid flexion
      3. Atonic: complete loss of tone of antigravity muscles
      4. Myoclonic: muscle jerking
   B. Nonconvulsive (petit mal) seizure
      1. Impaired consciousness the only sign
      2. Poorly documented in animals

Diagnosis

I. Diagnostic goals include the following.
   A. Determine an etiology.
   B. Evaluate prognosis for seizure recurrence.
   C. Establish whether medical therapy is necessary.
II. Obtain historical information.
   A. Pedigree information, vaccination status, and recent travel
   B. Trauma and potential toxin exposure
   C. Previous medical and surgical problems
   D. Drug history
III. Tabulate seizure information to evaluate progression and changes.
   A. Dates and times
   B. Description
   C. Duration
   D. Postictal changes
IV. Identify interictal changes that may indicate underlying forebrain disease.
   A. Mentation: changes in behavior, such as being more withdrawn or attention seeking, any unusual episodes of aggression or irritability, or failure to follow simple commands
   B. Vision: bumping into objects on one side
   C. Gait: evidence of mild conscious proprioceptive disturbances, such as stumbling up and/or down stairs
   D. Sleep/wake cycle disturbances: restless sleep patterns or looking tired
V. Obtain a minimum database.
   A. Complete blood count
   B. Serum chemistry profile
   C. Urinalysis
VI. Consider advanced diagnostic testing.
   A. Metabolic screening may be performed but may not reveal a diagnosis.
      1. Liver function testing
         a) Serum bile acid study
         b) Fasting plasma ammonia concentration
         c) Definitive testing for portosystemic shunts (see Chap. 34)
      2. Serial fasting blood glucose and insulin concentrations (see Chap. 45)
      3. Specific serum antibody titers for infectious

diseases, e.g., neosporosis, toxoplasmosis, fungal infections
      4. Blood lead concentration
   B. EEG in dogs mainly helps identify underlying cerebrocortical disease.
      1. The EEG may also be used as a prognostic indicator in idiopathic epileptic dogs.
      2. The presence of interictal epileptic activity may correlate with an increased risk of seizure recurrence.
   C. Cerebrospinal fluid collection and analysis (see Chaps. 3 and 21) is most helpful in identifying inflammatory conditions of the brain.
      1. Collect fluid from the cerebellomedullary cistern.
      2. This is a relatively nonspecific yet sensitive test for the identification of intracranial neoplasia.
   D. The most specific test for the identification of malformations, mass effects, or other changes in brain architecture is neuroimaging.
      1. Computed tomography
      2. Magnetic resonance imaging

Differential Diagnosis

I. Epidemiology approach (Podell et al., 1995)
   A. Dog (Fig. 22–1)
      1. The probability of primary (idiopathic) epileptic seizures increases with the following.
         a) The dog is between 1 and 5 years of age at the first seizure.
         b) The dog is a large breed (>15 kg).
         c) The dog is a purebred dog documented to have a hereditary component for epilepsy.
         d) The interval between the first and second seizure events is long (>4 weeks).
      2. The probability of secondary epileptic seizures increases with the following.
         a) The dog is <1 or >7 years old at the first seizure.
         b) The first seizure is a partial seizure.
         c) The interval between the first and second seizure events is brief (<4 weeks).
      3. The probability of reactive epileptic seizures increases when the interval between the first and second seizure events is brief (<4 weeks).
   B. Cat
      1. No epidemiologic data are available to predict accurately which cats are more prone to a particular seizure etiology.
      2. All cats are regarded as having secondary or reactive epileptic seizures until definitively proved otherwise.
II. Age-related approach
   A. Dog
      1. <1 year of age
         a) The most common causes of seizures are developmental and inflammatory diseases (Oliver, 1980).

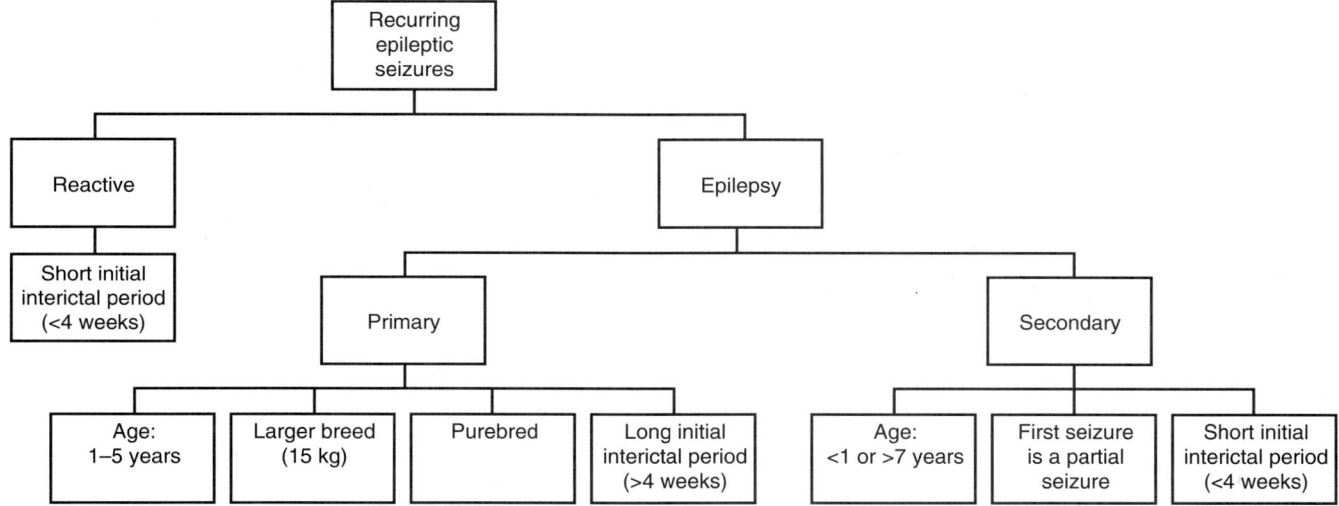

Figure 22–1. Flow chart of an epidemiologic approach to the differential diagnosis of epileptic seizures in the dog. Primary epilepsy represents an idiopathic cause, and secondary epilepsy represents a structural lesion of the brain. Reactive epileptic seizures imply that a normal brain is reacting adversely to a change in systemic metabolism. The boxes underneath each of these categories are risk factors that have been shown to be associated with that particular diagnosis.

  b) Specific diseases to consider are canine distemper encephalitis and hydrocephalus.
  c) Although specific breeds such as the Maltese, Chihuahua, Yorkshire terrier, and the brachycephalic breeds are prone to congenital hydrocephalus, any dog may suffer from this disease (Becker and Selby, 1980).
  d) Congenital portosystemic shunting is always ruled out for this age group.
 2. 1–5 years of age
  a) The most common cause of seizures is primary epilepsy.
  b) A proportion of dogs in this age category may suffer from a congenital brain anomaly that is progressive in nature.
 3. >5 years of age: brain tumors more prevalent
B. Cat
 1. <1 year of age
  a) Inflammatory disease: feline infectious peritonitis, protozoal infection, other viral meningoencephalitides
  b) Developmental anomalies of the brain
  c) Metabolic disease
 2. 1–7 years of age
  a) Inflammatory disease
  b) Trauma
  c) Toxicities
  d) Vascular accidents: feline ischemic encephalopathy
 3. >7 years of age
  a) Neoplasia
  b) Metabolic disease
  c) Vascular accidents: feline ischemic encephalopathy

Treatment

 I. Principles of therapy (Podell, 1996)
  A. Ultimate goal: seizure-free status without adverse effects
  B. Realistic goals
   1. Seizure control, not necessarily seizure elimination
   2. Decrease in frequency and severity of seizures
   3. Prevention of cluster seizure events
   4. Decrease in postictal severity
  C. Realistic expectations by owners
   1. Lifelong commitment
   2. Daily medication commitment
   3. Potential for emergency treatment
   4. Inherent risks of therapy
 II. Reasons to start monotherapy
  A. Identifiable structural lesion is present (secondary epileptic seizures).
  B. Status epilepticus has occurred.
  C. More than three generalized seizures have occurred within a 24-hour period.
  D. Two or more cluster seizure events (two or more seizures) have occurred within a 12-week period.
  E. Two or more isolated seizure events have occurred within an 8-week period.
  F. The first seizure was within 1 week of head trauma.
  G. Prolonged, severe, or unusual postictal periods occur.
 III. Monotherapy options (Table 22–1)
  A. Dog: generalized seizures
   1. Phenobarbital is the drug of choice.
    a) Phenobarbital is given initially at 2.5 mg/kg PO BID, with subsequent increases within 30 days to maintain a trough thera-

Table 22–1. **Summary of Antiepileptic Drug Therapy in the Dog**

Monotherapy phenobarbital as the first choice
Indications
- Identification of a structural lesion
- Status epilepticus
- Two or more isolated seizures within an 8-wk period
- Two or more cluster seizure episodes within a 12-wk period
- First observed seizure within 1 week of head trauma
- Prolonged, severe, or unusual postictal periods

Pharmacokinetics
- Initial elimination half-life of 42–89 h
- Steady-stage elimination half-life of 24–30 h
- Steady-state serum concentration and total body clearance stable by 30 days

Mechanisms of action
- Facilitation of inhibitory neurotransmission via GABA receptors
- Inhibition of postsynaptic potentials produced by glutamate
- Inhibition of voltage-gated calcium channels

Administration
- 2.5 mg/kg PO BID
- IV loading dose: total mg IV = body weight (kg) × 0.8 L/kg × 25 μg/ml

Monitoring
- Measure trough serum phenobarbital concentrations at 14, 45, 90, 180, and 360 days and every 6 mo thereafter
- Therapeutic range is 20–40 μg/ml
- Evaluate serum chemistry panel at 45 days and every 6 mo

Adverse effects
- Transient: lethargy, behavior change
- Persistent: Polyuria, polydipsia, polyphagia, weight gain, excessive sedation, splenomegaly, hepatomegaly, elevation in serum alkaline phosphatase, decrease in serum thyroxine and urine specific gravity
- Severe: hepatotoxicity
- Functional tolerance

Potassium bromide as add-on second drug
Indications
- Persistent seizure activity with steady-state trough serum phenobarbital concentration ≥30 μg/ml for at least 1 mo
- Hepatotoxicity from phenobarbital or primary hepatic disease (e.g., portosystemic shunt)
- Severe cluster seizures

Pharmacokinetics
- Average biologic elimination half-life of 25–46 days
- Time to achieve steady-state kinetics: 120 days

Mechanisms of action
- Competitive interaction with chloride to hyperpolarize neuronal membranes
- Synergistic effect with drugs that enhance chloride conductance (e.g., barbiturates)

Administration
- Potassium bromide dissolved in double distilled water as 200 mg/ml solution
- Dose: 20–40 mg/kg/day PO in food as initial dose
- Dose can be given once a day or divided every 12 h

Monitoring
- Measure trough serum concentrations 30 and 120 days after initiation and then every 6 mo
- Therapeutic range is 100–200 mg/dl (1000–2000 μg/ml) with concurrent phenobarbital administration to maintain trough serum phenobarbital concentration at 25–30 μg/ml
- Decrease phenobarbital if signs of hepatotoxicity occur or if dog is seizure free for 6 mo

Adverse effects
- Lethargy
- Polydipsia, polyuria
- Pancreatitis
- Ataxia
- Stupor

Felbamate
Indications
- Complex partial seizures
- Refractory to phenobarbital and bromide therapy

Pharmacokinetics
- Elimination half-life of about 6 h
- Renal excretion (90%)
- Causes a 25% increase in current phenobarbital levels

Mechanisms of action
- Reduces excitatory neurotransmission
- Prevents seizure spreading in brain

Administration
- Dogs <10 kg: 200 mg PO TID; increase 200 mg/wk up to a maximum dose of 600 mg PO TID or until seizure control is obtained
- Dogs >10 kg: 400 mg PO TID; increase 400 mg/wk to a maximum dose of 1200 mg PO TID or until seizure control is obtained

Monitoring and adverse effects
- No active drug metabolites are commercially measurable
- Monitor complete blood counts every 8–12 wk to check for bone marrow suppression
- Monitor liver enzymes every 8–12 wk to check for hepatotoxicity

peutic serum concentration (see Patient Monitoring).

b) Phenobarbital is rapidly absorbed within 2 hours, with a maximal plasma concentration obtained 4–8 hours after oral administration. Thus, peak serum concentrations are measured 6 hours after the last dose if toxicity is suspected.

c) It may compete with other drugs for protein-binding sites in the blood.

(1) The higher the unbound portion of serum phenobarbital, the higher the brain concentration.

(2) Concomitant use of certain highly protein-bound drugs (e.g., digoxin) may cause signs of phenobarbital neurotoxicity.

d) Phenobarbital is an autoinducer of hepatic microsomal enzymes (p450 system), which can progressively reduce its elimination half-life with chronic dosing.

e) Initial steady-state serum phenobarbital

concentrations are achieved in approximately 14 days.

f) At 5 mg/kg/day dosing, steady-state serum phenobarbital concentration and total body clearance are stable by 30 days.

2. Potassium bromide (KBr)

a) KBr is administered as a 200 mg/ml solution dissolved in double distilled water at 20–40 mg/kg/day PO.

b) KBr has an elimination half-life in the dog of about 25 days. Steady-state concentrations may not be obtained for over 3 months. Serum concentrations may fluctuate during this time.

c) Monotherapy KBr is most effective in the epileptic dog after seizures have been controlled with concomitant phenobarbital and KBr.

B. Dog: partial seizures

1. Felbamate (Felbatol) is a dicarbamate that is believed to increase the seizure threshold and prevent seizure spreading by reducing excitatory neurotransmission in the brain.

a) It is most successful in treating partial seizure activity.

b) Dosing in dogs <10 kg is as follows.

(1) Initially give 200 mg PO TID.

(2) Increase by 200 mg per week up to a maximum dose of 600 mg PO TID or until seizure control is obtained.

c) Use the following doses in dogs >10 kg.

(1) Initially give 400 mg PO TID.

(2) Increase by 400 mg per week up to a maximum dose of 1200 mg PO TID or until seizure control is obtained.

2. Clorazepate is a longer-acting benzodiazepine with active metabolites.

a) Monotherapy dose is 2 mg/kg PO BID.

b) No benefit is attained from use of the sustained-release formulation.

C. Cat: generalized seizures

1. Diazepam 2.5 mg PO TID

a) Increase by 2.5 mg per week if seizures are uncontrolled.

b) Maximum dose is 7.5 mg PO TID.

2. Clorazepate

a) Initial dose is 3.75 mg PO BID.

b) Titrate the dose up or down depending on response and excessive sedation.

3. Phenobarbital

a) Initial dose is 2.5 mg/kg PO SID.

b) Elimination half-life of 41–45 hours suggests that once-a-day dosing may be adequate, but twice-a-day dosing may be needed for seizure control.

c) A wide variation of response and adverse effects can occur in the cat.

d) A vitamin K–dependent coagulopathy can occur at higher, chronic dosing.

4. Potassium bromide at 30 mg/kg/day

a) Give in capsule formulation or in flavored syrup.

b) Elimination half-life is approximately 11–13 days.

c) Steady-state concentration is obtained in 7–8 weeks.

D. Cat: partial seizures

1. Benzodiazepines are the drugs of choice.

2. Use these drugs as for generalized seizures.

IV. Treatment of the refractory canine epileptic

A. Definition of refractory idiopathic epilepsy

1. Seizure etiology has not been identified.

2. Phenobarbital has been administered for at least 3 months, with all serum trough concentrations between 20 and 40 μg/ml and a trough, steady-state concentration >30 μg/ml without a subsequent change in dosage for at least 1 month prior to KBr initiation.

3. Seizure number and severity have not changed for at least 3 months, despite phenobarbital and other antiepileptic drug treatment.

B. Potassium bromide (Podell and Fenner, 1993)

1. KBr is the recommended second antiepileptic drug to be used in combination with phenobarbital.

2. Initial dose of 10 mg/kg PO BID is given in food.

a) This protocol allows for a gradual adaptation to the cumulative sedative effects of KBr and phenobarbital.

b) Dosages are then adjusted based on trough serum concentrations (see Patient Monitoring).

C. Long-acting benzodiazepines

1. Clorazepate 2 mg/kg PO BID may be tried.

2. Do not use oral diazepam, as this reduces the effectiveness of diazepam as an emergency treatment.

D. Felbamate as described for monotherapy

1. Decrease the existing phenobarbital dosage by 25% when starting felbamate therapy.

2. The combination of KBr and felbamate may be useful in dogs with refractory idiopathic epilepsy and/or underlying drug-induced hepatotoxicity.

V. Hospital emergency treatment for seizures

A. Criteria for bringing an animal to the hospital for emergency therapy

1. Excessive duration of a single seizure (>5 minutes)

2. One or more seizures per hour for 3 consecutive hours regardless of seizure length

3. Status epilepticus

4. Three or more seizures in a 24-hour period

B. Supportive therapy

1. Maintain a patent airway.

2. Administer thiamine (vitamin B$_1$) 25–50 mg IM.

a) Give it before any dextrose-containing solution is administered.

b) Thiamine is an essential coenzyme in glucose use by the brain.

3. Administer 50% dextrose 1 ml/kg IV over 10 minutes.

4. Administer isotonic saline IV at a maintenance rate (IV diazepam can precipitate in
other crystalloid solutions).
5. Maintain normal body temperature.
   a) Animals may become hyperthermic with
   continuous or recurrent seizure activity.
   b) All cooling measures are stopped when
   rectal temperature reaches 102°F (to prevent rebound hypothermia).
C. Phase 1 of specific seizure therapy
   1. This therapy consists of using short-acting
   anticonvulsants with minimal side effects to
   immediately control the active seizures, while
   rapidly establishing serum levels of a maintenance drug to preserve control.
   2. Administer a bolus dose of diazepam 0.5 mg/
   kg IV at a rate not exceeding 5 mg/minute.
   Diazepam is given if a seizure episode lasts
   at least 1 minute, there have been two or
   more seizures, or an underlying intracranial
   etiology is suspected.
   3. Administer phenobarbital simultaneously with
   diazepam to provide sustained antiepileptic effect as the serum levels of diazepam decline.
      a) A loading dose of phenobarbital is given
      to all drug-naive patients to rapidly estab-
      lish therapeutic drug levels using the for-
      mula: loading dose (total mg) = desired
      serum level (μg/ml) × body weight (kg)
      × 0.8 L/kg.
         (1) Use an IV injection at a rate not ex-
         ceeding 100 mg/minute.
         (2) For dogs, the desired serum level is
         25 μg/ml.
         (3) For cats, the desired serum level is 15
         μg/ml.
      b) For confirmed epileptics, evaluate serum
      phenobarbital level before administering
      more of the drug.
         (1) Give 1 mg/kg IV for each μg/ml of
         desired increase in the animal's se-
         rum level.
         (2) Raise the serum concentration in in-
         crements of 5 μg/ml.
         (3) If the phenobarbital level is ≥35 μg/
         ml, go to phase 2.
   4. Institute maintenance phenobarbital either PO
   or IM.
      a) Naive animals
         After the IV loading dose, initiate oral
         therapy at a dose of 2.5 mg/kg BID at the
         next time of administration.
      b) Established epileptic animals
         (1) Increase the dose to a level higher
         than that being administered on ad-
         mission.
         (2) Use the formula: (Desired level/estab-
         lished level) × total mg = new total
         mg/day.
         (3) Increase the desired level in the main-
         tenance-dose formula at increments of
         5 μg/ml up to 40 μg/ml (dog) or 30
         μg/ml (cat).

D. Phase 2 of specific seizure therapy
   1. If the seizures stop after phase 1 therapy,
   continue to administer maintenance phenobarbital PO or IM at the dose calculated.
   2. If the seizures continue, but at a lower frequency than before, administer an additional
   dose (0.5 mg/kg) of diazepam IV.
      a) Continue to administer maintenance phe-
      nobarbital PO or IM at the calculated
      dose.
      b) If the animal has more than three seizures
      after starting therapy, go to phase 3.
      c) If there is a continued high frequency of
      seizures, proceed directly to phase 3.
E. Phase 3 of specific seizure therapy
   1. This phase of therapy is designed for animals
   that fail to respond to the initial course of
   bolus doses of IV diazepam and phenobarbital.
   2. Begin a continuous IV diazepam infusion at
   an initial rate of 0.1 mg/kg/h in 2.5%
   dextrose/0.9% NaCl at a maintenance rate.
      a) The dose can be increased up to 0.5 mg/
      kg/h (dog) or 0.3 mg/kg/h (cat).
      b) Seizures can occur with benzodiazepine
      withdrawal, so the dosage rate should be
      decreased by 25% every 6 hours for at
      least two reductions before discontinuing
      the drug.
   3. If the animal has three or more seizures while
   on the diazepam infusion, administer pentobarbital or propofol IV.
      a) For pentobarbital, give an initial bolus to
      induce general anesthesia at 2 mg/kg IV
      slowly to effect (if the patient has been on
      phenobarbital prior to admission, a higher
      dose may be needed).
      b) For propofol, give a slow infusion of 4–8
      mg/kg IV to effect.
         (1) Advantages of propofol are that it is
         excreted primarily renally (therefore
         it is safer to use in dogs with liver
         disease), is rapidly metabolized to
         allow for rapid recovery, and does not
         induce any biochemical changes.
         (2) Disadvantages of propofol are that it
         can induce apnea, cause hypovolemia,
         and is relatively expensive for pro-
         longed use.
      c) Maintain the anesthesia for 4 hours.
      d) Provide supportive care.
         (1) Maintain a separate IV catheter to ad-
         minister maintenance fluid therapy.
         (2) Intubate the animal.
         (3) Provide a padded area for the animal
         to lie on.
         (4) Turn the animal every 4 hours.
         (5) Consider starting IV broad-spectrum
         antibiotic treatment at the time of in-
         tubation.
         (6) Monitor heart rate and temperature
         every hour.

4. After 4 hours, let the animal recover from the previous anesthesia; if any further seizures occur, start a continuous infusion of pentobarbital or propofol.
   a) After an initial bolus sufficient to induce general anesthesia, a continuous IV infusion of pentobarbital (5 mg/kg/h) or propofol (8–12 mg/kg/h) is started.
   b) If the animal has been on phenobarbital prior to admission, it may require much higher levels of pentobarbital or propofol to maintain a satisfactory plane of anesthesia.
   c) Once a dosage is found that maintains a satisfactory anesthesia, continue it for 12 hours.
   d) At the end of 12 hours, discontinue the anesthesia.
   e) The animal is maintained on pentobarbital or propofol for approximately 24 hours.
   f) Similar supportive care is initiated as for the previous pentobarbital or propofol therapy.
   g) Maintenance phenobarbital therapy is administered IM throughout the anesthesia.
F. Phase 4: gas anesthesia
   1. Indications include refractory seizures to all the earlier phases of therapy or contraindication to the use of benzodiazepine or barbiturate drugs (hepatotoxicity or hepatic encephalopathy).
   2. Isoflurane provides a rapid induction and adjustable anesthetic depth, with smooth emergence from anesthesia.
   3. Isoflurane also offers the advantages of no hepatotoxicity, fewer perfusion problems, and less effect on elevation of intracranial pressure than halothane.
   4. Provide anesthetic support for the animal.
      a) Endotracheal intubation is maintained.
      b) Optimal therapy dictates the use of a respirator throughout the anesthetic period to prevent atelectasis and to maintain adequate perfusion-ventilation.
      c) Pulse oximetry or arterial blood gases are monitored every 4–8 hours to ensure adequate oxygenation.
VI. At-home emergency treatment for seizures (Podell, 1995)
A. Indications
   1. Generalized cluster epileptic seizures
   2. Status epilepticus
B. Pharmacokinetics of rectal administration of diazepam
   1. Peak plasma concentrations within 15 minutes after administration
   2. Maintenance of antiepileptic plasma concentrations for up to 1 hour
C. Protocol for rectal administration of diazepam in dogs
   1. Give 1 mg/kg of diazepam parenteral solution (5 mg/ml) per rectum, up to a maximum of 2

mg/kg in one dose if phenobarbital is being used chronically.
   2. Administer at the onset of a seizure and up to three times in 24 hours.
D. Protocol for rectal administration of diazepam in cats
   1. No pharmacokinetic data are available for the cat.
   2. Give 0.5 mg/kg of diazepam parenteral solution (5 mg/ml) per rectum if the cat is on phenobarbital therapy.
   3. It is not recommended if the cat is already being treated with a benzodiazepine on a chronic basis.
E. Potential benefits and risks of rectal administration of diazepam
   1. Benefits
      a) Reduces or eliminates the need for emergency clinic visits
      b) Stops progression of cluster seizure activity
      c) Reduces adverse postictal effects
      d) Reduces owner anxiety
      e) Improves overall quality of life of epileptic animal
   2. Risks
      a) No known toxic effects in the dog
      b) Enhanced lethargy
      c) Undocumented effects in the cat

Patient Monitoring

I. Drug serum monitoring
A. The major advantage of monitoring serial serum trough drug concentrations is to individualize treatment by documenting that an adequate amount of the drug is being given while minimizing the potential for toxic effects.
B. The goal of any antiepileptic drug therapy is to achieve a therapeutic steady-state condition in which the serum concentration fluctuates within the established therapeutic range for that drug.
   1. The lower limit of the therapeutic range can be defined as the minimal concentration at which 50% of animals will have any therapeutic benefit.
   2. The upper limit can be defined as the maximal concentration at which 50% of animals will not have any toxic adverse effects.
C. Trough serum concentrations of an antiepileptic drug are monitored to determine whether a therapeutic value is present at the lowest serum concentration, as dogs are most susceptible to seizure at this time.
D. Specific therapeutic ranges are as follows.
   1. Monotherapy with phenobarbital: 20–40 μg/ml (dog) and 15–30 μg/ml (cat)
   2. KBr and phenobarbital therapy
      a) Optimal initial phenobarbital concentration: 25 μg/ml
      b) Optimal initial KBr concentration: 1500 μg/ml (150 mg/dl)

E. Trough serum phenobarbital concentrations are measured 14, 45, 90, 180, and 360 days after the initiation of treatment, at 6-month intervals thereafter, and if a dog has more than two seizure events between these times.

F. Trough KBr and phenobarbital levels are measured at 30 and 120 days after starting KBr and then every 6 months.

G. Phenobarbital adjustments of the trough concentration can be calculated with the following formula: (desired concentration / actual concentration) $\times$ total mg per day = new total mg phenobarbital per day (to be divided BID or TID).

H. No linear relationship exists to adjust KBr levels; gradual increases of 100–200 mg/wk allow for a better adaptation to the sedating effects.

I. When KBr approaches a steady-state serum concentration in the therapeutic range, a decrease in the total daily phenobarbital dose can be attempted.

   1. The ultimate goal is to achieve steady-state trough serum concentrations of 25 μg/ml and 150–200 mg/dl for phenobarbital and KBr, respectively.

   2. Further reductions in phenobarbital can be attempted if a seizure-free period is maintained for 6 months.

   3. Some dogs can be successfully weaned off phenobarbital when steady-state KBr serum concentrations are obtained, especially if the dog has been seizure free for 6 months and has a trough serum KBr concentration of $\geq$200 mg/dl.

II. Pitfalls in the treatment of epilepsy

A. It is essential that the correct seizure etiology be identified in all epileptic animals before the onset of therapy.

B. Correct selection of an antiepileptic drug at the start of therapy greatly improves the chance of successful therapy.

C. Inadequate serum concentration of antiepileptic drugs usually results in poor seizure control.

D. Adjustments in drug dosages should be based on serum drug concentrations when possible, and not on an amount-per-weight basis.

E. By determining the underlying etiology, choosing the correct drug from the start, and monitoring drug concentration on a regular basis, the clinician can determine whether a functional tolerance to the drug has developed early in the course of therapy.

F. The earlier that proper adjustments can be instituted in an epileptic animal's life, the better the chance for a successful outcome.

SLEEP DISORDERS

Definition

I. Cataplexy

A. Cataplexy is a brief, sudden episode of muscle weakness without loss of consciousness.

B. Signs are caused by motor inhibition, are short in duration, and are completely reversible.

C. Episodes may be initiated by periods of excitement.

D. It can occur in combination with narcolepsy.

II. Narcolepsy

A. Narcolepsy is a disorder of recurrent daytime somnolence.

B. It manifests as uncontrollable and excessive sleeping episodes.

Causes

I. Autosomal recessive inheritance: Doberman pinscher, Labrador retriever, poodle, and dachshund

II. Canine breeds reported with narcolepsy-cataplexy: Airedale, Afghan, Irish setter, malamute, Saint Bernard, rottweiler, English springer spaniel, Welsh corgi, and giant schnauzer

III. Rare in cats

Pathophysiology

I. Neurotransmitter imbalance is the principal problem.

A. Depressed serotonin metabolism

B. Excessive facilitation of the cholinergic system

II. Immune-mediated disease may be a contributing factor.

Clinical Signs

I. Onset: typically by 6 months of age

II. Sudden, paroxysmal generalized muscle atonia

III. Episodes often precipitated by excitement

IV. Conservation of consciousness with cataplexy

V. Intact respirations, cough and swallow reflexes

VI. Duration of event: seconds to 10–20 minutes

VII. Some animals aroused by external stimuli

VIII. Possible signs of rapid eye movement (REM) sleep with ocular motility, facial or eye muscle twitching, and whining

Diagnosis

I. Food-elicited test

A. Place 10 pieces of palatable food approximately 1 cm^3 in size in a row about 1 foot apart from each other.

B. Record the time required to eat all the pieces and the number, type, and duration of attacks.

C. A normal dog will eat the food in $\leq$1 minute and have no attacks.

D. Positive response occurs with any of the following.

   1. The dog takes >2 minutes to eat the food and has two or more attacks.

   2. The animal drops to the ground with flaccid paralysis (complete attack).

   3. Thoracic and/or pelvic limbs drop to the ground, but the head does not (partial attack).

II. Pharmacologic testing

A. Yohimbine response test

1. Administer 50 μg/kg yohimbine IV bolus.
2. A positive response is a 75% reduction in the number or severity (time reduction) of attacks.
3. The response is present within 30 minutes and may last up to 4 hours.
B. Physostigmine challenge
   1. Administer 0.025 mg/kg physostigmine salicylate IV bolus.
      a) Follow each injection with a food elicited test in 10 minutes.
      b) Repeat the test with additional 0.025-mg/kg increments up to 0.1 mg/kg.
   2. In affected animals, signs increase in severity and frequency in a dose-dependent manner.
   3. Total effect of each dose lasts 15–45 minutes.
C. Atropine response test
   1. Give atropine sulfate 0.1 mg/kg IV bolus, and follow each injection with a food elicited test in 10 minutes.
   2. In affected animals, signs decrease in severity and frequency.
D. Imipramine challenge
   1. Administer 0.5 mg/kg imipramine IV bolus.
   2. A positive response is general improvement in arousal.
   3. This test is not specific for the diagnosis of narcolepsy-cataplexy.
III. Electrophysiologic testing
   A. EEG recordings are consistent with the acute onset of REM sleep during an attack.
   B. Concurrent electromyographic recordings from appendicular muscles show complete loss of activity during an attack.

Differential Diagnosis

I. Syncope
II. Epileptic seizures
III. Metabolic disorders
   A. Hypoglycemia
   B. Electrolyte disorders: hypocalcemia, hypokalemia
   C. Glucocorticoid deficiency (Addison's disease)

Treatment

I. Yohimbine

A. The drug of choice
B. Dose: 50–100 μg/kg SQ BID–TID
II. Methylphenidate (Ritalin)
   A. Dose: 0.25 mg/kg PO SID or BID
   B. May be used alone or in combination with imipramine
III. Imipramine
   A. Dose: 0.5–1 mg/kg PO TID
   B. Titrated to effect

Patient Monitoring

I. Prognosis for a good quality of life is fair to good.
II. Improvement with increasing age may be seen.
III. Continuous daily therapy is often required.
IV. Alterations of lifestyle may be necessary to avoid precipitating events.

Bibliography

Becker SV, Selby LA: Canine hydrocephalus. Compend Contin Ed Pract Vet 4:647, 1980

Brown SA: Anticonvulsant therapy in small animals. Vet Clin North Am [Small Anim Pract] 18:1197, 1988

Dayrell-Hart B, Steinberg SA, Van Winkle TJ et al: Hepatotoxicity of phenobarbital in dogs: 18 cases (1985–1989). J Am Vet Med Assoc 199:1060, 1991

Fenner WR, Hass J: Mechanisms of seizure disorders. p. 501. In Indrieri R (ed): Problems in Veterinary Medicine: Epilepsy. JP Lippincott, Baltimore, 1989

Knecht CD, Sorjonen DC, Simpson ST: Ancillary tests in the diagnosis of seizures. J Am Anim Hosp Assoc 20:455, 1984

McNamara JO: The neurological basis of epilepsy. Trends Neurosci 15:357, 1992

Oliver JE: Protocol for the diagnosis of seizure disorders in companion animals. J Am Vet Med Assoc 172:822, 1980

Podell M: The use of diazepam per rectum at home for the acute management of cluster seizures in dogs. J Vet Intern Med 8:68, 1995

Podell M: Seizures in dogs. Vet Clin North Am [Small Anim Pract] 26:779, 1996

Podell M, Fenner WR: Bromide therapy in refractory canine idiopathic epilepsy. J Vet Intern Med 7:318, 1993

Podell M, Fenner WR, Powers JD: Seizure classification in dogs from a nonreferral-based population. J Am Vet Med Assoc 206:1721, 1995

23

Disorders of the Brain

Karen R. Muñana

CONGENITAL/DEVELOPMENTAL DISORDERS

Hydrocephalus

Definition

Hydrocephalus is an excessive accumulation of cerebrospinal fluid (CSF) within the ventricular system or subarachnoid space of the brain.

Causes

I. Primary or congenital
   A. Congenital hydrocephalus has multiple causes, many of which are not completely understood.
      1. Congenital malformation or obstruction of the CSF pathway may alter the flow of fluid during brain development.
      2. The presence of in utero infections, toxins, and/or nutritional imbalances may be predisposing factors.
   B. The cranial vault increases in size to compensate for the accumulation of fluid such that intracranial pressure is typically not increased.
II. Secondary or acquired: occurs secondary to other central nervous system (CNS) disease, such as trauma, inflammatory conditions, or neoplasia
III. Difficult to distinguish between congenital and acquired hydrocephalus, especially in young animals

Pathophysiology

I. The obstructive or noncommunicating form of hydrocephalus results from a blockage within the ventricular system.
   A. The usual site of obstruction is the mesencephalic aqueduct or the lateral foramina of the fourth ventricle.
   B. Obstructive hydrocephalus may be either congenital or acquired.
II. The communicating form of hydrocephalus results from either increased production (rare) or impaired absorption of CSF.

A. It is most commonly associated with the congenital form of the disease.
B. It may be acquired secondary to meningitis, subarachnoid hemorrhage, or neoplasia that interferes with the absorption of fluid by the arachnoid villa.

Clinical Signs

I. Hydrocephalus as a distinct clinical entity refers to the congenital form of the disease.
II. Small, toy, and brachycephalic breeds are at increased risk.
III. Clinical signs include seizures, altered mentation, visual deficits, and incoordinated gait.

Diagnosis

I. Compatible clinical signs in a young dog of a predisposed breed
II. Physical examination findings
   A. Enlarged, dome-shaped calvarium
   B. Palpable open fontanelles
III. Radiologic findings
   A. Skull radiographs may reveal the calvarium to be of a homogeneous density, referred to as having a "ground-glass" appearance.
   B. A dilated ventricular system may be demonstrated with ultrasonographic imaging through an open fontanelle or with computed tomography (CT) or magnetic resonance imaging (MRI).
IV. Electroencephalography
   High-amplitude, slow wave activity is characteristically seen.

Differential Diagnosis

I. Metabolic encephalopathies
   A. Hepatic encephalopathy
   B. Hypoglycemia
II. Lissencephaly
III. Encephalitis
IV. Other congenital or developmental defects of the brain

Treatment

I. Corticosteroids
  A. Are believed to act by decreasing CSF production
  B. Are initially given BID (prednisone 0.25–0.5 mg/kg PO, dexamethasone 0.05 mg/kg PO) and gradually tapered to QOD
  C. May be discontinued in some dogs with no recurrence of signs
II. Diuretics to decrease CSF volume
  A. Furosemide 1–2 mg/kg PO BID
  B. Acetazolamide 0.1 mg/kg PO TID
III. Surgical shunting of CSF
  A. Placement of a ventriculoperitoneal shunt has proved beneficial in some cases refractory to medical management.
  B. CSF is shunted from the ventricular system of the brain to the abdominal cavity.
IV. Anticonvulsants
  A. Anticonvulsant therapy is indicated in animals with seizures.
  B. Phenobarbital at 2.2 mg/kg PO BID is the treatment of choice.
  C. Side effects include sedation, polyuria, polydipsia, and polyphagia.

Patient Monitoring

I. Prognosis is fair with early diagnosis and treatment.
II. Subtle neurologic deficits may persist, and the animal may be difficult to housebreak or train.
III. Avoid episodes likely to cause decompensation, such as general anesthesia and excessive IV fluid administration.

Lissencephaly

Definition and Causes

I. Lissencephaly is a condition in which the normal cerebrocortical folding that produces gyri and sulci is absent, resulting in a smooth appearance to the brain surface.
II. The disease is seen most commonly in the Lhasa apso breed, in which a genetic mechanism is presumed.
III. The condition has also been reported in wire-haired fox terriers, Irish setters, and a cat.

Pathophysiology

I. Lissencephaly is believed to result from a defect in neuronal migration and proliferation during development.
II. This developmental defect, which selectively affects the cerebral cortex, causes forebrain dysfunction.

Clinical Signs

I. Clinical signs are usually detected early in life.
II. Characteristic signs include behavioral abnormalities, seizures, and visual deficits.

Diagnosis

I. Compatible clinical signs in a Lhasa apso <1 year old are highly suggestive.
II. Absence of sulci and gyri may be visualized with MRI.
III. Characteristic electroencephalographic findings include the following.
  A. Irregular random slow waves
  B. Lack of symmetry between cortical areas on both sides of the brain
IV. Definitive diagnosis is made on necropsy.

Differential Diagnosis

I. Hydrocephalus
II. Metabolic encephalopathies
III. Encephalitis
IV. Other developmental or congenital defects of the brain

Treatment and Monitoring

I. No definitive treatment is available.
II. Seizures are managed with anticonvulsants.
III. Prognosis is fair; the disease is not progressive, but seizures may be difficult to control.

Cerebellar Hypoplasia

Definition

Cerebellar hypoplasia refers to a condition in which the cerebellum does not develop normally because of an absence of cells.

Causes

I. Occurs most commonly in cats and is associated with in utero infection with feline panleukopenia virus
II. Has been reported in dogs secondary to in utero infection with canine herpesvirus
III. Is a presumed genetic malformation in wire-haired fox terriers, Irish setters, and chow chows

Pathophysiology

I. In utero or perinatal infection with panleukopenia or herpesvirus causes destruction of the rapidly dividing cells in the germinal layer of the cerebellum.
II. Purkinje's cells may also be destroyed.

Clinical Signs

I. Symmetrical nonprogressive cerebellar signs are seen at the onset of ambulation.
II. Hypermetria, truncal sway, ataxia, and intention tremor are usually observed.

Diagnosis

I. The presumptive diagnosis is based on characteristic signs in a young animal.

II. Other causes are excluded based on the history and laboratory findings.
III. Diagnosis can be confirmed only on necropsy.

Differential Diagnosis

I. Lysosomal storage disorders
II. Encephalitis
III. Cerebellar abiotrophy

Treatment and Monitoring

I. No treatment is available.
II. The disease is not progressive.
III. Although never normal, many affected animals make acceptable pets.

Malformation of Foramen Magnum

Definition

I. It is a disorder of toy-breed dogs in which a defect in the development of the occipital bone results in enlargement of the foramen magnum.
II. The clinical significance of the defect has been questioned; some believe that the clinical signs in affected dogs are attributable to the presence of other congenital abnormalities.

Cause and Pathophysiology

I. The cause of this developmental disorder is unknown.
II. The malformation can cause compression of the cerebellum and spinal cord.
III. It may also result in the obstruction of CSF flow, producing hydrocephalus.

Clinical Signs

I. Signs become apparent between 2 and 6 months of age.
II. Seizures, personality changes, and cervical pain have been described in affected dogs.

Diagnosis

I. Frontal radiographs of the skull reveal an enlarged and misshapen foramen magnum.
II. Evaluate the animal for other congenital disorders, such as hydrocephalus.

Differential Diagnosis

I. Hydrocephalus
II. Metabolic encephalopathies
III. Lysosomal storage disorder
IV. Infectious encephalitis
V. Atlantoaxial subluxation (causing cervical pain)

Treatment and Monitoring

I. No definitive treatment is available.
II. The prognosis in most cases is fair to guarded.
III. Clinical signs may progress.

Dysmyelinogenesis and Hypomyelinogenesis

Definition

I. Dysmyelinogenesis refers to abnormal myelination of the nervous system.
II. Hypomyelinogenesis refers to lack of myelin in the nervous system.

Causes

I. Congenital form
  A. Welsh springer spaniels: only breed in which a genetic basis for the disease has been proved
  B. Chow chows
  C. Weimaraners
  D. Samoyeds
  E. Bernese mountain dogs
  F. Lurchers
  G. Dalmatians
II. Possible in utero exposure to a virus or toxin

Pathophysiology

I. There is a defect in the number or function of oligodendrocytes (the myelin-producing cells of the CNS).
II. Primary axonal abnormalities can also prevent myelination.

Clinical Signs

I. Tremor of the head, body, and limbs is seen in puppies 1–4 weeks of age.
II. Ataxia and hypermetria may also be noted.
III. There is no evidence of weakness.
IV. Tremors worsen with excitement and activity and often abate with rest.

Diagnosis

I. A presumptive diagnosis is based on characteristic signs in a dog of a predisposed breed.
II. MRI may reveal lack of white matter in the brain.
III. Diagnosis is confirmed on necropsy.

Differential Diagnosis

I. Toxins
  A. Metaldehyde
  B. Organophosphates
  C. Chlorinated hydrocarbons
  D. Fluoroacetate
II. Diffuse encephalitis
III. Metabolic disturbances
  A. Hypocalcemia
  B. Hypoglycemia
IV. Generalized tremor syndrome of dogs: seen in mature small-breed dogs, especially those with white hair coats

Treatment and Monitoring

I. No specific treatment exists.
II. Prognosis is variable.
III. Affected chow chows, Weimaraners, and Bernese mountain dogs typically improve such that they are clinically normal by 1 year of age, but in Welsh springer spaniels the disease tends to remain static over time.
IV. Tremors may be severe enough in some dogs to interfere with normal eating; these dogs must be hand fed.

Leukoencephalomyelopathy

Definition and Causes

I. This is a demyelinating disorder of the brain and spinal cord in rottweiler dogs.
II. The cause is unknown, but genetic, toxic, metabolic, nutritional, vascular, and infectious causes have been proposed (Gamble and Chrisman, 1984).

Pathophysiology

I. The clinical dysfunction is caused by demyelination of the white matter tracts in the cervical spinal cord.
II. Histopathologic lesions can also be identified in the thoracic and lumbar spinal cord, the spinal tract of the trigeminal nerve, the white matter of the cerebellum, and the optic nerves (Chrisman, 1992).

Clinical Signs

I. The typical presenting complaint is of a slowly progressive ataxia of all four limbs, first noted in dogs between 1.5 and 4 years of age.
II. Additional neurologic signs include the following.
A. Thoracic limb hypermetria
B. Tetraparesis
C. Conscious proprioceptive deficits
D. Exaggerated patellar reflexes
E. Crossed extensor reflexes

Diagnosis

I. Characteristic clinical signs in a young rottweiler dog are very suggestive.
II. Diagnosis is by exclusion; other causes of cervical myelopathy must be ruled out.
III. Diagnosis is confirmed on necropsy.

Differential Diagnosis

I. Cervical spondylomyelopathy
II. Intervertebral disk disease
III. Neoplasia
IV. Myelitis

Treatment and Monitoring

I. There is no effective treatment.
II. Signs are progressive.

Congenital Vestibular Disease

Definition

Dysfunction of the peripheral vestibular system is seen in young dogs and cats and is believed to be caused by a congenital defect.

Causes

I. The disorder is presumed to be inherited.
II. It has been reported in the following breeds.
A. Dogs
1. Doberman pinschers
2. American cocker spaniels
3. German shepherd dogs
4. Akita dogs
5. Beagles
B. Cats
1. Siamese
2. Burmese

Pathophysiology

Aggregates of lymphocytes have been identified within the inner ear of affected Doberman puppies (Forbes and Cook, 1991), but the significance of these lesions remains unclear.

Clinical Signs

I. Onset of signs usually occurs between 3 and 12 weeks of age.
II. Head tilt, ataxia, circling, and deafness may be seen.
III. Nystagmus is not a feature of this disorder.

Differential Diagnosis

I. Otitis media/interna
II. Ototoxicity
A. Aminoglycoside antibiotics
B. Topical antiseptics: iodophors, chlorhexidine

Treatment and Monitoring

I. No treatment is available.
II. Signs of vestibular dysfunction may improve over several weeks.
III. Improvement is the result of compensation rather than resolution.
IV. Deafness is permanent.

DEGENERATIVE DISORDERS

Lysosomal Storage Disease

Definition and Causes

I. This group of disorders consists of inborn errors in metabolism in which specific enzyme deficiencies cause substrate accumulation within cells of the nervous system, with resultant clinical dysfunction.
II. The enzyme deficiency is usually inherited as an autosomal recessive trait.

III. The disorders are named and classified according to the nature of the substrate that accumulates (Table 23–1).

Pathophysiology

I. Most of the diseases cause substrate accumulation within neurons, which results in progressive neurologic dysfunction.
II. Neurons are unable to divide to lessen the amount of accumulated substrate and are therefore more susceptible to dysfunction than cells capable of mitosis.
III. One disease (globoid cell leukodystrophy) causes myelin degradation in the central and peripheral nervous system, and its subsequent accumulation in macrophages.

Clinical Signs

I. Animals are usually normal at birth and develop signs of neurologic dysfunction within the first year of life.
II. Specific diseases are known to be present in certain breeds.
III. All the storage disorders are progressive and fatal.

IV. Neurologic signs often reflect cerebellar involvement.
V. The spinal cord is also frequently involved in the disease process.
VI. Visual deficits can occur from dysfunction of either neurons in the visual cortex or the ganglion cell layer of the retina.

Diagnosis

I. Progressive neurologic deficits in a young animal of a predisposed breed are suggestive of the diagnosis.
II. Substrate accumulation may be identified in several organs, most commonly in cells of the reticuloendothelial system.
III. Biochemical confirmation of the nature of the accumulated substrate verifies the diagnosis.

Differential Diagnosis

I. Hypomyelinogenesis, dysmyelinogenesis
II. Cerebellar abiotrophy
III. Encephalitis
IV. Hydrocephalus

Table 23–1. **Lysosomal Storage Diseases of Dogs and Cats**

Disease	Enzyme Deficiency	Clinical Signs	Breeds
GM$_1$ gangliosidosis	β-Galactosidase	Tremors, incoordination, paresis, visual deficits	Beagle, English springer spaniel, Portuguese water dog Siamese, Korat, domestic shorthair cat
GM$_2$ gangliosidosis	Hexosaminidase	Ataxia, impaired vision, dementia, tremors, incoordination, paresis	German shorthaired pointer, Japanese spaniel Siamese, domestic shorthair cat
Sphingomyelin lipidosis			
Niemann-Pick type A	Sphingomyelinase	Ataxia, tremors, hypermetria	Miniature poodle Siamese, Balinese, domestic shorthair cat
Niemann-Pick type C	Unknown	Tremors, incoordination	Domestic shorthair cat
Ceroid lipofuscinosis	Unknown	Behavioral changes, visual loss, dementia, ataxia, seizures	English setter, Chihuahua, saluki, dachshund, English cocker spaniel, border collie, Austrialian cattle dog, blue heeler Siamese cat
Glucocerebrosidosis	Glucocerebrosidase	Ataxia, tremors, hypermetria	Australian silkie terrier Abyssinian cat
Globoid cell leukodystrophy	β-Galacotosidase (galactocerebrosidase)	Ataxia, tremors, hypermetria, paresis, impaired vision	Cairn terrier, West Highland white terrier, beagle, blue tick hound, poodle, Pomeranian, basset hound, dalmatian Domestic shorthair cat
Fucosidosis	α-L-Fucosidase	Ataxia, behavioral changes, dysphonia, dysphagia, seizures	English springer spaniel
Mannosidosis	α-Mannosidase	Ataxia, tremors, hyermetria	Persian, domestic shorthair cat
Glycogenosis type II	α-Glucosidase	Exercise intolerance, seizures	Lapland dog
Mucopolysaccharidosis type VI	Arylsulfatase B	Paresis, seizures	Siamese cat
Metachromatic leukodystrophy	Arylsulfatase	Progressive motor dysfunction, seizures, opisthotonus	Domestic shorthair cat

Treatment and Monitoring

   I. There is currently no effective treatment.

   II. The prognosis is poor, as the disease is always progressive.

Cerebellar Abiotrophy

Definition and Causes

   I. This disorder is characterized by a progressive degeneration of cells within the cerebellum.

   II. The abiotrophy is assumed to have a genetic cause.

   III. It has been reported in Kerry blue terriers, Gordon setters, rough-coated collies, Airedale terriers, Finnish harriers, Bernese mountain dogs, Akitas, beagles, Border collies, Brittany spaniels, Labrador retrievers, golden retrievers, American cocker spaniels, Cairn terriers, Great Danes, smooth-haired fox terriers, and miniature poodles.

Pathophysiology

   I. Abiotrophy literally means lack of a vital substance necessary for the nutritional life of a cell.

   II. The disease is believed to be caused by an intrinsic abnormality in the metabolic capabilities of Purkinje's cells in the cerebellum, resulting in their death.

Clinical Signs

   I. Affected animals are normal at birth and when ambulation begins but develop signs of cerebellar disease at an early age.

   II. The disease in Gordon setters manifests later in life, with the onset of signs typically occurring between 6 and 36 months of age.

   III. Cerebellar signs commonly include ataxia, dysmetria, and intention tremor, with no evidence of weakness.

   IV. The disease is slowly progressive.

Diagnosis

   I. Progressive cerebellar signs in a predisposed breed

   II. Exclusion of other diagnoses with brain imaging (CT, MRI) and CSF analysis

Differential Diagnosis

   I. Lysosomal storage disease

   II. Encephalitis

   III. Cerebellar hypoplasia

Treatment and Monitoring

   I. There is presently no effective treatment.

   II. Cerebellar signs may become severe enough over time to hamper the animal's ambulation and ability to prehend food.

   III. Signs are progressive in all cases, but the rate of progression varies among breeds.

Canine Neuroaxonal Dystrophy

Definition and Causes

   I. This is a degenerative disease of rottweilers characterized by swelling of distal axons throughout the CNS.

   II. The disease is believed to be inherited as an autosomal recessive trait.

Pathophysiology

   I. Distal portions of axons show accumulations of smooth membranes and tubulovesicular elements, which result in microscopically visible axonal swelling.

   II. The cause of the axonal accumulations is unknown; it has been postulated that a defect in axonal transport may exist.

Clinical Signs

   I. Affected pups may be judged to be clumsier than normal.

   II. Abnormal gait is usually noted by 1 year of age.

   III. Gait deficits include ataxia of all limbs, usually with some hypermetria of the thoracic limbs.

   IV. Strength and conscious proprioception are normal throughout the course of the disease.

   V. Menace deficit, with preserved vision and pupillary light reflexes, and head tremors may be seen as the disease progresses.

Diagnosis

   I. A diagnosis of neuroaxonal dystrophy may be suspected based on the signalment, history, and clinical findings.

   II. Ancillary diagnostic tests rule out other causes of disease.

   III. Conjunctival biopsy from severely affected dogs may reveal the presence of reduced numbers of sensory nerve endings (Chrisman et al., 1984).

   IV. Diagnosis is confirmed with the demonstration of characteristic neuropathologic findings.

     A. Large numbers of axonal spheroids are seen throughout the neuraxis.

     B. The dorsal horn of the spinal cord, nucleus gracilis, and nucleus cuneatus are most severely affected.

Differential Diagnosis

   I. Cervical spondylomyelopathy

   II. Encephalomyelitis

   III. Congenital vertebral malformation

   IV. Cerebellar abiotrophy

   V. Lysosomal storage disease

Treatment and Monitoring

   I. No effective therapy is available.

   II. The disease slowly progresses over several years.

III. Incoordination may become so severe as to hamper ambulation.

INFECTIOUS DISORDERS

Encephalitis

Definition

I. Encephalitis refers to inflammation of the brain.
II. The meninges are often concomitantly involved, resulting in a meningoencephalitis.

Causes

I. Viral infections
   A. Canine distemper virus: most common cause of viral encephalitis in dogs
   B. Feline infectious peritonitis (FIP) virus: most common cause of viral encephalitis in cats
   C. Feline immunodeficiency virus (FIV)
   D. Rabies
   E. Pseudorabies
   F. Canine herpesvirus
   G. Canine parainfluenza virus
   H. Canine parvovirus
   I. Infectious canine hepatitis
   J. Central European tick-borne encephalitis
   K. Feline leukemia virus (FeLV)
II. Bacterial infections
   A. Aerobes
   B. Anaerobes
III. Protozoal infections
   A. Toxoplasmosis
   B. Neosporosis
   C. Encephalitozoonosis
   D. Acanthamebiasis
   E. *Sarcocystis*-like organism
   F. Trypanosomiasis
   G. Babesiosis
IV. Rickettsial infections
   A. Ehrlichiosis
   B. Rocky Mountain spotted fever
   C. Salmon poisoning disease
V. Fungal infections
   A. Cryptococcosis
   B. Blastomycosis
   C. Histoplasmosis
   D. Coccidioidomycosis
   E. Aspergillosis
   F. Phaeohyphomycosis
   G. Hyalohyphomycosis
VI. Algal infections: protothecosis

Pathogenesis

I. Infectious agents cause pathology in the CNS by both direct and indirect mechanisms.
   A. Direct invasion of neural cells by infectious organisms may result in impaired function or cell destruction.
   B. Indirect mechanisms of disease include the following.
      1. Ischemia secondary to vasculitis
      2. Edema and resultant brain swelling
      3. Toxic effects of inflammatory mediators on neural cells
II. Infectious agents may gain access to the CNS hematogenously or through local extension.

Clinical Signs

I. Affected animals characteristically have an acute onset of multifocal CNS disease.
   A. Forebrain involvement may present as seizures, dementia, visual deficits, facial hypoesthesia, and postural deficits in the limbs.
   B. Brain stem involvement may present as cranial nerve deficits, paresis, and depression of consciousness.
   C. Cerebellar involvement may present as ataxia of head and limbs, dysmetria, intention tremor, and menace deficits.
   D. Meningeal involvement results in cervical pain and rigidity.
II. Signs are generally progressive.
III. Associated systemic disease may be present, particularly fever and ophthalmic abnormalities (see Section XV).

Diagnosis

I. A minimum database (complete blood count, chemistry profile, and urinalysis) may suggest systemic or other organ involvement.
II. CSF analysis is the most useful test for establishing a diagnosis.
   A. White blood cell (WBC) count is characteristically elevated.
   B. The magnitude of WBC elevation and the differential count may help determine the cause of the inflammation.
      1. Viral disease typically results in mild lymphocytic inflammation, but neutrophilic inflammation can be seen with FIP.
      2. Bacterial infections usually cause a marked increase in neutrophils in the CSF (>500/μl). Neutrophils may show toxic changes in cellular morphology.
      3. Protozoal disease results in a mixed population of neutrophils and mononuclear cells.
      4. Rickettsial infections typically result in mild mononuclear inflammation, but neutrophilic inflammation may be seen with Rocky Mountain spotted fever.
      5. Fungal infections usually cause a neutrophilic inflammation.
         a) Neutrophil counts may be greatly elevated (>500/μl) in many cases.
         b) Eosinophilic inflammation may be seen with cryptococcosis.
      6. Protothecosis causes mixed inflammation,

with either neutrophils or lymphocytes predominating.

C. Elevated protein concentrations are usually found in association with the inflammation.
  1. Increased protein concentrations may be caused by breakdown of the blood-brain barrier, intrathecal immunoglobulin production, or both.
  2. FIP causes a marked increase in protein concentrations, which are often >2 g/dl.

D. Ancillary tests can be performed on the CSF based on findings of WBC and protein concentrations.
  1. Culture the CSF if bacterial infection is suspected. A negative culture does *not* rule out bacterial encephalitis.
  2. Antibody titers can be done on CSF for other infectious diseases.

III. Exposure to a specific infectious agent may be confirmed with serologic testing.

IV. Some cases of infectious encephalitis can be confirmed only histopathologically.

Differential Diagnosis

I. Inflammatory (noninfectious) encephalitis
II. Neoplasia
III. Parasitic encephalitis
IV. Toxic encephalopathy

Treatment

I. Provide definitive treatment for the infectious agent if possible.
  A. Antimicrobials are selected that are known to cross the blood-brain barrier (Table 23–2).
  B. IV therapy is preferred initially. After the clinical signs stabilize or improve, oral administration may be used.
  C. Long-term therapy (4–6 weeks minimum) is often required to eradicate the infection.
  D. See Section XV for guidelines on the treatment of specific infectious agents.

II. Provide supportive care as needed.
  A. IV fluid therapy
  B. Anticonvulsants for seizures: phenobarbital 2.2 mg/kg PO BID

III. Provide symptomatic treatment for brain swelling if the animal's neurologic status deteriorates rapidly.

A. Monitor for signs of increased intracranial pressure and brain herniation.
  1. Deterioration of level of consciousness to stupor or coma
  2. Absent pupillary light reflexes with abnormal pupil size
  3. Changes in respiratory or heart rate

B. If brain swelling is suspected, administer mannitol 1 g/kg IV over 20 minutes.

Patient Monitoring

I. Prognosis is dependent on the causative agent and the severity of neurologic deficits.
  A. Bacterial, protozoal, and rickettsial infections may resolve with long-term antimicrobial therapy.
  B. Viral infections are not treatable and carry a guarded prognosis; the majority of these infections are fatal.
  C. Mycotic infections of the CNS are typically difficult to treat.

II. Even if the infection can be eliminated, residual neurologic deficits may persist owing to irreversible damage to the brain parenchyma.

INFLAMMATORY DISORDERS

Granulomatous Meningoencephalomyelitis (GME)

Definition

This is an inflammatory disease of the CNS in dogs, characterized histologically by marked perivascular infiltrates of mononuclear cells, granuloma formation, and necrosis.

Causes

I. The cause is unknown.
II. Several etiologies have been proposed.
  A. Immune mediated
  B. Infectious
  C. Neoplastic, as a form of CNS lymphosarcoma
III. The disease is most common in middle-aged toy- to small-breed dogs, and poodles and terriers may be predisposed (Cuddon and Smith-Maxie, 1984).

Pathophysiology

I. Three clinicopathologic forms of GME exist (Braund, 1985).
  A. Focal form
    1. Clinical signs are suggestive of a single space-occupying mass.
    2. Focal lesions are most common in the pontomedullary region and cerebral white matter.
  B. Diffuse form
    1. Clinical signs are suggestive of a multifocal CNS disorder.
    2. The cerebrum, brain stem, cerebellum, and

Table 23–2. *Antimicrobial Penetration into the CNS*

High Penetration	Intermediate Penetration	Poor Penetration
Trimethoprim	Penicillin	Aminoglycosides
Metronidazole	Ampicillin	Cephalosporins
Enrofloxacin	Oxacillin	Erythromycin[a]
Chloramphenicol[a]	Tetracycline[a]	
Doxycycline[a]		

[a]Bacteriostatic; others are bactericidal.

cervical spinal cord are most commonly involved with this form of the disease.
  C. Ocular form
    1. There is an acute onset of visual impairment and dilated, unresponsive pupils.
    2. Ophthalmologic findings are indicative of optic neuritis.
 II. Histopathologically, the disease is characterized by perivascular accumulations of macrophages, lymphocytes, and plasma cells.
    1. The perivascular infiltrates can coalesce to form granulomas.
    2. CNS necrosis and edema may be seen secondary to granuloma formation.
    3. Meningeal involvement may also be seen.

Clinical Signs

  I. The disease typically has an acute onset and is progressive.
 II. Clinical signs reflect the area(s) of involvement in the brain.
    A. Cerebral disease manifests with seizures, behavioral changes, visual deficits, and postural deficits.
    B. Cerebellar disease manifests with dysmetria and intention tremors.
    C. Brain stem disease manifests with hemiparesis or tetraparesis, cranial nerve deficits (with vestibular signs being most common), and depression of consciousness.
 III. Cervical pain is often seen with meningeal involvement.

Diagnosis

  I. CSF analysis typically reveals mononuclear inflammation, with an associated increase in protein concentrations (Bailey and Higgins, 1986).
    A. Neutrophilic inflammation can also be seen.
    B. CSF may be normal with the focal form of the disease.
 II. Advanced imaging techniques, such as CT or MRI, may reveal abnormalities.
    A. Space-occupying lesions may be seen with the focal form.
    B. Diffuse disease may cause the brain parenchyma to have a patchy, heterogeneous appearance.
 III. GME can be confirmed only histopathologically.

Differential Diagnosis

  I. Infectious encephalitis
 II. Neoplasia

Treatment

  I. Corticosteroids are the mainstay of therapy.
    A. Immunosuppressive doses of prednisone (1–2 mg/kg PO BID) are initiated, and the dose is gradually decreased when signs stabilize or improve.

  B. Treatment is not curative, and lifelong therapy is often required.
 II. Radiation therapy has been shown to be helpful in a limited number of cases (Sisson et al., 1989).

Patient Monitoring

  I. Overall, the prognosis for dogs with GME is poor to guarded, as the disease is typically fatal.
 II. The diffuse form of the disease carries the worst prognosis, with usual survival times of weeks to months.
 III. Dogs with the focal form of the disease may survive for months to years.
 IV. The ocular form is not fatal, but the disease can progress to involve other regions of the brain.

Chronic Encephalitis of Pug Dogs

Definition and Causes

  I. It is a chronic, progressive necrotizing meningoencephalitis seen in pug dogs.
 II. The etiology of the disease is unknown.
 III. A familial tendency has been reported.
 IV. Several features of the disease are similar to those seen with alpha-type herpesvirus encephalitides in other species. It has been hypothesized that the disease may be caused by the recurrence of latent infection following an initial neonatal canine herpesvirus infection (Cordy and Holliday, 1989).

Pathophysiology

  I. Microscopic lesions consist of a nonsuppurative meningoencephalitis with extensive parenchymal necrosis.
 II. Lesions are typically most severe in the cerebral hemispheres.

Clinical Signs

  I. The disease is most commonly seen in young to middle-aged dogs.
 II. Clinical signs are referable to the forebrain.
    A. The most common presenting clinical sign is seizures.
    B. Other signs include altered mentation, circling, head pressing, and blindness.
 III. Cervical rigidity can be seen in association with meningeal inflammation.

Diagnosis

  I. CSF analysis typically reveals a marked increase in leukocytes, with lymphocytes predominating.
 II. Definitive diagnosis must be based on histopathology.

Differential Diagnosis

  I. Infectious encephalitis
 II. Granulomatous meningoencephalitis

III. Metabolic encephalopathies
IV. Toxic encephalopathies

Treatment

I. There is no specific therapy for this disease.
II. Empirical treatment with anticonvulsants and anti-inflammatories has been attempted, with poor results.

Patient Monitoring

I. The disease is progressive and carries a poor prognosis.
II. Most dogs die or are euthanized 1–6 months after the onset of signs.

Necrotizing Meningoencephalomyelitis

Definition and Causes

I. It is a chronic, progressive neurologic disorder of Yorkshire terriers and Maltese dogs with histologic similarities to chronic encephalitis of pug dogs.
II. The etiology is unknown.
III. A viral cause has been postulated based on characteristics of the lesions.

Pathophysiology

I. The disease causes a nonsuppurative meningoencephalitis with associated parenchymal necrosis.
II. The disease has a predilection for the cerebrum in Maltese dogs (Stalis et al., 1995).
III. Yorkshire terriers may show signs of cerebral and brain stem involvement (Tipold et al., 1993).

Clinical Signs

I. Neurologic signs are acute in onset and progressive.
II. Dogs with cerebral involvement display clinical signs compatible with forebrain disease.
   A. Seizures are the most common presenting sign.
   B. Other signs include behavioral changes, postural deficits, and visual deficits.
III. Dogs with brain stem involvement may show signs of paresis, depression of consciousness, and cranial nerve deficits. Vestibular signs are the most commonly identified abnormality.

Diagnosis

I. CSF analysis typically reveals lymphocytic inflammation.
II. Histopathology is required to make a definitive diagnosis.

Differential Diagnosis

I. Infectious encephalitis
II. Granulomatous meningoencephalomyelitis

III. Metabolic encephalopathies
IV. Toxic encephalopathies

Treatment and Monitoring

I. No treatment is available.
II. The disease is progressive and fatal.

Eosinophilic Meningoencephalomyelitis

Definition

I. It is an inflammatory condition of the CNS that is characterized by an increase in eosinophils in the CSF of affected animals.
II. The condition has been reported in both dogs and cats, with golden retrievers overrepresented in one report (Smith-Maxie et al., 1989).

Causes

I. The cause of this condition is unknown.
II. It has been postulated that the disease represents a hypersensitivity reaction, possibly an allergic response to an unidentified agent.

Pathophysiology

I. The presence of eosinophilic inflammation in the brain may lead to "eosinophil-induced neurotoxicity," in which neurons and myelinated axons suffer damage secondary to a toxic effect of proteins present in eosinophil granules.
II. Three neurotoxins have been identified within eosinophil granules: major basic protein, eosinophil cationic protein, and eosinophil-derived neurotoxin.

Clinical Signs

I. Neurologic signs reflect a diffuse or multifocal disease process.
   A. Disturbances of consciousness and abnormal behavior are common presenting signs.
   B. Other deficits that have been reported include circling, ataxia, paresis, hypermetria, head tremors, seizures, blindness, and facial nerve palsy.
II. The clinical course is variable; signs may improve, remain static, or worsen over time.

Diagnosis

I. Complete blood count may reveal the presence of a mild to moderate eosinophilia in some cases.
II. CSF analysis characteristically shows evidence of inflammation, with a dramatic increase in eosinophil numbers.
III. Other causes of eosinophilic inflammation in the CNS must be excluded (see Differential Diagnosis).

Differential Diagnosis

I. Infectious encephalitis
   A. Toxoplasmosis, neosporosis

B. Cryptococcosis
C. Prototomycosis
II. Parasitic encephalitis
III. Neoplasia
IV. Toxic encephalitis
V. Foreign body encephalitis

Treatment

I. The use of corticosteroids (prednisone 1 mg/kg PO BID initially; taper dose once signs abate) is advocated because of the presumed immunologic basis of the inflammation.
II. Infectious causes of CNS inflammation should be ruled out before initiating corticosteroid therapy.

Patient Monitoring

I. The disease carries a fair to guarded prognosis.
II. Because of the limited number of reported cases and their variable clinical course, no generalizations can be made regarding response to therapy and natural progression of disease.

Feline Polioencephalomyelitis

Definition and Causes

I. It is a chronic, progressive neurologic disease of cats characterized histologically by neuronal degeneration and perivascular accumulations of mononuclear cells.
II. The cause is unknown.
III. The pathologic changes characteristic of the disease suggest a viral etiology, although a causative viral agent has not been identified (Vandevelde and Braund, 1979).

Pathophysiology

The disease causes neuronal degeneration, which is most severe in the spinal cord but is also found in multiple areas of the brain.

Clinical Signs

I. The disease has been reported in cats of all ages.
II. Neurologic signs have a slow onset and a chronic, progressive course.
   A. Gait abnormalities, including incoordination, paresis, and hypermetria, are common.
   B. Seizures, intention tremors of the head, and abnormal pupillary light reflexes have been seen in some animals.

Diagnosis

I. Nonspecific systemic signs of disease may be present.
   A. Complete blood count may reveal leukopenia and anemia.

B. Ophthalmic examination may reveal areas of tapetal hyperreflectivity and subretinal infiltrates.
II. A mild increase in CSF protein concentration has been reported.
III. Definitive diagnosis can be made only by identifying characteristic lesions on necropsy.

Differential Diagnosis

I. Infectious encephalitis
II. Neoplasia

Treatment and Monitoring

I. There are no reported attempts at therapy.
II. The disease is slowly progressive.
III. Prognosis is guarded.

Canine Pyogranulomatous Meningoencephalomyelitis

Definition and Causes

I. It is an acute, progressive disease of the CNS that affects only mature pointers.
II. The cause is unknown.
III. A bacterial etiology has been proposed based on clinical and pathologic data (Braund, 1980).

Pathophysiology

The disease is characterized histologically by extensive areas of mononuclear and neutrophilic inflammation in the meninges and parenchyma of the brain and spinal cord.

Clinical Signs

I. Signs suggestive of meningitis predominate.
II. Affected dogs display cervical rigidity, kyphosis, and a reluctance to move.
III. Incoordinated gait, trigeminal and facial nerve paralysis, and Horner's syndrome may also be seen.

Diagnosis

I. CSF from affected dogs reveals a marked neutrophilic inflammation, with an associated increase in protein concentrations.
II. Other causes of neutrophilic CNS inflammation must be excluded.
III. Diagnosis can be confirmed only by finding characteristic histopathologic changes in an animal with a compatible history and signalment.

Differential Diagnosis

I. Infectious encephalitis
   A. Bacterial
   B. Fungal
   C. Rickettsial
II. Steroid-responsive meningitis

Treatment and Monitoring

I. There are no reports of successful treatment.
II. The disease is rapidly progressive, with a typical duration of 2–3 weeks.
III. The prognosis is poor.

IDIOPATHIC DISORDERS

Peripheral Vestibular Syndrome

Definition

This disorder of cats and older dogs is characterized by the acute onset of peripheral vestibular signs.

Causes and Pathophysiology

I. The etiology has not been determined.
II. No abnormalities have been identified on necropsy examination of affected animals.
III. This idiopathic disorder is a common cause of peripheral vestibular disease in both dogs and cats.

Clinical Signs

I. Acute onset of nonprogressive neurologic disease is typical.
II. The feline disease is seen in cats of all ages and is most common in spring to fall months.
III. The canine disease is seen year-round and typically affects older (geriatric) dogs.
IV. Neurologic signs are indicative of a peripheral vestibular disorder.
   A. Head tilt, falling, circling, rolling
   B. Horizontal or rotary nystagmus
   C. No depression of consciousness, postural deficits, or other cranial nerve deficits that would be suggestive of a central (brain stem) vestibular disorder
   D. Possibly bilateral lesions in cats, in which case no head tilt or spontaneous nystagmus is noted
V. Animals may display anorexia or vomiting due to the disequilibrium.

Diagnosis

I. Compatible history and examination findings are highly suggestive.
II. Rule out other causes of peripheral vestibular disease with the following diagnostic tests.
   A. Minimum database: complete blood count, chemistry profile
   B. Thorough otoscopic examination
   C. Radiographs or CT evaluation of the tympanic bulla

Differential Diagnosis

I. Otitis interna/media
II. Middle ear polyps (cats)
III. Trauma
IV. Neoplasia of middle ear or peripheral nerve
V. Endocrine-associated neuropathies
   A. Hypothyroidism
   B. Diabetes mellitus
   C. Hyperadrenocorticism
VI. Toxins
   A. Aminoglycoside antibiotics
   B. Topical chlorhexidine or iodophor compounds

Treatment

I. No definitive therapy is available.
II. Provide supportive therapy until the condition resolves.
   A. Administer fluid therapy if the animal is anorexic.
   B. Antihistamines such as meclizine (cat: 2 mg/kg PO SID; dog: 4 mg/kg PO SID) may be helpful in decreasing anorexia and vomiting associated with the disequilibrium.

Patient Monitoring

I. The prognosis is good, and the condition resolves on its own.
II. Recovery is usually seen within 1–3 weeks.
III. Residual head tilt or ataxia may persist.

Trigeminal Neuropathy

Definition

I. It is a disorder of dogs characterized by the acute onset of paralysis of the muscles of mastication, resulting in a dropped jaw.
II. The condition is also known as mandibular paralysis.

Causes and Pathophysiology

I. The etiology is unknown.
II. Pathologically, bilateral nonsuppurative inflammation is seen in all motor branches of the trigeminal nerve and ganglion.
III. The sensory branches of the trigeminal nerve remain normal.

Clinical Signs

I. Animals present with an acute inability to close the mouth.
II. Owners may report excessive drooling and difficulty prehending food.
III. Horner's syndrome may also be apparent.
IV. The remainder of the neurologic examination is normal.

Diagnosis

I. Compatible history and examination findings
II. No evidence of abnormalities on diagnostic work-up
   A. Minimum database: complete blood count, chemistry profile

B. Palpation of temporomandibular joint: no evidence of luxation or fracture associated with trauma
C. ± CSF analysis: normal

Differential Diagnosis

I. Trauma to the temporomandibular joint
II. Endocrine-associated neuropathies
A. Hypothyroidism
B. Diabetes mellitus
C. Hyperadrenocorticism
III. Rabies
A. Rabies must be considered in the acute stages of the disease.
B. Rabies is a progressive disease, and other neurologic deficits typically become apparent within 5–7 days after the onset of signs.

Treatment

I. No definitive treatment is available.
II. Provide supportive care until the condition resolves.
A. Instruct the owner to feed the dog "meatballs" made from canned food and to place the food in the dog's mouth manually.
B. Offer water with a syringe.

Patient Monitoring

I. The prognosis is excellent, and the condition resolves on its own.
II. Recovery usually takes 2–3 weeks.

Idiopathic Facial Paralysis

Definition and Causes

I. It is a disorder of mature dogs, characterized by the acute onset of facial nerve paralysis.
II. The cause is unknown.
III. American and English cocker spaniels appear to be predisposed to this condition.

Pathophysiology

Pathologic studies reveal active demyelination of large diameter fibers within the facial nerve (Braund, 1987).

Clinical Signs

I. Characteristic findings include ear droop, lip droop, inability to blink the eye, and excessive salivation.
II. Decreased tear production may be seen due to involvement of facial nerve fibers that innervate the lacrimal gland.
III. Signs may be either unilateral or bilateral.

Diagnosis

I. Minimum database
II. Thyroid function tests

III. Adrenal function tests
IV. Radiographs of the tympanic bulla

Differential Diagnosis

I. Otitis media/interna
II. Endocrine-associated neuropathies
A. Hypothyroidism
B. Hyperadrenocorticism
C. Diabetes mellitus
III. Neoplasia of the facial nerve or surrounding tissues
IV. Trauma

Treatment

I. No definitive treatment is available.
II. Treatment for keratoconjunctivitis sicca may be necessary in cases with lacrimal gland involvement (see Chap. 95).

Patient Monitoring

I. Prognosis for recovery of function is fair and varies from case to case.
II. If improvement is going to occur, it usually does so within 1–2 months.

Generalized Tremor Syndrome

Definition and Causes

I. This is a disorder characterized by the acute onset of rhythmic involuntary contractions of muscles of the body, head, and limbs.
II. The cause is unknown.
III. The condition is seen primarily in Maltese and other small white dogs.

Pathophysiology

Pathophysiologic mechanisms that have been proposed include the following.
I. Defect in neurotransmission
II. Immune-mediated disorder
III. Underlying encephalitis/meningitis

Clinical Signs

I. Signs are initially noted between 6 months and 5 years of age.
II. The presence of generalized tremors is the most notable examination finding.
III. Other neurologic deficits may be found.
A. Absent menace response
B. Nystagmus or disconjugate, jerky eye movements
C. Ataxia
D. Paresis
E. Head tilt

Diagnosis

I. Characteristic signs in a young, small-breed, white dog allow a presumptive diagnosis.

II. Obtain a minimum database (complete blood count, chemistry profile) to rule out metabolic disturbances.

III. CSF analysis reveals mild lymphocytic inflammation in most cases, with or without concurrent elevation in protein concentration (Bagley et al., 1993b); infectious causes of lymphocytic inflammation must be ruled out.

Differential Diagnosis

I. Dysmyelinogenesis, hypomyelinogenesis
II. Toxicoses
   A. Organophosphates
   B. Hexachlorophene
   C. Bromethalin
   D. Metaldehyde
III. Metabolic imbalances
   A. Hypocalcemia
   B. Hypoglycemia
   C. Azotemia
   D. Hyperammonemia

Treatment

I. Most tremors resolve or lessen on immunosuppressive therapy with prednisone 1–2 mg/kg PO BID.
II. After remission of signs, the prednisone is decreased to the lowest dosage that controls the tremors.
III. Symptomatic therapy may also be attempted to decrease the tremors.
   A. Diazepam 0.25 mg/kg PO TID-QID
   B. Propranolol 1 mg/kg PO TID

Patient Monitoring

I. Prognosis for medical control of the tremors is fair to good.
II. Disease course is variable; some animals remain free of clinical signs after the cessation of corticosteroids, and others need to be maintained on low-dose therapy to control signs.
III. Recurrence of tremors is possible.

Scotty Cramp

Definition and Causes

I. Scotty cramp is a paroxysmal disorder seen in Scottish terriers characterized by hyperkinetic episodes.
II. A similar condition has been seen in young dalmation dogs.
III. The disease is believed to be inherited, with a recessive mode of transmission.

Pathophysiology

I. The disease involves a functional defect in the neural pathways that control or moderate muscle contraction.
II. An imbalance of the neurotransmitter serotonin has been suggested by pharmacologic studies.
III. No structural abnormalities in neural tissue or muscle are noted on histopathologic examination.

Clinical Signs

I. Signs are initially seen between 6 weeks and 18 months of age.
II. The episodes are stimulated by exercise, excitement, or stress.
III. Abnormalities suggest muscle cramping or spasms.
   A. Stiff "goose-stepping" gait, characterized by hyperflexion and hyperextension of the limbs
   B. Hypertension of the pelvic limbs, causing the dog to fall over
   C. Spasms in the cervical and facial muscles
IV. Mental status remains normal during the episodes.
V. Signs are alleviated by a short period of rest (approximately 10 minutes).

Diagnosis

I. Characteristic signs in a young Scottish terrier are very suggestive.
II. Minimum database (complete blood count, chemistry profile), creatine kinase levels, and CSF analysis are all normal.
III. Pharmacologic testing can be performed to support a diagnosis.
   A. Methysergide (0.3 mg/kg PO) is given, and the animal is exercised 2 hours later.
   B. This drug is a serotonin antagonist and induces clinical signs.
   C. This provocative testing is most useful in mildly affected dogs.

Differential Diagnosis

I. Primary muscle disease (see Chap. 80)
   A. Myotonia
   B. Polymyositis
   C. Myopathy
II. Hypocalcemia

Treatment

I. Symptomatic therapy may be tried with either of the following.
   A. Diazepam 0.5 mg/kg PO TID
   B. Acepromazine 0.1–0.75 mg/kg PO BID
II. Vitamin E (125 IU/kg/day) has also been recommended (Clemmons et al., 1980); it does not reduce the severity of an episode but reduces the likelihood that an episode will occur.
III. Change the environment to reduce exposure to precipitating events.

Patient Monitoring

I. The disease can be managed with treatment but cannot be cured.
II. The disorder is not progressive.

PARASITIC DISORDERS

CNS Larva Migrans

Definition

Aberrant migration of parasite larvae through the CNS results in tissue damage and subsequent clinical signs.

Causes

   I. *Toxocara canis*
   II. *Ancylostoma caninum*
   III. *Angiostrongylus cantonensis*
   IV. *Dirofilaria immitis*

Pathophysiology

   I. Migrating larvae damage neural tissue by two mechanisms.
     A. Necrosis of tissue along the pathway of the migration
     B. Evoking an inflammatory response, which causes ischemia, edema, and toxic injury to myelin, axons, and neurons
   II. Neuronal necrosis may be seen with *D. immitis*, as a result of the migration of larvae within the neurovascular system, causing cerebral infarction.

Clinical Signs

   I. Signs are typically acute in onset and rapidly progressive.
   II. Neurologic signs reflect the anatomic structures the parasite has invaded.
     A. Forebrain: seizures, blindness, circling, behavioral changes, postural deficits
     B. Brain stem: paresis, depression of consciousness, cranial nerve deficits, including head tilt and nystagmus
     C. Cerebellum: ataxia, hypermetria, intention tremor
   III. Neurologic signs may reflect focal or multifocal involvement.

Diagnosis

   I. CSF analysis characteristically reveals eosinophilic inflammation. Neutrophilic inflammation may also be seen, secondary to tissue necrosis associated with the parasitic migration.
   II. The presence of *Dirofilaria* in the peripheral blood supports a diagnosis of aberrant *D. immitis* migration.
   III. Definitive diagnosis requires histologic demonstration of the parasite within the CNS.

Differential Diagnosis

   I. Infectious encephalitis
     A. Protozoal infections, cryptococcosis, and protothecosis have been associated with eosinophilic inflammation in CSF.
     B. Bacterial encephalitis should be considered in cases with neutrophilic inflammation.
   II. Other parasitic encephalitis
   III. Eosinophilic meningoencephalomyelitis
   IV. Granulomatous meningoencephalomyelitis

Treatment and Monitoring

   I. No successful therapy has been reported to date.
   II. The prognosis is guarded.

Intracranial Cuterebral Myiasis

Definition and Causes

Aberrant migration of *Cuterebra* larvae within the CNS parenchyma of an abnormal host for the parasite, such as a dog or a cat

Pathophysiology

   I. Proposed routes of entry into the brain for the larvae include the following.
     A. Migration through the foramina of the skull
     B. Penetration of the ethmoid bone and cribriform plate
     C. Passage through the general circulation following penetration of a major vessel
     D. Migration through the external and middle ear, with penetration of the mastoid region and invasion of the venous sinuses and meninges
   II. Typical microscopic findings consist of multifocal areas of necrosis surrounded by mixed inflammatory infiltrates.

Clinical Signs

   I. Cases of intracranial cuterebriasis most commonly occur from June through October, corresponding to when adult female flies deposit their ova.
   II. Affected animals usually present with acute onset of progressive neurologic dysfunction.
   III. The clinical signs reflect the neuroanatomic structures invaded by the parasitic migration.
   IV. Many animals present with disorientation, depression, and behavioral changes, reflective of forebrain involvement.

Diagnosis

   I. CSF analysis characteristically reveals a mixed inflammatory reaction, with the predominant cell type being neutrophils or eosinophils.
   II. Definitive diagnosis requires identification of the parasite within the nervous tissue.

Differential Diagnosis

   I. Infectious encephalitis
     A. Protozoal infections, cryptococcosis, and protothecosis have been associated with eosinophilic inflammation on CSF analysis.

   B. Bacterial encephalitis should be considered in cases with neutrophilic inflammation.
 II. Other parasitic encephalitis
III. Eosinophilic meningoencephalomyelitis
IV. Granulomatous meningoencephalomyelitis

Treatment and Monitoring

  I. Experimental therapy with ivermectin (0.3 mg/kg SQ QOD for three treatments) has been used in cases of suspected intracranial *Cuterebra* infection (Hendrix et al., 1989) but has not yet been proved effective.
 II. The prognosis is guarded.
III. Even if appropriate treatment can be instituted, neurologic dysfunction may persist because of tissue necrosis associated with the parasite migration and destruction of the parasite.

METABOLIC AND TOXIC DISORDERS

Metabolic Encephalopathy

Definition

This disturbance in brain function is caused by disorders of metabolism and typically manifests as bilateral, diffuse cerebral dysfunction.

Causes

   I. Hypoxia
     A. Myocardial failure
     B. Disturbances in hemoglobin function
       1. Carbon monoxide poisoning
       2. Methemoglobinemia
     C. Cellular hypoxia: cyanide poisoning
  II. Hypoglycemia
     A. Pancreatic beta-cell tumor
     B. Insulin overdose
     C. Liver failure
     D. Sepsis
 III. Acidosis
 IV. Alkalosis
  V. Hyperosmotic states
     A. Hyperglycemia: diabetes mellitus
     B. Hypernatremia
       1. Dehydration
       2. Diabetes insipidus
       3. Hyperaldosteronism
 VI. Hypo-osmostic states, hyponatremia
     A. Addison's disease
     B. Water intoxication
     C. Inappropriate secretion of antidiuretic hormone
VII. Alterations in calcium homeostasis
     A. Hypercalcemia
       1. Paraneoplastic syndrome
       2. Rodenticide toxicity
       3. Hyperparathyroidism
     B. Hypocalcemia
       1. Eclampsia

       2. Hypoparathyroidism
VIII. Endogenous neurotoxins
     A. Hepatic insufficiency (see Hepatic Encephalopathy, later)
     B. Renal insufficiency
     C. Pancreatitis
 IX. Endocrine disorders
     A. Hyperthyroidism
     B. Hypothyroidism

Pathophysiology

   I. Energy deprivation (glucose, oxygen) leads to alterations in the resting membrane potential and disturbances in neurotransmitter function and metabolism. Certain toxins and metabolic disturbances may interfere with energy metabolism in the brain.
  II. Electrolyte imbalances may affect neuronal excitability and neurotransmission. Calcium plays an essential role in the release of neurotransmitter at the synapse.
 III. Changes in serum osmolality and water balance lead to altered osmotic balance in neural cells, which may result in either brain edema or dehydration. Shrinking of endothelial cells may lead to disruption of the blood-brain barrier.
 IV. Endogenous toxins may result in the production of "false neurotransmitters."

Clinical Signs

   I. Metabolic encephalopathies cause diffuse, bilaterally symmetrical signs of forebrain disease.
  II. Onset of signs may be acute or chronic; signs may wax and wane with certain conditions.
 III. The primary clinical signs are as follows.
     A. Altered mentation
       1. Confusion, disorientation
       2. Dementia
       3. Aimless pacing, circling, head pressing
     B. Altered consciousness
       1. Obtundation
       2. Stupor
       3. Coma
     C. Seizures
     D. Motor deficits
       1. Tremors
       2. Myoclonus
       3. Paresis to paralysis

Diagnosis

   I. Other evidence of metabolic disturbances may be identified from the history or on physical examination.
  II. Minimum database (complete blood count, chemistry profile, urinalysis) and serum bile acid levels are indicated in all cases.
 III. Other diagnostic tests to be considered based on history, physical findings, and results of initial blood tests include the following.

A. Blood gases
B. Serum osmolality
C. Resting ammonia/ammonia tolerance test
D. Thyroid function tests
E. Cardiac work-up: electrocardiogram, blood pressure measurements, cardiac radiographs and ultrasonography
F. Abdominal radiographs and ultrasonography

Differential Diagnosis

I. Diffuse encephalitis
II. Hydrocephalus
III. Midline thalamic mass lesion (brain tumor)

Treatment and Monitoring

I. Ensure adequate airway, breathing, and circulation if the animal's condition has progressed to a comatose state.
II. Correct the underlying metabolic disturbance.
III. Treat seizures.
   A. Administer dextrose if hypoglycemia is a possibility.
   B. Diazepam 1 mg/kg IV is the anticonvulsant drug of choice.
   C. Use barbiturates with caution.
      1. Metabolism may be compromised with liver disease.
      2. Acidosis causes increased penetration of barbiturates into the brain.
   D. In general, seizures are difficult to control until the underlying metabolic imbalance is corrected.
IV. In most cases, normal neurologic function is restored once the metabolic disturbance is corrected.

Hepatic Encephalopathy

Definition

I. Hepatic encephalopathy is a clinical syndrome in which neurologic dysfunction occurs secondary to advanced liver disease, which causes the accumulation of substances that have toxic effects on the CNS.
II. It is a frequently encountered metabolic encephalopathy in small animals.

Causes

I. Congenital portocaval shunts
II. Acute fulminant hepatic failure
III. Chronic liver disease, with associated acquired portosystemic shunts
IV. Congenital deficiency of urea cycle enzymes, resulting in the accumulation of ammonia

Pathophysiology

I. The pathogenesis of hepatic encephalopathy is not completely understood, but current theories fall into four categories (Maddison, 1992).
II. Several toxins have been shown to act synergistically with ammonia to induce an encephalopathic state, including short chain fatty acids, mercaptans, phenols, and bile salts.
III. Alterations in amino acid metabolism result in increased concentrations of aromatic amino acids and decreased concentrations of branched chain amino acids.
   A. This can result in alterations in the synthesis of neurotransmitters or the formation of false neurotransmitters.
   B. The amino acid tryptophan has a direct neurotoxic effect.
IV. Imbalance occurs between the excitatory neurotransmitter glutamine and the inhibitory neurotransmitter gamma-aminobutyric acid (GABA).
V. Increased cerebral concentrations of an endogenous benzodiazepine-like substance may also occur.

Clinical Signs

I. Systemic signs of liver failure (see Chap. 34)
II. Diffuse, symmetrical signs of forebrain dysfunction
   A. Behavioral changes
   B. Alterations in consciousness
   C. Seizures
   D. Tremors
III. Neurologic signs
   A. May wax and wane
   B. Characteristically worsen following a high-protein meal

Diagnosis

I. Minimum database: complete blood count, chemistry profile, urinalysis
II. Serum bile acid levels: fasting and postprandial
III. Abdominal radiographs and ultrasonography

Differential Diagnosis

I. Other metabolic or toxic encephalopathies
II. Diffuse encephalitis
III. Hydrocephalus
IV. Midline, thalamic mass lesion (brain tumor)

Treatment

I. Control the production and absorption of toxic products from the gut.
   A. Stop all oral food intake until neurologic signs abate.
   B. Resume feeding with a high-quality, low-protein diet.
   C. Decrease urease-producing colonic bacteria.
      1. 10% povidone-iodine enema (instill into colon, drain 10–15 minutes later; may be repeated every 4–6 hours)
      2. Metronidazole 7.5 mg/kg PO TID
   D. Acidify the colonic contents to favor conversion of ammonia to ammonium ion (which is not absorbed) by administering lactulose.
      1. By stomach tube, 20–60 ml every 4–6 hours

2. By enema, 300–450 g diluted in 200–300 ml of water
3. 5 ml per 5–10 kg PO divided TID

II. Correct any acid–base, electrolyte, or fluid imbalance that may precipitate an encephalopathic episode.
III. Treat seizures symptomatically.
IV. Correct the underlying liver disorder, if possible.

Patient Monitoring

I. In most cases, clinical signs abate with appropriate therapy; however, the long-term prognosis is poor unless hepatic dysfunction is reversible.
II. Avoid factors that may precipitate hepatic encephalopathy.
   A. High-protein meals
   B. Gastrointestinal bleeding
   C. Azotemia, alkalosis
   D. Administration of anesthetics or sedatives
   E. Constipation

Lead Poisoning

See Chap. 127.

VASCULAR DISORDERS

Feline Ischemic Encephalopathy

Definition and Causes

I. Ischemic necrosis of cerebral tissue may occur spontaneously in adult cats.
II. The cause is unknown.
III. There is no evidence of cardiomyopathy in affected cats.

Pathophysiology

I. The histopathologic lesion consists of a variable degree of ischemic necrosis of one or, less commonly, both cerebral hemispheres.
II. The infarcted tissue is frequently in the area of brain supplied by the middle meningeal artery.
III. Actual vascular lesions are rarely identified.

Clinical Signs

I. Onset of signs is peracute and suggestive of a forebrain lesion.
   A. Behavioral changes
   B. Alterations in mentation
   C. Seizures
   D. Postural deficits
   E. Blindness
II. Bilateral blindness with dilated, unresponsive pupils may be caused by ischemic necrosis of the optic chiasm.
III. Signs are nonprogressive, and some improvement is typically noted within a few days.

Diagnosis

I. CSF analysis often reveals a mildly elevated protein concentration with no increase in WBC numbers.
II. Advanced imaging techniques, such as CT or MRI, may demonstrate the necrotic focus in severe cases.

Differential Diagnosis

I. Infectious encephalitis
II. Neoplasia
III. Cerebral infarct secondary to cardiomyopathy

Treatment

I. No definitive treatment is available.
II. Anticonvulsants are administered to cats with seizures (see Chap. 22).

Patient Monitoring

I. The prognosis is favorable, as many of the initial signs ameliorate within a few days.
II. Neurologic deficits, most typically behavioral changes and seizures, may persist.

Vascular Injury

Definition

I. Damage to the blood vessels of the brain results in an area of either hemorrhage or infarct.
II. The incidence of vascular disease is low compared with other causes of brain dysfunction in dogs and cats.

Causes

I. Infarcts most commonly result from either primary vascular disease or thromboembolism.
   A. Primary vascular disease
      1. Atherosclerosis secondary to hypothyroidism
      2. Vasculitis
         a) Rickettsial disease (Rocky Mountain spotted fever)
         b) Immune-mediated disease
      3. Hypertension
   B. Thromboembolism
      1. Cardiomyopathy
      2. Bacterial endocarditis
      3. Sepsis
      4. *D. immitis* infection
      5. Severe polycythemia
      6. Disseminated intravascular coagulopathy
      7. Hypercoagulable disorders
II. Hemorrhage may occur from alterations in vessel integrity or secondary to bleeding disorders.
   A. Alterations in vascular integrity
      1. Arteriovenous malformations
      2. Hypertension
      3. Trauma
   B. Bleeding disorders

1. Thrombocytopenia
2. Vitamin K–dependent rodenticide toxicity
3. Disseminated intravascular coagulopathy
4. Coagulation factor deficiencies

Pathophysiology

I. Development of clinical signs secondary to vascular injury is dependent on the size and location of the vessel involved, the rapidity with which the injury develops, and the susceptibility of the affected area of brain to energy deprivation.
II. Of the general divisions of the brain, the cerebral cortex and cerebellum are the most susceptible to injury.
III. Energy deprivation results in malacia of the brain tissue, characterized histologically by necrosis and capillary proliferation.

Clinical Signs

I. Acute onset of asymmetrical neurologic dysfunction is typical.
II. Signs are nonprogressive and may slowly improve.
III. Neurologic signs reflect the location of the lesion.
  A. Forebrain: seizures, blindness, circling, behavioral changes, postural deficits
  B. Cerebellum: ataxia, intention tremor, vestibular signs
  C. Brain stem: cranial nerve deficits, paresis, depression of consciousness, pupillary abnormalities, respiratory and cardiac disturbances
IV. Evidence of cardiovascular, metabolic, or bleeding disorders may also be seen.

Diagnosis

I. CSF may be normal or show only mild changes.
  A. Increased protein may be noted.
  B. Erythrophagocytosis and xanthochromia indicate previous hemorrhage.
  C. Collection of CSF may be contraindicated in animals with bleeding disorders, as the procedure itself may induce hemorrhage.
II. Advanced imaging modalities (CT and MRI) can reveal changes characteristic of vascular infarct or hemorrhage.

Differential Diagnosis

I. Trauma
II. Neoplasia
III. Focal encephalitis

Treatment

I. Specific treatment for any underlying disease
II. Prednisone 0.5–1 mg/kg PO BID for several days, with a tapering dose thereafter to decrease edema and inflammation
III. General supportive care

Patient Monitoring

I. Prognosis is variable and dependent on the underlying cause, severity of signs, and location of the lesion.
  A. Brain stem lesions carry a fair to guarded prognosis.
  B. Prognosis is fair to good with forebrain and cerebellar lesions.
II. Clinical improvement may take weeks to months.

NUTRITIONAL DISORDERS

Thiamine Deficiency

See Chap. 120.

NEOPLASTIC DISORDERS

Brain Tumors

Definition

I. Primary brain tumors arise from neuroectodermal or mesodermal cells that are normally present in or associated with the brain.
II. Secondary tumors may originate from surrounding tissues and locally extend into the brain, or they may arise from hematogenous metastasis of primary tumors in other tissues.

Causes

I. Classification of brain tumors is based primarily on characteristics of the constituent cell type.
II. Primary tumors include the following (Bagley et al., 1993a).
  A. Tumors of neuroepithelium
    1. Astrocytoma
    2. Oligodendroglioma
    3. Glioblastoma
    4. Medulloblastoma
    5. Ependymoma
    6. Choroid plexus tumors
  B. Tumors of meninges: meningioma
  C. Tumors of lymphoid tissue: lymphosarcoma
  D. Tumors of nerve sheaths
    1. Schwannoma
    2. Neurofibroma
  E. Tumors of pituitary gland and craniopharyngeal duct
    1. Pituitary adenoma
    2. Craniopharyngioma
III. Secondary tumors are as follows.
  A. Metastatic tumors
    1. Hemangiosarcoma
    2. Prostatic carcinoma
    3. Mammary gland adenocarcinoma
    4. Bronchial adenocarcinoma
    5. Malignant melanoma
  B. Primary tumors from nearby structures

1. Osteosarcoma
2. Chondrosarcoma
3. Fibrosarcoma
4. Nasal adenocarcinoma

Pathophysiology

I. Direct effects of tumor growth include compression and invasion of normal brain parenchyma.
II. Indirect effects of tumor growth are often more significant than direct effects.
   A. Damage to the blood-brain barrier, with resultant edema
   B. Obstruction to CSF flow, causing secondary hydrocephalus
   C. Brain herniation caused by increased intracranial pressure from an enlarging space-occupying mass within the rigid cranial cavity
   D. Hemorrhage

Clinical Signs

I. Breed predispositions have been reported for several tumor types.
   A. Brachycephalics, especially boxers and Boston terriers
      1. Glial cell tumors
      2. Pituitary tumors
   B. Dolichocephalics: meningiomas
II. Onset of disease may be acute or insidious, depending of the location, rate of growth, and indirect effects of the tumor.
III. Neurologic signs reflect the location of the tumor, with the following typical clinical patterns.
   A. Forebrain tumors cause seizures, circling, behavioral abnormalities, visual deficits, and postural deficits.
   B. Brain stem tumors cause cranial nerve deficits, paresis, and depression of consciousness.
   C. Cerebellar tumors cause dysmetria and intention tremor.
   D. "Cavernous sinus syndrome" is seen with tumors involving the floor of the calvarium.
      1. Cranial nerves III (oculomotor), IV (trochlear), VI (abducens), and branches of V (trigeminal) traverse the cavernous sinus on the floor of the calvarium.
      2. Characteristic signs include ophthalmoplegia, mydriasis with absent pupillary light reflexes, ptosis, decreased corneal sensation, and decreased retractor oculi reflex (Theisen et al., 1996).
IV. Signs are usually lateralizing, although midline tumors may cause symmetrical deficits.
V. Metastatic tumors usually involve multiple areas within the CNS, which may result in multifocal signs.

Diagnosis

I. Obtain a minimum database to look for any evidence of systemic disease.
   A. Particularly useful when seizures are the only presenting sign
   B. As a screening for metastatic disease
II. Ophthalmoscopic examination may reveal the presence of papilledema, suggestive of increased intracranial pressure.
III. Thoracic radiography is used to evaluate for evidence of metastasis.
   A. Most primary brain tumors do not metastasize.
   B. Many tumors that metastasize to the brain also spread to the lungs.
IV. Diagnosis is usually based on advanced imaging modalities (CT, MRI). Images are evaluated for the presence of mass lesions, contrast enhancement, compression of normal brain structures, and secondary hydrocephalus.
V. CSF analysis may provide additional information.
   A. Brain tumors typically cause an increased protein concentration with normal cell counts.
   B. Increased WBC counts may be seen with specific tumor types.
      1. Lymphoma: increased lymphocytes or lymphoblasts
      2. Meningioma: increased neutrophils secondary to tumor necrosis
   C. CSF analysis may not be performed in many cases when mass lesions are identified on CT or MRI, owing to the increased risk of brain herniation associated with the collection of CSF in these cases.

Differential Diagnosis

I. Infectious/inflammatory granulomas
   A. Toxoplasmosis
   B. Fungal encephalitis
   C. Granulomatous meningoencephalomyelitis
   D. Brain abscess
II. Vascular disorder
   A. Hematoma
   B. Infarct

Treatment

I. Decrease edema associated with the tumor with prednisone 0.5–1 mg/kg PO BID initially, then slowly tapering to QOD.
II. Treat seizures with phenobarbital 2.2 mg/kg PO BID.
III. Treat for increased intracranial pressure if a sudden, dramatic worsening of neurologic status is seen with mannitol 1 g/kg IV, given over 20 minutes.
IV. Options for definitive tumor treatment include surgery and radiation therapy.
   A. Surgery allows for tumor resection or cytoreduction and also provides a histologic diagnosis.
   B. Surgery is often reserved for tumors that are superficial and therefore more easily approachable.
   C. Radiation therapy, either alone or in combination with surgery, has been shown to increase survival time (Heidner et al., 1991).

Patient Monitoring

I. Overall prognosis is fair to guarded and is dependent on the location and type of the tumor.

II. In most instances, the goal of therapy is remission of signs and increased survival time rather than cure.

TRAUMATIC DISORDERS

Cranial Trauma

Definition and Causes

I. Neurologic dysfunction secondary to head trauma, resulting from edema and hemorrhage within the brain

II. Usually caused by a fall, automobile accident, blunt trauma to the head, or penetrating missile injuries

Pathophysiology

Neurologic dysfunction secondary to cranial trauma can occur by several mechanisms.

I. Depressed skull fractures, with compression and injury to underlying brain parenchyma

II. Angular acceleration of the brain, causing diffuse axonal injury

III. Impact of the brain against the skull, resulting in coup injuries (occurring under the area of impact) and countrecoup injuries (occurring in the opposite location)

IV. Hemorrhage and hematoma formation

V. Vasogenic edema

Clinical Signs

I. There is an acute onset of neurologic dysfunction, the signs of which may be focal or diffuse.

II. Forebrain damage may result in loss of consciousness if it is diffuse and severe, but it more frequently causes circling, altered mentation, blindness, and postural deficits. (Post-traumatic seizures may occur weeks to months after the injury.)

III. Brain stem injury frequently results in depression of consciousness (often to a comatose state).

A. Pupil size and responsiveness, and the presence or absence of normal physiologic nystagmus, are assessed in these cases.

B. Dilated, unresponsive pupils and the absence of physiologic nystagmus are poor prognostic indicators.

IV. Cerebellovestibular injury can result in dysmetria, ataxia, disequilibrium, head tilt, and nystagmus.

V. Clinical signs are monitored frequently for at least 24 hours following injury.

A. In most cases, the clinical signs are most severe within a short time of the injury.

B. Evidence of a worsening clinical state indicates brain swelling or hematoma formation.

Diagnosis

I. Signs of brain dysfunction in an animal known to have suffered an injury

II. Presence of abrasions, penetrating wounds, or other evidence of cranial trauma

III. Radiographs revealing evidence of skull fractures

IV. Advanced imaging techniques identifying areas of hemorrhage, hematoma formation, and severe edema

Differential Diagnosis

I. Other disorders should be considered when the presumed trauma was not observed and signs of trauma are not evident upon examination.

II. Consider metabolic encephalopathies, toxic encephalopathies, and vascular disorders.

Treatment

I. Provide emergency care to ensure airway patency, adequate ventilation, and stable cardiovascular function.

II. Treat brain edema and increased intracranial pressure.

A. Hyperoxygenate to prevent further tissue hypoxia.

B. Hyperventilate to decrease pCO_2 and promote cerebral vasoconstriction, thereby reducing intracranial pressure.

C. Administer one of the soluble glucocorticoids.

1. Prednisolone sodium succinate 10–30 mg/kg IV, followed by tapering doses every 6–8 hours for the next 48–72 hours

2. Dexamethasone sodium phosphate 2–4 mg/kg IV; repeat in 6–8 hours, then administer tapering doses every 6–8 hours for the next 48–72 hours

3. Effectiveness of glucocorticoid therapy controversial

D. Mannitol should be used cautiously and only in cases with severe neurologic compromise or a deteriorating condition despite aggressive medical therapy.

1. Recommended dose is 1 g/kg IV given over 20 minutes; may be repeated every 4–8 hours for 1–2 more doses.

2. It is contraindicated in hypovolemic animals.

3. Ongoing, undetectable intracranial hemorrhage may be exacerbated by the administration of mannitol.

III. High-dose methylprednisolone therapy has been shown experimentally to decrease tissue ischemia and necrosis and improve neurologic outcome following brain and spinal cord injury (Brown and Hall, 1992).

A. Recommended dose of methylprednisolone sodium succinate is 30 mg/kg IV initially, 15 mg/kg IV at 2 and 6 hours later, then 2.5 mg/kg/hour for 42 hours.

B. The drug is most effective if given within the first few hours after trauma and may be ineffective if given more than 8 hours after injury.

IV. Surgery is indicated if depressed skull fractures are present or if the animal's condition deteriorates despite aggressive medical management.

V. Provide supportive care.
   A. Administer fluid therapy and nutritional support.
   B. Turn recumbent animals every 6 hours and keep them clean, dry, and well padded.

Patient Monitoring

I. Prognosis depends on the severity and location of the injury.
II. For comatose animals, recovery is unlikely if no improvement is seen within 48–72 hours after injury.
III. Recovery of function may take weeks to months, although the majority of improvement is seen within 4 weeks of the injury.
IV. Long-term sequelae of cranial trauma include seizures and persistent neurologic deficits.

Bibliography

Bagley RS, Kornegay JN, Page RL et al: Central nervous system. p. 2137. In Slatter D (ed): Textbook of Small Animal Surgery. 2nd Ed. WB Saunders, Philadelphia, 1993a

Bagley RS, Kornegay JN, Wheeler SJ et al: Generalized tremors in Maltese dogs: clinical findings in seven cases. J Am Anim Hosp Assoc 29:141, 1993b

Bailey CS, Higgins RJ: Characteristics of cerebrospinal fluid associated with canine granulomatous meningoencephalomyelitis: a retrospective study. J Am Vet Med Assoc 188:418, 1986

Braund KG: Encephalitis and meningitis. Vet Clin North Am [Small Anim Pract] 10:31, 1980

Braund KG: Granulomatous meningoencephalomyelitis. J Am Vet Med Assoc 186:138, 1985

Braund KG: Diseases of peripheral nerves, cranial nerves, and muscle. p. 364. In Oliver JE, Hoerlein BF, Mayhew IG (eds): Veterinary Neurology. WB Saunders, Philadelphia, 1987

Brown SA, Hall ED: Role of oxygen-derived free radicals in the pathogenesis of shock and trauma, with focus on central nervous system injuries. J Am Vet Med Assoc 200:1849, 1992

Chrisman CL: Neurological diseases of rottweilers: neuroaxonal dystrophy and leukoencephalomalacia. J Small Anim Pract 33:500, 1992

Chrisman CL, Cork LC, Gamble DA: Neuroaxonal dystrophy of Rottweiler dogs. J Am Vet Med Assoc 184:464, 1984

Clemmons RM, Peters RI, Meyers KM: Scotty cramp: a review of cause, characteristics, diagnosis and treatment. Compend Contin Educ Pract Vet 2:385, 1980

Cordy DR, Holliday TA: A necrotizing meningoencephalitis of pug dogs. Vet Pathol 26:191, 1989

Cuddon PA, Smith-Maxie L: Reticulosis of the central nervous system in the dog. Compend Contin Educ Pract Vet 6:23, 1984

Forbes S, Cook JR: Congenital peripheral vestibular disease attributed to lymphocytic labyrinthitis in two related litters of Doberman pinscher dogs. J Am Vet Med Assoc 198:447, 1991

Gamble DA, Chrisman CL: A leukoencephalomyelopathy of Rottweiler dogs. Vet Pathol 21:274, 1984

Heidner GL, Kornegay JN, Page RL et al: Analysis of survival in a retrospective study of 86 dogs with brain tumors. J Vet Intern Med 5:219, 1991

Hendrix CM, DiPinto MN, Cox NR et al: Aberrant intracranial myiasis caused by larval *Cuterebra* infection. Compend Contin Educ Pract Vet 11:550, 1989

Maddison JE: Hepatic encephalopathy: current concepts of the pathogenesis. J Vet Intern Med 6:341, 1992

Sisson AF, LeCouteur RA, Dow SW: Radiation therapy of granulomatous meningoencephalomyelitis of dogs. Proc Am Coll Vet Intern Med 7:1031, 1989

Smith-Maxie LL, Parent JP, Rand J et al: Cerebrospinal fluid analysis and clinical outcome of eight dogs with eosinophilic meningoencephalomyelitis. J Vet Intern Med 3:167, 1989

Stalis IH, Chadwick B, Dayrell-Hart B et al: Necrotizing meningoencephalomyelitis of Maltese dogs. Vet Pathol 32:230, 1995

Theisen SK, Podell M, Schneider T et al: A retrospective study of cavernous sinus syndrome in 4 dogs and 8 cats. J Vet Intern Med 10:65, 1996

Tipold A, Fatzer R, Jaggy A et al: Necrotizing encephalitis in Yorkshire terriers. J Small Anim Pract 34:623, 1993

Vandevelde M, Braund KG: Polioencephalomyelitis in cats. Vet Pathol 16:420, 1979

24 Disorders of the Spinal Cord

William B. Thomas

CONGENITAL AND DEVELOPMENTAL DISORDERS

Spinal Arachnoid Cyst

Definition

I. Benign dilatation of the spinal subarachnoid space that is lined by an arachnoidal membrane and filled with cerebrospinal fluid (CSF)
II. Synonyms: subarachnoid cyst, meningeal cyst, leptomeningeal cyst

Causes and Pathophysiology

I. Some cases arise congenitally and may be associated with other developmental disorders of the spine.
II. They may be acquired secondary to arachnoid adhesions caused by trauma or meningitis, which alter CSF flow and cause dilatation of the subarachnoid space.
III. Lesions have been reported in the dorsal aspect of the cranial cervical and caudal thoracic regions.
IV. Neurologic deficits, if they occur, are caused by compression of the spinal cord.

Clinical Signs

I. Signalment: reported in immature and mature dogs and cats
II. May be an incidental finding
III. Progressive para- or tetraparesis
IV. May or may not be painful

Diagnosis

I. Plain radiography: usually normal; may show expansion of the vertebral canal
II. Myelography
   A. Focal, usually teardrop-shaped dilatation of the dorsal subarachnoid space

B. Variable attenuation of the adjacent portion of the spinal cord

Differential Diagnosis

I. Other developmental disorders
II. Neoplasia
III. Intervertebral disk disease
IV. Meningomyelitis

Treatment

I. Medical therapy
   A. Short-term administration of prednisone 0.5 mg/kg/day PO
   B. Cage rest
II. Surgery
   A. Drainage and excision of cyst
   B. Allows histopathologic diagnosis

Patient Monitoring

I. Medical therapy may be successful in mildly affected dogs (Dyce et al., 1991).
II. The prognosis is good with surgery (Bentley et al., 1991; Dyce et al., 1991).

Atlantoaxial Subluxation

Definition

Instability of the atlantoaxial joint that permits C2 to luxate dorsally, causing compression of the spinal cord

Causes

I. In toy breed dogs, it is usually caused by abnormal development or degeneration of the atlantoaxial joint.
II. It may occur as a component of occipitoatlantoaxial malformation in dogs and cats.

252

III. It can occur in any breed of dog or cat as a result of trauma.

Pathophysiology

I. In toy breeds, instability may be caused by abnormal development of the atlantoaxial joint or by avascular necrosis of the dens. Abnormalities include one or more of the following.
   A. Aplasia, hypoplasia, or dorsal angulation of the dens
   B. Separation of the dens from C2
   C. Absence of the transverse atlantoaxial ligament
II. Many cases are caused by relatively minor trauma superimposed on congenital instability.
III. Neurologic deficits are caused by compression of the cranial cervical spinal cord segments or caudal aspect of the brain stem. This occurs with dorsal displacement of the atlas when the neck is flexed ventrally.

Clinical Signs

I. Age of onset varies.
   A. Signs associated with congenital malformations are most common in toy breed dogs <1 year of age but can occur at any age.
   B. Trauma can be a cause in animals of any age or breed.
II. Onset is often acute.
III. Signs may progress or wax and wane.
IV. Neck pain is present in about 60% of cases.
V. Gait dysfunction occurs in about 85% of cases and ranges from ataxia to tetraplegia, with normal or exaggerated spinal cord reflexes.
VI. Death from respiratory paralysis can occur in severe cases.

Diagnosis

I. Radiography usually confirms the diagnosis.
II. Flexion of the neck is avoided initially.
III. Lateral view may show increased space between the arch of C1 and the spinous process of C2, or dorsal displacement of C2 relative to C1.
IV. Ventrodorsal and oblique views are helpful in evaluating the dens, which may be normal, hypoplastic, absent, separated, or dorsally angulated. Open mouth views are avoided because they require marked flexion of the neck.
V. Gentle flexion of the atlantoaxial joint may be necessary to identify instability in mild cases but is performed only if standard views are normal.

Differential Diagnosis

I. Trauma
II. Intervertebral disk disease
III. Meningomyelitis

Treatment

I. Animals with mild signs may recover with 6 weeks of cage rest and application of a neck brace that maintains extension of the atlantoaxial joint.

II. Surgical therapy is indicated for most cases to decompress the spinal cord and immobilize the atlantoaxial joint.
   A. There are several techniques.
      1. Ventral fixation using pins, screws, or a plate, with or without bone graft (Wheeler and Sharp, 1994; McCarthy et al., 1995)
      2. Dorsal fixation using wire, suture, the nuchal ligament, bone cement, pins, or atlantoaxial retractor (Wheeler and Sharp, 1994; McCarthy et al., 1995)
   B. There is a relatively high rate of complications.
      1. Surgical trauma to the spinal cord
      2. Upper respiratory problems from retraction of the trachea during the ventral approach
      3. Implant failure
   C. Postoperative care includes the use of external support and cage rest for 2–6 weeks.

Patient Monitoring

I. Dogs with congenital instability may relapse after conservative treatment.
II. Surgery is successful in about 60% of cases (Thomas et al., 1991; McCarthy et al., 1995).
III. Radiographs taken 6–8 weeks later are helpful in evaluating joint fusion or bony healing.

Multiple Cartilaginous Exostoses

Definition

I. Multiple cartilaginous exostosis (MCE) is a benign, proliferative disorder of bone characterized by the formation of multiple cartilage-capped exostoses that arise from the surfaces of bones formed by endochondral ossification.
II. Synonyms include osteochondromatosis, osteocartilaginous exostoses, and multiple exostoses.

Causes

I. The cause is unknown.
II. A hereditary component is involved in some dogs.
III. The feline leukemia virus may be involved in feline MCE.

Pathophysiology

I. Exostoses may arise from displacement of chondrocytes.
II. Any bone formed by endochondral ossification may be affected.
III. Lesions consist of cortical bone covered with hyaline cartilage. There is a center of cancellous bone containing nodules of cartilage undergoing endochondral ossification.
IV. Growth of exostoses stops at skeletal maturity.
V. Neoplastic transformation is uncommon but can occur in older animals.
VI. Clinical signs, if they occur, are caused by compression of the spinal cord or spinal nerves.

Clinical Signs

I. Signalment: immature dogs and cats
II. May be asymptomatic
III. Vertebral exostoses: pain or signs of a progressive, focal spinal cord lesion

Diagnosis

I. Plain radiography
   A. Lesions are radiodense with smooth borders.
   B. During growth, lesions may have a mottled appearance owing to hyaline cartilage.
II. Myelography: useful in defining the location and extent of any spinal cord compression

Differential Diagnosis

I. Neoplasia
II. Vertebral malformation

Treatment

I. Asymptomatic lesions do not require treatment.
II. Surgical excision is performed promptly in animals with neurologic deficits caused by spinal cord compression to prevent permanent spinal cord damage.

Patient Monitoring

I. Prognosis is generally good.
II. Recurrence or development of other lesions is possible in immature animals.
III. Development of neoplasia at the site of MCE has been reported in dogs older than 7 years of age (Owen and Bostock, 1971).

Myelodysplasia

Definition

I. Myelodysplasia refers to a variety of related malformations of the spinal cord.
II. In Weimaraners, it has been called spinal dysraphism or dysraphia, but these terms imply abnormal closure of the neural tube, which is not apparent.

Causes

I. In Weimaraners, it is probably inherited as a codominant gene with variable penetrance that is lethal in homozygotes.
II. It occurs sporadically in other breeds of dog.

Pathophysiology

I. Myelodysplasia usually affects thoracolumbar segments.
II. In the developing spinal cord of affected Weimaraner embryos, there is abnormal migration of the mantle layer of cells, which interferes with development of the basal plate.

III. Resulting abnormalities may include the following.
   A. Dilatation of the central canal (hydromyelia)
   B. Cavitation of the spinal cord (syringomyelia)
   C. Absent or duplicated central canal
   D. Abnormal distribution or migration of gray matter
   E. Abnormal formation of the ventral median fissure

Clinical Signs

I. Breeds: Weimaraner; sporadically in other breeds (Samoyed, dalmatian, rottweiler, and mixed-breed dogs)
II. Age: signs usually observed by 4–6 weeks of age, abnormal flexor reflex possibly identified shortly after birth
III. Nonprogressive neurologic dysfunction
   A. Simultaneous protraction of the pelvic limbs (''bunny hopping'')
   B. Ataxia and paresis of the pelvic limbs
   C. Bilateral flexor reflex in the pelvic limbs (when a flexor reflex is initiated in one limb, both limbs flex)
IV. Other possible abnormalities
   A. Scoliosis
   B. Abnormal hair patterns in the dorsal neck region
   C. Depression of the sternum in the median plane (kilosternia)

Diagnosis

I. Diagnosis is based on clinical signs and exclusion of other causes.
II. Ancillary tests, such as radiography, myelography, and CSF analysis, are usually normal.

Differential Diagnosis

I. Vertebral malformation
II. Spina bifida
III. Myelitis

Treatment and Monitoring

I. There is no treatment.
II. Signs do not worsen or resolve.
III. Mildly affected animals may have an acceptable quality of life.

Vertebral Malformations

Definition

I. Congenital malformation of one or more vertebra
II. Types of vertebral malformations
   A. Hemivertebra: wedge-shaped vertebra, with the base oriented dorsally, ventrally, or medially
   B. Block vertebrae: partial or complete fusion of adjacent vertebrae
   C. Butterfly vertebra: cleft in the sagittal plane of the vertebra
   D. Transitional vertebrae

1. These occur at the junction of major divisions of the spine and have the characteristics of two types of vertebrae.
2. For example, a lumbosacral transitional vertebra has characteristics of both lumbar and sacral vertebrae.

Causes

I. Often unknown
II. Inherited in some cases
   A. Hemivertebra is an autosomal recessive disorder in German shorthaired pointers and is inherited in English bulldogs and Yorkshire terriers (Bailey and Morgan, 1992).
   B. There is a high incidence of hemivertebra and butterfly vertebra in French and English bulldogs, pugs, and Boston terriers, suggesting a genetic component.

Pathophysiology

I. Most vertebral malformations occur in the embryo during the stage of resegmentation and are related to abnormal distribution of intersegmental arteries (Bailey and Morgan, 1992).
II. Spinal cord compression can occur as a result of stenosis of the vertebral canal, malalignment of vertebrae, or instability of the spine.
III. Vertebral malformations may coexist with malformations of the spinal cord.

Clinical Signs

I. Most vertebral malformations are incidental radiographic findings not associated with clinical signs.
II. Hemivertebrae are the most common malformations to cause clinical signs.
III. Neurologic deficits are referable to a focal myelopathy.
   A. Onset is usually, but not always, in immature animals.
   B. Signs may progress as the animal grows.

Diagnosis

I. Plain radiography may reveal several abnormalities.
   A. Malformed vertebrae appear to be formed of normal bone with smooth borders.
      1. Vertebral end plates are smooth with normal or increased opacity (sclerosis).
      2. Osteophytes may develop secondary to instability or abnormal distribution of stress.
   B. Hemivertebrae have wedge-shaped vertebral bodies with varying degrees of scoliosis.
   C. Block vertebrae appear as partially or completely fused vertebrae, often with a remnant of the intervertebral disk.
   D. On ventrodorsal views of butterfly vertebrae, vertebral end plates are triangular, with the apex toward the center of the vertebral body.
   E. With transitional vertebrae, abnormalities include

the transverse processes of C7 resembling ribs, a transverse process instead of a rib present on a caudal thoracic vertebra, and the last lumbar vertebra having a transverse process that is fused with the sacrum.
II. Myelography is indicated to define any spinal cord compression in animals with neurologic deficits.

Differential Diagnosis

I. Vertebral fracture, especially compression fracture or healed fracture/luxation
II. Healed diskospondylitis
III. Other developmental disorders
IV. Vertebral neoplasia

Treatment and Monitoring

I. Surgical decompression and/or stabilization is performed if necessary.
II. Prognosis is guarded, although animals with mild neurologic deficits may recover.

Spina Bifida

Definition

I. Spina bifida is an anomaly characterized by a midline cleft in the vertebral arch.
II. The term spina bifida occulta indicates that the adjacent spinal cord and soft tissue are normal.
III. Meningocele is protrusion of the meninges through the vertebral cleft.
IV. Meningomyelocele is protrusion of the meninges and spinal cord through the vertebral cleft.

Causes

I. Possibly inherited in bulldogs
II. Can also be caused by a variety of teratogens (e.g., griseofulvin) and nutritional deficiencies

Pathophysiology

I. Spina bifida is probably related to abnormal development of the neural tube.
II. It may be associated with other malformations, including hydrocephalus, myelodysplasia, and vertebral malformations such as hemivertebrae.
III. As the animals grows, there is normally a relatively greater increase in the length of the vertebral column compared with the spinal cord. Spina bifida may result in abnormal tension on the spinal cord by the meningeal attachment at the site of malformation (tethered cord syndrome), which can cause progressive neurologic dysfunction.
IV. There may be an abnormal communication between the subarachnoid space and skin (fistulated meningocele), which predisposes to bacterial meningitis.

Clinical Signs

I. Breed: most common in English and French bulldogs, Boston terriers, and pugs

II. Age: neurologic deficits usually apparent by 4–6 weeks

III. Often an incidental radiographic finding

IV. Neurologic deficits referable to a focal spinal cord lesion, most commonly involving the lumbosacral segments

V. Abnormalities of the overlying skin, including dimpling and abnormal direction of hair growth

VI. Possible cutaneous leakage of CSF

Diagnosis

I. Plain radiography: cleft in one or more vertebral arches

II. Myelography: meningocele or meningomyelocele

Differential Diagnosis

Other congenital spinal cord disorders

Treatment and Monitoring

I. Not necessary for spina bifida occulta

II. Surgical repair for meningoceles

III. Surgical excision of filum terminale for treatment of tethered cord syndrome

IV. No effective treatment for meningomyeloceles or associated myelodysplasia

V. Prognosis poor for animals with severe neurologic deficits

Sacrocaudal Dysgenesis

Definition

I. Malformation of the sacrocaudal vertebrae and spinal cord segments

II. Associated abnormalities
A. Aplasia or hypoplasia of the caudal and sacral vertebrae, spinal cord segments, and nerves
B. Spina bifida with or without meningocele or meningomyelocele
C. Myelodysplasia

Causes

I. Hereditary
A. Manx cats: dominant gene with incomplete penetrance; may be lethal in homozygotes
B. English bulldogs: probably inherited

II. Unknown cause in sporadic cases

Pathophysiology

Neurologic deficits are caused by abnormal or absent spinal cord segments, causing lower motor neuron signs to the pelvic limbs, bladder, urinary and anal sphincters, and perineum.

Clinical Signs

I. Breed
A. Manx or other tailless cats
B. English bulldogs, pugs, Boston terriers

II. Age: signs usually apparent by 4–6 weeks of age

III. Short or absent tail

IV. Dimple in skin overlying sacrum

V. Palpable vertebral defects

VI. Neurologic dysfunction
A. Incontinence: most common presenting sign
1. Urine dribbling, enlarged atonic bladder that is easily expressed
2. Fecal retention, absent anal reflex
B. Pelvic limb dysfunction
1. "Bunny-hopping" gait
2. Ataxia or paraparesis
3. Weak or absent flexor reflexes
4. Muscle atrophy

Diagnosis

I. Plain radiography: dysgenesis or agenesis of sacral and caudal vertebrae

II. Myelography: possible meningocele

Differential Diagnosis

I. Other congenital vertebral malformations

II. Myelitis

Treatment and Monitoring

I. Meningoceles in animals with minimal neurologic deficits may be treated surgically.

II. Management of urinary and fecal incontinence with manual bladder expression and enemas may be necessary.

III. There is no effective treatment for animals with substantial neurologic deficits.

DEGENERATIVE DISORDERS

Degenerative Myelopathy

Definition

I. Degenerative myelopathy is a slowly progressive, noninflammatory degeneration of the white matter of the spinal cord.

II. Synonyms include German shepherd myelopathy and chronic degenerative radiculomyelopathy.

III. See Table 24–1 for other degenerative diseases that affect the spinal cord.

Causes

I. The cause is unknown.

II. A genetic basis is suspected in German shepherd dogs.

Pathophysiology

I. Some affected dogs have altered cell-mediated immune response and elevated circulating immune complexes, suggesting the possibility of an immune-mediated cause (Clemmons, 1989).

Table 24–1. **Degenerative Diseases of the Spinal Cord**

Disease	Inheritance	Age of Onset	Clinical Features	Pathologic Findings
Demyelinating myelopathy of miniature poodles	Unknown	2–5 mo	Paraparesis progressing over several weeks to tetraplegia, normal or exaggerated spinal cord reflexes	Degeneration of myelin, most prominent in the cervical segments
Leukoencephalomyelopathy of rottweilers	Unknown	1.5–3.5 yr	Ataxia, UMN tetraparesis, progressive over about 1 yr	Primary demyelination, most prominent in the cervical segments
Neuroaxonal dystrophy of rottweilers	Unknown	4–18 mo	Initially ataxia of trunk and limbs progressing over several years to head tremor and nystagmus	Axonal swelling (spheroids) in the gray matter of the brain stem and spinal cord
Hereditary ataxia in smooth fox terriers and Jack Russell terriers	Autosomal recessive in smooth fox terriers	2–6 mo	Slowly progressive ataxia, most prominent in the pelvic limbs, intention tremor	Axonal degeneration with wallerian-type demyelination
Nervous system degeneration in Ibizan hounds	Autosomal recessive (presumed)	4–6 wk	Ataxia, hypermetria of all limbs, absent patellar reflexes, occasionally seizures	Axonal degeneration with spheroid formation throughout the spinal cord
Labrador retriever axonopathy	Autosomal recessive (presumed)	4–6 wk	Ataxia and tetraparesis, hypermetria, variable rate of progression, usually nonambulatory by 5 mo	Severe degeneration of axons and myelin in the spinal cord white matter
Hereditary myelopathy of Afghan hounds	Autosomal recessive (presumed)	3–13 mo	Rapidly progressive UMN paraparesis, may progress to tetraparesis	Severe demyelination with cavitation, most prominent in the midthoracic segments

UMN = upper motor neuron.

II. A diffuse, noninflammatory degeneration of myelinated axons in the spinal cord (most prominent in the thoracolumbar segments) results in decreased proprioception and upper motor neuron (UMN) deficits in the pelvic limbs.
III. In a few cases, the lumbar dorsal nerve roots are involved, resulting in weak or absent patellar reflexes.

Clinical Signs

I. Breed
  A. It is most common in German shepherd and German shepherd–mix dogs.
  B. A similar condition occasionally affects other breeds, including boxers, Chesapeake Bay retrievers, collies, Kerry blue terriers, Labrador retrievers, Old English sheepdogs, Siberian huskies, Pembroke Welsh corgis, and pugs.
  C. It occurs rarely in cats.
II. Age: >5 years old
III. Onset insidious
IV. Slowly progressive ataxia and paresis of the pelvic limbs
  A. Deficits are bilateral but may be asymmetrical.
  B. Decreased proprioceptive positioning is an early feature and is helpful in differentiating this disease from orthopedic disease.
  C. Spinal reflexes are usually normal or exaggerated, but in about 10% of cases, the patellar reflexes are weak or absent.
  D. Incontinence and thoracic limb deficits develop only in very advanced cases.
V. Not painful

Diagnosis

I. Diagnosis is based on clinical findings and exclusion of other potential causes.
II. Plain radiography may show spondylosis deformans or ossification of the dura mater, but these are rarely significant and are unrelated to degenerative myelopathy.
III. Myelography is normal but is performed to exclude compressive causes of spinal cord disease.
IV. Analysis of CSF collected from the cerebellomedullary cistern is normal, but lumbar samples often contain mildly elevated protein content and normal number of cells.

Differential Diagnosis

I. Intervertebral disk protrusion
II. Neoplasia
III. Myelitis
IV. Lumbosacral stenosis
V. Orthopedic disease, such as hip dysplasia and cruciate ligament injuries

Treatment

I. A program consisting of exercise, vitamin E 2000 IU/day PO, vitamin B complex, and aminocaproic acid 500 mg PO TID has been reported to help, but controlled trials are lacking (Clemmons et al., 1995).

II. *N*-Acetylcysteine 70 mg/kg PO TID for 2 weeks then TID every other day has also been suggested (Clemmons et al., 1995).

III. Supportive care to aid in walking and to prevent decubitus ulcers is important.

Patient Monitoring

I. Affected dogs usually deteriorate, often in a stepwise fashion.

II. Neurologic disability usually leads to euthanasia within 6–12 months.

Intervertebral Disk Disease

Definition

I. Intervertebral disk disease is extrusion or protrusion of the intervertebral disk, resulting in compression of the spinal cord, spinal nerve, or nerve root.

II. Extrusion is tearing of the annulus fibrosus and rupture of the nucleus pulposus into the vertebral canal (type I disk herniation).

III. Protrusion is partial tearing of the annulus fibrosus and bulging of the dorsal aspect of the disk into the vertebral canal (type II disk herniation).

Causes

I. Extrusion or protrusion is usually secondary to disk degeneration.

II. An otherwise normal disk can extrude as a consequence of major external trauma.

Pathophysiology

I. Type I disk disease
   A. It is most common in chondrodystrophoid breeds of dog, such as dachshunds.
   B. Biochemical and morphologic changes in the disks start at about 4 months of age and are advanced by 1–3 years of age.
   C. There is a loss of water content in the nucleus and replacement with chondroid tissue that mineralizes. The disk loses its ability to adequately dissipate stress, which can lead to degeneration of the annulus fibrosus and extrusion of the disk through the torn annulus.
   D. Disk extrusion is often acute, resulting in more severe spinal cord injury compared with chronic disk protrusion. This is a result of the dynamic component of the disk material striking the cord, persistent compression, and vascular compromise.
   E. Secondary biochemical changes in the spinal cord lead to further spinal cord damage. In severe cases, these secondary changes can lead to pro-

gressive ascending and descending malacia of the spinal cord (see Trauma).

II. Type II disk disease
   A. It is most common in nonchondrodystrophoid breeds, especially larger dogs.
   B. At about 5 years of age, degeneration starts in the annulus fibrosus with disruption of the normal lamellar structure, fragmentation, and fibroid metaplasia and slowly progresses.
   C. The disk bulges, but the nucleus is still confined by the outer fibers of the annulus.

III. Pain associated with disk disease
   A. Radicular pain: compression or stretching of nerve root
   B. Diskogenic pain: stretching or tearing of the annulus
   C. Meningeal pain: stretching or inflammation of the meninges

Clinical Signs

I. Type I disk disease
   A. Breed: dachshunds, beagles, Pekingese, French bulldogs, cocker spaniels, Shih Tzus, Lhasa apsos
   B. Age: 1–10 years; peak incidence at 3–6 years

II. Type II disk disease
   A. Breed: nonchondrodystrophoid breeds, especially large dogs
   B. Age: >5 years
   C. Clinical signs rare in cats

III. Cervical disk disease
   A. Onset is often acute.
   B. Neck pain is the most common sign and is manifested as cervical rigidity, muscle spasms, and reluctance to move the neck.
   C. Unilateral or bilateral thoracic limb lameness may occur from radicular pain (root signature).
   D. Neurologic deficits are usually bilateral but may be asymmetrical.
      1. Severity ranges from ataxia to tetraparesis.
      2. Tetraplegia is uncommon.
      3. Normal (acute) or exaggerated (chronic) spinal cord reflexes are present.
      4. Horner's syndrome rarely occurs.
      5. Respiratory paresis is rare.

IV. Thoracolumbar disk disease
   A. Type I disk extrusion: onset often acute
   B. Type II disk extrusion: onset usually chronic and progressive
   C. Thoracolumbar pain
      1. Kyphosis, stilted gait, reluctance to move
      2. Paraspinal and abdominal muscle rigidity (may be confused with abdominal pain)
   D. Unilateral or bilateral pelvic limb lameness with lesions caudal to L2-L3
   E. Neurologic deficits
      1. Tend to be more severe, compared with cervical disk disease
      2. Usually bilateral but may be asymmetrical
      3. Range from mild ataxia of pelvic limbs to paraplegia

4. Spinal cord reflexes
   a) Lesion cranial to L3-L4: normal to exaggerated spinal reflexes
   b) Lesions caudal to L3-L4: decreased to absent patellar, flexor, and/or perineal reflexes
5. Cutaneous trunci (panniculus) reflex possibly lost caudal to lesion
6. Urinary and fecal incontinence
7. In severe cases, deep pain perception lost caudal to lesion

Diagnosis

I. Plain radiography
   A. General anesthesia is necessary for precise positioning.
   B. Radiographic signs of intervertebral disk disease include the following.
      1. Radiopaque mass within the vertebral canal
      2. Narrowed or wedge-shaped disk space
      3. Narrowed or abnormally shaped intervertebral foramen
      4. Narrowed joint space between articular processes
   C. A calcified disk in situ indicates only disk degeneration, not protrusion or extrusion.
   D. Survey radiographs allow an accurate diagnosis in about 70% of cases (Kirberger et al., 1992; Olby et al., 1994).
II. Myelography
   A. Myelography is indicated if plain radiographs do not conclusively identify a lesion that correlates with clinical signs in an animal in which surgery is being considered.
   B. In thoracolumbar disk disease, myelography is often useful in determining on which side of the vertebral canal the disk material lies, which is helpful in planning surgery.
   C. Extradural compression is usually evident on lateral, ventrodorsal, or oblique views.
   D. With acute type I extrusions, there may be loss of the contrast columns over several spinal cord segments owing to spinal cord swelling or diffuse extradural compression.
   E. Myelography is accurate in 85–97% of cases (Kirberger et al., 1992; Olby et al., 1994).
III. Computed tomography (CT) or magnetic resonance imaging (MRI): helpful in the diagnosis of lateral disk extrusions, which may not be evident on myelography
IV. CSF analysis
   A. Lumbar samples are more likely to be abnormal than cerebellomedullary samples.
   B. Acute disk extrusion may cause moderate elevations in protein content and mild mononuclear pleocytosis (Thomson et al., 1989).

Differential Diagnosis

I. Acute type I disk extrusion
   A. Trauma
   B. Meningomyelitis
   C. Diskospondylitis
   D. Atlantoaxial subluxation
   E. Fibrocartilagenous embolic myelopathy
II. Chronic type II disk protrusion
   A. Neoplasia
   B. Degenerative myelopathy
   C. Myelitis
   D. Orthopedic disease

Treatment

I. Nonsurgical therapy is indicated for an initial episode of neck or back pain with no or mild neurologic deficits.
   A. Cage rest
      1. Strict confinement to a small cage is the most important aspect of nonsurgical therapy.
      2. Daily observation is indicated to identify any deterioration in neurologic status.
      3. Confinement should continue for 2–3 weeks.
   B. Anti-inflammatory or analgesic medications as needed for pain relief
      1. Prednisone 0.5 mg/kg PO SID
      2. Butorphanol 0.2–0.4 mg/kg IM or SQ q 2–6 h
   C. Medication without concurrent cage confinement: absolutely contraindicated, as increased activity may lead to further disk extrusion and worsening of neurologic dysfunction
II. Surgery is indicated when substantial neurologic deficits are present, there is failure of nonsurgical treatment, or episodes are recurrent.
   A. The more severe the neurologic deficits, the more urgent the need for surgery.
   B. Techniques for treating cervical intervertebral disk disease are as follows.
      1. Ventral decompression (ventral slot) is usually the procedure of choice (Fry et al., 1991).
      2. Rare cases of lateral extrusion may require hemilaminectomy.
      3. Adjacent disks may be fenestrated prophylactically.
   C. Thoracolumbar intervertebral disk disease may be treated as follows.
      1. Dorsolateral hemilaminectomy is usually the procedure of choice (Muir et al., 1995).
      2. Adjacent disks may be fenestrated prophylactically.
III. Animals with acute onset of severe neurologic deficits may benefit from administration of methylprednisolone (see Trauma, later in this chapter), although medication is not a substitute for surgery.
IV. Management of urinary incontinence is necessary to prevent retention cystitis and detrusor muscle damage caused by bladder distention in animals with neurogenic incontinence (see Chap. 50).

Patient Monitoring

I. Cervical disk disease
   A. Dogs may recover with nonsurgical therapy, but relapse is fairly common (about 35%).

B. Ventral slotting is associated with an excellent prognosis, although residual neurologic deficits are possible in severely affected dogs (Seim and Prata, 1982).

II. Thoracolumbar disk disease
 A. Mildly affected dogs often recover with nonsurgical therapy, although 30–40% relapse later (Davies and Sharp, 1983; Levine and Caywood, 1984).
 B. Surgical decompression is associated with a good prognosis in dogs with acute disk extrusion and intact deep pain perception (Muir et al., 1995). Most show improvement within 2 weeks, although 6–8 weeks may be required for full recovery.
 C. In paraplegic animals, the presence or absence of deep pain perception is the single most important prognostic indicator.
  1. Dogs with absent deep pain perception have a 40–50% recovery rate if surgery is performed within 24–48 hours (Muir et al., 1995; Duval et al., 1996).
  2. One to 6 months may be required for recovery.
  3. If surgery is delayed longer than 48 hours, the prognosis is poor.
 D. The prognosis for recovery from chronic type II disk protrusion is guarded, as surgical removal of protruded disk material may be difficult without causing iatrogenic spinal cord trauma.

Lumbosacral Stenosis

Definition

I. Narrowing of the lumbosacral vertebral canal resulting in compression of the cauda equina or lumbosacral nerves
II. Similar terms: cauda equina syndrome, lumbosacral spondylopathy, lumbosacral instability

Causes

I. Degenerative lumbosacral stenosis is the most common cause and likely results from cumulative stress on the lumbosacral disk, ligaments, and joints.
II. High prevalence in German shepherd dogs suggests a genetic component.
III. Congenital lumbosacral transitional vertebrae are associated with increased risk of degenerative lumbosacral stenosis (Morgan et al., 1993).
IV. Osteochondrosis of the sacral end plate may be involved.
V. Idiopathic lumbosacral stenosis may result from failure of the neural arch to develop normally.

Pathophysiology

I. Compression of the cauda equina or spinal nerves
II. Degeneration and protrusion or extrusion of the L7-S1 disk: most common finding
III. Thickening and infolding of the ligamentum flavum

IV. Narrowing of the intervertebral foramen secondary to collapse of the disk space
V. Instability and subluxation of the lumbosacral joint (minority of cases)

Clinical Signs

I. Signalment
 A. Degenerative lumbosacral stenosis is most common in large-breed dogs, especially German shepherd dogs.
 B. Small-breed dogs, especially poodles, beagles, and Lhasa apsos, may be predisposed to idiopathic lumbosacral stenosis.
 C. Most affected dogs are middle-aged or older.
 D. It is rare in cats.
II. Clinical findings
 A. Lumbosacral pain (most common finding)
  1. Difficulty rising
  2. Pain on palpation of the spinous processes of L7 and S1 or extension of the lumbosacral joint
 B. Unilateral or bilateral pelvic limb lameness
 C. Ataxia or paresis of the pelvic limbs
 D. Weak flexor reflex in the pelvic limbs
 E. Muscle atrophy
 F. Weakness and decreased sensation in tail
 G. Urinary or fecal incontinence
  1. Decreased anal tone and perineal reflex
  2. Atonic, easily expressed bladder
 H. Excessive licking or chewing of the tail, perineum, or pelvic limbs

Diagnosis

I. Plain radiography
 A. Spondylosis deformans
 B. Narrowing of the L7-S1 disk space
 C. Ventral displacement of the sacrum relative to L7
 D. Usually not sufficient for diagnosis
II. Myelography
 A. May be of limited value because of the reduced size of the subarachnoid space in the lumbosacral region
 B. May show extradural compression at the lumbosacral junction
III. Epidurography
 A. Obstruction to cranial flow of contrast medium at the lumbosacral junction
 B. Dorsal deviation of the ventral epidural space
 C. May have false-positives (Selcer et al., 1988)
IV. Diskography: demonstrates disk protrusion or extrusion (Sisson et al., 1992)
V. Intraosseous venography: unreliable
VI. CT and MRI: most definitive but not widely available (Adams et al., 1995)

Differential Diagnosis

I. Diskospondylitis
II. Neoplasia
III. Vertebral fracture/luxation

IV. Orthopedic disorders (hip dysplasia, cruciate ligament injury)

Treatment

I. Nonsurgical therapy
  A. Cage rest for 6 weeks
  B. Anti-inflammatory drugs
    1. Prednisone 0.5 mg/kg PO SID
    2. Aspirin 10–20 mg/kg PO BID
II. Surgery
  A. Indications
    1. Poor response to nonsurgical therapy
    2. Neurologic deficits, including incontinence
  B. Techniques
    1. Dorsal laminectomy with diskectomy and excision of the ligamentum flavum
    2. Facetectomy to decompress spinal nerve(s)
    3. Distraction and fusion for cases associated with redundant dorsal annulus fibrosus, but contraindicated in cases of disk protrusion (Slocum and Slocum, 1993)

Patient Monitoring

I. Six to 8 weeks of cage rest is recommended after surgery.
II. Decompressive surgery carries a good prognosis for dogs with pain or lameness (Chambers et al., 1988).
III. Working dogs have a more guarded prognosis.
IV. Incontinence often does not resolve completely.

Cervical Spondylomyelopathy

Definition

I. Cervical vertebral malformation or malarticulation resulting in compression of the cervical spinal cord segments
II. Synonyms: canine wobbler syndrome, cervical vertebral malformation-malarticulation

Causes

I. Genetic factors are established for the borzoi and suspected for the Doberman pinscher and Great Dane.
II. Overnutrition, especially excess calcium and calories, may contribute.

Pathophysiology

I. The C6-7 intervertebral joint is the most commonly affected; the C5-6 joint is the next most common site.
II. Compression of the spinal cord can be constant (static compression) or intermittent, depending on the position of the neck (dynamic compression).
II. Compression may be caused by one or more of the following.
  A. Stenosis of the vertebral canal, especially the cranial aspect of the vertebrae (most common in younger dogs)
  B. Intervetebral disk degeneration and protrusion (most common in older dogs)
  C. Hypertrophy of the ligamentum flavum and the joint capsule
  D. Malformation and degeneration of the articular processes
  E. Dorsal displacement of the cranial aspect of the vertebra owing to instability

Clinical Signs

I. Signalment
  A. Doberman pinschers 3–9 years old
  B. Great Danes <2 years old
  C. Other large-breed dogs and basset hounds occasionally affected
  D. Males more commonly affected, except in borzois (affected dogs have been females)
II. Clinical features
  A. Onset is usually insidious, but acute onset may be associated with minor trauma.
  B. Neurologic deficits are referable to a cervical lesion.
    1. Ataxia, paresis, and postural reaction deficits in all limbs, possibly more obvious in pelvic limbs
    2. Spinal cord reflexes
      a) Pelvic limbs: normal to exaggerated
      b) Thoracic limbs: normal, exaggerated, or decreased
    3. Atrophy of the supraspinatus and infraspinatus muscles
  C. Neck pain is variable and is more common with acute onset.

Diagnosis

I. Plain radiography
  A. Narrowed intervertebral disk space(s)
  B. Malalignment of vertebrae, especially dorsal displacement of the cranial aspect of the vertebral body
  C. Stenosis of the cranial aspect of the vertebrae
  D. Malformed vertebral body
  E. Usually does not fully characterize the lesions
II. Myelography
  A. Essential if surgery is a consideration
  B. Lateral and ventrodorsal views with the neck in a neutral position
  C. Stressed lateral views
    1. Helpful in characterizing lesions as dynamic (changes with different neck positions) or static (no change with different neck positions) and helpful in planning surgery
    2. Traction
      a) Performed if compression is seen on initial views
      b) Substantial decrease in the amount of compression: dynamic lesion
    3. Extended view
      a) Performed if no compression is seen on neutral views

  b) May identify mild, dynamic lesions
  c) Used cautiously if substantial compression is seen on neutral views because of the potential for exacerbating damage to the spinal cord
  D. Myelographic abnormalities: one or more sites of static or dynamic extradural compression
III. CT myelography and MRI
  Both accurately identify compression and may provide prognostic information by identifying spinal cord atrophy (Sharp et al., 1995).

Differential Diagnosis

  I. Intervertebral disk disease not associated with cervical spondylomyelopathy
  II. Neoplasia
  III. Myelitis
  IV. Trauma
  V. Diskospondylitis

Treatment

  I. Nonsurgical therapy
    A. Indicated in dogs with mild signs or those that are not acceptable candidates for general anesthesia and surgery
    B. Restricted activity
    C. Prednisone 0.5 mg/kg/day PO
  II. Surgery
    A. Indications include the following.
      1. Poor response to nonsurgical therapy
      2. Substantial neurologic deficits
      3. Substantial compression on myelography
    B. In addition to standard presurgical evaluations, the following diseases should be considered in Doberman pinschers that are candidates for surgery.
      1. Hypothyroidism
      2. Von Willebrand's disease
      3. Cardiomyopathy
    C. There are several surgical techniques.
      1. Choice of technique is based on type of lesion and individual surgeon's preference.
      2. Ventral decompression is indicated for static ventral compression.
      3. Ventral distraction-fusion is indicated for single or multiple dynamic lesions and involves screws or pins with bone cement, screws and intervertebral washers, or bone plates.
      4. Dorsal decompression is indicated for dorsal compression or multiple lesions.

Patient Monitoring

  I. Mildly affected dogs often improve temporarily with conservative therapy, but the long-term prognosis without surgery is poor (Denny et al., 1977).
  II. The prognosis with surgery is guarded (40–80% recovery rate) and difficult to predict in an individual animal.
  III. Prognosis is worse for dogs with more severe neuro-

logic dysfunction, with longer duration of clinical signs, or with multiple as opposed to single lesions.
  IV. Fusion of one or more intervertebral spaces may lead to increased stress on adjacent disk spaces, eventually causing a second lesion (domino effect).

Spondylosis Deformans

Definition

  I. Spondylosis deformans is a chronic noninflammatory disease characterized by the production of osteophytes on the spine.
  II. The term spondylitis should not be used, as this implies an inflammatory process, which is not present.

Causes and Pathophysiology

  I. It may develop as a consequence of aging or trauma.
  II. Breakdown of the outer annular fibers results in weakening of the attachment of the intervertebral disk to the vertebral end plate.
    A. Subsequent ventral protrusion of the disk stretches the ventral longitudinal ligament.
    B. Osteophytes develop at the sites of the vertebral attachment of these ligaments (Romatowski, 1986).
  III. Osteophytes grow by endochondral ossification.
  IV. Osteophytes typically develop along the ventral and lateral surface of the vertebral bodies, rarely extending dorsally to compress the spinal cord or spinal nerve; thus, clinical signs are rare.

Clinical Signs

  I. Most common in middle-aged and older dogs, especially large breeds
  II. Common in middle-aged to older cats
  III. Usually an incidental radiographic finding
  IV. Rarely, osteophytes encroaching on the vertebral canal or spinal nerve, causing pain and neurologic deficits

Diagnosis

  I. On plain radiography, smoothly marginated osteophytes are found at the ventral and lateral aspect of the vertebral end plates adjacent to a disk.
    A. They have a characteristic curved shape, with the concavity toward the disk.
    B. They may extend the length of the vertebral body and appear confluent along two or more vertebrae.
    C. Vertebral end plates are smooth but may be sclerotic
  II. One or multiple sites anywhere along the vertebral column may be affected.

Differential Diagnosis

  I. Diskospondylitis
  II. Trauma, especially healed fracture/luxation

Treatment

I. Treatment is usually not necessary.

II. Analgesics may be helpful in case of pain or stiffness.

Patient Monitoring

I. Radiographic lesions usually progress.

II. If pain or neurologic deficits are present, another condition is probably responsible.

INFLAMMATORY AND INFECTIOUS DISORDERS

Diskospondylitis and Vertebral Osteomyelitis

Definition

I. Diskospondylitis is infection of the intervertebral disk and adjacent vertebrae.

II. Vertebral osteomyelitis is infection of only the vertebra.

III. Vertebral physitis is osteomyelitis restricted to the physis.

Causes

I. Most cases are caused by bacteria.
   A. *Staphylococcus intermedius*: most common organism (Kornegay, 1993)
   B. *Brucella canis*
   C. *Streptococcus* spp.
   D. *Staphylococcus aureus, Pseudomonas* spp., *Escherichia coli, Pasteurella haemolytica,* and other bacteria

II. Fungal infections occur less frequently.
   A. *Aspergillus* spp.
   B. *Coccidioides immitis*

III. Plant awn migration with secondary infection of *Actinomyces* spp. can cause vertebral osteomyelitis, especially of the lumbar vertebrae.

Pathophysiology

I. Most cases are caused by hematogenous spread of organisms, which localize in the vascular loops of the vertebral epiphysis. Primary sites of initial infection include the skin, urinary tract, and heart.

II. Immunosuppression may play a role.

III. A few cases are secondary to foreign body migration, surgery, or local soft tissue infection.

IV. Diskospondylitis in cats is usually secondary to bite wounds adjacent to the spine.

V. Neurologic deficits may occur from proliferation of bone and fibrous tissue causing spinal cord compression. Less commonly, spinal cord damage is caused by pathologic fracture of the spine or extension of infection to the spinal cord.

Clinical Signs

I. Signalment
   A. Large and giant breeds of dogs, especially German shepherd dogs and Great Danes
   B. Male to female ratio: 2:1
   C. Vertebral physitis: dogs <2 years of age (Jimenez and O'Callaghan, 1995)
   D. Rare in cats

II. Clinical findings
   A. Focal hyperpathia is the most common sign.
   B. Stilted gait, kyphosis, or neck rigidity may also be noticed.
   C. Systemic illness, including fever, depression, and weight loss, can occur.
   D. Neurologic deficits range from ataxia to paralysis caudal to the lesion.
   E. Multiple sites can occur.

Diagnosis

I. Plain radiography
   A. Diskospondylitis causes lysis of vertebral end plates adjacent to the affected disk.
   B. Collapse of the disk space usually occurs.
   C. Sclerosis of the end plates with ventral and lateral spur formation is also common.
   D. Vertebral osteomyelitis is characterized by periosteal bone formation.
   E. Vertebral physitis causes lysis of the caudal physis with spondylosis.
   F. The most common sites are the midthoracic vertebrae, thoracolumbar vertebrae, C6-C7, and L7-S1 (Kornegay, 1993).

II. Myelography: indicated only in animals with substantial neurologic deficits that are potential candidates for surgery

III. Bone scintigraphy: helpful in identifying early cases

IV. Cultures
   A. Blood cultures are positive in 45–75% of untreated cases (Kornegay, 1993).
   B. Urine cultures are positive in 25–40% of cases (organisms other than *Staphylococcus* spp. may not be the cause of the vertebral infection).
   C. Culture of the bone or disk space is indicated in animals that fail to respond to initial therapy.

V. Serology for *B. canis*

VI. Hemogram: often normal, leukocytosis possible

VII. Urinalysis: ± concurrent urinary tract infection

Differential Diagnosis

I. Spondylosis deformans

II. Vertebral neoplasia

III. Intervertebral disk disease

IV. Meningomyelitis

V. Myositis

VI. Polyarthritis

Treatment

I. Antibiotics
  A. Choice of drugs is based on results of culture and sensitivity.
  B. If cultures are negative, *Staphylococcus* is assumed to be the cause.
    1. Give cephalexin 20 mg/kg PO TID, or cloxacillin 10 mg/kg PO QID.
    2. If no response within 5 days, reevaluate therapy or consider surgery.
    3. Antibiotic administration is continued for at least 6 weeks.
  C. For diskospondylitis caused by brucellosis, consider the following.
    1. Enrofloxacin 5–15 mg/kg PO BID (Kerwin et al., 1992)
    2. Minocycline 12 mg/kg PO BID and gentamicin 2.2 mg/kg IM TID
II. Cage rest until signs resolve
III. Analgesics
  A. Use oxymorphone 0.05–0.2 mg/kg SQ q 4–6 h or similar analgesics as needed.
  B. Analgesic treatment should be short term to allow determination of response to antibiotics.
IV. Surgery
  A. Surgical curettage of an affected disk space to obtain tissue for culture is occasionally necessary in animals refractory to antibiotics.
  B. Decompression of the spinal cord and possible internal stabilization may be necessary in animals with substantial neurologic deficits and myelographic evidence of spinal cord compression if there is no improvement with antibiotics.

Patient Monitoring

I. Dogs with minimal neurologic deficits usually respond within 5 days of treatment.
II. Prognosis for dogs with substantial neurologic deficits is guarded, although complete recovery is possible.
III. Recurrence is possible if antibiotics are discontinued prematurely or in dogs infected with *B. canis*.

Meningitis

Definition

I. Meningitis is inflammation of the meninges.
II. Myelitis is inflammation of the parenchyma of the spinal cord.
III. Meningomyelitis is inflammation of both the meninges and the spinal cord.

Causes

I. Bacteria: *Staphylococcus* spp., *Pasteurella multocida, Actinomyces, Nocardia* (Meric, 1988)
II. Idiopathic: steroid-responsive meningitis-arteritis (most common cause of meningitis in dogs)
III. Other diseases (see Chap. 23)
  A. Canine distemper
  B. Granulomatous meningoencephalomyelitis
  C. Feline infectious peritonitis
  D. Systemic fungi

Pathophysiology

I. Infectious meningitis
  A. Routes of infection include hematogenous; direct extension from adjacent tissue, such as paranasal sinuses and ears; and disruption of the meninges by trauma, such as skull fracture.
  B. Adverse effects arise largely from the release of endogenous cytokines into the CSF in response to the inciting organism. The end result is meningeal inflammation, increased permeability of the blood-brain barrier, brain edema, and alterations of blood flow to the brain.
II. Steroid-responsive meningitis-arteritis
  A. Underlying cause is unknown.
  B. There is inflammation of the meningeal arteries and, less commonly, the extraneural arteries.
  C. High levels of IgA in the serum and CSF of affected dogs suggest an immune-mediated cause (Tipold et al., 1995).
  D. Predisposition in boxers, beagles, and Bernese mountain dogs suggests a genetic component.

Clinical Signs

I. Signalment
  A. Infectious causes: any age or breed of dog or cat
  B. Steroid-responsive meningitis-arteritis: most common in young adult large-breed dogs (Tipold and Jaggy, 1994)
II. Clinical signs
  A. Generalized or focal spinal hyperpathia
    1. Most consistent sign
    2. Cervical rigidity
    3. Stiff, stilted gait; reluctance to move
    4. Pain on palpation/manipulation of the spine
    5. May seem painful all over
  B. Fever
  C. Neurologic deficits: ataxia or paresis, depression, seizures
  D. Signs of brain edema and increased intracranial pressure
    1. Deteriorating level of consciousness
    2. Tetraparesis progressing to tetraplegia, opisthotonus
    3. Cranial nerve abnormalities

Diagnosis

I. CSF analysis
  A. Indicated early in the evaluation of meningitis
  B. Cytology
    1. Bacterial meningitis
      a) Marked increase in cell count, predominantly neutrophils
      b) Degenerate appearance of neutrophils
      c) May be intracellular bacteria
    2. Steroid-responsive meningitis-arteritis

a) Acute cases have a moderate to marked neutrophilic pleocytosis; neutrophils are not degenerate.

b) Chronic cases usually have a moderate mononuclear pleocytosis (Tipold and Jaggy, 1994).

C. Protein: moderate to marked increase
D. Cultures
1. Aerobic and anaerobic cultures are submitted if there is an increase in neutrophils.
2. False-negatives are common.
II. Hematology: normal or inflammatory leukogram
III. Blood cultures: indicated if bacterial meningitis is a consideration

Differential Diagnosis

I. Polyarthritis
II. Polymyositis
III. Diskospondylitis
IV. Cervical intervertebral disk disease
V. Encephalomyelitis

Treatment

I. Bacterial meningitis
A. Antibiotic therapy (Table 24–2) is instituted as soon as CSF is collected. Antibiotics are not withheld if a delay in CSF collection is unavoidable.
1. Administer a parenteral antibiotic that the organism is sensitive to and that reaches bactericidal concentrations within the central nervous system.
2. Recommendations include the following.
a) Initial therapy consists of penicillin or amoxicillin.
b) If gram-negative organisms are seen on CSF cytology, start enrofloxacin or cefotaxime.
c) Therapy may need to be altered based on results of culture and sensitivity and clinical response.
d) Therapy is continued for at least 3 weeks after resolution of signs.
B. Mannitol is given at 1 g/kg IV slowly for increased intracranial pressure.

C. Anticonvulsants are instituted for seizures.
II. Steroid-responsive meningitis-arteritis
A. Give prednisone 4 mg/kg/day PO for 1–2 weeks.
B. Gradually taper dose until it reaches 0.5 mg/kg every other day, and continue this dose for at least 6 months.

Patient Monitoring

I. Clinical evidence of response includes resolution of pain and fever.
II. Repeat analysis of CSF is helpful in determining response to therapy.
III. Neurologic deficits often resolve with prompt therapy but may persist or progress despite treatment.
IV. Relapse may occur if therapy is discontinued prematurely.
V. Without treatment, steroid-responsive meningitis-arteritis may resolve spontaneously, only to recur later. Prompt treatment is usually effective in resolving clinical signs and preventing relapse.

VASCULAR DISORDERS

Fibrocartilaginous Embolic Myelopathy

Definition

Ischemia or infarction of the spinal cord caused by occlusion of spinal cord vasculature with fragments of fibrocartilage

Causes and Pathophysiology

I. The source of the embolism is presumed to be the nucleus pulposus of the intervertebral disk.
II. Several mechanisms have been proposed.
A. Extrusion of disk material directly into a spinal cord artery
B. Extrusion into the ventral vertebral venous plexus, with reflux back into the spinal cord vasculature
C. Abnormal persistence of embryonal arteries of the annulus fibrosus, with extrusion of disk material into these arteries
D. Extrusion into newly formed vessels in the

Table 24–2. *Antibiotic Therapy for Bacterial Meningitis in Dogs and Cats*

Drug	Indications	Dose	Route	Interval (h)
Penicillin G (aqueous)	Initial therapy, gram-positive and anaerobic infections	20–40,000 U/kg	IV	4–6
Ampicillin	Initial therapy, gram-positive and anaerobic infections	10–20 mg/kg	IV	6
Enrofloxacin	Gram-negative infections	2.5 mg/kg	IM	12
Cefotazime	Gram-negative infections	20–40 mg/kg	IV	8
Metronidazole	Anaerobic infections	10–20 mg/kg	PO	8
Trimethoprim/sulfa	Gram-positive and gram-negative infections	15–20 mg/kg	IM	12

annulus fibrosus, with retrograde flow into the spinal cord vasculature (Neer, 1992)

III. Trauma or vigorous exercise may play a role in some cases.

IV. The result is occlusion of arterial and/or venous blood flow and ischemia of the spinal cord.

Clinical Signs

I. Signalment
   A. Large- and giant-breed dogs are most commonly affected.
   B. Miniature schnauzers and Shetland sheepdogs may also be predisposed (Neer, 1992).
   C. This condition does not affect chondrodystrophic breeds.
   D. Most dogs are 3–7 years old.
   E. It is rare in cats.

II. Clinical features
   A. Onset is invariably sudden; signs rarely progress beyond the first 24 hours.
   B. A history of trauma or vigorous exercise may be noted.
   C. Neurologic deficits reflect a focal, often asymmetrical spinal cord lesion.
      1. Any area of the spinal cord can be affected.
      2. Severity varies from mild ataxia to paralysis with loss of deep pain perception.
      3. Hyperesthesia is uncommon, although the dog may cry out at onset.

Diagnosis

I. Based on clinical signs and exclusion of other possible causes

II. Plain radiography
   A. Usually normal
   B. May show narrowed disk space

III. Myelography
   A. Usually normal
   B. May show intramedullary enlargement, indicating spinal cord swelling

IV. CSF analysis
   A. May be normal
   B. Mild neutrophilic pleocytosis and increased protein possible within first 24 hours
   C. Mild mononuclear pleocytosis and increased protein possible after first 24 hours

Differential Diagnosis

I. Trauma
II. Intervertebral disk extrusion
III. Myelitis
IV. Neoplasia
V. Spinal cord hemorrhage secondary to coagulopathy

Treatment

I. Supportive care
   A. Prevention of decubitus

   B. Management of incontinence, including manual bladder expression or urethral catheterization

II. Glucocorticoids
   A. Have been recommended, but no data exist to show that they are beneficial
   B. Methylprednisolone: administered within the first 8 hours of onset (see Trauma, later in chapter)

Patient Monitoring

I. Animals with mild signs often improve within 7–14 days.
II. Full recovery may take several weeks, and persistent deficits are possible.
III. Prognosis is poor if deep pain perception is absent or if no improvement is seen within 14 days.

NUTRITIONAL DISORDERS

Hypervitaminosis A

See Chap. 79.

NEOPLASIA

Definition and Causes

I. Spinal neoplasia includes primary and secondary tumors of the vertebrae, meninges, spinal nerve roots, and/or spinal cord.

II. In general, causes are unknown.

III. Lymphoma in cats is associated with the feline leukemia virus.

Classification

I. Extradural tumors: located outside the dura mater
   A. Primary vertebral tumors
      1. Osteosarcoma: most common spinal tumor in dogs
      2. Chondrosarcoma
      3. Fibrosarcoma
      4. Hemangiosarcoma
      5. Myeloma
   B. Secondary (metastatic) vertebral tumors
      1. Mammary carcinoma
      2. Prostatic carcinoma
      3. Thyroid carcinoma
      4. Osteosarcoma
      5. Others
   C. Epidural tumors
      1. Lymphoma: most common spinal tumor in cats
      2. Metastatic tumors

II. Subarachnoid tumors: located within the subarachnoid space
   A. Nerve sheath tumor
   B. Meningioma
   C. Nephroblastoma

III. Intramedullary tumors: located within the parenchyma of the spinal cord
   A. Ependymoma
   B. Astrocytoma
   C. Oligodendroglioma

Clinical Signs

I. Signalment
  A. Breed
    1. Any breed dog, but large breeds predisposed (Luttgen et al., 1980)
    2. German shepherd dogs and golden retrievers predisposed to spinal nephroblastoma (Summers et al., 1988)
  B. Age
    1. Median age for spinal tumors in dogs is 6 years (Luttgen et al., 1980).
    2. Dogs with spinal nephroblastoma are usually 5–36 months old (Summers et al., 1988).
    3. Median age for spinal lymphoma in cats is 2–3 years (Spodnick et al., 1992; Lane et al., 1994).
II. Clinical features
  A. Hyperesthesia
    1. Most common initial sign
    2. May initially present with vague discomfort or lameness
    3. May progress to severe, focal pain
    4. Intramedullary tumors possibly nonpainful
  B. Neurologic deficits
    1. Usually chronic and progressive
    2. Acute onset: intramedullary tumors or vertebral tumors with pathologic fracture
    3. Ataxia and paresis caudal to lesion
    4. May be asymmetrical

Diagnosis

I. Plain radiography
  A. Vertebral tumor may cause lytic and/or productive changes.
  B. Nerve sheath tumor may cause enlargement of the intervertebral foramen.
  C. Epidural, subarachnoid, and intramedullary tumors may cause enlargement of the vertebral canal.
II. Myelography
  A. Most useful diagnostic technique
  B. Myelographic patterns (see also Chap. 4)
    1. Extradural tumor causes the adjacent contrast medium column to deviate away from the tumor. The column opposite the tumor may be thinned or deviate away from the tumor.
    2. With subarachnoid tumors, there is usually a filling defect in the column containing the tumor, and contrast medium may outline the tumor. The column adjacent to the tumor is often widened (golf tee sign). The column opposite the tumor may be thinned or deviate away from the tumor.
    3. With intramedullary tumors, all columns may be thinned or diverge away from the spinal cord.
III. CSF analysis
  A. It is often normal.
  B. Increased protein with normal cells is the most common abnormality.
  C. Neoplastic cells are rarely seen in the CSF, the major exception being dogs with spinal lymphoma.
IV. CT and CT myelography also useful
V. MRI especially useful for intramedullary tumors
VI. Surgical biopsy often required for definitive diagnosis
VII. Ancillary diagnostic procedures
  A. Thoracic radiography is indicated to detect pulmonary metastasis.
  B. Feline leukemia virus testing is positive in 84–94% of cats with spinal lymphoma (Spodnick et al., 1992; Lane et al., 1994).
  C. Bone marrow cytology detects lymphoma in 69% of cats with spinal lymphoma (Spodnick et al., 1992).

Differential Diagnosis

I. Intervertebral disk disease
II. Diskospondylitis/vertebral osteomyelitis
III. Meningomyelitis
IV. Degenerative myelopathy
V. Trauma

Treatment

I. Medical therapy
  A. Anti-inflammatory dosages of corticosteroids (prednisone 0.5 mg/kg PO SID) may provide temporary improvement for many spinal tumors.
  B. Chemotherapy is indicated for spinal lymphoma (see also Chap. 67).
II. Surgery
  A. Surgical excision is possible for some epidural and subarachnoid tumors.
  B. Surgery is rarely successful in malignant vertebral and intramedullary tumors.
III. Radiation therapy: helpful in some cases (Siegel et al., 1996)

Patient Monitoring

I. Vertebral tumors: poor prognosis
II. Epidural tumors
  A. Prognosis is guarded.
  B. For cats with spinal lymphoma treated with chemotherapy, the complete remission rate is 50%, with a median duration of remission of 14 weeks (Spodnick et al., 1992).
III. Subarachnoid tumors
  A. Complete surgical excision is possible for some meningiomas, spinal nephroblastomas, and nerve sheath tumors.
  B. Most, however, have a guarded prognosis.
IV. Intramedullary tumors: poor prognosis

TRAUMA

Definition and Causes

I. Acute spinal cord injury can be caused by external trauma, such as motor vehicle accidents, or by internal injury, such as disk extrusion.

II. Spinal cord injury caused by external trauma is usually associated with vertebral column injury, such as fracture or luxation.

III. Causes of external injury include motor vehicle accidents, falls, bite wounds, and gunshot wounds.

Pathophysiology

I. Acute spinal cord injury
   A. Primary injury
      1. Concussive injury is spinal cord damage caused by a sudden, dynamic force applied to the spinal cord, for example, a bullet striking the spinal cord.
      2. Compressive injury is caused by persistent attenuation of the spinal cord, for example, spinal luxation causing compression of the spinal cord. The severity of spinal cord damage is related to the degree and duration of compression.
   B. Secondary injury
      1. It is caused by metabolic processes that lead to further spinal cord injury beyond that caused by the primary injury.
      2. Mechanisms of secondary injury include the following.
         a) Release of free radicals, calcium, lipases, and other substances that lead to cell membrane damage (Brown and Hall, 1992; Battle and Northrup, 1993)
         b) Release of agents that cause vasoconstriction, platelet aggregation, thrombosis, and ischemia
      3. These processes begin within minutes of injury, causing hemorrhage and edema, and can lead to necrosis of the spinal cord within 24–48 hours.
II. Vertebral injury
   A. Dorsal compartment injury
      1. Damage to the pedicles, lamina, or articular processes
      2. Usually caused by hyperextension
      3. Relatively stable injury
   B. Ventral compartment injury
      1. Damage to vertebral body, intervertebral disk, or dorsal longitudinal ligament
      2. Usually caused by hyperflexion or axial loading
      3. Relatively stable injury
   C. Combined compartment injury
      1. Damage to dorsal and ventral components
      2. Most common vertebral injury
      3. Usually caused by flexion and rotational forces
      4. Unstable injury

Clinical Signs

I. Onset is usually immediate and nonprogressive. Progressive signs can occur when there is further displacement of unstable vertebral injuries.
II. Signs of other injuries may be present.
   A. Cardiovascular shock
   B. Chest injury
   C. Abdominal injury
   D. Head injury
   E. Other orthopedic injuries
III. Neurologic signs must be evaluated with care.
   A. Do not assess postural reactions in a nonambulatory animal until unstable vertebral injury has been excluded based on radiographs.
   B. Neuroanatomic localization is usually possible based on assessment of voluntary movement, spinal reflexes, cranial nerves, spinal palpation, and deep pain perception. The presence or absence of deep pain perception caudal to the injury is the most important prognostic finding.
   C. Focal hyperesthesia occurs and may be severe.
   D. Certain clinical syndromes may accompany the injury.
      1. Spinal shock
         a) Transient (usually <1 hour) in dogs and cats
         b) Flaccid paralysis with absent reflexes caudal to lesion
      2. Schiff-Sherrington posture
         a) Associated with acute thoracolumbar lesions
         b) Paraplegia with increased extensor tone in the thoracic limbs
         c) Does *not* indicate that recovery is impossible
      3. Progressive myelomalacia
         a) Occurs in a minority of severe spinal cord injuries
         b) Caused by progression of secondary injury leading to ascending and descending necrosis of the spinal cord
         c) Often not evident until several days after injury
         d) Flaccid paraplegia progressing to flaccid tetraplegia
         e) Fever, generalized hyperesthesia, and depression common
         f) Usually leads to death from respiratory paralysis within 3–7 days

Diagnosis

I. History or physical evidence of trauma
II. Plain radiography
   A. Perform lateral view first. Dorsoventral views are best obtained by horizontal beam view if an unstable vertebral injury is suspected.

B. Radiography determines location of injury and degree of displacement and allows estimation of stability.

C. In general, radiographic findings correlate poorly with prognosis, which is based primarily on the neurologic examination (Feeney and Oliver, 1980).

III. Myelography

    A. Indications

        1. If plain radiographs are normal or do not correlate with clinical assessment

        2. To determine whether there is persistent spinal cord compression if surgical decompression is being considered

    B. Myelographic abnormalities

        1. Extradural compression is the most common pattern.

        2. Intramedullary swelling can occur from spinal cord edema or hemorrhage.

        3. Pooling of contrast medium within the spinal cord is caused by myelomalacia.

Differential Diagnosis

    I. Acute intervertebral disk extrusion

    II. Pathologic fracture from neoplasia or infection

    III. Orthopedic injury, such as pelvic fracture

    IV. Meningomyelitis

    V. Fibrocartilaginous embolism

    VI. Neoplasia

    VII. Ischemic neuromyopathy (cats)

Treatment

    I. Treat any life-threatening injuries, such as shock.

    II. Immobilize the spine to prevent further displacement of unstable vertebral injuries. Strap or tape patient to a rigid board or gurney.

    III. Institute medical therapy for acute spinal cord injury.

    A. Corticosteroids

        1. Methylprednisolone sodium succinate (Solu-Medrol)

           a) Improves neurologic outcome in experimental animal studies and human clinical trials if given within 8 hours of injury (Hoerlein et al., 1985; Bracken et al., 1990)

           b) Indicated for severe neurologic deficits within 8 hours of acute spinal cord injury

           c) Dosage schedule

               (1) 30 mg/kg IV loading dose, then

               (2) 15 mg/kg IV 2 and 6 hours later, then

               (3) 15 mg/kg IV every 6 hours for 24–48 hours

        2. Dexamethasone

           a) Less effective than methylprednisolone (Hoerlein et al., 1983)

           b) Associated with a risk of serious, even fatal, gastrointestinal ulceration and pancreatitis (Moore and Withrow, 1982; Toombs et al., 1986)

           c) Dose: 1–2 mg/kg IV

    B. Dimethyl sulfoxide (DMSO)

        1. Some experimental studies have shown DMSO to be beneficial in spinal cord injury, but clinical trials are lacking (Brayton, 1986).

        2. Dose is 1 g/kg IV of 40% concentration in 5% dextrose/water SID for 3–4 days (Brayton, 1986).

    C. Mannitol is probably not effective and may be deleterious in spinal cord injury (Hoerlein et al., 1983).

    D. Nonsteroidal anti-inflammatory drugs are not beneficial in spinal cord injury and are associated with substantial risk of gastrointestinal ulceration.

    E. Analgesics are indicated for relief of pain, especially in vertebral injury.

        1. Morphine 0.5–1 mg/kg IM or SQ every 4–6 hours for dogs

        2. Butorphanol 0.2–0.5 mg/kg IV, IM, or SQ every 1–2 hours for dogs, every 2–4 hours for cats

IV. Nonsurgical treatment is indicated when there are no or mild neurologic deficits (e.g., the animal can walk)

    A. Cage rest for 4–6 weeks

    B. Clean, well-padded surface

    C. External splints

        1. Fairly effective for cervical and thoracolumbar injuries, but do not provide much stability for lumbosacral injuries (Patterson and Smith, 1992)

        2. Meticulous nursing care required to prevent pressure sores under the splint or straps

V. Surgery is indicated for severe or progressive neurologic deficits and radiographic evidence of an unstable vertebral injury or persistent spinal cord compression.

    A. Decompression

        1. Performed as soon as possible in animals with severe neurologic deficits and radiographic or myelographic evidence of spinal cord compression

        2. Hemilaminectomy or dorsal laminectomy

    B. Stabilization

        1. Indicated for unstable vertebral injury

        2. Preceded by decompression

        3. Techniques: pins or screws and bone cement, plating, and modified spinal instrumentation (Wheeler and Sharp, 1994)

Patient Monitoring

    I. Prognosis depends largely on the severity of the neurologic deficits.

    A. Voluntary movement: good prognosis

    B. Paralysis but intact deep pain perception: guarded prognosis

    C. Paralysis and loss of deep pain perception: poor prognosis

    II. Evaluate neurologic status daily for the first 10 days. Any deterioration indicates the possibility of instability.

    III. Improvement in neurologic function, if it is to occur,

is usually apparent within 2–3 weeks, although 6–12 weeks may be required for full recovery, and persistent deficits are possible.

Bibliography

Adams WH, Daniel GB, Pardo AD, Selcer RR: Magnetic resonance imaging of the caudal lumbar and lumbosacral spine in 13 dogs (1990–1993). Vet Radiol Ultrasound 36:3, 1995

Bailey CS, Morgan JP: Congenital spinal malformations. Vet Clin North Am [Small Anim Pract] 22:985, 1992

Battle FJ, Northrup BE: Pathophysiology of acute spinal cord injury. Traum Q 9:29, 1993

Bentley JF, Simpson ST, Hathcock JT: Spinal arachnoid cyst in a dog. J Am Anim Hosp Assoc 27:549, 1991

Bracken MB, Shepard MJ, Collins WF et al: A randomized, controlled trial of methylprednisolone or naloxone in the treatment of acute spinal-cord injury. New Engl J Med 322:1405, 1990

Brayton CF: Dimethyl sulfoxide (DMSO): a review. Cornell Vet 76:61, 1986

Brown SA, Hall ED: Role of oxygen-derived free radicals in the pathogenesis of shock and trauma, with focus on central nervous system injuries. J Am Vet Med Assoc 200:1849, 1992

Chambers JN, Selcer BA, Oliver JE: Results of treatment of degenerative lumbosacral stenosis in dogs by exploration and excision. Vet Comp Ortho Traumatol 3:130, 1988

Clemmons RM: Degenerative myelopathy. p. 830. In Kirk RW (ed): Current Veterinary Therapy X. WB Saunders, Philadelphia, 1989

Clemmons RM, Wheeler S, LeCouteur RA: How do I treat degenerative myelopathy? Prog Vet Neurol 6:71, 1995

Davies JV, Sharp NJH: A comparison of conservative treatment and fenestration for thoracolumbar disc disease in the dog. J Small Anim Pract 24:721, 1983

Denny HR, Gibbs C, Gaskell CJ: Cervical spondylopathy in the dog—a review of thirty-five cases. J Small Anim Pract 18:117, 1977

Duval J, Dewey C, Roberts R, Aron D: Spinal cord swelling as a myelographic indicator of prognosis: a retrospective study in dogs with intervertebral disc disease and loss of deep pain. Vet Surg 25:6, 1996

Dyce J, Herrtage ME, Houlton JEF, Palmer AC: Canine spinal "arachnoid cysts." J Small Anim Pract 32:433, 1991

Feeney DA, Oliver JE: Blunt spinal trauma in the dog and cat: neurologic, radiologic, and therapeutic correlations. J Am Anim Hosp Assoc 16:664, 1980

Fry TR, Johnson AL, Hungerford L, Toombs J: Surgical treatment of cervical disc herniations in ambulatory dogs: ventral decompression vs. fenestration, 111 cases (1980–1988). Prog Vet Neurol 2:165, 1991

Hoerlein BF, Redding RW, Hoff EJ, McGuire JA: Evaluation of dexamethasone, DMSO, mannitol, and solcoseryl in acute spinal cord trauma. J Am Anim Hosp Assoc 19:218, 1983

Hoerlein BF, Redding RW, Hoff EJ, McGuire JA: Evaluation of naloxone, crocetin, thyrotropin releasing hormone, methylprednisolone, partial myelotomy, and hemilaminectomy in the treatment of acute spinal cord trauma. J Am Anim Hosp Assoc 21:67, 1985

Jacobson LS, Kiberger RM: Canine multiple cartilagenous exostoses: unusual manifestations and a review of the literature. J Am Anim Hosp Assoc 32:45, 1996

Jimenez MM, O'Callaghan MW: Vertebral physitis: a radiographic diagnosis to be separated from discospondylitis. Vet Radiol Ultrasound 36:188, 1995

Kerwin SC, Lewis DD, Hribernik TN et al: Diskospondylitis associated with *Brucella canis* infection in dogs: 14 cases (1980–1991). J Am Vet Med Assoc 201:1253, 1992

Kirberger RM, Roos CJ, Lubbe AM: The radiological diagnosis of thoracolumbar disc disease in the dachshund. Vet Radiol Ultrasound 33:255, 1992

Kornegay JN: Discospondylitis. p. 1087. In Slatter D (ed): Textbook of Small Animal Surgery. 2nd Ed. WB Saunders, Philadelphia, 1993

Lane SB, Kornegay JN, Duncan JR, Oliver JE: Feline spinal lymphosarcoma: a retrospective evaluation of 23 cats. J Vet Intern Med 8:99, 1994

Levine SH, Caywood DD: Recurrence of neurological deficits in dogs treated for thoracolumbar disk disease. J Am Anim Hosp Assoc 20:889, 1984

Luttgen PJ, Braund KG, Brawner WR, Vandevelde M: A retrospective study of twenty-nine spinal tumours in the dog and cat. J Small Anim Pract 21:213, 1980

McCarthy RJ, Lewis DD, Hosgood G: Atlantoaxial subluxation in dogs. Compend Contin Educ Pract Vet 17:215, 1995

Meric SM: Canine meningitis: a changing emphasis. J Vet Intern Med 2:26, 1988

Moore RW, Withrow SJ: Gastrointestinal hemorrhage and pancreatitis associated with intervertebral disk disease in the dog. J Am Vet Med Assoc 180:1443, 1982

Morgan JP, Bahr A, Franti CE, Bailey CS: Lumbosacral transitional vertebrae as a predisposing cause of cauda equina syndrome in German shepherd dogs: 161 cases (1987–1990). J Am Vet Med Assoc 202:1877, 1993

Muir P, Johnson KA, Manley PA, Dueland RT: Comparison of hemilaminectomy and dorsal laminectomy for thoracolumbar intervertebral disc extrusion in dachshunds. J Small Anim Pract 26:360, 1995

Neer TM: Fibrocartilaginous emboli. Vet Clin North Am [Small Anim Pract] 22:1017, 1992

Olby NJ, Dyce J, Houlton JEF: Correlation of plain radiographic and lumbar myelographic findings with surgical findings in thoracolumbar disc disease. J Small Anim Pract 35:345, 1994

Owen LN, Bostock DE: Multiple cartilaginous exostoses with development of a metastasizing osteosarcoma in a Shetland sheepdog. J Small Anim Pract 12:507, 1971

Patterson RH, Smith GK: Backsplinting for treatment of thoracic and lumbar fracture/luxation in the dog: principles of application and case series. Vet Comp Ortho Traumatol 5:179, 1992

Romatowski J: Spondylosis deformans in the dog. Compend Contin Educ Pract Vet 8:531, 1986

Seim HB, Prata RG: Ventral decompression for the treatment of cervical disk disease in the dog: a review of 54 cases. J Am Anim Hosp Assoc 18:233, 1982

Selcer BA, Chambers JN, Schwensen K, Mahaffey MB: Epidurography as a diagnostic aid in canine lumbosacral compressive disease: 47 cases (1981–1986). Vet Comp Ortho Traumatol 2:97, 1988

Sharp NJH, Cofone M, Robertson ID et al: Computed tomography in the evaluation of caudal cervical spondylomyelopathy of the Doberman pinscher. Vet Radiol Ultrasound 36:100, 1995

Siegel S, Kornegay JN, Thrall DE: Postoperative irradiation of spinal cord tumors in 9 dogs. Vet Radiol Ultrasound 37:150, 1996

Sisson AF, LeCouteur RA, Ingram JT et al: Diagnosis of cauda equina abnormalities by using electromyography, discography, and epidurography in dogs. J Vet Intern Med 6:253, 1992

Slocum B, Slocum TD: L7-S1 fixation-fusion for cauda equina compression—an alternative view. p. 1105. In Slatter D (ed): Textbook of Small Animal Surgery. 2nd Ed. WB Saunders, Philadelphia, 1993

Spodnick GJ, Berg J, Moore FM, Cotter SM: Spinal lymphoma in cats: 21 cases (1976–1989). J Am Vet Med Assoc 200:373, 1992

Summers BA, deLahunta A, McEntee M, Kuhajda FP: A novel intradural extramedullary spinal cord tumor in young dogs. Acta Neuropathol (Berl) 75:402, 1988

Thomas WB, Sorjonen DC, Simpson ST: Surgical management of atlantoaxial subluxation in 23 dogs. Vet Surg 20:409, 1991

Thomson CE, Kornegay JN, Stevens JB: Canine intervertebral disc disease: changes in the cerebrospinal fluid. J Small Anim Pract 30:685, 1989

Tipold A, Jaggy A: Steroid responsive meningitis-arteritis in dogs: long-term study of 32 cases. J Small Anim Pract 35:311, 1994

Tipold A, Vandevelde M, Zurbriggen A: Neuroimmunological studies in steroid-responsive meningitis-arteritis in dogs. Res Vet Sci 58:103, 1995

Toombs JP, Collins LG, Graves GM et al: Colonic perforation in corticosteroid-treated dogs. J Am Vet Med Assoc 188:145, 1986

Wheeler SJ, Sharp NJH: Small Animal Spinal Disorders: Diagnosis and Surgery. Mosby-Wolfe, London, 1994

25

Disorders of Peripheral Nerves

Karen Dyer Inzana
Christiane Massicotte

CONGENITAL/ DEVELOPMENTAL DISORDERS

Probable Inherited Disorders of the Peripheral Nervous System
(Table 25–1)

Definition

Congenital neuropathies are disorders of the ventral horn cell (motor neuron), peripheral axon, or Schwann cell that occur with predictable pathology in specific breeds.

Cause and Pathophysiology

I. Genetic inheritance patterns are known or suspected for most of these conditions.
II. Pathology varies with the different diseases.
III. The underlying biochemical defect is known for only a few syndromes.

Clinical Signs

I. Clinical signs occur most commonly in young dogs and cats. Breed and age vary with the syndrome (see Table 25–1).
II. Clinical features are as follows.
   A. Rate of onset (acute vs. chronic) varies with syndrome.
   B. Most animals present with pelvic limb weakness that progresses to generalized weakness, muscle atrophy, and diminished or absent spinal reflexes.
   C. Laryngeal paralysis is a common manifestation of many peripheral neuropathies.
   D. Sensory neuropathies may present with self-mutilation as the initial clinical sign.

Diagnosis

I. Electromyography shows spontaneous electrical activity.
II. Motor and sensory nerve conduction velocity may be abnormal.
III. Muscle biopsy shows neurogenic atrophy.
IV. Nerve biopsy shows pathology typical of the syndrome (i.e., axonal loss or demyelination).

Differential Diagnosis

I. Other congenital or acquired nerve or muscle diseases
II. Toxic neuropathies
III. Metabolic neuropathies
IV. Infectious diseases of spinal cord, peripheral nerve, or muscle

Treatment and Monitoring

I. No therapy is recognized for any of the congenital neuropathies
II. Repeat breeding of parents as well as siblings of affected animals should be discouraged.
III. Most are progressive in nature and result in death or euthanasia.

INFECTIOUS DISORDERS

Protozoan Polyradiculoneuritis
Definition and Cause

I. Protozoan infections are discussed in detail in Chapter 114.
II. In addition to the more generalized clinical signs associated with protozoan infections, pups infected at <3 months of age often develop polyradiculoneuritis.

Table 25–1. Congenital/Developmental Disorders of Peripheral Nerves

Disorder/Breeds	Cause/Pathology	Clinical Signs/Progression	References
I. Inherited Neuropathies Characterized by Loss of Motor Neuron (Ventral Horn Cell)			
Progressive neuronopathy in Cairn terriers	Both sexes affected; genetics uncertain. Chromatolysis of neurons in spinal ventral gray matter, numerous brain stem nuclei, and spinal, autonomic, and myenteric ganglia.	Pelvic limb weakness begins between 12 and 24 weeks of age and progresses to tetraparesis over 2 months. Head tremor is a consistent finding. Nystagmus, head tilt, and cataplexy reported in a single case.	Cummings et al., 1988 Palmer and Blakemore, 1989 Cummings et al., 1991
Focal spinal muscular atrophy in German shepherd dogs	Both sexes affected; genetics uncertain. Asymmetrical loss of motor neurons in cervical intumescence.	Forelimb weakness beginning around 2 weeks of age. One case euthanized; the other case reached a plateau around 8 weeks.	Cummings et al., 1989
Hereditary progressive spinal muscle atrophy in pointers	Both sexes affected; probable autosomal recessive condition. Lipid accumulation in spinal motor neurons and brain stem neurons.	Pelvic limb weakness begins between 18 and 23 weeks of age and progresses to tetraparesis over 3–4 months.	Inada et al., 1978
Spinal muscular atrophy in rottweilers	Only affected females have been reported; genetics uncertain. Chromatolysis and perikaryal swelling noted in spinal motor neurons and neurons in brain stem.	Paraparesis at 4 weeks of age progressing to tetraparesis within 1–2 weeks with pelvic limb rigidity. Megaesophagus is present in some.	Shell et al., 1987
Spinal muscular atrophy in Brittany spaniels	Both sexes affected; autosomal dominant inheritance with variable penetrance. Motor neurons have chromatolysis secondary to internodal swellings in proximal axons. Swellings contain massive accumulations of neurofilaments. Neurofilaments are also present in cell body and proximal dendrites of some motor neurons. Nerves that innervate proximal muscle groups are preferentially affected.	Paraparesis that progresses to tetraparesis. Late features include respiratory muscle paresis, causing dyspnea and ineffective thermoregulation, and cranial nerve involvement, causing difficulty grasping food and swallowing. There are three variants of the disease. 1. Accelerated form occurs in homozygotes. Onset occurs between 6 and 8 weeks with tetraparesis by 3–4 months of age. 2. Intermediate form occurs in heterozygotes. Onset between 6 and 12 months, with tetraparesis by 2–3 years. 3. Chronic form occurs in heterozygotes with onset during adulthood with mild clinical signs that are gradually progressive	Cork et al., 1979, Cork et al., 1982 Sack et al., 1984
Neuronal abiotrophy in Swedish Lapland dogs	Both sexes affected; probable autosomal recessive. Chromatolysis of spinal motor neurons, neurons in dorsal root ganglia, cerebeller Purkinje cells, and other brain stem nuclei.	Thoracic or pelvic limb weakness at 5–7 weeks of age that progresses to tetraparesis within 1–2 weeks.	Sandefelt et al., 1973
II. Inherited Neuropathies Characterized by Loss of Motor Axon			
Giant axonal neuropathy in Alsatians (German shepherd dogs)	Both sexes affected; probable autosomal recessive. Giant axonal swelling containing masses of neurofilaments found in distal segments of myelinated and unmyelinated axons. Both central and peripheral nervous systems involved.	Paraparesis at 14–15 months, with gradual progression to thoracic limbs. Megaesophagus and laryngeal paralysis are also features of the disease.	Griffiths et al., 1980b Duncan and Griffiths, 1981
Hereditary polyneuropathy in Alaskan malamutes	Both sexes affected; probable autosomal recessive. Axonal loss of both motor and sensory fibers in peripheral nerves and in spinal nerve roots, and white matter degeneration in spinal cord and brain stem.	Paraparesis between 7 and 18 months of age, with gradual progression to thoracic limbs. Megaesophagus is a prominent feature.	Moe, 1992

Table continued on following page

Table 25–1. **Congenital/Developmental Disorders of Peripheral Nerves** (Continued)

Disorder/Breeds	Cause/Pathology	Clinical Signs/Progression	References
II. Inherited Neuropathies Characterized by Loss of Motor Axon (Continued)			
Neuropathy in Birman cats	Only affected females have been reported; genetics uncertain. Diffuse loss of myelinated fibers in peripheral nerves, spinal cord, and cerebellum, with a predominantly distal distribution.	Paraparesis between 8 and 10 weeks of age. Insufficient data to report progression.	Moreau et al., 1991
Polyneuropathy in rottweilers	Both sexes affected; possible autosomal recessive. Distal axonal degeneration in both motor and sensory fibers with secondary demyelination.	Paraparesis in adult dogs (1.5–4 years) that gradually progresses over 1 year to tetraparesis.	Braund et al., 1994
Progressive axonopathy in boxers	Both sexes affected; autosomal recessive inheritance. Paranodal axonal swellings containing accumulations of disorganized neurofilaments and vesiculotubular structures are present in spinal nerve roots and lateral and ventral funiculi of spinal cord. This is associated with reduced axonal diameter in distal segments of peripheral nerves.	Pelvic limb ataxia with paraparesis at 1–3 weeks, with gradual progression to involve the thoracic limbs by 1 year of age and then reach a plateau. Head bobbing and ocular tremor seen in a few cases.	Griffiths et al., 1980a Griffiths, 1985
III. Inherited Neuropathies Characterized by Schwann Cell Dysfunction			
Hypomyelinating neuropathy in golden retrievers	Both sexes affected; genetics uncertain. Reduced myelination in peripheral nerves.	Pelvic limb ataxia between 5 and 7 weeks of age with minimal progression.	Matz et al., 1990 Braund et al., 1989
Hypertrophic neuropathy in Tibetan mastiffs	Both sexes affected; probable autosomal recessive. Recurrent demyelination and remyelination create thickening of peripheral nerves. Schwann cells have accumulations of 6–7 nm filaments.	Paraparesis by 7.5–10 weeks of age that rapidly progresses over a few days to tetraplegia. Clinical signs improve over the following 4–6 weeks, but animals remain weak.	Cummings et al., 1981a Cooper et al., 1984a, 1984b
IV. Inherited Neuropathies Characterized by Loss of Sensory Neuron or Axon			
Sensory neuronopathy in long-haired dachshunds	Both sexes affected; probable autosomal recessive. Loss of axons in distal peripheral nerve segments (including vagus nerve) and terminal regions of primary sensory axons in fasciculus gracillis suggests a distal axonopathy of primary sensory neurons.	Generalized ataxia noted around 8 weeks of age. Diminished pain perception noted over whole body. Urinary and fecal incontinence and genital self-mutilation are prominent features. Disease appears nonprogressive.	Duncan and Griffiths, 1982 Duncan et al., 1982
Acral mutilation in English pointers and German shorthaired pointers	Both sexes affected; probable autosomal recessive. Reduction in the size of neurons in dorsal root ganglia and degeneration of primary sensory neurons in peripheral nerves and spinal cord are accompanied by a loss of substance P immuno-reactivity in spinal cord.	Onset between 2 and 12 months of age. Loss of pain perception and mutilation of feet are most prominent signs.	Cummings et al., 1981b, 1983
V. Inherited Neuropathies Associated with Inborn Errors of Metabolism			
Hyperchylomicronemia in cats (domestic shorthair, Himalayan, Persian, Siamese breeds)	Both sexes affected; probable autosomal recessive condition. Deficiency in lipoprotein lipase activity causes hyperlipidemia, xanthomas with infiltration and entrapment of peripheral nerves near intervertebral foramen and other bony prominences.	Clinical signs of dysfunction of one or more peripheral nerves usually begin around 8 months of age. Loss of sympathetic supply to the eye (Horner's syndrome) and tibial and radial nerve paralysis are common.	Jones, 1993

Table 25–1. Congenital/Developmental Disorders of Peripheral Nerves (Continued)

Disorder/Breeds	Cause/Pathology	Clinical Signs/Progression	References
V. Inherited Neuropathies Associated with Inborn Errors of Metabolism (*Continued*)			
Hyperoxaluria in domestic shorthaired cats	Both sexes affected; autosomal recessive condition. Deficiency in D-glycerate dehydrogenase. Peripheral nerve changes are characterized by marked accumulations of neurofilaments in proximal axons of motor and sensory axons.	Animals develop acute signs of renal failure and generalized weakness between 5 and 9 months of age.	McKerrell et al., 1989
α-L-Fucosidosis in English springer spaniels	Both sexes affected; autosomal recessive deficiency in the lysosomal enzyme α-L-fucosidase. Proximal enlargements of multiple cranial and spinal nerves due to infiltration by foamy macrophages and fibroedematous tissue containing fructose-containing substances. There is extensive cytoplasmic vacuolation in neurons and glia in central nervous system.	Behavioral changes may be noted as early as 4–6 months of age and progress slowly over 2–3 years. Aphonia, depressed gag reflex, and dysphagia reflect cranial neuropathies. Spinal nerves are affected during the terminal stages.	Taylor et al., 1987 Barker et al., 1988
Globoid cell leukodystrophy in West Highland white terriers, Cairn terriers, Pomeranians, basset hounds, bluetick hounds, domestic shorthaired cats	Both sexes affected; probable autosomal recessive deficiency of lysosomal enzyme galactocerebroside β-galactosidase. Accumulations of lipid-laden macrophages (globoid cells) are found in both peripheral and central nervous systems, accompanied by a loss of myelination and a decrease in oligodendrocyte and Schwann cell numbers.	Pelvic limb ataxia and generalized tremor typically begin between 3 and 5 months of age. This progresses to paraplegia, then tetraplegia, hyporeflexia, and eventually blindness and dementia by 1 year of age.	Blakemore et al., 1974 Vicini et al., 1988
Niemann-Pick disease in Siamese cats	Both sexes affected; probable autosomal recessive deficiency of sphingomyelinase. Sphingomyelin and other lipids accumulate in liver, renal tubular cells, bone marrow cells, neurons, and glia. Siamese cats also have demyelinating peripheral neuropathy.	Pelvic limb ataxia and generalized tremor typically begin between 2 and 5 months of age.	Cuddon et al., 1989
Glycogen storage disease type IV in Norwegian forest cats	Both sexes affected; probable autosomal recessive deficiency in glycogen branching enzyme. Intracytoplasmic storage of glycogen in nervous system and cardiac and skeletal muscle with loss of spinal motor neurons.	Generalized tremors, weakness, and fever begin at 5 months of age and progress to tetraplegia by 8 months of age.	Fyfe et al., 1990 Coates et al., 1996
VI. Inherited Neuropathies Associated with Laryngeal Paralysis			
Laryngeal paralysis in Bouviers des Flandres	Both sexes affected; autosomal dominant. Degeneration of recurrent laryngeal nerves, with loss of neurons in nucleus ambiguus and occasional axonal loss in tibial nerve.	Inspiratory dyspnea, laryngeal stridor, and exercise intolerance between 4 and 6 months of age. Progression of the syndrome is not reported.	Venker-van Haagen et al., 1978, 1981
Laryngeal paralysis in Siberian husky dogs and their crosses	Both sexes affected; genetics not determined. Degeneration reported only in recurrent laryngeal nerve. Spontaneous activity may occur in other muscles as well.	Inspiratory dyspnea, laryngeal stridor, and exercise intolerance noted between 2 and 6 months of age. Progression of this syndrome has not been reported.	O'Brien and Hendriks, 1986
Laryngeal paralysis in dalmatians	Both sexes affected; inheritance uncertain. Distal axonal degeneration of medium and large diameter fibers in all peripheral nerves, including the recurrent laryngeal nerves. Megaesophagus was also present in more than 50% of cases.	Inspiratory dyspnea, laryngeal stridor, exercise intolerance, and regurgitation first noticed between 2 and 6 months of age. Clinical signs of more generalized polyneuropathy may develop before, concurrently, or after laryngeal paralysis. Aspiration pneumonia resulted in death within a year of diagnosis in most cases.	Braund et al., 1994

III. Previous reports incriminated *Toxoplasma gondii* in neonatal radiculoneuritis, but recent reports suggest that *Neospora caninum* is a more common pathogen in these cases (Dubey et al., 1990).

Pathophysiology

I. Both intense inflammatory changes and organisms at various stages in the life cycle may be found in multiple tissues including brain, spinal cord, and skeletal muscle.

II. The most intense inflammatory reaction in neonatal pups occurs in the nerve roots of the lumbosacral spinal cord.

III. Macrophages, lymphocytes, and plasma cells are found infiltrating nerve roots with evidence of axonal necrosis and Schwann cell loss.

Clinical Signs

I. Clinical signs are characterized by pelvic limb weakness that progresses over days to weeks to paraplegia with the limbs fixed in rigid extension.

II. Muscle atrophy is marked, and spinal reflexes are absent.

III. Sensation is preserved in most cases, and the animals appear hyperpathic on manipulation of the limbs.

IV. Other evidence of multifocal neurologic disease may also be present, including cranial nerve deficits and seizures.

Diagnosis

I. Serologic tests are available that will identify serum antibodies to both toxoplasmosis and neosporosis (see Chap. 114).

II. Organism culture and isolation, transmission in laboratory species, immunocytochemistry, and identification of the organism in biopsy specimens have been helpful in confirming active infection.

Treatment and Monitoring

I. Both organisms are sensitive to clindamycin at 10 mg/kg PO TID × 2 weeks.

II. Sulfonamide 30 mg/kg PO BID and pyrimethamine 0.5 mg/kg PO BID have also been effective in extinguishing the infection.

III. Pelvic limb rigidity is not reversible.

IV. Multiple litters born to previously infected dams are at risk of developing polyradiculoneuritis.

INFLAMMATORY/IMMUNE-MEDIATED DISORDERS

Acute Polyradiculoneuritis (Coonhound Paralysis)

Definition

I. By definition, polyradiculoneuritis is an inflammatory condition of multiple nerve roots.

II. Coonhound paralysis is the most common form of acute polyradiculoneuritis in dogs.

III. It was first described in 1954 as occurring in dogs after exposure to raccoon saliva (Kingma and Catcott, 1954).

IV. However, an identical syndrome has been described in dogs with no known exposure to raccoons and is commonly referred to as idiopathic polyradiculoneuritis.

V. A syndrome similar to idiopathic polyradiculoneuritis also has been reported in cats (Luttgen, 1987).

Causes

I. An antigen in raccoon saliva is thought to stimulate an immune reaction against peripheral nerve myelin.

II. The antigenic stimulation in animals without raccoon exposure is unknown, but it may be viral, toxic, or infectious.

III. An immunologic etiology is proposed because of the following.
   A. Not all dogs bitten by the same raccoon develop clinical signs of weakness.
   B. Once affected, dogs are susceptible to repeat episodes, and repeat episodes can be induced with injections of raccoon saliva.
   C. Dogs with an acute onset of clinical signs shortly after known exposure have antibodies against an antigen in raccoon saliva (Cuddon, 1990).
   D. Inflammatory cell infiltrate occurs after demyelination, suggesting antibody-mediated damage to peripheral nerve myelin.

Pathophysiology

I. All regions of the peripheral nerves are injured; however, ventral roots are most severely affected.

II. Segmental demyelination with milder degrees of axonal degeneration is the most prominent pathologic change.

III. Inflammatory cell infiltrate, primarily mononuclear cells, is also a prominent pathologic feature (Cummings et al., 1982).

Clinical Signs

I. Signs consist of generalized flaccid paralysis with diminished or absent spinal reflexes.

II. Signs often begin in the rear limbs and ascend to the thoracic limbs. In severe cases, cranial nerve deficits and respiratory paralysis may occur.

III. Animals often retain voluntary tail movement and voluntary control of urination and defecation.

IV. Pain perception remains intact, and animals may seem hyperpathic.

V. Signs begin 7–10 days after raccoon exposure and may progress for 2–10 days after the onset of symptoms.

VI. Spontaneous recovery may begin as early as 1 week after the onset of clinical signs, or it may be delayed for several months. Recovery may take several months and is often incomplete.

Diagnosis

I. Clinical signs and history of raccoon exposure are highly suggestive of the disease.
II. Abnormal electromyogram (EMG) spontaneous activity occurs 5–7 days after the onset of clinical signs.
III. Motor nerve conduction velocity is usually slow, and the muscle action potential may be prolonged.
IV. Small motor potentials that normally occur after the initial muscle action potential during motor nerve conduction studies (F wave) may be delayed, and the potential may appear dispersed (Cuddon, 1990).
V. Lumbar cerebrospinal fluid (CSF) typically contains increased protein without an increase in white blood cells (albuminocytologic dissociation).

Differential Diagnosis

I. Tick paralysis
II. Botulism
III. Myasthenia gravis

Treatment and Monitoring

I. There is no specific therapy.
II. Immunosuppressive therapy usually increases the incidence of secondary infections and muscle atrophy.
III. Supportive care is important during recovery.
   A. Maintain soft bedding that is kept dry and clean.
   B. Turn and bathe the animal frequently.
   C. Ensure adequate hydration and nutrition in animals that cannot move the head and neck.
   D. Passive limb manipulation, muscle massage, and hydrotherapy help maintain normal range of motion in paralyzed limbs.
   E. Monitor the animal for pneumonia, urinary tract infections, and decubital ulcers.

Brachial Plexus Neuritis

Definition and Cause

I. Brachial plexus neuritis (BPN) is an inflammatory neuritis involving primarily the ventral nerve roots that give rise to the brachial plexus.
II. It is a rare condition that has been reported in both dogs and cats.
III. The cause is unknown, but thought to be associated with a hypersensitivity reaction.
   A. Dogs have experienced urticarial reactions prior to the onset of clinical signs (Cummings et al., 1973).
   B. One case occurred shortly after ingestion of horse meat, and the dog showed a positive intradermal reaction to horse meat allergens (Cummings et al., 1973).
   C. There are similarities to an immunologic reaction in humans referred to as brachial plexus neuropathy.

Pathophysiology

I. Histologically there is axonal degeneration in nerves of the brachial plexus with associated chromatolysis in both motor and sensory neurons. Mast cell infiltration is prominent in reported cases.
II. Lesions are often asymmetrical and may involve all or only portions of the brachial plexus.

Clinical Signs

I. Signs consist of an acute onset of flaccid paralysis of the brachial plexus with diminished or absent spinal reflexes. Sensory nerves may be affected as well, causing anesthesia of the distal limb.
II. Pelvic limb function remains unaffected.

Diagnosis

I. History and clinical signs are suspicious.
II. Electrophysiologic evidence of axonal loss is seen in forelimb nerves.
   A. EMG evidence of diffuse spontaneous activity occurs 5–7 days after the onset of clinical signs.
   B. Motor and sensory nerve conduction velocities may be mildly slow, but the amplitude of the muscle or nerve action potential is small and prolonged.
III. CSF was normal in two dogs evaluated (Cummings et al., 1973).

Differential Diagnosis

I. Brachial plexus avulsion
II. Injury to spinal cord at cervical intumescence

Treatment and Monitoring

I. There is no specific treatment.
II. Supportive care consists of passive limb manipulation, muscle massage, and hydrotherapy to maintain normal range of motion in paralyzed limbs.
III. Clinical recovery has occurred spontaneously between 4 days and 4 months (Bright et al., 1978).
IV. No improvement was noted in another case 45 days after the onset of clinical signs (Cummings et al., 1973).

Sensory Ganglioradiculoneuritis

Definition and Cause

I. This is a poorly defined sensory neuropathy that affects young adult dogs of various breeds.
II. The etiology is unknown, but immune-mediated, toxic, and viral causes have been considered (Wouda et al., 1983; Steiss et al., 1987).

Pathophysiology

I. Pathology is characterized by a non-suppurative inflammation of dorsal root ganglia and cranial sensory ganglia with loss of sensory neuron cell bodies.

II. There is concomitant loss of larger diameter sensory axons in both peripheral nerves and sensory tracts in the spinal cord.

Clinical Signs

I. The onset of clinical signs may be subacute, acute, or chronic, with an equally variable rate of progression.
II. Initial signs consist of rear limb ataxia, which may progress over weeks or months to generalized ataxia.
III. Facial hypalgesia, dysphagia, and regurgitation secondary to megaesophagus have been seen in some cases.
IV. Limb muscle tone and strength are preserved, but tendon reflexes are diminished to absent.

Diagnosis

I. There is electrophysiologic evidence of loss of sensory axons.
   A. EMG is normal or shows minimal evidence of muscle denervation.
   B. Motor nerve conduction is usually normal to slightly decreased.
   C. Sensory nerve conduction is usually not recordable.
II. Axonal atrophy of large diameter fibers is found on biopsy of a mixed or primary sensory peripheral nerve.
III. CSF is normal or may show mild increases in protein and white blood cell (WBC) count.

Differential Diagnosis

I. Doxorubicin, methylmercury, or pyridoxine intoxication
II. Congenital sensory neuropathy

Treatment and Monitoring

I. There is no treatment.
II. Self-mutilation has been reported in a few cases.
III. Recovery from this condition has not been reported.

Myasthenia Gravis

Definition and Causes

I. Myasthenia gravis (MG) is a disorder characterized by failure in neuromuscular transmission secondary to a reduction in acetylcholine receptors on the postsynaptic muscle membrane.
II. There are two forms of myasthenia gravis—congenital and acquired.
   A. In congenital MG, the deficiency in acetylcholine receptors may be caused by reduced or imperfect synthesis or accelerated degradation.
   B. In acquired MG, there is antibody-mediated destruction of acetylcholine receptors.
III. Congenital MG is an autosomal recessive condition in Jack Russell terriers, smooth-haired fox terriers, English springer spaniels, and Samoyeds. It has also

been reported in Siamese and domestic short-haired cats (Indrieri et al., 1983).
IV. Acquired MG is associated with immune dysfunction that in occasional cases has been linked to thymomas or other forms of neoplasia in the cat and dog.

Pathophysiology

I. Normal neuromuscular transmission requires the following.
   A. Acetylcholine released from the nerve terminal crosses the synaptic cleft and binds to acetylcholine receptors.
   B. These receptors are cation channels that, when stimulated, induce an action potential in the muscle fiber.
   C. Acetylcholine action is terminated by esterases located near the acetylcholine receptors on the muscle membrane.
II. Either a relative or actual decrease in the number of receptors causes inefficient neuromuscular transmission and clinical signs of weakness.

Clinical Signs

I. Generalized muscle weakness that worsens with exercise
II. Congenital form
   A. Signs typically begin between 6 and 8 weeks in puppies and 4 and 5 months in kittens.
   B. Megaesophagus is infrequent but has been reported in smooth-haired fox terriers (Miller et al., 1983).
III. Acquired form
   A. Signs have a bimodal age association with peaks occurring between 2 and 4 years and again at >9 years.
   B. All breeds of dogs are susceptible; however, German shepherd dogs, golden retrievers, and Labrador retrievers are overrepresented. Abyssinians and Somalis appear overrepresented in cats.
   C. Megaesophagus is common with acquired MG.
   D. In some cases, clinical signs may be confined to weakness of esophageal, pharyngeal, and facial muscles (Shelton et al., 1990).
   E. In addition to generalized weakness and megaesophagus, cats frequently exhibit dysphonia and cervical ventroflexion.

Diagnosis

I. Administration of a short-acting acetylcholinesterase inhibitor, edrophonium chloride, at a dosage of 0.2–5 mg IV, results in temporary improvement in most cases.
II. Repetitive stimulation of motor neurons results in successively smaller muscle action potentials.
III. Circulating antibodies to acetylcholine receptors can be demonstrated in the serum of at least 85% of cases.
IV. Antibodies can be identified immunocytochemically

bound to the postsynaptic muscle membrane (Pflugfelder et al., 1981).

Treatment

I. Administration of a longer acting acetylcholinesterase inhibitor, pyridostigmine bromide, at 0.2–2 mg/kg PO BID-TID, results in improvement in skeletal muscle weakness in most cases of acquired MG.

II. Neostigmine may be administered IM at a dose of 0.05 mg/kg, 3–4 times a day, initially if regurgitation precludes oral anticholinesterase therapy.

III. With any acetylcholinesterase inhibitor, clinical signs of overdosage such as increased weakness, bradycardia, respiratory distress, and gastrointestinal hypermotility may mimic signs of the disease. A test injection of edrophonium may help determine whether weakness is the result of a cholinergic crisis or insufficient response to therapy.

IV. With congenital MG, acetylcholinesterase inhibitors may improve clinical signs but are not as effective as in acquired cases.

V. Immunosuppressive therapy remains controversial in cases of acquired MG.
  A. Corticosteroids are known to cause exacerbation of weakness in humans with MG (Shelton, 1996).
  B. Polydipsia, polyphagia, and immunosuppression are undesirable side effects of steroids in animals with aspiration pneumonia.
  C. Immunosuppression reduces the level of circulating antibody and can shorten the course of the disease.
  D. It has been recommended to administer lower doses of prednisone initially (0.25 mg/kg) and to gradually increase to immunosuppressive levels (2 mg/kg) over 2–3 weeks (Shelton, 1996).
  E. Azathioprine (2 mg/kg PO SID-QOD) has been recommended in refractory cases (Luttgen and LeCouteur, 1992).

VI. Plasmapheresis resulted in improvement in a single case (Bartges et al., 1990).

VII. Thymectomy is helpful in cats with thymomas or other thymic disease (Scott-Moncrieff et al., 1990).

Patient Monitoring

I. Esophageal motility does not respond to anti-acetylcholinesterase therapy as readily as skeletal muscle, and aspiration pneumonia is the most common cause of death in MG.

II. Esophageal function often improves with remission of the disease.

III. Spontaneous remission occurs but may take months in some cases.

IV. Exact percentages of dogs and cats that recover from acquired MG have not been reported. In this author's experience, roughly 50% of animals succumb to the disease.

IDIOPATHIC DISORDERS

Distal Denervating Disease

Definition and Cause

I. Ten dogs with similar clinical signs and degenerative changes in distal peripheral nerve segments were described as having distal denervating disease (Griffiths and Duncan, 1979b).

II. The cause is unknown, but an unidentified toxin is considered likely (Duncan and Griffiths, 1984).

Pathophysiology

I. It is a distal motor neuropathy characterized by axonal degeneration in terminal nerve branches.

II. Proximal axons are preserved, and there is no evidence of reaction in nerve cell bodies.

Clinical Signs

I. There is no obvious age, breed, or sex predilection.

II. There is a variable rate of onset, with clinical signs developing over the course of days or over more than 1 month.

III. Tetraparesis is the predominant clinical sign, with variable degrees of cranial nerve dysfunction.
  A. Muscle atrophy is marked in proximal extensor groups.
  B. Spinal reflexes are depressed or absent, but pain sensation is preserved.
  C. Voluntary control of tail movement, urination, and defecation is maintained.

Diagnosis

I. Electrophysiologic abnormalities suggest a distal motor neuropathy.
  A. EMG shows spontaneous activity in all muscles.
  B. Motor nerve conduction velocity is normal or slightly reduced.
  C. The amplitude and duration of the muscle action potential evoked by stimulation of peripheral nerves are small and prolonged.
  D. Sensory nerve conduction is normal.

II. Muscle and nerve biopsy confirms a distal axonopathy with denervation atrophy of muscle.

Differential Diagnosis

I. Cases with an acute onset could be confused with acute polyradiculoneuritis (coonhound paralysis), tick paralysis, myasthenia gravis, or botulism.

II. Metabolic and paraneoplastic neuropathies should be considered in cases with a more gradual onset.

Treatment and Monitoring

I. There is no treatment.

II. Supportive care includes physical therapy, soft bedding, and hand feeding and watering.

III. Recovery occurs in 4–6 weeks, presumably from collateral axonal sprouting of nerve terminals.

Distal Symmetrical Neuropathy

Definition and Cause

I. Numerous adult large breeds of dogs have been described as developing a distal sensorimotor polyneuropathy that has been classified as distal symmetrical neuropathy (Braund, 1995).
II. The cause is unknown.

Pathophysiology

I. Pathologic changes are characterized by degeneration of large diameter axons in distal portions of appendicular and laryngeal nerves.
II. Variable degrees of segmental demyelination may also be observed.
III. No changes are present in the central nervous system.

Clinical Signs

I. Clinical signs are insidious in onset and gradually progressive over 1–2 months.
II. Pelvic limb paresis is the initial presenting sign, but tetraparesis and atrophy of muscles of mastication eventually develop.
III. Distal limb muscles are more profoundly affected.

Diagnosis

I. Electrophysiologic changes suggest a distal axonopathy.
  A. EMG shows spontaneous activity in all muscles.
  B. Motor nerve conduction velocity is normal or slightly reduced.
  C. The amplitude and duration of the muscle action potential evoked by stimulation of peripheral nerves are small and prolonged.
II. Muscle and nerve biopsy confirms a distal axonopathy with denervation atrophy of muscle.

Differential Diagnosis

I. Metabolic or endocrine neuropathies
II. Toxin exposure
III. Paraneoplastic neuropathy

Treatment and Monitoring

I. No treatment has been described.
II. The syndrome is chronic and progressive in nature.

Chronic Relapsing Neuropathy

Definition and Cause

I. Chronic relapsing neuropathy is a generalized polyradiculoneuropathy identified in mature dogs and cats and characterized by a chronic remitting and relapsing clinical course (Cummings and de Lahunta, 1974; Shores et al., 1987; Malik et al., 1991).
II. The cause is unknown.

Pathophysiology

I. Histologically, variable degrees of mononuclear cell infiltrates are found in peripheral nerves and nerve roots.
II. The inflammatory response varies markedly between nerves but is characterized by macrophages, monocytes, and lymphocytes.
III. Primary demyelination is most prominent, with lesser degrees of axonal necrosis involving both motor and sensory nerves.

Clinical Signs

I. Clinical signs may develop over weeks or months and typically follow a waxing and waning course.
II. Initial signs consist of weakness in one or more limbs.
III. With increasing chronicity, muscle atrophy, depressed spinal reflexes, and sensory deficits are more obvious.
IV. Cranial nerves are affected as well.

Diagnosis

I. Cerebrospinal fluid may contain increased protein concentrations without concomitant pleocytosis (albuminocytologic dissociation).
II. Electrophysiologic changes are most consistent with demyelination.
  A. EMG shows spontaneous activity in denervated muscles.
  B. Motor and sensory nerve conduction is slowed, with more variable degrees of reduction in amplitude and dispersion of the evoked muscle action potential.
III. Muscle and nerve biopsy reveals denervation of muscle and demyelination and remyelination of peripheral nerve fibers. The presence of inflammatory cell infiltrates in biopsy specimens is variable and is probably dependent on the stage of disease.

Differential Diagnosis

I. Other chronic progressive neuropathies should be considered, including those with metabolic and toxic etiologies.
II. Toxoplasmosis may have similar clinical signs in some cats.

Treatment and Monitoring

I. Prednisolone at immunosuppressive doses (2 mg/kg PO BID) improved clinical signs in both cats in which it was administered (Shores et al., 1987; Malik et al., 1991).
II. Supportive care including physical therapy, soft bed-

ding, attention to cleanliness, and hand watering and feeding is essential.

III. Long-term prognosis is fair in cats but poor in dogs.

Dancing Doberman Disease

Definition and Cause

A progressive neuromuscular disorder that occurs primarily in the pelvic limbs of young adult Doberman pinschers (Chrisman, 1990).

Pathophysiology

I. The pathophysiology of this disorder is unknown.

II. Some dogs have multifocal pelvic limb muscular atrophy and hypertrophy, focal necrosis, and endomysial/perimysial fibrosis suggestive of a form of myotonic myopathy (Braund, 1995).

III. Other dogs have peripheral nerve changes suggestive of a distal neuropathy (Chrisman, 1990).

IV. A single case with neuronal degeneration and gliosis in the spinal cord and lumbosacral nerve roots has been reported (Chrisman, 1990).

Clinical Signs

I. To date, this syndrome has been reported only in Doberman pinschers.

II. Both males and females are affected.

III. Clinical signs begin between 6 months and 7 years of age and consist initially of persistent flexion of one pelvic limb while standing.

IV. The opposite pelvic limb becomes affected in most cases within 3 to 6 months, causing a shifting limb lameness and increased tendency to sit rather than stand.

V. Conscious proprioceptive deficits have been reported in two dogs 5 and 6 years, respectively, after the disease was diagnosed.

VI. Exaggerated pelvic limb reflexes and atrophy of the gastrocnemius muscle are also common signs.

Diagnosis

I. History and clinical signs are most helpful.

II. Electrophysiologic abnormalities consist of a mixture or myopathic and neuropathic changes.

A. EMG shows spontaneous electrical activity in affected muscles.

B. Motor and sensory nerve conduction velocity are usually normal.

C. Muscle and nerve biopsy may show evidence of myopathy or neuropathy.

Differential Diagnosis

I. Lumbosacral stenosis

II. Intervertebral disk disease of the lower lumbar spine

III. Neoplasia of the lower lumbar spinal cord or nerve roots

Treatment and Monitoring

I. No treatment has proved beneficial.

II. The syndrome is slowly progressive, but affected animals remain functional pets for years.

METABOLIC/TOXIC NEUROPATHIES

Diabetes Mellitus–Induced Neuropathy

Definition and Cause

I. Peripheral neuropathies have been identified in both dogs and cats with diabetes mellitus.

II. The cause of diabetic neuropathy remains controversial in all species examined.

Pathophysiology

I. Current theories suggest that multiple mechanisms play a role in the pathogenesis.

II. Thickening and hyalinization of peripheral nerve vasculature suggest that ischemia may play a role in the genesis of diabetic neuropathy.

III. Metabolic derangements cause increased sorbitol accumulation and depletion of *myo*-inositol content, which reduces Na^+, K^+-ATPase activity.

IV. Amino acid uptake and protein synthesis are reduced in dorsal root ganglia of diabetic rats, and axonal transport is reduced. This suggests that distal axonal changes may result from reduced delivery of molecules from neuronal cell bodies.

V. Immunologic mechanisms have also been implicated in some cases of diabetic neuropathy after identification of autoantibodies and inflammatory infiltrates into autonomic ganglia of diabetic patients.

VI. Diabetic neuropathy in animals is characterized by both segmental demyelination and axonal necrosis (Braund and Steiss, 1982).

Clinical Signs

I. In dogs, clinical signs are usually subclinical. Occasionally dogs present with a relatively acute onset of pelvic limb weakness, generalized muscle atrophy, and normal to mildly depressed spinal reflexes.

II. Clinical signs are more common in diabetic cats. Plantigrade stance, depressed patellar reflexes, and pelvic limb weakness are common.

Diagnosis

I. The diagnosis of diabetes mellitus is described in Chapter 43.

II. Electrophysiologic changes associated with diabetic neuropathy include the following (Steiss et al., 1981).

A. EMG shows diffuse spontaneous activity.

B. Motor and sensory nerve conduction is mildly slowed, and the muscle action potential is reduced in amplitude.

III. Nerve and muscle biopsy shows both demyelination and distal axonal loss with evidence of denervation in muscle sections.

Differential Diagnosis

I. Other endocrine neuropathies
II. Paraneoplastic neuropathy
III. Toxic neuropathies

Treatment and Monitoring

I. Improved glycemic control results in resolution of clinical signs in both dogs and cats.
II. Neurologic improvement occurs over weeks to months after insulin therapy.

Hypoglycemic Neuropathy

Definition

Several dogs with peripheral neuropathy and hypoglycemia secondary to functional insulin-secreting tumors have been reported (Schrauwen, 1991; Bergman et al., 1994).

Cause and Pathophysiology

I. Peripheral nerves from affected dogs show variable degrees of axonal degeneration and segmental demyelination.
II. The pathogenesis of the neuropathy is unknown. Theories include metabolic defects induced by hyperinsulinism or hypoglycemia and a paraneoplastic phenomenon.

Clinical Signs

I. In most cases, cerebral signs of seizures and disorientation overshadow subclinical peripheral nerve changes.
II. Paraparesis or tetraparesis combined with muscle atrophy and diminished spinal reflexes has been reported in occasional cases (Schrauwen, 1991; Bergman et al., 1994).

Diagnosis

I. Fasting hypoglycemia and hyperinsulinemia with an amended insulin/glucose ratio > 30 are usually indicative of an insulinoma (see Chap. 45).
II. Electrophysiologic changes include the following.
  A. EMG shows spontaneous activity.
  B. Motor nerve conduction is slightly slowed, with dispersion and reduced amplitude of the muscle action potential induced by sciatic nerve stimulation (Bergman et al., 1994).
III. Peripheral nerve and muscle biopsy shows variable degrees of axonal degeneration and primary demyelination with neurogenic atrophy of muscles.

Differential Diagnosis

I. Other endocrine neuropathies
II. Paraneoplastic neuropathy
III. Toxic neuropathies

Treatment and Monitoring

I. Treatment of insulinomas is described in Chapter 45.
II. Successful recovery from neuropathy has not been described.

Hypothyroid Neuropathy

Definition and Cause

I. There is a high association of neuromuscular disease (both neuropathy and myopathy) and hypothyroidism in dogs.
II. Both the incidence of concurrent disease and resolution of clinical signs with thyroid supplementation support a causal relationship between hypothyroidism and neuromuscular disease.

Pathophysiology

I. The pathophysiologic basis of hypothyroid-induced neuromuscular disease is unknown.
II. In humans and experimental animals, hypothyroidism has been associated with changes in both Schwann cells and axons (Pollard, 1993).
  A. Histologically, both axonal necrosis and demyelination are features of hypothyroid neuropathy.
  B. Excessive glycogen aggregates have been observed in the cytoplasm of Schwann cells and axons.
    1. In Schwann cells, glycogen aggregates were associated with mitochondrial aggregates, lamellar bodies, and lipid droplets.
    2. Remaining axons often appear to have shrunken axons with inappropriately thick myelin sheaths suggesting axonal atrophy.
  C. Axonal transport studies suggest slow axonal transport is reduced in hypothyroid rats.

Clinical Signs

I. Most recognized cases occur in middle-aged or older large-breed dogs.
  A. Clinical signs of chronic progressive generalized weakness, muscle atrophy, and diminished spinal reflexes are most common (Indrieri et al., 1987; Jaggy et al., 1994; Braund, 1995).
  B. Laryngeal paralysis is often associated with hypothyroidism and may represent an early indicator of generalized peripheral neuropathy.
II. Cranial nerve dysfunction has been reported in both large- and small-breed mature dogs (Jaggy et al., 1994).
  A. Facial nerve paralysis
  B. Vestibular dysfunction with head tilt, ataxia, and nystagmus
  C. Trigeminal nerve dysfunction
III. There is also a high association between myasthenia gravis and hypothyroidism (Dewey et al., 1995).

Diagnosis

I. Low resting thyroid levels and inappropriate response to thyroid-stimulating hormone administration support the diagnosis of hypothyroidism (see Chap. 41).

II. Electrophysiologic studies support neuromuscular disease.
   A. EMG shows diffuse spontaneous activity.
   B. Motor and sensory nerve conduction velocity may be slowed.

III. Nerve and muscle biopsy may reveal axonal degeneration, demyelination, and myopathy.

Differential Diagnosis

I. Other endocrine neuropathies
II. Paraneoplastic neuropathy
III. Toxic neuropathies

Treatment and Monitoring

I. Thyroid supplementation is administered as outlined in Chapter 41.
II. Clinical signs usually improve with supplementation, but improvement may take several months.

Paraneoplastic Polyneuropathies

Definition and Cause

I. Cancer can present as a multisystemic disease, affecting tissues well removed from the site of the tumor.
II. Many animals with chronic progressive peripheral neuropathies have tumors, and animals with cancer have clinical or subclinical evidence of nervous system dysfunction (Dyer et al., 1986; Braund et al., 1987).

Pathophysiology

I. The pathogenesis of paraneoplastic neuropathies is unknown; however, several theories have been proposed.
   A. Production of a biologically active compound by the neoplasm has toxic effects on peripheral nerves. Insulinomas may be an example.
   B. Competition between the tumor and the host for essential metabolites may cause a secondary nutritional deficiency. There is little evidence to support this theory.
   C. Immunosuppression associated with neoplasia may predispose the animal to opportunistic infections. There is little evidence to support this theory.
   D. An immune-mediated disorder produces autoantibodies against antigens shared by both the tumor and peripheral nerves.
      1. Shared neural antigens have been noted in many types of human cancer (Dropcho, 1988).
      2. The high association between neoplasia and acquired myasthenia gravis, a recognized immune disorder in animals, supports this pathogenesis.
II. Both axonal necrosis and primary segmental demye-

lination have been found in peripheral nerves of dogs with presumed paraneoplastic neuropathy.

Clinical Signs

I. In most cases, clinical signs remain subclinical.
II. A few cases may present with generalized weakness, muscle atrophy, and diminished to absent spinal reflexes.

Diagnosis

I. Diagnosis is dependent on ruling out other causes of chronic progressive neuropathies, including other metabolic and toxic causes, and identifying the presence of a primary neoplasm.
II. Electrophysiologic changes are most suggestive of axonopathy.
   A. EMG shows diffuse spontaneous activity.
   B. Motor and sensory nerve conduction velocity may be slowed.
III. Nerve and muscle biopsy may reveal axonal degeneration, demyelination, and myopathy.

Differential Diagnosis

I. Other endocrine neuropathies
II. Toxic neuropathies

Treatment and Monitoring

I. Successful treatment has not been reported.
II. Successful elimination of the underlying neoplasm may ameliorate clinical signs.

Botulism

Definition and Cause

I. Botulism is an acute, rapidly progressive, generalized lower motor neuron paralysis that results from ingestion of the exotoxin produced by *Clostridium botulinum* (Barsanti, 1990).
II. Eight antigenically different types of botulinus neurotoxins (types A, B, C1, C2, D, E, F, and G) have been identified.
III. Most cases of botulism in animals are caused by type C, with occasional cases caused by type D reported.
IV. The toxin is produced under anaerobic conditions by the gram-positive rod, *C. botulinum*.
V. *C. botulinum* is a saprophytic organism, found worldwide in soil.
VI. Clinical cases are usually due to ingestion of preformed toxin, typically in decayed carrion.

Pathophysiology

I. Once ingested, the toxin is absorbed from the gastrointestinal tract and is carried to cholinergic nerve terminals, where it prevents the release of acetylcholine.
II. The toxin binds to presynaptic nerve terminals.

III. The toxin moves inside the cell during acetylcholine release.

IV. Once inside the nerve terminal, the toxin prevents release of acetylcholine presumably by inhibition of the calcium ion flux necessary for transmitter release.

Clinical Signs

I. Clinical signs may occur within hours of toxin ingestion or may be delayed for up to 6 days.

II. Blockage of acetylcholine release results in generalized lower motor neuron paralysis and parasympathetic dysfunction.

A. Signs may begin in the pelvic limbs and ascend to thoracic limbs and cranial nerves. Voluntary tail movement is usually maintained.

B. Facial nerve paralysis, pharyngeal dysfunction, and megaesophagus are common.

C. Evidence of parasympathetic dysfunction includes mydriasis and decreased lacrimation.

D. Respiratory paralysis occurs in severe cases secondary to intercostal and diaphragmatic paralysis.

Diagnosis

I. Botulism is confirmed by identifying toxin in serum, stomach contents, or feces.

A. A neutralization mice test is performed by injecting toxin alone and in combination with specific antitoxins. It identifies both the type and potency of the botulinus toxin.

B. Radioimmunoassay, enzyme-linked immunosorbent assay (ELISA), and passive hemagglutination identify toxin and type but do not evaluate potency.

C. Recovery of *C. botulinum* from fecal culture is presumptive evidence of intoxication, as the organism rarely colonizes the canine intestine.

II. Typical electrophysiologic changes in affected patients include the following.

A. EMG is usually normal unless the case is unusually severe.

B. Motor conduction velocities are normal or slightly decreased.

C. The muscle action potential induced by peripheral nerve stimulation is unusually small, but repetitive stimulation does not cause a decrementing response.

Differential Diagnosis

I. Polyradiculoneuritis
II. Tick paralysis
III. Myasthenia gravis

Treatment and Monitoring

I. The antitoxin must be specific for the type of botulinus toxin. A polyvalent toxin that contains type C is recommended for dogs.

A. Recommended antitoxin dosage is 10,000– 15,000 units IV or IM, administered twice at 4-hour intervals.

B. Anaphylaxis is possible, so a test injection of 0.1 ml interdermally 20 minutes prior to administration is recommended.

C. The antitoxin is effective at inactivating circulating and bound toxin prior to being taken up by the nerve terminal.

D. The antitoxin is ineffective once the toxin is inside the axon.

II. Recovery once clinical signs appear requires regeneration of nerve terminals, which usually occurs in 2–3 weeks. Supportive care during this time is critical.

A. Passive flexion and extension of the limbs 2–3 times daily maintains joint and muscle flexibility.

B. Soft bedding and frequent turning together with frequent bathing prevent decubital ulcers.

C. Alimentation and hydration must be maintained. The presence of megaesophagus may necessitate holding the animal upright during feeding, or placement of a gastric feeding tube.

III. Antibiotics are indicated if secondary infections occur.

A. There is little evidence that antibiotics are necessary to control *C. botulinum* infections.

B. Common sites for secondary infections include the urinary and respiratory tracts.

Tick Paralysis

Definition and Cause

I. Tick paralysis is an acute, rapidly progressive, generalized lower motor neuron paralysis caused by a neurotoxin released from several species of ticks.

II. Although several species are capable of producing the syndrome, *Dermacentor andersoni* (the Rocky Mountain wood tick) and *Dermacentor variabilis* (the American dog tick) are most often incriminated in North America, and *Ixodes holocyclus* is most often incriminated in Australia (Malik and Farrow, 1991).

Pathophysiology

I. The engorged female tick is believed to secrete a neurotoxin that prevents release of acetylcholine from cholinergic nerve terminals.

II. Several neurotoxins may be released from *Ixodes* ticks, one of which is holocyclotoxin, which is thought to interfere with calcium entry in nerve terminal necessary for acetylcholine release.

Clinical Signs

I. Clinical signs develop 5–9 days after tick attachment.

II. Weakness may begin in the pelvic limbs and ascend to thoracic limbs over 24–48 hours.

A. Spinal reflexes are absent.

B. Pain perception is normal.

C. Autonomic dysfunction is rare in North American cases but common in Australia.

D. Death may result from respiratory paralysis in 1–5 days if ticks are not removed.

Diagnosis

I. Improvement in clinical signs within 24 hours of tick removal provides firm evidence of tick paralysis.
II. Electrophysiologic abnormalities are as follows.
  A. EMG is normal in all cases. Animals usually recover or die before EMG abnormalities occur.
  B. Motor nerve conduction may be normal or slightly slowed.
  C. The muscle action potential induced by peripheral nerve stimulation may be small or nonexistent (Chrisman, 1975).
  D. Repetitive nerve stimulation does not produce a decremental response in the evoked muscle action potential.

Differential Diagnosis

I. Polyradiculoneuritis
II. Botulism
III. Myasthenia gravis

Treatment and Monitoring

I. Clinical signs improve within 24 hours and the animals are normal within 48 hours of tick removal.
  A. All ticks may be difficult to find. Careful examination of ears and interdigital spaces and the clipping of long-haired dogs are indicated.
  B. Organophosphates eliminate ticks but may potentiate ineffective neuromuscular transmission if the diagnosis is incorrect.
II. In Australia, clinical signs may progress for 24–48 hours after tick removal. Administration of hyperimmune serum at 0.5–1 ml/kg IV has been advocated (Malik and Farrow, 1991).

Miscellaneous Toxins

Definition and Causes

Many toxic compounds are recognized to cause injury to both the central and peripheral nervous systems in domestic animals (Table 25–2).

Pathophysiology

I. Pathophysiology varies with different toxins.
II. For many toxins, the exact pathogenesis is unknown.
III. Disturbances in neuromuscular transmission, neural metabolism, and axonal transport may be components of many toxic neuropathies.

Clinical Signs

I. Clinical signs may begin acutely or more insidiously.
II. Generalized lower motor signs of weakness, muscle atrophy, and hyporeflexia may be combined with central nervous system dysfunction and gastrointestinal disturbances.

Table 25–2. **Possible Causes of Toxic Neuropathy in Animals**

Chemical Agents	Heavy Metals
Organophosphorus compounds	Arsenic
Parathion	Lead
Malathion	Gold
Triorthocresyl phosphate	Thallium
Diisopropyl fluorophosphate	Mercury
Acrylamide	**Drugs**
Lindane	Vincristine
Polychlorinated biphenyls	Vinblastine
Carbon tetrachloride	Doxorubicin
Methyl butyl ketone	Chloramphenicol
Zinc pyridinethione	Ampicillin
Carbon disulfide	Erythromycin
N-Hexane	Tetracycline
Chlorophenothane	Nitrofurantoin
	Diphenylhydantoin

From Shell LG, Dyer KR: Peripheral nerve disorders. P. 1171. In Birchard SJ, Sherding RG (eds): Saunders Manual of Small Animal Practice. WB Saunders, Philadelphia, 1994, with permission.

Diagnosis

I. History of possible exposure
II. Toxicologic identification of suspicious agents

Treatment and Monitoring

I. Remove animal from source of intoxication.
II. Heavy metal and organophosphate intoxication are discussed further in Chapters 124 and 127.

VASCULAR DISORDERS

Definition and Causes

I. The most common vascular neuropathy occurs secondary to aortic thromboembolism in cats with cardiac disease.
II. Thromboembolization of the caudal aorta has also been reported in dogs with heartworm disease.
III. Occlusion of the terminal aorta causes ischemic injury to the sciatic nerve near its bifurcation into tibial and peroneal nerves as well as the muscles of the thigh region.

Pathophysiology

I. Thromboembolization of the terminal aorta physically limits blood flow to the pelvic limbs, but experimental ligation of the aorta does not reproduce clinical signs.
II. Vasoactive substances released from the clot, such as serotonin and thromboxane, also limit collateral blood flow to the affected region (Sisson and Thomas, 1995).
III. Axonal necrosis occurs in the center of nerve fascicles in the distal sciatic nerve and its branches (Griffiths and Duncan, 1979a).

IV. In peripheral areas that maintain perfusion, paranodal demyelination is evident.

Clinical Signs

I. Clinical signs of paraplegia are typically peracute in onset.
II. Femoral pulses are undetectable, the limb muscles are hard and cold, and nailbeds are cyanotic and do not bleed if cut.
III. Complete absence of all rear limb reflexes and nociception is common.
IV. Voluntary motor control is usually preserved to the tail, bladder, and rectum.

Diagnosis

I. Diagnosis of feline cardiac disease is discussed in Chapter 10.
II. Motor nerve conduction through the sciatic tibial nerve is usually absent, or the few remaining axons produce an extremely small muscle action potential.

Treatment and Monitoring

I. Treatment is discussed in detail in Chapter 10.
II. Neurologic function improves in at least 50% of cats within 2–3 weeks (Fox, 1987).
III. Unfortunately, the potential for additional thromboembolic events remains high.

NEOPLASIA

Primary Peripheral Nerve Tumors

Definition and Cause

I. Peripheral nerve sheath tumors have been referred to as schwannoma, neurilemmoma, neurofibroma, and neurofibrosarcoma.
II. Most canine primary nerve sheath tumors are poorly differentiated neoplasms in which the cell of origin is difficult to identify.
III. Most authors prefer the term nerve sheath tumors to reflect the uncertain cell origin.
IV. The cause of these tumors is unknown.

Pathophysiology

I. These tumors may arise along the course of any peripheral nerve, including cranial nerves and spinal nerve roots.
II. Although any peripheral nerve may be affected, most occur in proximal nerve segments involving the brachial plexus or its associated nerve roots (Brehm et al., 1995).
III. Proliferation of neoplastic cells within the nerve sheath causes compression and destruction of peripheral axons.

Clinical Signs

I. Most affected animals present as adults (range of 2–13 years, with median of 8–9 years).
II. All breeds and both sexes are equally affected.
III. Clinical signs vary with the area affected.
   A. Most occur in the cervical spinal cord or brachial plexus.
      1. Chronic progressive forelimb lameness, muscle atrophy, pain in the axillary area, and a palpable mass may be present.
      2. Horner's syndrome and loss of ipsilateral panniculus response reflect loss of T1, T2 proximal nerve roots, which contain preganglionic sympathetic fibers that supply the face, and give rise to the lateral thoracic nerve, respectively.
      3. Ipsilateral hemiparesis that progresses to paraparesis occurs with extension of neoplastic tissue into the spinal canal and secondary spinal cord compression.
      4. Invasion of surrounding tissues and pulmonary metastasis are rare sequelae (Uchida et al., 1992).
   B. Occasional cases involving the spinal nerve roots of the thoracolumbar spinal cord have been reported that cause progressive paraparesis to paralysis (Bradley et al., 1982).
   C. Tumors involving multiple cranial nerves have also been reported (Zachary et al., 1986).
      1. Signs consist of trigeminal, facial, and vestibular nerve paralysis.
      2. Signs may progress to hemiparesis and dysphagia as the brain stem and glossopharyngeal nerves are compressed.
   D. Tumors of the lumbar plexus may lead to progressive rear limb lameness, muscle atrophy, and pain (Brehm et al., 1995).

Diagnosis

I. EMG shows evidence of denervation in affected muscle groups.
II. Survey radiographs may show enlarged intervertebral foramen and myelography may show an intradural extramedullary mass if neoplastic cells have invaded the nerve roots.
III. Computed tomography has been helpful in identifying neoplastic nerve roots (McCarthy et al., 1993).
IV. Surgical exploration and biopsy of nerve or plexus may be necessary to confirm the diagnosis.

Differential Diagnosis

I. Initially, these tumors may present as a musculoskeletal injury.
II. Peripheral nerves may be compressed by other neoplastic processes.
III. Rarely, asymmetrical intervertebral disk herniation may compress spinal nerve roots and present as a monoparesis.

Treatment and Monitoring

I. Surgical excision has been curative in a few isolated cases (Bailey 1990; Brehm et al., 1995).
II. Inability to completely resect all neoplastic cells results in recurrence in most cases.
III. Median survival intervals after diagnosis in dogs with tumors of the brachial plexus or nerve roots are 12 and 5 months, respectively (Brehm et al., 1995).
IV. Although proposed as a treatment, efficacy of radiation therapy is unknown.

Secondary Peripheral Nerve Tumors

Definition and Cause

I. Tumors arising from non-neural cells may occasionally invade or compress peripheral nerves.
II. Infiltration of peripheral and cranial nerves by neoplastic myeloid cells has been documented with both lymphosarcoma and myelomonocytic leukemia (Carpenter et al., 1987; Hobbs and Cobb, 1990).
III. Sarcomas and carcinomas can incorporate peripheral nerves in their growth (Braund, 1995).

Clinical Signs

I. Cranial nerve V has been most often affected with lymphosarcoma and leukemia.
II. Other clinical signs vary with the nerves affected.

Diagnosis

I. Evidence of myeloid neoplasia on lymph node aspirate, bone marrow cytology, peripheral blood smears
II. Biopsy of affected nerves

Treatment and Monitoring

I. Combination chemotherapy may result in temporary improvement in overall clinical signs in cases of myeloid neoplasia (see Chaps. 64 and 67).
II. Recovery from the peripheral neuropathy associated with myeloid neoplasia has not been reported.

TRAUMATIC NEUROLOGIC DISORDERS

Definition and Causes

I. Peripheral nerves may be injured by a number of means, including compression, laceration, or chemical irritation (injection injuries).
II. Complete functional transection of a nerve is referred to as neurotmesis.
III. Dysfunction of a nerve that occurs in the absence of structural damage is referred to as neuropraxia.
IV. Neuropraxia is often reversible over time, neurotmesis is not.
V. Clinically, neuropraxia is impossible to distinguish

from neurotmesis; therefore, it is best to wait at least 7 days after acute peripheral nerve injury before rendering a hopeless prognosis.

Pathophysiology

I. Most macromolecules or their precursors are synthesized in the cell body and transported to distal sections of peripheral nerves by axonal transport system.
II. Separation of the axonal cell process from its cell body results in a predictable pattern of axonal degeneration and secondary demyelination referred to as wallerian degeneration.
III. Peripheral nerves attempt to regenerate if the distal axon is severed.
IV. Regrowth occurs at a rate of approximately 1–2 mm/day, and regenerating axons have better success at reinnervating their appropriate target if guided by the original connective tissue framework of the axons.
V. Regenerating peripheral axons that fail to reach their target often appear histologically as maloriented whorls or axons, Schwann cells, and fibroblasts referred to as neuromas.
VI. Although the exact mechanism is speculative, neuromas are often a source of painful stimuli.

Clinical Signs

I. Signs vary with the peripheral nerve affected (Table 25–3).
II. Typically there is an acute loss of motor and sensory function supplied by affected nerves.
III. This is followed by rapid muscle atrophy.
IV. The specific cutaneous regions (autonomous zones) supplied by each peripheral nerve in the thoracic and pelvic limb have been identified, and mapping the distribution of cutaneous anesthesia can help identify the specific nerves involved (Bailey et al., 1982; Haghighi et al., 1991).

Diagnosis

I. History and clinical signs are most helpful.
II. EMG shows spontaneous activity in denervated muscles 5–7 days after peripheral nerve injury.
III. Nerve conduction velocity is absent with complete transection of the nerve.

Treatment and Monitoring

I. Techniques have been described for reanastomosing severed nerves.
II. Compression or entrapment should be surgically corrected.
III. Prognosis for recovery depends on the length regenerating axons must travel to successfully reinnervate their target and on the alignment of connective tissue supportive structures in the transected end.
 A. Peripheral axons regenerate at a rate of 1–2 mm/day, or approximately 1 in./mo. Proximal nerve injuries in large breeds of dogs would require many months for regeneration to occur, and mus-

Table 25–3. Traumatic Neurologic Disorders

Nerve	Spinal Cord Segment	Function	Cutaneous Distribution	Signs of Dysfunction
Nerves of the Brachial Plexus				
Suprascapular	C6-C7	Extension and lateral support of the shoulder	None	Minor gait abnormality
Axillary	C6-C8	Flexion of shoulder	Dorsolateral brachium—behind scapular spine	Minor gait abnormality; incomplete withdrawal reflex
Musculocutaneous	C6-C8	Flexion of elbow	Medial forelimb—medial humeral condyle	Minor gait abnormality; unable to raise paw to tabletop
Radial	C6-T2	Extension of elbow, carpus, and digits	Dorsolateral forelimb—dorsal surface of paw	Loss of weight bearing; unable to fix limb in extension
Median and ulnar	C8-T2	Flexion of carpus and digits	Palmar surface of paw, caudal forelimb	Minor gait abnormality; incomplete withdrawal reflex
Nerves of the Pelvic Plexus				
Obturator	L4-L6	Adduction of pelvic limb	None	Minor gait abnormality; limb may slide laterally on slick floor
Femoral	L3-L6	Extension of stifle	Saphenous branch supplies medial thigh and digit	Inability to extend stifle
Sciatic	L6-S3	Flexion and extension of hip	Caudal and lateral surfaces of limb	Cannot flex or extend digits and hock or flex stifle
Peroneal	L6-S3	Flexion of hock, extension of digits	Dorsal aspect of paw, hock, and distal limb	Cannot extend paw, therefore knuckles on dorsum, poor hock flexion
Tibial	L6-S3	Extension of hock, flexion of paw	Plantar surface of paw	Unable to fix hock in extension

cle contraction may preclude return to function even if reinnervation is successful.
B. Growth cones of regenerating axons must be directed to their target by the remaining connective tissue framework in the distal stump, or they grow in maloriented whorls referred to as neuromas.
C. Crushing or compression injuries generally have a better prognosis than transection injuries, even with surgical reanastomosis, because the connective tissue framework is better preserved.
IV. Physical therapy is imperative during the regenerative period to prevent joint and muscle contracture.
A. Passively flex and extend the limb 2–3 times daily.
B. Prevent injury to desensitized areas with protective bandaging.

Brachial Plexus Avulsions

Definition and Cause

I. These are caused by injury to all or portions of the C6-T2 nerve roots secondary to traction of the thoracic limb.
II. The most common site of injury of both dorsal and ventral roots is intradural, presumably because nerve roots lack a perineurium at this site (Griffiths, 1974).

III. Nerve roots from at least two spinal cord segments must be avulsed in order to appreciate clinical signs.

Pathophysiology

I. Injury to nerve roots causes wallerian degeneration in axons separated from their cell bodies.
II. In peripheral nerves, motor axons degenerate, whereas sensory axons are preserved.
III. In spinal cord segments, central projections from primary sensory neurons degenerate.

Clinical Signs

I. Clinical signs vary depending on which nerve roots are injured.
II. Flaccid paralysis of the affected limb, with loss of sensation distal to the elbow, is most common (Griffiths et al., 1974).
III. Injury to T1-T2 nerve roots results in loss of preganglionic sympathetic neurons to the face as well as loss of the lateral thoracic nerve.
A. Horner's syndrome
B. Loss of the ipsilateral panniculus
IV. Injury to C5, C6, and C7 nerve roots results in ipsilateral paralysis of the diaphragm.

Diagnosis

I. History and clinical signs are most helpful.
II. EMG 5–7 days after the injury is helpful in delineating the distribution of muscles denervated by the injury.
III. Motor nerve conduction is absent, whereas sensory fibers in peripheral nerve can still conduct an action potential because they are still in contact with their cell body in dorsal root ganglia. There is no conscious perception of pain, because sensory fibers are interrupted as they enter the spinal cord.

Treatment and Monitoring

I. There is no treatment for complete avulsions.
II. Salvage procedures for partial injuries have been described, including arthrodesis of the carpus, translocation of the biceps tendon, and sliding skin grafts to provide cutaneous sensation to small areas of the limb (Griffiths et al., 1974).
III. Cases with complete analgesia distal to the elbow respond poorly to these techniques because of repeated injury to areas devoid of sensation, and the limb must often be amputated.
IV. Partial or mild injuries may show evidence of improvement within 1–2 weeks.
V. Horner's syndrome associated with complete brachial plexus injury is usually irreversible.

Bibliography

Bailey CS: Long term survival after surgical excision of a schwannoma of the sixth cervical spinal nerve in a dog. J Am Vet Med Assoc 196:754, 1990

Bailey CS, Kitchell RL, Johnson RD: Spinal nerve root origins of the cutaneous nerves arising from the canine brachial plexus. Am J Vet Res 43:820, 1982

Barker CG, Herrtage ME, Shanahan F et al: Frucosidosis in English springer spaniels: results of a trial screening programme. J Small Anim Pract 29:623, 1988

Barsanti JA: Botulism. p. 515. In Greene CE (ed): Infectious Diseases of the Dog and Cat. WB Saunders, Philadelphia, 1990

Bartges JW, Klausner JS, Bostwick EF et al: Clinical remission following plasmapheresis and corticosteroid treatment in a dog with acquired myasthenia gravis. J Am Vet Med Assoc 196:1276, 1990

Bergman PJ, Bruyette DS, Coyne BE et al: Canine clinical peripheral neuropathy associated with pancreatic islet cell carcinoma. Prog Vet Neurol 5:57, 1994

Blakemore WF, Mitten RW, Palmer AC et al: Value of a nerve biopsy in diagnosis of globoid cell leucodystrophy in the dog. Vet Rec 93:70, 1974

Bradley RL, Withrow SJ, Snyder SP: Nerve sheath tumors in the dog. J Am Anim Hosp Assoc 18:915, 1982

Braund KG: Disorders of peripheral nerves. p. 701. In Ettinger SJ, Feldman EC (eds): Textbook of Veterinary Internal Medicine. 4th Ed. WB Saunders, Philadelphia, 1995

Braund KG, Steiss JE: Distal neuropathy in spontaneous diabetes mellitus in the dog. Acta Neuropathol (Berl) 57:263, 1982

Braund KG, McGuire JA, Amling KA et al: Peripheral neuropathy associated with malignant neoplasms in dogs. Vet Pathol 24:16, 1987

Braund KG, Mehta JR, Toivio-Kinnucan M et al: Congenital hypomyelinating polyneuropathy in two golden retriever littermates. Vet Pathol 26:202, 1989

Braund KG, Shores A, Cocrane S et al: Laryngeal paralysis-polyneuropathy complex in young dalmatians. Am J Vet Res 55:534, 1994

Brehm DM, Vite CH, Steinberg HS et al: A retrospective study of 51 cases of peripheral nerve sheath tumors in the dog. J Am Anim Hosp Assoc 31:349, 1995

Bright RM, Carbtree BJ, Knecht C: Brachial plexus neuropathy in the cat; a case report. J Am Anim Hosp Assoc 14:612, 1978

Carpenter JL, King NW, Abrams KL: Bilateral trigeminal nerve paralysis and Horner's syndrome associated with myelomonocytic neoplasia in a dog. J Am Vet Med Assoc 191:1594, 1987

Chrisman CL: Differentiation of tick paralysis and acute idiopathic polyradiculoneuritis in the dog using electromyography. J Am Anim Hosp Assoc 11:455, 1975

Chrisman CL: Dancing doberman disease: clinical findings and prognosis. Prog Vet Neurol 1:83, 1990

Coates JR, Paxton R, Cox NR et al: A case presentation and discussion of type IV glycogen storage disease in a Norwegian forest cat. Prog Vet Neurol 7:5, 1996

Cooper BJ, de Lahunta A, Cummings JF et al: Canine inherited hypertrophic neuropathy: clinical and electro-diagnostic studies. Am J Vet Res 45:1172, 1984a

Cooper BJ, Duncan I, Cummings JF et al: Defective Schwann cell function in canine inherited hypertrophic neuropathy. Acta Neuropathol (Berl) 63:51, 1984b

Cork LC, Griffin JW, Choy C et al: Pathology of motor neurons in accelerated hereditary canine spinal muscular atrophy. Lab Invest 46:89, 1982

Cork LC, Griffin JW, Munnell JF et al: Hereditary canine spinal muscular atrophy. Neuropathol Exp Neurol 37:209, 1979

Cuddon PA: Electrophysiological and immunological evaluation in coonhound paralysis. Proc Am Coll Vet Intern Med 8:1009, 1990

Cuddon PA, Higgins RJ, Duncan ID et al: Polyneuropathy in feline Niemann-Pick disease. Brain 112:1429, 1989

Cummings JF, de Lahunta A: Chronic relapsing polyradiculoneuritis in a dog. A clinical, light- and electron-microscopic study. Acta Neuropathol (Berl) 28:191, 1974

Cummings JF, Lorenz MD, de Lahunta A et al: Canine brachial plexus neuritis: a syndrome resembling serum neuritis in man. Cornell Vet 63:589, 1973

Cummings JF, Cooper BJ, de Lahunta A, Van Winkle TJ: Canine inherited hypertropic neuropathy. Acta Neuropathol (Berl) 53:137, 1981a

Cummings JF, de Lahunta A, Winn SS: Acral mutilation and nociceptive loss in English pointer dogs. A canine sensory neuropathy. Acta Neuropathol (Berl) 53:119, 1981b

Cummings JF, de Lahunta A, Holmes DF et al: Coonhound paralysis. Further clinical studies and electron microscopic observations. Acta Neuropathol (Berl) 56:167, 1982

Cummings JF, de Lahunta A, Braund KG et al: Animal model of human disease. Hereditary sensory neuropathy. Nociceptive loss and acral mutilation in pointer dogs: canine hereditary sensory neuropathy. Am J Pathol 112:136, 1983

Cummings JF, de Lahunta A, Moore JJ: Multisystemic chromatolytic neuronal degeneration in a Cairn terrier pup. Cornell Vet 78:301, 1988

Cummings JF, Georges C, de Lahunta A et al: Focal spinal muscular atrophy in two German shepherd pups. Acta Neuropathol 79:113, 1989

Cummings JF, de Lahunta A, Gasteiger EL: Multisystemic chromatolytic neuronal degeneration in Cairn terriers: a case with generalized cataplectic episodes. J Vet Intern Med 5:91, 1991

Dewey CW, Shelton GD, Bailey CS et al: Neuromuscular dysfunction in five dogs with acquired myasthenia gravis and presumptive hypothyroidism. Prog Vet Neurol 6:117, 1995

Dropcho EJ: The remote effects of cancer on the nervous system. Neurol Clin 7:579, 1988

Dubey JP, Greene CE, Lappin MR: Toxoplasmosis and neosporosis. p. 818. In Greene CE (ed): Infectious Diseases of the Dog and Cat. WB Saunders, Philadelphia, 1990

Duncan ID, Griffiths IR: Canine giant axonal neuropathy; some aspects of its clinical, pathological and comparative features. J Small Anim Pract 22:491, 1981

Duncan ID, Griffiths IR: A sensory neuropathy affecting long-haired Dachshund dogs. J Small Anim Pract 23:381, 1982

Duncan ID, Griffiths IR: Peripheral neuropathies of domestic animals. p. 707. In Dyck PJ, Thomas PK, Lambert EH, Bunge R (eds): Peripheral Neuropathy. 2nd Ed. WB Saunders, Philadelphia, 1984

Duncan ID, Griffiths IR, Munz M: The pathology of a sensory neuropathy affecting long haired Dachshund dogs. Acta Neuropathol (Berl) 58:141, 1982

Dyer KR, Duncan ID, Hammang JP et al: Peripheral neuropathy in two dogs: correlation between clinical, electrophysiological and pathological findings. J Small Anim Pract 27:133, 1986

Fox PR: Feline thromboembolism associated with cardiomyopathy. Proc Am Coll Vet Intern Med 5:714, 1987

Fyfe JC, Giger U, Van Winkle T et al: Familial glycogen storage disease type IV in Norwegian forest cats. Proc Am Coll Vet Intern Med 8:1129, 1990

Gaber CE, Amis TC, LeCouteur RA: Laryngeal paralysis in dogs: a review of 23 cases. J Am Vet Med Assoc 186:377, 1985

Griffiths IR: Avulsion of the brachial plexus - 1. Neuropathology of the spinal cord and peripheral nerves. J Small Anim Pract 15:165, 1974

Griffiths IR: Progressive axonopathy: an inherited neuropathy of Boxer dogs. 1. Further studies of the clinical and electrophysiological features. J Small Anim Pract 26:381, 1985

Griffiths IR, Duncan ID: Ischaemic neuromyopathy in cats. Vet Rec 104:518, 1979a

Griffiths IR, Duncan I: Distal denervating disease: a degenerative neuropathy of the distal motor axon in dogs. J Small Anim Pract 20:579, 1979b

Griffiths IR, Duncan ID, Lawson DD: Avulsion of the brachial plexus - 2. Clinical aspects. J Small Anim Pract 15:177, 1974

Griffiths IR, Duncan ID, Barker J: A progressive axonopathy of Boxer dogs affecting the central and peripheral nervous system. J Small Anim Pract 21:29, 1980a

Griffiths IR, Duncan ID, McCulloch MC et al: Further studies of the central nervous system in canine giant axonal neuropathy. Neuropathol Appl Neurobiol 6:421, 1980b

Haghighi SS, Kitchell RL, Johnson RD et al: Electrophysiologic studies of the cutaneous innervation of the pelvic limb of male dogs. Am J Vet Res 52:352, 1991

Hobbs SL, Cobb MA: A cranial neuropathy associated with multicentric lymphosarcoma in a dog. Vet Rec 127:525, 1990

Inada S, Sakamoto H, Haruta K et al: A clinical study on hereditary progressive neurogenic muscular atrophy in Pointer dogs. Jpn J Vet Sci 40:539, 1978

Indrieri RJ, Creighton SR, Lambert EH et al: Myasthenia gravis in two cats. J Am Vet Med Assoc 182:57, 1983

Indrieri RJ, Whalen LR, Cardinet GH et al: Neuromuscular abnormalities associated with hypopthyroidism and lymphocytic thyroiditis in three dogs. J Am Vet Med Assoc 190:544, 1987

Jaggy A, Oliver JE, Fergurson DC et al: Neurological manifestations of hypothyroidism: A retrospective study of 29 dogs. Vet Intern Med 8:328, 1994

Jones BR: Inherited hyperchylomicronaemia in the cat. J Small Anim Pract 34:493, 1993

Joseph RJ, Carrillo JM, Lennon VA: Myasthenia gravis in the cat. J Vet Intern Med 2:75, 1988

Kingma FJ, Catcott EJ: A paralytic syndrome in coonhounds. North Am Vet 35:115, 1954

Luttgen PJ: Polyradiculoneuritis in a cat. Proc Am Coll Vet Intern Med 5:842, 1987

Luttgen PJ, LeCouteur RA: Disorders of peripheral nerves. p. 303. In Morgan RV (ed): Handbook of Small Animal Practice. 2nd Ed. Churchill Livingstone, New York, 1992

Malik R, Farrow BRH: Tick paralysis in North America and Australia. Vet Clin North Am [Small Anim Pract] 21:157, 1991

Malik R, France MP, Churcher R et al: Prednisolone responsive neuropathy in a cat. J Small Anim Pract 32:529, 1991

Matz ME, Shell LG, Braund K: Peripheral hypomyelinization in two golden retriever littermates. J Am Vet Med Assoc 197:228, 1990

McCarthy RJ, Feeney DA, Lipowits AJ: Preoperative diagnosis of tumors of the brachial plexus by use of computed tomography in three dogs. Am Vet Med Assoc 202:291, 1993

McKerrell RE, Blakemore WF, Heath MF et al: Primary hyperoxaluria (L-glyceric aciduria) in the cat: a newly recognised inherited disease. Vet Rec 125:31, 1989

Miller LM, Lennon VA, Lambert EH et al: Congenital myasthenia gravis in 13 smooth fox terriers. J Am Vet Med Assoc 182:694, 1983

Moe L: Hereditary polyneuropathy of Alaskan malamutes. p. 1038. In Kirk RW, Bonagura JD (eds): Current Veterinary Therapy XI: Small Animal Practice. WB Saunders, Philadelphia, 1992

Moreau PM, Vallat JM, Hugon J et al: Peripheral and central distal axonopathy of suspected inherited origin in Birman cats. Acta Neuropathol 82:143, 1991

O'Brien JA, Hendriks J: Inherited laryngeal paralysis: analysis in the Husky cross. Vet Q 8:301, 1986

Palmer AC, Blakemore WF: A progressive neuronopathy in the young Cairn terrier. J Small Anim Pract 30:101, 1989

Pflugfelder CM, Cardinet GH III, Lutz H et al: Acquired canine myasthenia gravis: immunocytochemical localization of immune complexes at neuromuscular junctions. Muscle Nerve 4:289, 1981

Pollard JD: Neuropathy in diseases of the thyroid and pituitary glands. p. 1266. In Dyck PJ, Thomas PK, Griffin JW et al (eds): Peripheral Neuropathy. 3rd Ed. WB Saunders, Philadelphia, 1993

Sack GH, Cork LC, Morris JM et al: Autosomal dominant inheritance of hereditary canine spinal muscular atrophy. Ann Neurol 15:369, 1984

Sandefelt E, Cummings JF, de Lahunta A et al: Hereditary neuronal abiotrophy in the Swedish lapland dog. Cornell Vet 63 (Suppl 3):7, 1973

Schrauwen E: Clinical peripheral neuropathy associated with canine insulinoma. Vet Rec 128:211, 1991

Scott-Moncrieff JC, Cook JR, Lantz GC: Acquired myasthenia gravis in a cat with thymoma. J Am Vet Med Assoc 196:1291, 1990

Shell LG, Jortner BS, Leib MS: Spinal muscular atrophy in two Rottweiler littermates. J Am Vet Med Assoc 190:878, 1987

Shelton GD: Myasthenia gravis—1000 cases later. Proc Am Coll Vet Intern Med 14:658, 1996

Shelton GD, Willard MD, Cardinet GH III et al: Acquired myasthenia gravis: selective involvement of esophageal, pharyngeal, and facial muscles. J Vet Intern Med 4:281, 1990

Shores A, Braund KG, McDonald RK: Chronic relapsing polyneuropathy in a cat. J Am Anim Hosp Assoc 23:569, 1987

Sisson DD, Thomas WP: Myocardial diseases. p. 995. In Ettinger SJ, Feldman EC (eds): Textbook of Veterinary Internal Medicine. 4th Ed. WB Saunders, Philadelphia, 1995

Steiss JE, Orsher AN, Bowen JM: Electrodiagnostic analysis of peripheral neuropathy in dogs with diabetes mellitus. Am J Vet Res 42:2061, 1981

Steiss JE, Pook HA, Clark EG et al: Sensory neuronopathy in a dog. J Am Vet Med Assoc 190:205, 1987

Taylor RM, Farrow BRH, Healy PJ: Canine fucosidosis: clinical findings. J Small Anim Pract 28:291, 1987

Uchida K, Nakayama H, Sasaki N et al: Malignant schwannoma in the spinal root of a dog. J Vet Med Sci 54:809, 1992

Venker-van Haagen AJ, Hartman W, Goldegebuure SA: Spontaneous laryngeal paralysis in young Bouviers. J Am Anim Hosp Assoc 14:714, 1978

Venker-van Haagen AJ, Bouw J, Hartman W: Hereditary transmission of laryngeal paralysis in Bouviers. J Am Anim Hosp Assoc 17:75, 1981

Vicini DS, Wheaton LG, Zachary JF et al: Peripheral nerve biopsy for diagnosis of globoid cell leukodystrophy in a dog. J Am Vet Med Assoc 192:1087, 1988

Wouda W, Vandevelde M, Oettli P et al: Sensory neuronopathy in dogs: a study of four cases. J Comp Path 183:437, 1983

Zachary JF, O'Brien DP, Ingles BW et al: Multicentric nerve sheath fibrosarcomas of multiple cranial nerve roots in two dogs. J Am Vet Med Assoc 188:723, 1986

Digestive System

26

Introduction

Albert E. Jergens

DIAGNOSTIC APPROACH

I. Disorders of the digestive system in dogs and cats are commonly encountered by the veterinary practitioner.
II. Salient clinical signs associated with gastrointestinal disorders include dysphagia, regurgitation, vomiting, and diarrhea.
III. A problem-oriented approach to the diagnosis and treatment of gastrointestinal diseases is recommended.
  A. Gather information.
    1. Obtain a thorough history.
    2. Perform a physical examination.
  B. Identify and list all problems.
  C. Establish rule-outs for each problem.
  D. Design a plan to diagnose each problem.
    1. Complete blood count (CBC), biochemical profile, fecal flotation, and urinalysis
    2. Radiographic imaging
    3. Endoscopic examination with biopsy
    4. Laparotomy with biopsy
    5. Additional diagnostic procedures as needed (Table 26–1)
  E. Initiate therapy and reassess each problem.
IV. Initial diagnostic testing is directed at lesion localization within the digestive system.

LESION LOCALIZATION

Oropharynx

I. Oropharyngeal disorders cause derangements in prehension, mastication, and bolus formation.
II. Clinical signs are variable but may include halitosis, ptyalism, gagging, dysphagia, and pawing at the mouth or face.
III. Immediate regurgitation of food is sometimes seen.

Esophagus

I. The esophagus functions to transport ingesta from the pharynx to the stomach.
II. Upper and lower esophageal sphincters prevent laryngotracheal aspiration of esophageal contents and gastroesophageal reflux of gastric contents, respectively.
III. Esophageal disorders usually result in regurgitation and difficulty in swallowing food and/or water (dysphagia).
IV. Respiratory signs (nasal discharge, moist cough, dyspnea) are common and are attributable to laryngotracheal aspiration.
V. Clearly differentiate regurgitation from vomiting to prevent erroneous diagnostic work-up and potential misdiagnosis.

Stomach

I. The stomach performs a variety of major functions that promote nutrient digestion and absorption.
  A. The proximal stomach acts as a storage reservoir for food and fluids.
  B. The distal stomach is involved with vigorous motor activity, which grinds ingesta (trituration) and regulates its passage into the small intestine.
  C. It secretes hydrochloric acid and pepsinogen, which play important roles in the initial digestion of proteins.
  D. The gastric mucosa secretes mucus, which lubricates ingesta and facilitates its movement into the intestine. Mucus also protects the mucosal surface from intrinsic chemical injury.
II. Vomiting is usually present if the lesion is in the stomach.
  A. Vomiting is a centrally mediated reflex involving neural pathways that synapse in the medulla at the vomiting center.
  B. It may be caused by the following.
    1. Mucosal inflammation, as seen with gastritis
    2. Interference with normal gastric emptying, as

Table 26–1. Dignostic Procedures for the Detection of Gastrointestinal Disease

Procedure	Utility
Dietary trial	Food intolerance, IBD
Complete blood count	Pneumonia, hypoadrenocorticism, anemia, parasites, hydration, PLE, IBD (eosinophilia)
Biochemistries	Renal/liver disease, hypoadrenocorticism, PLE, electrolytes
Urinalysis	Renal/liver disease, hydration status
Fecal flotation	Parasitic ova
Fecal smear	Giardiasis, other protozoa
Fecal cytology	Bacterial colitis, clostridial spores
Fecal culture	Bacterial enterocolitis
Fecal enterotoxin	Clostridial enteritis
Trypsin-like immunoreactivity assay	Exocrine pancreatic insufficiency, feline acute pancreatitis
Duodenal aspirate	Giardiasis, SIBO
Serum folate/cobalamin	SIBO (?), mucosal disease
Survey radiographs	Foreign body, masses, organomegaly
Upper GI series	Foreign body, masses, mucosal ulceration
Barium-impregnated plastic spheres (BIPs)	Gastric emptying, intestinal transit
Ultrasonography	Foreign body, masses, bowel wall thickening, pancreatitis, intussusception
Serology	FeLV, FIV, fungal agents
Serum thyroxine	Feline hyperthyroidism
Bile acids	Hepatobiliary function
ACTH stimulation test	Hypoadrenocorticism
Endoscopy	Foreign body, mucosal disease
Laparotomy	Mucosal/parenchymal biopsy

IBD = inflammatory bowel disease; PLE = protein-losing enteropathy; SIBO = small intestinal bacterial overgrowth; FeLV = feline leukemia virus; FIV = feline immunodeficiency virus; ACTH = adrenocorticotropic hormone.

Adapted from Strombeck DR, Guilford WG: Approach to clinical problems in gastroenterology. p. 56. In Strombeck DR, Guilford WG (eds): Small Animal Gastroenterology. 2nd Ed. Stonegate Publishing, Davis, 1990.

seen with motility disturbances or pyloric outflow obstruction
C. The color and consistency of the vomitus may provide important diagnostic clues.
   1. Bile-stained vomitus implies intestinal reflux of bile.
   2. Blood in the vomitus (hematemesis) is seen with upper gastrointestinal hemorrhage. Vomited blood may appear as fresh clots or may have a ''coffee grounds'' appearance owing to digestion.
   3. Vomiting >10 hours after eating is suggestive of gastric retention.
III. Other signs of gastric disease include anorexia, weight loss, abdominal discomfort/distention, and melena.
IV. Potential consequences of severe vomiting include dehydration with prerenal azotemia, electrolyte deficiencies, and acid–base imbalances.

Intestines

I. The intestinal tract acts primarily to digest and absorb nutrients and to move luminal contents aborally.
II. Major functions of the small intestine are as follows.
   A. Secretion for nutrient digestion
   B. Secretion and absorption of fluid and electrolytes
   C. Absorption of vitamins and minerals
   D. Motility
      1. Segmental (mixing) contractions mix ingesta and slow its passage through the intestine, which facilitates digestion and absorption.
      2. Peristaltic (propulsive) contractions propel ingesta aborally.
   E. Maintenance of local (intestinal) immunity via mucosal secretion of immunoglobulin A (IgA)
III. Major functions of the large intestine are as follows.
   A. Absorption of water and electrolytes from the proximal colon
   B. Reservoir for fecal storage
   C. Bacterial degradation of nutrients
   D. Motility
      1. The proximal colon exhibits retrograde peristalsis, which thoroughly mixes ingesta.
      2. The middle colon shows coordinated peristalsis aborally.
      3. The distal colon shows strong peristaltic contractions that empty the colon.
IV. Clinical signs of intestinal disease are variable.
   A. Diarrhea is defined as increased fecal volume, fluidity, or frequency of defecation.
   B. There are several mechanisms by which diarrhea may arise.
      1. Osmotic diarrhea caused by nutrient maldigestion or malabsorption
      2. Hypersecretion of fluid and electrolytes caused by bacterial toxins and other secretagogues

3. Increased permeability caused by structural defects in the gut wall
4. Alterations in intestinal transit (uncommon)

C. Other signs associated with intestinal disease include alterations in appetite, weight loss, vomiting, and constipation.

D. Attempt to localize diarrhea to either the small or the large bowel, because that will determine the direction of subsequent diagnostic evaluations.

CONCLUSION

I. Acute causes of gastroenteritis are often self-limited and respond favorably to symptomatic therapy.

II. Chronic causes of gastrointestinal dysfunction usually require a definitive diagnosis so that specific therapy can be instituted.

III. Current diagnostic techniques and the latest therapeutic principles are found in the subsequent chapters of this section.

27

Diseases of the Oral Cavity and Pharynx

Debra L. Zoran
Mark E. Hitt
Linda J. DeBowes

CONGENITAL/ DEVELOPMENTAL DISORDERS

Debra L. Zoran

See Table 27–1.

INFECTIOUS/INFLAMMATORY DISORDERS

Debra L. Zoran

Stomatitis/Gingivitis/Glossitis

Definition

I. These include inflammatory processes of the oral mucosa, tongue, and gingiva that result in ulceration, necrosis, and secondary infection.
   A. Stomatitis: inflammation of the mucous membranes of the mouth
   B. Glossitis: inflammatory lesions of the tongue
   C. Gingivitis: inflammation of the gingiva
   D. Faucitis: inflammatory lesions of the glossopalatine folds or angles of the mouth
   E. Cheilitis: inflammatory lesions of the lips
   F. Periodontitis: lesions of the periodontal membrane, gingiva, and alveolar bone
II. Many oral inflammatory diseases are secondary to a variety of systemic diseases or disorders and may involve multiple oral soft tissue structures.
III. These inflammatory conditions are a frequent problem in cats.

Causes

I. Dental plaque/calculus (see Small Animal Dental Diseases later)

II. Immune-mediated diseases
   A. Pemphigus diseases: pemphigus foliaceus, pemphigus erythematosus, and pemphigus vulgaris
   B. Systemic lupus erythematosus
   C. Drug eruptions/toxic epidermal necrolysis
   D. Food hypersensitivity
   E. Discoid lupus erythematosus, bullous pemphigoid
   F. Allergic contact dermatitis (plastic)
   G. Idiopathic vasculitis
   H. Ulcerative gingivitis-stomatitis of Maltese terriers
III. Idiopathic disorders
   A. Feline gingivitis-stomatitis-pharyngitis complex
   B. Feline eosinophilic granuloma complex
   C. Eosinophilic granuloma of Siberian huskies
   D. Ulcerative eosinophilic stomatitis of Cavalier King Charles spaniels
IV. Immunodeficiency
   A. Neutrophil function defects
   B. Neutropenia
   C. Prolonged immunosuppressive drug therapy
V. Infectious diseases
   A. Bacteria
      1. Major anaerobic species: *Bacteroides* spp., *Fusobacterium*, *Propionibacterium*, *Peptostreptococcus*, and *Clostridium*.
      2. Gram-positive aerobes: *Streptococcus*, *Staphylococcus* spp., *Corynebacterium*, and *Actinomyces*.
      3. Gram-negative aerobes: *Escherichia coli*, *Pseudomonas*, *Proteus*, and *Pasteurella* spp.
      4. Spirochetes
         a) Acute necrotizing ulcerative gingivitis (ANUG, Vincent's stomatitis, trench mouth)
         b) Leptospirosis: *Leptospira canicola*, *Leptospira icterohaemorrhagiae*

Table 27–1. Congenital/Developmental Disorders

Defect	Causes	Clinical Characteristics	Diagnosis	Treatment	Comments
Primary cleft palate (lip)	May be secondary to intrauterine trauma or insult. Affected pups are born to affected parents.	Often associated with secondary cleft palate in the dog. May occur unilaterally or bilaterally. No signs other than the physical defect.	Physical examination	Surgical lip reconstruction	Animals should not be bred. Higher incidence in brachycephalic breeds, beagles, cockers, and dachshunds.
Secondary cleft palate (hard and soft palate)	Inherited or secondary to developmental insult. Occurs in both dogs and cats.	Inability to nurse, poor growth, milk drainage from nares, coughing, gagging, and sneezing during nursing. Nasal discharge due to rhinitis may occur with time. Aspiration pneumonia may be fatal.	Physical examination of mouth reveals abnormal division of hard/soft palate.	Surgical reconstruction of palate when animal is 2–4 months of age; nutritional and medical supportive care until then.	Higher incidences in brachycephalic breeds, Shetland sheepdogs, schnauzers, Labrador retrievers, and German shepherd dogs.
Malocclusion: Prognathism	Genetic factors: normal in brachycephalic dogs and Persian cats. Abnormal dentition (position of teeth or retained teeth). Trauma	Clinical appearance: long mandible with short maxilla. May predispose to periodontal and gingival disease.	Physical examination	Early removal of retained supernumerary, or malpositioned deciduous teeth. Orthodontic or orthopedic procedures can be used to correct the anatomy.	Maltese terriers are predisposed to retained teeth.
Malocclusion: Brachynathism	Genetic factors: long-haired dachshunds, Shar pei. Abnormal in any breed, but no known cause.	Physical finding of shortened mandible with a long maxilla. If severe, may prevent normal jaw function and eating.	Physical examination	No specific treatment is available.	Note: Undershot jaw is the breed standard for the Brussels griffon.
Microcheilia	Unknown cause	Physical finding of a reduced oral fissure.	Physical examination	None	Reported in miniature schnauzers.
Lip-fold dermatitis	Congenital trait resulting in abnormal conformation of the lip fold in spaniel breeds.	Chronic moist, fetid dermatitis of lip folds	Physical examination	Resection of skin folds	Affected animals should not be bred. Breed with a higher incidence: Brittany spaniel.
Elongated soft palate	Brachycephalic breeds are predisposed.	Associated with exercise and heat intolerance, and abnormal oropharyngeal function	Physical examination, radiography	Surgical removal of offending tissue	Breeds with a higher incidence: Affenpinscher, chow chow, English and French bulldogs, Pekingese, and pugs.
Craniomandibular osteopathy	Developmental condition	Proliferation of bones of skull and mandible, painful swelling of mandible, reduced jaw motion results in reluctance to eat, and depression.	Physical examination and radiographic changes (exostosis of mandible, tympanic bulla and, calvarium).	Corticosteroids and nonsteroidal anti-inflammatory drugs may relieve signs but are not curative. Surgery is of limited success in most cases.	Breeds that may be affected: West Highland white, Scottish and Cairn terriers, Labradors, Great Danes, and Dobermans.

Data from Clark, RW, 1992; Norden DM, 1992; Clark RW, 1994.

B. Viral diseases
  1. Feline calicivirus (most common)
  2. Feline immunodeficiency virus (FIV)
  3. Feline herpesvirus (FHV-1)
  4. Feline leukemia virus (FeLV)
  5. Canine adenovirus (CAV-2)
  6. Canine distemper virus/feline panleukopenia virus
  7. Feline syncytium-forming virus
  8. Papovavirus
  9. Feline infectious peritonitis (FIP) virus (rare)
C. Fungal diseases
  1. Blastomycosis (*Blastomyces dermatitidis*)
  2. Candidiasis (*Candida albicans*)
  3. Cryptococcosis (*Cryptococcus neoformans*)
  4. Others: histoplasmosis, sporotrichosis, and coccidioidomycosis
VI. Metabolic diseases
  A. Diabetes mellitus
  B. Hypoparathyroidism
  C. Uremia (most common cause)
  D. Hypothyroidism
VII. Neoplasia (see later)
VIII. Nutritional disorders
  A. Hypervitaminosis A: oral lesions in conjunction with bony exostosis

B. Niacin deficiency (pellagra)
C. Protein-calorie malnutrition
D. Riboflavin deficiency (Roe, 1991)
E. Calcium imbalances: periodontal disease
IX. Physiochemical/traumatic causes
   A. Caustic or irritant chemicals
      1. Acids/alkalis
      2. Phenols
      3. Petroleum products
      4. Benzalkonium chloride
   B. Anti-neoplastic therapies
      1. Chemotherapeutic drugs
      2. Radiation treatment
   C. Dilantin (diphenylhydantoin)
   D. Foreign bodies
      1. Plant material
      2. Fiberglass
      3. Bone fragments
      4. Quills, claws
      5. Rubber bands, string, or Christmas tree tinsel
   E. Heavy metals: thallium, mercury
   F. Insect bites/stings: bees, spiders, scorpions, ants, etc.
   G. Irritant plants: dieffenbachia, poinsettia, philodendron
   H. Electric cord burns
   I. Persistent overgrooming (cats)
   J. Trauma

Pathophysiology

I. A variety of factors influence the pathogenesis of inflammatory oral disease, including the multitude of microorganisms in the mouth and the fact that the oral cavity is subject to trauma, abrasion, and frequent changes in hydration and temperature.
II. The primary defenses against oral disease are the epithelial surface, saliva, and the local (inflammatory) and systemic immune responses (humoral and cell-mediated immunity).
III. Depression of oral defense mechanisms, both locally and systemically, allows secondary infections by organisms that are not normally pathogenic (Tenorio et al., 1991).
   A. Acquired immunodeficiency diseases, such as FIV, and chronic corticosteroid use are important causes.
   B. Long-term antibiotic treatment can alter the normal microflora, creating resistant species and allowing the overgrowth of bacteria, *Candida* spp., or spirochetes.
   C. Chronic systemic diseases alter the replication, exfoliation, and maturation of epithelial cells, predisposing these tissues to disease.
IV. Uremia causes oral ulceration by several mechanisms.
   A. Oral microbes degrade urea to ammonia, and the high systemic concentration of urea leads to production of cytotoxic levels of ammonia.
   B. Hyperammonemia results in decreased rates of tissue repair, reduced platelet function (increased bleeding and ulcerations), and reduced immune function.

V. Animals with diabetes often develop oral infections from immune compromise, which is exacerbated by the presence of xerostomia or dehydration.
VI. Immune-mediated diseases cause oral lesions by production of autoantibodies to the normal epithelial components, resulting in destruction of normal mucosa with concurrent ulcers, erosions, blisters, and inflammation.

Clinical Signs

I. A careful history of the signalment, onset, and duration of clinical signs is important. It is also important to distinguish whether the disease process is localized to the oral cavity or is a manifestation of systemic disease.
II. The most common presenting complaints that may be associated with stomatitis, gingivitis, and/or glossitis include the following.
   A. Anorexia or reduced appetite
   B. Abnormal or exaggerated chewing motions, "chattering" teeth
   C. Halitosis
   D. Pytalism (drooling)
   E. Bleeding from the mouth or gums
   F. Dysphagia
   G. Vomiting, retching, gagging, or regurgitation
   H. Face rubbing or head shaking
   I. Nasal discharge, sneezing
   J. Fever, depression, or regional lymphadenopathy

Diagnosis

I. General anesthesia may be required to achieve a complete examination if the animal is fractious or in pain.
   A. Feline gingivitis-stomatitis-pharyngitis complex
      1. Generalized hyperemia of mucous membranes and lips
      2. Severe gingival recession and resorptive lesions of teeth and surrounding bone (teeth may be loose)
      3. Severe oral ulceration
      4. Fever, depression, and weight loss from inappetence
      5. Pain when opening the mouth, especially with faucitis
   B. Feline eosinophilic granuloma complex (see later)
   C. Eosinophilic granuloma of Siberian huskies
      1. Proliferative eosinophilic lesions of the tongue occurring primarily in young dogs
      2. Other signs: difficult prehension or swallowing, drooling, and oral pain
   D. Acute necrotizing ulcerative gingivitis (ANUG) (Pedersen, 1992)
      1. Acute onset of severe halitosis, gingivitis, and oral ulceration of tongue, buccal mucosa, and palate
      2. Lesions possibly covered with a gray pseudo-membrane of necrotic tissue and purulent exudate

3. Localized or systemic immunodeficiency probably necessary for development
   E. Leptospirosis
   1. *L. canicola*: severe generalized hyperemia of mucous membranes, oral ulceration and hemorrhage, gingival petechiae, glossitis, and lingual necrosis
   2. *L. icterohaemorrhagiae*: severe generalized hyperemia of mucous membranes, oral hemorrhage, and gingival petechiae
   F. FHV-1
   1. Acute vesicular to ulcerative glossitis and stomatitis
   2. Rhinitis, conjunctivitis or keratoconjunctivitis, and pharyngitis
   3. Persistent infections with recrudescence
   G. Calicivirus (Harbour et al., 1991; Waters et al., 1993)
   1. Oral vesiculation and ulceration of the tongue, palate, and fauces are the most common clinical manifestations.
   2. Transient fever, limping, and focal interstitial pneumonia occur in some infected cats (Pedersen, 1992).
   H. FeLV: chronic proliferative gingivitis, stomatitis, and oral ulceration
   I. FIV
   1. Chronic gingivitis, stomatitis, and periodontitis
   2. Acute, rapidly progressive gingival necrosis
   3. More severe and persistent with concurrent calicivirus
   J. Candidiasis
   1. Creamy, plaque-like lesions on the tongue, oral mucosa, lips, and mucocutaneous junctions
   2. Inflammation and ulceration of mucosa beneath lesions
   K. Blastomycosis: ulcerative, granulomatous plaques on tongue, gingiva, and palate
   L. Cryptococcosis: fleshy, proliferative lesions on the palate, gingiva, lips, or tongue
   M. Phycogranulomatosis
   1. It is a chronic, localized to diffuse glossitis surrounding embedded plant material.
   2. In cats, the lingual frenulum is a common location for awns or burrs to lodge.
   N. Diphenylhydantoin (Dilantin): gingival hyperplasia in both cats and dogs
II. Hematology is usually nonspecific but an important part of the database.
   A. Anemia: chronic oral hemorrhage, anemia of chronic disease, FIV/FeLV
   B. Leukocytosis: chronic inflammation or infection
   C. Eosinophilia: eosinophilic granuloma complex
III. Other laboratory tests to differentiate cause
   A. Biochemical profile
   B. Thyroid function tests (see Chap. 41)
   C. Virologic testing for FIV/FeLV, etc.
   D. Immunologic testing (see Chap. 89)
   E. Cytology
   1. Bacterial agents, especially spirochetes, can be identified.

2. Fungal elements from *Blastomyces* or *Histoplasma* spp. may be found.
3. Neoplasia may be detected.
   F. Culture
   1. Routine bacterial culture of oral lesions is not recommended, because most cultures reveal normal microbial flora.
   2. If routine antimicrobial therapy is ineffective, culture and sensitivity testing can be used to select antibiotics that are not resistant.
IV. Biopsy
   A. Histopathology is necessary for differentiation.
   B. Other specialized analysis of histopathologic specimens can be carried out to diagnose immune-mediated disorders.

Differential Diagnosis

I. Oral neoplasia
II. Other inflammatory oral or dental diseases

Treatment

I. Primary objective: identify, remove or treat the underlying cause
II. Antibiotic therapy
   A. Rarely are bacteria alone the primary cause of oral disease.
   B. Because secondary bacterial overgrowth is a common problem, symptomatic therapy is indicated.
   1. Amoxicillin 22 mg/kg PO, SQ, IM TID
   2. Amoxicillin/clavulanic acid
      a) Dogs: 12.5–25 mg/kg PO, BID
      b) Cats: 62.5 mg PO BID
   3. Clindamycin 10 mg/kg PO BID
   4. Cephalexin 22 mg/kg PO, IM, SQ TID
   5. Tetracycline 22 mg/kg PO, IM BID-TID
   6. Doxycycline 2.5–5 mg/kg PO BID
   7. Metronidazole 15 mg/kg PO BID-TID, SID to maintain remission
III. Antifungal therapy
   A. Ketoconazole 10–15 mg/kg PO BID
   B. Itraconazole 5–10 mg/kg PO SID
   C. Fluconazole 2.5–10 mg/kg PO BID
IV. Antiviral therapy
   It has not been demonstrated as clinically beneficial in dogs or cats.
V. Immunosuppressive or anti-inflammatory therapy: see Lymphoplasmacytic Stomatitis later
VI. Nutritional support
   A. Canned diets or soft, blenderized foods may be tolerated best.
   B. Vitamin supplementation with vitamins A and C may be useful to promote epithelial regeneration and healing.
   C. Taurine and potassium supplementation may be needed in cats that are not eating a complete diet.
   D. Nutritional support in the form of percutaneous endoscopic gastrostomy (PEG) tube placement or nasogastric tube feeding may be necessary in cats or dogs with prolonged anorexia.

VII. Oral hygiene
    A. It is maintained through frequent dental scaling (every 3–6 months) and oral cleansing, especially in cats with recurrent or poorly controlled disease.
    B. Oral cleansing to remove necrotic tissue and debris enhances recovery.
    C. Preparations that may be used in oral washes include the following.
        1. Chlorhexidine (0.2%)
        2. Hydrogen peroxide (1%)
        3. Povidone-iodine (1:10)

Patient Monitoring

I. Adequate nutrition and hydration are essential for normal healing and successful management of oral disease.
II. Prolonged antibiotic therapy or frequent changing of antibiotics must be avoided to prevent development of candidiasis and/or resistant bacterial species.
III. Maintenance of oral hygiene through dental care and oral washes is very important.

Tonsillitis

Definition

I. It is inflammation of the tonsils and surrounding pharyngeal structures, with secondary lymphoid hyperplasia.
II. Primary tonsillitis is rare in dogs and is usually seen in young, small-breed dogs.
III. Secondary tonsillitis follows some chronic insult, such as vomiting, coughing, or gagging.

Causes

I. Primary tonsillitis is believed to be a manifestation of the normal development of pharyngeal defense mechanisms as the tonsil is exposed to infectious agents.
II. Secondary tonsillitis can be caused by a variety of insults.
    A. Chronic vomiting or regurgitation
    B. Chronic coughing, gagging, or retching
    C. Chronic nasopharyngeal disease or nasal discharge
    D. Foreign body penetration

Pathophysiology

I. Microorganisms that penetrate the tonsillar epithelium are phagocytized and processed by macrophages, presented to B and T lymphocytes, and subsequently stimulate both the humoral and cell-mediated immune system responses.
II. Lymphoid hyperplasia and reactivity occur with neutrophilic infiltrates when chronic infection overwhelms the tonsillar defense mechanisms.

Clinical Signs

I. Fever, depression
II. Head shaking
III. Dysphagia, repeated attempts to swallow
IV. Anorexia

Diagnosis

I. Clinical signs, history, and direct visualization of enlarged, hyperemic, friable tonsils, and pharyngitis are suggestive; however, the tonsils do not always protrude from the crypts.
II. Cultures are of questionable value because the most common organisms associated with tonsillitis are also the normal microflora of the mouth (*E. coli, Staphylococcus aureus, Staphylococcus albus*, hemolytic streptococci, diplococci, *Proteus*, and *Pseudomonas*).
III. Cytology may be useful to rule out neoplasia and other differential diagnoses.
IV. Radiography may help identify penetrating radiopaque foreign bodies (e.g., bone fragments, etc.).
V. Endoscopic evaluation of the nasopharynx, esophagus, and larynx may be necessary.
VI. Sonography of adjacent lymph nodes and salivary glands may be helpful.

Differential Diagnosis

I. Neoplasia: squamous cell carcinoma, lymphosarcoma
II. Underlying disorders that cause chronic vomiting, regurgitation, or coughing

Treatment and Monitoring

I. Where possible, identify and correct the underlying disorder.
II. Broad-spectrum antibiotic treatment for 5–7 days is curative in most cases of primary tonsillitis.
    A. Amoxicillin, amoxicillin/clavulanic acid, tetracycline/doxycycline, clindamycin, or metronidazole may be administered.
    B. Long-term antibiotic therapy or frequent changes in antibiotics are avoided because they may promote bacterial resistance and fungal overgrowth.
III. Tonsillectomy is rarely indicated unless the enlarged tonsils interfere with chewing or swallowing, or if tonsillar neoplasia has not been ruled out.

IDIOPATHIC DISEASES

Mark E. Hitt

Lymphoplasmacytic Stomatitis

Definition

I. It is a chronic proliferative inflammatory disorder of oropharyngeal mucosa variably affecting the gingiva, palatoglossal arches (faucitis), base of the tongue, larynx, and the palatine, nasal, and caudal pharynx.
II. Mature cats (>12 months of age) are most frequently affected. Dogs are diagnosed with similar pathology, but less often.
III. Synonyms include plasma cell gingivitis and stomatitis, lymphoplasmacytic glossopharyngitis, and lymphocytic laryngopharyngitis.

Causes and Pathophysiology

I. It is considered an idiopathic condition after chronic viral, bacterial, and mechanical/traumatic factors have been ruled out.

II. A hypersensitivity reaction to oral or dental tissues with bacterial antigens has been hypothesized as the pathogenesis.

Clinical Signs

I. Signs are related to inflammation and proliferation of tissue.

II. Predominant signs are distorted masticatory movements, halitosis, inappetence, bleeding from gums, and ptyalism.

III. Oral examination reveals variable degrees of raised, erosive, proliferative, or erythematous lesions that may have concurrent ulcerative and nodular appearances.

    A. Usually lesions are found at the palatoglossal arches, around the teeth, and along the caudal aspects of the frenulum of the tongue.

    B. Additional affected areas may include the caudal pharynx, nasopharynx, laryngeal mucosa, commissure of the buccal mucosa, and tongue.

Diagnosis

I. Diagnosis is based on biopsy and histopathologic evaluation of the lesions.

    A. Surgical, endoscopic, and rongeur-cup type biopsies are acceptable.

    B. Cytologic samples are often non-diagnostic owing to the abundant cellular and bacterial debris on the surface of the lesions.

II. Histologic findings are an intense mixture of lymphocytes and plasma cells with variable predominance of lymphoid cells under an eroded epithelium.

    A. Additional inflammatory cells including eosinophils, macrophages, and neutrophils can be present.

    B. Repeated biopsy of chronic or relapsing cases is advised because of concerns for oral neoplasia.

III. Clinical pathologic information is often more helpful with evaluation of the differential diagnosis.

    A. A complete blood count (CBC) may reveal variable patterns of leukocytosis and mild anemia of chronic inflammatory disease.

    B. Elevation of serum globulins and serum electrophoresis may support a polyclonal gammopathy reflective of a chronic lymphoid inflammatory response.

    C. Bacterial cultures for aerobes and anaerobes and gram staining are not initially performed because of overlap between normal flora and pathogenic organisms; however, they may be helpful in chronic cases.

Differential Diagnosis

I. Eosinophilic granuloma complex: lesions more localized to the hard palate, philtrum, lips, and tongue

II. Neoplasia: especially squamous cell carcinoma and lymphosarcoma

III. Linear foreign body wrapped at the base of the tongue and penetrating foreign bodies lodged in the mucosa, e.g., plant awns and burrs

IV. Severe pyorrhea associated with various bacterial infections and periodontitis

V. Chronic viral infections: FeLV, FIV, caliciviruses

VI. Adverse drug reactions

VII. Immune-mediated systemic syndromes: systemic lupus erythematosus, pemphigoid disorders

VIII. Inflammation from persistent vomition or reflux of gastric acid and bile

IX. Eosinophilic granuloma of Siberian huskies

Treatment

I. Treatment involves aggressive anti-inflammatory or immunosuppressive medications.

II. The disorder is a persistent condition requiring long-term control.

III. Formulation of medications into liquids may be preferable.

IV. Oral hygiene is helpful for treating halitosis and removing superficial debris.

V. Anti-inflammatory and immunosuppressive drugs include the following.

    A. Prednisone/prednisolone 2 mg/kg PO SID-BID

    B. Methylprednisolone acetate 2–4 mg/kg IM at 2–6-week intervals in cats as tolerated

    C. Megestrol acetate 2.5 mg per cat PO QOD for 3 doses, then once or twice weekly as needed; not to be used in unspayed females, diabetics, or concurrently with corticosteroids

    D. Azathioprine 0.3 mg/kg PO QOD in cats; 1–2 mg/kg PO SID-QOD in dogs

    E. Chlorambucil 0.25–0.33 mg/kg PO q 72 h in cats; 1–2 mg/m² PO QOD in dogs

    F. Aurothioglucose 1 mg/kg IM weekly for 10–20 weeks, then tapered to once monthly; response may be delayed for 1–3 months

VI. Antibiotics are often helpful initially, and intermittently as secondary infections recur (see Stomatitis earlier).

VII. Dental extraction is a last resort for treatment and may be helpful by removing sites for immunogenic/antigenic stimulation between natural tissues and bacterial antigens.

VIII. Response to treatment is variable.

    A. Response to therapy may take weeks to assess.

    B. This is a chronic condition that is most often kept in remission, not cured.

    C. Combinations of corticosteroids and immunosuppressive agents have usually provided the most success.

Patient Monitoring

I. Clients should be advised that frequent reassessments every few weeks to months are necessary to adjust medications.

II. Monitoring of complete blood count (CBC), platelet counts, serum chemistries, and urinalyses are advised at 1–3-month intervals to assess for potential adverse effects of medication and chronic inflammation that may include anemia, leukopenia, thrombocytopenia, hepatopathy, and increased risk of bacterial infections.

Oral Feline Eosinophilic Granuloma Complex

Definition and Cause

I. Two forms of eosinophilic granuloma complex (EGC) affect the oral cavity.
   A. Indolent or "rodent ulcer" type erosions, often on the upper lip
   B. Eosinophilic granulomas anywhere in the oral cavity
II. These lesions are idiopathic.
III. They involve an accumulation of a dense matrix of mixed inflammatory cells, which may have a predominance of eosinophils in fibroproliferative tissue.
IV. They present as erosions, plaques, or proliferative lesions.

Clinical Signs

I. The clinical signs are the same as those of idiopathic lymphoplasmacytic stomatitis and include prehensile discomfort, halitosis, and ptyalism.
II. Lesions are generally more focal than those seen in lymphoplasmacytic disease.

Diagnosis

I. Diagnosis is based on biopsy and histopathologic evaluation (see Table 85–1).
II. Surgical, endoscopic, and rongeur-cup type biopsies are acceptable.
III. Cytologic samples are often non-diagnostic owing to abundant cellular and bacterial debris on the surface of the lesions.

Differential Diagnosis

I. Squamous cell carcinoma
II. Linear string foreign body
III. Lymphoplasmacytic oropharyngeal disease

Treatment

I. Corticosteroids are used initially (prednisone, dexamethasone, triamcinolone) orally and/or intralesionally (see Chap. 85).
II. Megestrol acetate may be tried at 0.25–0.5 mg/kg PO SID for 3 days then once or twice weekly for several weeks until resolution.
III. Radiation or cryotherapy may be effective for nonresponsive rodent ulcers.

PHARYNGEAL AND SWALLOWING DISORDERS

Mark E. Hitt

Oropharyngeal Dysphagia Disorders

Definition

I. Dysphagia is defined as difficulty in swallowing.
II. An abnormal oropharyngeal phase of swallowing can occur at several points.
   A. Oral stage: prehension in the oral cavity, bolus formation at the base of the tongue, and initiation of swallowing reflex
   B. Pharyngeal stage: rapid contractions of pharynx to direct the bolus aborally toward the cricopharyngeal passage
   C. Cricopharyngeal stage: coordinated relaxation of the upper esophageal sphincter (UES), propulsion of the bolus by the tightened pharynx into the proximal esophagus, and re-tightening of the UES and relaxation of the pharynx

Causes and Pathophysiology

I. Dysphagia is clinically difficult to separate into the specific stages.
   A. Visual observation can be difficult to assess.
   B. There are many overlapping causes involving more than one phase of swallowing.
II. Oral and pharyngeal dysphagia may arise from the following.
   A. Hypoglossal nerve dysfunction
      1. Hydrocephalus or other causes of increased intracranial pressure
      2. Trauma to the hypoglossal nerves (central or peripheral)
   B. Systemic neuromuscular disease
      1. Myasthenia gravis focal or generalized
      2. Endocrine neuropathies
         a) Hypothyroidism
         b) Hyperadrenocorticism
         c) Hypoadrenocorticism
      3. Myopathies
         a) Familial myopathies (see Chap. 80)
         b) Muscular dystrophy–like disease of Bouviers des Flandres
      4. Immune-mediated myositis
         a) Masticatory myositis
         b) Eosinophilic myositis
         c) Systemic lupus erythematosus–associated
   C. Infectious causes
      1. Rabies virus
      2. Submucosal abscess: foreign bodies, bite wounds
   D. Traumatic and physical obstruction
      1. Skeletal disorders and fractures
      2. Dental disease
      3. Craniomandibular osteopathy
      4. Tumors of the oropharynx
      5. Pharyngeal mucocele
      6. Inflammatory nasopharyngeal polyps in cats
      7. Retropharyngeal lymphadenopathy from regional infection or metastasis (e.g., tonsillar carcinoma, thyroid carcinoma)
      8. Pharyngeal mucosal laxity associated with hyperadrenocorticism in small and toy breeds of dogs
      9. Brachycephalic syndrome (see Chap. 14)
      10. Oropharyngeal foreign bodies
III. The etiology of cricopharyngeal dysphagia is variable.
   A. Failure to coordinate (asynchronous) the relaxation of the UES (achalasia) with cricopharyn-

geal contraction as an idiopathic congenital condition
  B. Acquired or congenital strictures in the region of the cricopharynx and UES
IV. The mechanism of dysphagia varies with the individual cause and may be a dysfunction of anatomy or an asynchronous coordination of events or arise from obstruction.

Clinical Signs

I. Oral dysphagia
  A. Prehensile dysfunction may be noted.
    1. Drooling, dropping food from mouth
    2. Exaggerated efforts to toss food back into the oral cavity
  B. Tongue fails to propel material aborally and has poor retractile strength when grasped.
  C. Any asymmetry of muscular or skeletal anatomy may be noted on examination.
II. Pharyngeal dysphagia
  A. Prehension is normal, but there are repeated efforts at swallowing.
  B. Gagging and coughing of saliva or a food bolus may occur.
  C. Liquids may be swallowed more easily, but a post-swallowing cough or "clearing of the throat" is often reported in the history.
  D. Rhinitis and nasal discharge are often noted.
  E. Aspiration pneumonia with associated coughing, fever, or chronic pulmonary disease may be present.
  F. Complete history and physical and neurologic examinations may identify systemic disorders.
III. Cricopharyngeal dysphagia
  A. Puppies are most commonly reported to be affected (achalasia) at the time of weaning.
  B. Repeated efforts are made to swallow the same bolus of food.
  C. Aspiration pneumonia is a common complication.

Diagnosis

I. Complete neurologic and musculoskeletal examinations are imperative.
II. Carefully take a history from the owner and observe any swallowing attempts.
III. Evaluate standard hematologic and biochemical tests to identify predisposing disorders.
IV. Serologic evaluation of antinuclear antibody (ANA), acetylcholine receptor antibody (AChR-Ab), and masticatory myositis antibody tests may be helpful in identifying immune-mediated disorders.
V. Electromyography can also be helpful in identifying cranial nerve dysfunction but may be difficult to perform and interpret.
VI. Radiography and imaging techniques may be indicated.
  A. Positive contrast swallow videofluoroscopy is an ideal technique for evaluation of dysphagia. Iohexol is an isosmotic agent that is nonirritating to the airway if aspirated and can be used as an alternative to barium suspensions.

  B. Cervical region soft tissue and musculoskeletal abnormalities may be detected on survey radiographs.
  C. Thoracic radiography may identify megaesophagus or detect mass lesions (e.g., thymoma, lymphosarcoma, heart base tumors).
  D. Abdominal radiography may identify causes of gastric acid reflux or reveal evidence of more widespread dysautonomic gastrointestinal function.
  E. Magnetic resonance imaging and computed tomography are helpful in localizing tumors.

Differential Diagnosis

I. See Causes listed earlier
II. Megaesophagus (see Chap. 29)
III. Retropharyngeal lymphadenopathy or abscess
IV. Meningitis with neck pain
V. Musculoskeletal disorders: temporomandibular joint disease, fractures
VI. Trigeminal neuralgia
VII. Retrobulbar abscess
VIII. Idiopathic polyneuropathy of dalmations and other breeds

Treatment

I. Treatment for dysphagia relies on determining the underlying causes.
II. Symptomatic treatment includes nutritional support.
  A. Elevated feeding using varied textures of foods is often unrewarding for dysphagia.
  B. Percutaneous endoscopic gastrostomy (PEG) tubes are superior to nasoesophageal and pharyngoesophageal tubes.
  C. Myotomy of the UES may be performed for cricopharyngeal achalasia, but for other dysphagias it may increase risk of aspiration pneumonia.
III. See Chap. 18 for treatment of aspiration pneumonia.

Patient Monitoring

I. Spontaneous improvement has been noted in a few cases of cranial nerve neuropathies, but neuropraxias and musculoskeletal injuries may require months.
II. Prognosis is guarded to poor if a specific cause cannot be identified and treated because of the risk of aspiration pneumonia and the debilitation that ensues from malnutrition.

NEOPLASIA

by Debra L. Zoran

Epulis

Definition and Cause

I. An epulis is a benign mesenchymal tumor that arises from the periodontal connective tissue and is often located in the gingival tissue near the incisors.
II. Classification of epulides is controversial, but they are most commonly grouped as ossifying epulis, fi-

bromatous epulis, or squamous or acanthomatous epulis.

   A. Acanthomatous epulis may be a form of basal cell carcinoma (White, 1991).
   B. Synonyms for acanthomatous epulis are adamantinoma and amelioblastoma.
III. Epulides are common in dogs (20% of oral tumors) but are rare in cats (White and Gorman, 1989).
IV. No known cause or risk factors have been identified.

Pathophysiology

   I. Ossifying and fibromatous epulides are firm or pedunculated, nonulcerating and noninvasive tumors that can occur as single or multiple growths. Epulides are usually 1–4 cm and variably fixed to the bone at the gum line.
   II. Acanthomatous epulis is locally aggressive, often associated with marked bony lysis, and more commonly affects the mandible (Thrall, 1984). Distant metastasis of epulis is not reported.

Clinical Signs

   I. Because of their location, masses are often discovered before signs develop; however, dogs may be presented for anorexia, drooling, oral hemorrhage, dysphagia, and halitosis.
   II. Epulis is most commonly observed in geriatric dogs, but it can occur at any age (Diebielzig et al., 1979).

Diagnosis

   I. Surgical biopsy of the oral mass is diagnostic, but fine-needle aspirate or scraping may also be useful to rule out other malignant tumor types.
   II. Histologically, acanthomatous epulis may closely resemble squamous cell carcinoma. Regional metastasis is more common with squamous cell carcinoma, and thus, careful examination of regional lymph nodes (aspirate) is important (Verstraete et al., 1992).

Differential Diagnosis

   I. Severe gingival hypertrophy
   II. Oral papillomas
   III. Squamous cell carcinoma
   IV. Fibrosarcoma
   V. Other neoplasms: chondroma, osteoma, hemangioma, lipoma

Treatment and Monitoring

   I. Fibromatous and ossifying epulides are treated with surgical excision.
   II. Because epulides arise from the periodontal ligament, excision at the level of the gingiva often is incomplete and the tumor may regrow.
   III. Partial maxillectomy or mandibulectomy is often necessary to prevent local recurrence of acanthomatous epulis.
   A. The prognosis is guarded to good (White and Gorman, 1989).
   B. Cryosurgery is not recommended because local recurrence is common.

   C. Radiation therapy is also an effective treatment method for acanthomatous epulis.
IV. Successful use of chemotherapy to treat epulides using doxorubicin and cyclophosphamide has been reported (Gorman et al., 1984).

Oral Papillomatosis

Definition and Causes

   I. Multiple, benign cauliflower-like growths arising from squamous epithelium affect the lips, buccal mucosa, gingiva, tongue, and pharyngeal structures.
   II. Papillomas are seen primarily in young dogs (<1 year) with no breed or sex predilection.
   III. The tumors are induced by canine oral papillomavirus (papovavirus) and are contagious.
   IV. They are not related to the nonviral, cutaneous papillomas that are common in geriatric dogs.

Pathophysiology

   I. The incubation period following viral infection is approximately 4–8 weeks.
   II. Tumor growth lasts 1–5 months.
   III. Spontaneous regression of the growths follows over 6–12 weeks (Calvert, 1990).
   IV. Regression of the growths is accompanied by lifelong immunity.

Clinical Signs

   I. The disease may be asymptomatic, but in dogs with multiple or large papillomas, dysphagia, ptyalism, and halitosis, or other signs of oral disease (inappetence, face rubbing, etc.), may be observed.
   II. Lesions vary in appearance from the typical large, gray, pedunculated masses to small, white, smooth nodules. Regressing lesions appear dark and shriveled.

Diagnosis

   I. Clinical signs and gross appearance in a young dog are suggestive.
   II. Surgical biopsy and histopathology confirm the diagnosis.

Differential Diagnosis

   I. Transmissible venereal tumor (TVT)
   A. Lesions are typically present on external genitalia as well as the mouth.
   B. TVT is usually sessile and more often ulcerated.
   C. Biopsy is diagnostic.
   II. Squamous cell carcinoma: often presents as sessile, ulcerated masses with bony lysis
   III. Epulis

Treatment and Monitoring

   I. Treatment is usually not recommended if only a few papillomas are present.
   II. If large or multiple growths cause persistent clinical signs or do not regress, treatment is indicated.

III. Several methods are effective, including surgical excision, cryotherapy, and electrosurgery.

IV. The efficacy of autologous wart vaccines is questionable, and they are not recommended.

Squamous Cell Carcinoma (SCC)

Definition

I. SCC is a malignant neoplasm of squamous epithelium.

II. It is the most common oral neoplasm of cats (70% of all oral tumors) and the second most common (20–30%) oral tumor in dogs (Stebbins et al., 1989; Withrow, 1995).

III. Although tumors of the tongue are rare, SCC of the tongue is the most common form.

IV. It is most commonly seen on the ventrolateral surface of the tongue in cats and in the tonsillar crypt or gingival mucosa in dogs.

V. Gingival SCC usually arises adjacent to the incisors and premolars of the lower jaw or near the molars in the upper jaw (Guilford, 1996).

Causes

I. There is no known cause for SCC.

II. Conditions that may be associated with an increased incidence of SCC include the following.
   A. Chronic periodontal disease
   B. Eosinophilic ulcer
   C. Oral papillomatosis

III. Dogs living in an urban environment have a higher incidence (10:1) of tonsillar SCC.

Pathophysiology

I. The biologic behavior of SCC varies by the species affected and the location within the oral cavity.
   A. SCC of the tongue and tonsil are aggressive forms that tend to metastasize early to regional (retropharyngeal or mandibular lymph nodes) and distant (lungs) sites (Carpenter et al., 1993).
   B. SCC of the gingival tissues is locally aggressive (bony invasion in 75%) and superficially ulcerative but is slowly progressive (10% regional metastasis, and 3% to distant sites) (White, 1991).
   C. Small, rostrally located, gingival SCCs tend to have the best prognosis (Ogilvie and Moore, 1995).

II. Generally, SCC tends to occur with greater frequency in white dogs and cats, even though lack of protective pigment may have less effect in the mouth (Withrow, 1995).

Clinical Signs

I. SCC of the tongue
   A. In cats, the tumor arises at the base of the tongue and may initially appear as a small, raised ulcer.
   B. Canine SCC of the tongue is more likely to arise on the dorsal surface.
   C. The animal may be asymptomatic or show severe dysphagia, difficulty in prehension of food, oral hemorrhage, excessive licking movements, ptyalism, and gagging.

D. Lingual forms are usually seen in older dogs and cats.

II. SCC of the tonsil (Evans and Shoter, 1988)
   A. They are most often seen in old (mean age, 10–12 years), male (2:1) dogs (Spodnick and Page, 1995).
   B. Palpation of enlarged mandibular or retropharyngeal lymph nodes in an older dog indicates the need for a careful examination of the tonsils and caudal oropharynx.
   C. The tumor typically presents as a unilateral, firm mass deeply attached in the tonsillar crypt and may be associated with subcutaneous swelling, severe dysphagia, and pain.
   D. It rapidly metastasizes to the retropharyngeal lymph nodes, so the disease should be considered systemic at the time of diagnosis.

III. SCC of the gingiva
   A. The mean age of occurrence is slightly younger (7–9 years) than for tonsillar SCC.
   B. Lesions may present as non-healing ulcers in the gingiva adjacent to teeth or as proliferative, expansile masses without ulceration.
   C. Both single and multiple masses are reported.

Diagnosis

I. Surgical biopsy of the mass and enlarged lymph nodes with histopathology is required for diagnosis.
   A. Cytologic exam of oral neoplasms is often not rewarding as a result of the accompanying necrosis and inflammation.
   B. Any non-healing, ulcerated region in the oral cavity should be biopsied to rule out SCC.

II. All animals with oral masses are staged using blood tests, radiography, and cytology/histopathology.

Differential Diagnosis

I. SCC of the tongue
   A. Sublingual foreign body
   B. Eosinophilic granuloma complex
   C. Other less common neoplasms: granular cell myoblastomas (second most common tongue tumor), fibrosarcoma, malignant melanoma, mast cell tumor, lymphosarcoma

II. SCC of the tonsil
   A. Lymphosarcoma
   B. Salivary gland adenocarcinoma (rare)
   C. Tonsillitis or tonsillar abscess

III. SCC of the gingiva
   A. Chronic gingivitis and periodontitis
   B. Eosinophilic granuloma complex
   C. Epulis
   D. Other neoplasms: fibrosarcoma, osteosarcoma, or malignant melanoma
   E. Osteomyelitis (especially in cats)

IV. SCC of the palatine mucosa
   A. Plasmacytic gingivitis-stomatitis complex
   B. Salivary gland adenocarcinoma

Treatment

I. Attempt to rule out metastatic disease first, because many forms of SCC have metastasized at the time of diagnosis.

II. Surgical excision is the initial treatment of choice for debulking and tumor removal but may be difficult because of extensive invasion of underlying tissue and bone.
   A. Hemimandibulectomy or total maxillectomy/ mandibulectomy has the greatest success rates for gingival SCC (80% survival for 1 year) (Spodnick and Page, 1995). When the tumor mass is large and surgical margins are incomplete, concurrent radiation therapy is indicated (Ogilvie and Moore, 1995).
   B. SCC of the tongue is amenable to surgical removal in 40–60% of canine cases, but the percentage is lower in cats owing to its usual location on the ventral surface of the base of the tongue (Guilford, 1996).
   C. For tonsillar SCC, surgical debulking is only palliative and is typically used in conjunction with radiation therapy. Radiation therapy with concurrent hyperthermia following surgical debulking of the tumor mass appears to give the best long-term results (Ogilvie and Moore, 1995).
III. Adjuvant or neoadjuvant chemotherapy may improve survival time in cases with systemic metastasis.
   A. The BAC protocol (bleomycin, doxorubicin, and cyclophosphamide) has been recommended for feline SCC, but the results are not well documented (Jeglum and Sadanaga, 1996).
   B. Cisplatin combined with doxorubicin may also be useful (Brooks et al., 1988).

Patient Monitoring

I. Oral and thoracic radiographs are periodically monitored to assess disease progression.
II. Because of the rapid growth of tonsillar SCC, owners should be made aware of the potential for airway obstruction.
III. Nutritional support of the animal is an important part of treatment.
   A. Aggressive forms of nutritional support, such as PEG tube insertion, are often utilized for SCC or any oral malignancy.
   B. Special diets such as soft, blenderized foods or canned diets may improve food consumption.

Malignant Melanoma

Definition and Causes

I. It is a neoplasm of melanocytes within the epidermis.
II. Melanoma is the most commonly reported oral tumor in dogs (30–40%); however, the tumor is rare in cats (Goldschmidt, 1985).
III. There is no known cause for the disease.
IV. Certain breeds appear to be more susceptible, especially black-coated breeds such as the black cocker spaniel and Scottish terrier; the tumor is also common in poodles, dachshunds, and golden retrievers (Goldschmidt, 1985).

Pathophysiology

I. Most oral melanomas (90%) are malignant.
II. Major sites are the pigmented gingiva, buccal mucosa, and palate. The tongue is a less common site.

III. Melanomas are locally aggressive tumors.
   A. Smaller tumor sizes (<2 cm diameter) are associated with longer survival times (Harvey et al., 1981).
   B. Metastasis to regional sites (lymph nodes) occurs early in most dogs.
   C. The time to metastasis of melanoma to distant sites (lungs, brain, kidney) is more variable and often occurs late in the course of the disease (Todoroff and Brodey, 1979).

Clinical Signs

I. The mean age for melanoma in dogs is 10–12 years (Spodnick and Page, 1995).
II. There is no apparent sex predilection for oral melanoma in dogs (Hahn et al., 1994).
III. Female cats may be predisposed, but the numbers reported are small.
IV. The clinical signs depend on location and size of the tumor and include halitosis, dysphagia, difficulty chewing or painful chewing, face rubbing, oral hemorrhage, drooling, and inappetence.
V. Melanomas are typically pigmented, but the less common amelanotic melanomas have a pinkish-white appearance. The latter tumors are friable and necrotic and bleed very easily.
VI. Local invasion of bone is common (>50%).

Diagnosis

I. Excisional biopsy with histopathology is diagnostic, although amelanotic melanomas are often reported histologically as anaplastic sarcomas.
II. A complete work-up includes a hemogram, biochemical profile, urinalysis, thoracic and oral radiography, and regional lymph node aspirates or biopsy for staging of the disease.

Differential Diagnosis

I. Fibrosarcoma
II. Squamous cell carcinoma
III. Other less common oral neoplasms: fibrosarcoma, hemangiosarcoma

Treatment and Monitoring

I. The prognosis is guarded to poor, because the tumor may have metastasized to distant sites by the time of diagnosis (1-year survival is 25%).
II. Radical surgical excision, with maxillectomy or mandibulectomy, is the most common treatment.
III. Radiation therapy may be useful, but large doses may be required (McChesney et al., 1989).
   A. Concurrent hyperthermia enhances the effectiveness of radiation therapy.
   B. Radiation therapy appears to be most effective with small tumors.
IV. Chemotherapy for metastatic disease is generally unrewarding (<25% response rate).
   A. Cisplatin 60 mg/m^2 IV every 3 weeks
   B. Carboplatin 300 mg/m^2 IV every 3 weeks (Ogilvie and Moore, 1995)

V. Immunotherapy may be considered along with chemotherapy for control of metastatic disease.
   A. Cimetidine: role in dogs with melanoma unknown
   B. *Corynebacterium parvum*
   C. Liposome-encapsulated muramyl-tripeptide–phosphatidylethanolamine (L-MTP-PE)

Oral Fibrosarcoma

Definition and Cause

   I. It is a malignant tumor of fibrocytes.
   II. Fibrosarcoma is the second most common tumor of the oral cavity in cats (20%) (Spodnick and Page, 1995).
   III. In dogs, oral fibrosarcoma is the third most commonly reported malignant tumor (10–20%), after melanoma and SCC (Spodnick and Page, 1995).
   IV. The median age of occurrence is 8 years, with large-breed dogs being overrepresented, especially golden retrievers and Doberman pinschers (Ciekot et al., 1994). Males may be predisposed.
   V. Cats are usually older (mean age, 10 years).
   VI. No known causes or viral associations; it is not related to feline sarcoma virus.

Pathophysiology

   I. It is a solid, fleshy tumor that arises from the gingival connective tissue or the periodontal bone; gingival origin is the most common.
   II. The most common sites are the maxillary gingiva and the hard palate in the area between the canine and carnassial teeth.
   III. Fibrosarcomas are locally aggressive but only occasionally metastasize in cats or old dogs. In young dogs, the tumor tends to act more aggressively and metastasize to distant sites.

Clinical Signs

   I. The presenting signs depend on the location and size of the tumor and may include dysphagia, ptyalism, anorexia or inappetence, halitosis, exaggerated chewing motions or difficulty chewing, or pawing at the mouth.
   II. Fibrosarcomas may grow to be very large (>4 cm diameter) (Todoroff and Brodey, 1979).

Diagnosis

   I. Diagnosis is suggested by the age, breed, sex, and location.
   II. Definitive diagnosis is made by excisional biopsy and histopathologic examination.
   III. Staging of the tumor is important.
      A. Oral radiography often underestimates the tumor margins.
      B. Computed tomography is more accurate for determining the extent of bony involvement.

Differential Diagnosis

   I. Squamous cell carcinoma
   II. Malignant melanoma
   III. Hemangiosarcoma

   A. Low incidence of occurrence in the oral cavity (5%)
   B. Breeds affected: German shepherd dogs, golden retrievers
IV. Other oral neoplasms
   A. Osteosarcoma
   B. Salivary gland adenocarcinoma
   C. Mast cell tumors
   D. Lymphosarcoma
   E. Epulis
   F. Undifferentiated carcinomas and sarcomas

Treatment

   I. Wide surgical excision (partial or complete maxillectomy) is required to prevent local recurrence.
   II. Radiation therapy as a single treatment modality is disappointing, unless large doses (>50 Gy) are used.
      A. Megavoltage radiation may be more effective than orthovoltage radiation (Ogilvie and Moore, 1995).
      B. Radiation combined with hyperthermia appears to improve local control (Brewer and Turrel, 1982).
   III. Fibrosarcoma is unresponsive to cryotherapy.
   IV. Combination therapy with surgical debulking, radiation, and/or chemotherapy (doxorubicin, dacarbazine, cisplatin) may give the best long-term results.

Patient Monitoring

   I. Local recurrence occurs in 50% of the cases (Withrow, 1995).
   II. Some fibrosarcomas are very slow growing, so 6- to 18-month survival times with good quality of life are possible.
   III. Metastatic disease is slow to develop, but regional lymph node aspirates and thoracic radiographs are monitored to assess disease progression and treatment success.
   IV. If radiation therapy is considered, side effects that will likely occur include keratoconjunctivitis sicca, moist desquamation/mucositis, cataracts, and xerostomia.

SMALL ANIMAL DENTAL DISEASES

Linda J. DeBowes

Developmental Disorders
See Table 27–2.

Periodontal Disease

Definition

   I. Periodontal disease commonly refers to microbial-induced inflammatory diseases of the periodontium.
   II. The periodontium includes the supporting structures of the tooth: the gingiva, alveolar bone, periodontal ligament, and cementum.
   III. Gingivitis is periodontal disease that is confined to the gingiva.

Table 27–2. Developmental Disorders of the Teeth

Condition/Disorder	Cause	Clinical Signs	Treatment
Retained deciduous teeth	Genetic, developmental	Deciduous tooth present after eruption of succeeding permanent tooth.	Extract deciduous tooth (crown and root) as soon as identified.
Discolored teeth	Enamel/dentin discolored secondary to tetracyclines administered during tooth development or pulpal hemorrhage/necrosis	No clinical signs associated with tetracycline staining; tooth may be painful if pulp inflammation or periapical disease present.	Vital tooth, no treatment necessary unless causing pain; non-vital tooth may be treated by various endodontic procedures or extraction.
Enamel hypoplasia	Hypomineralization of the dental enamel during the developmental and maturation phases caused by damage to ameloblasts by infectious, inflammatory, or nutritional factors	I. Dogs: rough, mottled appearance to crown, stained crown, or focal areas of enamel loss II. Cats: yellowish or rough tooth crown III. Pain may be present if significant loss of enamel exposes the dentin; the tooth may be painful/sensitive on exposure to hot or cold.	None if teeth are not sensitive or painful; sensitive or painful teeth, dentinal sealer applied as needed.

IV. Periodontitis is periodontal disease that results in destruction of the supporting structures of the tooth (periodontium) with concurrent gingivitis.

Cause

I. Dental plaque is a yellow-grayish substance that adheres to the tooth surface.
II. Dental plaque is primarily composed of bacteria, salivary glycoproteins, and extracellular polysaccharides.
III. Plaque bacteria initiate an inflammatory response in adjacent tissues.

Pathophysiology

I. Pellicle
   A. Invisible glycoprotein layer that forms within hours on a recently cleaned tooth
   B. Bacteria established on the pellicle within 24 hours
II. Supragingival microbial plaque accumulation
   A. Initially, primarily gram-positive, non-motile bacteria are present.
   B. Marginal gingivitis develops first, as an acute inflammatory response to the bacteria.
   C. Established gingivitis is associated with a lymphocytic, plasmacytic infiltrate and breakdown of gingival connective tissue.
III. Subgingival microbial plaque
   A. Accumulates when supragingival plaque leads to alterations in the marginal gingival epithelium, allowing for subgingival progression of bacteria
   B. Increased proportion of gram-negative, anaerobic, motile bacteria that progress apically in the gingival sulcus/periodontal pocket
IV. Dental calculus (tartar)
   A. Mineralized plaque
   B. Has a rough surface that enhances plaque accumulation

Clinical Signs

I. Gingivitis
   A. Halitosis
   B. Gingival inflammation
      1. Erythema of marginal gingiva
      2. Edema, thickening and rounding of gingival margin
      3. Gingival bleeding as severity of inflammation increases
II. Periodontitis
   A. Signs of attachment loss: periodontal pockets, gingival recession, mobile teeth
   B. Concurrent gingivitis
   C. Other associated problems
      1. Facial swelling
      2. Nasal discharge, sneezing
      3. Periodontal or periapical abscesses
      4. Oronasal fistulas

Diagnosis

I. Oral and dental examination is performed under anesthesia.
II. Gingivitis is diagnosed when gingival inflammation is present.
   A. Gingival erythema, edema, inflammatory infiltrate
   B. Loss of sharp gingival margin
   C. Marginal gingival epithelium altered, allowing for easier placement of periodontal probe in gingival sulcus
   D. Pseudopocket formation
   E. Gingival bleeding on probing (in more severe disease)
III. Periodontitis is diagnosed with loss of tissues making up the periodontium.
   A. Periodontal pockets: >3 mm in dogs; >0.5 mm in cats
   B. Gingival recession

C. Alveolar bone loss: noticeable on dental examination and dental radiographs
IV. Dental radiographs help confirm the diagnosis and extent of disease.
  A. Gingivitis: no evidence of alveolar bone loss
  B. Periodontitis
    1. Horizontal and/or vertical alveolar bone loss
    2. Secondary endodontic disease may occur

Differential Diagnosis

I. Immune-mediated oral disease
  A. Pemphigus vulgaris
  B. Bullous pemphigoid
II. Neoplasia
III. Infectious disease: feline immunodeficiency virus (FIV)

Treatment

I. Antimicrobial therapy may be advised in patients with severe periodontitis or at risk for distant site infections secondary to bacteremia associated with dental procedures.
  A. Single dose, preoperatively for prevention of bacteremia in dogs and cats (Harvey, 1996)
  B. Amoxicillin 20–25 mg/kg IV, ampicillin 20–25 mg/kg IV, amoxicillin-clavulanic acid 11–22 mg/kg PO, 1 hour prior to procedure
II. Scale teeth to remove calculus and plaque.
  A. Mechanical methods: ultrasonic, sonic, rotary scaler
  B. Hand instruments
    1. Scalers: for supragingival use only
    2. Curettes: for supragingival and subgingival use
III. Polish teeth to remove remaining plaque and smooth the tooth surface.
  A. Scaling creates "scratches" on tooth surface.
  B. Rough tooth surface enhances plaque accumulation.
  C. Perform on all tooth surfaces.
  D. Use a slow-speed handpiece with prophy angle attached, a rubber prophy cup, and fine grit polishing paste.
  E. Rinse and clean debris from gingival sulcus and oral cavity as final step.
IV. Institute oral hygiene program at home.
  A. Goal is to decrease plaque accumulation.
  B. Brush teeth ideally every day, or a minimum of 3 times weekly.
    1. Not recommended if pet is likely to injure person brushing the teeth or if it causes oral pain.
    2. Mechanical devices used to remove plaque include toothbrushes (veterinary design or a pediatric, junior, soft bristle type), finger toothbrushes, and gauze pads or gauze wrapped around a finger.
    3. Use dentifrices designed for animals.
    4. Demonstrate technique to owners and recommend initially that they brush only the buccal and labial surfaces while holding the mouth closed.

C. Use dietary means to help decrease plaque accumulation.
  1. Hill's Science Diet, t/d
  2. Removes supragingival plaque only on teeth that are used to chew the kibble
  3. Recommended after teeth are scaled and polished to supplement daily tooth brushing
D. Chew "toys" and rawhides may provide some oral health benefits; hard "toys" that may damage tooth or soft tissue structures should be avoided.
E. Antibacterial products such as chlorhexidine have an antimicrobial effect and may be part of the oral health care at home for patients with severe periodontitis.

Patient Monitoring

I. Recheck schedule is dependent on the extent of periodontal disease, home oral hygiene performed, and owner's interest in decreasing progression of disease.
II. Patients with disease limited to gingivitis may need professional teeth cleaning on an annual basis or more or less frequently depending on home oral hygiene.
III. Patients with periodontitis may require professional teeth cleaning every 3–6 months to remove subgingival plaque and calculus and slow progression of disease.

Odontoclastic Resorptive Lesions

Definition and Cause

I. Non-carious odontoclastic resorption of tooth substance
II. Etiology undetermined

Pathophysiology

I. Odontoclasts stimulated and mediate tooth resorption
II. Loss of tooth structure usually beginning at cemento-enamel junction
  A. Progressive resorption horizontally, coronally, apically
  B. Stages/Grades
    1. Stage 1: resorption limited to enamel
    2. Stage 2: resorption of enamel and dentin, pulp not involved
    3. Stage 3: resorption extends into pulp, majority of tooth intact
    4. Stage 4: resorption extends into pulp, extensive loss of tooth structure
    5. Stage 5: root(s) present, crown missing, variable amount of gingiva extending over retained roots
III. Increased incidence and number of lesions in older cats

Clinical Signs

I. Loss of tooth substance
II. Gingival changes
  A. Hyperplastic gingiva extends coronally and covers the resorptive lesion
  B. Gingival inflammation at resorptive site

III. Oral pain
  A. Reluctance to eat dry cat food
  B. Altered mastication
  C. Behavior changes: aggression, reclusive attitude

Diagnosis

I. Oral examination
  A. Loss of tooth substance may be evident.
  B. Gingival changes may be suggestive.
II. Dental examination
  A. Use periodontal explorer.
  B. Examine subgingivally for lesions.
III. Dental radiography
  A. Resorptive lesions identified as radiolucencies of tooth root/crown
  B. May identify lesions not diagnosed on dental examination

Differential Diagnosis

I. Loss of tooth crown: fractured tooth
II. Gingival inflammation, hyperplasia: periodontal disease, neoplasia

Treatment

I. Stage I
  A. Scale, polish teeth.
  B. Fluoride varnish treatment or a dentinal sealer has been recommended; however, a documented benefit has not been established for these treatments.
II. Stage II
  A. Extraction
  B. Restoration: reported success rate of 33–36% after 12–16 months (Lyon, 1992; Zetner and Steurer, 1995)
III. Stage III, IV: extraction
IV. Stage V
  A. Extraction of retained roots/root fragments is indicated when associated with gingival inflammation or radiographic evidence of a bony reaction.
  B. Retained roots do not need to be extracted if healthy gingiva covers root and there is no radiographic evidence of inflammation/infection.

Patient Monitoring

I. Schedule regular appointments every 6–12 months to evaluate for clinical signs of resorptive lesions and, if needed, to scale and polish the teeth.
II. Monitor for clinical signs of resorptive lesions; if present, anesthetize for complete oral evaluation and treatment.

Periapical and Periodontal Abscesses

Definition

I. A periapical abscess involves the periapical/apical portion of a tooth.
II. A periodontal abscess involves the periodontal/subgingival portion of the tooth.

Cause and Pathophysiology

I. Periapical abscess
  A. Endodontic (pulpal) bacterial infection extending beyond the apex leading to abscess formation
    1. Trauma causing pulpitis
    2. Fractured tooth with pulp exposure
  B. Extension of periodontal disease
II. Abscess in periodontal pocket
  A. Periodontal disease
  B. Foreign body
  C. Subgingival fracture
III. Neutrophilic response to local inflammation/infection

Clinical Signs

I. Periapical abscess
  A. Maxillary fourth premolar most common
  B. Pain on biting, malaise
  C. Swelling or fistula
    1. Usually with the fourth maxillary premolar there is external drainage below medial canthus of eye and occasionally drainage through the buccal mucosa or into the nose (palatal root).
    2. Maxillary first molars may cause retrobulbar swelling, pain on opening the mouth, or exophthalmos.
    3. Mandibular teeth may cause mandibular swellings and drain externally on the ventral aspect of the mandible or drain intraorally.
II. Periodontal abscess
  A. Gingival inflammation
  B. Purulent exudate from gingival sulcus
  C. Oral fistula usually at or coronal to mucogingival junction

Diagnosis

I. Oral/dental examination
  A. Tooth discoloration or pulp exposure may be identified with periapical abscess; gingiva may look healthy.
  B. Periodontal pockets with purulent material, foreign debris, or associated dentition problem (e.g., subgingival fracture) may be noted.
II. Dental radiographs
  A. Periapical lucency may be present with chronic periapical abscess, as well as apical destruction/loss of roots.
  B. Periodontal abscess is identified clinically and may have associated radiographic changes as with periodontitis.

Differential Diagnosis

I. Neoplasia
II. Other causes of intraoral or facial fistulas

Treatment and Monitoring

I. Periapical abscess
  A. Endodontic therapy

Evaluate dental radiographs to determine whether a root canal is an option and whether a conventional or surgical root canal is required.
B. Extraction of affected tooth
C. Antibiotics
1. Administered prior to endodontics or extraction to resolve acute signs and continue empirically for 7–14 days following the procedure.
2. Amoxicillin-clavulanic acid 11–22 mg/kg PO BID or clindamycin 5–11 mg/kg PO BID (Harvey, 1996)
II. Periodontal abscess
A. Periodontal therapy is required to remove subgingival plaque, calculus, and foreign debris.
B. Extraction is indicated for severe periodontitis, for predisposing factors (e.g., subgingival root fracture), or for continued periodontal abscess.
C. Antibiotics are generally not required after definitive periodontal treatment; chlorhexidine may be applied daily until inflammation has resolved.
III. Postoperative care
A. Following a root canal, perform dental radiographs to evaluate success initially at 6 months, then yearly.
B. Following extractions, monitor gingival healing for 10–14 days.

Oronasal Fistulas

Definition and Cause

I. A communication between the oral cavity and nasal passage
II. Usually caused by periodontal disease of the maxillary canine tooth
A. Inapparent fistula: canine tooth present with communication between oral cavity and nasal passage on palatal aspect of tooth
B. Apparent fistula: canine tooth missing

Pathophysiology

I. Only a thin layer of bone exists between the palatal aspect of the maxillary canine tooth and nasal mucosa.
II. This bone may be destroyed by periodontal disease, iatrogenically during extraction, or by neoplasia or trauma.

Clinical Signs

I. Nasal discharge: serous, serosanguineous, or hemorrhagic
II. Sneezing with or without an obvious nasal discharge (see earlier)

Diagnosis

I. Visualization of oronasal fistula upon oral examination
II. Blood from ipsilateral nostril on probing an inapparent oronasal fistula

Differential Diagnosis

I. Other causes of sneezing, nasal discharge (see Chap. 14)
II. Other causes of deep, erosive oral lesions, e.g., neoplasia, bite wounds

Treatment

I. Single flap procedure to repair fistula (Harvey and Emily, 1993)
A. It is usually successful.
B. Tension on flaps may result in failure.
II. Double flap repair procedure (Harvey and Emily, 1993)
A. Used for large defects
B. Used if single flap procedure failed
III. Small defects with no associated clinical signs: no treatment

Patient Monitoring

I. Animals should not chew on any objects that may pull out sutures or disrupt the repair for the first 10–14 days, until rechecked.
II. Evaluate for success of repair at 2 weeks postoperatively and again at 4 weeks if not completely healed at 2-week recheck.
III. Repair is most likely to fail if flaps are sutured under tension, have inadequate blood supply, or are not of sufficient size (Harvey and Emily, 1993).

Trauma—Loss of Tooth Crown

Definition

I. Dental attrition: physiologic loss of tooth substance that occurs in the course of normal use
II. Dental abrasion: unusual or mechanical processes causing the wearing away of tooth substance
III. Fracture: breakage of a part of the tooth

Causes

I. Attrition: malocclusion resulting in abnormal contact between teeth during mastication
A. Congenital, hereditary jaw, skull abnormalities
B. Malaligned fracture repairs
C. Temporomandibular joint luxation(s)
II. Abrasion
A. Chewing on hard objects, abrasive surfaces: cage materials, rocks, sticks, hard chew toys, etc.
B. Self-trauma (pruritic skin diseases)
III. Fracture
A. Chewing on hard objects (as discussed earlier)
B. Direct trauma, e.g., hit with baseball bat, hit by car
C. Resorptive lesions (cat)

Pathophysiology

I. Attrition, abrasion
A. Odontoblasts are stimulated to produce "reparative" dentin.

B. If loss of tooth structure progresses slowly, "reparative" dentin protects the pulp from exposure.
II. Fracture: pulpal exposure common

Clinical Signs

I. Attrition, abrasion
   A. Loss of crown with dark brown area ("reparative" dentin) visible on worn surface
   B. Severe, rapid loss of crown structure without signs of "reparative" dentin and potential pulp exposure
II. Fracture
   A. Loss of crown structure, sharp edges
   B. Pulp exposure, pulp may be vital or nonvital, bleeding on probing of the pulp with an explorer indicates a vital pulp, necrotic pulp dark brown/black

Diagnosis

I. Oral and dental examination
II. Periodontal explorer used to detect pulp (root canal) exposure

Treatment

I. Attrition
   A. Follow the American Veterinary Medical Association (AVMA) principles of professional ethics and be aware of the American Kennel Club rules when considering orthodontic correction of malocclusions.
   B. For selected extractions to remove teeth in malocclusion, consult veterinary dentist for appropriate treatment planning.
   C. For pulp exposure, consider the following.
      1. Endodontics if sufficient crown remaining to be a functional tooth (see later discussion under fracture)
      2. Extraction of tooth if minimal crown remaining, owners decline endodontics
   D. Bacteremias may occur during extraction, and antibiotics are recommended in animals at risk for distant site infection (e.g., immune system compromise).
II. Abrasion
   A. Correct dermatologic problem if self-trauma is the problem.
   B. Remove objects causing the abrasion.
   C. Treat pulp exposure as described later.
III. Fracture with pulp exposure: treat to prevent potential periapical disease
   A. Deciduous tooth: extraction
   B. Permanent tooth, open apex
      1. Perform endodontics.
         a) Vital pulp: vital pulpotomy performed as soon as possible and up to 2 weeks after exposure to allow for continued root growth and development of a mature root apex (apexogenesis) (Harvey and Emily, 1993; Lobprise, 1993)
         b) Non-vital pulp: endodontic procedure performed to stimulate closure of the apex by cementum formation (apexification), followed by conventional endodontic therapy performed (Harvey and Emily, 1993)
         c) Antibiotics recommended (Harvey and Emily, 1993)
      2. Consider extraction.
   C. Permanent tooth, closed apex, <18 months old, recent fracture
      1. Vital pulpotomy may be attempted to allow for continued root development. A potential for failure exists and may require additional treatment via root canal or extraction (Harvey and Emily, 1993).
      2. Conventional root canal may be performed if vital pulpotomy is not desired.
      3. Extraction is also an option.
   D. Permanent tooth, closed apex, >18 months old
      1. Root canal
      2. Extraction

Patient Monitoring

I. Evaluate extraction sites for healing 10–14 days postoperatively.
II. Dental radiographs are taken following endodontic procedures to monitor for treatment success and signs of failure.
   A. Permanent tooth, open apex, vital pulp with vital pulpotomy performed
      Monitor with dental radiographs at 3–6-month intervals for apex closure and dentinal bridge formation (Harvey and Emily, 1993).
   B. Permanent tooth, open apex, non-vital pulp treated to induce apexification
      Monitor with dental radiographs at 3–6-month intervals until apexification is complete (Harvey and Emily, 1993).
   C. Permanent tooth, root canal performed
      1. Perform dental radiographs at 6–12 months after the procedure.
      2. Repeat x-rays when the animal is anesthetized for dental cleanings (i.e., annually).
      3. Evaluate for periapical lucency indicating periapical disease and root canal treatment failure, and retreat tooth if possible.
III. Instruct owners to monitor for clinical signs of endodontic failure, such as reluctance to chew or bite on "toys" or retrieve objects, altered eating behavior, facial swelling, or altered attitude (i.e., less active).

Bibliography

Beck ER, Withrow SJ, McChesney AE et al: Canine tongue tumors: a retrospective review of 57 cases. J Am Anim Hosp Assoc 22:525, 1986
Braund KG: Laryngeal paralysis-polyneuropathy complex in young dalmation dogs. p. 1136. In Kirk RW, Bonagura J (eds): Current Veterinary Therapy. WB Saunders, Philadelphia, 1995
Brewer WG Jr, Turrel JM: Radiotherapy and hyperthermia in

treatment of fibrosarcoma in the dog. J Am Vet Med Assoc 181:146, 1982

Brooks MB, Matus RE, Leifer CE et al: Chemotherapy versus chemotherapy plus radiotherapy in the treatment of tonsillar squamous cell carcinoma in the dog. J Vet Intern Med 2:206, 1988

Calvert CA: Canine viral papillomatosis. p. 288. In Greene CE (ed): Infectious Diseases of the Dog and Cat. WB Saunders, Philadelphia, 1990

Carpenter LG, Withrow SJ, Powers BE et al: Squamous cell carcinoma of the tongue in 10 dogs. J Am Anim Hosp Assoc 29:17, 1993

Ciekot PA, Powers BE, Withrow SJ et al: Histologically low-grade, yet biologically high-grade, fibrosarcomas of the mandible and maxilla in dogs: 25 cases (1982–1991). J Am Vet Med Assoc 204:610, 1994

Clark RW (ed): Medical Genetic and Behavioral Aspects of Purebred Cats. Forum Publications, Fairway, Kansas, 1992

Clark RW (ed): Medical Genetic and Behavioral Aspects of Purebred Dogs. Forum Publications, Fairway, Kansas, 1994

DeBowes L: Palatal defect and draining fistula at mucogingival junction secondary to malocclusion. Proc World Vet Dental Congress 8:109, 1994

Diebielzig RR, Goldschmidt MH, Brodey RS: The nomenclature of periodontal epulides in dogs. Vet Pathol 16:209, 1979

Diehl K, Rosychuk RAW: Feline gingivitis-stomatitis-pharyngitis. Vet Clin North Am [Small Anim Pract] 23:139, 1993

Evans SM, Shoter F: Canine oral nontonsillar squamous cell carcinoma. Vet Radiol 29:3, 1988

Goldschmidt MH: Benign and malignant neoplasms of domestic animals. Am J Dermatopathol 7 (Suppl):203, 1985

Gorman NT, Bright RM, Mays MB, Thrall DE: Chemotherapy of a recurrent acanthomatous epulis in a dog. J Am Vet Med Assoc 184:1158, 1984

Greene CE: Gastrointestinal and intra-abdominal infections. p. 125. In Greene CE (ed): Infectious Diseases of the Dog and Cat. WB Saunders, Philadelphia, 1990

Guilford WG: Diseases of the oral cavity and pharynx. p. 189. In Guilford WG, Center SA, Strombeck D et al (eds): Strombeck's Small Animal Gastroenterology. 3rd Ed. WB Saunders, Philadelphia, 1996

Hahn KA, DeNicola DB, Richardson RC et al: Canine oral malignant melanoma: prognostic utility of an alternative staging system. J Small Anim Pract 35:251, 1994

Harbour DA, Howard PE, Gaskell RM: Isolation of feline calicivirus and feline herpesvirus from domestic cats: 1980 to 1989. Vet Rec 128:77, 1991

Harvey CE: Inflammatory oral diseases in cats. J Am Anim Hosp Assoc 27:585, 1991

Harvey CE: Plasmacytic-lymphocytic stomatitis. p. 59. In August JR (ed): Consultations in Feline Internal Medicine. 2nd Ed. WB Saunders, Philadelphia, 1994

Harvey CE: Oral and pharyngeal infections in dogs and cats. Proc West Vet Conf 21, 1996

Harvey CE, Emily PP: Small Animal Dentistry. CV Mosby, Philadelphia, 1993

Harvey HJ, MacEwen EG, Braum D et al: Prognostic criteria for dogs with oral melanomas. J Am Vet Med Assoc 178:580, 1981

Jeglum KA, Sadanaga K: Oral tumors: the surgeon and the medical oncologist. Vet Clin North Am [Small Anim Pract] 26:145, 1996

Joffe DJ, Allen AL: Ulcerative eosinophilic stomatitis in three Cavalier King Charles spaniels. J Am Anim Hosp Assoc 31:34, 1995

Lobprise HB: Pedodontics. Proc Vet Dentistry Forum 7:25, 1993

Lyon KF: Subgingival odontoclastic resorptive lesions. Vet Clin North Am [Small Anim Pract] 22:1417, 1992

McChesney SL, Withrow SJ, Gillette EL et al: Radiotherapy of soft tissue sarcomas in dogs. J Am Vet Med Assoc 194:60, 1989

McKeever PJ, Klausner JS: Plant awn, candidal, nocardial, and necrotizing ulcerative stomatitis in the dog. J Am Anim Hosp Assoc 22:1, 1986

Norden DM: Normal development and congenital defects in the cat. p. 1248. In Kirk RW, Bonagura JD (eds): Current Veterinary Therapy XI: Small Animal Practice. WB Saunders, Philadelphia, 1992

Ogilvie GK, Moore AS: Tumors of the oral cavity. p. 320. In Ogilvie GK, Moore AS (eds): Managing the Veterinary Cancer Patient: A Practice Manual. Veterinary Learning Systems, Trenton, NJ, 1995

Page RL, Thrall DE: Clinical indications and applications of radiotherapy and hyperthermia in veterinary oncology. Vet Clin North Am [Small Anim Pract] 20:1075, 1990

Pedersen NC: Inflammatory oral cavity diseases of the cat. Vet Clin North Am [Small Anim Pract] 22:1323, 1992

Roe DA: Riboflavin deficiency: mucocutaneous signs of acute and chronic deficiency. Semin Dermatol 10:293, 1991

Spodnick GJ, Page RL: Canine and feline oropharyngeal neoplasms. pp 691–695. In Bonagura JD (ed): Current Veterinary Therapy XII: Small Animal Practice. WB Saunders, Philadelphia, 1995

Stebbins KE, Morse CC, Goldschmidt MH: Feline oral neoplasia: a ten year survey. Vet Pathol 26:121, 1989

Suter PF, Watrous BJ: Oropharyngeal dysphagias in the dog: a cinefluorographic analysis of experimentally induced and spontaneously occurring swallowing disorders. I. Oral and pharyngeal stage dysphagias. Vet Radiol 24:11, 1983

Tenorio AP, Franti CE, Madewell BR et al: Chronic oral infections of cats and their relationship to persistent oral carriage of feline calici, immunodeficiency or leukemia viruses. Vet Immunol Immunopathol 29:1, 1991

Thrall DE: Orthovoltage radiotherapy of acanthomatous epulides in 39 dogs. J Am Vet Med Assoc 184:826, 1984

Todoroff RJ, Brodey RS: Oral and pharyngeal neoplasia in the dog: a retrospective study of 361 cases. J Am Vet Med Assoc 175:567, 1979

Verstraete FJM, Ligthelm AJ, Weber A: The histological nature of epulides in dogs. J Comp Path 106:169, 1992

Waters L, Hopper CD, Gruffydd-Jones TJ et al: Chronic gingivitis in a colony of cats infected with feline immunodeficiency virus and feline calcivirus. Vet Rec 132:340, 1993

White RAS: The alimentary system. p. 237. In White RAS (ed): Manual of Small Animal Oncology. British Small Animal Veterinary Association, Cheltenham, England, 1991

White RAS, Gorman NT: Wide local excision of acanthomatous epulides in the dog. Vet Surgery 18:1, 1989

White SD, Rosychuk RAW, Janik TA et al: Plasma cell stomatitis-pharyngitis in cats: 40 cases (1973–91). J Am Vet Med Assoc 200:1377, 1992

Williams CA, Aller MS: Gingivitis/stomatitis in cats. Vet Clin North Am [Small Anim Pract] 22:1361, 1992

Withrow SJ: Tumors of the gastrointestinal system. A. Cancer of the oral cavity. p. 227. In Withrow SJ, MacEwen EG (eds): Small Animal Clinical Oncology. WB Saunders, Philadelphia, 1995

Wolf AM: Feline gingivitis, stomatitis and pharyngitis. p. 568. In Kirk RW, Bonagura JD (eds): Current Veterinary Therapy XI: Small Animal Practice. WB Saunders, Philadelphia, 1992

Zetner K, Steurer I: Long-term results of restoration of feline resorptive lesions with micro-glass-composite. J Vet Dent 12:15, 1995

28

Diseases of the Salivary Glands

Ronald M. Bright

INFLAMMATORY DISORDERS

Hypersialism

Definition

I. Excessive secretion of saliva usually secondary to other causes

II. Synonyms: sialorrhea, "drooling," ptyalism, hypersialosis

Causes

I. A congenital form exists.
   A. Giant-breed dogs have a lower lip conformation that allows saliva to escape from the oral cavity via the commissures.
   B. It has rarely been reported as a primary disorder of the parotid gland (Bedford, 1980; Harvey, 1981).

II. Cats are very sensitive to some oral, otic, or ophthalmic medications and may drool excessively.

III. Anxiety or marked contentment may initiate excessive drooling in cats.

IV. Ptyalism is an important sign in cats with congenital portosystemic shunts.

V. Other causes include the following.
   A. Inflammation of oral structures
   B. Esophageal or oropharyngeal foreign bodies
   C. Oropharyngeal neoplasia
   D. Feline viral diseases affecting the mouth: herpesvirus, calici virus
   E. Toxins such as organophosphates
   F. Mandibular gland infarction and necrosis (Kelly et al., 1979; Mawby et al., 1991; Spangler and Culbertson, 1991; Cooke and Guilford, 1992; Brooks et al., 1995)

Pathophysiology

I. Primary disease has been reported in dogs with parotid gland enlargement (hyperplasia) causing excessive salivation.

II. Secondary diseases cause salivation in several ways.
   A. Drooping lower lips of Newfoundland and St. Bernard dogs promote saliva flow from the oral cavity.
   B. Oral or esophageal inflammatory processes causing pain reduce swallowing and cause hypersalivation.
   C. Saliva production is stimulated by viruses that cause stomatitis and gingivitis and by organophosphates.
   D. Mechanical obstruction (neoplasia, foreign body) of the oral cavity or upper esophagus can lead to insufficient swallowing of saliva.
   E. Mandibular gland infarction results in necrosis of the gland, with drooling being one of the responses to injury.

Clinical Signs

I. The parotid glands are enlarged with primary disease.

II. Ropy saliva hangs from the commissures of lips in giant-breed dogs.

III. Excessive salivation begins immediately after application of topical medication around the head and neck, or following the oral administration of certain medications (cats).

IV. Signs of toxemia or uremia may be present.

V. Inappetence can accompany the primary signs.

VI. Additional signs of salivary gland infarction and necrosis are listed under Adenitis.

Diagnosis

I. Large parotid lymph nodes are palpated.

II. There is a painful response to mandibular gland palpation (necrosis).

III. Signalment includes giant-breed dogs.

IV. There is known exposure to organophosphates.

V. Oral examination findings may include masses (neoplasia), ulcerations, erosions, or foreign objects.

VI. Laboratory findings may be consistent with congenital portosystemic shunt.
VII. Systemic signs of viral diseases may be seen.

Treatment

I. Symptomatic short-term therapy with anticholinergic drugs can be tried.
   A. Glycopyrrolate 0.01 mg/kg SQ PRN
   B. Atropine 0.02–0.04 mg/kg SQ PRN
II. Ligation of the parotid duct (Gunn, 1985) has been advocated.
III. In giant-breed dogs, surgical correction of the lip deformity is palliative.
   A. Cheiloplasty
   B. Extirpation of mandibular and sublingual glands (bilateral)
IV. Treatment of oropharyngeal disease (foreign bodies, oral tumors) may ameliorate the signs.
V. Administer atropine and 2-PAM for organophosphate toxicity (see Chap. 124).
VI. In cats, discontinue medications that evoke excessive salivation.
VII. Anxiety-related drooling can be corrected by removing the stimulus.

Patient Monitoring

I. Atrophy of gland follows ligation of ducts after a short postoperative period of pain and swelling.
II. Dryness of oral cavity may be seen.
III. Surgery to correct anatomic defects in show dogs is unethical.

Adenitis

Definition

An inflammatory reaction involving a salivary gland

Causes

I. Penetration of a foreign body (usually sharp) may allow progression to an abscess (Lammerding, 1983).
II. Adenitis may be concurrent with a mucocele (Knecht, 1990).
III. Viral diseases may initiate an inflammatory response.
   A. Paramyxovirus (mumps) in a household with human mumps (Harvey, 1985)
   B. Secondary to systemic virus such as distemper or rabies (Spangler and Culbertson, 1991)
IV. Dog bites can result in trauma to a specific salivary gland.
V. It may be secondary to carnassial tooth infection (Harvey, 1989).
VI. Infarction can result in an inflammatory response.
   A. Primarily of mandibular salivary gland
   B. Sublingual gland in beagle (Spangler and Culbertson, 1991)

Pathophysiology

I. Virus, bacteria, or trauma can initiate an inflammatory response.

II. The parotid gland is vulnerable to traumatic injury because of its location and proximity to the ear canal.
III. Glandular swelling can result in pain (sometimes severe). The mandibular gland has a tight fibrous capsule.
   A. Pressure from the gland within a closed capsule resulting in ischemic necrosis or secondary metaplasia (Harvey, 1985; Brooks et al., 1995)
   B. Painful and hard salivary gland and mandibular lymph node enlargement
   C. Infarction involving the mandibular salivary gland in dogs (Spangler and Culbertson, 1991)
   D. Bacterial infection secondary to the inflammation
   E. Abscessation of the zygomatic salivary gland leading to retrobulbar abscessation and swelling

Clinical Signs

I. The parotid or sublingual/mandibular glands are involved most often.
   A. Painful, firm swelling of salivary gland
   B. Local heat
   C. Draining or enlarged lymph nodes
   D. Ptyalism
   E. Fever, anorexia
   F. Vomiting, nausea, gagging
   G. Pain with manipulation of the head and neck (Brooks et al., 1995)
   H. Mucopurulent discharge from duct opening
   I. Abscessation with cutaneous fistula
II. Zygomatic gland involvement occurs less often because of its protected location.
   A. Anorexia
   B. Reluctance or pain when attempting to open mouth
   C. Exophthalmos

Diagnosis

I. Clinical signs often provide a tentative diagnosis.
II. History of virus (mumps) in household occurs only rarely.
III. History of trauma or tooth abscess is variable.
IV. Fever and swelling just caudal to last upper molar are suggestive of (zygomatic) gland involvement.
V. Aspiration of the retrobulbar space with cytology reveals inflammation but is not specific for salivary adenitis.
VI. Ultrasonography helps define the retrobulbar lesion.
VII. Sialography is likely to be of little benefit.
VIII. Definitive diagnosis is difficult and may require histopathologic examination of an excised gland.

Differential Diagnosis

I. Salivary gland neoplasia is rarely seen (Carberry et al., 1988).
II. Abscessation of surrounding tissue may extend to a salivary gland.
III. A salivary mucocele or fistula is an important alternative to consider.

IV. Other causes of retrobulbar cellulitis must be considered (see Chap. 103).

Treatment

I. Systemic antibiotics against gram-positive organisms are given for 7–10 days, pending culture and sensitivity results.
II. Extract the carnassial tooth if it is thought to be the cause of the parotid adenitis or abscess.
III. Hot packs may be applied to the parotid gland area.
IV. Surgical excision of the gland may be needed in cases of unresponsive adenitis.

Patient Monitoring

I. A fistula may form despite appropriate therapy, especially if a foreign body is present.
II. Lack of response to antibiotic therapy suggests the presence of a foreign body or inappropriate choice of antibiotic.
III. Chronic lagophthalmos may occur if the zygomatic gland remains persistently enlarged.

SALIVARY GLAND FISTULA

Definition

A non-healing wound with a continuous thin serous discharge that sometimes increases with feeding

Causes

I. A traumatic event can lead to everted fistula formation.
   A. Sharp or blunt trauma
   B. Ear surgery or surgical drainage of an abscess
II. Infection and necrosis of the parotid salivary gland may result from extension of a neoplastic disease involving the mandibular lymph nodes.

Pathophysiology

I. A salivary duct can become traumatized as a result of a bite wound or surgery (parotid). Saliva then flows through the injured area and leaks through an opening in the skin.
II. Sharp or blunt trauma to the zygomatic gland can cause leakage into the periorbital space and may result in exophthalmos.
III. Continuous flow of saliva does not allow the fistula to scar over and heal.
IV. Secondary bacterial infection often occurs from devitalization and necrosis of glandular tissue.
V. A carnassial tooth abscess can involve adjacent structures, including the zygomatic salivary gland.

Clinical Signs

I. There is swelling in the neck region that is usually nonpainful.

II. There are open draining wounds with serous, sometimes foul-smelling fluid that increases in volume after eating.
III. Swelling under the eye is seen with zygomatic gland involvement.

Diagnosis

I. A history of blunt or sharp trauma to the face and neck area is suggestive.
II. Cytology of the fluid leaking from the fistula may help confirm salivary gland origin.
III. Sialography demonstrates contrast material escaping through the fistula.
IV. Pilocarpine given orally increases the flow of saliva through the fistulous tract(s).
V. Surgical exploration of the fistulous tract confirms its relationship with a salivary gland.

Differential Diagnosis

I. Tonsillar squamous cell carcinoma with metastasis to cervical lymph nodes may result in a similar clinical presentation.
II. Foreign bodies such as grass awns or wood splinters can form draining tracts.
III. Chronic infection secondary to previous ear surgery may be an underlying cause of a fistula forming on the lateral face.

Treatment

I. Salivary gland extirpation is the treatment of choice.
II. Ligation of the duct proximal to the fistula (when the mandibular and sublingual salivary glands are involved) causes cessation of flow.
III. Broad-spectrum antibiotics are given for secondary bacterial involvement for a 2–3 week period of time.

Patient Monitoring

I. Usually there is an immediate response to surgery.
II. Duct ligation may result in transient swelling.
III. The effect of empirical antibiotic therapy must be monitored carefully, because a lack of response may dictate a change in antibiotics or indicate the need for a culture and sensitivity test.

SALIVARY MUCOCELE

Definition and Causes

I. It is a collection of saliva in a nonepithelium-lined swelling that causes an inflammatory response in the surrounding tissues.
II. The exact cause is often unknown.
   A. Local trauma
   B. Occlusion of the duct (sialolith)
   C. Developmental defect
   D. Migration of plant materials through sublingual papilla
   E. Invasion of duct or gland by tumor

Pathophysiology

I. Following damage to a salivary gland or duct, saliva leaks out into tissues along the path of least resistance.
   A. Most commonly affects the sublingual gland
   B. May occasionally involve the mandibular or zygomatic gland
II. The most frequent site for collection of extravasated saliva is the ventral neck region.
III. Swelling may also occur in the pharyngeal area or under the tongue (ranula).
IV. Occasionally saliva may accumulate in the retrobulbar space from a zygomatic mucocele.
V. Saliva stimulates the formation of a sac lined with granulation and connective tissue.
VI. Rarely, the lining becomes mineralized.
VII. Sialoadenitis may precede the formation of a mucocele (Spangler and Culbertson, 1991).

Clinical Signs

I. The owner reports a slow development of a soft, fluctuant, non-inflamed, cool, nonpainful cervical mass.
II. Pain may possibly precede the swelling.
III. Swelling under the tongue (ranula) may occur alone or concurrently with a cervical swelling.
   A. Mastication difficulties
   B. Tongue carriage affected
   C. Excessive licking
   D. May be painful or bleed if traumatized by teeth
IV. Pharyngeal location may cause the following (Harvey, 1981; Weber et al., 1986).
   A. Dysphagia
   B. Inspiratory dyspnea: may be severe
V. Retrobulbar location (zygomatic mucocele) may induce the following.
   A. Exophthalmos
   B. Reluctance or difficulty in opening mouth (very uncommon)

Diagnosis

I. History of a slow developing cervical mass is a consistent finding.
II. Signalment is of some importance.
   A. More common in poodles and German shepherd dogs (Knecht, 1990)
   B. More common in dogs <3 years of age
   C. Occasionally seen in cats
III. Palpation of a soft, fluctuant, cool swelling (cervical location) is a typical finding.
IV. Cytology of a fine-needle aspirate may be helpful in confirming presence of saliva.
   A. Blood-tinged
   B. Tenacious, stringy, thick fluid
   C. Mucus, red blood cells seen with periodic acid–Schiff (PAS) stain
V. Radiography may be helpful but is generally unnecessary to reach a definitive diagnosis.
   A. Sialography is difficult and usually unnecessary.
   B. Ultrasonography may help differentiate mucocele from a granulomatous or neoplastic lesion.
VI. Histopathology demonstrates a nonepithelial lining with no secretory component.

Differential Diagnosis

I. A cervical or intermandibular abscess usually appears over a shorter period of time.
II. A branchial cyst (Clark et al., 1989) is a rarely seen cause of swelling in the neck region.
III. Neoplasms most likely to occur in this region include a cystadenoma or lymphoma.
IV. Thyroglossal duct cysts (Dallman and Johnson, 1986) are rare but can have some clinical similarities.
V. Other causes of pharyngeal obstruction must be considered when evaluating the pharyngeal form of a salivary mucocele.
   A. Neoplasia
   B. Foreign body
VI. Hematoma or seroma (following trauma) must also be ruled out.

Treatment

I. Drainage options are available and should be considered in some rare instances.
   A. Fine-needle aspirate
      1. High-risk animals unable to undergo anesthesia and surgery
      2. As a temporary measure in dogs with inspiratory distress related to a pharyngeal mucocele
   B. May have to be repeated every 2–3 weeks
II. Surgical extirpation is the procedure of choice.
   A. Removal of mandibular and sublingual glands and their corresponding ducts as far rostral as possible is preferred.
   B. Although the monostomatic portion of the sublingual gland is most often involved, the mandibular gland is removed concurrently because it shares a common capsule.
   C. Mandibular mucoceles are usually lateralized but can occasionally be located on the midline (intermandibular).
      1. To determine which gland needs to be removed, place the animal in dorsal recumbency and gently push on the fluid-filled mass.
      2. The fluid usually moves to the side of the affected gland and forms a protrusion just below the angle of the mandible.
      3. A ranula is sometimes present, and its location (left or right) helps determine which glands need to be removed.
      4. If doubt still exists as to which gland is involved, a cervical midline incision allows access to both sides.
      5. Alternatively, separate lateral incisions overlying the mandibular and sublingual glands on both sides can be used for the approach.
      6. Drainage of the cyst and excision of redundant skin can be done at the time of extirpation.

D. Treatment of zygomatic mucoceles may require exploration of the orbit via a lateral orbitotomy.

Patient Monitoring

I. If drains are placed in the cyst, they are usually removed in 48 hours.
II. The recurrence rate is low.
   A. If recurrence of a mucocele occurs, it may be necessary to remove the remaining and more cranially located polystomatic portions of the sublingual gland via an oral approach.
   B. Prognosis is good following extirpation of the affected gland.

SIALOLITHIASIS

Definition

I. It is a stone or concretion in the salivary duct.
II. The composition includes magnesium carbonate, calcium carbonate, and/or calcium phosphate (Gunn, 1985).
III. They are rare but can occur in the parotid duct.
IV. Soft calculi or mineralized structures (mucocele stones) may be found in a mucocele (Harvey, 1985).

Causes

I. The cause of actual stone formation is unknown, but stones are thought to occur secondary to inflammation.
II. Precipitations of fibrin and mucin form ''soft stones,'' which may be found in mucoceles.
III. ''Mucocele stones'' are actually sloughed fragments of the mucocele lining that have become mineralized.

Pathophysiology

I. A sialolith causes obstruction of the salivary duct.
II. The gland swells because of the lodgment of a stone in the duct.
III. Over time, the gland atrophies and ceases to function unless the stone is removed.
IV. Sialoliths do not cause mucoceles (Gunn, 1985; Harvey, 1985).

Clinical Signs

I. Swelling overlying the parotid gland may be present.
II. Pain on palpation of the salivary gland may be noted.

Diagnosis

I. Subcutaneous palpation of the stone through the oral mucosa or beneath the skin may be possible.
II. Stones may be visible on plain radiography (Harvey, 1985).
III. Retrograde sialography may be helpful in locating the site of obstruction.

Differential Diagnosis

I. Foreign body
II. Salivary adenitis
III. Salivary neoplasia

Treatment

I. Incise through the oral mucosa and wall of the duct if the sialolith is felt under the mucosa.
II. Resuturing of the duct or oral mucosa is not done, but rather healing by secondary intention is allowed.

Patient Monitoring

I. Although an open stoma may result in a fistula, suturing the duct may cause scarring and eventual stenosis and obstruction.
II. Complete obstruction of the duct by a stone may result in atrophy of the gland and loss of function if it is allowed to persist for a prolonged period of time.

NEOPLASIA

Definition and Causes

I. Neoplasia is rare in the dog and cat.
II. Benign lesions seem to be exclusive to the cat (Spangler and Culbertson, 1991).
III. Most tumors are malignant and are found much more frequently in the dog (Carberry et al., 1988).
   A. Adenocarcinomas are the most common type.
   B. Parotid and mandibular glands are more frequently affected.
   C. Occasionally the zygomatic gland is involved.

Pathophysiology

I. Tissue within the superficial submucosa of the oropharynx is the origin of these tumors (Spangler and Culbertson, 1991).
II. Regional lymph node involvement is common, but distant metastasis is slow to develop.

Clinical Signs

I. There is no breed or sex predilection, and most affected animals are older.
II. Often a tumor can develop within the salivary gland with minimal signs.
III. Salivary gland tumors are usually unilateral.
IV. Tumors may be detected early on routine physical examinations by palpating swelling of the gland.
V. Pain may be elicited on palpation of the affected gland.
VI. If the swelling is extensive, then other signs may be seen as a result of encroachment on surrounding tissues.
VII. A mucocele may also develop.
VIII. Exophthalmos may result from zygomatic gland tumors.

Diagnosis

I. Fine-needle aspirates may be diagnostic.
II. If fine-needle aspirates are negative, an incisional or excisional biopsy may be required.
III. Lymph node aspirates and thoracic radiography are done to stage the tumor.

Differential Diagnosis

I. Adenitis may cause similar clinical signs but is often bilateral.
II. Neoplasia of the mandibular lymph node would be the most common differential diagnosis to consider.
III. An abscess of the salivary gland may occur alone or in conjunction with a tumor.
IV. Myxosarcoma of the face or orbit should also be considered.

Treatment

I. Wide excision of the gland and associated lymph node is recommended.
   A. The parotid gland is difficult to remove because of its anatomic relationship with surrounding structures.
   B. Recurrence is common because of the inability to remove all neoplastic tissue.
II. Radiation therapy is considered an effective adjunctive treatment (Carberry et al., 1988).
III. Chemotherapy thus far is an unproven modality.

Patient Monitoring

I. Complete excision is unlikely but may rarely be curative if performed early and before local or distant metastasis occurs.
II. Lymph node palpation and examination of the original surgery site are performed 3 months after the original surgery.
III. If the 3-month examination reveals no recurrence, then monitoring every 6 months is advised.
IV. Prognosis is poor regardless of the treatment modality(ies) used.

Bibliography

Bedford PGC: Unilateral parotid hypersialism in a dachshund. Vet Rec 107:557, 1980

Brooks GC, Hottinger HA, Dunstan RW: Canine necrotizing sialometaplasia: a case report and review of the literature. J Am Anim Hosp Assoc 31:21, 1995

Carberry CA, Flanders JA, Harvey HJ, Ryan AM: Salivary gland tumors in dogs and cats: a literature and case review. J Am Anim Hosp Assoc 24:561, 1988

Clark DM, Kostolich M, Mosier D: Branchial cyst in a dog. J Am Vet Med Assoc 194:67, 1989

Cooke MM, Guilford WG: Salivary gland necrosis in a wire-haired fox terrier. NZ Vet J 40:69, 1992

Dallman MJ, Johnson EO: Thyroglossal duct cyst in a dog. J Am Anim Hosp Assoc 22:195, 1986

Gunn C: Lips, oral cavity and salivary glands. p. 221. In Gourley IM, Vasseur PB (eds): Textbook of Small Animal Surgery. JP Lippincott, Philadelphia, 1985

Harvey CE: Pharyngeal mucoceles in dogs. J Am Vet Med Assoc 178:1282, 1981

Harvey CE: Salivary gland disease. p. 188. In Harvey CE (ed): Veterinary Dentistry. WB Saunders, Philadelphia, 1985

Harvey CE: Oral, dental, pharyngeal, and salivary gland disorders. p. 1203. In Ettinger SJ (ed): Textbook of Veterinary Internal Medicine. 3rd Ed. WB Saunders, Philadelphia, 1989

Harvey CE: Oral cavity. p. 510. In Slatter DH (ed): Textbook of Small Animal Surgery. WB Saunders, Philadelphia, 1993

Kelly DF, Lucke VM, Lane JG et al: Salivary gland necrosis in dogs. Vet Rec 104:268, 1979

Knecht CD: Salivary glands. p. 197. In Bojrab MJ (ed): Pathophysiology in Small Animal Surgery. Lea & Febiger, Philadelphia, 1990

Lammerding JJ: Salivary glands. p. 126. In Bojrab MJ (ed): Current Techniques in Small Animal Surgery. 2nd Ed. Lea & Febiger, Philadelphia, 1983

Mawby DI, Bauer MS, Lloyd-Bauer PM, Clark EG: Vasculitis and necrosis of the mandibular salivary glands and chronic vomiting in a dog. Can Vet J 32:562, 1991

Schmidt GM, Betts CW: Zygomatic salivary mucoceles in the dog. J Am Vet Med Assoc 172:940, 1978

Spangler WL, Culbertson MR: Salivary gland disease in dogs and cats: 245 cases (1985–1988). J Am Vet Med Assoc 198:465, 1991

Weber WJ, Hobson HP, Wilson SR: Pharyngeal mucoceles in dogs. Vet Surg 15:5, 1986

29

Diseases of the Esophagus

Albert E. Jergens

CONGENITAL DISORDERS

Vascular Ring Anomalies

See Chap. 6.

Disorders of Motility

Definition

I. Congenital idiopathic megaesophagus (CIM), esophageal hypomotility in Shar peis, and deranged esophageal motility in puppies and kittens result in abnormal peristaltic function of the esophageal body.
II. Functional defects in the upper and lower sphincters are absent.

Causes

I. Congenital megaesophagus is inherited in the wire-haired fox terrier and miniature schnauzer.
II. Increased incidence of CIM is seen in German shepherd dogs, Great Danes, Irish setters, Labrador retrievers, and Shar peis (Knowles et al., 1990; Strombeck and Guilford, 1990).
III. Esophageal dysfunction in Shar peis may also result from segmental hypomotility and esophageal redundancy (Stickle et al., 1992).
IV. Canine CIM is believed to be caused by immaturity of esophageal innervation (Leib and Hall, 1984).
V. Congenital megaesophagus in cats is rare, but Siamese cats may be predisposed (Hoenig et al., 1990).

Pathophysiology

I. Alterations in motor function cause esophageal dilatation and defective esophageal transport of ingesta and liquids.
II. Degrees of severity vary from segmental hypomotility to generalized dilatation with complete paralysis.

III. Dogs may show improvement in function with age as the esophagus matures.

Clinical Signs

I. Regurgitation of food and water through the mouth or nares (primary sign)
   A. Timing of regurgitation episodes after eating is extremely variable.
   B. Frequency of regurgitation is variable and implies no specific cause.
II. Profuse salivation with dysphagia
III. Fetid breath with ingesta fermentation
IV. Weight loss with failure to thrive
V. Respiratory distress (cough, dyspnea, tachypnea) as a consequence of aspiration pneumonia

Diagnosis

I. Survey radiography of the neck and thorax
   A. It confirms the presence of a dilated air-, fluid-, or ingesta-filled esophagus.
   B. Luminal air is not pathognomonic for dysmotility and may accumulate as a consequence of aerophagia or during anesthesia (Stickle and Love, 1989).
   C. Pulmonary alveolar opacities are seen with aspiration pneumonia.
II. Contrast radiography: esophagram
   A. It is indicated if survey films are questionable.
   B. Barium contrast agents are rapidly cleared from the normal esophagus via peristaltic waves.
   C. Intraluminal retention of contrast material is abnormal and implies defective motility.
   D. Fluoroscopy (if available) provides useful information concerning the magnitude of esophageal hypomotility.

Differential Diagnosis

I. Other causes for esophageal dysmotility in young animals include obstructive lesions (common) and acquired diseases (uncommon).

II. Esophageal obstruction may be caused by foreign bodies, strictures, and vascular ring anomalies.

III. See Table 29–1 for acquired causes of esophageal hypomotility.

Treatment

I. Medical therapy is largely symptomatic because the cause for hypomotility remains ill defined.
   A. Feed animals from an elevated platform to allow gravity to assist in ingesta movement.
   B. Feed multiple small meals daily to minimize esophageal dilatation and pulmonary aspiration.
   C. Vary consistency of the food (slurry vs. bulk) to see which diet is best tolerated.
   D. Cachectic/debilitated animals are best fed via gastrostomy tube.
   E. Aspiration pneumonia is treated with broad-spectrum antibiotics.
   F. Use of promotility drugs is controversial.
      1. Cisapride (Propulsid) 0.5 mg/kg PO BID may augment peristalsis in cats (Washabau and Hall, 1995).
      2. Cisapride is less likely to be of benefit with canine hypomotility.

II. Surgical therapy for CIM is not warranted.
   A. Achalasia of the lower sphincter is not present and does not contribute to megaesophagus (Sokolvsky, 1972; Strombeck and Troya, 1976).
   B. Complications of lower sphincter myotomies include gastroesophageal reflux and gastric herniation.

Table 29–1. *Some Diseases Associated with Megaesophagus and Esophageal Hypomotility*

Neuromuscular
- Congenital megaesophagus
- Idiopathic megaesophagus (hereditary?)
- Myasthenia gravis
- Systemic lupus erythematosus
- Polymyositis/polymyopathy
- Botulism
- Tetanus
- Canine distemper
- Dysautonomia

Toxicity
- Lead
- Thallium
- Anticholinesterase

Miscellaneous
- Hypoadrenocorticism
- Hypothyroidism
- Pyloric stenosis
- Gastric dilatation or volvulus
- Esophagitis

Adapted from Jones BD, Jergens AE, Guilford WG: Diseases of the esophagus. p. 1262. In Ettinger SJ (ed): Textbook of Veterinary Internal Medicine. 3rd Ed. Philadelphia, WB Saunders, 1989.

Patient Monitoring

I. Reevaluate at 1–2 month intervals to monitor disease progression and nutritional status.

II. Repeat thoracic radiographs (± esophagram) to assess esophageal dilatation.

III. Prognosis with CIM is guarded to poor.
   A. Response to medical therapy is best when diagnosed and treated early (<6 months old).
   B. Esophageal function spontaneously improves in some animals as they mature (Diamant et al., 1974).
   C. Many animals die from recurrent aspiration pneumonia.

IV. Shar peis with hypomotility warrant a guarded to good prognosis because esophageal function often improves with age.

Hiatal Hernia

Definition

I. Sliding hiatal hernia is an abnormal protrusion of the abdominal esophagus, gastroesophageal junction, and/or stomach into the thoracic cavity through the esophageal hiatus in the diaphragm (Ellison et al., 1987).

II. Both congenital and acquired forms of hiatal hernia are recognized.

III. Congenital hiatal hernias are most common and are best recognized in young Shar peis (Callan et al., 1993).

Causes

I. Congenital hiatal hernias occur as developmental defects to the esophageal hiatus or phrenicoesophageal ligament.

II. Acquired hiatal hernias usually result from trauma.

Pathophysiology

I. Displacement of the gastroesophageal junction occurs secondary to stretching of the phrenicoesophageal ligament, and the hiatus must be of adequate diameter to permit protrusion.

II. Inspiration (negative intrathoracic pressure) may contribute to intrathoracic herniation.

III. Most sliding hernias are intermittent.

Clinical Signs

I. Signs of reflux esophagitis predominate.
   A. Persistent regurgitation
   B. Vomiting, occasional hematemesis
   C. Hypersalivation

II. Respiratory distress may occur as a consequence of herniation and aspiration pneumonia.

III. Some animals are asymptomatic, presumably because of absence of reflux esophagitis.

Diagnosis

I. Thoracic radiography
   A. Survey radiographs often reveal a caudodorsal soft tissue opacity.
   B. Barium positive contrast studies confirm herniation of the stomach into the distal esophagus.
   C. Esophageal dilatation and alveolar infiltrates may also be seen.
II. Endoscopy
   A. Evidence of reflux esophagitis (mucosal erythema, erosions) may be observed.
   B. Gastroscopy reveals cranial displacement of the gastroesophageal junction and an enlarged esophageal hiatus.

Differential Diagnosis

I. Congenital megaesophagus
II. Miscellaneous esophageal motility disturbances
III. Esophageal obstruction caused by foreign body, stricture, or vascular ring anomaly
IV. Periesophageal hiatal hernia, gastroesophageal intussusception

Treatment

I. Institute medical therapy for reflux esophagitis if present (see Esophagitis).
II. Treat aspiration pneumonia with broad-spectrum antibiotics.
III. Consider surgical stabilization of the esophageal hiatus.
   A. Recommended techniques include transabdominal diaphragmatic crural apposition, esophagopexy, and left fundic tube gastropexy (Ellison et al., 1987).
   B. Fundoplication is generally not necessary.

Patient Monitoring

I. Perform postsurgical thoracic radiography to assess esophageal dilatation and aspiration pneumonia if present.
II. Continue medical therapy for reflux esophagitis and aspiration pneumonia as needed.
III. A good prognosis is warranted in animals with successful surgery.
IV. A more guarded prognosis is given to animals with concurrent esophageal motility disturbances.

DEGENERATIVE DISORDERS

Adult-Onset Megaesophagus

Definition

I. It is a generalized esophageal dilatation and aperistalsis that manifests in animals after maturity.
II. Adult-onset idiopathic megaesophagus is a dilatation of unknown cause.

III. Adult-onset acquired megaesophagus is dilatation where a cause can be identified.
IV. Adult-onset megaesophagus is a common cause for regurgitation in dogs but is uncommon in cats.

Causes

I. Etiopathogenesis in many cases is unknown, leading to a classification of idiopathic.
II. Numerous disease conditions have been associated with, or hypothesized to cause, esophageal dilatation.
III. These acquired (secondary) causes include neuromuscular diseases, immune-mediated disorders, hormonal imbalances, toxicities, and inflammation (Guilford, 1990) (see Table 29–1).

Pathophysiology

I. Any disruption of the esophageal musculature or of the central (swallowing center), afferent, or efferent pathways that control esophageal motility may predispose to megaesophagus. Some dogs with acquired megaesophagus appear to have defects in the afferent neural pathway (Washabau and Gaynor, 1996).
II. The absence of sufficient primary and secondary esophageal peristaltic waves leads to accumulation of ingesta, esophageal dilatation, and esophageal dysphagia.

Clinical Signs

I. Regurgitation of food and liquids occurs, but there is considerable variability in the timing of regurgitation episodes following meal ingestion.
II. Odynophagia (painful swallowing) is seen with inflammation or excessive dilatation and is evidenced by hypersalivation, repeated swallowing attempts, and postural changes in neck position.
III. Halitosis is associated with fermentation of retained ingesta.
IV. Respiratory distress (moist cough, respiratory crackles, dyspnea) may occur as a consequence of aspiration pneumonia.
V. Severe cachexia/debilitation may result from malnutrition.
VI. Signs associated with secondary causes may be seen.
   A. Muscle pain and stiff gait with polymyositis
   B. Weakness with neuromuscular disease
   C. Gastrointestinal signs with lead toxicity or Addison's disease

Diagnosis

I. An accurate patient history is extremely important.
   A. Failure to distinguish regurgitation from vomiting results in misdiagnosis.
   B. Suspect megaesophagus in any adult animal, particularly dogs, with a history of regurgitation.
II. Physical examination may provide clues of secondary causes of megaesophagus.
   A. Note muscle pain, weakness, neurologic deficits, and altered states of mentation.

B. Dermatologic abnormalities may be seen with hypothyroidism.

III. Radiography is warranted.

A. Survey radiographs of the neck and thorax usually reveal the presence of a dilated air-, fluid-, or ingesta-filled esophagus.

B. Pulmonary alveolar opacities are seen with aspiration pneumonia.

C. Barium contrast radiography (esophagram) confirms dilatation and provides evidence of other structural abnormalities (i.e., redundancy).

D. Fluoroscopy (if available) provides useful information concerning the magnitude of esophageal dysfunction.

IV. Laboratory tests may be helpful.

A. A minimum laboratory database includes a complete blood count, serum biochemical profile, and urinalysis.

B. Perform creatine kinase assay to rule out myopathy/myositis and serum cholesterol measurement to rule out hypothyroidism.

C. An acetylcholine receptor antibody titer is performed in all cases of unexplained megaesophagus when focal myasthenia gravis is suspected (Shelton et al., 1990).

D. Additional laboratory tests are performed on the basis of clinical suspicion (Table 29–2).

V. Esophagoscopy is rarely required for the diagnosis of megaesophagus except when neoplasia or other obstructive disorders are suspected.

Differential Diagnosis

I. Obstruction caused by foreign bodies, granulomas, strictures, or periesophageal masses

Table 29–2. *Suggested Diagnostic Tests in Animals with Megaesophagus*

First Choice Tests
- Complete blood count
- Serum biochemistries (include cholesterol)
- Urinalysis
- Thoracic radiographs
- Esophagram

Second Choice Tests
- Antinuclear antibodies
- Acetylcholine receptor antibody titer[a]
- T$_4$; thyroid-stimulating hormone/adrenocorticotropic hormone stimulation tests
- Creatine kinase

Tertiary Tests
- Electromyelogram
- Muscle/nerve biopsy
- Toxicology
- Cerebrospinal fluid tap/analysis
- Central nervous system imaging

[a]Comparative Neuromuscular Laboratory, Basic Science Building, Room B200, University of California, San Diego, La Jolla, CA 92093-0614.

Adapted from Twedt DC: Diseases of the esophagus. p. 1130. In Ettinger SJ, Feldman EC (eds): Textbook of Veterinary Internal Medicine. 4th Ed. Philadelphia, WB Saunders, 1995.

II. Severe esophagitis, diverticulum (rare)

III. Esophageal neoplasia

Treatment

I. Animals with acquired forms of megaesophagus are treated specifically for the disorder causing the esophageal dilatation whenever possible, and some may show improvement in esophageal motor function.

II. Idiopathic forms of megaesophagus and those acquired forms that fail to respond to specific medical therapy are managed symptomatically.

A. Feed from an elevated position to assist passage of ingesta to the stomach.

B. Frequent, small meals are fed to meet daily caloric requirements.

C. Vary consistency of the food (gruel vs. bulky boluses) to see which diet is best tolerated. In general, solid boluses are more likely to stimulate better peristaltic contractions.

D. Animals with severe aspiration pneumonia require special attention.

1. Gastrostomy tube feedings provide nutritional support and lessen the risk for aspiration.

2. Broad-spectrum antibiotics are used to combat bacterial pathogens.

E. Promotility drugs (cisapride, metoclopramide) are currently of unproven benefit.

1. Cisapride (Propulsid) 0.5 mg/kg PO BID may improve esophageal hypomotility in cats.

2. Anecdotal reports indicate possible clinical improvement in some dogs with megaesophagus (Tams, 1994).

F. Surgical therapy for adult-onset megaesophagus is not recommended.

Patient Monitoring

I. Reevaluate at 1–2 month intervals to monitor disease progression.

II. Repeat thoracic radiographs to assess esophageal dilatation and aspiration pneumonia.

III. Prognosis with adult-onset megaesophagus is generally poor.

A. Animals with idiopathic disease usually die or are euthanized because of their disease.

B. Animals with acquired disease may respond to specific drug therapy.

C. The prognosis in dogs with megaesophagus caused by focal myasthenia gravis is favorable. Up to one half of affected dogs respond to supportive therapy (Shelton et al., 1990).

Diverticula

Definition

I. These are pouch-like dilatations of the esophageal wall.

II. Diverticula are rare in both the dog and cat.

III. Diverticula may be congenital or acquired in origin.

IV. Acquired diverticula are classified as either pulsion or traction forms (Duda et al., 1985).

Causes

I. Congenital diverticula are attributable to developmental abnormalities of the esophagus.
II. Pulsion diverticula result from conditions of increased esophageal intraluminal pressure (such as stricture or foreign body).
III. Traction diverticula result from periesophageal inflammatory processes. Contraction of postinflammatory fibrosis leads to eversion and outpouching of the esophageal wall.

Pathophysiology

I. Accumulation of ingesta (impaction) within diverticula leads to esophageal inflammation.
II. Large diverticula disturb normal esophageal motility.
III. Small diverticula may be subclinical.

Clinical Signs

I. Signs are most often seen with large, multilobulated diverticula.
II. Postprandial regurgitation results from mechanical obstruction and motility disturbances.
III. Odynophagia and retching are common.
IV. Severe cases with mucosal ulceration may eventually perforate and cause signs of mediastinitis and respiratory distress.

Diagnosis

I. Thoracic radiography
   A. Survey films show an air or soft tissue opacity adjacent to the esophagus.
   B. Barium contrast procedures show pooling of contrast material within the diverticulum.
II. Endoscopy
   A. Confirms the size of the defect and degree of food impaction
   B. Allows for critical assessment of associated mucosal defects such as ulceration

Differential Diagnosis

I. Normal esophageal redundancy
   A. It is especially seen in young brachycephalic breeds and Shar peis.
   B. Repeated radiography with the neck extended removes the esophageal ''slack.''
II. Esophageal foreign body
III. Periesophageal abscess, granuloma, or neoplasm

Treatment

I. Surgical resection
   A. Diverticulectomy is the preferred therapy.
   B. Large diverticula require greater excision and reconstruction of the esophageal wall.

II. Medical therapy
   A. Traction diverticula are treated with broad-spectrum antibiotics, and pulsion diverticula are treated for their specific cause (see Esophagitis, Stricture).
   B. Feed frequent meals from an upright position.
   C. Provide animals with a semi-liquid or liquid diet to minimize ingesta impaction in the lesion.
   D. Postoperative antibiotics decrease ingesta leakage and bacterial contamination.

Patient Monitoring

I. Monitor body temperature, white blood cell count, and demeanor for postoperative complications such as mediastinitis, pleuritis, and esophagopulmonary fistula formation.
II. Esophageal stricture may result from esophageal resection.
III. Repeat survey and contrast radiographs postoperatively to evaluate for additional morphologic and functional defects.
IV. Animals with esophageal hypomotility are treated symptomatically as for megaesophagus (see earlier).

INFLAMMATORY DISORDERS

Esophagitis

Definition

I. Inflammation of the esophageal wall ranges from mild mucosal inflammation to severe transmural involvement.
II. Lesions may occur from both acute and chronic insults.
III. Reflux esophagitis appears to be common in brachycephalic breeds as a consequence of their narrowed upper airways (Twedt, 1995).

Causes

I. Gastroesophageal (GE) reflux with lower sphincter incontinence may be caused by general anesthesia, hiatal defects, persistent vomiting, and anticholinergic therapy (Strombeck and Harrold, 1985; Dent et al., 1988).
II. Reflux may also occur around malpositioned nasogastric and pharyngostomy tubes that extend through the lower sphincter and into the stomach.
III. Ingestion of caustic agents such as acids, alkalis, or corrosive drugs such as pills or capsules that are retained in the esophagus may be a cause.
IV. Other causes include the following.
   A. Acute or persistent vomiting
   B. Thermal burns
   C. Physical trauma from esophageal foreign bodies
   D. Infectious agents (uncommon)

Pathophysiology

I. Esophageal injury secondary to GE reflux occurs from the following.

A. Refluxed gastric fluid usually contains acid, pepsin, trypsin, and bile salts, which are directly injurious to the mucosa.

B. Prolonged acidification of the esophageal mucosa and reduced or absent esophageal clearance (often associated with anesthesia) contribute to the pathogenesis of inflammation (Strombeck and Guilford, 1990).

C. Reflux of alkaline duodenogastric contents and bile also produces inflammatory changes in the wall of the esophagus.

II. Drug/chemical-induced esophagitis is affected by other factors.

A. Esophageal damage is caused by changes in mucosal pH, hyperosmolarity, and unknown mechanisms.

B. It is compounded in animals with concurrent esophageal motility disturbances.

III. Mild esophagitis is usually limited to the mucosa and heals quickly without fibrosis.

IV. Severe esophagitis extends into the muscular layer and may cause persistent ulceration, stricture formation, and esophageal perforation.

V. Focal or generalized disturbances in esophageal motility may accompany esophagitis.

Clinical Signs

I. Signs vary with the severity of esophageal inflammation.

A. Mild esophagitis may be asymptomatic.

B. Moderate to severe esophagitis causes anorexia, dysphagia, odynophagia, and hypersalivation.

II. Regurgitation is usually intermittent, but it may be persistent. Thick, ropey saliva that is blood-tinged is often expelled.

III. Occasional vomiting may be noted.

IV. Gradual weight loss occurs with chronicity.

Diagnosis

I. History

A. Consistent with a history of recent anesthesia, ingestion of foreign material, vomiting, or other factors associated with decreased lower esophageal sphincter tone

B. Progressive dysphagia with severe esophagitis

II. Physical examination

A. May be non-contributory with mild disease

B. Pain on cervical neck palpation

C. Evidence of glossitis/pharyngitis following ingestion of caustic substances

III. Radiography

A. Survey radiographs are often unremarkable.

1. Small accumulations of air within the lumen secondary to motility disturbances

2. Caudodorsal soft tissue opacity in the thorax indicative of hiatal herniation

B. Barium contrast procedures are usually required.

1. Liquid barium pools at sites of deranged motility and outlines mucosal irregularities.

2. Narrowing of esophageal lumen is seen with stricture.

3. Contrast examination with fluoroscopy (if available) allows visualization of defective bolus transport and gastroesophageal reflux.

IV. Endoscopy

A. Endoscopic examination is the most reliable means to diagnose esophagitis (Tams, 1990).

B. Lesions are most prominent in the distal esophagus, adjacent to and including the lower esophageal sphincter.

C. Mild cases often appear normal, but subtle lesions such as mild erythema and focal petechiae may be seen.

D. More advanced cases show marked erythema, multifocal petechiae, erosions, and mucosal irregularity (granularity).

E. Presence of GE reflux and a dilated lower esophageal sphincter are suggestive of a reflux disorder.

Differential Diagnosis

I. Megaesophagus and other acquired causes for esophageal hypomotility

II. Esophageal stricture

III. Constriction from vascular ring or periesophageal mass

IV. Hiatal hernia

V. Gastritis, gastric ulceration

Treatment

I. Immediate treatment for caustic or thermal insults

A. Eliminate offending agent.

B. Do not induce emesis.

C. Orally administer neutralizing compounds, followed by suction evacuation of gastric contents if possible.

1. Use magnesium oxide solution (1:25 dilution with warm water) or milk of magnesia for unabsorbed acids.

2. For caustic alkalis, use vinegar (diluted 1:4 with water) or lemon juice.

D. Contact the National Animal Poison Control Center (217-333-2053) for specific instructions.

E. Anesthesia-related GE reflux is manually suctioned from the esophageal lumen.

II. Dietary modification

A. With acute esophagitis, promote esophageal rest by withholding food and/or water for 24–48 hours.

B. Once feeding resumes, provide small frequent meals of a low-fat, high-protein diet to maximize lower esophageal sphincter tone (Jones et al., 1989).

C. Severe esophagitis necessitates gastrostomy tube placement for nutritional support and to bypass the inflamed esophagus.

III. Mucosal protectants

A. They are indicated following ingestion of caustic agents and with esophageal erosions.

B. Topical sucralfate (Carafate) promotes esophageal healing and mucosal cytoprotection (Katz et al., 1988).

C. Crush sucralfate 1 g and mix with 10 ml water to make a slurry; give 5–10 ml of slurry PO TID-QID.

IV. Histamine H$_2$-receptor antagonists or proton pump inhibitors to reduce gastric acidity and the effects of GE reflux (Tytgat et al., 1990)

  A. Cimetidine (Tagamet) 1–4 mg/kg PO TID-QID

  B. Ranitidine (Zantac) 2 mg/kg PO BID-TID

  C. Famotidine (Pepcid) 0.5–1 mg/kg PO SID-BID

  D. Omeprazole (Prilosec) 2 mg/kg PO SID

  E. H$_2$-blockers and omeprazole not used concurrently

  F. Omeprazole for severe cases of esophagitis

V. Promotility drugs to enhance gastric emptying and increase lower esophageal sphincter tone (Washabau and Hall, 1995)

  A. Metoclopramide (Reglan) 0.2–0.4 mg/kg PO TID-QID

  B. Cisapride (Propulsid) 0.1 mg/kg PO BID-TID

  C. Administered 30 minutes before feeding

VI. Surgical therapy uncommonly required (except for repair of hiatal hernia)

Patient Monitoring

I. Continue bland diet for 3–4 weeks.

II. Duration of drug therapy is empirical and varies with severity of signs and endoscopic lesions.

  A. Mild lesions are treated for 5–7 days.

  B. Moderate to severe esophagitis is treated for 3–4 weeks.

III. Complications may arise with severe disease.

  A. Segmental or generalized esophageal hypomotility may occur.

  B. Strictures may develop.

IV. Prognosis in most cases of esophagitis (including GE reflux) is good with appropriate medical management.

Fistula

Definition

I. Fistula is an abnormal communicating tract between the esophagus and usually the respiratory system (esophagopulmonary, esophagotracheal, and esophagobronchial fistula).

II. Leakage of esophageal contents into adjacent tissues results in their contamination.

III. It is relatively uncommon in the dog and cat.

Causes

I. Usually results from esophageal foreign bodies that cause perforation of the esophagus

II. Less commonly seen as a consequence of ruptured diverticulum, neoplasia, or periesophageal inflammation

Pathophysiology

I. Chronic mural pressure by an intraluminal foreign body induces mucosal ischemia and eventual necrosis.

II. Healing leads to development of a fibrous tract that invades the adjacent tissue.

III. A communicating tract develops, with resultant airway contamination from esophageal contents.

IV. The most common locations for acquired fistulas are the right caudal lung lobe in dogs and the left caudal and accessory lobes in cats (Park, 1984).

Clinical Signs

I. Coughing and respiratory distress occur during swallowing. Coughing is most pronounced after the ingestion of fluids.

II. Dysphagia and regurgitation are associated with intraluminal foreign bodies.

III. Anorexia, lethargy, weight loss, and fever are seen with mediastinitis and/or bronchopneumonia.

IV. Crackles may be auscultated over affected lung regions.

Diagnosis

I. Survey thoracic radiographs may reveal a radiodense foreign object in the esophagus, alveolar pulmonary opacities, or pulmonary consolidation.

II. Positive contrast esophagram confirms the esophago-airway communication. Avoid iodinated contrast agents that are hyperosmolar and that might promote pulmonary edema.

III. Endoscopic examination is of limited value in confirming a small fistula. It may be useful in detecting mucosal inflammation or retained foreign material.

IV. Laboratory tests (hemogram) may reflect inflammation and non-regenerative anemia.

Differential Diagnosis

I. Aspiration or lobar pneumonia, pulmonary abscess, or granuloma

II. Esophageal foreign body or diverticulum

III. Various causes of oropharyngeal dysphagia

Treatment

I. Surgical correction of the fistulous tract is required.

II. Lobectomy may be necessary as a result of pulmonary consolidation or foreign material contained within the airways.

III. Symptomatic medical therapy includes esophageal rest, dietary manipulation, and broad-spectrum antibiotics for aspiration pneumonia.

Patient Monitoring

I. Postoperatively monitor temperature and respiratory signs, and repeat thoracic radiographs.

II. Complications include dehiscence, sepsis, stricture,

pneumothorax, and pulmonary abscessation and warrant a guarded prognosis for recovery.

III. A good prognosis is given to animals following successful surgery.

NEOPLASIA

Definition

I. Primary tumors of the esophagus are rare in the dog and cat.

II. Neoplasms may also occur as metastatic lesions or as periesophageal masses.

III. Both benign and malignant tumors are seen.

Causes

I. Malignant tumors
   A. Fibrosarcoma in the dog and squamous cell carcinoma in the cat are most common (Withrow, 1989).
   B. Osteosarcomas, undifferentiated carcinomas, and leiomyosarcomas occur less frequently.
   C. Esophageal sarcoma in dogs may be associated with *Spirocerca lupi* infection.

II. Benign tumors
   A. Leiomyomas are the most common benign tumors.
   B. Leiomyomas may be incidental findings and frequently occur near the lower esophageal sphincter.

III. Periesophageal tumors arising from a variety of adjacent structures
   A. Lymph nodes
   B. Thyroid
   C. Thymus and heart base

Pathophysiology

I. Esophageal and periesophageal tumors usually encroach into the esophageal lumen, causing progressive intrinsic or extrinsic obstruction.

II. Primary and metastatic tumors may also invade the esophageal wall, disrupting esophageal motility.

III. Both mechanical obstruction and dysmotility may contribute to progressive esophageal dysphagia.

Clinical Signs

I. Most animals are middle-aged or older.

II. Signs are consistent with a slowly progressive stenosis.
   A. Regurgitation, dysphagia, and vomiting with lower sphincter involvement
   B. Anorexia, weight loss, and depression with advanced disease

III. Palpable neck mass or cervical dilatation may be associated with megaesophagus.

IV. Dyspnea or cough is caused by airway impingement or aspiration pneumonia.

Diagnosis

I. History of progressive esophageal dysphagia in middle-aged or older animals

II. Physical examination
   A. Palpable neck mass, cervical dilatation
   B. ± Crackles on thoracic auscultation

III. Survey radiography
   A. Cervical tumors cause tracheal deviation away from the mass.
   B. Intrathoracic tumors appear as soft tissue opacities ± mineralization within the mediastinum.
   C. Intraluminal air may be present and facilitate recognition of mass lesions, or generalized esophageal dilatation may be visible.
   D. Pulmonary opacities may occur secondary to metastatic disease or aspiration pneumonia.
   E. Hypertrophic osteopathy is reported in dogs with esophageal fibrosarcoma.

IV. Contrast radiography
   A. It is useful in detecting mucosal irregularities and stenosis caused by intrinsic/extrinsic compression.
   B. Fluoroscopy confirms deranged esophageal motility.

V. Endoscopy
   A. Esophagoscopy allows visual inspection of esophageal mucosa and permits selection of a biopsy site.
   B. Endoscopic biopsy of the esophagus is difficult because the mucosa is tough and it is difficult to position the biopsy instrument perpendicular to the mucosa.
   C. Biopsies with small pinch forceps often provide only superficial epithelia. Better specimens are obtained with a suction capsule biopsy instrument.

VI. Ultrasonography: helpful in localizing and performing biopsies on some cervical tumors

VII. Surgical biopsy: definitive diagnosis

Differential Diagnosis

I. Esophagitis

II. Esophageal hypomotility of varied causes

III. Hiatal hernia

IV. Foreign body granuloma

V. Benign periesophageal obstruction caused by reactive lymphadenopathy, granuloma, or abscess

Treatment

I. Treatment options are extremely limited for malignant tumors.
   A. Many tumors are quite advanced at the time of diagnosis.
   B. Their locally aggressive nature precludes successful surgical removal.
   C. Chemotherapy, radiation therapy, and surgery all tend to provide poor results.

II. Benign esophageal tumors, such as leiomyoma, generally have a good prognosis after successful surgery (Rolfe et al., 1994).

Patient Monitoring

I. Prognosis is grave for malignant neoplasia.
II. Symptomatic therapy with upright feedings, gastrostomy tube placement, and antibiotics for aspiration pneumonia is palliative at best.

TRAUMA

Foreign Bodies

Definition

I. The ingestion of foreign bodies is a common cause of dysphagia in the dog, but is uncommon in cats.
II. Foreign bodies lodge most commonly at points of minimal esophageal distention, including the thoracic inlet, base of the heart, and diaphragmatic hiatus (Roudebush et al., 1986).

Causes

I. Objects ingested often include bones, fish hooks, needles, sticks, and toys.
II. Severity of clinical signs is related to the size of the foreign body and duration of esophageal obstruction.

Pathophysiology

I. Retained foreign bodies cause partial or complete mechanical obstruction.
II. Esophageal muscle spasm and tissue edema occur around the foreign body, making passage more difficult.
III. Mucosal abrasion, laceration, and perforation may occur with sharp or angular objects.
IV. Sustained pressure necrosis may also cause fistula formation, stricture, and perforation.

Clinical Signs

I. Small foreign bodies may be easily passed, and signs are not observed.
II. Other objects cause signs of partial to complete esophageal obstruction.
  A. Regurgitation of food and water
  B. Hypersalivation
  C. Dysphagia, odynophagia
  D. Persistent gulping or swallowing movements
  E. Anorexia from esophageal pain
  F. Respiratory signs from airway impingement, mediastinitis, or aspiration pneumonia

Diagnosis

I. History of foreign body ingestion
II. Physical examination
  A. Variable, ranging from unremarkable to the presence of halitosis as a consequence of tissue necrosis
  B. Large cervical foreign bodies possibly palpable
  C. Respiratory crackles with aspiration pneumonia
  D. Fever with mediastinal/pulmonary infections
  E. Oral cavity evaluation for linear foreign bodies under the base of the tongue
  F. May be extremely painful
III. Laboratory tests
  A. Hemogram reveals leukocytosis with infection.
  B. Serum chemistries are usually normal.
IV. Survey radiography
  A. Abnormal accumulations of gas or fluid may occur cranial to the obstruction.
  B. Radiopaque foreign bodies (bones, fish hooks) are readily visualized.
  C. Pneumomediastinum, pneumothorax, or evidence of mediastinitis is found with perforation.
  D. Alveolar pulmonary opacities are seen with aspiration pneumonia.
V. Contrast radiography
  A. It is required to visualize radiolucent foreign bodies and to detect perforations.
  B. If a perforation is suspected, use an iodinated contrast agent to avoid barium-induced pleuritis.
VI. Esophagoscopy
  A. Allows direct visualization of the foreign body
  B. Allows assessment of mucosal damage
  C. Provides means of endoscopic removal (Tams, 1990)

Differential Diagnosis

I. Other esophageal or periesophageal masses
II. Mediastinitis/pleuritis of varied causes
III. Severe esophagitis of various causes

Treatment

I. Esophageal foreign bodies are medical emergencies!
II. Endoscopic removal with retrieval instruments is indicated.
  A. Either rigid or flexible esophagoscopy may be performed.
  B. Larger grasping forceps, normally used with rigid endoscopes, may be passed along the side of the flexible endoscope.
  C. Distal esophageal foreign bodies may be pushed into the stomach.
    1. Digestible objects need not be removed.
    2. Non-digestible materials may require removal via gastrotomy.
  D. Thoroughly evaluate the mucosa after foreign body extraction to check for esophageal laceration or large perforations.
  E. Obtain postoperative thoracic radiographs to assess for pneumomediastinum/pneumothorax.
III. Institute medical therapy for esophagitis (see Esophagitis).
IV. Surgery is indicated if endoscopic removal of the foreign body fails, to repair large defects in the esophageal wall, or to permit thoracic drainage of fluid.

Patient Monitoring

I. One third of animals with esophageal foreign bodies develop complications (Strombeck and Guilford, 1990).
   A. Minor trauma, such as lacerations, carries a good prognosis.
   B. Significant esophageal necrosis with large perforation carries a guarded prognosis.
   C. Permanent sequelae may include fistula, diverticulum, or stricture formation, and local defects in motility.
II. If signs of esophageal dysfunction persist, perform an esophagram to rule out obstructive esophageal disease such as stricture.
III. Stricture is treated by balloon dilatation procedures (see next section).

Stricture

Definition

I. A stricture is a circumferential narrowing of the esophageal lumen caused by muscular inflammation and resultant scar tissue formation.
II. Strictures may occur at any point along the length of the esophagus.

Causes

I. Esophageal strictures have been reported secondary to general anesthesia and gastroesophageal reflux.
II. Predisposing factors for anesthesia-induced reflux include a ''head down'' position and the use of preanesthetic agents that reduce lower esophageal sphincter tone (Pearson et al, 1978).
III. Other causes of stricture formation include foreign bodies, esophageal surgery, and malignant neoplasia.

Pathophysiology

I. Severe esophageal mucosal inflammation extends into the muscle layer and heals by fibrosis.
II. Fibrotic changes (maturation with contraction) in the wall of the esophagus cause luminal narrowing.
III. The time period from severe mucosal damage to esophageal stenosis is approximately 1–3 weeks (Zawie, 1989).

Clinical Signs

I. Classic for esophageal dysfunction
   A. Regurgitation, dysphagia
   B. Tolerance of oral liquids better than solids
   C. Tendency of signs to be progressive
II. Weight loss in spite of a good appetite

Diagnosis

I. Often suggested by clinical history
II. Thoracic radiography
   A. Survey radiographs are often unremarkable.

B. Esophagram (liquid barium ± barium mixed with food) demonstrates esophageal luminal stenosis.
   C. Contrast studies delineate the number and location of strictures.
III. Endoscopic examination
   A. Esophagoscopy confirms stricture and may permit differentiation of benign from malignant stricture via mucosal biopsy.
   B. Endoscopy does not identify extrinsic causes for esophageal stenosis such as periesophageal masses, vascular ring anomalies, or adhesions that constrict the lumen from outside its wall.

Differential Diagnosis

I. Periesophageal masses: neoplasia, lymphadenopathy, granuloma
II. Vascular ring anomalies: unlikely except in young dogs
III. Extraluminal adhesions caused by previous thoracic trauma

Treatment

I. Benign strictures are best treated by balloon catheter dilatation under endoscopic guidance.
   A. It is safer and more effective than rigid bougienage procedures.
   B. Flexible endoscopy is required.
   C. A technique for balloon catheter dilatation in both dogs and cats has been previously described (Burk et al., 1987; Hardie et al., 1987).
      1. A special polyethylene catheter (Rigiflex Dilators, Microvasive Inc., Milford, MA) is advanced and positioned in the stricture under endoscopic guidance.
      2. Once inflated, the catheter applies stationary, radial force to mechanically dilate the strictured site.
      3. Multiple (2–4) dilatation procedures (each requiring a separate anesthetic procedure) are generally required (Harai et al., 1995).
      4. Complications of balloon dilatation include iatrogenic esophagitis and esophageal perforation.
   D. Medical therapy is needed after dilatation.
      1. Withhold feeding for 24 hours, or place a gastrostomy tube for enteral feeding in animals requiring multiple dilatation procedures.
      2. Use of corticosteroids to prevent reformation of fibrous tissue is sometimes advocated (Zawie, 1989). Prednisone, 1–2 mg/kg PO divided BID for 10–14 days, is effective.
      3. Prevent further injury to the esophageal mucosa from gastroesophageal reflux by administering H_2-blockers and/or drugs to enhance lower esophageal sphincter tone (see Esophagitis).
II. Surgical resection of benign strictures is less desirable.

A. Success rates are less than with balloon dilatation procedures.

B. Restricture at the surgical site is a common sequela.

III. Malignant esophageal strictures are treated with a combination of surgical resection (if possible), balloon dilatation (if needed), and appropriate postsurgical irradiation and/or chemotherapy.

Patient Monitoring

I. Continue dietary management and medical therapy of gastroesophageal reflux for 10–14 days after balloon dilatation.

II. Repeat esophagram 2 weeks after dilatation to assess for restricturing.

III. Gradually taper corticosteroids over a 2-week period.

IV. Additional dilatation procedures are required in animals in whom there is failure to maintain adequate luminal diameter.

V. The prognosis for benign strictures is good to excellent with successful dilatation.

VI. The prognosis is poor in all animals with malignant causes for esophageal stricture.

Bibliography

Burk RL, Zawie DA, Garvey MS: Balloon catheter dilatation of intramural esophageal strictures in the dog and cat: a description of the procedure and a report of six cases. Semin Vet Med Surg 2:241, 1987

Callan MB, Washabau RJ, Saunders HM, et al: Congenital esophageal hiatal hernia in the Chinese Shar Pei dog. J Vet Intern Med 7:210, 1993

Dent J, Dodds WJ, Hogan WJ et al: Factors that influence induction of gastroesophageal reflux in normal human subjects. Dig Dis Sci 33:270, 1988

Diamant N, Szczepanski M, Mui H: Idiopathic megaesophagus in the dog: reasons for spontaneous improvement and a possible method of medical therapy. Can Vet J 15:66, 1974

Duda M, Sery Z, Vojacek K et al: Etiopathogenesis and classification of esophageal diverticula. Int Surg 70:291, 1985

Ellison GW, Lewis DD, Phillips L et al: Esophageal hiatal hernia in small animals: literature review and a modified surgical technique. J Am Anim Hosp Assoc 23:391, 1987

Guilford WG: Megaesophagus in the dog and cat. Semin Vet Med Surg 5:37, 1990

Harai BH, Johnson SE, Sherding RG: Endoscopically guided balloon dilation of benign esophageal strictures in 6 cats and 7 dogs. J Vet Intern Med 9:332, 1995

Hardie EM, Greene RT, Ford RB: Balloon dilatation for treatment of esophageal stricture: a case report. J Am Anim Hosp Assoc 23:547, 1987

Hoenig M, Mahaffey MB, Parnell PG et al: Megaesophagus in two cats. J Am Vet Med Assoc 196:763, 1990

Jones BD, Jergens AE, Guilford WG: Diseases of the esophagus. p. 1255. In Ettinger SJ (ed): Textbook of Veterinary Internal Medicine. WB Saunders, Philadelphia, 1989

Katz PO, Geisinger KR, Hassan M et al: Acid-induced esophagitis in cats is prevented by sucralfate but not synthetic prostaglandin E. Dig Dis Sci 33:217, 1988

Knowles KE, O'Brien DP, Amann JF: Congenital idiopathic megaesophagus in a litter of Chinese Shar Peis: clinical, electrodiagnostic and pathological findings. J Am Anim Hosp Assoc 26:313, 1990

Leib MS, Hall RL: Megaesophagus in the dog: II. Clinical aspects. Compend Contin Educ Pract Vet 6:11, 1984

Park RD: Bronchoesophageal fistula in the dog: literature survey, case presentations and radiographic manifestations. Compend Contin Educ Pract Vet 6:669, 1984

Pearson H, Darke PG, Gibbs C et al: Reflux esophagitis and stricture formation after anesthesia: a review of seven cases in dogs and cats. J Small Anim Pract 19:507, 1978

Rolfe DS, Twedt DC, Seim HB: Chronic regurgitation or vomiting caused by esophageal leiomyoma in three dogs. J Am Anim Hosp Assoc 30:425, 1994

Roudebush P, Jones BD, Vaughan RW: Medical aspects of esophageal disease. p. 81. In Jones BD (ed): Canine and Feline Gastroenterology. WB Saunders, Philadelphia, 1986

Shelton GD, Willard MD, Cardinet GH III et al: Acquired myasthenia gravis. Selective involvement of esophageal, pharyngeal, and facial muscles. J Vet Intern Med 4:282, 1990

Sokolvsky V: Achalasia and paralysis of the canine esophagus. J Am Vet Med Assoc 260:943, 1972

Stickle RL, Love NE: Radiographic diagnosis of esophageal diseases in dog and cats. Semin Vet Med Surg 4:179, 1989

Stickle RL, Sparschu G, Love N et al: Radiographic evaluation of esophageal function in Chinese Shar Pei pups. J Am Vet Med Assoc 201:81, 1992

Strombeck DR, Guilford WG: Diseases of swallowing. p. 140. In Strombeck DR, Guilford WG (eds): Small Animal Gastroenterology. Stonegate Publishing, Davis, California, 1990

Strombeck DR, Harrold D: Effects of atropine, acepromazine, meperidine and xylazine on gastroesophageal sphincter pressure in the dog. Am J Vet Res 46:963, 1985

Strombeck DR, Troya L: Evaluation of lower motor neuron function in two dogs with megaesophagus. J Am Vet Med Assoc 169:411, 1976

Tams TR: Esophagoscopy. p. 47. In Tams TR (ed): Small Animal Endoscopy. Mosby–Year Book, St. Louis, 1990

Tams TR: Cisapride: clinical experience with the newest GI prokinetic drug. Proc Am Coll Vet Intern Med 12:100, 1994

Twedt DC: Diseases of the esophagus. p. 1124. In Ettinger SJ, Feldman EC (eds): Textbook of Veterinary Internal Medicine. 4th Ed. WB Saunders, Philadelphia, 1995

Tytgat GN, Nio CY, Schotborgh RH: Reflux esophagitis. Scand J Gastroenterol (Suppl) 175:1, 1990

Washabau RJ, Gaynor A: Pathogenesis of canine megaesophagus: neuropathy. Proc Am Coll Vet Intern Med 14:583, 1996

Washabau RJ, Hall JE: Cisapride. J Am Vet Med Assoc 207:1285, 1995

Withrow SJ: Esophageal cancer. p. 190. In Withrow SJ, MacEwen EG (eds): Clinical Veterinary Oncology. JB Lippincott, Philadelphia, 1989

Zawie DA: Esophageal strictures. p. 904. In Kirk RW (ed): Current Veterinary Therapy X: Small Animal Practice. WB Saunders, Philadelphia, 1989

30

Diseases of the Stomach

Christine C. Jenkins
Robert C. DeNovo, Jr.

CONGENITAL/ DEVELOPMENTAL DISORDERS

Antral Pyloric Hypertrophy

Definition

I. Antral pyloric hypertrophy is an obstructive narrowing of the pyloric canal caused by hypertrophy of the pyloric circular smooth muscle or hyperplasia of the pyloric mucosa or both.
II. Two types occur.
    A. Congenital pyloric hypertrophy (synonym: congenital pyloric stenosis)
    B. Acquired pyloric hypertrophy (adult-onset)

Causes

I. The exact causes are unknown.
II. Neural dysfunction may be the underlying cause of abnormal antral motility.
III. Endocrine causes such as hypergastrinemia from chronic distention are also suspected to play a role.

Pathophysiology

I. Pyloric antral hypertrophy causes partial or complete obstruction of the pyloric outflow tract, which manifests as gastric retention.
II. Chronic gastric retention causes gastric distention, which stimulates gastrin release resulting in hypergastrinemia.
III. Gastrin is trophic to antral tissues; chronic hypergastrinemia causes mucosal hyperplasia (Dodge and Karim, 1976).
IV. Congenital pyloric stenosis occurs in some dogs and cats without pyloric thickening; in such instances, functional obstruction from a motility disorder may be the underlying cause.

Clinical Signs

I. Signalment is as follows.
    A. Congenital antral hypertrophy

    1. It occurs in brachycephalic dogs, with Boston terriers and boxers the most commonly affected.
    2. Most cats are Siamese.
    B. Acquired antral hypertrophy
    1. Middle-aged small breeds most commonly affected: Lhasa apso, Shih Tzu, miniature poodle
    2. Large breeds reported: German shepherd dogs, Doberman pinschers
    3. Sex predilection: males
II. Vomiting is the most common clinical sign observed.
III. In congenital pyloric antral hypertrophy, vomiting occurs shortly after weaning, with the introduction of solid food.
IV. In acquired pyloric antral hypertrophy, progressive chronic intermittent vomiting is most commonly reported.
    A. Vomiting usually occurs 8–10 hours after eating.
    B. Vomiting immediately after eating is also reported.
V. Projectile vomiting is common with pyloric obstruction.
VI. Postprandial abdominal distention and discomfort, relieved by vomiting, may be observed.
VII. Other signs include weight loss, increased appetite, and regurgitation from concurrent esophagitis or gastroesophageal reflux disease.

Diagnosis

I. Signalment
II. History of chronic vomiting
III. Laboratory findings
    A. Hemogram (complete blood count [CBC]) is usually normal.
    B. Serum chemistries are usually normal except for acid–base imbalances.
    C. Acute or mild vomiting may result in normal acid–base or metabolic acidosis due to dehydration.

D. Electrolytes may be normal, slightly decreased, or severely decreased.
E. Severe vomiting or pyloric obstruction may result in a net loss of hydrogen chloride (HCl).
F. Subsequent severe hypokalemia and hypochloremia may result in metabolic alkalosis.

IV. Imaging techniques
   A. Survey abdominal radiographs may be normal or show gastric dilation.
   B. Barium contrast study may show the following.
      1. Gastric outflow narrowing described as a "beak sign" or presence of an obstructive mass in the pyloric antrum
      2. Hypertrophic mucosal folds that appear as a focal polyp or mass in the antrum
   C. Fluoroscopy may be used in conjunction with contrast radiographs to evaluate peristaltic function.
   D. Abdominal ultrasonography may detect an abnormally thickened antral wall.
   E. Scintigraphy may be used to evaluate gastric emptying (see Gastric Motility Disorders).
   F. Gastroscopy may be normal.
      1. Gastric retention due to pyloric dysfunction or obstruction is suspected if liquid and food in the stomach are still present following fasting before anesthesia.
      2. Redundant or thickened antral mucosa may be observed.
      3. The pyloric sphincter may appear misshapen or be obscured from view by the antral hypertrophy.
      4. The antrum may be difficult to insufflate.
   G. Exploratory laparotomy and biopsy of the pyloric antrum are necessary for a definitive diagnosis.
      1. Gastric antrum and pylorus may be thickened upon palpation.
      2. Biopsy is recommended to rule out neoplasia.
   H. Histopathologic findings may show variable degrees of mucosal hyperplasia or hypertrophy of pyloric smooth muscle or mucosal hyperplasia.

Differential Diagnosis

I. Intrinsic lesions: infiltrative disease of the antral wall including inflammatory, neoplastic, or granulomatous
II. Extrinsic lesions: compression of the gastric outflow tract from extramural structures such as neoplastic or granulomatous lesions involving the pancreas, liver, and serosal surface of the stomach
III. Obstructive lesions: foreign bodies, antral ulcers, or polyps
IV. Metabolic diseases associated with chronic vomiting: hepatic, renal, and adrenal insufficiencies, pancreatitis, diabetes mellitus

Treatment

I. Medical therapy may be used for early or mild cases and for postoperative care; however, surgery is the treatment of choice.
II. The surgical objective is to improve gastric outflow by removal of hypertrophied mucosa and to widen the gastric outflow tract by pyloromyotomy and pyloroplasty (Heineke-Mikulicz or Y to U pyloroplasty). Gastroduodenostomy may also be required if the pyloric antrum must be removed because of severe disease.
III. Prokinetic drugs may decrease gastric distention and enhance pyloric emptying.
   A. Metoclopramide
      1. Dogs: 0.2–0.4 mg/kg PO TID, 0.5 hour before meals
      2. Cats: 0.1–0.2 mg/kg PO TID, 0.5 hour before meals
   B. Cisapride in dogs: 2.5–5 mg PO TID or 0.08–1.25 mg/kg PO TID (0.5 hour before meals)
IV. Small frequent feedings of a highly digestible diet such as rice or pasta, or a commercial prescription diet for gastrointestinal disease such as Iams' Low Residue or Hill's i/d are suggested.

Patient Monitoring

I. 80% of dogs improve postoperatively.
II. Some suffer severe distention/dilation resulting in irreversible motility dysfunction, which may require long-term prokinetic therapy and additional surgery.

INFLAMMATORY DISORDERS

Acute Gastritis

Definition

Inflammation and mucosal damage occur in response to gastric mucosal insult.

Causes

I. Exogenous causes
   A. Dietary indiscretion: most common cause in dogs
   B. Drugs: nonsteroidal anti-inflammatory drugs (NSAIDs), e.g., aspirin, indomethacin, phenylbutazone, flunixin meglumine, ibuprofen
   C. Foreign object ingestion
   D. Toxins: ethylene glycol, lead, arsenic, poisonous plants
   E. Infectious diseases
      1. Viruses: canine distemper, parvovirus, coronavirus
      2. Feline panleukopenia
      3. Mycoses: histoplasmosis, phycomycosis (usually chronic in nature)
      4. Parasites
         a) *Physaloptera* spp. in dogs
         b) *Ollulanus tricuspis* in cats
      5. Bacteria: *Helicobacter* spp. (also associated with chronic gastritis)
II. Endogenous causes
   A. Systemic diseases that cause gastric erosions or ulceration
   B. Hepatic, renal, or adrenal insufficiency
   C. Pancreatitis, ketoacidotic diabetes mellitus
   D. Decreased gastric perfusion: shock, sepsis, stress

Pathophysiology

I. Endogenous or exogenous agents cause damage to the gastric mucosa, resulting in increased permeability to gastric acid.

II. Once acid penetrates the gastric epithelial cell lining, the subepithelium is damaged.

III. Acid stimulates mast cell degranulation and histamine release from mast cells located in the submucosa and lamina propria.

IV. Local inflammation, edema formation, and vascular damage occur, and further stimulate inflammation via neutrophils and lymphocytes.

Clinical Signs

I. Vomiting is the most common clinical sign associated with acute gastritis.

II. Other signs include variable appetite, increased salivation, polydipsia, abdominal pain.

III. Diarrhea may occur concurrently if enteritis is present.

Diagnosis

I. Historical findings such as exposure to exogenous factors are suggestive.

II. Pertinent physical findings such as abdominal pain or fever are supportive.

III. Serum chemistries and electrolytes are often normal.
   A. Abnormalities in serum chemistries and electrolytes either parallel the severity and duration of vomiting or may indicate systemic causes of gastritis.
   B. CBC is usually normal, or a stress leukogram may be noted.
   C. Leukopenia suggests parvovirus infection.

IV. Serology or virus identification may indicate viral causes (see Chap. 110).

V. Examination of feces or vomitus may diagnose parasitic causes (see Chap. 32).

VI. Imaging techniques may be considered.
   A. Survey abdominal radiographs may be normal or may reveal gastric distention and/or gas- or liquid-filled bowel.
   B. Barium contrast study with or without fluoroscopy may indicate obstructive disease but is usually normal in most cases of acute gastritis.
   C. Other nonspecific findings include flocculation of barium and changes in gastrointestinal transit time.

VII. Gastroscopy may be helpful.
   A. It may be normal or show nonspecific mucosal changes such as erythema, petechiation, frank or digested blood, or evidence of erosion or ulceration.
   B. Gastric foreign bodies or *Physaloptera* may be visualized.

Treatment

I. Most cases of acute gastritis are self-limiting and do not require therapy.

II. Dietary modifications are indicated.
   A. Withhold food or water for 8–12 hours.
   B. Once vomiting stops, offer a small amount of water initially.
   C. If the animal does not vomit after several hours, offer small amounts of highly digestible food such as a high-carbohydrate diet.
   D. If vomiting persists for 12–24 hours and the animal is becoming dehydrated, further evaluation and fluid therapy are recommended.

III. If vomiting persists or if it is profuse, intravenous fluid therapy is necessary.
   A. Normal saline or lactated Ringer's solution are the fluids of choice.
   B. Potassium is supplemented in the fluids because hypokalemia is common in acute vomiting animals.
   C. Before adding potassium, the presence of hyperkalemia should be determined if acute renal failure, post-obstructive uropathy, or Addison's disease is suspected.
   D. If a foreign body is diagnosed, it should be removed within 24–48 hours (if it cannot pass through the gastrointestinal tract without harm). Removal may be done endoscopically or surgically.

IV. Antiemetics are reserved for refractory vomiting only.
   A. Antiemetics can mask underlying diseases and delay proper therapy.
   B. Phenothiazine derivatives may be used.
      1. Chlorpromazine (Thorazine) may be given as follows.
         a) 0.1–2.2 mg/kg PO SID-QID
         b) 0.25–0.5 mg/kg IM SID-QID
         c) 0.05–0.1 mg/kg IV SID-QID
      2. Avoid their use in dehydrated animals, as they can be hypotensive.
   C. Prokinetic drugs may also be used.
      1. Metoclopramide at 0.2–0.4 mg/kg PO, SQ TID-QID or 1–2 mg/kg/24 h as a continuous IV infusion
      2. Contraindicated in gastric obstructive disease and may cause central nervous system (CNS) depression

Patient Monitoring

I. Animals who do not improve should be reevaluated.

II. If signs recur or become chronic in nature, causes of chronic vomiting should be ruled out (see Chronic Gastritis).

Chronic Gastritis

Definition

Chronic inflammation of the stomach results from continued insult or damage to the gastric mucosa.

Causes and Classifications

I. Chronic gastritis is classified according to several types depending on cause, type of inflammatory cell infiltrate, and/or pathologic changes.

II. The underlying cause may not be determined.

III. Repeated exposure to drugs, toxins, infectious causes, and dietary antigens may be responsible for the development of chronic gastritis (see Causes of Acute Gastritis).

IV. In some cases, chronic gastritis may occur from an abnormal immune response to ubiquitous agents or to a one-time insult.

V. Immune-mediated disease can result in atrophic gastritis or hypertrophic gastritis.

VI. Experimentally, chronic gastritis can be induced with intradermal injections of homologous gastric juice stimulating both humoral and cell-mediated immunity (Krohn and Finlayson, 1973).

VII. *Helicobacter* infection is recognized as a cause of chronic gastritis in dogs and cats.

VIII. *Helicobacter*-associated gastritis, characterized by lymphocytic plasmacytic infiltrate and milder neutrophilic and eosinophilic infiltrate, is also seen in dogs and cats.

IX. Histologic classifications are as follows.

A. Chronic superficial gastritis

1. It is the most common form of chronic gastritis.

2. Superficial chronic gastritis may be an early change and is characterized by inflammatory cell infiltrate in the interstitium between gastric pits.

3. Plasma cells predominate, with some lymphocytic and neutrophilic infiltrates.

4. Other possible lesions include erosions, hemorrhage, and edema.

B. Chronic atrophic gastritis

1. More severe lesions are present than in superficial gastritis, with more lymphocytes and plasma cell infiltrate extending deeper into the mucosa.

2. Mucosa may appear discolored and thinner than normal from loss of normal gastric glands.

3. Decrease in parietal cells in gastric glands results in decreased hydrochloric acid production or achlorhydria.

4. If achlorhydria exists, then gastrin production increases, resulting in hypergastrinemia.

C. Chronic hypertrophic gastritis

1. It is characterized by thickened gastric mucosa with prominent rugal folds.

2. Gastric mucosal hypertrophy occurs when interstitial edema or cystic gastric glandular formation increases mucosal thickening.

3. Gastric mucosal hypertrophy can occur secondary to hypergastrinemia when gastric acid secretion is inhibited for prolonged periods, from antacid administration, or from hypersecretory conditions (i.e., Zollinger-Ellison syndrome).

4. Hypertrophic gastritis may also occur secondary to chronic inflammation.

5. It is also reported in basenjis with immunoproliferative small bowel disease.

D. Eosinophilic gastritis

1. It is characterized by a diffuse eosinophilic infiltration and granulation tissue formation.

2. It may also occur in a nodular form and be confused with neoplasia.

3. An immune-mediated etiology is suspected, possibly secondary to allergy or parasites.

4. Mild eosinophilic infiltrates are also found in some cases of *Helicobacter* infection.

Pathophysiology

Chronic gastritis occurs when excessive inflammatory cell infiltrates lead to fibrosis of the mucosa and submucosa, which predisposes to erosions, edema, and hemorrhage of the gastric mucosa.

Clinical Signs

I. Intermittent vomiting: most common

II. Vomitus: mucus, bile, or blood (if erosions or ulcers present)

III. Appetite variable

IV. Weight loss

V. Abdominal pain

VI. Polydipsia

VII. Pica

VIII. Melena

Diagnosis

I. History of chronic vomiting

II. Laboratory findings

A. Hemogram

1. It is normal in most cases.

2. If there is significant acute hemorrhage with anemia, the hemogram may be regenerative.

3. If there is chronic blood loss, a microcytic hypochromic anemia may be present.

4. White blood cell count is usually normal.

5. In some cases of eosinophilic gastritis, an eosinophilia may be present.

B. Serum chemistries and electrolytes

1. They are usually normal unless vomiting is severe or prolonged.

2. Electrolyte abnormalities include hyponatremia, hypokalemia, and hypochloremia.

3. If vomiting is chronic, metabolic acidosis may occur secondary to dehydration, or metabolic alkalosis may arise secondary to hypochloremia, hypokalemia, and loss of HCl.

III. Contrast radiography and ultrasonography

They are insensitive indicators of this disease unless there is significant mucosal hypertrophy or nodular lesion(s) secondary to eosinophilic gastritis, mycotic disease, or neoplasia.

IV. Endoscopy and gastric biopsy

A. Definitive diagnosis requires mucosal biopsy.

B. The esophagus is evaluated visually for signs of inflammation secondary to vomiting or gastric reflux.

C. The duodenum is examined and biopsy performed because inflammation may also involve the small intestine.

D. Grossly there may be no obvious lesions, or there may be evidence of a thin or thickened mucosa, erosions, ulcerations, or signs of hemorrhage.

E. *Helicobacter*-associated gastritis may reveal the following.
   1. Grossly the mucosa may appear normal, or there may be evidence of edema, punctate irregularities, erosions, or ulcerations.
   2. In some cases there are diffuse nodular lesions, occasionally with eroded surfaces.
   3. Gastric mucosa may bleed easily on contact with the endoscope.
   4. Histopathologic evaluation may reveal spiral organisms in gastric mucus, in the gastric pits, or adhered to gastric epithelial cells.
   5. Microbiologic tests on gastrointestinal biopsies include a urease test and silver stains (Warthin-Starry) to evaluate the presence of spiral organisms.
   6. Some *Helicobacter* species can be grown in culture from gastric biopsies; however, *H. helmannii* and *H. felis* are difficult to isolate.

Differential Diagnosis

I. Other causes of chronic intermittent vomiting, including metabolic diseases such as hepatic, renal, or adrenal insufficiency
II. Neoplasia of the gastrointestinal tract
III. Gastric motility disorders
IV. Gastrinoma or systemic mastocytosis
V. Pancreatitis
VI. Lead poisoning
VII. Phycomycosis

Treatment

I. Treat the underlying cause.
II. Institute an elimination diet for 6–8 weeks to rule out food allergy.
   A. Bland diets high in carbohydrates and with one source of protein, preferably novel to that animal
   B. Home-made diets: lamb and rice
   C. Commercial diets: Hill's d/d, Iams' Low Residue
III. If there is evidence of ulceration based on clinical signs or endoscopy, H_2-receptor blocker or proton-pump inhibitors may be indicated for short-term therapy.
   A. Cimetidine 5–10 mg/kg PO TID (dogs)
   B. Ranitidine 2 mg/kg PO BID-TID (dogs); 2.5 mg/kg PO BID (cats)
   C. Omeprazole 0.7 mg/kg PO SID
IV. If spiral organisms are documented, treatment of *Helicobacter*-associated gastritis may be warranted.
   A. Empirical or dual therapy: Amoxicillin 10 mg/kg PO TID and H_2-receptor blocker or omeprazole for 14–21 days
   B. Triple therapy: Amoxicillin, metronidazole 15 mg/kg PO TID, and bismuth subsalicylate 0.25 ml/kg PO q 4–6 h for 14–21 days (tetracycline or clarithromycin can be substituted for bismuth).

V. Immunosuppressive therapy may be necessary to decrease inflammation if severe lymphocytic-plasmacytic or eosinophilic gastritis is present, especially if it is not responsive to the previous therapies.
   A. Corticosteroids such as prednisone or prednisolone are drugs of choice.
      1. Dogs: prednisone 1–2 mg/kg/day PO for 5–10 days, then decrease by 25% weekly if animal is asymptomatic (low-dose QOD therapy may be necessary for 4–6 weeks)
      2. Cats: prednisone 2–4 mg/kg/day PO, then taper as for dogs
   B. If the animal is unresponsive or intolerant to corticosteroids, other immunosuppressive agents such as azathioprine can be considered.
      1. Dogs: 2 mg/kg PO SID for 2 weeks, then decrease to 2 mg/kg QOD
      2. Cats: 0.2 mg/kg PO SID-QOD
      3. CBC monitored weekly for 4 weeks to avoid leukopenia and thrombocytopenia, then monthly

Patient Monitoring

I. If an underlying cause can be identified and treated, the prognosis is very good.
II. Some animals require long-term dietary modification and/or maintenance steroid therapy.

Gastric Erosive or Ulcer Disease

Definition

I. Gastric erosions are superficial mucosal defects that do not penetrate the lamina muscularis mucosae.
II. Gastric ulcers penetrate deeper into the muscularis mucosae layer.

Causes

I. Drugs
   A. Nonsteroidal anti-inflammatory drugs
      1. Aspirin, indomethacin, phenylbutazone
      2. Ibuprofen, piroxicam
      3. Meclofenamic acid
      4. Flunixin meglumine
   B. Corticosteroids, usually in combination with other factors
II. Diminished gastric blood flow
   A. Hypotension
   B. Shock
   C. Sepsis
III. Hypersecretory conditions with increased HCl production by gastric parietal cells
   A. Gastrin-secreting tumor of pancreas (Zollinger-Ellison syndrome) has been documented in dogs and cats.
   B. Systemic mastocytosis causes increased histamine release, which may produce increased HCl secretion by gastric parietal cells.
IV. Metabolic diseases
   A. Hepatic insufficiency is associated with hypergastrinemia and hyperhistaminemia, which results in increased gastric acid production.

B. Renal insufficiency can also result in increased gastrin levels from decreased renal clearance.

C. Uremic toxins can also damage the gastrointestinal mucosa predisposing to erosions and ulcerations.

D. Hypoadrenocortism may cause ulceration secondary to decreased mucosal blood flow from hypotension and decreased vascular tone.

V. Mechanical injury

VI. Gastrointestinal foreign bodies: stones, metal objects, bones, etc.

VII. Infections: *Helicobacter* and *Helicobacter*-like species

VIII. Stress: possibly from release of catecholamines, endogenous steroids, or serotonin

Pathophysiology

I. Gastric ulceration occurs when one or more of the previously listed factors injure the protective gastric mucosal barrier, allowing damaging elements such as gastric acid, bile, and pepsin to cause further damage to the submucosa.

II. Ulceration can also result from mechanical injury, e.g., foreign bodies.

Clinical Signs

I. Vomiting: most common sign

II. ± Evidence of gastric hemorrhage: frank blood, "coffee-ground"-like vomitus, or melena

III. ± Pale mucous membranes

IV. Abdominal pain

V. Variable appetitite

VI. Weight loss

VII. No apparent signs ("silent" disease)

VIII. Signs of shock with gastrointestinal perforation

Diagnosis

I. History of chronic vomiting, hematemesis, or melena

II. Laboratory findings
A. CBC may be normal.
B. If severe acute hemorrhage occurs, a regenerative anemia may be present.
C. Chronic gastrointestinal bleeding causing a microcytic hypochromic anemia is more likely.
D. White blood cell count may be normal or indicative of stress.
E. Serum biochemistries may be normal or indicative of underlying metabolic diseases.
F. Panhypoproteinemia may be present from blood loss.
G. Electrolytes are usually normal.

III. Imaging techniques
A. Survey abdominal radiographs may be normal or may reveal radiopaque foreign objects, gastric distention, or evidence of gastrointestinal perforation and peritonitis.
B. Barium contrast study may reveal gastrointestinal ulceration; however, false-negative results are common.

C. If perforation is suspected, organic iodides are used for contrast radiography (see Chap. 4).

IV. Gastroscopy
A. Discrete small erosions are seen as punctate or linear lesions in the stomach and duodenum.
1. Ulcerations may be single or multiple.
2. Fresh or digested blood may be seen in the stomach or duodenum.
3. Despite the presence of blood, gross erosions or ulcerations are not always evident endoscopically.
B. Multiple biopsy specimens are taken whether or not gross lesions are evident. If an ulcer is found, the biopsy is performed at the periphery to avoid perforation through a necrotic center.
C. If gastrointestinal perforation or peritonitis is suspected, surgical exploration is indicated. Biopsies are performed to determine underlying causes of ulceration.
D. Measurement of gastrin level is required to diagnose a gastrinoma.
1. Provocative testing can be done using secretin and calcium.
2. Secretin and calcium stimulate release of gastrin from gastrinomas, whereas animals without the tumor have minimal response.

Differential Diagnosis

I. Causes of acute and chronic gastritis

II. Neoplasia

III. Phycomycosis

IV. Gastric foreign body

V. Intestinal ulceration

Treatment

I. Antiulcer drugs are indicated if hematemesis and/or melena are present.
A. H₂-receptor blockers
1. Cimetidine 5–10 mg/kg PO TID
2. Ranitidine 2 mg/kg PO BID-TID
3. Famotidine 0.5–1 mg/kg PO SID
B. Proton-pump inhibitors
1. Omeprazole 0.7 mg/kg PO SID
2. Most potent gastric antisecretory drug available
C. Protectants: sucralfate 0.5–1 tablet PO TID-QID

II. Synthetic prostaglandins (misoprostol 3–5 μg/kg PO TID) are used to prevent ulceration from NSAID use.

III. Antibiotic therapy using either dual or triple drug therapy is recommended for *Helicobacter*-associated ulceration.
A. Dual therapy: amoxicillin 22 mg/kg PO TID, omeprazole 0.7 mg/kg PO SID
B. Triple therapy: amoxicillin, metronidazole 25–30 mg/kg divided PO BID-TID, and bismuth subsalicylate 0.25 ml/kg PO TID-QID

IV. Perforated ulcers and peritonitis require stabilization of shock and subsequent surgical exploration (see Chaps. 37 and 38).

V. Significant gastrointestinal hemorrhage may require whole blood transfusions (see Chap. 69).

Patient Monitoring

I. Most animals improve following treatment of the underlying cause.

II. Malignant gastric ulcers warrant a poor prognosis.

III. Animals with a gastrointestinal perforation have a better prognosis if the perforation is surgically corrected before significant peritonitis occurs.

IV. Any animal that suffers severe gastrointestinal hemorrhage should also be evaluated for a coagulopathy.

V. Animals with gastric ulceration from systemic mastocytosis or gastrinoma require life-long antiulcer medications.

GASTRIC MOTILITY DISORDERS AND DELAYED GASTRIC EMPTYING

Definition

I. Abnormal gastric motor function is present and usually results in delayed gastric emptying.

II. These disorders may be mild and transient, or persistent, resulting in gastric retention of stomach contents.

III. The stomach is normally empty in <8 hours following a meal.

Causes

I. Neurologic influences
   A. The sympathetic nervous system inhibits gastric motility.
   B. Under conditions such as stress, severe pain, trauma, psychogenic disorders, and abdominal or spinal surgery, sympathetic influence predominates.

II. Electrolyte and acid–base abnormalities
   A. Hypokalemia
   B. Hypocalcemia and hypercalcemia
   C. Acidosis

III. Metabolic diseases
   A. Uremia
   B. Hypothyroidism
   C. Hepatoencephalopathy
   D. Diabetes mellitus
   E. Hypoadrenocorticism

IV. Inflammatory diseases
   A. Acute or chronic gastritis/gastroenteritis
   B. Acute pancreatitis
   C. Peritonitis

V. Drugs
   A. Anticholinergics
   B. Narcotics
   C. Beta-adrenergic agonists

VI. Pyloric outflow obstruction
   A. Mechanical obstruction: foreign body, tumor, granuloma, inflammatory polyps
   B. Functional obstruction: pylorospasm

VII. Idiopathic causes
   A. Tachyarrhythmia and dysrhythmia from abnormal gastric slow-wave activity or abnormal gastric pacemaker activity
   B. Bilious vomiting syndrome characterized by early morning vomiting in young hyperactive, small-breed dogs

VIII. Gastric dilatation-volvulus syndrome

Pathophysiology

I. Normal gastric motility
   A. Normal gastric motor function is required for proper storage, mixing, and processing of food into a size that will pass through the pyloric sphincter into the duodenum.
   B. These processes require proper synchrony of motor activities of the fundus (responsible for food storage) and the distal fundus and pyloric antrum (responsible for grinding of foodstuffs and gastric emptying).
   C. Myogenic control involves the gastric pacemaker, which generates continuous slow-wave activity and the fast-wave potentials that occur during contractions.
   D. Coordination of smooth muscle contraction occurs by extrinsic and instrinsic nervous innervation.
   E. Gastric smooth muscle activity is also under endocrine control and is affected by gastrin, secretin, cholecystokinin, and other hormones.
   F. Gastric emptying in the postprandial state is affected by certain characteristics of the meal.
      1. The rate of emptying of liquids is determined primarily by volume; the greater the volume, the slower the emptying rate.
      2. The rate of emptying for solids is determined primarily by caloric density; the higher the caloric density, the slower the gastric emptying rate.

II. Decreased motility of the stomach
   A. May result in gastric paresis and gastric retention
   B. Secondary chronic gastric distention and vomiting

Clinical Signs

I. Chronic intermittent vomiting: usually >8 hours after eating

II. Gastric distention: frequently after a meal, often relieved by vomiting

III. ± Weight loss

Diagnosis

I. History and clinical signs suggestive of gastric retention

II. Laboratory findings
   A. Electrolytes are often normal.
   B. Hyponatremia, hypokalemia, and hypochloremia may be present secondary to chronic or profuse

vomiting (occurs most frequently from pyloric outflow obstruction).
C. Acid–base status is often normal.
1. Metabolic acidosis may be present if dehydration occurs.
2. Metabolic alkalosis may be present if there is concurrent hypokalemia and hypochloremia.
D. CBC is usually normal unless the animal is dehydrated.

III. Imaging techniques
A. Survey films may reveal gastric distention or may be normal.
B. Barium contrast study may indicate abnormal gastric emptying.
C. Fluoroscopy may indicate abnormal peristalsis, abnormal filling of the pylorus, and delayed gastric emptying.

IV. Other tests
A. Endoscopy may be done to evaluate for gastritis and obstructive disease. In cases of functional motility disorders, endoscopy is nondiagnostic.
B. Surgical exploration to evaluate for mechanical cause of obstruction and to perform biopsy of gastric tissues may be done if noninvasive techniques are nondiagnostic.
1. If the animal is unresponsive to medical management, or with possible gastropexy in cases of chronic bloat, pyloroplasty may be considered.
2. Some animals may still require prokinetic drugs and small frequent feedings postoperatively.
C. Other specialized techniques to consider include the following.
1. Scintigraphy using radiolabeled food to measure gastric emptying
2. Barium-impregnated polyspheres (BIPS) technique to measure passage of different sized beads
3. Electrophysiologic evaluation of stomach contractions

Differential Diagnosis

Other causes of chronic vomiting, gastritis, and gastric outflow obstruction

Treatment

I. Dietary modification: small, frequent meals consisting of low-fat, low-protein, high-carbohydrate foods (pasta, rice, cottage cheese)
II. Prokinetic agents
A. Metoclopramide
1. Is indicated for treatment of gastroesophageal reflux, gastroduodenal reflux, and gastric motility disorders
2. Adverse effects: nervousness, anxiety, and depression
3. Contraindication: pyloric or intestinal obstruction suspected

4. Dogs: 0.2–0.4 mg/kg PO TID (0.5 hour before meals)
5. Cats: 0.1–0.2 mg/kg PO TID (0.5 hour before meals)
B. Cisapride
1. Can be used in gastroesophageal reflux, gastroduodenal reflux, gastric motility disorders, and for the treatment of constipation and feline megacolon
2. Dose: 2.5–5 mg PO TID or 0.08–1.25 mg/kg PO TID (0.5 hour before meals)
C. Erythromycin
Stimulates gastric motility by increasing release of motilin in cats and by unknown mechanisms in dogs

Patient Monitoring

I. Response to therapy depends on the underlying cause of the motility disorder.
II. Some animals do not improve with medical and/or surgical therapy.

NEOPLASIA

Definition and Causes

I. Primary and benign gastric tumors occur infrequently, accounting for approximately 1% of all malignancies in dogs.
II. Causes of gastric neoplasia in dogs and cats are unknown.
III. In humans, gastric adenocarcinoma and some gastric lymphomas are associated with *Helicobacter pylori* infection; similar association in dogs and cats is unknown at this time.
IV. Gastric lymphosarcoma is associated with feline leukemia virus in the cat (25–30% are positive).

Classification

I. Malignant tumors
A. Adenocarcinoma is the most common malignant gastric tumor in dogs.
1. It can be a scirrhous, polypoid, or ulcerated mass.
2. It usually affects older dogs (mean age, 8 years).
3. It is commonly found in the lesser curvature of the stomach.
4. Metastasis to regional lymph nodes, liver, and lungs is common.
B. Lymphosarcoma is the most common gastric tumor in cats; it occurs less frequently in dogs.
1. May appear as multiple discrete masses or as diffusely thickened mucosa with or without ulcerations
2. May also affect other regions of the gastrointestinal tract
C. Other malignant tumors include fibrosarcoma, leiomyosarcomas, and metastatic tumors from other sites.

II. Benign tumors
 A. Leiomyomas
  1. Second most common gastric tumor in the dog; typically occurs in dogs >10 years of age
  2. Sometimes deeply ulcerated
  3. May cause pyloric outflow obstruction syndrome
  4. Sometimes an incidental finding
 B. Benign adenomatous polyps
  1. Appear as pedunculated nodules (multiple or single) usually in pyloric antrum, but may extend into duodenum
  2. May cause pyloric outflow obstruction syndrome
  3. Occur in dogs and cats
  4. Histologically appear as mucosal hypertrophy

Pathophysiology

I. Gastric tumors may obstruct pyloric outflow, alter normal motility, or cause bleeding from ulceration.
II. Benign tumors frequently cause no clinical signs.
III. Malignant tumors often metastasize to regional lymph nodes, liver, lungs, and occasionally to the adrenal glands.

Clinical Signs

I. Chronic progressive vomiting is the most common sign.
II. Gastric distention may be observed if there is impaired gastric emptying.
III. Signs of anemia may be present if there is significant bleeding from an ulcerated mass
IV. Other signs include melena, hematemesis, and weight loss.

Diagnosis

I. Chronic vomiting and weight loss in an older animal (in some cases vomiting can be of acute onset) are suggestive.
II. Abdominal palpation may reveal a mass in rare cases.
III. Laboratory findings are usually nonspecific.
 A. CBC
  1. Normocytic, normochromic anemia is the most frequent laboratory abnormality.
  2. Microcytic, hypochromic anemia from chronic blood loss is common.
 B. Serum chemistries
  1. Serum chemistries are usually normal unless there is concurrent disease or metastasis of tumor to the liver.
  2. Prerenal azotemia may be present from dehydration.
  3. Metabolic acidosis may arise from chronic vomiting.
  4. Serum electrolytes may be normal, or hypokalemia, hyponatremia, and hypochloremia may be detected.
IV. Imaging techniques are indicated.

 A. Survey abdominal films may be normal. Thoracic films may indicate pulmonary metastasis.
 B. Contrast barium study may indicate thickening of the stomach wall, a mass in the stomach, or pyloric outflow obstruction.
  1. Distortion of gastric lumen or rugal folds
  2. Filling defects
  3. Ulceration
  4. Delayed gastric emptying
 C. Abdominal ultrasonography may indicate a thickened stomach wall or mass lesion(s).
V. Endoscopy is often helpful.
 A. Mass lesion(s) may be evident, and frank or digested blood may be visualized in the stomach.
 B. Other lesions include thickened irregular mucosa, with or without evidence of ulceration or erosions.
 C. Biopsy samples are taken from the periphery of ulcerated lesions to avoid the necrotic center. It can be difficult to perform a biopsy with pinch biopsy forceps on scirrhous carcinomas.
VI. Laparotomy and gastrotomy may reveal masses or a thickened gastric wall (with or without ulceration). Biopsy samples are taken to rule out benign tumors and inflammatory lesions.

Differential Diagnosis

I. Eosinophilic granuloma
II. Inflammatory infiltrate, phycomycosis, fungal granuloma
III. Antral pyloric hypertrophy

Treatment

I. Surgical resection is the treatment of choice for some masses, especially polyps and leiomyomas.
II. Most malignant tumors are not completely resectable at the time of diagnosis.
III. Partial gastrectomy is sometimes required, followed by gastroduodenostomy or gastrojejunostomy (Bright, 1994).
IV. Palliative surgery for malignancies may increase survival for several months (Theilen and Madewell, 1987).
V. Chemotherapy can be attempted for gastrointestinal lymphoma. Response is variable depending on extent of disease (see Chap. 67).
 A. Solitary lymphosarcoma masses are removed surgically, followed by chemotherapy.
 B. Some cats with gastric lymphosarcoma respond well to chemotherapy, with disease remission lasting for >12 months.

Patient Monitoring

I. Prognosis for benign neoplasia is good.
II. Prognosis for gastric malignant neoplasia is poor.
III. Postoperative complications from partial gastrectomy are common.
 A. Acute: leaking from incision site can cause peritonitis

B. Chronic
  1. Post-prandial discomfort, vomiting, and diarrhea from "dumping syndrome" can occur as a result of decreased storage capacity of the stomach.
  2. Alkaline reflux esophagitis may result from abnormal pyloric function (Bright, 1994).

Bibliography

Birchard SJ, Couto CG, Johnson S: Non-lymphoid intestinal neoplasia in 32 dogs and 14 cats. J Am Anim Hosp Assoc 22:533, 1986

Bright RM: Surgery of the stomach. p. 676. In Birchard SJ, Sherding RG (eds): Saunders Manual of Small Animal Practice. WB Saunders, Philadelphia, 1994

DeNovo RC: Pyloric antral hypertrophy syndrome. p. 918. In Kirk RW (ed): Current Veterinary Therapy X: Small Animal Practice. WB Saunders, Philadelphia, 1989

Dodge JA, Karim AA: Induction of pyloric hypertrophy by pentagastrin. Gut 17:280, 1976

Guilford WG, Center SA, Strombeck DR et al: Acute gastritis: chronic gastric diseases. p. 261. In Strombeck DR (ed): Small Animal Gastroenterology. 3rd Ed. WB Saunders, Philadelphia, 1996

Hall JA, Twedt DC, Burrows CF: Gastric motility in dogs. II. Disorders of gastric motility. Compend Contin Educ Pract Vet 12:247, 1990

Henry GA, Long PH, Burns JL et al: Gastric spirillosis in beagles. Am J Vet Res 48:831, 1987

Jenkins CC, DeNovo RC, Patton CS et al: Comparison of effects of cimetidine and omeprazole on mechanically created gastric ulceration and on aspirin-induced gastritis in dogs. Am J Vet Res 52:658, 1991

Krohn KJE, Finlayson NDC: Interrelations of humoral and cellular immune responses in experimental canine gastritis. Clin Exp Immunol 14:237, 1973

Lavelle JP, Landas S, Mitros FA et al: Acute gastritis associated with spiral organisms from cats. Dig Dis Sci 39:744, 1994

Lee A, Krakowka S, Fox JG et al: Role of *Helicobacter felis* in chronic canine gastritis. Vet Pathol 29:487, 1992

Magne ML, Twedt DC: Diseases of the stomach. p. 217. In Tams TR (ed): Handbook of Small Animal Gastroenterology. WB Saunders, Philadelphia, 1996

Moreland KJ: Ulcer disease of the upper gastrointestinal tract in small animals: pathophysiology, diagnosis, and management. Compend Contin Educ Pract Vet 10:1265, 1988

Murtaugh RJ, Matz ME, Labato MA et al: Use of synthetic-prostaglandin-E₁ (misoprostol) for prevention of aspirin-induced gastroduodenal ulceration of arthritic dogs. J Am Vet Med Assoc 202:251, 1993

Stanton ME, Bright RM, Toal R et al: Chronic hypertrophic pyloric gastrophaty as a cause of pyloric obstruction in the dog. J Am Vet Med Assoc 186:157, 1985

Theilen GH, Madewell BR: Tumors of the digestive tract. p. 499. In Theilen GH, Madewell BR (eds): Veterinary Cancer Medicine. 2nd Ed. Lea & Febiger, Philadelphia, 1987

31

Acute Gastric Dilatation-Volvulus

Michael E. Matz

Definition

I. Gastric dilatation is overdistention of the stomach with gas, fluid, or ingesta.
  A. Normally dilatation is relieved by eructation or vomiting.
  B. Overdistention of the stomach may result in gastric atony, causing a more prolonged state of gastric dilatation.
II. Gastric volvulus is a twisting of the stomach on its long axis. The stomach usually rotates in a clockwise direction (ventrodorsal view) and effectively occludes the elimination of gastric contents through either the esophagus or duodenum.
III. Gastric dilatation-volvulus (GDV) is overdistention of the stomach in combination with volvulus of the stomach.
  A. Which event occurs first is unknown.
  B. It is probable that dilatation can cause volvulus, just as volvulus can cause dilatation.
IV. Gastric dilatation-volvulus is an acute, life-threatening condition in which survival is dependent on early recognition by the owner, as well as prompt and accurately initiated emergency treatment.

Causes

I. The prevalence of acute GDV in the general canine population is low.
  A. Acute GDV is most common in large and/or deep-chested breeds of dogs such as the Great Dane, German shepherd dog, standard poodle, Doberman pinscher, and Irish setter, but it has been observed in smaller breeds of dogs and cats.
  B. Gastric dilatation-volvulus is most often noted in middle-aged to older dogs (reported mean ages of 5.2 and 7.5) but can occur at any age (Muir, 1982a; Brockman et al., 1995).
II. A number of risk factors have been identified, but none has emerged as the single most important cause of GDV.
  A. It appears that GDV results from the combined interaction of multiple risk factors.

B. Identified risk factors include the following.
  1. Age: risk increasing with age
  2. Conformation: deep chested
    a) May increase likelihood of volvulus
    b) Altered anatomic relationship at gastroesophageal sphincter possibly impairs normal eructation
  3. Laxity of gastric ligaments (hepatogastric and hepatoduodenal): possibly increases likelihood of volvulus
  4. Intake of large volume of food or water
    a) Rapid intake leads to gastric dilatation.
    b) Large volumes of food take longer to empty than small volumes.
    c) Overdistention may result in abnormal myoelectric activity and impaired gastric emptying.
  5. Composition of diet
    a) No causal relationship proven for types of food (dry vs. canned)
    b) Effects of feeding frequency (free choice vs. intermittent feeding) unknown
  6. Postprandial exercise: may physically displace the stomach, increasing the chance of volvulus
  7. Accumulation of gastric gas
    a) Aerophagia: rapid eating or drinking, excitement, anxiety, or abnormal esophageal motility
    b) Carbon dioxide: interaction of gastric bicarbonate and acid, bacterial fermentation
  8. Impaired eructation
    a) Functionally abnormal gastroesophageal junction
    b) Impaired eructation reflex
  9. Delayed gastric emptying

Pathophysiology

I. Gastric effects
  A. Gastric hypoxia and ischemia
    1. Result from impaired gastric blood flow

a) Gas and fluid accumulation, which increase transmural pressure, resulting in venous stasis and congestion
b) Obstruction of gastric venous outflow from volvulus
c) Infarction and avulsion of short gastric and epiploic arteries and veins
d) Thrombosis of gastric microvasculature
e) Increased tissue hydrostatic pressure from interstitial edema with decreased capillary blood flow
f) Increased sympathetic tone
g) Reduced cardiac output
2. Causes a third-space shift of fluid and protein from the intravascular space into the gastric lumen
3. Results in the production (arachidonic acid pathway) and release of various cytokines that induce vascular and inflammatory changes
B. Gastric ulceration
1. Gastric hypoxia and ischemia compromise epithelial integrity, allowing back diffusion of hydrogen ions in the gastric mucosa resulting in acid-induced gastric ulceration.
2. It may lead to hemorrhage that is exacerbated when coagulation factors are consumed by disseminated intravascular coagulation.
C. Altered gastric motility
1. Ischemia and overdistention of the gastric wall may cause myonecrosis and/or damage to the myenteric plexus resulting in gastric dysrhythmias.
2. It may persist for several days following recovery.
II. Hemodynamic effects
A. Reduced venous return
1. Gastric distention occludes or partially occludes the caudal vena cava.
2. Collateral blood flow through the azygos vein and vertebral sinuses attempts to compensate for reduced flow through the vena cava.
B. Decreased cardiac output
1. Decreased venous return
2. Endotoxemia
3. Myocardial ischemia
4. Release of cardiodepressant substances
a) Tumor necrosis factor
b) Myocardial depressant factor
5. Arrhythmias and biventricular systolic and diastolic dysfunction
C. Reduced portal blood flow due to gastric dilatation
D. Reduced splanchnic blood flow
1. Decreased cardiac output
2. Gastric distention
a) Compresses adjacent large veins
b) Increases intra-abdominal pressure compressing distant veins and vascular beds
3. Caudal vena caval and portal hypertension
4. Increased sympathetic venous tone
E. Shock
1. Hypovolemia secondary to vascular pooling results in decreased blood volume, cardiac output, and arterial pressure with subsequent inadequate tissue perfusion.
2. Endotoxemia and sepsis result from breakdown of the gastric and intestinal mucosal barrier, and reduced portal blood flow prevents removal of the endotoxins and bacteria by the reticuloendothelial system.
3. Tissue hypoxia and endotoxins activate vasoactive and cytotoxic substances that perpetuate inadequate tissue perfusion.
F. Cardiac arrhythmias
1. Myocardial ischemia
2. Electrolyte and acid–base disorders
3. Autonomic imbalance
G. Disseminated intravascular coagulation
1. Vascular stasis
2. Endothelial damage
3. Platelet activation
4. Endotoxins
III. Respiratory effects
   Pressure applied to the diaphragm and thorax by the dilated stomach restricts pulmonary function, resulting in reduced blood oxygen tension.
IV. Potential effects on abdominal organs
A. Spleen: impaired splenic venous drainage, splenic congestion, possible thrombosis and necrosis
B. Liver: congestion, hemorrhage, and necrosis
C. Pancreas: edema and necrosis
D. Intestine: edema, hemorrhage, and mucosal injury
E. Kidney: eventual renal failure
V. Reperfusion injury
A. It appears that significant tissue damage may occur when ischema is relieved and tissues are reperfused.
B. Tissue damage during reperfusion occurs mainly from the release of oxygen free radicals from affected tissues and neutrophils.
C. Oxygen free radicals initiate lipoperoxidation of cell and organelle membranes, destroy intracellular enzyme systems, and cleave DNA strands.
D. It may result in multiorgan failure.
E. The role of reperfusion injury in GDV has not been completely elucidated.
VI. Severity of these changes variable in individual dogs

Clinical Signs

I. Acute, nonproductive retching
II. Excessive salvation
III. Abdominal distention and discomfort
IV. Restlessness or depression
V. Tachypnea or dyspnea
VI. Cranial abdominal distention
VII. Possible weakness or collapse

Diagnosis

I. Suspicious history and clinical signs
II. Compatible physical examination findings

A. Tympanic sound from gas-filled stomach with abdominal percussion
B. Abdominal pain
C. Splenomegaly
D. Evidence of circulatory shock
   1. Tachycardia
   2. Muddy mucous membranes
   3. Prolonged capillary refill time
   4. Weak femoral pulses
III. Laboratory findings
   A. Hemoconcentration is typical.
   B. Hypokalemia is the most common electrolyte disorder.
   C. Acid–base status is variable.
      1. Metabolic acidosis (most common) occurs because of decreased circulating blood volume, arterial hypoxemia, and lactic acid accumulation.
      2. Metabolic alkalosis mainly results from sequestration of hydrogen ions in the gastric lumen.
      3. Normal pH is noted when these changes offset each other.
IV. Radiographic findings
   A. Radiology is used to confirm the diagnosis of GDV.
   B. Preferred view is obtained with the animal in right lateral recumbency
   C. Gastric dilatation is identified by a large gas-, fluid-, and/or ingesta-filled stomach.
   D. Identification of GDV requires the following.
      1. Observation of a soft tissue fold that appears to compartmentalize the stomach.
      2. The fold results from the displacement of the pylorus in a cranial, dorsal, and leftward direction.
      3. Splenomegaly may be observed.
      4. Abdominal fluid or free abdominal gas may indicate gastric perforation.
   E. Radiography after gastric decompression can be misleading because spontaneous gastric repositioning may occur.
   F. It is often unnecessary and may cause added stress.
   G. Consider radiography after fluid therapy and temporary decompression have been initiated.

Differential Diagnosis

I. Gastric dilatation (alone)
II. Splenic torsion
III. Intestinal volvulus
IV. Diaphragmatic hernia
V. Peritonitis

Treatment

I. Goals
   A. Successful management of GDV depends on anticipating potential complications and initiating appropriate prophylactic therapy.
   B. Initial management begins with aggressive fluid therapy followed by gastric decompression to avoid the risk of cardiovascular collapse.
   C. Decompression precedes fluid therapy only if the animal is in respiratory distress.
   D. After stabilization, surgical repositioning of the stomach and gastropexy are performed.
II. Medical management—presurgical
   A. Place a large-bore catheter in either the cephalic or jugular vein. A second catheter may be used to provide rapid fluid delivery.
   B. During catheter placement, blood samples are obtained.
      1. Immediate evaluation of hematocrit (PCV)/total solids (TS), platelet count, electrolytes, blood glucose, serum urea nitrogen, urine specific gravity, and if available, activated clotting time and blood gases
      2. Complete blood count, serum biochemical profile, urinalysis, and coagulation profile
   C. Crystalloids such as lactated Ringer's solution or Normosol-R are started at an initial rate of 60–90 ml/kg/h IV.
      1. Monitoring of clinical parameters (i.e., heart rate, pulse quality) and measurement of arterial blood pressure (if available) determine end point of volume replacement.
      2. Cardiovascular and hydration status dictate subsequent fluid administration rates following initial volume replacement.
   D. Colloids may be considered if oncotic support will help maintain blood pressure (see Chaps. 69 and 131).
   E. Hypertonic saline may be given to a rapidly deteriorating, hypovolemic animal when significant hemorrhage is absent.
      1. Use a 7.5% NaCl solution or 7% NaCl in 6% dextran 70.
      2. Administer 5 ml/kg IV over 5–10 minutes.
      3. Follow with crystalloids.
   F. If fluid therapy fails to maintain mean arterial pressure above 80 mm Hg or good pulse quality, consider the following.
      1. Dobutamine 5–20 µg/kg/min IV
      2. Dopamine 5–10 µg/kg/min IV
   G. Potassium chloride is added to maintenance fluids after the initial rapid volume replacement at 20–40 mEq/L or ideally based on actual serum potassium measurement (see Chap. 47).
   H. Routine addition of sodium bicarbonate is not recommended and is only administered if the pH is <7.2 or if the base deficit is >12 mEq/L (dosage 1–2 mEq/kg IV). Sodium bicarbonate is not added to calcium-containing fluids.
   I. Dextrose is added to maintenance fluids to a concentration of 2.5–5% if hypoglycemia from endotoxemia or sepsis is present.
   J. Corticosteroids are routinely administered because of their postulated beneficial effects in the treatment of shock (see Chap. 131).
      1. Choices
         a) Prednisolone sodium succinate 11–30 mg/kg IV

b) Dexamethasone sodium phosphate 1–2 mg/kg IV
   2. May be best given prior to gastric decompression

K. Oxygen-derived free radical inhibitors or scavengers
   1. They are used for treatment of reperfusion injury.
   2. They must be given prior to reperfusion to be effective.
   3. Desferrioxamine, dimethyl sulfoxide (DMSO), allopurinol, and deferoxamine have been studied in the dog.
   4. The role and effectiveness of these drugs must be better clarified before they can be recommended.

L. Antibiotics and antiarhythmics (see under Postoperative medical management)

III. Gastric decompression
A. Trocarization
   1. It is less stressful than passing a stomach tube.
   2. Use a 16–18-gauge 2-inch needle or over the needle catheter.
   3. Percuss the abdomen to ensure that the spleen is not in the path of the needle.
   4. Partial decompression by trocarization may facilitate passage of an orogastric tube.

B. Orogastric tube
   1. Use a large-bore, well-lubricated tube.
   2. Measure the tube (from end of nose to last rib) to avoid advancing the tube too far and damaging or perforating a weakened gastric wall.
   3. If the tube is difficult to pass, rotating the tube or placing the dog in a sitting or elevated head position may facilitate passage.
   4. Excessive force on the tube may result in esophageal or gastric perforation.
   5. Narcotics may facilitate passage of the tube in noncompliant animals.
      a) Oxymorphone 0.1–0.2 mg/kg IV
      b) Meperidine 0.5 mg/kg IV
   6. After decompression of the stomach is achieved, lavage the stomach with warm water to remove remaining contents.
   7. Inability to pass the tube does not confirm volvulus, and passage of the tube does not rule it out.

C. Temporary gastrostomy
   1. Used in animals too unstable to undergo surgery.
   2. Use if gastric decompression cannot be achieved by trocarization or via a stomach tube.

D. Importance and timing
   1. It is essential that gastric decompression is achieved prior to surgery.
   2. Following gastric decompression, spontaneous repositioning of the stomach may occur. In most cases, however, surgical correction of the volvulus and gastropexy to prevent recurrence are still required.

IV. Surgical management
A. General principles
   1. Surgical intervention should occur as soon as the patient is stabilized by appropriate fluid and decompression therapy.
      a) The incidence of complications appears to increase the longer surgery is delayed.
      b) Patient stabilization is usually accomplished within 2–4 hours of presentation.
   2. Longer periods of stabilization maybe necessary in animals with marked electrolyte or acid–base imbalances or cardiac arrhythmias or in animals that require transport to a referral center for surgery and postoperative care. Decompression can be maintained during this time with a nasogastric, pharyngostomy, or esophagostomy tube or via temporary gastrostomy.
   3. Radiographic evidence of perforation or the presence of blood during gastric lavage indicates the need for immediate surgery.
   4. Goals of surgery include the following.
      a) Anatomic repositioning of the stomach
      b) Assessment of gastric and splenic viability
      c) Gastropexy to prevent recurrence
         Without surgical gastropexy, recurrence rates are as high as 71–80% (Meyer-Lindenberg et al., 1993; Eggertsdottir and Moe, 1995).

B. Anesthesia
   1. Preanesthetics
      a) Oxymorphone 0.1–0.2 mg/kg IM, IV
      b) Meperidine 0.5 mg/kg IM, IV
   2. Induction with agents that spare the cardiovascular system
      a) Combination agents
         (1) Diazepam 0.25 mg/kg and ketamine 2.5 mg/kg IV
         (2) Diazepam 0.25 mg/kg and oxymorphone 0.1–0.2 mg/kg IV
      b) Mask down with inhalant agents
   3. Maintenance with inhalant agents
      a) Isoflurane: anesthetic of choice
      b) Halothane
   4. Assisted ventilation recommended
   5. Patient monitoring
      a) Mucous membrane color and peripheral pulse
      b) Direct or indirect blood pressure, maintain above 60 mmHg
      c) Pulse oximetry
      d) End tidal CO_2
      e) Electrocardiography
      f) Blood gases
      g) PCV/TS in any actively bleeding patient

C. Surgical procedures
   1. Derotation of stomach/spleen
      a) Passage of a stomach tube after induction of anesthesia allows continuous gastric decompression.
      b) The stomach typically rotates such that

the pylorus moves dorsally, cranially, and to the left; the fundus moves ventrally, caudally, and to the right.

   c) Rotation is usually 90–360° in a clockwise direction with the animal in a ventrodorsal position.

2. Assessment of stomach and splenic viability

   a) Infarction and necrosis are most commonly found along the greater curvature of the body and fundus.

   b) Gastric wall viability is most often based on subjective clinical evaluation of serosal color, perfusion, and vascular patency.

     (1) Greenish to grayish serosa indicates arterial injury and probable necrosis.

     (2) Blue-black to black serosa represents venous occlusion.

     (3) Dark red serosa usually represents a reversible lesion.

     (4) Lack of active bleeding after incision of gastric wall indicates devitalized tissue.

     (5) Evaluation of the gastric mucosa is a poor indicator of gastric mural viability.

   c) Suspect areas are reevaluated after gastric repositioning.

   d) Use of intravenous fluorescein is not as accurate as the other clinical criteria in assessing gastric wall viability.

   e) Nuclear imaging may be valuable in assessing gastric wall viability postoperatively.

3. Partial gastrectomy

   a) It is performed when gastric wall necrosis is evident.

   b) A stapling instrument allows the procedure to be performed rapidly while preserving a closed lumen.

4. Partial gastric invagination

   a) It is simple and efficient to perform and does not require opening of the gastric lumen.

   b) It is used when gastric wall viability is difficult to assess or when it is essential to reduce surgical time.

   c) Large invaginations are avoided because of the potential for severe hemorrhage when the tissues slough.

5. Complete or partial splenectomy

   a) They are performed only when vessel infarction and/or avulsion lead to splenic necrosis.

   b) They do not influence the recurrence of gastric volvulus.

   c) Other abdominal organs are also inspected for pathology.

6. Gastropexy

   a) It is performed to prevent recurrence of volvulus.

   b) Most methods involve pexy of the gastric antrum to the right side of the dog to

prevent the pylorus and duodenum from moving to the left as the stomach rotates.

   c) The technique used depends on surgeon preference and time involved.

   d) Recurrence rates are similar for all gastropexy techniques.

   e) Tube gastrostomy/gastropexy can be performed easily and rapidly and allows for gastric decompression and/or a route enteral nutrition postoperatively.

     (1) Appears to have a higher morbidity rate associated with premature tube removal, cellulitis around tube, and alterations in gastric myoelectric activity

     (2) Usually reserved for the most critically ill dogs

     (3) Recommended when significant gastric resection is required

     (4) May be used in combination with another gastropexy technique

   f) For incisional gastropexy, incisions are made in the abdominal wall and gastric antrum and are sutured together (Betts, 1976).

   g) During circumcostal gastropexy, a rectangular flap is created in the gastric antrum and sutured around the caudal most complete rib on the right side (Fallah et al., 1982).

   h) Muscular flap gastropexy involves suturing a transversus abdominis muscle flap to the edge of an incision in the seromuscular layer of the pyloric antrum (Schulman et al., 1986).

   i) For a belt-loop gastropexy, a tongue-shaped flap is created in the gastric antrum, passed through a tunnel created in the transversus abdominis muscle, and reattached to the antrum (Whitney, 1989a).

   j) Median gastropexy is when the gastric antrum is incorporated into the cranial suture of the abdominal wall during closure (Meyer-Lindenberg et al., 1993). Formed adhesions may complicate future abdominal surgery.

7. Tube placement for postoperative decompression and care

   a) Gastrostomy tube (see earlier)

   b) Nasogastric tube

     (1) When gastric resection not required

     (2) Placed intraoperatively to ensure proper positioning

   c) Jejunostomy tube if gastric resection is necessary or significant pancreatic pathology exists

V. Postoperative medical management

  A. Fluid therapy

   1. Maintain isotonic fluids at a rate that meets maintenance requirements and replaces potential continuing losses from vomiting and/or diarrhea (see Appendix I).

2. Maintain normal serum potassium levels with 20–30 mEq of KCl added to each liter of maintenance fluids in animals with normal serum potassium levels (because of a likely total body potassium deficit). Increase dosage in animals with lower serum potassium levels.
3. Colloids may be used in combination with crystalloid at 20 ml/kg/day to reduce the amount of crystalloids needed.
4. Fluids can be discontinued over a 36–48-hour period after institution of oral alimentation.

B. Alimentation
1. Withhold food and water for 24–48 hours.
2. Gradually start oral alimentation.
   a) Offer small amounts of water.
   b) Introduce food in another 12–24 hours if no vomiting occurs.
      (1) Easily digestible diet of low fat and protein content (e.g., Prescription Diet i/d)
      (2) Small amounts every 4–6 hours
      (3) No more than ½ of the daily caloric requirement on the first day
      (4) Quantity of food increased and the frequency of feedings decreased over next 2–3 days
3. Enteral (jejunostomy tube) or parenteral nutrition is considered in animals with prolonged postoperative vomiting or other complications that prevent oral alimentation.

C. Treatment of cardiac arrhythmias
1. Arrhythmias occur in approximately 50% of the cases.
2. Most occur 12–36 hours after presentation, so constant electrocardiographic (ECG) monitoring is required.
3. Most are ventricular in origin.
   a) Ventricular premature contractions (VPCs)
   b) Ventricular tachycardia (most common)
4. Indications for treatment of ventricular arrhythmias are as follows.
   a) Clinical signs of decreased cardiac output
   b) Greater than 20–30 VPCs per minute
   c) Multifocal QRS configuration
   d) R wave falls close to T wave (R on T phenomenon)
   e) Repetitive or persistent ventricular tachycardia
   f) Failure to subside with correction of hypoxia, hypovolemia, electrolyte and acid–base abnormalities
5. Lidocaine hydrochloride is the drug of choice.
   a) Initially, give slow bolus of 1–2 mg/kg IV.
   b) If the arrhythmia recurs, begin continuous IV infusion of 25 µg/kg/min, and increase up to 75 µg/kg/min based on clinical need.
   c) Side effects include vomiting, tremors, seizures, and hypotension.
6. Procainamide hydrochloride (8–20 mg/kg IM, PO TID-QID) is useful for maintaining control of the arrhythmia following successful therapy with lidocaine.
   a) If the arrhythmia remains controlled, taper the lidocaine infusion over 24–48 hours and maintain on oral procainamide.
   b) Procainamide can also be used as a first line antiarrhythmic or if the arrhythmia is refractory to lidocaine.
      (1) Initially, give slow IV bolus of 6–12 mg/kg over 5 minutes.
      (2) Follow with a continuous IV infusion beginning at 20 µg/kg/min, and adjust dosage upward to 50 µg/kg/min based on clinical need.
7. Other antiarrhythmmics may be considered.
   a) Mexiletine and tocainide are orally active synthetic analogues of lidocaine.
   b) They can be used in place of procainamide for continued antiarrhythmic therapy in lidocaine-responsive ventricular arrhythmias.
      (1) Dosage for tocainide is 10–20 mg/kg PO TID.
      (2) Dosage for mexiletine is 5–8 mg/kg PO BID-TID.
8. Ventricular arrhythmias may be refractory to all treatments and may become life-threatening, or they may resolve on their own.

D. Antibiotics
1. They are often administered because of predisposition to sepsis.
2. They should be effective against gram-positive and gram-negative aerobes and anaerobes.
   a) Ampicillin 22 mg/kg IV TID
   b) Cephalexin 22 mg/kg IV TID
3. For severely affected dogs (septic shock or gastric necrosis evident), consider additional antibiotics.
   a) Ampicillin/cephalexin plus enrofloxacin at 2.5 mg/kg IV BID
   b) Ampicillin/cephalexin plus gentamicin at 2.2 mg/kg IV TID
   c) Gentamicin is administered with extreme caution and only after initial fluid volume replacement because it is nephrotoxic in the face of hypovolemia. It is usually reserved for postoperative administration.

E. Disseminated intravascular coagulation (DIC): see therapy in Chap. 66

F. Gastric acid inhibitors
1. Indicated in animals with moderate to severe gastric mucosal injury
2. Cimetidine 10 mg/kg IV, PO TID-QID
3. Ranitidine 1–2 mg/kg IV, PO BID-TID

G. Prokinetic agents
1. Indicated for persistent postoperative vomiting or delayed gastric emptying and ileus
2. Immediate postoperative period: metoclopramide 0.5 mg/kg IV, SQ, TID-QID or 1–2 mg/kg/day continuous IV infusion
3. For long-term management

a) Metoclopramide 0.5 mg/kg PO TID
b) Cisapride 0.5 mg/kg PO TID
c) Erythromycin 1–5 mg/kg PO TID

Patient Monitoring

I. Close monitoring is essential owing to the high incidence of complications.
II. Repeat physical examinations every 4–6 hours, paying attention to the following.
  A. Attitude
  B. Hydration status
  C. Body temperature
  D. Appearance of mucous membranes
  E. Pulse quality
  F. Heart rate and rhythm
  G. Presence of tympany or pain on abdominal palpation
III. Assess fluid therapy via measurement of body weight, packed cell volume/total solids, electrolytes, and blood gases (if considered necessary) every 12–24 hours.
IV. Monitor hemodynamic status with the following.
  A. Pulse quality, indirect blood pressure, urine output, central venous pressure
  B. Continuous ECG
V. Monitor for presence of anemia and hypoproteinemia.
  A. PCV/TS, biochemical profile
  B. PCV < 20%: transfusion of packed red cells or whole blood
  C. Total protein <3–3.5 g/dl: colloidal support
VI. Assess for sepsis via measurement of complete blood count and blood glucose every 24 hours.
VII. Gastric necrosis, gastric rupture, and peritonitis account for most postoperative deaths.
  A. If suspected, confirm by abdominocentesis, radiography (plain, contrast), ultrasonography, or diagnostic peritoneal lavage.
  B. Onset of peritonitis requires immediate surgical intervention.
VIII. Assessment of organ damage is done via repeated blood chemistries and urinalysis.
IX. Presence of disseminated intravascular coagulation is confirmed by coagulation profile (see Chap. 66).
X. Mortality associated with GDV is as high as 60%.
XI. Factors associated with higher mortality rates include the following.
  A. Delayed diagnosis
  B. Non-aggressive treatment
  C. Compromised cardiovascular function
  D. Depressed mentation
  E. Coagulation abnormalities
  F. Need for partial gastrectomy

Prevention

I. Diet and feeding change may be tried.
  A. No specific type of diet is recommended.
  B. Feed multiple (2–4) small meals per day.
  C. Limit exercise postprandially.
  D. Minimize consumption of large amounts of water.
II. Gastropexy is performed in animals with simple gastric dilatation to prevent volvulus that may accompany subsequent episodes.

Bibliography

Allen DA, Schertel ER, Muir WW III, Valentine AK: Hypertonic saline/dextran resuscitation of dogs with experimentally induced gastric dilatation-volvulus shock. Am J Vet Res 52:92, 1991

Andrews FJ, Malcontenti C, O'Brien PE: Sequence of gastric mucosal injury following ischemia and reperfusion. Role of reactive oxygen metabolites. Dig Dis Sci 37:1356, 1992

Badylak SF, Lantz GC, Jeffries M: Prevention of reperfusion injury in surgically induced gastric dilatation-volvulus in dogs. Am J Vet Res 51:294, 1990

Berardi C, Wheaton LG, Twardock AR et al: Nuclear imaging to evaluate gastric mucosal viability following surgical correction of gastric dilatation/volvulus. J Am Anim Hosp Assoc 29:239, 1993

Betts CW: "Permanent" gastropexy—as a prophylactic measure against gastric-volvulus. J Am Anim Hosp Assoc 12:177, 1976

Brockman DJ, Washabau RJ, Drobatz KJ: Canine gastric dilatation/volvulus syndrome in a veterinary critical care unit: 295 cases (1986–1992). J Am Vet Med Assoc 207:460, 1995

Burrows DF, Bright RM, Spencer CP: Influence of dietary composition on gastric emptying and motility in dogs: potential involvement in acute gastric dilatation. Am J Vet Res 46:2609, 1985

Caldwell CB, Ricota JJ: Changes in visceral blood flow with elevated intraabdominal pressure. J Surg Res 43:14, 1987

Clark GN, Pavletic MM: Partial gastrectomy using an automatic stapling instrument for treatment of gastric necrosis secondary to gastric dilatation-volvulus. Vet Surg 20:61, 1991

Crowe DT: Use of a nasogastric tube for gastric and esophageal decompression in the dog and cat. J Am Vet Med Assoc 188:1178, 1986

Eggertsdottir AV, Moe L: A retrospective study of conservative management of gastric-dilatation volvulus in the dog. Acta Vet Scand 36:175, 1995

Ellison GW: Gastric dilatation-volvulus. Surgical prevention. Vet Clin North Am [Small Anim Pract] 23:513, 1993

Fallah AM, Lumb WV, Nelson AW et al: Circumcostal gastropexy in the dog—a preliminary study. Vet Surg 11:9, 1982

Flanders JA, Harvey HJ: Results of tube gastrostomy as treatment for gastric volvulus in the dog. J Am Vet Med Assoc 185:74, 1984

Forman MB, Virmani R, Puett DW: Mechanisms and therapy of myocardial reperfusion injury. Circulation 81:69, 1990

Glickman LT, Glickman NW, Perez MS et al: Analysis of risk factors for gastric dilatation and gastric dilatation-volvulus in dogs. J Am Vet Med Assoc 204:1465, 1994

Hall JA, Solie TN, Seim HB et al: Acute gastric dilatation alters gastric electromechanical activity in the dog. Gastroenterology 95:869, 1988

Hall JA, Twedt DC, Curtis CR: Relationship of plasma gastrin immunoreactivity and gastroesophageal sphincter pressure in clinically normal dogs and in dogs with previous gastric dilation-volvulus. Am J Vet Res 50:1228, 1989

Hall JA, Willer RL, Seim HB et al: Gastric emptying of nondigestible radiopaque markers after circumcostal gastropexy in clinically normal dogs and dogs with gastric dilatation-volvulus. Am J Vet Res 53:1964, 1992

Harvey RC: Anesthetic management for canine gastric dilatation-volvulus. Semin Vet Med Surg (Small Anim) 1:230, 1986

Hathcock JT: Radiographic view of choice for the diagnosis of gastric volvulus: the right lateral recumbent view. J Am Anim Hosp Assoc 20:967, 1984

Horne WA, Gilmore DR, Dietze AE et al: Effects of gastric distention-volvulus on coronary blood flow and myocardial oxygen consumption in the dog. Am J Vet Res 46:98, 1985

Hosgood G: Gastric dilatation-volvulus in dogs. J Am Vet Med Assoc 204:1742, 1994

Jennings PB, Mathey WS, Ehler WJ: Intermittent gastric dilatation after gastropexy in a dog. J Am Vet Med Assoc 200:1707, 1992

Johnson RG, Barrus J, Greene RW: Gastric dilatation-volvulus: recurrence rate following tube gastrostomy. J Am Anim Hosp Assoc 20:33, 1984

Komtebedde J, Guilford WG, Haskins SC et al: Evaluation of systemic and splanchnic visceral oxygen variables in dogs with surgically induced gastric dilatation-volvulus. Vet Crit Care 1:5, 1991

Lantz GC: Oxygen free radicals and reperfusion injury. p. 64. In Bonagura JD (ed): Kirk's Current Veterinary Therapy XII: Small Animal Practice. WB Saunders, Philadelphia, 1995

Lantz GC, Badylak SF: Treatment of reperfusion injury in dogs with experimentally induced gastric dilatation volvulus. Am J Vet Res 53:1594, 1992

Lantz GC, Bottoms GD, Carlton WW et al: The effect of 360 gastric volvulus on the blood supply of the nondistended normal dog stomach. Vet Surg 13:189, 1984

Leib MS: Circumcostal gastropexy for preventing recurrence of gastric dilatation-volvulus in the dog: an evaluation of 30 cases. J Am Vet Med Assoc 187:245, 1985

Leib MS, Blass CE: Gastric dilatation-volvulus in dogs: an update. Compend Contin Educ Pract Vet 6:961, 1984

Leib MS, Martin RA: Therapy of gastric dilatation-volvulus in dogs. Compend Contin Educ Pract Vet 9:225, 1987

Leib MS, Wingfield WE, Twedt DC et al: Plasma gastrin immunoreactivity in dogs with acute gastric dilation-volvulus. J Am Vet Med Assoc 185:205, 1984

Matthiesen DT: Partial gastrectomy as treatment of gastric volvulus. Results in 30 dogs. Vet Surg 14:185, 1985

Matthiesen DT: Indications and techniques of partial gastrectomy in the dog. Semin Vet Med Surg 2:248, 1987

Matthiesen DT: Pathophysiology of gastric dilatation-volvulus. p. 220. In Bojarb MJ (ed): Disease Mechanisms in Small Animal Surgery. Lea and Febiger, Philadelphia, 1993a

Matthiesen DT: Gastric dilatation-volvulus syndrome. p. 580. In Slatter D (ed): Textbook of Small Animal Surgery. W B Saunders, Philadelphia, 1993b

McCord JM: Oxygen derived free radicals in postischemic tissue injury. N Engl J Med 312:159, 1985

McCoy DM: Partial invagination of the canine stomach for treatment of infarction of the gastric wall. Vet Surg 15:237, 1986

Meyer-Lindenberg A, Harder A, Fehr M et al: Treatment of gastric dilatation-volvulus and a rapid method for prevention of relapse in dogs: 134 cases (1988–1991). J Am Vet Med Assoc 203:1303, 1993

Millis DL, Hauptman JG, Fulton RB: Abnormal hemostatic profiles and gastric necrosis in canine gastric dilatation-volvulus. Vet Surg 22:93, 1993

Muir WW: Acid-base and electrolyte disturbances in dogs with gastric dilatation-volvulus. J Am Vet Med Assoc 182:229, 1982a

Muir WW: Gastric dilatation-volvulus in the dog, with emphasis on cardiac arrhythmias. J Am Vet Med Assoc 180:739, 1982b

Muir WW: Small-volume resuscitation using hypertonic saline. Cornell Vet J 80:7, 1990

Muir WW, Bonagura JD: Treatment of cardiac arrhythmias in dogs with gastric dilatation-volvulus. J Am Vet Med Assoc 184:1366, 1984

Muir WW, Lipowitz AJ: Cardiac dysrhythmias associated with gastric dilatation-volvulus in the dog. J Am Vet Med Assoc 172:683, 1978

Muir WW, Weisbrode SE. Myocardial ischemia in dogs with gastric dilatation-volvulus. J Am Vet Med Assoc 181:363, 1982

Orton EC, Muir WW: Isovolumetric indices and humoral cardioactive substance bioassay during clinical and experimentally induced gastric dilatation-volvulus in dogs. Am J Vet Res 44:1516, 1983a

Orton EC, Muir WW: Hemodynamics in experimental gastric dilatation-volvulus in dogs. Am J Vet Res 44:1512, 1983b

Pfeiffer CJ, Keith JC, April M: Topographic localization of gastric lesions and key role of plasma bicarbonate concentration in dogs with experimentally induced gastric dilatation. Am J Vet Res 48:262, 1987

Sanan S, Sharma G, Singh B et al: Evaluation of desferrioxamine mesylate on survival and prevention of histopathological changes in the liver, in hemorrhagic shock: an experimental study in dogs. Resuscitation 17:63, 1989

Schulman AJ, Lusk R, Lippincott CL et al: Muscular flap gastropexy: a new technique to prevent reoccurrences of gastric dilatation-volvulus syndrome. J Am Anim Hosp Assoc 22:339, 1986

Stampley AR, Burrows CF, Ellison GW et al: Gastric myoelectric activity after experimental gastric dilatation-volvulus and tube gastrostomy in dogs. Vet Surg 21:10, 1992

Strombeck DR, Harrold D: Effect of gastrin, histamine, serotonin, and adrenergic amines on gastroesophageal sphincter pressure in the dog. Am J Vet Res 46:1684, 1985

Van Kruiningen HJ, Wojan LD, Stake PE et al: The influence of diet and feeding frequency on gastric function in the dog. J Am Anim Hosp Assoc 23:145, 1987

Wheaton LG, Thacker HL, Caldwell S: Intravenous fluorescein as an indicator of gastric viability in gastric dilatation-volvulus. J Am Anim Hosp Assoc 22:197, 1986

Whitney WO: Belt-loop gastropexy: technique and results of surgery in 20 dogs. J Am Anim Hosp 25:75, 1989a

Whitney WO: Complications associated with the medical and surgical management of gastric dilatation-volvulus in the dog. Probl Vet Med 1:268, 1989b

Wingfield WE, Betts CW, Rawlings CA: Pathophysiology associated with gastric dilatation-volvulus in the dog. J Am Anim Hosp Assoc. 12:126, 1976

Wingfield WE, Twedt DC, Moore RW et al: Acid-base and electrolyte values in dogs with acute gastric dilatation-volvulus. J Am Vet Med Assoc 180:1070, 1982

Diseases of the Small Intestines

David A. Williams

32

CONGENITAL/ DEVELOPMENTAL DISORDERS

Selective Cobalamin Malabsorption in Giant Schnauzers and Border Collie Dogs

Definition and Cause

I. Selective inability to absorb cobalamin (vitamin B_{12})
II. Possibly inherited as an autosomal recessive trait to a specific defect in ileal mucosal function

Pathophysiology

I. In giant schnauzers, a defect has been demonstrated in transport of intrinsic factor/cobalamin complex receptor to the ileal brush border membrane and is caused by defective glycosylation during synthesis of the receptor.
II. All other nutrients are absorbed normally.

Clinical Signs

I. Anorexia and lethargy at 7–12 weeks of age; later in Border collies
II. Failure to gain weight, cachexia
III. Normal linear growth of bone

Diagnosis

I. Characteristic signalment and history
II. Severely low serum cobalamin concentration
   A. Use assay method validated for use in dog serum.
   B. Normal concentration is 348 ± 88 pg/ml.
III. Hematologic findings (see Chap. 63)
   A. Mild nonregenerative anemia
   B. Neutropenia, hypersegmented neutrophils
   C. Occasionally enlarged platelets

D. Rare megaloblastic changes in red cell precursors in bone marrow
IV. Methylmalonic aciduria: reflects metabolic defect secondary to cobalamin deficiency

Differential Diagnosis

I. Rule out other causes of anorexia and lethargy in young dogs, e.g., other vitamin deficiencies, portosystemic shunts, certain toxins, and infectious diseases.
II. Rule out other causes of failure to thrive, e.g., severe intestinal parasitism, malnutrition, other malaborptive diseases, and immunodeficiencies.

Treatment and Monitoring

I. Give cyanocobalamin 0.25–1 mg SQ, IM weekly for 1 month, then every 3–6 months.
II. Dogs should be normal within 1 month after onset of treatment.
III. Assay serum cobalamin every 6–12 months or if signs recur.
IV. Do not breed affected animals.

Wheat-Sensitive Enteropathy in Irish Setters

Definition and Cause

I. It is a hereditary defect in small intestinal mucosal function associated with dietary sensitivity to gluten in wheat.
II. Underlying abnormal permeability of the small intestines may play a role in the development of sensitivity to gluten.

Pathophysiology

I. Challenge of affected dogs with gluten results in changes in the intestinal mucosa that interfere with the normal digestive–absorptive process.

353

A. Changes in brush border enzyme activities
B. Increased permeability of the intestine to low-molecular-weight markers such as ethylenediaminetetraacetic acid (EDTA)
C. Increased numbers of intraepithelial lymphocytes
D. Decreased villous height
II. An abnormal immune reaction to gluten or its breakdown products appears to mediate epithelial cell destruction.
III. Withdrawal of wheat from the diet results in improvement of mucosal abnormalities.

Clinical Signs

I. Diarrhea (semiformed feces) beginning at 4–7 months of age
II. Weight loss or poor weight gain
III. Small stature

Diagnosis

I. Suspicious signs in a young Irish setter should be investigated.
II. Serum folate concentration may be subnormal, reflecting dysfunction of the upper small intestine.
III. Xylose absorption test results may also be subnormal.
IV. Intestinal biopsy often reveals villous atrophy with increased intraepithelial lymphocytes.
V. Resolution of clinical signs after withdrawal of dietary sources of gluten supports the diagnosis.
VI. Return of clinical signs and abnormalities in jejunal mucosa after challenge with diets containing gluten is definitive.

Differential Diagnosis

I. Other malabsorptive diseases of the small intestines (see later)
II. Intestinal parasitism
III. Inflammatory bowel disease

Treatment and Monitoring

I. Feed only diets that contain no wheat products.
A. Most commercial pet foods contain gluten.
B. Commercial gluten-free diets are available.
II. Dogs should be normal within 4–6 weeks of changing the diet.
III. Assay serum folate and cobalamin every 6–12 months or if signs recur.
IV. Do not breed affected animals.

INFECTIOUS DISEASES

Viral Infections

Definition

Numerous viruses have been implicated as pathogens causing infectious enteritis in dogs and cats.

Causes

I. Canine intestinal viruses include parvoviruses, coronavirus, rotavirus, astrovirus, paramyxo-like virus, adenovirus, picornavirus, and distemper virus.
II. Feline intestinal viruses include panleukopenia virus (parvovirus), enteric coronavirus, rotavirus, astrovirus, feline immunodeficiency virus, and feline leukemia virus.

Pathophysiology

I. Most commonly the virus invades and kills the enterocytes lining the villi or crypts.
II. The severity of clinical signs reflects the degree and site of enterocyte loss.
A. Villus cell damage (e.g., by coronavirus) is relatively well tolerated because enterocytes are soon replaced as crypt proliferation continues.
B. Crypt cell damage (e.g., by parvovirus) results in severe clinical signs because normal enterocyte proliferation is disrupted with subsequent massive loss of villous absorptive and barrier functions.

Clinical Signs

Tremendous variation exists in the spectrum and severity of signs (see also Chap 110).
I. Canine parvovirus
A. Initial lethargy and inappetence, commonly followed by fever, depression, dehydration, vomiting, and diarrhea
B. Diarrhea, tinged with blood
C. Hypothermia and endotoxic shock terminally
D. Doberman pinschers, rottweilers: increased susceptibility, even after routine vaccination
E. Subclinical disease in older animals
II. Canine coronavirus
A. Similar to parvovirus, but signs less severe
B. Pyrexia and hemorrhagic diarrhea less common
III. Rotavirus: mild self-limiting diarrhea in puppies and kittens
IV. Canine distemper
A. Severe diarrhea with vomiting, dehydration, and rapid weight loss
B. Intestinal signs often before respiratory and other signs
V. Feline panleukopenia virus
A. Varies from mild diarrhea, anorexia, and depression to severe hemorrhagic diarrhea, fever, and vomiting
B. More severe in kittens
VI. Feline enteric coronavirus
A. Infection often subclinical but may cause mild to moderate diarrhea with vomiting and fever
B. Predominantly affects young kittens 4–12 weeks of age
VII. Feline leukemia virus
A. Occasionally associated with a panleukopenia-like syndrome accompanied by diarrhea and weight loss

B. May cause signs of bowel obstruction or malabsorption from lymphosarcoma of the bowel

VIII. Feline immunodeficiency virus: chronic diarrhea with or without weight loss

Diagnosis

I. Infection with viruses is common in recently acquired (nonvaccinated) puppies and other nonvaccinated dogs.

II. Littermates are often affected simultaneously in kennel or cattery situations.

III. Hematologic tests may provide clues as to the cause.
   A. Leukopenia (neutropenia) is common with parvovirus or panleukopenia virus.
   B. Distemper virus causes lymphopenia, atypical reactive lymphocytes, and viral inclusion bodies in red and white blood cells (most commonly seen in buffy coat smears).
   C. Canine and feline coronaviruses do not usually cause significant changes in the hemogram.
   D. Neutrophilia may develop during the recovery phase.
   E. Neutrophils may show signs of toxic change.

IV. Commercial enzyme immunoassays for parvovirus and rotavirus antigen in feces are reliable, rapid, and inexpensive.

V. Electron microscopic detection of virus particles in feces is a rapid and inexpensive diagnostic method available at some specialized laboratories. Consider this test to confirm viral involvement when simple screening tests are negative.

VI. Virus isolation is diagnostic but is also expensive, time consuming, and not widely available.

VII. Serodiagnosis requires demonstration of seroconversion (two samples, 2–4 weeks apart) or the presence of immunoglobulin M (IgM), which is found only during the few weeks immediately after infection (see Chap. 110).

VIII. Necropsy and light microscopy are diagnostic in most cases of canine distemper and parvovirus infection, but other methods such as electron microscopy are required to confirm coronavirus, rotavirus, and other infections.

Differential Diagnosis

I. Nonspecific enteritis
II. Bacterial enteritis
III. Toxin-induced intestinal disease
IV. Gastrointestinal foreign bodies and obstruction
V. Acute pancreatitis

Treatment

I. Outpatient supportive care is adequate in mild cases.
   A. Rest the intestinal tract by withholding food for 24–72 hours.
   B. Introduce small, frequent meals of a bland, low-fat diet (e.g., rice, pasta, potato) after resolution of vomiting and diarrhea.
   C. Reintroduce a regular maintenance diet over several days.
   D. Oral fluid therapy may be given, such as Enterolyte or Pedialyte at a rate of 40–80 ml/kg/day.

II. Parenteral fluid therapy is required if clinical signs are severe and dehydration is present.
   A. Lactated Ringer's or 0.9% sodium chloride can be given at a rate of 40–80 ml/kg/day SQ, IV, with additional volume to replace ongoing losses.
   B. Add potassium chloride (10–20 mEq/L) to the fluids if anorexia, vomiting, and diarrhea are severe or if hypokalemia is demonstrated.
   C. Young animals may become hypoglycemic and may benefit from oral or IV glucose solutions.
   D. Subcutaneous fluid administration is avoided in leukopenic animals because of the risk of secondary infections.
   E. Acid–base abnormalities are variable, because vomiting may lead to alkalosis, and diarrhea to acidosis. Treat acid–base disorders only as indicated by blood gas analysis.
   F. Plasma, whole blood transfusion, or hetastarch is indicated if hypoalbuminemia is severe (albumin <1.5 g/dl).

III. Isolate animals with suspected viral gastroenteritis to prevent infection of other animals.

IV. Antibiotics are not usually needed in mild cases of viral gastroenteritis. However, parenteral antibiotic therapy is warranted in animals with severe viral gastroenteritis (hemorrhagic diarrhea, vomiting, leukopenia) when bacteremia and endotoxemia are likely. Suitable antibiotics include the following.
   A. Ampicillin 11–22 mg/kg SQ, IM, IV TID-QID and gentamicin 2 mg/kg SQ, IM, IV TID
   B. Enrofloxacin, dog: 2–4 mg/kg PO, SQ BID; cat: 1–2 mg/kg PO, SQ BID

V. Motility modifiers such as loperamide (Imodium) are not recommended for symptomatic control of diarrhea in viral gastroenteritis. Exceptions may be made for mildly affected patients treated on an outpatient basis.

VI. Antiemetics are indicated when vomiting is severe.
   A. Chlorpromazine 0.5 mg/kg SQ TID-QID
   B. Metoclopramide 0.3–0.5 mg/kg SQ TID-QID or as a continuous IV drip at 0.01–0.02 mg/kg/h

Patient Monitoring

I. Re-examine hospitalized animals several times a day to assess hydration and evaluate complications such as septic shock and intestinal intussusception.

II. Monitor laboratory parameters.
   A. Determine packed cell volume (PCV) and total solids SID-BID to evaluate the state of hydration and determine the progression of hypoproteinemia.
   B. Evaluate serum electrolytes and acid–base status SID-QOD as clinical signs warrant.

III. Consider vaccination of all potentially exposed animals.

IV. In cases of parvovirus infection, disinfect the environment with household bleach at a 1:32 dilution.

V. Prognosis for most patients with viral gastroenteritis is good.
A. Patients with parvovirus enteritis may require aggressive and expensive supportive care.
B. The prognosis is more guarded in young animals.
C. Some dogs develop potentially reversible dietary sensitivity following recovery from acute disease. This sensitivity may resolve spontaneously if the offending antigen(s) is removed from the diet for several weeks by feeding an appropriate elimination diet.

Bacterial Infections

Definition

I. Bacterial enteritis is caused by a number of bacteria that either invade the intestinal mucosa or produce enterotoxins.
II. Documentation of the role of bacterial pathogens causing diarrhea in dogs and cats is still limited.

Causes

I. *Escherichia coli* is a normal organism in the ileum and large bowel, but both invasive and enterotoxigenic isolates may potentially cause diarrhea in dogs and cats.
II. *Salmonella* spp. are frequently isolated from feces of clinically normal dogs and cats. Impaired immunity from malnutrition, malignancy, and immunosuppressive therapy may increase the incidence of clinical disease.
III. *Yersinia enterocolitica* and *Yersinia pseudotuberculosis* may be found in asymptomatic dogs and cats but have also been associated with enterocolitis in dogs and cats.
IV. *Bacillus piliformis* (Tyzzer's disease) rarely causes chronic hemorrhagic enterocolitis with hepatic necrosis in dogs and cats.
V. *Campylobacter jejuni* is a motile microaerophilic thermophilic bacterium that can cause enteritis in both people and animals.
VI. *Clostridium* spp. are involved with some intestinal diseases.
A. *C. difficile* and its cytotoxin have been associated with antibiotic-responsive diarrhea.
B. *C. perfringens* type A enterotoxin has been associated with outbreaks of diarrhea in hospitalized dogs.
C. *Clostridium* spp. have been implicated in canine hemorrhagic gastroenteritis (see later).

Pathophysiology

I. Toxigenic diarrhea is due to the release of enterotoxins produced by the bacteria.
A. Enterotoxin stimulates cyclic adenosine monophosphate, which increases sodium-dependent chloride secretion from crypt cells, thereby causing loss of water, bicarbonate, and potassium into the gut lumen.

B. Included in this group are *E. coli* and *C. perfringens.*
II. Invasive organisms cause enteritis by their ability to invade intestinal epithelium, especially that of the lower bowel (distal ileum and colon).
A. Local inflammation disrupts the mucosal barrier and results in exudative loss of plasma and/or blood, with increased mucus production. Bacteremia is common.
B. *Salmonella, Y. enterocolitica,* and *Campylobacter* are invasive organisms.
III. Antibiotics can alter the resident microbial flora and allow invasion of antibiotic-resistant strains of bacterial pathogens.

Clinical Signs

I. Toxigenic diarrhea is watery and voluminous, with little evidence of an inflammatory response or systemic illness.
A. The diarrhea leads to dehydration, acidosis, and potassium depletion.
B. Animals are weak and dehydrated, with little evidence of tenesmus, mucus, or blood in the stool.
C. It occurs less commonly than invasive diarrhea.
II. Invasive diarrheas are often acute and hemorrhagic in nature.
A. Affected animals have dysentery with abdominal pain, fever, vomiting, and anorexia.
B. The diarrhea varies from watery to mucoid with fresh blood in severe cases.
C. Coincident with the diarrhea may be signs of septicemia (i.e., fever, collapse, shock, and coagulopathies).
III. Some organisms (e.g., *Campylobacter* and *Y. enterocolitica*) may cause a combination of the two syndromes.
A. *Y. enterocolitica* usually produces a self-limiting diarrhea in the dog.
B. *C. jejuni* causes hemorrhagic diarrhea, although signs of chronic colitis may also be seen.

Diagnosis

I. A tentative diagnosis may be based on compatible history and clinical signs.
II. Differentiation from viral enteritis is often not possible, and the two can coexist.
III. Laboratory tests may be difficult to interpret.
A. Organisms may be cultured from feces.
1. Clinicians must be cautious in linking isolation of a microorganism from stool cultures with causation of the diarrhea.
2. Significance of bacterial culture in cases of diarrhea must take into account history (environment and diet of affected animals) as well as results of other tests (for viral and parasitic enteritis), because normal animals may harbor organisms such as *Salmonella* spp. and *Campylobacter* spp.
3. Specific culture media and conditions may be

required to identify some bacteria such as *Campylobacter*.
4. Identification of a pathogenic or nonpathogenic *E. coli* requires specific typing and/or studies of toxin production.
B. *C. difficile* or *C. perfringens* type A toxins may be identified in feces using specific immunoassays.
C. Microscopic examination of feces may be helpful.
   1. The presence of leukocytes suggests a severe inflammatory process such as with invasive bacteria, and this finding should be followed by bacteriologic culture.
   2. A skilled observer may recognize the characteristic seagull-shaped forms of *Campylobacter* spp.
   3. Sporulating *Clostridium* spp. and spores may be seen.
D. Bacterial enteritis may be associated with either peripheral leukocytosis or leukopenia.
IV. Diagnosis of *B. piliformis* is based on histologic examination of intestinal and liver specimens.

Differential Diagnosis

I. Viral enteritis
II. Parasitic enteritis
III. Toxin-induced enteritis
IV. Dietary indiscretion
V. Nonspecific enteritis
VI. Acute pancreatitis

Treatment and Monitoring

I. Provide supportive care until normal food intake is resumed.
   A. Institute fluid therapy as for viral enteritis, as described previously.
   B. Local intestinal protectants may be used.
      1. Bismuth subsalicylate (Pepto-Bismol) 1–2 ml/kg PO TID-QID may reduce duration of clinical signs.
      2. They are often unpalatable and difficult to give.
   C. Motility modifiers are specifically contraindicated in bacterial diarrhea.
II. Consider antibacterial therapy for specific pathogens identified (controversial for *Campylobacter* and *Salmonella* spp.).
   A. Ampicillin 11 mg/kg SQ, IM, IV QID
   B. Gentamicin 2.2 mg/kg SQ, IM, IV TID
      1. For *Campylobacter* and *Yersinia*
      2. Combined with cephalothin for systemic salmonellosis
   C. Trimethoprim/sulfadiazine 15 mg/kg PO, SQ BID
      1. Give for 60 days to eliminate carrier state of salmonellosis.
      2. *Yersinia* is usually sensitive to this combination.

D. Erythromycin 10 mg/kg PO TID $\times$ 5–7 days for *Campylobacter*
E. Enrofloxacin for gram-negative bacteria and salmonellosis carrier states
   1. Dog: 2–4 mg/kg PO, SQ BID
   2. Cat: 1–2 mg/kg PO, SQ BID
III. Remove potential sources of infection (e.g., contaminated food products).
IV. Prevent zoonotic infection of in-contact humans.
V. Patient monitoring is similar to that discussed under Viral Infections.

Parasitic Enteropathies

Definition

I. Enteric parasites vary in their pathogenicity, depending on the burden of parasites and virulence of the strain, as well as host factors such as local immune status.
II. Transmission occurs by various routes.
   A. Usually by ingestion of water or other material contaminated with infected feces
   B. Ingestion of an intermediate or paratenic (transport) host
   C. Pre- or postnatal transmission from the mother

Causes

I. Ascarids
   A. *Toxocara canis, Toxascaris leonina:* dogs
   B. *Toxocara cati, Toxascaris leonina:* cats
II. Hookworms
   A. *Ancylostoma caninum:* dogs; *Ancylostoma tubaeforme:* cats
   B. *Ancylostoma braziliense, Uncinaria stenocephala:* dogs, cats
III. Whipworms
   A. *Trichuris vulpis:* dogs
   B. *Trichuris campanula:* cats
IV. *Strongyloides*
   A. *Strongyloides stercoralis:* dogs
   B. *Strongyloides tumefaciens:* cats
V. *Giardia* spp.
VI. *Pentatrichomonas* spp.
VII. Protozoa: *Isospora* spp., *Toxoplasma* spp., *Cryptosporidium* spp.
VIII. Tapeworms
   A. *Dipylidium caninum:* dogs, cats
   B. *Taenia pisiformis:* dogs
   C. *Taenia taenaeformis:* cats

Pathophysiology

I. Parasite-induced inflammatory changes and immunologic sequelae lead to mucosal dysfunction and malabsorption.
II. *A. caninum* is a voracious bloodsucker and more pathogenic than other less hematophagous hookworms.
III. Young animals often have the most severe clinical signs because of relatively high parasite burden.

IV. Mixed infections are common in young animals.
V. Poor environmental conditions can allow parasites to become enzootic problems in specific geographic areas or in collections of animals.
VI. Immunosuppressed animals may be prone to develop clinical signs when infected with parasites such as *Cryptosporidium* spp. that usually cause mild self-limiting disease.

Clinical Signs

I. Many infections are subclinical.
II. Infections may be self-limiting in immunocompetent animals.
III. The pathogenicity of some parasites (e.g., *Pentatrichomonas,* Coccidia) that are found in both healthy animals and those with diarrhea is questionable.
IV. Diarrhea, weight loss, anorexia, and vomiting are common.
V. Tenesmus with fresh blood and mucus in feces may be seen if there is large bowel involvement.
VI. Ascarid-infected animals often pass worms in vomitus or diarrhea.
VII. Whipworms are predominantly large bowel parasites (see Chap. 33).
VIII. *A. caninum* infection can cause life-threatening anemia in puppies and may cause iron deficiency anemia in older, heavily parasitized animals.

Diagnosis

I. Diagnosis is most commonly made by identification of the organism in the feces.
  A. Ascarids—ova or worms
  B. Hookworms—ova
  C. Whipworms—ova
  D. *Strongyloides* spp.—larvae, ova
  E. *Giardia* spp.—trophozoites, cysts
  F. *Pentatrichomonas* spp.—trophozoites
  G. Coccidia—oocysts
  H. Tapeworms—ova, proglottids
II. Examination of multiple fecal samples is recommended, because occult infections are possible, particularly with whipworms and in young puppies and kittens.
III. Detection of *Giardia* can be difficult.
  A. Zinc sulfate centrifugal flotation is the best technique for recovery of cysts.
  B. Prompt microscopic examination of a wet mount of fresh feces is required to observe motile trophozoites before they encyst.
  C. Lugol's 2% iodine stains cysts and trophozoites.
  D. Direct examination of juice aspirated from the duodenum at endoscopy or exploratory laparotomy is more reliable.
  E. A commercial enzyme immunoassay is available to detect specific *Giardia* antigen in feces.
IV. Use of a Baermann procedure facilitates identification of *Strongyloides* larvae.
V. *Cryptosporidium* spp. may be seen on histologic or cytologic examination of intestinal biopsy specimens.

Differential Diagnosis

I. Chronic inflammatory, obstructive, and neoplastic diseases of the stomach and small intestine
II. Exocrine pancreatic insufficiency
III. Systemic diseases that can cause gastrointestinal signs (e.g., feline hyperthyroidism and canine hypoadrenocorticism)

Treatment

I. To rule out occult infection, broad-spectrum parasiticidal therapy is warranted in many animals with unexplained diarrhea, weight loss, or other signs consistent with parasitic infection, even though specific evidence of infection is lacking.
II. Parasiticidal drugs that are available include the following (see Appendix IV for dosages).
  A. Ascarids: fenbendazole, mebendazole, piperazine, pyrantel pamoate
  B. Hookworms: fenbendazole, ivermectin, mebendazole, pyrantel pamoate
  C. Whipworms: febantel + praziquantel, fenbendazole, ivermectin, mebendazole, pyrantel pamoate
  D. *Strongyloides:* ivermectin
  E. *Giardia:* furazolidone, metronidazole, quinacrine
  F. *Pentatrichomonas:* metronidazole
  G. Protozoa
    1. *Isospora:* amprolium sulfadimethoxine
    2. *Toxoplasma:* clindamycin
    3. *Cryptosporidium:* spiramycin, paramomycin
  H. Tapeworms: epsiprantel, praziquantel

Patient Monitoring

I. Reinfection and/or failure to eradicate the infection with a single treatment may necessitate repeated treatments.
II. Prophylactic treatment of puppies and kittens is warranted in view of the frequency of occult maternally acquired infections.
III. *Giardia* is a potential zoonotic agent.

Mycotic Diseases

Definition

I. Mycotic infections of the small bowel are uncommon.
II. With the exception of histoplasmosis, they tend to be opportunistic infections associated with lowered resistance from malnutrition, immunosuppression, or disturbed endogenous flora secondary to antimicrobial therapy.

Causes

I. *Histoplasma capsulatum*
II. Phycomycosis: *Pythium* spp., others

III. *Candida albicans*
IV. *Aspergillus* spp.

Pathophysiology

I. Invasion varies from superficial mucosal involvement (*Candida*) to full-thickness infection that may produce a chronic malabsorption syndrome (*Histoplasma*).
II. Phycomycetes cause granulomatous inflammatory lesions, most commonly in the small intestine, with clinical signs of intestinal obstruction.

Clinical Signs

I. Histoplasmosis
   A. Chronic weight loss, anorexia, and diarrhea are common.
   B. Hematochezia and mucoid feces occur with colonic involvement.
   C. Fever, lymphadenopathy, hepatosplenomegaly, icterus, ascites, cough, and dyspnea reflect systemic involvement.
II. Phycomycetes
   A. These organisms are associated with weight loss, anorexia, vomiting, diarrhea, and palpable abdominal masses.
   B. Large bowel and/or small bowel diarrhea may be present, depending on the location and degree of fungal invasion.
III. Candidiasis and aspergillosis
   A. These conditions cause chronic diarrhea with ulcerative lesions.
   B. Vascular invasion and systemic involvement are more common with aspergillosis.

Diagnosis

I. Histoplasmosis
   A. Definitive diagnosis is made by identification of organisms on cytologic examination of macrophages in large or small intestine or of mononuclear cells in bone marrow or lymph nodes, or culture of *Histoplasma* from blood or other tissue.
   B. Hematologic abnormalities are variable and nonspecific but may include anemia, leukocytosis, leukopenia, monocytosis, and thrombocytopenia.
   C. Hypoalbuminemia, hypoglobulinemia or hyperglobulinemia, decreased concentrations of serum cobalamin and folate, and increased activities of serum liver enzymes may be noted.
   D. Affected animals usually have lived in regions bordering the Mississippi River or in Texas.
II. Phycomycosis
   A. Definitive diagnosis is made by identification of organisms (fungal hyphae) on histopathologic examination and fungal culture of intestinal biopsies.
   B. It is most prevalent in states bordering the Gulf of Mexico, especially Louisiana.
III. Aspergillosis and candidiasis

Definitive diagnosis requires identification of organisms in cytologic or histologic preparations of intestinal tissue.

Differential Diagnosis

I. Lymphocytic-plasmacytic, eosinophilic, or granulomatous enteritis
II. Intestinal neoplasia
III. Intussusception
IV. Intestinal foreign body
V. Villous atrophy
VI. Other diffuse enteropathies causing malabsorption

Treatment

I. Histoplasmosis
   A. Itraconazole (5 mg/kg PO SID-BID for 3–4 months) is often effective.
   B. Amphotericin B and/or ketoconazole may be tried (see Chap. 109).
      1. For severe cases, treat initially with amphotericin 0.5 mg/kg IV QOD to a cumulative dose of 4 mg/kg.
      2. Ketoconazole (10 mg/kg PO BID) is effective in mild cases and is used as follow-up therapy to amphotericin.
   C. Chronic treatment may be required.
   D. Relapses are possible if treatment is stopped.
II. Phycomycosis
   A. Itraconazole or ketoconazole may be effective in isolated cases.
   B. Amphotericin B and sodium iodide have not been effective.
   C. Surgical resection of obstructive mass lesions is advisable.
   D. Most cases fail to respond to medical and/or surgical therapy.
III. Candidiasis: itraconazole, ketoconazole
IV. Aspergillosis: itraconazole; ketoconazole with or without concurrent 5-flucytosine
V. Supportive care
   A. Parenteral vitamin supplements are given if serum cobalamin, folate, or other vitamin concentrations are subnormal.
   B. Parenteral fluid therapy may be indicated as outlined earlier for viral infections.

Patient Monitoring

I. The prognosis for mycotic small intestinal disease is poor to guarded.
II. Long-term therapy is often required, and relapses are common if medication is withdrawn.
III. Adverse side effects of drug administration are possible.
IV. Measurements of body weight, appetite, fecal consistency, and serum cobalamin and folate concentrations are the best indices of response to treatment.

Canine Hemorrhagic Gastroenteritis (HGE)

Definition and Cause

I. It is a peracute hemorrhagic enteritis of dogs characterized by sudden onset of vomiting, severe bloody diarrhea, and rapid dehydration.
II. The exact etiology is unknown, although enterotoxemia caused by *Clostridium* spp. has been implicated.

Pathophysiology

I. Physiologic abnormalities may reflect effects of a clostridial enterotoxin.
II. Certain pathologic features suggest that immune-mediated mechanisms may cause mucosal hemorrhage, ischemia, and necrosis.
III. Water and electrolyte losses into the gut lumen are often dramatic.

Clinical Signs

I. Signalment
   A. Prevalent in young adult toy and miniature breeds, particularly schnauzers and poodles
   B. Can affect all ages and breeds of dogs
II. Usually peracute and severe
III. Severe hematochezia and melena
   A. Enteric blood loss can occur so rapidly that it is not apparent until a rectal examination is performed or a rectal thermometer is used.
   B. Acute hypovolemia and shock are possible.
IV. Anorexia and depression
V. Vomiting (may be bloody)
VI. Abdominal pain
VII. Fever (rarely)

Diagnosis

I. Presumptive diagnosis is based on characteristic history and clinical signs in a previously healthy animal.
II. Hemoconcentration is often marked; packed cell volume (PCV) = 50–80%.
III. Tests for parvovirus, parasites, and other pathogens are negative.
IV. Abdominal radiographs show no abnormalities supporting obstructive enteropathy or other abdominal disease.
V. Evidence for a bleeding disorder is lacking.
VI. Prompt response to symptomatic care is supportive.

Differential Diagnosis

I. Parvovirus enteritis
II. Bacterial enteritis, especially salmonellosis
III. Acute obstructive disorders
IV. Endotoxic or hypovolemic shock from other causes
V. Pancreatitis
VI. Intestinal neoplasia
VII. Coagulopathies

Treatment

I. Fluid therapy is administered.
   A. Severe volume depletion is common, and intensive IV therapy is often required.
   B. Balanced electrolyte solutions are given at a rate of up to 40–60 ml/kg/h IV until the PCV is <50% and then decreased to 60–80 ml/kg/day.
II. Hypoproteinemia may be severe when rehydration is complete, and colloid therapy is warranted if serum albumin is <1.5 g/dl.
III. Antibiotics are given because of the possible role of clostridial infection and the potential for septicemia.
   A. Ampicillin is adequate unless there are signs of septicemia.
   B. Gentamicin may be added if septicemia is suspected.
IV. Short-acting glucocorticoids are given to dogs in shock.
   A. Hydrocortisone sodium succinate 10 mg/kg IV
   B. Dexamethasone sodium phosphate 0.5–1 mg/kg IV

Patient Monitoring

I. Monitor PCV and total solids every 6–24 hours as needed.
II. Modify rate and route of fluid therapy as appropriate.
III. Monitor urine output and central venous pressure in animals with severe shock.
IV. Withhold food and water for 1–2 days and then gradually reintroduce them.
V. The prognosis is good if adequate supportive care is given.

MALABSORPTIVE DISORDERS

Definition

I. Malabsorption refers to deficiency in the absorption of one or more nutrients as a result of disruption of the normal processes of digestion and absorption.
II. The distinction between malabsorption and maldigestion is not absolute, because diseases that cause primarily malabsorption usually also involve some impairment of digestion, and vice versa.

Causes

I. Chronic inflammatory bowel diseases
   A. Lymphocytic-plasmacytic enteritis
   B. Eosinophilic enteritis
   C. Neutrophilic enteritis
   D. Granulomatous enteritis
II. Villous atrophy
   A. Idiopathic
   B. Resembling tropical sprue in human beings
   C. Dietary sensitivity (e.g., wheat-sensitive enteropathy)
III. Intestinal neoplasia: lymphosarcoma, adenocarcinoma, leiomyosarcoma

IV. Small intestine bacterial overgrowth (not recognized in cats)
   A. Associated with enteropathy of German shepherd dogs
   B. Associated with exocrine pancreatic insufficiency
   C. Secondary to intestinal obstruction or pseudo-obstruction
   D. Idiopathic forms
V. Chronic infectious enteropathies
   A. Histoplasmosis and other fungal enteropathies
   B. Giardiasis and other parasitic enteropathies
VI. Short bowel syndrome: massive bowel resection
VII. Others: amyloidosis, lymphangiectasia

Pathophysiology

I. Multiple mechanisms may contribute to malabsorption.
   A. Reduced or impaired activities of enzymes in the brush border membrane of the intestinal mucosa
   B. Decreased mucosal absorptive surface area secondary to villous atrophy
   C. Disruption of normal enterocyte function by inflammatory changes within the mucosa
   D. Obstruction to flow of lymph secondary to local inflammation
II. Independent of cause, the end result is decreased transport of nutrients.

Clinical Signs

I. Tremendous variation in spectrum and severity of signs
II. Abnormal bowel movements
   A. Occasional soft stool to severe watery diarrhea
   B. Greasy stools with severe steatorrhea (rare)
   C. Stools containing obviously undigested food
III. Increased frequency of defecation and stool volume
IV. Weight loss
V. Appetite: increased or decreased
VI. Depression, abdominal discomfort
VII. Borborygmus, flatulence
VIII. Vomiting

Diagnosis

I. Serum tests may indicate that there is intestinal disease, pancreatic disease, or malabsorption.
   A. Trypsin-like immunoreactivity (TLI)
      1. Trypsinogen is a specific pancreatic acinar cell marker enzyme normally present in serum of dogs at a concentration of 5.2–35 μg/L.
      2. A commercial canine specific assay is available (Canine TLI Assay, Diagnostic Products Corp., Los Angeles, CA).
      3. Assay of feline TLI is currently available from the GI Laboratory, 1248 Lynn Mall, Room 1321, Purdue University, West Lafayette, IN 47907-1248.
      4. TLI is normal in animals with small intestinal disease but markedly subnormal in those with exocrine pancreatic insufficiency.
      5. Serum is collected after food has been withheld for at least 6 hours.
      6. Serum TLI is very stable and can be mailed for analysis without any special requirements.
   B. Folate and cobalamin (vitamin B$_{12}$)
      1. These water-soluble vitamins are plentiful in commercial pet foods; therefore dietary insufficiency is highly improbable.
      2. They are absorbed in the upper (folate) and lower (cobalamin) small intestine, so serum concentrations reflect the absorptive capacity of the respective segments of bowel.
      3. Different assay methods (bioassay, radioassays) give different results.
         a) Many commercial radioassay kits are not suitable for use with canine and feline samples.
         b) It is essential that laboratories derive their own control ranges in pet (not experimental) animals and use methods validated in that species.
      4. Serum is collected after food has been withheld for at least 12 hours.
      5. Serum folate and cobalamin are stable and can be mailed for analysis without any special packing requirements. Avoid exposure of samples to light.
      6. Red blood cell folate concentration is very high, therefore values obtained in hemolyzed serum may be falsely elevated.
      7. The functional impairment of the intestines must be severe enough and of sufficient duration to deplete endogenous stores for serum values to be abnormal.
      8. Low serum folate concentration indicates disease of the upper small intestine.
      9. Subnormal serum cobalamin concentration indicates disease of the lower small intestine.
      10. Subnormal levels of both serum folate and cobalamin often occur with severe intestinal disease affecting the entire small intestine.
      11. With exocrine pancreatic insufficiency or bacterial overgrowth in the upper small intestine, increased serum folate and low serum cobalamin levels are expected.
      12. Because serum vitamin concentrations can be abnormal in both exocrine pancreatic insufficiency and small intestinal disease, pancreatic function (serum TLI or fecal proteolytic activity) should always be evaluated before or at the same time.
   C. D-Xylose absorption test
      1. Measurement of this poorly metabolized sugar reflects absorptive capacity of the small intestine.
      2. The test has low sensitivity for detection of small intestinal disease. Extensive disease must be present before abnormal test results are obtained.
      3. The test is impractical in most clinical situations, and more information is obtained by assay of serum folate and cobalamin.

D. Oral fat absorption test or plasma turbidity test
   1. Failure to develop lipemia after oral administration of fat supposedly reflects fat malabsorption.
   2. The test is very insensitive and is not recommended for diagnosis of small intestinal diseases. Steatorrhea, if present at all, is usually modest in small intestinal disease.
E. Hemogram
   1. Findings are nonspecific and may include eosinophilia, lymphopenia, neutrophilia, and anemia of chronic disease.
   2. Eosinophilia does not necessarily indicate eosinophilic gastroenteritis.
F. Serum biochemical profiles
   1. Cholesterol and triglyceride levels are often subnormal in malnourished patients.
   2. Albumin and globulin levels may be low, reflecting protein-losing enteropathy, although this is uncommon.
   3. Liver enzymes can be mildly to moderately increased.
   4. Serum bile acid concentrations may be abnormally increased in some patients, and usually these changes resolve after treatment of the underlying enteropathy.

II. Fecal evaluation may indicate that there is intestinal disease, pancreatic disease, or malabsorption.
   A. Fecal proteolytic assay using radial enzyme diffusion or azoprotein substrate (or specific assay of trypsin or chymotrypsin) is useful for diagnosis of exocrine pancreatic insufficiency when serum TLI assay is not available.
   B. Examination for evidence of intestinal parasites is always warranted.
   C. Bacteriologic culture may be considered, especially for *Salmonella*.
   D. Quantitative analysis of fecal fat output is required to document steatorrhea. This is usually impractical and expensive and rarely helps with patient management.
   E. Examination for fat droplets (Sudan III stain, with modifications to detect ''split'' or hydrolyzed fat) is subjective and imprecise.
      1. Only if steatorrhea is massive (a very rare occurrence with small intestinal disease) will increased numbers of fat droplets be consistently seen.
      2. Many false diagnoses of steatorrhea are made using this method.
   F. Examinations for starch granules and muscle fibers (if present in the diet) are also subjective and imprecise.
   G. Other diagnostic tests are listed under the specific causes.

III. Radiography is indicated, but results are often nonspecific.
   A. Survey radiographs may show thickened loops of bowel.
   B. Upper gastrointestinal contrast studies may reveal gastric and/or small intestinal ulcers, masses, or an infiltrative bowel pattern (diffuse mucosal irregularity).

IV. Endoscopic examination often reveals coexistent gastric abnormalities (retained food, hemorrhagic lesions, reflux of bile, hyper- or hypomotility). Duodenoscopy often shows similar findings with a granular, cobblestone, or ulcerated appearance to the mucosa.

V. Definitive diagnosis requires examination of intestinal biopsies.
   A. Full-thickness biopsies are most definitive.
      1. Endoscopic mucosal biopsies (partial thickness) are adequate in most cases.
      2. Endoscopic biopsies often miss intestinal lymphosarcoma and cannot show the submucosal lymphatic dilation indicative of lymphangiectasia.
   B. Cytology of impression smears or squash preparations may give a rapid diagnosis of neoplastic, infectious, or inflammatory disease.
   C. Histologic examination is essential to document villous atrophy and may confirm neoplastic, infectious, inflammatory, or other disease; however, morphologic abnormalities are often mild, and many pathologists are reluctant to make specific diagnoses.
   D. There may be no morphologic abnormalities in some dogs with significant intestinal disease, because the underlying problem may be functional in origin.
   E. Tissue assay for marker enzymes (lactase, sucrase, maltase, alkaline phosphatase, peptidase) in intestinal biopsies is a more sensitive method to detect and classify intestinal diseases but is neither practical nor widely available.

Differential Diagnosis

   I. Exocrine pancreatic insufficiency
   II. Hyperthyroidism in cats
   III. Diabetes mellitus
   IV. Hypoadrenocorticism
   V. Protein-losing enteropathy

Treatment

   I. Directed at underlying cause, if known
   II. Exocrine pancreatic insufficiency: see Chap. 35
   III. Lymphocytic-plasmacytic, eosinophilic, and neutrophilic enteritis, granulomatous enteritis, villous atrophy
      A. Prednisolone 1–2 mg/kg PO BID for 7–14 days, then tapered over 2–3 months to minimal effective dose (e.g., 0.5 mg/kg PO QOD)
      B. Dietary therapy: highly digestible, low-fat, or elimination diets
      C. Antibiotic therapy for bacterial overgrowth (see later)
      D. Immunosuppressive therapy with azathioprine if response to above measures is inadequate or if side effects of steroid administration are unacceptable

1. Initial doses: dog, 2–2.5 mg/kg PO SID; cat, 0.2–0.3 mg/kg PO SID
   2. For maintenance control: QOD ± prednisone
IV. Intestinal neoplasms: see Neoplasia, later
V. Antibiotic therapy for bacterial overgrowth
   A. Tetracycline 10–20 mg/kg PO BID for 1 month
   B. Trimethoprim/sulfadiazine 15 mg/kg PO BID for 1 month
   C. Tylosin for 1 month as needed
      1. Dogs: 40–80 mg/kg PO SID in food
      2. Cats: 10–20 mg/kg PO SID in food
   D. Metronidazole for 2–3 weeks
      1. Dogs: 20–40 mg/kg PO SID
      2. Cats: 10 mg/kg PO SID
   E. Tylosin and metronidazole
      1. They are not initial drugs of choice for the broad spectrum of organisms often present in small intestine bacterial overgrowth in dogs.
      2. They have relatively narrow spectra and are particularly effective against obligate anaerobic bacteria such as those present in the colon.
      3. Response to these antibiotics does not necessarily indicate bacterial overgrowth.
VI. Parasitic or fungal enteropathies: see earlier
VII. Short bowel syndrome
   A. Highly digestible, low-fat, or elemental diet or parenteral nutrition
   B. Frequent small meals
   C. Antibiotic therapy for bacterial overgrowth
   D. Cholestyramine 200–300 mg/kg PO BID in dogs, to bind bile acids
   E. Parenteral vitamin supplements
   F. H_2-receptor or proton pump blockers for gastric hypersecretion
   G. Motility-modifying antidiarrheals, such as loperamide 0.08 mg/kg PO TID (dog)
VIII. Lymphangiectasia: see later
IX. Obstruction and pseudo-obstruction
   A. Resection of limited local lesions
   B. Antibiotic therapy for bacterial overgrowth
   C. Trial therapy with metoclopramide
   D. Parenteral vitamin supplements
   E. Enteral or parenteral nutrition
X. Nonspecific management
   A. If diarrhea is present without weight loss, then low-fat or highly digestible (non-fermentable, low-fiber) diets are fed for 2–3 weeks on a trial basis.
   B. If weight loss accompanies the diarrhea, then highly digestible (non-fermentable, low-fiber) or elimination diets alone are fed for 2–3 weeks.
      1. Homemade elimination diets (lamb and rice) are often low in fat and fiber content.
      2. Challenge diets to document specific sensitivities (wheat/gluten, soybean, beef, pork, chicken) are recommended after apparent improvement occurs when feeding an elimination diet.
   C. Vitamin supplementation is suggested, but avoid overdosing, especially with long-term usage.
      1. Cobalamin 250 μg/day SQ, IM weekly for 1–3 months

   2. Folic acid 1–5 mg PO SID for 2–4 weeks
   3. Tocopherol 100–500 IU IM, PO SID with food for 1 month
   4. Thiamine for anorexic cats: 10 mg/kg SQ, IM SID × 3–4 days
   5. Vitamin K to normalize prothrombin or activated partial thromboplastin time
   D. If all treatments are ineffective, symptomatic therapy can be tried.
      1. Metronidazole for diarrhea
      2. Narcotic antidiarrheals (e.g., loperamide)
      3. Metoclopramide and cimetidine to reduce vomiting
   E. Avoidance of stress may be beneficial in some patients.

Patient Monitoring

I. Client communication is important because immediate success is not always possible, and some degree of trial and error is required before optimal management is attained.
II. Monitor body weight at 3- to 4-week intervals.
III. Repeat physical and laboratory examinations if the disease lingers, because the detection of masses and biochemical or hematologic abnormalities may become more apparent with time.
IV. If serum vitamin, protein, or lipid concentrations are subnormal, repeat the assay to monitor response to therapy.

INFLAMMATORY DISORDERS

Eosinophilic Enteritis

Definition and Causes

I. Eosinophilic enteritis is characterized by an infiltration of the wall of the stomach, small intestine, and/or colon with eosinophils.
II. The etiology is unknown, but suggested causes include parasite migration and an abnormal sensitivity to dietary or bacterial antigens in the intestine.

Pathophysiology

I. Infiltration by eosinophils probably occurs in association with an immune response to an antigen.
II. If accompanied by defects in digestive and absorptive function or lymphatic obstruction from inflammation, malabsorption may occur.
III. Protein loss occurs with inflammatory exudation, lymphatic obstruction, or ulceration of the bowel.

Clinical Signs

I. Anorexia, vomiting
II. Large and/or small bowel diarrhea with melena and/or hematochezia
   A. Dogs: signs of gastroenteritis
   B. Cats: signs of enterocolitis
III. Weight loss

IV. ± Thickened loops of bowel and mesenteric lymph-adenopathy on physical examination

Diagnosis

I. Diagnostic tests to consider were outlined under Malabsorptive Disorders, earlier.
II. Hematologic findings vary.
  A. ± Peripheral eosinophilia
  B. Blood loss anemia (microcytic, hypochromic) or anemia of chronic disease
III. Definitive diagnosis requires demonstration of eosinophilic infiltrates on multiple biopsy specimens.

Differential Diagnosis

I. Lymphocytic-plasmacytic enteritis
II. Granulomatous enteritis
III. Intestinal parasitism
IV. Neoplasia
V. Other causes of malabsorption
VI. Hypereosinophilic syndrome of cats (Neer, 1991)
  A. It is characterized by eosinophilic infiltrates in multiple organs, especially bone marrow, small intestines, liver, spleen, and mesenteric lymph nodes.
  B. Presenting signs mimic malabsorptive diseases and include vomiting, diarrhea, anorexia, and weight loss. Dermatologic signs and splenomegaly may also be noted.
  C. Eosinophils appear mature, unlike the immature forms seen with eosinophilic leukemia.
  D. Response to prednisone is poor; survival is usually ≤6 months.

Treatment and Monitoring

I. The use of controlled diets may improve clinical signs but only infrequently cures the problem.
  A. Cottage cheese, rice, and chicken
  B. Numerous commercial restricted-antigen diets
II. Treat for potential parasite infestations.
  A. Dogs: fenbendazole 55 mg/kg PO SID × 3 days
  B. Cats: pyrantel pamoate 10 mg/kg PO once, repeat in 3 weeks
III. Prednisolone therapy is usually required.
  A. Initial dose is 1 mg/kg PO BID in dogs and 2–3 mg/kg PO BID in cats, for 1–2 weeks.
  B. Taper over 2–3 months to minimal effective QOD dose.
IV. Azathioprine (dogs) or chlorambucil (cats) may be tried for unresponsive cases but is rarely necessary.
V. Prognosis is good; therapy can normally be withdrawn in several weeks.

Lymphocytic-Plasmacytic Enteritis

Definition

I. Lymphocytic-plasmacytic enteritis is a disorder characterized by an infiltration of the wall of the stomach, small intestine, and/or colon with lymphocytes and plasma cells.

II. In the basenji breed, there is a genetic susceptibility to a specific "immunoproliferative" enteropathy characterized by lymphocytic-plasmacytic inflammation.

Causes

I. The etiology is unknown, but suggested causes include abnormal sensitivity to dietary, parasitic, or bacterial antigens in the intestine.
II. Bacterial overgrowth in the small intestine may also be a cause.

Pathophysiology

I. Infiltration by inflammatory cells probably arises in association with an immune response to an antigen.
II. Malabsorption develops from defects in brush border digestive and absorptive function.
III. Protein loss may occur from inflammatory exudation, lymphatic obstruction, or ulceration of the bowel.

Clinical Signs

I. Tremendous variation in severity
II. Vomiting, anorexia
III. Diarrhea: large bowel and/or small bowel in origin
IV. Weight loss, anorexia
V. Thickened loops of bowel and mesenteric lymphadenopathy on physical examination

Diagnosis

I. See diagnostic tests outlined under Malabsorptive Disorders.
II. Hemogram is usually normal.
III. Hypoalbuminemia and hyperglobulinemia eventually develop in affected basenjis.
IV. In other breeds, serum protein concentrations are usually normal, although there may be panhypoproteinemia in severe cases.
V. Definitive diagnosis is based on finding diffuse infiltration of lymphocytes and plasma cells in the lamina propria.

Differential Diagnosis

I. Eosinophilic enteritis
II. Granulomatous enteritis
III. Other causes of malabsorption and protein-losing enteropathy
IV. Neoplasia

Treatment

I. See Malabsorptive Disorders for dietary advice.
II. Treat for potential parasitic infections.
III. Prednisone therapy is usually required, as described for Eosinophilic Enteritis.
IV. Some cases respond to antimicrobial therapy, as for bacterial overgrowth, in combination with corticosteroid therapy.

V. Azathioprine is reserved for cases refractory to prednisone.
  A. Severe hypoproteinemia may indicate that immunosuppressive therapy with azathioprine will be required in addition to prednisolone, at least in the short term.
  B. Azathioprine therapy is also warranted if the side effects of prednisolone therapy are severe and unacceptable.

Patient Monitoring

I. Prognosis for the disease varies.
  A. Many animals apparently recover from some transient insult.
  B. Other cases can be successfully managed only by long-term dietary or glucocorticoid therapy.
II. Immunoproliferative enteropathy in the basenji is progressive in most cases and often fatal within months to years.
III. Owners must be warned that in some animals the disease is chronic.
  A. There is currently no way to predict which animals will require long-term therapy.
  B. Symptoms may be refractory or progressive, but this is rare.

Protein-Losing Enteropathies

Definition

I. Protein-losing enteropathy is characterized by excessive loss of plasma and other proteins into the gastrointestinal tract.
II. These disorders may be primary or caused by numerous other diseases.

Causes

I. Any acute or chronic inflammatory disease that results in increased permeability of the mucosa to protein
  A. Eosinophilic gastroenteritis
  B. Plasmacytic-lymphocytic enteritis
  C. Granulomatous enteritis
  D. Histoplasmosis
  E. Villous atrophy: gluten enteropathy, certain viral and bacterial enteritides
  F. Parasitic enteritis in young animals
  G. Chronic obstruction or intussusception
  H. Ulcerative small intestinal disease
  I. Intestinal neoplasia, particularly lymphosarcoma
  J. Intestinal blood loss from any cause
II. Diseases affecting intestinal lymphatic drainage
  A. Lymphangiectasia is any condition characterized by dilated submucosal, subserosal, and/or mesenteric lymphatics.
  B. Congenital intestinal lymphangiectasia is a rare defect of lymphatics present from birth. It has been reported to be common in the Norwegian Lundehunde.
  C. Acquired lymphangiectasia occurs in older animals and is often idiopathic.

1. It may also develop from mechanical lymphatic obstruction caused by neoplasia or inflammation in lymphatics, lymph nodes, or adjacent tissue.
2. It may also arise with functional lymphatic obstruction from increased pressure in the vena cava secondary to cardiovascular disease.

Pathophysiology

I. Protein is normally lost into the small intestine. Most of the proteins are subsequently digested, absorbed, and reused to make new protein.
II. Protein loss is accelerated in inflammatory or lymphatic obstructive disorders.
III. Hepatic capacity to synthesize protein is limited, and when this is exceeded by the rate of enteric protein loss, hypoproteinemia results.
IV. Severe hypoproteinemia causes decreased plasma oncotic pressure and may lead to peripheral edema, ascites, or pleural effusion.

Clinical Signs

I. Commonly chronic diarrhea
  A. Intermittent or continuous
  B. Sometimes accompanied by hematochezia
II. Vomiting, anorexia
III. Possibly severe weight loss
IV. ± Edema of dependent areas, ascites, and hydrothorax

Diagnosis/Differential Diagnosis

I. Gastrointestinal symptoms such as diarrhea and vomiting may not always occur.
II. Hypoalbuminemia and hypoglobulinemia, often accompanied by hypocholesterolemia and lymphopenia, are classic findings.
III. Hepatic and renal disease must be excluded as causes of hypoalbuminemia.
  A. Serum globulins are rarely decreased with renal or hepatic disease.
  B. Perform a urinalysis and determine urine protein: creatinine ratio to quantify proteinuria (see Chap. 47).
  C. Measure serum bile acids to assess hepatic function (see Chap. 34).
IV. Analysis of ascitic fluid reveals a pure or modified transudate.
V. In the author's experience, the fecal concentration of the plasma protein α_1-protease inhibitor is increased in dogs with protein-losing enteropathy.
  A. This is an extremely sensitive and specific test for protein-losing enteropathy in human patients.
  B. Species-specific immunoassays must be used.
  C. A canine assay is not readily available at this time.
VI. Perform other gastrointestinal function and morphologic testing to rule out infectious and inflammatory disorders as discussed earlier.

VII. Attempts should be made to histologically diagnose the underlying disease by techniques less invasive than laparotomy, because malnutrition and hypoproteinemia may lead to anesthetic and postoperative complications.
  A. Endoscopy is preferred.
  B. Careful surgical technique and use of nonabsorbable sutures are recommended because of hypoproteinemia.
  C. Biopsy specimen should always be taken, even if the small intestine appears grossly normal.

Treatment

I. Specifically treat the underlying enteropathy if possible.
II. Feed low-fat diets to minimize lymphatic absorption.
  A. Low-fat cottage cheese and rice
  B. Numerous commercial low-fat diets
III. If necessary, supplement with medium-chain triglyceride oil to increase caloric intake.
  A. Medium-chain triglycerides are not absorbed via lymphatics but are transported directly to the liver in portal blood.
  B. Add 0.5 tsp to each meal, increasing to a maximum 1 tbsp per meal or 0.5 oz/10 kg PO divided TID-QID to minimize side effects.
  C. Hyperosmolality of the product can worsen diarrhea, so the dose should be increased gradually.
IV. Administer hetastarch 20 ml/kg/day IV and possibly plasma at 10–20 ml/kg IV as needed.

Patient Monitoring

I. Monitor body weight, serum protein concentration, and clinical course every 7–14 days.
II. Prognosis for protein-losing enteropathy is guarded because the underlying primary disease is often chronic and cannot be cured.
III. Clinical signs can often be controlled, however, using symptomatic and rather nonspecific therapy as outlined earlier.

Ulcers

Definition

I. Ulcers are physical disruptions in the epithelium lining the mucosal surface of the small intestine.
II. They are uncommon in dogs and cats.

Causes

I. Mastocytosis and mast cell tumors
II. Gastrin-secreting tumors (gastrinomas) usually of pancreatic origin: Zollinger-Ellison syndrome
III. Drugs
  A. Aspirin, indomethacin, phenylbutazone, flunixin, other nonsteroidal anti-inflammatory agents
  B. Corticosteroids
IV. Hepatic and renal failure
V. Neoplasia

VI. Hyperadrenocorticism
VII. Idiopathic causes

Pathophysiology

I. Hypergastrinemia or hyperhistaminemia results in increased secretion of gastric acid, which damages duodenal mucosa.
II. Mucosal prostaglandins mediate a cytoprotective effect that is inhibited by nonsteroidal anti-inflammatory drugs.
III. Corticosteroid excess or deficiency may impair mucus production and other mucosal cell protective mechanisms, predisposing to injury.

Clinical Signs

I. Diarrhea with gross melena or occult blood
II. Vomiting with hematemesis of "coffee grounds" fluid
III. Pale mucous membranes if anemic
IV. Nausea, variable appetite, weight loss
V. May adopt "prayer position" if there is severe abdominal pain
VI. Peritonitis, if the ulcer perforates

Diagnosis

I. Suggestive clinical signs: melena, hematemesis, anemia, or cutaneous mast cell tumors
II. Laboratory tests
  A. Anemia arises for two reasons.
    1. Acute blood loss: normochromic, normocytic initially, becoming regenerative after 4–5 days
    2. Chronic blood loss leading to iron deficiency: hypochromic, microcytic
  B. Hypoproteinemia may be found with decreases in both serum albumin and globulin.
  C. High serum gastrin concentrations occur with gastrinomas and chronic renal failure.
  D. Fecal examination is positive for gross or occult blood (difficult to interpret if fed meat-based diets).
  E. Other tests may suggest hepatic or renal disease, hyperadrenocorticism, or mast cell tumors.
III. Radiography
  A. Plain radiographs are usually unremarkable unless peritonitis is present.
  B. An upper gastrointestinal contrast study may reveal gastrointestinal mucosal defects.
IV. Duodenoscopy may allow visualization of the bleeding lesion(s).

Differential Diagnosis

I. Neoplasia
II. Intestinal parasites
III. Gastric disease, especially gastric outlet obstruction and gastric ulcers
IV. Other inflammatory or infiltrative small intestinal diseases

Treatment

I. Transfuse with whole blood if there is severe anemia.
II. Withdraw any inciting medications.
III. Use H_2-receptor antagonists or protein pump inhibitors to decrease gastric acid secretion.
    A. Cimetidine 5–10 mg/kg PO, IV, SQ TID-QID
    B. Ranitidine 2.2–4.4 mg/kg PO BID
    C. Famotidine 0.5 mg/kg PO SID
    D. Omeprazole 0.6–1 mg/kg PO SID
    E. See also Chap. 30.
IV. Administer sucralfate 1 g/25 kg PO BID-TID as a protective agent.
V. Antacids are relatively ineffective and are not palatable to most dogs and cats.
VI. Withhold food for 24–48 hours to decrease acid secretion. Subsequently feed a bland, carbohydrate-rich diet (cottage cheese, pasta, potatoes, rice).
VII. Treat mastocytosis with corticosteroids after stabilization of the animal and pretreatment with an H_2-receptor antagonist (see Chap. 64).
VIII. Surgical intervention may be needed to resect tumors, to excise bleeding ulcers, or when there is perforation and peritonitis.

Patient Monitoring

I. Monitor clinical signs as well as PCV and total protein SID-BID.
II. Change to a regular diet after 7–10 days if clinical signs suggest ulcers are resolving.
III. Continue H_2 antagonist therapy until a normal diet is fed, and then withdraw after 7–10 symptom-free days. Long-term therapy may be needed for ulcers associated with an underlying chronic disease.

INTESTINAL OBSTRUCTION

Definition

Partial or complete obstructions of the small intestine are caused by mechanical, neurogenic, or myogenic lesions that slow or prevent passage of the intestinal contents.

Causes

I. Intraluminal causes include tumors, polyps, foreign bodies, and intussusceptions.
II. Intramural obstructions include tumors, hematomas, abscesses, granulomas, congenital stenosis and atresia, and inflammatory lesions.
III. Extramural lesions include adhesions, strangulation through mesenteric tears, strictures secondary to surgery, incarceration of the bowel in hernias, volvulus, and abnormalities of adjacent organs (e.g., lymphadenopathy and pancreatic masses).
IV. Functional obstructions also can arise.
    A. Pseudo-obstructions of the small intestine are functional obstructions caused by hypomotility and ileus.
        1. Many pseudo-obstructions are idiopathic in nature.
        2. Intestinal sclerosis is a rare cause of pseudo-obstruction.
        3. Hypokalemia and acute viral infections can inhibit intestinal motility.
    B. Linear foreign bodies such as strings and cords cause functional obstructions by "pleating" of the small intestine.

Pathophysiology

I. Small intestinal obstructions produce dehydration, hypovolemia, and electrolyte imbalances.
II. Fluids and electrolytes are lost by emesis, diarrhea, and/or sequestration in the obstructed bowel loops. Fluid, electrolyte, and acid–base imbalances vary with the site and severity of obstruction.
    A. High small intestinal obstruction
        1. Early onset of vomiting and rapid dehydration
        2. Hypochloremic metabolic alkalosis
        3. Hypokalemia
    B. Low small intestinal obstruction
        1. Slower onset of vomiting and dehydration
        2. Metabolic acidosis
        3. Hypokalemia, hyponatremia, hypochloremia
III. Stasis secondary to small intestinal obstruction causes bacterial overgrowth, with subsequent endotoxin and bacterial absorption leading to endotoxemia and septicemia.
IV. Partial low obstruction may be chronic and cause malabsorption because of secondary bacterial overgrowth.
V. Strangulation of the intestines interferes with the vascular integrity of the obstructed bowel loop; this occurs with volvulus, intussusception, and incarcerated hernias.

Clinical Signs

I. The clinical manifestations and consequences of an obstruction depend on its location, completeness, and duration, as well as the vascular integrity of the bowel segment.
II. Vomiting, diarrhea, anorexia, and weight loss are common.
    A. Upper small intestinal obstructions are associated with immediate and frequent vomiting and with severe dehydration and electrolyte imbalances, especially if the obstruction is complete.
    B. Lower small intestinal obstructions are associated with intermittent vomiting, anorexia, and weight loss.
III. Diarrhea may be seen with lower small intestinal obstruction; bloody diarrhea is common with intussusception.
IV. Abdominal pain and distention, panting, and abnormal "praying" positions may be noted.

Diagnosis

I. Compatible clinical signs
II. Physical examination
    A. Palpation may reveal a mass in the small intes-

tine or fluid and gas-filled loops of bowel proximal to the obstruction.
- B. Sedation can facilitate a thorough examination if the animal is fractious or in pain.
- C. Pendulous kidneys, enlarged mesenteric lymph nodes, feces, other abdominal masses, and the spleen may be mistaken for small intestinal obstructions.

III. Laboratory findings
- A. Hemogram
  1. Often normal
  2. ± Neutrophilia with left shift, anemia of chronic disease
- B. Serum biochemical profile
  1. Hypokalemia, hyper-, or hyponatremia may occur, with variable chloride concentrations.
  2. It helps to rule out disorders that cause similar symptoms (e.g., pancreatitis and liver and renal disease).
  3. Prerenal azotemia and hepatic enzyme leakage are common secondary to small intestinal obstructive lesions.

IV. Radiology
- A. Survey radiographs may reveal the following.
  1. Dilation of the small intestine with gas and fluid proximal to the obstruction
  2. Foreign bodies, intraluminal filling defects, or abnormal locations of an organ
  3. Distinct radiographic pleated bunching of the bowel and multiple gas bubbles through affected loops with linear foreign bodies
  4. Massively dilated bowel loops without evidence of a physically obstructive lesion
     a) Pseudo-obstruction
     b) Stasis caused by viral or nonspecific enteritis
- B. Horizontal beam radiographs show an interface of fluid and gas. With complete obstruction, gas-capped fluid is seen in intestinal loops at different horizontal levels.
- C. Upper gastrointestinal positive contrast studies may confirm or reveal obstructive lesions, especially those that are low or partial (see Chap. 4).
  1. Delayed transit of contrast medium through the small intestine
  2. Dilution of barium in the gastrointestinal tract and dilation of loops cranial to obstruction
  3. Contrast medium outlining foreign bodies or annular lesions or revealing pleating or beading of the intestine

V. Exploratory laparotomy
Occasionally obstructions are only confirmed at surgery.

Differential Diagnosis

- I. Pancreatitis
- II. Hypoadrenocorticism
- III. Renal disease
- IV. Hepatic disease
- V. Infectious and inflammatory small intestinal diseases
- VI. Intestinal parasitism

VII. Toxin ingestion
VIII. Other causes of "acute abdomen" syndrome (see Chap. 37)

Treatment

- I. Stabilization of fluid and electrolyte abnormalities and secondary complications, followed by surgical correction of the intestinal obstruction, are the primary goals.
- II. Parenteral fluid therapy is started with lactated Ringer's or normal saline (40–80 ml/kg/day IV). Potassium supplementation (10–20 mEq/L fluids) is usually needed.
- III. Parenteral broad-spectrum antibiotic therapy is used to combat bacterial overgrowth, endotoxemia, and peritonitis if present.
- IV. Short-acting corticosteroids may be indicated for shock.
- V. Antiemetics (metoclopramide) may provide symptomatic relief if vomiting is severe but are contraindicated if there is total upper intestinal obstruction.
- VI. No food or fluids are given by mouth before surgery.
- VII. Surgical therapy depends on the nature and site of the obstruction.
  - A. Enterotomy and removal of foreign bodies
  - B. Intestinal resection and anastomosis
  - C. Reduction of intussusceptions with subsequent plication of the bowel
  - D. Repair of hernias, correction of extraintestinal lesions
  - E. Intestinal biopsy if there is pseudo-obstruction

Patient Monitoring

- I. Postoperative care involves the following.
  - A. Delay oral intake for 24–48 hours.
  - B. Monitor temperature, capillary refill time, and vital signs BID-QID.
  - C. Monitor PCV and total solids BID-SID.
  - D. Monitor electrolytes and abnormal serum chemistries every 24–72 hours.
  - E. Resume oral fluids first, and then introduce small meals of bland food.
  - F. Continue fluid therapy until normal oral intake has resumed and vomiting has stopped.
- II. Prognosis is variable depending on the cause, duration of obstruction, and presence of complicating factors (e.g., peritonitis or septicemia).

NEOPLASIA

Definition

- I. Intestinal adenocarcinomas and gastrointestinal lymphosarcoma are the most common malignant tumors of the small intestine.
- II. Other malignancies include mast cell tumors (cats), leiomyosarcomas, and carcinoid tumors.
- III. Leiomyomas are the most common benign tumors of the small intestine.

IV. Other benign tumors include polyps, fibromas, lipomas, and glandular adenomas.

Causes

I. Cause is usually unknown.
II. Intestinal adenocarcinomas are more common in Siamese cats than other breeds.
III. Gastrointestinal lymphosarcoma is caused by feline leukemia virus in cats.
  A. Most cases involve B lymphocytes of the gut-associated lymphoid tissue.
  B. Both lymphoblastic and chronic lymphocytic forms of the disease may be found.

Pathophysiology

I. Small intestinal adenocarcinomas typically are annular, stenotic constrictions that can be found in any segment of the intestinal tract but are most common in the large bowel of the dog and the jejunum and ileum of the cat.
II. Gastrointestinal lymphosarcoma may be either a diffuse infiltrative disease causing mural thickening and signs of malabsorption or a nodular disease causing obstructive signs.
III. Leiomyosarcomas and leiomyomas often cause iron deficiency anemia before classic clinical signs of small intestinal disease are evident.
IV. Mast cell tumors may be associated with excessive histamine release and hypersecretion of gastric acid.

Clinical Signs

I. Intestinal adenocarcinomas often cause signs of chronic intestinal obstruction (i.e., diarrhea and vomiting), with or without blood.
  A. Clinical signs may persist for months, owing to the slowly progressive obstruction caused by these tumors.
  B. Weight loss is usually noted.
  C. Metastasis is common, and secondary signs of liver, lymph node, peritoneal, or pulmonary involvement may precede or accompany signs of gastrointestinal disease.
II. Signs associated with gastrointestinal lymphosarcoma vary from acute disease to a prolonged history of vague illness depending on the site and type of intestinal involvement.
  A. Anorexia, vomiting, and diarrhea may be seen with solitary mass lesions.
  B. Signs of malabsorption and maldigestion with weight loss and diarrhea may be seen with diffuse lymphosarcoma (most common in cats).
  C. Dogs tend to have a more acute history than cats.
  D. Systemic involvement with pyrexia, icterus, and anemia may be seen with either type.
III. Other tumors usually cause obstructive clinical signs except for leiomyosarcoma, which often causes an iron deficiency anemia because of chronic, often subclinical, blood loss.
IV. Systemic mastocytosis in cats is associated with vomiting, diarrhea, anorexia, weight loss, and anemia.

Diagnosis

I. Suspicious symptoms in an older animal
II. Physical examination
  A. Small intestinal adenocarcinoma may be palpable with or without mesenteric lymph node involvement.
  B. Diffuse lymphosarcoma may produce gross thickening of the entire small intestine.
  C. It may also be unremarkable except for weight loss.
III. Laboratory findings
  A. A feline leukemia virus test is positive in a minority of cats with alimentary lymphosarcoma.
  B. Hemogram findings are variable and nonspecific.
    1. Nonresponsive anemia of chronic disease is common with lymphosarcoma and other malignancies of long duration.
    2. Iron deficiency anemia is highly suggestive of leiomyoma or other slowly growing intestinal neoplasms.
    3. Occasionally malignant lymphocytes or mast cells are identified.
  C. Biochemical profile shows the following.
    1. Panhypoproteinemia may occur if there is protein-losing enteropathy, which is most common with lymphosarcoma.
    2. Other abnormalities usually reflect invasiveness of the primary tumor or metastases.
IV. Radiology
  A. Survey radiographs are often unremarkable.
    1. Thoracic views should be included to search for metastasis.
    2. Hepatosplenomegaly often accompanies lymphosarcoma and mast cell tumors.
  B. A positive contrast study is usually necessary to demonstrate filling defects, intraluminal masses, and/or obstruction.
V. Biopsy of small intestinal lesion or mass
  A. It is often required for definitive diagnosis and usually requires exploratory laparotomy.
  B. Lymphosarcoma can sometimes be diagnosed via endoscopic biopsy or biopsy of other affected tissues.
  C. Excisional biopsy is appropriate with mass lesions causing obstruction.
  D. Cytologic examination of needle aspirates from thickened bowel loops or mass lesions may reveal neoplastic cells.

Differential Diagnosis

I. Annular adenocarcinoma or mass-like lymphosarcoma
  A. Foreign body
  B. Intussusception
  C. Granulomatous inflammatory disease
II. Diffuse lymphosarcoma
  A. Malabsorption-maldigestion syndromes

B. Other infiltrative diseases of the bowel
C. Other infectious diseases of the bowel

Treatment

I. Intestinal adenocarcinoma
A. Surgical excision is preferred.
B. Postoperative chemotherapy has had limited success.
II. Lymphosarcoma
A. It is often diagnosed late in the course of the disease, and nutritional status is often poor.
B. See chemotherapeutic protocols in Chap. 67.
C. Cats with chronic lymphocytic lymphosarcoma (CLL) often respond to chlorambucil and prednisone therapy (see Table 64–4).
III. Mast cell tumor
A. It is commonly treated with resection and glucocorticoids.
B. Chemotherapy with vincristine or doxorubicin may be tried in resistant cases (see Chaps. 64 and 70).
IV. Benign intestinal masses
Surgery is curative.

Patient Monitoring

I. Intestinal adenocarcinoma
A. The prognosis for adenocarcinomas is poor, particularly if there is evidence of metastasis or unresectable tumor at the time of diagnosis.
B. After resection of the primary mass, many animals gain weight and are asymptomatic for several months, especially cats.
C. Recurrence or metastatic disease often necessitates euthanasia within 3–9 months.
II. Lymphosarcoma
A. The prognosis for most forms of intestinal lymphosarcoma is poor.
B. Some animals with solitary intestinal lymphomas do well for several months with surgical excision and prednisone therapy alone.
C. Combination chemotherapy may induce remission in some animals.
1. Many animals are in a very poor nutritional state (cachexic) at the time of diagnosis, and chemotherapy is not particularly successful.
2. Euthanasia is a reasonable option for many of these cases.
D. The prognosis for cats with CLL is better, as survival for 2–3 years is possible if remission is achieved for chemotherapy.
E. Alimentary lymphosarcoma should always be considered a systemic disease that will eventually recur.

Bibliography

Baldwin S: Feline enteric viruses. p. 1168. In Kirk RW (ed): Current Veterinary Therapy VIII. WB Saunders, Philadelphia, 1983

Batt RM: Bacterial overgrowth associated with naturally occurring enteropathy in German shepherd dogs. Res Vet Sci 35:42, 1983

Batt RM, Morgan J: Role of serum folate and vitamin B_{12} concentration in differentiation of small intestinal abnormalities in the dog. Res Vet Sci 32:17, 1982

Burrows CF: Canine hemorrhagic gastroenteritis. J Am Anim Hosp Assoc 13:451, 1977

Cornelius LM, Roberson EL: Treatment of gastrointestinal parasitism. p. 921. In Kirk RW (ed): Current Veterinary Therapy IX. WB Saunders, Philadelphia, 1986

DeNovo RC: Therapeutics of gastrointestinal diseases. p. 862. In Kirk RW (ed): Current Veterinary Therapy IX. WB Saunders, Philadelphia, 1986

Dillon AR: Bacterial entritis. p. 872. In Kirk RW (ed): Current Veterinary Therapy IX. WB Saunders, Philadelphia, 1986

Fyfe JC, Ramanujam KS, Ramaswamy K et al: Defective brush-border expression of intrinsic factor-cobalamin receptor in canine inherited intestinal cobalamin malabsorption. J Biol Chem 266:4489, 1991

Gilson SD, Parker BB, Twedt DC: Evaluation of two commercial test kits for detection of blood in feces of dogs. Am J Vet Res 51:1385, 1990

Greene CE (ed): Infectious Diseases of the Dog and Cat. WB Saunders, Philadelphia, 1990

Hendrix CM, Blagburn BL: Common gastrointestinal parasites. Vet Clin North Am 13:627, 1983

Moore R, Carpenter J: Intestinal sclerosis with pseudo-obstruction in three dogs. J Am Vet Med Assoc 184:830, 1984

Neer TM: Hypereosinophilic syndrome in cats. Compend Contin Educ Pract Vet 13:549, 1991

Pollock R: Canine viral enteritis. p. 1164. In Kirk RW (ed): Current Veterinary Therapy VIII. WB Saunders, Philadelphia, 1983

Roberson EL, Cornelius LM: Gastrointestinal parasitism. p. 797. In Kirk RW (ed): Current Veterinary Therapy IX. WB Saunders, Philadelphia, 1986

Rutgers HC, Batt RM, Kelly DF: Lymphocytic-plasmacytic gastroenteritis associated with bacterial overgrowth in a dog. J Am Vet Med Assoc 192:1739, 1988

Sherding RG: Diseases of the small bowel. p. 1323. In Ettinger SJ (ed): Textbook of Veterinary Internal Medicine. 3rd Ed. WB Saunders, Philadelphia, 1989

Straw RC: Tumors of the intestinal tract. p. 200. In Withrow SJ, MacEwen EG (eds): Veterinary Clinical Oncology. JB Lippincott, Philadelphia, 1989

Tams TR, Twedt DC: Canine protein-losing gastroenteropathy. Compend Contin Educ Pract Vet 3:105, 1981

Williams DA: Malabsorption, small intestinal bacterial overgrowth, and protein-losing enteropathy. p. 367. In Guilford WG, Center SA, Strombeck DR et al (eds): Small Animal Gastroenterology. 3rd Ed. WB Saunders, Philadelphia, 1996

Williams DA, Guilford WG: Procedures for the evaluation of pancreatic and gastrointestinal tract diseases. p. 77. In Guilford WG, Center SA, Strombeck DR et al (eds): Small Animal Gastroenterology. 3rd Ed. WB Saunders, Philadelphia, 1996

Zimmer J: Clinical management of acute gastroenteritis including virus induced enteritis. p. 1171. In Kirk RW (ed): Current Veterinary Therapy VIII. WB Saunders, Philadelphia, 1983

33

Diseases of the Large Intestine

Susan E. Bunch

DEGENERATIVE DISORDERS

Megacolon

Definition and Causes

I. Megacolon arises from loss of normal colonic function and leads to infrequent evacuation of feces and colonic distention.
II. Any mechanical or functional source of obstruction can cause it.
   A. Pelvic nerve or sacral spinal cord disease
   B. Dysautonomia
   C. Pelvic canal stenosis
      1. Pelvic fracture or sacroiliac luxation
      2. Severe prostatomegaly
      3. Severe subiliac lymphadenomegaly
      4. Colonic foreign body
      5. Expansile pelvic neoplasm
   D. Annular rectal adenocarcinoma
   E. Dietary indiscretion rendering the feces impassable: bone, rock, sand impaction
   F. Fibrous stricture subsequent to chronic colitis/proctitis (rare)
III. Although it can arise as a rare congenital condition, it most often occurs in cats, as an acquired form.
   A. It is caused by generalized, permanent dysfunction of colonic smooth muscle, believed to be associated with abnormal activation of smooth muscle myofilaments.
   B. This disruption of colonic motility results in intractable constipation.

Pathophysiology

I. Persistent distention leads to loss of coordinated colonic motility and smooth muscle hypotony.
II. Water continues to be absorbed from the fecal matter, creating feces the consistency of concrete, which are difficult to pass.

III. Mucosal injury may result from prolonged direct intraluminal pressure.

Clinical Signs

I. History
   A. Repeated, nonproductive attempts to defecate are typical, regardless of the underlying cause.
   B. A small amount of liquid feces with fresh blood may be passed.
   C. Hints as to an underlying cause may include indiscriminant eating habits, recurrent urinary infection in an intact male dog, previous pelvic trauma, or signs of illness in other parts of the gastrointestinal tract.
   D. Cats with idiopathic megacolon have repeated episodes of severe constipation relieved only by manual extraction of feces.
   E. Anorexia and vomiting may also be noted in animals that have a more protracted, untreated course.
II. Physical examination
   A. A distended, firm colon is detected by abdominal palpation.
   B. Rectal examination is essential to discover an underlying cause (Table 33–1).
   C. Animals with a protracted course may be depressed, dehydrated, and thin; cats often have an unkempt hair coat.

Diagnosis

I. A thorough physical examination (including neurologic and rectal examinations) with abdominal radiography often confirms the presence of a distended colon and the inciting cause.
II. If there is no radiographic evidence of a cause, consider colonoscopy under heavy sedation or anesthesia.

Table 33–1. Digital Rectal Examination Findings in Animals with Signs of Large Intestinal Disease

Presence of pain
 1. Tail
 2. Perirectal
 3. Rectal
Fecal character
 1. Fresh blood or mucus
 2. Melena: indicating upper gastrointestinal involvement
 3. Abrasive foreign material: bones, plastic, sand, rocks
 4. Size and consistency
Perineal, anal abnormalities (see Chap. 36)
 1. Perianal fistula
 2. Hernia
 3. Anal sac abscess
 4. Proctitis
 5. Poor anal tone
 6. Perianal/anal neoplasm
Rectal abnormalities
 1. Focal constrictive or proliferative lesions
 2. Diffuse ''corrugated'' mucosal pattern
Extraintestinal abnormalities
 1. Malaligned, healed pelvic fracture
 2. Prostatomegaly
 3. Subiliac lymphadomegaly
 4. Mass associated with the pelvis or sacrum: osteosarcoma, fibrosarcoma
 5. Urethral mass or calculus: stranguria mistaken for intestinal tenesmus

Differential Diagnosis

 I. Possibilities include any cause of persistent tenesmus (especially in a female dog), including tenesmus of urinary origin (i.e., pollakiuria, dysuria, stranguria).
 II. Colitis or proctitis, in which there are frequent attempts to defecate and small amounts of feces are passed, must also be considered.

Treatment

 I. Specific treatment depends on the underlying cause of constipation.
 II. Supportive care is usually needed initially.
  A. Fluid therapy is indicated for dehydrated, electrolyte-depleted animals.
  B. Removal of impacted fecal material may be achieved by several means.
   1. Serial warm-water enemas may be successful if the fecal mass is relatively soft.
   2. Sedation, colonic lubrication (water-soluble jelly in a dose syringe, or diluted with water (1:1) and infused through a large-gauge red rubber catheter), and digital evacuation may be tried.
   3. Anesthesia and forceps-assisted extraction may be necessary if the fecal material is of cement-like consistency.
 III. To prevent recurrence, or for management while specific treatment for an underlying cause is initiated, keep the feces soft and the colon empty.
  A. Supplement the diet with fiber (soluble or insolu-

ble) in the form of psyllium, oat bran, or canned pumpkin.
  B. Encourage frequent defecation by regular walks for dogs and clean litter boxes for cats.
  C. Add a laxative to the diet.
   1. Lactulose 2–10 ml PO TID in a dosage to maintain soft stools
   2. Dioctyl sodium sulfosuccinate 50 mg PO SID-BID
  D. Administer a smooth muscle prokinetic agent, such as cisapride (Propulsid).
   1. In vitro studies of normal feline colons indicate that cisapride effectively stimulates longitudinal contractions.
   2. The dosage in cats is 2.5–5 mg PO BID-TID; an effective dosage is not known for dogs, although a dosage of 0.5 mg/kg PO BID-TID may be tried.
   3. Cisapride may not be beneficial in severe cases.
 IV. Animals with idiopathic or irreversible megacolon, especially cats, that fail medical management are candidates for subtotal colectomy (Bright et al., 1986; Rosin et al., 1988; Holt and Johnston, 1991).
  A. Complications are unusual.
  B. Most cats are considerably improved after surgery, have normal enteric function, and require minimal continued medical management.
  C. The procedure is done less frequently in dogs, so there is little available information as to its expected outcome.

Patient Monitoring

 I. Regular physical examinations are done on a weekly basis initially to detect recurrence of constipation.
 II. Aggressive medical management of idiopathic megacolon in cats, including early use of cisapride, may delay the need for surgery.

INFECTIOUS DISEASES

Protothecosis, Amebiasis, and Balantidiasis

See Chap. 114.

ACUTE LARGE INTESTINAL DIARRHEA

Dietary Indiscretion, Intolerance, or Sensitivity

Definition and Causes

 I. It involves ingestion of excess quantities of a normal diet or of matter not considered to be part of the animal's normal diet.
 II. This could include abnormal foodstuffs (table scraps or garbage), foreign matter (bones or rocks), or abrupt exposure to a different diet.

III. Because of more discriminatory eating habits, cats are less often affected than dogs.

Pathophysiology

I. Ingestion of excessive quantities of osmotically active particles favors movement of water into the lumen, overwhelming the reserve absorptive capacity of the colon.

II. Bacterial action on ingested particles yields fermentation products such as ammonia and hydrogen sulfide and hydrogenated fatty acids, which stimulate excess secretion and hypomotility.

III. Spoiled food may contain bacteria that generate enterotoxins.

IV. Completely undigested foreign material such as bone fragments is abrasive, causing direct mucosal injury.

V. Some individuals may be sensitive to a particular dietary protein or food additive, resulting in release of inflammatory mediators, such as kinins and prostaglandins.

Clinical Signs

I. History
  A. The history most often includes markedly increased frequency of defecation of small volumes of feces, which typically contain mucus, fresh blood, and perhaps foreign matter.
  B. Defecation may be accompanied by sustained straining (rectal tenesmus) and/or signs of pain (dyschezia).
  C. Dogs that live outdoors or are poorly supervised are especially likely to develop this condition.
  D. There may be an identifiable temporal association between feeding of a different diet and sudden onset of large intestinal signs.
  E. There also may be signs of upper gastrointestinal involvement (vomiting, small intestinal diarrhea).

II. Physical examination
  A. Generally, there are few signs of systemic illness.
  B. Mild depression or vague abdominal discomfort may be detected by abdominal palpation.
  C. Dehydration is not usually present unless the upper gastrointestinal tract is also involved.
  D. Rectal examination is essential (see Table 33–1).
    1. The perineum may be stained with blood and mucus.
    2. Digital examination may elicit pain.
    3. Foreign matter mixed in with semi-liquid feces is often easily recognized, but there may be only bloody fluid and mucus.
    4. The remainder of the rectal examination is normal.

Diagnosis

I. It is based primarily on characteristic history and lack of other detectable causes.

II. If the history is questionable, fecal flotation is done to rule out parasitic causes of acute large intestinal diarrhea (Table 33–2).
  A. *Trichuris vulpis*: dogs only in the United States

Table 33–2. *Common Disorders of the Large Intestine in Dogs and Cats*

	Disorders That Cause Diarrhea	Disorders That Cause Constipation
Acute	Dietary indiscretion/ intolerance[a] Trichuriasis[a] *Clostridium perfringens* enterotoxicosis[a]	Foreign body lodged in the pelvic canal[a]
Chronic	Lymphocytic- plasmacytic colitis Idiopathic large intestinal diarrhea[a]	Idiopathic megacolon[b] Malaligned, healed pelvic fracture Prostatomegaly[a] Distal spinal cord injury[b] Perineal hernia[a]

[a]Common in dogs.
[b]Common in cats.

  B. *Ancylostoma* spp. or *Uncinaria stenocephala*: occasionally in the large intestine of dogs and cats

III. Signs usually resolve rapidly after removal of the offending substance and supportive care.

Differential Diagnosis

I. If signs do not improve within 3–5 days after removal of the offending substance and provision of simple supportive care (especially if there are other signs of illness), other diagnoses must be considered.

II. These include other primary enteritides (Table 33–3).
  A. Infectious enteritis
  B. Early manifestations of a systemic illness

Treatment

I. Remove offending substance, e.g., stop feeding the new diet.

II. Withhold food for 24 hours initially.

III. Allow access to water, if the animal is not vomiting.

IV. If the animal is dehydrated, restore fluid balance with a replacement fluid such as lactated Ringer's solution over 24–48 hours.
  A. Calculate needs (replacement + maintenance + ongoing losses; see Appendix I).
  B. Fluids are given in divided amounts subcutaneously, since most affected animals are ≤5% dehydrated.

V. After the period of food withdrawal, provide small amounts of a low-fat, highly digestible diet, such as rice with boiled chicken or uncreamed cottage cheese, or prescription diets such as Purina CNM EN-Formula and Hill's i/d, 3–4 times daily.

VI. The animal's normal diet may be slowly reinstituted after about 3 days.

VII. Symptomatic medications may be needed to relieve pain, encourage rest, and decrease excess intestinal secretion.
  A. Motility modifiers
    1. Narcotic analgesics increase desirable rhyth-

Table 33–3. **Miscellaneous, Uncommon Disorders of the Large Intestine in Dogs and Cats**

Disorders That Cause Acute Diarrhea	Diagnosis	Treatment
Infectious agents		
Giardiasis	Fecal smear, ZnSO₄ concentration	Fenbendazole
Salmonella spp.	Blood and fecal culture (special media)	Chloramphenicol, amoxicillin, trimethoprim/sulfa
Campylobacter spp.	Fecal smear, culture (special media)	Erythromycin, aminoglycosides
Yersinia enterocolitica	Blood and fecal culture (special media)	Chloramphenicol, aminoglycosides, cephalosporin
Entamoeba histolytica	Fecal smear with methylene blue	Metronidazole
Balantidium coli	ZnSO₄ concentration, fecal smear	Metronidazole, tetracycline
Heterobilharzia americana	Fecal smear, biopsy	Fenbendazole ± praziquantel
Cryptosporidium spp.	Fecal smear with special stainᵃ	Controversial—tylosin?
Corticosteroid-associated ulceration in dogs with neurologic disease	Physical examination, colonoscopy	Discontinue corticosteroid therapy as soon as possible; abdominal surgery may be needed
Secondary to severe pancreatitis	Physical examination, ultrasonography	Manage pancreatitis aggressively

Disorders That Cause Chronic Diarrhea	Diagnosis	Treatment
Congenital abnormalities		
Vascular ectasia	Colonoscopy, biopsy	Surgical resection of the affected area
Short colon	Colonoscopy, barium enema	Low-residue diet
Enterocyst	Ultrasonography, exploratory surgery	Surgical resection
Histoplasmosis	Rectal scraping for cytology, biopsy	Itraconazole (see Chap. 109)
Ileocolic intussusception	Ultrasonography, exploratory surgery	Surgical resection
Cecal inversion	Ultrasonography, exploratory surgery	Surgical resection
Extramedullary plasmacytoma	Ultrasonography, exploratory surgery	Melphalan, prednisone

Disorders That Cause Constipation	Diagnosis	Treatment
Congenital abnormalities		
Atresia, stenosis	Physical examination	Reconstructive surgery
Dysautonomia	Physical examination, pharmacologic ocular function testing, plasma catecholamine levels	Supportive care (see Chaps. 25 and 102)
Colorectal diverticulum	Rectal examination, barium enema	Surgical resection
Benign colorectal stricture	Colonoscopy, biopsy	Surgical resection; treat underlying cause

ᵃCarbol-fuchsin, crystal violet.

mic segmentation contractions and promote fluid and electrolyte resorption, thereby decreasing the frequency and volume of defecation.

2. These agents should be used for only 24–48 hours.
    a) Loperamide: 0.08–0.2 mg/kg PO TID-QID for dogs, 0.04 mg/kg PO SID-BID *cautiously* for cats
    b) Diphenoxylate (with atropine to discourage abuse): 0.05–0.1 mg/kg PO TID-QID for dogs, 0.063 mg/kg PO TID for cats
    c) Contraindicated in diarrhea associated with endotoxin or enterotoxin, because they delay evacuation of toxic substances

B. Antisecretory agents
    1. Antiprostaglandin activity decreases fluid and electrolyte secretion.
    2. Consider bismuth subsalicylate 1–2 ml/kg PO TID for dogs only.
    3. Warn owners that this medication may give the feces a very dark color.
    4. This product is avoided in cats because of their inherent sensitivity to salicylates.

Patient Monitoring

I. Signs are resolved in 3–5 days.
II. Recurrences can be prevented by eliminating exposure to garbage and inciting diets.

Trichuriasis

Definition and Causes

I. *Trichuris vulpis* causes acute, and potentially chronic, mucosal and submucosal inflammation of the cecum in dogs.
II. Heavy infestation may also involve the ileum and entire colon.
III. The organism is one of the most common nematode parasites of urban and rural dogs in North America.

Pathophysiology

I. Ingested infective eggs hatch into first-stage larvae in the small intestine; they then penetrate the mucosa and eventually mature in the cecum.
II. There they burrow into the submucosa and cause varying degrees of mononuclear cell inflammation.
III. Parasite burden and location (focal vs. diffuse), as well as the health status of the host, contribute to the degree of illness; heavy infestation may result in anemia caused primarily by mucosal bleeding.
IV. Owing to the hardiness of *Trichuris* ova in the environment (and likelihood of reinfection), intermittent shedding of ova, long prepatent period (70–100 days), longevity of the adult organism (months to years), variation in host response, and interaction with other parasites, trichuriasis may be responsible for either acute or chronic large intestinal diarrhea.

Clinical Signs

I. Signs are typical of most causes of acute or chronic large intestinal diarrhea (see Tables 33–2 and 33–3).
   A. Infection may be inapparent, or there may be signs of systemic illness.
   B. Parasite burden does not necessarily correlate with severity of clinical manifestations.
II. History is often nonspecific.
   A. Most dogs have signs of large intestinal diarrhea.
   B. Additional signs of illness may include weight loss and abdominal discomfort.
   C. Some animals with trichuriasis may be presented for problems resembling mineralocorticoid insufficiency, e.g., weakness, anorexia, large intestinal diarrhea, and polydipsia.
III. Physical examination findings are variable.
   A. Many affected dogs have no abnormalities.
   B. Dehydration, bradycardia, and hypothermia are detected in some animals.
   C. Rectal examination is always performed to rule out a focal nonobstructive lesion, such as a polyp, that could cause hematochezia or mucoid stools.

Diagnosis

I. Diagnosis is made by finding large, oval, brown, double-operculate eggs in a direct fecal smear or by centrifugal flotation; usually no other tests are needed.

II. Ova must be distinguished from swallowed ova of other less common trichinelloid species, such as *Eucoleus aerophilus* and *E. bohemi,* which infect the respiratory tract.
III. Response to empirical treatment in animals with typical history, signs, and environmental risk for trichuriasis but serial negative results of fecal flotation tests may also be diagnostic.
IV. Adult parasites can be visualized grossly during colonoscopy, but other tests are performed (including empirical deworming) before this procedure is considered.
V. Animals with trichuriasis and signs similar to mineralocorticoid insufficiency may have hypochloremia, hyperkalemia, azotemia, poor urine concentrating ability, and metabolic acidosis. Such animals have been found to have normal adrenal responsiveness (both cortisol and aldosterone) after ACTH administration.

Differential Diagnosis

I. Any other cause of acute or chronic large intestinal diarrhea (see Tables 33–2 and 33–3)
II. Hypoadrenocorticism
III. Other trichinelloid infections

Treatment

I. Fenbendazole is safe and effective, has no known contraindications, and is useful against other intestinal parasites.
   A. The dose is 50 mg/kg PO SID for 3 consecutive days.
   B. Treatment is repeated in 3 weeks if other common gastrointestinal parasites are present, and again 3 months later for *T. vulpis.*
II. Other supportive care is given, e.g., fluid therapy for dehydration, as necessary.

Patient Monitoring

I. Signs of improvement in fecal character are usually apparent within 2–3 days after treatment.
II. Because of intermittent shedding of ova, post-treatment fecal flotation cannot be used to judge treatment efficacy.
III. Re-treatment is recommended if signs return, with or without a positive fecal flotation result.
IV. If reinfection is likely from environmental sources that cannot be adequately cleaned or eliminated, switching to a heartworm preventive product that is also efficacious for *T. vulpis* is recommended.
   A. Milbemycin oxime (Interceptor) 0.5 mg/kg PO once monthly
   B. Diethylcarbamazine with oxibendazole (Filaribits Plus) 6 mg/kg PO SID
      Some dogs may develop adverse hepatic idiosyncratic reactions to this product.

Clostridium perfringens–Associated Enterotoxicosis

Definition and Causes

I. Colonization by *Clostridium perfringens* type A (a normal intestinal anaerobic inhabitant), sporulation, and production/release of enterotoxin are stimulated by unknown means.

II. Large intestinal diarrhea can develop as a result of an acute hospital-associated infection (by ingestion of organisms) or as a more insidious chronic, naturally occurring disease.

III. Isolation of the organism from feces does not necessarily indicate a causal relationship with illness; identification of both high spore counts and enterotoxin is necessary.

Pathophysiology

I. No single factor that encourages proliferation of the organism and ultimate release of enterotoxin has been identified; it is likely that a blend of host and intestinal mucosal and luminal factors is involved.

II. The enterotoxin causes excess intestinal fluid and electrolyte secretion, brush-border mucosal epithelial injury, and hypomotility.

III. Proliferation of *C. perfringens* has been described in association with other intestinal conditions, such as parvovirus enteritis and hemorrhagic gastroenteritis.

IV. Involvement of this organism in other conditions such as irritable bowel syndrome, inflammatory bowel disease, stress-associated diarrhea, and fiber-responsive large intestinal diarrhea is yet to be determined.

Clinical Signs

I. History
   A. Signs of acute large intestinal diarrhea often develop during or soon after a hospital stay (primarily in dogs).
   B. Some dogs have a more chronic course, with intermittent bouts of diarrhea that seem to resolve spontaneously.
   C. Other systemic signs of illness, e.g., vomiting, are unusual.

II. Physical examination
   A. Generally unremarkable
   B. Possibly fresh blood and mucus in the feces

Diagnosis

I. A presumptive diagnosis can be made on the basis of the onset of acute large intestinal diarrhea closely associated with a hospital stay.

II. Thin fecal smears are made and stained to identify the presence of high numbers of clostridia and spores, which is supportive of the diagnosis.
   A. Special stains for spores are available, but they are often unnecessary as the spores can usually be seen microscopically with routine staining procedures.
   B. Gram's or Wright-Giemsa stain demonstrates excess numbers of a uniform population of positively stained rods.
   C. Spores do not take up stain, but rather become evident as clear vacuoles in association with gram-positive vegetative rods.
   D. It may be necessary to repeat the smear if there is any question about the number of organisms or spores; >3–4 spores/high power field is abnormal.

III. Identification of fecal enterotoxin during an episode of diarrhea is diagnostic.
   A. A reverse passive latex agglutination assay (PET-RPLA, Oxoid Toxin Detection Kit, Unipath, Ogdensburg, NY) is readily available.
   B. The assay was developed for use in people but can be used without modification in animals, because the enterotoxin is antigenically similar.
   C. Only a small volume of fresh feces is needed; it is suspended in buffered saline, and 25 μl of the supernatant is used to detect enterotoxin.
   D. The degree of agglutination is measured; the result is reported on a scale from negative to 3+.

Differential Diagnosis

I. Any cause of acute large intestinal diarrhea (see Tables 33–2 and 33–3)

II. Stress-induced diarrhea (poorly defined)

Treatment

I. Many animals with mild signs recover spontaneously within 3 days.

II. For animals with nosocomial, more severe, or persistent signs, antibiotic administration for about 5 days is recommended to reduce clostridial populations.
   A. Ampicillin or amoxicillin 22 mg/kg PO TID
   B. Metronidazole 10 mg/kg PO BID
   C. Tylosin tartrate (2.27 g of tylosin per teaspoon) 10–20 mg/kg BID mixed in food (may also be useful long term for dogs with chronic clostridial enterotoxicosis)

III. Changing to a high-fiber diet may also be of long-term benefit by changing the pH of the feces, thereby inhibiting sporulation or altering bacterial growth.

Patient Monitoring

I. Most animals recover rapidly with antibiotic treatment.

II. Identification of other underlying intestinal diseases, such as inflammatory bowel disease, is worthwhile in animals with recurrent episodes.

III. Some animals are best managed by lower daily doses of antibiotics given long term (assuming there is no concurrent intestinal disease).

CHRONIC INFLAMMATORY DISORDERS

Colitis

Definition and Causes

I. It is a collection of diseases characterized by diffuse mucosal infiltration of the large intestine with inflammatory cells.

II. The term "inflammatory bowel disease," which specifically refers to two immune-mediated large intestinal disorders of people (Crohn's disease and ulcerative colitis), is often used loosely for this disorder.

III. In dogs and cats, lymphocytic-plasmacytic colitis is the most common form, eosinophilic and histiocytic ulcerative colitis are less common, and granulomatous, plasmacytic, and suppurative colitis are least common.

IV. Mucosal inflammation can develop as a nonspecific response to several local and systemic conditions and intraluminal events, including parasitic infection, bacterial adherence or overgrowth, and dietary allergy.

V. Some forms of chronic colitis appear to have a familial basis, e.g., histiocytic ulcerative colitis in boxers and French bulldogs.

VI. An immunologic basis has been postulated because of the character of the most common cellular infiltrates, as well as a positive response to treatment with immunosuppressive drugs or hypoallergenic diets.

VII. Immunologic studies have not been done in dogs and cats; the cause in most cases is unknown.

Pathophysiology

I. Inflammatory cell infiltrates in the lamina propria disrupt cell-to-cell associations, interfering with normal colonic motility and function (e.g., absorption of water and electrolytes). The submucosa and muscularis may be involved in severe cases.

II. Goblet cell hyperplasia leads to excess mucus production. The mucosa is friable and easily damaged, with resulting hematochezia.

III. Inflammatory cell infiltrates can occur only in the large intestine or can involve the stomach and small intestine (see Chaps. 30 and 32). With distal involvement of the colon, straining and dyschezia are more likely.

IV. The degree and type of cellular infiltrate do not seem to correlate with severity of clinical signs.

Clinical Signs

I. History
   A. Signs are typical of any cause of acute large bowel diarrhea, but they are of several weeks' duration.
   B. Anorexia, vomiting, and dehydration are unusual but can be present if the large intestinal disease is especially severe or if there is gastric and/or small intestinal involvement.
   C. Except for certain familial tendencies (basenji dog and purebred cats for lymphocytic-plasmacytic colitis; boxer and French bulldog for histiocytic ulcerative colitis), there is no particular breed predisposition.
   D. Most affected dogs and cats are young to middle-aged.
   E. Some studies have shown a male gender predisposition, but others have not.

II. Physical examination
   A. It is normal in most cases, except for results of digital rectal examination.
   B. Rectal examination is necessary to rule out other causes of large intestinal signs (see Tables 33–1, 33–2, and 33–3).
   C. Occasionally, the large intestine may be thickened and/or painful upon abdominal palpation.

Diagnosis

I. Unless there are historical or physical examination findings that are inconsistent with diffuse large intestinal disease, all dogs and cats should undergo a sequence of treatment trials before more detailed diagnostic tests are done (Fig. 33–1).
   A. A complete blood count (CBC), chemistry profile, urinalysis, and rectal cytology are obtained.
      1. Laboratory test results are usually unremarkable.
      2. The only helpful finding might be eosinophilia, which may indicate trichuriasis or the eosinophilic form of inflammatory infiltrate in dogs, or the more disseminated hypereosinophilic syndrome of cats.
      3. Monoclonal gammopathy may accompany eosinophilic or plasmacytic enterocolitis.
      4. High serum alanine transaminase activity is often reported, especially in cats.
      5. Rectal cytology may identify a causative agent (e.g., *Histoplasma, Prototheca, Cryptosporidium* spp.) or an excessive number of certain inflammatory cells.
   B. Cats are also tested for feline leukemia virus (FeLV) and feline immunodeficiency virus (FIV).
   C. Dogs are dewormed empirically for trichuriasis.
   D. Dogs, and perhaps cats, are also treated empirically for clostridial enterotoxicosis.
   E. All dogs and cats are switched to a different, restrictive diet for 4–6 weeks.
      1. High-quality, easily digestible protein
         a) Dogs: Hill's Prescription Diet i/d, Iams Eukanuba Low Residue, Purina PRO PLAN CNM Intestinal
         b) Cats: Hill's c/d
      2. High fiber
         a) Dogs and cats: Hill's Prescription Diet w/d or r/d
         b) Dogs and cats: soluble fiber, such as oat

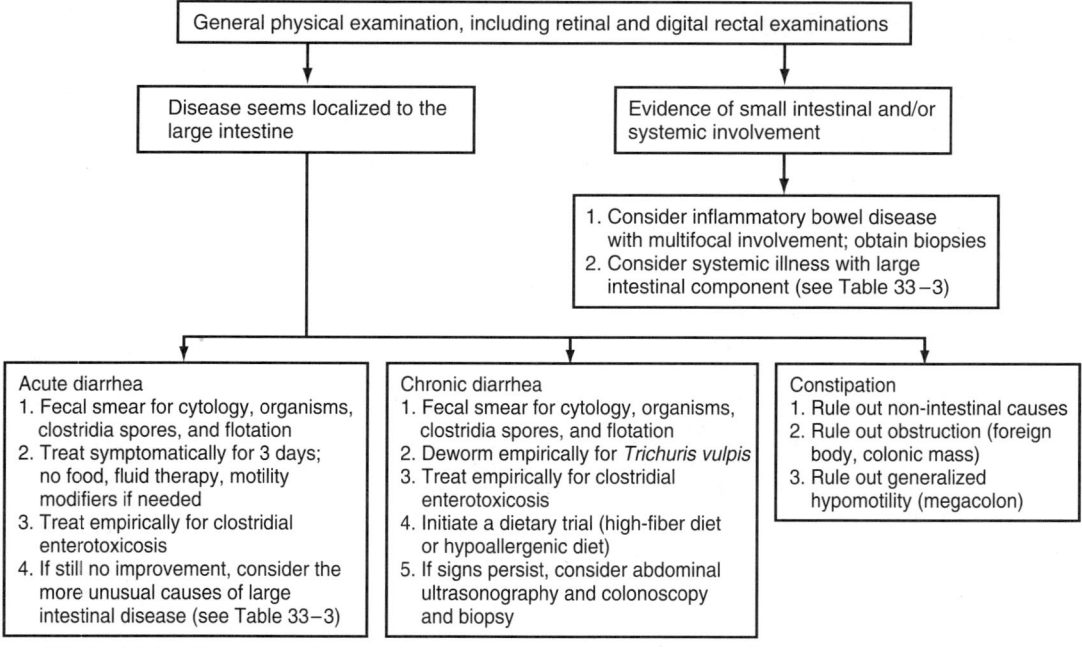

Figure 33–1. Diagnostic approach for animals with a history consistent with large intestinal disease.

bran or psyllium, 1–3 tablespoons/day added to the regular diet

3. Elimination diet: containing protein and carbohydrate sources not commonly found in commercial foods
   a) Dogs and cats: Hill's Prescription Diet d/d, Iams Eukanuba Response Formula FP
   b) Other hypoallergenic commercially available diets (Brown et al., 1995)

II. A more aggressive diagnostic approach is needed for animals that have failed empirical treatment trials.
   A. Radiography is recommended to rule out focal lesions, including masses (neoplasm, granuloma).
      1. Survey abdominal radiographs are not usually helpful.
      2. A barium enema can be performed.
      3. Abdominal ultrasonography usually provides more information about the large and small intestine and regional lymph nodes.
   B. Colonoscopy allows direct visualization of the entire large intestinal mucosal surface, identification of mass lesions, and acquisition of multiple biopsy specimens.
      1. The animal must be prepared adequately before colonoscopy.
         a) Withhold food for 24 hours.
         b) Administer an oral lavage solution (50–80 ml/kg divided in two doses 2–4 hours apart) the afternoon before.
            (1) Colyte (Reed and Carnick, Piscataway NJ)
            (2) GoLytely (Braintree Laboratories Inc., Braintree, MA)
            (3) Homemade generic solution
               Chemicals are premixed, then added to 1 L of deionized water before administration: 59 g polyethylene glycol, 1.46 g sodium chloride, 0.745 g potassium chloride, 1.68 g sodium bicarbonate, 5.68 g sodium sulfate (anhydrous).
         c) Give a warm-water enema the morning of colonoscopy.
      2. Most animals require heavy sedation or general anesthesia. Administration of a narcotic (oxymorphone 0.05 mg/kg IM, SQ) and an anticholinergic (atropine 0.04 mg/kg SQ) stimulates colonic tone and facilitates colonoscopy.
      3. Position the animal in left lateral recumbency.
      4. Use of a flexible fiberoptic endoscope permits the most complete examination. The rectum, entire length of the colon, cecum, and terminal ileum are accessible with this instrument.
      5. Multiple biopsy specimens are obtained from any area that appears granular, proliferative, friable, or ulcerative. Specimens are also collected even if the mucosa appears normal or changes seem minimal.

Differential Diagnosis

I. Any cause of chronic large intestinal diarrhea (see Tables 33–2 and 33–3)
II. Systemic disease with a large intestinal component, e.g., histoplasmosis, prototheocosis, lymphoma

Treatment

I. Additional, more aggressive treatment is needed for animals that have failed dietary management alone (see earlier).

II. Sulfasalazine is the drug of choice for dogs with lymphocytic-plasmacytic, histiocytic-ulcerative, and suppurative colitis.
   A. The initial dosage is 15–20 mg/kg PO TID.
   B. Severely affected dogs may need 50 mg/kg PO TID (maximum: 3 g/day).
   C. The dosage may be reduced after signs are controlled for at least 1–2 weeks (usually a total of 3–4 weeks of treatment).

III. Prednisone is often chosen for cats with lymphocytic-plasmacytic colitis, because of their sensitivity to salicylate-containing compounds.
   A. The dosage is 2 mg/kg/day PO.
   B. The dosage may be reduced after signs are controlled for at least 1–2 weeks (usually a total of 3–4 weeks of treatment).
   C. For cats in which the use of prednisone is less desirable, e.g., those with diabetes mellitus, sulfasalazine can be tried.
      1. The dosage is lower than that for dogs (10 mg/kg PO SID-BID).
      2. An oral suspension is available to permit accurate dosing.

IV. Other drugs can be added to or tried in place of sulfasalazine in dogs if signs persist.
   A. Prednisone 2 mg/kg PO may be effective and allow the sulfasalazine dosage to be reduced further.
   B. Metronidazole may also be used, because it has beneficial effects other than its antimicrobial activity against anaerobes.
      1. Immunosuppressive effects include altered neutrophil chemotaxis and diminished cell-mediated response.
      2. Dosage is 10–15 mg/kg PO BID-TID.
   C. The use of tylosin tartrate (2.27 g of tylosin per teaspoon) is controversial, and its mechanism of action is unknown.
      1. Dosage is 10–20 mg/kg BID mixed in food.
      2. It is safe for long-term use (weeks to months).

V. Prednisone is the drug of choice for eosinophilic, plasmacytic, and granulomatous (regional) colitis in dogs and cats.
   A. Dogs: 2 mg/kg/day PO
   B. Cats: 4 mg/kg/day PO

Patient Monitoring

I. Clinical signs usually begin to resolve soon after initiation of drug therapy.

II. Drug therapy (sulfasalazine or prednisone) may be tapered after signs have been resolved for at least 2 weeks.

III. Some animals require drug therapy for life; others may be controlled with diet changes alone after drug discontinuation.

IV. Keratoconjunctivitis sicca is a common adverse reaction to sulfonamide use; it may be reversed if detected early. Tear production is assessed every 2–4 weeks in dogs receiving sulfasalazine long term.

Idiopathic Large Intestinal Diarrhea

Definition and Causes

I. It is large intestinal diarrhea for which no underlying cause can be found, and no histologic abnormalities are identified in the colon.

II. It resembles irritable bowel syndrome in people, which is characterized by episodes of large intestinal diarrhea often associated with stressful events and is believed to have a neurologic component.

III. No studies of irritable bowel syndrome have been conducted in dogs and cats, so it is not known whether the disorder represents undiagnosed *Clostridium* enterotoxicosis.

Pathophysiology

I. This condition often responds to dietary fiber supplementation.

II. Fiber administration has several beneficial effects on the colon.
   A. Soluble fiber traps water and delays intestinal transit time, allowing excess water to be absorbed, and it is fermented by intestinal bacteria, yielding more bacterial by-products.
   B. These effects increase fecal bulk, as does insoluble fiber, which is not digested.
   C. Increased fecal bulk stimulates rhythmic segmental contractions, further prolonging fecal transit time.
   D. Both types of fiber bind bile acids, some of which are injurious to colonic mucosa.
   E. Anaerobic bacteria in the colon metabolize fiber, yielding short chain fatty acids (SCFAs) such as butyric acid. Most SCFAs are absorbed, but some remain in the intestinal lumen to participate in several metabolic functions that maintain mucosal epithelial health.

Clinical Signs

I. Recurrent episodes of large intestinal diarrhea

II. History
   A. Signs are intermittent.
   B. A relationship with stressful events, e.g., boarding, travel, grooming, new members of the household, separation, or visits to the veterinarian, may be delineated by careful questioning of the owner.
   C. Affected animals may not outwardly appear excitable or overly anxious.
   D. There is no evidence of systemic illness.

III. Physical examination
   A. Results of general physical examination are normal.
   B. Results of digital rectal examination are normal, other than findings consistent with large intestinal diarrhea (pain, hematochezia, excess mucus).

Diagnosis

I. It is based on a compatible history and an absence of physical, laboratory, or histologic abnormalities.
II. Animals must have failed several treatment trials, including empirical deworming for *Trichuris* spp. treatment for *Clostridium* enterotoxicosis, and use of a bland or hypoallergenic diet.

Differential Diagnosis

See Tables 33–2 and 33–3.

Treatment

I. Identify, minimize, or eliminate stressful events, if possible.
II. Add soluble fiber.
  A. Supplement the existing diet with psyllium 1–3 tablespoons/day.
  B. Change to a specially formulated high-fiber diet, such as Hill's Prescription Diet w/d or r/d.
III. If necessary, motility modifying agents can be given to control acute episodes (see earlier).
IV. Perceived abdominal pain may be relieved by the use of antispasmodic agents.
  A. Propantheline 0.25 mg/kg PO BID-TID
  B. Hyoscyamine 0.003–0.006 mg/kg PO BID-TID
V. A common antianxiety agent often used in people and, to a limited extent, in dogs is Librax (Roche Products), a combination of a sedative (5 mg chlordiazepoxide hydrochloride) and an anticholinergic (2.5 mg clidinium bromide). Dosage is 0.10–0.25 mg/kg of clidinium PO BID-TID.

Patient Monitoring

I. Unless specific initiating events can be identified and eliminated, repeat episodes are to be expected.
II. The disorder is not life-threatening but may be challenging to control.

MISCELLANEOUS DISORDERS

See Table 33–3.

NEOPLASIA

Definition and Causes

I. Primary tumors of the cecum, colon, and rectum are uncommon (dogs) to rare (cats).
II. At least twice as many colonic tumors are malignant as are benign in dogs; virtually all are malignant in cats.
III. Most primary tumors are solitary and occur in the colon and rectum.
  A. Benign
    1. Mucosal adenomas (polyps) are most common.

    2. Small polyps are unlikely to represent premalignant lesions, although they can be multiple.
    3. Leiomyomas and other tumors have been reported sporadically.
  B. Malignant
    1. Adenocarcinoma is the most common primary tumor and often occurs in pedunculated or annular intraluminal forms in the rectum.
    2. Gastrointestinal lymphoma most often involves the small and possibly the large intestine.
     a) The large intestine may also be affected in multicentric lymphoma.
     b) Lesions may be focal nodular or diffuse infiltrative.
    3. Other primary tumors include leiomyosarcoma (especially cecal), carcinoid, extramedullary plasmacytoma, and mast cell tumor.
IV. No causative factors have been identified in large intestinal cancer of dogs and cats. Most cats with gastrointestinal lymphoma are FeLV-negative.

Pathophysiology

I. Most benign tumors are slowly progressive with persistent, intermittent signs for as long as 1 year before diagnosis, whereas malignant tumors are detected within 3 months.
II. Hematochezia is most often associated with benign and malignant tumors that involve the mucosa.
III. Annular adenocarcinoma often causes intestinal tenesmus and constipation.

Clinical Signs

I. History
  A. Signs are typical of any cause of chronic large intestinal diarrhea or constipation.
  B. Persistent intestinal tenesmus can cause rectal prolapse; prolapsed polypoid tumors can be visualized directly in the anus.
  C. Rectal bleeding independent of defecation may be observed.
  D. Some tumors, especially of the cecum, result in perforation, with septic peritonitis as the first presenting sign.
  E. Malignant large intestinal tumors are most often seen in male, medium- to large-breed dogs or domestic short-haired cats of either gender over 9 years of age.
II. Physical examination
  A. Large colonic tumors are identifiable by abdominal palpation. In diffuse intestinal lymphoma, the colon may be generally thickened.
  B. Digital rectal examination is very important in distinguishing intestinal from extraintestinal causes of large intestinal diarrhea, tenesmus, hematochezia, and dyschezia.
  C. A rectal annular constrictive lesion is most commonly adenocarcinoma, but occasionally it results from an inflammatory condition (proctitis, colitis).

D. The presence of systemic signs, e.g., vomiting, dehydration, anemia, is variable.

Diagnosis

I. Because signs of large intestinal neoplasia are similar to those of chronic colitis, a similar diagnostic plan is recommended.
II. Results of CBC, chemistry profile, and urinalysis are usually normal. Paraneoplastic leukocytosis (extreme neutrophilia) has been reported in a dog with a rectal adenomatous polyp (Thompson et al., 1992).
III. Abdominal ultrasonography is useful.
   A. Focal vs. diffuse lesions
   B. Findings compatible with dissemination, e.g., enlarged lymph nodes, hepatic nodules
IV. Gastrointestinal contrast studies can be done if colonoscopy is not available.
V. The most common malignant large intestinal tumors do not disseminate to the lungs, so thoracic radiography is performed primarily if multicentric lymphoma is suspected.
VI. Lesions of gastrointestinal lymphoma in dogs are often surrounded by marked lymphocytic-plasmacytic infiltrates, so multiple deep (submucosal) biopsies may be needed.
VII. Exploratory celiotomy can be undertaken to obtain biopsy specimens or resect focal lesions.

Treatment

I. Specific treatment is determined from biopsy results.
II. Surgical resection is recommended for the following tumors.
   A. Rectal adenoma (polyp)
   B. Distal rectal polypoid adenocarcinoma
   C. Solitary cecal or colonic tumor of any cell type (with wide margins), especially if there is perforation or obstruction
III. Chemotherapy may be attempted for lymphoma.
   A. Gastrointestinal lymphoma is not as responsive as the multicentric form (see Chap. 67).
   B. Chemotherapy is instituted following resection of a solitary mass.
IV. Successful treatment protocols have not been established for luminal annular rectal adenocarcinoma.
   A. Local resection and cryosurgery may offer longer survival times than radical resection.
   B. Radiation therapy has been successful in a small number of dogs (Straw, 1996).
   C. Palliative therapy with stool softeners or colostomy may be tried, as distant metastasis is unusual, and local recurrence is the most common cause for euthanasia.
   D. The gross appearance of the tumor may offer some prognostic information; single polypoid masses have the best prognosis, and annular lesions have the worst.

Patient Monitoring

I. Local recurrence within 8–10 weeks is common for malignant tumors and occurs occasionally with polyps.
II. Return of clinical signs (hematochezia, dyschezia, intestinal tenesmus, mucoid stools) warrants repeat investigation.

Bibliography

Birchard SJ, Couto CG, Johnson SE: Nonlymphoid intestinal neoplasia in 32 dogs and 14 cats. J Am Anim Hosp Assoc 22:533, 1986

Boothe DM: GI pharmacology update. Vet Preview 1:2, 1994

Bowman DE: Hookworm parasites of dogs and cats. Compend Contin Educ Pract Vet 14:585, 1992

Bright RM, Burrows CF, Goring R et al: Subtotal colectomy for treatment of acquired megacolon in the dog and cat. J Am Vet Med Assoc 188:1412, 1986

Brown CM, Armstrong PJ, Globus H: Nutritional management of food allergy in dogs and cats. Compend Contin Educ Pract Vet 17:637, 1995

Burrows CF: Evaluation of a colonic lavage solution to prepare the colon of the dog for colonoscopy. J Am Vet Med Assoc 195:1719, 1989

Burrows CF: Canine colitis. Compend Contin Educ Pract Vet 14:1347, 1992

Campbell BG: Trichuris and other trichinelloid nematodes of dogs and cats in the United States. Compend Contin Educ Pract Vet 13:769, 1991

Church EM, Melhaff CJ, Patnaik AK: Colorectal adenocarcinoma in dogs: 78 cases (1973–1984). J Am Vet Med Assoc 191:727, 1987

Couto CG, Rutgers HC, Sherding RG et al: Gastrointestinal lymphoma in 20 dogs. J Vet Intern Med 3:73, 1989

Dennis JF, Kruger JM, Mullaney TP: Lymphocytic/plasmacytic colitis in cats: 14 cases (1985–1990). J Am Vet Med Assoc 202:313, 1993

DiBartola SP, Rogers WA, Boyce JT et al: Regional enteritis in two dogs. J Am Vet Med Assoc 181:904, 1982

DiBartola SP, Johnson SE, Davenport DJ et al: Clinicopathologic findings resembling hypoadrenocorticism in dogs with primary gastrointestinal disease. J Am Vet Med Assoc 187:60, 1985

Diehl KJ, Lappin MR, Jones RL et al: Monoclonal gammopathy in a dog with plasmacytic gastroenterocolitis. J Am Vet Med Assoc 201:1233, 1992

Fluke MH, Hawkins EC, Elliott GS et al: Short colon in two cats and a dog. J Am Vet Med Assoc 195:87, 1989

Gibbons GC, Murtaugh RJ: Cecal smooth muscle neoplasia in the dog: report of 11 cases and literature review. J Am Anim Hosp Assoc 25:191, 1989

Graves TK, Schall WD, Refsal K et al: Basal and ACTH-stimulated aldosterone concentrations are normal or increased in dogs with trichuriasis-associated pseudohypoadrenocorticism. J Vet Intern Med 8:287, 1994

Guilford WG: Adverse reactions to foods: a gastrointestinal perspective. Compend Contin Educ Pract Vet 16:957, 1994

Hart JR, Shaker E, Patnaik AK et al: Lymphocytic-plasmacytic enterocolitis in cats: 60 cases (1988–1990). J Am Anim Hosp Assoc 30:505, 1994

Holt D, Johnston DE: Idiopathic megacolon in cats. Compend Contin Educ Pract Vet 13:1411, 1991

Jackson MW, Helfand SC, Smedes SL et al: Primary IgG secreting plasma cell tumor in the gastrointestinal tract of a dog. J Am Vet Med Assoc 204:404, 1994

Jergens AE: Rational use of antimicrobials for gastrointestinal disease in small animals. J Am Anim Hosp Assoc 30:123, 1994

Jergens AE, Moore FM, Haynes JS et al: Idiopathic inflammatory bowel disease in dogs and cats: 84 cases (1987–1990). J Am Vet Med Assoc 201:1603, 1992

Johnson SE: Canine eosinophilic gastroenterocolitis. Semin Vet Med Surg (Small Anim) 7:145, 1992

Kruth SA, Prescott JF, Welch MK et al: Nosocomial diarrhea associated with enterotoxigenic *Clostridium perfringens* infection in dogs. J Am Vet Med Assoc 195:331, 1989

Kudisch M, Pavletic MM: Subtotal colectomy with surgical stapling instruments via a transcecal approach for treatment of acquired megacolon in cats. Vet Surg 22:457, 1993

Leib MS, Matz ME: Diseases of the large intestine. p. 1232. In Ettinger SJ, Feldman EC (eds): Textbook of Veterinary Internal Medicine. 4th ed. WB Saunders, Philadelphia, 1995

Leib MS, Sponenberg DP, Wilcke JR et al: Suppurative colitis in a cat. J Am Vet Med Assoc 188:739, 1986

Leib MS, Hay WH, Roth L: Plasmacytic-lymphocytic colitis in dogs. p. 939. In Kirk RW (ed): Current Veterinary Therapy X: Small Animal Practice. WB Saunders, Philadelphia, 1989

Leib MS, Monroe WE, Codner EC: Performing rigid or flexible colonoscopy in dogs with chronic large bowel diarrhea. Vet Med 86:900, 1991

Malik R, Hunt GB, Hinchliffe JM et al: Severe whipworm infection in the dog. J Small Anim Pract 31:185, 1990

McPherron MA, Withrow SJ, Seim HB III et al: Colorectal leiomyomas in seven dogs. J Am Anim Hosp Assoc 28:43, 1992

Miller WW, Hathcock JT, Dillon AR: Cecal inversion in eight dogs. J Am Anim Hosp Assoc 20:1009, 1984

Moon HW: Mechanisms in the pathogenesis of diarrhea: a review. J Am Vet Med Assoc 172:443, 1978

Morgan RV, Bachrach A: Keratoconjunctivitis sicca associated with sulfonamide therapy in dogs. J Am Vet Med Assoc 180:432, 1982

Murdoch DB: Diarrhoea in the dog: causes, investigation and management. Vet Int 1:2, 1991

Nelson RW, Stookey LJ, Kazacos E: Nutritional management of idiopathic chronic colitis in the dog. J Vet Intern Med 2:133, 1988

Papageorges M, Higgins R, Gosselin Y: *Yersinia enterocolitica* enteritis in two dogs. J Am Vet Med Assoc 182:618, 1983

Richter KP, Cleveland MV: Comparison of an orally administered gastrointestinal lavage solution with traditional enema administration as preparation for colonoscopy in dogs. J Am Vet Med Assoc 195:1727, 1989

Rogers KS, Butler LM, Edwards JF et al: Rectal hemorrhage associated with vascular ectasia in a young dog. J Am Vet Med Assoc 200:1349, 1992

Rosin E: Megacolon in cats: the role of colectomy. Vet Clin North Am [Small Anim Pract] 23:587, 1993

Rosin E, Walshaw R, Melhaff C et al: Subtotal colectomy for treatment of chronic constipation associated with idiopathic megacolon in cats: 38 cases (1979–1985). J Am Vet Med Assoc 193:850, 1988

Runyon CL, Merkley DF, Hagemoser WA: Intussusception associated with a paracolonic enterocyst in a dog. J Am Vet Med Assoc 185:443, 1984

Seiler RJ: Colorectal polyps of the dog: a clinicopathologic study of 17 cases. J Am Vet Med Assoc 174:72, 1979

Simpson JW: Role of nutrition in aetiology and treatment of diarrhoea. J Small Anim Pract 33:167, 1992

Spodnick GJ, Kyles AE, Cullen JM et al: Surgical management of a large colorectal diverticulum in a dog. J Am Vet Med Assoc 208:72, 1996

Straw RC: Tumors of the intestinal tract. p. 252. In Withrow SJ, MacEwen EG (eds): Small Animal Clinical Oncology. 2nd Ed. WB Saunders, Philadelphia, 1996

Tams TR: Irritable bowel syndrome. p. 604. In Kirk RW, Bonagura JD (eds): Current Veterinary Therapy XI: Small Animal Practice. WB Saunders, Philadelphia, 1992

Thompson JP, Christopher MM, Ellison GW et al: Paraneoplastic leukocytosis associated with a rectal adenomatous polyp in a dog. J Am Vet Med Assoc 201:737, 1992

Trevor PB, Saunders GK, Waldron DR et al: Metastatic extramedullary plasmacytoma of the colon and rectum in a dog. J Am Vet Med Assoc 203:406, 1993

Twedt DC: *Clostridium perfringens*–associated enterotoxicosis in dogs. p. 602. In Kirk RW, Bonagura JD (eds): Current Veterinary Therapy XI: Small Animal Practice. WB Saunders, Philadelphia, 1992

Twedt DC: Dietary fiber in gastrointestinal disease. Proc Am Coll Vet Intern Med 11:225, 1993

van der Gaag I: The histological appearance of large intestinal biopsies in dogs with clinical signs of large bowel disease. Can J Vet Res 52:75, 1988

van der Gaag I, Happé RP: Follow-up studies by large intestinal biopsies and necropsy in dogs with clinical signs of large bowel disease. Can J Vet Res 53:473, 1989

Washabau RJ, Hall JA: Cisapride. J Am Vet Med Assoc 207:1285, 1995

Washabau RJ, Sammarco J: Effects of cisapride on feline colonic smooth muscle function. Am J Vet Res 57:541, 1996

Washabau RJ, Stalis IH: Alterations in colonic smooth muscle function in cats with idiopathic megacolon. Am J Vet Res 57:580, 1996

Willard MD: Inflammatory bowel disease: perspectives on therapy. J Am Anim Hosp Assoc 28:27, 1992

Wylie KB, Hosgood G: Mortality and morbidity of small and large intestinal surgery in dogs and cats: 74 cases (1980–1992). J Am Anim Hosp Assoc 30:469, 1994

Zajac AM: Developments in the treatment of gastrointestinal parasites of small animals. Vet Clin North Am [Small Anim Pract] 23:671, 1993

34

Diseases of the Hepatobiliary System

Cynthia R. Leveille-Webster

VASCULAR ANOMALIES

Portosystemic Shunts

Definition

A portosystemic shunt (PSS) is an abnormal vascular communication between the portal and systemic circulation.

Causes

I. Congenital vascular anomalies
   A. These occur in both dogs and cats but are more common in the former.
   B. Predisposition exists in Irish wolfhounds (polygenic inheritance), dachshunds, Yorkshire terriers, Maltese, miniature schnauzers, and Australian cattle dogs (Johnson et al., 1987; Maddison, 1988; Bostwick and Twedt, 1995).
   C. Most often a single shunting vessel is present.
      1. Intrahepatic shunts are more common in large-breed dogs. Patent ductus venosus is the most common type of intrahepatic shunt.
      2. Extrahepatic shunts are more common in small-breed dogs and cats.
         a) Portal–azygous
         b) Portal–abdominal vena cava
         c) Left gastric vein to abdominal vena cava (most common in cats)
         d) Atresia of portal vein (often multiple shunts)
II. Acquired PSSs
   A. They result from increased resistance to portal blood flow, most often secondary to chronic fibrotic liver disease; they are rare in cats.
   B. See Chronic Canine Inflammatory Hepatic Disease (later).

Pathophysiology

I. The shunting vessel diverts portal blood flow directly into the systemic circulation, bypassing removal of potential toxins by the liver and leading to the development of hepatic encephalopathy (HE). In addition, the liver atrophies from lack of exposure to hepatotrophic factors normally present in portal blood.
II. HE is the reversible alteration of mental status and neurologic function associated with impaired extraction and/or metabolism of neuroactive metabolites, most likely of gut origin, which collectively cause neural inhibition (Maddison, 1992).
   A. The etiology of HE has not been identified, but it is believed that multiple factors are involved and that these factors are derived from the gut, because therapeutic measures that minimize interaction between enteric bacterial and nitrogenous substances in the gut ameliorate the clinical signs of HE.
      1. Ammonia is the most studied of the toxins involved.
         a) Sources of ammonia include the following.
            (1) Bacterial splitting of urea in the colon and ileum
            (2) Bacterial deamination of dietary proteins
            (3) Glutamine metabolism in the kidney and small intestine
            (4) Skeletal muscle catabolism of proteins for energy
         b) Normally, ammonia is delivered to the liver via the portal circulation, is converted to urea, and undergoes urinary excretion.
         c) In the presence of a PSS, ammonia is diverted to the systemic circulation, and blood and brain ammonia concentrations increase.
         d) Ammonia is likely a direct neurotoxin, although the mechanisms underlying this toxicity are not fully understood.
      2. Mercaptans, derived from bacterial metabolism of sulfur-containing amino acids such as

methionine, are synergistic with ammonia in causing HE.

3. Short chain fatty acids, derived from enteric bacterial digestion of medium chain triglycerides, carbohydrates, and protein, and from incomplete hepatic metabolism of long chain fatty acids, are also synergistic with ammonia.

4. Imbalances of excitatory and inhibitory neurotransmitters occur.
   a) Gamma-aminobutryic acid (GABA) is the major inhibitory neurotransmitter in the brain, and studies have shown increased GABA concentrations in the brains of encephalopathic animals.
   b) Increased cerebral concentrations of endogenously generated benzodiazepams (inhibitory) have been demonstrated in HE.
   c) Brain concentrations of glutamate, the major excitatory neurotransmitter in the brain, are decreased.
   d) The concentration of aromatic amino acids increases, with a concomitant decrease in branched chain amino acids. This increase is associated with generation of aromatic amines, which may act as false neurotransmitters.

B. Factors that can precipitate HE in a predisposed animal are as follows.
   1. Gastrointestinal protein loading
      a) Excessive dietary intake of protein
      b) Gastrointestinal bleeding
   2. Catabolic conditions with increased protein mobilization from muscle
      a) Infection
      b) Neoplasia
      c) Corticosteroid excess
   3. Increased renal ammonia production in response to metabolic acidosis and hypokalemia
   4. Increased generation of HE toxins in the colon
      a) Constipation
      b) Azotemia
   5. Synergistic neural inhibition by concurrent administration of drugs
      a) Benzodiazepams
      b) Barbiturates
      c) Other anesthetic/sedative agents

Clinical Signs

I. Signs are usually seen in animals <3 years old.
II. The primary clinical signs are referable to neural inhibition in the central nervous system.
   A. Behavioral changes: personality changes, loss of training
   B. Seizures
   C. Depression, stupor, coma
   D. Blindness
III. Other systems may also be involved.
   A. Gastrointestinal signs
      1. Ptyalism (especially in cats)

2. Intermittent anorexia, vomiting, and/or diarrhea
   B. Urinary signs
      1. Polyuria/polydipsia
      2. Stranguria, hematuria: associated with ammonium urate urolithiasis
   C. Other signs
      1. History of intolerance to anesthetic agents
      2. Poor body stature
      3. Fever
      4. Copper-colored irises in cats

Diagnosis

I. Supportive findings are as follows.
   A. Hematology
      1. Mild microcytic, hypochromic anemia, the etiology of which is poorly understood (it does not appear to be associated with iron deficiency)
      2. Poikilocytosis (cats)
   B. Serum biochemistry
      1. Low blood urea nitrogen
      2. Hypoalbuminemia
      3. Hypoglycemia (especially in small-breed dogs)
      4. Hypocholesterolemia
      5. Normal to mildly increased serum alanine aminotransferase (ALT) and alkaline phosphatase (SAP)
   C. Diagnostic imaging
      1. Microhepatica
      2. Renomegaly
      3. Ammonium biurate urolithiasis: not radiodense, but detectable by ultrasonography
   D. Urinalysis
      1. Ammonium biurate crystals
      2. Hematuria, pyuria, bacteriuria
      3. Isosthenuria
   E. Ancillary diagnostic testing
      1. Increased blood ammonia concentrations
      2. Increased postprandial serum bile acids, with or without increased preprandial serum bile acids
      3. Rectal portal scintigraphy
         a) Radioactive ^{99m}technetium pertechnetate placed in the colon is absorbed across the colonic mucosa and enters the portal circulation.
         b) In the presence of a normal portal circulation, gamma camera scintigraphy detects radioactivity in the liver before its appearance in the heart.
         c) If a PSS is present, a greater fraction is seen in the heart initially than in the liver.
         d) It is a sensitive, specific, noninvasive technique to detect PSS and to quantitate the fraction of blood shunting away from the liver (Daniel et al., 1991; Koblik and Hornof, 1995; Forster-van Hijfte et al., 1996)
      4. Typical changes on hepatic biopsy: hepatic

atrophy with attenuation of the portal vasculature, proliferation of portal arterioles, and occasionally the presence of periportal lipogranulomas
II. Definitive diagnosis requires visualization of the shunting vessel.
  A. Ultrasonographic visualization of shunting vessel
    1. Highly operator dependent
    2. Reported sensitivity of 100% and 80% for intra- and extrahepatic shunts, respectively (Holt et al., 1995)
  B. Exploratory laparotomy
    1. Direct visualization of shunting vessel
    2. Angiography of the portal circulation

Differential Diagnosis

I. Hepatic failure
  A. Exposure to hepatotoxic agents
  B. Infectious/inflammatory hepatitis (see later)
  C. Hepatobiliary neoplasia
  D. Hepatic lipidosis (cats; see later)
II. Congenital urea cycle enzyme deficiency (rare)
III. Other hepatic vascular disorders
  A. Microvascular dysplasia
  B. Intrahepatic arteriovenous fistula
IV. Other causes of seizure disorders in young animals (see Chap. 22)

Treatment

I. Acute management is aimed at decreasing the enteric bacterial production of potential toxins and correcting predisposing factors.
  A. Nothing by mouth (NPO)
  B. IV fluid therapy: 0.9% NaCl or 0.45% NaCl with 2.5% dextrose and potassium supplementation, as needed
  C. Cleansing enemas every 4–6 hours as needed, warmed to body temperature
    1. Saline
    2. Betadine: 10 ml/kg of a 1:10 dilution retained for 15 minutes
    3. Lactulose: 10 ml/kg of a 1:3 dilution retained for 15 minutes
  D. Oral antibiotics once the animal is able to swallow
    1. Neomycin 10–20 mg/kg BID-TID
    2. Amoxicillin 10 mg/kg BID
    3. Metronidazole 7.5 mg/kg TID
  E. Infusion of branched chain amino acid solutions: marginally effective and expensive
  F. Benzodiazepam receptor antagonist (flumazenil): experimental, expensive
II. Chronic management consists of either surgical ligation or medical therapy.
  A. Surgical ligation of the shunting vessel (Lawrence et al., 1992; Komtebedde et al., 1995; Smith et al., 1995)
    1. Single extrahepatic shunts are usually easier to ligate than intrahepatic shunts, which can be difficult to localize.

2. The degree of ligation depends on the resultant increase in portal pressure. Portal pressure after ligation should not exceed 16–18 cm H_2O.
3. Multiple shunts do not respond to surgical management, because they are usually associated with portal hypertension.
4. Anesthesia is complicated by abnormal liver function and increased sensitivity to many anesthetic agents. Avoid diazepams, barbiturates, and acepromazine.
  B. Some animals do very well with long-term medical management, although it is difficult to predict which ones.
    1. Lactulose
      a) It is a nonabsorbable disaccharide that passes to the colon, where it is fermented by bacteria to organic acids.
      b) These acids lower colonic pH and promote the conversion of NH_3 to the nonabsorbable ion NH_4^+.
      c) It alters enteric bacterial metabolism to increase their incorporation of ammonia into endogenous proteins, which are subsequently passed in the feces.
      d) It also accelerates intestinal transit time so that the time for production and absorption of toxins is decreased.
      e) Dosage is empirical, starting with 0.25–0.5 ml/kg PO BID-TID. The goal is to produce no more than 2–3 soft stools a day.
    2. Oral antibiotics, as in acute management; synergistic with lactulose
    3. Dietary modifications
      a) The optimum protein requirements for animals with HE is unknown.
        (1) Aggressive protein restriction has been recommended but may lead to a negative nitrogen balance.
        (2) Protein requirements should be individualized for each animal, but in general, one should start with diets containing at least 16% or 30% protein on a dry-matter basis for dogs or cats, respectively.
        (3) If HE is not controlled, medical management can be instituted and, if necessary, additional dietary protein restriction recommended.
        (4) Protein sources with high biologic value are used, such as eggs and dairy products.
        (5) Meat-source proteins are avoided, because they are more likely to precipitate HE.
        (6) Vegetable-source proteins are beneficial, possibly owing to their increased fiber content (see later).
      b) It is imperative that daily caloric needs be met with simple, easily digestible carbo-

hydrate sources such as cooked white rice or pasta.

   c) Dietary fiber promotes fecal nitrogen excretion.

     (1) Colonic fermentation of fiber results in luminal acidification, which decreases ammonia absorption.

     (2) Fiber also increases the incorporation of nitrogen into enteric bacteria.

     (3) Fiber must be used cautiously in animals with poor nutritional status.

   d) There is no need to restrict fats unless steatorrhea develops.

Patient Monitoring

I. Monitoring after surgical ligation
  A. Continue IV fluids.
  B. Watch for signs of portal hypertension within the first 24 hours after surgery.
    1. Hypovolemia
    2. Vomiting, diarrhea
    3. Prolonged recovery from surgery
    4. Requires emergency laparotomy to remove ligature
  C. Monitor blood glucose.
  D. Postoperative seizures may occur up to 3 days after surgery. The etiology is unknown, but they may be more common in older animals (Hardie et al., 1990; Matushek et al., 1990).
II. Monitoring animals on chronic medical therapy
  A. Body weight, serum albumin, and total protein are monitored as indicators of nitrogen balance, initially every month and then every 4–6 months.
  B. Blood ammonia is monitored as an indicator of the efficacy of treatment for HE, initially every month and then every 4–6 months.
  C. Serum bile acids and albumin are monitored as indicators of overall hepatic function, initially every month and then every 4–6 months.
III. Prognosis
  A. Postoperatively, some animals have a normal life expectancy.
    1. If liver function tests normalize (bile acids return to normal), medical management can be withdrawn.
    2. Improvement usually occurs within the first 6 months after surgery.
  B. Despite a successful surgery with complete occlusion of the shunting vessel, some animals may not return to normal hepatic function, and medical management will be necessary for the animal's life.
  C. Some animals develop a progressive hepatopathy.
  D. Some information exists on prognostic indicators of surgical success.
    1. The earlier clinical signs start, the worse the prognosis, possibly related to a greater shunting fraction in younger animals.
    2. Alternatively, dogs >2 years of age at the time of surgery have a poorer prognosis.

    3. Intrahepatic shunts carry a worse prognosis than extrahepatic shunts.
  E. The prognosis varies widely with nonsurgical management of PSS.

Hepatoportal Microvascular Dysplasia

Definition and Cause

I. The presence of multiple microscopic intrahepatic shunts
II. Occurs in the same breeds that have macroscopic shunts
III. Possible inherited disorder in Cairn terriers

Clinical Signs

I. Many dogs are asymptomatic, probably because only a small amount of blood is shunted away from the liver.
II. When signs are present, they are identical to those seen in dogs with macroscopic PSS, with the exception that dogs with microvascular dysplasia usually present at an older age (Phillips et al., 1993; Schermhorn et al., 1996).

Diagnosis

I. Increased serum bile acids
II. No ultrasonographic, surgical, or portographic evidence of a shunt
III. Normal rectal portal scintigraphy
IV. Other causes of hepatic insufficiency ruled out with hepatic biopsy
  A. Portal arteriolar proliferation with dilated portal veins and decreased size of smaller portal vessels
  B. Histopathologic changes identical to those reported for macroscopic shunts

Differential Diagnosis

I. Congenital PSS
II. Congenital urea cycle enzyme deficiency
III. Other causes of seizures

Treatment

I. Medical management is the same as for congenital PSS.
II. Asymptomatic dogs with increased bile acids as their only abnormality do not require treatment.

Urea Cycle Enzyme Defects

Definition and Cause

I. Congenital deficiency in one or more of the activities of the hepatic enzymes involved in the conversion of ammonia to urea in the liver
II. Rare, but reported in the dog

Pathophysiology

I. There are several enzymes involved in the hepatic urea cycle that converts ammonia to urea.
II. Deficiency in arginosuccinate has been reported in two dogs.
III. Hyperammonemia and HE develop.

Clinical Signs

I. HE
II. Intermittent vomiting and diarrhea
III. Poor body stature

Diagnosis

I. Normal serum biochemistry and bile acids in a young dog with increased postprandial ammonia concentrations (fasting blood ammonia may be normal) are suggestive findings.
II. Exclude the presence of a PSS.
III. Definitive diagnosis is based on liver biopsy and determination of hepatic urea cycle enzyme concentrations.

Treatment and Monitoring

I. Institute supportive therapy to prevent signs of HE.
II. No specific therapy is available.
III. Monitor blood ammonia as needed.

Intrahepatic Arteriovenous Fistula

Definition and Cause

I. A precapillary anastomosis between the hepatic artery and portal vein
II. Reported as a congenital malformation in both cats and dogs

Pathophysiology

I. Arterialization of the portal circulation results in chronic portal hypertension.
II. Multiple extrahepatic PSSs develop.
III. Ascites is a common sequela.

Clinical Signs

I. Ascites
II. HE
III. Intermittent anorexia, vomiting, and diarrhea
IV. Abdominal bruit

Diagnosis

I. Supportive findings
   A. Young animal with ascites and HE
   B. Hypoalbuminemia
   C. Large hypoechoic structures within the liver on ultrasonography
II. Definitive diagnosis

A. Visualization of large vessel associated with one or more liver lobes at surgery
B. Abdominal arteriography via femoral vein catheterization

Differential Diagnosis

I. The list of differentials is the same as for PSS.
II. Young animals with PSS usually do not have ascites.
III. Fibrotic hepatopathies in young dogs must also be considered (see later).

Treatment and Monitoring

I. Surgical removal of involved hepatic lobe or ligation of the fistula
II. Medical management of ascites and HE (see earlier)

Other Hepatic Vascular Disorders

See Table 34–1.

INFLAMMATORY DISORDERS

Hepatic Abscessation

Definition

I. Focal infection of the liver may occur with bacteria, fungi, or other agents.
II. Infections may be primary or secondary.

Causes

I. Routes of infection
   A. Hematogenous spread via the portal vein, hepatic artery, or umbilical vein (neonates)
   B. Direct extension from surrounding area, such as might occur with a pancreatic abscess or peritonitis
   C. Ascending from the biliary tree
II. Underlying disease that predisposes to infectious disease (Farrar et al., 1996)
   A. Long-term corticosteroid excess
   B. Diabetes mellitus
   C. Pancreatitis
   D. Neoplasia
   E. Sepsis

Clinical Signs

I. Nonspecific signs most common: anorexia, lethargy, vomiting, diarrhea
II. Fever
III. Abdominal pain
IV. Hepatomegaly
V. Coagulopathy

Diagnosis

I. Supportive clinicopathologic findings
   A. Neutrophilic leukocytosis with a left shift, with or without a monocytosis

Table 34–1. Hepatic Vascular Disease

Hepatic Lesion	Species	Presenting Signs	Accompanying Histologic Lesions	Concurrent Disease or Drug Therapy	Reference
Portal vein thrombosis	Dog	Abdominal effusion Vomiting Anorexia	Intestinal infarcts Pancreatic necrosis Steroid hepatopathy Amyloidosis Neoplasia	Immune-mediated hemolytic anemia Pancreatitis Peritonitis Corticosteroids	van Winkle and Bruce, 1993
Peliosis hepatis	Dog	Variable	Glomerulonephritis Interstitial nephritis Cirrhosis	Heartworm disease Renal failure Diabetes mellitus Corticosteroids	Brown et al., 1994 Ioune et al., 1988
	Cat	Hepatomegaly Hemorrhagic abdominal effusion Anemia Icterus	None	None	
Budd-Chiari syndrome (varying degrees of centrilobular congestion, sinusoidal dilatation, and perivenular fibrosis)	Dog	Abdominal effusion Hepatomegaly Abdominal pain	Cor triatriatum dexter Neoplasia "Kinking" of the caudal vena cava		Crowe et al., 1984 Cornelius and Mahaffey, 1985 Macintire et al., 1995 Otto et al., 1991
	Cat	Abdominal effusion	Congenital stenosis of the caudal vena cava		

B. Increased SAP and ALT

C. Hypoalbuminemia, with or without hypoproteinemia

D. Hyperbilirubinemia

E. Coagulation abnormalities: thrombocytopenia, prolonged prothrombin time and partial thromboplastin time

II. Diagnostic imaging

A. Radiography: hepatomegaly, with or without abdominal effusion, concurrent bronchopneumonia

B. Ultrasonography: hypoechoic, hyperechoic, or heteroechoic mass, with or without abdominal effusion

III. Definitive diagnosis: based on biopsy and culture

A. Most commonly isolated organisms are enteric gram-negatives and anaerobes. Mixed infections are common.

B. Ultrasonography may be used to obtain material from the abscess for culture.

1. Fine-needle aspirate of the abscess is a safe method to obtain material for culture and cytology.

2. Guided biopsies are generally not recommended, because of possible seeding of the abdomen with infection.

C. Look for concurrent sites of infection from which material for culture can be obtained.

Treatment and Monitoring

I. Surgical débridement, resection, and biopsy are indicated, with follow-up antibiotics based on culture and sensitivity.

II. Medical management with the following may be considered.

A. Long-term antibiotic therapy alone (4–6 months)

B. Long-term antibiotic therapy combined with periodic ultrasound-guided percutaneous drainage of the abscess

C. Response to therapy monitored with ultrasonographic evaluation of the abscess

III. Treat any underlying disorders.

Chronic Canine Inflammatory Hepatic Disease (CCIHD)

Definition

I. Previously referred to as chronic active hepatitis

II. A histologic term for a group of chronic progressive hepatic diseases that share several common histologic abnormalities

A. Presence of inflammatory infiltrates dominated by lymphocytes and plasmacytes

B. Bile duct proliferation

C. Areas of nodular hepatic regeneration

D. Fibrosis: initially periportal, but progressing to interconnect portal areas (bridging fibrosis)

E. Varying degree of hepatocellular necrosis/degeneration

F. Progresses histologically to cirrhosis

Causes

I. Idiopathic: most common

II. Infectious

A. Viral: infectious canine hepatitis
B. Bacterial: leptosporosis
C. Canine acidophil hepatitis
III. Hepatotoxins (see later)
IV. Autoimmune
  A. Little direct evidence exists in dogs to support this cause.
  B. Most dogs do not have hypergammaglobulinemia and/or high circulating levels of non–organ-specific autoantibodies such as antinuclear antibodies (Anderson and Sevelius, 1992).
  C. Some evidence exists for the presence of liver-specific antibodies in the serum of dogs with CCIHD (Weiss et al., 1995).
V. Genetic factors: breed-specific hepatopathies reported in Doberman pinschers, cocker spaniels, West Highland white terriers, and Skye terriers

Pathophysiology

I. Most often, the initiating event is not identified, but once injury occurs, pathologic progression to cirrhosis and hepatic failure often results.
II. Several factors are implicated in pathologic progression.
  A. Abnormal immune responses, including loss of normal T suppressor function and development of autoantibodies to previously sequestered hepatic cytosolic and membrane proteins (exposed secondary to hepatocellular necrosis)
  B. Hepatic retention of toxic substances
    1. Hydrophobic bile acids
    2. Leukotrienes
    3. Cholesterol
    4. Copper (see later)
    5. Iron
    6. Endotoxin
  C. Stimulation of hepatic fibrogenesis
    1. The replacement of normal hepatic parenchyma by fibrous tissue destroys normal architectural relationships within the liver and leads to the development of portal hypertension (Leveille and Arias, 1993).
    2. Although many factors are likely involved in stimulating hepatic fibrogenesis, the presence of hepatic inflammation is a major factor.
III. Hepatic inflammation, regeneration, and fibrosis result in the development of portal hypertension and the establishment of multiple extrahepatic PSSs, which in turn promote the development of ascites and HE.

Clinical Signs

I. Clinical signs are generally nonspecific and wax and wane until late in the course of the disease.
  A. Polyuria and polydipsia
  B. Intermittent anorexia, vomiting, and diarrhea
II. Specific signs of liver dysfunction may arise.
  A. Jaundice
  B. HE
  C. Ascites

D. Hemorrhagic tendencies
  1. Melena or hematemesis may occur secondary to gastrointestinal ulceration.
  2. Several abnormalities in coagulation may accompany chronic hepatic disease.
    a) Vitamin K deficiency may develop in chronic cholestatic disorders, owing to intestinal fat malabsorption from lack of bile acids.
    b) Alternatively, with severe hepatic parenchymal disease, there may be abnormal activation of vitamin K or aberrant vitamin K–dependent carboxylation of coagulation factors.
    c) The liver is the site of production of most clotting factors, and with severe hepatic failure, these may become deficient.
    d) Because the liver is important in removing circulating activated clotting factors and fibrin degradation products, a hypercoagulable state may develop, predisposing to disseminated intravascular coagulation.
    e) Both quantitative and qualitative platelet defects may be present.
III. Common factors have been identified in breed-specific hepatopathies.
  A. Doberman pinschers
    1. It is most commonly seen in middle-aged females.
    2. Occasionally, there is excess copper accumulation in periportal hepatocytes, but this is likely an effect of decreased biliary copper excretion from cholestasis rather than a cause of the hepatopathy.
  B. Cocker spaniels
    1. It occurs in all ages but is more common in older dogs.
    2. There is an increased incidence in males.
    3. Dogs often present with ascites and hypoalbuminemia.
  C. Bedlington terriers (see Copper Toxicosis, later)
  D. West Highland white terriers
    1. It is often associated with excessive accumulation of copper in hepatocytes in young dogs.
    2. Copper accumulation may not be progressive and is not always associated with hepatic disease.
  E. Skye terriers
    1. It occurs at all ages, with no predilection.
    2. Increased hepatic copper stores have not been reported in all affected dogs.

Diagnosis

I. Supportive signs
  A. Consistent elevation of serum ALT and SAP
  B. Abnormal liver function tests
    1. Hyperbilirubinemia
    2. Increased serum bile acids
    3. Hypoglycemia
    4. Decreased blood urea nitrogen

5. Hypoalbuminemia
6. Hyperammonemia
7. Low-protein ascitic fluid transudate
C. Hepatomegaly initially, then microhepatica on radiography
II. Definitive diagnosis: hepatic biopsy
   A. Assess coagulation status before obtaining the biopsy, because postbiopsy bleeding is the most common complication.
   B. Techniques include ultrasound-guided laparoscopy and laparotomy.

Treatment

I. There are four goals in the treatment of CCIHD.
II. Eliminate etiologic agents.
   A. Treat with antibiotics for infectious disease.
   B. Discontinue hepatotoxic drugs.
   C. It may not be possible in most cases, because an etiologic factor is usually not identified.
III. Provide an optimum environment for hepatic regeneration.
   A. Dietary management as described for PSS
   B. Adequate rest
IV. Control complications.
   A. Most therapy is directed at controlling complication such as ascites, HE, gastroduodenal ulceration, coagulopathies, and secondary bacterial infections.
   B. Institute therapy for HE (see earlier).
   C. Treat ascites with the following.
      1. Sodium restriction
      2. Diuretics
         a) The goal is slow mobilization of fluid to prevent the development of dehydration, metabolic alkalosis, and/or hypokalemia, all of which can precipitate HE.
         b) It is best to use a combination of spironolactone (1–2 mg/kg PO BID) and furosemide (0.25–0.5 mg/kg PO BID-TID).
      3. Abdominal paracentesis seldom necessary unless dyspnea, abdominal pain, or compromised renal function is present
   D. Prevent gastrointestinal ulceration.
      1. H$_2$ receptor antagonists
         a) Give famotidine 0.5–1 mg/kg PO SID or SQ BID.
         b) Avoid cimetidine, because it can suppress hepatic CP450 enzyme activity.
      2. Cytoprotective agents: sucralfate
   E. Treat any secondary bacterial infections.
      1. Animals with chronic hepatic disease are predisposed to develop bacterial infections.
      2. Secondary infection is suspected when the following are found.
         a) Fever
         b) Neutrophilic leukocytosis with a left shift on complete blood count
         c) Extensive neutrophilic infiltrates on hepatic biopsy
      3. Treatment is based on culture and sensitivity of hepatic tissue, bile, or blood.

a) Usually gram-negatives or anaerobes of gastrointestinal origin are isolated.
b) Avoid the use of antibiotics metabolized or excreted by the liver (chloramphenicol or erythromycin) or those associated with hepatotoxic reactions in the dog (trimethoprim-sulfa).
V. Control factors involved in disease progression. (There is no proven therapy to slow the progression of CCIHD, but several drugs have been used because of their success in treating people with chronic hepatopathies.)
   A. Corticosteroids
      1. Consider corticosteroids if the following criteria are met.
         a) Serum hypergammaglobulinemia
         b) Positive autoantibody titers
         c) Evidence of extrahepatic autoimmune disease
         d) Hepatic biopsy with significant plasma cell infiltrates
         e) Elimination of an infectious etiology
      2. Carefully weigh potential side effects against benefits.
         a) May potentiate ascites (owing to sodium retention) or HE (from enhanced tissue catabolism)
         b) May increase the possibility of gastrointestinal ulceration and secondary infections
         c) May promote the development of steroid hepatopathy
      3. Prednisone 1 mg/kg PO BID is tapered to alternate-day therapy with 0.25–0.5 mg/kg PO when remission is obtained.
      4. Monitoring is complicated by corticosteroid induction of serum ALT and SAP.
      5. If intolerance to corticosteroids develops, replace with azathioprine 1 mg/kg PO SID tapered to QOD.
   B. Ursodeoxycholate
      1. Ursodeoxycholate is a relatively hydrophilic bile acid that, when administered orally, replaces the more hydrophobic hepatotoxic bile acids and potentially protects hepatocytes from the adverse effects of the latter.
      2. It is also a choleretic and has immune modulatory actions.
      3. Limited information is available in the veterinary literature on its efficacy in CCIHD (Anwer and Meyer, 1995).
      4. The dose extrapolated from human medicine is 10–15 mg/kg PO SID. It is rarely associated with vomiting.
   C. Colchicine
      1. Dose is 0.03 mg/kg PO SID.
      2. Side effects include hemorrhagic diarrhea.
      3. Some limited reports exist of success in dogs.
      4. It is used primarily in noninflammatory fibrotic hepatopathies.
   D. Zinc supplementation

1. The zinc status of dogs with chronic hepatic disease is unknown.
2. Zinc inhibits collagen production, limits the intestinal absorption of copper, and functions as an antioxidant. Zinc deficiency may also interfere with the urea cycle in the liver and potentiate HE.
3. Dose is 50–200 mg elemental zinc PO SID given as zinc acetate.
4. Side effects include hemolytic anemia, iron deficiency, and vomiting.
5. Serum zinc levels are monitored and maintained at 200–400 μg/dl.

Patient Monitoring

I. Evaluate serum ALT, SAP, bilirubin, and albumin concentrations every month for the first 6 months and then every 4–6 months.
II. Evaluate serum bile acids every 6 months.
III. In ascitic animals, monitor body weight and abdominal girth and, if on diuretics, monitor serum acid–base status and potassium levels.
IV. In animals with HE, monitor mental status and blood ammonia.
V. The best way to assess response to therapy is with repeated hepatic biopsy.
   A. Look for inflammatory infiltrates to become attenuated and confined to the portal triads.
   B. Do not expect much to change in <6 months.

Canine Granulomatous Hepatitis

Definition

Granulomatous hepatitis is recognized histologically by the presence of histiocytic inflammation (macrophages) often in association with concurrent lymphoplasmacytic or neutrophilic infiltrates.

Causes and Pathophysiology

I. Often associated with a systemic disease
   A. The underlying disease leads to T-lymphocyte sensitization and subsequent granuloma formation.
   B. The sensitizing agent may be an infectious agent, drug, immune complex, or neoplastic cell (Chapman et al., 1993).
II. Infectious causes
   A. Bacteria: *Actinomyces, Nocardia, Mycobacterium* spp.
   B. Fungal: histoplasmosis, aspergillosis, paecilomycosis, sporotrichosis, cryptococcosis
   C. Parasitic: dirofilariasis, visceral larva migrans, capillariasis, hepatozoonosis
   D. Protozoal: prototheocosis, toxoplasmosis
III. Noninfectious causes
   A. Autoimmune disorders: systemic lupus erythematosus
   B. Neoplasia: malignant histiocytosis
   C. Inflammatory disorders: inflammatory bowel disease, lymphangiectasia
   D. Drugs
IV. Idiopathic disease

Clinical Signs

I. Lethargy, anorexia, weight loss
II. Episodic or persistent fever
III. Hepatomegaly
IV. Signs of underlying systemic disorder

Diagnosis

I. Hepatic biopsy
   A. Special stains for mycotic and microbial agents are performed.
   B. Aerobic and anaerobic cultures of hepatic tissue are indicated.
II. Serologic testing for fungal pathogens, dirofilariasis, and, if indicated, antinuclear antibody titers.

Treatment and Monitoring

I. Primary therapy is for the underlying etiology.
II. Manage the complications of decreased hepatic function as outlined earlier.
III. Prognosis depends on the etiology.

Feline Cholangitis-Cholangiohepatitis Syndrome

Definition

I. Cholangitis pertains to inflammation in the biliary tree, whereas cholangiohepatitis refers to inflammation that extends into the hepatic parenchyma.
II. This syndrome describes a complex of related inflammatory hepatobiliary diseases in the cat.
III. It is characterized histologically according to the predominant inflammatory cellular infiltrate (Day, 1995).
   A. Suppurative (neutrophilic)
   B. Nonsuppurative
      1. Lymphocytic, plasmacytic
      2. Lymphocytic
   C. Biliary cirrhosis with fibrosis of the extra- and intrahepatic biliary system

Causes and Pathophysiology

I. Suppurative cholangitis
   A. Ascending infection from the intestine: rare unless predisposing cause of biliary stasis such as cholelithiasis, biliary fluke infestation, or pancreatitis exists
   B. Blood-borne infections: secondary to bacterial septicemia or infection with hepatotrophic agents such as toxoplasmosis or feline infectious peritonitis (FIP)
II. Nonsuppurative cholangitis/cholangiohepatitis
   A. The intense lymphoplasmacytic infiltrate suggests a role for immune dysregulation, but there is little evidence to document this.

B. Some evidence supports the idea that it represents the end result of repeated bouts of suppurative inflammation secondary to chronic pancreatitis or inflammatory bowel disease (Weiss et al., 1996).

C. A pre-neoplastic state is possible in cases with intense lymphocytic infiltrates.

D. The vast majority of cases are idiopathic.

Clinical Signs

I. Occurs in cats of all breeds, usually middle-aged to older.

II. Initial clinical signs are nonspecific; therefore, cats often present with late-stage disease.
  A. Intermittent vomiting and/or diarrhea
  B. Intermittent anorexia or occasionally polyphagia
  C. Weight loss
  D. Fever, especially with the suppurative form

III. Specific signs of hepatic disease may be seen.
  A. Icterus is present in many cats.
  B. Signs of HE may be present.
  C. Ascites is rare, even with end-stage disease.

Diagnosis

I. Supportive findings
  A. Neutrophilic leukocytosis, especially in the suppurative form
  B. Serum hyperbilirubinemia and bilirubinuria
  C. Increased serum ALT and SAP
  D. Increased pre- and postprandial bile acids
  E. Hypergammaglobulinemia
  F. Hyperammonemia
  G. Coagulation abnormalities

II. Ultrasonography: hepatomegaly, even with end-stage disease

III. Definitive diagnosis: hepatic biopsy

Differential Diagnosis

I. Feline idiopathic hepatic lipidosis

II. Hepatobiliary neoplasia, particularly feline lymphoma

III. FIP

IV. Feline leukemia virus (FeLV)–associated disease

V. Toxoplasmosis

VI. Biliary fluke infestation

VII. Acute pancreatitis with secondary bile duct obstruction/infection

VIII. Exposure to hepatotoxins

Treatment

I. Suppurative disease
  A. Antibiotic therapy for 8 weeks, based on culture and sensitivity of hepatic biopsy or bile
    1. Amoxicillin/clavulanic acid
    2. Cephalosporins
    3. Metronidazole (anaerobes only; undergoes hepatic metabolism)
    4. Fluoroquinolones
    5. Aminoglycosides
  B. Supportive care
    1. Correct abnormalities in hydration, electrolytes, and acid–base status.
    2. Treat HE.
    3. Provide nutritional support.
      a) The use of benzodiazepam appetite stimulants is *not* recommended, because of their ability to precipitate or aggravate HE.
      b) If concurrent pancreatitis exists, partial or total parenteral nutrition is considered.
      c) Enteral nutrition is not usually needed.
      d) Long-term nutritional requirements of cats with chronic hepatic disease are unknown. Follow the recommendations for HE, earlier, paying particular attention to the cat's high-protein and B vitamin requirements and its need for the essential amino acids taurine and arginine.
    4. Choleretics may be initiated in the absence of signs of extrahepatic biliary obstruction.
      a) There are limited reports of therapeutic efficacy in the cat, but they appear safe in normal cats (Nicholson et al., 1993; Day et al., 1994).
      b) The dose is 10–15 mg/kg PO SID.

II. Nonsuppurative disease
  A. Aggressively rule out the possibility of secondary infection.
  B. Although there is no proven efficacy, immunosuppressive therapy is recommended.
    1. Prednisone 2 mg/kg PO SID tapered to alternate-day therapy
    2. Azathioprine not recommended in the cat
  C. Ursodeoxycholate is used for its choleretic, immune-modulating, and hepatoprotective properties, although its efficacy in this syndrome is unproved.

Patient Monitoring

I. Monitor serum ALT, SAP, albumin, and total protein every 4 weeks for the first 6 months and then every 4–6 months.

II. Monitor body weight and appetite.

III. Repeated hepatic biopsy is the best way to assess response to therapy.

INFILTRATIVE DISEASES

Feline Idiopathic Hepatic Lipidosis

Definition

I. Hepatic lipidosis is the accumulation of fat, usually in the form of triglycerides, within the cytoplasm of the hepatocyte.

II. Primary (idiopathic) hepatic lipidosis (IHL) is seen in cats and is associated with hepatic failure.

III. Secondary hepatic lipidosis occurs with a number

of disease states and is usually not associated with liver disease.

Causes and Pathophysiology

I. Secondary hepatic lipidosis occurs in both dogs and cats when an abnormality in hepatic lipid metabolism is present.
   A. Increased mobilization of fatty acids to the liver
      1. Diabetes mellitus
      2. Starvation or conditions associated with malnutrition, such as chronic pancreatitis or inflammatory bowel disease
      3. Obesity
   B. Decreased mitochondrial oxidation of fatty acids
      1. Mitochondrial damage
      2. Carnitine deficiency
      3. Primary hepatobiliary disease
   C. Abnormality in the packaging and/or secretion of lipoproteins
      1. Interference with hepatic protein synthesis
      2. Disruption of the hepatic urea cycle, leading to buildup of metabolic intermediates that interfere with lipoprotein production
      3. Malnutrition
II. The nature of the defect in hepatic lipid metabolism in cats with IHL is unknown. This disease is associated with acute hepatic failure (Center et al., 1993; Dimski and Taboada, 1995).
   A. Ultrastructural analysis of hepatocytes from affected cats shows some evidence of damage to mitochondria and peroxisomes (an additional site of fatty acid oxidation).
   B. The hepatic lesion, but not the syndrome of liver failure, can be reproduced by prolonged caloric restriction in overweight cats.

Clinical Signs

I. Complete or partial anorexia, particularly in obese cats that have recently undergone a stressful event
II. Icterus
III. Signs of HE
IV. Vomiting and ptyalism
V. ±Concurrent pancreatitis (Akol et al., 1993)

Diagnosis

I. History is often suggestive.
II. Supportive findings include the following.
   A. Hyperbilirubinemia and bilirubinuria
   B. Marked increase in SAP, with smaller elevations in ALT
   C. Hyperammonemia
   D. Increased pre- and postprandial bile acids
   E. Ultrasonography
      1. Hepatomegaly with a diffusely hyperechoic liver
      2. Evidence of pancreatic inflammation
III. Definitive diagnosis requires hepatic biopsy.
   A. Hepatocellular vacuolation, with evidence of

cholestasis, and minimal, if any, inflammation or necrosis are present.
   B. Cytologic evaluation of a fine-needle aspirate may be useful in establishing a diagnosis, but occasionally hepatic lipidosis develops secondary to inflammatory hepatic disease, which may not be readily apparent on cytology.
   C. Anticipate complications of the biopsy procedure.
      1. Assess coagulation before the biopsy.
         a) Give parenteral vitamin K.
         b) If coagulation abnormalities exist, consider a whole blood transfusion or fresh frozen plasma before the biopsy.
         c) Monitor packed cell volume after the biopsy.
      2. Use sedation cautiously, as these cats may be encephalopathic and thus extremely sensitive to sedatives and anesthetics.

Differential Diagnosis

I. Feline cholangitis-cholangiohepatitis syndrome
   A. Cats with this syndrome usually have a more chronic, insidious course than those with IHL and often present in a poor nutritional state, as opposed to cats with IHL, which usually have a recent history of obesity.
   B. The ALT is usually more elevated in cats with this syndrome, reflecting the greater hepatocellular necrosis and degeneration seen on hepatic biopsy.
II. Other differentials are the same as for feline cholangitis-cholangiohepatitis syndrome (see earlier).

Treatment

I. Feline IHL is reversible.
II. Begin with correction of fluid, electrolyte, and acid–base disturbances.
   A. Supplement fluid therapy with B vitamins and glucose.
   B. Provide potassium as needed.
III. Institute therapy for HE (see earlier).
IV. Provide aggressive nutritional support.
   A. Institute total or partial parenteral nutrition, especially if concurrent pancreatitis exists.
   B. Nasogastric tubes may be placed for short-term administration of liquid diets.
   C. Percutaneous endoscopic gastrostomy or surgical gastrostomy tubes are placed for long-term management. Feed gruels of cat food to meet nutritional needs.
   D. A recent study showed that a high-protein, calorie-dense diet was best at mobilizing lipids from the liver (Biourge et al., 1993). This potential beneficial action should be weighed against the risk of precipitating HE.
   E. Monitor for the development of hypophosphatemia and hemolytic anemia, which may occur in the immediate (12 to 72 hours) refeeding period (Justin and Hohenhaus, 1995).

F. Vomiting is best controlled with metoclopramide (0.2–0.4 mg/kg PO, SQ TID) and/or famotidine (0.5–1 mg/kg PO SID) if evidence of gastrointestinal ulceration (melena, hematemesis) is present.

G. Supplementation with taurine (500 mg/day), carnitine (150–500 mg/day), zinc (7–8 mg/day), thiamine (100–200 mg/day), and fish oils has been advocated, although there is little experimental evidence to suggest beneficial effects.

V. Consider appetite stimulants.

A. Do *not* use benzodiazepams, as they may potentiate HE.

B. Cyproheptadine is a serotonin antagonist that has been advocated as an appetite stimulant.
1. Dose is 2 mg/kg/day.
2. Side effects include excitability and aggression.
3. It is metabolized in the liver and excreted in urine.

VI. Do *not* use corticosteroids, because they promote peripheral lipolysis with increased delivery of fats to the liver, and their catabolic actions may potentiate HE.

Patient Monitoring

I. Send cats home as soon as they are stable to avoid the stress of hospitalization.

II. Continue to have the owners offer food daily.

A. Once the cat's appetite returns, tube feedings can be slowly weaned.

B. Once the cat is consuming all of it nutritional requirements by mouth, which may take several weeks, the gastrostomy tube can be removed.

III. Monitor serum liver enzymes and bilirubin weekly until the cat begins to eat normally.

IV. With aggressive nutritional support, approximately 50–60% of cats diagnosed with IHL survive (Jacobs et al., 1989; Center et al., 1993).

V. Once the cat is cured, there is no tendency for the disease to recur.

FIBROTIC HEPATOPATHIES

Definition

Hepatic fibrosis in the absence of significant inflammation has been recognized in young to middle-aged dogs (Rutgers et al., 1993).

Causes and Pathophysiology

I. Three histologic lesions have been reported.
A. Periportal fibrosis
B. Perisinusoidal fibrosis (reticulofibrosis)
C. Central perivenular fibrosis (idiopathic veno-occlusive disease)

II. The etiology of these diseases is unknown.

Clinical Signs

I. Primarily young dogs: mean age, 24 months; range, 4 months to 7 years

II. Increased incidence in German shepherd dogs

III. Ascites, weight loss, anorexia, signs of HE

Diagnosis

I. Supportive signs
A. Erythrocyte microcytosis
B. Mild to moderate increases in SAP and ALT
C. Hypoproteinemia
D. Increased blood ammonia and serum bile acids
E. Microhepatica

II. Definitive diagnosis: hepatic biopsy

Treatment

I. Manage the complications of hepatic failure as described for CCIHD, earlier.

II. Try colchicine 0.03 mg/kg PO SID.

TOXIC HEPATOPATHIES

Copper Toxicosis

Definition

I. Copper balance in the body is maintained by biliary excretion.

II. The accumulation of copper within hepatocytes results in the development of a chronic inflammatory hepatopathy that ultimately progresses to cirrhosis and hepatic failure (Rolfe and Twedt, 1995).

Causes

I. Bedlington terriers have an autosomal recessive defect in hepatic copper metabolism.
A. Expression of an abnormal hepatic copper-binding protein leads to copper sequestration.
B. Copper accumulation is progressive and precedes the development of hepatic injury.
C. Without treatment, hepatic copper levels can approach 30 times normal.

II. Increased hepatic copper accumulation has been reported in canine breed-specific hepatopathies.

III. It is not known if the increased concentrations are the cause or the result of hepatic disease, because cholestasis by itself limits biliary excretion of copper and can result in increased hepatic copper concentrations.
A. In West Highland white terriers, a familial trait leads to excess hepatic copper accumulation (up to 5 times normal). Copper accumulation is not progressive, however, and is not always associated with the development of hepatic pathology (Thornberg and Crawford, 1986).
B. Increased hepatic copper concentrations have been reported in some, but not all, Skye terriers and Doberman pinschers with chronic liver disease.

Pathophysiology

I. Copper is a direct hepatotoxin.

II. Increased cytoplasmic copper concentrations are toxic to hepatic mitochondria and peroxisomes, which leads to the increased generation and release of cytotoxic free radicals. Lysosomal membrane damage results in the release of proteolytic enzymes.

III. Early hepatocyte lesions consist of scattered areas of focal necrosis and inflammation. Progressive injury leads to a histologic picture similar to that described earlier for CCIHD.

IV. Acute copper release from the liver can lead to an acute hemolytic crisis owing to red blood cell oxidant damage.

Clinical Signs

I. In the early stages of copper accumulation in Bedlington terriers, the dogs are asymptomatic.

II. Acute hepatic failure, occasionally accompanied by acute hemolytic anemia, may develop.
  A. Depression, lethargy, anorexia
  B. Jaundice, signs of HE
  C. Pale mucous membrane, weakness

III. Signs of chronic hepatic insufficiency as described earlier for CCIHD may be noted.

Diagnosis

I. Supportive findings are as follows.
  A. Evidence of liver disease in a predisposed breed
  B. Increased ALT, SAP, bile acids, or blood ammonia; hypoalbuminemia; microhepatica

II. Definitive diagnosis depends on determination of hepatic copper concentrations.
  A. Copper concentrations can be estimated with special copper stains with rubeanic acid or rhodamine. These methods correlate well with quantitative determination when the values are >1000 ppm (ppm = μg/g dry liver weight).
  B. Quantitative determination by atomic absorption analysis requires at least 1 g of tissue and can usually be performed on needle biopsy samples.
  C. Normal canine values are <400 ppm.
  D. In Bedlington terriers, values >2000 ppm are consistently associated with hepatocellular damage.

Treatment

I. Treatment is aimed at enhancing copper excretion by the use of copper chelating agents and limiting further copper absorption from the gastrointestinal tract.
  A. Use of copper chelators is the treatment of choice.
    1. Penicillamine 10–15 mg/day PO
    2. 2,3,2 Trientine 10–15 mg/kg/day PO
  B. Decrease intestinal absorption with elemental zinc 50–200 mg/day PO.

II. Supportive management for hepatic insufficiency is indicated in symptomatic animals (see earlier).

Patient Monitoring

I. All Bedlington terriers are screened at 1 year of age with quantitative determination of hepatic copper levels. If the disease in this breed is detected early and treated appropriately, the dogs have a normal life expectancy.

II. Repeated hepatic biopsy for monitoring of hepatic copper levels may be warranted.

III. Monitor biochemical indicators of hepatocellular damage every 4–6 months.

Glucocorticoid-Induced Hepatopathy

Definition

I. Glucocorticoid-induced hepatopathy is a condition in dogs that is characterized by glycogen deposition in hepatocytes and resultant hepatomegaly.

II. It is a rare disease in the cat.

Causes

I. Pharmacologic administration of glucocorticoids

II. Hyperadrenocorticism as a result of a functional pituitary or adrenal tumor

III. Chronically ill or stressed animals

Pathophysiology

I. The exact mechanism whereby glucocorticoids cause the accumulation of glycogen in canine hepatocytes is unknown, but it may involve a glucocorticoid-induced alteration in the balance between glycogen production and breakdown.

II. Moderate to marked increases in SAP and mild increases in ALT may be seen in dogs with glucocorticoid-induced hepatopathy. These elevations are most often associated with induction, although they may occur secondary to hepatocellular damage (Dillon et al., 1980).

Clinical Signs

I. Most dogs have no signs of hepatic dysfunction except for hepatomegaly.

II. Concurrent signs of glucocorticoid excess may be present.
  A. Polyuria, polydipsia
  B. Obesity, distended abdomen, weakness
  C. Bilateral symmetrical alopecia

III. Rarely, dogs have signs of hepatic failure, such as ascites, HE, hypoalbuminemia, hyperbilirubinemia, or increased pre- and postprandial bile acids.

Diagnosis

I. Supportive findings include the following.
  A. History of glucocorticoid therapy
  B. Clinical signs of hyperadrenocorticism
  C. Hepatomegaly with a diffusely hyperechoic texture on ultrasonography
  D. Marked increases in SAP, with lesser degrees of elevation in ALT

E. Positive diagnostic testing for hyperadrenocorticism
F. Increases in serum bile acids
G. Determination of the glucocorticoid isoenzyme of SAP seldom helpful
II. Definitive diagnosis requires hepatic biopsy.

Differential Diagnosis

I. Inflammatory hepatic disease
II. Infectious hepatic disease
III. Hepatotoxicity
IV. Hepatobiliary neoplasia
V. Drug-induced elevations in hepatic enzymes

Treatment

I. Discontinue glucocorticoid therapy and/or treat for hyperadrenocorticism.
II. Institute supportive care if signs of hepatic failure are present.

Patient Monitoring

I. Check hepatic enzyme levels every 1–3 months. They should return to normal within 6 months.
II. If enzyme values do not normalize, look for concurrent cause of hepatic pathology.
III. Glucocorticoid-induced hepatopathy is usually a reversible lesion.

Anticonvulsant-Induced Hepatotoxicity

Definition and Causes

I. Therapy with several anticonvulsant medications has been associated with hepatic disease in both dogs and cats.
II. In dogs, long-term administration of primidone, phenytoin, and phenobarbital, especially in combination, can result in chronic progressive inflammatory hepatic disease (Bunch et al., 1985; Dayrell-Hart et al., 1991).
III. Short-term administration of diazepam in cats has been associated with fulminant hepatic failure (Center et al., 1996).

Pathophysiology

I. The exact mechanisms whereby anticonvulsants cause hepatic disease in dogs and cats are unknown.
  A. The findings that the hepatic lesions associated with chronic primidone and phenytoin administration can be reproduced in laboratory beagles and that phenobarbital hepatotoxicity appears to be dose related suggest that these drugs are direct hepatotoxins.
  B. The relatively low incidence of disease in dogs on long-term anticonvulsant therapy, however, is more consistent with an idiosyncratic reaction.

II. Two syndromes have been associated with anticonvulsant administration in dogs.
  A. Chronic inflammatory hepatic disease
  B. Cholestatic disease
III. Diazepam reactions in the cat appear to be idiosyncratic.

Clinical Signs

I. Clinical signs in dogs on phenobarbital, primidone, and phenytoin are the same as those of chronic hepatic insufficiency (see earlier).
II. Clinical signs in cats on diazepam are those of acute hepatic insufficiency (see Feline Idiopathic Hepatic Lipidosis, earlier) and appear 3–9 days after starting therapy.

Diagnosis

I. Phenobarbital, primidone, and phenytoin in dogs
  A. History of chronic use of anticonvulsants is suggestive.
  B. Elevations of serum ALT and SAP are common.
    1. All the anticonvulsants can induce hepatic enzyme activity in the absence of morphologic lesions.
    2. Evaluate liver function tests such as bile acids, bilirubin, blood ammonia, or serum albumin to discriminate induction from injury.
  C. Evidence of chronic inflammatory hepatic disease or cirrhosis is found on liver biopsy.
  D. Definitive diagnosis is not possible, but signs of hepatic failure combined with improvement after discontinuation of the drug are highly suggestive.
II. Diazepam toxicosis in cats
  A. Marked increases in ALT, with moderate elevations in SAP
  B. Hyperbilirubinemia, bilirubinuria
  C. Hepatic encephalopathy
  D. Coagulopathy
  E. Acute hepatic necrosis on biopsy

Differential Diagnosis

I. Anticonvulsant hepatotoxicity in dogs
  A. Concurrent exposure to other hepatotoxic drugs
  B. Idiopathic chronic inflammatory hepatic disease
  C. Infectious hepatopathies
  D. Hepatobiliary neoplasia
II. Diazepam hepatotoxicity in cats
  A. IHL
  B. Cholangiohepatitis syndrome
  C. Other drug toxicity
  D. Infectious disease
    1. FeLV
    2. FIP
    3. Toxoplasmosis
    4. Biliary flukes
  E. Acute pancreatitis
  F. Hepatobiliary neoplasia

Treatment

I. Canine anticonvulsant hepatotoxicity
   A. Gradually reduce the dose of phenytoin, primidone, and phenobarbital and begin potassium bromide for seizure control (see Chap. 22)
   B. Hepatic disease may be progressive, even if anticonvulsant therapy is eliminated.
   C. Provide supportive care for chronic hepatic insufficiency (see earlier).
II. Feline diazepam hepatotoxicity
   A. Stop diazepam therapy.
   B. Provide supportive care for acute hepatic failure (see Feline Idiopathic Hepatic Lipidosis, earlier).
   C. Prognosis is guarded.
   D. In cats on diazepam therapy, monitor serum ALT every 2–3 days and stop therapy immediately if any increase occurs.

Patient Monitoring

I. Phenytoin is not used as an anticonvulsant in dogs because of its unfavorable pharmacokinetics.
II. Primidone is used with caution, because hepatotoxicity has been reproduced experimentally.
III. Avoid combinations of phenobarbital, primidone, and/or phenytoin.
IV. Perform yearly monitoring of hepatic function.
V. Monitor serum phenobarbital levels periodically, and institute alternative anticonvulsant therapy if adequate seizure control requires concentrations above the therapeutic range, i.e., >45 μg/dl (see Chap. 22).

Miscellaneous Hepatotoxic Drugs

See Table 34–2.

HEPATOBILIARY NEOPLASIA

Definition

I. Primary hepatobiliary neoplasms (Hammer and Sikkema, 1995)
   A. Hepatocellular adenoma and carcinoma
   B. Bile duct adenoma and carcinoma: may be intrahepatic (more common in dogs) or extrahepatic (more common in cats)
   C. Hemangiosarcoma: may also be metastatic
   D. Lymphoma: usually part of multicentric disease
   E. Miscellaneous (rare): hepatic carcinoids, fibrosarcoma, leiomyosarcoma, osteosarcoma
II. Metastatic spread of cancer
   A. Splenic hemangiosarcoma
   B. Mammary gland adenocarcinoma
   C. Pancreatic carcinoma
   D. Intestinal adenocarcinoma

Causes

I. Except for hepatic lymphoma associated with FeLV and feline immunodeficiency virus (FIV), the etiology of primary hepatobiliary neoplasm in cats and dogs is unknown.
II. The liver is a frequent site of metastasis of intraabdominal neoplasia.

*Table 34–2. **Pharmacologic Agents Associated with Hepatotoxicity***

Agent	Species	Type of Toxicity[a]	Histologic Lesion	Reference
Thiacetarsamide	Canine	Intrinsic	Acute necrosis	Carlisle et al., 1974
Metofane	Canine	Idiosyncratic	Acute necrosis	Nidiritu and Weigel, 1977
Halothane	Canine	Idiosyncratic	Acute necrosis	Meuten and Pecquet-Goad, 1984
Mebendazole	Canine	Idiosyncratic	Acute necrosis	Polzin et al., 1981
Oxibendazole	Canine	Idiosyncratic	Subacute to chronic inflammatory	Hardy et al., 1989
Primidone	Canine	? Idiosyncratic	Chronic inflammatory	Bunch et al., 1985
Phenytoin	Canine	? Idiosyncratic	Chronic cholestatic	Bunch et al., 1985
Phenobarbital	Canine	? Intrinsic	Chronic inflammatory	Dayrell-Hart et al., 1991
Diazepam	Feline	Idiosyncratic	Acute fulminant necrosis	Center et al., 1996
Trimethoprim/sulfa	Canine	Idiosyncratic	Acute necrosis Subacute inflammatory	Toth and Derwelis, 1980; Cribb, 1989; Rowland et al., 1992
Glucocorticoids	Canine	Intrinsic	Vacuolar	Rogers and Ruebner, 1977
Ketoconazole	Canine, feline	Idiosyncratic	Reversible increases in liver enzymes	Legendre, 1995
Griseofulvin	Feline	Idiosyncratic	Not reported	Helton et al., 1986
Methotrexate	Canine	Idiosyncratic	Subacute necrosis and fibrosis	Pond and Morrow, 1982

[a]Intrinsic toxins cause predictable dose-dependent hepatic damage. Idiosyncratic hepatotoxins are associated with an individual's unique susceptibility and are independent of dose or duration of therapy.

Clinical Signs

I. May be unrelated to hepatic function and associated more with a mass effect
   A. Cranial abdominal organomegaly
   B. Acute collapse associated with rupture of mass
   C. Sepsis associated with abscessed mass
II. Nonspecific signs of weight loss, polyuria/polydipsia, vomiting, diarrhea
III. Signs of hepatic failure such as icterus, HE, or ascites (especially with invasive bile duct carcinomas)
IV. Signs of hypoglycemic paraneoplastic syndrome (see Chap. 71)

Diagnosis

I. Elevations in liver enzymes or hyperbilirubinemia may be present.
II. Diagnostic imaging (radiography and ultrasonography) is used to confirm and characterize the mass (Whitely et al., 1989).
   A. Hepatocellular carcinoma and hemangiosarcoma typically present as a large solitary mass.
      1. The former has a predilection for the left lateral lobe.
      2. The masses may be cavitary, owing to the presence of necrotic cores or vascular channels, and therefore may be difficult to differentiate from a hepatic abscess.
   B. Bile duct adenomas or carcinomas may present as a solitary mass in the biliary tract, often leading to bile duct obstruction.
   C. In older cats, benign biliary cystadenomas appear as solitary (occasionally multiple) fluid-filled cysts within the hepatic parenchyma.
   D. Hepatic lymphosarcoma usually presents as a diffusely hyperechoic liver.
   E. Metastatic disease often appears as hyper- or hypoechoic nodules.
III. Perform thoracic radiography to look for metastatic disease.
IV. Elevated serum levels of alpha-fetoprotein, an embryonic protein whose expression re-emerges with malignant transformation, have been reported with hepatocellular carcinoma in dogs.
V. Definitive diagnosis is established by biopsy of the mass.

Differential Diagnosis

I. Nodular hepatic hyperplasia (Stowater et al., 1990)
   A. This is not a neoplastic lesion but is often difficult to distinguish from one.
   B. It usually appears as multiple nodules in the hepatic parenchyma and is a common asymptomatic postmortem lesion in older dogs.
   C. Histologically, it is composed of well-organized cords of hepatocytes and may be accompanied by mild hepatocellular necrosis, which might be reflected as a mild increase in liver enzymes on a biochemical profile.
II. Hepatic cirrhosis with regenerative nodules

Treatment and Monitoring

I. Treatment depends on the type of neoplasia present and the location and extent of disease.
II. Hepatic lymphosarcoma is treated with chemotherapy.
III. Hepatocellular adenoma or carcinoma is usually amenable to surgical removal via hepatic lobectomy.
   A. Surgery is curative for adenoma.
   B. Most carcinomas have metastasized by the time they are diagnosed, but because the tumors are slow-growing, surgical resection may minimize adverse effects associated with necrotic cores and functional impairment of other abdominal viscera.
IV. Hepatic hemangiosarcoma usually has metastasized at the time of diagnosis; surgical removal in combination with ancillary chemotherapy to prevent emergence of metastatic disease is recommended.
V. Surgical resection of intrahepatic bile duct adenoma (via hepatic lobectomy) or solitary extrahepatic masses (with concurrent cholecystoduodenostomy, if necessary) may be curative.
VI. Bile duct carcinomas (extrahepatic or intrahepatic) are typically not surgically resectable and are highly aggressive, with over 90% showing evidence of metastasis at the time of diagnosis.

EXTRAHEPATIC BILIARY DISORDERS

Extrahepatic Bile Duct Obstruction

Definition

The presence of an intraluminal lesion or extraluminal compression that interferes with the emptying of bile into the intestinal lumen (Neer, 1992)

Causes

I. Intraluminal lesions
   A. Cholelithiasis (Kirpenstein et al., 1993)
      1. Rare in cats and dogs
      2. Usually a mixture of cholesterol, bilirubin, calcium, magnesium, and oxalates
      3. Usually an incidental lesion, but may become symptomatic when associated with concurrent biliary infection or obstruction
   B. Biliary neoplasia: most common cause in the cat
   C. Cholangitis or cholecystitis: infection of the gallbladder
      1. Ascending infection from the biliary tree or blood borne
      2. Usually gram-negative enteric bacteria or anaerobes
      3. Emphysematous cholecystitis associated with gas formation within the wall or lumen of the gallbladder; reported in diabetic and nondiabetic dogs

D. Parasitic disease: biliary flukes

II. Extraluminal lesions: pancreatitis (most common cause in the dog) (Fahie and Martin, 1995)

Pathophysiology

I. Obstruction results in increased intraluminal pressure that secondarily damages biliary epithelial cells, leading to the regurgitation of luminal contents into the circulation.

II. Chronic inflammation or infection in the biliary tree typically ascends into progressively smaller ducts and ultimately results in extension of inflammation in the portal triads. Long-standing biliary obstruction eventually leads to biliary cirrhosis.

III. Bile duct obstruction for longer than 7–10 days can result in fat malabsorption, steatorrhea, and fat-soluble vitamin deficiencies. The latter is most often clinically manifested as a coagulopathy owing to vitamin K malabsorption.

IV. Rupture of the biliary tract is possible, especially when concurrent disease decreases the integrity of wall, e.g., severe infectious/necrotizing inflammation.

V. If infection is present, bile duct rupture results in septic peritonitis, but even if the bile is sterile, a chemical peritonitis will develop (Parchman and Flanders, 1990).

Clinical Signs

I. Icterus

II. Steatorrhea, acholic stools

III. Bleeding tendencies

IV. Abdominal pain

V. Signs of concurrent pancreatitis

VI. Fever with primary or secondary cholecystitis or cholangitis

VII. Septic shock associated with necrotizing cholecystitis

Diagnosis

I. Suggestive signs
   A. Hyperbilirubinemia, bilirubinuria
   B. Moderate to marked increases in SAP, with mild to moderate increases in ALT
   C. Prolonged bleeding time that responds to parenteral vitamin K administration
   D. Neutrophilic leukocytosis with left shift with infectious disease
   E. Dilated, distended gallbladder, with concurrent dilatation of the common bile duct and the intrahepatic bile duct
      1. It may be difficult to make the diagnosis with ultrasonography early in the course of obstruction, because intrahepatic ducts may not become distended until 4–5 days after total obstruction occurs (Parthington and Biller, 1995).
      2. In suggestive cases, repeated ultrasonography is indicated.
   F. Hepatobiliary scintigraphy (experimental)
   G. Fecal sediment analysis for fluke ova

II. Definitive diagnosis: exploratory laparotomy with manual expression of the gallbladder

Differential Diagnosis

I. Intrahepatic cholestasis associated with a variety of acute and chronic hepatopathies

II. Bile duct peritonitis secondary to rupture of the biliary system from blunt abdominal trauma or a penetrating abdominal wound
   A. Associated with a bile-stained abdominal effusion
   B. Chemical peritonitis due to bile leakage not evident for 5–15 days after rupture

Treatment and Monitoring

I. Therapy depends on the etiology.

II. Bile duct obstruction caused by inflammation of the pancreas usually resolves with medical management of the pancreatitis.

III. Infectious causes may require surgical decompression, especially in the presence of significant biliary sludging.
   A. Culture and sensitivity of bile and gallbladder wall are obtained at surgery.
   B. Empirical treatment with antibiotics pending culture is instituted.

IV. Biliary stones and neoplasia are treated with surgical removal and decompression; be prepared to create a biliary diversion at the time of surgery, if needed.

V. Biopsy the liver at the time of surgical exploration to rule out concurrent hepatobiliary disease.

VI. Prognosis depends on the specific etiology.

Bibliography

Akol K, Washabau R, Saunders H et al: Acute pancreatitis in cats with hepatic lipidosis. J Vet Intern Med 7:205, 1993

Anderson M, Sevelius E: Circulating autoantibodies in dogs with chronic liver disease. J Small Anim Pract 33:389, 1992

Anwer MS, Meyer DJ: Bile acids in the diagnosis, pathology and therapy of hepatobiliary diseases. Vet Clin North Am [Small Anim Pract] 25:503, 1995

Berger B, Whiting PG, Breznock EM et al: Congenital feline portosystemic shunts. J Am Vet Med Assoc 188:517, 1986

Biourge V, Massat B, Groff J et al: Protein reduces liver lipid accumulation during rapid weight loss in obese cats. Proc Am Coll Vet Intern Med 11:948, 1993

Bostwick DR, Twedt DC: Intrahepatic and extrahepatic portal venous anomalies in dogs: 52 cases (1982–1992). J Am Vet Med Assoc 206:1181, 1995

Brown PJ, Henderson JP, Galloway P et al: Peliosis hepatis and telangiectasis in 18 cats. J Small Anim Pract 35:73, 1994

Bunch SE, Castleman WL, Baldwin BH et al: Effects of long-term primidone and phenytoin administration on canine hepatic function. Am J Vet Res 46:195, 1985

Bunch SE, Jordan HL, Sellon RK et al: Characterization of iron status in young dogs with portosystemic shunt. Am J Vet Res 56:853, 1995

Carlisle CH, Prescott CW, McCosler PJ et al: The toxic effects of thiacetarsamide sodium in normal dogs and dogs infested with *Dirofilaria immitis*. Aust Vet J 50:204, 1974

Center S, Crawford M, Guida L et al: A retrospective study

of 77 cats with severe hepatic lipidosis. J Vet Intern Med 7:349, 1993

Center S, Elston TE, Rowland PH et al: Fulminant hepatic failure associated with oral administration of diazepam in 11 cats. J Am Vet Med Assoc 209:618, 1996

Chapman BL, Hendrick MJ, Washabau RJ: Granulomatous hepatitis in dogs: nine cases (1987–1990). J Am Vet Med Assoc 203:680, 1993

Cornelius L, Mahaffey M: Kinking of the intrathoracic caudal vena cava in five dogs. J Small Anim Pract 26:67, 1985

Crawford MA, Schall WD, Jensen RK et al: Chronic active hepatitis in 26 Doberman pinschers. J Am Vet Med Assoc 187:1343, 1985

Cribb AE: Idiosyncratic reactions to sulfonamides. J Am Vet Med Assoc 195:1612, 1989

Crowe DT, Lorenz M, Hardie EM et al: Chronic peritoneal effusion due to partial caudal vena caval obstruction following blunt trauma: diagnosis and successful surgical treatment. J Am Anim Hosp Assoc 20:231, 1984

Daniel GB, Bright R, Ollis P et al: Per rectal portal scintigraphy using ^{99m}technetium pertechnetate to diagnose portosystemic shunts in dogs and cats. J Vet Intern Med 5:23, 1991

Day DG: Feline cholangiohepatitis complex. Vet Clin North Am [Small Anim Pract] 25:375, 1995

Day DG, Meyer DJ, Johnson SE et al: Evaluation of total serum bile acids concentration and bile acid profiles in healthy cats after oral administration of ursodeoxycholic acid. Am J Vet Res 55:1474, 1994

Dayrell-Hart B, Steinberg SA, VanWinkle TJ, Farnbach GC: Hepatotoxicity of phenobarbital in dogs: 18 cases (1985–1989). J Am Vet Med Assoc 199:1060, 1991

Dillon AT, Spano JS, Powers RD: Prednisone induced hematologic, biochemical and histologic changes in the dog. J Am Anim Hosp Assoc 16:831, 1980

Dimski D, Taboada J: Feline idiopathic hepatic lipidosis. Vet Clin North Am [Small Anim Pract] 25:337, 1995

Doige CE, Lester S: Chronic active hepatitis in dogs—a review of fourteen cases. J Am Anim Hosp Assoc 17:725, 1981

Fahie M, Martin RA: Extrahepatic biliary tract obstruction: a retrospective study of 45 cases (1983–1993). J Am Anim Hosp Assoc 31:478, 1995

Farrar ET, Washabau RJ, Saunder HM: Hepatic abcesses in dogs: 14 cases (1982–1994). J Am Vet Med Assoc 208:243, 1996

Fittschen C, Bellamy EC: Prednisone induced morphologic and chemical changes in the liver of dogs. Vet Pathol 21:399, 1984

Forster-van Hijfte MA, McEvoy FJ, White RN et al: Per rectal portal scintigraphy in the diagnosis and management of feline congenital portosystemic shunts. J Small Anim Pract 37:7, 1996

Hammer AS, Sikkema DA: Hepatic neoplasia in the dog and cat. Vet Clin North Am [Small Anim Pract] 25:419, 1995

Hardie EM, Kornegay JN, Cullen JM: Status epilepticus after ligation of portosystemic shunts. Vet Surg 19:412, 1990

Hardy RM: Chronic hepatitis in cocker spaniels—another syndrome. Proc Am Coll Vet Intern Med 11:256, 1993

Hardy RM, O'Brien T, Adams LG et al: Periportal hepatitis associated with the use of the heartworm-hookworm preventative (diethylcarbamazine-oxibendazole) in thirteen dogs. J Am Anim Hosp Assoc 25:419, 1989

Helton KA, Nesbitt GH, Caciolo PL: Griseofulvin toxicity in cats: literature review and report of seven cases. J Am Anim Hosp Assoc 22:453, 1986

Holt DE, Schelling CG, Saunder M et al: Correlation of ultrasonographic findings with surgical, portographic and necropsy findings in dogs and cats with portosystemic shunts: 63 cases (1987–1993). J Am Vet Med Assoc 207:1190, 1995

Ioune S, Matsunuma N, Ono KI et al: Five cases of canine peliosis hepatis. Jpn J Vet Sci 50:565, 1988

Jacobs G, Cornelius L, Keene B et al: Treatment of idiopathic hepatic lipidosis in cats: 11 cases (1986–1987). J Am Vet Med Assoc 195:635, 1989

Johnson CA, Armstrong PJ, Hauptman JG: Congenital portosystemic shunts in dogs: 46 cases (1979–1986). J Am Vet Med Assoc 191:1478, 1987

Johnson GF, Zawie DA, Gilbertson SR et al: Chronic active hepatitis in Doberman pinschers. J Am Vet Med Assoc 180:1438, 1982

Justin RB, Hohenhaus AE: Hypophosphatemia associated with enteral alimentation in cats. J Vet Intern Med 9:228, 1995

Kirpenstein J, Fingland RB, Ulrich T et al: Cholelithiasis in dogs: 29 cases (1980–1990). J Am Vet Med Assoc 202:1137, 1993

Koblik PD, Hornof WJ: Transcolonic sodium pertechnetate Tc 99m scintigraphy for diagnosis of macrovascular portosystemic shunts in dogs, cats and potbellied pigs: 176 cases (1988–1992). J Am Vet Med Assoc 207:729, 1995

Komtebedde J, Koblik PD, Breznock EM et al: Long-term clinical outcome after partial ligation of single extrahepatic vascular anomalies in 20 dogs. Vet Surg 24:379, 1995

Laflamme DP, Mahaffey EA, Allen SA et al: Microcytosis and iron status in dogs with surgically induced portosystemic shunts. J Vet Intern Med 8:212, 1994

Lawrence D, Bellah JR, Diaz R: Results of surgical management of portosystemic shunts in dogs: 20 cases (1985–1990). J Am Vet Med Assoc 201:1750, 1992

Legendre AM: Anti-mycotic drug therapy. p. 327. In Bonagura JD (ed): Kirk's Current Veterinary Therapy XII. WB Saunders, Philadelphia, 1995

Leveille CR, Arias IM: Pathophysiology and pharmacologic modulation of hepatic fibrosis. J Vet Intern Med 7:73, 1993

Macintire DK, Henderson RH, Banfield C: Budd-Chiari syndrome in a kitten caused by membranous obstruction of the caudal vena cava. J Am Anim Hosp Assoc 31:484, 1995

Maddison JE: Canine congenital portosystemic encephalopathy. Aust Vet J 65:245, 1988

Maddison JE: Hepatic encephalopathy: current concepts of the pathogenesis. J Vet Intern Med 6:341, 1992

Matushek KJ, Bjorling D, Matthews K: Generalized motor seizures after portosystemic shunt ligation in dogs: five cases (1981–1988). J Am Vet Med Assoc 196:2014, 1990

Meuten DJ, Pecquet-Goad ME: Hepatic necrosis associated with use of halothane in a dog. J Am Vet Med Assoc 184:478, 1984

Neer TM: A review of disorders of the gallbladder and extrahepatic biliary tract in the dog and cat. J Vet Intern Med 6:186, 1992

Nidiritu CG, Weigel J: Hepatorenal injury in a dog associated with methoxyflurane. Vet Med Small Anim Clin 72:545, 1977

Nicholson BT, Center SA, Rowland PJ et al: Evaluation of the safety of ursodeoxycholic acid in healthy cats. Proc Am Coll Vet Intern Med 11:949, 1993

Otto CM, Mahaffey M, Jacobs C et al: Cor triatrium dexter with Budd-Chiari syndrome and a review of ascites in young dogs. J Small Anim Pract 31:385, 1991

Parchman MB, Flanders JA: Extrahepatic biliary tract rupture: evaluation of the relationship between the site of rupture and the cause of rupture in 15 dogs. Cornell Vet 80:267, 1990

Parthington BP, Biller DS: Hepatic imaging with radiology and ultrasound. Vet Clin North Am [Small Anim Pract] 25:305, 1995

Phillips L, Tappe J, Lyman R: Hepatic microvascular dysplasia with demonstrable macroscopic shunts. Proc Am Coll Vet Intern Med 11:438, 1993

Polzin DJ, Stowe CM, O'Leary TP et al: Acute hepatic necrosis associated with the administration of mebendazole to dogs. J Am Vet Med Assoc 179:1013, 1981

Pond EC, Morrow D: Hepatotoxicity associated with methotrexate therapy in a dog. J Small Anim Pract 23:659, 1982

Rogers WA, Ruebner BH: A retrospective study of probable glucocorticoid-induced hepatopathy in dogs. J Am Vet Med Assoc 170:603, 1977

Rolfe DS, Twedt DC: Copper-associated hepatopathies in dogs. Vet Clin North Am [Small Anim Pract] 25:399, 1995

Rowland PH, Center SA, Dougherty SA: Presumptive trimethoprim sulfa related hepatotoxicity in a dog. J Am Vet Med Assoc 200:348, 1992

Rutgers HC, Haywood S, Kelly DF: Idiopathic hepatic fibrosis in 15 dogs. Vet Rec 133:115, 1993

Scavelli TD, Hornbuckle WE, Roth L et al: Portosystemic shunts in cats: seven cases (1976–1984). J Am Vet Med Assoc 189:317, 1986

Schermhorn T, Center SA, Dykes A et al: Characterization of hepatoportal microvascular dysplasia in a kindred of Cairn terriers. J Vet Intern Med 10:219, 1996

Smith KR, Bauer M, Monnet E: Portosystemic communications: follow-up of 32 cases. J Small Anim Pract 36:435, 1995

Stanton ME, Bright RM: Gastroduodenal ulceration in dogs: retrospective study and review of the literature. J Vet Intern Med 3:238, 1989

Stowater JL, Lamb CR, Schelling SH: Ultrasonographic features of canine hepatic nodular hyperplasia. Vet Radiol 31:268, 1990

Strombeck DR, Miller LM, Harrold D: Effects of corticosteroid treatment on survival time in dogs with chronic hepatitis: 151 cases (1977–1985). J Am Vet Med Assoc 193:1109, 1988

Swalec KM, Smeak DD: Partial versus complete attenuation of single portosystemic shunts. Vet Surg 19:406, 1990

Thornberg LP, Crawford SJ: Liver disease in West Highland white terriers. Vet Rec 4:110, 1986

Toth DM, Derwelis SK: Drug-induced hepatitis in a dog. Vet Med Small Anim Clin 75:421, 1980

van den Ingh TS, Rothuizen J, Cupery R: Chronic active hepatitis with cirrhosis in the Doberman pinscher. Vet Q 10:84, 1988

Van Winkle TJ, Bruce E: Thrombosis of the portal vein in eleven dogs. Vet Pathol 30:28, 1993

Weiss DJ, Armstrong PJ, Mruthyunjaya A: Anti-liver membrane protein antibodies in dogs with chronic hepatitis. J Vet Intern Med 9:267, 1995

Weiss DJ, Gagne JM, Armstrong PJ: Relationship between inflammatory hepatic disease and inflammatory bowel disease, pancreatitis and nephritis in cats. J Am Vet Med Assoc 209:1114, 1996

Whitely MB, Feeney DA, Whitely LO et al: Ultrasonographic appearance of primary and metastatic canine hepatic tumors—a review of 48 cases. J Ultrasound Med 8:621, 1989

Wrigley RH, Konde LJ, Park R et al: Ultrasonographic diagnosis of portacaval shunts in young dogs. J Am Vet Med Assoc 191:421, 1987

35

Diseases of the Exocrine Pancreas

Jean A. Hall

INFLAMMATORY DISEASES (PANCREATITIS)

Acute Pancreatitis in Dogs

Definition

I. It is an acute condition of the pancreas that develops when the normal glandular defense mechanisms have been overwhelmed by activated pancreatic enzymes.

II. Acute pancreatitis can range from a mild self-limited illness to a rapidly fulminant, fatal disorder.
   A. Mild: edematous interstitial involvement
      1. No multisystemic organ involvement
      2. Self-limiting disease
      3. Uncomplicated recovery
   B. Severe: hemorrhagic or necrotizing
      1. Progression of mild edematous pancreatitis to hemorrhagic or necrotizing pancreatitis
      2. Multisystemic organ failure
      3. Self-perpetuating disease
      4. Complications common, e.g., pseudocyst, abscess
      5. Guarded prognosis
   C. Acute and recurrent acute disease commonly diagnosed

Causes

I. Factors that cause or contribute to acinar cell injury include the following.
   A. Nutritional considerations
      1. Pancreatitis is more common in obese dogs.
      2. Low-protein, high-fat diets may induce pancreatitis.
   B. Hyperlipidemia
      1. It may be a cause of pancreatitis via action of pancreatic lipase on abnormally high concentrations of triglycerides in pancreatic capillaries, resulting in release of fatty acids that cause localized acidosis and vasoconstriction.
      2. There is a high frequency of pancreatitis in miniature schnauzers with idiopathic hyperlipoproteinemia.
      3. It may also be the result of pancreatitis, as a result of abdominal fat necrosis.
   C. Drugs
      1. Drugs suspected of causing acute pancreatitis include azathioprine, L-asparaginase, thiazide diuretics, furosemide, sulfonamides, and tetracycline.
      2. Corticosteroids may induce pancreatitis; however, no experimental evidence exists for this association.
         a) Glucocorticoids in association with spinal trauma may predispose to pancreatitis.
         b) Dogs with naturally occurring or iatrogenic hypercortisolism may be predisposed to pancreatitis.
      3. Cholinesterase inhibitors and cholinergic agonists have been associated with pancreatitis.
      4. Histamine H_2-receptor antagonists may induce pancreatitis.
   D. Ischemia of pancreas
      1. It may arise from hypovolemia, fat embolism, or sympathetic stimulation causing vasoconstriction.
      2. Temporary occlusion of venous outflow during abdominal surgery in the anterior abdomen may be responsible for postoperative pancreatitis.
   E. Biliary tract disease: extension of inflammatory disease from one organ to the other
   F. Duct obstruction (rare)
      1. Compression, spasm, or edema of the duct or duodenal wall
      2. Underlying causes: neoplasia, parasite migration, trauma, or surgical damage
   G. Duodenal reflux (rare)
      1. Enteropeptidase, activated proteases, bile, and bacteria entering the pancreatic duct

403

2. Requires high duodenal pressure, e.g., with vomiting
H. Trauma
   1. Surgical trauma or accidental abdominal trauma (automobile accident)
   2. Rarely, pancreatic biopsy
I. Hypercalcemia, as seen with hyperparathyroidism
II. Risk factors associated with acute pancreatitis in dogs are outlined in Table 35–1 (Cook et al., 1993; Hess et al., 1996).

Pathophysiology

I. Pancreatitis develops when zymogens are activated within the gland with subsequent pancreatic autodigestion.
II. Enzyme activation may be initiated by reflux of enterokinase or bile from the duodenum, by abnormal fusion of zymogens with lysosome exposing them to lysosomal proteases, or by other causes.
III. Free radical damage may be important in the progression of pancreatitis.
IV. Once trypsin is activated, it then activates other zymogens resulting in the following.
   A. Local changes
      1. Direct pancreatic cell membrane disruption and destruction of supporting stroma
      2. Pancreatic arteriolar vasodilation and increased vascular permeability followed by interstitial edema and hemorrhage
      3. Pain
      4. Leukocytic infiltration
      5. Peripancreatic fat necrosis
   B. Systemic alterations
      1. Arterial hypotension, capillary vasodilation

Table 35–1. **Risk Factors of Acute Pancreatitis in Dogs**

A. Spayed dogs and castrated male dogs >7 years old
B. Overweight body condition (obesity)
C. Breeds
   1. Small body size
   2. Terriers—Yorkshire terrier, Airedale, and Cairn terrier
   3. Non-sporting breeds—miniature poodle, toy poodle, Lhasa apso, schipperke, miniature schnauzer
D. Intercurrent diseases
   1. Prior gastrointestinal disease
   2. Diabetes mellitus
   3. Hyperadrenocorticism
   4. Hypothyroidism
   5. Chronic renal failure
   6. Congestive heart failure
   7. Autoimmune disorders
E. Recent drug treatment
   1. Antibiotics, e.g., trimethoprim/sulfa
   2. Corticosteroids
   3. Chemotherapeutic agents
   4. Organophosphate insecticides
F. Anesthesia
G. Surgery

---

2. Portal venous blood pooling
3. Hypovolemia subsequent to loss of fluid from the vascular space
4. Compensatory mechanism of peripheral vasoconstriction, further reducing pancreatic arterial blood flow and promoting continued pancreatic injury
5. Leakage of digestive enzymes and vasoactive amines into the abdominal cavity and blood stream, causing similar injury to the peritoneum, liver, lungs, kidneys, and heart
V. Changes remain relatively mild as long as there are sufficient plasma protease inhibitors (α_1-protease inhibitor and α-macroglobulins) to neutralize active proteases.

Clinical Signs

I. Clinical signs of acute pancreatitis are extremely variable; there are no pathognomonic signs.
II. Common signs and physical examination findings are as follows.
   A. Acute vomiting, often after a fatty meal
   B. Depression, dehydration
   C. Abdominal pain
      1. Indicated by restlessness, assumption of the ''position of relief'' or ''praying position''
      2. Localization of discomfort to the right cranial quadrant of the abdomen with palpation
   D. Fever (usually caused by inflammation, not infection)
III. Unusual signs and physical examination findings are the following.
   A. Weakness, tachypnea, tachycardia, dehydration, hepatomegaly, and hyperemia of mucous membranes (20–40%)
   B. Diarrhea (possibly hemorrhagic), abdominal mass, jaundice, abdominal distention, cachexia, coagulopathy, muscle fasciculations, or tetany (20%)
   C. Multiple, nonpruritic, draining skin lesions (Paterson, 1994)
      1. Sterile nodular panniculitis associated with a bile duct carcinoma
      2. Direct enzymatic necrosis of subcutaneous fat hypothesized

Diagnosis

I. There is no single test, other than direct examination of the pancreas, that is definitively diagnostic for acute pancreatitis.
II. A presumptive diagnosis of acute pancreatitis can be made based on information learned from the history, physical examination, selected laboratory test results, and ultrasonographic findings.
III. History and physical examination often reveal typical predisposing factors (see Table 35–1).
IV. Laboratory tests may denote the following.
   A. Complete blood count
      1. Commonly neutrophilia with or without a left shift

2. Neutropenia with a degenerative left shift from severe necrosis, peritonitis, sepsis, or endotoxemia
3. Increased packed cell volume from dehydration
4. Red blood cell (RBC) fragments consistent with subclinical disseminated intravascular coagulopathy (DIC) (see Chap. 66)

B. Serum chemistries
   1. Azotemia often present
      a) Prerenal: urine concentrated
      b) Renal: isosthenuria present
   2. Serum alkaline phosphatase and alanine transaminase often increased
   3. Elevated total bilirubin from severe hepatocellular damage and intrahepatic or extrahepatic obstruction of bile flow
   4. Hyperglycemia probably from increased glucagon secretion and stress-related increases in catecholamines and cortisol
   5. Hypocalcemia (mild to moderate) secondary to altered membrane integrity with an acute shift of calcium into soft tissues
   6. Hypercholesterolemia and hypertriglyceridemia

C. Assays of pancreatic enzymes and zymogens in serum
   1. Hyperamylasemia
      a) Magnitude of increase does not correlate with severity of pancreatitis, and value must be interpreted in light of renal function (involved in degradation) and other tissue sources of amylase.
      b) Values are increased within 3 hours of onset of pancreatitis and usually return to normal within 6–8 days.
      c) Normal values do not exclude the diagnosis of pancreatitis, especially if hypertriglyceridemia is present.
   2. Hyperlipasemia
      a) Serum lipase values generally parallel amylase values in pancreatitis.
      b) There are other sources of lipase other than the pancreas, but high values are associated primarily with pancreatitis.
      c) Up to threefold elevations of lipase activity may be noted in dogs with renal failure.
      d) Parenteral dexamethasone and prednisone or manipulation of the pancreas during exploratory laparotomy increases serum lipase activity without causing pancreatitis.
      e) It has been reported to be a more reliable marker for pancreatitis than that of amylase in dogs.
   3. Hyperamylasemia and hyperlipasemia
      a) Combined with characteristic clinical features, these abnormalities establish the diagnosis of pancreatitis until proved otherwise.

      b) Values do not, however, correlate with the severity of pancreatic inflammation.
   4. Elevated serum trypsin-like immunoreactivity (TLI)
      a) Increases earlier and decreases sooner than other enzymes, perhaps reflecting its shorter half-life
      b) Pancreas-specific in origin
      c) Concentrations >35 μg/L consistent with pancreatitis
      d) Elevated TLI and serum lipase most likely to identify dogs with pancreatitis
      e) Does not change in response to prednisone administration (Williams et al., 1995)

D. Acid–base and electrolyte disturbances
   1. Metabolic acidosis: proportionate to the severity of vomiting
   2. Hyponatremia, hypokalemia, hypochloremia

V. The following radiographic findings support a tentative diagnosis of pancreatitis, but the absence of abnormal findings does not rule out pancreatitis.
   A. Increased density, diminished contrast, and granularity in the right cranial abdomen ("ground-glass" appearance)
   B. Displacement of the stomach to the left and the descending duodenum to the right
   C. Widening of the angle between the pyloric antrum and the proximal duodenum
   D. Presence of a mass medial to the descending duodenum
   E. Static gas pattern in the duodenum or transverse colon
   F. Caudal displacement of the transverse colon
   G. Gastric distention suggestive of gastric outlet obstruction and delayed gastric emptying of barium with corrugation of the duodenal wall consistent with abnormal peristalsis

VI. Ultrasonographic findings reported with pancreatitis include the following.
   A. Nonhomogeneous mass effect with loss of echodensity or mottled echogenicity in the area of the pancreas
   B. Pancreatic pseudocysts or abscesses: cystic masses

VII. Abdominocentesis for fluid analysis and amylase and lipase measurement may be performed.
   A. Abdominal fluid has characteristics of an exudate, i.e., protein content >2.5 g/dl, nucleated cell count of 3000–5000 cells/μl with predominantly nondegenerate neutrophils.
   B. Amylase and lipase activities are higher than serum values.

VIII. Exploratory laparotomy or laparoscopy may be considered if the diagnosis remains questionable.

Differential Diagnosis

I. Diseases of the digestive tract
   A. Systemic infections: canine distemper, infectious canine hepatitis, parvovirus, leptospirosis

B. Intestinal obstruction, e.g., foreign body, volvulus
C. Intestinal infarction
D. Acute cholecystitis
E. Bacterial enterotoxemia
F. Hemorrhagic gastroenteritis

II. Nondigestive tract diseases
A. Pyometra, acute metritis
B. Acute prostatitis
C. Testicular torsion
D. Acute pyelonephritis
E. Renal failure
F. Ruptured bladder
G. Peritonitis
H. Ketoacidotic diabetes mellitus
I. Hypoadrenocorticism

III. Other causes of acute abdomen syndrome (see Chap. 37)

Treatment

I. Goals
A. To maintain fluid and electrolyte balance while the pancreas is allowed to rest and recover from the inflammatory event
B. To reestablish the integrity of the circulatory system, i.e., correct shock, dehydration, and hypovolemia
C. To reduce pancreatic secretions
D. To relieve pain
E. To manage complications

II. Medical management of simple or mild pancreatitis
A. Eliminate any predisposing factors, e.g., drugs.
B. Maintain pancreatic microcirculation by fluid volume replacement.
1. Administer a balanced electrolyte solution (e.g., lactated Ringer's solution) to replace deficits and to meet the needs for maintenance and continuing losses.
2. Administer via SQ route if signs are mild.
3. Use IV route if dehydration is severe and vomiting is persistent.
4. Routinely add 20 mEq KCl per liter of maintenance fluids.
5. Administer bicarbonate if necessary to correct metabolic acidosis.
C. Antiemetics can be used for 24–48 hours if vomiting is severe.
1. Consider chlorpromazine (Thorazine) 0.25–0.5 mg/kg IM TID-QID. Ensure adequate volume expansion to avoid hypotension.
2. Metoclopramide (Reglan) may also be given at 0.2–0.5 mg/kg SQ TID-QID or 1–2 mg/kg/24 h as a constant-rate IV infusion.
D. Corticosteroids are indicated only for shock and only short term (see Chap. 131).
E. Allow nothing per os (NPO) for 48–96 hours to reduce stimuli for pancreatic secretion.
1. Offer water 1–2 days after vomiting has stopped.
2. If water is tolerated, then gradually reintroduce food, initially feeding a high-carbohy-drate diet (e.g., rice, pasta) that is restricted in fat and protein to minimize pancreatic secretion.
3. If vomiting resumes, return to NPO for 24–48 hours.
4. Gradually institute a high-carbohydrate, fat-restricted, balanced diet.
5. Emphatically discourage feeding table scraps or unsupervised eating.
6. Avoid anticholinergics, because they are of questionable value and potentiate ileus.
F. Relieve abdominal pain with analgesics.
1. Butorphanol (Torbugesic) 0.2–0.4 mg/kg SQ q 4–6 h
2. Meperidine HCl (Demerol) 5–10 mg/kg IM TID
3. A trial period of pancreatic enzyme supplements (Viokase) to induce feedback inhibition
G. Manage acute complications.
1. Routine use of antibiotics is not recommended, because bacteria do not play a primary role.
2. Administer parenteral antibiotics when toxic changes are present in the hemogram or when the dog is febrile.
3. To control sepsis and prevent pancreatic abscessation, consider a cephalosporin, e.g., cephalothin 20 mg/kg IV TID-QID.

III. Medical management of complicated or severe pancreatitis
A. Use the same approach as for mild pancreatitis, except be more aggressive.
B. Begin intensive fluid therapy, because the major causes of death are hypovolemia and shock.
1. To treat shock, give crystalloids at ≤85 ml/kg IV in the first hour.
2. Consider transfusion of plasma or whole blood (10–20 ml/kg) to replace albumin and restore plasma oncotic pressure.
3. A blood transfusion may reduce pancreatic edema, pulmonary edema, and pleural effusion.
4. Fresh or fresh frozen plasma also provides α-macroglobulins, which may be exhausted as a result of an overabundance of free trypsin.
C. Allow nothing per os for 3–5 days beyond termination of vomiting.
1. Maintenance of NPO is necessary in some dogs for 7–14 days.
2. Consider feeding by an alternative route if food is withheld >5 days or if >10% of body weight is lost.
3. Feeding an elemental diet by jejunostomy catheter or total parenteral nutrition may be required.
D. Administer analgesics as outlined earlier.
E. Manage complications.
1. If sepsis or peritonitis occurs, consider a cephalosporin with or without an aminoglycoside.
2. Control DIC (see Chap. 66).
3. See other acute complications later.

IV. Surgical therapy

A. Surgical intervention is indicated for management of septic peritonitis (lavage and drainage).
B. Some late complications of pancreatitis require surgical intervention, e.g., abscess formation, granuloma, or stricture formation with obstruction of the common bile duct.
C. Peritoneal dialysis can be performed using a dialysis catheter to remove toxic material from the peritoneal cavity (see Chap. 47).

Patient Monitoring

I. The following complications should be anticipated and treated accordingly with severe acute pancreatitis.
  A. Acute renal failure (see Chap. 47)
  B. DIC
  C. Sepsis, pancreatic abscess, infected pseudocyst
    1. Devitalized pancreatic tissue may become infected with gram-negative bacteria.
    2. A pseudocyst (cyst of pancreatic secretions surrounded by granulation tissue) or abscess may cause recurrence of clinical signs after the initial recovery period.
    3. Ultrasonography is helpful in identifying a pancreatic mass.
    4. Surgical drainage with bacterial culture is needed for treatment of pseudocysts and abscesses.
  D. Pulmonary insufficiency (unusual)
    1. Circulating pancreatic enzymes, vasoactive substances, and free fatty acids may injure capillary alveolar membranes, causing fluid extravasation, thromboembolism, edema, or pleural effusion.
    2. Monitor respiratory rate, arterial blood gases, thoracic radiographs, and central venous pressure (CVP), especially when giving high volumes of fluid therapy.
    3. A radionuclide lung perfusion scan may be performed to support a diagnosis of pulmonary thromboembolism.
    4. See treatment outlined in Chap. 18.
  E. Cardiac arrhythmias
    1. Ventricular arrhythmias and conduction disturbances may occur.
    2. See treatment outlined in Chap. 7.
  F. Rarely, diabetes mellitus or exocrine pancreatic insufficiency from repeated episodes of pancreatitis
  G. Jaundice
    1. Toxic substances or obstruction of the extrahepatic bile duct may be the cause.
    2. Ultrasonography may be helpful in documenting a large common bile duct and dilated intra- and extrahepatic bile ducts associated with biliary obstruction.
    3. Progressive or persistent jaundice in the face of aggressive medical management indicates the need for exploratory laparotomy.
II. The unpredictable nature of pancreatitis makes it difficult to give an accurate prognosis.

A. Most patients with mild, uncomplicated pancreatitis recover spontaneously and do well if high-fat foods are avoided.
B. Severe acute pancreatitis, especially the hemorrhagic type, requires intensive care, commonly develops complications, and has a guarded to grave prognosis.
C. Respiratory distress, cardiac abnormalities, bleeding disorders, and acute renal failure all are poor prognostic signs.

Acute Pancreatitis in Cats

Definition

I. It is an inflammatory process involving the exocrine pancreas.
II. Unlike in the dog, the diagnosis is often missed ante mortem, because "classic" pancreatitis is rare in cats.

Causes

I. The cause is usually not known.
II. Some cases have been associated with the following.
  A. Severe abdominal trauma (high-rise syndrome)
  B. Infectious diseases
    1. Herpesvirus I
    2. Feline infectious peritonitis
    3. *Toxoplasma gondii*
    4. Parasite infestation (*Amphimerus pseudofelineus*)
  C. Hepatic lipidosis
    1. 38% of cats with hepatic lipidosis had acute pancreatitis (Akol et al., 1993).
    2. 59% of cats with acute pancreatitis had fatty change in their liver (Van Winkle and Hill, 1989).
    3. Acute pancreatitis may be a cause, consequence, or coincident disease.
  D. Cholangitis/cholangiohepatitis (questionable relationship [Hill and Van Winkle, 1993])
  E. Organophosphate or drug toxicity
  F. Ascending infection from the small intestine
  G. Malnutrition rather than overnutrition (Hill and Van Winkle, 1993)

Pathophysiology

I. Trypsinogen is activated within acinar cells, leading to activation of other proteases, phospholipases, and cascade systems.
II. In a retrospective study of 40 cats with necropsy-confirmed acute pancreatitis (Hill and Van Winkle, 1993), the following histologic classification was made.
  A. Acute pancreatic necrosis was the dominant feature in 32 of 40 cats.
  B. Suppurative inflammation predominated and necrosis was minimal in 8 of 40 cats, which were characterized by being underweight, hypoglycemic, younger in age, and dying acutely.

Clinical Signs

I. Clinical signs are vague and nonspecific.
II. In one study, the following clinical signs were reported (Hill and Van Winkle, 1993).
   A. Lethargy (100%), anorexia (97%), dehydration (92%)
   B. Hypothermia (68%)
   C. Vomiting (35%), abdominal pain (25%)
   D. Palpable abdominal mass (23%)
   E. Dyspnea (20%), ataxia (15%), diarrhea (15%)
III. Clinical course of the disease varied (Hill and Van Winkle, 1993).
   A. 38% had acute cardiovascular shock.
   B. 62% had two stages of disease.
      1. Protracted period of anorexia, lethargy, weight loss, and occasional vomiting
      2. Acute deterioration, shock, and a moribund state, despite fluid therapy
IV. Clinical course of the disease in cats with concurrent hepatic lipidosis is as follows (Akol et al., 1993).
   A. Cats are more likely to be cachectic and have coagulation abnormalities.
   B. Peritoneal effusion was present in all cats.
   C. Only 20% recovered when both disorders were present, whereas there was 50% recovery with hepatic lipidosis alone.

Diagnosis

I. A thorough diagnostic evaluation, a high index of clinical suspicion, and abdominal ultrasonography are necessary for pancreatitis to be diagnosed ante mortem.
II. Cats of all ages (3 weeks to 16 years), of either sex, and of any breed may be affected. Siamese cats may be over-represented.
III. Hematologic changes are uncommon and nonspecific.
   A. Neutrophilia (30%)
   B. Anemia terminally (55%)
   C. Nucleated red blood cells without evidence of a responsive anemia (sign of systemic disease in the cat)
IV. Serum biochemical abnormalities are common (Hill and Van Winkle, 1993).
   A. Hypoglycemia (75% of cats with suppurative pancreatitis)
   B. Increased alanine aminotransferase (68%)
   C. Increased bilirubin (64%)
   D. Hyperglycemia (64% of cats with acute pancreatic necrosis)
   E. Hypercholesterolemia (64%)
   F. Hypokalemia (56%)
   G. Increased alkaline phosphatase (50%)
   H. Hypocalcemia (45%)
   I. Hypophosphatemia (14%)
V. Pancreatic enzymes (serum amylase and lipase) are unreliable, because both may be within normal limits.
VI. Vitamin K–responsive coagulopathy may occur from fat and vitamin K malabsorption (Simpson KW et al., 1994).

VII. Radiographic abnormalities may include the following.
   A. Decreased contrast in the cranial abdomen
   B. Dilated and gas-filled small intestines
   C. Transposition of the duodenum, stomach, and transverse colon
   D. Changes subtle and nonspecific
VIII. Abdominal ultrasonography may be the most useful technique for detecting pancreatic lesions ante mortem (Simpson KW et al., 1994).
   A. A hypoechoic pancreas or a mass may be observed in the cranial abdomen.
   B. A heterogeneous mass with hypoechoic and hyperechoic components may also be seen.
   C. Peritoneal effusion may occur in cats with concurrent hepatic lipidosis and acute pancreatitis.
IX. Serum trypsin-like immunoreactivity (TLI) is a promising diagnostic test.
   A. In a study of 12 cats with severe pancreatitis, TLI ranged from 14.8–540 µg/L, with a mean of 100.1 µg/L (Parent et al., 1995).
   B. The normal range for serum TLI is 17–49 µg/L.
X. Consider serologic evaluation for toxoplasmosis if multiple cats are symptomatic or evidence is present for multiple organ involvement (see Chap. 2).
XI. Histologic examination is the definitive test.

Differential Diagnosis

I. Other causes of acute vomiting: foreign bodies, panleukopenia
II. Other causes of gastrointestinal symptoms with abdominal pain: diffuse infiltrative bowel diseases and neoplasia, peritonitis, steatitis
III. Other causes of acute jaundice: hepatic lipidosis, cholangiohepatitis, feline leukemia virus (FeLV)–related diseases, hemolytic anemias
IV. Other causes of pleural and peritoneal effusions

Treatment

I. It is the same as for acute pancreatitis in dogs (see earlier).
II. Opposing nutritional strategies exist for hepatic lipidosis and concurrent acute pancreatitis.
   A. Hepatic lipidosis is treated by providing adequate caloric intake.
   B. Acute pancreatitis is treated by restricting oral intake.
   C. Toxoplasmosis is difficult to treat successfully (see Chap. 114); chronic recurrent pancreatitis may develop.
III. Total parenteral nutrition or feeding via jejunostomy catheter may be essential if cats are to be kept NPO for a prolonged length of time.
IV. Low-fat, balanced diets with vitamin supplementation are then fed.

Patient Monitoring

I. Fluid therapy must be monitored carefully to avoid pulmonary edema. Monitor respiratory rate, packed cell volume (PCV), total solids (TS), and, if needed, CVP.

II. Cats with concurrent hepatic lipidosis and acute pancreatitis have a worse prognosis, which is in part related to coagulation abnormalities and pulmonary thrombosis.

III. Serious complications are rare, but transient or permanent diabetes mellitus may occur.

Chronic Pancreatitis

Definition and Causes

I. Chronic pancreatitis may occur as a result of undetected acute pancreatitis.

II. It may occur with improper home management of previously diagnosed acute pancreatitis.

III. It may be a subclinical disease of older cats, often diagnosed at necropsy, and characterized by the presence of fibrosis on histopathologic examination.

IV. It may accompany another systemic illness, such as the following.
  A. Dogs: diabetes mellitus, hyperadrenocorticism, idiopathic hyperlipidemia
  B. Cats: toxoplasmosis, feline infectious peritonitis (FIP), panleukopenia, cholangiohepatitis

Pathophysiology

I. Chronic pancreatitis is characterized by recurrent episodes or persistent signs.
  A. There is progressive destruction of pancreatic parenchyma.
  B. It may lead to permanent impairment of pancreatic or hepatic function.
    1. Exocrine pancreatic insufficiency
    2. Diabetes mellitus
    3. Extrahepatic bile duct obstruction
  C. When the disease is mild, minimal morphologic changes occur and there is subclinical loss of exocrine function.
  D. With severe disease, morphologic damage occurs with clinical exocrine pancreatic insufficiency or diabetes mellitus and marked pancreatic fibrosis.

II. Hepatic lipidosis or cholangiohepatitis and pancreatic disease coexist in cats because the common bile duct joins the major pancreatic duct for a short distance before entering the duodenum.

Clinical Signs

I. Anorexia, chronic intermittent vomiting
II. Diarrhea, weight loss
III. Palpable irregularity of pancreas or peripancreatic fat (cats)

Diagnosis

I. History and clinical signs are nonspecific.
II. Results of laboratory tests are quite variable, as listed earlier for acute pancreatitis in dogs and cats.
III. Rule out toxoplasmosis and FIP (cats).

IV. Ultrasonography may reveal a pancreatic pseudocyst (cavitated pancreatic mass containing sterile liquefied necrotic debris) in dogs (Wolfsheimer et al., 1991) or cats (Hines et al., 1996).

Treatment and Monitoring

I. Treatment during active symptomatology is the same as that for acute pancreatitis.

II. Prophylactic measures include permanent dietary management with high-carbohydrate, fat-restricted, balanced diets.

III. The prognosis is fair to good if predisposing factors (e.g., hyperlipoproteinemia) can be controlled.

NONINFLAMMATORY DISEASES

Exocrine Pancreatic Insufficiency (EPI) in Dogs

Definition

I. Progressive loss of exocrine pancreatic acinar cells results in failure to secrete adequate amounts of pancreatic enzymes with clinical signs of malabsorption.

II. Clinical signs do not develop until more than 85–90% of the secretory capacity of the pancreas has been lost.

Causes

I. The most common cause is noninflammatory pancreatic acinar atrophy of young dogs.
  A. Many breeds can be affected, especially large breeds.
  B. There is a high prevalence in German shepherd dogs, and the disease may be inherited in an autosomal recessive manner.

II. Chronic pancreatitis is a less common cause, because the end stage of chronic relapsing pancreatitis is fibrosis and atrophy.

III. Pancreatic neoplasia (rare) and congenital pancreatic hypoplasia or aplasia are much less common causes.

IV. EPI can occur with nonpancreatic diseases, e.g., severe protein-calorie malnutrition and duodenal hyperacidity.

Pathophysiology

I. Reduced secretion of digestive enzymes leads to nutrient malabsorption from a failure of digestion in the small intestine.

II. In addition, changes in small intestinal mucosal function and morphology lead to nutrient malabsorption.
  A. Altered mucosal enzyme activities have been documented, i.e., abnormal transport of sugars, amino acids, and fatty acids.
  B. Factors that may contribute to impaired mucosal function include the following.

1. Loss of the trophic influence of pancreatic secretions and products of digestion on the small intestinal mucosa
2. Bacterial overgrowth in the small intestine
3. Malnutrition's direct effects on gastrointestinal mucosa

III. In animals with EPI secondary to chronic pancreatitis, diabetes mellitus may occur as a result of islet cell destruction and leads to glucose intolerance.

Clinical Signs

I. Signalment
   A. Onset of signs occurs often before 2 years of age, in large-breed dogs (predominantly German shepherd dogs), and with no sex predilection.
   B. Pancreatitis-induced EPI can occur at any age but most often occurs in middle-aged and older dogs, often smaller breeds, and with no sex predilection.

II. Common clinical signs and physical examination findings
   A. Dogs are active, bright, and alert despite chronic history of weight loss.
   B. There is mild to marked weight loss.
      1. Weight loss occurs despite a ravenous appetite and increased food intake.
      2. Pica and coprophagia may be observed because of a voracious appetite.
      3. Some dogs are emaciated at presentation, with severe muscle wasting and absence of body fat.
   C. Diarrhea is common.
      1. Maldigestion and malabsorption lead to an increased quantity of osmotically active carbohydrate and protein products in the intestinal lumen that are fermented by bacteria.
      2. Diarrhea is characterized by large volumes of soft, semi-formed fatty feces with a rancid odor.
      3. It often improves or resolves in response to fasting or after introducing a low-fat diet or a highly digestible diet.
   D. There may be a history of vomiting.
   E. Borborygmus and flatulence may occur.
   F. Intestinal loops may be distended with ingesta and gas.
      1. Owners may report episodes of abdominal discomfort.
      2. There may be discomfort on abdominal palpation.
   G. Poor quality hair coat with oily staining of the perineum may be noted.
   H. Polyuria and polydipsia may occur alone or in association with diabetes mellitus.

Diagnosis

I. Characteristic history and clinical signs may suggest a diagnosis of EPI, although these are nonspecific and do not distinguish EPI from other causes of maldigestion.

II. Many laboratory tests have been used for the diagnosis of EPI.
   A. Hematology, serum chemistries, urinalysis, and abdominal radiographs are usually unremarkable.
   B. Chymotrypsin activity in the proximal small intestine may be assayed in vivo by the oral administration of the synthetic substrate bentiromide or bentiromide-PABA (BT-PABA).
      1. It offers similar sensitivity and specificity to the assay for fecal proteolytic activity.
      2. BT-PABA is administered orally after an 18-hour fast (16.7 mg/kg PO). In the small intestine in the presence of chymotrypsin, PABA is released and absorbed.
      3. Plasma samples are obtained at 0, 30, 60, 90, and 120 minutes after administration.
      4. Dogs with EPI secrete very little chymotrypsin and, therefore, have very little rise in plasma PABA at 60 and 90 minutes.
      5. In normal dogs, peak PABA is ≥ 5 µg/ml.
      6. This assay offers no advantages over serum TLI or fecal proteolytic activity, and its use is not widespread.
   C. Microscopic examination of feces for excessive fat or undigested starch, assessment of fecal proteolytic activity by gelatin digestion, and plasma turbidity tests all have a significant proportion of false-negative and false-positive results, and their use even as crude screening tests is not recommended.

III. The most reliable and widely used test currently available is assay of serum trypsin-like immunoreactivity (TLI).
   A. Serum TLI concentration is both highly sensitive and specific for the diagnosis of EPI.
   B. Sample collection is as follows.
      1. Withhold food for 12 hours.
      2. A single serum sample is obtained.
      3. Serum TLI is stable, so samples can be mailed to an appropriate laboratory for analysis.
      4. Prior administration of oral pancreatic extracts (usually of porcine origin) does not affect canine-specific assays of serum TLI.
      5. The radioimmunoassay used must be specific for canine TLI.
      6. Samples can be submitted to Dr. David Williams, Dept. of Veterinary Clinical Sciences, 1248 Lynn Hall, Purdue University, West Lafayette, IN 47907.
   C. Interpretation is usually straightforward.
      1. TLI concentrations are markedly reduced in EPI (<2 µg/L).
      2. Dogs with small intestinal disease have normal TLI concentrations (5–35 µg/L).
      3. A reduction of TLI may precede signs of weight loss, diarrhea, and abnormalities in the fecal proteolytic activity assay or bentiromide absorption test.

IV. Low fecal proteolytic activity is consistent with EPI.
   A. Fecal proteolytic activity is best measured using dyed protein substrates such as azocasein or by

radial enzyme diffusion into agar gels containing casein substrate.

B. Because dogs with normal pancreatic function occasionally pass feces with low proteolytic activity, repeated determinations must be made, or the test can be performed on a single sample collected after feeding crude soybean meal for 2 days.

C. Feces is collected on each of 3 consecutive days and immediately frozen for shipment to the laboratory.
   1. Normal 3-day mean azocasein hydrolysis is 19–200 azocasein U/g.
   2. Normal 3-day mean radial enzyme diffusion is 6–24 mm.

D. Because the serum TLI assay is more reliable and practical, it is preferred over fecal proteolytic assays for diagnosis of EPI.

V. Measurement of serum folate and cobalamin (vitamin B_{12}) is indicated.
   A. Serum folate levels may be increased as a result of increased synthesis of folate by excessive numbers of bacteria and intestinal acidification. Normal serum folate levels are 6.7–17.4 µg/L.
   B. Cobalamin levels may be decreased because bacteria can utilize or bind the vitamin, making it unavailable for absorption. Normal serum cobalamin levels are 225–660 ng/L.

Differential Diagnosis

I. The major considerations in the differential diagnosis for EPI are the small intestinal malabsorptive diseases, in particular diffuse, infiltrative diseases (see Chap. 32).

II. Serum TLI can be used to distinguish EPI from malabsorptive disorders.

Treatment

I. Goals
   A. To replace pancreatic digestive enzymes
   B. To restore nutritional balance

II. Digestive enzyme replacement
   A. Give 2 teaspoonfuls of powdered non–enteric-coated preparation per 20 kg with each meal (as a starting dose).
      1. Preincubation of food with enzyme powder for 30 minutes prior to feeding does not improve the effectiveness.
      2. Enteric-coated preparations have generally been ineffective or less effective than powdered pancreatic extracts.
      3. Addition of bile salts, antacids, or sodium bicarbonate to the enzyme supplement does not improve fat absorption.
      4. Tablet formulations of pancreatic enzymes should be crushed prior to feeding.
   B. Enzymes are mixed with a maintenance dog food immediately prior to feeding.
   C. Two meals a day are usually adequate to promote weight gain.

1. Dogs often gain 0.5–1 kg per week.
2. Diarrhea often disappears within a few days.
3. Maintenance of a strict dietary routine is imperative.

D. Once clinical improvement is noticed, a minimum effective dose of enzyme supplement is determined that will prevent return of clinical signs.
   1. This varies from dog to dog and also between batches of enzyme replacement.
   2. Most large dogs require at least 1 teaspoonful of enzyme supplement per meal.
   3. One meal per day may be adequate in some dogs.

III. Nutritional support
   A. Regular maintenance dog food is usually adequate for long-term feeding when given with appropriate enzyme replacement.
   B. A low-fat (below 20 g/1000 kcal metabolizable energy), highly digestible diet also has been recommended (Simpson JW et al., 1994).
      1. This type of diet may be helpful for the initial stabilization period (4 months) and for long-term maintenance if response to enzyme supplementation is incomplete.
      2. A recent study showed that feeding a low-fat diet did not significantly alleviate clinical signs (Westermarck et al., 1995).
   C. High-fiber diets are avoided because dietary fiber impairs pancreatic enzyme activity in vitro.
   D. Consider fat-soluble vitamin supplementation.
      1. Tocopherol 500 IU PO SID with food for 1 month
      2. Cobalamin 250 µg IM, SQ every 7 days for several weeks
   E. Medium-chain triglyceride oil (1–2 ml/kg/day) may be given with a severely restricted-fat diet if steatorrhea persists or if weight gain does not occur in response to therapy.

IV. Reduction of gastric acid secretion
   A. Not recommended for routine use (expensive)
   B. May inhibit the activity of gastric lipase
   C. Cimetidine 10 mg/kg PO or ranitidine 2 mg/kg PO 30 minutes preprandially

V. Antibiotic therapy
   A. Bacterial overgrowth causing persistent diarrhea may improve after antimicrobial therapy with tetracycline, tylosin, or metronidazole (see Chap. 32).
   B. Bacterial overgrowth that has persisted for some time may be only partially reversible even with prolonged antibiotic therapy.

VI. Glucocorticoid therapy
   A. If there is a poor response to the previously mentioned treatments, prednisolone at 1–2 mg/kg PO BID for 7–14 days may be beneficial.
   B. Lymphocytic-plasmacytic gastroenteritis may coexist with EPI.

Patient Monitoring

I. Monitor body weight weekly.

II. Frequency of bowel movements decreases and fecal

consistency improves within the first week of effective therapy.

III. EPI may never be adequately controlled in some dogs despite all these measures.

IV. If response to treatment is incomplete, consider the following.
   A. Change to a low-fat, highly digestible diet and to a different brand of pancreatic enzymes.
   B. Administer antibiotics for small intestinal bacterial overgrowth.
   C. Administer an oral H$_2$-receptor blocker.
   D. Reconsider diagnosis and/or rule out concurrent disease by endoscopic biopsies of the small intestine.

V. Lifelong treatment is usually required.

VI. Prognosis is generally good.
   A. Because EPI develops mostly in large breeds and requires lifelong treatment, the costs of treatment are of great importance to the owner.
   B. Some dogs may fail to regain full body weight, although signs of diarrhea and polyphagia resolve.
   C. A high prevalence (10%) of fatal mesenteric torsion has been observed in German shepherd dogs with EPI in Finland (Westermarck and Rimaila-Parnanen, 1989).

VII. Management of concurrent EPI and diabetes mellitus as a result of chronic pancreatitis is difficult.

Exocrine Pancreatic Insufficiency in Cats

Definition and Causes

I. Exocrine pancreatic insufficiency (EPI) results from inadequate secretion of digestive enzymes by the pancreas.

II. Most of the feline cases result from loss of acinar cells because of end-stage chronic pancreatitis.

III. Other causes are rare.
   A. Idiopathic pancreatic acinar atrophy
   B. Obstruction of the pancreatic duct by a pancreatic or other abdominal mass
   C. Iatrogenic, following proximal duodenal resection and cholecystoduodenostomy
   D. Pancreatic fluke infestation (*Eurytrema procyonis*)

Pathophysiology

I. Insufficient enzyme secretion results in similar changes as noted for canine EPI.

II. Because the most common cause of EPI in cats is chronic pancreatitis, feline EPI may be accompanied by diabetes mellitus.

III. Because the pancreas is the major source of intrinsic factor, serum levels of cobalamin are markedly decreased in the cat as compared with the dog.

Clinical Signs

I. Polyphagia
II. Weight loss and/or emaciation

III. Diarrhea
   A. Large amounts of semiformed feces
   B. Severe watery diarrhea possible
   C. Tan to gray feces

IV. Steatorrhea with greasy soiling of the hair coat

V. Vitamin K responsive coagulopathy (rare)

Diagnosis

I. Clinical signs are nonspecific and may occur with malabsorption due to any cause.

II. Physical exam reveals poor body condition.

III. Routine hematology, serum chemistries, urinalysis, and abdominal radiographs are usually unremarkable.
   A. Alanine aminotransferase and alkaline phosphatase may be mildly increased.
   B. Serum cholesterol and/or triglyceride levels may be mildly decreased.

IV. A significant laboratory finding is severely low serum cobalamin concentrations in most cases.
   A. The reference range for healthy pet cats is 200–1680 ng/L.
   B. Serum cobalamin was undetectable (<27 ng/L) in 10 of 11 cats with low feline TLI concentrations (≤8 μg/L).

V. Diagnostic tests to assess pancreatic function include the following.
   A. Feline-specific trypsin-like immunoassay
      1. A radioimmunoassay for the determination of feline trypsin-like immunoreactivity has been established and validated.
      2. The reference range for healthy cats is 17–49 μg/L.
      3. Cats with feline TLI concentrations ≤8 μg/L have a presumptive diagnosis of EPI.
   B. Fecal proteolytic activity measured by an azoprotein or radial enzyme diffusion method
      1. As in dogs, fecal proteolytic activity is consistently low in most cats with EPI.
      2. At least three fecal samples are assayed, preferably from consecutive days.
      3. Samples must be frozen immediately and shipped overnight to avoid falsely low readings.
      4. This test is more widely available for the diagnosis of EPI in cats.

VI. Histopathologic examination is the only way to definitively confirm EPI.

Differential Diagnosis

I. Diabetes mellitus (± present concurrently)
II. Hyperthyroidism
III. Primary enteropathies
   A. Intestinal lymphosarcoma
   B. Inflammatory bowel disease

Treatment

I. Most cats can be managed successfully by dietary supplementation with pancreatic enzymes.

A. A powdered, non–enteric-coated form of pancreatic enzymes is recommended.

B. The initial dose is 0.5 teaspoon per 5 kg body weight mixed with maintenance food.

C. As soon as clinical improvement is noted, the dose is decreased to the minimum effective dose.

D. Diarrhea usually resolves in 2–3 days.

E. The cat's daily caloric needs are calculated and fed as 2–3 meals per day.
   1. Up to 20% more than calculated maintenance requirements are fed initially.
   2. The quantity fed is then adjusted to maintain an ideal body weight.

II. If weight gain or control of diarrhea is suboptimal, consider these measures.

A. Antibiotic trial for small intestinal bacterial overgrowth
   1. Oxytetracycline 50–100 mg PO BID for 14 days
   2. Metronidazole 25–100 mg PO BID for 14 days

B. Dietary modification
   1. Consider low-fat diet; avoid high-fiber diet.
   2. Consider adding MCT oil if EPI is unresponsive to other treatments.

C. Vitamin supplementation
   1. Oral supplementation with fat-soluble vitamins
   2. Parenteral vitamin K_1 5–20 mg SQ BID for coagulopathy
   3. Tocopherol 30–100 IU/day PO with food
   4. Cobalamin 100 μg SQ every 7 days for 1 month

D. Glucocorticoid therapy for associated small intestinal disease
   1. Endoscopic small intestinal biopsies can help in the diagnosis of concurrent enteropathy.
   2. Consider a prednisolone trial at 5 mg PO BID for 4–6 weeks.

Patient Monitoring

I. Lifelong treatment is required.

II. Monitoring and response to treatment are similar as for dogs with EPI.

PARASITES

Definition and Causes

I. Pancreatic flukes in cats are the result of infection with *Eurytrema procyonis*, a parasite of the pancreatic duct of the raccoon.

II. Cats may contract *E. procyonis* via ingestion of an intermediate host, e.g., a snail or a grasshopper.

Pathophysiology

I. Early reports in domestic cats suggested that these trematodes were generally non-pathogenic.

II. However, they may cause dilatation and obstruction of the pancreatic ducts in cats, leading to atrophy and fibrosis.

III. Duct obstruction together with atrophy and fibrosis of the pancreas may severely decrease pancreatic secretory capacity.

Clinical Signs

I. Low levels of infection may be clinically imperceptible.

II. Weight loss and intermittent vomiting, consistent with pancreatitis, have been reported in one cat (Anderson et al., 1987).

Diagnosis

I. Infection may be an incidental finding based on observation of characteristic eggs in the feces, i.e., dicrocoeliid eggs with a single operculum.

II. Histologic evidence of trematodes in pancreatic tissue biopsies is diagnostic.

Differential Diagnosis

I. Chronic pancreatitis

II. Exocrine pancreatic insufficiency

Treatment and Monitoring

I. Treatment with fenbendazole (30 mg/kg/day PO for 6 days) has been effective.

II. Praziquantel 40 mg/kg PO SID for 3 days is also a logical choice.

III. The infected cat is not a significant zoonotic risk.

NEOPLASIA

Definition and Causes

I. Tumors of the exocrine pancreas are rare in both dogs and cats.
   A. Benign and malignant neoplasms occur with similar frequency (5.5% of nonhematopoietic tumors) in cats (Bunch, 1992).
   B. In dogs, malignant tumors constitute 0.6% of all tumors (Bunch, 1992).
   C. Pancreatic tumors are a solitary mass in 50% of affected dogs (Anderson and Johnson, 1967). The remaining dogs have numerous nodules throughout the pancreas.

II. Benign tumors include the following.
   A. Nodular hyperplasia
   B. Adenoma (rare)

III. Malignant tumors are adenocarcinomas (rare in cats).
   A. Duct cell origin
   B. Acinar cell origin (most common in cats)

IV. Functional islet cell tumors (insulinoma) are discussed in Chap. 45.

V. Metastatic neoplasms are very rare.

VI. The etiology of pancreatic tumors is unknown.

Pathophysiology

I. Benign pancreatic neoplasms usually do not cause clinical signs and are incidental findings.
II. Malignant neoplasms are very aggressive.
   A. They have often metastasized to the duodenal wall, liver, regional lymph nodes, mesentery, stomach, or lungs (less common) at the time of presentation.
   B. Affected animals often have abnormalities in liver enzyme activities because of associated obstruction of the bile ducts or widespread hepatic metastasis.
   C. Expansive growth of the neoplasm may cause duodenal invasion and obstruction of gastric outflow or obstruction of the common bile duct with jaundice.
III. Occasionally, dogs have concurrent signs of diabetes mellitus or exocrine pancreatic insufficiency (Bright, 1985).

Clinical Signs

I. Signalment
   A. Aged dogs and cats, possible predilection in Airedale and spaniel breeds
   B. No obvious gender predilection
II. Clinical signs and physical examination findings
   A. Nonspecific signs: weight loss, depression, anorexia, dehydration, fever, and abdominal pain
   B. Vomiting uncommon, often terminal occurrence
   C. ± Palpable mass in the right cranial abdomen and ascites
   D. ± Jaundice
   E. Rarely panniculitis with subcutaneous swellings and shifting lameness (Brown et al., 1994)
   F. Progressive, nonscarring, alopecic dermatologic disease with acinar adenocarcinoma in cats (Brooks et al., 1994)

Diagnosis

I. History and clinical signs are often nonspecific.
II. Hemogram may be indistinguishable from that of acute pancreatitis.
III. Biochemical test results reveal pancreatic and hepatic abnormalities.
   A. Serum lipase levels may be extremely elevated in dogs; a level 25 times normal is probably diagnostic for exocrine pancreatic carcinoma (Fineman et al., 1994).
   B. Pancreatic carcinoma (metastatic and localized) has been reported in association with diabetes mellitus in cats.
IV. Small pancreatic masses are often missed on survey radiographs and ultrasonography because of overlying gas-filled small intestinal loops.
   A. Large pancreatic masses may cause ventrolateral displacement of the duodenum and separation of the transverse colon and gastric body by an increased soft tissue opacity.
   B. The displaced duodenum can be seen only if air or barium contrast material fills the intestinal lumen.
   C. Liver metastases also may be detected.
   D. Thoracic radiographs may indicate pulmonary metastases.
V. Rarely, analysis of abdominal effusion reveals carcinoma cells.
VI. Exploratory celiotomy with biopsy and histopathology is necessary for a definitive diagnosis.

Differential Diagnosis

I. Rule out chronic pancreatitis.
II. Pancreatic paraneoplastic alopecia in cats must be differentiated from feline hyperadrenocorticism, feline symmetrical alopecia, self-induced alopecia, and telogen defluxion.

Treatment and Monitoring

I. Surgical extirpation is indicated for a single mass.
II. Surgical salvage procedures may be performed.
   A. Nonresectable but obstructive tumors
      1. Cholecystojejunostomy for obstruction of common bile duct
      2. Gastrojejunostomy to redirect gastric outflow
   B. May transiently improve the quality of life (<6 months)
III. Chemotherapy has not been described in cats and dogs.
IV. The prognosis for animals with carcinomas is extremely poor; survival for >1 year after diagnosis has not been reported.

Bibliography

Akol KG, Washabau RJ, Saunders HM, Hendrick MJ: Acute pancreatitis in cats with hepatic lipidosis. J Vet Intern Med 7:205, 1993

Anderson NV, Johnson KH: Pancreatic carcinoma in the dog. J Am Vet Med Assoc 150:286, 1967

Anderson WI, Georgi ME, Car BD: Pancreatic atrophy and fibrosis associated with Eurytrema procyonis in a domestic cat. Vet Rec 120:235, 1987

Beechey-Newman N, Simpson KW, Rae D et al: Specific diagnosis of canine acute pancreatitis by an ELISA for trypsinogen activation peptide. J Vet Intern Med 8:151, 1994

Bellah JR, Bell G: Serum amylase and lipase activities after exploratory laparotomy in dogs. Am J Vet Res 50:1638, 1989

Boari A, Williams DA, Famigli-Bergamini P: Observations on exocrine pancreatic insufficiency in a family of English setter dogs. J Small Anim Pract 35:247, 1994

Bright JM: Pancreatic adenocarcinoma in a dog with maldigestion syndrome. J Am Vet Med Assoc 187:420, 1985

Brooks DG, Campbell KL, Dennis JS et al: Pancreatic paraneoplastic alopecia in three cats. J Am Anim Hosp Assoc 30:557, 1994

Brown PJ, Mason KV, Merrett DJ et al: Multifocal necrotizing steatitis associated with pancreatic carcinoma in three dogs. J Small Anim Pract 35:129, 1994

Bunch SE: Diseases of the exocrine pancreas. p. 459. In Morgan RV (ed): Handbook of Small Animal Practice. 2nd Ed. Churchill Livingstone, New York, 1992

Cook AK, Breitschwerdt EB, Levine JF et al: Risk factors associated with acute pancreatitis in dogs: 101 cases (1985–1990). J Am Vet Med Assoc 203:673, 1993

Dill-Macky E: Pancreatic diseases of cats. Compend Contin Educ Pract Vet 15:589, 1993

Edwards DF, Bauer MS, Walker MA et al: Pancreatic masses in seven dogs following acute pancreatitis. J Am Anim Hosp Assoc 26:189, 1990

Fineman L, DeNicola D, Bruyette D et al: Serum lipase concentrations in dogs with pancreatic carcinoma. Proc Vet Cancer Soc 14:16, 1994

Fittschen C, Bellamy JEC: Prednisone treatment alters the serum amylase and lipase activities in normal dogs without causing pancreatitis. Can J Comp Med 48:136, 1984

Fox JN, Mosley JG, Vogler GA et al: Pancreatic function in domestic cats with pancreatic fluke infection. J Am Vet Med Assoc 178:58, 1981

Fyfe JC: Feline intrinsic factor (IF) is pancreatic in origin and mediates ileal cobalamin (cbl). J Vet Intern Med 7:133, 1993

Georgi JR, Georgi ME: Trematodes. p. 101. In Georgi JR, Georgi ME (eds): Canine Clinical Parasitology. Lea & Febiger, Philadelphia, 1992

Hall EJ, Bond PM, McLean C et al: A survey of the diagnosis and treatment of canine exocrine pancreatic insufficiency. J Small Anim Pract 32:613, 1991

Hall JA, Macy DW, Husted PW: Acute canine pancreatitis. Compend Contin Educ Pract Vet 10:403, 1988

Hansen JF, Carpenter RH: Fatal acute systemic anaphylaxis and hemorrhagic pancreatitis following asparaginase treatment in a dog. J Am Anim Hosp Assoc 19:977, 1983

Harrington DP, Jones BD, Gross ME et al: Laparoscopic biopsy of the normal canine pancreas. J Vet Intern Med 10:156, 1996

Hess RS, Washabau RJ, Van Winkle TJ, Shofer FS: Risk factor analysis of canine acute pancreatitis. J Vet Intern Med 10:156, 1996

Hill RC, Van Winkle TJ: Acute necrotizing pancreatitis and acute suppurative pancreatitis in the cat. A retrospective study of 40 cases (1976–1989). J Vet Intern Med 7:25, 1993

Hines BL, Salisbury SK, Jakovljevic S, DeNicola DB: Pancreatic pseudocyst associated with chronic-active necrotizing pancreatitis in a cat. J Am Anim Hosp Assoc 32:147, 1996

Keller ET: High serum trypsin-like immunoreactivity secondary to pancreatitis in a dog with exocrine pancreatic insufficiency. J Am Vet Med Assoc 196:623, 1990

Medinger TL, Burchfield T, Williams DA: Assay of trypsin-like immunoreactivity (TLI) in feline serum. J Vet Intern Med 7:133, 1993

Moriello KA, Bowen D, Meyer DJ: Acute pancreatitis in two dogs given azathioprine and prednisone. J Am Vet Med Assoc 191:695, 1987

Murtaugh RJ, Herring DS, Jacobs RM et al: Pancreatic ultrasonography in dogs with experimentally induced acute pancreatitis. Vet Radiol 26:27, 1985

Nemzek JA, Walshaw R, Hauptman JG: Mesenteric volvulus in the dog: a retrospective study. J Am Anim Hosp Assoc 29:357, 1993

Ogilvie GK, Moore AS: Tumors of the exocrine pancreas. p. 365. In Ogilvie GK, Moore AS (eds): Managing the Veterinary Cancer Patient. Veterinary Learning Systems, Trenton, New Jersey, 1995

Parent C, Washabau RJ, Williams DA et al: Serum trypsin-like immunoreactivity, amylase and lipase in the diagnosis of feline acute pancreatitis. J Vet Intern Med 9:194, 1995

Parent J: Effects of dexamethasone on pancreatic tissue and on serum amylase and lipase activities in dogs. J Am Vet Med Assoc 180:743, 1982

Paterson S: Panniculitis associated with pancreatic necrosis in a dog. J Small Anim Pract 35:116, 1994

Perry LA, Williams DA, Pidgeon GL et al: Exocrine pancreatic

insufficiency with associated coagulopathy in a cat. J Am Anim Hosp Assoc 27:109, 1991

Roudebush P, Schmidt DA: Fenbendazole for treatment of pancreatic fluke infection in a cat. J Am Vet Med Assoc 180:545, 1982

Rutgers C, Herring DS, Orton EC: Pancreatic pseudocyst associated with acute pancreatitis in a dog: ultrasonographic diagnosis. J Am Anim Hosp Assoc 21:411, 1985

Salisbury SK, Lantz GC, Nelson RW et al: Pancreatic abscess in dogs: six cases (1978–1986). J Am Vet Med Assoc 193:1104, 1988

Sheldon WG: Pancreatic flukes (*Eurytrema procyonis*) in domestic cats. J Am Vet Med Assoc 148:251, 1966

Simpson JW, Maskell IE, Quigg J, Markwell PJ: Long term management of canine exocrine pancreatic insufficiency. J Small Anim Pract 35:133, 1994

Simpson KW: Current concepts of the pathogenesis and pathophysiology of acute pancreatitis in the dog and cat. Compend Contin Educ Pract Vet 15:247, 1993

Simpson KW, Morton DB, Batt RM: Effect of exocrine pancreatic insufficiency on cobalamin absorption in dogs. Am J Vet Res 50:1233, 1989

Simpson KW, Shiroma JT, Biller DS et al: Ante mortem diagnosis of pancreatitis in four cats. J Small Anim Pract 35:93, 1994

Steiner JM, Williams DA: Validation of a radioimmunoassay for feline trypsin-like immunoreactivity (FTLI) and serum cobalamin and folate concentrations in cats with exocrine pancreatic insufficiency (EPI). J Vet Intern Med 9:193, 1995

Steiner JM, Williams DA: Feline trypsinlike immunoreactivity in feline exocrine pancreatic disease. Compend Contin Educ Pract Vet 18:543, 1996

Stewart AF: Pancreatitis in dogs and cats: cause, pathogenesis, diagnosis, and treatment. Compend Contin Educ Pract Vet 16:1423, 1994

Strombeck DR, Farver T, Kaneko JJ: Serum amylase and lipase activities in the diagnosis of pancreatitis in dogs. Am J Vet Res 42:1966, 1981

Van Winkle TJ, Hill RC: Pancreatic necrosis and pancreatitis in domestic cats: a retrospective of 47 cases. Proc Am Coll Vet Pathol 40:218, 1989

Westermarck E, Rimaila-Parnanen E: Mesenteric torsion in dogs with exocrine pancreatic insufficiency: 21 cases (1978–1987). J Am Vet Med Assoc 195:1404, 1989

Westermarck E, Batt RM, Vaillant C, Wiberg M: Sequential study of pancreatic structure and function during development of pancreatic acinar atrophy in a German shepherd dog. Am J Vet Res 54:1088, 1993

Westermarck E, Junttila JT, Wiberg ME: Role of low dietary fat in the treatment of dogs with exocrine pancreatic insufficiency. Am J Vet Res 56:600, 1995

Whitney MS: The laboratory assessment of canine and feline pancreatitis. Vet Med 88:1045, 1993

Williams DA: Acute pancreatitis. p. 631. In Kirk RW (ed): Current Veterinary Therapy XI: Small Animal Practice. WB Saunders, Philadelphia, 1992

Williams DA: Diagnosis and management of pancreatitis. J Small Anim Pract 35:445, 1994

Williams DA: Exocrine pancreatic disease. p. 1372. In Ettinger SJ, Feldman EC (eds): Textbook of Veterinary Internal Medicine. 4th Ed. WB Saunders, Philadelphia, 1995a

Williams DA: Feline exocrine pancreatic insufficiency. p. 732. In Bonagura JD (ed): Kirk's Current Veterinary Therapy XII. WB Saunders, Philadelphia, 1995b

Williams DA, Minnich F: Canine exocrine pancreatic insufficiency: a survey of 640 cases diagnosed by assay of serum trypsin-like immunoreactivity. J Vet Intern Med 4:123, 1990

Williams DA, Reed SD, Perry LA: Fecal proteolytic activity in clinically normal cats and in a cat with exocrine pancreatic insufficiency. J Am Vet Med Assoc 197:210, 1990

Williams DA, Waters CB, Adams LG et al: Serum trypsin-like immunoreactivity, amylase and lipase following administration of prednisone to dogs. J Vet Intern Med 9:193, 1995

Williams DA, Melgarejo T, Henderson J, Kazacos E: Serum trypsin-like immunoreactivity (TLI), trypsinogen activation peptides (TAP), amylase and lipase in canine experimental pancreatitis. J Vet Intern Med 10:159, 1996

Wolfsheimer KJ, Hedlund CS, Pechman RD: Pancreatic pseudocyst in a dog with chronic pancreatitis. Canine Pract 16(1):6, 1991

36

Diseases of the Anus and Perineum

D. J. Krahwinkel, Jr.

CONGENITAL DISORDERS

Atresia Ani

Definition

I. It is a congenital disease of puppies and kittens in which the rectum does not communicate with the anal opening, resulting in fecal retention.
II. Anatomically, there are several different configurations possible, but all result in the same physiologic disease (Matthiesen and Marretta, 1993).

Pathophysiology

I. Failure of fecal material to exit the rectum
II. Constipation and obstipation, resulting in megacolon
III. Bowel stasis
IV. Severe abdominal enlargement

Clinical Signs

I. Signs begin to develop at 2–4 weeks of age.
II. Abdominal distention occurs, often with bulging of the perineum.
III. Anorexia and failure to grow may be noted.
IV. Absence of defecation is classic.

Diagnosis

I. It is based on age of the animal and clinical signs.
II. Physical examination fails to locate a perforate anal opening.
III. Radiographs reveal a megacolon.

Treatment

I. The goal is to restore continuity of the rectum and anal canal, regardless of the type of atresia.
II. Incise the skin over the anus, being careful to preserve the anal sphincter.
III. Locate the blind end of the rectal pouch and mobilize it.
IV. Advance the rectal pouch to the level of the anal opening.
V. Open the terminal end of the rectal pouch.
VI. Suture the opened rectum to the skin at the anal opening.

Patient Monitoring

I. Fecal incontinence is common, despite meticulous technique.
II. Anal stricture can occur at the new mucocutaneous junction.
III. Megacolon may not resolve, despite surgical correction.
IV. Infection and dehiscence of the suture line can occur.

Anogenital Cleft

Definition

I. An embryologic deformity involving the anus and the urogenital tract
II. Failure of cleavage of the embryonic caudal cloaca, resulting in a common fecal and urine opening

Clinical Signs

I. Urine and feces pass through a common skin opening.
II. Affected animals are predisposed to urinary tract infections.
III. Frequent soiling of the perineum is common.
IV. If there is urinary and fecal continence, there may be minimal clinical signs.

Diagnosis

I. Physical examination of the perineal region reveals a mucosal-lined cleft containing both the urethra and the anus.

II. Probe or catheterize the rectal and urethral openings to confirm their location.
III. Check the animal for other congenital defects, such as hernias or cleft palate.

Treatment

I. Confirm competence of the anal sphincter.
II. Confirm location of the urethral opening.
III. Surgically create laterally based, bilateral skin flaps (Bellenger and Canfield, 1993).
IV. Incise tissue between the rectal tube and the urethra.
V. Advance skin flaps medially and suture on the midline to re-form the perineum.

Patient Monitoring

I. Fecal incontinence or anal stricture may occur postoperatively.
II. Incisional infection and dehiscence are often problems.
III. Recurrent urinary tract infections occur if the urethra and anal canal are not separated.
IV. Urine scalding and/or dermatitis from fecal soiling occur in animals that are incontinent.

DEGENERATIVE DISORDERS

Perineal Hernia

Definition

I. It occurs from breakdown of the muscular diaphragm of the pelvis (coccygeus, levator ani, external anal sphincter muscles).
II. Pelvic and abdominal tissues and organs (fat, prostate, urinary bladder, rectum) herniate into the perineum.

Causes

I. Gonadal hormone imbalance (Mann, 1993)
   A. Excess estrogen from aging testes causes relaxation of musculature.
   B. Deficiency of androgenic steroids results in weakening of musculature.
II. Muscular atrophy resulting from increased age, nerve damage, or rudimentary tail
III. Prostatic hypertrophy with tenesmus
IV. Rectal diseases such as deviation, sacculation, or diverticulum, resulting in constipation and tenesmus (Krahwinkel, 1983)
V. Combinations of the preceding causes

Pathophysiology

I. Poorly established sequence of events
II. Weakening or breakdown of pelvic muscles, usually between external anal sphincter and levator ani muscles (can occur between levator ani and coccygeus muscles)

III. Retroperitoneal fat pushing through muscle defect
IV. Loss of support of rectal wall by pelvic muscles
V. Increased incidence of straining to defecate and resulting constipation
VI. Deviation, sacculation, or diverticulation of the rectum
VII. Complete breakdown of musculature, with herniation of fat, prostate, bladder, rectum

Clinical Signs

I. It occurs most frequently in older male dogs (rarely in females or in cats).
II. The Boston terrier, boxer, collie, corgi, Old English sheepdog, Pekingese, and kelpie are predisposed (Bellenger and Canfield, 1993).
III. Common signs are constipation, tenesmus, obstipation, and dyschezia.
IV. Bilateral or unilateral reducible perineal swelling develops; unilateral lesions affect the right side in 68% of cases and the left side in 32% of cases (Bellenger and Canfield, 1993).
V. Stranguria and hematuria may develop when the urinary bladder is trapped in the hernia.
VI. In cats, it may be associated with perineal urethrostomy, megacolon, and perineal masses (Welches et al., 1992).

Diagnosis

I. Species, age, and breed of animal
II. Presence of reducible perineal mass
III. Rectal exam revealing absence of muscular pelvic diaphragm
IV. Barium enema showing rectal contents within hernia
V. Retrograde urethrocystogram displaying urinary bladder within hernia

Differential Diagnosis

I. Perineal tumors
II. Hematoma, seroma, or prostatic cyst
III. Rectal sacculation or deviation without perineal hernia

Treatment

I. Medical management is used preoperatively or in animals that are poor surgical risks.
   A. Low-residue diet for reduced fecal volume
   B. Fecal softeners and/or enemas to promote bowel evacuation (dioctyl sodium sulfosuccinate 100–200 mg PO daily)
   C. Catheterization of bladder if retroflexed into hernia
   D. Manual emptying of rectum as needed
   E. Supportive care of nutrition and prevention of geriatric diseases
II. Surgical treatment is preferred in most cases.
   A. Preoperative preparation
      1. Obtain a complete blood count, chemistry panel, and urinalysis.

2. Start fecal softeners 1–2 days before surgery.
3. Empty the rectum manually, place a cotton ball in it, and place a pursestring suture around the anus.
4. Give IV cefoxitin (20 mg/kg) at the time of anesthetic induction; repeat after 90 minutes.
5. Catheterize the urinary bladder.

B. Standard herniorrhaphy
1. A curved incision is made from the base of the tail ventrally over the hernia.
2. The hernia sac is opened to reveal hernia contents.
3. Necrotic fat is excised, and contents of the hernia are reduced into the pelvic and abdominal cavities.
4. Monofilament absorbable sutures are preplaced dorsally between coccygeus and anal sphincter muscles (usually 3–5 sutures).
5. Sutures are preplaced ventrally between the anal sphincter and internal obturator medially and the coccygeus and internal obturator laterally (usually 3–5 additional sutures).
6. Pudendal nerve and vessels are identified on the surface of the internal obturator muscle and avoided during suture placement.
7. The urethra (with catheter in place) is palpated and pushed toward the opposite side to avoid ligation.
8. Sutures are all tied, and the hernia opening is evaluated.
9. If necessary, sutures can be placed through the sacrotuberous ligament (being careful to avoid the sciatic nerve).
10. Interrupted absorbable sutures are placed in the deep subcutaneous fascia to reinforce the primary closure.
11. Skin is closed with interrupted monofilament sutures. (Excess skin can be excised).
12. Bilateral hernias can be repaired simultaneously or sequentially, 4–6 weeks apart.
13. Castration may be performed at the time of herniorrhaphy, but there is no conclusive evidence that castration is of value, except for the treatment of prostatomegaly.

C. Internal obturator muscle transposition
1. It is the preferred procedure because of the decreased rate of reherniation.
2. A standard approach is used as described earlier.
3. The internal obturator muscle attachment to the caudal ischium is severed.
4. The caudal half of muscle belly is elevated from the floor of the pelvis (to the level of the obturator foramen).
5. Muscle is used as a flap and sutured into the defect between the anal sphincter and the coccygeus (Fig. 36–1) (Bellenger and Canfield, 1993).
6. Suturing materials and techniques are as described previously.

D. Postoperative care
1. Low-residue diet to reduce fecal volume

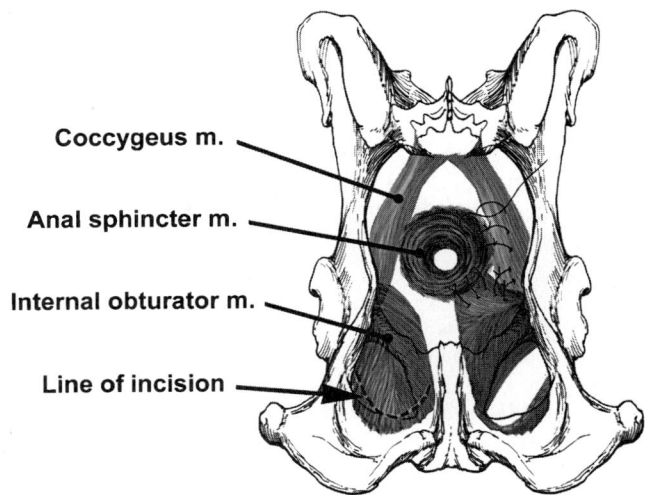

Coccygeus m.
Anal sphincter m.
Internal obturator m.
Line of incision

Figure 36–1. Obturator muscle is used as a flap and sutured to the external anal sphincter and coccygeus muscles to repair a perineal hernia. (Courtesy of University of Tennessee College of Veterinary Medicine.)

2. Fecal softeners for 4–6 weeks to reduce straining
3. Local warm compresses to reduce swelling

Patient Monitoring

I. Potential postoperative complications are as follows.
A. Femoral and tibial nerve paralysis from hyperextension of stifle and pressure at surgery
B. Infection from contaminated surgical site
C. Fecal incontinence from damage of pudendal or caudal rectal nerves
D. Urinary obstruction from sutures placed around or through pelvic urethra
E. Sciatic paralysis as a result of damage to sciatic nerve when sutures were placed around the sacrotuberous ligament
F. Straining owing to retention of fecal balls in rectal sacculation
G. Rectal prolapse when rectal sacculations are inverted during surgery
H. Hernia recurrence from poor technique, poor healing, or additional tissue breakdown
I. Herniation of opposite side (a common occurrence)
II. The recurrence rate can be as high as 45% (Bellenger and Canfield, 1993).

INFLAMMATORY DISEASES

Perianal Fistula (Anal Furunculosis)

Definition

A chronic and debilitating ulcerative disease of the perianal region characterized by the formation of sinus and fistulous tracts

Causes

I. Several theories, but none have been proved
II. Moist, contaminated environment created by a broad-based, low-slung tail carriage
III. Hypothyroidism (Killingsworth et al., 1988)
IV. Immunologic defect (Day, 1993)
V. Bacterial pyodermatitis

Pathophysiology

I. Inflammation of the perianal epidermis (Washabau and Brockman, 1995)
II. Progression of disease into the adnexal structures
III. Secondary superficial necrosis and ulceration
IV. Progressive involvement, resulting in deep inflammation and creation of subcutaneous sinus tracts
V. Deeper extension of inflammation and necrosis, causing formation of fistulas from perianal area into the anal mucosa
VI. Anal sacs secondarily involved

Clinical Signs

I. Most common in German shepherd dogs; also in other breeds, especially Irish setters
II. Anorexia, weight loss, chronic debilitation
III. Tenesmus, dyschezia, hematochezia
IV. Fecal incontinence in severe cases
V. Malodorous anorectal discharge
VI. Very painful upon examination (may require sedation or anesthesia)

Diagnosis

I. History of suspicious clinical signs in a predisposed breed
II. Examination revealing mild to severe lesions
   A. Small draining sinuses
   B. Fistulous tracts from perianal skin to anal mucosa
   C. Ulceration and erosion of perianal skin
   D. Any or all of the preceding in various stages
III. Rectal palpation of anal structure
IV. Histopathologic exam: hidradenitis and necrotizing pyogranulomatous inflammation

Differential Diagnosis

I. Perianal adenocarcinoma
II. Ruptured anal sac
III. Granulomas secondary to *Pythium insidiosum* (Ellison, 1995)

Treatment

I. Medical therapy
   A. Not usually successful
   B. Hair removal, cleansing with antibacterial solution (povidone-iodine or chlorhexidine), and hydrotherapy
   C. Anti-inflammatory doses of prednisolone (1 mg/kg PO daily) in combination with oral antibiotics (cephalexin 20 mg/kg TID)
   D. Immunosuppression by cyclosporine for 4 weeks in combination with oral cephalexin (Matthews and Sukhiami, 1996)
   E. Elevation of tail to permit aeration
II. Surgical therapy (Ellison, 1995)
   A. The goal is to expose and remove the lining of sinuses and fistulas and debride ulcerative lesions.
   B. Many cases require multiple treatments for success.
   C. A variable success rate occurs with different treatments.
   D. Chemical cauterization may be effective in mild cases.
      1. Agents include Lugol's solution, silver nitrate, or phenol.
      2. It requires opening of all sinuses and fistulas.
   E. Deroofing and fulguration are recommended.
      1. Anal sacculectomy is performed.
      2. Tracts are probed and opened by removing the roof of each tract.
      3. The lining of each lesion is electrofulgurated or electrocoagulated.
      4. Incisions are left to heal by second intention.
   F. Cryosurgery has been used successfully.
      1. All tracts are probed and surgically opened.
      2. Nitrous oxide or liquid nitrogen is used to freeze all ulcerative lesions and the lining of all tracts.
      3. Healing is by second intention.
   G. Laser excision is a relatively new treatment.
      1. Sinuses and fistulas are probed and opened.
      2. Carbon dioxide or Nd:YAG laser is used to excise tract linings and cauterize all ulcerative lesions.
      3. It has a higher success rate (95%) than some other treatments.
   H. Surgical excision is used on superficial lesions.
      1. A circular incision is made peripheral to diseased tissue.
      2. A second circular incision is made in the margin of healthy anal mucosa.
      3. All diseased tissue between the two incisions is excised; care is taken to preserve the anal sphincter muscle.
      4. Anal sacs are removed.
      5. Skin margins are sutured to the anal mucosa.
      6. There is a high rate of fecal incontinence postoperatively.
   I. Rectal pull-through is used for severe cases (Matthiesen and Marretta, 1993).
      1. Salvage procedure for severe disease and for rectal stricture
      2. Circular incision peripheral to all diseased margins
      3. Second circular incision at anal mucosa margin
      4. Dissection around anal opening and forward along the outside of the caudal rectal wall

5. Amputation of all diseased tissue of anorectal tube
6. Closure of skin to rectal wall
7. Results in fecal incontinence

J. Tail amputation can be used.
1. Reduces moist, contaminated environment
2. May be effective alone in minor disease, but most commonly used as an adjunct to other modalities
3. High amputation at level of second or third coccygeal vertebra

K. Postoperative care is as follows.
1. Hydrotherapy and antimicrobial cleaning of perineum
2. Periodic clipping of perineal hair
3. Fecal softeners and low-residue diet
4. Prevention of self-mutilation with Elizabethan collars or side braces

Patient Monitoring

I. Mild cases heal with no complications.
II. Severe cases have frequent complications, including anal stricture, fecal incontinence, and dehiscence of suture lines.
III. Recurrence of fistulas is common.

Anal Sac Disease

Definition

I. Anal sac disease involves three different entities.
A. Impaction
B. Infection
C. Abscess
II. The conditions are probably three separate phases of the same disease (Washabau and Brockman, 1995).

Causes

I. Large quantity of thick secretions (Nesbitt, 1989)
II. Small duct system
III. Changes in anal muscle tone or fecal form
IV. Sequelae to diarrhea or estrus
V. Bacterial infection with *Streptococcus fecalis, Escherichia coli, Clostridium welchii, Proteus* spp., and *Staphylococcus* spp.

Pathophysiology

I. Initially, the anal sacs become impacted.
II. Impacted sacs become secondarily infected.
III. Increased inflammation and irritation result.
IV. Abscess formation then occurs, with or without sac rupture.

Clinical Signs

I. Scooting, licking or biting at the perineum
II. Tail chasing
III. Tenesmus, painful defecation
IV. More common in small dog breeds; rare in cats

Diagnosis

I. Palpation of distended, obstructed anal sacs is suggestive.
II. Palpation may be painful.
III. Expressed material is thick and pasty, or purulent and hemorrhagic with a fetid odor.
IV. Perianal region may be inflamed, with or without a draining wound.
V. Cytology, culture, and bacterial sensitivity of sac contents reveal inflammation and infection.

Differential Diagnosis

I. Perianal fistula
II. Perianal neoplasia
III. Anal pruritus

Treatment

I. Impaction
A. Manually express the sacs.
B. If the material is too tenacious to express, flush the sac with warm saline through a feline urinary catheter.
C. Recurrent disease is treated by sacculectomy (Matthiesen and Marretta, 1993).
1. Sacs flushed with antimicrobial solution
2. Duct and sac opened with scalpel or scissors
3. Lining of sac grasped with hemostats
4. Scalpel or small scissors used to peel away sac (Fig. 36–2)
5. Care taken to avoid caudal rectal nerves deep to sac
6. Closure of incised sphincter muscle and skin
II. Infection
A. Sac lavage with antimicrobial solution (0.5% chlorhexidine or 10% povidone-iodine)

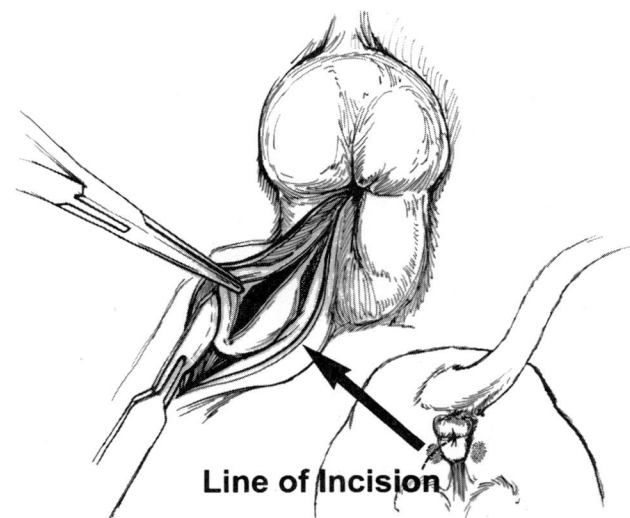

Line of Incision

Figure 36–2. The anal sac is opened and grasped with hemostats. The lining of the sac is removed by careful dissection with scalpel or fine scissors. (Courtesy of University of Tennessee College of Veterinary Medicine.)

B. Instillation of antibiotic-corticosteroid ointment (e.g., Panolog or Otomax)
C. Systemic antibiotics (amoxicillin 20 mg/kg PO BID) for 7 days
D. Warm compresses or hydrotherapy
E. Recurrent infections treated by sacculectomy
III. Abscess
   A. Abscessed sac opened and drained (if not spontaneously draining)
   B. Treated as described for infection
   C. Permitted to heal by second intention
   D. Recurrent abscesses treated with sacculectomy

Patient Monitoring

I. Recurrence of anal sac diseases is common.
II. Surgical excision can result in temporary or permanent fecal incontinence.
III. Draining fistulas develop if pieces of sacs are left after sacculectomy.

Anal and Rectal Prolapse

Definition

I. Prolapse of anal mucosa through anal opening
II. Prolapse of rectum through anal opening

Causes

I. Tenesmus resulting from gastrointestinal diseases causing diarrhea
II. Dystocia
III. Secondary to perianal hernia with rectal sacculation
IV. Secondary to urethral obstruction

Pathophysiology

I. Predisposing cause results in straining.
II. Initial straining produces protrusion of anal mucosa.
III. Continued straining causes prolapse of all layers of rectal wall.
IV. Environmental exposure results in edema, hyperemia, trauma, and necrosis of rectal tissue.

Clinical Signs

I. Usually a young dog or cat
II. Previous period of tenesmus
III. Protrusion of small section of anal mucosa
IV. Protrusion of a tubular segment of bowel

Diagnosis

I. Protrusion of normal anal mucosa
II. Protrusion of a tubular segment of bowel
III. Palpation of fornix of the prolapse: little to no space present

Differential Diagnosis

I. Anorectal neoplasia
II. Prolapsed ileocolic intussusception

Treatment

I. Correction of predisposing cause of prolapse
II. Medical therapy
   A. Lubricate and replace prolapsed tissue.
   B. Topical applications of antibiotic-steroid ointments (e.g., Panolog, Otomax) help reduce swelling.
   C. A pursestring suture at the anal opening is tied tight enough to prevent re-prolapse but loose enough to permit fecal passage. Remove the suture after 7 days.
   D. With pursestring treatment, stool softeners such as dioctyl sodium sulfosuccinate (100–200 mg PO daily) are given.
   E. Low-residue diet may be used to reduce frequency of bowel movements.
III. Surgical therapy
   A. Colopexy (Popovitch et al., 1994)
      1. It is used for recurrent rectal prolapses.
      2. A caudal ventral midline laparotomy is performed.
      3. The prolapse is reduced by traction on the colon.
      4. The descending colon is sutured to the left ventral abdominal wall.
   B. Amputation of prolapse (Matthiesen and Marretta, 1993)
      1. It is necessary when there is marked trauma or necrosis of the prolapsed tissue.
      2. Stay sutures are placed through the prolapsed segment at the anal opening.
      3. Prolapsed tissue is resected 1–2 cm distal to the anus.
      4. Two layers of prolapsed stump are sutured using absorbable monofilament suture and a simple interrupted pattern (Fig. 36–3).
      5. The amputated stump is replaced, and a pursestring suture is placed around the anal opening as described earlier.

Patient Monitoring

I. Prolapses commonly recur.
II. It is important to identify and correct any underlying cause.
III. Resection of a prolapse can result in major complications such as dehiscence, leakage, and rectal stricture.
IV. Treatment by colopexy usually prevents recurrence.

NEOPLASIA

Definition and Classification

I. Perianal gland adenomas (circumanal gland or hepatoid cell adenomas)
II. Perianal gland adenocarcinomas

Pathophysiology

I. Adenomas
   A. Development and growth of adenomas are related to androgen levels.

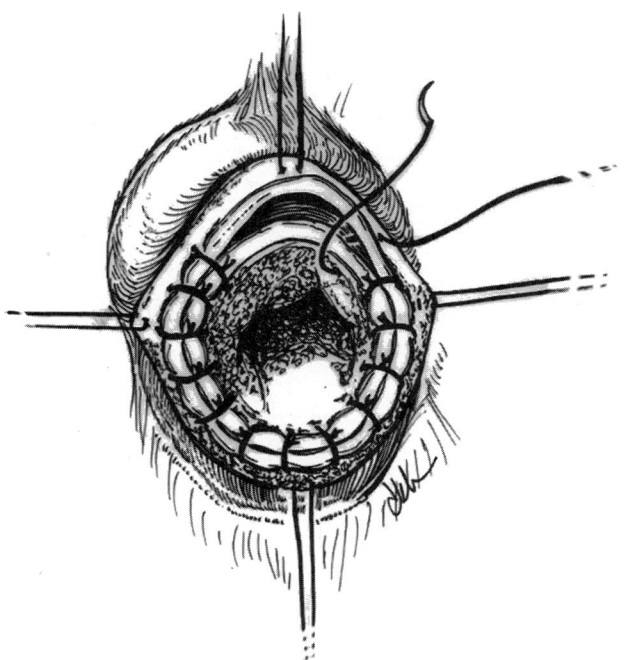

Figure 36–3. The prolapsed rectum is secured with 3–4 stay sutures at the base of the prolapse. The amputation is performed 1 cm distal to the stay sutures, and the two layers of the prolapse stump are sutured. (Courtesy of University of Tennessee College of Veterinary Medicine.)

  B. Most occur in older intact male dogs.
  C. Metastasis is rare.
 II. Adenocarcinoma
  A. Adenocarcinoma often occurs in older female dogs and may produce a parathyroid hormone–related protein, causing hypercalcemia and hypophosphatemia (Ogilvie and Moore, 1995).
  B. Metastasis is common.

Clinical Signs

 I. Singular or multiple masses are noted, usually in the perianal area, but occasionally in the inguinal region, thighs, or ventral tail.
 II. Nodular masses of variable sizes may be found.
 III. Masses eventually ulcerate, bleed, and become necrotic.
 IV. Tenesmus and constipation are occasionally present.
 V. Deep invasion and metastasis to sublumbar nodes are common with adenocarcinoma (Ross et al., 1991).

Diagnosis

 I. Age and sex of affected dogs are suggestive.
 II. Location and visual appearance of lesions are supportive.
 III. Hypercalcemia and hypophosphatemia are present in about one quarter of animals with adenocarcinoma (Ross et al., 1991).
 IV. Rectal palpation reveals perianal and sublumbar masses.

 V. Tumor cells are seen on cytology.
 VI. Biopsy and histopathologic evaluation are required for a definitive diagnosis.
 VII. Radiographic or ultrasonographic detection of enlarged sublumbar lymph nodes often indicates metastasis.

Differential Diagnosis

 I. Anal sac abscess
 II. Perianal fistula
 III. Other types of cutaneous neoplasms

Treatment

 I. Adenoma
  A. Surgical excision of masses is usually curative.
  B. External beam radiation and cryotherapy are also effective.
  C. Castration is performed.
  D. Estrogen therapy may be considered but is normally contraindicated because of deleterious effects on bone marrow (Washabau and Brockman, 1995).
 II. Adenocarcinoma
  A. Primary excision is advised but may not be possible because of the invasive nature of the neoplasm.
  B. The role of chemotherapy is not yet defined.
  C. Excision followed by external beam radiation and cisplatin chemotherapy may be effective (Ogilvie and Moore, 1995).

Patient Monitoring

 I. Metastasis of carcinoma is common and occurs early in the disease.
 II. Local recurrence of carcinoma occurs in many dogs.
 III. Prognosis is guarded for long-term survival with carcinomas, despite treatment (Ross et al., 1991; Ogilvie and Moore, 1995).
 IV. Surgical complications include wound infection, dehiscence, and fecal incontinence.
 V. Excision and castration effectively control adenomas.

Bibliography

Bellenger CR, Canfield RB: Perineal hernia. p. 471. In Slatter DH (ed): Textbook of Small Animal Surgery. WB Saunders, Philadelphia, 1993

Day MJ: Immunopathology of anal furunculosis in the dog. J Small Anim Pract 34:381, 1993

Ellison GW: Treatment of perianal fistulas in dogs. J Am Vet Med Assoc 206:1680, 1995

Killingsworth CR, Walshaw R, Reimann KA et al: Thyroid and immunologic status of dogs with perianal fistula. Am J Vet Res 49:1742, 1988

Krahwinkel DJ: Rectal diseases and their role in perineal hernia. Vet Surg 12:160, 1983

Mann FA: Perineal herniation. p. 92. In Bojrab MJ (ed): Disease Mechanisms in Small Animal Surgery. 2nd Ed. Lea & Febiger, Philadelphia, 1993

Matthews KA, Sukhiami RS: OL27-400 (cyclosporin) treatment of canine perianal fistulas. Proc Am Coll Vet Surg 31:14, 1996

Matthiesen DT, Marretta SM: Diseases of the anus and rectum.

p. 627. In Slatter DH (ed): Textbook of Small Animal Surgery. WB Saunders, Philadelphia, 1993

Nesbitt GH: Diseases of the anal sacs: a review. Vet Forum 1:16, 1989

Ogilvie GK, Moore AS: Managing the Veterinary Cancer Patient. Veterinary Learning Systems, Trenton, NJ, 1995

Popovitch CA, Holt D, Bright R: Colopexy as a treatment for rectal prolapse in dogs and cats: a retrospective study of 14 cases. Vet Surg 23:115, 1994

Ross JT, Scavelli TD, Matthiesen DT, Patnaik AK: Adenocarcinoma of the apocrine glands of the anal sac in dogs: a review of 32 cases. J Am Anim Hosp Assoc 27:349, 1991

Washabau RJ, Brockman DJ: Recto-anal disease. p. 1398. In Ettinger SJ, Feldman EC (eds): Textbook of Veterinary Internal Medicine. 4th Ed. WB Saunders, Philadelphia, 1995

Welches CD, Scavelli TD, Aronsohn MG, Matthiesen DT: Perineal hernia in the cat: a retrospective study of 40 cases. J Am Anim Hosp Assoc 28:431, 1992

37

Acute Abdomen Syndrome

Rebecca Kirby

Definition and Causes

I. Acute abdomen syndrome is a complex of disorders that result in the animal experiencing acute and severe pain from the abdominal cavity, the abdominal organs, or the nerves, muscles, fascia, or skin associated with the abdomen.

II. Many etiologies of this syndrome lead to complications that can be immediately life-threatening, such as the systemic inflammatory response syndrome (SIRS).

III. Causes include infection, ischemia, acute distention, or inflammation of one or more abdominal organs, the peritoneal space, or tissues constituting the abdominal wall (see Differential Diagnosis, later).

Pathophysiology

I. Location of pain fibers
   A. Submucosa and muscularis layers of hollow viscera: urinary bladder, gallbladder, uterus, stomach, and bowel
   B. Peritoneal lining
   C. Capsule of solid organs: liver, spleen, kidneys, pancreas, and prostate

II. Initiation of pain
   A. Tension of the peritoneal lining, or the capsule or muscularis of abdominal organs
      1. Severe dilatation with fluid, air, or both: obstruction, pyometra, urinary bladder obstruction, acute splenic torsion, ileus
      2. Active contractions of the muscle layers: hypersegmentation of the bowel
      3. Traction on the peritoneum or muscular layers: adhesions
   B. Inflammation
      1. Infectious processes: parvovirus enteritis, hemorrhagic gastroenteritis
      2. Trauma
      3. Toxins: lead, corrosive agents
      4. Severe hyperthermia: heatstroke

C. Combination of tension and inflammation
   1. Ischemia: bowel infarct, mesenteric volvulus
   2. Fluid accumulation: septic peritonitis

Clinical Signs

I. Significant historic information
   A. Vaccination and internal parasite history
   B. Past medical problems or medications administered, e.g., nonsteroidal anti-inflammatory drugs and corticosteroids
   C. Sudden changes or excessive fat content in the diet
   D. Access to garbage, bones, or moldy food
   E. Availability of string, small toys, balls, garbage, corncobs, panty hose, bones, or other small, frequently ingested items
   F. Recent trauma
   G. Exposure to toxins

II. Assessment of vomiting
   A. Yellow- or green-tinted vomitus is indicative of true vomiting vs. regurgitation.
   B. Vomiting that occurs shortly after eating suggests irritation or inflammation of the stomach.
   C. Vomiting of large amounts of undigested food 4–6 hours after eating is typical of gastric retentive disorders such as motility abnormalities or outflow obstruction.
   D. Projectile vomiting indicates pyloric outflow obstruction.
   E. The character of the vomitus may reflect the origin of the problem or severity of the disorder.
      1. Blood in the vomitus (hematemesis) implies esophageal, gastric, or duodenal hemorrhage.
      2. White, mucoid fluid is probably of gastric origin or may be swallowed saliva.
      3. Fetid green or brown fluid is usually duodenal in origin.
      4. Yellow or green vomitus indicates biliary reflux.

425

III. Other clinical signs
   A. Restlessness or reluctance to lie down
   B. Abdominal distention or arched back
   C. Fever
   D. Anorexia
   E. Depression, malaise

Diagnosis

I. Physical examination
   A. Perfusion and hydration status
      1. Poor perfusion is suggested by prolonged capillary refill time, weak pulses, tachycardia or bradycardia, and pale mucous membranes.
      2. Hydration is estimated by skin turgor and mucous membrane moisture.
      3. Hydration may appear normal with peracute fluid loss until fluid shifts occur from the interstitial to intravascular fluid compartments.
   B. Abdominal palpation
      1. Detection of ascites, abdominal distention, bowel or mass lesions, organ enlargement, or bowel distention
      2. Localization and severity of pain
         a) Focal pain suggests involvement of nearby structures.
         b) Generalized pain implies a diffuse disorder of the abdominal cavity.
         c) Severe pain suggests visceral and parietal peritoneal involvement.
         d) Dull, poorly localized pain suggests a diffuse inflammatory process.
         e) Intermittent pain is often associated with gastroenteritis, partial mechanical small bowel obstruction, and, occasionally, subacute pancreatitis.
         f) Palpation that causes retching or vomiting implies irritation of regional organs.
   C. Abdominal auscultation
      1. Presence of gastric or bowel sounds implies that gastrointestinal (GI) motility is present.
      2. A silent abdomen suggests hypomotility, ileus, fluid accumulation, or diffuse peritonitis.
   D. Rectal examination
      1. The prostate and other palpable pelvic structures are evaluated by rectal examination.
      2. Feces are evaluated for melena associated with upper GI bleeding.
   E. Cardiovascular system
      1. Poor perfusion is often present.
      2. Arrhythmias may be detected.
   F. Nervous system
      1. Any change in mentation requires that special care be taken to prevent aspiration of vomitus.
      2. Careful examination is made for evidence of back pain, which may lead to signs of an acute abdomen.
   G. Muscles, fascia, and skin of the abdomen
      1. Look for evidence of fasciitis, cellulitis, myositis, steatitis, or other pathology that can result in signs of an acute abdomen.

      2. Petechiation, ecchymosis, or bruising of the skin suggests underlying coagulation disorders.
      3. Bruising, abrasion, and lacerations can be seen with trauma-related acute abdomen.
II. Laboratory data
   A. Immediate tests
      1. Packed cell volume (PCV) and total protein
      2. Serum color for icterus, lipemia, or hemolysis
      3. Serum for glucose, electrolytes, blood urea nitrogen
      4. Platelet estimate, activated clotting time
      5. Urine specific gravity and examination for glucose, protein, bacteria, white blood cells, and renal tubular cell casts
   B. Complete database
      1. Complete blood count, biochemical profile, amylase, lipase
      2. Coagulation profile, antithrombin III, arterial blood gases
   C. Electrocardiogram
III. Specific diagnostic procedures
   A. Abdominal radiographs are evaluated for generalized loss of detail as a sign of diffuse peritoneal disease, gas in the intestinal lumen or free within the abdomen, signs of foreign bodies, intestinal obstruction, volvulus, ileus, mass lesions, and changes in organ size and shape, etc.
   B. Abdominal paracentesis is done to evaluate any free peritoneal fluid.
      1. Assess cytologic preparations, bacterial cultures, hematocrit, total protein, cell count, and amylase, creatinine, and potassium content.
      2. Rule out septic peritonitis, bowel perforation, hemorrhage, acute pancreatitis, and urine peritonitis (Table 37–1).
   C. Abdominal ultrasonography is helpful to detect subtle organ enlargement, mass lesions, meta-

*Table 37–1. **Parameters to Evaluate on Free Abdominal Fluid Samples or Diagnostic Peritoneal Lavage (DPL) Fluid Samples***

Test	Interpretation
PCV (free fluid)	Actual PCV of fluid
PCV (DPL fluid)	Every 1% per 500 ml fluid is equivalent to 10–20 ml free blood
Cytology	
Bacteria, fibers	Hollow viscus rupture
Neutrophils	Peritonitis
Bacteria in WBCs	Septic peritonitis
Bilirubin	Biliary or upper GI rupture
Amylase	>1000 sigU/ml suggests pancreatitis or GI disruption
Creatinine	> serum suggests urinary tract rupture
WBCs	>500/mm^3 = peritonitis; 0–500/mm^3 = repeat aspirate

PCV = packed cell volume; WBCs = white blood cells; GI = gastrointestinal.

static disease, vascular occlusion, free abdominal fluid, and pancreatitis.
  D. Diagnostic peritoneal lavage is done when the diagnosis is uncertain and emergency surgical intervention is anticipated (Crowe, 1976).
    1. A peritoneal catheter is placed, and 10–20 ml/kg of sterile isotonic saline is infused into the abdomen; the animal is rolled and gently palpated to move the fluid.
    2. A sample is withdrawn and evaluated as described earlier for abdominal paracentesis.

Differential Diagnosis

  I. GI tract lesions
    A. Gastric ulceration, pyloric outflow obstruction, gastric dilatation-volvulus, perforation
    B. Intestinal obstruction, volvulus, ulceration, perforation, infection, intussusception
    C. Mesenteric thrombosis, volvulus, avulsion of mesenteric vessels
    D. Lymph node neoplasia or infection
    E. Pancreatitis, infarction of the pancreas
  II. Reproductive tract
    A. Uterine infection, torsion, rupture
    B. Intra-abdominal testicular torsion, infarct, abscess
    C. Prostatic infection, cyst, infarct, abscess
  III. Reticuloendothelial system (liver and spleen)
    A. Splenic tumors, torsion, fracture, infection, thrombosis, enlargement secondary to systemic disease
    B. Liver abscess, infection, tumor, biliary obstruction, rupture
  IV. Urinary tract
    A. Kidney swelling, renal calculi, fracture, hematoma, avulsion
    B. Ureteral obstruction, rupture, passage of calculi
    C. Urinary bladder obstruction, trauma, rupture
    D. Urethral obstruction, rupture
  V. Peritoneal space and surfaces
    A. Hemoperitoneum
    B. Pneumoperitoneum
    C. Bile peritonitis
    D. Septic peritonitis
  VI. External abdominal structures
    A. Steatitis
    B. Myositis
    C. Fasciitis
    D. Nerve root irritation from disk disease or neoplasia
    E. Hernias with strangulated viscera
      1. Umbilical
      2. Inguinal
      3. Perineal
      4. Abdominal wall

Treatment

  I. Immediate goals of treatment are as follows.
    A. Ventilation and oxygenation
      1. Aspiration of vomitus requires the following.
        a) Immediate evacuation of particles by suction
        b) Intubation, ventilation, oxygenation, and removal of obstruction from large bronchi if significant respiratory compromise
      2. Animals with cyanosis, difficulty breathing, or poor perfusion require oxygen support.
        a) Consider oxygen delivery via a face mask, transtracheal catheter, nasal catheter (see Chap. 3), hood, or cage.
        b) Persistent hypoxemia requires increased oxygen delivery, possibly via tracheal intubation and ventilation and oxygenation with 100% oxygen.
    B. Fluid therapy for poor perfusion
      1. Immediate intravascular volume replacement is required.
        a) One or more large-bore indwelling intravenous (IV) catheters are placed.
        b) Pre-treatment blood samples and urinalysis are obtained.
        c) Fluid replacement is initiated.
          (1) Crystalloids at shock rate if used alone or at half the shock rate if used with plasma expanders or blood products (see Chap. 131)
          (2) Plasma expanders such as hetastarch (if SIRS is suspected) or dextran-70 at 20 ml/kg IV in the dog and 10–15 ml/kg IV very slowly to effect in the cat
          (3) Whole blood or packed red blood cell therapy for blood loss (see Chap. 69)
      2. Identify and treat any cause of shock, such as blood loss, vasovagal reflex and bradycardia, cardiac arrhythmias, hypovolemia, and sepsis.
        a) Shock associated with hemoperitoneum, hematemesis, melena, or hematochezia suggests significant hemorrhage.
        b) Whole blood or packed red cell transfusions are given if significant anemia or shock occurs.
        c) Resuscitation from shock should bring blood pressure back to low-normal range (helps avoid exacerbation of bleeding).
        d) Consider rear limb and abdominal counterpressure to tamponade bleeding occurring within the peritoneal or retroperitoneal space.
        e) Severe gastric hemorrhage may require gastric lavage with cool tap water, blood transfusions, and surgical intervention.
    C. Analgesia
      1. Injectable analgesics such as butorphanol (0.1 mg/kg IV) or oxymorphone (0.05–0.1 mg/kg IV in dogs; 0.02 mg/kg IV in cats, given with a tranquilizer) are administered.
      2. They may be combined with a tranquilizer such as diazepam (0.2–0.6 mg/kg IV) or acepromazine (0.05 mg/kg IV in dogs and 0.025 mg/kg IV in cats once blood volume and pressure are normal).

D. Evaluation of mental status
1. Assess for hypoglycemia, severe shock, or trauma.
2. Precautions are taken to avoid aspiration.
3. Glucose supplementation (see Chap. 45) and resuscitation for shock are implemented as required.
II. Determine the need for immediate abdominal decompression or surgical intervention (Table 37–2).
A. Several diseases require emergency surgical intervention.
B. Surgical conditions include total intestinal obstruction, perforation of bowel, septic peritonitis, intussusception, linear foreign bodies, ruptured splenic tumor, renal abscess, pyometra, prostatic abscess, and splenic, gastric, or intestinal volvulus.
C. The animal must be rapidly stabilized prior to anesthesia.
III. Maintenance therapy involves the following.
A. Hydration and oncotic pressure
1. These animals require larger volumes for rehydration and maintenance because of rapid fluid shifts into third body fluid spaces (i.e., GI tract, peritoneal space, uterus).
2. Balanced electrolyte solutions are given initially.
a) Dehydration with poor perfusion requires volume replacement in 1–3 hours.
b) Dehydration with adequate perfusion requires replacement over 2–6 hours.
3. Maintain albumin above 2 g/dl.
B. Hypoglycemia
1. Blood glucose values <60 mg/dl require immediate supplementation (0.1–0.5 g/kg IV).

Table 37–2. **Indications for Surgical Exploration of Affected Area in an Animal with Acute Abdomen Syndrome**

Lack of diagnosis in a deteriorating animal
Free abdominal air
Bacteria seen within WBCs in free abdominal or DPL fluid
Plant fibers and bacteria seen in free abdominal or DPL fluid
Bilirubin seen in free abdominal or DPL fluid
Significant or continued abdominal hemorrhage
Torsion or volvulus of abdominal organ(s)
Evidence of organ ischemia
Penetrating abdominal foreign bodies
Evidence of mass lesion or abscess
Evidence of pyometra
Failure of medical therapy for pancreatitis
Total or partial gastric or intestinal obstruction
Rupture of an abdominal organ
Intussusception
Profound ileus not caused by drugs or electrolyte disorders
Hernia: diaphragmatic, peritoneal, perineal
Entrapped abdominal organ(s)
Débridement of infected wounds, muscles, fascia
Need for a feeding tube that bypasses the stomach
Obtain biopsies by direct visualization of site

WBCs = white blood cells; DPL = diagnostic peritoneal lavage.

2. Maintain glucose with 2.5–5% dextrose in electrolyte solution.
3. Persistent or recurring low glucose suggests sepsis or septic shock.
C. Electrolytes
1. Potassium values <3 mEq/L require supplementation, especially if acidosis is present.
2. Rate of potassium administration does not exceed 0.5 mEq/kg/h IV.
3. Hypernatremia (values >160 mEq/L) are corrected over 12–24 hours.
D. Acid–base status
1. Fluid replacement is the primary means of treating acid–base imbalances.
2. Rarely, IV sodium bicarbonate may be required for severe metabolic acidosis. The amount to administer slowly is determined by the formula: $0.3 \times$ kg body weight $\times$ (18 − measured plasma bicarbonate value) = mEq/L of sodium bicarbonate.
3. Alkalosis is treated by volume replacement with 0.9% saline.
E. Antiemetics
1. Administer if the animal is debilitated by the physical act of vomiting or if uncontrolled fluid losses are occurring.
2. They are selected based on the likely mechanism of vomiting and potential side effects of the drug.
a) Metoclopramide 0.2–0.4 mg/kg SQ TID-QID or 1–2 mg/kg/day IV by continuous rate infusion
b) Chlorpromazine 0.05 mg/kg IV in dogs and 0.01–0.025 mg/kg IV in cats after fluid and blood pressure resuscitation
3. Anticholinergics are not used.
F. Nasogastric tube (see Chap. 3)
1. Allows decompression of the stomach and evacuation of gastric fluids
2. Allows slow enteral feeding early in therapy
G. GI protectants for hematemesis
1. Cimetidine 4 mg/kg IV, SQ TID-QID
2. Sucralfate 250 mg/15 kg PO TID once vomiting is controlled
H. Antibiotics
1. Translocation of gram-positive and gram-negative aerobes and anaerobes may occur.
2. Institute broad-spectrum antibiotics after samples of blood, urine, and/or septic focus are taken for culture.
a) Cefazolin 40 mg/kg IV, then 20 mg/kg IV TID-QID
b) Metronidazole 7–10 mg/kg IV given over 30 minutes TID
I. Coagulation
1. Monitor for disseminated intravascular coagulation (DIC) early.
2. Trends in changes may be more important than actual values.
3. Treat DIC early with plasma and heparin at 50–100 U/kg SQ TID (see Chap. 66).

J. Nutrition
   1. Ensure that the animal is getting nutritional support within the first 24 hours of hospitalization.
   2. Nutrition can be provided by several methods.
      a) Partial parenteral nutrition can be given while weaning the animal onto enteral feeding.
      b) Microenteral nutrition is initiated within hours of admission, once vomiting is controlled. This consists of giving small quantities of a glucose and electrolyte solution orally or by feeding tube.
      c) Placement of a gastrotomy or jejunostomy tube is considered if abdominal exploratory surgery is required.
      d) Placement of a nasogastric tube, esophagostomy tube, or gastrotomy tube is considered in the anorexic, nonsurgical animal.
      e) Total parenteral nutrition is reserved for animals that cannot tolerate enteral feeding through the stomach or when a jejunostomy tube cannot be placed.
   3. Animals are given their caloric requirements by gradually increasing the concentration of the diet and then increasing the quantity.

Patient Monitoring

I. Apply the rule of 20 (Kirby, 1995).
   A. Careful evaluation of these 20 parameters is necessary 1–2 times daily during this critical stage of the animal's disease.
   B. Establishing a check-off list ensures that complications are detected and treated early.
   C. The rule of 20 includes monitoring the following parameters: fluid balance, oncotic pressure, albumin, blood pressure, heart rate and function, ventilation and oxygenation, electrolytes, renal function, red cell mass/hemoglobin, mentation, glucose, immune status and function, liver function, drug dosages, nutrition, coagulation, wound care and bandages, analgesia, GI function and motility, and level of nursing care.

II. Worsening of the animal's condition is indicated by the following.
   A. Failure to maintain blood pressure and fluid volume
   B. Appearance of multiple organ dysfunction
   C. Increase in pain intensity or distribution
   D. Development of shock in a previously stable animal
   E. Failure of respiratory system
   F. Death

Bibiliography

Crowe DT: Diagnostic abdominal paracentesis and lavage in the evaluation of abdominal injuries in dogs and cats: clinical and experimental investigations. J Am Anim Hosp Assoc 168:700, 1976

Crowe DT, Devey JJ: Assessment and management of the hemorrhaging patient. Vet Clin North Am [Small Anim Pract] 24:1095, 1994

Dillon AR, Spano JS: The acute abdomen. Vet Clin North Am [Small Anim Pract] 13:461, 1983

Kirby R: Septic shock. p. 139. In Bonagura JD (ed): Kirk's Current Veterinary Therapy XII. WB Saunders, Philadelphia, 1995

Plumb DC: Veterinary Drug Handbook. PharmaVet Publishing, White Beak Lake, MN, 1991

Purvis D, Kirby R: Systemic inflammatory response syndrome: septic shock. Vet Clin North Am [Small Anim Pract] 24:1225, 1994

Rudloff E, Kirby R: Hypovolemic shock and resuscitation. Vet Clin North Am [Small Anim Pract] 24:1015, 1994

Saxon WD: The acute abdomen. Vet Clin North Am [Small Anim Pract] 24:1207, 1994

38

Diseases of the Peritoneum

Frances M. Moore

Definition

I. Primary peritonitis
   A. By strict definition, primary peritonitis is limited to inflammatory processes that involve the peritoneum and are not the result of extension from primary disease elsewhere (MacCoy, 1981; Julian, 1985).
   B. Primary peritonitis is rare, and, in small animals, the most common example is feline infectious peritonitis (FIP) caused by the FIP coronavirus.
II. Secondary peritonitis
   A. Secondary peritonitis is an extension of inflammation from other organs or may result from contamination of the abdominal cavity with contents of the digestive or urogenital tract (Crowe and Bjorling, 1985; Hosgood and Salisbury, 1988, 1989; Salisbury and Hosgood; 1989; Hosgood, 1993).
   B. Rarely, penetrating wounds may result in abdominal contamination and secondary peritonitis.
   C. Peritonitis may be localized or diffuse, with the inflammation confined by the body's defense mechanisms in localized infections.
III. Chyloabdomen
   A. Chylous abdominal effusions are rare in cats and dogs.
   B. In cats, hemangiosarcoma, especially involving the root of the mesentery, is the most common condition associated with chyloabdomen. The abdominal effusion is usually both sanguineous and chylous (Gores et al., 1994).
   C. In dogs with chyloabdomen, the etiology has varied (Crowe and Bjorling, 1985; Fossum et al., 1987, 1992; Gores et al., 1994; Myers et al., 1996).
      1. In one, a ruptured mesenteric lymphatic led to chylous peritoneal effusion, and in two other dogs, lymphatic obstruction caused the chyloabdomen.
      2. An occluding thrombus of a mesenteric lym-

phatic was found in one animal, whereas in the other dog, the chyloabdomen occurred after surgical ligation of the thoracic duct was performed to alleviate chylothorax.
      3. Another report revealed chyloabdomen occurring in a dog with chylothorax and mediastinal lymphangiosarcoma.
      4. Trauma has also been cited as a cause of chyloabdomen in dogs and cats.
      5. Intestinal lymphangiectasia and protein-losing enteropathy have been associated with chyloabdomen in dogs.
IV. Hemoabdomen
   Trauma, ruptured tumors (especially splenic tumors), and bleeding diatheses may result in hemoabdomen.
V. Neoplastic abdominal effusions
   A. Tumors from many different sites may have intra-abdominal/peritoneal metastases.
   B. Carcinomas and adenocarcinomas may manifest as carcinomatosis, in which the omentum is often displaced cranially, forming a mass lesion adjacent to the greater curvature of the stomach.
   C. Primary peritoneal neoplasia (mesothelioma) is rare, but it has been reported in cats and dogs (Carpenter et al., 1987; Leisewitz and Nesbit, 1992; DiPinto et al., 1995).

Causes and Pathophysiology

I. Septic peritonitis
   A. Although both viral and bacterial infectious agents may induce septic peritonitis, bacterial peritonitis is, by far, the most common.
      1. FIP coronavirus may induce primary peritonitis in cats.
      2. In dogs, localized peritonitis may accompany certain viral infections, but the primary lesions do not involve the peritoneum, and clinical signs relate to the primary organs affected.

a) Infectious canine hepatitis viral infection may be associated with localized peritonitis.

b) Canine parvoviral infection may be accompanied by localized peritonitis of the involved intestine (Julian, 1985).

B. Septic bacterial peritonitis may result from peritoneal bacterial contamination from the digestive or urogenital tracts.

1. The digestive tract is the most common source for bacterial peritonitis. Intestinal bacteria may enter the peritoneum from rupture of the bowel wall secondary to intestinal neoplasia and foreign body penetration.

2. Devitalization of the intestinal wall from ischemia relating to intestinal volvulus, intussusception, and venous thrombosis may result in transmigration of luminal bacteria into the peritoneum with subsequent bacterial peritonitis.

3. Uterine rupture associated with pyometra or abdominal contamination during ovariohysterectomy for pyometra may cause septic peritonitis.

4. Bacterial peritonitis, especially peritonitis associated with *Actinomyces* and *Nocardia* infection in dogs, may occur without known source of the bacterial contamination (Julian, 1985; Hosgood, 1993).

a) These lesions may represent external contamination of the abdominal cavity in which the site of penetration cannot be found or may represent so-called spontaneous bacterial peritonitis.

b) Usually, dogs with peritoneal actinomycosis do not have historical evidence of preexistent ascites or the nephrotic syndrome.

II. Chemical peritonitis

A. Pancreatitis, gallbladder or bile duct rupture, and urine leakage into the abdominal cavity may result in chemical peritonitis (MacCoy, 1981; Crowe and Bjorling, 1985).

B. In pancreatitis, pancreatic enzymes break down fat and cause necrotizing purulent steatitis and peritonitis.

1. Omental adhesions often develop, and a large mass of adhesions forms adjacent to the pancreas.

2. Extrahepatic biliary obstruction may occur secondarily.

C. Steatitis in association with relative dietary deficiency of vitamin E and excessive polyunsaturated fat occurs occasionally in cats and is known as yellow fat disease.

1. Lesions of yellow fat disease involve both subcutaneous and abdominal fat deposits and may be associated with generalized peritonitis.

2. The yellow color of fat in this condition results from the accumulation of lipofuscin in macrophages within the inflamed areas (Julian, 1985).

D. Bile leakage from gallbladder or extrahepatic biliary duct may induce localized or diffuse necrotizing purulent peritonitis.

E. Barium produces intense chemical peritonitis and potentiates peritonitis induced by bowel wall rupture (Crowe and Bjorling, 1985).

F. Uroperitoneum is often associated with peritonitis; however, the chemical irritant effect of sterile urine in the abdomen is debated (Hardie, 1989).

1. In critical cases of uroabdomen, it is difficult to determine the mechanism of peritonitis.

2. The animal may have numerous problems contributing to peritonitis, including leakage of infected urine, abdominal trauma, inflammation of the urogenital tract, and decreased abdominal defense mechanisms resulting from a variety of conditions such as preexistent abdominal effusion.

III. Nonseptic peritonitis

A. Trauma and uncomplicated abdominal surgery result in mild nonseptic peritonitis.

B. Peritonitis may also be induced by talcum powder from surgical gloves.

C. Sterile gauze used in surgical procedures induces localized foreign body granulomatous peritonitis if left in the abdomen (Crowe and Bjorling, 1985).

D. Omental pansteatitis from vitamin E deficiency in cats results in peritonitis.

E. Migrating larval forms of some tapeworms (*Mesocestoides* and *Spirometra*) may cause peritonitis in dogs.

IV. Sclerosing encapsulating peritonitis

A. Sclerosing encapsulating peritonitis (SEP) is a chronic form of peritonitis in which abdominal organs become encased in connective tissue.

B. This unusual condition is rare and has been reported in both dogs and cats (Hardie et al., 1994).

C. The initiating cause of the peritonitis is varied.

D. These cases characteristically have profuse abdominal effusion associated with generalized peritonitis with abundant peritoneal collagenous connective tissue with numerous adhesions.

E. The prognosis for recovery is guarded.

V. Nonseptic hemorrhagic exudates

A. May result from abdominal trauma or rupture of abdominal neoplasms, especially splenic neoplasms

B. May reflect a generalized bleeding diathesis (Prasse, 1992)

Clinical Signs

I. Because peritonitis is often secondary to other disease conditions, clinical signs are often the result of the primary disease process.

II. Fever, tachycardia, dehydration, and hypovolemia may accompany septic peritonitis and septicemia.

III. Abdominal effusion and enlargement may be de-

tected on physical examination or by radiography or ulstrasonagraphy in cases of chronic peritonitis.
   IV. Occasionally an animal may assume an unusual stance, such as the ''praying position'' with the sternum lowered and the hind legs raised, whereas others may appear tucked up (Crowe and Bjorling, 1985).

Diagnosis and Differential Diagnosis

   I. Detection and confirmation of abdominal effusion
      A. Ultrasonography and radiography aid in the detection of abdominal effusion.
      B. Abdominocentesis or peritoneal lavage can be used to obtain fluid for analysis and cytology.
      C. Fluid analysis and cytology are the definitive tests for the diagnosis of peritonitis.
   II. Transudates (low-protein ascites)
      A. Abdominal transudates are colorless, transparent effusions with protein content <2.5 g/dl and nucleated cell counts <500/μl.
      B. These effusions can result from cirrhosis and from portal or hepatic hypertension, especially in hypoproteinemic animals (Greene, 1979; Prasse, 1992).
      C. Transudates may also be seen with hepatic arteriovenous fistulas, a rare condition reported in dogs and cats.
   III. Modified transudates (high-protein ascites)
      A. Modified transudates (high-protein ascites) have >2.5 g/dl protein.
      B. These effusions frequently accompany cardiac disease, hepatic venous hypertension (with escape of fluid through the hepatic capsule), and intra-abdominal neoplasia.
      C. Cirrhosis and portal hypertension may result in modified transudates in the animal with normal serum protein.
      D. Chronic fluid administration may complicate clinical assessment of the animal's condition.
   IV. Peritoneal exudates
      A. Abdominal exudates usually have protein levels >3.0 g/dl. The cell count in the fluid varies with the cause and ranges from <1000 to >100,000/μl (Prasse, 1992).
      B. Nonseptic hemorrhagic exudates contain blood, nondegenerate neutrophils, histiocytes, and occasional reactive mesothelial cells.
      C. Nonseptic, inflammatory exudates contain either nondegenerate or degenerate neutrophils, histiocytes, and reactive mesothelial cells.
         1. Degenerate neutrophils without bacteria typify the effusion associated with pancreatitis. Fluid amylase levels may also be increased over normal serum levels.
         2. Bile peritonitis is often dull green, and bile pigment may be found in histiocytes in the effusion. As time progresses, the effusion becomes increasingly purulent with degenerate neutrophils. Tests for bilirubin are positive (Prasse, 1992).

      3. Early cases of uroperitoneum have minimal cellular exudate, consisting predominantly of histiocytes with progressively increasing numbers of neutrophils over time (Hardie, 1989; Prasse, 1992).
         a) Fluid urea nitrogen and creatinine levels may be markedly increased compared with serum levels.
         b) Uroperitoneum may be associated with a disproportionate rise in serum urea nitrogen values relative to creatinine because of diffusion of urea back into serum from intra-abdominal urine.
      D. The distinctive effusion associated with feline infectious peritonitis viral infection is an exudate of moderate cellularity (3000–15,000/μl) with nondegenerate neutrophils predominating and total solids of >3.5 g/dl.
         1. Fluid is often straw-colored and viscous and may contain clots.
         2. Some cases of feline infectious peritonitis do not demonstrate the characteristic effusion, and others have no abdominal effusion.
      E. Chyloabdomen is diagnosed by the typical cloudy (lactescent) appearance of the fluid and high fluid level of triglyceride relative to cholesterol values (fluid cholesterol: triglyceride levels <1) (Fossum et al., 1992). Nondegenerate neutrophils, vacuolated histiocytes, and blood are found in these effusions, which may be positive with Sudan stain for fat.
      F. Septic, inflammatory exudates are high-protein effusions (usually >3.0 g/dl) with degenerate neutrophils predominating.
         1. Fewer histiocytes and occasional reactive mesothelial cells are common findings.
         2. Sepsis may develop in previously sterile abdominal effusions, because peritoneal immune defenses are compromised as a result of the prolonged effusion or debilitated state of the animal.
   V. Neoplastic effusions
      A. Most effusions associated with intra-abdominal neoplasia are modified transudates or exudates.
      B. Carcinomas tend to exfoliate into accompanying effusions, whereas sarcomas do not.
      C. Malignant lymphoma may also be diagnosed in abdominal effusions.
      D. Mesotheliomas are rare tumors, and the neoplastic mesothelial cells may be difficult to distinguish from reactive mesothelial cells.
   VI. Other laboratory findings
      A. Serum biochemical and hematologic assays may reflect the primary disease process, but these tests are not specific indicators of peritonitis.
      B. Hypoglycemia may reflect systemic sepsis in cases of septic peritonitis.
      C. Chronic peritoneal exudation can result in hypoproteinemia, hypoalbuminemia, and hyponatremia because of the dynamics of third space fluid loss (MacCoy, 1981; Harvey, 1990).

Treatment and Monitoring

I. Therapy for animals with peritonitis is directed at the primary disease process.
  A. Abdominal exploratory surgery is frequently indicated to find the source of the peritonitis, to remove necrotic tissue, and to perform abdominal lavage (Salisbury and Hosgood, 1989).
  B. Treatment of septic peritonitis depends on the cause, severity, and duration of the problem and whether the peritonitis is localized or diffuse (Crowe and Bjorling, 1985). Intravenous antibiotic therapy is indicated.
  C. The reader is referred to Chap. 37 for treatment and monitoring of the disease processes associated with peritonitis.
II. Prognosis depends on the type of primary disease process.
  A. Prognosis for secondary peritonitis is guarded.
  B. Neoplastic abdominal effusions warrant a poor prognosis.
  C. Sclerosing, encapsulating peritonitis signals a poor prognosis.

Bibliography

Carpenter JL, Andrews LK, Holzworth J: Tumors and tumor like lesions. p. 583. In Holzworth J (ed): Diseases of the Cat: Medicine and Surgery. WB Saunders, Philadelphia, 1987

Crowe DT, Bjorling DE: Peritoneum and peritoneal cavity. p. 571. In Slatter DH (ed): Textbook of Small Animal Surgery. WB Saunders, Philadelphia, 1985

DiPinto MN, Dunstan RW, Lee C: Cystic peritoneal mesothelioma in a dog. J Am Anim Hosp Assoc 31:385, 1995

Fossum TW, Sherding RG, Zach PM et al: Intestinal lymphangiectasia associated with chylothorax in two dogs. J Am Vet Med Assoc 190:61, 1987

Fossum TW, Hay WH, Boothe HW et al: Chylous ascites in three dogs. J Am Vet Med Assoc 1:70, 1992

Gores BR, Berg J, Carpenter JL et al: Chylous ascites in cats: nine cases (1978–1993). J Am Vet Med Assoc 205:1161, 1994

Greene CE: Ascites: diagnostic and therapeutic considerations. Compend Contin Educ Pract Vet 1:712, 1979

Hardie EM: Peritonitis from urogenital conditions. Probl Vet Med 1:36, 1989

Hardie EM, Rottman JB, Levy JK: Sclerosing encapsulating peritonitis in four dogs and a cat. Vet Surg 23:107, 1994

Harvey HJ: Complications of small intestinal biopsy in hypoalbuminemic dogs. Vet Surg 19:289, 1990

Hoefs JC, Runyon BA: Spontaneous bacterial peritonitis. Dis Mon Jan/Dec, 1–48, 1985

Hosgood G: Drainage of the peritoneal cavity. Compend Contin Educ Pract Vet 15:1605, 1993

Hosgood G, Salisbury SK: Generalized peritonitis in dogs: 50 cases (1975–1986). J Am Vet Med Assoc 193:1448, 1988

Hosgood GL, Salisbury SK: Pathophysiology and pathogenesis of generalized peritonitis. Probl Vet Med 1:159, 1989

Julian RJ: The peritoneum, retroperitoneum, and mesentery. p. 323. In Jubb KVF, Kennedy PC, Palmer N (eds): Pathology of Domestic Animals. Academic Press, New York, 1985

Leisewitz AL, Nesbit JW: Malignant mesothelioma in a seven-week-old puppy. J S Afr Vet Assoc 63:70, 1992

MacCoy D: Peritonitis. p. 142. In Bojrab MJ (ed): Pathophysiology in Small Animal Surgery. Lea & Febiger, Philadelphia, 1981

Myers NC, Engler SJ, Jakowski RM: Chylothorax and chylous ascites in a dog with mediastinal lymphangiosarcoma. J Am Anim Hosp Assoc 32:263, 1996

Prasse DW: Diseases of the peritoneum. p. 489. In Morgan RV (ed): Handbook of Small Animal Practice. 2nd Ed. Churchill Livingstone, New York, 1992

Salisbury SK, Hosgood GL: Management of the patient with generalized peritonitis. Probl Vet Med 1:68, 1989

Endocrine and Metabolic System

39

Introduction

C. B. Chastain

GENERAL CONSIDERATIONS

I. The endocrine system is a group of organs that secrete messenger substances (hormones) directly into the bloodstream to affect other distant organs in the body.

II. Actions of hormones include the following.
  A. To maintain homeostasis
  B. To coordinate response to stresses
  C. To control growth
  D. To control processes of reproduction

III. The secretion rate of one hormone is usually controlled by a "closed-loop" feedback secretory product, often another hormone, produced by the first hormone's target organ.
  A. Negative closed loop
    1. It is the most common type.
    2. Hormone (or substance) A stimulates hormone B secretion, but B inhibits A.
  B. Positive closed loop
    1. It occurs only in the ovary-pituitary loop.
    2. Hormone A stimulates hormone B secretion, and B stimulates A.

IV. The organs generally considered part of the (nonreproductive) endocrine system, and their major known hormone products, are as follows.
  A. Hypothalamus
    1. Thyrotropin-releasing hormone (TRH)
    2. Corticotropin-releasing hormone (CRH)
    3. Growth hormone–releasing hormone
    4. Growth hormone–inhibiting hormone (somatostatin)
    5. Antidiuretic hormone (ADH)
  B. Hypophysis
    1. Thyrotropin (thyroid-stimulating hormone [TSH])
    2. Corticotropin (adrenocorticotropic hormone [ACTH])
    3. Growth hormone (GH)
  C. Thyroid
    1. Thyroxine (T_4)
    2. Triiodothyronine (T_3)
    3. Calcitonin
  D. Parathyroids
    Parathyroid hormone (PTH)
  E. Pancreatic islets and gastrointestinal tract
    1. Insulin
    2. Glucagon
    3. Gastrin
  F. Adrenals
    1. Cortisol
    2. Aldosterone
    3. Adrenal androgens
    4. Epinephrine
    5. Norepinephrine
  G. Kidney
    1. Vitamin D (1,25-dihydroxycholecalciferol)
    2. Erythropoietin
  H. Heart
    Atrial natriuretic peptide

V. Signs of endocrine diseases are generally nonspecific and present as a dysfunction of a hormone's target organ.

INCIDENCE OF ENDOCRINE DISEASE

I. A survey of 2540 veterinarians in small animal practice revealed an apparent incidence of endocrine disease in 7% of small animals seen.

II. The definitive diagnosis of endocrine disorders is hampered by several factors.
  A. Many interrelationships occur between endocrine glands and their compensatory mechanisms.
  B. The effects produced by neoplastic endocrine disorders are often not proportionate to the size of the tumor.
  C. Physiologic adaptation is frequently difficult to differentiate from endocrine disease.
  D. Endocrine disorders can occur as multiple concurrent disorders.
  E. Laboratory tests may be unavailable, or insensitivity and errors can occur.

III. Age influences the incidence of small animal endocrine disorders (Table 39–1).

437

Table 39–1. **Typical Age of Onset for Endocrine Disorders**

0 to 1 Year	1 to 5 Years	5 to 10 Years	More Than 10 Years
Familial diabetes mellitus	Hypoadrenocorticism	Hypothyroidism	Diabetes insipidus
Pituitary dwarfism	Hypercalcemia resulting from	Diabetes mellitus	Primary hyperparathyroidism
Cretinism	lymphosarcoma	Hyperadrenocorticism	Hypercalcemia resulting from
Nutritionally induced secondary	Hypoparathyroidism	Insulinomas	apocrine gland
hyperparathyroidism	Hypothyroidism	Secondary hyperparathyroidism	adenocarcinomas of the anal
Hypervitaminosis D		resulting from acquired renal	sacs
Secondary hyperparathyroidism		disease	Secondary hyperparathyroidism
resulting from congenital			resulting from acquired renal
renal disease			disease

BASIC CAUSES OF ENDOCRINE DISEASE

I. Primary hyperfunction
   A. Autonomy occurs when a hormone is produced in amounts exceeding normal production because it is no longer affected by feedback mechanisms.
   B. Autonomous hyperfunction is usually caused by neoplasia or, sometimes, hyperplasia.
II. Secondary hyperfunction
   Hypersecretion of a hormone can result from over-stimulation of its organ of production by a tropic (stimulatory) hormone or by a persistent metabolic stimulus.
III. Primary hypofunction
   A. Failure of proper structural or biochemical development or destructive processes in an endocrine gland can reduce its secretion capability.
   B. Destructive processes are often related to a breakdown in immunity, but trauma, drug induction, and neoplasia can also impair endocrine gland function.
IV. Secondary hypofunction
   Deficiency of a tropic hormone impairs the target endocrine gland's ability to produce normal quantities of its secretory product.
V. Ectopic hypersecretion of hormones or hormone-like substances
   A. Neoplasms in nonendocrine glands are sometimes able to synthesize hormones, especially peptide hormones.
   B. The abnormal secretion may be excessive, mimicking that of primary hyperfunction in an endocrine organ.
VI. Failure of target cell response
   A. Hormones mediate their effects on target organs by attaching to receptors and modifying intracellular activities.
   B. The failure of a hormone to produce a normal effect can result from a lack in the quantity or quality of target cell receptors or from a failure in the target cell's intracellular response.
VII. Abnormal degradation of a hormone
   A. Disorders of organs necessary for degradation and elimination of hormones can lead to excessive accumulation of hormone levels.
   B. Some drugs are known to decrease the degradation of hormones, whereas other drugs can induce an increased rate of hormone degradation.
VIII. Iatrogenic hormone excess
   When hormones are administered at any dose in excess of that necessary for replacement of a hormone deficiency, excessive hormone effects can result.

BASIC PRINCIPLES OF ENDOCRINE DIAGNOSTICS

I. Concentration of hormones in the bloodstream
   A. Changes in secretion rates
      1. Most hormones are secreted continuously, with severalfold increases possible when appropriate stimuli are present.
      2. Many hormones fluctuate in concentration at rhythmic intervals.
         a) Weekly, monthly, or seasonal rhythms are called infradian rhythms.
         b) Circadian (diurnal) rhythms are those episodic, rhythmic, or pulsatile changes that occur within a day (hour or minute).
   B. Hormone transport in the bloodstream
      1. Thyroid and steroid hormones bind to plasma proteins while being transported in the bloodstream.
      2. Small percentages of the total amount of the hormone in the bloodstream, called the free hormone, are not protein bound.
      3. Free hormones are generally thought to be the only portion in circulation capable of binding target cell receptors.
      4. Drugs can affect the hormone-binding affinity or the quantity of a specific hormone-binding plasma protein, thereby altering the total hormone measured.
II. Effects of hormones mediated through cell receptors
   A. The concentration of hormone receptors is affected by genetics, the stage of growth, the stage of the target cell cycle, and the degree of differentiation or transformation of the target cell.
   B. Frequently, the concentration of a hormone and its homologous receptor are in an inverse rela-

tionship, especially with polypeptide hormones and catecholamines.

1. When a target cell is exposed to high concentrations of its homologous hormone, it decreases the concentration of its receptors (downregulation).
2. In some cases, the desensitivity may be caused by limited postreceptor events.
3. A few hormones increase the number of receptors (upregulation).

III. Measurements of hormone concentrations
   A. Following screening assessments, the definitive diagnosis of an endocrinopathy is usually based on measuring an abnormal concentration of a hormone in the bloodstream or, less commonly, in the urine.
   B. Immunoassays, such as radioimmunoassays and enzyme-linked assays, are the most sensitive and specific hormone assays for clinical diagnostics.
   C. Dynamic (stimulation and suppression) tests are frequently indicated.
      1. Measurement of the serum or plasma baseline (resting) levels of hormones cannot always separate normalcy from an endocrinopathy.
      2. Administration of stimuli or suppressants of the secretion of a hormone can be used to evaluate whether the response and the degree of the response are within normal limits.
         a) Suppression tests can demonstrate whether partial or complete autonomy is present in hyperfunctional endocrinopathies.
         b) Stimulation tests can help confirm the diagnosis of a hypofunctional endocrinopathy and assess the degree of hypofunction.
   D. Inappropriate hormone levels are usually significant.
      1. Stimulation or suppression of endocrine organs occurs continuously in vivo.

   2. When the level of the primary endogenous stimulus or suppressant can be measured concurrently with the level of the affected hormone, a comparison of the two values can be of diagnostic value (e.g., high plasma levels of PTH are inappropriate if the serum calcium level is high).

IV. Sensitivity, specificity, and predictive value of endocrine function tests
   A. A clinical diagnosis of endocrine disease should be based on a composite of patient history, physical findings, routine laboratory findings, and endocrine function tests.
   B. No single endocrine function test is 100% reliable; the diagnostic value of an endocrine test is estimated by its sensitivity, specificity, and predictive value. An ideal test would have 100% sensitivity, specificity, and predictive values.
      1. Sensitivity indicates the percentage of patients with the disease having the abnormal test result.
      2. Specificity indicates the percentage of patients without the disease being free of the abnormal test result.
      3. Predictive value indicates the percentage of patients with the disease among all patients with the abnormal test result.

Bibliography

Anonymous: How veterinarians spend time in their practices. Am Anim Hosp Assoc Trends 1:16, 1985

Jubiz W: Endocrinology. A Logical Approach for Clinicians. 2nd Ed. McGraw-Hill, New York, 1985

Rijnberk A, de Vries HW: Medical History and Physical Examination in Companion Animals. Kluwer Academic Publishers, Boston, 1995

Watts NB, Keffer JH: Practical Endocrine Diagnosis. 2nd Ed. Lea & Febiger, Philadelphia, 1989

40

Diseases of the Pituitary Gland

Rhett Nichols
Robert K. McDonald
Leland Thompson

PITUITARY HYPOFUNCTION (HYPOPITUITARISM): PITUITARY DWARFISM

Robert K. McDonald
(Revised by Rhett Nichols)

Definition

I. Hypopituitarism is a deficiency of one, several, or all pituitary hormones leading to decreased synthesis and secretion of target organ hormones, e.g., cortisol, thyroxine (T_4), or growth hormone (GH)–dependent peptides.
II. In the young dog, the term hypopituitarism is associated with a primary GH deficiency, with or without a deficiency of other pituitary hormones.
  A. Referred to as pituitary dwarfism
  B. Most common in the German shepherd dog, but also reported in the spitz, toy pinscher, Karelian bear dog, and an inbred colony of immunodeficient Weimaraners

Causes

I. Simple autosomal recessive trait in the German shepherd dog and Karelian bear dog
II. Contributing factors
  A. Failure of oropharyngeal ectoderm to differentiate into the trophic hormone-secreting cells of the pars distalis
  B. Progressive formation of multilobulated mucin-filled pituitary cysts that enlarge and compress the pars nervosa and infundibular stalk
  C. Lack of peripheral action of GH caused by abnormal structure of the hormone or nonresponsive target tissues

  D. Benign tumor of Rathke's cleft (craniopharyngioma)
III. Adult-onset disease most frequently associated with primary pituitary neoplasia

Pathophysiology

I. Growth is regulated by a variety of factors, including inheritance, nutrition, and humoral agents.
II. Normal growth is dependent on humoral growth factors and the ability of target tissues to respond to them.
  A. Insulin-like growth factors (IGFs)
    1. Also called somatomedins, IGFs have marked growth-promoting effects on bone, cartilage, connective tissue, and skeletal and cardiac muscle.
    2. IGF-1, also called somatomedin C, is a hepatic insulin-like peptide.
    3. Unlike other growth factors, IGFs are GH dependent.
  B. Fibroblast growth factor
  C. Nerve growth factor
  D. Epidermal growth factor
III. Normal thyroid hormone levels are also important.
  A. Thyroid hormone acts synergistically with GH and somatomedins to promote chondrogenesis.
  B. Thyroid hormone is required for normal GH messenger RNA synthesis.
IV. Secondary hypoadrenocorticism and hypogonadism may develop following decreased secretion of adrenocorticotropic hormone (ACTH) and follicle-stimulating or luteinizing hormones, respectively.

Clinical Signs

I. Short stature compared to littermates
II. Dermatologic abnormalities (see also Chap. 88)

A. Soft, woolly hair coat caused by retention of the lanugo or secondary hairs and lack of primary or guard hairs
B. Gradual bilaterally symmetrical alopecia sparing the head and extremities
C. Progressive hyperpigmentation
D. Skin becomes thin, inelastic, and scaly
III. Musculoskeletal abnormalities
A. Delayed closure of growth plates
B. Delayed eruption of permanent dentition and retained deciduous teeth
IV. Reproductive abnormalities
A. Hypogonadism may develop, although normal reproductive function has been reported.
B. In the male, small testicles, azoospermia, and a flaccid penile sheath are seen.
C. In the female, an absence of the estrous cycle is noted.
V. Shortened life expectancy
VI. May retain a shrill, puppy-like bark

Diagnosis

I. Presumptive diagnosis is based on breed, history, clinical signs, and the results of an insulin response test.
II. In the past, definitive diagnosis required a GH stimulation test using clonidine or xylazine as GH-stimulating agents, but the assay for GH is not currently available.
III. Routine laboratory evaluation (complete blood count [CBC], urinalysis, serum chemistries, fecal flotation) is performed to rule out other causes of dwarfism, e.g., gastrointestinal, kidney, or liver disorders.
IV. Results of laboratory testing are usually normal with uncomplicated pituitary dwarfism. Abnormalities that may be seen are mild anemia, hypoalbuminemia, hypophosphatemia, and azotemia.
V. Insulin response test may be considered.
A. Because GH has anti-insulin properties, animals with deficient GH are very sensitive to the hypoglycemic effects of insulin.
B. After a 12-hour fast, administer regular insulin at 0.05 U/kg IV.
C. Collect blood glucose samples before and 15, 30, 45, 60, and 90 minutes after insulin administration.
D. Glucose levels are expected to fall to ≤50% of fasting values and return to normal levels more slowly than controls.
E. This test may cause *serious* hypoglycemia, especially during the first hour, and is sometimes difficult to interpret.
VI. GH stimulation test is not currently available.
A. Administer clonidine (Catapres) 10 μg/kg or xylazine (Rompun) 300 μg/kg IV.
B. Collect serum before and 15, 30, 45, 60, and 90 minutes after stimulation and freeze samples until assayed.
C. Pituitary dwarfs demonstrate either little or no GH stimulation compared with normal controls.

VII. Serum IGF-1 (somatomedin C) levels can be quantitated by radioimmunoassay to indirectly assay GH status.
A. Serum IGF-1 levels parallel body size in dogs; production is impaired by glucocorticoids and estrogens.
B. They are expected to be low or undetectable in GH-deficient states.
VIII. Skin biopsy changes are consistent with endocrinopathy.
IX. Assessment of thyroid and adrenal function may be performed.
A. Thyroid-stimulating hormone (TSH) and ACTH stimulation tests are usually normal in dogs with uncomplicated hypopituitarism.
B. In some cases of hypopituitarism, secondary hypothyroidism and/or secondary hypoadrenocorticism are seen, characterized by low basal hormone levels (T_4 and cortisol), a poor stimulation response to exogenous TSH and ACTH, and low endogenous ACTH and canine TSH levels.

Differential Diagnosis

Rule out other potential causes of short stature.
I. Malnutrition: decreased caloric intake, maldigestion/malabsorption syndromes, heavy intestinal parasitism
II. Congenital heart or kidney disease
III. Congenital liver disease, including portosystemic shunts
IV. Congenital hypothyroidism (cretinism)
V. Hyper- or hypoadrenocorticism
VI. Diabetes mellitus
VII. Metabolic storage diseases
VIII. Skeletal dysplasia

Treatment

I. GH replacement
A. Give dog 0.1 IU/kg SQ three times weekly for 4–6 weeks.
B. Human, porcine, and bovine GH are biologically active in the dog.
C. Only human GH is available commercially, but it is difficult to obtain and is expensive.
II. Thyroid replacement
A. Pituitary dwarfs may have secondary hypothyroidism.
B. Because of the synergistic influence of GH and thyroid hormone on the growth process, decreased thyroid hormone levels may diminish the effectiveness of GH therapy.
C. Give thyroxine 20 μg/kg/day PO for the remainder of the animal's life.
D. If hypoadrenocorticism is also present, replace adrenocortical hormones first.
III. Cortisone replacement
A. Secondary hypoadrenocorticism may also be seen in pituitary dwarfs.
B. In those cases with grossly abnormal ACTH response tests, replace cortisone using physiologic doses.

Patient Monitoring

I. Most pituitary dwarfs are presented for short stature, lethargy, and alopecia.
   A. Response to GH therapy can easily be assessed by monitoring changes in the dermatologic abnormalities (see Chap. 88).
   B. GH therapy is usually stopped after the initial 4–6 weeks, at which time hair growth should be visible.
   C. If hair coat abnormalities recur, GH treatment may be repeated.
II. Because most pituitary dwarfs are presented when their growth plates are closed or about to close, body height does not greatly increase with therapy.
III. Some dogs become nonresponsive or refractory to GH replacement therapy. It is believed that these dogs develop antibodies to GH, thereby diminishing the biologic activity of the hormone.
IV. Potential adverse reactions to GH therapy include diabetes mellitus and hypersensitivity reactions.

ACROMEGALY

Leland Thompson
(Revised by Rhett Nichols)

Definition

Acromegaly is the clinical syndrome caused by chronic hypersecretion of growth hormone (GH, somatotropin), resulting in overgrowth of connective tissue, bone, and viscera.

Causes

I. In cats, acromegaly usually results from excessive secretion of GH by a pituitary adenoma.
II. Causes in dogs include prolonged progesterone therapy or increased endogenous progesterone concentrations during diestrus and, rarely, pituitary neoplasia.
III. Progesterone stimulates the ectopic production of GH from mammary gland tissue.

Pathophysiology

I. GH is a single-chain polypeptide (approximately 22,000 daltons) produced by the pituitary.
II. It has both anabolic and catabolic effects and is necessary for normal somatic growth.
   A. Anabolic effects
      1. Effects are mediated by somatomedins or insulin-like growth factors (IGFs) synthesized and released from the liver in response to GH.
      2. IGFs have weak insulin-like activity and also promote growth in bone, cartilage, connective tissue, and skeletal and cardiac muscle.
   B. Catabolic effects
      1. Effects are mediated directly by the GH peptide itself, which has anti-insulin activity.
      2. GH promotes lipolysis and hyperglycemia and restricts glucose transport.

3. Diabetes mellitus associated with acromegaly results from the anti-insulin effects of GH.

Clinical Signs

I. Affected cats are usually middle-aged to old (8 to 14 years), mixed breed, and male.
II. Diabetes mellitus associated with GH excess tends to occur in aged intact female dogs.
III. Altered facial appearance and body size are often the first clinical signs observed.
   A. Broad, blunt face
   B. Thickened skin; excessive folds around face and neck
   C. Increased body weight
   D. Abdominal enlargement
   E. Hypertrophied organs: heart, liver, kidneys
   F. Enlarged interdental spaces
   G. Inspiratory stridor
IV. Insulin-resistant diabetes mellitus can occur because excessive GH decreases the number of insulin receptors and causes postreceptor insulin defects.
   A. Initially, hyperglycemia is associated with high serum insulin values (insulin resistance).
   B. As the disease progresses, pancreatic beta-cell exhaustion may occur, resulting in low serum insulin concentrations.
   C. Diabetes mellitus associated with GH excess is often refractory to insulin therapy, requiring high doses of exogenous insulin.
   D. Dogs treated with exogenous GH for hormone-responsive dermatosis are at risk for developing diabetes mellitus.
V. Cardiomyopathy may occur in cats.
   A. Systolic murmur
   B. Gallop rhythm
   C. Congestive heart failure (pleural effusion, pulmonary edema)
VI. Polyuria and polydipsia may develop from renal hypertrophy with increased glomerular filtration rates, or secondary to diabetes mellitus.
VII. Central nervous system signs caused by extrasellar growth of a pituitary neoplasm are uncommon but may include head pressing, dull behavior, or anorexia.

Diagnosis

I. History of prolonged progestogen therapy or diestrus in dogs
II. Characteristic signs of acromegaly, especially in the insulin-resistant diabetic animal
III. Laboratory abnormalities
   A. Hyperglycemia, glucosuria
   B. Mildly elevated serum alkaline phosphatase and alanine transaminase
   C. Hyperphosphatemia
   D. Hypercholesterolemia
   E. Hyperproteinemia
   F. Mild erythrocytosis (cats)
IV. Radiography
   A. Enlarged soft tissue structures in cervical region
   B. Cardiomegaly

V. Definitive diagnosis
  A. It is established by demonstrating elevated circulating GH concentrations or by evaluating pituitary GH responsiveness to a glucose load.
  B. A validated assay for GH is not currently available.
VI. Computed tomography (CT) scanning or magnetic resonance imaging (MRI)
  A. Identification of a mass lesion in the pituitary region supports the diagnosis.
  B. Determination of the location and size of a pituitary tumor may aid in selecting therapy.

Differential Diagnosis

I. Other causes of inspiratory stridor
  A. Elongated soft palate
  B. Laryngeal paralysis
  C. Foreign body
  D. Upper airway neoplasia
II. Simple diabetes mellitus
III. Hyperadrenocorticism

Treatment

I. Withdrawal of progestogen therapy, ovariohysterectomy for estrous control
II. Therapy for pituitary neoplasms
  A. Surgical excision of pituitary adenomas has not been evaluated in veterinary medicine. Large pituitary tumors may not be amenable to surgery.
  B. Pituitary-directed radiation therapy has limited availability in veterinary medicine.
  C. Medical therapy in humans includes estrogen therapy, the dopaminergic agonists bromocriptine and levodopa, and a long-acting somatostatin analogue (SMS 201–995).
    1. Experience is limited, but attempts to treat feline acromegalics with bromocriptine or somatostatin have been unsuccessful (CD Lothrop, personal communication).
    2. Further work is needed to determine whether dosage or dosage intervals need to be altered.

Patient Monitoring

I. With successful therapy, soft tissue abnormalities usually resolve in 6–8 weeks.
II. GH-induced diabetes mellitus may be either permanent or reversible.
  A. Various factors affect reversibility.
    1. Dose of progestogen
    2. Duration of progesterone influence
    3. Individual animal's response to GH
  B. Close monitoring of diabetic animals following withdrawal of progestogen or ovariohysterectomy is advised, because insulin requirements may decrease or cease completely.
  C. Feline acromegalics with severe insulin-resistant diabetes mellitus usually can be controlled with high insulin doses (NPH BID).

III. Survival time for feline acromegalics has been 8–30 months. Most affected cats die or are euthanized as a result of complications associated with congestive heart failure, renal failure, or neurologic signs from tumor expansion.

DIABETES INSIPIDUS

Rhett Nichols

Definition

I. Diabetes insipidus (DI) is a disorder of water metabolism characterized by polyuria, urine of low specific gravity or osmolality, and polydipsia.
II. DI can result from any of three basic defects.
  A. Nephrogenic diabetes insipidus (NDI): partial or complete renal insensitivity to the antidiuretic hormone arginine vasopressin (ADH)
  B. Central diabetes insipidus: partial or complete primary deficiency in the secretion of ADH
  C. Excessive intake of water: also referred to as dipsogenic diabetes insipidus, primary polydipsia, psychogenic polydipsia, or compulsive water drinking

Causes

I. Central DI results from lesions of the hypothalamus and neurohypophysis.
  A. Idiopathic
  B. Neoplasia
  C. Trauma
  D. Congenital defects
  E. Infection or inflammation
II. Nephrogenic DI is most often caused by a variety of acquired renal and metabolic disorders; congenital NDI is rare. Common examples of acquired NDI include the following.
  A. Hyperadrenocorticism
  B. Hypercalcemia
  C. Pyometra
  D. Liver disease
  E. Chronic renal disease, e.g., pyelonephritis
  F. Hypokalemia
  G. Hyperthyroidism
III. Excessive water drinking (primary polydipsia) can result from a defect in the thirst mechanism, or it may be a manifestation of a behavioral problem.

Pathophysiology

I. The production and release of ADH is controlled by a variety of factors.
  A. Plasma osmolality is the most important factor.
  B. Other factors include blood volume or pressure, hypoglycemia, pain, emotion, physical exercise, and certain pharmacologic agents, e.g., barbiturates and morphine.
II. ADH exerts its primary action by binding to specific receptor sites on the distal convoluted tubules and collecting ducts of the kidney.

A. ADH-sensitive adenyl cyclase is then stimulated, resulting in the generation of cAMP within the cell.
B. Increased intracellular cAMP causes an increase in permeability of the tubular epithelial cells to water; as a result of the concentration gradient created by the renal medullary interstitium, water moves across the epithelial cells from the tubular lumen to the interstitium.
C. The final urine concentration (urine specific gravity or osmolality) is dependent on the presence and quantity of ADH and ADH receptors and the tonicity of the renal medullary interstitium.
D. Lack of ADH or ADH receptors, interference with the ability of ADH to bind to its receptors, or a ''washed-out'' renal medullary interstitium will result in urine of low specific gravity and polyuria.

Clinical Signs

I. Age: variable, depending on cause
   A. Idiopathic DI has no specific age predilection.
   B. Animals with congenital NDI are <1 year of age.
   C. Animals with central nervous system (CNS) neoplasia are usually older (>8 years).
II. Sex and breed: no predisposition
III. Major presenting complaint: polyuria (PU) and polydipsia (PD)

Diagnosis

I. History: profound polyuria and polydipsia
II. Physical examination
   A. Weight loss may be observed if the animal is preoccupied with drinking.
   B. Dehydration may be present if water is unavailable for as little as 4–6 hours.
   C. Neurologic signs, e.g., disorientation, seizures, or blindness, may develop in animals with pituitary or hypothalamic neoplasia or trauma.
III. Complete blood count (CBC) and serum chemistry profiles
   A. These are usually unremarkable with central DI, congenital NDI, and primary polydipsia.
   B. With the more common causes of PU/PD (cases of acquired NDI and diabetes mellitus), specific and obvious abnormalities are present.
IV. Urinalysis
   A. Most dogs have a urine specific gravity <1.007, and cats usually have a urine specific gravity of 1.008–1.012.
   B. Animals with partial deficiencies of ADH may produce partially concentrated urine.
V. Modified water deprivation test (modified WDT)
   A. This test is designed to determine whether endogenous ADH is released in response to dehydration and whether the kidneys can respond to ADH.
   B. The modified WDT may differentiate the three types of DI when performed properly.

C. The test is contraindicated in animals that are already dehydrated or have other laboratory abnormalities. Rule out all other more common causes of PU/PD first.
D. The modified WDT is performed in two stages: an abrupt water deprivation test, followed by a vasopressin (ADH) response test.
   1. Abrupt water deprivation test
      a) Obtain baseline data, including body weight, urine specific gravity, blood urea nitrogen (BUN), estimated skin elasticity, and, if possible, urine and serum osmolality.
      b) Remove all water and food and empty the urinary bladder.
      c) Stop the test when any of the following occur.
         (1) Urine specific gravity >1.025 (900 mOsm/L)
         (2) Abnormally elevated BUN (>50 mg/dl)
         (3) Loss of body weight >5%
         (4) Estimated dehydration >5% based on decreased skin turgor and/or significant elevations in hematocrit, total solids
      d) Begin monitoring at 2 hours after initiating the test and at 1- to 4-hour intervals.
      e) Interpret results as follows.
         (1) Animals with complete central DI and NDI fail to concentrate their urine above 1.008.
         (2) Animals with partial central DI usually have urine specific gravities of 1.010–1.020.
         (3) Animals with primary (psychogenic) polydipsia usually concentrate their urine >1.025 unless renal medullary washout is severe.
   2. Exogenous vasopressin (ADH) response test
      a) If the WDT suggests DI, an ADH response test can be performed to help determine the exact cause of the disorder.
      b) Immediately following the abrupt water deprivation test, aqueous ADH (Pitressin, Parke-Davis) is administered at 0.5 U/kg IM (maximum 5 U).
      c) Empty the bladder and collect urine at 30, 60, and 90 minutes for determining specific gravity and/or osmolality.
      d) Interpretation is as follows:
         (1) Urine specific gravity >1.015 suggests central DI (complete or partial)
         (2) Urine specific gravity <1.015 suggests NDI or renal medullary washout.
VI. ADH trial
   A. An alternative to the modified WDT is to perform a closely monitored therapeutic trial with desmopressin acetate (DDAVP, Rhone-Poulenc Rorer Pharmaceuticals, Inc.), a synthetic analogue of ADH.

B. The owner measures the animal's water intake 2–3 days before the test is initiated.
C. Several dosage forms may be tried.
  1. DDAVP 2–4 drops BID into nose or conjunctival sac for 3–5 days
  2. DDAVP 1–2 μg SQ BID for 3–5 days
D. Dramatic reduction in water intake or an increase in urine concentration >50% strongly suggests ADH deficiency and a diagnosis of central DI.
E. Animals with NDI and some with severe medullary washout do not respond to ADH.

Differential Diagnosis

Numerous disease processes may cause PU/PD. Many of these disorders are characterized by other systemic signs, in addition to specific abnormalities in serum biochemical and electrolytes, that help differentiate them from DI. Some other causes of polyuria and polydipsia are as follows.
  I. Diabetes mellitus
  II. Hyperadrenocorticism
  III. Hyperthyroidism
  IV. Hypertension (severe)
  V. Liver disease
  VI. Hypercalcemia
  VII. Chronic renal disease
  VIII. Pyelonephritis
  IX. Pyometra
  X. Hypokalemia
  XI. Hyperviscosity syndromes

Treatment

  I. Hormone replacement with desmopressin (DDAVP) is the most effective treatment of complete or partial central DI but is not effective for NDI.
    A. Dosage: 2–4 drops of topical preparation administered in the conjunctival sac, nose, prepuce, or vulva BID–TID
    B. Duration of action: 8–12 hours
    C. Advantages: easy to administer
    D. Disadvantages: short duration of action, expensive
  II. Nonhormonal therapy includes the use of chlorpropamide and thiazide diuretics. These drugs can be used alone, in combination, or as an adjunct to hormone therapy.
    A. Chlorpropamide (Diabinese)
      1. Oral sulfonylurea agent that appears to potentiate the renal tubular effects of ADH and may also stimulate ADH release
      2. Requires the presence of some ADH to be effective and thus is effective only in animals with partial ADH deficiency
      3. Dosage: 10–40 mg/kg/day PO
      4. Advantages: further reduction of polyuria
      5. Disadvantages: not effective in the treatment of complete central DI or NDI; also may cause hypoglycemia
    B. Thiazide diuretics
      1. With a low-sodium diet, thiazides can be used to treat both central and nephrogenic DI
      2. Hydrochlorothiazide 2.5–5 mg/kg PO BID
      3. Chlorothiazide 20–40 mg/kg PO BID
      4. Advantages: reduction of polyuria in some cases of DI; only effective treatment for complete NDI other than salt restriction
      5. Disadvantages: secondary hypokalemia
  III. Restoration of the renal hypertonic medullary interstitium may resolve some cases of primary polydipsia.
    A. Gradual water restriction, over several days, prevents excessive dehydration while attempting to restore urine-concentrating ability.
    B. Behavior modification may be necessary in many cases.
  IV. Pet owners sometimes choose no therapy. The untreated animal with idiopathic or congenital DI appears to survive well so long as water is always available and the thirst center remains intact.

Patient Monitoring

  I. During the initial course of therapy, monitor for overhydration and dehydration.
    A. If overhydration occurs, reduce availability of water until the animal adapts.
    B. Dehydration can be avoided so long as water is available at all times and the animal is able and willing to drink.
  II. Long-term monitoring is best done by the owner. Optimal dosage and frequency of medication are based on monitoring water consumption and polyuria.

Bibliography

Bell PM, Atkinson AB, Hadden DR, et al: Bromocriptine reduced growth hormone in acromegaly. Arch Intern Med 146:1145, 1986

Campbell KL: Growth hormone-related disorders in dogs. Compend Contin Educ Pract Vet 10:477, 1988

Capen CC, Martin SL: Disorders of the pituitary gland. p. 1523. In Ettinger SJ (ed): Textbook of Veterinary Internal Medicine. 2nd Ed. WB Saunders, Philadelphia, 1983

Eigenmann JE: Disorders associated with growth hormone oversecretion: diabetes mellitus and acromegaly. In Kirk RW (ed): Current Veterinary Therapy IX. WB Saunders, Philadelphia, 1986

Eigenmann JE, Peterson ME: Diabetes mellitus associated with other endocrine disorders. Vet Clin North Am 14:837, 1984

Eigenmann JE, Venker-van Hagen AJ: Progestin-induced and spontaneous acromegaly due to reversible growth hormone over-production. J Am Anim Hosp Assoc 17:813, 1981

Feldman EC, Nelson RW: Disorders of growth hormone. p. 38. In: Canine and Feline Endocrinology and Reproduction. 2nd Ed. WB Saunders, Philadelphia, 1996a

Feldman EC, Nelson RW: Hyperadrenocorticism (Cushing's syndrome). p. 187. In: Canine and Feline Endocrinology and Reproduction. 2nd Ed. WB Saunders, Philadelphia, 1996b

Jackson IMD, Barnard LB, Lamberton P: Role of a long-acting somatostatin analogue (SMS201–995) in the treatment of acromegaly. Am J Med 81:94, 1986

Lamberts SWJ, Uitterlinden P, Verschoor L, et al: Long term treatment of acromegaly with the somatostatin analogue SMS 201–995. N Engl J Med 313:1576, 1985

Lothrop CD: Canine growth hormone responsive dermatosis. p. 978. In Kirk RW (ed): Current Veterinary Therapy X: Small Animal Practice. WB Saunders, Philadelphia, 1989

McKnight JA, McChance DR, Sheridan B, et al: A long term dose-response study of somatostatin analogue (SMS 201–995, ectreotide) in resistant acromegaly. Clin Endocrinol (Oxf) 34:119, 1991

Müller GH, Kirk RW, Scott DW: Cutaneous endocrinology. p. 575. In: Small Animal Dermatology. 4th Ed. WB Saunders, Philadelphia, 1989

Nichols R: Diabetes insipidus. p. 973. In Kirk RW (ed): Current Veterinary Therapy IX. WB Saunders, Philadelphia, 1986

Nichols R, Hohenhaus AE: Use of the vasopressin analogue desmopressin for polyuria and polydipsia and bleeding disorders. J Vet Med Assoc 205:168, 1994

Peterson ME: Effects of megestrol acetate on glucose tolerance and growth hormone secretion in the cat. Res Vet Sci 42:254, 1987

Peterson ME: Feline acromegaly (growth hormone excess). p. 981. In Kirk, RW (ed): Current Veterinary Therapy X: Small Animal Practice. WB Saunders, Philadelphia, 1989

Peterson ME, Taylor RS, Greco DS, et al: Acromegaly in 14 cats. J Vet Intern Med 4:192, 1990

Randolph JF, Miller CL, Cummings JF, et al: Delayed growth in two German shepherd dog littermates with normal serum concentrations of growth hormone, thyroxine, and cortisol. J Am Vet Med Assoc 196:77, 1990

Scott DW, Kirk RW, Hampshire J, Altzuler N: Clinicopathologic findings in a German shepherd dog with pituitary dwarfism. J Am Anim Hosp Assoc 14:183, 1983

Scott DW, Walton DK: Hyposomatotropism in the mature dog: a discussion of 22 cases. J Am Anim Hosp Assoc 22:467, 1986

41

Diseases of the Thyroid Glands

David L. Panciera
David M. Vail

HYPOTHYROIDISM

David L. Panciera

Definition

Hypothyroidism is a deficiency of thyroxine (T_4) and 3,5,3'-triiodothyronine (T_3) resulting in clinical signs involving almost all organ systems.

Causes

I. Primary hypothyroidism is dysfunction of the thyroid gland.
   A. Accounts for the vast majority of cases
   B. Two major types in dogs
      1. Lymphocytic thyroiditis
         a) Lymphocytic infiltrate associated with destruction of thyroid parenchyma
         b) Accounts for approximately 50% of cases
         c) Gradual destruction of the thyroid over months to years
         d) Antibodies present against thyroglobulin and a second colloid antigen, but not thyroid peroxidase
         e) Relative importance of these antibodies unknown
      2. Idiopathic follicular atrophy
         a) Characterized by loss of thyroid parenchyma with replacement by connective tissue without an inflammatory infiltrate
         b) Cause unknown, but may be a primary degenerative disorder
         c) Accounts for about 50% of cases
   C. Other causes of primary hypothyroidism
      1. Iodine deficiency or excess
      2. Secondary to neoplasia or infection
      3. Congenital thyroid dysgenesis or defective hormone synthesis

II. Secondary hypothyroidism occurs when pituitary gland secretion of bioactive thyrotropin (TSH) is inadequate.
   A. Subsequent thyroid follicle atrophy
   B. Rare
   C. Causes
      1. Congenital malformation of the pituitary
      2. Destruction of pituitary gland: neoplasia, infection
      3. Suppression of pituitary TSH secretion by drugs and possibly by illness or malnutrition
   D. Frequently occurs with other pituitary deficiencies or excesses

III. Tertiary hypothyroidism arises from decreased hypothalamic thyrotropin-releasing hormone (TRH).
   A. Results in reduced pituitary TSH secretion with subsequent atrophy of the thyroid follicles
   B. Not proven to occur in the dog

IV. Feline hypothyroidism is uncommon (Rand et al., 1993).
   A. Iatrogenic hypothyroidism following treatment for hyperthyroidism is the most common cause.
   B. Clinical signs may go unrecognized.

Clinical Signs and Pathophysiology

I. Signalment
   A. Most common in purebred, mid- to large-sized dogs
   B. Breed predisposition: boxer, cocker spaniel, dachshund, Doberman pinscher, English bulldog, golden retriever, Great Dane, Irish setter, miniature schnauzer, poodle, Shetland sheepdog, and beagle
   C. Age usually 3–8 years
   D. Females more often affected than males

II. Clinical signs
   A. Very gradual in onset

B. General signs
1. Cold intolerance
2. Weight gain despite normal food intake
3. Lethargy and mental dullness
4. Exercise intolerance
C. Dermatologic signs
1. Most common abnormalities
2. Drying of the skin and hair coat
3. Alopecia
   a) Often begins on the tail and becomes generalized
   b) Bilateral alopecia of the trunk of the body (see Chap. 88)
   c) Remaining hair is dull, dry, brittle, easily epilated, possibly lighter in color
   d) Slow hair growth, especially where previously shaved
4. Hyperpigmentation, hyperkeratosis, dry or oily seborrhea
5. Myxedema with "tragic" facial expression
6. Increased incidence of pyoderma
D. Immune system
1. Both neutrophil and lymphocyte function may be impaired.
2. Pyoderma results from both abnormal systemic immune responses and alterations in local immunity from seborrhea.
E. Cardiovascular signs
1. Heart rate, stroke volume, contractility, pre-ejection period, and velocity of circumferential fiber shortening are decreased.
2. Cardiac dysfunction from direct cardiac effects and peripheral vascular effects results in the following.
   a) Slowing of the heart rate
   b) Weak pulses and apex beat
   c) Electrocardiographic (ECG) abnormalities: low voltage R-wave, bradycardia, arrhythmias
   d) Echocardiographic abnormalities
      (1) Mild to moderate decreases in fractional shortening
      (2) Decreased thickness of left ventricular posterior wall, interventricular septum, and excursion of the left ventricular posterior wall
F. Neuromuscular signs (Jaggy et al., 1994)
1. Generalized peripheral neuropathy (uncommon)
   a) Most common complaint: weakness
   b) Spinal reflexes: hyporeflexic or normal
   c) Hypotonic muscles
   d) Accompanies other signs of hypothyroidism
2. Localized peripheral neuropathies
   a) Facial nerve paralysis and vestibular nerve palsy are the most common peripheral neuropathies.
   b) Unilateral forelimb lameness has also been reported (Budsberg et al., 1993).
   c) The relationship between hypothyroidism and laryngeal paralysis is not well established.
3. Myopathy: stiff, stilted gait, weakness, and dragging of the limbs
4. Central nervous system (CNS) signs
   a) Cerebrovascular atherosclerosis and associated hypoxia or infarction
   b) Metabolic axonopathy
   c) Ataxia, hemiparesis, hypermetria, head tilt, nystagmus, circling, and dysfunction of multiple cranial nerves
5. Thyroid hormone replacement therapy: usually results in improvement or resolution of signs
G. Gastrointestinal signs
1. Constipation, possibly diarrhea
2. Megaesophagus reported, but poorly documented
H. Hematologic signs
1. Von Willebrand factor and bleeding time are not affected by hypothyroidism (Panciera et al., 1996).
2. Nonregenerative anemia is common.
I. Reproductive signs
1. Infertility
2. Shortened duration of estrus
3. Prolonged anestrus
4. Prolonged or excessive estrual bleeding
5. Inappropriate galactorrhea in intact females
6. Decreased libido
J. Ocular signs
1. Secondary to hyperlipidemia
   a) Corneal lipid deposits
   b) Anterior uveitis, lipemic aqueous
2. Possibly keratoconjunctivitis sicca
K. Myxedema stupor or coma (Kelly, 1989)
1. Life-threatening consequence of severe hypothyroidism
2. Accompanied by other typical signs of hypothyroidism
3. Hypothermia without shivering
4. Severe depression, stupor, coma
5. Bradycardia despite hypotension
6. Nonpitting edema
L. Congenital hypothyroidism (Greco et al., 1991)
1. Also typical signs of adult-onset hypothyroidism
2. Impaired mental development: mental dullness, lethargy, difficulty in training, hypermetria
3. Dwarfism with poor epiphyseal calcification of the long bones and vertebrae, joint laxity
4. Macroglossia, delayed dental eruption
M. Feline hypothyroidism (Rand et al., 1993)
1. Transient hypothyroidism following thyroidectomy generally causes no signs of hypothyroidism.
2. Incidence is very rare.
3. Signs expected with severe, prolonged hypothyroidism are similar to those in the dog, such as lethargy, seborrhea, poor hair coat, obesity, hypothermia, and bradycardia.

Diagnosis

I. Routine laboratory tests
  A. Complete blood count: mild, normocytic, normochromic anemia in 25–30% of cases
  B. Serum chemistries
    1. Hypercholesterolemia in 50–75% of cases
    2. Elevated creatine kinase activity in 10–50% of cases
    3. Mild elevations in alkaline phosphatase
    4. Hyponatremia, lipemia, hypercholesterolemia, hypercarbia, hypoglycemia, and hypocortisolemia in dogs with myxedema coma
  C. Urinalysis: usually normal
II. Thyroid function tests
  A. Necessary to confirm a diagnosis of hypothyroidism
  B. Resting thyroid hormone concentrations
    1. Normal canine T_4 is 20–52 nmol/L (15–40 ng/ml).
    2. Normal canine T_3 is 1.2–3.1 nmol/L (0.8–2 ng/ml).
    3. Resting serum T_4 concentration is more reliable than T_3.
    4. Resting serum T_4 and T_3 concentrations in hypothyroid dogs can overlap those found in normal dogs.
      a) T_3 is frequently normal in hypothyroid dogs.
      b) T_4 is usually below normal in hypothyroidism.
    5. Numerous factors can affect resting serum T_4 and T_3 concentrations, making their interpretation difficult (Table 41–1).
  C. Serum-free T_3 and T_4 concentrations
    1. Thyroid hormones are highly protein bound (>99%).
    2. Non-protein-bound or free T_4 (fT_4) and T_3 (fT_3) are the metabolically active fractions of thyroid hormone.
    3. Measurement of fT_4 by equilibrium dialysis is superior to other assay methods because it is less affected by nonthyroidal illness and drug administration.
  D. Serum canine thyroid-stimulating hormone (cTSH)
    1. Endogenous cTSH can now be measured.
    2. Serum cTSH is elevated in primary hypothyroidism.
      a) As T_4 and T_3 secretions decrease, the reduction in negative feedback results in an increase in cTSH secretion.
      b) Serum cTSH is markedly elevated in severe hypothyroidism.
        (1) Serum cTSH may be normal in 20–40% of hypothyroid dogs.
        (2) Serum cTSH is elevated, whereas serum T_4 and T_3 may be normal in early or mild hypothyroidism in humans.
    3. Elevated cTSH and subnormal serum T_4 are diagnostic of hypothyroidism in a dog with typical clinical signs.

Table 41–1. Factors Affecting Resting Serum T_4 and T_3 Concentrations

Factors That Decrease T_4 and T_3	Factors That Increase T_4 and T_3
Normal hourly fluctuation	Normal hourly fluctuation
Nonthyroidal illness	Nonthyroidal illness (usually during recovery from illness)
Prolonged fasting (>48 h)	
General anesthesia	Diestrus and pregnancy
Age >7 yr	Age <3 mo
Breed (greyhounds have low T_4)	T_4 and T_3 autoantibodies
T_4 and T_3 autoantibodies (interfere with immunoassays)	Pharmaceuticals estrogens progesterone insulin narcotic analgesics
Pharmaceuticals glucocorticoids sulfonamides diphenylhydantoin phenobarbital primidone diazepam salicylates phenylbutazone iodinated radiographic contrast agents o,p'-DDD furosemide	

    4. fT_4 by equilibrium dialysis should be used in conjunction with serum cTSH in dogs with atypical signs, nonthyroidal illness, or concurrent drug administration.
    5. Serum cTSH measurement combined with serum thyroid hormones replaces the TSH response test.
    6. It may be useful in differentiating primary hypothyroidism from secondary and tertiary hypothyroidism.
  E. TSH response test
    1. Largely replaced by measurement of serum cTSH
    2. Expensive and often not available
  F. TRH response test
    1. Administration of TRH causes secretion of TSH, which then stimulates thyroid hormone synthesis and secretion.
    2. Protocol is as follows.
      a) Administer synthetic TRH (Relefact, Hoechst-Roussel) 0.5–1 mg IV (0.2–0.4 mg in small animals).
      b) Obtain blood samples before and 6 hours after injection for T_4 assay.
    3. Inadequate responses are not diagnostic.
      a) When compared with the TSH response test, a much smaller increase in T_4 (5–25 nmol/L) occurs.
      b) Some normal dogs do not respond to TRH administration with a significant rise in serum T_4 concentration.
    4. Accuracy of the test may improve with post-

TRH measurement of serum cTSH rather than T_4.
5. It can cause cholinergic side effects.
G. Response to thyroid hormone administration
 1. Therapeutic trial with thyroid hormone can cause an unnecessary delay in reaching a proper diagnosis.
 2. Results can be misleading. Thyroid hormone administration may result in improvement of clinical signs in a euthyroid dog because of its anabolic effects.
 3. Concurrent treatment with corticosteroids, antibiotics, or topical medications may result in improvement unrelated to thyroid supplementation.
 4. If a positive response to thyroid hormone occurs, withdraw treatment.
  a) If signs recur, hypothyroidism is confirmed and treatment can be reinstituted.
  b) If signs do not recur, hypothyroidism is not present and an alternative diagnosis should be sought.

Treatment

I. Sodium levothyroxine (T_4)
 A. Hormone of choice
  1. Best mimic of normal thyroid hormone secretion
  2. Rapidly converted to T_3, thereby providing an adequate source of T_3
  3. Thyrotoxicosis less likely
 B. Dog dosage: 22 μg/kg or 0.5 mg/m² PO BID
  1. Dosage interval may be reduced in most dogs to SID after resolution of clinical signs.
  2. Increase to BID again if signs recur.
 C. Cat dosage: 0.05–0.1 mg PO SID
 D. Alteration of initial dosage with certain concurrent diseases
  1. Cardiac disease, diabetes mellitus, hypoadrenocorticism, or in aged dogs: initially treat with 25% of usual dose, then increase by 25% every 2 weeks to 22 μg/kg
  2. Concurrent hypoadrenocorticism: begin glucocorticoid replacement before starting thyroid hormone treatment
  3. Diabetes mellitus: monitor blood glucose concentrations closely, because insulin requirements may change with thyroid hormone supplementation
  4. Renal failure or liver insufficiency: lower dosage required because of decreased hormone metabolism and excretion
II. Sodium liothyronine (T_3)
 A. Not used routinely
  1. Results in normal serum T_3 but low T_4
  2. Increased incidence of thyrotoxicosis
 B. Indicated if inadequate absorption of T_4 occurs
  1. T_3 has a higher oral bioavailability than T_4.
  2. Suspect poor absorption if the animal has no increase in *both* serum T_4 and T_3 after oral administration of T_4.

C. Suggested defects in the conversion of T_4 to T_3
 1. This has not been documented in the dog.
 2. Low serum T_3 and normal serum T_4 concentrations may occur from the following.
  a) Decreased conversion of T_4 to T_3 from nonthyroidal illness or the concurrent use of certain drugs
  b) Autoantibodies to T_3
D. Dog dosage: 4–6 μg/kg PO TID
E. Cat dosage: 4 μg/kg PO BID-TID
III. T_4/T_3 combinations: no advantage over T_4 alone and not recommended
IV. Treatment of myxedema coma
 A. Intravenous thyroid hormone
 B. Glucocorticoids
 C. Antibiotics
 D. Passive warming
 E. Supportive care
 F. Treatment of any concurrent disease

Patient Monitoring

I. Treat for 8 weeks before evaluating response to therapy.
II. Improved alertness and activity usually occur within 1–3 weeks.
III. Improvement in dermatologic changes and weight often takes several weeks to months.
IV. If response does not occur within 6–8 weeks, reevaluate diagnosis and perform postpill testing. Possible causes of therapeutic failure include the following.
 A. Misdiagnosis
 B. Poor owner compliance with hormone administration
 C. Inadequate dosage or frequency of administration
 D. Poor absorption of the compound
 E. Use of an outdated product
 F. Presence of T_4 or T_3 autoantibodies (unlikely)
 G. T_4 to T_3 conversion defect (unproved)
V. Postpill testing involves the following.
 A. Indications
  1. Response to treatment is inadequate.
  2. Thyrotoxicosis is suspected.
  3. A change in the brand of the supplement has occurred.
  4. The animal has been given drugs known to alter thyroid hormone concentrations.
 B. Protocol
  1. Test 6–8 weeks after initiating treatment.
  2. Measure serum T_4 and T_3 3–4 hours after T_4 administration.
  3. Measurement of serum cTSH in dogs may be useful in addition to T_4. Serum cTSH should be in the normal range if the dosage is correct.
  4. Measure only serum T_3 2–4 hours after T_3 administration.
 C. Interpretation
  1. Serum T_4 and T_3 are normal to high-normal.
   a) Continue at same dose if clinical response is good.
   b) Reevaluate diagnosis if clinical response is inadequate.

2. T_4 and T_3 are both low.
  a) Check client compliance.
  b) Increase dose.
  c) Change from T_4 to T_3 if higher doses of T_4 do not increase postpill T_3.
  d) Thyroid hormone autoantibodies may be interfering with assay, causing low or undetectable hormone concentrations.
3. T_4 is normal, T_3 is low.
  a) If clinical response is good, do not change treatment.
  b) Rule out concurrent disease, drug administration, or T_3 autoantibodies.
  c) Reevaluate diagnosis.
  d) Change to T_3 supplementation if all other causes are excluded and clinical response to T_4 is inadequate.
4. Decrease dose if T_4 and/or T_3 are greatly elevated or if signs of thyrotoxicosis are present.
VI. Thyrotoxicosis is rare because dogs and cats metabolize thyroid hormones rapidly.
  A. Signs include polydipsia, polyuria, polyphagia, weight loss, diarrhea, tachycardia, pruritus, anxiety, and pyrexia.
  B. Diagnosis is confirmed by demonstrating elevated serum T_4 and T_3.
  C. Search for the underlying cause before further treatment is administered.
    1. Inappropriate dosing
    2. Decreased metabolism of hormones
    3. Misdiagnosis of hypothyroidism
  D. Discontinue treatment until signs resolve and then reinstitute at a lower dose or decreased frequency of administration.

FELINE HYPERTHYROIDISM

David L. Panciera

Definition

Hyperthyroidism is induced by excessive concentrations of circulating thyroid hormones.

Causes

I. Adenomatous hyperplasia (functional thyroid adenoma)
  A. Most common cause of feline hyperthyroidism (98%)
  B. Usually bilateral (>70%)
II. Thyroid carcinoma: rare in the cat (<2%)

Clinical Signs and Pathophysiology

I. Signalment
  A. Age: mean, 12–13 years; range, 4–22 years
  B. No breed or sex predilection
II. General signs
  A. Palpable thyroid glands

1. Detectably enlarged glands are present in 80% of cats.
2. Thyroid tissue may be at the thoracic inlet or in the cranial mediastinum and may not be palpable.
B. Weight loss with polyphagia
  1. Weight loss (>95%)
  2. Polyphagia (50%)
  3. From inadequate caloric intake to meet the increased energy expenditure present in the thyrotoxic state
C. Behavioral changes
  1. Hyperkinetic behavior, nervousness, and aggressiveness (30%)
  2. May be secondary to a direct effect of thyroid hormone on the central nervous system (CNS)
D. Muscle weakness (12%)
III. Gastrointestinal signs
  A. Diarrhea or large fecal volume (15%)
    1. From increased food intake, increased gastrointestinal motility, and malassimilation
    2. Feces unformed and voluminous
  B. Vomiting (35–50%)
    1. Rapid intake of large quantities of food
    2. Direct effects of thyroid hormone on the chemoreceptor trigger zone
  C. Anorexia (7–20%)
  D. Hepatic dysfunction
    1. Elevated serum hepatic enzyme activity
    2. From liver hypoxia secondary to increased utilization of oxygen by the intestinal tract
    3. Secondary to congestive heart failure
    4. Direct toxic effect of thyroid hormones on the liver
IV. Renal signs
  A. Polyuria and polydipsia (35–50%)
    1. From increased renal blood flow, glomerular filtration rate, and renal tubular reabsorptive and secretory capacities
    2. Also primary polydipsia from CNS effects of thyroid hormones
    3. Concurrent renal insufficiency in some cases
  B. Prerenal azotemia or increased tissue catabolism with increased urea and creatinine
  C. Deterioration of renal function following correction of hyperthyroidism from decreased renal blood flow (Graves et al., 1994)
V. Skeletal signs
  A. Hyperphosphatemia: increased mineral resorption from bone
  B. Increased serum alkaline phosphatase activity possibly of bony origin
VI. Cardiovascular signs
  A. Cardiac murmur and/or gallop rhythm (50%)
  B. Cardiac hypertrophy
    1. Increased cardiac output, heart rate, and stroke volume
    2. Increased peripheral vascular resistance
    3. Increased adrenergic responsiveness
    4. Direct effects of thyroid hormones on the heart
  C. Heart failure (<5%)

1. Generally reversible with treatment
2. Cardiac dilatation and poor contractile function (rare)
    a) Heart failure may persist following treatment for hyperthyroidism.
    b) Prognosis is guarded.
D. ECG abnormalities
    1. Sinus tachycardia (10%)
    2. Increased R-wave amplitude in lead II (35%)
    3. Left axis deviation or left anterior fascicle block
    4. Atrial and ventricular premature contractions
E. Radiography
    1. Cardiomegaly (50%)
    2. Pulmonary edema or pleural effusion
F. Echocardiography
    1. Mild to moderate left ventricular and ventricular septal hypertrophy
    2. Increased fractional shortening
    3. Atrial enlargement
G. Systemic arterial hypertension (common) with hypertensive retinopathy
VII. Erythrocytosis (slightly elevated hematocrit)
A. Present in about 45% of cases
B. Elevated mean corpuscular volume (45%)
C. From increased erythropoietin production and a direct effect on the bone marrow mediated by $beta_2$-adrenergic receptors

Diagnosis

I. Routine laboratory tests
A. Complete blood count: erythrocytosis, stress leukogram
B. Serum chemistries
    1. Elevated liver enzymes (>90%)
    2. Elevated urea and creatinine (20–30%)
    3. Hyperglycemia (20%)
    4. Hyperphosphatemia
C. Urinalysis: specific gravity <1.035 in 50% of cases
II. Thyroid hormone concentrations
A. Serum T_4 concentration (normal, 15–55 nmol/L; 12–43 ng/ml)
    1. Elevated in 98% of affected cats: T_4 >55 nmol/L (43 ng/ml)
    2. Fluctuates during the day and may be normal at a given time
    3. Occasionally multiple samples required for a definitive diagnosis
B. Serum T_3 concentration (normal, 0.6–1.9 nmol/L; 0.4–1.2 ng/ml)
    1. More variable than T_4
    2. Normal in 10–30% of hyperthyroid cats
C. Serum fT_4 concentration by equilibrium dialysis
    1. Elevated in some hyperthyroid cats with a normal serum total T_4
    2. Indicated when total T_4 is repeatedly normal
D. T_3 suppression test
    1. Useful if repeated T_4 concentrations are normal
    2. Rationale

a) T_3 normally suppresses TSH secretion, thus decreasing T_4 secretion.
b) Thyroid function is autonomous in hyperthyroid cats and is not dependent on TSH for secretion; therefore, T_4 secretion is minimally affected by T_3 administration.
3. Protocol
    a) Obtain blood for T_4, then begin T_3 at 25 µg PO TID for 7 doses.
    b) Assay T_4 and T_3 again on the morning of the third day, 2–4 hours after the last dose of T_3.
4. Normal response: a decrease in T_4 to <20 nmol/L (15 ng/ml)
5. Hyperthyroidism: T_4 fails to suppress to <20 nmol/L
E. TRH stimulation test (Peterson et al., 1994)
    1. Indications similar to T_3 suppression test
    2. Rationale
        a) TRH causes TSH secretion, which in turn causes secretion of T_4.
        b) Thyroid function is autonomous in hyperthyroidism, so the increase in TSH results in a subnormal or no increase in T_4.
    3. Protocol
        a) Obtain blood for T_4 analysis, then administer 0.1 mg/kg TRH IV.
        b) Obtain second blood sample 4 hours later.
    4. Normal response: increase in T_4 >60% of baseline concentration
    5. Hyperthyroidism: increase in T_4 <50% of baseline concentration
    6. Cholinergic signs, including transient vomiting, defecation, salivation, and tachypnea
III. Radionuclide imaging with ^{99m}Tc pertechnetate
A. Allows localization of functional and abnormal thyroid tissue
B. Determines if disease is unilateral or bilateral
C. Locates any ectopic tissue
D. Identifies presence of metastasis (rare)
IV. Biopsy
A. Fine-needle aspiration identifies thyroid tissue but is not usually necessary for diagnosis.
B. Excisional biopsy allows differentiation of benign from malignant neoplasia.

Differential Diagnosis

I. Weight loss in spite of good appetite
A. Malassimilation
    1. Infiltrative small intestinal disease: neoplasia, inflammation
    2. Pancreatic exocrine insufficiency
B. Diabetes mellitus
C. Neoplasia
II. Other primary diseases
A. Chronic renal failure
B. Hepatic disease
C. Cardiomyopathy

Treatment

I. Antithyroid drugs (Table 41–2)
   A. May be used as sole treatment or to correct hyperthyroidism before surgery
   B. Methimazole (Peterson et al., 1988)
      1. Drug of choice: incidence of severe side effects much less than propylthiouracil
      2. Dose: 5 mg/cat PO SID-TID, with higher dose (15 mg/day) reserved for severe hyperthyroidism; reduced to lowest effective dose for long-term treatment
      3. Side effects
         a) Occur in about 20% of cats treated: usually within the first 12 weeks of treatment
         b) Anorexia, vomiting, and lethargy: most common side effects but generally do not require discontinuation of drug
         c) Pruritus with excoriations: requires discontinuation of drug
         d) Reversible hepatotoxicity
         e) Hematologic abnormalities
            (1) Eosinophilia, lymphocytosis, and leukopenia: transient, and cessation of treatment not necessary
            (2) Serious hematologic side effects: agranulocytosis (2%); thrombocytopenia (3%); usually resolve within 1 week of stopping drug
            (3) Antinuclear antibody: develops in 20%, but not associated with clinical disease
   C. Carbimazole (Mooney et al., 1992)
      1. Metabolized methimazole
      2. May have fewer side effects than methimazole
      3. Dose: 5 mg PO BID-TID
      4. Not available in the United States
   D. Propylthiouracil
      1. Not recommended because of severe side effects

      a) Immunomediated hemolytic anemia and thrombocytopenia (8%)
      b) Persistent pancytopenia
      2. Dose: 10 mg/kg PO TID initially
II. Propranolol
   A. Beta-adrenergic antagonist
   B. Does not affect thyroid hormone concentrations
   C. Used in combination with antithyroid agents
   D. Useful to control cardiac complications, especially tachycardia, arrhythmias, and hypertension
      1. Use if the heart rate exceeds 240 beats/minute and if tachyarrhythmias are present.
      2. It can be used in the presence of heart failure unless myocardial contractility is severely impaired.
   E. Dose: 2.5 mg PO BID-TID initially; can be doubled if response is inadequate
III. Radioactive iodine treatment: treatment of choice if available (Peterson and Becker, 1995)
   A. Iodine-131 is concentrated in the adenomatous thyroid gland.
   B. Normal thyroid tissue is spared.
   C. Dose (3–5 μCi) is based on severity of clinical signs, serum T_4 concentration, and size of thyroid gland.
   D. Recurrence rate is <3%.
   E. Thyroid carcinoma is most effectively treated with a combination of surgery and a higher dose of radioiodine than used for adenomas.
IV. Surgery
   A. Anesthesia
      1. Attain euthyroid state for 2–4 weeks before surgery.
      2. Avoid anticholinergics, xylazine, ketamine, and other drugs that are arrhythmogenic.
      3. Minimize stress with preoperative narcotic analgesics, butorphanol, or acepromazine.
   B. Surgical procedure
      1. Intracapsular or extracapsular techniques
         a) Intracapsular thyroidectomy is less likely to disturb parathyroid tissue but more

Table 41–2. **Advantages and Disadvantages of Treatment Options for Feline Hyperthyroidism**

Treatment	Advantages	Disadvantages
Methimazole	Ease of therapy	Lack of owner compliance
	Availability	Continuous administration necessary
	Inexpensive	Frequent side effects
	Anesthesia and surgery not required	Does not control tumor growth
Propylthiouracil	Similar to methimazole	Frequent occurrence of serious side effects
Radioactive iodine	Minimal side effects	Availability limited
	Destroys all affected thyroid tissue regardless of location	Requires prolonged hospitalization
	Retreatment necessary in <10%	
Surgery	Effective	Risk of general anesthesia
	Usually curative	Ectopic thyroid tissue not removed
	Readily available	Hypoparathyroidism following bilateral thyroidectomy
	Recurrence rate similar to that after radioactive iodine	Laryngeal paralysis, Horner's syndrome occur rarely
		Lifelong supplementation required following bilateral procedures

likely to incompletely remove adenomatous tissue.
- b) Extracapsular thyroidectomy completely removes abnormal thyroid tissue, but damage to the parathyroid glands is more likely to occur.
- c) Combined intracapsular and extracapsular techniques can be performed.
  - (1) Extracapsular dissection on caudal portion of gland to ensure optimal removal of thyroid tissue
  - (2) Intracapsular dissection on the cranial portion to spare parathyroid glands and vasculature
2. Although one thyroid may be normal in size at the time of surgery, more than 70% of cats have bilateral disease.
3. Staged thyroidectomy involves two unilateral thyroidectomies at least 4 weeks apart.
   - a) Reduces incidence of hypoparathyroidism
   - b) Requires two periods of anesthesia and surgery

Patient Monitoring

I. Methimazole therapy
   - A. Measure serum T_4 every 2 weeks.
     1. T_4 is normal in most cats within 2–4 weeks.
     2. Increase dose 5 mg/day if T_4 remains elevated after 4 weeks of treatment.
     3. Reduce dose if T_4 is subnormal.
     4. A dosage of 5 mg PO SID-BID is generally required to maintain euthyroidism.
   - B. Obtain a complete blood count every 2–3 weeks for the first 3 months and every 3–4 months thereafter. Stop treatment if agranulocytosis or thrombocytopenia occurs.
II. Radioactive iodine
   - A. Euthyroidism is attained within 1–2 weeks after treatment.
   - B. Recheck T_4 2 and 6 months after treatment. Transient hypothyroidism can persist for several months after treatment.
   - C. Consider retreatment if serum T_4 is elevated 6 months after treatment.
III. Surgery
   - A. Monitor serum Ca^{2+} at least daily for 3–5 days postoperatively when bilateral thyroidectomy is performed, as hypoparathyroidism and hypocalcemia can occur from damage to the parathyroid glands during surgery.
   - B. Hypocalcemia is treated with intravenous and/or oral calcium and oral vitamin D as described in Chap. 42.
IV. Iatrogenic hypothyroidism
   - A. It occurs infrequently following surgery or radioiodine.
   - B. Treatment is indicated only when low serum T_4 is accompanied by clinical signs of hypothyroidism.

THYROID TUMORS IN THE DOG

David M. Vail

Definition

I. Thyroid tumors account for 10–15% of all head and neck tumors in the dog.
II. Signalment
   - A. Neoplasia of the thyroid affects primarily aged dogs (mean, 9 years).
   - B. Benign adenomas may be overrepresented in boxers.
   - C. Malignant carcinomas may be overrepresented in boxers, old English sheepdogs, Shetland sheepdogs, and golden retrievers.
   - D. No sex predilection is known.

Causes

I. Usually unknown
II. Incidence initially believed to be higher in areas of endemic goiter secondary to iodine deficiency, but no evidence of this in the dog

Pathophysiology

I. Malignant carcinoma (65–87% of all canine thyroid tumors)
   - A. Three histologic types exist: follicular (most common), compact, or papillary.
   - B. Most are present in the area of the normal thyroid gland.
   - C. Two thirds are unilateral.
   - D. Ectopic sites, such as the cranial mediastinum and the base of the tongue, do occur.
   - E. Most tumors are invasive into surrounding tissues such as muscle, esophagus, trachea, larynx, blood vessels (carotid, jugular), and nerves (sympathetic chain, recurrent laryngeal).
   - F. Status of thyroid function in affected dogs varies.
     1. Most are euthyroid.
     2. Roughly 15% are hypothyroid from the following.
        - a) Destruction of normal thyroid tissue
        - b) Production of inactive thyroid hormones that suppress pituitary–thyroid axis
     3. Less than 5% are hyperthyroid because of a functional tumor.
   - G. Metastatic potential is high.
     1. They can metastasize hematogenously to lungs or via lymphatics to regional lymph nodes.
     2. Roughly one third have metastasized by the time of diagnosis; likelihood of metastasis increases in proportion to the volume of the primary tumor.
     3. Brain, spine, and ocular metastases are rarely reported.
   - H. Chronic disseminated intravascular coagulation

(DIC) has been reported as an accompanying paraneoplastic syndrome.

II. Medullary carcinoma (less common)
  A. Arises from the calcitonin-producing C cells of the thyroid gland
  B. Rarely produces active calcitonin with clinical hypocalcemia
  C. May be associated with the multiple endocrine neoplasia syndrome
  D. Possesses gross and histologic characteristics of a less malignant nature than thyroid carcinoma (Carver et al., 1995)
III. Benign adenomas
  A. Less common than their malignant counterpart and typically of little clinical importance
  B. Most diagnosed incidentally at necropsy
  C. Well-encapsulated, noninvasive

Clinical Signs

I. The presence of a ventral cervical mass is often the only clinical sign, because the majority of these tumors are nonfunctional and can attain a large size before diagnosis.
II. Signs related to pressure on or infiltration of surrounding structures can occur late in the course of disease.
  A. Dysphagia
  B. Dyspnea
  C. Precaval syndrome (edema of face, neck, and forelimbs)
III. Signs of hypocalcemia can occur rarely with thyroid medullary carcinoma (most are eucalcemic).

Diagnosis

I. History and physical exam
  A. Cervical mass present
  B. Regional lymph node assessment
II. Radiology
  A. Plain cervical radiography, xeroradiography, or computed tomography help delineate extent of local disease.
  B. Thoracic radiographs are indicated to identify metastasis and ectopic mediastinal tumors.
III. Fine-needle aspirate
  A. Thyroid tumors tend not to exfoliate well, and aspirates are commonly diluted secondary to blood admixture.
  B. Neoplastic endocrine cells can usually be identified on the feathered edge of the smear, but the cell of origin may be difficult to determine.
  C. Modify the technique by using a needle without the syringe and holding a finger over the hub while repeatedly penetrating the mass to "core" a sample and minimize dilution with blood.
  D. Also aspirate suspicious regional lymph nodes.
IV. Biopsy
  A. Cutting needle biopsies are diagnostic if attainable.
  B. Surgical wedge biopsies may be necessary.
  C. Significant biopsy-induced hemorrhage can occur

because of the high vascularity of these tumors and the possibility of chronic DIC.
V. Nuclear medicine
  A. It is not as widely used for canine thyroid tumors because they are often nonfunctional.
  B. ^{99m}Tc or ^{123}I can help establish the extent of primary or metastatic disease and provide insight into the degree of possible function of the tumor.
  C. In 29 cases, ^{99m}Tc scans were no more beneficial than thoracic radiographs for detecting pulmonary metastasis (Marks et al., 1994)
VI. Thyroid function tests
  A. Baseline thyroid hormone assays or a TSH stimulation test may be used to determine thyroid function.
  B. "Thyroid storm," that is, a massive release of excess thyroid hormone following TSH stimulation, has not been reported in dogs with thyroid tumors.

Differential Diagnosis

I. Other malignancies
  A. Chemodectoma (carotid body tumors)
  B. Lymphosarcoma
  C. Metastatic tonsillar squamous cell carcinoma
  D. Regional soft tissue sarcoma
  E. Thyroglossal duct neoplasia
  F. Miscellaneous primary or metastatic tumor types
II. Benign disease
  A. Abscess
  B. Granuloma
  C. Salivary mucocele
  D. Thyroglossal duct remnants

Treatment

I. Surgical excision, if possible, is the therapy of choice.
  A. Median survivals of 36 months have been reported for mobile thyroid carcinomas following surgical excision in 20 cases (Klein et al., 1995).
  B. Obtain presurgical coagulation panel and be prepared for the possibility of intraoperative transfusion therapy.
  C. Ideally, perform enbloc excision without disrupting the tumor; unilateral ligation of the common carotid and jugular vein is well tolerated in the dog.
  D. Educate the owner about the possibility of postoperative Horner's syndrome or unilateral laryngeal paralysis.
  E. The single most important prognostic factor for survival is whether the tumor can be surgically excised; this decision is based on its size and adherence to surrounding and underlying structures.
II. Chemotherapy is inconsistently effective.
  A. Doxorubicin
    1. When used alone, no complete responses and only a few partial responses have been reported (Klein et al., 1995), and median sur-

vival has not been significantly different from that of dogs that did not receive therapy.
  2. Dosage is 30 mg/m² IV every 3 weeks, to a maximum cumulative dose of 250 mg/m².
  B. Cisplatin or mitoxantrone
   1. Partial responses have been reported in dogs receiving 60 mg/m² of cisplatin (Knapp et al., 1988).
   2. Mitoxantrone resulted in a partial response in 1 of 10 dogs treated (Ogilvie et al., 1991).
  C. Ultimately, effective chemotherapeutics may be used in four settings.
   1. Primary therapy for nonresectable tumors
   2. Adjuvant therapy for incompletely excised tumors
   3. To decrease tumor volume before surgical excision
   4. To palliate clinical signs
 III. The efficacy of radiation therapy is uncertain, but it has been used as primary therapy or to reduce tumor volume before surgical excision.
 IV. Iodine 131 (^{131}I) therapy may have minimal value.
  A. As most thyroid tumors in dogs are nonfunctional, ^{131}I uptake by the tumor would be expected to be inadequate; iodine uptake studies should precede this therapy if it is being considered as a primary or adjuvant therapy.
  B. Reversal of clinical signs and a partial response have been reported in a functional thyroid carcinoma in the dog (Peterson, 1989).
  C. Much higher doses of ^{131}I are required in dogs with carcinomas than in cats with adenomas.

Patient Monitoring

 I. Surgical follow-up
  A. Evaluate surgical margins histologically.
  B. Monitor for hypoparathyroidism subsequent to surgery; life-threatening hypocalcemia can occur ≥3 days after surgery.
  C. Schedule rechecks at 1 month following surgery and then every 3 months, including a physical exam, regional lymph node assessment, and thoracic radiography.
 II. Thyroid function
  A. Perform thyroid function studies 1 month after surgery and periodically thereafter if necessary.
  B. Thyroid supplementation may be required for postoperative hypothyroidism.

Bibliography

Bichsel P, Jacobs G, Oliver JE Jr: Neurologic manifestations associated with hypothyroidism in four dogs. J Am Vet Med Assoc 192:1745, 1988

Broussard JD, Peterson ME, Fox PR: Changes in clinical and laboratory findings in cats with hyperthyroidism from 1983 to 1993. J Am Vet Med Assoc 206:302, 1995

Budsberg SC, Moore GE, Klappenbach K: Thyroxine-responsive unilateral forelimb lameness and generalized neuromuscular disease in four hypothyroid dogs. J Am Vet Med Assoc 202:1859, 1993

Carver JR, Kapatkin A, Patnaik AK: A comparison of medullary thyroid adenocarcinoma in dogs: a retrospective study of 38 cases. Vet Surg 24:315, 1995

Chastain CB, Young DW, Kemppainen RJ: Anti-triiodothyronine antibodies associated with hypothyroidism and lymphocytic thyroiditis in a dog. J Am Vet Med Assoc 194:531, 1989

Feldman EC, Nelson RW: Canine and Feline Endocrinology and Reproduction. 2nd Ed. WB Saunders, Philadelphia, 1996

Ferguson DC (ed): Thyroid disorders. Vet Clin North Am [Small Anim Pract] 24:431, 1994

Graves TK, Olivier B, Nachreiner RF et al: Changes in renal function associated with treatment of hyperthyroidism in cats. Am J Vet Res 55:1745, 1994

Greco, DS, Feldman EC, Peterson ME et al: Congenital hypothyroid dwarfism in a family of giant schnauzers. J Vet Intern Med 5:57, 1991

Jaggy A, Oliver JE, Ferguson DC et al: Neurological manifestations of hypothyroidism: a retrospective study of 29 dogs. J Vet Intern Med 8:328, 1994

Kelly MJ: Canine myxedema stupor and coma. p. 998. In Kirk RW (ed): Current Veterinary Therapy X: Small Animal Practice. WB Saunders, Philadelphia, 1989

Klein MK, Powers BE, Withrow SJ et al: Treatment of thyroid carcinoma in dogs by surgical resection alone: 20 cases (1981–1989). J Am Vet Med Assoc 206:1007, 1995

Knapp DW, Richardson RC, Bonney PL et al: Cisplatin therapy in 41 dogs with malignant tumors. J Vet Intern Med 2:41, 1988

Mooney CT, Thoday KL, Doxey DL: Carbimazole therapy of feline hyperthyroidism. J Small Anim Pract 33:228, 1992

Marks SL, Koblik PD, Hornof WJ, Feldman EC: ^{99m}Tc-pertechnetate imaging of thyroid tumors in dogs: 29 cases (1980–1992). J Am Vet Med Assoc 204:756, 1994

Nachreiner RF, Refsal KR, Ravis WR et al: Pharmacokinetics of L-thyroxine after its oral administration in dogs. Am J Vet Res 54:2091, 1993

Ogilvie GK, Obradovich JE, Elmsie RE et al: Efficacy of mitoxantrone against various neoplasms in dogs. J Am Vet Med Assoc 198:1618, 1991

Panciera DL: Hypothyroidism in dogs: 66 cases (1987–1992). J Am Vet Med Assoc 204:761, 1994

Panciera DL, Johnson GS: Plasma von Willebrand factor antigen concentration and buccal mucosal bleeding time in dogs with experimental hypothyroidism. J Vet Intern Med 10:60, 1996

Peterson ME: Feline hypothyroidism. p. 1000. In Kirk RW (ed): Current Veterinary Therapy X: Small Animal Practice. WB Saunders, Philadelphia, 1989

Peterson ME, Becker DV: Radioiodine treatment of 524 cats with hyperthyroidism. J Am Vet Med Assoc 207:1422, 1995

Peterson ME, Broussard JD, Gamble DA: Use of the thyrotropin releasing hormone stimulation test to diagnose mild hyperthyroidism in cats. J Vet Intern Med 8:279, 1994

Peterson ME, Graves TK, Gamble DA: Triiodothyronine (T3) suppression test. An aid in the diagnosis of mild hyperthyroidism in cats. J Vet Intern Med 4:233, 1990

Peterson ME, Kintzer PP, Hurvitz AI: Methimazole treatment of 262 cats with hyperthyroidism. J Vet Intern Med 2:150, 1988

Rand JS, Levine J, Best SJ et al: Spontaneous adult-onset hypothyroidism in a cat. J Vet Intern Med 7:272, 1993

Swalec KM, Birchard SJ: Recurrence of hyperthyroidism after thyroidectomy in cats. J Am Anim Hosp Assoc 26:433, 1990

Turrel JM, Feldman EC, Nelson RW et al: Thyroid carcinoma causing hyperthyroidism in cats: 14 cases (1981–1986). J Am Vet Med Assoc 193:359, 1988

Vail DM, Panciera DL, Ogilvie GK: Thyroid hormone concentrations in dogs with chronic weight loss, with special reference to cancer cachexia. J Vet Intern Med 8:122, 1994

42

Diseases of the Parathyroid Glands

William E. Monroe

HYPOPARATHYROIDISM

Definition

I. Hypoparathyroidism is a condition caused by a failure of production or secretion of parathyroid hormone (PTH), or a failure of target tissues to respond to PTH (pseudohypoparathyroidism).

II. It is characterized by hypocalcemia and hyperphosphatemia with normal renal function.

Causes

I. Conditions associated with low plasma PTH (true hypoparathyroidism)
   A. Iatrogenic
      1. Following surgical thyroidectomy/parathyroidectomy
      2. Most common in cats after surgical removal of thyroid neoplasia
   B. Parathyroid atrophy from prolonged hypercalcemia
      1. Signs occur following removal of a functional parathyroid neoplasm.
      2. Rarely, it may develop with inappropriate oversupplementation with calcium (Ca) and vitamin D.
   C. Lymphocytic/plasmacytic parathyroiditis and atrophy
      1. Thought to be immunomediated
      2. Most common cause for naturally acquired hypoparathyroidism in adult dogs
      3. Atrophy of unknown cause in adult cats
   D. Idiopathic, possibly familial parathyroid atrophy or dysgenesis in St. Bernard dogs (Jones and Alley, 1985)
   E. Parathyroid hypoplasia or agenesis: congenital, life-threatening
   F. Severe hypomagnesemia
      1. Inhibits PTH secretion and causes peripheral resistance to PTH

2. May be seen with diabetes mellitus or gentamicin toxicity
   G. Viral-induced: canine distemper

II. Conditions associated with failure to respond to PTH (pseudohypoparathyroidism): not documented in dogs or cats

Pathophysiology

I. Because of a lack of PTH action on the kidney, Ca excretion is increased, phosphorus (P) excretion is reduced, and magnesium (Mg) resorption is reduced.

II. Without PTH, mobilization of calcium from bone in response to hypocalcemia is severely impaired.

III. Ca and P absorption from the intestine is decreased indirectly because of a relative deficiency of calcitriol (vitamin D_3) from its reduced synthesis in the absence of PTH.

IV. The net effect is hypocalcemia, hyperphosphatemia, occasionally mild hypomagnesemia, increased renal fractional excretion of Ca, and reduced renal fractional excretion of P.

V. Hypocalcemia decreases nerve cell membrane stability, leading to hyperexcitability and tetany.

Clinical Signs

I. Occur with serum Ca <6–7 mg/dl

II. Usually episodic, with hours to days between episodes, and often associated with excitement or physical activity

III. Generalized seizures

IV. Focal muscle twitching to generalized muscle tremors

V. Ataxia, stiff gait

VI. Excessive panting

VII. Hyperthermia; cats occasionally hypothermic

VIII. Weakness and lethargy

IX. Polyuria and polydipsia

X. Behavioral aberrations
   A. Disorientation, aggression, excessive scratching

B. Restlessness, excitement
XI. Anorexia; ptyalism and/or dysphagia occasionally in cats
XII. Cataracts
XIII. Electrocardiographic abnormalities
  A. Prolonged Q–T interval
  B. Ventricular premature depolarizations

Diagnosis

I. Primary hypoparathyroidism
  A. Suspicious clinical signs with a history of recent thyroid/parathyroid surgery
  B. Laboratory findings
    1. Hypocalcemia with hyperphosphatemia
    2. Normal renal function
    3. Normal or only slightly reduced serum Mg
    4. Low plasma PTH concentration
      a) See Primary Hyperparathyroidism, later, for discussion of PTH assays.
      b) PTH is often undetectable in these cases.
  C. Biopsy of parathyroid gland
    1. Not necessary in most cases
    2. Requires surgical removal of one intact gland
II. Pseudohypoparathyroidism
  A. Laboratory findings are similar to those for primary hypoparathyroidism, except that plasma PTH is elevated.
  B. Administration of exogenous PTH does not increase urinary fractional P excretion.

Differential Diagnosis

I. Neuromuscular and behavioral abnormalities
  A. Metabolic disorders
    1. Hypoglycemia
    2. Hypercalcemia
    3. Severe disturbances of serum potassium and sodium
    4. Liver dysfunction or failure
    5. Renal failure or severe azotemia
  B. Cardiac disease: episodic tachy- or bradyarrhythmias
  C. Primary neurologic disease
    1. Cerebral diseases
    2. Polyneuropathy or polyneuritis
  D. Toxicities
    1. Metaldehyde
    2. Caffeine
    3. Organophosphates and carbamates
    4. Ethylene glycol
II. Other causes of hypocalcemia
  A. Hypoalbuminemia (see correction formula for Ca under Primary Hyperparathyroidism)
  B. Chronic or acute renal failure
  C. Puerperal tetany
  D. Acute pancreatitis
  E. Phosphate enemas or laxatives (hyperphosphatemia)
  F. Soft tissue trauma
  G. Intestinal malabsorption
  H. Dietary deficiency: hypocalcemia develops late

  I. Massive blood transfusion with citrated blood
  J. Rapid intravenous infusion of phosphates or Ca-free solutions
  K. Hypovitaminosis-D
  L. Osteoblastic bone tumor
  M. Laboratory error
  N. Hypercalcitoninism from functional thyroid medullary carcinoma

Treatment

I. Therapy for hypocalcemic tetany
  A. Rapid 10% Ca gluconate (~ 10 mg/ml elemental Ca) infusion
    1. Give 0.5–1.5 ml/kg up to 10 ml (5–15 mg/kg elemental Ca) diluted in 5% dextrose/water (D/W) slowly over 20–30 minutes to effect.
    2. Monitor ECG for bradycardia, shortening of the Q–T interval, or ST elevation, and stop infusion if these occur.
  B. Slow 10% Ca gluconate administration
    1. Begin once tetany is controlled at a rate to keep serum Ca concentration normal.
    2. Dosage is approximately 20 mg/kg Ca over 6–8 hours IV diluted in a maintainence volume of 5% D/W (22 ml/kg every 8 hours).
    3. Alternatively, give the dose of 10% Ca gluconate required to stop tetany TID-QID SQ.
    4. Caution: Do not give Ca chloride SQ.
II. Maintenance therapy
  A. Oral vitamin D
    1. Vitamin D_2 (ergocalciferol)
      a) Dosage is initially 4000–6000 U/kg/day PO.
      b) Then reduce to 1000–2000 U/kg once daily to once weekly to maintain serum Ca at 8–10 mg/dl.
      c) Maximal effect occurs within 5–21 days.
      d) Toxicity from overdose subsides in 1–18 weeks.
    2. Dihydrotachysterol (Hytakeral)
      a) Give 0.03 mg/kg/day PO for 2 days, then 0.02 mg/kg/day for 2 days, then 0.01 mg/kg/day or adjusted as needed.
      b) Maximal effect is within 1–7 days.
      c) Toxicity subsides in 1–3 weeks.
    3. Calcitriol (Rocaltrol)
      a) Give 0.03–0.06 μg/kg/day PO.
      b) Maximal effect occurs in 1–4 days.
      c) Toxicity subsides in 1 day to 2 weeks.
    Note: Vitamin D can usually be withdrawn within 8–12 weeks for hypoparathyroidism secondary to thyroid/parathyroid surgery.
  B. Oral calcium
    1. Can be given as carbonate (40% Ca), gluconate (9% Ca), lactate (13% Ca), or acetate (25% Ca) salts
    2. Carbonate preferred
    3. Dose: 50–75 mg elemental Ca/kg/day PO divided TID-QID

4. Can usually be tapered and withdrawn as vitamin D reaches maximal effect
C. Decreased access to phosphorus
    1. Low-P diets (kidney diets) and oral phosphate binders such as aluminum hydroxide may be needed to keep serum P concentration normal and serum Ca $\times$ P product <70 to avoid soft tissue mineralization.
    2. Dose of aluminum hydroxide is 100 mg/kg/day initially, with or before meals, adjusted every 10–14 days until serum P is normal.
    3. Because Ca carbonate is also a P binder, when it is used for Ca supplementation, additional P binders may not be required.

Patient Monitoring

I. Monitor serum Ca daily until it has stabilized (8–10 mg/dl) for several days, then weekly until vitamin D and Ca therapy is regulated, then every 1–3 months indefinitely or until therapy is no longer needed.
II. Monitor serum P weekly until normal and until the serum Ca $\times$ P product remains <70, then every 1–3 months.
III. For iatrogenic cases, monitor plasma PTH concentration monthly.
    A. Vitamin D and calcium therapy may be tapered and stopped when PTH values are normal.
    B. Cats that have undergone bilateral thyroid/parathyroidectomy may recover the ability to maintain a normal serum Ca concentration in spite of persistent hypoparathyroidism (Flanders et al., 1991).
IV. Advise the owner to monitor for polyuria/polydipsia as a sign of hypercalcemia.
V. If hypercalcemia develops, withdraw medications until Ca is normal for 2–3 days, then restart vitamin D at a lower dose. Treat hypercalcemia aggressively if Ca is >16 mg/dl or if clinical signs are present, as outlined for Primary Hyperparathyroidism.

PRIMARY HYPERPARATHYROIDISM

Definition

I. Primary hyperparathyroidism is a clinical disorder caused by excessive unregulated production of PTH without another disease that secondarily stimulates overproduction of PTH.
II. It is characterized by hypercalcemia and in some cases by skeletal demineralization.

Causes

I. Functional parathyroid gland neoplasm (most common cause)
    A. Adenoma: most common tumor
    B. Cystadenoma: occasionally in cats
    C. Carcinoma: rarely

II. Neonatal parathyroid hyperplasia: reported in two German shepherd pups (Thompson et al., 1984)
III. Parathyroid hyperplasia associated with multiple endocrine neoplasia
IV. Primary, idiopathic, parathyroid hyperplasia
    A. More than one gland (usually all four) are grossly and microscopically hyperplastic.
    B. Rule out causes of secondary parathyroid hyperplasia.

Pathophysiology

I. PTH is normally secreted in response to a low serum ionized Ca concentration, with secretion inhibited by a high Ca concentration.
II. Excessive secretion of PTH occurs because of failure to respond to Ca concentration (neoplasia) or because of an increased parenchymal mass (hyperplasia) with normal sensitivity to Ca concentration (Martin et al., 1987).
III. PTH has several functions.
    A. Renal Ca excretion is inhibited, and P excretion is enhanced.
    B. Bone resorption occurs because of an increased number and activity of osteoclasts, secondarily increasing serum Ca and P concentrations.
    C. Absorption of Ca and P from the intestine is enhanced by increased conversion of 25-hydroxycholecalciferol to calcitriol.
IV. Net effect of hyperparathyroidism is hypercalcemia, low-normal or hypophosphatemia (with impaired renal function, hyperphosphatemia may be present), reduced renal fractional Ca excretion, increased renal fractional P excretion, and bone resorption.
V. Hypercalcemia has deleterious effects, including the inhibition of neuromuscular activity, direct cellular toxicity (especially hypercalcemic nephropathy), and soft tissue mineralization.

Clinical Signs

I. Signalment
    A. Middle-age or older: dogs 6–13 years, cats 8–15 years
    B. Slightly higher incidence in females
    C. Siamese cats and keeshonds overrepresented
II. Signs of hypercalcemia
    A. Subtle or no signs
        1. Hypercalcemia often noted fortuitously on chemistry profiles
        2. Mild or unremarkable signs noted by the owner
    B. Renal abnormalities
        1. Polyuria and polydipsia from inhibition of antidiuretic hormone (ADH) activity
        2. Azotemia $\pm$ renal failure from mineralization, and glomerular arteriolar vasoconstriction
        3. Calcium urolithiasis
    C. Neuromuscular dysfunction
        1. Muscular weakness, lethargy
        2. Seizures, stiff gait, shivering

D. Gastrointestinal disorders (depressed motility)
   1. Anorexia
   2. Vomiting, constipation, obstipation
E. Electrocardiographic abnormalities
   1. Shortened Q–T interval
   2. Atrioventricular block
   3. Ventricular premature depolarizations
F. Paradoxical signs of acute hypoparathyroidism
   1. These occur after infarction of functional parathyroid adenoma.
   2. See section on Hypoparathyroidism.

III. Skeletal signs (uncommon)
   A. Demineralization and loss of radiographic bone density, particularly of the maxillary and mandibular lamina dura dentes
   B. Fibrous osteodystrophy, especially of the mandible and maxilla
   C. Pathologic fractures

IV. Parathyroid findings
   A. Palpable cervical mass: rare except in cats
   B. Mediastinal mass: occasionally in dogs with mediastinal parathyroid carcinoma

Diagnosis

I. A major objective of the diagnostic work-up is to rule out secondary causes of hypercalcemia, which are generally more common than primary hyperparathyroidism.

II. Document persistent hypercalcemia (Ca >12 mg/dl).
   A. Correct calcium for albumin concentration in dogs; corrected Ca = measured Ca − albumin + 3.5.
   B. The formula is not dependable for cats (Flanders et al., 1989).

III. From the history rule out the following.
   A. Severe hypothermia
   B. Disuse osteoporosis
   C. Vitamin D intoxication

IV. Physical examination is usually normal.
   A. Palpate lymph nodes, spleen, liver for evidence of lymphosarcoma.
   B. Perform ophthalmic exam for evidence of lymphosarcoma.
   C. On rectal palpation, check for the presence of anal sac adenocarcinoma.
   D. Palpate bones for pain to help rule out bony neoplasia, multiple myeloma, osteomyelitis, and pathologic fractures.

V. Review chemistry profile.
   A. Low sodium (Na), high potassium (K), with Na:K ratio <26:1 and azotemia: possible hypoadrenocorticism
   B. Hyperphosphatemia, azotemia, and Na:K ratio >26:1
      1. Primary renal failure; azotemia usually severe
      2. Vitamin D intoxication
      3. Renal failure secondary to hypercalcemia
         a) Azotemia is usually mild.
         b) It occurs uncommonly at presentation with primary hyperparathyroidism.
         c) Ionized calcium is usually normal or low.
   C. Hyperglobulinemia
      1. Obtain a serum protein electrophoresis.
      2. Monoclonal gammopathy is consistent with myeloma.

VI. Hematology is usually normal with primary hyperparathyroidism.

VII. Radiography may be helpful to delineate the cause.
   A. Skull radiography
      1. Demineralization of maxilla and mandible, especially the lamina dura dentes, with primary hyperparathyroidism or renal failure
      2. Fibrous osteodystrophy of maxilla and mandible with primary hyperparathyroidism or renal failure
   B. Thoracic radiography
      1. Normal with primary hyperparathyroidism
      2. Mediastinal mass or enlarged lymph nodes with lymphosarcoma
      3. ± Metastatic nodules with other neoplasms
   C. Abdominal radiography or ultrasonography
      1. Usually normal with primary hyperparathyroidism but may show renal mineralization or urinary calculi
      2. Organomegaly or masses with hypercalcemia of malignancy
   D. Radiography of long bones
      1. Pathologic fractures occasionally seen with primary hyperparathyroidism
      2. Primary bone tumor
      3. Osteomyelitis (solitary or multiple)
      4. Multiple lytic lesions: myeloma or metastatic solid tumor
   E. Adenomas or hyperplastic glands detected in 70% of dogs with primary hyperparathyroidism using cervical ultrasonography (Wisner et al., 1993)

VIII. Lymph node aspiration cytology of any abnormally large nodes is performed to rule out lymphosarcoma and hypercalcemia of malignancy.

IX. Documentation of elevated serum PTH concentration in the face of hypercalcemia, without evidence of causes of secondary hyperparathyroidism, confirms primary hyperparathyroidism (use an assay validated for the species being examined).
   A. Commercially available assays valid for canine sera
      1. PTH-MM RIA kit, Incstar Corp (Torrance and Nachreiner, 1989a)
         a) Little clinical use with canine cases
         b) Canine normal range not known
      2. Allegro Intact PTH, Nichols Institute (Torrance and Nachreiner, 1989a, 1989b)
         a) The best-studied assay for use with canine sera
         b) Normal range, 16–136 pg/ml
   B. PTH assay for cats
      1. A two-site intact PTH assay, Allegro Intact PTH, Nichols Institute, has been validated for cats (Barber et al., 1993).
      2. Normal range is 3.3–22.5 pg/ml.

C. Interpretation
  1. High PTH without azotemia confirms primary hyperparathyroidism.
  2. Normal PTH is suggestive of primary hyperparathyroidism.
  3. Low PTH is indicative of hypercalcemia of malignancy.
  4. A high PTH and azotemia are not diagnostic, because renal failure secondarily elevates PTH.
  5. A normal or low PTH with azotemia is indicative of hypercalcemia of malignancy.
X. PTH-related peptide (PTH-rP) may be detected in the serum in some cases of hypercalcemia of malignancy, and the assay is available commercially (Animal Health Diagnostic Lab. Michigan State University).
XI. Surgically explore cervical area for parathyroid lesions.

Differential Diagnosis

I. Hypercalcemia with low-normal or hypophosphatemia
  A. Primary hyperparathyroidism (elevated PTH)
  B. Hypercalcemia of malignancy (low or normal PTH)
  C. Severe hypothermia (Ross and Goldstein, 1981)
II. Hypercalcemia with hyperphosphatemia
  A. Atypical primary renal failure
    1. In acute renal failure, it may occur during the polyuric phase from mobilization of Ca and P previously deposited in soft tissue during the oliguric phase.
    2. Hypercalcemia may occur in 5–10% of dogs with chronic renal failure.
    3. Ionized calcium is low or normal.
  B. Severe primary hypoadrenocorticism
  C. Hypervitaminosis D (vitamin D rodenticides)
  D. Active, lytic bony lesions
    1. Primary bone neoplasia
    2. Metastatic neoplasia
    3. Osteomyelitis
    4. Disuse osteoporosis
III. Hypercalcemia with variable (near normal) P concentration
  A. Artifact: hyperlipidemic sample
  B. Bone growth in young dogs
  C. Associated with dehydration and hyperalbuminemia
  D. Usually has no clinical significance

Treatment

I. Medical therapy for reducing hypercalcemia while awaiting surgery
  A. Medical therapy to attempt to increase Ca excretion is indicated when there are neurologic signs, cardiac arrhythmias, azotemia, dehydration, Ca >16 mg/dl, and/or Ca × P product >70.
    1. Normal saline IV
      a) Correct fluid deficit: % dehydration × kg body weight, replaced in 6 hours
      b) Saline diuresis with additional 130–200 ml/kg/day IV
    2. Diuretics
      a) Give furosemide 2 mg/kg IV, SQ, PO BID-TID.
      b) Do *not* use thiazide diuretics; they reduce Ca excretion.
  B. More aggressive therapy is indicated if fluid and diuretic therapy is ineffective.
    1. Prednisolone 2 mg/kg PO, SQ BID
    2. Calcitonin 4–6 IU/kg SQ, IM every 8–12 hours
    3. Diphosphonates
      a) Etidronate disodium 7.5 mg/kg/day IV for 3 days diluted in 250 ml 0.9% NaCl over several hours (human dose)
      b) Contraindicated in severe renal failure
    4. Mithramycin 25 μg/kg IV (Rosol et al., 1994)
  C. The following drugs may be tried for refractory, life-threatening hypercalcemia, but they must be used cautiously because of their high toxicity.
    1. Phosphate IV
      a) Appropriate dosage not well documented
      b) Worsens tissue mineralization
    2. Sodium EDTA 25–75 mg/kg/hour IV diluted to a 3% solution in 5% D/W or 0.9% saline
II. Maintenance medical therapy for animals not amenable to or awaiting surgery
  A. Furosemide 2 mg/kg PO BID-TID
  B. Prednisolone 2 mg/kg PO BID
III. Surgical therapy
  A. Definitive treatment requires removal of abnormal parathyroid tissue.
    1. Surgical removal of parathyroid neoplasms
    2. Surgical removal of at least three of the four glands with hyperplasia
  B. Surgical technique/precautions are described elsewhere (Black and Peterson, 1983).
    1. A cystic mass may be an embryonic remnant or a thyroid adenocarcinoma.
    2. If the external parathyroid gland is involved, it is removed alone. If the internal parathyroid gland or glands are involved, the thyroid gland with its parathyroid tissues is removed (Berger and Feldman, 1987).
    3. Clinically apparent hypocalcemia is common postoperatively within 3–6 days.

Patient Monitoring

I. Measure serum Ca and P daily while attempting to reduce severe hypercalcemia. The goals of therapy include the following.
  A. Ideally, reduction of serum Ca into the normal range
  B. Elimination of the clinical signs of hypercalcemia
  C. Reduction of the Ca × P product to <70
II. Postoperative monitoring requires repeated evaluation of serum Ca.

A. Keep the animal hospitalized and measure serum Ca daily for 7 days.

B. If signs of hypocalcemia develop, institute therapy as outlined under Hypoparathyroidism.

C. If serum Ca is <8 mg/dl without clinical signs, begin vitamin D or one of its analogues and oral Ca as for hypoparathyroidism.

D. Adjust therapy so that Ca stabilizes in the range of 8–10 mg/dl.

E. Measure serum Ca every 1–2 weeks. If hypercalcemia occurs, stop all medication until Ca is <8 mg/dl.

F. After the Ca concentration has stabilized (8–10 mg/dl), gradually withdraw vitamin D therapy at a rate of 25% every 1–2 weeks while continuing to monitor serum Ca.

G. When vitamin D therapy has been eliminated and serum Ca remains normal, gradually eliminate Ca supplementation.

H. Generally, all therapy can be withdrawn by 8–12 weeks.

I. Monitoring plasma PTH concentration monthly may also aid in determining when vitamin D and Ca therapy may be stopped, but it may be of limited use in cats that have had a thyroid/parathyroidectomy (see Hypoparathyroidism).

PSEUDOHYPERPARATHYROIDISM

See Chap. 71.

Bibliography

Barber PJ, Elliot J, Torrance AG: Measurement of feline intact parathyroid hormone: assay validation and sample handling studies. J Small Anim Pract 34:614, 1993

Berger B, Feldman EC: Primary hyperparathyroidism in dogs: 21 cases (1976–1986). J Am Vet Med Assoc 191:350, 1987

Black AP, Peterson ME: Thyroid biopsy and thyroidectomy. p. 388. In Bojrab MJ (ed): Current Techniques in Small Animal Surgery. 2nd Ed. Lea & Febiger, Philadelphia, 1983

Bruyette DS, Feldman EC: Primary hypoparathyroidism in the dog—report of 15 cases and review of 13 previously reported cases. J Vet Intern Med 2:7, 1988

Feldman EC: Disorders of the parathyroid glands. p. 1437. In Ettinger SJ, Feldman EC (eds): Textbook of Veterinary Internal Medicine. 4th Ed. WB Saunders, Philadelphia, 1995

Feldman EC, Nelson RW: Hypercalcemia and primary hyperparathyroidism. p. 455. In: Canine and Feline Endocrinology and Reproduction. 2nd Ed. WB Saunders, Philadelphia, 1996a

Feldman EC, Nelson RW: Hypocalcemia and primary hypoparathyroidism. p. 497. In: Canine and Feline Endocrinology and Reproduction. 2nd Ed. WB Saunders, Philadelphia, 1996b

Flanders JS, Neth S, Erb HN et al: Functional analysis of ectopic parathyroid activity in cats. Am J Vet Res 52:1336, 1991

Flanders JA, Scarlett JM, Blue JT, Neth S: Adjustment of total serum calcium concentration for binding to albumin and protein in cats: 291 cases (1986–1987). J Am Vet Med Assoc 194:1609, 1989

Jones BR, Alley MR: Primary idiopathic hypoparathyroidism in St. Bernard dogs. N Z Vet J 33:94, 1985

Kallet AJ, Richter KP, Feldman EC et al: Primary hyperparathyroidism in cats: seven cases (1984–1989). J Am Vet Med Assoc 199:1767, 1991

Klausner JS, O'Leary TP, Osborne CA: Calcium urolithiasis in two dogs with parathyroid adenomas. J Am Vet Med Assoc 191:1423, 1987

Kornegay JN, Greene CE, Martin C et al: Idiopathic hypocalcemia in four dogs. J Am Anim Hosp Assoc 16:723, 1980

Martin TJ, Raisz LG, Rodan G: Calcium regulation and bone metabolism. p. 1. In Martin TJ, Raisz LG (eds): Clinical Endocrinology of Calcium Metabolism. Marcel Dekker, New York, 1987

Meuten DJ, Chew DJ, Capen CC, Kociba GJ: Relationship of serum total calcium to albumin and total protein in dogs. J Am Vet Med Assoc 180:63, 1982

Peterson ME, James KM, Wallace M et al: Idiopathic hypoparathyroidism in five cats. J Vet Intern Med 5:47, 1991

Richter KP, Kallet AJ, Feldman EC, Brum D: Primary hyperparathyroidism in seven cats. Proc Am Coll Vet Intern Med 8:1117, 1990

Rosol TJ, Chew DJ, Hammer AS et al: Effect of mithramycin on hypercalcemia in dogs. J Am Anim Hosp Assoc 30:244, 1994

Rosol TJ, Nagode LA, Couto CG et al: Parathyroid hormone (PTH)-related protein, PTH, and 1,25-dihydroxyvitamin D in dogs with cancer-associated hypercalcemia. Endocrinology 131:1157, 1992

Ross LA, Goldstein M: Biochemical abnormalities associated with accidental hypothermia in a dog and cat. Proc Am Coll Vet Intern Med 1:66, 1981

Sherding RG, Meuten DJ, Chew DJ et al: Primary hypoparathyroidism in the dog. J Am Vet Med Assoc 176:439, 1980

Thompson KG, Jones LP, Smylie WA et al: Primary hyperparathyroidism in German shepherd dogs: a disorder of probable genetic origin. Vet Pathol 21:370, 1984

Torrance AG, Nachreiner R: Human-parathormone assay for use in dogs: validation, sample handling studies, and parathyroid function testing. Am J Vet Res 50:1123, 1989a

Torrance AG, Nachreiner R: Intact parathyroid hormone assay and total calcium concentration in the diagnosis of disorders of calcium metabolism in dogs. J Vet Intern Med 3:86, 1989b

Wisner ER, Nyland TG, Feldman EC et al: Ultrasonographic evaluation of the parathyroid glands in hypercalcemic dogs. Vet Radiol Ultrasound 34:108, 1993

43

Diseases of the Endocrine Pancreas (Islet Cells)

Michael Schaer

DIABETES MELLITUS

Definition

I. A complex metabolic disorder caused by multivariable factors that is characterized by insulin deficiency or impaired insulin action, resulting in carbohydrate intolerance and abnormal protein and lipid metabolism

II. Signalment
   A. Adult (middle-aged and older) dogs and cats most commonly affected
   B. Dogs <1 year of age uncommonly affected (<1.5%)
   C. Intact and neutered female dogs more commonly affected than males
   D. More common in adult male cats
   E. All canine breeds affected, but most common in poodle and dachshund

Classification

I. Type I
   A. Similar to insulin-dependent or juvenile-onset in humans
   B. Can occur at young age (≤1 year) but more common in middle-aged and older dogs and cats
   C. Ketoacidosis common
   D. Markedly deficient endogenous insulin production, only occasional insulin resistance
   E. Insulin treatment always necessary
   F. Breeds at higher risk: keeshond, golden retriever, poodle, old English sheepdog, Doberman pinscher, German shepherd dog, Labrador retriever, and mixed-breed dogs

II. Type II
   A. Comparable to non–insulin-dependent or adult-onset in humans
   B. Often occurs in the cat, but rarely in the dog; obesity a risk factor
   C. Pathophysiological defects involved
      1. Secretory activity of beta cell
      2. Interaction between gastrointestinal tract and liver
      3. Receptor and postreceptor intracellular events
   D. Measurable amounts of endogenous insulin present
   E. Can be managed in humans with dietary therapy, oral hypoglycemics, and weight loss; use of this approach in cats is only partially successful
   F. Overt diabetes in animals best treated with injectable insulin
   G. Spontaneous resolution in cats possible

III. Secondary diabetes
   A. Associated with other diseases
   B. Known to occur with pancreatic disease, certain endocrine disorders (especially hyperadrenocorticism and acromegaly), insulin receptor abnormalities, and specific genetic syndromes (in humans)
   C. May also be drug induced (corticosteroids, megestrol acetate)
   D. Requires insulin treatment; insulin resistance common

Causes

I. Multifactorial disorder
   A. Genetic predisposition
   B. Environmental influences: high-carbohydrate diets
   C. Chemicals and drugs: glucocorticoids, megestrol acetate, and other progestogens
   D. Immune destruction of beta cells
   E. Acquired hormonal abnormalities
      1. Deficiency in insulin receptor numbers
      2. Deficient insulin adherence to receptors

3. Commonly associated with excess glucocorticoid and growth hormone (GH) production or administration in dogs and cats

II. Pancreatic disease
   A. Pancreatitis
      1. Transient insulin deficiency occurs during acute episodes.
      2. Permanent diabetes occurs when ≥90% of beta cells are destroyed by a massive episode or chronic recurrent events.
   B. Pancreatic adenocarcinoma or other diffuse neoplastic diseases: rarely associated with diabetes

Pathophysiology

I. Consequences of insulin deficiency or resistance
   A. Increased hepatic glucose output (gluconeogenesis)
   B. Decreased glucose utilization peripherally
   C. Increased proteolysis, glycogenolysis, lipolysis
   D. Impaired glycogenesis
II. Consequences of hyperglycemia
   A. Hyperosmolality
   B. Glycosuria causes osmotic diuresis with loss of Na^+, K^+, P, Cl^-, and water with compensatory polydipsia
   C. Dehydration
   D. Glucose toxicity: impaired insulin secretion induced by prolonged, severe hyperglycemia
III. Weight loss from catabolic reactions (as outlined earlier)

Clinical Signs

I. Polydipsia and polyuria
II. Polyphagia prior to ketoacidosis and other complications
III. Eventual weight loss
IV. Hepatomegaly (hepatic triglyceride accumulation—''fatty liver'')
V. Cataracts: sudden onset common in dogs; seldom occur in cats

Diagnosis

I. Sustained hyperglycemia
   A. Repeated fasting blood sugar >150 mg/dl

B. Repeated postprandial blood sugar >200 mg/dl
II. Sustained glycosuria
   A. Do not confuse with primary renal glycosuria (see Chap. 47).
   B. Some drugs such as vitamin C and copper-reducing agents can cause false-positive urine glucose test results, depending on methodology.
   C. Diagnosis is confirmed with the detection of marked hyperglycemia (>300 mg/dl) and concomitant glycosuria.
III. Transient stress hyperglycemia ruled out
   A. Rarely exceeds 175 mg/dl in the dog; commonly 200–250 mg/dl or higher in the cat (ketones absent)
   B. Does not usually require insulin treatment
   C. Lasts for only a few hours to days
IV. Compatible clinical signs
V. Other clinicopathologic abnormalities (in the nonketotic patient)
   A. Elevated liver enzymes: serum alkaline phosphatase (SAP) and serum aminotransferases (SALT, SAST)
   B. Elevated plasma lipids: cholesterol and triglycerides

Treatment

I. Intermediate- or ultra-long-acting insulin for maintenance or for stabilization of uncomplicated cases
   A. See Table 43–1 for types of insulin.
   B. Dosage and frequency for intermediate- and prolonged-acting insulins are as follows.
      1. Isophane (NPH) and Lente in dogs often begins at 0.5 U/kg SQ SID; can be given as split morning and evening dosages to provide a more even availability.
      2. Ultralente is the preferred maintenance insulin for the cat.
         a) Begin dose at 0.5 U/kg SQ SID; can also be given as split dose.
         b) At least 20% of diabetic cats that show difficulty with regulation might respond to NPH or Lente insulin given twice daily.
      3. See also the section on problem diabetics, later.
II. Oral hypoglycemics
   A. These are commonly used in humans with type

Table 43–1. **Insulin Preparations: General Types**

Type of Insulin	Appearance	Type of Action	Peak Activity[a,b]	Duration (h)[b]	Available Concentration	Species Available	Modifying Agent	Mixes with Regular Insulin	Route of Administration
Crystalline zinc insulin (regular)	Clear	Rapid	2–4	5–8	U-100 U-500	Beef/pork/human	None	—	SQ, IM, IV
NPH	Cloudy	Intermediate	8–12	18–26	U-100	Beef/pork/human	Protamine	Yes	SQ
Mixture NPH and regular	Cloudy	Rapid and intermediate	2–12	18–26	U-100	Human	None	Yes	SQ
Lente	Cloudy	Intermediate	8–16	18–28	U-100	Beef/pork/human	None	Yes	SQ
Ultralente	Cloudy	Prolonged	16–24	24–36	U-100	Beef/human	None	Yes	SQ

[a]Hours after administration.
[b]These data are from human studies. Peak activity and duration times in dogs and cats can be shorter.

II diabetes, but use has been restricted to cats in veterinary medicine.

B. Actions depend on presence of preformed insulin in the beta cells.

C. Glipizide and glyburide have been tried in some dogs and cats, but their effects require further critical evaluation.

D. Glipizide at 5 mg PO BID has been shown to be effective in approximately 50% of mildly diabetic cats. Use is restricted to the nonanorexic, nonketoacidotic cat.

E. Most cats receiving glipizide eventually require insulin treatment.

F. Most oral hypoglycemics can cause hypoglycemia, elevated liver enzymes, and occasional vomiting.

III. Diet

A. Keep consistent; feed a balanced ration.
   1. Avoid high fat and high sugar content.
   2. Moderate- to high-fiber diets may decrease the insulin dose requirement and improve glycemic control.

B. Feed dogs twice daily.

C. Sometimes a midday snack helps avoid hypoglycemia.

D. Free-choice feeding for cats is acceptable; however, obesity should be avoided.

E. To avoid obesity, use weight-reduction or commercially available ''light'' diets.

IV. Exercise

A. Regular exercise is recommended and is easier to provide for dogs.

B. Exercise decreases the insulin requirement because of decreased insulin dependency of muscle for glucose transport.

C. Vigorous exercise necessitates lower insulin dosages and readily available provisions (carbohydrates or glucagon) for counteracting hypoglycemia. This is especially important for unavoidable excessive weekend exercise.

Patient Monitoring

I. Home urine monitoring

A. It has been used effectively to monitor diabetic dogs and cats, but results can be misleading.

B. It does not represent moment-to-moment blood glucose fluctuations but may provide glycemic trends.

C. Discrepancy between blood and urine glucose values occurs because of the following.
   1. Variability in renal threshold for glucose
   2. Various time intervals over which the urine sample may have accumulated before being voided
   3. Semiquantitative nature of urine glucose tests

D. At blood glucose levels below the renal threshold, a negative urine value cannot distinguish euglycemia, hypoglycemia, and moderate hyperglycemia.

E. Tests used include Test-Tape, Keto-Diastix, and Clinitest.

F. The daily protocol for a single injection of insulin is as follows.
   1. First, check the urine glucose level in the morning.
   2. Next, administer adjusted insulin dose SQ according to criteria in Table 43–2.
   3. Then, feed one half of the day's total intake (free-choice feeding for cats is satisfactory).
   4. If possible, measure the urine glucose in the early afternoon.
      a) Large amounts of glycosuria in the morning accompanied by no glycosuria in the afternoon can suggest the need for decreased insulin or split dosage.
      b) Persistently large amounts of glycosuria call for increased insulin dosage.
      c) Negative glycosuria calls for insulin dosage reduction.
   5. In the evening, feed the other half of the daily ration.
   6. Be aware that the urine sugar level does not necessarily parallel the blood level at any given time. For a more accurate assessment, serial blood glucose measurements throughout the day are recommended.
   7. Urine extracted from soaked gravel can be used to detect negative or large amounts of glycosuria (Schaer, 1994).

G. The daily protocol for split injection of insulin is as follows.
   1. Feedings and urine monitoring are the same as earlier.
   2. Give one half of the calculated total day's insulin dose in the morning and the other half approximately 12 hours later.
   3. This protocol provides a more physiologically normal delivery of insulin.

II. Blood glucose monitoring

A. Sequential determinations are required over an 8- to 24-hour period to compose a glucose curve.

B. For insulin dosage adjustment based on blood glucose, see Table 43–3.

C. A blood glucose curve is recommended when the urine glucose levels are erratic, the animal is

*Table 43–2. **Morning Urine Glucose Monitoring for the Diabetic Pet***

Urine Glucose	Adjusted NPH or Ultralente Insulin Dose
2%	Increase 1 U (2–3 U, large dog) above previous day's dose
1%	Increase 0.5 U (2–3 U, large dog) above previous day's dose
0.1%, 0.25%. 0.5%	Repeat previous day's dose (increase 1–2 U for large dog if 0.5%)
Negative	Decrease 2 U (2–4 U, large dog) from previous day's dose

Table 43–3. *Blood Glucose Curve Monitoring After the Morning NPH or Ultralente Injection*

Blood Glucose Level (mg/dl)			NPH and Ultralente Insulin Adjustment for Following Day
Morning	Late Morning/ Early Afternoon	Evening	
150–200	100–200	100–250	Repeat previous dose
>250	>250	>250	Increase insulin 1 U (cat or small dog) or 2 U (large dog) above previous day's dose
>200	<150	>200	Reduce dose by 25–30% and begin split-dosage technique, especially if insulin has short-term effect
<100	<100	<100	Omit dose until glucose >150; reassess animal's need for daily insulin treatment

having repeated hypoglycemic reactions, or the animal shows persistent marked glycosuria.

   D. A blood glucose curve showing all points between 150 and 250 mg/dl is satisfactory.

   E. Reliance solely on single blood glucose measurements once or twice a month can cause dysregulation and is not recommended.

   F. Although determination of blood glucose is much more accurate than urine monitoring, daily urine monitoring is also recommended to detect sudden increases or decreases in insulin demands (before the animal shows metabolic decompensation).

III. Glycosylated hemoglobin and fructosamine values

   A. These are useful for monitoring monthly blood glucose trends.

   B. They can be used in dogs and cats, although they may not be readily available.

   C. High blood glucose levels irreversibly bind to hemoglobin (Hb), thereby raising amounts of glycosylated Hb in the blood (normal values vary with methodology).

   D. Fructosamine is formed by the binding of blood glucose to serum proteins, particularly albumin. Fructosamine concentrations reflect blood glucose levels over the preceding 2 to 3 weeks.

Problem Diabetics

I. Transient insulin response (shortened duration of action)

   A. This usually occurs with NPH and Lente insulins in dogs and cats and occasionally with Ultralente in cats.

   B. It is characterized by early onset and peak action times of the insulin and a decreased duration of action.

   C. Blood glucose declines, often to hypoglycemic levels, within a few hours after injection, followed by persistent hyperglycemia for the remainder of the 24-hour period.

   D. Indications and detection are as follows.

     1. Marked morning glycosuria, often with minimal or no glycosuria in afternoon sample

     2. Subsequent or sequential increased insulin dosing

     3. Hypoglycemic episodes 2–6 hours after the injection

     4. Can confirm with a blood glucose curve

   E. Treat by reducing insulin dose by 25–30% and splitting it into two equal portions given 12 hours apart. Subsequent amounts are titrated to effect.

II. Posthypoglycemic hyperglycemia (Somogyi reaction)

   A. Insulin overdosage causes hypoglycemia with subsequent hyperglycemic compensatory response via increased secretion of glucagon, epinephrine, cortisol, and GH.

   B. Excess insulin dose is often caused by faulty client–veterinarian communication or undetected transient insulin response.

   C. Characteristics and detection are as follows.

     1. Early-morning hyperglycemia with marked glycosuria

     2. Late-morning or afternoon hypoglycemia with minimal glycosuria

     3. Rebound hyperglycemia persisting until next insulin injection

   D. Treat by reducing the insulin dose by 25–50% or by using a split-dose technique if the animal shows transient insulin response after trying a reduced dose.

III. Insulin resistance

   A. It occurs when a normal amount of insulin produces a subnormal biologic response.

   B. Suspect it in dogs and cats when the insulin dose exceeds 2 U/kg and 0.2–1 U/kg, respectively.

   C. Rule out and treat any coexisting disorder.

     1. Hyperadrenocorticism (see Chap. 44)

     2. Diestrus in the dog

       a) Markedly elevated insulin requirements can occur.

       b) This may be caused by mammary gland production of GH.

       c) It is best managed with immediate ovariohysterectomy.

       d) Anticipate need for dramatic insulin reductions (50–75%) by 24 hours postoperatively.

       e) Recommend that all intact female diabetic dogs be spayed soon after diabetes is diagnosed and the animal is stabilized.

     3. Acromegaly (see Chap. 40)

       a) This can cause markedly increased insulin requirements, along with characteristic acromegalic physical features.

       b) Treatment entails removing the source of the stimulus responsible for elevated GH levels, if possible.

       c) Insulin requirements should be titrated to effect. Dosages can exceed 6 U/kg BID.

       d) Cats can require insulin doses in excess of 30–40 U BID.

4. Infections
    a) Infections cause insulin resistance through endogenous production of the stress hormones, e.g., cortisol, epinephrine, and GH.
    b) Effective management requires prompt diagnosis and treatment consisting of surgical drainage (when indicated), bacterial culture and sensitivity determinations, and the use of the appropriate bactericidal antibiotic.
5. Pancreatic exocrine insufficiency
    a) Animals are insulin sensitive because of deficiencies in available food substrate.
    b) Expect increased insulin needs associated with improved food substrate availability once replacement enzyme therapy is started.
6. Significant anti-beef, -pork, -human insulin antibody development is considered rare.
D. Insulin dose should be titrated according to the animal's need as long as hypoglycemia does not occur and hyperglycemia is persistent.
    1. Cat dosages may exceed 20–30 U of insulin a day.
    2. Large dogs might require in excess of 200 U/day.
    3. There is no such thing as "maximum" dosage with persistent hyperglycemia; the animal should receive as much as it needs as long as hypoglycemia does not occur.

IV. Postinsulin hypoglycemia
A. A decline in the blood glucose to <70 mg/dl
B. Caused by insulin excess, food substrate unavailability (anorexia, vomiting, malabsorption), and/or excessive exercise
C. Clinical signs: weakness, anxiety, behavioral changes, muscle twitching, generalized seizures, and coma
D. Detection
    1. Presence of suspicious signs usually within projected peak action time
    2. Increased occurrence after removal of physiologic stresses or with the onset of chronic liver disease or certain hypoendocrinopathies
    3. Recent trend of decreased glycosuria often accompanied by hypoglycemic signs
E. Treatment
    1. Temporarily withhold insulin.
    2. If the animal is conscious, give carbohydrates orally.
        a) Karo syrup (15 g carbohydrate/15 ml) at 0.5–1 ml/kg PO
        b) 50% dextrose 1–2 ml/kg PO
    3. If the animal is unconscious, give the following.
        a) 50% dextrose 1 ml/kg IV and maintain on 5% dextrose solution
        b) Glucagon 0.03 mg/kg IM, IV, SQ
    4. Readjust further insulin doses in accordance with the animal's needs.

DIABETIC KETOACIDOSIS (DKA)

Definition

I. A severe stage of diabetes mellitus characterized by hyperglycemia, hyperketonemia, and metabolic acidosis
II. Frequently a metabolic emergency requiring prompt diagnosis and treatment

Pathophysiology

I. Often considered a bihormonal disorder
A. Hypoinsulinemia and hyperglucagonemia
B. Resulting in overproduction and underutilization of glucose and ketoacids
II. Consequences of insulin deficiency and glucagon excess
A. Peripheral lipolysis with massive influx of fatty acids into the liver
B. Activation of hepatic mitochondrial ketogenic pathway by increased carnitine acyltransferase activity
    1. An enzyme responsible for mitochondrial uptake of fatty acids
    2. Fatty acids metabolized by β-oxidation to organic ketone acids, acetoacetate, and β-hydroxybutyrate
C. Acceleration of ketogenesis and gluconeogenesis
III. Metabolic acidosis
A. This is caused by overproduction of acetoacetate and β-hydroxybutyrate.
    1. Released into the circulation, where they reduce the body buffer base, i.e., bicarbonate
    2. Body unable to compensate, leaving animal with metabolic acidosis with an increased anion gap
B. Other possible contributing factors to acidosis include renal failure and lactic acid generation.
IV. Ketone detection
A. Plasma and urinary ketones are detected semi-quantitatively with nitroprusside reagent (Ketostix, Acetest).
B. These products detect acetoacetate and acetone but not β-hydroxybutyrate, which requires special laboratory techniques.
C. Acetone imparts a Juicy Fruit odor to the breath.
D. Shock may cause a disproportionate formation of β-hydroxybutyrate.
    1. β-Hydroxybutyrate is not detected by the nitroprusside test reaction.
    2. This explains why some acidotic diabetics initially test negative for ketones.
    3. β-Hydroxybutyrate in the urine can be converted to detectable acetoacetate by adding 3 drops of H_2O_2 to the urine sample.
    4. With treatment, β-hydroxybutyrate is metabolized to acetoacetate, which is then metabolized to CO_2 and water, explaining why some animals show a stronger ketone reaction on

the second and third days despite their overall clinical improvement.

Clinical Signs

I. History
   A. Acute or chronic onset
   B. May have precipitating factor(s), such as bacterial or viral infection
   C. Early signs: polydipsia, polyuria, weight loss, ±polyphagia
   D. Late signs: mental depression, vomiting, anorexia, dehydration, tachypnea; animal obviously ill
II. Physical examination
   A. Be thorough to detect other coexisting disorders, such as acute pancreatitis or any infectious processes.
   B. Extent or severity of signs varies, depending on the stage of disease.

Diagnosis

I. History and physical examination findings
II. Clinicopathologic criteria
   A. Blood glucose >250 mg/dl
   B. Plasma pH <7.3 with anion gap
   C. Plasma bicarbonate <15 mEq/L
   D. Ketonemia, ketonuria, glycosuria
III. Other diagnostic findings
   A. Elevated serum alkaline phosphatase and liver transaminase enzymes, usually from hepatic lipidosis
   B. Normo- or hyponatremia
   C. Normo- or hypokalemia
   D. Normo- or hypophosphatemia
   E. Renal function
      1. Blood urea nitrogen (BUN) and creatinine levels range from normal to elevated.
      2. Elevations are caused by either prerenal volume depletion or overt renal failure.
      3. Dilute urine might be misleading, because glycosuria can cause a water diuresis that does not necessarily reflect renal tubular damage.
   F. Hemogram
      1. Variable: normal or stress leukocytosis or hemoconcentration
      2. Left shift and toxic changes signal bacterial infection: check urine, especially, for presence of bacteria and white blood cells (WBCs).
      3. Possible mild to moderate anemia, perhaps from Heinz body formation in cats.
   G. Anion gap (AG) associated with metabolic acidosis
      1. Occurs from lowered plasma bicarbonate
      2. AG >30 mEq/L very significant
   H. Radiography
      1. Hepatomegaly
      2. Rarely emphysematous cystitis
      3. Presence of other coexisting problems, such as acute pancreatitis, pyometra, emphysematous cholecystitis

Treatment

I. Fluid therapy
   A. Replacement needs equal the sum of the following.
      1. Dehydration deficit = % dehydration × kg body weight (BW) × 1000 ml
      2. 24-hour maintenance needs
         a) With normal urine output: 60 ml/kg/day
         b) With oliguria: equals the amount of urine output plus insensible losses (20 ml/kg/day)
         c) With anuria: provide insensible losses; begin dialysis
      3. Extra ongoing losses (vomiting or diarrhea)
   B. Give one half of the estimated dehydration deficit over the first 2–4 hours if the animal is not markedly hypotensive.
   C. With hypovolemic shock, the IV fluid rate in the first hour of treatment should be 70–90 ml/kg for a dog and 35–45 ml/kg for a cat.
   D. Hydration alone can decrease the blood glucose level and make the response to insulin more predictable; therefore, insulin treatment is sometimes delayed for the first 1–2 hours, especially when the serum potassium level is <3.0 mEq/L.
   E. Fluids of choice are as follows.
      1. Rehydration and initial 24–48 hours maintenance: 0.9% saline and lactated Ringer's solutions
      2. Maintenance fluids: 0.45% saline or half-strength lactated Ringer's solution with potassium chloride supplementation
      3. Dextrose solutions (2.5–5%): reserved for when blood glucose <250 mg/dl
II. Insulin therapy
   A. If the animal is alert, well hydrated, and eating, begin with intermediate (NPH, Lente) or long-acting (Ultralente) insulins. All intermediate- and long-acting insulins are usually given SQ and never IV.
   B. Use regular crystalline insulin if the animal is clinically decompensated (mentally depressed, dehydrated, anorectic, vomiting).
      1. Rapid onset of action: immediately with IV and IM administration; usually within 30–60 minutes after SQ
      2. Short duration of action (assuming normal renal function)
         a) IV: 40 minutes to 1 hour
         b) IM: approximately 2–4 hours
         c) SQ: approximately 6–8 hours
   C. IV continuous low-dose technique
      1. For large dog: initial dose of 0.2 U/kg followed by 0.1 U/kg/h
      2. For small dog and cat: 0.5–1 U/h
      3. Requires two separate IV lines and delivery through a pediatric infusion set or an infusion pump
      4. Safe and efficacious, but labor intensive
   D. IM technique
      1. Safe and efficacious; rapidly absorbed

Table 43–4. Adjustment of Insulin in the Ketoacidotic Cat and Dog

| Blood Glucose | Units of Subcutaneous Regular Insulin Every 6–10 h | | IV Fluid Supplement |
	Cat or Small Dog	Medium/Large Dog	
>400 mg/dl	Increase 1–2 U above previous dose	Increase 2–4 U above previous dose	Continue maintenance fluids
240–400 mg/dl	Repeat previous dose	Increase 1–2 U above previous dose	2.5% dextrose when blood glucose <250 mg/dl
180–240 mg/dl	Decrease 2 U from previous dose	Decrease 4 U from previous dose	2.5% dextrose
<180 mg/dl	Omit insulin for 4–6 h	Omit insulin for 4–6 hours	2.5–5% dextrose

2. For animals <10 kg: 2 U followed by 1 U hourly
3. For dogs >10 kg: 0.25 U/kg followed by 0.1 U/kg hourly

E. SQ technique
1. Slower onset and longer duration of action
2. Inadequately absorbed in hypotensive animals; therefore not recommended until fluids have been administered
3. Initial dose: 0.5 U/kg titrated to effect every 4–8 hours

F. Goals and monitoring
1. Do not be overly concerned by ketones in the urine; they will spontaneously diminish over 48–72 hours.
2. Rate of blood glucose decline should not exceed 100 mg/dl/hour.
3. Check blood glucose hourly with IM and IV insulin techniques and every 4–6 hours when using the SQ method.
4. Add glucose to fluids (2.5–5%) when blood glucose <250 mg/dl. Note that each 12.5 ml of 50% dextrose added to 250 ml of lactated Ringer's solution or 0.9% NaCl yields a $2\frac{1}{2}$% solution.
5. Temporarily omit insulin treatment if blood glucose <150 mg/dl; reinstitute when level reaches or exceeds 200–250 mg/dl.
6. Give 50% dextrose 1 ml/kg IV bolus if overt hypoglycemia occurs.
7. Convert to SQ route with regular insulin when animal is clinically improved (Table 43–4).
8. Begin NPH or Ultralente when the animal is eating and appears clinically improved.

III. Electrolyte supplementation
A. Sodium (normal, 137–147 mEq/L)
1. Hyponatremia can be factitious from hyperlipidemia and marked hyperglycemia, or real from urinary or gastrointestinal sodium ion loss.
2. Treat hyponatremia with 0.9% saline solution and reassess the serum sodium level on the following day.
B. Potassium (normal, 3.5–5.5 mEq/L)
1. Hypokalemia is the most important electrolyte disturbance in DKA.
2. Treat with KCl solution added to IV maintenance fluids (Table 43–5).
3. All ketoacidotic animals should receive daily potassium supplementation unless they are oliguric or anuric.
C. Phosphorus (normal, 2.5–5 mg/dl)
1. In DKA, phosphorus depletion is usually clinically silent, but hypophosphatemia-induced hemolysis is possible.
2. Treat with potassium phosphate solution at 0.01–0.03 mmol/kg/h, followed by serial serum phosphorus measurements; discontinue when serum phosphorus = 2.5 mg/dl.
3. Risks of causing secondary hyperphosphatemia and feasibility of therapy must be weighed against its benefit.
D. Bicarbonate (normal, 17–25 mEq/L)
1. True need for supplementation is controversial.
2. In most situations, the metabolic acidosis reverses without supplemental treatment following cessation of ketogenesis; metabolic conversion of ketones to CO_2, H_2O, and HCO_3^-; improved renal function; and dilution of acids with fluid therapy.
3. Reserve use of bicarbonate for when blood pH <7.0.
4. Bicarbonate need (mEq) = base deficit × 0.3 × kg BW.

Patient Monitoring

I. Postinsulin (secondary) hypoglycemia
A. Give 50% dextrose 1 ml/kg IV push.
B. Provide 2.5–5% dextrose maintenance infusion IV.
C. Decrease or omit next insulin dose.

II. Hypokalemia
A. Monitor serum potassium at least once daily.
B. Provide KCl in IV fluids as shown in Table 43–5.

Table 43–5. Recommended Potassium Chloride Supplementation

Serum Potassium Deficit (mEq/L)	KCl Added to 24-h Infusion
Mild, K$^+$ = 3.0–3.5	2–3 mEq/kg BW
Moderate, K$^+$ = 2.5–3.0	3–5 mEq/kg BW
Severe, K$^+$ ≤2.5	5–10 mEq/kg BW

BW = body weight.

III. Cerebral edema
 A. It is caused by rapid decline in blood glucose level.
 B. Osmotic dysequilibrium occurs with water shifting into the brain.
 C. It can be avoided by allowing for a more gradual blood glucose reduction over a 6- to 12-hour period at ≤100 mg/dl/h.
 D. Treat with mannitol 1 g/kg IV over a 5- to 30-minute period to counteract brain edema in severe cases.
IV. Metabolic alkalosis
 A. Avoid bicarbonate use; correct hypokalemia.
 B. Switch fluids to 0.9% NaCl.
 C. Treat any specific cause of vomiting.
 V. Paradoxic cerebrospinal fluid acidosis
 A. It is caused by too rapid and excessive bicarbonate infusion.
 B. Animal dies suddenly.
 C. Avoid overly zealous use of bicarbonate.
VI. Sepsis
 A. Maintain strict IV catheter asepsis and avoid using indwelling urinary catheters.
 B. Culture any site of suspected infection.
 C. Use bactericidal antibiotics according to sensitivity results.
 D. Avoid nephrotoxic antibiotics (i.e., aminoglycosides) in the presence of renal failure.

Bibliography

Chastain CB: Intensive care of dogs and cats with diabetic ketoacidosis. J Am Vet Med Assoc 179:972, 1981

Chastain CB, Ganjam VK: Clinical Endocrinology of Companion Animals. Lea & Febiger, Philadelphia, 1986

Feldman EC, Nelson RW: Canine and Feline Endocrinology and Reproduction. WB Saunders, Philadelphia, 1996

Ford SL: NIDDM in the cat: treatment with the oral hypoglycemic medication, glipizide. Vet Clin North Am [Small Anim Pract] 25:599, 1995

Foster DW, McGarry JD: The metabolic derangements and treatment of diabetic ketoacidosis. N Engl J Med 309:159, 1983

Ihle SL: Nutritional therapy for diabetes mellitus. Vet Clin North Am [Small Anim Pract] 25:585, 1995

Kitabchi AE: Low-dose insulin therapy in diabetic ketoacidosis: fact or fiction? Diabetes Metab Rev 5:337, 1989

Kitabchi AE, Murphy MB: Diabetic ketoacidosis and hyperosmolar hyperglycemic nonketotic coma. Med Clin North Am 72:1545, 1988

Kozak GP, Rolla AR: Diabetic comas. p. 109. In Kozak GP (ed): Clinical Diabetes Mellitus. WB Saunders, Philadelphia, 1982

Lever E, Jaspar JB: Sodium bicarbonate therapy in severe diabetic ketoacidosis. Am J Med 75:263, 1983

Macintire DK: Emergency therapy of diabetic crises: insulin overdose, diabetic ketoacidosis, and hyperosmolar coma. Vet Clin North Am [Small Anim Pract] 25:139, 1995

Miller E: Long-term monitoring of the diabetic dog and cat: clinical signs, serial blood glucose determinations, urine glucose, and glycosylated blood proteins. Vet Clin North Am [Small Anim Pract] 25:571, 1995

Morris L, Murphy MB, Kitabchi AE: Bicarbonate therapy in severe diabetic ketoacidosis. Ann Intern Med 105:836, 1986

Schaer M: Insulin treatment for the diabetic dog and cat. Compend Contin Educ Pract Vet 5:579, 1983

Schaer M: A method for detecting glucosuria in urine-soaked cat litter. Fel Pract 22:6, 1994

Willard MD, Zerbe CA, Schall WD et al: Severe hypophosphatemia associated with diabetes mellitus in six dogs and one cat. J Am Vet Med Assoc 190:1007, 1987

44

Diseases of the Adrenal Gland

Rhett Nichols
Mark E. Peterson
Leland Thompson

HYPOADRENOCORTICISM

Rhett Nichols and Mark E. Peterson
(Revised by Rhett Nichols)

Definition

I. Hypoadrenocorticism is a syndrome that results from deficiency of glucocorticoid and/or mineralocorticoid secretion from the adrenal cortex.
II. Primary adrenocortical insufficiency (Addison's disease) results from a disease process of the adrenal gland itself; this usually causes a deficiency of both classes of corticosteroids.
III. Secondary adrenocortical insufficiency refers to insufficient pituitary adrenocorticotropic hormone (ACTH) secretion with resultant glucocorticoid deficiency. Mineralocorticoid concentrations usually remain normal in secondary hypoadrenocorticism.

Causes

I. Primary adrenocortical insufficiency is the result of atrophy or destruction of all layers of the adrenal cortex. Causative factors include the following.
   A. Idiopathic (probably immune-mediated)
   B. Mitotane therapy for hyperadrenocorticism (mineralocorticoid concentrations usually normal)
   C. Granulomatous (fungal) infections, viral diseases, neoplasia, or hemorrhage from any cause
II. Secondary hypoadrenocorticism can be caused by the following.
   A. Abrupt withdrawal of long-term and/or high-dose exogenous corticosteroid therapy
   B. Lesions of the hypothalamus or pituitary gland, e.g., tumors
   C. Idiopathic ACTH deficiency (rare)

Pathophysiology

I. Glucocorticoid deficiency causes the following effects.
   A. Decreased gluconeogenesis and glycogenolysis
   B. Impaired energy metabolism
   C. Decreased vascular sensitivity to catecholamines
   D. Decreased alertness
   E. Diminished stress tolerance
   F. Impaired renal ability to excrete free water
II. Mineralocorticoid deficiency causes the following effects.
   A. Renal wasting of sodium, chloride, and water
   B. Renal retention of potassium and hydrogen ions
III. The following metabolic abnormalities are seen with varying degrees of severity.
   A. Hypotension and reduced cardiac output from depletion of circulating blood volume caused by hyponatremia and poor vascular tone
   B. Poor tissue perfusion with weakness, depression, prerenal azotemia, and eventually shock
   C. Hyperkalemia and metabolic acidosis from mineralocorticoid deficit and reduced glomerular filtration rate
   D. Increased plasma antidiuretic hormone (ADH) concentrations secondary to extracellular fluid volume depletion causing dilutional hyponatremia, worsened by renal sodium wasting
   E. Abnormalities in sodium and potassium concentrations with muscle weakness, central nervous system (CNS) depression, and abnormal cardiac function

Clinical Signs

Hypoadrenocorticism has been referred to as the "great pretender," with clinical signs resembling those seen in other disorders.

I. Signalment
A. Breeds at higher risk: Great Dane, Portuguese water dog, rottweiler, standard poodle, West Highland white terrier, and wheaten terrier
B. Age: most are <7 years; range, 4 months to 14 years
C. Sex: female predilection (as high as 70%)
II. Acute or end-stage adrenocortical insufficiency
A. Weakness and depression progressing to collapse
B. Bradycardia and other hyperkalemia-associated arrhythmias
C. Hypovolemia and shock
III. Subacute or chronic adrenocortical insufficiency
A. Intermittent anorexia, vomiting, and diarrhea may be seen.
B. Muscle weakness, lethargy, and depression are common.
C. Clinical signs may transiently respond to fluid and/or corticosteroid administration.
D. Exacerbations of clinical signs are often associated with stress.

Diagnosis

I. History and clinical signs
A high index of suspicion is necessary because both history and clinical signs are compatible with other common disorders.
II. Hemogram
A. Absolute eosinophilia and lymphocytosis may occur.
B. Increased packed cell volume (PCV) and total solids may result from dehydration.
C. Mild anemia is present in some cases.
III. Serum biochemical and electrolyte abnormalities
A. Hyperkalemia and hyponatremia are seen in most cases of primary hypoadrenocorticism.
1. Animals with early primary hypoadrenocorticism may have normal serum electrolyte concentrations.
2. Iatrogenic hypoadrenocorticism from mitotane is usually associated with normal serum electrolyte concentrations.
3. Serum electrolyte concentrations are generally normal in secondary hypoadrenocorticism.
B. Azotemia develops from renal or prerenal causes.
C. Hypercalcemia is seen in 30% of affected animals, possibly caused by decreased renal calcium excretion.
D. Mild hypoalbuminemia is present in some cases.
E. Hypoglycemia occurs rarely.
IV. Urine specific gravity
A. Urine specific gravity is usually <1.030.
B. This urine-concentrating defect probably results from medullary washout secondary to renal sodium wasting.
V. Electrocardiographic (ECG) abnormalities
ECG changes are primarily dependent on the degree of hyperkalemia. Acid–base balance and serum sodium and calcium concentrations also play a role.
A. Widening and flattening of P waves, increased duration of P–R interval

B. Increased T-wave amplitude
C. Decreased amplitude and prolongation of QRS complexes
D. Bradycardia
E. Sinoventricular rhythm and atrial standstill
VI. Radiographic findings
A. Microcardia, hypoperfusion of lungs
B. Megaesophagus (rare)
VII. ACTH stimulation test
A. It is required for a definitive diagnosis.
B. Animals with hypoadrenocorticism show a "blunted" or no serum cortisol response to ACTH administration.
1. Primary hypoadrenocorticism: pre- and post-ACTH serum cortisol concentrations are usually <1 μg/dl (<30 nmol/L).
2. Secondary hypoadrenocorticism: the serum cortisol response to exogenous ACTH is blunted; however, post-ACTH cortisol concentrations are usually >2.5 μg/dl (>75 nmol/L).
C. See Hyperadrenocorticism, later, for a description of the testing protocol.
D. False elevations of cortisol concentrations may occur with administration of prednisone, prednisolone, cortisone, or fludrocortisone.
1. These drugs are discontinued 24–48 hours before the test.
2. Dexamethasone and desoxycorticosterone pivalate (DOCP) do not interfere with the cortisol assay; however, dexamethasone is a potent steroid and suppresses endogenous ACTH secretion.
VIII. Endogenous plasma ACTH concentrations
A. Elevated with primary hypoadrenocorticism
B. Very low or undetectable with secondary hypoadrenocorticism

Differential Diagnosis

I. Primary gastrointestinal disorders
II. Primary renal failure
III. Cardiovascular, neurologic, muscular, and metabolic causes of acute collapse or muscular weakness
IV. Other causes of hypercalcemia

Treatment

I. Specific blood samples and diagnostic testing are necessary before instituting therapy.
A. Obtain blood for hematology, serum chemistries, and basal cortisol concentration.
B. Obtain a urine sample for a complete urinalysis.
C. The ACTH stimulation test can be performed simultaneously (best to use IV cosyntropin [Cortrosyn]) with initial therapy.
D. Use dexamethasone for initial glucocorticoid replacement (see later) because it does not influence the cortisol assays.
II. Acute hypoadrenocorticism
Treatment is directed toward correcting hypotension and hypovolemia, improving vascular integrity, pro-

viding an immediate source of glucocorticoids, and correcting electrolyte imbalances and acidosis.
  A. Hypovolemia
     1. Rapidly infuse normal saline 40–80 ml/kg/h IV over the first 1–2 hours, followed by reduced rate.
     2. Give dexamethasone sodium phosphate 0.5–2 mg/kg IV; repeat in 2–6 hours if needed.
     3. Convert to maintenance prednisone, prednisolone, or cortisone acetate (see later) over the following 3–5 days.
  B. Hyperkalemia
     1. It can usually be successfully treated with parenteral fluid therapy (normal saline) alone.
        a) In some cases, more aggressive therapy may be needed.
        b) Indications for more aggressive therapy for hyperkalemia include severe bradyarrhythmias and sinoatrial standstill.
     2. Insulin-dextrose therapy
        a) Give regular insulin 0.5 U/kg IV bolus.
        b) Administer 1–1.5 g of dextrose per unit of insulin (as 50% dextrose) IV bolus.
        c) Give 1–1.5 g of dextrose per unit of insulin added to IV fluids over the next 4–6 hours.
     3. Alternative therapy for severe hyperkalemia includes parenteral calcium gluconate or sodium bicarbonate.
        a) Give 10% calcium gluconate 0.5–1.5 ml/kg IV over 10–20 minutes to antagonize the effect of potassium on the myocardium.
        b) *Cautiously* give sodium bicarbonate 1–2 mEq/kg IV over 10–20 minutes to cause temporary transcellular shift of potassium.
        c) The ECG should be monitored closely during calcium or bicarbonate administration.
  C. Acidosis
     1. Consider sodium bicarbonate therapy if severe acidosis is present (pH <7.1).
     2. Give 25% of calculated dose IV during the first 6 hours of therapy if serum bicarbonate concentration is <12 mEq/L.
  D. Supportive care
     1. Correct hypothermia with passive warming methods.
     2. If hypoglycemia is present, give 50% dextrose 0.5–1.5 ml/kg IV slowly.
III. Chronic or subacute adrenocortical insufficiency
  A. Fluid therapy
     1. Give normal saline 60–80 ml/kg/day IV.
     2. Decrease the fluid volume over 48–96 hours based on return to normal of clinical and laboratory abnormalities.
  B. Glucocorticoid supplementation (one of the following)
     1. Prednisone or prednisolone 0.2–0.4 mg/day PO
     2. Cortisone acetate 1 mg/kg/day PO
  C. Mineralocorticoid supplementation (one of the following)

     1. Fludrocortisone acetate (Florinef) 0.02 mg/kg/day PO, with dosage adjusted on basis of serial electrolyte determinations
     2. DOCP 1–2 mg/kg IM or SQ every 25–28 days
        a) DOCP is a long-acting injectable mineralocorticoid.
        b) It is not currently approved for use in small animals; client waiver forms may be obtained from the manufacturer.

Patient Monitoring

Animals with primary hypoadrenocorticism require chronic supplementation of glucocorticoid and mineralocorticoid and sometimes the addition of salt to the diet. Animals with secondary hypoadrenocorticism can be managed with glucocorticoid supplementation only.
  I. Mineralocorticoid therapy
    A. Initially monitor serum electrolytes, blood urea nitrogen (BUN), and creatinine every 1–2 weeks; when stabilized, reevaluate every 3–4 months.
    B. Adjust mineralocorticoid dosage based on serum potassium and sodium concentrations; serum potassium frequently remains 4.5–5.2 mEq/L.
      1. Fludrocortisone acetate
         a) Change dose by 0.05–0.10 mg/day.
         b) The average dose to control disease is 0.1 mg/5 kg/day (1 tablet/10 lb).
      2. DOCP
         a) The recommended dose by the manufacturer is 2.2 mg/kg IM every 25 days.
         b) Most dogs are controlled on 1–1.5 mg/kg IM or SQ every 3–4 weeks.
         c) Some may require 2–3 mg/kg IM or SQ every 3–4 weeks.
  II. Sodium chloride
    A. Dose is 1–5 g/day PO.
    B. It may be needed to help normalize serum sodium concentrations.
  III. Glucocorticoid therapy
    A. Many dogs also require glucocorticoid supplementation to prevent signs of glucocorticoid deficiency.
    B. Persistent mild azotemia may respond to glucocorticoid administration.
    C. Give prednisolone or prednisone 0.2–0.4 mg/kg/day PO or cortisone acetate 1 mg/kg/day PO.
    D. Extra glucocorticoid (2–10 times basal levels) is given during periods of illness or stress.

HYPERADRENOCORTICISM

Rhett Nichols and Mark E. Peterson
(Revised by Rhett Nichols)

Definition

Spontaneous canine hyperadrenocorticism (Cushing's syndrome) refers to the clinical signs and biochemical abnormalities that result from chronic exposure to glucocorticoid excess.

Causes

I. Pituitary-dependent hyperadrenocorticism
  A. This is the most common form (85% of naturally occurring cases).
  B. Excessive secretion of ACTH, usually from a pituitary microadenoma, causes bilateral adrenocortical hyperplasia.
II. Functional adrenocortical tumors
  A. These account for 15% of the cases of canine Cushing's syndrome.
  B. Of adrenocortical tumors, 50% are benign.
III. Iatrogenic hyperadrenocorticism
  A. It is caused by excessive or prolonged administration of oral, parenteral, or topical corticosteroids.
  B. Clinical signs and physical exam findings are similar to those seen in the natural disease.
  C. The adrenal cortex is atrophied in this condition.

Clinical Signs and Pathophysiology

I. Signalment
  A. Hyperadrenocorticism is a disease of primarily middle-age to aged dogs; however, age may range from 6 months to 17 years or older.
  B. Poodles, dachshunds, Boston terriers, and boxers are predisposed, but all breeds can be affected.
  C. No sex predilection is seen in the pituitary-dependent form.
II. Urinary system
  A. Polyuria (PU) and polydipsia (PD) are noted in the majority of cases, because glucocorticoids decrease renal tubular reabsorption of water, increase glomerular filtration rate and renal blood flow, and inhibit the action of ADH.
  B. Pollakiuria, hematuria, and stranguria are sometimes present from lower urinary tract infection.
III. Cardiovascular system
  A. Panting is quite common and may result from decreased pulmonary compliance, pulmonary hypertension, or the direct effects of cortisol on the respiratory center.
  B. Severe respiratory distress can be caused by pulmonary thromboembolism, a potential complication.
  C. Systemic hypertension is common. Causes include increased renin substrate and the permissive effects of glucocorticoids with catecholamines.
IV. Endocrine system
  A. Some dogs also develop diabetes mellitus with signs of PU, PD, weight loss, and polyphagia.
  B. Many of these are insulin resistant (requiring >2 U/kg/day).
  C. Cortisol antagonizes the actions of insulin by interfering with its action at the cellular level and by promoting gluconeogenesis.
V. Central nervous and neuromuscular systems
  A. Lethargy is a common CNS disturbance and may be associated with high levels of ACTH and/or the effects of excessive cortisol on cerebral enzymes and neurotransmitter synthesis.
  B. Expansion of a pituitary tumor may cause subtle signs such as restlessness, inappetence, and disorientation, which may progress to more definitive signs such as stupor, ataxia, tetraparesis, and aimless wandering.
  C. Muscle weakness and atrophy are quite common and result from muscle wasting secondary to catabolic effects.
  D. Pendulous, distended, or "pot-bellied" abdomen results from hepatomegaly, a redistribution of abdominal fat, and abdominal muscle weakness.
  E. Unilateral or bilateral facial nerve paralysis occasionally develops; the cause is unclear.
  F. Increased joint laxity with bilateral ruptured cruciate ligaments or carpal dislocation sometimes occurs.
VI. Integument system (see also Chap. 88)
  A. Bilaterally symmetrical alopecia with dull, dry hair coat
    1. It is most noticeable around the neck, flanks, sides, and perineum.
    2. The head and extremities are classically spared.
    3. Clipped areas fail to regrow hair.
    4. The cause is atrophy of the epidermis and pilosebaceous apparatus with onset of telogen phase or lack of hair growth.
  B. Thin skin
    1. It is best noted over the abdomen, where the skin appears wrinkled.
    2. It results from protein catabolism of dermal structures and inhibition of fibroblast proliferation and collagen deposition.
  C. Mineralization of skin (calcinosis cutis)
    1. Not common; usually develops in dorsal thoracic, neck, or inguinal areas
    2. Probably caused by rearrangement of collagen and elastin matrix that attracts and binds calcium
  D. Hyperpigmentation
    1. Cause unclear; circulating ACTH metabolites with a similar structure to melanocyte-stimulating hormone (MSH) may play a role
    2. May occur secondary to concurrent hypothyroidism
VII. Reproductive system
  A. In the male, testicular atrophy may develop because of low circulating concentrations of pituitary follicle-stimulating hormone (FSH) and luteinizing hormone (LH) resulting from feedback inhibition by cortisol.
  B. Anestrus may occur secondary to reduced concentrations of FSH or LH.
  C. Clitoral hypertrophy sometimes develops from elevated adrenal androgen concentrations produced by the hypertrophied adrenal cortex.

Diagnosis

I. History may identify exposure to exogenous glucocorticoids; the presence of PU, PD, polyphagia, or muscle weakness; or, less commonly, the development of insulin-resistant diabetes mellitus.

II. Physical examination reveals many of the clinical signs listed earlier.

III. Routine laboratory tests are often abnormal.

A. Marked elevations in serum alkaline phosphatase (SAP) occur in >90% of cases.

1. Elevations in SAP activity >1000 IU/dl are common.

2. Use of SAP isoenzyme assays may be helpful to differentiate steroid-induced increases from increases in SAP activity caused by primary hepatic disease.

B. Elevations in serum concentrations of cholesterol (>280 mg/dl) and alanine transferase occur in more than half of cases.

C. Mild elevations in blood glucose are common, with overt diabetes mellitus (>300 mg/dl) occurring in 10%.

D. Urine often has a low specific gravity (<1.030).

E. Mild proteinuria is common, but a protein:creatinine ratio >3 is usually from glomerular disease or secondary urinary tract infection.

F. The hemogram may reveal a stress leukogram (neutrophilia, lymphopenia, eosinopenia), mild erythrocytosis (PCV >55), and sporadic nucleated red blood cells.

IV. Radiography is often helpful.

A. Plain films

1. Hepatomegaly is often seen.

2. Approximately 30% of adrenal tumors are calcified.

3. Calcification of bronchial walls may occur.

B. Ultrasonography

1. Bilaterally enlarged adrenal glands (bilateral adrenal hyperplasia) or unilateral adrenal masses (adrenal neoplasia) can sometimes be imaged.

2. The liver appears diffusely hyperechoic in most cases. Metastasis from adrenal adenocarcinoma (if present) can usually be imaged.

C. Computed tomography (CT) or magnetic resonance imaging (MRI)

1. Pituitary tumors >1 cm in diameter (macroadenomas or macroadenocarcinomas) are relatively easy to delineate.

2. Pituitary microadenomas may be defined if they are ideally positioned or approach 1 cm in diameter.

3. CT and MRI are the most accurate and reliable methods to evaluate adrenal glands, followed by diagnostic ultrasonography and plain radiography.

4. The location of the adrenal tumor and evidence of metastasis can be identified in most cases.

5. Both procedures are expensive.

V. Adrenal function tests are required to further define the abnormality (Table 44–1).

A. Basal plasma or serum cortisol concentrations
These are not very useful because of constant fluctuations throughout the day.

B. ACTH stimulation test

1. Most commonly used test

2. Pituitary-dependent hyperadrenocorticism: 85% have an exaggerated response

3. Iatrogenic hyperadrenocorticism: "blunted" or no response

4. Adrenocortical tumors: 50% show an exaggerated response

5. Protocols

a) Plasma or serum for cortisol analysis is obtained before and 2 hours after 2.2 U/kg ACTH gel IM.

b) Plasma samples are obtained before and 1 hour after 0.25 mg of synthetic ACTH (Cortrosyn) IV or IM. A lower dosage (0.125 mg IV) can be used in cats.

C. Low-dose dexamethasone suppression test (LDDST)

1. Useful in confirming the diagnosis

2. Sensitivity approaches 90%

3. Does not differentiate pituitary-dependent hyperadrenocorticism from adrenal neoplasia in most cases

4. Specificity poor if applied to animals that are suffering from nonadrenal illness

*Table 44–1. **Pituitary-Adrenal Function Tests: Normal Ranges***

Test	Unit	Dog	Cat
Serum or plasma cortisol[a]			
Basal cortisol (serum or plasma)	nmol/L	25–125	15–150
Post–ACTH cortisol	nmol/L	200–550	130–450
Post–low-dose dexamethasone	nmol/L	≤40	≤40
Post–high-dose dexamethasone[b]	nmol/L	≤40	≤40
Urine cortisol[a]			
Urine cortisol:creatine ratio	nmol/L and mmol/L,[c] respectively	≤35	—
Plasma ACTH	pmol/L[d]	2–15	1–20

[a] To convert cortisol unit from μg/dl to nmol/L, divide value by 27.59.

[b] This test is used, after adrenocortical hyperfunction has been confirmed, to differentiate adrenal tumor (no suppression) from pituitary-dependent adrenal hyperplasia (suppression usually occurs).

[c] To convert creatinine from mg/dl to mmol/L, multiply value by 0.088.

[d] To convert pg/ml to pmol/L, multiply value by 0.220.

5. Protocol
    a) Plasma or serum samples for cortisol analysis are obtained before and 4 and 8 hours after 0.015 mg/kg dexamethasone IV or IM.
    b) In normal dogs, circulating cortisol concentrations fall below 1 μg/dl (30 nmol/L) by 2–4 hours and remain suppressed for the full 8 hours of the test period.
    c) In most dogs with spontaneous hyperadrenocorticism, serum cortisol concentrations may fall (see later) but remain >1 μg/dl (30 nmol/L) at 4 and 8 hours.
    d) In about a third of dogs with pituitary-dependent hyperadrenocorticism, serum cortisol concentrations are suppressed <1 μg/dl 2–4 hours after administration of dexamethasone but then "escape" from suppression, with cortisol concentration increasing >1 μg/dl by 6–8 hours after administration.
    e) Functional adrenal masses do not show cortisol suppression and therefore do not exhibit this escape phenomenon.
    f) Cats require a higher dose of dexamethasone (0.1 mg/kg) to demonstrate normal suppression.
D. High-dose dexamethasone suppression test (HDDST).
    1. This test is used to differentiate pituitary-dependent hyperadrenocorticism from adrenocortical neoplasia.
    2. Adrenal tumors do not suppress, so cortisol concentrations do not fall below 1.5 μg/dl (40 nmol/L) during the testing period.
    3. Some dogs with pituitary-dependent hyperadrenocorticism, especially those with large pituitary tumors, also fail to suppress.
    4. Protocol: A serum or plasma sample for cortisol analysis is obtained before and 4 and 8 hours after 0.1–1 mg/kg dexamethasone IV or IM.
E. Endogenous plasma ACTH concentration
    1. It can be used to distinguish pituitary-dependent hyperadrenocorticism from adrenocortical tumors.
    2. In theory, dogs with pituitary-dependent hyperadrenocorticism have normal to high ACTH concentrations, and dogs with functional adrenal tumors have low concentrations of ACTH.
    3. This test is expensive, and the specifics of sample handling are difficult.
        a) ACTH is a very labile peptide.
        b) Plasma samples should be collected, centrifuged, separated, and transferred immediately to a cold plastic tube for storage at −70°C.
        c) Alternatively, aprotinin (Trasylol), a protease inhibitor, can be added to the plasma sample to prevent breakdown of ACTH.

Samples can be stored at 4°C and sent to the laboratory by 2-day mail.
F. Urinary cortisol:creatinine ratio
    1. This test is a highly sensitive screening test, but it has low specificity. (It may rule out hyperadrenocorticism, but it cannot confirm the diagnosis of hyperadrenocorticism.)
    2. Protocol is as follows.
        a) Fresh urine is submitted to the laboratory for urine cortisol and urine creatinine determinations.
        b) When urine cortisol is expressed as nmol/L and urine creatinine is expressed as mmol/L, a cortisol:creatinine ratio >35 is suggestive of hyperadrenocorticism.
        c) To convert cortisol concentrations from μg/dl to nmol/L, multiply by 28; to convert creatinine from mg/dl to mmol/L, multiple by 0.088.
    3. Urine cortisol:creatinine ratios are also valid in cats.
VI. Ancillary laboratory tests to consider include the following.
    A. Thyroid function tests
        1. Serum T_3 and T_4 and free T_4 concentrations are low in many cases, but the response to exogenous thyroid-stimulating hormone (TSH) parallels that of normal.
        2. Low circulating thyroid hormone concentrations probably result from cortisol-induced depression of pituitary TSH and altered thyroid hormone protein binding.
        3. The low thyroid hormone concentrations appear to be a secondary condition that resolves with treatment of the primary disease.
    B. Bile acids
        1. May be increased from "steroid hepatopathy"
        2. Often return to normal with treatment
    C. Liver biopsy
        1. Specific changes compatible with glucocorticoid hepatopathy
        2. Serves as a diagnostic aid but does not differentiate endogenous from iatrogenic steroid hepatopathy
    D. Systemic blood pressure measurement
        1. Many dogs are hypertensive secondary to high cortisol concentrations.
        2. Hyperadrenocorticism is associated with high concentrations of renin substrate.

Differential Diagnosis

I. Diabetes mellitus
II. Renal disease
III. Liver disease
IV. Hypothyroidism
V. Pyelonephritis
VI. Hypercalcemia
VII. Diabetes insipidus
VIII. Psychogenic polydipsia
IX. Hyperthyroidism
X. Acromegaly

Treatment

I. Mitotane (*o,p'*-DDD; Lysodren) therapy of pituitary-dependent hyperadrenocorticism

  A. Causes selective necrosis of the zona fasciculata and zona reticularis of the adrenal cortex

  B. Initial therapy: the loading period

   1. Give mitotane 30–50 mg/kg/day PO for 5–10 days.

   2. One of the earliest side effects during the initial phase of therapy is decreased appetite. Other common side effects include lethargy, vomiting, weakness, and diarrhea.

   3. If adverse effects occur, stop the drug and administer prednisone or prednisolone (0.2–0.4 mg/kg PO SID).

   4. The effectiveness of therapy is best monitored using the ACTH stimulation test.

    a) The goal of therapy is to achieve subclinical hypoadrenocorticism whereby pre- and post-ACTH serum cortisol concentrations are in the basal cortisol range (1–5 μg/dl or 25–150 nmol/L).

    b) If basal and post-ACTH serum cortisol concentrations become <1 μg/dl (or <10 nmol/L), stop the mitotane and supplement glucocorticoids as needed until circulating cortisol concentrations normalize.

    c) If basal or post-ACTH serum cortisol concentrations are above the normal resting range, continue this daily mitotane treatment and repeat the ACTH stimulation tests at 5- to 10-day intervals until cortisol concentrations fall within the normal resting range.

   5. Dogs with concurrent diabetes mellitus and insulin resistance are usually given less mitotane during the loading period. Dogs that are receiving low daily insulin dosages can be treated as described earlier.

    a) Mitotane is started after the animal is regulated with insulin.

    b) Dose is 25 mg/kg PO daily for 7–10 days.

    c) Monitor blood glucose at least twice daily, and adjust insulin dosage appropriately with blood glucose levels.

  C. Maintenance therapy

   1. When serum cortisol concentrations normalize, begin a maintenance dosage of 25 mg/kg PO twice weekly.

   2. If adverse side effects occur, stop the drug and begin glucocorticoid supplementation.

   3. In most cases, mitotane can be resumed 2–6 weeks later, when plasma cortisol concentrations have returned to the normal resting range.

   4. Iatrogenic hypoadrenocorticism with the associated electrolyte changes of hyponatremia and hyperkalemia develops in about 5% of dogs.

   5. Many dogs relapse within 12 months of therapy, requiring increased dosages of mitotane.

II. Mitotane therapy of adrenocortical tumors

  A. Remission of clinical signs has been achieved for more than 24 months in some dogs with adrenocortical adenomas and carcinomas.

  B. The majority of dogs have a good to excellent response to treatment.

  C. Administer 50–75 mg/kg/day PO and perform ACTH stimulation testing weekly until pre- and post-ACTH serum cortisols are <1 μg/dl (<30 nmol/L).

  D. Initial maintenance dose is 75–100 mg/kg/week in divided doses; maintenance doses as high as 200–300 mg/kg/week may be required.

  E. Common side effects include anorexia, weakness, and lethargy. If they develop, stop the drug and start again later at a lower dosage.

III. Ketoconazole therapy of pituitary-dependent hyperadrenocorticism

  A. Ketoconazole (Nizoral) reversibly inhibits adrenal steroidogenesis.

  B. The initial dosage is 5–10 mg/kg PO BID.

  C. Perform an ACTH stimulation test after 7–10 days.

  D. Once adequate control is achieved, lifelong BID therapy must be maintained for proper management.

  E. Side effects include anorexia, vomiting, and, rarely, icterus. If they occur, stop the drug and provide supportive care if needed.

  F. Disadvantages of ketoconazole therapy include high cost, continuous BID administration, possible hepatopathy, and sporadic lack of efficacy, possibly from poor gastrointestinal absorption.

IV. L-Deprenyl (Eldepryl) therapy for pituitary-dependent hyperadrenocorticism has shown some success.

  A. It is a monoamine oxidase type B inhibitor.

  B. It normalizes dopamine levels in the brain, thereby lowering ACTH production.

  C. Initial dosage in dogs is 1 mg/kg/day PO.

  D. Monitor clinical signs and LDDST; if no improvement in 30–60 days, raise dosage to 2 mg/kg/day PO.

  E. There are no reported side effects, but it should not be given with other monoamine oxidase B inhibitors.

  F. Efficacy is reported to be as high as 80% (Bruyette et al., 1996).

  G. Major disadvantage is its expense.

V. Surgical therapy

  A. Pituitary-dependent hyperadrenocorticism

   1. Bilateral adrenalectomy is not recommended in dogs; however, it may be the only effective, practical treatment in cats.

   2. Although hypophysectomy has long been performed in Europe, the surgery is difficult, expensive, and rarely performed in the United States.

   3. Many animals are also poor surgical candidates.

B. Adrenal tumors
  1. Adrenalectomy is the treatment of choice in many cases, especially when metastasis is not evident.
  2. Preoperative radiography, ultrasonography, or CT are performed to identify which adrenal gland is affected and any possible metastases.
  3. Postoperative care is complicated.
    a) Treat for hypoadrenocorticism because the contralateral adrenal will be atrophied. Give glucocorticoids at five times the maintenance dosage; mineralocorticoid therapy is rarely needed.
    b) Once stable, taper supplemental glucocorticoid therapy over 2–3 months to allow the contralateral adrenal to regain normal function.
VI. Radiation therapy
  A. Radiation therapy may be useful in cases caused by a pituitary macrotumor.
  B. The total dose of radiation (54 Gy) is delivered in fractions (300 cGy/fraction) over 4–6 weeks.
  C. Potential complications (rare) include deafness, cataracts, trigeminal neuropathy, seizures, and panhypopituitarism.
  D. Dogs with a pituitary macrotumor and severe neurologic signs warrant a grave prognosis.
  E. The disadvantages of radiation therapy include high cost, limited availability, and need for repetitive anesthesia.
  F. Elevated serum cortisol concentrations may not fall to normal for several months following pituitary radiation.

Patient Monitoring

I. The long-term prognosis is always guarded because of the many complications associated with the disease. The average life span after diagnosis is 2 years. Complications include the following.
  A. Thromboembolism
  B. Infection
  C. Hypertension
  D. Congestive heart failure
  E. Recurrence of symptoms
  F. Progression of pituitary tumor growth
II. Overdosage and underdosage with either mitotane or ketoconazole can complicate therapy, so persistent monitoring is necessary.
  A. Owners should observe for recurrence of symptoms, especially polyuria and polydipsia.
  B. The ACTH response test is done every 3–6 months to assess adrenal reserve.
    1. If post-ACTH serum cortisol concentrations are >5 μg/dl or >150 nmol/L, increase the dosage of mitotane or increase daily dosage of ketoconazole.
    2. Suspend therapy with any signs of hypoadrenocorticism or with post-ACTH cortisols <1 μg/dl (<25 nmol/L).
    3. Lifelong therapy is usually required.

PHEOCHROMOCYTOMA

Leland Thompson
(Revised by Rhett Nichols)

Definition and Causes

I. Pheochromocytoma is a tumor of chromaffin cells. Most arise from the adrenal medulla, but extra-adrenal pheochromocytomas may occur along sympathetic chains.
II. Pheochromocytoma may be inherited as an autosomal dominant trait in 10% of human patients, but heritability has not been determined in animals.

Pathophysiology

I. Pheochromocytomas can be locally invasive, causing tumor thrombosis of the posterior vena cava. Metastasis is uncommon.
II. The clinical manifestations of pheochromocytoma arise from overproduction of catecholamines (epinephrine or norepinephrine), with resultant systemic hypertension.
  A. Absence of normal feedback controls for catecholamine production and release may allow oversecretion.
  B. The mechanism of release of catecholamines from pheochromocytomas is poorly understood.
    1. Release may be stimulated by direct pressure (sudden movement or strain), altered tumor blood flow, or chemical mediators.
    2. Secretion may be constant or paroxysmal.
    3. Varying concentrations of epinephrine or norepinephrine may be released.
III. The tissue response to excess catecholamines depends on several factors.
  A. The number and class of receptors (alpha or beta).
  B. The potency of catecholamines at specific receptors.
  C. The threshold of response of specific receptors.

Clinical Signs

I. Signs of pheochromocytoma are often vague, nonspecific, and easily confused with more common disorders. Thus, pheochromocytoma is rarely diagnosed ante mortem.
II. Affected animals are usually older dogs; there is no sex or breed predisposition.
III. Signs associated with space-occupying mass include weight loss and lethargy.
IV. Ascites and peripheral edema in the hind legs may occur with thrombosis of the posterior vena cava.
V. Signs associated with catecholamine excess are variable.
  A. Signs may be acute, chronic, or episodic.
  B. Common presenting signs such as retinal hemorrhages or heart failure are related to sustained systemic hypertension.
  C. Chronic episodic signs are most common.

1. Depression, weakness
2. Tachypnea, dyspnea
3. Polydipsia, polyuria
4. Restlessness, irritability
5. Seizures, ataxia, syncope
6. Flushing of the skin and mucous membranes
7. Epistaxis

D. Acute hypertensive crisis may result in sudden collapse.
  1. Shock
  2. Ventricular fibrillation
  3. Severe vomiting and diarrhea
  4. Cerebral hemorrhage

E. Hypovolemic shock may result from rupture of intra-abdominal vascular tumor.

Diagnosis

I. Most pheochromocytomas are diagnosed as incidental findings at necropsy.
II. Physical examination may suggest an abdominal mass or systemic hypertension.
  A. Palpable mass
  B. Ascites, rear limb edema
  C. Tachycardia or other arrhythmias
  D. Retinal hemorrhages
  E. Harsh lung sounds
  F. Dilated pupils
III. Routine laboratory tests show no consistent abnormalities. The following may be observed.
  A. Hemoconcentration (increased hematocrit and total protein)
  B. Mature neutrophilia resulting from catecholamine-induced demargination
  C. Proteinuria or hematuria resulting from hypertensive glomerulopathy
IV. Diagnostic imaging is important to confirm the diagnosis.
  A. Plain radiography
    1. Adrenal mass, possibly calcified, displacing the adjacent kidney
    2. Cardiomegaly
    3. Pulmonary edema
  B. Contrast studies
    1. Intravenous urography may demonstrate displacement of a kidney by an adrenal mass.
    2. Venography may demonstrate compression or thrombosis in the posterior vena cava.
  C. Abdominal ultrasonography may demonstrate an adrenal mass. Catecholamine release can be induced by pressure on the sonogram transducer.
  D. CT and MRI are the diagnostic imaging procedures of choice.
V. Blood pressure concentrations may document hypertension.
  A. Multiple pressure determinations are indicated because of the paroxysmal release of catecholamines by many pheochromocytomas.
  B. Evidence of systemic hypertension indicates a need for further diagnostic screening.
VI. Catecholamine concentrations may be elevated.

A. Assays for plasma or urinary catecholamines or their metabolites are technically difficult, expensive, and not routinely available.
B. Release of catecholamines in affected dogs is often episodic, and normal dogs may exhibit elevated catecholamine levels with stress of venipuncture. Determination of urinary concentrations on 24-hour samples may be more reliable.
C. Normal values vary and should be determined by the particular laboratory used.

VII. Provocative or suppressive pharmacologic tests may be indicated when basal catecholamine determinations are equivocal.
  A. Provocative or suppressive pharmacologic tests block or stimulate catecholamine effects, resulting in profound blood pressure changes in affected dogs compared with normal dogs.
  B. These tests can be dangerous and should be used only when clinical findings strongly suggest pheochromocytoma, and radiographic and ultrasonographic findings are equivocal.
    1. Phentolamine suppression test
    2. Histamine test

Differential Diagnosis

I. Other causes of systemic hypertension
  A. Chronic renal disease
  B. Hypothyroidism
  C. Hyperadrenocorticism
II. Other metabolic or systemic disorders
  A. Cardiovascular diseases
  B. Neurologic disorders
  C. Pulmonary disease

Treatment

I. The therapy of choice is surgical excision. Medical therapy is used to stabilize cardiovascular and metabolic status before surgery.
II. Presurgical stabilization includes the following.
  A. Alpha-adrenergic blocking agents to lower blood pressure
    1. Phenoxybenzamine hydrochloride 0.2–1.5 mg/kg PO BID is given for 10–14 days before surgery.
    2. Begin with low dose and gradually increase until the desired decrease in blood pressure in achieved.
  B. Beta-adrenergic blocking agents to control cardiac arrhythmias and hypertension
    1. Propranolol 0.15–0.5 mg/kg PO TID
    2. Must be used in conjunction with phenoxybenzamine to prevent severe hypertension
III. The anesthetic regimen must be carefully chosen.
  A. Narcotic agents combined with glycopyrrolate are preferred preanesthetics.
  B. Isoflurane with concurrent use of nitrous oxide is preferred.
  C. Avoid alpha-blocking phenothiazines that may cause a hypotensive crisis.

D. Avoid atropine, which may cause profound tachyarrhythmias.

E. Short-acting barbiturates and halothane may be arrhythmogenic.

IV. Careful monitoring during surgery is mandatory.

A. Place an intra-arterial catheter for measuring blood pressure and a jugular catheter for monitoring central venous pressure.

B. Monitor cardiac rhythm with an electrocardiogram.

C. Tumor manipulation may induce hypertension, which is best treated with phentolamine (0.02–0.1 mg/kg IV).

D. Ventricular arrhythmias can be managed with propranolol (0.03–0.1 mg/kg IV).

E. Hypotension resulting from tumor removal is managed with fluid administration while monitoring central venous pressure.

V. Consider the following when planning surgery.

A. Most tumors lie in the retroperitoneal space in or around the adrenal gland or near the aorta.

B. Tumor vascularity and potential for vena cava invasion necessitate caution in dissection.

1. Noninvasive tumors usually can be excised completely.

2. Complete exploration of the abdomen to identify metastases is indicated.

Patient Monitoring

I. Complete resection without evidence of metastases has a good prognosis.

II. If no decrease in blood pressure is observed following surgery, an additional tumor is likely present.

III. Urinary catecholamines and their metabolites return to normal within days of surgery with adequate resection.

IV. Monitor for recurrence of clinical signs.

Bibliography

Benowitz NL: Pheochromocytoma. Adv Intern Med 35:195, 1990

Bruyette DS, Darling LA, Griffin D, Ruehl WW: L-Deprenyl for canine pituitary dependent hyperadrenocorticism: pivotal clinical trial (abstract). J Vet Intern Med 10:192, 1996

Duesberg CA, Feldman EC, Nelson RW et al: Magnetic resonance imaging for diagnosis of pituitary macrotumors in dogs. J Am Vet Med Assoc 206:657, 1995

Feldman EC: Adrenal gland disease. p. 1721. In Ettinger SJ (ed): Textbook of Veterinary Internal Medicine: Diseases of the Dog and Cat. 3rd Ed. WB Saunders, Philadelphia, 1989

Feldman EC, Nelson RW: Pheochromocytoma and multiple endocrine neoplasia. p. 306. In: Canine and Feline Endocrinology and Reproduction. 2nd Ed. WB Saunders, Philadelphia, 1996

Kemppainen RJ: Non-dexamethasone-suppressive, pituitary-dependent hyperadrenocorticism in a dog. J Am Vet Met Assoc 187:276, 1985

Kintzer PP, Peterson ME: Use of o,p'-DDD in treatment of canine hyperadrenocorticism caused by hyperfunctional adrenal neoplasia. p. 1034. In Kirk RW (ed): Current Veterinary Therapy X: Small Animal Practice. WB Saunders, Philadelphia, 1989

Kintzer PP, Peterson ME: Mitotane (o,p'-DDD) treatment of 200 dogs with pituitary-dependent hyperadrenocorticism. J Vet Intern Med 5:182, 1991

Kintzer PP, Peterson ME: Mitotane (o,p'-DDD) treatment of dogs with cortisol-secreting adrenocortical neoplasia: 32 cases (1980–1992). J Am Vet Med Assoc 205:54, 1994

Peterson ME, Gilbertson SR, Drucker WD: Plasma cortisol response to exogenous ACTH in 22 dogs with hyperadrenocorticism caused by adrenocortical neoplasia. J Am Vet Med Assoc 180:542, 1982

Peterson ME, Greco DS, Orth DN: Primary hypoadrenocorticism in ten cats. J Vet Intern Med 3:55, 1989

Peterson ME, Kintzer PP, Kass PH: Pretreatment clinical and laboratory findings in dogs with hypoadrenocorticism: 225 cases (1979–1993). J Am Vet Med Assoc 208:85, 1996

Rakich PM, Lorenz MD: Clinical signs and laboratory abnormalities in 23 dogs with spontaneous hypoadrenocorticism. J Am Anim Hosp Assoc 20:647, 1984

Rogers W, Strauss J, Chew D: Atypical hypoadrenocorticism in three dogs. J Am Vet Med Assoc 179:155, 1981

Samaan NA, Hickey RC, Shutts PE: Diagnosis, localization, and management of pheochromocytoma. Cancer 62:2451, 1988

Scavelli TD, Peterson ME, Matthiesen DT: Results of surgical treatment for hyperadrenocorticism caused by adrenocortical neoplasia in 25 dogs. J Am Vet Med Assoc 189:1360, 1986

Smiley LE, Peterson ME: Evaluation of a urine cortisol:creatinine ratio as a screening test for hyperadrenocorticism in dogs. J Vet Intern Med 7:163, 1993

Twedt DC, Wheeler SL: Pheochromocytoma in the dog. Vet Clin North Am [Small Anim Pract] 14:767, 1984

Wheeler SL: Pheochromocytoma. p. 977. In Kirk RW (ed): Current Veterinary Therapy IX. WB Saunders, Philadelphia, 1986

45

Miscellaneous Endocrine and Metabolic Disorders

Albert E. Jergens
Mark E. Hitt

HYPERLIPIDEMIA

Albert E. Jergens

Definition

I. Hyperlipidemia is an increased concentration of lipids in the blood.
   A. Hyperlipidemia includes both hypertriglyceridemia and hypercholesterolemia.
   B. Lactescence (lipemia) is grossly apparent when triglyceride concentration exceeds 400 mg/dl.
   C. Physiologic or postprandial lipemia may persist up to 12 hours after a fat-containing meal.
   D. Fasting hyperlipidemia always indicates abnormal lipid metabolism.
II. Hyperlipidemia results from either increased synthesis or reduced degradation of lipoproteins.
   A. Primary: idiopathic or genetic defects in lipoprotein metabolism
   B. Secondary: associated with underlying metabolic disorders

Laboratory Classification

I. Lipoproteins
   A. Hyperlipidemia may result from increased serum triglyceride and/or cholesterol concentrations.
   B. Lipoproteins are protein–lipid complexes that facilitate lipid transport in plasma.
      1. Lipoproteins contain both triglycerides and cholesterol, but in varying amounts.
      2. Four major lipoprotein classes are based on differences in electrophoretic mobility and density.
         a) Chylomicrons
            (1) Derived from dietary fat and synthesized within the intestinal mucosa
            (2) Rich in triglyceride
         b) Very low-density lipoprotein (VLDL)
            (1) Synthesized in the liver
            (2) Rich in triglyceride
         c) Low-density lipoprotein (LDL)
            (1) Formed from VLDL following removal of triglyceride by lipoprotein lipase
            (2) Rich in cholesterol
         d) High-density lipoprotein (HDL)
            (1) Synthesized in the liver
            (2) Cholesterol rich, functions as major cholesterol carrier
            (3) Major lipoprotein class present in the fasting dog and cat
   C. Hyperlipidemia is clinically significant when triglyceride concentrations exceed 500 mg/dl or cholesterol exceeds 300 mg/dl.
   D. In general, hyperlipidemia caused by increased serum triglycerides is of greater clinical importance.
II. Chylomicron test
   A. Overnight (8–12 hours) refrigeration of plasma or serum is required.
   B. Chylomicrons float to top and form a cream layer above a clear serum infranatant (hyperchylomicronemia).
   C. Diffuse serum lactescence signifies VLDL.
   D. It provides quick assessment as to the nature of hypertriglyceridemia.
III. Lipoprotein lipase activity
   A. Lipoprotein lipase from vascular endothelium hydrolyzes triglycerides peripherally and removes them from serum.

B. Hyperlipidemia is assessed in dogs before and 15 minutes after heparin administration of 100 IU/kg IV.

C. Measure cholesterol and triglycerides before and after heparin administration.

D. Failure to reduce lipid concentrations suggests decreased lipoprotein lipase activity.

IV. Effect on serum biochemistries

A. Hyperlipidemia interferes with many serum biochemical tests.

1. Concentrations of sodium, potassium, and chloride are falsely decreased by lipid displacement of the aqueous phase.

2. Concentrations of total protein, albumin, globulin, glucose, calcium, phosphorus, and bilirubin are falsely elevated (DeBowes, 1987).

B. The degree of biochemical abnormalities depends on the severity of the hyperlipidemia.

Causes and Pathophysiology

I. Postprandial hyperlipidemia

A. Most common cause of hyperlipidemia

B. Characterized by hyperchylomicronemia subsequent to a recent meal

II. Secondary hyperlipoproteinemia

A. Diabetes mellitus

1. Increased mobilization of stored triglycerides from adipose tissue

2. Increased hepatic production of VLDL (triglycerides)

3. Reduced lipoprotein lipase activity that impairs removal of circulating lipoproteins

4. Typified by hypertriglyceridemia with less severe hypercholesterolemia

B. Hypothyroidism

1. Impaired removal of circulating lipoproteins

2. Reduced hepatic degradation of cholesterol

3. Commonly severe hypercholesterolemia and moderate hypertriglyceridemia

C. Pancreatitis

1. The association between pancreatitis and hyperlipidemia is incompletely understood.

a) It remains unclear which of the two is the primary disorder.

b) One theory suggests that hyperlipidemia precedes pancreatitis.

2. This disease usually produces both hypertriglyceridemia and hypercholesterolemia.

D. Hyperadrenocorticism

1. Reported with naturally occurring and iatrogenic hyperadrenocorticism in both the dog and the cat

2. Glucocorticoid stimulation of peripheral lipolysis

3. Increased hepatic secretion of VLDL

4. Reduced lipoprotein lipase activity secondary to insulin antagonism

5. Characterized by hypertriglyceridemia and mild hypercholesterolemia

E. Cholestatic liver disease

1. Hypercholesterolemia caused by impaired cholesterol excretion in bile

2. Production of abnormal lipoprotein (lipoprotein X)

3. Commonly hypercholesterolemia only

F. Nephrotic syndrome

1. Decreased plasma oncotic pressure (hypoalbuminemia) stimulates hepatic lipoprotein (VLDL) synthesis.

2. Defective lipoprotein lipase occurs from urinary loss of plasma cofactors that regulate its function.

3. Hypercholesterolemia is a predominant feature.

G. Miscellaneous causes

1. Drugs

a) Glucocorticoids, estrogens

b) Megestrol acetate in cats

2. Obesity

3. Late pregnancy

III. Primary hyperlipoproteinemia

A. Idiopathic canine hyperlipoproteinemia

1. Reported in miniature schnauzers

2. Decreased activity of lipoprotein lipase

B. Juvenile hyperchylomicronemia

1. Reported in the following animals

a) Four-week-old puppy (Baum et al., 1969)

b) Eight-month-old cat (Jones et al., 1983)

c) Two 3-week-old kitten siblings (Bauer and Verlander, 1984)

2. Suspected autosomal recessive mode of inheritance

Clinical Signs

I. Secondary

A. Extremely variable, depending on the cause

B. Associated with hypertriglyceridemia

1. Acute abdominal pain

2. Seizures

3. Vomiting

4. Diarrhea

5. Lipid-laden aqueous humor

6. Lethargy

7. Cutaneous xanthomas: accumulation of lipid in macrophages, forming lipid granulomas

C. Associated with hypercholesterolemia

1. Atherosclerosis (rare)

2. Lipemia retinalis: milky appearance to retinal veins and arteries

3. Crystalline corneal opacification

II. Primary

A. Hyperlipoproteinemia of miniature schnauzers

1. Abdominal pain

a) Vague, nonlocalizing discomfort of unknown cause

b) Acute pancreatitis not documented

2. Diarrhea

3. Vomiting

4. Depression, behavioral changes

5. Episodes of polydipsia

6. Seizures

B. Juvenile hyperchylomicronemia
   1. Lipemia retinalis
   2. Subcutaneous xanthomas
   3. Peripheral neuropathy, compression from xanthomas

Diagnosis

I. Postprandial hyperlipidemia
   Rule out by withholding food from the animal for at least 12 hours (Fig. 45–1).
II. Secondary hyperlipoproteinemia
   A. Perform routine database (complete blood count, serum biochemistries, urinalysis) to help identify metabolic disturbances.
   B. Determine cholesterol and triglyceride concentrations.
   C. Perform appropriate endocrine function testing.
III. Primary hyperlipoproteinemia
   A. A definitive diagnosis requires that secondary causes be ruled out.
   B. Common laboratory abnormalities in miniature schnauzers with hyperlipoproteinemia include the following.
      1. Fasting hyperlipidemia
      2. Positive chylomicron test: both cream layer and lactescence (VLDL)
      3. Severe hypertriglyceridemia and moderate hypercholesterolemia
      4. No lipolytic activity after heparin administration, suggesting that absolute lipoprotein lipase deficiency is not the cause

C. Diagnostic features of juvenile hyperchylomicronemia include the following.
   1. Fasting hyperlipidemia is noted.
   2. Blood resembles "cream of tomato soup."
   3. Severe hyperchylomicronemia and hypercholesterolemia are present.
   4. Reduced lipolytic activity after heparin administration suggests deficient lipoprotein lipase activity.

Treatment

I. Secondary hyperlipoproteinemia
   A. Treat underlying metabolic disorder.
   B. Nutritional therapy is also advisable (see later).
II. Primary hyperlipoproteinemia
   A. Therapeutic intervention is warranted to reduce the risks associated with elevated triglycerides such as abdominal pain, diarrhea, seizures, peripheral neuropathies, and cutaneous xanthomas.
   B. If acute gastroenteritis is present, provide supportive therapy.
      1. Nothing by mouth (NPO)
      2. Intravenous fluid therapy to correct hydration and electrolyte abnormalities
      3. Antiemetics to control vomiting
   C. Long-term therapy requires dietary management.
      1. Goals are to reduce triglyceride levels to <500 mg/dl and decrease secondary clinical signs.
      2. Commercially available low-fat diets include Prescription Diet r/d or w/d.

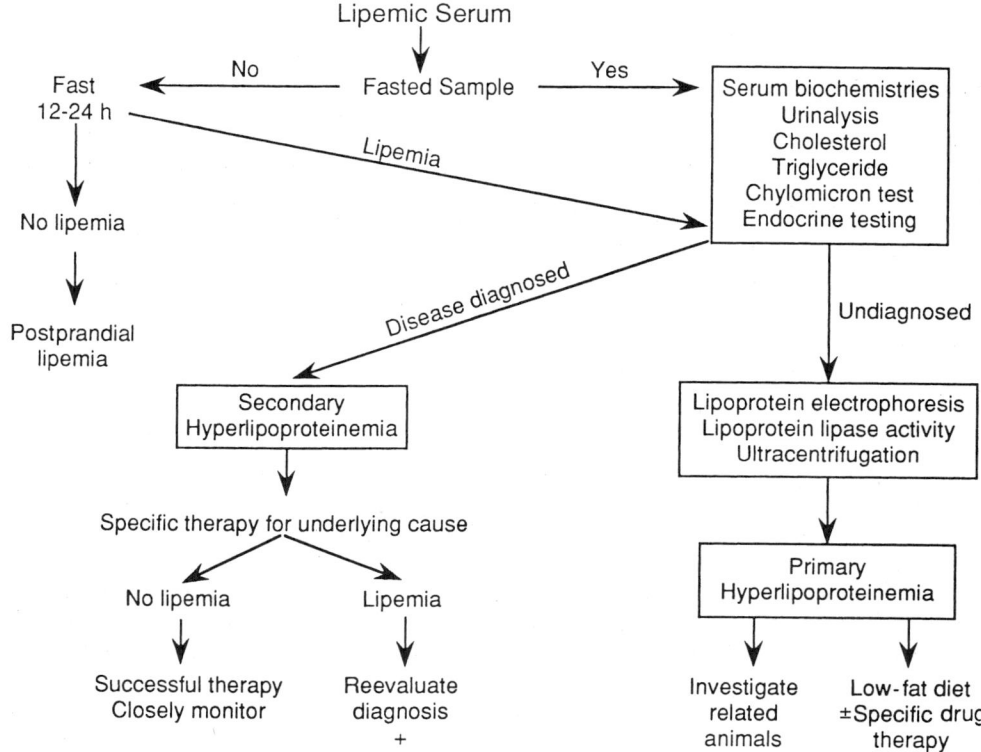

Figure 45–1. Diagnostic approach to the dog or cat with hyperlipidemia. (Modified from Jones and Manella, 1990, with permission.)

3. Homemade diets consisting of low-fat cottage cheese, lean ground beef, or skinless poultry may be substituted.
4. If response to diet changes is poor, try adding fish oils rich in omega-3 fatty acids.

D. Lipid-lowering drugs have not been widely used.
   1. Although extensively used in humans, these agents have not been approved for use in the dog and cat.
   2. Nicotinic acid may be tried; niacinamide is ineffective.

Patient Monitoring

I. Continue to monitor the primary disease and consider additional dietary fat restriction if lipemia fails to improve.
II. Dietary therapy of affected miniature schnauzers usually results in marked clinical improvement.
   A. Normalization of serum triglyceride concentrations can usually be achieved with low-fat rations.
   B. If fat-restricted diets result in excessive weight loss, provide caloric supplementation with medium-chain triglycerides.
   C. Therapy is required for the life of the animal.
III. Primary hyperchylomicronemia of cats can be treated as follows.
   A. Feeding a low-fat diet lowers blood lipid levels over 2–3 months.
   B. Dietary therapy can be expected to reverse peripheral neuropathy over 2–3 months.
   C. Therapy is required for the life of the animal.

ERYTHROPOIETIN ABNORMALITIES

Albert E. Jergens

Definition

I. Erythropoietin is a glycoprotein hormone that regulates normal erythropoiesis by modulating red blood cell precursors in the bone marrow.
II. It is produced by primarily renal interstitial cells.
III. Renal hypoxia is the major stimulus for erythropoietin secretion.

Causes

I. Causes of reduced serum erythropoietin
   A. Chronic renal failure
   B. Polycythemia vera
II. Stimuli for appropriately increased serum erythropoietin
   A. Right-to-left cardiovascular shunts
   B. Chronic pulmonary disease
   C. High altitudes
   D. Hemoglobinopathy
   E. Respiratory center depression
III. Causes of inappropriately increased serum erythropoietin

A. Tumors secreting erythropoietic substances
   1. Renal carcinoma
   2. Hepatoma
   3. Uterine leiomyoma
   4. Ovarian carcinoma
   5. Pheochromocytoma
   6. Adrenocortical neoplasms
   7. Renal lymphosarcoma
   8. Nasal fibrosarcoma
B. Parenchymal renal disease
   1. Renal cysts
   2. Hydronephrosis
   3. Polycystic kidneys
C. Hormonal stimulation
   1. Androgen therapy
   2. High dosages of adrenocortical steroids

Pathophysiology

I. Reduced erythropoietin secretion
   A. Chronic renal failure
      1. Inadequate production from nephron loss
      2. Characterized by nonregenerative anemia
   B. Polycythemia vera
      1. It is a myeloproliferative disorder resulting from clonal proliferation of erythroid precursors.
      2. Erythropoiesis is autonomous and is independent of erythropoietin stimulation.
      3. Normal erythropoietin production is suppressed by the elevated hematocrit.
      4. Absolute primary polycythemia occurs.
II. Appropriately increased erythropoietin secretion
   A. Production is increased to compensate for inadequate tissue oxygenation.
   B. Absolute secondary polycythemia occurs.
III. Inappropriately increased erythropoietin secretion
   A. Production increases without systemic tissue hypoxia.
   B. Production of erythropoietin or erythropoietin-like substances by neoplastic tissues occurs autonomously and for unknown reasons.
   C. The paradoxic overproduction of erythropoietin with certain renal diseases is poorly understood, but may be autonomous.
   D. Absolute secondary polycythemia occurs.

Clinical Signs

I. Reduced erythropoietin secretion
   A. Chronic renal failure (see Chap. 47)
   B. Polycythemia vera (see Chap. 63)
II. Appropriately increased erythropoietin secretion
   A. Clinical signs of cardiopulmonary disease
   B. Signs of hyperviscosity
III. Inappropriately increased erythropoietin secretion
   A. Clinical signs of parenchymal renal disease
   B. Other manifestations of occult neoplasia
   C. Signs of hyperviscosity

Diagnosis

I. Reduced erythropoietin secretion
  A. Chronic renal failure (see Chap. 47)
  B. Polycythemia vera
    1. Rule out dehydration as a cause for relative polycythemia.
    2. Confirm increased total red cell mass.
      a) Hematocrit >60%
      b) Total red blood cell (RBC) count $\geq 12 \times 10^6/\mu l$
    3. Exclude secondary causes for absolute polycythemia.
    4. Serum erythropoietin concentrations are low or absent.
II. Increased erythropoietin secretion
  A. Appropriate secretion caused by hypoxia
    1. Confirm increased RBC mass.
    2. Rule out relative polycythemia.
    3. Determine arterial blood oxygen saturation; value <92% suggests hypoxia.
    4. Obtain thoracic radiographs to assess cardiopulmonary disease.
    5. Perform electrocardiography and echocardiography to assess cardiac function.
    6. Serum erythropoietin concentrations are normal to increased.
  B. Inappropriate secretion without hypoxia
    1. Confirm increased RBC mass.
    2. Rule out relative polycythemia.
    3. Perform a thorough physical exam to identify any neoplasms.
    4. Urinalysis and biochemistry results may support renal disease.
    5. Renal imaging studies (survey radiography, ultrasonography, intravenous pyelography) may be needed to identify structural lesions.
    6. Arterial oxygen saturation is normal.
    7. Serum erythropoietin concentrations are normal to increased.

Differential Diagnosis

I. Differential considerations for increased hematocrit in the dog and cat include relative and absolute polycythemia.
II. With relative polycythemia, the packed cell volume (PCV) is elevated with a normal RBC mass; disorders causing absolute polycythemia have both increased PCV and total RBC mass.

Treatment

I. Reduced erythropoietin secretion
  A. For advice on the use of supplemental erythropoietin therapy for chronic renal failure, see Chap. 47.
  B. For specific therapy of polycythemia vera, see Chap. 63.
II. Increased erythropoietin secretion
  A. Medical therapy for patients with cardiopulmonary disease is outlined in Section II.

B. Surgical removal of erythropoietin-secreting tumors or renal cysts results in reduction of serum erythropoietin concentration and normalization of PCV and total RBC mass.
C. Phlebotomy is indicated for animals with clinically detrimental absolute polycythemia (see Chap. 63).

Patient Monitoring

I. Prognosis for animals with chronic renal failure and reduced erythropoietin secretion is guarded, and they require lifelong therapy.
II. Prognosis for animals having inappropriately increased erythropoietin secretion varies, based on the cause and severity of polycythemia.
  A. Complications of severe polycythemia result from hyperviscosity and vascular accidents.
  B. Polycythemia caused by renal disease has a good prognosis with successful removal of renal cysts. PCV and total RBC mass should be monitored for several months after surgery.
  C. Tumor-associated polycythemia has a variable prognosis.
    1. Prognosis is good with complete surgical removal of tumor.
    2. There is a guarded prognosis for large tumor burdens not amenable to complete excision.
    3. PCV and total RBC mass should be monitored for several months after surgery.
    4. Return of elevated PCV and RBC mass suggests tumor recurrence and/or metastatic disease.

HYPOGLYCEMIA

Mark E. Hitt

Definition

I. Resting blood glucose (BG) is <50 mg/dl (2.77 mmol/L).
II. Clinical signs are related to neuroglycopenia (reduced level of glucose available for passive diffusion to the brain).
III. Glucose provides the primary substrate for energy used to maintain normal cellular function in the central nervous system (CNS).

Causes

I. Juvenile-onset (Table 45–1)
  A. Neonatal hypoglycemia
  B. Transient juvenile hypoglycemia
  C. Portosystemic anomalies (see Chap. 34)
  D. Glycogen storage diseases (see Chap. 23)
II. Adult-onset
  A. Exertional or "hunting dog" hypoglycemia
  B. Insulinoma
  C. Paraneoplastic disorder (see Chap. 71)
  D. Hepatocellular insufficiency (see Chap. 34)
  E. Cachexia-associated

Table 45–1. Common Hypoglycemia-Related Diseases

Disorder	Pathophysiology	Incidence	Clinical Features	Treatment	Prevention
Neonatal hypoglycemia	Limited glycogen reserves and gluconeogenic enzymes	Common in dogs and cats <21 days old	Depression Seizures	Oral glucose Orogastric intubation	Feed QID
Transient juvenile hypoglycemia	Limited glycogen reserves and gluconeogenic enzymes Concurrent stress or disease Less able to utilize ketones or fatty acids	Common in immature, toy, or miniature breeds	Ataxia Seizures Decreased menace response	See text	Assess diet Decrease stress
Hunting dog hypoglycemia	Fasted dogs with 1–8 h of exercise Improper conditioning	Common in hunting dogs	Disorientation Ataxia Hunger Seizures	Feed simple sugar diet Give IV dextrose if warranted	Provide proper conditioning before hunting Carry meal or candy bar while hunting
Insulinoma (beta-cell tumor)	Functional beta-cell carcinoma May or may not have insulin release in response to normal feedback from blood glucose	Most common cause of hypoglycemia in dogs >5 yr old Standard poodles, boxers, Irish setters, fox terriers at greater risk	Episodic weakness, disorientation, ataxia, seizures, behavioral changes, polyphagia Variable blood glucose at time of presentation	See text	None
Sepsis-associated	Complex Undetermined	Common with severe bacteremia	Cardiovascular signs and septic shock	IV dextrose, fluids IV bactericidal antibiotics	None

III. Age-independent
  A. Sepsis-associated (bacteremia)
  B. Hypoadrenocorticism (see Chap. 44)
  C. Drug-related
    1. Insulin overdosage (''insulin shock'')
    2. Ethylene glycol
    3. Ethanol
    4. Salicylates
    5. Sulfonylureas
  D. Hypopituitarism
  E. Spurious

Pathophysiology

I. Euglycemia
  A. Glucose homeostasis
    It relies on the balance of glucose availability and glucose utilization.
  B. Glucose availability
    1. Glucose from dietary intake and intestinal absorption
    2. Gluconeogenesis from amino acids (especially alanine), lactate, fatty acids; glycerol and glycogenolysis from hepatic and muscle glycogen
    3. Glucagon
      a) Released from alpha cells of the pancreatic islets in response to low BG
      b) Promotes gluconeogenesis
    4. Glycogen reserves
      a) These provide the only significant form of carbohydrate storage in the body.
      b) Hepatic glycogen is depleted by a fast of 24–72 hours in adult dogs and 6 hours in puppies.
  C. Glucose utilization
    1. Glucose is the primary substrate for cellular energy.
    2. Insulin facilitates entry of glucose into cells, *except* for RBCs, hepatocytes, renal tubules, pancreatic beta islet cells, and most of the brain.
  D. Glucose influence on the brain
    1. Glucose deprivation results in impaired oxygen utilization.
    2. Cerebrum (especially the occipital visual cortical region) is most sensitive to neuroglycopenia.
II. Normal response to decreasing blood glucose
  A. Glucagon is released, stimulating gluconeogenesis and glycogenolysis.
  B. Graduated release of counterregulatory hormones occurs.
    1. Epinephrine and cortisol stimulate glucagon release, glycogenolysis, and lipolysis.
    2. Growth hormone inhibits the action of insulin and promotes lipolysis.
  C. Oxidation of fatty acids results in ketone production as an alternative cellular energy source.
  D. Neural adaptation to the use of fatty acids and ketones occurs in a few days if BG remains depressed.

E. Normal adult dogs have been fasted for 30 days without their developing hypoglycemia.

Clinical Signs

I. Signs and their intensity depend on the following.
  A. Rate of BG decline and time for neural adaptation
    1. These factors are as important as is the actual BG value.
    2. Adaptation to a chronic, slowly progressive disease may delay clinical signs, despite BGs of 20–50 mg/dl (1.1–2.7 mmol/L).
    3. Types of presentation include both hypoglycemic crises or milder episodic signs.
  B. Duration of hypoglycemic episode: influences severity
  C. Repetitive nature of seizures (can result in neural hypoxic damage and development of epilepsy)
  D. Concurrent stress or disease: complicates diagnosis and treatment
II. Catecholamine-related signs
  A. Trembling
  B. Nervousness
  C. Anxiety
  D. Hunger
III. Neuroglycopenic signs
  A. Ataxia
  B. Episodic weakness
  C. Visual or menace response deficit
  D. Bizarre behavior
  E. Shaking, trembling
  F. Collapse, seizures, coma

Diagnosis

I. Clinical signs, signalment, and history consistent with hypoglycemia
II. Laboratory confirmation
  A. Resting BG <50 mg/dl
  B. Fasting BG <50 mg/dl following carefully supervised fast (1–48 hours)
III. Fulfillment of Whipple's triad of clinical findings
  A. Clinical signs of hypoglycemia
  B. Laboratory hypoglycemia
  C. Resolution of clinical signs following administration of intravenous glucose
IV. Diagnostic tests for suspected insulinoma
  A. Presence of serum or urinary ketones, concurrent with hypoglycemia, eliminates the diagnosis of insulinoma (insulin prevents ketogenesis).
  B. Fulfill Whipple's triad (not pathognomonic) and rule out other causes of hypoglycemia.
  C. *Supervised* fast results in a BG <60 mg/dl with an inappropriate plasma immunoreactive insulin (IRI) level in the normal or high range; contact the selected laboratory concerning handling and shipping requirements before collecting the sample for IRI.
  D. Determine an amended insulin:glucose ratio (AIGR).

1. Supervise a fast for 1–48 hours (measure BG every 1–4 hours).
2. Obtain a sample for IRI level at nadir of the BG (<60 mg/dl or end of fast).
3. An alternative is to sample BG and IRI at the time of clinical signs.
4. Formula is as follows:
   a) $\dfrac{\text{Plasma IRI } (\mu U/ml) \times 100}{\text{Blood glucose } (mg/dl) - 30}$
   b) Results: normal <30; abnormal >30
5. Repeat tests if results are still suspicious but not definitive.
6. Both false-positive and false-negative results can occur.
   E. In some instances, an exploratory laparotomy may be necessary to confirm a diagnosis.
V. Ancillary tests
   A. Urinalysis
   B. Complete blood count
   C. Serum chemistries for hepatic or other organ disorders
   D. Thoracic and abdominal radiography for evaluation of organ size and for possible metastasis
   E. Abdominal ultrasonography, computed tomography, magnetic resonance imaging
      1. Look for a pancreatic mass.
      2. Search for primary or metastatic neoplasia in liver or other abdominal organs.

Differential Diagnosis

I. Spurious hypoglycemia
   A. Failure to promptly centrifuge and separate serum from cells
   B. Incorrect technique or expired reagents
   C. Ruled out with repeated testing
II. Neurologic manifestations (see also Chap. 22)
   A. Neurologic canine distemper
   B. Idiopathic epilepsy
   C. Hypocalcemia
   D. Hepatic encephalopathy
   E. Thiamine deficiency
   F. Poisoning
      1. Insecticides: organophosphates, carbamates, organochlorines
      2. Pesticides: strychnine, metaldehyde
      3. Lead toxicosis
III. Episodic weakness
   A. Hypoadrenocorticism
   B. Hypocalcemia
   C. Myasthenia gravis
   D. Hypokalemia
   E. Primary brain disorders
   F. Congenital or hereditary myopathies
   G. Syncope (arrhythmias, CNS hypoxia)
   H. Hepatic encephalopathy

Treatment

I. Hypoglycemic crisis
   A. Feed animal if, or when, it can eat.

B. Provide oral glucose.
   1. Monosaccharide can be absorbed from oral cavity mucous membranes using gentle digital massage and prevention of aspiration.
   2. Common oral monosaccharides used to treat hypoglycemia include the following.
      a) Glucose
         (1) Dextrose (D-glucose monohydrate)
         (2) Corn syrup
         (3) Fruit juices
      b) Fructose
         (1) Converted to glucose in the liver
         (2) Honey
         (3) Fruit juices
   C. Orogastric intubation can be used to administer 10–20 ml/kg of 20% dextrose, depending on the status of the animal.
   D. Consider IV dextrose.
      1. Initially 5–10 ml/kg of 20% dextrose to improve mental status or stop seizure activity
      2. Follow by 10–20 ml/kg/h of 10% dextrose until neurologically stable
   E. Monitor BG frequently.
II. Episodic hypoglycemia
   A. Identify specific cause.
   B. Treat as for hypoglycemic crisis.
   C. Prevent by feeding a well-balanced diet every 4–6 hours.
III. Specific therapy for insulinoma (beta-cell tumor)
   A. Hypoglycemic crisis
      1. Administer IV dextrose (as earlier) with caution, because it may stimulate further release of insulin.
      2. Maintain BG at >60 mg/dl with a combination of food and IV dextrose so that the animal is neurologically normal.
      3. If mental status does not improve, assess for possible cerebral edema and consider use of IV mannitol, diazepam, and prednisolone.
   B. Medical therapy
      1. Frequent meals
         a) Make sure these are rich in protein, fats, and complex carbohydrates.
         b) If this is adequate for maintenance of euglycemia, the addition of medications may not be immediately necessary.
      2. Glucocorticoids
         a) Antagonize the effects of insulin
         b) Prednisolone-sodium-succinate 1–2 mg/kg IV (before the animal returns to eating)
         c) Oral prednisolone starting at 0.5 mg/kg and increasing to 4 mg/kg in divided doses, as clinically warranted to maintain euglycemia
      3. Diazoxide
         a) Promotes hyperglycemia by inhibiting secretion of insulin from islet cells and inhibiting peripheral cellular uptake of glucose
         b) Does *not* treat the cancer
         c) Used after glucocorticoids and diet no longer maintain euglycemia
         d) Initial dosage of 5–10 mg/kg PO BID,

increasing only as necessary up to 40 mg/kg in divided doses

    e) Expensive; may not prolong survival time

   4. Hydrochlorothiazide

    a) May potentiate the effects of diazoxide

    b) Dose of 1–4 mg/kg PO BID

   5. Octreotide acetate

    a) Somatostatin analogue that may reduce insulin secretion

    b) May be tried before diazoxide

    c) Dose of 10–20 μg PO, SQ BID–TID

   6. Antineoplastic drugs

    a) Streptozotocin

      (1) It is an antineoplastic agent with some specificity for the pancreatic islet cells.

      (2) Inconsistent results and a high frequency of adverse reactions and renal toxicities dictate its use only as a last resort.

      (3) It is administered as a slow IV injection at 20 mg/kg once weekly for 4 weeks.

    b) Alloxan

      (1) May be helpful in dogs

      (2) Very nephrotoxic

      (3) Given as single IV dose of 65 μg/kg with concurrent fluids

C. Surgical therapy

   1. It is the preferred means of treatment for an insulinoma.

   2. An extensive pancreatectomy can result in exocrine pancreatic insufficiency and diabetes mellitus.

   3. Metastasis is common, and examination of the liver and regional lymph nodes should be done at the time of surgery.

    a) Animals may sometimes live 6–24 months as a result of combined management.

    b) Recurrence of hypoglycemia from metastasis is common within 3–12 months.

   4. Biopsy pancreas to assess beta cells if no tumor is evident at surgery.

   5. Transient diabetes mellitus may occur postoperatively until atrophied non-neoplastic islet cells recover their function; crystalline insulin may be required initially, changing to intermediate-acting or long-acting insulin as warranted.

   6. Pancreatitis may occur postoperatively and require symptomatic treatment (see Chap. 35).

IV. Supportive care

  A. Specific treatment of concurrent diseases

  B. Stress reduction

   1. Quiet environment

   2. Frequent nursing attendance

   3. Warm environment or circulating warm-water blanket

  C. IV fluid maintenance as required

Patient Monitoring

  I. Evaluate vital signs frequently.

  II. Evaluate neurologic and mental status frequently.

III. Monitor the following.

  A. Maintain BG at >90 mg/dl.

   1. Measure BG in postsurgical insulinoma cases every 4 hours.

    a) Persistent hypoglycemia indicates metastasis is probably present or the tumor was incompletely resected.

    b) Hyperglycemia >300 mg/dl requires insulin therapy.

   2. For juvenile animals, monitor BG every 1–6 hours.

   3. In adult animals, measure BG as often as it is clinically warranted by the specific diagnosis.

  B. Reevaluate serum electrolytes (especially potassium) if values are initially abnormal.

IV. Monitor for metastasis of insulinoma at 3- to 6-month intervals by performing the following.

  A. Hepatic function tests and serum enzymes

  B. Abdominal radiography and ultrasonography

  C. Thoracic radiography

  D. Measurement of a fasting BG and AIGR

Bibliography

Armstrong PJ, Ford RB: Hyperlipidemia. p. 1046. In Kirk RW (ed): Current Veterinary Therapy X: Small Animal Practice. WB Saunders, Philadelphia, 1989

Atkins CE: Disorders of glucose homeostasis in neonatal and juvenile dogs: hypoglycemia—Part I. Compend Contin Educ Pract Vet 6:197, 1984a

Atkins CE: Disorders of glucose homeostasis in neonatal and juvenile dogs: hypoglycemia—Part II. Compend Contin Educ Pract Vet 6:353, 1984b

Bauer JE, Verlander JW: Congenital lipoprotein lipase deficiency in hyperlipemic kitten siblings. Vet Clin Pathol 13:7, 1984

Baum D, Schweid AL, Porte D et al: Congenital lipoprotein lipase deficiency and hyperlipemia in the young puppy. Proc Soc Exp Biol Med 131:183, 1969

Campbell KL: Diagnosis and management of polycythemia in dogs. Compend Contin Educ Pract Vet 12:543, 1990

Crispin SM, Barnett KC: Arcus lipoides corneae secondary to hypothyroidism in the Alsatian. J Small Anim Pract 19:127, 1978

Cuoto CG, Boudrieau RJ, Zanjani ED: Tumor-associated erythrocytosis in a dog with nasal fibrosarcoma. J Vet Intern Med 3:183, 1989

DeBowes LJ: Lipid metabolism and hyperlipoproteinemia in dogs. Compend Contin Educ Pract Vet 9:727, 1987

Ford RB: Idiopathic hyperchylomicronemia in miniature schnauzers. J Small Anim Pract 34:488, 1993

Johnson RK: Canine hyperlipidemia. p. 203. In Ettinger SJ (ed): Textbook of Veterinary Internal Medicine. 3rd Ed. WB Saunders, Philadelphia, 1989

Jones BR, Johnstone AC, Cahill JI et al: Peripheral neuropathy in cats with inherited primary hyperchylomicronemia. Vet Rec 119:268, 1986

Jones BR, Manella C: Some aspects of hyperlipidemia in the dog and cat. Aust Vet Pract 20:136, 1990

Jones BR, Wallace A, Harding DRK et al: Occurrence of idiopathic, familial hyperchylomicronemia in a cat. Vet Rec 112:543, 1983

Kern TJ, Riis RC: Ocular manifestations of secondary hyperlipidemia associated with hypothyroidism and uveitis in a dog. J Am Anim Hosp Assoc 16:907, 1980

Leifer CE, Peterson ME, Matus RE et al: Hypoglycemia associated with nonislet cell tumor in 13 dogs. J Am Vet Med Assoc 186:53, 1985

Leifer CE, Peterson ME, Matus RE: Insulin-secreting tumor: diagnosis and medical and surgical management in 55 dogs. J Am Vet Med Assoc 188:60, 1986

Nelson RW, Hager D, Zanjani ED: Renal lymphosarcoma with inappropriate erythropoietin production in a dog. J Am Vet Med Assoc 182:1396, 1983

Peterson ME, Randolf JF: Diagnosis of canine primary polycythemia and management with hydroxyurea. J Am Vet Med Assoc 180:415, 1982

Peterson ME, Randolf JF: Diagnosis and therapy of polycythemia. p. 406. In Kirk RW (ed): Current Veterinary Therapy VIII. WB Saunders, Philadelphia, 1983

Peterson ME, Zanjani ED: Inappropriate erythropoietin production from a renal carcinoma in a dog with polycythemia. J Am Vet Med Assoc 179:995, 1981

Phillipson BE, Rothrock DW, Connor WE et al: Reduction of plasma lipids, lipoproteins, and apoproteins by dietary fish oils in patients with hypertriglyceridemia. New Engl J Med 312:1210, 1985

Rogers WA, Donovan EF, Kociba GJ: Idiopathic hyperlipoproteinemia in dogs. J Am Vet Med Assoc 166:1087, 1975a

Rogers WA, Donovan EF, Kociba GJ: Lipids and lipoproteins in normal dogs and in dogs with secondary hyperlipoproteinemia. J Am Vet Med Assoc 166:1092, 1975b

Scott RC, Patnaik AK: Renal carcinoma with secondary polycythemia in the dog. J Am Anim Hosp Assoc 8:275, 1972

Steiner JM, Bruyette DS: Canine insulinoma. Compend Contin Educ Pract Vet 18:13, 1996

Turnwald GH, Troy GC: Hypoglycemia. Part I. Carbohydrate metabolism and laboratory evaluation. Compend Contin Educ Pract Vet 5:932, 1983

Turnwald GH, Troy GC: Hypoglycemia. Part II. Clinical aspects. Compend Contin Educ Pract Vet 6:115, 1984

Waters DJ, Prueter JC: Secondary polycythemia associated with renal disease in the dog: two case reports and review of the literature. J Am Anim Hosp Assoc 24:109, 1988

Whitney MS: Evaluation of hyperlipidemias in dogs and cats. Semin Vet Med Surg (Small Anim) 7:292, 1992

Urinary System

46

Introduction

Gregory F. Grauer

ASSESSMENT OF RENAL FUNCTION

Azotemia

I. Blood urea nitrogen (BUN)
   A. BUN is produced in the liver from two ammonia molecules.
   B. It is excreted via glomerular filtration and tubular reabsorption.
   C. Concentration depends on several nonrenal factors; therefore, it is only a crude estimate of glomerular filtration rate (GFR).
      1. Conditions associated with increased BUN concentration
         a) Increased production
            (1) High dietary protein
            (2) Postprandial measurement
            (3) Gastrointestinal hemorrhage
            (4) Increased protein catabolism: fever, corticosteroid administration, prolonged inadequate caloric intake
         b) Decreased excretion
            (1) Prerenal factors: decreased cardiac output, dehydration, hypotension
            (2) Renal dysfunction: BUN elevated only after three fourths or more of all nephrons are nonfunctional
            (3) Postrenal factors: urethral obstruction, ruptured urinary bladder
      2. Conditions associated with decreased BUN concentration
         a) Decreased production
            (1) Low dietary protein
            (2) Hepatic dysfunction
         b) Increased excretion associated with prolonged diuresis/polyuria and decreased tubular reabsorption of urea nitrogen
II. Serum creatinine (SC)
   A. Produced constantly on a daily basis as an end product of normal muscle metabolism
   B. Excreted via glomerular filtration
   C. Concentration less dependent on nonrenal factors compared with BUN.
      1. The inverse of SC (1/SC) may be used to predict the probable range of GFR (Finco et al., 1995).
      2. Conditions associated with increased SC concentration include the following.
         a) Decreased excretion
            (1) Prerenal factors: decreased cardiac output, dehydration, hypotension
            (2) Renal dysfunction: SC elevated only after three fourths or more of all nephrons are nonfunctional
            (3) Postrenal factors: urethral obstruction, ruptured urinary bladder
         b) Increased postprandial absorption (Evans, 1987)
      3. Conditions associated with decreased SC include decreased production owing to severe muscle atrophy or wasting (rare).

Glomerular Filtration Rate

Clearance tests measure the volume of plasma that is completely cleared of a substance per unit of time; this value represents GFR.
I. Creatinine clearance (CrCl)
   A. Endogenous CrCl is best performed over a 24-hour period. The technique is described in Finco et al., 1993.
      1. Advantages
         a) It does not require special drugs.
         b) SC and urine creatinine concentrations can be measured in most clinical laboratories.
      2. Disadvantages
         a) Noncreatinine chromogens in serum are measured by the commonly used Jaffe reaction and cause significant error if SC is within normal range or only slightly elevated.
         b) A peroxidase-coupled kinetic enzymatic procedure (PAP) is necessary to avoid measurement of noncreatinine chromogens in serum (Finco et al., 1993).

493

c) Significant error may also be caused by incomplete urine collection.
  3. Normal values
    a) Dogs: 2–5 ml/min/kg
    b) Cats: 1.6–4 ml/min/kg
  B. Exogenous CrCl can be performed by constant intravenous infusion of a creatinine solution (Finco et al., 1991) or by the subcutaneous administration of one large dose of a creatinine solution (Finco et al., 1982).
    1. Advantage: High serum and urine creatinine concentrations minimize laboratory (noncreatinine chromogens) and urine collection (volume) errors.
    2. Disadvantages
      a) Requires a creatinine solution that is not available commercially
      b) Requires passing a stomach tube and rinsing the bladder via a urinary catheter
    3. Normal values
      a) Dogs: 3–5 ml/min/kg
      b) Cats: 2–4 ml/min/kg
II. Measurement of plasma/serum disappearance of substances after intravenous administration
  A. Creatinine (Labato and Ross, 1991): correlates well with exogenous CrCl
  B. Sodium sulfanilate (Maddison et al., 1984): may not be as well correlated with exogenous CrCl and is not readily available to practitioners
  C. Iohexol (Brown et al., 1996): provides a reliable estimate of GFR, but the analyzer is expensive and not readily available

Proteinuria

I. Classification
  A. Physiologic
    1. Strenuous exercise
    2. Seizures
    3. Exposure to extreme heat or cold
    4. Fever
  B. Pathologic
    1. Nonurinary
      a) Bence Jones proteins
      b) Hemoglobinuria/myoglobinuria
      c) Congestive heart failure
      d) Genital tract inflammation
    2. Urinary
      a) Nonrenal: lower urinary tract inflammation (e.g., bacterial cystitis, cystourolithiasis)
      b) Renal
        (1) Glomerular
        (2) Tubular
        (3) Renal parenchymal inflammation (e.g., pyelonephritis, renal tumor)
II. Measurement
  A. Interpret urine protein screening tests (dipstick or sulfosalicylic acid) in light of the following.
    1. Urine specific gravity (USG)
      a) A 2+ dipstick reaction for protein with a USG of 1.010 suggests greater proteinuria

than does the same 2+ reaction with a USG of 1.045.
      b) Significant proteinuria is suggested with a trace or 1+ protein reaction with a USG <1.020 or a ≥2+ protein reaction with any USG as long as the urine sediment examination is normal (see the following).
    2. Urine sediment examination
      If there is evidence of urinary tract inflammation (e.g., pyuria, hematuria, bacteriuria) in the urine sediment, the inflammation usually causes proteinuria as well.
  B. If screening tests demonstrate persistent, significant proteinuria and the urine sediment examination is normal, proteinuria should be quantitated.
    1. 24-hour urine protein excretion
      a) Either a metabolism cage or an indwelling urinary catheter is used to collect all the urine produced over a 24-hour period.
      b) This procedure is labor intensive, can be complicated by urinary tract infection (indwelling catheters), and can result in errors with incomplete 24-hour urine collection.
    2. Urine protein/creatinine ratio (UP/C)
      a) Its predictive value is based on the fact that protein and creatinine are excreted proportionately and relatively constantly through the glomerular capillary walls.
      b) It has been validated in dogs and cats under variable activity levels and times of collection.
      c) Fasted or nonfasted samples may be used.
      d) Urine may be obtained by cystocentesis, catheter, or voiding.
      e) The ratio is not accurate in the face of the following.
        (1) A rapidly changing GFR (e.g., acute renal failure)
        (2) An abnormal urine sediment (Bagley et al., 1991)
      f) A ratio >1.0 indicates significant proteinuria.
      g) There is a rough correlation between the severity of the glomerular lesions and the magnitude of the proteinuria. In general, dogs with amyloidosis have greater proteinuria than do dogs with glomerulonephritis, and dogs with glomerulonephritis usually have greater proteinuria than do dogs with end-stage renal failure.

Tubular Function

I. Urine concentration measured by USG or osmolality
  A. Definitions
    1. Hypersthenuria
      a) Dogs: USG ≥1.030 or urine osmolality ≥1500 mOsm/kg
      b) Cats: USG ≥1.035 or urine osmolality ≥1800 mOsm/kg

2. Minimally concentrated urine
   a) Dogs: USG between 1.013 and 1.029 or urine osmolality between 350 and 1500 mOsm/kg
   b) Cats: USG between 1.013 and 1.034 or urine osmolality between 350 and 1800 mOsm/kg
3. Isosthenuria: USG between 1.008 and 1.012 or urine osmolality between 250 and 350 mOsm/kg for dogs and cats
4. Hyposthenuria: USG ≤1.007 or urine osmolality ≤250 mOsm/kg for dogs and cats

B. Production of hypersthenuric urine
  1. Requires adequate concentrations of antidiuretic hormone (ADH)
  2. Requires tubular responsiveness to ADH
    a) Functional presence of one third or more of total nephrons
    b) Hypertonic renal medullary interstitium

II. Tests of urine concentrating ability (Fig. 46–1)
  A. Modified/gradual water deprivation test
   1. This test is used to ensure that renal medullary hypertonicity exists. Renal medullary solute washout can occur secondary to any prolonged diuresis/polyuria.
   2. Measure the animal's 24-hour water consumption to confirm polydipsia. Normal is <100 ml/kg/24 hours.
   3. Reduce water consumption gradually (by 10% every other day) until patient is consuming 80–90 ml/kg/24 hours; this usually takes 10–14 days.
   4. Feed a high-protein diet and lightly salt the food.
   5. Interpretation of results is as follows.
    a) Hypersthenuric urine is produced: primary polydipsia

    b) Hypersthenuric urine is not produced
     (1) Diabetes insipidus: either central/pituitary or nephrogenic
     (2) Insufficient impetus for urine concentration (dehydration)

B. Water deprivation test
  1. This test is used to differentiate primary polydipsia from primary polyuria in patients that have failed to produce hypersthenuric urine during a modified/gradual water deprivation test.
  2. The water deprivation test is contraindicated in patients that are initially dehydrated or azotemic.
  3. Baseline measurements are taken as follows.
   a) Remove all urine from the bladder by voluntary voiding or by catheterization and determine the USG or osmolality.
   b) Weigh the animal and measure total solids, BUN, SC, and serum/plasma osmolality.
  4. Withdraw food and water.
  5. Empty the bladder every 2–6 hours and measure USG or osmolality; also weigh the animal and measure total solids, BUN, SC, and serum/plasma osmolality.
  6. Stop the test when any of the following occur.
   a) Hypersthenuric urine is produced.
   b) The animal loses >5% of body weight from dehydration or there is a large increase in plasma total solids.
   c) Serum/plasma osmolality is >320 mOsm/kg.
   d) The animal becomes azotemic.
  7. Interpretation of results is as follows.
   a) Hypersthenuric urine is produced: primary polydipsia

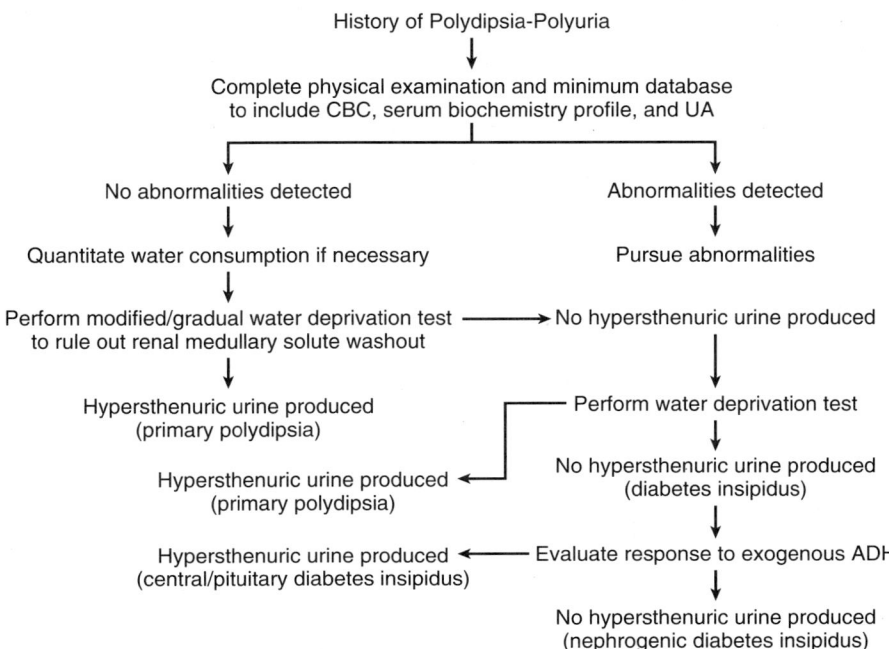

History of Polydipsia-Polyuria
↓
Complete physical examination and minimum database to include CBC, serum biochemistry profile, and UA

No abnormalities detected   Abnormalities detected
↓   ↓
Quantitate water consumption if necessary   Pursue abnormalities
↓
Perform modified/gradual water deprivation test ⟶ No hypersthenuric urine produced
to rule out renal medullary solute washout
↓
Hypersthenuric urine produced   ⟵ Perform water deprivation test
(primary polydipsia)
↓
Hypersthenuric urine produced ⟵   No hypersthenuric urine produced
(primary polydipsia)   (diabetes insipidus)
↓
Hypersthenuric urine produced ⟵ Evaluate response to exogenous ADH
(central/pituitary diabetes insipidus)
↓
No hypersthenuric urine produced
(nephrogenic diabetes insipidus)

Figure 46–1. Diagnostic algorithm for animals with polyuria and polydipsia. CBC = complete blood count; UA = urinalysis; ADH = antidiuretic hormone.

b) Hypersthenuric urine is not produced: diabetes insipidus—either central/pituitary or nephrogenic

C. Exogenous ADH response test

1. This test is used to differentiate central/pituitary diabetes insipidus from nephrogenic diabetes insipidus in patients that fail to produce hypersthenuric urine in response to a water deprivation test.

2. The exogenous ADH response test is contraindicated in azotemic and pregnant patients.

3. Perform the test immediately after the water deprivation test when there is still impetus for urine concentration.

4. Remove all urine from the bladder.

5. Administer desmopressin acetate (DDAVP, USV Laboratories, Tarrytown, NY).

   a) 2–4 drops (2 μg/dog) intranasally or conjunctivally

   b) 2–5 μg/dog subcutaneously

6. Empty the bladder and measure USG or osmolality hourly for 2–4 hours.

7. Interpretation of results is as follows.

   a) Hypersthenuric urine is produced: central/pituitary diabetes insipidus

   b) Hypersthenuric urine is not produced: nephrogenic diabetes insipidus

III. Phenolsulfonphthalein (PSP) excretion (see also Chap. 2)

A. The test is actually a more valid reflection of renal plasma flow than of tubular function.

B. It is not a valid measure of renal function in the cat (Ross and Finco, 1981).

C. The normal dog has a >30% excretion at 20 minutes after injection.

IV. Urinary electrolyte excretion

A. The quantity of electrolytes in the urine is the net result of tubular reabsorption and secretion.

B. Tubular function can be evaluated by calculating the fractional clearance (FCl) of electrolytes.

C. FCl is defined as a ratio of the clearance of the electrolyte to that of creatinine as follows: FCl of electrolyte $x = (U_x/S_x)/(U_{Cr}/S_{Cr})$, where U_x, S_x, U_{Cr}, and S_{Cr} represent the respective urine and serum concentrations of electrolyte (x) and creatinine (Cr).

D. The ratio is usually multiplied by 100 and expressed as a percentage.

E. FCls are best calculated using an aliquot of a 24-hour urine sample, because random urine samples may not accurately reflect 24-hour urinary electrolyte excretion (Vaden et al., 1989; Adams et al., 1991).

F. Normal values are as follows (DiBartola, 1992).

1. Sodium (Na): <1% (dogs and cats)

2. Chloride: <1% (dogs) and <1.3% (cats)

3. Potassium: <20% (dogs) and <24% (cats)

4. Phosphorus: <39% (dogs) and <73% (cats)

G. The FCl of Na may be helpful in differentiating prerenal from renal azotemia.

1. Prerenal azotemia should be associated with an FCl of Na <1%.

2. Renal azotemia is usually associated with an FCl of Na >1%.

Bibliography

Adams LG, Polzin DJ, Osborne CA et al: Comparison of fractional excretion and 24-hour urinary excretion of sodium and potassium in clinically normal cats and cats with induced chronic renal failure. Am J Vet Res 52:718, 1991

Bagley RS, Center SA, Lewis RM et al: The effect of experimental cystitis and iatrogenic blood contamination on the urine protein/creatinine ratio in the dog. J Vet Intern Med 5:66, 1991

Brown SA, Finco DR, Boudinot FD et al: Evaluation of a single injection method, using iohexol, for estimating glomerular filtration rate in cats and dogs. Am J Vet Res 57:105, 1996

DiBartola SP: Clinical evaluation of renal function. Proc Waltham Symp Treat Small Anim Dis 16:10, 1992

Evans GO: Post-prandial changes in canine plasma creatinine. J Small Anim Pract 28:311, 1987

Finco DR, Brown SA, Crowell WA et al: Exogenous creatinine clearance as a measure of glomerular filtration rate in dogs with reduced renal mass. Am J Vet Res 52:1029, 1991

Finco DR, Brown SA, Vaden SL, Ferguson DC: Relationship between plasma creatinine concentration and glomerular filtration rate in dogs. J Vet Pharmacol Ther 18:418, 1995

Finco DR, Coulter DB, Barsanti JA: Procedure for a simple method of measuring glomerular filtration rate in the dog. J Am Anim Hosp Assoc 18:804, 1982

Finco DR, Tabaru H, Brown SA et al: Endogenous creatinine clearance measurement of glomerular filtration rate in dogs. Am J Vet Res 54:1575, 1993

Labato MA, Ross LA: Plasma disappearance of creatinine as a renal function test in the dog. Res Vet Sci 50:253, 1991

Maddison JE, Pascoe PJ, Jansen BS: Clinical evaluation of sodium sulfanilate clearance for the diagnosis of renal disease in dogs. J Am Vet Med Assoc 185:961, 1984

Ross LA, Finco DR: Relationship of selected clinical renal function tests to glomerular filtration rate and renal blood flow in cats. Am J Vet Res 42:1704, 1981

Vaden SL, Babineau C, Ford RB: Comparison of methods to evaluate urine electrolyte concentrations in normal dogs. J Vet Intern Med 3:138, 1989

47

Diseases of the Kidney

Scott A. Brown
Gregory F. Grauer

CONGENITAL/ DEVELOPMENTAL DISORDERS

See Table 47–1.

DEGENERATIVE DISORDERS

Scott A. Brown

Feline Perirenal Cysts

Definition and Cause

I. Perirenal cysts are an idiopathic condition of older (usually >8 years of age) male or neutered male cats characterized by perirenal cyst-like structures that may occur unilaterally or bilaterally.
II. The cyst may be intra- or extracapsular.

Clinical Signs

I. A large abdominal mass
   A. Progressive abdominal enlargement as a historic complaint
   B. Palpable abdominal mass on physical examination
II. Uremia
   A. Renal dysfunction may be caused by compression from cyst.
   B. Cyst may also occur as an incidental finding in a cat with renal failure from parenchymal renal disease.

Diagnosis

I. Abdominal radiographs reveal large fluid density in the area of the kidney(s).
II. Excretory urography reveals normal to small kidneys. Kidney, pelvis, and ureter are normal, and contrast material does not enter the cyst.

III. Ultrasonography reveals fluid-filled structure perirenally.
IV. Aspirate of cyst reveals a hypocellular, low-protein fluid (transudate).

Differential Diagnosis

I. Hydronephrosis
II. Neoplasia
III. Polycystic kidney disease (congenital)

Treatment

I. It is generally presumed that surgical drainage and excision of the cyst wall will improve renal function, but that is not always the case, and a renal biopsy should be obtained at the time of the initial surgery.
II. Prognosis is good if renal biopsy is normal.
III. In uremic cats, a cyst can be decompressed percutaneously.
   A. In animals with bilateral perirenal cysts, this procedure may restore adequate renal function to allow surgical cystectomy.
   B. However, aspiration risks laceration of the renal artery, vein, and ureter, necessitating emergency surgery and possibly nephrectomy.
IV. Unless contralateral renal function is proved adequate, nephrectomy is contraindicated.

Patient Monitoring

I. If the cyst is decompressed percutaneously, cyst size is reassessed 4–6 weeks later to ascertain rate of fluid accumulation.
II. If the cat is not azotemic following cyst removal, the prognosis is good. Otherwise, the prognosis is similar to that for any cat with renal failure.

*Table 47–1. **Examples of Familial Nephropathies in Dogs and Cats***

Breed	Primary Defect	Clinical Findings
Abyssinian	Amyloidosis	Azotemia
Basenji	Proximal tubule dysfunction	Glucosuria
		Metabolic acidosis
		Azotemia
Bernese mountain dog	Glomerulopathy	Proteinuria
		Azotemia
Bull terrier	Glomerulopathy	Proteinuria
	Interstitial fibrosis	Azotemia
Cocker spaniel	Glomerulopathy	Azotemia
Chow chow	Glomerulopathy	Azotemia
	Interstitial fibrosis	
Doberman pinscher	Glomerulopathy	Proteinuria
		Azotemia
Lhasa apso	Glomerulopathy	Hyposthenuria
	Interstitial fibrosis	Azotemia
Norwegian elkhound	Proximal tubule dysfunction	Hyposthenuria
		Glucosuria
		Azotemia
Pembroke Welsh corgi	Telangiectasia	Hematuria
Samoyed	Glomerulopathy	Proteinuria
		Azotemia (males)
Shar pei	Amyloidosis	Azotemia
Shih Tzu	Glomerulopathy	Hyposthenuria
		Azotemia
Soft-coated wheaten terrier	Glomerulopathy	Proteinuria
	Interstitial fibrosis	Azotemia

INFECTIOUS AND INFLAMMATORY DISEASES

Gregory F. Grauer

Leptospirosis

Definition and Causes

I. Acute interstitial nephritis can be caused by infection with one of the serovars of *Leptospira interrogans* (see also Chap. 111).
II. Dogs are susceptible to infection by several serovars.
  A. *Leptospira icterohaemorrhagiae* and *Leptospira canicola* are the most common isolates.
  B. *Leptospira grippotyphosa, Leptospira pomona,* and *Leptospira bratislava* have also been incriminated in recent studies (Rentko et al., 1992).
III. Although cats can be affected, clinical disease is rare.

Pathophysiology

I. Leptospires usually enter the body through mucous membranes.
  A. Invasion of a susceptible host results in leptospiremia, which terminates in 4–7 days with the appearance of specific antibodies and phagocytosis.
  B. Multiplication of the organism occurs in renal tubular cells.
  C. Direct transmission between animals usually involves contact with infected urine.
  D. Indirect transmission may occur via contact with stagnant or slow-moving water.
II. The most commonly affected organs are the liver and kidneys.
  A. Leptospires persist and multiply within renal tubular cells, even in the presence of high serum neutralizing antibody titers.
  B. Inflammation within the kidney is associated with replication of the spirochete and the production of toxic lipid by-products.
  C. Disseminated intravascular coagulation can contribute to renal as well as systemic pathology.
  D. Carriers shed the organism in urine and may be seronegative.

Clinical Signs

I. Depend on the age and immunity of the host, environmental factors affecting the organism, and the virulence of the infecting serovar (Greene, 1995)
II. Peracute infections: massive leptospiremia, shock, and death
III. Acute and subacute infections
  A. General: fever, depression, dehydration
  B. Dermatologic: icterus, petechiae/ecchymosis
  C. Gastrointestinal
    1. Anorexia
    2. Vomiting, diarrhea
    3. Pharyngitis, tonsillitis
    4. Melena, hematochezia
    5. Intestinal intussusception
  D. Musculoskeletal: muscle pain owing to myositis, with reluctance to move
  E. Ophthalmic: ocular discharge, anterior uveitis

F. Respiratory
 1. Dyspnea, cough, adventitial lung sounds
 2. Nasal discharge
 G. Urinary: renal pain, progressive renal dysfunction

IV. Chronic infections
 A. The majority of canine infections are chronic and may be subclinical.
  1. Fever
  2. Anterior uveitis
  3. Anorexia, weight loss
 B. Although acute interstitial nephritis occurs with leptospirosis, data do not support leptospirosis as a cause of chronic interstitial nephritis.
  1. Chronic interstitial nephritis occurs in geographic regions where leptospirosis does not.
  2. Dogs that recover from leptospirosis usually have no residual renal effects.

Diagnosis

I. Suspicious history and clinical signs: no vaccinations, potential exposure, fever of unknown origin, and renal and/or hepatic dysfunction
II. Laboratory assessment
 A. Hematology
  1. Leukopenia possibly present early in the infection
  2. Leukocytosis, often with a left shift later in the course of the disease
  3. Thrombocytopenia
  4. Normocytic, normochromic anemia
  5. Increased fibrinogen and fibrin degradation products
 B. Serum biochemistry profile
  1. Azotemia, hyperphosphatemia
  2. Electrolyte alterations associated with vomiting and/or diarrhea
  3. Increased serum alanine aminotransferase (ALT), aspartate aminotransferase (AST), alkaline phosphatase (ALP), and bilirubin concentrations with hepatic involvement
  4. Hypoalbuminemia
 C. Urinalysis
  1. Proteinuria
  2. Bilirubinuria
  3. Pyuria, hematuria
  4. Granular casts
  5. Leptospires occasionally seen in urine by darkfield or fluorescent microscopy techniques
 D. Identification of leptospires in renal or hepatic biopsy tissue with silver stains or fluorescent antibody microscopy
 E. Serology
  1. Microscopic agglutination
   a) Detects antibody to specific serovars
    (1) It will detect IgM 7–9 days after the onset of clinical signs.
    (2) Because the test is serovar specific, multiple antigens must be tested.
    (3) Large doses of antibiotics early in the disease may cause low antibody pro-

duction and false-negative serology results.
    (4) Natural carriers, such as dogs with *L. canicola,* may not have detectable serum agglutinins even though infection and shedding are present.
   b) Demonstration of a fourfold rise in titer over 2–4 weeks is indicative of active infection.
   c) A titer cannot be used to distinguish between infection and vaccine-induced antibody; however, titers >1:800 are usually associated with infection.
  2. Complement fixation
   a) Broader cross-reactivity
   b) Useful as a screening test
  3. Genus-specific enzyme-linked immunosorbent assay (ELISA)
   a) Can detect IgG and IgM, making differentiation between acute and chronic infections possible
   b) Cannot differentiate between vaccine-induced and disease-induced titers with certainty

Differential Diagnosis

I. Other causes of acute renal failure
 A. Ethylene glycol and other nephrotoxicants
 B. Acute pyelonephritis
 C. Borreliosis
II. Other causes of acute hepatitis
 A. Infectious canine hepatitis
 B. Other bacterial infections
 C. Hepatotoxicants

Treatment

I. Supportive care/fluid therapy (see Acute Renal Failure later in the chapter)
II. Specific therapy
 A. Elimination of the leptospiremia: procaine penicillin G 20,000–50,000 U/kg IM, SQ BID for 2 weeks
 B. Elimination of the carrier state
  1. Dihydrostreptomycin sulfate 10–15 mg/kg IM BID is given for 2 weeks *after* renal function has returned to normal.
  2. Tetracycline 20 mg/kg PO TID or doxycycline 10 mg/kg PO SID is also thought to be effective. Doxycycline should be considered in animals with decreased renal function.

Patient Monitoring

I. Renal function is monitored as described later under Acute Renal Failure.
II. Serum agglutination titers are measured during the acute illness, 2–4 weeks later, and 4–6 weeks after dihydrostreptomycin or tetracycline treatment.
III. Dogs should be immunized after recovery to prevent infection by a different serovar.

IV. Prevention involves the following measures.
   A. Provide adequate sanitation, especially in kennels. Drain any standing water.
   B. Try to decrease exposure to wild or domestic animal carriers. Remove carrier dogs from kennel.
   C. Vaccination is important (Broughton and Scarnell, 1985).
      1. Vaccination reduces shedding of the organism in urine.
      2. It does not protect against infection but does protect against disease.
      3. Vaccine reactions have been reduced but are still common.
      4. Risk of disease vs. vaccine reaction must be weighed.
      5. Vaccines
         a) Inactivated whole cell bacterins of *L. canicola* and *L. icterohaemorrhagiae*
         b) Pentavalent bacterins
         c) Three immunizations at least 3 weeks apart
         d) Protection for only 3–6 months
V. Leptospirosis is a zoonotic disease.
   A. Animals with leptospirosis should be isolated during treatment.
   B. Urine shedding of leptospires can occur for longer than 6 months.
   C. Transmission to humans often involves contact with infected cattle or wild rodents (Songer and Thiermann, 1988).

Borreliosis
See Chap. 111.

Pyelonephritis

Definition

   I. Pyelonephritis is inflammation of the renal pelvis and renal parenchyma. The inflammation is usually associated with a bacterial infection.
   II. Pyelitis is inflammation of the renal pelvis alone. Pyelitis is more common than pyelonephritis.

Causes

   I. Bacteria in descending order of frequency are *Escherichia coli*, *Staphylococcus aureus*, *Proteus mirabilis*, *Streptococcus* spp., *Klebsiella pneumoniae*, *Pseudomonas aeruginosa*, *Enterobacter* spp. (Barsanti et al., 1994).
   II. Fungi, viruses, and parasites are rarely associated with bacterial pyelonephritis.

Pathophysiology

   I. Route of infection (Crowell et al., 1995)
      A. Ascending infection from the lower urinary tract is by far the most common route.
      B. Hematogenous/embolic infection may also occur, but rarely.
         1. The renal parenchyma may be infected from bacterial emboli from extrarenal sources (e.g., bacterial endocarditis, diskospondylitis, periodontal disease).
         2. The resulting embolic nephritis may be focal or diffuse, neutrophilic or lymphoplasmacytic, mild or severe.
         3. Occasionally the lesions progress to involve the renal pelvis and appear similar to those associated with ascending pyelonephritis.
   II. Factors that may enhance the susceptibility of the kidney to infection
      A. Anatomic abnormalities that may result in urine stasis or easy ascension of bacteria
         1. Congenital anomalies (e.g., ectopic ureters, vaginal strictures)
         2. Acquired abnormalities
            a) Neoplasia/granulomatous disease
            b) Urolithiasis
            c) Development of fibrous scar tissue and stenosis
         3. Indwelling urinary catheter
      B. Functional and metabolic abnormalities
         1. Vesicoureteral reflux
         2. Disorders of micturition (see Chap. 50)
            a) Big bladder disorders (urine stasis)
               (1) Decreased detrusor contractility
               (2) Increased outflow resistance
            b) Small or normal-sized bladder disorders (urine leakage)
               (1) Increased detrusor contractility
               (2) Decreased outflow resistance
         3. Glucosuria
         4. Systemic immunosuppression: chronic renal failure, hyperadrenocorticism
      C. Bacterial infection of the lower urinary tract
   III. Progression of disease leading to acute or chronic renal failure
      A. *E. coli* infection of the renal parenchyma can result in vasoconstriction and ischemia.
      B. Leukocyte infiltration can result in renal tissue damage associated with release of lysosomal enzymes and oxygen radicals.
      C. Immune responses may become directed against Tamm-Horsfall proteins and allow tissue damage to persist and even continue in the absence of bacterial pathogens.
      D. Nephrolithiasis may develop.
      E. Renal scarring and atrophy may lead to end-stage kidney disease.

Clinical Signs

   I. Acute pyelonephritis
      A. Fever, depression, anorexia
      B. Arched back or abnormal gait associated with lumbar/renal pain
      C. Polydipsia/polyuria
      D. Vomiting, especially if the animal is uremic
   II. Chronic pyelonephritis
      A. Nonspecific signs: anorexia, lethargy, exercise intolerance, weight loss

B. Polydipsia/polyuria
C. Frequently asymptomatic

Diagnosis

I. History and physical examination findings
II. Laboratory evaluation
    A. Hemogram: leukocytosis with left shift possible with acute pyelonephritis
    B. Serum biochemistry profile
        1. Azotemia and hyperphosphatemia occur with renal dysfunction.
        2. Hyperglobulinemia may be observed with chronic pyelonephritis.
    C. Urinalysis
        1. Bacteriuria
        2. Pyuria/hematuria
        3. ±Cellular/granular casts; white blood cell casts.
        4. Low urine specific gravity
    D. Urine culture
        1. Urine for culture is best obtained by cystocentesis.
        2. Positive culture indicates urinary tract infection but does not localize the infection to a specific portion of the urinary tract.
III. Imaging techniques (Neuwirth et al., 1993)
    A. Excretory urography is often used to diagnose pyelonephritis, but it is neither sensitive nor specific for pyelonephritis. Abnormalities compatible with a diagnosis of pyelonephritis include the following.
        1. Renal pelvic and proximal ureteral dilatation
        2. Decreased nephrographic and pyelographic opacity
        3. Blunting or distortion of the renal pelvic diverticula
        4. Prolonged retention of dye in the renal pelvis
        5. None of the above: excretory urography may be normal in both acute and chronic pyelonephritis
    B. Ultrasonographic findings may include the following.
        1. Dilatation of renal pelvis and proximal ureter
        2. Changes in renal parenchymal echogenicity
        3. Increased prominence of the pelvic and ureteral mucosa
    C. Excretory urogram and ultrasonographic changes may persist after infection has been eliminated.
IV. Renal histopathologic evaluation
    Together with culture of renal biopsy specimens, it is the only definitive method of diagnosis, but with focal disease, renal histology may be normal and culture negative.

Differential Diagnosis

I. Other causes of fever, leukocytosis, and painful abdomen (e.g., peritonitis, pancreatitis)
II. Nephrolithiasis and ureterolithiasis
III. Lower urinary tract infections
IV. Bacterial prostatitis and metritis

Treatment and Monitoring

I. Correction of any underlying predisposing factors (e.g., ectopic ureter, urachal remnants, urolithiasis, prostatitis)
II. Antibiotic therapy selected on the basis of bacterial culture and sensitivity of urine or renal tissue
    A. Antibiotics that achieve high concentrations in the renal medullary interstitium are recommended.
        1. Ampicillin, amoxicillin, amoxicillin–clavulanic acid
        2. Trimethoprim/sulfa drugs
        3. Cephalosporins
        4. Chloramphenicol
        5. Fluoroquinilones
        6. Aminoglycosides: should be used only as a last resort because of potential nephrotoxicity
    B. Antibiotics with the highest in vitro efficacy against common urinary pathogens based on anticipated urine concentrations of the antibiotic (from the Colorado State University, Veterinary Diagnostic Laboratory) are as follows.
        1. *E. coli*: enrofloxacin, first-generation cephalosporins, amoxicillin–clavulanic acid
        2. *Staphylococcus* spp.: amoxicillin–clavulanic acid, first-generation cephalosporins, enrofloxacin, trimethoprim/sulfa
        3. *Proteus* spp.: amoxicillin–clavulanic acid, enrofloxacin, first-generation cephalosporins
        4. *Streptococcus* spp.: amoxicillin–clavulanic acid, amoxicillin, chloramphenicol
        5. *Klebsiella* spp.: enrofloxacin, amoxicillin–clavulanic acid, first-generation cephalosporins
        6. *Pseudomonas* spp.: tetracyclines, aminoglycosides
        7. *Enterobacter* spp.: tetracyclines, aminoglycosides, enrofloxacin
    C. Antibiotics are administered for a minimum of 4 weeks.
        1. Urine culture is performed after 3–5 days of antibiotic therapy to assess the in vivo efficacy of the selected antibiotic.
            a) No growth: Continue treatment with the same antibiotic.
            b) Bacterial growth: Change antibiotic based on sensitivity; repeat urine culture after another 3–5 days.
        2. Urine culture is performed 5–7 days after termination of antibiotic treatment.
            a) If infection is still present, continue antibiotic treatment based on bacterial sensitivity for 6–8 weeks. Reculture urine after completion of the second antibiotic cycle.
            b) If there is no bacterial growth, discontinue antibiotics. Repeat urine cultures at 6- to 8-week intervals until three consecutive negative cultures are obtained. A positive culture signals the need for another 6- to 8-week course of antibiotics.
    D. Infection may persist in some animals despite repeated courses of antibiotics.

1. Consider chronic (>6 months) low-dose antibiotic treatment to control the infection.
2. One half to one third of the total daily dose of an antibiotic that is excreted in the urine is given at bedtime.

III. Ancillary treatments
   A. Induction of diuresis/polyuria may be helpful in washing organisms out of the renal medulla.
      1. Lightly salt the diet.
      2. Use low doses of a diuretic.
      3. Encourage liquid intake with broth or bouillon.
   B. Alter urine pH to maximize antibiotic efficacy.
      1. Acidify the urine with ammonium chloride for penicillins and tetracyclines.
      2. Alkalinize the urine with potassium citrate or sodium bicarbonate for aminoglycosides and fluoroquinilones.
      3. Efficacy of chloramphenicol, sulfonamides, and cephalosporins does not seem to be affected by urine pH.
   C. Acute or chronic renal failure, if present, is treated as described later.

PARASITES

Scott A. Brown

Capillaria plica

Definition

I. Adults are thread-like yellow nematodes up to 6 cm in length.
II. They invade the urinary bladder, ureteral submucosa, and renal pelvis.

Pathophysiology

I. Bipolar ova are passed in the urine.
   A. The ova embryonate and are ingested by the intermediate host (earthworms).
   B. Ingestion of earthworms leads to infection of dogs.
   C. The fox and raccoon may be natural hosts and reservoirs.
II. The adults produce a mild superficial inflammatory response.

Clinical Signs

I. Dysuria, pollakiuria
II. No clinical signs
III. Hematuria and/or pyuria

Diagnosis

I. Diagnosis is by identification of the characteristic ova in the urine sediment.
II. False diagnoses can result from contamination of feces with urine containing *C. plica* ova or from contamination of urine with feces containing *Trichuris vulpis* ova.

Treatment and Monitoring

I. Disease is usually self-limiting; within 3–4 months, animals develop negative ovum counts.
II. Ivermectin may be administered at 200 μg/kg PO once; not safe in collies.
III. Fenbendazole 50 mg/kg PO SID for 3–10 days can be tried.
IV. Albendazole at 50 mg/kg PO BID for 10–14 days may be effective, but may cause anorexia.
V. Control in kennels with a high prevalence rate relies on discontinuation of use of soil and grass surfaces.

Capillaria feliscati

Definition

I. Adults are thread-like nematodes up to 4.5 cm in length.
II. They invade the urinary bladder of cats.
III. The parasite is uncommon in the United States but may have a prevalence rate as high as 34% in Australia.

Pathophysiology

I. Bipolar ova are passed in the urine.
II. Urine contamination of feces can produce a false-positive result on fecal flotation.
III. The adults produce a mild superficial inflammatory response.

Clinical Signs

I. Clinical signs are usually absent.
II. Dysuria, pollakiuria, hematuria, and/or pyuria are occasionally observed.

Diagnosis

Diagnosis is by identification of the characteristic ova in urine sediment.

Treatment

I. The disease is usually self-limiting, and within 3–4 months animals develop negative ova counts.
II. Medical therapy can also be tried.
   A. Ivermectin 200 μg/kg PO once
   B. Fenbendazole 25 mg/kg PO BID for 3–10 days

Dioctophyma renale

Definition

I. Adults are red in color and up to 1 m in length.
II. They most often reside in the peritoneal cavity or the kidney (7:1 predilection for the right kidney).
III. They have also been reported in the bladder, urethra, ovary, uterus, and pericardium.

Pathophysiology

I. Frequently, infections in dogs are "dead-end," because the infection is single sex or present in a site where ova do not pass to the external environment.

A. In renal infections with a gravid female worm, which accounts for about 40% of infections, bipolar mamillated ova are passed in the urine.

B. The ova embryonate and are ingested by the intermediate host, an aquatic annelid.

C. The infective annelid is then passed to the dog via ingestion of a paratenic host (ingestion of raw fish or frogs).

II. The adults produce gradual renal parenchymal destruction.

Clinical Signs

I. Clinical signs are often absent.
II. Bilateral infections can lead to uremia.
III. Clinical signs may be referable to an abnormal site of infection.

Diagnosis

I. Diagnosis is by identification of the characteristic ova in urine or abdominal fluid.
II. Diagnosis may also occur with identification of adult worms upon surgical exploration.

Treatment

I. Treatment involves surgical removal of adult worms via unilateral nephrectomy if a kidney is involved and renal parenchymal destruction is complete.
II. Thorough exploratory surgery is indicated to identify and remove all adult worms.

Patient Monitoring

I. Control is difficult, as ova can live in the environment for years.
II. Ingestion of raw fish and frogs should be prevented.
III. *D. renale* is a public health concern; human infections are rare and require ingestion of infective larvae via raw fish or frogs.

NEPHROTOXICOSIS

Gregory F. Grauer

Definition

Nephrotoxicity is an adverse structural or functional alteration in the kidney caused by chemical (toxicants) or biologic products (toxins) that are inhaled, ingested, or absorbed through the skin.

Causes

I. Nephrotoxicants are a major cause of acute renal failure (ARF). Currently, therapeutic agents, rather than poisons and industrial chemicals, represent the most common source of nephrotoxicant-induced ARF.

II. Potential nephrotoxicants are numerous and varied.
   A. Therapeutic agents
      1. Antimicrobials
         a) Aminoglycosides
         b) Cephalosporins
         c) Polymixins
         d) Sulfonamides
         e) Tetracyclines (excessive dosages)
         f) Amphotericin B
      2. Anthelmintics: thiacetarsamide
      3. Intravenous radiographic contrast agents
      4. Anesthetics: methoxyflurane, enflurane
      5. Analgesics/nonsteroidal anti-inflammatory drugs (NSAIDs)
         a) Aspirin
         b) Acetaminophen
         c) Ibuprofen
         d) Phenylbutazone
      6. Chemotherapeutic agents
         a) Cisplatin
         b) Methotrexate
         c) Daunorubicin
         d) Azathioprine
         e) Adriamycin
         f) Cyclosporine
         g). Doxorubicin (cats)
      7. Gold salts
   B. Heavy metals
      1. Lead
      2. Mercury
      3. Cadmium
      4. Chromium
      5. Arsenic
      6. Thallium
   C. Organic compounds
      1. Ethylene glycol
      2. Carbon tetrachloride
      3. Chloroform
      4. Pesticides
      5. Herbicides
      6. Solvents
   D. Pigments
      1. Hemoglobin
      2. Myoglobin
   E. Toxins: snake and bee venoms
   F. Miscellaneous causes/conditions
      1. Vitamin D_3–containing rodenticides/hypercalcemia
      2. Hypokalemia
      3. Hypomagnesemia

Pathophysiology

I. Nephrotoxicant-induced tubular injury is usually the result of direct effects on epithelial cells.
   A. Toxicants can attach at luminal or basolateral membrane sites or to intracellular organelles.
   B. Cellular function is then disrupted by membrane and transport system damage and interference with energy production and cellular respiration. This leads to calcium influx, cell swelling, and death.

C. Toxicants that disrupt tubular function also indirectly affect glomerular function by tubuloglomerular feedback mechanisms, in which local generation of angiotensin II and other mediators leads to hemodynamic and mesangial cell alterations.

D. Nephrotoxic injury to the glomerulus includes the loss of capillary surface area (e.g., aminoglycosides), disruption of endothelial integrity and surface barriers by cationic substances (e.g., doxorubicin), and mesangial cell proliferation and hypertrophy (e.g., azathioprine).

II. The duration of exposure, quantity, and type of nephrotoxicant have a role in determining the severity and potential reversibility of nephrotoxicant-induced renal damage.

III. There are additional factors that can potentiate nephrotoxicant-induced renal damage.
A. Old age/renal insufficiency
B. Fever/sepsis
C. Dehydration
D. Hypokalemia (Brinker et al., 1981)
E. Liver disease/dysfunction
F. Decreased dietary protein intake (Grauer et al., 1994)
G. Concurrent use of potentially nephrotoxic drugs
1. Concurrent use of furosemide and gentamicin in dogs has been associated with increased risk for and severity of ARF.
2. Dogs appear to be fairly resistant to the effects of methoxyflurane exposure of short duration; however, the administration of flunixin meglumine with methoxyflurane anesthesia has resulted in acute tubular necrosis.
3. NSAIDs are risk factors for ARF as well as potential nephrotoxicants.
a) NSAIDs in single doses and with chronic use inhibit renal prostaglandin synthesis by inhibiting cyclooxygenase activity.
b) Prostaglandins, particularly of the E and I series, serve important vasodilatory functions in the kidney and influence glomerular filtration rate (GFR) and solute excretion.
4. Intravenous radiographic contrast agents may cause renal vasoconstriction and should be administered with care to those animals under anesthesia or receiving NSAIDs or other potentially nephrotoxic drugs.

Clinical Signs

I. Clinical signs develop secondary to renal functional and structural abnormalities.
A. Hypercalcemia interferes with the antidiuretic hormone (ADH)/ADH receptor interaction, resulting in polyuria. In addition, hypercalcemia can cause tubular cell necrosis and mineralization, leading to ARF.
B. Nephrotoxicants may interfere with proximal tubular cell reabsorptive function, resulting in normoglycemic glucosuria and proteinuria.

C. Tubular cell necrosis can result in renal epithelial cells, granular casts, red blood cells, and white blood cells in the urine sediment.

II. Systemic clinical signs associated with uremia secondary to ARF may predominate.

Diagnosis/Differential Diagnosis

I. History of exposure to a potential nephrotoxicant is an important aspect of diagnosis.

II. Clinical and laboratory findings in many cases are consistent with ARF (see the later section).

III. Trough serum gentamicin concentrations (Riviere et al., 1984) and urine enzyme/creatinine excretion ratios (Grauer et al., 1995) are excellent early markers of gentamicin-induced nephrotoxicosis.

IV. Vitamin D_3 intoxication is usually associated with severe hypercalcemia.

V. The early stages of ethylene glycol intoxication usually result in the following clinicopathologic abnormalities.
A. Measurable concentrations of ethylene glycol in serum and urine
B. Marked increases in plasma osmolality with large osmolar gap
C. Moderate to severe metabolic acidosis with large anion gap
D. Central nervous system abnormalities: polydipsia/polyuria, disorientation, ataxia, seizures
E. Vomiting
F. Monohydrate calcium oxalate crystalluria

VI. Ultrasonography may be helpful in detecting abnormalities.
A. Increased echogenicity is compatible with renal tissue mineralization or deposition of calcium oxalate crystals.
B. Decreased echogenicity is associated with renal swelling.

VII. Renal histopathology confirms acute tubular damage and may help identify the etiology and establish a prognosis.

Treatment and Monitoring

I. Fluid, electrolyte, and acid-base treatment considerations: see Acute Renal Failure

II. Specific antidotal treatment for nephrotoxicants: see Section XVIII

IMMUNE-MEDIATED DISEASES

Gregory F. Grauer

Glomerulonephritis (GN)

Definition

Inflammation of the glomerulus associated with the presence of immune complexes in the glomerular capillary walls

Causes

I. Deposition of preformed circulating immune complexes occurs because of the large blood supply to the kidney and the filtration forces across the glomerular capillary wall.
  A. Immune complexes are most pathogenic when formed with roughly equal numbers of antigen and antibody molecules.
  B. Complexes are deposited in a random fashion along the glomerular capillary wall, resulting in a "lumpy-bumpy" appearance when examined by immunocytochemical, immunofluorescent, or electron microscopy.
II. In situ immune complex formation occurs when antibody reacts with "planted" antigens within the glomerular capillary wall.
  A. Antigen can be incorporated in the glomerular basement membrane (GBM) as a result of electrical charge or glycoprotein-carbohydrate interactions.
  B. It often results in a smooth, linear appearance when examined by immunocytochemical, immunofluorescent, or electron microscopy.
  C. It has also been shown to occur in dogs with GN associated with heartworm disease (Grauer, 1992).
III. Antigens associated with immune complex GN are often difficult to identify, but numerous diseases and disorders have been associated with GN in dogs and cats (Table 47–2).
IV. Immune complex GN is termed idiopathic when an underlying disease process cannot be identified. True autoimmune GN, where antibody is directed against normal capillary wall structures, has not been documented in dogs and cats.

Pathophysiology

I. The presence of immune complexes within the glomerulus initiates a complex inflammatory reaction involving complement, neutrophils, macrophages, platelets, the coagulation system cascade, and resident mesangial, epithelial, and endothelial glomerular cells.
II. Increased production of thromboxane by resident glomerular cells and platelets has a major role in the inflammatory response (Grauer, 1992).
III. The glomerular inflammation causes thickening of the capillary walls (membranous GN), cellular hyperplasia (proliferative GN), or both (membranoproliferative GN).
IV. Proteinuria is the hallmark clinicopathologic abnormality associated with GN and occurs from the following.
  A. Decreased permselectivity of the capillary walls
  B. Loss of the negative charge (glycosaminoglycans and proteoglycans) normally associated with the GBM, which allows filtration of negatively charged proteins such as albumin
V. The nephrotic syndrome occurs secondary to severe, prolonged proteinuria.

Table 47–2. **Diseases/Disorders Associated with Glomerulonephritis in Dogs and Cats**

Infectious
  Bacteria
    Endocarditis
    Brucellosis
    Pyometra
    Borreliosis
    Mycoplasmal polyarthritis
    Septicemia
  Viruses
    Infectious canine hepatitis
    Feline leukemia virus/feline immunodeficiency virus
    Feline infectious peritonitis
    Chronic feline upper respiratory disease complex
  Rickettsia
    Ehrlichiosis
    Rocky Mountain spotted fever
  Dirofilariasis
  Protozoa
    Trypanosomiasis
    Leishmaniasis
Neoplasia: all types
Inflammatory disorders
  Pancreatitis
  Systemic lupus erythematosus/systemic immune-mediated disease
  Prostatitis
  Chronic skin disease
Miscellaneous conditions
  Hyperadrenocorticism
  Diabetes mellitus
  Familial glomerular disease
    Doberman pinschers
    Samoyeds
    Rottweilers
    Greyhounds
    Bernese mountain dogs
    Softcoated wheaten terriers
    Cats

  A. Nephrotic syndrome is a descriptive term and does not imply an etiologic diagnosis.
  B. By definition, it includes proteinuria, hypoalbuminemia, hypercholesterolemia, and edema or ascites.
  C. Systemic hypertension and hypercoagulability are also often present.
VI. Primary glomerular disease is often progressive, leading to chronic renal insufficiency/failure.

Clinical Signs and Diagnosis

I. Mild to moderate proteinuria
  A. Asymptomatic or nonspecific signs
  B. Lethargy, mild weight loss, decreased muscle mass
  C. Serum albumin <3.0, but >1.5 g/dl
II. Marked proteinuria (>3.5 g/day)
  A. Severe muscle wasting
  B. Edema/ascites (may result in weight gain)
  C. Serum albumin <1.5 g/dl

D. Hypercholesterolemia, hyperlipidemia

III. Hypercoagulability resulting in pulmonary thrombo-embolism
  A. Acute dyspnea or panting
  B. Sudden death
  C. Mild or no pulmonary parenchymal radiographic abnormalities
  D. Hypoxia with normal or low PCO_2
  E. Fibrinogen concentrations >300 mg/dl and antithrombin III concentrations <70% of normal

IV. Renal insufficiency/failure
  A. Lethargy, anorexia, weight loss
  B. Nausea, vomiting
  C. Polydipsia/polyuria
  D. Azotemia with minimally concentrated or isosthenuric urine
  E. Hyperphosphatemia
  F. Nonregenerative anemia

V. Diagnostic tests
  A. If routine screening tests for proteinuria demonstrate persistent, significant proteinuria, quantitation of proteinuria is indicated (see Chap. 46).
  B. Confirm GN and rule out renal amyloidosis with a renal biopsy.

Differential Diagnosis

I. Proteinuria (see also Chap. 46)
  A. Physiologic: compatible history, low-magnitude proteinuria
  B. Pathologic nonurinary
    1. It is usually associated with lymphoma (Bence Jones proteinuria) or hemoglobinuria/myoglobinuria.
    2. Proteinuria associated with congestive heart failure is usually low in magnitude.
    3. Proteinuria associated with genital tract inflammation is accompanied by an active urine sediment.
  C. Pathologic urinary
    1. Nonrenal proteinuria is usually associated with lower urinary tract inflammation and an active urine sediment.
    2. Renal proteinuria
      a) Tubular proteinuria is usually accompanied by normoglycemic glucosuria.
      b) Renal parenchymal inflammation results in proteinuria with an active urine sediment.
      c) Glomerular proteinuria is usually high in magnitude with an inactive urine sediment (hyaline casts may be observed).
        (1) Immune complex GN
        (2) Amyloidosis

II. Hypoproteinemia
  A. Decreased production
    1. Hepatic insufficiency
    2. Prolonged malnutrition
  B. Increased loss
    1. Gastrointestinal: protein losing enteropathy
    2. Chronic blood loss

III. Other causes of generalized edema and/or ascites
  A. Vasculitis
  B. Other causes of hypoalbuminemia
  C. Heart failure
  D. Liver disease with chronic portal hypertension
  E. Caudal vena caval obstruction

Treatment

I. The most important aspect of treatment is identification and correction of the underlying disease process.

II. If an underlying disease process cannot be identified or corrected, consider immunosuppressive therapy.
  A. There are no controlled clinical trials that demonstrate the efficacy of immunosuppressive drugs in the treatment of canine and feline GN.
  B. Corticosteroids may be more efficacious in cats than in dogs. Corticosteroids are not recommended in dogs unless the underlying disease is steroid responsive (e.g., systemic lupus erythematosus).
    1. There appears to be an association between long-term high-dose corticosteroid use and GN in dogs (Center et al., 1987).
    2. There may also be an association between long-term high-dose corticosteroid use and pulmonary thromboembolism in dogs.
  C. Cyclophosphamide 50 mg/m² PO SID for 3 or 4 days, then discontinued for 4 or 3 days, has been recommended.
  D. Azathioprine 2 mg/kg PO SID–QOD is given to dogs only.
  E. Cyclosporine 15 mg/kg PO SID may be tried in dogs but was of no benefit in one GN study (Vaden et al., 1995).

III. Anti-inflammatory/hypercoagulability treatment decreases glomerular inflammation and the tendency for the development of thromboemboli.
  A. Low-dose aspirin 0.5–5 mg/kg PO SID–BID (dogs)
  B. Specific thromboxane synthetase inhibitors or receptor antagonists (Grauer, 1992)
  C. Warfarin: titrate dose based on prothrombin time

IV. Supportive care
  A. Dietary
    1. Reduce sodium intake.
    2. Reduce protein intake.
      a) High dietary protein enhances proteinuria.
      b) High-quality, reduced-quantity protein diets are recommended.
  B. Systemic hypertension
    1. Dietary sodium reduction
    2. Enalapril
      a) Dose is 0.5 mg/kg PO SID–BID.
      b) Enalapril also has potential antiproteinuric effects (Grodecki et al., 1995).
  C. Edema and/or ascites
    1. Dietary sodium reduction
    2. Cage rest
    3. Low-dose furosemide as needed if necessary (volume contraction and reduced renal function may result from overzealous diuretic use)

4. Abdominocentesis for patients with tense ascites and/or respiratory distress
5. Plasma transfusions
   a) Provide only transient relief
   b) Not routinely recommended

Patient Monitoring

I. Proteinuria
  A. Monitor the urine protein/creatinine ratio to assess response to treatment and/or progression of disease every 2–4 weeks.
  B. Serum albumin and animal body weight are assessed every 2–4 weeks.
II. Renal insufficiency/failure (see Chronic Renal Failure later in the chapter)

Amyloidosis

Definition

I. Amyloid refers to a group of diseases characterized by extracellular deposition of chemically inert fibrillar glycoproteins.
II. Amyloid glycoproteins are deposited in a β-pleated sheet conformation, which results in its unique appearance and chemical properties (e.g., insolubility and resistance to proteolysis in vivo).
III. Amyloid deposition in the kidney can result in proteinuria and/or renal insufficiency/failure.

Causes

I. Four types of amyloidosis have been described in human beings: reactive, immunoglobulin-associated, heredofamilial, and localized.
II. Reactive (secondary) amyloidosis is the most common form in animals (DiBartola and Benson, 1989).
  A. Reactive amyloidosis is a systemic syndrome characterized by tissue deposition of amyloid A protein.
    1. Amyloid A protein is an amino-terminal fragment of the acute-phase reactant serum amyloid A protein (SAA).
    2. Cytokines (e.g., interleukins, tumor necrosis factor) released from macrophages during tissue injury stimulate hepatocytes to produce SAA.
    3. The biologic function of SAA is unknown. SAA binds to high-density lipoproteins, displacing other apolipoproteins.
  B. Reactive amyloidosis is most common in the dog (DiBartola et al., 1989).
  C. Amyloidosis is uncommon in cats, with the exception of Abyssinians.
  D. Diseases that have been associated with reactive amyloidosis include the following.
    1. Chronic infectious inflammation
    2. Chronic noninfectious inflammation
    3. Neoplasia
    4. Cyclic hematopoiesis in gray collies
    5. Ciliary dyskinesia and recurrent respiratory infections in dogs

E. Most reactive amyloidosis, however, occurs in the absence of a discernible underlying cause.
F. Familial reactive amyloidosis has been documented.
  1. Dogs
    a) Shar pei (DiBartola et al., 1990)
    b) Beagle (Bowles and Mosier, 1992)
  2. Cats
    a) Abyssinian (Boyce et al., 1984)
    b) Oriental shorthair
    c) Siamese

Pathophysiology

I. In most dogs, amyloid is deposited in the glomerulus, resulting in proteinuria.
  A. Progressive deposition of amyloid may interfere with glomerular blood flow and cause subsequent tubular and interstitial disease.
  B. In most cases, chronic end-stage renal failure is the outcome.
II. In cats and Shar pei dogs, medullary amyloidosis without discernible glomerular involvement may occur.

Clinical Signs

I. In most dogs, clinical signs are the same as those listed earlier for GN.
  A. In general, glomerular deposition of amyloid results in more severe proteinuria than does immune complex GN.
  B. Nephrotic syndrome and pulmonary thromboemboli are more common in dogs with amyloidosis than in dogs with GN.
  C. Progression to renal insufficiency/failure is also common.
II. Proteinuria is often mild or absent in cats and Shar pei dogs with medullary amyloidosis, but renal failure is common.

Diagnosis

I. Proteinuria is the hallmark of glomerular amyloidosis.
  A. Commonly affected breeds include beagles, collies, and walker hounds.
  B. Most dogs with amyloidosis are >5 years old.
II. Renal insufficiency/failure is the hallmark of familial amyloidosis in Abyssinian cats and Shar pei dogs.
  A. Renal failure usually occurs in animals <6 years old.
  B. Many affected Shar pei dogs have a history of episodic joint swelling (most commonly the tibiotarsal joint) and fever that resolve within several days, regardless of treatment.
  C. This syndrome has also been observed in Shar pei dogs without amyloidosis and appears to be similar to familial Mediterranean fever in humans (Majeed and Barakat, 1989).

Differential Diagnosis

I. Most dogs: immune complex GN
II. Cats and Shar pei dogs: other causes of chronic renal insufficiency/failure

Treatment

I. Identify and correct the underlying disease process if possible.
II. Specific treatment for amyloidosis is usually unrewarding.
  A. Aggressive use of cytotoxic drugs such as chlorambucil, cyclophosphamide, and methotrexate has been beneficial in some human beings with reactive amyloidosis, but these drugs have not been studied in animals with amyloidosis.
  B. Dimethyl sulfoxide (DMSO) has been used in dogs with amyloidosis but is often associated with adverse side effects (Grauer and DiBartola, 1995) and remains controversial.
  C. Similar to its use in human beings with familial Mediterranean fever (Majeed and Barakat, 1989), colchicine has been recommended for use in Shar pei dogs that have had tibiotarsal joint swelling and fever to prevent subsequent amyloidosis.
    1. There are no controlled clinical trials that demonstrate the efficacy of colchicine in preventing renal amyloidosis in animals.
    2. Colchicine would not be expected to be beneficial once renal failure has become established.
III. Supportive treatment for hypoproteinemia and chronic renal failure is also instituted.

Patient Monitoring

I. Proteinuria
  A. Monitor the urine protein/creatinine ratio to assess response to treatment and/or progression of disease every 2–4 weeks.
  B. Serum albumin and patient body weight are assessed every 2–4 weeks.
II. For renal insufficiency/failure, see Chronic Renal Failure later in the chapter.
III. Prognosis is poor because the disease is progressive and no specific treatment has proved to be effective.

ACUTE RENAL FAILURE

Gregory F. Grauer

Definition

I. Acute renal failure (ARF) results from an abrupt decline in glomerular filtration rate (GFR) and is usually caused by an ischemic or toxic insult.
  A. Ischemic or toxicant-induced injury frequently damages the metabolically active proximal tubule and thick ascending loop of Henle epithelial cells, causing impaired regulation of water and solute balance.

B. The degree of renal dysfunction is usually life threatening if treatment is not initiated.
II. ARF is an important clinical syndrome because it is common and frequently results in death.
III. In some cases, after expensive and intense supportive care, ARF may be reversible, and adequate renal function may be regained.

Causes

I. Potential ischemic events
  A. Shock: hypovolemic, hemorrhagic, hypotensive, septic
  B. Decreased cardiac output
    1. Congestive heart failure
    2. Arrhythmias
    3. Cardiac arrest
    4. Cardiac tamponade
  C. Deep anesthesia/extensive surgery
  D. Trauma
  E. Hyperthermia/hypothermia
  F. Extensive cutaneous burns
  G. Transfusion reactions
  H. Renal vessel thrombosis, microthrombus formation, disseminated intravascular coagulation
  I. Hyperviscosity/polycythemic syndromes
  J. NSAID drug administration
II. Nephrotoxicant-induced tubular injury (see Nephrotoxicosis)
III. Miscellaneous conditions
  A. Immune-mediated diseases
    1. Glomerulonephritis/amyloidosis
    2. Systemic lupus erythematosus
    3. Vasculitis
  B. Hypercalcemia
  C. Infectious diseases: pyelonephritis, leptospirosis, borreliosis
  D. Urinary tract obstruction
  E. Diabetes mellitus

Pathophysiology

I. Ischemic injury occurs when renal blood flow is attenuated by decreased blood pressure or by renal vasoconstriction.
II. Decreased renal blood flow results in reduced amounts of oxygen and metabolic substrates presented to tubular cells, and this "cellular starvation" initiates a cycle of events (Grauer and Lane, 1995).
  A. The adenosine triphosphate (ATP) cellular energy pool is depleted.
  B. Decreased cell transport function results in increased intracellular solute concentrations and cell swelling.
  C. Membrane damage results in excessive calcium influx into renal tubular epithelial cells and vasoconstriction.
  D. Persistent vasoconstriction and cell swelling create vascular stasis and platelet and red blood cell aggregation.
  E. Energy substrate delivery remains impaired, and ATP restoration cannot occur.

F. Generation of leukotrienes and thromboxanes results in further vasoconstriction.

III. Nephrotoxic injury (see Nephrotoxicosis) also commonly results in ARF.

IV. The induction phase is the time between the renal insult and the development of azotemia and defective urine concentrating capacity.
   A. Therapeutic intervention at this time may prevent progression of renal damage and development of established ARF.
   B. Clinical detection of the induction phase of ARF is difficult.
      1. Cellular damage initially may be sublethal, but without intervention, more and more cells sustain lethal injury.
      2. Clinicopathologic signs may include a progressive decline in GFR and urine concentrating ability, and a progressive increase in proteinuria, enzymuria, and cylindruria.

V. The maintenance phase of ARF develops when renal tubular lesions are established.
   A. Reduced renal blood flow and GFR are common to all forms of ARF, although reductions in GFR are usually greater than the reduction in renal blood flow.
   B. At the individual nephron level, reduced GFR occurs in ARF owing to a combination of tubular obstruction, tubular backleak, afferent arteriolar vasoconstriction, and decreased glomerular capillary permeability.
   C. It is likely that a combination of these factors contributes to the decreased GFR of ARF.
   D. Therapeutic intervention during the maintenance phase, although often life-saving, usually does little to diminish existing renal lesions or improve renal function.

VI. The recovery phase of ARF is associated with improved renal function.
   A. GFR increases as nephron repair and compensation occur.
   B. Even if recovery is incomplete, adequate but subnormal function may be reestablished.
   C. Tubular lesions may be repaired if the tubular basement membrane is intact and sufficient viable epithelial cells are present.
   D. Although additional nephrons cannot be produced and irreversibly damaged nephrons cannot be repaired, functional and morphologic hypertrophy of surviving nephrons may adequately compensate for the decrease in nephron numbers.

Clinical Signs

I. Depression, lethargy, collapse
II. Anorexia, uremic and/or acidotic odor to breath
III. Vomiting and diarrhea, with or without melena
IV. Evidence of other organ dysfunction
   A. Icterus
   B. Petechiae, ecchymoses
   C. Tachypnea, tachycardia
   D. Hypo- or hyperthermia
   E. Brick red or muddy mucous membranes

Diagnosis

I. History of exposure to a potential nephrotoxicant or of an ischemic episode is suggestive.
II. Acute onset of azotemia and hyperphosphatemia is suggestive.
III. Oliguria/anuria is more common with ischemic insults; nonoliguric ARF occurs with mild to moderate gentamicin- and cisplatin-induced ARF.
IV. Lumbar/renal pain is infrequently identified on abdominal palpation.
V. Renal biopsy is indicated when any of the following is true.
   A. A definitive diagnosis is lacking.
   B. Significant and persistent proteinuria is present.
   C. Diffuse systemic disease is suspected.
   D. Conservative methods of treatment have failed.
      1. Oliguria persists beyond 2–3 days of therapy.
      2. Severe uremia or hyperkalemia persists for 4–5 days.
   E. Histologic assessment is necessary to determine prognosis.
      1. Histologic evidence of tubular regeneration and intact tubular basement membranes is considered a good prognostic indicator of reversibility.
      2. Extensive tubular necrosis and interstitial mineralization with disrupted basement membranes are poor prognostic signs and suggest irreversible damage.
VI. Because therapeutic intervention is most successful when initiated in the induction phase of ARF, early recognition of renal dysfunction can be life saving.
   A. Physical examination of the patient at risk for ARF should include assessment of cardiovascular function, blood pressure, and hydration status.
   B. Urine output is monitored in all critically ill animals and is quantified in high-risk patients undergoing anesthesia by use of a closed indwelling urine collection system.
      1. Normal urine output is approximately 1–2 ml/h/kg; significant increases or decreases from normal may signal the onset of ARF.
      2. Oliguria or anuria requires prompt attention and treatment.
   C. Urinalysis and the urine sediment are examined daily for red blood cells, white blood cells, casts, renal epithelial cells, or cellular debris in patients receiving potentially nephrotoxic drugs.
      1. Enzymes such as gamma-glutamyl transpeptidase (GGT) and *N*-acetyl-beta-D-glucosaminidase (NAG) are too large to be normally filtered by the glomerulus.
         a) GGT and NAG enzymuria indicates cell leakage and is usually caused by tubular damage or necrosis (Greco et al., 1985).
         b) Urine enzyme/creatinine ratios have been shown to accurately reflect 24-hour urinary enzyme excretion in early gentamicin nephrotoxicosis in dogs (Grauer et al., 1995).
         c) Interpretation of enzymuria is aided by

Table 47–3. Indices That May Help Differentiate Prerenal Azotemia from ARF

Index	Prerenal Azotemia	ARF
Urine specific gravity	Hypersthenuric	Isosthenuric or minimally concentrated
Urine sodium (mEq/L)	<10–20	>25
Fractional excretion of sodium (%)	<1	>1
Urine creatinine to plasma creatinine ratio	>20:1	<10:1
Renal failure index (urine sodium/ urine to plasma creatinine ratio)	<1	>2
Response to fluid therapy	Marked	Minimal

comparison with baseline values obtained prior to a potential renal insult.

2. The development of glucosuria or increases in the fractional excretion of sodium and chloride are additional early signals of tubular dysfunction.

Differential Diagnosis

I. Prerenal azotemia (Table 47–3)
II. Chronic renal failure (Table 47–4)

Treatment

I. Prerenal and postrenal factors contributing to renal dysfunction need to be quickly identified and treated.
II. If renal damage is suspected, all potentially nephrotoxic drugs are discontinued.
III. Underlying diseases must be identified and managed if possible (e.g., hypoadrenocorticism, pyometra, hepatic disease).
IV. Treatable intrinsic renal disorders (e.g., leptospirosis, pyelonephritis) are identified, and appropriate management is initiated.

V. General treatment considerations include the following.
   A. Goals are to correct renal hemodynamic disorders and alleviate water and solute imbalances to allow time for nephron regeneration and compensation.
   B. Positive response to treatment is evidenced by the following.
      1. Increase in glomerular filtration as measured by a decrease in serum creatinine concentrations
      2. Increase in urine production (if the animal has oliguria or anuria)
         a) An increase in urine production facilitates management of ARF by decreasing serum urea nitrogen and potassium concentration (with increased tubular flow rates and volumes, reabsorption of urea and potassium is decreased) and by lessening the tendency for overhydration to occur.
         b) In most cases, increased urine production occurs as a result of decreased tubular reabsorption of filtrate, not an increase in glomerular filtration.

VI. Specific treatment recommendations involve the following.
   A. Fluid therapy remains the mainstay of treatment for ARF. The goals of fluid therapy are to correct fluid and electrolyte imbalances, improve renal hemodynamics, and initiate diuresis.
      1. Fluid deficits are replaced intravenously over the first 4–6 hours of treatment. The fluid rate should, however, be reduced in animals with known or suspected cardiovascular dysfunction.
      2. Use 0.45% saline and 2.5% dextrose solutions or 0.9% saline solutions initially.
      3. In addition to deficit needs, maintenance and continuing fluid losses must be provided for.
      4. During the rehydration phase, urine produc-

Table 47–4. Parameters That May Help Differentiate Acute from Chronic Renal Failure

Parameter	Acute Renal Failure	Chronic Renal Failure
History	Ischemic episode or toxicant exposure	Previous renal disease or renal insufficiency Long-standing polydipsia/polyuria Chronic weight loss, vomiting, diarrhea
Physical examination	Good body flesh Smooth, swollen, painful kidneys Relatively severe clinical signs for level of dysfunction	Poor body condition Small, irregular kidneys Relatively mild clinical signs for level of dysfunction Osteodystrophy
Clincopathologic findings	Normal or increased hematocrit Active urine sediment Normal to increased serum potassium More severe metabolic acidosis	Nonregenerative anemia Inactive urine sediment Normal to low serum potassium Less severe metabolic acidosis

tion is measured and the animal is monitored for overhydration.

  a) Frequent assessment of body weight, central venous pressure, packed cell volume, and plasma total solids will detect early overhydration.

  b) If overhydration occurs, slow the rate of fluid administration and treat with diuretics and/or vasodilators.

5. If urine production is <1 ml/lb/h and there are no signs of overhydration after initial fluid therapy, further fluid therapy to expand the extracellular fluid volume is indicated.

  a) An additional fluid volume (3–5% of the animal's body weight in kg) is given, because dehydration <5% cannot be detected clinically.

  b) If this volume expansion is attempted, observe the animal closely for signs of overhydration.

6. Significant decreases in serum creatinine concentration that occur secondary to fluid therapy are usually associated with correction of prerenal dehydration.

B. If oliguria persists after fluid therapy, initiate one or more of the following.

1. Furosemide 2–6 mg/kg IV TID

  a) Although furosemide is easy to administer, an infusion of mannitol or use of a dopamine infusion in combination with furosemide is likely to be more effective than furosemide alone.

  b) Furosemide has been shown to exacerbate gentamicin toxicity and should be avoided in ARF caused by aminoglycosides.

2. Mannitol (10% or 20%) 0.5–1 g/kg slowly IV over 15–20 minutes

  a) Urine output improves within 1 hour if the treatment is effective.

  b) A second bolus may be attempted, but the potential for volume overexpansion and complications such as pulmonary and tissue edema increases considerably.

  c) Mannitol should not be used in overhydrated patients, as the increase in intravascular volume may precipitate pulmonary edema.

3. Low-dose dopamine 2–10 μg/kg/min IV infusion

  a) When furosemide therapy is combined with dopamine infusion, the likelihood of inducing diuresis is enhanced.

  b) Although the recommended dosage has minimal systemic effects, dopamine can be arrhythmogenic, and electrocardiographic monitoring is advised.

  c) If an arrhythmia or tachycardia is observed, discontinuation of the dopamine infusion should result in rapid improvement.

C. Treatment of hyperkalemia involves primarily fluid therapy.

1. Moderate hyperkalemia (<6 mEq/L) is largely resolved with administration of potassium-free fluids (dilution) and improved urine flow (increased excretion).

2. Severe hyperkalemia (>6–8 mEq/L) or hyperkalemia resulting in cardiotoxicity is specifically treated.

  a) Sodium bicarbonate 0.5–2 mEq/kg IV over 20–30 minutes

  b) Regular insulin 0.1–0.25 U/kg IV followed by a glucose bolus of 1–2 g per unit of insulin

  c) 10% calcium gluconate 0.5–1 ml/kg IV over 10–15 minutes (while monitoring the animal's ECG) to counteract the cardiotoxic effects of excess potassium

3. The effects of these treatments are short-lived, and therapy to initiate and maintain diuresis is important to maintain potassium excretion and normokalemia.

D. Treatment of metabolic acidosis is proportional to its severity.

1. Mild to moderate metabolic acidosis commonly resolves with fluid therapy, and specific treatment is usually not necessary unless the blood pH is <7.1–7.15 or total CO_2 measures <10–12 mEq/L.

2. Bicarbonate requirements can be calculated using the base deficit as determined from arterial blood, or by using an estimated base deficit [body weight (kg) × 0.5 × base deficit (or 20 − total CO_2) = mEq bicarbonate required].

3. Optimally, one half the calculated bicarbonate dosage is administered slowly IV over 15–30 minutes, and then acid-base parameters are reassessed.

4. Overzealous bicarbonate administration may result in ionized calcium deficits, paradoxic cerebrospinal fluid acidosis, and cerebral edema.

E. Maintenance fluid therapy is tailored in nonoliguric ARF, or once diuresis has been established, to match urine volume and insensible losses (Table 47–5).

1. The volume of ongoing fluid loss from vomiting and/or diarrhea is estimated, and that amount is added to the 24-hour fluid needs of the patient.

Table 47–5. Hypothetical Daily Fluid Requirements

	Normal Patient	Oliguric ARF Patient	Nonoliguric ARF Patient
Insensible fluid loss (ml/kg/day)	20	20	20
Urine production (ml/kg/day)	40	4	175
Total maintenance fluid needs (ml/kg/day)	60	24	195

2. If hyperkalemia is not present and diuresis has been established, polyionic maintenance fluids (e.g., Normosol) are used.
3. In the recovery phase of ARF, urine volume and electrolyte losses can be great.
4. Potassium supplementation may actually be necessary, especially if the patient is vomiting or anorexic (Table 47–6).
    F. Supportive care is often needed.
1. Gastrointestinal complications are among the most frequent systemic signs in acute uremia (see Chronic Renal Failure for specific therapy).
2. Critically ill uremic patients are highly susceptible to infection; therefore, early diagnosis and specific treatment based on culture and sensitivity are important.

Patient Monitoring

I. Monitor serum urea nitrogen, creatinine, and phosphorus concentrations at least daily during fluid, diuretic, and vasodilator therapy.
II. A positive response to treatment is indicated by the following.
    A. A significant decrease in azotemia following initial fluid therapy (i.e., correction of prerenal dehydration)
    B. Establishment of diuresis and subsequent significant decreases in blood urea nitrogen (BUN), serum potassium, and metabolic acidosis
    C. Control of nausea, vomiting, and gastrointestinal bleeding, so that adequate caloric intake is maintained
III. Increases in GFR (not associated with correction of pre- or postrenal complications) result from nephron repair and compensation and typically occur within 10–21 days in cases of reversible ARF.
IV. Monitor serum urea nitrogen, creatinine, and phosphorus concentrations every 2–3 days once diuresis is established.

CHRONIC RENAL FAILURE

Scott A. Brown

Definition

I. Renal failure is the presence of persistent azotemia (see Chap. 46) of renal origin.

Table 47–6. *Fluid Therapy Potassium Supplementation Guidelines*

Measured Serum Potassium Concentration (mEq/L)	Amount of Potassium Chloride (mEq) to Be Added to Each Liter of Fluid[a]
3.0–3.5	28
2.5–3.0	40
2.0–2.5	60
<2.0	80

[a]Do not exceed a rate of 0.5 mEq/kg/h.

II. Chronic renal failure (CRF) is renal-origin azotemia that is of prolonged duration, generally more than 2 weeks.

Causes

I. Tubulointerstitial disorders
    A. Congenital/familial disorders: basenji nephropathy (Brown, 1989)
    B. Immune-mediated conditions: some forms of chronic interstitial nephritis
    C. Amyloidosis: Abyssinian or Shar pei nephropathy
    D. Neoplasia
        1. Renal adenocarcinoma
        2. Lymphosarcoma
        3. Metastases
    E. Degenerative disease: chronic interstitial nephritis
    F. Hydronephrosis
    G. Nephrocalcinosis
    H. Idiopathic disease
II. Glomerular disorders
    A. Congenital/familial disorders: Samoyed nephropathy (Jansen et al., 1987)
    B. Immune-mediated diseases: immune complex glomerulonephritis
    C. Amyloidosis (DiBartola et al., 1989)
    D. Parasites: *D. renale*
    E. Degenerative disorders: glomerulosclerosis (Diamond and Karnovsky, 1988)
    F. Vascular abnormalities: hemolytic-uremic syndrome
    G. Idiopathic disease
III. Vascular disorders
    A. Infarction
        1. Disseminated intravascular coagulation
        2. Intrarenal endothelial injury and coagulopathy: hemolytic-uremic syndrome
        3. Embolization: bacterial endocarditis
    B. Hypertension
        1. Glomerular (Brown et al., 1990)
        2. Systemic (Snyder, 1991; Littman, 1994)
    C. Hypotension
        1. Chronic hypotension is not generally recognized as a cause of CRF in dogs and cats.
        2. In animals with CRF, any decline in systemic arterial blood pressure can acutely decrease GFR and thus worsen azotemia.

Pathophysiology

I. Uremic syndrome
    A variety of changes are observed in animals with CRF, producing a constellation of clinically identifiable abnormalities commonly referred to as the uremic syndrome.
II. Urinary system
    A. Reduced numbers of nephrons result in a high obligatory solute load per nephron, interfering with the renal concentrating mechanism.
    B. The result is polyuria (and secondary polydipsia)

caused by a urine specific gravity that approaches isosthenuria as the renal failure worsens.

   C. A low urine specific gravity may predispose to the development of urinary tract infection.

III. Gastrointestinal system

   A. Accumulation of nitrogenous wastes, metabolic acidosis, and changes in the gastrointestinal tract can lead to anorexia, weight loss, and/or vomiting.

   B. Accumulation of dental tartar and development of associated gingival disease occur rapidly, possibly from alterations in oral flora caused by the local presence of uremic toxins, which serve as a substrate for ammoniagenesis in urease-producing bacteria.

   C. Necrosis of the distal portions of the tongue is observed with severe uremia, especially after a sudden superimposition of a prerenal condition in an animal with CRF.

IV. Endocrine system

   A. Secondary hyperparathyroidism is usually observed.

   B. Contributory factors include the following.

     1. Phosphate retention leading to calcium-phosphate deposition within tissues (metastatic mineralization) and subsequent reduction of plasma ionized calcium stimulate release of parathyroid hormone (PTH).

     2. Loss and/or inhibition of the renal 1-alpha hydroxylase enzyme, causing reduced generation of 1,25 dihydroxyvitamin D (calcitriol), results in increased synthesis of PTH.

   C. Clinical abnormalities attributed to the presence of excess PTH include uremic osteodystrophy, anemia, arthritis, cardiomyopathy, encephalopathy, glucose intolerance, hyperlipidemia, immunosuppression, myopathy, pancreatitis, pruritus, skin ulcerations, and soft tissue calcification.

V. Hematologic changes

   A. Anemia of chronic renal disease

     1. From decreased production of erythropoietin

     2. From depressed erythrogenesis and shortened erythrocyte life span to an accumulation of toxins

   B. Coagulopathies

     1. Platelet abnormality is functional and almost always subclinical; circulating numbers of platelets are generally normal.

     2. Markedly proteinuric animals may develop thromboembolism, attributed to a deficiency of antithrombin III owing to urinary loss (Green and Kabel, 1982).

VI. Nervous system

   A. The accumulation of nitrogenous wastes, metabolic acidosis, disorders in potassium and sodium homeostasis, anemia, and inadequate caloric intake contribute to lethargy and inactivity.

   B. Seizures (presumably from accumulation of a uremic toxin) have been observed in animals with severe uremia, most frequently in young animals.

   C. Hypothermia, attributed to effects of uremic toxins on the hypothalamic thermoregulatory center, is generally observed only with severe uremia.

VII. Cardiovascular system

   A. The most frequently observed abnormality is systemic hypertension. It may be multifactorial in cause, although altered renal handling of sodium and enhanced generation of angiotensin II appear to play an important role in dogs.

   B. Systemic hypertension can lead to retinal hemorrhages and/or detachment, seizures, cardiac hypertrophy, and progressive renal injury.

   C. Cardiac arrhythmias and pericardial effusion are rarely observed.

VIII. Other systems

   A. Immune suppression may occur, although it is subtle and subclinical in most animals.

   B. Abnormalities of the respiratory system, such as pneumonitis, are rare in dogs and cats.

IX. Progression of renal disease

   A. Frequently, animals with renal disease suffer progressive decrements of renal function until terminal uremia ensues (Brown, 1994).

   B. Possible causes of this progression include the following.

     1. Primary renal disease

     2. Secondary factors that are self-perpetuating and operate independently of the primary disease

       a) Dietary phosphate excess

       b) Glomerular hyperfiltration, hypertension, and hypertrophy

       c) Systemic hypertension

       d) Glomerular inflammatory injury

       e) Progressive tubulointerstitial fibrosis mediated by local production of growth factors

Clinical Signs

  I. Chronic history of polyuria and polydipsia

 II. Lethargy, inactivity, weakness

III. Anorexia, weight loss

IV. Vomiting, oral ulcerations, stomatitis, glossitis

 V. Uremic osteodystrophy

VI. Seizures, hypothermia

Diagnosis

  I. Clinical signs compatible with uremia

 II. Laboratory confirmation of renal azotemia

   A. Urine specific gravity usually <1.020 (some cats with renal failure retain urinary concentrating ability)

   B. Absence of clinical evidence of a prerenal disorder such as dehydration, systemic hypotension, or hypoadrenocorticism

   C. Evidence of a normal excretory pathway (patency of both ureters, urethra, and urinary bladder)

III. Laboratory evidence of chronicity (see Table 47–4)

   A. The presence of a normocytic, normochromic, nonregenerative anemia is the major laboratory

finding that supports the presence of chronic rather than acute renal failure.
  B. Detection of small, irregular kidneys via palpation, radiography, or ultrasonography is suggestive of chronic disease.
  C. Radiographic evidence of osteodystrophy and/or clinical findings referable to renal osteodystrophy (e.g., flexible, enlarged, demineralized mandible) are also important.
  D. Glomerulopathies are rarely acute in animals.
IV. Serum biochemical abnormalities
  A. Serum total calcium concentration is often a poor reflection of the physiologic level of calcium in the bloodstream (free or ionized calcium) in animals with CRF.
    1. Serum total calcium concentration is usually normal. Perhaps one third of affected animals have mild hypocalcemia, as reflected by reduced serum ionized calcium concentrations.
    2. Serum total calcium concentration may be elevated in some animals. These animals generally have a normal ionized calcium concentration with increased levels of complexed calcium.
    3. Hypocalcemia (reduced ionized calcium) is most frequently observed in the terminal phases of CRF. These animals may have normal, high, or low total serum calcium concentrations.
  B. Serum phosphate concentration is often elevated, and the extent is directly related to the degree of renal dysfunction and the level of dietary phosphate.
  C. Serum potassium concentration is often abnormal.
    1. Hypokalemia is most often observed in polyuric animals. It is common in feline patients, in which it reflects inadequate potassium intake and/or the effects of an acidifying diet that promotes kaliuresis.
    2. Hyperkalemia is uncommon except in the terminal phases of CRF and is often associated with oliguria or anuria.
  D. Metabolic acidosis is frequently observed.
    1. The acidosis is generally associated with an increased anion gap owing to the accumulation of unmeasured anion.
    2. Although uncommon, a normal anion gap metabolic acidosis may be present in an animal with renal tubular acidosis.
V. Delineation of the underlying cause
  A. Signalment
  B. History: toxicant exposure
  C. Evidence of other organ involvement: polysystemic illness
  D. Renal biopsy

Differential Diagnosis

I. Prerenal azotemia from dehydration and/or hypotension: hypoadrenocorticism

II. Postrenal azotemia: bladder rupture or ureteral avulsion

Treatment

I. Specific therapy directed against any primary renal disease (e.g., pyelonephritis)
II. Supportive therapy
  A. Adequate fresh water must be available at all times.
  B. Avoid vasoactive agents that decompensate renal function, such as nonsteroidal anti-inflammatory agents.
  C. Provide adequate water-soluble vitamins, which may be depleted in polyuric animals.
III. Nutritional modifications
  A. Nutritional modifications are not indicated in nonazotemic or geriatric animals.
  B. To slow progression of renal failure, dietary phosphate restriction is used in all azotemic cats and dogs.
    1. Dogs: low-phosphorus diet with approximately 0.25% phosphorus on a dry matter basis (supplying 34–42 mg/kg/day)
    2. Cats: reduced-phosphorus diet containing approximately 0.5% phosphorus on a dry matter basis (supplying 65–85 mg/kg/day)
    3. Goal: normophosphatemia
  C. After an initial dietary trial with a low-phosphorus diet for 2–4 weeks, begin intestinal phosphorus binders dosed to effect (initial dose of 30–180 mg/kg/day with meals).
    1. Either aluminum- or calcium-containing salts can be used as phosphorus binders at the same initial doses, but the former may be associated with osteodystrophy or encephalopathy, and the latter is causally associated with hypercalcemia in some dogs and cats.
    2. Mix the phosphorus binder with moistened or canned food and change doses gradually to limit food aversion.
  D. To reduce the clinical signs of uremia in dogs, dietary protein restriction is instituted once BUN levels reach 60–75 mg/dl.
    1. At that time, the diet should contain approximately 14–17% protein on a dry matter basis (supplying 2–2.5 g/kg/day).
    2. Adequate caloric intake should be ensured and facilitated by gradual diet changes and trials with various commercially available preparations or formulations.
  E. In cats, dietary protein restriction is considered when BUN levels are elevated. The diet should contain approximately 28–31% protein on a dry matter basis (supplying 3.8–4.5 g/kg/day).
  F. Because of its benefit in slowing the rate of progression of renal failure, dietary phosphorus restriction is begun earlier in renal failure than is dietary protein restriction.
IV. Therapy for secondary hyperparathyroidism
  A. Oral calcitriol therapy at 0.025–0.05 μg/kg/day

PO SID (separately from meals) lowers PTH in most dogs.

B. Similar effects occur in cats with renal failure.

V. Therapy for anemia

A. Recombinant erythropoietin 50–100 U/kg SQ 2–3 times weekly increases the hematocrit in most affected animals (Cowgill, 1991).

B. Because the prevalence of antibody production causes many animals to respond to erythropoietin for only 6–12 months, it is used only in those animals with a hematocrit <20% and clinical signs attributable to anemia.

C. Supplement animals with oral ferrous sulfate.

D. Goal is to reach the low end of the normal range for hematocrit (30–35%).

E. Anabolic steroids and blood transfusions are of limited usefulness.

VI. Therapy for acidosis

A. Goal is to keep total carbon dioxide or bicarbonate concentrations within the normal range.

B. Initially, give sodium bicarbonate 15 mg/kg PO TID; it should be used cautiously in hypertensive patients.

C. Potassium citrate may also be given at an initial dose of 30 mg/kg PO BID.

VII. Therapy for vomiting

A. H$_2$-receptor antagonists
  1. Cimetidine 4 mg/kg PO BID–TID
  2. Ranitidine 1–2 mg/kg PO BID

B. Other antiemetics as required to control vomiting

VIII. Therapy for hypokalemia (particularly in cats)

A. Potassium gluconate 2–6 mEq/cat/day PO mixed with food

B. Other potassium salts not as well tolerated

C. Diet with high potassium, low acid content

IX. Therapy for hypertension

A. Therapy for hypertension must be based on measurement of blood pressure.
  1. Measurement must be accomplished in a quiet setting with a minimum of five consistent readings.
  2. Preferred indirect methods are an oscillometric measurement using the coccygeal artery or ultrasonic Doppler technique using the tarsal artery in dogs, and the ultrasonic Doppler technique using the median artery in cats

B. Treatment is instituted if systolic pressure exceeds 200 mmHg and/or diastolic pressure exceeds 110 mmHg.

C. Goal of therapy is to reduce arterial pressure by at least 25–50 mmHg while sustaining adequate renal function. Ideally, blood pressure is in the normal range during treatment.

D. A variety of adverse effects of lowering blood pressure may be observed, including a decrement in renal function, weakness, syncope, and enhanced kaliuresis leading to hypokalemia.

E. Antihypertensive measures to consider include the following.
  1. Low-sodium diet (efficacy)
  2. Angiotensin-converting enzyme (ACE) inhibitors
      a) Enalapril 0.5 mg/kg PO SID–BID
      b) Benazepril 0.25 mg/kg PO SID–BID
  3. Amlodipine (effective in cats)
      a) Cat: 0.625 mg/cat PO SID
      b) Dog: 0.5–1 mg/kg PO SID
  4. Alpha-1 antagonist: prazosin 1 mg/10 kg PO SID–TID
  5. Beta antagonists
      a) Atenolol (cardiospecific) 2 mg/kg PO SID–BID
      b) Propranolol (nonspecific)
          (1) Dog: 5–80 mg PO BID–TID
          (2) Cat: 2.5–10 mg PO BID–TID
  6. Diuretics
      a) Hydrochlorothiazide
          (1) Dog: 0.5–5 mg/kg PO BID
          (2) Cat: 1–2 mg/kg PO BID
      b) Furosemide 1 mg/kg PO SID–BID
      c) Spironolactone 1–2 mg/kg PO SID–BID

F. Antihypertensive therapy usually starts with a low-sodium diet and may use multiple agents simultaneously. There is no contraindication to the coadministration of agents, although two agents from the same class (e.g., atenolol plus propranolol) are not generally beneficial.

X. Therapy for progressive renal disease

A. Dietary phosphorus restriction with or without intestinal phosphorus restriction

B. Dietary protein restriction: no apparent benefit in dogs, controversial in cats

C. Dietary supplementation with omega-3 polyunsaturated fatty acids (PUFA)
  1. The goal is an omega-6/omega-3 PUFA ratio between 1:1 and 5:1.
  2. Commercial diets are available that lie within or close to this range for PUFA ratios, and manufacturers generally supply this information on their products.
  3. As an alternative, dietary supplements containing eicosapentaenoic or docosahexaenoic acid (both are omega-3 PUFA) are available at health food stores.

D. Use of an ACE inhibitor
  1. Enalapril 0.5 mg/kg PO SID–BID
  2. Benazepril 0.25 mg/kg PO SID–BID

E. Antihypertensive therapy as described earlier

Patient Monitoring

I. Nonazotemic renal failure

A. Monitor urinalysis, urine culture, serum creatinine, hematocrit, and blood pressure every 6 months.

B. Perform a biochemical profile and complete blood count annually.

II. Azotemic renal failure

A. Obtain a urinalysis and urine culture, and measure serum creatinine, hematocrit, and blood pressure every 3–6 months.

B. Test more frequently if renal function is unstable (creatinine >4 mg/dl) or systemic hypertension is documented.

C. Perform a biochemical profile and complete blood count annually.
III. Uremic renal failure
  A. Measure serum creatinine, BUN, electrolytes, calcium, and phosphate every 1–3 days until animal becomes nonuremic.
  B. Then manage as azotemic renal failure.
IV. Measure serum calcium every 2–4 weeks in animals on calcitriol and alter therapy as needed to avoid hypercalcemia.
V. Measure blood pressure every 2–3 weeks following onset of antihypertensive therapy until blood pressure stabilizes, then every 3–6 months.

PERITONEAL DIALYSIS

Gregory F. Grauer

Definition

I. Dialysis is the diffusion of solutes from one solution to another across a semipermeable membrane.
II. One solution is the animal's plasma and interstitial fluid, and the second solution is the dialysate fluid placed within the peritoneal cavity.
III. The semipermeable membrane is the peritoneum.

Pathophysiology

I. Dynamics of fluid and solute exchange across the peritoneum (Cowgill, 1995)
  A. Diffusion
    1. Large molecules such as proteins cross the peritoneum very slowly or not at all.
    2. Smaller molecules such as urea and glucose and electrolytes such as sodium and potassium easily cross the peritoneum. These solutes move from the side with the highest concentration to the opposite side until equilibrium is reached.
  B. Ultrafiltration and convective transport
    1. Water moves across the peritoneum toward the side with higher osmolality until no osmotic pressure gradient exists.
    2. As water passes through the peritoneum, solutes capable of passing through the ultrafiltration channels are dragged along (solvent drag or convective transport).
  C. Various solutes as well as water can be added to, or removed from, the animal's plasma and interstitial fluid by altering the solute and osmolality composition of the dialysate solution.
II. Other factors influencing peritoneal dialysis
  A. Peritoneal blood flow
    1. It is usually sufficient to permit excellent diffusion of solutes and water unless the animal is in shock.
    2. Warming the dialysate solution 2–3° above the animal's body temperature increases peritoneal blood flow.
  B. Volume of dialysate solution infused into the animal
    1. Large volumes
      a) Provide a greater amount of surface area for diffusion but also require longer equilibration times
      b) May decrease cardiac output and cause increased peripheral resistance associated with increased intra-abdominal pressure and decreased venous return
      c) May cause abdominal discomfort and dyspnea/respiratory distress by decreasing movement of the diaphragm
    2. Small volumes
      a) Equilibration time is shorter, and cardiovascular complications are minimized.
      b) More fluid exchanges must be performed, increasing technical time and the chances of infection.

Clinical Considerations

I. Indications
  A. Acute renal failure
    1. Failure of fluid, diuretic, and vasodilator therapy to induce a diuresis in oliguric/anuric patients
    2. Failure of fluid, diuretic, and vasodilator therapy to control the biochemical and clinical manifestations of uremia
    3. Life-threatening fluid overload/pulmonary edema
    4. Life-threatening electrolyte and/or acid–base disturbance
  B. Chronic renal failure
    1. Uremia that is unresponsive to conventional dietary/medical management
    2. Long-term peritoneal dialysis for irreversible, end-stage renal disease rarely practical in animals
  C. Miscellaneous conditions
    1. Severe pulmonary edema that is refractory to conventional medical therapy
    2. Acute intoxication/drug overdose when the toxicant is dialyzable (e.g., ethylene glycol)
    3. To provide core warming for profound hypothermia
II. Contraindications
  A. Diaphragmatic hernia
  B. Severe intra-abdominal adhesions
  C. Recent abdominal surgery (a relative contraindication)
    1. Volume and flow of dialysate solution may contribute to breakdown of suture lines in stomach, intestines, or urinary bladder.
    2. Distention of the abdomen with dialysate solution may result in leakage through a ventral midline incision and increase the possibility of peritonitis.
III. Factors to consider before initiating peritoneal dialysis
  A. Time commitment
    1. A great deal of time is required by both veterinary and technical staff.

2. 24-hour monitoring is necessary.
3. Owners considering chronic ambulatory peritoneal dialysis for animals with end-stage renal disease need to understand that it takes several hours each day to perform the exchanges.
B. Economic commitment
  1. Costs for catheters, administration sets, and dialysate solution
  2. Professional and technical time fees
C. Extensive and accurate patient records necessary
D. Most commonly performed on ARF patients with severe excretory dysfunction and poor response to conventional medical management
E. Histologic evidence of reversibility of renal damage: important as a prognostic indicator

IV. Choice of dialysate solution
A. Glucose concentration
  1. The solution must contain at least 1.5% glucose to prevent rapid diffusion of dialysate water into the plasma.
  2. Standard commercial dialysate solutions have glucose concentrations of 1.5, 2.5, 3.5, and 4.25%.
  3. Sources of dialysate solutions are as follows.
    a) Baxter Healthcare Corp., Renal Division, McGraw Park, IL 60015 (Dianeal)
    b) Fresenius USA, Inc., Walnut Creek, CA 94598 (Impersol)
    c) McGaw, Inc., Irvine CA 92713 (Dialyte)
  4. Lactated Ringer's solution (LRS) with 1.5% glucose can be used in an emergency situation (add 30 ml of 50% glucose to 1 L LRS).
  5. The glucose concentration of the dialysate is based on individual requirements for fluid removal.
    a) For routine dialysis, 1.5% glucose concentrations are used.
    b) For overhydrated animals, 4.25% glucose concentrations are used.
B. Electrolyte composition of dialysate solutions can be altered as needed.
  1. Commercially available polyionic dialysate solutions are recommended (see earlier sources).
  2. Commercial solutions lack potassium, as hyperkalemia is common in oliguric ARF patients.
  3. Potassium may be added to dialysate solutions if hypokalemia occurs.

V. Dialysate dwell time and exchange cycles
A. Acute renal failure
  1. Each cycle should have a 10-minute inflow time, a 30- to 40-minute dialysate dwell time, and a 20- to 30-minute drain time.
  2. For the initial 10–12 cycles following catheter placement, dialysate volumes of 15–20 ml/kg may result in less leakage around the catheter site.
  3. Heparin (100–500 U/L) can be added to the dialysate during the initial sessions to prevent fibrin occlusions of the catheter.
  4. Goals of peritoneal dialysis include the following.
    a) BUN in the 60–100 mg/dl range
    b) Serum creatinine in the 4–6 mg/dl range
    c) Serum potassium, bicarbonate, sodium, and phosphorus within normal ranges
  5. Initial dialysis is likely to extend beyond 48 hours; check serum electrolytes, urea nitrogen, and creatinine every 12–24 hours. Dialysate volumes of 30–40 ml/kg can be used after the initial 10–12 cycles.
  6. Following the initial 24–48 exchanges, progressive increases in dwell time to 3–6 hours are indicated.
B. Continuous ambulatory peritoneal dialysis (CAPD)
  1. Dialysate can remain in the peritoneal cavity for 3–6 hours.
  2. Three or four exchanges are performed daily.

Technique

I. Peritoneal dialysis catheter
A. An indwelling catheter is recommended because of the repeated dialysate exchanges.
B. Ideal catheters have the following characteristics.
  1. Efficient fluid inflow and outflow
  2. Biocompatibility
  3. Resistance to infection of the subcutaneous tunnel and peritoneal cavity
  4. Little fluid leakage at the peritoneal interface
C. Two major catheter types are available.
  1. Straight tube catheters (Parker peritoneal dialysis cannulas and Tenckhoff catheters)
    a) Advantages
      (1) Relatively inexpensive
      (2) Can usually be inserted with local anesthesia
    b) Disadvantages
      (1) Catheter holes easily plugged with fibrin and omentum, causing fluid outflow obstruction
      (2) Greater potential for dialysate leakage at catheter placement site
  2. Column disk catheters (Lifecath, Quinton Instrument Co., Seattle, WA)
    a) Advantages
      (1) Less prone to outflow obstruction
      (2) Less prone to leakage at catheter site
    b) Disadvantages
      (1) Expensive but can be resterilized and reused
      (2) Usually requires general anesthesia and surgery to insert

II. Dialysis procedure (Cowgill, 1995)
A. Weigh the animal.
B. Warm the dialysate solution to 2–3° F above the animal's body temperature.
C. Infuse the desired volume of dialysate into the abdomen.
  1. Follow strict aseptic technique to prevent infection.

a) Sterile gloves with surgical cap and mask
b) Thorough scrubbing of tubing connections with povidone-iodine (Betadine) before disconnecting and reconnecting
2. If possible, do not disconnect the empty bag during the dwell time.
D. Allow the dialysate to remain in the abdomen for the desired period of time.
E. Drain fluid out of the abdomen into the original bag.
F. Measure the volume of fluid recovered.
G. Reweigh the animal.
H. Repeat the cycle at the desired frequency.
I. Dialysis is continued until the animal is producing normal volumes of urine.

III. Problems and complications
A. Catheter insertion problems (most commonly associated with straight tube catheters)
1. Penetration of bowel or urinary bladder
2. Laceration of a major vessel
B. Paracatheter fluid leakage
C. Catheter failure
1. The most common problem
2. Characterized by an inability to retrieve all the infused fluid
3. Corrective measures
a) Flush the catheter rapidly with 20 ml heparinized saline in an attempt to dislodge blood and/or fibrin clots and omentum.
b) Reposition the animal.
c) Try to reposition the catheter within the abdomen by external manipulation.
d) Placement of a new catheter may be necessary.
D. Peritonitis: Septic and aseptic peritonitis are common complications but are not necessarily indications to stop dialysis.
1. Diagnosis
a) Systemic signs (e.g., fever, abdominal pain, vomiting) may or may not be present.
b) Retrieved dialysate has a cloudy appearance.
c) Analysis of retrieved dialysate shows large numbers of neutrophils; bacteria may also be observed.
d) Bacterial culture and sensitivity are performed on the retrieved dialysate.
2. Prevention
a) Flush abdomen with 1 L of normal saline once daily.
b) Instill a saline-iodine solution (0.2 ml of 2% iodine USP in 1 L of saline) for 4 minutes and then drain (Thornhill, 1983).
3. Treatment
a) Dialysis can usually be continued.
b) Systemic and intraperitoneal antibiotic treatment is based on bacterial culture and sensitivity of the retrieved dialysate.
(1) Cephalothin is given as a loading dose of 1 g/L of dialysate, followed by a maintenance dose of 250 mg/L of dialysate.
(2) Aminoglycoside is given as a loading dose of 4 mg/kg IM, followed by a maintenance dose of 6 mg/L of dialysate (Thornhill, 1983).
(3) Heparin (500 U/L) is added to the dialysate to prevent fibrin occlusion of the catheter.
c) Treatment should be continued for 10–14 days.
d) If after 96 hours of aggressive treatment no clinical improvement occurs, the peritoneal access catheter should be removed.
E. Hypoalbuminemia
1. This occurs as a result of the relative permeability of albumin to the peritoneal membrane.
2. The rate of albumin loss is accelerated with peritonitis.
F. Pleural effusion
1. May develop associated with the combination of overhydration and hypoalbuminemia
2. May necessitate occasional thoracocentesis

Patient Monitoring

I. Hydration status: animal weighed before and after each exchange
II. Electrolytes, acid–base, osmolality, and renal function
A. With acute dialysis, serum urea nitrogen, creatinine, sodium, potassium, chloride, blood gases, and osmolality are measured at least twice daily.
B. With chronic dialysis, the parameters in (A) are measured daily for the first 3–4 days, then every other day if values remain stable.
C. Patients with end-stage renal disease that are being dialyzed at home with CAPD are monitored at least every 2 weeks.
III. Exchange volumes
A. These volumes are recorded at each retrieval.
B. Dialysate volume retrieved should be at least 90% of the volume infused (with the exception of the first few exchanges, when only 25–50% of the infused volume is recovered). The remaining volume is termed priming fluid.
C. With the exception noted in (B), never continue to infuse dialysate if the previous exchange volume has not been recovered. Respiratory and overhydration problems may result.

HEMODIALYSIS

Scott A. Brown

Definition

Use of artificial kidney for extracorporeal countercurrent flow of dialysate and blood to remove solutes from the bloodstream.

Uses

I. In chronic renal failure as an intermittent supplement to remove accumulated uremic toxins in animals with marginal renal function
II. Maintain animal with acute renal failure for 30–60

days to allow for compensatory hyperfunction to restore adequate renal function to sustain life

III. Remove toxin (e.g., ethylene glycol) following acute exposure

Disadvantages

I. Requires vascular access, artificial kidney, and sophisticated hemodialysis delivery system

II. Not generally available to veterinary practitioners except at specialized referral hospitals

III. Complications associated with the dialysis period more likely

Advantages

I. For some solutes, exchange is improved.

II. Relatively normal interdialytic period (up to 7 days) is possible with use of intensive intermittent hemodialysis in patients with marginal renal function.

RENAL TRANSPLANTATION

Scott A. Brown

Definition

I. Kidney from an unrelated donor animal is placed in a recipient (allograft).

II. A matched allograft shares similar cell surface antigens with the recipient's cells.

III. Rejection is graft destruction by the recipient's immune system.
  A. Acute rejection occurs 1–2 weeks after transplantation.
  B. Chronic rejection occurs over months to years.

Patient Selection

I. Cats with end-stage renal failure that are stable and nonuremic
  A. Acute rejection is uncommon in cats.
  B. Allograft may survive for 1–4 years, and the quality of life during this time is generally good to excellent (Gregory, 1995).
  C. Immunosuppressive therapy with cyclosporine is required. Because of variable gut absorption, trough levels of cyclosporine must be measured on a periodic basis.

II. Dogs with end-stage renal failure that are stable and nonuremic
  A. Acute rejection episodes are common in dogs.
  B. Allograft rarely survives for 6 months.
  C. Immunosuppressive therapy and intensive medical management are required.
    1. This generally involves combination therapy with cyclosporine, corticosteroids, azathioprine, and/or antilymphocytic sera.
    2. Because of variable gut absorption, trough levels of cyclosporine must be measured.
  D. Renal transplantation in dogs is not a practical alternative at this time, but newer immunosuppressive agents and antilymphocyte globulin hold promise for the future.

Donor Selection

I. The donor must be a healthy adult with normal complete blood count, urinalysis, and biochemical panel; negative urine culture; and kidneys that appear normal on excretory urography.

II. Recipient cats should be negative for feline leukemia and immunodeficiency viruses and free of oxalate urolithiasis and urinary tract infection.

III. A cross-matched allograft is used, especially in dogs.

IV. Unilateral nephrectomy poses no known long-term risk to the donor.

Treatment and Monitoring

I. The surgery is performed at referral centers with considerable experience in the procedure.

II. Intensive long-term follow-up is required.
  A. Serial urinalyses
  B. Serial BUN and creatinine determinations
  C. Evaluation of patient for development of complications, including infections secondary to immunosuppression
  D. Serial blood cyclosporine determinations

Complications

I. Acute rejection
  A. It is characterized by depression, fever, and vomiting.
  B. No change in serum creatinine occurs until very late in the rejection process.
  C. Treatment is adjustment of the immunosuppressive regimen.

II. Infections
  A. Urinary tract infections may occur, and treatment is dictated by urine culture and sensitivity testing.
  B. Fungal infections may occur in association with high plasma concentrations of cyclosporine.
  C. In cats, viral upper respiratory infections may develop and are treated with supportive therapy.

III. Ureteral obstruction at site of implantation
  A. It most often occurs 1–2 weeks postoperatively.
  B. It requires corrective surgery.

NEPHROLITHS

Scott A. Brown

Definition

I. Presence of calculus within the kidney

II. Prevalence of different mineral types (Ling, 1995; Osborne et al., 1995)
  A. Male dogs: struvite (38%), calcium oxalate (33%), urate (33%), calcium phosphate (32%), silica (9%), cystine (1%)
  B. Female dogs: struvite (58%), calcium phosphate (38%), calcium oxalate (35%), urate (12%), silica (5%)
  C. Cats (male and female): calcium oxalate (73%), calcium phosphate (34%), struvite (6%), urate (1%)

Pathophysiology

I. Diet, breed, and intercurrent disease (e.g., infection) lead to predisposition to mineral type.
   A. Struvite nephroliths are associated with pyelonephritis.
   B. Urate nephroliths are more common in dalmatians and animals with a portosystemic shunt.
   C. Dogs with a renal defect for cystine reabsorption are predisposed to formation of cystine uroliths.
II. Nephroliths often do not interfere with kidney function but may serve as a nidus for bacterial infection.

Clinical Signs

I. Hematuria
II. Flank pain
III. Evidence of azotemia: elevated BUN and/or creatinine inconsistently present
IV. Evidence of urinary tract infection (e.g., pollakiuria, stranguria) or secondary nidus of infection (e.g., diskospondylitis)
V. Evidence of intercurrent disease: hepatoencephalopathy in dogs with portosystemic shunting and urate nephroliths

Diagnosis

I. Radiographic and/or ultrasonographic studies
   A. Identify presence, site, and extent of calculus.
   B. Entire tract must be studied to determine whether stones are present in multiple sites.
   C. Excretory urography assists in determining patency of urinary tract.
   D. Ultrasonography may help identify nephroliths and characterize accompanying kidney disease.
II. Evaluation of renal function and structure
   A. Measure serum urea nitrogen and creatinine.
   B. If nephrectomy or nephrotomy is contemplated, kidneys should be assessed by dye excretion during excretory urography or (preferably) individual renal scintigrams.
   C. Perform a urinalysis and culture to detect urinary tract infection that may be primary (struvite) or secondary (any mineral type).

Differential Diagnosis

I. Traumatic renal injury
II. Renal neoplasia
III. Pyelonephritis
IV. Dystrophic or metastatic renal mineralization

Treatment

I. Surgical removal may be required in some cases.
   A. Nephrolithotomy, pyelolithotomy, or nephrectomy can be used.
   B. Surgery significantly compromises the function of the affected kidney in the short run and (possibly) also in the long run.
   C. With bilateral nephroliths, staged unilateral procedures 2–4 weeks apart are preferred.

D. Perform quantitative stone analysis of any retrieved calculi.
II. Lithotripsy is stone fragmentation by application of external forces.
   A. Principal advantages are as follows.
      1. More rapid dissolution than medical therapy
      2. Less patient risk than surgery
      3. May produce less short-term and long-term renal injury than nephrotomy
   B. Shock-wave lithotripsy has frequently been used for nephroliths in people but has rarely been applied to animals.
III. Medical management involves the following.
   A. It may be the best alternative in patients with a patent urinary tract and preexisting renal disease when there is a clear suspicion of mineral type (see Chap. 49).
   B. For struvite nephroliths, institute the following.
      1. Eradicate urinary tract infection, if present.
      2. Feed an acidifying diet that is low in protein, phosphate, and magnesium, with dietary sodium supplementation to promote diuresis.
      3. It may take many months to a year for the stone to dissolve.
   C. Treatment of urate nephroliths is as follows.
      1. Eradicate urinary tract infection, if present.
      2. Correct portosystemic shunt, if present.
      3. In dogs without shunts, feed a diet that is low in protein and purine content and is also alkalinizing.
      4. Administer allopurinol 10 mg/kg/day PO to dalmatians; use with caution if hepatic disease is present.
      5. It may require many months to a year for stone dissolution.
   D. Calcium oxalate nephroliths cannot be effectively dissolved by medical therapy.

Patient Monitoring

I. Radiographic or other imaging studies at 2- to 6-month intervals to assess size and recurrence of nephrolith
II. Serial serum urea nitrogen and creatinine determinations
III. Urinalysis and urine culture every 3 months until stone dissolved

RENAL NEOPLASIA

Gregory F. Grauer

Definition

I. Primary renal neoplasia is rare in the dog and cat, accounting for <2.5% and 1.7% of all tumors in dogs and cats, respectively.
II. Most primary renal tumors in dogs (85%) are epithelial in origin, and over 90% are malignant (Klein et al., 1988).
III. The following tumor types and incidence were ob-

served in a retrospective review of 54 canine primary renal neoplasms (Klein et al., 1988).
   A. Renal carcinoma, 69%
   B. Transitional cell carcinoma, 9%
   C. Renal adenoma and papilloma, 7%
   D. Sarcoma, 7%
   E. Nephroblastoma, 4%
   F. Lymphoma, 2%
   G. Fibroma, 2%
IV. Lymphoma is the most common renal tumor in the cat, but controversy exists as to whether feline renal lymphoma is a primary disease process.
V. Renal cell carcinomas (40%) and nephroblastomas (20%) are the most common nonlymphoma feline renal tumors.
VI. Metastatic renal tumors are more common than primary tumors (Hammer and LaRue, 1995) and may occur through hematogenous or lymphatic routes or by direct extension from nearby organs (e.g., adrenal gland neoplasia).
   A. Osteosarcoma
   B. Hemangiosarcoma
   C. Lymphoma
   D. Mast cell tumor
   E. Melanoma
   F. Lung, mammary, and gastrointestinal carcinomas

Causes

I. The cause of canine primary renal tumors is unknown.
II. Cats with renal lymphoma test positive for feline leukemia virus (FeLV) about 50% of the time.
III. Renal cystadenocarcinoma appears to be inherited in an autosomal dominant manner in the German shepherd dog (Lium and Moe, 1985).

Pathophysiology

I. Benign neoplasia
   A. Approximately 10% of primary renal tumors in dogs are benign.
   B. Adenomas, papillomas of transitional cells, lipomas, hemangiomas, fibromas, and hamartomas have been reported.
II. Renal cell carcinomas (renal adenocarcinoma, hypernephroma, Grawitz's tumor)
   A. Arise from tubular epithelial cells
   B. Occur in middle-aged and older dogs (7–9 years)
   C. More common in male than in female dogs
   D. Right and left kidneys at equal risk
   E. Invasion and destruction of the entire kidney common
   F. Extrarenal invasion of surrounding epaxial muscles, adrenal gland, and vena cava common
   G. Metastasize to lungs (30% at time of diagnosis), contralateral kidney, skin, lymph nodes, liver, spleen, heart, brain, bone, and eyes
III. Multifocal cystadenocarcinomas
   A. Can be accompanied by nodular dermatofibrosis and uterine leiomyomas

   B. Reported only in German shepherd dogs (Lium and Moe, 1985)
IV. Nephroblastoma (embryonal nephroma, Wilms' tumor, embryonal nephroblastoma)
   A. It is believed to arise from nephrogenic mesenchyma.
   B. The tumor is composed of metanephric blastoma, stroma, and epithelial derivatives at various stages of differentiation.
   C. 60% of reported cases occur in dogs <1 year of age.
   D. It may occur in older dogs, perhaps as a result of malignant transformation of nests of renal tissue with embryonal potential.
   E. The tumor may grow to a large size, resulting in abdominal distention.
   F. Metastatic disease occurs about 65% of the time.
V. Renal transitional cell carcinomas
   A. Arise from tissue in the renal pelvis
   B. Locally invasive and can result in urine outflow obstruction
   C. Increased incidence in male dogs
VI. Renal lymphoma
   A. Renal involvement is often associated with alimentary or multicentric lymphosarcoma.
   B. Bilateral renal involvement is common.
   C. 50% of cats are FeLV positive.
   D. Renal lymphoma also occurs in dogs.

Clinical Signs

I. Many dogs do not have clinical signs referable to the urinary tract.
   A. Depression, inappetence
   B. Weight loss
   C. Abdominal distention
   D. Less commonly, vomiting and fever
II. Classic signs of renal neoplasia are less commonly observed.
   A. Abdominal mass
   B. Renal/lumbar pain
   C. Hematuria
III. Paraneoplastic syndromes may be detected.
   A. Anemia: chronic disease, destruction of erythropoietin sources, blood loss
   B. Azotemia: destruction of renal tissue
   C. Hypertrophic osteopathy
   D. Polycythemia: increased production of erythropoietin, tumor-induced renal hypoxia
   E. Polydipsia/polyuria: destruction of renal tissue, polycythemia
   F. Leukocytosis: tumor necrosis and inflammation
   G. Cancer cachexia
IV. Multiple skin nodules occur on the head, neck, and extremities with cystadenocarcinomas.

Diagnosis

I. Suspicious physical examination and laboratory findings
   A. Enlarged kidneys/cranial abdominal mass
   B. Renal/lumbar pain

C. Hematuria: microscopic or macroscopic

D. Neoplastic renal tubular cells in the urine sediment (rare)

E. Cytology of fine-needle aspirates (lymphoma)

II. Imaging techniques

  A. Plain radiographs

  B. Excretory urography

  C. Ultrasonography

III. Histopathology necessary for definitive diagnosis

Differential Diagnosis

I. Other causes of renomegaly: hydronephrosis, polycystic kidneys, perinephric and renal cysts, abscesses, granulomas

II. Other causes of retroperitoneal or cranial abdominal masses: adrenal, pancreatic, ovarian, hepatic neoplasia; retroperitoneal hemangiosarcoma

Treatment

I. Nephroureterectomy is the treatment of choice for unilateral, nonmetastatic renal tumors.

  A. Rule out pulmonary metastasis with thoracic radiographs. Consider ultrasonography or computed tomography (CT) to rule out abdominal metastasis.

  B. Evaluate contralateral kidney function by excretory urography or nuclear medicine scans prior to nephrectomy.

  C. Surgical recommendations involve the following.

    1. Ligation of the renal artery and vein as soon as possible

    2. Complete removal of kidney and ureter

    3. Removal of as much perirenal fat as possible

    4. Excision of all regional lymph nodes

    5. Histologic evaluation of all tissues

II. Chemotherapy and radiation therapy may be tried (see Chap. 70).

Patient Monitoring

I. If metastasis or vascular invasion has occurred, the prognosis is poor.

II. Following nephrectomy, mean survival time in dogs is 6–12 months (Klein et al., 1988).

TRAUMATIC DISORDERS

Scott A. Brown

Definition

I. A renal contusion is a bruise resulting from external compression with intraparenchymal disruption of blood vessels and associated hemorrhage. If severe, crushing injuries can disrupt the function of tubular elements and/or large vascular structures.

II. Lacerations occur when there is gross tearing of renal parenchyma.

III. In some cases, an extensive laceration may sever the renal artery, vein, and/or ureter, causing an injury referred to as avulsion of the renal pedicle.

Causes

I. Severe blunt trauma: automobile accident

II. Sharp, penetrating wound

Pathophysiology

I. Renal contusions are usually self-limiting and generally inapparent unless hematuria is observed.

II. Crushing injury from severe blunt trauma or penetrating injury to the renal pedicle or parenchyma may lead to significant hemorrhage, disruption of renal parenchyma, and/or urine leakage.

III. Lacerations or pedicle avulsions can lead to marked hemorrhage and/or dysfunction of a substantial portion of the affected kidney(s).

Clinical Signs

I. History or evidence of trauma is present in most but not all animals.

II. Hematuria is often present.

  A. It may be marked.

  B. It may be missed in some animals.

III. Signs of hypovolemia may be present in cases of severe, acute blood loss.

IV. Flank pain may be present from intracapsular renal parenchymal swelling or local accumulation of blood or urine.

  A. Urine accumulation, if sterile, generally produces only mild irritation.

  B. Animal may present with marked abdominal distention from uroperitoneum.

V. Uremia can occur with urine leakage or with bilateral renal parenchymal injuries.

Diagnosis

I. History of trauma is suggestive.

II. Detectable retroperitoneal or abdominal mass, especially if progressively enlarging, can be evidence of blood or urine extravasation.

III. Abdominal radiography is required.

  A. Plain radiographs are rarely diagnostic, but the following may be observed.

    1. Poor visualization or abnormal position of renal shadow

    2. Retroperitoneal mass

    3. Loss of intra-abdominal contrast

  B. Excretory urography usually identifies extravasation of contrast material and generally indicates the site of rupture of the kidneys.

    1. Nonvisualization of one kidney or poor visualization of both kidneys may indicate the presence of poor renal function (preexisting renal failure) or systemic hypotension.

    2. Excretory urography also identifies trauma to other areas of the urinary tract.

IV. Ultrasonography may be helpful in evaluating certain

renal injuries with hematoma formation or in identifying intravesicular blood clots.

V. Abdominal paracentesis and fluid analysis are often helpful. With urine leakage into the abdomen, the creatinine concentration in abdominal fluid, when compared with that in simultaneously obtained plasma, is usually several-fold greater.

Differential Diagnosis

I. Traumatic injury to other abdominal organs
II. Renal neoplasia with secondary disruption of renal tubular and vascular elements

Treatment

I. With the exception of life-threatening hemorrhage, injuries to the kidney should not receive priority over emergency therapy of cardiorespiratory abnormalities.
II. Appropriate therapy is dependent on the type and site of injury.
III. Prior to any surgical therapy, thorough evaluation of the integrity of the entire urinary tract should be performed using radiographic studies.

Patient Monitoring

I. Abdominal radiographic or ultrasonographic studies
II. Serial evaluation of mucous membranes, hematocrit, and/or blood pressure level to assess the severity of blood loss
III. Serial BUN and/or creatinine determinations to assess adequacy of renal function

Bibliography

Adams L, Polzin DJ, Osborne CA et al: Influence of dietary protein/calorie intake on renal morphology and function in cats with 5/6 nephrectomy. Lab Invest 70:347, 1994

Barsanti JA, Finco DR, Brown SA: Disease of the lower urinary tract. p. 1769. In Sherding RG (ed): The Cat: Diseases and Clinical Management. 2nd Ed. Churchill Livingstone, New York, 1994

Bernard MA, Valli VE: Familial renal disease in Samoyed dogs. Can Vet J 18:181, 1977

Bowles MH, Mosier DA: Renal amyloidosis in a family of beagles. J Am Vet Med Assoc 201:569, 1992

Boyce JT, DiBartola SP, Chew DJ, Gasper PW: Familial renal amyloidosis in Abyssinian cats. Vet Pathol 21:33, 1984

Brinker KR, Bulger RE, Dolgan DC et al: Effect of potassium depletion on gentamicin nephrotoxicity. J Lab Clin Med 98:292, 1981

Broughton ES, Scarnell J: Prevention of renal carriage of leptospirosis in dogs by vaccination. Vet Rec 117:307, 1985

Brown CA, Crowell WA, Brown SA et al: Suspected familial renal disease in chow chows. J Am Vet Med Assoc 196:1279, 1990

Brown SA: Fanconi's syndrome. p. 1163. In Kirk RW (ed): Current Vet Therapy X. WB Saunders, Philadelphia, 1989

Brown SA: Canine renal disease. p. 313. In Wills J, Simpson K (eds): The Waltham Book of Clinical Nutrition of the Dog & Cat. Elsevier Ltd., Oxford, 1994

Brown SA: Primary diseases of glomeruli. p. 368. In Osborne CA, Finco DR (eds): Canine and Feline Nephrology and Urology. Williams & Wilkins, Baltimore, 1995a

Brown SA: Reassessment of the use of calcitriol in chronic renal failure. p. 963. In Kirk RW, Bonagura JD (eds): Current Vet Therapy XII: Small Animal Practice. WB Saunders, Philadelphia, 1995b

Brown SA, Finco DR, Crowell WA, et al: Single-nephron adaptations to partial renal ablation in the dog. Am J Physiol 258:F495, 1990

Brown SA, Prestwood AK: Parasites of the urinary tract. p. 1153. In Kirk RW (ed): Current Veterinary Therapy IX: Small Animal Practice. WB Saunders, Philadelphia, 1986

Center S, Smith C, Wilkinson E et al: Clinicopathologic, renal immunofluorescent, and light microscopic features of glomerulonephritis in the dog: 41 cases (1975–1985). J Am Vet Med Assoc 190:87, 1987

Chew DJ, DiBartola SP, Boyce JT, Gasper PW: Renal amyloidosis in related Abyssinian cats. J Am Vet Med Assoc 181:139, 1982

Cook SM, Lothrop CD: Serum erythropoietin concentrations measured by radioimmunoassay in normal, polycythemic, and anemic dogs and cats. J Vet Intern Med 8:18, 1994

Cowgill LD: Systemic hypertension. p. 360. In Kirk RW (ed): Current Veterinary Therapy IX. WB Saunders, Philadelphia, 1986

Cowgill LD: Clinical experience and the use of recombinant human erythropoietin in uremic dogs and cats. Proc Am Coll Vet Intern Med 9:147, 1991

Cowgill LD: Application of peritoneal dialysis and hemodialysis in the management of renal failure. p. 573. In Osborne CA, Finco DR (eds): Canine and Feline Nephrologoy and Urology. Williams & Wilkins, Baltimore, 1995

Cowgill LD, Kallet AJ: Recognition and management of hypertension in the dog. p. 1025. In Kirk RW (ed): Current Veterinary Therapy VIII. WB Saunders, Philadelphia, 1983

Crowell WA, Neuwirth L, Mahaffey MB: Pyelonephritis. p. 484. In Osborne CA, Finco DR (eds): Canine and Feline Nephrology and Urology. Williams & Wilkins, Baltimore, 1995

Diamond JR, Karnovsky MJ: Focal and segmental glomerulosclerosis: analogies to atherosclerosis. Kidney Int 33:917, 1988

DiBartola SP, Benson MD: The pathogenesis of reactive systemic amyloidosis. J Vet Intern Med 3:31, 1989

DiBartola SP, Tarr MJ, Parker AT et al: Clinicopathologic findings in dogs with renal amyloidosis: 59 cases (1976–1986). J Am Vet Med Assoc 195:358, 1989

DiBartola SP, Tarr MJ, Webb DM, Giger U: Familial renal amyloidosis in Chinese shar-pei dogs. J Am Vet Med Assoc 197:483, 1990

Finco DR, Brown SA, Crowell WA et al: Effects of phosphorous/calcium-restricted and phosphorous/calcium-replete 32% protein diets in dogs with chronic renal failure. Am J Vet Res 53:157, 1992a

Finco DR, Brown SA, Crowell WA et al: Effects of dietary phosphorus and protein in dogs with chronic renal failure. Am J Vet Res 53:2264, 1992b

Gaber L, Walton C, Brown S, Bakris G: Effects of antihypertensive agents on the morphologic progression of diabetic nephropathy in dogs. Kidney Int 46:161, 1994

Gertz MA: Secondary amyloidosis (AA). J Intern Med 232:517, 1988

Grauer GF: Glomerulonephritis. Semin Vet Med Surg (Small Anim) 7:187, 1992

Grauer GF, DiBartola SP: Glomerular disease. p. 1760. In Ettinger SJ, Feldman EC (eds): Textbook of Veterinary Internal Medicine. 4th Ed. WB Saunders, Philadelphia, 1995

Grauer GF, Greco DS, Behrend EN et al: Effects of dietary protein conditioning on gentamicin-induced nephrotoxicosis in healthy male dogs. Am J Vet Res 55:90, 1994

Grauer GF, Greco DS, Behrend EN et al: Estimation of quantitative enzymuria in dogs with gentamicin-induced nephrotoxicosis using urine enzyme/creatinine ratios from spot urine samples. J Vet Intern Med 9:324, 1995

Grauer GF, Lane IF: Acute renal failure. p. 1720. In Ettinger SJ, Feldman EC (eds): Textbook of Veterinary Internal Medicine. 4th Ed. WB Saunders, Philadelphia, 1995

Greco DS, Turnwald GH, Adams R et al: Urinary gamma-glutamyl transpeptidase activity in dogs with gentamicin-induced nephrotoxicity. Am J Vet Res 46:2332, 1985

Green R, Kabel A: Hypercoagulable state in 3 dogs with nephrotic syndrome: role of acquired antithrombin III deficiency. J Am Vet Med Assoc 181:914, 1982

Greene CE: Bacterial diseases. p. 367. In Ettinger SJ, Feldman EC (eds): Textbook of Veterinary Internal Medicine. 4th Ed. WB Saunders, Philadelphia, 1995

Gregory CR: Clinical renal transplantation. p. 597. In Osborne CA, Finco DR (eds): Canine and Feline Nephrology and Urology. Williams & Wilkins, Baltimore, 1995

Grodecki K, Gaines M, Jacobs R et al: ACE inhibitor treatment of chronic renal failure in a canine model of hereditary nephritis. Vet Pathol 32:555, 1995

Hammer AS, LaRue S: Tumors of the urinary tract. p. 1788. In Ettinger SJ, Feldman EC (eds): Textbook of Veterinary Internal Medicine. 4th Ed. WB Saunders, Philadelphia, 1995

Jansen B, Valli V, Thorner P et al: Samoyed hereditary glomerulopathy: serial, clinical and laboratory (urine, serum biochemistry and hematology) studies. Can J Vet Res 51:387, 1987

Jones BR, Gething MA, Badcoe LM et al: Familial progressive nephropathy in young bull terriers. N Z Vet J 37:79, 1989

Klein MK, Cockerell GL, Harris CK et al: Canine primary renal neoplasms: a retrospective review of 54 cases. J Am Anim Hosp Assoc 24:443, 1988

Ling GV: Nephrolithiasis: prevalence of mineral type. p. 980. In Kirk RW, Bonagura JD (eds): Current Veterinary Therapy XII: Small Animal Practice. WB Saunders, Philadelphia, 1995

Littman MP: Spontaneous systemic hypertension in 24 cats. J Vet Intern Med 8:79, 1994

Lium B, Moe L: Hereditary multifocal renal cystadenocarcinomas and nodular dermatofibrosis in the German shepherd dog: macroscopic and histopathologic changes. Vet Pathol 22:447, 1985

Majeed HA, Barakat M: Familial Mediterranean fever (recurrent polyserositis) in children: analysis of 88 cases. Eur J Pediatr 148:636, 1989

Morgan RV: Systemic hypertension in four cats: ocular and medical findings. J Am Anim Hosp Assoc 22:615, 1986

Nagode LA, Chew DJ: Nephrocalcinosis caused by hyperparathyroidism in progression of renal failure: treatment with calcitriol. Semin Vet Med Surg (Small Anim) 7:202, 1992

Nash A: Familial renal disease in dogs. J Small Anim Pract 30:178, 1989

Neuwirth L, Mahaffey M, Crowell W et al: Comparison of excretory urography and ultrasonography for detection of experimentally-induced pyelonephritis in dogs. Am J Vet Res 54:660, 1993

Osborne CA, Unger L, Lulich JP: Canine and feline nephroliths. p. 981. In Kirk RW, Bonagura JD (eds): Current Veterinary Therapy XII: Small Animal Practice. WB Saunders, Philadelphia, 1995

Rentko VT, Clark N, Ross LA, Schelling SH: Canine leptospirosis: a retrospective study of 17 cases. J Vet Intern Med 6:235, 1992

Reusche VT, Liehs M, Bren G: A new familial membranoproliferative glomerulonephritis in Bernese mountain dogs. J Vet Intern Med 6:120, 1992

Riviere JE, Carver MP, Coppoc GL et al: Pharmacokinetics and comparative nephrotoxicity of fixed-dose versus fixed-interval reduction of gentamicin dosage in subtotal nephrectomized dogs. Toxicol Appl Pharmacol 75:496, 1984

Ross LA, Finco DR, Crowell WA: Effect of dietary phosphorus restriction on the kidneys of cats with reduced renal mass. Am J Vet Res 43:1023, 1982

Snyder PS: Canine hypertensive disease. Compend Contin Educ Pract Vet 13:1785, 1991

Snyder PS, Henik RA: Feline systemic hypertension. Proc Am Coll Vet Intern Med 12:126, 1994

Songer JG, Thiermann AB: Leptospirosis. J Am Vet Med Assoc 193:1250, 1988

Thornhill JA: Peritonitis associated with peritoneal dialysis: diagnosis and treatment. J Am Vet Med Assoc 182:721, 1983

Vaden SL, Breitschwerdt EB, Armstrong PJ et al: The effects of cyclosporin versus standard care in dogs with naturally occurring glomerulonephritis. J Vet Intern Med 9:259, 1995

Wilcock B, Patterson J: Familial glomerulonephritis in Doberman pinscher dogs. Can Vet J 20:244, 1979

48

Diseases of the Ureter

Jody P. Lulich
Carl A. Osborne

CONGENITAL ABNORMALITIES

Ectopic Ureter

Definition and Cause

I. Ectopic ureters occur when one or both ureters fail to terminate normally in the trigone of the urinary bladder.
II. They arise from an abnormal origin or sustained migration of the embryonic ureter before inserting into the urogenital tract.

Pathophysiology

I. Normal ureters enter the dorsolateral caudal serosal surface of the urinary bladder, obliquely traverse the bladder wall, and terminate at the trigone.
II. Intramural ectopic ureters enter the serosal surface of the bladder wall at its normal site and continue through the wall past the trigone to terminate in the urethra or vagina.
  A. They open at the trigone, but also continue and open at a second more distal site.
  B. Ureteral troughs are intramural ectopic ureters that continue beyond the trigone as an incomplete structure (trough).
  C. Ureters without a terminal orifice may be associated with hydroureter and hydronephrosis.
III. Extramural ureters bypass the bladder wall and enter into the urethra, vagina, or uterus.
  A. Common in cats
  B. Less commonly recognized in dogs
IV. Associated conditions include ureteral ectasia, urogenital tract infection (pyelonephritis, ureteritis, cystitis, urethritis, vaginitis), impaired renal function, primary urethral incompetence, bladder hypoplasia, hydronephrosis, and vaginal pooling of urine.

Clinical Signs

I. Clinical signs associated with ectopic ureters depend on their site of termination and on the presence of other congenital and acquired abnormalities.
II. Urinary incontinence is the most commonly recognized clinical sign; it is usually detected at the time of weaning.
III. The severity of incontinence may vary.
  A. Constant dribbling
    1. More common in females than males
    2. More common in dogs than cats
    3. Common with ureters that terminate in the vagina
    4. Typical with ureters that terminate in more distal portions of the urethra
    5. Also associated with defects in urethral sphincter competence
  B. Intermittent incontinence
    1. It may also be associated with vaginal pooling of urine that gravitates out of the vagina with changes in body position.
    2. In males, the longer urethra and strong external sphincter control may account for the intermittent nature of incontinence.
    3. Some animals with constant dribbling may exhibit intermittent incontinence following pharmacologic management to increase urethral sphincter tone.
  C. Perineal (perivulvar) fur often stained by urine
  D. Perineal urine scald dermatitis
IV. The normal voiding phase of micturition is usually present. Even with bilateral ectopic ureters, sufficient urine usually refluxes to fill the bladder, although bladder capacity may be reduced.
V. Progressive destruction of renal parenchyma of the associated kidney may occur as a result of ascending infection and may be associated with progressive decrease in function as the kidney becomes sclerotic.
VI. Urinary incontinence may be absent on the rare occasion that the ectopic ureter has no distal orifice.

Diagnosis

I. Suspicious clinical signs
   A. Recognition of urinary incontinence at an early age
   B. Urine-stained perineum
   C. Signs of renal failure and sepsis with bilateral generalized renal infection
II. Urinalysis results
   A. Nonlocalizing inflammation
   B. May have evidence of pyuria and hematuria
   C. Loss of concentrating ability with development of renal failure
III. Bacterial urine culture results
   A. Bacterial urinary tract infections are commonly associated with ectopic ureters in dogs.
   B. Ectopic ureters are not common underlying causes for bacterial infection in cats.
IV. Radiography
   A. Knowledge of exact sites of ectopic ureter termination and concomitant urinary tract abnormalities has prognostic and therapeutic significance.
   B. Survey abdominal films are usually normal.
   C. Contrast procedures provide the best visualization of urinary tract anatomy.
   D. Contrast urethrocystograms and vaginograms can be used to assess ureter termination sites.
   E. Excretory urography is also useful but may be associated with poor visualization if the ureter is not dilated, if there is poor excretion of contrast medium as a result of reduced kidney function, or if there is interference caused by concomitant accumulation of contrast medium in the ureter and urinary bladder.
   F. A combination of procedures may be most helpful.
      1. Simultaneous pneumocystography can reduce interference resulting from accumulation of contrast medium in bladder.
      2. Fluoroscopy can be used to follow progressive antegrade or retrograde filling of the urinary tract with contrast agents.
V. Other tests
   A. Cystoscopy and vaginoscopy are useful in revealing the site of ureter termination and ureteral troughs.
   B. Exploratory celiotomy can also be used to determine the site of ureter termination.
   C. Urethral pressure profiles are used to detect concomitant defects in urethral competence mechanisms.

Differential Diagnosis

I. Urinary incontinence from urethral incompetence
II. Overflow incontinence
III. Partial urethral obstruction

Treatment

I. Medical management of ectopic ureters is not consistently effective in controlling urinary incontinence.

II. Eradicate and control any urinary tract infection (UTI) prior to ureteral surgery.
III. Choice of surgical technique depends on the number of ectopic ureters, their termination sites, the functional status of ureters and kidneys, and the presence of concomitant abnormalities.
   A. Indications favoring reconstructive surgery
      1. Normal function of kidney drained by ectopic ureter
      2. Extravesicular termination of both ureters
      3. Functional capacity of both kidneys reduced
   B. Surgical correction of neostoma in situ (Caywood and Lipowitz, 1989)
      1. This technique is ideal for intramural ectopic ureter.
      2. Without transecting the ureter, urine is diverted into the urinary bladder by creating an opening between the transmural section of ureteral and bladder mucosa.
      3. The segment of ureter distal to neostoma is ligated.
      4. Advantages include the following.
         a) Ureteral blood and nerve supply are preserved.
         b) Postsurgical outflow obstruction is minimized.
         c) Postsurgical vesicoureteral reflux is minimized.
   C. Ureteroneocystotomy (Caywood and Lipowitz, 1989)
      1. Ideal for extramural ectopic ureter
      2. Involves transecting the ectopic ureter near the bladder and reimplanting the ureter through a submucosal antireflux tunnel surgically created in the bladder wall
      3. Considerations
         a) Transecting the ureter may interrupt its blood and nerve supply.
         b) Strictures may form at the anastomosis site.
   D. Ureteral branching distal to trigone (Caywood and Lipowitz, 1989)
      1. Ectopic ureter opens normally at the trigone and at a second site distal to the trigone.
      2. Ureteral segment distal to normal site or termination is ligated.
   E. Closure of ureteral troughs (Caywood and Lipowitz, 1989)
   F. Nephrectomy and ureterectomy
      1. Considered when the associated kidney has generalized and severe irreversible disease
      2. Considered only if contralateral kidney has adequate function to maintain homeostasis

Patient Monitoring

I. Some degree of temporary occlusion of the ureteral lumen at the site of anastomosis is common and is caused by inflammatory swelling of tissues following surgery. It usually persists for several weeks.
II. Urinary incontinence may persist following surgical

correction of ectopic ureters in animals with concomitant primary urethral dysfunction.
   A. It may be controlled by alpha adrenergic agonists (i.e., phenylpropanolamine) alone or in combination with diethylstilbestrol.
   B. Improvement in the animal's urethral pressure profile prior to surgery with alpha adrenergic treatment is a positive prognostic sign.
III. Control of UTI is managed by urine cultures and administration of appropriate antimicrobial drugs.

Ureterocele

Definition

Ureterocele is a cystic dilation of the terminal submucosal segment of the intravesicular ureter.

Causes and Pathophysiology

   I. Most are detected in female dogs.
  II. Development of an acquired ureterocele was reported following surgical correction of an ectopic ureter.
 III. Several different types have been reported.
   A. Orthotopic (simple) ureterocele
     1. Distal ureter orifice is in the normal position.
     2. Ureterocele is located at the trigone of the urinary bladder.
   B. Ectopic ureteroceles are ureteroceles with concomitant ectopic ureter.
 IV. Associated conditions include ureteral ectasia, urogenital tract infection, reduced renal function, and hydronephrosis.

Clinical Signs

   I. Some animals may be asymptomatic.
  II. When present, signs are usually observed in young animals.
   A. Dysuria
   B. Urinary incontinence
   C. Urinary tract infection
 III. As orthotopic ureteroceles enlarge, they can be associated with dysuria and outflow obstruction.
 IV. Ectopic ureteroceles may be associated with urinary incontinence.

Diagnosis

   I. Ureterocele should be considered as a cause of dysuria, urinary incontinence, and recurrent urinary tract infections in young animals.
  II. Radiography is required to confirm the diagnosis.
   A. Survey abdominal films are usually normal.
   B. Contrast radiography (intravenous urogram, retrograde urethrocystography) may reveal a filling defect in the bladder or urethra.
   C. Ultrasonography may reveal cystic structures in the bladder or urethra.
   D. Hydroureter and hydronephrosis may indicate urinary tract obstruction.

Differential Diagnosis

   I. Radiolucent uroliths
  II. Blood clots in the trigone

Treatment

   I. Goals are as follows
   A. Prevent urinary obstruction
   B. Preserve renal function
   C. Control UTI
   D. Control clinical signs
  II. Obstructive orthotopic ureteroceles can be managed by cystoscopy and incision of the ureterocele.
 III. For ectopic ureteroceles, ureterocelectomy and ureteral transplantation are considered if the ipsilateral kidney is functional.
 IV. With severe hydronephrosis, ureteronephrectomy is considered, provided that renal function can be sustained by the contralateral kidney.

Patient Monitoring

   I. Control of UTI is managed by repeated urine cultures and administration of appropriate antimicrobial drugs.
  II. Postsurgical contrast radiography is indicated to evaluate surgical success in the event of continued clinical signs.

VESICOURETERAL REFLUX

Definition

Retrograde flow of urine from the urinary bladder into the ureters and renal pelves

Causes

    I. Vesicoureteral inflammation
   II. Surgical altering of the trigone of the urinary bladder, including urine diversion procedures
  III. Obstruction (mechanical or functional) below the bladder neck
  IV. Ectopic ureters
   V. Ureteral ectasia
  VI. Urinary tract infection
 VII. Urinary bladder compression
   A. Induced micturition and manual compression
   B. Voiding urohydropropulsion
VIII. Urinary bladder overfilling
   A. Retrograde contrast radiography
   B. Retrograde urohydropropulsion

Pathophysiology

   I. Unidirectional flow of urine from the ureters into the bladder associated with the ureterovesical flap valve normally protects the kidneys from contamination by bladder urine.
  II. Factors affecting the functional competence of the ureterovesical valve are as follows.

A. Length of the submucosal (intravesical) segment of the distal ureter
B. Diameter of the intravesical ureter
C. Pliability of the roof of the intravesical portion of the distal ureter that functions as the flap valve
D. Integrity of the detrusor (bladder wall) muscle, which supports the intravesical portion of the ureter
E. Ureteral peristalsis
F. Intraluminal pressures in the ureters and urinary bladder

III. There are several classifications of vesicoureteral reflux.
A. Primary vesicoureteral reflux denotes an intrinsic maldevelopment of the vesicoureteral junction.
   1. Self-resolving primary vesicoureteral reflux has been reported in young dogs (7–12 weeks old).
   2. It is not commonly recognized in older dogs.
   3. It occurs more frequently in females.
B. Secondary vesicoureteral reflux implies an acquired disorder of the vesicoureteral junction.

IV. The following are potential consequences associated with vesicoureteral reflux.
A. Upper urinary tract infection
B. Recurring lower urinary tract infection from prevention of complete bladder emptying
C. Reflux nephropathy
   1. Renal parenchyma is damaged by antigenic proteins derived from the lower urinary tract.
   2. Renal damage may also arise from excessive parenchymal pressures.
   3. Hypertension associated with renal scarring can occur.

Clinical Signs

I. Signs related to secondary renal disease
II. Evidence of renal failure
III. Signs of persistent urinary tract infections

Diagnosis

I. Radiography is needed to confirm the diagnosis.
II. Compression cystourethrography is preferred.
A. The animal is maintained in a light plane of anesthesia.
B. The bladder is filled with a radiocontrast agent.
C. With the animal in lateral recumbency, external pressure is applied to the urinary bladder in an attempt to induce voiding.
D. As voiding of urine begins, the radiograph is taken and evaluated for vesicoureteral reflux.
E. Ideally, the vesicoureteral junction is observed fluoroscopically for reflux of contrast agents.
F. Pharmacologically induced micturition (bethanechol chloride) may provide an alternative to manual expression of the urinary bladder.
III. Other radiographic procedures can be performed.
A. Voiding contrast cystourethrography (Lage, 1992)

B. Maximal distention retrograde cystourethrography
C. Factors affecting results
   1. Anesthetic agent and depth of anesthesia
   2. Patient positioning
   3. Degree of urinary bladder distention
   4. Age of animal
IV. Other diagnostic procedures that may be helpful include cystoscopy and radionuclide cystography (King, 1992).

Treatment

I. The major goals of treatment are to preserve renal function and control UTI.
II. Vesicoureteral reflux may spontaneously resolve in young dogs as they mature.
III. An endoscopic procedure has been used to correct experimentally induced vesicoureteral reflux in dogs (Kohri et al., 1988).
IV. To prevent iatrogenic infection of the upper urinary tract, urine is cultured and bacteriuria eradicated prior to manual compression or bladder distention, if possible. Otherwise, consider periprocedural antimicrobials.

Patient Monitoring

I. Control of UTI is managed by repeated urine cultures and administration of appropriate antimicrobial drugs.
II. Periodic evaluation of serum concentrations of creatinine and urea nitrogen and urine specific gravity is used to detect onset of renal failure.

URETERAL OBSTRUCTION

Definition

I. Obstruction of ureter(s) may be partial or complete and results from a variety of causes.
II. Unilateral obstruction is more common than bilateral.

Causes

I. Intraluminal
A. Ureteroliths
   1. Migrate from kidney
   2. Calcium oxalate and calcium phosphate uroliths: most common
B. Blood clots
   1. Usually associated with severe hematuria
   2. Of greatest concern following acute trauma, especially renal biopsy
C. Fungal bezoar
   1. More common with fungi that form hyphae or pseudohyphae
   2. Examples: *Aspergillus, Candida*
II. Intramural
A. Primary neoplasia
B. Metastatic neoplasia

C. Ectopic ureters with no terminal orifice
III. Extramural
  A. Compression
    1. Prostatic enlargement: inflammation, infection, neoplasia, hypertrophy
    2. Perineal hernia
    3. Uterine stump granuloma
    4. Neoplasia of trigone of the urinary bladder
    5. Neoplasia of other adjacent structures
      a) Adrenals
      b) Pelvis or vertebral column
      c) Lymph nodes
  B. Inadvertent surgical ligation
  C. Ureteral neocystotomy

Pathophysiology

I. Factors influencing outcomes
  A. Degree of obstruction
    1. Most available information pertains to complete obstruction.
    2. Pathophysiology of partial obstruction has not been extensively investigated.
  B. Duration of obstruction and urine flow rate
    1. Longer periods of obstruction are more harmful to kidneys than shorter periods.
    2. Rapid flow rates (polyuria) accentuate renal damage.
II. Effects of obstruction on glomerular filtration rate (GFR)
  A. Increased pressure in Bowman's space opposes glomerular filtration.
  B. Vasoactive mediators as a result of ureteral obstruction tend to decrease GFR.
  C. GFR decreases progressively with duration of complete unilateral ureteral obstruction (Vaughan and Gillenwater, 1971; Yarger and Griffith, 1974)
    1. 43% of normal after 24-hour obstruction
    2. 17% of normal after 1-week obstruction
    3. 14% of normal after 2-week obstruction
    4. 3% of normal after 4-week obstruction
  D. Recovery of GFR depends on duration of unilateral obstruction (Kerr, 1956).
    1. 100% recovery after 1-week obstruction
    2. 70% recovery after 2-week obstruction
    3. 30% recovery after 4-week obstruction
    4. 0% recovery after 7-week obstruction
    5. Time for maximum recovery: 26 weeks
  E. Complete bilateral obstruction may rapidly lead to death from uremia and its complications.
III. Effects of obstruction on tubular function
  A. Postobstructive diuresis
    1. The ability of the kidney to concentrate urine is markedly impaired, while the ability to dilute urine is less affected.
    2. Impaired concentrating ability results from the following.
      a) Increased medullary blood flow and medullary solute washout
      b) Impaired response of collecting ducts to antidiuretic hormone

      c) Initial diuresis attributed to homeostatic mechanisms designed to resolve systemic positive balance in water, electrolytes and nitrogenous waste
  B. Impaired distal tubule proton (acid) excretion
  C. Increased fractional excretion of potassium, even with concomitant development of hypokalemia
IV. Renal and ureteral structural changes
  A. Mild hydroureter and hydronephrosis may not be noted with acute obstruction.
  B. Hydroureter and hydronephrosis are often the result of chronic partial or unilateral complete obstruction.
  C. Unilateral obstruction is associated with compensatory hypertrophy of the contralateral kidney.

Clinical Signs

I. Most animals are asymptomatic unless obstruction is accompanied by infection, uremia, or pain associated with passage of renoliths into the ureter.
II. Renomegaly may be detected during physical examination.

Diagnosis

I. Contrast intravenous urography results in a delayed and prolonged pyelogram phase and accumulation of contrast medium proximal to obstruction.
II. Ultrasonography is usually less sensitive than contrast intravenous urography for detection and localization of early obstruction.

Treatment

I. Treatment goals are as follows.
  A. Prevent urinary obstruction
  B. Preserve renal function
  C. Control UTI
  D. Control clinical signs
II. If hyperkalemia, dehydration, cardiovascular shock, and metabolic acidosis are present, they are managed first (see Acute Renal Failure in Chap. 47).
III. Bacterial urinary tract infection may lead to life-threatening septicemia.
IV. If the kidney retains function, remove the obstruction and repair the ureter surgically (if possible).
V. If kidney damage is severe and the contralateral kidney can sustain renal function, perform unilateral ureteronephrectomy.
VI. Ureteral stents may be needed to maintain a patent lumen following repair and during ureteral healing.

Patient Monitoring

I. Control of UTI is managed by repeated urine cultures and administration of appropriate antimicrobials.
II. Contrast intravenous urography is performed 4 weeks postoperatively to assess patency of the ureter following repair.

URETEROLITHIASIS

See Chaps. 47 and 49.

Bibliography

Caywood DD, Lipowitz AJ: Ureter. p. 229. In Caywood DD, Lipowitz AJ (eds): Atlas of General Small Animal Surgery. CV Mosby, St Louis, 1989

Kerr WS: Effects of complete ureteral obstruction in dogs on kidney function. Am J Physiol 184:521, 1956

King LR: Vesicoureteral reflux, megaureter, and ureteral reim-plantation. p. 1689. In Walsh PC, Retik AB, Stamey TA, Vaughn ED (eds): Campbell's Urology. 6th Ed. WB Saunders, Philadelphia, 1992

Kohri K, Kataoka K, Akyama T et al: Treatment of vesicoureteral reflux by endoscopic injection of blood. Urol Int 43:324, 1988

Lage AL: Diseases of the ureter. p. 585. In Morgan RV (ed): Handbook of Small Animal Practice. 2nd Ed. Churchill Livingstone, New York, 1992

Vaughan ED, Gillenwater JY: Recovery following complete chronic unilateral ureteral occlusion: functional, radiologic and pathologic alterations. J Urol 106:27, 1971

Yarger WE, Griffith LD: Intrarenal hemodynamics following chronic unilateral ureteral obstruction in the dog. Am J Physiol 227:816, 1974

49

Diseases of the Urinary Bladder

Jody P. Lulich
Carl A. Osborne

CONGENITAL DISEASES

Anatomic Abnormalities

Definition

I. Some anatomic abnormalities result from congenital aberrations in bladder development.

II. Others (vesicourachal diverticula, pelvic bladder) are thought to develop as a consequence of urinary tract disease.

III. Common anatomic abnormalities of the bladder include the following.
   A. Persistent (patent) urachus
   B. Vesicourachal diverticula
   C. Urachal cyst
   D. Bladder hypoplasia
   E. Bladder duplication
   F. Pelvic bladder

Causes and Pathophysiology

I. Persistent urachus is synonymous with a patent urachus and occurs when the urachal canal remains functionally patent between the bladder and umbilicus after birth.

II. Vesicourachal diverticula occurs when a portion of the urachus at the bladder vertex fails to close, resulting in an outward protrusion of the bladder lumen at the vertex.
   A. Congenital macroscopic diverticula appear to be uncommon.
   B. They must be distinguished from acquired macroscopic diverticula that develop after the onset of lower urinary tract diseases associated with increases in intraluminal pressure, e.g., urethral obstruction, urolithiasis, reflex dyssynergia (Osborne et al., 1989).

C. Microscopic urachal remnants that persist in the vertex of the bladder following birth represent a risk factor for development of macroscopic diverticula in adult cats.

D. Many diverticula per se do not result in clinical symptoms; diverticula-associated urinary tract infection occurs more frequently in dogs.

III. Urachal cyst develops if secreting urachal epithelium persists in isolated segments of the urachus after birth.

IV. Bladder hypoplasia is a potentially reversible reduction in bladder capacity that is commonly associated with conditions in which urine storage is bypassed, e.g., ectopic ureters.

V. Bladder duplication is a rare congenital disorder reported in dogs (Kruger et al., 1996).

VI. Pelvic bladder is the term used to describe the radiographic detection of >10% of the bladder in the pelvic canal.
   A. It is uncertain whether a pelvic bladder is congenital or acquired.
   B. Increased urge and force to empty an inflamed bladder may predispose to its caudal displacement.

VII. Detection of congenital abnormalities is an indication that other portions of the urinary tract and/or the genital tract may also be anomalous.

VIII. Anatomic abnormalities of the urinary bladder may contribute to persistent and recurrent urinary tract infections (UTI), urinary incontinence, and urinary obstruction.

Clinical Signs

I. These conditions are often asymptomatic in the absence of urinary tract infection or urinary tract obstruction.

II. Dysuria and hematuria may be associated with infections.

III. Urinary incontinence has been associated with persistent urachus (urine accumulation at the umbilicus) and pelvic bladder.

Diagnosis

I. Suspicious clinical signs
   A. Recurring UTI, dysuria, pollakiuria, and/or hematuria, especially in young animals
   B. Appearance of urine at the umbilicus (persistent urachus), omphalitis
II. Evidence of pyuria, hematuria, and sometimes bacteriuria
III. Positive bacterial urine culture results (uncommon in cats)
IV. Radiographic studies
   A. Survey radiographs may identify bladder duplication or a pelvic bladder.
   B. Positive contrast cystography, pneumocystography, or double contrast cystography is usually required to verify most anatomic abnormalities of the bladder.
V. Other tests
   A. Ultrasonography and cystoscopy are beneficial; however, their usefulness as a diagnostic tool is often operator-dependent.
   B. Some abnormalities may be detected only during exploratory laparotomy and cystotomy.

Differential Diagnosis

I. Urocystoliths and blood clots adhered to the bladder wall
II. Benign polyps
III. Neoplastic tissue proliferation

Treatment and Monitoring

I. To better assess the necessity of correcting anatomic abnormalities, first eliminate associated diseases, e.g., UTI, urolithiasis, urinary tract obstruction.
II. Bladder hypoplasia and acquired vesicourachal diverticula usually resolve spontaneously following correction of associated diseases.
III. Persistent urachus, persistent symptomatic diverticula, and symptomatic urachal cysts are surgically excised.
IV. Radiographic evaluation of any surgical repair is done postoperatively, especially if clinical signs recur.

INFLAMMATORY DISORDERS

Bacterial Cystitis

Definition

I. Bacterial cystitis occurs when sufficient numbers of bacteria adhere, grow, replicate, and invade the urinary bladder.

II. Uncomplicated (simple) UTIs represent acute, previously untreated infections in which underlying structural or functional abnormalities in host defense mechanisms cannot be identified. These infections are usually self-limiting, and prognosis for complete recovery is very good.

III. Complicated UTIs are infections in which a predisposing cause can be identified.

IV. Recurrent UTIs are those that return following withdrawal of therapy; they can be divided into two general types: relapses and reinfections.
   A. Relapse is a persistence of the original invading organism and is likely to result from inappropriate use of antimicrobials (ineffective agent, wrong dosage schedule, inappropriate duration, ineffective administration).
   B. Reinfections are recurrent infections caused by a different pathogen from that which caused the original infection. They are likely to result from failure to eliminate underlying predisposing causes.

V. Bacterial colonization of the urinary bladder indicates a transient or permanent disruption in normal host defenses.

Causes and Pathophysiology

I. Frequently isolated bacteria
   A. *Escherichia coli*
   B. *Staphylococcus intermedius*
   C. *Streptococcus* spp.
   D. *Proteus mirabilis*
   E. *Klebsiella pneumoniae*
   F. *Pseudomonas aeruginosa*
II. Routes of infection
   A. Ascending through the urethra (most common)
   B. Descending from the kidney and/or prostate
   C. Lymphatic extension
III. Common predisposing factors
   A. Administration of glucocorticoid or other immunosuppressive agents
   B. Instrumentation of the urinary tract, especially catheterization
   C. Surgical alteration of normal urinary tract anatomy: perineal urethrostomy, prescrotal urethrostomy, antepubic urethrostomy, partial urethrectomy, trigonal colonic anastomosis
   D. Urolithiasis
   E. Outflow obstruction
IV. Potential sequelae to infection
   A. Extension to other organs: pyelonephritis, prostatitis, septicemia
   B. Struvite urolith formation
   C. Granulomatous urethrocystitis
   D. Emphysematous cystitis
   E. Polyp formation
   F. Urinary incontinence

Clinical Signs

I. Pollakiuria: frequent voiding of small amounts of urine

II. Dysuria: difficult or painful urination
III. Stranguria: straining to urinate
IV. Hematuria

Diagnosis

I. Clinical signs that localize disease to the lower urinary tract (but are not specific for bacterial urinary tract infection)
   A. Pollakiuria, dysuria, and stranguria are typical.
   B. Bacteriuria and pyuria may be noted.
   C. Bacteriuria may not be detected in some cases of UTI.
      1. Bacteria are not detected in urine sediment evaluations until organisms exceed 10^5 per milliliter (coccal forms).
      2. It may be difficult to detect bacteria in dilute urine samples.
   D. Pyuria may be absent in animals with endogenous (hyperadrenocorticism) or exogenous (glucocorticoid and chemotherapy administration) sources of immunosuppression.
II. Bacterial urine culture and susceptibility results
   A. Collect urine prior to antimicrobial therapy.
      1. Cystocentesis is the preferred method of collection.
      2. Midstream samples may also be used.
      3. Avoid obtaining urine samples by transurethral catheterization.
         a) May introduce new bacteria into susceptible bladder
         b) May damage protective urothelial surface
   B. Culture urine immediately, if possible, or transport samples in appropriate transport media.
   C. Interpretation of quantitative results depends on method of collection (Table 49–1).
      1. Bacterial counts $>10^5$/ml are indicative of urinary tract infection.
      2. Any bacterial counts from animals currently receiving antibacterials may be significant, and they warrant investigation as to appropriateness of therapy.
      3. Identification of more than one bacterial species is more likely to represent improper urine collection and contamination than a true multispecies infection.
III. Radiography/ultrasonography
   A. May be helpful for identifying underlying causes, e.g., urolithiasis, neoplasia

   B. Help rule out sequelae of infections, e.g., urolithiasis, pyelonephritis
   C. Performed in animals with recurrent infections
IV. Other tests
   A. Anaerobic bacterial infections are rare, so anaerobic cultures are not usually performed.
   B. Mycoplasmal infections have been reported, but they are apparently uncommon.

Differential Diagnosis

I. Other causes of dysuria
   A. Urethritis
   B. Neoplasia of the bladder, especially in older dogs
   C. Idiopathic hematuria and dysuria of cats
   D. Urolithiasis
II. Other causes of bacteriuria
   A. Prostatitis
   B. Pyelonephritis

Treatment

I. Eliminate underlying cause and restore normal host defenses, if possible.
II. Use of antimicrobials is best achieved when selection is based on bacterial susceptibility results.
   A. Use antimicrobials that achieve high concentrations in urine, such as the penicillins, sulfonamides, and fluoroquinolones.
   B. Uncomplicated UTIs are often successfully treated with antimicrobials based on Gram staining properties.
      1. Gram-positive bacteria: use penicillins or clavulanate-potentiated penicillins
      2. Gram-negative bacteria: use fluoroquinolones or sulfonamides
III. General guidelines
   A. Uncomplicated UTI
      1. Treat with appropriate antibiotic for 7–14 days.
      2. Clinical signs should resolve in 1–2 days.
   B. Complicated UTI
      1. Treat with appropriate antibiotic for 7–14 days after resolution of clinical signs.
      2. Correct any underlying defect.
   C. First-time relapsing UTI: 4–6 weeks of antibiotics
   D. Subsequent relapsing UTI: 6–8 weeks of antibiotics

Table 49–1. **Interpretation of Quantitative Urine Culture in Dogs and Cats**

Collection Method	Contaminant		Suspicious		Significant	
	Dog	*Cat*	*Dog*	*Cat*	*Dog*	*Cat*
Cystocentesis	≤ 100	≤ 100	100–1000	100–1000	≥ 1000	≥ 1000
Catheterization	≤ 1000	≤ 100	1000–10,000	100–1000	≥ 10,000	≥ 1000
Voluntary voiding	≤ 10,000	≤ 1000	10,000–90,000	1000–10,000	≥ 100,000	≥ 10,000
Manual compression	≤ 10,000	≤ 1000	10,000–90,000	1000–10,000	≥ 100,000	≥ 10,000

Numbers indicate colony-forming units per milliliter of urine.

E. Reinfections
1. Treat for 7–14 days following remission of clinical signs.
2. Continue antimicrobial therapy for another 3–6 months at ⅓ the daily dose administered after the animal's last voiding of the day (bedtime).

Patient Monitoring

I. To ensure proper antimicrobial selection, adequate dosage, and appropriate administration, culture the urine via cystocentesis 3–5 days after initiation of the antibiotic.
II. To ensure adequate duration of antimicrobial therapy, urine cultures are performed 3–5 days after the drugs are discontinued.
III. To minimize development of resistant bacteria, urine cultures are performed just prior to reducing the antimicrobial dosage to a subtherapeutic level (once nightly dose), and once each month the subtherapeutic dose is administered.
IV. To monitor recurrent reinfections, urine may need to be cultured every 3–6 months.
V. To monitor the development of UTI in animals with known aberrations in natural host defenses, urine is cultured as follows.
A. During and following persistent catheterization
B. Every 1–2 months in dogs with endogenous or exogenous glucocorticoid excess
C. Every 1–2 months in dogs receiving chemotherapy
D. Every 1–3 months in dogs with diabetes mellitus
E. Every 3–6 months in cats with perineal urethrostomies

Fungal Cystitis

Definition

I. Fungal cystitis occurs when pathogenic fungi adhere, grow, replicate, and invade the urinary bladder.
II. Fungal infections of the urinary tract appear to be uncommon.
III. Fungi are not found in the urine of healthy animals.
A. When present, they usually indicate disruption of local and systemic host defenses.
B. They may also be an indication of systemic fungal infection that has extended to the urinary tract.
IV. Asymptomatic funguria occurs when fungi are found in the urine of otherwise healthy animals (without clinical signs of lower urinary tract disease).
V. Symptomatic fungal UTIs are associated with signs of urethritis, cystitis, and/or systemic illness.

Causes and Pathophysiology

I. Most frequently isolated fungi
A. *Torulopsis*
B. *Candida*
C. *Cryptococcus*
D. *Blastomyces*
E. *Aspergillus*
II. Routes of infection
A. Ascending through the urethra
B. Hematogenous route
III. Predisposing factors
A. Systemic fungal infection
B. Administration of glucocorticoids or other immunosuppressive agents
C. Prolonged antibacterial therapy
D. Alteration of normal urinary tract anatomy
E. Urolithiasis

Clinical Signs

I. Variable, some asymptomatic
II. Dysuria, pollakiuria
III. ± Urethral obstruction

Diagnosis

I. Any evidence of systemic fungal disease
II. Evidence of funguria (budding yeast or elongated hyphae) in properly collected urine samples
A. Red and white blood cells are not always observed.
B. Absence of pyuria is not synonymous with infection by nonpathogenic fungi.
III. Fungal urine culture results
A. Fungi require special conditions for growth, so consult a diagnostic laboratory for proper storage and transport.
B. Unlike bacteriuria, the clinical significance of funguria cannot be reliably predicted by counting the number of colony-forming units per milliliter of urine.
IV. Bladder biopsy
Demonstration of fungal tissue invasion on histology provides undisputed evidence of pathogenic colonization of fungi.
V. Radiography/ultrasonography
A. Survey radiography is usually unremarkable.
B. Contrast radiography/ultrasonography may be needed to identify underlying causes and bezoar formation.

Differential Diagnosis

I. Urine contaminated by fecal or genital tract fungi
II. Fungal contamination of containers used to collect, store, or analyze urine

Treatment and Monitoring

I. Eliminate any underlying cause and restore normal host immunocompetence, if possible.
II. Some asymptomatic infections may spontaneously resolve.
III. Therapy is indicated for those animals with symptomatic funguria or asymptomatic animals with debilitating disease or receiving cytotoxic chemotherapy.

IV. If possible, use antifungal agents that achieve high concentrations in urine (flucytosine, fluconazole).
  A. Flucytosine is effective against urinary *Candida, Torulopsis,* and *Cryptococcus* spp.
  B. Ketoconazole and itraconazole are not commonly used, because little active drug is excreted in urine.
V. Therapy is continued until two successive negative urine cultures are obtained at 2-week intervals.
VI. Surgery may be needed to mechanically remove bezoars.

Other Forms of Cystitis

See Table 49–2.

Idiopathic Hematuria and Dysuria in Cats

Definition

I. Hematuria and dysuria, with or without urethral obstruction, are common lower urinary tract problems in cats that can result from a wide array of causes.
II. A cause of the lower urinary tract disease often cannot be identified.
III. Synonymous syndromes
  A. Feline urologic syndrome
  B. Idiopathic feline lower urinary tract disease
  C. Interstitial cystitis

Causes

I. The cause(s) may be singular, multiple, interacting, or unrelated.
II. Theoretical causes include the following.
  A. Crystalluria
  B. Viral infections

C. Mycoplasmal infections
D. Defective glycosaminoglycans
E. Neurogenic mediators (substance P)
III. The following may be contributing factors.
  A. Crystalluria
  B. Urethral swelling, spasms, or strictures
  C. Stress
  D. Products of bladder inflammation
  E. Alkaline urine or concentrated urine
  F. Dry diets
  G. Gender: male cats affected more often

Clinical Signs

I. Straining to urinate, pollakiuria, visible hematuria
II. Urinating outside the litter box in abnormal places
III. Frequent licking of urogenital area
IV. Signs of postrenal uremia, if urethra obstructed
  A. Anorexia, vomiting, and dehydration
  B. Depression, collapse

Diagnosis

I. Successful diagnosis and management depend on elimination of known treatable causes of lower urinary tract disease in cats (see Differential Diagnosis later).
II. Characteristic clinical signs are suggestive.
III. Physical examination findings are variable.
  A. Nonobstructed cat
    1. Bladder is small, empty, and may be painful.
    2. Cat may attempt to urinate following bladder palpation.
  B. Cat with urethral obstruction (primarily male cats)
    1. Distended, turgid, painful bladder
    2. May attempt to urinate unsuccessfully following bladder palpation

Table 49–2. *Some Infrequent Causes of Cystitis*

Type	Definition	Cause	Diagnosis	Treatment
Emphysematous Cystitis	Intraparenchymal gas within the bladder wall	Bacterial fermentation of glucose within devitalized bladder wall	Survey radiography: mottling of bladder wall with small gas bubbles	Eradicate UTI and control glucosuria
Polypoid Cystitis	Mucosal polypoid projections of the bladder urothelium	Chronic irritation (e.g., UTI, uroliths) to the urinary bladder, promoting mucosal hyperplasia	Contrast radiography or ultrasonography	Spontaneously regress with eradication of underlying cause
Drug-induced Cystitis	Bacteriologically sterile cystitis resulting from drug toxicity	Retrograde flushing solutions or metabolites of cyclophosphamide	History of drug administration and elimination of other causes	Discontinue drug, promote diuresis, and treat secondary UTI
Idiopathic Cystitis	Cystitis in which structural abnormalities, infections, cystotoxic drug administration, and trauma to the urinary bladder have been eliminated as causes	Unknown	This diagnosis is surmised by excluding known causes of bladder inflammation	Antispasmotics (propantheline, oxybutynin, phenoxybenzamine), urinary analgesics (phenazopyridine in dogs only), and sedatives (diazepam, amitriptyline) can be used to minimize dysuria.

3. Inability to express urine
4. Mucoid/crystalline material protruding from penile urethra
5. May be depressed, in shock, comatose, and hypothermic

IV. Radiography is often helpful.
   A. Include distal urethra in film.
   B. If there is urethral obstruction, bladder is distended and urethral plug may be visible.
   C. If there is no obstruction, bladder is usually small.

V. Urinalysis is indicated.
   A. Hematuria is common.
   B. Pyuria is less common.
   C. Bacteriuria is rare with first-time occurrences.

VI. Serum biochemistry values may denote varying degrees of azotemia, hyperkalemia, acidosis, and hyperphosphatemia with urethral obstruction or bladder rupture.

Differential Diagnosis

I. Urolithiasis
II. Bacterial urinary tract infection
III. Neoplasia
IV. Behavioral marking

Treatment

I. Depressed cat in cardiovascular shock
   A. Restore effective circulating volume (see Chaps. 47 and 131).
   B. Correct serum biochemical abnormalities.
      1. Perform decompressive cystocentesis to aid elimination of waste products and hyperkalemia (repeat as needed).
      2. Peritoneal dialysis may be needed if bladder is ruptured.
   C. Perform urinalysis, radiography, and serum biochemistries to determine cause and disease severity.
   D. Delay alleviation of obstruction or sedation, and perform decompressive cystocentesis until animal is stable.

II. Correction of intraluminal urethral obstruction
   A. Sedation may be needed.
      1. Inhalation anesthetics are best.
      2. Propofol provides good short-term sedation.
      3. Other intravenous agents (e.g., diazepam, midazolam, ketamine, acepromazine) are also effective.
   B. Attempt to dislodge urethral plug.
      1. Massage distal urethra to dislodge or disrupt plug.
      2. Next, attempt to induce voiding with gentle compression of the urinary bladder.
      3. If unsuccessful, decompress the bladder via cystocentesis so that retrograde flushing does not result in additional bladder overdistention. Save this urine sample for diagnostic purposes.
      4. Using a physiologic solution, flush the urethra

with an open-ended catheter to disrupt and dislodge the plug.
      5. Alternate with gentle compression of the urinary bladder in an attempt to further dislodge obstruction, and save any material for analysis.
      6. Repeat these steps as needed.
      7. If obstruction persists, flush intraluminal obstructing material retrograde into bladder lumen.
   C. After relieving obstruction, promote diuresis through administration of IV or SQ crystalloid solutions (lactated Ringer's solution, saline) to promote formation of dilute urine with the goal of dispersing and dissolving inflammatory and crystalline precipitates.
   D. Consider indwelling catheterization for the following animals.
      1. Animals with a poor urine stream following urethral flushing
      2. Uremic cats
      3. Cats with detrusor atony
      4. High-risk animals that cannot be observed during the next 12–24 hours for reobstruction
      5. History of recent obstruction (within last week)
   E. Attempt to prevent reobstruction.
      1. Manually express the bladder (3–5 times per day) to expel solids aggregating in the bladder and to disrupt any early less organized urethral obstruction.
      2. Submit matrix/crystalline plugs for quantitative mineral analysis, and provide therapy to minimize crystal formation.
      3. Promote diuresis through administration of additional crystalloid solutions.

III. The nonobstructed cat
   A. Perform diagnostic tests to identify and eliminate treatable causes.
   B. Many forms of therapy have been used as single agents or combined with others (Kruger et al., 1996), but none are of proven value in idiopathic disease.
      1. Antibacterial agents
      2. Urinary antiseptics, analgesics, acidifiers
      3. Smooth and skeletal muscle antispasmotics
      4. Anti-inflammatory agents
      5. Mood altering drugs, sedatives
      6. Urohydrodistention
      7. Urothelial débridement
      8. Special diets
   C. Clinical signs often subside within 5–7 days with or without therapy.
      1. Signs may recur after variable periods of time and again subside without therapy.
      2. Idiopathic hematuria and dysuria tend to decrease in frequency and severity as cats age.

IV. Understanding client concerns
   A. Urethral obstruction can be minimized by providing therapy to decrease crystal formation and to promote formation of less concentrated urine.
      1. Feed canned diet.

2. Provide flavored water in addition to regular water.
3. Feed diets that minimize concomitant crystalluria.
B. Patient pain and discomfort can be managed with the following.
   1. Diazepam 1–2 mg/cat PO SID-BID
   2. Alprazolam 0.1–0.2 mg/cat PO SID-BID
   3. Amitriptyline 5–12.5 mg/cat PO SID
   4. Prednisolone 1–2 mg/kg PO SID
C. House soiling can be managed by confining cats for brief periods (5 days) in a large portable kennel.

Patient Monitoring

I. Serum biochemistry tests are performed daily until postrenal azotemia and hyperkalemia normalize.
II. Culture urine for bacteria immediately following urinary catheter removal and 5 days after cessation of antibiotic therapy.
III. Urine samples are evaluated for crystals monthly and then every 2–3 months.

Urocystolithiasis

Definition

I. The preferred term for microscopic precipitates in urine is crystals.
II. Macroscopic precipitates are referred to as uroliths.
III. Uroliths are polycrystalline concretions that typically contain 90–95% crystalloids and <5–10% organic matrix.
IV. Urolithiasis is the formation of uroliths from less soluble crystalloids of urine.
V. Unlike urethral plugs, uroliths are usually hard and brittle.
VI. Uroliths are commonly recognized in dogs and cats.

Classification

I. Magnesium ammonium phosphate (struvite)
II. Calcium oxalate
   A. Monohydrate
   B. Dihydrate
III. Purines
   A. Ammonium acid urate
   B. Sodium acid urate
   C. Uric acid
   D. Calcium sodium urate
   E. Xanthine
IV. Cystine
V. Calcium phosphate
   A. Carbonate calcium apatite
   B. Calcium phosphate (hydroxyapatite)
   C. Calcium hydrogen phosphate dihydrate
   D. Tricalcium phosphate
VI. Silica
VII. Compound types
VIII. Mixed types
IX. Matrix

Causes and Pathophysiology

I. Struvite uroliths
   A. Urine must be supersaturated with magnesium, ammonium, and phosphate ions for uroliths to form.
   B. Metabolic, dietary, and familial factors are involved in struvite formation.
   C. Risk factors are listed below.
      1. Urinary tract infection with urease-producing bacteria
         a) Common in dogs, especially females
         b) Rare in cats, especially males
         c) *Staphylococcus* and *Proteus* spp. common
      2. Alkaline urine promoting formation of phosphate ions
      3. Concentrated urine with supersaturation of crystalloids
      4. Diets high in magnesium and phosphorus with increased urine excretion of magnesium and phosphorus
      5. Diets high in protein
II. Calcium oxalate uroliths risk factors
   A. Hypercalciuria
      1. Metabolic factors promoting hypercalciuria, including intestinal hyperabsorption of calcium, metabolic acidosis, and hypercalcemia (Sutton et al., 1979)
      2. Drugs promoting hypercalciuria, including glucocorticoids, furosemide, and vitamin and mineral supplements (e.g., sodium chloride)
   B. Hyperoxaluria
      1. Familial defect (primary hyperoxaluria) (McKerrell et al., 1989)
      2. Pyridoxine deficiency (Bai et al., 1989)
      3. Fat malabsorption
   C. Hypocitraturia
   D. Defective macromolecular crystal growth inhibitors
   E. Concentrated urine with supersaturation of crystalloids
   F. Breeds commonly affected: Yorkshire terrier, miniature schnauzer, Lhasa apso, miniature poodle, bichon frisé, Persian, and Himalayan
   G. Gender: males more often than females
III. Urate uroliths
   A. Hyperuricosuria is an important risk factor.
      1. Hypoxanthine, xanthine, uric acid, and allantoin represent the final pathway of purine metabolism
      2. Decreased concentration or availability of uricase results in excessive uric acid excretion and subsequent urate urolith formation.
      3. Proximal renal tubular reabsorption of uric acid minimizes the concentration of uric acid in urine.
   B. Dalmatians are at risk for urate urolithiasis because of incomplete oxidation of available uric acid.
   C. Some English bulldogs may have similar aberrations in urate metabolism as dalmatians
   D. Other breeds with urate uroliths usually have

evidence of liver dysfunction, with the most common liver disease being a portosystemic shunt.

IV. Cystine uroliths
  A. An inborn error of cystine metabolism is present and characterized by decreased renal tubular reabsorption of cystine and/or cysteine (the immediate precursor of cystine).
  B. Excessive urinary excretion of lysine, glycine, ornithine, and arginine has also been observed.
  C. It is reported most often in male English bulldogs, mastiffs, dachshunds, basset hounds, and rottweilers.
  D. Many other breeds have been affected.
  E. Not all cystinuric dogs form uroliths.

V. Calcium phosphate uroliths
  A. This mineral is commonly found as a minor component of struvite or calcium oxalate uroliths.
  B. Uroliths composed principally of calcium phosphate are uncommon and are usually associated with metabolic disorders such as primary hyperparathyroidism, renal tubular acidosis, and excessive dietary calcium and phosphorus.

VI. Silica uroliths
  A. A link exists between dietary ingredients and urolith formation. Diets containing substantial quantities of corn gluten feed or soybean hulls are especially suspect.
  B. Male dogs are affected more often than females.
  C. Large-breed dogs are at greater risk, especially German shepherd dogs, golden retrievers, and Labrador retrievers.

VII. Compound uroliths
  A. Compound uroliths form because factors promoting precipitation of one type of urolith have been superseded by factors promoting precipitation of another mineral.
  B. Administration of urinary acidifiers to manage struvite uroliths may promote hypercalciuria resulting in a shell of calcium oxalate or calcium phosphate.
  C. All uroliths predispose to urinary tract infection. If infections by microorganisms that produce urease persist, it is likely that struvite will precipitate over preexisting uroliths.

VIII. Rare and unusual uroliths
  A. Although crystalluria has been reported with a variety of drugs, urolith formation in dogs and cats has been associated only with sulfonamide administration.
    1. If conditions favor sulfonamide precipitation (acidic and concentrated urine), preexisting uroliths may become surrounded by precipitated drug metabolites rendering them less amenable to medical dissolution.
    2. For this reason, sulfonamide antimicrobials are not to be routinely administered to dogs or cats with uroliths.
  B. Foreign material in the lumen of the urinary tract may predispose to urolith formation by serving as a template for heterogeneous nucleation of crystals or by promoting urinary tract infection.

Clinical Signs

I. Dysuria and hematuria
II. Urinary incontinence
III. Inappropriate urination
IV. Stranguria or inability to urinate
V. Voiding of uroliths
VI. Systemic signs of urinary obstruction: anorexia, lethargy, vomiting, depression

Diagnosis/Differential Diagnosis

I. Urocystoliths must be considered in animals with signs of dysuria and hematuria.
II. Urinalysis, urine culture, radiography, and ultrasonography may be required to identify and differentiate uroliths from urinary tract infection, urinary tract neoplasia, polyps, blood clots, and urogenital anomalies.
III. Clinical signs associated with uroliths are not specific for their mineral composition. A variety of methods are used to evaluate the composition of uroliths, including their gross appearance, crystalluria, radiographic appearance, quantitative analysis, and bacterial culture (Table 49–3).
IV. Quantitative analysis of uroliths provides the most definitive diagnostic, prognostic, and therapeutic information.

Treatment

I. Struvite uroliths can be dissolved medically or removed surgically (Osborne et al., 1990).
  A. Eradicate and control UTI, if present.
    1. When uroliths are dissolved, antimicrobials are administered for the entire period of dissolution (usually 2–3 months).
    2. When uroliths are surgically removed, antimicrobials are given 1–3 days prior to surgery and for 2–4 weeks following surgery.
  B. Acetohydroxamic acid at 12.5 mg/kg PO BID is administered to those dogs in which eradication and control of UTI are not well managed with antimicrobials.
  C. Diets to dissolve uroliths include commercially prepared diets such as Hill's Prescription Diet s/d.
    1. Diet is usually fed for a prolonged period of time.
      a) 3–4 months in dogs and cats with infection-induced uroliths
      b) 1–2 months in cats with sterile struvite uroliths
    2. Diet is usually continued for 30 days beyond radiographic dissolution of uroliths.
  D. Prevention of struvite uroliths involves the following.
    1. Control and early eradication of UTI
    2. Dietary prevention

Table 49–3. Predicting Mineral Composition of Common Canine Uroliths

	Predictors								
Mineral Type	Typical Urine pH	Crystal Appearance	Urine Culture	Radiographic Density	Radiographic Contour	Serum Abnormalities	Breed Predisposition	Gender Predisposition	Common Ages
Magnesium ammonium phosphate	Neutral to alkaline	3–8-sided colorless prisms	Urease-producing bacteria (*Staphylococcus, Proteus, Ureaplasma*)	+ to + + + + (sometimes laminated)	Smooth, round, or faceted; may assume shape of renal pelvis, ureter, bladder, or urethra	None	Miniature schnauzer, miniature poodle, bichon frisé, cocker spaniel	Female (>80%)	2–9 years
Calcium oxalate	Acid to neutral	Dihydrate salt: colorless envelope or octahedral shape Monohydrate salt: spindles or dumbbell shape	Negative	+ + to + + + +	Rough or spiculated (dihydrate salt) Small smooth, round (monohydrate salt) Sometimes jackstone	Usually normocalcemic, occasionally hypercalcemic	Miniature schnauzer, standard schnauzer, Lhasa apso, Yorkshire terrier, miniature poodle, Shih Tzu, bichon frisé	Male (>70%)	5–12 years
Urate	Acid to neutral	Yellow-brown amorphous spherical shapes (ammonium urate)	Negative	– to + +	Smooth (occasionally irregular), round or oval	Low urea nitrogen and serum albumin in dogs with hepatic disease and portosystemic shunts	Dalmatian, English bulldog, miniature schnauzer, Yorkshire terrier, Shih Tzu	Male (>90%)	1–5 years
Calcium phosphate	Alkaline to neutral (brushite forms in acid urine)	Amorphous, or long thin prisms	Negative	+ + to + + + + +	Smooth or irregular; round or faceted	Occasional hypercalcemia	Yorkshire terrier, miniature schnauzer, Shih Tzu	Male (>55%)	<1 year; 6–10 years
Cystine	Acid to neutral	Flat, colorless, hexagonal plates	Negative	+ to + +	Smooth (occasionally irregular; round to oval	None	English bulldog, dachshund, basset hound, Newfoundland	Male (>98%)	1–7 years
Silica	Acid to neutral	None observed	Negative	+ + to + + +	Round center with radial spoke-like projections (jackstone)	None	German shepherd dog, golden retriever, Labrador retriever, miniature schnauzer, Cavalier King Charles spaniel	Male (>95%)	3–10 years

a) Canned diets are considered better than dry formulations.

b) Commercially prepared diets are available for dogs (Hill's Prescription Diet c/d for dogs) and cats (many brands).

II. Effective dissolution protocols for calcium oxalate uroliths have yet to be established.

A. Removal of urolith is recommended.

1. Voiding urohydropropulsion

2. Catheter retrieval

3. Cystotomy

4. Lithotripsy (not as effective for urocystoliths as for nephroliths)

B. Prevention involves the following.

1. Correct hypercalcemia, if present.

2. Commercially prepared diets are available to help prevention.

a) Dog: Hill's Prescription Diet u/d or w/d if hyperlipidemia is a concern

b) Cats: diets designed for renal failure that promote an alkaline urine such as Hill's Prescription Diet k/d

c) Canned foods better than dry formulations

3. Provide additional water to reduce urine saturation of calculogenic minerals by promoting formation of less concentrated urine.

4. Promoting diuresis with NaCl is contraindicated because it also promotes calcium excretion.

5. Potassium citrate (40–75 mg/kg PO BID to achieve a urine pH of 7) can be given to animals that do not consistently produce neutral or alkaline urine.

III. Treatment of urate uroliths involves medical dissolution and physical removal.

A. Dietary principles include reducing purine content to minimize purine excretion, increasing urine pH to reduce purine saturation, and diluting urine to reduce purine saturation.

1. Commercially prepared foods are available for dogs (Hill's Prescription Diet u/d).

2. Canned foods are better than dry formulations.

B. Allopurinol binds to and inhibits the action of xanthine oxidase and thereby decreases production of uric acid by inhibiting its conversion from hypoxanthine and xanthine.

1. It may not be as effective in dogs with portosystemic shunts because of decreased hepatic metabolism of drug.

2. Dosage is 15 mg/kg PO BID.

3. Other than formation of xanthine uroliths, adverse reactions to allopurinol are apparently uncommon in dogs.

4. No studies are available on its effectiveness or adverse effects in cats.

C. Urine alkalization reduces renal ammonia production (ammonium ion and hydrogen ions precipitate urate ions).

1. Potassium citrate 40–75 mg/kg PO BID to achieve a urine pH of approximately 7–7.5

2. Sodium bicarbonate 10–90 grains/day PO to achieve a urine pH of approximately 7–7.5

D. Eradication and control of UTI are important because ammonia generated by microorganisms may promote ammonium urate urolith formation.

E. Augment urine volume by adding additional water to food or feeding reduced protein diets, which decrease renal medullary urea concentration.

F. Additional sodium chloride is avoided because it may promote sodium urate precipitation or calcium excretion and subsequent calcium urate precipitation.

G. Mechanical urolith removal may be accomplished by voiding urohydropropulsion, catheter retrieval, or cystotomy.

H. Prevention of urate uroliths is difficult.

1. Genetic aberrations in dalmatians and English bulldogs are lifelong.

2. If benefits outweigh risks, correct portosystemic shunts in affected dogs (see Chap. 34).

3. Dietary recommendations are similar to those for dissolution.

4. Allopurinol is considered if diet alone does not prevent recurrence; however, in some dogs, allopurinol results in xanthine urolith formation.

IV. Treatment of cystine uroliths can involve medical dissolution and physical removal.

A. Dietary principles are as follows.

1. It is believed that most urinary cystine results from endogenous metabolism of sulfur-containing amino acids and is not diet-derived.

2. The effect of reducing sulfur-containing amino acids (methionine) in the diet may be minimal.

3. Nonacidify the urine to reduce purine saturation.

4. Promote less concentrated urine to reduce cystine saturation.

5. Commercially prepared foods are available for dogs (Hill's Prescription Diet u/d).

6. Canned foods are better than dry formulations.

B. *N*-(2-Mercaptopropionyl)-glycine (2-MPG) decreases the concentration of cystine by a thiol disulfide exchange reaction resulting in a compound, cysteine-2-MPG disulfide, that is more soluble in urine than cystine.

1. Dosage is 15–25 mg/kg PO BID.

2. Combine with Hill's Prescription Diet canned u/d.

3. Dissolution occurred in an average of 85 ± 45 days.

C. D-Penicillamine (dimethylcysteine) combines with cysteine to form cysteine-D-penicillamine disulfide; this compound has been reported to be 50 times more soluble than free cystine.

1. The most common dosage for dogs is 15 mg/kg PO BID.

2. It is associated with a higher incidence of

adverse effects that are more severe than those with 2-MPG.
  - D. Augment urine volume.
  - E. Mechanical urolith removal can be accomplished by voiding urohydropropulsion, catheter retrieval, or cystotomy.
  - F. Prevention may be attempted.
    1. Dietary recommendations are similar to dissolution measures.
    2. 2-MPG can be added if diet alone is unsuccessful.
- V. Dissolution protocols have yet to be established for calcium phosphate uroliths.
  - A. Physical removal is indicated for animals with clinically active disease.
    1. Voiding urohydropropulsion
    2. Catheter retrieval
    3. Cystotomy
    4. Lithotripsy (not as effective for urocystoliths as for nephroliths)
  - B. Prevention may be attempted.
    1. Correct underlying metabolic defect, if possible.
    2. Diet changes that minimize calcium oxalate excretion are recommended, but efficacy has not been proved.
    3. Canned foods are considered better than dry formulations.
- VI. Effective protocols to dissolve silica have yet to be developed.
  - A. Mechanical methods of urolith removal are necessary for animals with clinically active disease.
  - B. For prevention, avoid diets containing substantial levels of plant proteins, and increase urine volume by enhancing water consumption.
- VII. Dissolution of compound uroliths may be tried.
  - A. Any uroliths refractory to current methods of medical dissolution should be removed surgically or by voiding urohydropropulsion.
  - B. Preventive protocols are designed principally to minimize recurrence of minerals composing the nucleus, rather than the shell, of compound uroliths.

Patient Monitoring

- I. Postsurgical radiography is performed.
  - A. It is required to assess complete surgical removal of uroliths.
  - B. Depending on the skill of the surgeon, uroliths remain in the bladder following surgery in 20–80% of affected animals.
  - C. Retrograde and antegrade flushing of the urethra as well as passage of urethral catheters are apparently inadequate methods of evaluating successful urolith removal.
- II. When medically dissolving uroliths, monthly evaluations are ideal.
  - A. Radiography is needed to assess urolith size and position.
  - B. Urinalyses can be used to assess reductions in crystal number, reductions in inflammatory cells, and owner compliance.
    1. Dogs consuming canned Hill's Prescription Diet u/d usually have specific gravities <1.017.
    2. Dogs consuming canned Hill's Prescription Diet s/d usually have specific gravities <1.010.
  - C. Urine culture can be used to assess the correct choice, dosage, and duration of antimicrobials, owner's ability to administer the drugs, and appearance of new or resistant bacteria.
  - D. Serum chemistry profiles can be used to assess owner compliance, because dogs consuming canned Hill's Prescription Diet u/d or Prescription Diet s/d usually have serum urea nitrogen concentrations <10 mg/dl.
- III. When preventing urolith recurrence, monitor more frequently (usually every 1–3 months) initially, until desired effect and stability of results are noted.
  - A. Urine cultures can be used to assess resolution of UTI and pattern of recurrent infections. They are also essential in preventing infection-induced struvite urolith recurrence.
  - B. Urinalyses can be used to assess absence of crystals.
    1. Crystals indicate that urine is supersaturated and can support urolith formation and growth.
    2. Consider additional therapy if crystalluria is persistently observed in properly collected samples.
  - C. Radiography can be used to assess early urolith recurrence prior to clinical signs so that small uroliths can be removed nonsurgically via voiding urohydropropulsion.

NEOPLASIA

Definition

- I. Prevalence is greater in dogs than cats.
- II. Tumors are identified more commonly in females than males.
- III. Transitional cell carcinoma is the most frequently identified tumor.
- IV. Rhabdomyosarcomas are typically identified in young large-breed dogs.
- V. Secondary bladder tumors are uncommon and, when present, usually arise from the urethra or prostate.

Causes

- I. Chemical carcinogens: tryptophan metabolites (dogs), cyclophosphamide, nitrosamines
- II. Industrial carcinogens: tobacco, dyes, paint, rubber
- III. Chronic irritation
- IV. Idiopathic factors

Clinical Signs

- I. Hematuria, dysuria, pollakiuria, stranguria
- II. Signs of ureteral or urethral obstruction

III. Evidence of chronic recurrent UTI
IV. Signs related to metastasis

Diagnosis

I. Rectal palpation may reveal changes in bladder or urethral symmetry, consistency, and texture.
II. Cytologic evaluation of urine sediment may reveal elevated numbers of epithelial cells with a variety of anaplastic features.
III. Filling defects are commonly identified via radiography or ultrasonography.
IV. Hypertrophic osteopathy or metastatic neoplasia may occur at other locations and be identified radiographically.
V. Light microscopic evaluation of biopsy samples is needed to confirm the diagnosis.

Differential Diagnosis

I. Inflammatory polyps
II. Blood clots, urocystoliths, chronic UTI
III. Neoplasia of adjacent organs

Treatment and Monitoring

I. Complete surgical excision is the best treatment, but it is not always possible.
  A. Partial cystectomy can be performed for tumors not invading the urethra or trigone.
  B. Total cystectomy and urinary diversion have been associated with unacceptable complications such as metabolic acidosis, pyelonephritis, renal failure, and septicemia.
  C. Prepubic catheterization and indwelling catheters may provide short-term alleviation of urethral obstruction associated with inoperable tumors.
II. Chemotherapy or radiation therapy may help minimize clinical signs, but remission is usually short (weeks to months).
III. Piroxicam has been helpful in providing comfort through its analgesic and anti-inflammatory properties.
  A. A nonsteroidal anti-inflammatory agent
    1. Inhibits prostaglandin synthesis
    2. Superoxide inhibition
  B. Dosage in dogs: 0.3 mg/kg PO SID
IV. Antimicrobials are necessary to control secondary UTI.
V. Prognosis is as follows.
  A. Prognosis is good for benign tumors and malignant tumors that are completely excised.
  B. Because most transitional cell carcinomas are associated with extensive wall invasion and extension to other locations, long-term prognosis is poor.

BLADDER TRAUMA

Definition and Causes

I. Injury to the urinary bladder may be caused by blunt (automobiles, kicks, or falls) or penetrating abdominal trauma (knives, scalpels, needles, bullets, or fractured bone fragments).
II. The bladder may also be injured by overzealous palpation or expression when devitalized (particularly in association with prolonged obstruction), by overinsertion of rigid urinary catheters, and by overdistention of the bladder lumen during retrograde contrast urethrocystography or bladder flushing procedures.
III. Improper placement of peritoneal dialysis catheters containing stylets, improper cystocentesis technique, careless celiotomy incisions, or careless abdominal trocarization may also injure the bladder.

Pathophysiology

I. Overdistention without mucosal tearing is usually associated with hemorrhage and mild dysuria.
II. Small rents in the bladder wall may spontaneously heal, and urine spilled into the abdominal cavity is rapidly reabsorbed.
III. Transient intraperitoneal extravasation of urine from the bladder as a result of overdistention or cystocentesis is usually self-limiting and resolves quickly (hours to a day).
IV. Larger rents in the bladder wall often require surgical correction and, subsequent, constant bladder decompression.
  A. These injuries usually result in azotemia, acidemia, hyperkalemia, ascites, and/or infection.
  B. If appropriate therapy is not initiated, severe peritonitis, postrenal azotemia, and death typically occur in 3–5 days.
V. Displacement of the urinary bladder (bladder herniation) can result in urethral obstruction and bladder wall devitalization.
  A. Extraperitoneal extravasation of urine from the urinary bladder may not be associated with localizing signs during early stages.
  B. Continuous loss of urine eventually causes signs related to cellulitis including fever, depression, dysuria, and fistulous tracts.
VI. Peritonitis may develop with penetrating wounds or concomitant UTI.

Clinical Signs

I. Hematuria is common.
II. Voluntary urination does not eliminate the possibility of a bladder tear.
III. Ascites and/or peritonitis can occur.
IV. Anorexia, depression, fever, abdominal pain, and vomiting may occur as azotemia and peritonitis develop.
V. In the case of extraperitoneal herniation, a distended bladder may be palpated in the herniated sac.

Diagnosis

I. Suspicious historical and clinical signs
  A. Suspect bladder rupture in all animals with a history of abdominal or pelvic injury.

B. Development of the previously described clinical signs is highly suggestive.

II. Radiography

A. Survey radiographs may reveal loss of abdominal contrast resulting from fluid accumulation or displacement of the bladder.

B. Pelvic bone fractures are the most common injury associated with bladder rupture.

C. Ultrasonography identifies free fluid in the abdomen.

D. Positive contrast urethrocystography is the procedure of choice to identify rents in the bladder.

1. Using a balloon catheter eliminates the need to insert the catheter beyond the distal urethra and, therefore, minimizes the chance of further catheter-induced trauma or infection.

2. Use diluted (2.5–5%) contrast agents designed for intravenous urography (see Chap. 4).

3. Conventional ventrodorsal, lateral, and oblique views are obtained.

4. If possible, fluoroscopic evaluation is done during injection of contrast agent.

5. The fundus of the bladder is the site most commonly ruptured.

III. Abdominal paracentesis

A. Aspirated fluid is typically bloody.

B. Abdominal fluid creatinine concentrations are higher than simultaneously sampled serum creatinine concentrations.

C. Abdominal fluid cultures are needed to detect bacterial peritonitis.

IV. Other tests

A. Serum concentrations of urea nitrogen, creatinine, potassium, phosphorus, and total carbon dioxide are needed to assess, manage, and monitor sequelae of urine retention.

B. Peripheral white blood cell counts become elevated as peritonitis occurs.

Differential Diagnosis

I. Urine leakage from sites other than the bladder
II. Other abdominal organ trauma
III. Ascites from other mechanisms
IV. Urinary obstruction from causes other than trauma: urethroliths, urethral plugs, or urethral neoplasia
V. Ruptured cysts of other abdominal organs
VI. Other causes of peritonitis (see Chap. 38)

Treatment

I. Treatment of urinary tract trauma depends on the cause, location, and severity of lesions.
II. If present, treat life-threatening shock and metabolic sequelae first.
III. Depending on the severity of disease, urinary diver-

sion (urinary catheterization, tube cystostomy) and/or peritoneal lavage (dialysis) may be needed.

IV. Small rents can be managed nonsurgically.
A. Correct any underlying obstruction.
B. Keep urinary bladder empty with continuous urinary catheterization (closed system) for approximately 3–10 days.

V. Surgical repair is the treatment of choice for large traumatic rents in the urinary bladder.
A. Correct any underlying obstruction.
B. Once metabolic abnormalities have abated, surgical exploratory laparotomy and bladder repair are performed.

VI. Antimicrobial agents may be used to prevent or control infections caused by commensal microbes.

VII. Herniated bladders are decompressed and then surgically secured in their original position.

Patient Monitoring

I. After removal of urinary catheter, monitor voluntary voiding to eliminate the possibility of unresolved urinary obstruction.

II. Culture urine following urinary catheter removal and healing.

III. Abnormal concentrations of serum electrolytes should return to normal in approximately 1–3 days following restoration of bladder integrity.

IV. Positive contrast radiography is repeated if clinical signs persist.

Bibliography

Bai SC, Sampson DA, Morris JG, Rogers QR: Vitamin B-6 requirement of growing kittens. J Nutr 119:1020, 1989

Kruger JM, Osborne CA, Lulich JP: Management of nonobstructive idiopathic feline lower urinary tract disease. Vet Clin North Am [Small Anim Pract] 26:571, 1996

Linda M, Shortkiffe D, Stamey TA: Infections of the urinary tract: introduction and general principles. p. 738. In Walsh PC, Gittes RF, Perlmutter AD, Stamey TA (eds): Campbell's Urology. WB Saunders, Philadelphia, 1986

Lulich JP, Osborne CA: Catheter-assisted retrieval of urocystoliths from dogs and cats. J Am Vet Med Assoc 201:111, 1992

Lulich JP, Osborne CA, Unger LK et al: Nonsurgical removal of urocystoliths by voiding urohydropropulsion. J Am Vet Med Assoc 203:660, 1993

McKerrell RE, Blakemore WF, Heath MF et al: Primary hyperoxaluria (L-glyceric aciduria) in the cat: a newly recognized inherited disease. Vet Rec 125:31, 1989

Osborne CA, Kroll RA, Lulich JP et al: Medical management of vesicourachal diverticula in 15 cats with lower urinary tract disease. J Small Anim Pract 30:608, 1989

Osborne CA, Lulich JP, Kruger JK et al: Medical dissolution of feline struvite urocystoliths: prospective clinical study of 30 cases. J Am Vet Med Assoc 196:1053, 1990

Sutton RA, Wong NL, Dirks J: Effects of metabolic acidosis and alkalosis on sodium and calcium transport in the dog kidney. Kidney Int 15:520, 1979

50

Disorders of Micturition

India F. Lane

GENERAL INFORMATION

Definition

I. Micturition includes both a storage phase and an emptying phase.

II. Disturbances in either phase result in loss of voluntary, coordinated, or complete micturition.

III. Disorders of storage result in pollakiuria, nocturia, and urinary incontinence.

IV. Disorders of emptying result in urine retention, incomplete voiding, and overflow urinary incontinence.

V. Micturition disorders may be classified according to origin (neurogenic vs. non-neurogenic), frequency (intermittent vs. continuous), or residual volume (distended bladder vs. non-distended bladder).

VI. The most useful classification of urinary incontinence is based on the functional status of the urine ''pump'' (urinary bladder) and urinary outlet (bladder neck and urethra).
   A. Hypocontractile bladder: detrusor atony, detrusor hyporeflexia, hypercompliance
   B. Hypercontractile bladder: hypocompliance, detrusor hyperreflexia, detrusor instability, urge incontinence
   C. Hypotonic urethra: urethral incompetence, urethral hypoplasia
   D. Hypertonic urethra: increased outlet resistance, functional urethral obstruction

Causes

I. Disorders of micturition are caused by neurogenic, anatomic, and functional disorders.

II. Urine retention has numerous causes (Table 50–1).

III. Urinary incontinence may arise from a variety of causes (Table 50–2).

Pathophysiology

I. Anatomy
   A. Urinary bladder
      1. Detrusor muscle is composed of an interwoven network of smooth muscle bundles.
      2. Tight cellular junctions between smooth muscle cells allow rapid transmission of neuromuscular impulses.
   B. Urethra
      1. Urethral smooth muscle is an extension of detrusor smooth muscle with both longitudinal and circular or spiral fibers.
      2. A striated muscle zone (external urethral sphincter) is located primarily in the prostatic urethra in male dogs and in the mid-urethra in female dogs.
      3. In the cat, the striated muscle zone is located primarily in the post-prostatic urethra in the male and in the distal urethra in the female.

II. Neurophysiology
   A. Local neuromuscular receptors, peripheral nerves, spinal pathways, and input from higher centers are required for voluntary, coordinated micturition.
   B. The pelvic nerve originates from sacral spinal cord segments (S1–S3) and projects parasympathetic impulses to ganglia in the urinary bladder wall and cholinergic (muscarinic) receptors in the detrusor muscle.
   C. The hypogastric nerve originates from the lumbar spinal cord, synapses in the caudal mesenteric ganglion, and supplies sympathetic input to adrenergic receptors.
      1. Beta-adrenergic receptors in the detrusor muscle
      2. Alpha-adrenergic receptors in the smooth muscle of the bladder neck and urethra
   D. The pudendal nerve originates from the sacral spinal cord segments and provides somatic innervation to striated urethral muscle.
   E. Supraspinal organization of the micturition reflex involves the micturition center located in the pons, the cerebral cortex, and additional modulatory input from the cerebellum, basal ganglia, and hypothalamus.

III. Storage phase
   A. The urinary bladder is relaxed and fills against an appropriate degree of outlet resistance.

Table 50-1. *Major Causes of Urine Retention in Small Animals*

Disorder	Characteristics	Management
Lesions of sacral spinal cord—lower motor neuron	1. Distended, flaccid urinary bladder 2. Bladder easily expressed 3. Depressed genitoanal reflexes 4. Overflow incontinence	1. Correct primary lesion 2. Keep bladder small 3. Consider bethanechol 4. Manage urinary tract infection
Lesions of suprasacral spinal cord—upper motor neuron	1. Distended, firm urinary bladder 2. Bladder not easily expressed 3. Incomplete reflex voiding may develop (autonomic bladder) 4. Proprioceptive deficits	1. Correct primary lesion 2. Keep bladder small 3. Reduce outlet resistance (phenoxybenzamine) 4. Consider bethanechol once outflow resistance is normal/reduced
Detrusor atony	1. Distended bladder 2. Expressibility variable 3. Weak or no detrusor activity 4. Overflow incontinence	1. Keep bladder small 2. Bethanechol trial 3. ± Phenoxybenzamine
Anatomic urethral obstruction	1. Distended urinary bladder 2. Dysuria and stranguria 3. Overflow incontinence 4. Difficult to pass catheter and express 5. ± Hematuria	1. Alleviate obstruction 2. Ensure urine flow
Functional urethral obstruction	1. History of obstruction, inflammation 2. Distended bladder, difficult to express 3. Catheterization usually easy	1. Catheterize to keep bladder small 2. Phenoxybenzamine/prazosin 3. Skeletal muscle relaxants
Detrusor-urethral dyssynergia	1. Distended bladder 2. Voiding initiated, then interrupted	1. Keep bladder small 2. Phenoxybenzamine/prazosin

Table 50-2. *Major Causes of Urinary Incontinence in Small Animals*

Disorder	Characteristics	Management
Ectopic ureters	1. Severe or continuous incontinence 2. Non-distended bladder 3. Affected since birth	1. Surgical intervention 2. Manage urinary tract infection 3. ± Alpha agonists
Congenital urethral incompetence/hypoplasia	1. Severe incontinence 2. Non-distended bladder 3. Neurologically intact	1. Alpha agonist trial 2. Concurrent reproductive hormone administration 3. Surgical reconstruction?
Urinary bladder storage dysfunction	1. Intermittent urine dribbling 2. Pollakiuria 3. Non-distended bladder	1. Manage urinary tract infection or other underlying cause 2. Oxybutynin/propantheline
Urethral incompetence	1. Older, neutered animal 2. Non-distended bladder 3. Neurologically intact 4. Intermittent resting incontinence 5. Normal voluntary voiding	1. Manage urinary tract infection 2. Alpha agonists 3. Reproductive hormone replacement
Paradoxic incontinence/overflow incontinence	1. Distended urinary bladder 2. Urine dribbling 3. ± Dysuria, stranguria	1. Alleviate obstruction 2. Keep bladder empty 3. See Table 50-1
FeLV-associated incontinence	1. Intermittent urine dribbling 2. Non-distended bladder 3. Anisocoria common 4. Feline leukemia positive	1. Anticholinergic trial

B. This phase is characterized by sympathetic dominance.

C. Activation of beta receptors in the urinary bladder facilitates relaxation of the detrusor muscle.

D. Activation of alpha receptors in the urethra facilitates smooth muscle contraction and outlet resistance.

E. Striated urethral muscle reflexively contracts if intra-abdominal pressure is increased, or it may be voluntarily contracted.

IV. Voiding phase

A. Afferent impulses from stretch receptors in the bladder wall are transmitted to the brain stem and cerebral sensory areas via the pelvic nerve and spinal pathways.

B. Voluntary relaxation via the pudendal nerve is required for initiation of voiding.

C. Efferent parasympathetic motor impulses are transmitted via reticulospinal pathways and the pelvic nerve to initiate bladder contraction.

D. Sympathetic and somatic input is reflexively inhibited to facilitate urethral opening.

E. Input from the micturition center is required for sustained contraction, sustained inhibition of outlet sphincters, and complete emptying.

F. Following voiding, sympathetic nervous system dominance resumes.

Diagnosis

I. Signalment

A. Congenital anatomic and neurologic abnormalities are likely in young animals.

B. Older animals may be affected by underlying neurologic, urologic, or systemic disease.

C. Reproductive hormone–responsive urethral incompetence is common in neutered animals.

D. Prostatic disease should be considered in intact male dogs.

E. In cats, neurologic injuries, congenital abnormalities, and incontinence associated with feline leukemia virus (FeLV) are the most common disorders.

II. History

A. Reproductive status, age at neutering, age at onset of incontinence

B. Characterization of any previous urogenital or other medical problems

C. Characterization of voiding: frequency, posture, urine volume, initiation and maintenance of urine stream

D. Characterization of urine: color, smell, presence of blood

E. Pattern of urinary incontinence

1. Continuous or intermittent
2. Small volumes or large volumes
3. During periods of resting or during activity or movement
4. Initiated by positional changes (e.g., urine pooling)

F. Previous traumatic injuries to spine, pelvis, tail, limbs

G. Difficulty in walking, standing, defecating

H. Estimated daily water consumption

III. Physical examination

A. General appearance, including attitude, mental status, ambulation, gait, and conformation

B. Examination of external genitalia for conformational abnormalities, lesions, masses, urine staining

C. Abdominal palpation, including urinary bladder size, tone, and expressibility; presence of pelvic masses; pain

D. Digital rectal palpation to assess anal tone, prostate, and prostatic urethra in males; pelvic canal, urethra, and bladder neck in females

E. Digital vaginal examination to evaluate conformation and to detect vaginal bands, strictures, masses

F. Neurologic assessment

1. Pudendal nerve integrity and sacral spinal cord reflex arcs are assessed by evaluating anal tone, perineal sensation, and bulbospongiosus reflexes.
2. Pressure on the bulbus glandis in the male or the vulva in the female should elicit a visible contraction of the anal sphincter.
3. The sacral spinal cord is further assessed by evaluating tail tone and tail carriage and by palpating for lumbosacral pain.
4. Thoracolumbar spinal cord integrity is evaluated by proprioception, placing responses, and postural reactions in the hindlimbs.

G. Observation of voiding: assessment of posture, urine stream, initiation, and completion

H. Measurement of urine residual volume

1. The bladder may be catheterized after voiding to determine residual volume.
2. Normal residual volume in the dog is 0.2–0.4 ml/kg.

IV. Laboratory analysis

A. A urinalysis is indicated in all cases.

1. Physiochemical and urine sediment examination
2. Culture and antibiotic susceptibility testing of urine

B. Serum urea and creatinine measurements are indicated if any upper urinary tract dysfunction is likely (e.g., urine retention, urinary obstruction, congenital abnormalities).

C. A complete minimum database is indicated in polydipsic-polyuric or ill animals.

D. FeLV and feline immunodeficiency virus (FIV) testing may be indicated in cats.

V. Survey radiography

A. Urinary bladder size, position

B. Prostate gland

C. Pelvic conformation

D. Radiodense urocystoliths or urethroliths

VI. Contrast radiography

A. Indications

1. Disorders of micturition in juvenile animals
2. Continuous urinary incontinence or urine leakage from abnormal anatomic sites

3. Urinary incontinence or urine retention observed shortly after ovariohysterectomy or other surgical procedures
B. Excretory urography
  1. Renal morphology
  2. Renal function (qualitative)
  3. Hydroureter
  4. Ureteral terminations
C. Cystourethrography
  1. Filling defects in the urinary bladder or bladder neck
  2. Uroliths
  3. Urachal diverticuli
  4. Abnormalities of the bladder wall/mucosa
  5. Bladder or urethral hypoplasia/dysplasia
D. Retrograde vaginourethrography
  1. Retrograde filling of ectopic ureters
  2. Vesicovaginal fistulas and ureterovaginal fistulas
  3. Urethral length and urinary bladder neck position
  4. Urethral mucosal lesions
  5. Urethral rupture
  6. Urethral or bladder neck masses
  7. Vaginal anomalies (e.g., strictures, masses)
VII. Urodynamic procedures
A. Available at many veterinary referral centers
B. General indications
  1. Diagnosis undetermined
  2. Multiple abnormalities suspected
  3. Poor response to appropriate medical management
  4. Functional assessment of congenital anatomic abnormalities
C. Cystometrography
  1. The cystometrogram is completed by recording intravesicular pressure as the bladder is slowly distended with air, carbon dioxide, saline, or water.
  2. A graph of intravesicular pressure vs. volume infused provides a curve depicting the filling and contractile phases of micturition.
  3. Urinary bladder capacity, elasticity, and contractile function can be objectively evaluated.
  4. Indications are as follows.
    a) Neurogenic disorders of micturition in which contractile function is in question
    b) Suspected detrusor atony
    c) Refractory urinary incontinence
    d) Assessment of functional storage capacity in animals with multiple disorders, urinary bladder damage, or ectopic ureters
    e) Evaluation of pharmacologic agents acting on urinary bladder
D. Urethral pressure profilometry (UPP)
  1. Intraurethral pressure measurements are made by recording resistance to infusion of fluid through a urinary catheter or via catheter-mounted transducers.
  2. The ''profile'' is completed by plotting pressures measured along the length of the urethra.

3. Indications for UPP are as follows.
  a) Diagnostic evaluation of urinary incontinence
  b) Localization of urethral obstructions
  c) Identification of increased urethral resistance or urethral spasm
  d) Assessment of urethral responses to pharmacologic agents
  e) Evaluation of urethral function in dogs with anatomic abnormalities such as ectopic ureters and vaginal anomalies
  f) Perioperative evaluation of urologic procedures
E. Electromyography (EMG)
  1. Recording electrodes are inserted percutaneously or mounted on a urinary catheter to record urethral striated muscle activity.
  2. Indications for EMG include neurogenic disorders of urethral function, incomplete or interrupted voiding with suspected dyssynergia, and urinary incontinence.
F. Uroflowmetry
  1. Measurement of urine flow in small animals is difficult because of the need to ''command'' urine flow and to collect urine in a designated reservoir.
  2. With simultaneous intravesicular pressure measurement, premature leakage of urine, interrupted voiding, and detrusor-urethral dyssynergia may be detected (Moreau et al., 1983).
  3. Indications include the following.
    a) Dysuria or obstructed voiding patterns
    b) Urinary incontinence
    c) Urinary bladder dysfunction or incomplete voiding
    d) Neurogenic disorders of micturition

DISORDERS OF URINE RETENTION

Neurogenic Disorders—Lower Motor Neuron (LMN) Deficits

Definition and Pathophysiology

I. These disorders result from lesions of the sacral spinal cord, peripheral pelvic nerve, and detrusor muscle.
II. Loss of most afferent and all efferent input to the bladder and urethral sphincters results in loss of bladder sensory and contractile responses and the spinal micturition reflex.
III. Urethral sphincters also are hypocontractile.

Causes

I. Congenital malformation of the sacral spinal column
II. Cauda equina compression
III. Lumbosacral disk disease
IV. Sacral or sacrococcygeal fractures

V. Traumatic or degenerative lesions of pelvic nerves
VI. Overdistention of bladder (atony)

Clinical Signs

I. Paraparesis or paralysis
II. Decreased anal tone and perineal reflexes
III. Depressed bulbocavernosus reflexes
IV. Fecal incontinence
V. Tail pain or loss of tail tone
VI. Distended, flaccid urinary bladder
VII. Overflow incontinence

Diagnosis

I. Abnormal neurologic findings
II. Distended urinary bladder that is easily expressed
III. Myelogram, epidurogram, magnetic resonance imaging

Differential Diagnosis

I. Other neurogenic disorders
II. Other causes of detrusor atony (Fig. 50–1)

Treatment

I. Correct the primary lesion, if possible.
II. Keep the bladder small via manual expression or urethral catheterization.
III. Pharmacologic manipulation may facilitate bladder emptying (see Bladder Dysfunction—Detrusor Atony).
IV. Manage concurrent urinary tract infection (UTI) and urine scald.

Patient Monitoring

I. Monitor bladder size and residual volume.
II. Monitor urine sediment for signs of inflammation. Culture urine if indicated.
III. Acute reversible or partial neurologic lesions have the best prognosis.
IV. Chronically, pharmacologic management may be ineffective, and long-term bladder expression or catheterization may be required.

Neurogenic Disorders—Upper Motor Neuron (UMN) Deficits

Definition and Pathophysiology

I. These result from lesions of the suprasacral spinal cord.
II. Sensory and motor pathways to the urinary bladder are interrupted; bladder function is lost, but sphincter tone usually remains.
III. Uninhibited pudendal nerve activity may create a hypertonic striated muscle sphincter and excessive outlet resistance.

Causes

I. Thoracolumbar disk disease
II. Fractures
III. Tumors

Clinical Signs

I. Initially characterized by a distended, firm urinary bladder that is difficult to express.
II. Over time, some urinary bladder contractile function

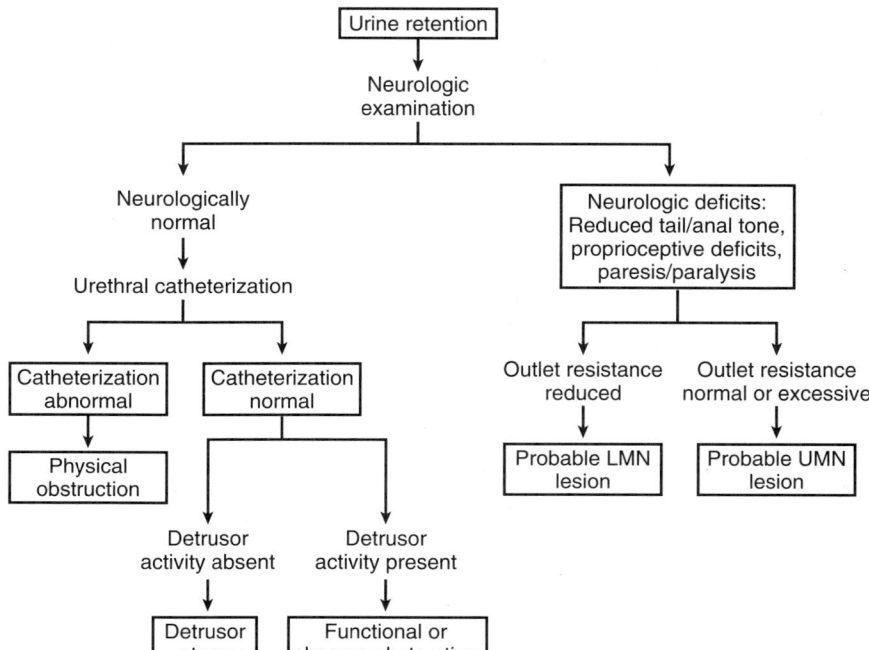

Figure 50–1. Algorithm for the approach to urine retention in small animals. (Data from Lane IF: Functional urine retention. In Tilley LP, Smith FWK Jr [eds]: Five Minute Veterinary Consult. Williams & Wilkins, Baltimore, in press.)

may return with emergence of a purely sacral reflex (autonomic bladder).
III. Voiding is usually involuntary, incomplete, and poorly coordinated.
IV. The urinary bladder may contract against inappropriate outlet resistance (detrusor-urethral dyssynergia), and detrusor atony may result.
V. Other signs include proprioceptive deficits, paraparesis or tetraparesis, ataxia, and hyperreflexia.

Diagnosis

I. Neurologic findings
II. Large, turgid urinary bladder that is difficult to express
III. Radiography or myelography

Differential Diagnosis

I. Other causes of detrusor atony
II. Functional or physical urethral obstruction
III. Detrusor-urethral dyssynergia

Treatment

I. Correction of the primary lesion
II. Urethral catheterization to keep bladder small
III. Pharmacologic manipulation to reduce outlet resistance (see Urethral Dysfunction—Increased Outlet Resistance)
IV. Pharmacologic manipulation to improve urinary bladder emptying (see Bladder Dysfunction—Detrusor Atony)
V. Management of any concurrent UTI

Patient Monitoring

I. Monitor bladder size and residual volume.
II. Monitor urine sediment for signs of inflammation. Culture urine if indicated.
III. Monitor return of neurologic function.
IV. Prognosis depends on the extent of the cord lesion.

Bladder Dysfunction—Detrusor Atony

Definition and Pathophysiology

I. Hypocontractility of the urinary bladder associated with primary failure of smooth muscle function
II. Usually characterized by a distended, flaccid bladder that is fairly easy to express (unless increased outflow resistance has caused overdistention and atony is secondary)

Causes

I. Neurogenic disorders
II. Acute or chronic overdistention of the urinary bladder
III. Dysautonomia
IV. Generalized muscle weakness

Clinical Signs

I. The animal may posture to urinate or apply an abdominal press and fail to produce an adequate stream.
II. Alternatively, few or no attempts to urinate may be observed.
III. Overflow incontinence may be observed.
IV. Abdominal pain or signs of uremia may be observed with acute urine retention.

Diagnosis

I. Urine retention with distended urinary bladder
II. Outlet resistance usually normal, although increased outflow resistance can lead to bladder overdistention and detrusor atony
III. Cystometrography

Treatment

I. Frequent manual expression, intermittent urinary catheterization, or temporary indwelling urinary catheterization may be required to keep the bladder small.
II. Parasympathomimetic (cholinergic) agents are frequently used to increase parasympathetic input and stimulate contraction, but urethral resistance must be minimized before initiating therapy.
   A. Bethanechol chloride is often administered.
      1. Starting doses of 2.5 mg for cats, 5 mg for small dogs, and 10 mg for larger dogs are recommended.
      2. The dosage may be slowly increased in 2.5- to 5-mg increments.
      3. Total dosages range from 5–25 mg PO BID-TID in dogs and 1.25–7.5 mg PO SID-TID in cats.
   B. Potential adverse effects include ptyalism, lacrimation, abdominal cramping, vomiting, and diarrhea.
III. Alternative pharmacologic agents used to improve urinary bladder contractile function include cholinesterase inhibitors, beta antagonists, dopamine antagonists, and selected prostaglandins.

Patient Monitoring

I. Monitor bladder size and residual volume.
II. Monitor urine sediment for UTI. Culture urine if indicated.
III. Atony from acute overdistention is usually reversible if the bladder is kept small.
IV. Prognosis for return of function in chronically atonic bladders is poor.

Urethral Dysfunction—Increased Outlet Resistance

Definition and Pathophysiology

I. Anatomic obstruction prevents urine flow during voiding.
II. Functional obstruction results from excessive smooth or striated muscle resistance in the urethra.

III. Inappropriate urethral resistance during voiding (detrusor-urethral dyssynergia) also interrupts voiding and results in urine retention.

Causes

I. Anatomic urethral obstruction
 A. Urolithiasis
 B. Mucoprotein-crystalloid plugs (cats)
 C. Bladder neck or urethral neoplasia
 D. Prostatic disease (usually neoplasia)
 E. Urethral strictures
II. Functional urethral obstruction (inappropriate urethral resistance or muscular urethral spasm)
 A. Neurogenic disorders
 B. Post-urethral or pelvic surgery
 C. Post-urethral obstruction
 D. Urethral inflammation or granulomatous urethritis
III. Detrusor-urethral dyssynergia
 A. Defined as a lack of coordination between urinary bladder contraction and urethral relaxation
 B. May be a consequence of neurologic lesions, local or idiopathic causes

Clinical Signs

I. The urinary bladder is distended and difficult or impossible to express.
II. Dysuria and stranguria are usually observed.
III. An attenuated urine stream may be observed with partial anatomic or functional obstructions.
IV. A normal initial urine stream that rapidly tapers may be observed with detrusor-urethral dyssynergia.
V. Paradoxic urinary incontinence may be observed in between attempts to void if intravesicular pressure exceeds outlet resistance and obstruction is not complete.

Diagnosis

I. Anatomic obstruction is diagnosed or ruled out by attempting urethral catheterization and is confirmed by contrast radiography or ultrasonography.
II. Catheterization is usually easy if obstruction is solely functional.
III. Gentle attempts to manually express the urinary bladder may trigger detrusor activity and allow subjective assessment of urethral resistance.
IV. If the animal initiates voiding but the urine stream is rapidly interrupted, functional obstruction or detrusor-urethral dyssynergia should be considered.
V. Urethral spasm may be detected by a urethral pressure profile.
VI. Confirmation of dyssynergia requires urodynamic studies, which simultaneously provide information regarding urinary bladder activity and urine flow.

Differential Diagnosis

I. Primary detrusor atony
II. UMN disorders

Treatment

I. Physical obstructions require hydropropulsion techniques or surgical intervention.
II. Smooth muscle relaxation may be accomplished pharmacologically.
 A. Phenoxybenzamine 0.25 mg/kg (2.5–5 mg PO SID–BID in cats and 5–20 mg PO BID in dogs)
 B. Prazosin (alternative agent) 1 mg/15 kg PO BID–TID
 C. Potential adverse effects: hypotension, reflex tachycardia, gastrointestinal irritation
 D. Avoided or used cautiously in animals with cardiovascular disease
III. Striated muscle relaxants such as diazepam may be used in addition to alpha antagonists and may be indicated in UMN lesions in which striated muscle activity is likely to be uninhibited.
 A. Diazepam may be administered several times daily to facilitate voiding or manual expression.
  1. Dosages are 1–2.5 mg PO TID–QID in cats and 2–10 mg PO TID–QID in dogs.
  2. The major side effect of diazepam is sedation, although vertigo and paradoxic excitement are observed occasionally.
 B. Dantrolene (1 mg/kg IV) has been effective in reducing feline striated urethral tone in experimental and clinical settings (Strater-Knowlen et al., 1995).
  1. The agent inhibits calcium movement in muscle cells.
  2. Oral preparations are administered at a dosage of 0.5–2 mg/kg PO TID (cats).
  3. It is contraindicated in animals with cardiac, pulmonary, or hepatic disease.
IV. Other muscle relaxants that may reduce urethral resistance include baclofen, calcium channel inhibitors, and acepromazine (Mawby et al., 1990; Marks et al., 1993).

Patient Monitoring

I. Monitor bladder size, residual volume, and urine stream.
II. Most causes of functional obstruction resolve with time and appropriate medical management.
III. Phenoxybenzamine reliably improves voiding in most cases of dyssynergia in dogs.

CONGENITAL DISORDERS OF URINARY INCONTINENCE

Ectopic Ureters

Definition and Pathophysiology

I. The termination of one or both ureters bypasses the normal reservoir of the urinary bladder.
II. Additional anatomic or functional abnormalities are usually observed concurrently.
 A. Renal dysplasia or aplasia
 B. Hydroureter, hydronephrosis

C. Vaginal anomalies
D. Urethral incompetence
E. Urinary bladder storage dysfunction

Clinical Signs

I. Continuous urinary incontinence is usually observed from birth or a very early age.
II. Intermittent or positional incontinence also has been described.
III. Urine-soaked fur along the perineum or hindlimbs may be observed.

Diagnosis

I. History of continuous incontinence, small bladder size
II. Abnormal ureteral termination on excretory urography or retrograde vaginourethrography
III. Hydronephrosis and hydroureter detected by ultrasonography or excretory urography
IV. Preoperative urodynamic evaluation to detect concurrent urethral or bladder functional abnormalities

Differential Diagnosis

I. Congenital urethral incompetence or hypoplasia
II. Other anatomic abnormalities

Treatment

I. Surgical correction of ureteral termination (see Chap. 48)
II. Alpha agonist administration (Table 50–3) for concurrent urethral incompetence

Patient Monitoring

I. Monitor for UTI.
II. Postoperative urinary incontinence is observed in one half to two thirds of animals (Stone and Mason, 1990; McLaughlin and Miller, 1991; Lane et al., 1995).
III. Concurrent urethral incompetence is manageable in approximately half of affected dogs.
IV. Mild to moderate hydroureter usually resolves following successful surgery.

Congenital Urethral Incompetence/Hypoplasia

Definition and Pathophysiology

I. Functional and anatomic urethral incompetence may be observed.
II. The disorder is often associated with other anatomic abnormalities (ectopic ureter in dogs, vaginal aplasia in cats).
III. The urethra may be normal (functional incompetence) or grossly dilated, shortened, or absent (urethral hypoplasia).

Clinical Signs

I. Severe urinary incontinence since birth
II. Small, easily expressed urinary bladder

Diagnosis

I. History of incontinence with a non-distended bladder
II. Lack of neurologic deficits or malformations
III. Anomalous urethra on cystourethrography or retrograde urethrography
IV. Poor closure pressures on urethral pressure profile

Differential Diagnosis

I. Ectopic ureter
II. Reproductive hormone–responsive urinary incontinence
III. Vaginal anomalies

Treatment and Monitoring

I. The condition may improve or resolve after first estrus or puberty.
II. Alpha agonists may be effective in some cases; high dosages are usually required.
III. Combination therapy with reproductive hormones or anticholinergic agents may improve the response (see Table 50–3).
IV. Response to pharmacologic manipulation is usually poor if anatomy is abnormal.
V. Surgical bladder neck or urethral reconstruction may reduce incontinence in some cases (Holt, 1992; Holt, 1993).

Urinary Bladder Storage Dysfunction

Definition and Pathophysiology

I. Poor compliance/elasticity during the filling phase or urinary bladder hypercontractility
II. Characterized by involuntary voiding at low bladder volumes and pressures

Causes

I. Sensory causes
    A. UTI/urolithiasis
    B. Chronic inflammatory processes
    C. Infiltrative masses
II. Congenital urinary bladder hypoplasia
III. Neuropathic hypercontractility (detrusor hyperreflexia)
IV. Idiopathic hypercontractility (detrusor instability)
V. FeLV
VI. Chronic partial obstruction
VII. Prostatic disease

Clinical Signs

I. Urinary incontinence
II. Pollakiuria
III. Urine leakage with standing, barking, or jumping

Table 50-3. *Pharmacologic Agents Used in the Management of Micturition Disorders*

Agent	Action	Dosage	Adverse Effects	Contraindications
To Increase Bladder Contractility				
Bethanechol (Urecholine)	Parasympathomimetic	Dog: 5–25 mg PO TID Cat: 1.25–5 mg PO TID	Vomiting, cramping, ptyalism, anorexia	Urethral obstruction, GI disease, hyperthyroidism
To Decrease Bladder Contractility				
Oxybutynin (Ditropan)	Anticholinergic; antispasmodic	Dog: 1.25–5 mg PO BID–TID Cat: 0.5–1.25 mg PO BID–TID	Vomiting, diarrhea, urine retention, sedation	Glaucoma, cardiac disease, GI obstruction
Propantheline (Pro-Banthine)	Anticholinergic	Dog: 7.5–15 mg PO TID Cat: 5–7.5 mg PO TID or PRN	As for oxybutynin	As for oxybutynin
Dicyclomine (Bentyl)	Anticholinergic; smooth muscle relaxant	Dog: 10 mg PO TID Cat: not determined	As for oxybutynin	As for oxybutynin
Imipramine (Tofranil)	Tricyclic antidepressant; anticholinergic and adrenergic effects	Dog: 5–15 mg PO BID Cat: 2.5–5 mg PO TID	Tremors, seizures, tachycardia, excitability	—
To Increase Urethral Resistance				
Diethylstilbestrol (DES)	Reproductive hormone (female)	Dog: 0.1–1 mg PO SID for 5 days, followed by 0.1–1 mg q 5–14 days PRN	Signs of estrus, bone marrow suppression, pyometra	Immune-mediated disease, pregnancy
Stilbestrol	Reproductive hormone (female)	Dog: as for DES, or 0.01–0.02 mg SID (see text)	As for DES	As for DES
Testosterone propionate	Reproductive hormone (male)	Dog: 2.2 mg/kg SQ or IM q 2–3 days Cat: 5–10 mg IM PRN	Aggression, prostatic disease, perianal disease	Prostatic disorders
Testosterone cypionate (DEPO-Testosterone)	Reproductive hormone (male)	Dog: 2.2 mg/kg IM or 200 mg/dog IM q 30–60 days	As for testosterone propionate	Prostatic disease
Phenylpropanolamine (Propagest, Dexatrim)	Alpha agonist	Dog: 1.5 mg/kg PO BID–TID Cat: 1.5–2.2 mg/kg PO BID–TID	Tachycardia, hypertension, restlessness, anorexia	Cardiac disease, glaucoma, hypertensive disease
Ephedrine	Alpha agonist	Dog: 1.2 mg/kg PO TID Cat: 2–4 mg PO TID	As for phenylpropanolamine	—
To Decrease Urethral Resistance				
Phenoxybenzamine (Dibenzyline)	Alpha antagonist; urethral smooth muscle relaxant	Dog: 0.25 mg/kg PO BID Cat: 1.25–7.5 mg PO SID–BID	Hypotension, GI upset, tachycardia	Cardiac disease, glaucoma, diabetes mellitus, renal failure
Prazosin (Minipress)	Alpha antagonist; urethral smooth muscle relaxant	Dog: 1 mg/15 kg PO TID Cat: 0.5 mg PO TID or 0.03 mg/kg IV	As for phenoxybenzamine	As for phenoxybenzamine
Baclofen (Lioresal)	Skeletal muscle relaxant	Dog: 1–2 mg/kg PO TID Cat: not recommended	Weakness, pruritus, GI upset	—
Dantrolene (Dantrium)	Skeletal muscle relaxant	Dog: 1–5 mg/kg PO TID Cat: 0.5–2 mg/kg PO TID or 1 mg/kg IV	Weakness, GI upset, sedation, hepatotoxicity	Cardiopulmonary disease
Diazepam (Valium)	Benzodiazepine; skeletal muscle relaxant	Dog: 2–10 mg PO TID Cat: 1–2.5 mg PO TID or 0.5 mg/kg IV	Sedation, polyphagia, paradoxic excitement, hepatotoxicity	Hepatic disease, pregnancy

Diagnosis

I. Exclusion of other causes of incontinence
II. Urinalysis and urine culture
III. Ideally diagnosed by cystometrography

Treatment

I. Goals are to reduce contractile activity and improve bladder storage capacity.
II. Primary treatment is directed at underlying sensory or neurogenic disorders (e.g., UTI, urolithiasis).
III. Parasympatholytic (anticholinergic) agents may be helpful.
  A. Propantheline
    1. Cats: 5–7.5 mg PO as needed (frequency varies from TID to every 2–3 days)
    2. Dogs: 7.5–30 mg PO BID
  B. Oxybutynin
    1. Anticholinergic agent with antispasmodic and smooth muscle relaxant activity
    2. Dogs and cats: approximately 0.2 mg/kg PO BID–TID
      a) 0.5–1 mg PO BID–TID in cats and small dogs
      b) 1.25–5 mg PO BID–TID in larger dogs
IV. Tricyclic antidepressant agents possess anticholinergic, antihistaminic, sedative, and neurotransmitter effects.
  A. Both anticholinergic effects and mild adrenergic effects facilitate urine storage.
  B. Imipramine is recommended at a dosage of 5–15 mg PO BID in dogs and 2.5–5 mg PO BID in cats.
V. Alternative agents used to reduce urinary bladder contractility include beta agonists, calcium channel antagonists, and other smooth muscle relaxants.

Patient Monitoring

I. Response to treatment is usually good in idiopathic cases.
II. Response is less predictable with structural or mucosal abnormalities.

Urethral Dysfunction—Urethral Incompetence

Definition and Pathophysiology

I. It is the most common cause of urinary incontinence in adult female dogs.
II. Weakened closure responses of smooth or striated muscle of the urethra allow urine leakage during the storage phase of micturition.

Causes

I. Congenital urethral dysfunction has been described in young, intact animals and may be observed in conjunction with other congenital urogenital abnormalities.
II. The following factors may contribute to the development of acquired reproductive hormone–responsive urethral incompetence.
  A. Aging or altered urethral receptors
  B. Uterine stump adhesions
  C. Abnormal urethral length or conformation
  D. Unusual bladder neck position
  E. Vestibulovaginal anomalies
III. UTI and inflammation can result in transient urethral incompetence.
IV. Prostatic disorders and prostatic surgery may disrupt proximal urethral closure function in male dogs.

Clinical Signs

I. Urethral incompetence is most common in spayed female dogs but is occasionally encountered in male dogs.
II. Medium to large breed dogs are affected most often.
III. Intermittent urine leakage occurs, especially when resting or sleeping.
IV. Voluntary urination is usually normal, and bladder size is small.
V. Incidence may reach 20% in all spayed female dogs and 30% in spayed female dogs weighing ≥20 kg (Arnold, 1992b).

Diagnosis

I. Historical and physical examination findings, including a non-distended urinary bladder
II. Lack of neurologic abnormalities
III. Observation of normal voiding pattern
IV. Urinalysis, urine sediment examination, and urine culture
V. Urethral pressure profile

Differential Diagnosis

I. Overflow incontinence (Fig. 50–2)
II. Neurogenic incontinence
III. Nocturia (voluntary), polyuria
IV. Behavioral incontinence (inappropriate urination)

Treatment

I. UTIs must be identified and treated appropriately before the initiation of pharmacologic agents.
II. Reproductive hormone administration is often effective in minimizing incontinence.
  A. In the urethra, estrogens enhance mucosal sealing characteristics, collagen content, and vascularity.
  B. Estrogen administration also appears to increase the density and sensitivity of alpha receptors in the bladder neck and urethra.
  C. Diethylstilbestrol (DES) and stilbestrol are administered at 0.1–1 mg PO SID for 5–7 days, followed by a similar dosage administered every 5–14 days.

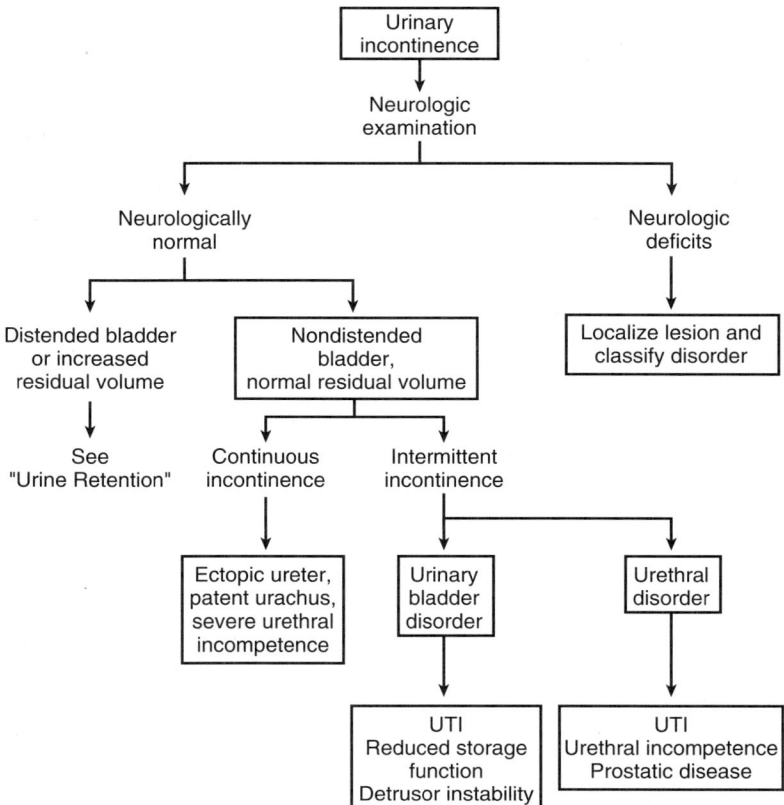

Figure 50–2. Algorithm for the approach to urinary incontinence in small animals. (Data from Lane IF: Urinary incontinence. In Tilley LP, Smith FWK Jr [eds]: Five Minute Veterinary Consult. Williams & Wilkins, Baltimore, in press.)

1. The dosage is adjusted to the minimal amount and frequency required.
2. Alternatively, stilbestrol may be administered at 0.04–0.06 mg PO SID for 1 week, then reduced at weekly intervals to 0.01 mg per day (Arnold, 1992a).
   a) After 4 weeks, treatment is discontinued, and a residual effect may be observed.
   b) Daily administration of 0.01–0.02 mg may be continued indefinitely if needed.
3. Potential side effects include bone marrow suppression, alopecia, behavioral changes, and signs of estrus.
4. Estrogen administration is not recommended in cats.

D. Testosterone propionate may be administered in males every 2–3 days for short-term effects.
   1. A longer duration of activity is provided by repository preparations such as testosterone cypionate or testosterone enanthate every 30–60 days.
   2. Dosages of 2.2 mg/kg IM are recommended; higher dosages of up to 200 mg/dog IM may be required (Barsanti et al., 1981).
   3. Testosterone propionate (5–10 mg IM/cat) may be effective in neutered male cats (Barsanti and Downey, 1984).
   4. Potential adverse effects include behavioral changes, aggression, prostatic disease, perianal adenomas, and perineal hernias.

III. Alpha-adrenergic agonists act at urethral alpha receptors to stimulate urethral smooth muscle contractile tone.
   A. Effective dosages of phenylpropanolamine in dogs range from 1–3 mg/kg PO BID–TID.
   B. Ephedrine or pseudoephedrine is administered at 5–15 mg PO TID or 1–2 mg/kg PO BID.
   C. Dosages can be slowly reduced to the minimum amount and frequency of administration required.
   D. Potential side effects include anxiety, hyperactivity, anorexia, tachycardia, hypertension, and gastrointestinal upset.
   E. Alpha-adrenergic agonists are contraindicated in animals with cardiac disease, hyperthyroidism, or other hypertensive disorders, such as renal failure, diabetes mellitus, or hyperadrenocorticism.
IV. A synergistic effect may be observed when alpha agonist administration is combined with reproductive hormone administration.
   A. Starting regimens are similar to those described for each agent.
   B. Final dosages of each agent are frequently lower than those required if either drug is used alone.
   C. The combination of an anticholinergic agent with alpha agonist or reproductive hormone administration may be valuable in some animals with concurrent bladder storage dysfunction.
V. Surgical management is considered when medical management is unsuccessful.

A. The goal is to increase urethral resistance by repositioning the urethra, increasing urethral pressure, or increasing urethral length.
B. Several methods have been described.
1. Seromuscular urethral sling (Bushby and Hankes, 1980)
2. Artificial mesh "sphincters" that encircle the urethra (Dean et al., 1989)
3. Polytetrafluoroethylene (Teflon) deposits injected into proximal urethral submucosa (Arnold et al., 1989)
4. Colposuspension techniques designed to reposition the intrapelvic bladder neck into a more intra-abdominal position (Holt, 1985b)
5. Bladder neck reconstruction (Holt, 1993)

Patient Monitoring

I. Periodic urinalyses are performed to monitor for UTI.
II. Periodic monitoring of complete blood count is recommended in animals receiving estrogen therapy.
III. Response to medical management in dogs with acquired urethral incompetence is generally good.
A. Excellent responses may be expected in 70–90% of dogs treated with alpha agonists.
B. Response to estrogen administration may be slightly lower; dogs may become refractory over time.
C. Neutered dogs that develop incontinence at a young age or shortly after neutering may have a poorer long-term response to medical treatment.
IV. Response is less favorable in dogs with congenital urethral incompetence or concurrent anatomic abnormalities.
V. Success of surgical techniques varies.
VI. In refractory cases, a thorough evaluation for exacerbating problems, such as UTI, polyuria, or subtle neurologic deficits, and a reevaluation of the diagnosis are indicated.

MISCELLANEOUS DISORDERS

Prostatic Disease

Definition and Causes

I. Prostatic disorders are the most common cause of urinary incontinence in adult male dogs.
II. Incontinence may be observed with suppurative inflammation, cystic hyperplasia, squamous metaplasia, and neoplasia of the prostate gland; however, it is most often associated with prostatic neoplasia.
III. Neoplasia may cause partial obstruction or severe destruction of the prostatic urethra.
IV. Urinary incontinence is a common complication of prostatic surgery, including prostatic biopsy, prostatic resection, and total prostatectomy (Basinger et al., 1987; Basinger et al., 1989; Goldsmid and Bellenger, 1991).

Clinical Signs

I. Prostatic disease may contribute to the development of several different disorders of micturition.
A. Inflammatory cystitis or urethritis
B. Urethral incompetence
C. Detrusor instability
D. Functional urethral obstruction
E. Partial obstruction with overflow incontinence and detrusor atony
II. Other clinical signs of prostatic disease may predominate.

Diagnosis

I. Abnormal prostatic contour or consistency on rectal palpation
II. Radiography and ultrasonography
III. Prostatic massage, brushing, or biopsy (see Chap. 52)
IV. Urodynamic procedures as needed

Treatment and Monitoring

I. Manage urinary obstruction by urethral catheterization.
II. Antimicrobials and castration may be required for primary prostatic disease.
III. Surgery may be indicated for staging of prostatic neoplasia or management of obstructive prostatic cysts.
IV. Response to alpha agonist administration is poor.
V. Prognosis for medical or surgical management of prostatic neoplasia is poor.

Feline Leukemia Virus–Associated Urinary Incontinence

Definition and Clinical Signs

I. Characterized by intermittent urine leakage and small residual urine volumes in FeLV-positive cats.
II. Other signs of illness are common (Barsanti and Downey, 1984; Barsanti and Finco, 1987).
A. Anorexia, weight loss, vomiting
B. Ptyalism, polydipsia
C. Infertility, abortion, and neonatal kitten death
III. Concurrent anisocoria may indicate multifocal autonomic dysfunction.
IV. Detrusor instability was identified by cystometrographic measurements in one cat (Lappin and Barsanti, 1987).

Treatment and Monitoring

I. Incontinence may resolve with anticholinergic agent administration (see Urinary Bladder Storage Dysfunction).
II. Response to other medical treatments is poor.

Bibliography

Abdel-Azim M, Sullivan M, Yalla SV: Disorders of bladder function in spinal cord disease. Neurol Clin 9:727, 1991

Adams WM, DiBartola SP: Radiographic and clinical features of pelvic bladder in the dog. J Am Vet Med Assoc 182:1212, 1983

Arnold S: Diagnosis and treatment of urinary incontinence. Proc Nephrol Urol Waltham Symp 16:75, 1992a

Arnold S: Relationship of incontinence to neutering. p. 875. In Kirk RW (ed): Current Veterinary Therapy XI: Small Animal Practice. WB Saunders, Philadelphia, 1992b

Arnold S, Jager P, DiBartola S et al: Treatment of urinary incontinence in dogs by endoscopic injection of Teflon. J Am Vet Med Assoc 195:1369, 1989

Barsanti JA: Urinary incontinence. p. 343. In Lorenz MD, Cornelius LM (eds): Small Animal Medical Diagnosis. Lippincott, Philadelphia, 1987

Barsanti JA, Downey R: Urinary incontinence in cats. J Am Anim Hosp Assoc 20:979, 1984

Barsanti JA, Edwards PD, Losonsky J: Testosterone responsive urinary incontinence in a castrated male dog. J Am Anim Hosp Assoc 17:117, 1981

Barsanti JA, Finco DR: Feline urinary incontinence. p. 1159. In Kirk RW (ed): Current Veterinary Therapy IX: Small Animal Practice. WB Saunders, Philadelphia, 1987

Basinger RR, Rawlings CA, Barsanti JA, Oliver JE: Urodynamic alterations associated with clinical prostatic diseases and prostatic surgery. J Am Anim Hosp Assoc 25:385, 1989

Basinger RR, Rawlings CA, Barsanti JA et al: Urodynamic alterations after prostatectomy in dogs without clinical prostatic disease. Vet Surg 16:405, 1987

Bradley WE, Timm GW: Physiology of micturition. Vet Clin North Am 4:487, 1974

Bushby PA, Hankes GH: Sling urethroplasty for the correction of urethral dilatation and urinary incontinence. J Am Anim Hosp Assoc 16:115, 1980

Dean PW, Novotny MJ, O'Brien DP: Prosthetic sphincter for urinary incontinence: results in three cases. J Am Anim Hosp Assoc 25:447, 1989

deGroat WC, Booth AM: Physiology of the bladder and urethra. Ann Intern Med 92:312, 1980

Frenier SL, Knowlen GG, Speth RC et al: Urethral response to alpha adrenergic agonist and antagonist drugs in anesthetized male cats. Am J Vet Res 53:1161, 1992

Goldsmid SE, Bellenger CR: Urinary incontinence after prostatectomy in dogs. Vet Surg 20:253, 1991

Gregory SP, Parkinson TJ, Holt PE: Urethral conformation and positioning in relation to urinary incontinence in the bitch. Vet Rec 131:167, 1992

Holt PE: Importance of urethral length, bladder neck position and vestibulovaginal stenosis in sphincter mechanism incompetence in the incontinent bitch. Res Vet Sci 39:364, 1985a

Holt PE: Urinary incontinence in the bitch due to sphincter mechanism incompetence: surgical treatment. J Small Anim Pract 26:237, 1985b

Holt PE: Pathophysiology and treatment of urethral sphincter mechanism incompetence in the incontinent bitch. Vet Int 3:15, 1992

Holt PE: Surgical management of congenital urethral sphincter mechanism incompetence in eight female cats and a bitch. Vet Surg 22:98, 1993

Holt PE, Gibbs C: Congenital urinary incontinence in cats: a review of 19 cases. Vet Rec 130:437, 1992

Labato MA: Disorders of micturition. p. 611. In Morgan RV (ed): Handbook of Small Animal Practice. 2nd Ed. Churchill Livingstone, New York, 1992

Lane IF: Disorders of micturition. p. 693. In Osborne CA, Finco DR (eds): Canine and Feline Nephrology and Urology. Williams & Wilkins, Baltimore, 1996

Lane IF: Pharmacologic management of feline lower urinary tract disorders. Vet Clin North Am [Small Anim Pract] 26:515, 1996

Lane IF, Lappin MR, Seim HB: Evaluation of results of preoperative urodynamic measurements in nine dogs with ectopic ureters. J Am Vet Med Assoc 206:1348, 1995

Lappin MR, Barsanti JA: Urinary incontinence secondary to idiopathic detrusor instability; cystometrographic diagnosis and pharmacologic management in 2 dogs and a cat. J Am Vet Med Assoc 191:1439, 1987

Leveille R, Atilola MAO: Retrograde vaginocystography: a contrast study for evaluation of bitches with urinary incontinence. Compend Contin Educ Pract Vet 13:934, 1991

Marks SL, Straeter-Knowlen IM, Knowlen G et al: The effects of phenoxybenzamine and acepromazine maleate on urethral pressure profiles of anesthetized healthy male cats (abstr.). J Vet Intern Med 7:122, 1993

Mawby DI, Meric SM, Crichlow EC, Papich MG: Pharmacologic relaxation of the urethra in male cats; a study of the effects of phenoxybenzamine, diazepam, nifedipine and xylazine. Can J Vet Res 55:28, 1990

McLaughlin R, Miller CW: Urinary incontinence after surgical repair of ureteral ectopia in dogs. Vet Surg 20:100, 1991

Moreau PM: Neurogenic disorders of micturition in the dog and cat. Compend Contin Educ Pract Vet 4:12, 1982

Moreau PM, Lappin MR: Pharmacologic manipulation of micturition. p. 1214. In Kirk RW (ed): Current Veterinary Therapy X: Small Animal Practice. WB Saunders, Philadelphia, 1989

Moreau PM, Lees GE, Gross DR: Simultaneous cystometry and uroflowmetry (micturition study) for evaluation of the caudal part of the urinary tract in dogs: studies of the technique. Am J Vet Res 44:1769, 1983

Oliver JE, Young WO: Air cystometry in dogs under xylazine-induced restraint. Am J Vet Res 34:1433, 1973

Richter KP: Use of urodynamics in micturition disorders in dogs and cats. p. 1145. In Kirk RW (ed): Current Veterinary Therapy X: Small Animal Practice. WB Saunders, Philadelphia, 1989

Richter KP, Ling GV: Clinical response and urethral pressure profile changes after phenylpropanolamine in dogs with primary sphincter incompetence. J Am Vet Med Assoc 187:605, 1985

Rosin AE, Barsanti JA: Diagnosis of urinary incontinence in dogs: role of the urethral pressure profile. J Am Vet Med Assoc 178:814, 1981

Stone EA, Mason LK: Surgery of ectopic ureters: types, method of correction, and postoperative results. J Am Anim Hosp Assoc 26:81, 1990

Straeter-Knowlen IM, Marks SL, Rishniw M et al: Urethral pressure response to smooth and skeletal muscle relaxants in anesthetized, adult male cats with naturally acquired urethral obstruction. Am J Vet Res 56:919, 1995

51

Diseases of the Urethra

Howard B. Seim, III

CONGENITAL DISORDERS

Hypospadias

See Chap. 58.

Urethrorectal Fistula

Definition and Causes

I. Urethrorectal fistula is a developmental anomaly of the fetal cloaca resulting in a permanent communication between the urethra and rectum.
II. The cause in dogs is unknown.
III. It is likely a result of failure of the urorectal septum to completely separate the cloaca into a cranial urethrovesical segment and a caudal rectal segment.

Clinical Signs

I. Signs are generally associated with abnormal micturition observed shortly after weaning.
II. Urine may pass through the anus or through the anus and urethra simultaneously.
III. Perineal urine scalding is often present.
IV. Cystitis is generally present.

Diagnosis

I. Diagnosis may be confirmed by visual examination of the rectum via speculum, proctoscope, or endoscope.
II. If the defect cannot be seen, a size 3–8 French soft plastic catheter may be used to explore the floor of the rectum.
III. If the defect cannot be visualized rectally, diagnosis is confirmed by positive contrast urethrography.

Differential Diagnosis

I. Traumatically induced rectovaginal fistula
II. Older age and history of previous trauma: suggestive of acquired, traumatic disease

Treatment

I. Surgical excision of the fistulous tract
   A. Ventral pubic symphysiotomy is performed, with exposure of the rectum and caudal urethra.
   B. Identify the fistula and pass umbilical tape around it for retraction.
   C. The fistula can be double ligated and transected between ligatures (Smith, 1993) or excised with the openings in the urethra and rectum sutured with 4–0 absorbable suture material using a simple interrupted pattern (Stone and Barsanti, 1992).
   D. The symphysis is stabilized using wire.
II. Concurrent treatment of urinary tract infection (UTI) (see Chap. 49)

Patient Monitoring

I. The surgical site is monitored for signs of wound infection.
II. Appropriate antimicrobial treatment for UTI is continued for at least 2 weeks.
III. Follow-up positive contrast urethrography is performed 4–6 weeks after surgery to confirm closure of the urethrorectal fistula.

INFLAMMATORY DISEASES

Urethral Prolapse

Definition and Causes

I. There is protuberance of 3–4 mm of urethral mucosa through the urethral orifice.
II. This disorder occurs only in male dogs and is most common in young brachycephalic breeds (e.g., English bulldogs and Boston terriers).
III. The cause is unknown, but prolonged sexual excitement and urethral infection have been suggested.

Clinical Signs

I. Excessive preputial and penile licking
II. Blood dripping from the prepuce

Diagnosis

I. Visual examination of the extruded penis is performed.

II. The prolapsed tissue is red to purple in color, is swollen, involves 360° of the urethral orifice, extrudes 3–4 mm from the tip of the penis, and looks like a rose.

Differential Diagnosis

I. Neoplasia of the tip of the penis or urethra (e.g., squamous cell carcinoma, transitional cell carcinoma)
   A. Tumors are generally asymmetrical and do not involve just the tip of the penis.
   B. Tumors usually occur in older animals (mean, 10 years) (Davies and Read, 1990b).

II. Transmissible venereal tumor
   A. This tumor may occur in young dogs.
   B. Tumor configuration and cytology may help identify it.

Treatment

I. Amputation of the prolapsed urethra is the treatment of choice.

II. Extrude the penis 3–4 cm and place a Penrose drain tourniquet around its base.

III. After inserting a urinary catheter, grasp the prolapsed portion of urethral mucosa and excise one fourth to one third of its circumference.

IV. Identify incised urethral mucosa and suture it to the incised penile epithelium.

V. Use 4–0 monofilament absorbable suture in a simple, continuous pattern.

VI. Continue to alternate incising and suturing until the prolapsed mucosa is completely excised.

Patient Monitoring

I. Hemorrhage is the most common immediate postsurgical complication; minor dripping from the prepuce may last up to 2 weeks after surgery.
   A. Apply an Elizabethan collar to prevent self-mutilation.
   B. Separate the animal from sources of excitation (e.g., other pets, bitch in heat).
   C. Use tranquilization to calm the dog.

II. If a UTI is present, treat as described in Chap. 49.

III. An indwelling catheter should *not* be used postoperatively, as this may irritate the surgical site, encourage hemorrhage, and promote UTI.

Urethritis

Definition and Causes

I. Inflammation of the urethra

II. Possible causes
   A. Epithelial neoplasia: squamous cell carcinoma, transitional cell carcinoma
   B. Idiopathic: chronic active granulomatous urethritis
   C. Trauma: calculi, catheterization, blunt nonpenetrating trauma
   D. Bacteria: associated with cystitis, vaginitis, prostatitis

Pathophysiology

I. Breakdown of the urothelial lining secondary to traumatic disruption or neoplastic infiltration of the urethral mucosa may result in erosion and ulceration.

II. Granulomatous urethritis is frequently associated with marked epithelial hyperplasia, probably related to elaboration and release of growth factors by inflammatory cells.

III. Mucosal defects created by any of the aforementioned causes may predispose to secondary bacterial infection.

Clinical Signs

I. Stranguria, hematuria, pollakiuria

II. Vaginal discharge, dripping blood from the prepuce

III. Evidence of complete urinary obstruction: distended bladder, painful abdomen, azotemia

Diagnosis

I. Suggestive signs of dysuria, stranguria, hematuria

II. Physical examination
   A. Rectal palpation may reveal a thick, irregularly shaped urethra.
      1. In female dogs, an irregularly shaped urethral papilla may be detected by vaginal examination.
      2. These findings are most common in granulomatous urethritis and urethritis secondary to neoplasia.
   B. It may be difficult to pass a urethral catheter in animals with luminal compromise.

III. Laboratory findings
   A. Urinalysis generally shows high numbers of red and white blood cells; infrequently, bacteria are seen.
   B. Serum urea nitrogen and creatinine are usually elevated with complete urethral obstruction.

IV. Radiographic findings
   A. Survey radiographs are normal or may reveal radiopaque calculi lodged in the urethra caudal to the os penis.
   B. Contrast retrograde urethrocystography may reveal multiple filling defects within the urethral lumen, marked irregular undulation of the mucosal border, or urethral stricture.

V. Urethral cytology (if a mass is palpable)
   A. Pass a flexible urethral catheter slightly cranial to the lesion.
   B. Inject 5 ml of sterile saline into the catheter using a 12-ml syringe.
   C. Aspirate the syringe while moving the catheter back and forth through the affected urethra.

D. If the mass is palpable rectally, the catheter is held against the lesion to facilitate aspiration of tissue and cells.

VI. Urethral biopsy (if a mass is palpable)
  A. In the female, biopsy specimens can be obtained by an episiotomy approach.
    1. Tissue located at the meatus is removed by sharp dissection.
    2. Specimens of tissue proximal to the meatus are obtained by passing a mosquito hemostat into the lumen.
  B. In the male, using either radiographs or fluoroscopy, a flexible biopsy forceps (i.e., as used in endoscopic biopsy) is passed into the urethra to the level of the lesion.
    1. If the mass is palpable rectally, the biopsy instrument is guided to the lesion by digital manipulation, and a specimen of tissue is removed.
    2. Biopsy must be done cautiously to avoid rupture of the urethra.
  C. To ensure representative samples for definitive diagnosis, multiple samples are recommended.

Differential Diagnosis

I. Neoplasia
II. Stricture
III. Calculi
IV. Trauma

Treatment

I. Treatment is based on the underlying cause.
  A. Epithelial neoplasia: see Neoplasia, later
  B. Idiopathic, chronic active granulomatous urethritis (Moroff et al., 1991)
    1. Prednisolone 1.1 mg/kg PO BID for 14 days, then decreased by 50% every 7 days to 0.07 mg/kg PO BID, with
    2. Cyclophosphamide for 4 consecutive days, then off 3 days, until remission
      a) Dogs up to 6.8 kg: 2.75 mg/kg/day PO
      b) Dogs 7.2–18.2 kg: 2.2 mg/kg/day PO
      c) Dogs >18.6 kg: 2 mg/kg/day PO
    3. Antibiotics for treatment of UTI for 4–6 weeks
      a) Cephalothin 20 mg/kg PO TID
      b) Trimethoprim-sulfadiazine 15–30 mg/kg PO BID
      c) Amoxicillin 20 mg/kg PO TID
    4. Maintenance of a urinary catheter until the dog can urinate
  C. Trauma
    1. Remove the traumatic focus (see Trauma, later).
    2. Calculi can be removed by retrograde hydropulsion into the bladder or by urethrotomy/urethrostomy (see Urethrolithiasis, later).
  D. Bacterial
    1. Determine the origin of infection and treat appropriately.

2. See Chaps. 49, 52, and 57 for the treatment of bacterial cystitis, prostatitis, and vaginitis, respectively.
II. Treatment of adjacent urinary tract structures may also be needed.

Patient Monitoring

I. Monitor ability to urinate and catheterize as necessary.
II. If surgery was performed (urethrotomy, urethrostomy), evaluate the surgical site 2–3 weeks postoperatively for healing.
III. Monitor urinalysis and urine culture in 2–4 weeks for persistent infection.
IV. Institute preventive measures for urolithiasis as outlined in Chap. 49.

URETHROLITHIASIS

Definition and Causes

I. Urolith is lodged in the urethra, causing partial or complete obstruction and urethritis.
II. See Chap. 49 for specific causes of calculi formation.
III. Generally, small cystic calculi migrate to the neck of the bladder during voiding and pass into the urethra.
  A. In the male, urethral calculi most commonly lodge caudal to the os penis.
  B. In the female, calculi may lodge at any location along the length of the urethra.
  C. Urethral obstruction is more common in males than females.

Clinical Signs

I. Stranguria, hematuria, pollakiuria, and occasionally blood dripping from the prepuce
II. Complete urinary obstruction: painful, distended abdomen; anuria; azotemia; hyperkalemia
III. Severity of signs dependent on degree and duration of obstruction

Diagnosis

I. Suspicious clinical signs
II. Inability to pass a catheter into the bladder
III. Survey radiography or positive contrast retrograde urethrocystography

Differential Diagnosis

I. Neoplasia
II. Urethral stricture
III. Urethritis (e.g., granulomatous)
IV. Urethral trauma

Treatment

I. Immediate care
  A. In animals with complete obstruction of a dura-

tion long enough to cause azotemia, temporary urinary diversion is provided by passing a urinary catheter alongside the calculus, performing a prepubic cystostomy, or performing frequent cystocenteses.

B. Treat azotemia with crystalloid IV therapy before calculus removal.

II. Calculus removal
   A. Retrograde hydropulsion is performed as follows.
      1. Thoroughly mix 45 ml of sterile saline and 15 ml of Surgilube in a 60-ml syringe and attach it to the largest high-density polyethylene urinary catheter that will pass through the os penis (5 to 8 French).
      2. Anesthetize the animal, extrude the penis, and pass the catheter up to and against the calculus. Place a gauze sponge around the tip of the penis and occlude the penis around the catheter by squeezing it with thumb and finger.
      3. Using a back and forth action on the catheter, simultaneously inject the saline/lubricant mix under pressure.
         a) The calculus and urethra are lubricated, and the viscosity of the mix encourages the calculus to dislodge and flush into the bladder.
         b) This technique is attempted regardless of how many stones are in the urethra.
      4. If this technique fails, place a finger in the rectum, palpate the urethra, and occlude its lumen; repeat step 3, and when maximum pressure is exerted on the urethra by the saline/lubricant mix, suddenly release digital urethral occlusion, allowing lodged calculi to flush into the bladder.
      5. A ventral midline celiotomy and cystotomy are then performed to remove all calculi.
   B. Urethrotomy (an incision over the calculi) may be performed to remove calculi that cannot be retropulsed. It is usually performed in the prescrotal or perineal region.
   C. Urethrostomy (a permanent opening to allow calculi to pass) may be indicated in animals that are chronic recurrent calculi formers (e.g., urate calculi in dalmatians). Scrotal urethrostomy is the technique of choice (Bilbrey et al., 1991).
   D. Treatment for UTI and dietary management are discussed in Chap. 49.

Patient Monitoring

I. Cystotomy
   A. Animals may pass small quantities of blood and blood clots for 2–3 days postoperatively.
   B. Animals presenting with complete urinary obstruction and postrenal azotemia are continued on crystalloid IV therapy until serum urea nitrogen and creatinine return to normal.
II. Urethrotomy/urethrostomy
   A. Hemorrhage from the urethral stoma is the most common immediate postsurgical complication.

B. It generally occurs 4–5 days postoperatively but occasionally lasts up to 2 weeks.
   C. Apply an Elizabethan collar to prevent self-mutilation.
III. Preventive measures for urolithiasis: see Chap. 49

NEOPLASIA

Definition

I. Primary neoplasia of the urethra in the dog is uncommon.
II. Transitional cell carcinoma and squamous cell carcinoma are most commonly reported.

Causes

I. The cause is unknown.
II. There is an increased incidence (1.5-fold risk) in female dogs (Davies and Read, 1990a).
III. Incidence also increases with age; affected dogs are generally 9–11 years old.

Pathophysiology

I. Urethral tumors are generally infiltrative in nature.
II. Urethral inflammation may be secondary to erosion or ulceration of the urethral mucosa by the invading neoplasm.
III. Neoplasms occasionally develop secondary to bacterial infection. It has been suggested that urethral neoplasia may arise from hyperplastic tissue associated with chronic cystitis.
IV. About one third of urethral neoplasms also involve the urinary bladder (Davies and Read, 1990b).

Clinical Signs

I. Stranguria, hematuria, pollakiuria
II. Vaginal discharge, dripping blood from the prepuce
III. Partial or complete urinary obstruction

Diagnosis

I. Suggestive clinical signs
II. Physical examination
   A. Rectal palpation may reveal a thick, irregularly shaped urethra. In female dogs, an irregularly shaped urethral papilla may be detected by vaginal examination.
   B. It is difficult to pass a urethral catheter in animals with luminal compromise.
III. Laboratory findings
   A. Urinalysis generally shows high numbers of red and white blood cells.
      1. Infrequently, bacteria are seen.
      2. Neoplastic cells are rarely seen.
   B. Systemic evidence of chronic urinary obstruction may occur (elevated serum urea nitrogen and creatinine).

IV. Radiographic findings
  A. Survey radiographs are generally normal.
  B. Positive contrast retrograde urethrocystography may reveal multiple filling defects within the urethral lumen, marked irregular undulation of the mucosal border, or stricture.
  C. Ultrasonography may reveal a mass near the bladder trigone or distal urethra but is difficult to perform on the pelvic urethra.
V. Urethral cytology
  A. It is often equivocal.
  B. Inflammation associated with the neoplasm may be secondary to erosion or ulceration.
  C. Urethritis is frequently associated with marked epithelial hyperplasia.
VI. Urethral biopsy
  A. It is recommended in all patients suspected of having urethral neoplasia.
  B. Limitations of urethral biopsy include inadequate tissue biopsied, subepithelial location of the neoplasm, or biopsy of associated necrotic tissue.
  C. To ensure representative samples for definitive diagnosis, multiple samples are recommended.

Differential Diagnosis

I. Urethritis (particularly granulomatous)
II. Transmissible venereal tumor
III. Stricture
IV. Calculi
V. Nonpenetrating trauma

Treatment

I. Immediate care
  A. If the neoplasia is causing urinary obstruction, temporary urinary diversion must be provided by passing a urethral catheter, performing frequent cystocenteses, or performing a prepubic cystostomy.
  B. Treat postrenal azotemia with intravenous fluids before surgical treatment.
II. Surgical treatment
  A. In males and females, tumors involving less than one third of the intrapelvic urethra are treated with wide surgical excision and anastomosis via sagittal pubic osteotomy (Davies and Read, 1990a).
  B. Males with distal urethral neoplasia are treated with wide surgical excision of the penis and scrotal or perineal urethrostomy.
  C. Animals with intrapelvic neoplasia involving greater than one third of the urethra are treated with wide surgical excision of the distal urethra and antepubic urethrostomy (Yoshioka and Carb, 1982).
  D. Animals with inoperable neoplasia may undergo palliative therapy with placement of a permanent prepubic cystostomy catheter, with or without chemotherapy (see Chemotherapy, later) (Smith et al., 1995).

E. Patients with proximal urethral involvement requiring complete urethral resection may be treated with trigonal-colonic anastomosis (Bovee et al., 1979) or ureterocolonic anastomosis (Stone et al., 1984). These urinary diversion techniques produce moderate to severe postoperative complications and should be considered only in select cases.
III. Chemotherapy
  A. Few drugs have been adequately tested for efficacy in treating urethral neoplasia.
  B. Preliminary reports suggest that cisplatin may cause a transient reduction in the size of urethral transitional cell carcinoma (Shapiro et al., 1988).
  C. Piroxicam exhibits antitumor activity on transitional cell carcinoma of the urinary bladder at 0.3 mg/kg PO SID (Knapp et al., 1994).

Patient Monitoring

I. Animals undergoing surgical resection and anastomosis have indwelling urinary catheters maintained for 5–14 days. Catheters are connected to a closed collection system to prevent development of UTI.
II. Animals undergoing urethrostomy (prescrotal, scrotal, perineal, or antepubic) are monitored for evidence of hemorrhage from the urethral stoma.
  A. This usually occurs 4–5 days postoperatively but occasionally occurs up to 2 weeks after surgery.
  B. Stricture or fistula formation is uncommon.
III. Animals with urinary diversion into the colon must be allowed to defecate 4–5 times daily and are evaluated daily for hydration, electrolyte, and acid–base abnormalities. In addition, excretory urography is performed at 3 and 6 months after surgery to evaluate the ureters and kidneys for signs of dilatation, stricture, and infection (Stone et al., 1984).
IV. Long-term prognosis for dogs with urethral neoplasia is guarded because of the invasiveness of the tumor at diagnosis.

TRAUMA

Definition and Causes

I. Traumatic lesions of the urethra include contusion, laceration, rupture, and obstruction.
  A. Contusions are generally caused by blunt trauma.
  B. Lacerations and ruptures are associated with pubic and os penis fractures, penetrating wounds (knife, gunshot, animal bite), and iatrogenic (catheterization, surgery) causes.
  C. Obstructions may occur with pubic or os penis fractures and calculi.
II. The most common cause of urethral trauma is vehicular accidents, with associated pelvic bone or os penis fractures.
III. Urethral trauma is more common in males.
IV. The overall incidence of urethral trauma is low (Selcer, 1982).

Clinical Signs

I. May be masked by other problems associated with trauma (shock, appendicular fractures, pneumothorax)
II. Vary depending on the location and degree of urethral injury
   A. Rupture or avulsion of the cranial portion of the urethra (abdominal) results in signs consistent with uroabdomen (see Chap. 49).
   B. Rupture of the intrapelvic and perineal portion of the urethra results in dysuria and hematuria, as well as local pain and cellulitis in the inguinal or perineal area. If subcutaneous infiltration of urine is not detected early, tissue necrosis may result.
   C. Rupture of the extrapelvic urethra may result in signs similar to those with intrapelvic trauma, but pain and cellulitis are evident in the parapreputial, scrotal, and caudal abdominal regions.
   D. Trauma resulting in urethral swelling without rupture may cause hematuria, dysuria, or anuria.

Diagnosis

I. Physical examination may reveal associated trauma (fractured pelvis) coupled with a distended abdomen, cellulitis, stranguria, or hematuria.
II. Urethral catheterization may be met with resistance, may not be possible, or may occur with ease.
III. Characteristic laboratory findings in animals with uroabdomen identify a rupture somewhere in the intra-abdominal portion of the urinary tract (see Chap. 49). Urethral rupture and subcutaneous urine leakage may also induce leukocytosis, azotemia, and hyperkalemia.
IV. Survey radiographs are rarely diagnostic.
V. Retrograde positive-contrast urethrocystography is necessary to identify the location and degree (complete or incomplete rupture) of urethral trauma.
   A. If contrast material reaches the bladder, the lesion is most likely incomplete (partial transection).
   B. If contrast material does not reach the bladder, the lesion is most likely complete (complete transection).

Differential Diagnosis

I. Periurethral hematoma or abscess
II. Neoplasia
III. Trauma to other areas of the urinary tract (bladder, ureters, kidney)

Treatment

I. Dependent on the location and severity of trauma
II. Urethral contusion without rupture
   A. Urethral catheterization only to relieve urinary obstruction
   B. Treatment of any underlying cause (e.g., stabilize fracture, treat UTI)
III. Incomplete rupture of the abdominal, intrapelvic, or extrapelvic urethra
   A. Pass a soft rubber or Silastic catheter across the ruptured urethra into the bladder.
   B. Consider a prepubic cystostomy catheter for urinary diversion (Dhein and Person, 1989).
IV. Avulsion of the urethra from the bladder neck
   A. Debride and suture the urethra.
   B. If primary suturing results in excessive tension, perform a distally based ventral tube flap (Fowler and Holmberg, 1987).
   C. Consider a prepubic cystostomy catheter for urinary diversion (Dhein and Person, 1989).
V. Complete rupture of the intrapelvic urethra
   A. Urethral anastomosis
      1. Perform a sagittal pubic osteotomy to approach the rupture (Davies and Read, 1990a).
      2. Identify the ruptured urethral ends using catheters passed normograde from the distal urethral orifice and retrograde from the urinary bladder.
      3. Debride the urethral ends and suture over an indwelling catheter.
      4. Place a prepubic cystostomy catheter for urinary diversion (Dhein and Person, 1989).
   B. Antepubic urethrostomy (Yoshioka and Carb, 1982)
      1. Through a ventral midline celiotomy, preserve as much distal urethra as possible, transect it, and suture it to the skin of the celiotomy incision just cranial to the pubis.
      2. Postoperatively, protect the skin around the urethral stoma from urine scalding with water-insoluble ointment (e.g., Vaseline, Desitin).
VI. Complete rupture of the extrapelvic urethra
   A. Urethral anastomosis: Identify the ruptured urethral ends, debride, and anastomose as described earlier.
   B. Urethrostomy: Consider urethrostomy just proximal to the urethral rupture.

Patient Monitoring

I. Urine diversion is continued during urethral healing.
   A. Indwelling catheters (urethral or cystostomy) that remain for 1–14 days postoperatively are attached to a closed collection system.
   B. Monitor catheter patency several times daily, and record urine output.
   C. Do not give prophylactic antibiotics, but treat any UTIs that develop (based on urine culture and sensitivity).
II. Follow-up contrast urethrocystography is performed if there is reason to suspect postoperative urine leakage.
III. The most serious postoperative complications are dehiscence and subsequent urine leakage.
IV. Positive-contrast urethrocystography is performed before catheter removal to document urethral healing.
V. Long-term follow-up includes positive-contrast urethrocystography at 3 and 6 months to rule out postoperative urethral stricture.

Bibliography

Bilbrey SA, Birchard SJ, Smeak DD: Scrotal urethrostomy: a retrospective review of 38 dogs (1973–1988). J Am Anim Hosp Assoc 27:560, 1991

Bovee KC, Pass MA, Wardley R et al: Trigonal-colonic anastomosis: urinary diversion procedure in dogs. J Am Vet Med Assoc 74:184, 1979

Davies JV, Read HM: Sagittal pubic osteotomy in the investigation and treatment of intrapelvic neoplasia in the dog. J Small Anim Pract 31:123, 1990a

Davies JV, Read HM: Urethral tumours in dogs. J Small Anim Pract 31:131, 1990b

Dhein CR, Person MW: Prepubic (suprapubic) catheterization of eight dogs with lower urinary tract disorders. J Am Anim Hosp Assoc 25:272, 1989

Fowler JD, Holmberg DL: Proximal urethral reconstruction using a distally based ventral bladder tube flap—an experimental study. Vet Surg 16:139, 1987

Knapp DW, Richardson RC, Chan TCK et al: Piroxicam therapy in 34 dogs with transitional cell carcinoma of the urinary bladder. J Vet Intern Med 8:273, 1994

Layton CE, Ferguson HR, Cook JE, Guffy MM: Intrapelvic urethral anastomosis—a comparison of three techniques. Vet Surg 16:175, 1987

Moroff SD, Brown BA, Matthiesen DT, Scott RC: Infiltrative urethral disease in female dogs: 41 cases (1980–1987). J Am Vet Med Assoc 199:247, 1991

Selcer BA: Urinary tract trauma associated with pelvic trauma. J Am Anim Hosp Assoc 18:785, 1982

Shapiro W, Kitchell BE, Fossum TW et al: Cisplatin for treatment of transitional cell and squamous cell carcinomas in dogs. J Am Vet Med Assoc 193:1530, 1988

Smith CW: Surgical diseases of the urethra. p. 1462. In Slatter D (ed): Textbook of Small Animal Surgery. 2nd Ed. WB Saunders, Philadelphia, 1993

Smith JD, Stone EA, Gilson SD: Placement of a permanent cystostomy catheter to relieve urine outflow obstruction in dogs with transitional cell carcinoma. J Am Vet Med Assoc 206:496, 1995

Stone EA, Barsanti JA: Urologic Surgery of the Dog and Cat. Lea & Febiger, Philadelphia, 1992

Stone EA, Goldschmidt MH, Walter MC: Urinary diversion. Vet Clin North Am 14:123, 1984

Waldron DR, Hedlund CS, Tangner CJ et al: The canine urethra—a comparison of first and second intention healing. Vet Surg 14:213, 1985

Yoshioka MM, Carb A: Antepubic urethrostomy in the dog. J Am Anim Hosp Assoc 18:290, 1982

52

Diseases of the Prostate Gland

Jeanne A. Barsanti

DEGENERATIVE DISORDERS

Benign Hyperplasia/Cystic Hyperplasia

Definition

I. Benign prostatic hyperplasia in dogs is an increase in epithelial cell number (hyperplasia) as well as epithelial cell size (hypertrophy), but the increase in number is more marked. It begins as glandular hyperplasia as early as 2.5 years of age (Berry et al., 1986).
II. Intraparenchymal fluid cysts may develop in association with hyperplasia. The tendency to cystic hyperplasia begins after 4 years of age (Lowseth et al., 1990).
  A. Intraparenchymal cysts may communicate with the urethra.
  B. The cysts vary in size and contour and contain a thin, clear to amber fluid.
III. Prostatic hyperplasia is the most common prostatic disease, with almost 100% of intact dogs developing histologic evidence of prostatic hyperplasia with aging. Most affected dogs are asymptomatic.
IV. The feline prostate does not undergo hyperplasia with aging.

Causes

I. Hyperplasia is associated with an altered androgen:estrogen ratio and requires the presence of the testes (Brendler et al., 1983).
II. Dihydrotestosterone within the gland probably serves as the main hormonal mediator for hyperplasia.

Pathophysiology

I. The vascularity of the prostate is increased with hyperplasia, and the gland has a tendency to bleed, which leads to the clinical signs of a hemorrhagic urethral discharge and hematuria.
II. The enlarged prostate may encroach on the rectal canal, causing tenesmus.

Clinical Signs

I. Intact, mature male dog
II. Most dogs asymptomatic
III. Usually alert, active, and afebrile
IV. Tenesmus associated with defecation (Table 52–1)
V. An intermittent hemorrhagic or clear, light yellow urethral discharge
VI. Intermittent or persistent hematuria
VII. Nonpainful, symmetrically enlarged prostate gland with a variable consistency (normal to mildly irregular)

Diagnosis

I. Laboratory findings are summarized in Table 52–2.
  A. Urine is normal or contains blood, either gross or microscopic.
  B. Semen and post-prostatic massage samples may be normal or hemorrhagic.
II. Imaging techniques are useful (Table 52–3).
  A. Survey abdominal radiography confirms mild to moderate prostatic enlargement with dorsal displacement of the colon and cranial displacement of the bladder.
  B. On distention retrograde urethrocystography, the prostatic urethra may be normal or may appear narrowed and undulant without mucosal irregularity, and urethroprostatic reflux may be greater than normal (Feeney et al., 1987a).
  C. On ultrasonography, the prostate may be diffusely hyperechoic with parenchymal cavities if intraparenchymal cysts have developed.
    1. The prostatic capsule is smooth, and the gland is symmetrically, mildly enlarged (Peter and Jakovljevic, 1992).

Table 52–1. **Clinical Signs Associated with Prostatic Diseases**

Fecal Tenesmus	Dysuria	Urethral Discharge	Systemic Signs[a]	Urinary Tract Infection
Hyperplasia	Cyst	Cystic hyperplasia	Acute bacterial prostatitis	Bacterial prostatitis
Cyst	Abscess	Cyst	Abscess	
Abscess	Neoplasia	Bacterial prostatitis	Cyst	
Neoplasia		Abscess	Neoplasia	
		Neoplasia		

[a]Including fever, depression, pain, anorexia, lethargy.

Adapted from Barsanti JA, Finco DR: Canine prostatic diseases. In Morrow DA (ed): Current Therapy in Theriogenology 2. WB Saunders, Philadelphia, 1986, with permission.

2. The cavitary areas are typically well defined and smoothly marginated (Feeney et al., 1989).
III. Definitive diagnosis is possible only by biopsy, but a biopsy-proven diagnosis is not needed to institute therapy if the clinical signs are typical.
IV. A presumptive diagnosis can be made by history and physical examination, with support from hematology, urinalysis, and prostatic fluid analysis in symptomatic dogs.
V. A positive response to castration can be used to help confirm the diagnosis.

Differential Diagnosis

I. Prostatic hyperplasia accompanies most other prostatic diseases in older, intact male dogs.
II. It may be difficult to distinguish from early neoplasia and from chronic infection on the basis of history and physical examination alone.
 A. Prostatic neoplasia does not respond to castration.
 B. Chronic prostatic infection results in urinary tract infection (UTI) and an inflammatory prostatic fluid.

Treatment

I. Treatment is required only if abnormal signs are present.
II. The most effective treatment is castration, which results in a 70% decrease in prostate size over 9 weeks (Juniewicz et al., 1993).

A. Involution begins within days, with a 50% reduction in size in 3 weeks (Cohen et al., 1995).
B. Prostatic secretion becomes minimal at 7–16 days after castration.
III. If castration is not feasible, low doses of estrogens can be used.
 A. Estrogens depress gonadotropin secretion by the pituitary gland, thereby reducing androgen concentrations and causing prostatic atrophy.
 B. Estrogens act primarily to decrease prostatic size by decreasing cellular mass. There may be no effect on intraparenchymal cysts.
 C. The potential side effects of estrogens must be weighed against their potential clinical benefit in each case before a decision is made to administer them.
  1. Severe bone marrow depression with resultant anemia, thrombocytopenia, and leukopenia can occur.
  2. Repeated administration and high doses can cause growth of the fibromuscular stroma of the prostate, metaplasia of prostatic glandular epithelium, and secretory stasis, with resultant prostatic enlargement and a predisposition to cyst formation, bacterial infection, and abscessation.
IV. Drugs that avoid the side effects of estrogens are the antiandrogens.
 A. Flutamide causes a significant decrease in prostatic size as detected by ultrasonography within 10 days (Cartee et al., 1990).
  1. When administered to research dogs at 5 mg/

Table 52–2. **Usual Laboratory Findings Associated with Prostatic Diseases**

Prostatic Disease	Leukocytosis	Hematuria	Pyuria	Bacteriuria	Hemorrhagic Prostatic Fluid	Purulent Prostatic Fluid	Bacteria in Prostatic Fluid
Cystic hyperplasia	No	Yes	No	No	Yes	No	No
Paraprostatic cysts	No	No	No	No	No	No	No
Acute prostatitis	Yes	Yes	Yes	Yes	NA	NA	NA
Chronic prostatitis	No	Yes	Yes	Yes	No	Yes	Yes
Prostatic abscessation	Yes	Yes	Yes	Yes	No	Yes	Yes
Prostatic neoplasia	No	Yes	Yes	No	Yes	Yes	No

NA = not applicable.

From Barsanti JA, Finco DR: Canine prostatic diseases. In Ettinger SJ (ed): Textbook of Veterinary Internal Medicine. WB Saunders, Philadelphia, 1986, with permission.

Table 52–3. **Radiographic and Ultrasonographic Findings Associated with Prostatic Diseases**

Disease	Radiographic Findings	Ultrasonographic Findings
Benign hyperplasia	Mild to moderate prostatomegaly	Diffusely hyperechoic, may contain focal hypoechoic areas (cysts)
Paraprostatic cyst	Asymmetrical prostatomegaly; caudal abdominal mass, may mineralize	Large hypoechoic or anechoic mass
Squamous metaplasia	Mild to moderate prostatomegaly; accentuated colliculus seminalis	Diffusely hyperechoic
Acute prostatitis	Normal to mild loss of detail in vicinity of prostate	Diffusely or focally hyperechoic
Chronic prostatitis	Normal or granular mineralization	Focally or diffusely hyperechoic
Abscessation	Asymmetrical prostatomegaly; sublumbar lymphadenopathy	Asymmetrical; diffusely hyperechoic with focal anechoic areas
Neoplasia	Asymmetrical prostatomegaly; may have granular mineralization; distortion of prostatic urethra; sublumbar lymphadenopathy; pelvic/vertebral osteolytic lesions	Multifocally hyperechoic; asymmetrical

Adapted from Barsanti JA, Finco DR: Prostatic diseases. In Ettinger SJ (ed): Textbook of Veterinary Internal Medicine. WB Saunders, Philadelphia, 1995; and from Barsanti JA: Diseases of the prostate gland. In Osborne CA, Finco DR (eds): Canine and Feline Nephrology and Urology. Williams & Wilkins, Philadelphia, 1995, with permission.

kg/day PO for 1 year, there was no change in libido or sperm production.

2. The drug is not approved for veterinary use and is expensive.

B. Delmadinone acetate (commonly used in Europe and Australia) is not as effective as castration (Read and Bryden, 1995).

V. Finasteride is a 5-alpha-reductase inhibitor (the final enzyme in the synthetic pathway for dihydrotestosterone) that is approved for use in men but can cause anomalies in male fetuses. Finasteride produces a dose-dependent decrease in prostatic size in dogs (Laroque et al., 1994).

VI. Progestagenic drugs may also be used.

A. Megestrol acetate at a dose of 0.55 mg/kg/day PO for 4 weeks resulted in resolution of clinical signs of hyperplasia with no decrease in sperm production (Olson et al., 1987), but it is not approved for use in male dogs.

B. Medroxyprogesterone acetate has also been used, but diabetes mellitus developed in one dog (Bamberg-Thalen and Linde-Forsberg, 1993).

Patient Monitoring

I. If the dog is asymptomatic, the owner is advised to watch for the development of typical clinical signs.

II. Palpate the dog's prostate gland 2–3 weeks after castration to be sure that it is involuting as expected. If it is not, a more serious prostatic disease such as neoplasia or abscessation may be present.

III. If medical therapy is chosen, the dog is monitored for changes in prostatic size and for development of adverse effects, according to the drug chosen.

Squamous Metaplasia
Definition and Causes

I. Squamous metaplasia is a change in the appearance of prostatic epithelium secondary to exogenous or endogenous hyperestrogenism. The major endogenous cause is a functional Sertoli cell tumor.

II. In addition to causing squamous metaplasia of the epithelial cells, estrogens cause secretory stasis.

Pathophysiology

I. The epithelial change, which can obstruct prostatic ducts and cause secretory stasis, predisposes to cyst formation, infection, and abscessation (O'Shea, 1963).

II. Prolonged exposure to estrogens results in mild to moderate prostatic enlargement, with possible secondary development of cysts or abscesses.

Clinical Signs

I. With endogenous hyperestrogenism, the testicles may be palpably abnormal, or one or both testicles may be cryptorchid.

A. The opposite testicle is usually atrophied.

B. With exogenous hyperestrogenism, both testicles may atrophy.

II. Other physical signs of hyperestrogenism include alopecia, hyperpigmentation, gynecomastia, and pendulous prepuce.

III. The prostate is enlarged to a variable degree.

Diagnosis

I. Laboratory results are variable.

A. Hematology may reflect estrogen toxicity.

1. Nonregenerative anemia

2. Thrombocytopenia

3. Granulocytosis followed by granulocytopenia

B. Hyperestrogenism does not directly affect biochemical parameters.

C. The urinalysis may indicate infection.

II. Prostatic fluid may show increased numbers of squamous epithelial cells and evidence of inflammation (Thrall et al., 1985).

III. Imaging techniques may be helpful (see Table 52–3).
   A. Survey radiographs indicate prostatomegaly.
   B. On retrograde urethrography, reflux of contrast material into cavities within the prostate gland and a persistent radiolucent filling defect in the prostatic urethra (enlarged colliculus seminalis) may be observed.
   C. Ultrasonography may identify filling defects within the prostate gland (cysts or abscesses).
IV. Definitive diagnosis is by biopsy, which shows that the prostatic ducts and acini are lined by squamous rather than columnar epithelium.
V. Presumptive diagnosis is based on the history of estrogen therapy or on the finding of a Sertoli cell tumor in association with prostatomegaly.

Differential Diagnosis

I. Diseases with similar appearances are hyperplasia and neoplasia.
II. The history of estrogen therapy or the finding of a Sertoli cell tumor makes metaplasia the more likely cause of prostatomegaly; however, a biopsy is necessary to definitively separate these conditions.

Treatment

I. Treatment requires removal of the source of estrogen.
   A. Castration in cases of endogenous hyperestrogenism
   B. Discontinuation of estrogen therapy
II. If the prostate is abscessed, treatment for abscessation is also required.

Patient Monitoring

I. Squamous metaplasia of the epithelium is reversible.
II. If the prostate is cystic but uninfected, monitoring includes repeated ultrasonic imaging approximately 1 month after treatment to ensure that the cysts are resolving.
III. If the prostate is abscessed, the animal is monitored as described later under Acute and Chronic Prostatitis, Abscessation.

Paraprostatic Cysts

Definition and Causes

I. Paraprostatic cysts are one or more large sacs of fluid found adjacent to the prostate and attached to it via a stalk (patent or nonpatent) or adhesions (White et al., 1987).
II. The cyst may or may not communicate with the urethra.
III. These large cysts may be prostatic in origin or may be remnants of the uterus masculinus (Weaver, 1978).
   A. During development, the uterus masculinus is a bi-horned structure with a stalk that opens on the dorsal wall of the urethra within the prostate gland.
      1. Normally the structure degenerates within the prostate gland as the fetus develops masculine traits.
      2. It is not known why cysts develop, but hyperestrogenism and a congenital defect have been suggested.
      3. Cystic uterus masculinus has been reported in cats.
   B. Paraprostatic cysts of prostatic origin may occur in the abdomen craniolateral to the prostate or in the pelvic canal (even extending to the perineum lateral to the anus).
      1. They can have a thin or thick wall with a smooth or calcified lining.
      2. Most do not communicate with the urethra.
      3. A cyst of apparently prostatic origin has been reported in a cat (Newell et al., 1992).

Pathophysiology

I. These cysts are often very large, which can lead to signs of tenesmus and abdominal or perineal distention.
II. Secondary infection may occur, especially if the cyst communicates with the urethra.

Clinical Signs

I. Clinical signs are related to cyst size, with encroachment on the urethra or colon resulting in dysuria or tenesmus (see Table 52–1).
II. Paradoxic urinary incontinence has also been noted, generally associated with bladder overdistention and partial urethral obstruction.
III. If the cyst is sufficiently large, abdominal distention may be seen.
IV. Alternatively, the cyst may extend into the perineal region, creating a swelling.
V. Hematuria or an intermittent hemorrhagic, serosanguineous, or yellow urethral discharge may be noted if the cyst communicates with the urethra.
VI. The cysts may be palpable in the caudal abdomen or perineal area; if calcified, they may feel firm.

Diagnosis

I. Urinalysis and urine culture (see Table 52–2)
   A. Urinalysis is usually normal, although hematuria is possible if hemorrhage occurs into the cyst and the cyst communicates with the urethra.
   B. UTIs are sometimes present, especially with infected cysts.
II. Hematology
   A. Hematologic findings are usually normal.
   B. A neutrophilic leukocytosis was noted in about 30% of cases in one series (Weaver, 1978).
III. Prostatic fluid
   A. If there is a urethral discharge that appears to be the same color as the dog's urine, the discharge

must be examined cytologically to differentiate prostatic fluid from urine.
  1. A ''urinalysis'' can be performed on both and compared.
  2. Cyst fluid usually has more protein than urine.
  B. Whether cyst fluid can be obtained by ejaculation or prostatic massage depends on whether the cyst communicates with the urethra. Alternatively, fluid can be aspirated under ultrasound guidance.
  C. Prostatic cyst fluid is usually yellow to serosanguineous to brown.
  1. It has low numbers of white blood cells (WBCs), variable numbers of red blood cells (RBCs), and variable numbers of epithelial cells, and it is usually sterile.
  2. If cyst fluid becomes infected, the cyst may become an abscess.
IV. Imaging techniques (see Table 52–3)
  A. On survey radiographs, there may be poor contrast in the caudal abdomen, with an asymmetrical or irregular prostatic shape (Johnston et al., 1991).
  1. Paraprostatic cysts may mineralize.
  2. With very large cysts, two bladder-like structures may be evident.
  B. A cystogram is often necessary to determine which structure is the bladder.
  C. On distention retrograde urethrocystography, the prostate may appear asymmetrical around the urethra, and the prostatic urethral lumen may be narrowed (Feeney et al., 1987a).
  1. Urethroprostatic reflux may be greater than normal.
  2. Contrast material often does not reflux into the cyst.
  D. Ultrasonography can confirm that the mass is cystic and can be used to direct fine-needle aspiration.
V. Definitive diagnosis
  A. Exploratory laparotomy with cyst drainage and excisional biopsy may be needed.
  B. Percutaneous needle biopsy of a cystic lesion is not recommended.

Differential Diagnosis

I. Abscessation
II. Neoplasia

Treatment

I. The recommended treatment for paraprostatic cysts is surgical drainage with excision or marsupialization (Stone and Barsanti, 1992).
II. Castration is also recommended.

Patient Monitoring

I. If the cyst was infected or is marsupialized, repeat a urinalysis and urine culture 1 week after discontinuing antibiotic therapy and monthly for 2–3 months to detect recurrence of infection.

II. Monitor the caudal abdomen for cyst recurrence with ultrasonography for several months.

INFLAMMATORY DISEASES

Acute and Chronic Prostatitis, Abscessation

Definition

I. These are inflammatory diseases of the prostate gland caused by bacterial infection.
II. Abscesses develop when the infection is severe and encapsulation of purulent material occurs.

Causes

I. The prostate gland can be predisposed to bacterial infection.
  A. Urethral diseases: urolithiasis, trauma, strictures, neoplasia
  B. UTI
  C. Prostatic diseases: cysts, squamous metaplasia, neoplasia
II. Several routes of infection are possible.
  A. Urethral (considered to be most common)
  B. Via infected urine
  C. Hematogenous
  D. Via the vas deferens
  E. From rectal flora by direct extension or lymphatics
III. The usual bacteria involved are *Escherichia coli* (most common), *Staphylococcus, Proteus, Klebsiella, Pseudomonas,* and *Streptococcus/Enterococcus* (Krawiec and Heflin, 1992).
IV. Infection by anaerobic bacteria, fungi, or mycoplasma is rare. Granulomatous chronic prostatitis may occur with blastomycosis and cryptococcosis.

Pathophysiology

I. Acute prostatitis
  A. There is little change in prostatic size associated with infection alone, but the gland may be enlarged owing to hyperplasia.
  B. Acute bacterial prostatitis can result in septicemia, which may be responsible for the severity of clinical signs in some cases.
II. Chronic prostatitis
  A. Chronic infection may be a sequela to an acute infection or may develop insidiously.
  B. There is little change in prostatic size associated with the infection, but the gland may be enlarged because of hyperplasia.
  C. Although inflammation is present, it is not severe enough to produce systemic symptoms.
  D. The prostate may serve as a nidus of infection for the urinary tract, and the prostatic infection may gradually abscess.
  E. The incidence in dogs is unknown, but chronic prostatitis is believed to be common (Krawiec and Heflin, 1992).

III. Prostatic abscessation
   A. Abscessation is thought to result from chronic infection of prostatic tissue, leading to accumulation of pockets of purulent material of varying size.
   B. It can also result from infection of prostatic cysts, whether intra- or extraparenchymal.
   C. Abscesses can become very large and may rupture, leading to peritonitis.

Clinical Signs

I. Acute prostatitis (see Table 52–1)
   A. Sexually mature, intact male dogs are at risk.
   B. Signs of systemic illness such as anorexia, lethargy, and fever are usually noted.
   C. Vomiting is possible.
   D. Dripping of fluid from the prepuce may be noted.
   E. Caudal abdominal pain that can be localized to the prostate gland by palpation may be present.
   F. The dog may walk stiffly in association with apparent pain.
   G. The size, symmetry, and contour of the prostate gland are normal, unless it is enlarged as a result of hyperplasia.
II. Chronic prostatitis
   A. Most often there are no signs directly referable to the prostate gland.
   B. The dog may be presented for recurrent episodes of cystitis.
   C. Affected dogs may be presented for a constant or intermittent urethral discharge or hematuria.
   D. Some dogs are lethargic.
   E. It is a consideration in male dogs presented for infertility.
   F. The prostate is not painful when palpated.
      1. Size is variable.
      2. Chronic infection by itself causes no increase in prostatic size (Barsanti et al., 1983).
   G. The prostate gland may vary in symmetry and consistency.
      1. Areas of fibrous tissue are more firm than areas of normal prostatic tissue.
      2. Areas of infection may be focal, multifocal, or diffuse.
III. Prostatic abscessation
   A. If the abscess or abscesses become very large, the dog may be presented with tenesmus or dysuria.
   B. Incursion on the urethra can lead to partial urethral obstruction with a chronically distended bladder, eventual detrusor dysfunction, and overflow urinary incontinence.
   C. Clinical signs related to infection include a constant or intermittent urethral discharge that may be hemorrhagic or purulent.
   D. If the abscess ruptures, a localized or generalized peritonitis results in lethargy, fever, pain, and possibly vomiting.
   E. The most common signs in one survey of cases were depression and lethargy (Mullen et al., 1990).

1. Evidence of septic shock (tachycardia, pale mucous membranes, delayed capillary refill, and weak pulse) was noted in about 10% of cases (Mullen et al., 1990).
2. Caudal abdominal pain was noted in 73% of cases (Mullen et al., 1990).
3. Icterus may be found in association with sepsis or endotoxemia (Hardie et al., 1984).
   F. On palpation, the prostate gland is abnormal.
      1. The prostate is usually enlarged, but the degree of enlargement is variable.
      2. The prostate gland is often asymmetrical and may vary in consistency from one part to another.

Diagnosis

I. Urinalysis and urine culture (see Table 52–2)
   A. Hematuria, pyuria, and bacteriuria are common.
   B. If the urinalysis indicates infection, perform a quantitative urine culture and sensitivity test on a sample collected by cystocentesis or catheterization.
II. Hematology and chemistry (see Table 52–2)
   A. In acute prostatitis and abscessation, a neutrophilic leukocytosis with or without a left shift often exists.
   B. In chronic prostatitis, the WBC count is usually normal (Barsanti and Finco, 1984).
   C. Serum chemistry is normal with acute and chronic prostatitis but may be abnormal with abscessation.
      1. Serum bilirubin and liver enzyme concentrations (especially alkaline phosphatase) may be increased.
      2. Even in the absence of icterus, liver function tests such as bromosulfophthalein (BSP) retention or bile acids may be abnormal.
      3. Hypoglycemia was noted in 40% of cases in one study (Mullen et al., 1990).
III. Prostatic fluid
   A. Prostatic fluid is usually not evaluated in dogs with acute prostatitis because ejaculation is too painful and because of the difficulty of interpreting prostatic massage samples when UTI is present.
   B. Assessment of prostatic fluid is essential to diagnose chronic prostatitis.
      1. Prostatic fluid collected by ejaculation is usually purulent and septic and may also be hemorrhagic. Quantitative culture of urine and prostatic fluid should yield significant numbers of the same organisms.
         a) Dogs with experimental chronic bacterial prostatitis had >1000 organisms/ml, but establishing a definitive number to separate infection from contamination is difficult (Barsanti et al., 1983).
         b) The finding of macrophages in the prostatic portion of semen correlates with prostatic infection and inflammation (Barsanti et al., 1983).

2. Prostatic fluid collected by ejaculation is preferred for the diagnosis of chronic prostatitis over prostatic fluid collected after prostatic massage.
   a) When prostatic massage is used in dogs with UTIs, the results are difficult to interpret because of the large number of bacteria already in the urinary tract.
   b) In order to use prostatic massage in diagnosing bacterial prostatitis, infection in the urine must be controlled first.
IV. Survey abdominal radiographs (see Table 52–3)
  A. They may be normal or show a loss of detail at the margins of the prostate gland in acute prostatitis.
  B. Granular parenchymal mineralization may be found with chronic prostatitis.
  C. Prostatic enlargement, which can be asymmetrical or irregular in outline, may be evident with abscessation.
   1. There may also be poor radiographic contrast of the caudal abdomen.
   2. The sublumbar lymph nodes may be enlarged.
V. Ultrasonography
  A. With acute and chronic prostatitis, the prostate gland may have focally to diffusely increased echogenicity (Feeney et al., 1987b).
  B. In chronic prostatitis, multifocal mineralization may also be seen, although mineralization is more common with neoplasia.
   1. Hypoechoic areas suggest abscessation.
   2. Ultrasonography cannot differentiate chronic prostatitis from hyperplasia or neoplasia.
  C. With abscessation, the prostate gland is usually hyperechoic with parenchymal cavities, irregular outline, and asymmetrical shape.
   1. The cavitary area(s) usually exhibit distal enhancement (Feeney et al., 1989).
   2. The internal margin of the cavity is often irregular, and the lumen may be septate.
VI. Distention retrograde urethrocystography
  A. This technique is not used in acute prostatitis, because the diagnosis can usually be made without it.
  B. In chronic prostatitis, results are normal except for urethroprostatic reflux in some cases.
  C. With abscessation, periurethral asymmetry and narrowing of the prostatic urethra are observed.
   1. The prostatic urethral lumen may appear undulant but is not distorted or destroyed.
   2. Reflux into the prostate gland may be noted if the abscess communicates with the urethra.
VII. Definitive diagnosis
  A. A definitive diagnosis of acute prostatitis is rarely made, because prostatic biopsy and tissue culture are usually not performed.
  B. Definitive diagnosis of chronic bacterial prostatitis is made by prostatic tissue culture and histopathology.
  C. The diagnosis of abscessation should be confirmed by fine-needle aspiration or exploratory celiotomy, because the current treatment of choice is surgical drainage.
   1. At surgery, the abscess contents are collected for aerobic and anaerobic culture, and a tissue specimen is obtained for microscopic examination and bacterial culture.
   2. The usual histologic finding is suppurative or chronic active prostatitis, although pyogranulomatous inflammation may also be noted.

Differential Diagnosis

I. In acute prostatitis, the major considerations are acute pyelonephritis and prostatic abscessation, which also present with systemic signs of illness, abdominal pain, and UTI.
II. Chronic prostatitis must be differentiated from other causes of chronic UTI, such as chronic pyelonephritis.
III. Abscessation, neoplasia, and paraprostatic cysts are the major diseases considered with marked prostatic enlargement.

Treatment

I. Acute prostatitis
  A. An antibiotic, based on urine culture and sensitivity, is administered for at least 28 days.
  B. If the presenting signs are severe, the antibiotic is initially given intravenously.
  C. An oral antimicrobial with prostatic penetrance (see later) is preferred for the remainder of therapy.
II. Chronic prostatitis
  A. Chronic bacterial prostatitis is difficult to treat effectively because the blood–prostatic fluid barrier is intact.
  B. The choice of an antimicrobial agent depends on whether a gram-positive or gram-negative organism is the infective agent.
   1. If the causative organism is gram-positive, erythromycin, clindamycin, chloramphenicol, or trimethoprim/sulfonamide can be chosen based on bacterial sensitivity.
   2. If the organism is gram-negative, chloramphenicol, enrofloxacin, or trimethoprim/sulfonamide is best.
  C. Antibiotics are continued for at least 6 weeks.
  D. Castration may be beneficial for chronic bacterial prostatitis (Cowan et al., 1991).
III. Prostatic abscessation
  A. Surgical drainage is currently the treatment of choice.
   1. There are many methods to accomplish this, including needle aspiration, tube or Penrose drains, or marsupialization.
   2. Complications are common with all methods (Hardie et al., 1984; Mullen et al., 1990).
   a) Drainage procedures often result in septic shock immediately after surgery.
   b) When drains are placed, ascending infec-

tion with antibiotic-resistant bacteria is possible.

    c) Marsupialization leaves a chronic draining stoma in some dogs.

    d) A common long-term complication is urinary incontinence.

B. With extensive prostatic involvement, removal of the prostate may be considered; however, serious complications also occur with prostatectomy, and the surgery is technically difficult.

C. If prostatic enlargement has resulted in partial urethral obstruction, bladder and urethral function are carefully assessed.

    1. Prolonged bladder distention may result in bladder atony. An indwelling urinary catheter may be necessary to let the detrusor muscle recover.

    2. If the bladder wall has been chronically distended and infected, it may be irreversibly damaged.

D. Castration is recommended as adjunctive therapy. Castration without abscess drainage leads to reduction of prostatic tissue but continuation of the abscess pocket(s).

E. Regardless of which surgical procedure is elected, affected dogs must receive antibiotic therapy.

    1. If the dog is systemically ill, intravenous antimicrobials are used initially.

    2. Based on prostatic penetration, the initial drugs of choice are chloramphenicol, trimethoprim, or a quinolone.

    3. The antibiotic choice is modified based on results of a culture and sensitivity and the presence or absence of bacteremia.

    4. After improvement of clinical signs, the dog is managed as a case of chronic bacterial prostatitis.

F. If an affected dog's condition stabilizes on antibiotic therapy and the owner declines surgery, the dog can be managed with long-term suppressive antibiotic therapy. (The owner must realize that the abscess usually persists and can potentially result in life-threatening infection.)

G. Prostatic abscesses are difficult and expensive to treat. Survival is approximately 50% at 1 year (Hardie et al., 1984; Mullen et al., 1990).

Patient Monitoring

I. Acute prostatitis

  A. Because acute infections may become chronic, re-examination is performed 7 days after completion of antibiotic therapy.

  B. This examination includes a physical examination, urinalysis, urine culture, and examination of prostatic fluid by cytology and culture.

II. Chronic prostatitis

  A. Urine and prostatic fluid are recultured 7 days and 1 month after discontinuing antibiotics to ensure that the infection has been eliminated (not merely suppressed).

B. Relapse within a few months after discontinuing therapy is common.

C. If initial therapy fails, a 3-month course of therapy is instituted, bearing in mind any potential adverse effects of the drug chosen.

III. Abscessation

  A. Failure to control prostatic infection and recurrent UTIs are common; the prostate may reabscess.

  B. Urinalysis and urine culture are evaluated monthly for several months after initial therapy is discontinued.

  C. The prostate gland is palpated and examined by ultrasonography at monthly intervals until abscess resolution is confirmed.

NEOPLASIA

Definition and Causes

I. The aging prostate gland is subject to neoplastic transformation, most commonly adenocarcinoma.

  A. Transitional cell carcinoma arising from the epithelium of the prostatic ducts also occurs.

  B. Other tumor types have been reported but are rare.

II. The prostate may also serve as a metastatic site for tumors that are primary elsewhere, such as lymphosarcoma, squamous cell carcinoma, and hemangiosarcoma.

III. Benign tumors of the prostate have not been reported, although one case of nodular, benign hyperplasia that appeared similar to a benign tumor has been reported (Gilson et al., 1992).

IV. The cause of primary prostatic neoplasia is unknown.

Pathophysiology

I. Prostatic neoplasia occurs in both intact and neutered male dogs. It is the most common prostatic disease diagnosed in dogs neutered prior to the onset of a prostatic disease (Krawiec and Heflin, 1992).

II. Prostatic neoplasia has been reported in cats.

III. Primary prostatic adenocarcinoma tends to metastasize through the external and internal iliac lymph nodes to vertebral bodies as well as to the lungs (Durham and Dietze, 1986).

  A. The tumor may grow into the neck of the bladder and obstruct the ureters.

  B. The colonic and pelvic musculature may be invaded via direct extension.

  C. The urethra may also become obstructed (Weaver, 1981).

  D. Cysts, abscesses, and areas of hemorrhage can be found in association with neoplasia.

IV. With transitional cell carcinomas, clinical signs are often related to partial urethral obstruction.

V. With any type of neoplastic invasion, the prostate becomes enlarged and often asymmetrical.

Clinical Signs

I. History and signalment (see Table 52–1)
  A. Signalment in dogs with adenocarcinoma
   1. Mean age of 9–10 years (Bell et al., 1991)
   2. Medium to large breeds
  B. Historical problems in dogs
   1. Tenesmus and dysuria
   2. Hemorrhagic urethral discharge
   3. Rear limb weakness, stiffness, and/or pain
   4. Chronic weight loss and anorexia
  C. Hematuria or urethral obstruction in cats
II. Physical examination (see Table 52–1)
  A. One or more firm, irregular nodules may be palpated prior to prostatic enlargement and clinical signs.
  B. In most cases, the gland is enlarged and asymmetrical, with increased firmness.
   1. It may be painful on palpation and is often unmovable.
   2. In determining whether the prostate is enlarged or not, the examiner must consider the dog's reproductive status.
    a) The prostate in a neutered dog involutes to a very small size.
    b) A prostate gland that would be normal for an intact dog is abnormal in a neutered dog.
  C. Systemic signs may include depression, cachexia, and pyrexia.

Diagnosis

I. Urinalysis and urine culture (see Table 52–2)
  A. Hematuria is the predominant abnormality.
  B. Pyuria may also be present.
  C. UTIs and prostatic infections occasionally occur concomitantly.
  D. Atypical cells are occasionally found in urine sediment.
II. Complete blood count and biochemical profile (see Table 52–2)
  A. Hemogram
   1. WBC counts are usually normal, but a neutrophilic leukocytosis with or without a left shift may be present owing to necrosis and inflammation associated with tumor growth.
   2. A mild nonregenerative anemia is found in about one fifth of cases (Bell et al., 1991).
  B. Biochemical profile
   1. Azotemia may be present as a result of obstruction of both ureters or of the urethra.
   2. Approximately 50% of affected dogs have an increase in serum alkaline phosphatase (Bell et al., 1991).
III. Prostatic fluid
  A. Semen samples are difficult to collect from dogs with advanced neoplasia.
  B. Abnormal epithelial cells may be detected after prostatic massage.
IV. Imaging techniques (see Table 52–3)
  A. Asymmetrical, irregular, and possibly marked prostatic enlargement may be evident on survey abdominal radiography.
   1. Occasionally, prostatic carcinomas are associated with multifocal or granular, poorly defined mineral densities.
   2. Examine the lumbar vertebral bodies and the pelvic bones for areas of lysis or proliferative changes suggestive of metastasis.
   3. Metastasis may also occur to long bones, scapula, ribs, and digits.
  B. Thoracic radiographs are indicated to check for metastasis to the lungs.
   1. Metastasis may appear as either a generalized increase in nodular interstitial density or single to multiple discrete nodules.
   2. Even if thoracic radiographs show no evidence of metastasis, there is a 40% chance that metastases are present (Bell et al., 1991).
  C. With distention retrograde urethrocystography, periurethral asymmetry and narrowing, distortion, or destruction of the prostatic urethra may be detected (Feeney et al., 1987a).
   1. Urethroprostatic reflux that is greater than normal is also common.
   2. Spread of the neoplasm into the bladder is possible.
  D. Ultrasonography usually shows focal or multifocal hyperechoic parenchyma with asymmetry and an irregular prostatic outline.
   1. Echogenicity tends to be very heterogeneous, with poorly defined hyperechoic foci that seem to coalesce (Johnston et al., 1991).
   2. There may be multifocal irregularly distributed areas of mineralization.
   3. Occasionally, cavitary lesions may also be noted, which can represent infarction, necrosis, hemorrhage, or edema.
V. Biopsy
  A. Unless metastatic disease is evident radiographically, the diagnosis of neoplasia should always be confirmed by aspiration or biopsy, because the prognosis is poor.
  B. A biopsy or aspirate is necessary to determine the type of neoplasm.
  C. If a surgical biopsy is obtained, a biopsy is also taken from the sublumbar lymph nodes.

Differential Diagnosis

I. Intact dogs
  A. When prostatomegaly is marked, neoplasia must be distinguished from prostatic abscessation and paraprostatic cysts.
  B. In early stages, neoplasia must be differentiated from hyperplasia.
   1. This is usually done by palpation and imaging, as the prostate tends to be irregular and asymmetrical in neoplasia and symmetrical and regular in hyperplasia.
   2. One case of nodular benign hyperplasia has been reported (Gilson et al., 1992).

3. Response to castration can also be used to differentiate these diseases.

II. Neutered dogs

A. If the dog was neutered before the development of signs related to prostatic disease, neoplasia is most likely.

B. Abscessation is possible, however, especially if the dog has had urinary tract disease.

Treatment

I. Radiation therapy is the treatment of choice for prostatic adenocarcinoma if metastatic disease is not evident (Turrel, 1987).

A. With intraoperative orthovoltage, median and mean survival times for 10 dogs were 114 and 196 days, respectively.

B. The usual goal is temporary control of the tumor and amelioration of clinical signs; cure is unlikely.

II. Prostatectomy is an alternative therapy, but the owner must be willing to accept the probable postsurgical development of urinary incontinence.

A. The longest reported postoperative survival in dogs with adenocarcinoma was 9 months (Hardie et al., 1984).

B. This dog had only a few small nodules in the prostate at the time of diagnosis.

III. Castration has no beneficial effect in dogs; however, lack of decrease in prostatic size after castration may help differentiate neoplasia from other prostatic diseases.

IV. The treatment of other prostatic tumors varies with type. Transitional cell carcinomas are currently treated with piroxicam at 0.3 mg/kg/day PO (Knapp et al., 1994).

Patient Monitoring

I. The owner must monitor the animal for quality of life.

A. Most animals are euthanized within 2 months of diagnosis because of progressive disease.

B. One animal survived 19 months without therapy, however (Bell et al., 1991).

II. If treatment is attempted, the size of the prostate is monitored and urinalysis and urine culture are performed to detect any secondary infection, approximately monthly.

Bibliography

Bamberg-Thalen B, Linde-Forsberg C: Treatment of canine benign prostatic hyperplasia with medroxyprogesterone acetate. J Am Anim Hosp Assoc 29:221, 1993

Barsanti JA, Finco DR: Evaluation of techniques for diagnosis of canine prostatic diseases. J Am Vet Med Assoc 185:198, 1984

Barsanti JA, Prasse KW, Crowell WA et al: Evaluation of various techniques for diagnosis of chronic bacterial prostatitis in the dog. J Am Vet Med Assoc 183:219, 1983

Bell FW, Klausner JS, Hayden DW et al: Clinical and pathologic features of prostatic adenocarcinomas in sexually intact and castrated dogs: 31 cases (1970–1987). J Am Vet Med Assoc 199:1623, 1991

Berry SJ, Coffey DS, Strandberg JD et al: Effect of age, castration and testosterone replacement on the development and restoration of canine benign hyperplasia. Prostate 9:295, 1986

Berry SJ, Strandberg JD, Saunders WJ et al: Development of canine benign prostatic hyperplasia with age. Prostate 9:363, 1986

Brendler CB, Berry SJ, Ewing LL et al: Spontaneous benign prostatic hyperplasia in the beagle. J Clin Invest 71:1114, 1983

Cartee RE, Pumph PF, Kenter DC et al: Evaluation of drug-induced prostatic involution in dogs by transabdominal B-mode ultrasonography. Am J Vet Res 51:1773, 1990

Cohen SM, Werrmann JG, Rasmusson GH et al: Comparison of the effects of new specific azasteroid inhibitors of steroid 5-alpha-reductase on canine hyperplastic prostate: suppression of prostatic DHT correlated with prostate regression. Prostate 26:55, 1995

Cowan LA, Barsanti JA, Crowell WA et al: Effects of castration on chronic bacterial prostatitis in dogs. J Am Vet Med Assoc 199:346, 1991

Dorfman M, Barsanti JA, Budsberg SC: Enrofloxacin concentrations in dogs with normal prostate and dogs with chronic bacterial prostatitis. Am J Vet Res 56:386, 1995

Durham SK, Dietze AE: Prostatic adenocarcinoma with and without metastasis to bone in dogs. J Am Vet Med Assoc 188:1432, 1986

Feeney DA, Johnston GR, Klausner JS et al: Canine prostatic disease—comparison of radiographic appearance with morphologic and microbiologic findings: 30 cases (1981–1985). J Am Vet Med Assoc 190:1018, 1987a

Feeney DA, Johnston GR, Klausner JS et al: Canine prostatic disease—comparison of ultrasonographic appearance with morphologic and microbiologic findings: 30 cases (1981–1985). J Am Vet Med Assoc 190:1027, 1987b

Feeney DA, Johnston GR, Klausner JS et al: Canine prostatic ultrasonography—1989. Semin Vet Med Surg 4:44, 1989

Gilson SD, Miller RT, Hardie EM, Spaulding KA: Unusual prostatic mass in a dog. J Am Vet Med Assoc 200:702, 1992

Hardie EM, Barsanti JA, Rawlings CA: Complications of prostatic surgery. J Am Anim Hosp Assoc 20:50, 1984

Hieble JP, Caine M: Etiology of benign prostatic hyperplasia and approaches to its pharmacological management. Fed Proc 45:2601, 1986

Hubbard BS, Vulgamott JC, Liska WD: Prostatic adenocarcinoma in a cat. J Am Vet Med Assoc 197:1493, 1990

Johnston GR, Feeney DA, Rivers B et al: Diagnostic imaging of the male canine reproductive organs. Vet Clin North Am [Small Anim Pract] 21:553, 1991

Juniewicz PE, Hoekstra SJ, Lemp BM et al: Effect of combination treatment with zanoterone (WIN 49596), a steroidal androgen receptor antagonist, and finasteride, a steroidal 5 alpha-reductase inhibitor, on the prostate and testes of beagle dogs. Endocrinology 133:904, 1993

Knapp DW, Richardson RC, Chan TCK et al: Piroxicam therapy in 34 dogs with transitional cell carcinomas of the urinary bladder. J Vet Intern Med 8:272, 1994

Krawiec DR, Heflin D: Study of prostatic disease in dogs: 177 cases (1981–1986). J Am Vet Med Assoc 200:1119, 1992

Laroque PA, Prahalada S, Gordon LR et al: Effects of chronic oral administration of a selective 5-alpha-reductase inhibitor, finasteride, on the dog prostate. Prostate 24:93, 1994

Lowseth LA, Gerlach RF, Gillett NA et al: Age-related changes in the prostate and testes of the beagle. Vet Pathol 27:347, 1990

Mullen HS, Matthiesen DT, Scavelli TD: Results of surgery and postoperative complications in 92 dogs treated for prostatic abscessation by a multiple Penrose drain technique. J Am Anim Hosp Assoc 26:369, 1990

Mulligan RM: Feminization in male dogs: a syndrome associated with carcinoma of the testes and mimicked by the administration of estrogen. Am J Pathol 20:865, 1944

Newell SM, Mahaffey MB, Binhazim A et al: Paraprostatic cyst in a cat. J Small Anim Pract 33:399, 1992

Obradovich J, Walshaw R, Goullaud E: The influence of castration on the development of prostatic carcinoma in the dog. J Vet Intern Med 1:183, 1987

Olson PN, Wrigley RH, Thrall MA, Husted PW: Disorders of the canine prostate gland: pathogenesis, diagnosis, and medical therapy. Compend Contin Educ Pract Vet 9:613, 1987

Osborne CA, Johnston GR, Polzin DJ et al: Feline urologic syndrome: a heterogeneous phenomenon? J Am Anim Hosp Assoc 20:17, 1984

O'Shea JD: Squamous metaplasia of the canine prostate gland. Res Vet Sci 4:431, 1963

Peter AT, Jakovljevic S: Real-time ultrasonography of the small animal reproductive organs. Compend Contin Educ Pract Vet 14:739, 1992

Read RA, Bryden S: Urethral bleeding as a presenting sign of benign prostatic hyperplasia in the dog: a retrospective study (1979–1993). J Am Anim Hosp Assoc 31:261, 1995

Schulman J, Levine SH: Pyometra involving uterus masculinus in a cat. J Am Vet Med Assoc 194:690, 1989

Stone EA, Barsanti JA: Urologic Surgery of the Dog and Cat. Lea & Febiger, Philadelphia, 1992

Thrall MA, Olson PN, Freemyer FG: Cytologic diagnosis of canine prostatic disease. J Am Anim Hosp Assoc 21:95, 1985

Turrel JM: Intraoperative radiotherapy of carcinoma of the prostate gland in 10 dogs. J Am Vet Med Assoc 190:48, 1987

Weaver AD: Discrete prostatic (paraprostatitic) cysts in the dog. Vet Rec 102:435, 1978

Weaver AD: Fifteen cases of prostatic carcinoma in the dog. Vet Rec 109:71, 1981

White RAS, Herrtage ME, Dennis R: The diagnosis and management of paraprostatic and prostatic retention cysts in the dog. J Small Anim Pract 28:551, 1987

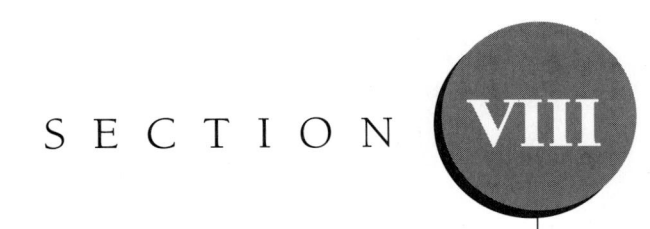

Reproductive System

53

Introduction

Janice L. Cain

ESTABLISHING A SMALL ANIMAL REPRODUCTION PRACTICE

Advantages of Developing Expertise

I. Expand services offered to current breeders
II. Attract new breeder clients
III. Learn new techniques and procedures
IV. Gain confidence in this area of veterinary medicine

Key Points for Ensuring Success

I. Extensive knowledge
   A. Breeders are becoming more informed about reproductive physiology and procedures.
   B. Often their interpretation of scientific information causes them to be misinformed.
   C. Breeders usually follow the advice offered by veterinarians when it is based on scientific fact and presented with confidence.
   D. Breeders appreciate a correctly informed professional opinion.
II. Expertise in performing procedures
   A. Most procedures are performed in the presence of the breeder.
   B. Do not be offended by breeders' suggestions or intimidated by their questions.
III. Availability
   A. Reproductive procedures may need to be conducted on weekends and holidays.
   B. Ensure that all situations are covered or backed up by a competent associate.
IV. Communication
   A. Often breeders are not sure what services are needed in a given situation.
   B. Many times a telephone discussion is necessary in advance of scheduled appointments.

Basic Equipment Needed

I. Microscope, slides and coverslips, Diff-Quik stain for evaluation of vaginal cytology and semen
II. Hemocytometer, Unopette dilution kits (see Chap. 60) for sperm counts
III. Rigid pediatric sigmoidoscope for vaginoscopy
IV. Ultrasonography for evaluation of uterus, ovaries, prostate, and testes
V. Latex artificial vaginas, collection tubes, and insemination pipettes for semen collection and vaginal insemination
VI. Slide warmer for proper evaluation of chilled-extended or frozen semen

REPRODUCTIVE TECHNIQUES

Timing of Ovulation

I. Indications
   A. Scheduling breedings for artificial insemination
   B. As a method to manage breeding in bitches with a history of infertility
   C. To increase the chance of conception when using poor-quality semen
   D. To increase conception rate and fecundity with natural breeding
II. Principles involved
   A. Follicular growth causes estrogen production, which causes cornification of vaginal epithelium.
   B. A spontaneous release of luteinizing hormone (LH) from the pituitary causes ovulation to occur approximately 48 hours later.
   C. From 4–6 days after the preovulatory LH peak, mature ova are within the oviducts and available for fertilization (peak fertile period).
   D. Behavioral sexual receptivity is usually longer than the peak fertile period.
   E. Serum progesterone concentration increases from <1 ng/ml to 1–2.5 ng/ml at the time of preovulatory LH peak (Concannon et al., 1977).
      1. The rate and amplitude of the early rise vary among bitches.
      2. At the time of ovulation, serum progesterone is 4–10 ng/ml.
      3. Progesterone continues to rise and peak

Table 53–1. *Ovulation Timing Protocols*

Progesterone Testing

1. Evaluate vaginal cytology every 1–2 days at the onset of proestrus.
2. Measure serum progesterone concentration every 1–2 days once the vaginal cytology indicates 50–70% superficial cells (i.e., 50–70% cornification).
3. The day the serum progesterone concentration increases above basal values is assigned as day 0.
4. Peak fertility is during days 4–6.
5. Evaluate vaginal cytology again near the end of the fertile period to determine the cytologic diestrual shift.
6. Progesterone evaluation is an estimation of the preovulatory LH peak; therefore, day 0 determined by this method may be inaccurate by 1–2 days.
7. Evaluation of the vaginal mucosal crenulation every 1–2 days during the time of progesterone testing can increase the accuracy of this protocol.

LH Testing

1. Evaluate vaginal cytology every 1–2 days at the onset of proestrus.
2. Evaluate serum LH level every 24 hours once the vaginal cytology indicates 50% superficial cells (i.e., 50% cornified).
3. A positive LH test identifies an LH peak.
4. Because false LH peaks can occur (although uncommon) before the preovulatory LH peak, measure serum progesterone concentration 2–3 days after the positive LH test to confirm the preovulatory LH peak.
5. Once a positive LH test is obtained, continue to draw serum daily and refrigerate; these samples can be run in the event the rise in LH was not the preovulatory LH peak.
6. Evaluate vaginal cytology again near the end of the fertile period to determine the cytologic diestrual shift.
7. Evaluation of the vaginal mucosal crenulation every 1–2 days during the time of LH testing can increase the accuracy of this protocol and aid in the determination of false LH peaks.

4. An abrupt change from nearly 100% superficial cells to >20% parabasal cells with or without white blood cells signifies the end of the fertile period.
  B. Serum progesterone concentration
    1. Begin to measure when 50–70% of vaginal cells are cornified.
    2. Measure every 24–48 hours to detect first rise above basal level.
    3. First rise occurs 1–3 days after preovulatory LH peak.
    4. Semiquantitative kits are available.
  C. Serum LH assay
    1. Determined daily when 50% of vaginal cells are cornified
    2. Can accurately determine preovulatory LH peak if measured daily
    3. False LH peaks possible, but not associated with progesterone rise
    4. Commercial kit available
  D. Vaginal mucosal crenulation
    1. It is a reliable but subjective indicator of ovulation.
    2. Onset of initial crenulation correlates to the preovulatory peak ± 24 hours.
    3. Crenulation continues after the LH peak, and mucosa becomes angulated with sharp profiles.
    4. Maximal angulation occurs at about the time of oocyte maturation (4–6 days after the preovulatory LH peak).

Artificial Insemination (AI)

I. Always evaluate the bitch for vaginal anomalies first.
II. Success is increased by combining AI with ovulation timing procedures (Table 53–2).
III. Semen collection is performed as described in Chap. 60.
IV. Vaginal insemination is performed as follows.
  A. An insemination pipette is placed in the cranial vagina as close to the cervix as possible.
  B. Elevate the bitch's rear quarters at least 45°.
  C. Semen is slowly deposited into the cranial vagina, followed by a small amount of air to clear the insemination pipette.
  D. Perform vaginal feathering for 2–5 minutes.

(15–80 ng/ml) about 15–20 days after the preovulatory LH peak.
    4. It returns to basal levels at the end of gestation or at the end of diestrus (60–70 days after the preovulatory LH peak).
  F. High serum estrogen causes edema of the vaginal mucosa, and as the edema recedes, the mucosa appears wrinkled or crenulated (Lindsay, 1990).
III. Parameters to evaluate (Table 53–1)
  A. Vaginal cytology
    1. Identification of cell types is as follows.
      a) Parabasal cells: smallest epithelial cells, round, high nucleus to cytoplasm ratio
      b) Superficial cells: squamous epithelial cells with keratinized cytoplasm, pyknotic or absent nuclei, angulated borders
      c) Intermediate cells: between parabasal and superficial cells in appearance, progressively larger cells with rounded borders
    2. Maximum cornification occurs 8 days before to 3 days after preovulatory LH peak (Concannon and Lein, 1989).
    3. It is most helpful to determine when serum progesterone and LH assays should be submitted.

Table 53–2. *Proposed Breeding Schedule Based on Ovulation Timing*

Day 0 = day of preovulatory LH peak
Natural breeding (unlimited): days 1, 3, 5, ±7
Natural breeding (limited): days 2 and 4
Artificial insemination: days 3 and 5 (or, alternatively, days 2 and 4)
Fresh-chilled semen: days 3 and 5 (or, alternatively, days 4 and 6)
Frozen semen—vaginal insemination: days 5 and 6
Frozen semen—surgical intrauterine insemination: day 5 or 6

E. Keep the bitch's rear quarters elevated for another 5–10 minutes.

Chilled-Extended Semen Collection and AI

I. Semen is collected, extended in a cryoprotectant buffer, and shipped to distant locations for insemination within 24 hours.
II. The American Kennel Club (AKC) allows registration of litters that result from these breedings, provided a veterinarian is involved with collection and insemination.
III. For a current list of approved semen freezing centers, write to the AKC at 5580 Centerview Drive, Raleigh NC 27606.
IV. Correct ovulation timing is necessary.
V. Only the sperm-rich fraction of the ejaculate is used (see Chap. 60).
VI. Vaginal insemination is performed as described earlier.

Insemination with Frozen Semen

I. Factors that affect freezability
  A. Dogs >7–9 years old may have semen that does not withstand the freezing process well, despite good initial semen quality.
  B. There is no difference in freezability among breeds.
  C. Libido greatly affects sperm count.
  D. Any concurrent illness can effect sperm quality, sperm quantity, and libido.
  E. Any drug administration at the time of or prior to semen collection may affect sperm production and libido.
  F. Because the interval since last ejaculation can effect semen quality, ejaculate the dog 1–2 weeks before semen collection for freezing.
II. Using frozen semen
  A. Whether the semen is deposited into the bitch by vaginal insemination or directly into the uterus via laparotomy depends on the post-thaw motility of the semen and the supply available from a particular dog.
  B. Consider intrauterine insemination (IUI) if motility is <50%.
  C. The insemination dose depends on the insemination route and post-thaw viability of the semen.
  D. Generally, 100 million live, motile, morphologically normal sperm are recommended.
  E. When to inseminate depends on ovulation timing.
    1. Vaginal inseminations are recommended on days 5 and 6 after the LH peak.
    2. If surgical IUI is done, a single insemination on day 5 or 6 is suggested.
  F. Handling and thawing of frozen semen require special considerations.
    1. Semen can be shipped in a specialized vessel that will keep it frozen for up to 2 weeks without the addition of liquid nitrogen.
    2. Request that the semen be shipped when the bitch has started proestrus and ovulation timing has begun.
    3. Semen is thawed according to the shipper's directions, which may vary, depending on the process used to freeze the semen.
    4. Insemination is performed immediately after thawing.
  G. Insemination may occur via two routes.
    1. For vaginal insemination, use the protocol described earlier.
    2. For IUI by means of a laparotomy, the uterus is exposed via a ventral midline incision.
      a) Semen is injected into the uterine lumen with a needle and syringe.
      b) During insemination, gentle fingertip clamping of the uterus distal to the uterine puncture ensures that the inseminant flows cranially.
      c) Low inseminant volume (1–3 ml) is required to prevent significant loss through the cervix.

Fertility Evaluation

See Chaps. 60 and 61.

Pregnancy Diagnosis and Periparturient Care

I. Ultrasonographic diagnosis of pregnancy
  A. Accurately diagnoses pregnancy as early as 21 days of gestation
  B. Determines fetal well-being
  C. Determines occurrence of fetal resorption
  D. Used to estimate litter size
II. Performing cesarean sections
  A. May be necessary in cases of dystocia (see Chap. 60)
  B. May be requested as an elective procedure for certain breeds
III. Neonatal care
  A. It is an often overlooked area of veterinary service.
  B. Generalized nursing care, with fluid therapy, may be necessary.
  C. Attempt to determine a diagnosis with "fading" puppies or kittens.
  D. Necropsy and histopathology of dead neonates may be needed.

Expertise in Feline Reproduction

See Chap. 61.

Treatment of Miscellaneous Conditions

I. For appropriate treatment of pyometra, see Chap. 56.
II. To induce abortion in cases of misalliance, see Chap. 60.

III. For information on contraception and estrus prevention, see Chap. 60.

IV. To correctly diagnose and treat diseases of the prostate, see Chap. 52.

Bibliography

Concannon PW, Hansel W, McEntee K: Changes in LH, progesterone and sexual behavior associated with preovulatory luteinization in the bitch. Biol Reprod 17:604, 1977

Concannon PW, Lein DH: Hormonal and clinical correlates of ovarian cycles, ovulation, pseudopregnancy, and pregnancy in dogs. p. 1269. In Kirk RW (ed): Current Veterinary Therapy X: Small Animal Practice. WB Saunders, Philadelphia, 1989

Lindsay FEF: Postuterine endoscopy in the bitch. p. 327. In Tams TR (ed): Small Animal Endoscopy. CV Mosby, St. Louis, 1990

Lindsay FEF, Concannon PW: Normal canine vaginoscopy. p. 112. In Burke T (ed): Small Animal Reproduction and Infertility. Lea & Febiger, Philadelphia, 1986

54

Diseases of the Ovaries

Steven J. Susaneck
Janice L. Cain

OVARIAN CYSTS

Definition

I. A cyst is a sac containing fluid or semisolid material.
II. Cysts are common in the ovaries of aging dogs and cats, and in some instances the fluid-filled cavities greatly enlarge the size of the organ.
III. Most ovarian cysts are small and clinically unimportant, however.
IV. There are four types of cysts found in the ovary.
   A. Follicular cysts
   B. Luteal cysts
   C. Epithelial tubular cysts
   D. Cysts of the rete ovarii

Causes and Pathophysiology

I. Follicular cysts
   A. They represent the failure of fluid to be absorbed from an incompletely developed follicle.
   B. They range from solitary, 1-cm nodules to confluent, cystic masses 10 cm in diameter.
   C. They appear on the surface of the ovary as pale blebs filled with clear watery fluid.
   D. Cysts are lined by layers of granulosa cells.
      1. Functional cysts produce estrogen.
      2. They may also contain some luteal cells that are progesterone secreting.
   E. Incidence may be ≥16% in mature bitches (Dow, 1960).
      1. Incidental finding at ovariohysterectomy in older bitches
      2. Clinically significant in younger bitches when causing abnormal estrous cycles
II. Luteal cysts
   A. They are solitary cysts lined by luteal tissue.
   B. They are found only rarely in older bitches.
   C. The corpus luteum in the dog shows central cavitation for a short time after ovulation.
      1. Generally, the cavitation disappears as the corpus luteum regresses.
      2. The cavitation may fill with fluid, however, forming a luteal cyst.
III. Epithelial tubular cysts
   A. They form from cells of the surface epithelium.
      1. The surface epithelium of the ovary in the growing animal consists largely of cuboidal cells and occasional cords and tubules.
      2. At puberty, proliferation of tubules begins to produce invaginations of the surface epithelium.
      3. After 5 years of age, there are numerous crypt-like infoldings of the epithelium, giving the surface of the ovary a palisade-like appearance.
      4. Because ovarian epithelial cells are secretory, obstructed tubules within the crypts may dilate and fill with fluid.
   B. They may enlarge to ≥1 cm.
   C. They closely resemble cystic follicles.
   D. Instead of being lined by granulosa cells, tubular cysts are lined by a single layer of flat cuboidal epithelium.
IV. Cystic rete ovarii
   A. The rete ovarii is a convoluted system of epithelial cell cords and tubules occupying part of the ovarian medulla.
   B. Because the rete often ends blindly and its epithelial cells are secretory, it is not surprising that cysts develop.
   C. Unlike other types of ovarian cyst, rete cysts are found in the hilar region of the ovary.
   D. Rete cysts have been reported in both dogs (Dow, 1960) and cats (Gelberg et al., 1984).

Clinical Signs

I. Most ovarian cysts of all types are clinically silent; there are usually no reproductive abnormalities associated with the condition.

II. Follicular cysts have these characteristics.
  A. They may be associated with prolonged proestrus behavior without sexual receptivity.
  B. Animals with estrogen-secreting follicular cysts may have a turgid vulva, a sanguineous vaginal discharge, and vaginal cytology typical of a bitch in proestrus.
  C. Behavioral estrus can result from cysts that produce estrogen and progesterone.
III. Prolonged anestrus has been reported in a dog with numerous enlarged tubular cysts (Andersen and Simpson, 1973).
IV. Extremely large ovarian cysts may produce a palpable abdominal mass.
V. Persistent nonseasonal estrus has been reported in older queens with cystic follicular hyperplasia (Stabenfeldt and Pedersen, 1991).

Diagnosis

I. Elevations in serum estradiol concentration may occur with follicular cysts in the dog (Schille et al., 1984).
  A. Normal concentrations are as follows.
    1. Anestrus: <15 pg/ml
    2. Proestrus: 15–100 pg/ml
  B. Follicular cysts may result in serum estrogen concentrations similar to those of proestrus.
II. Follicular cysts in queens can result in elevated serum estrogen concentrations (>20 pg/ml), with concurrent signs of estrus behavior for >3 weeks (Feldman and Nelson, 1996).
III. Abdominal radiography may be helpful.
  A. It is a useful diagnostic technique if the cyst is large.
  B. It may reveal a fluid-dense mass caudal to the kidney.
  C. Intravenous urography may be necessary to rule out involvement of the urinary system.
IV. Ultrasonography usually localizes fluid-filled cysts and differentiates an ovarian cyst from the kidney.
V. Because most ovarian cysts produce no clinical signs, diagnosis is usually made incidentally at the time of ovariohysterectomy.
VI. Histopathologic evaluation is necessary to distinguish among follicular, luteal, tubular, and rete cysts and to rule out neoplasia.

Differential Diagnosis

I. Polycystic kidneys
II. Neoplasia of the adrenals and kidneys
III. Ovarian neoplasia
IV. Any other cause of a midabdominal mass
V. Persistent estrus owing to overlapping waves of follicular activity in queens (Stabenfeldt and Pedersen, 1991)

Treatment and Monitoring

I. Most follicular cysts in small animals probably disappear spontaneously within a few months without treatment.

II. Human chorionic gonadotropin (HCG)
  A. It can be used to produce luteinization of a persistent follicular cyst.
  B. A dose of 500–1000 IU is given intramuscularly and repeated 48 hours later.
  C. If successful, conversion from proestrus to estrus occurs in 1–2 days.
  D. Within 2 weeks the animal should cease sexual behavior completely.
III. Gonadotropin-releasing hormone (GnRH)
  A. Produces luteinization of persistent follicular cyst
  B. Dose: 50–100 μg IM/day for 1–3 treatments (Olson et al., 1989)
IV. Ovariohysterectomy should be considered for any ovarian cyst.
  A. Animals with functional follicular cysts are likely to have estrogen-induced changes in the endometrium and are at risk for development of the cystic endometrial hyperplasia/pyometra complex.
  B. Dogs treated with HCG or GnRH are also prone to pyometra during the resulting luteal phase, so they must be monitored closely for 60–80 days after treatment.

PREMATURE OVARIAN FAILURE

Definition and Causes

I. It is a defect in the development of normal gonads and/or gametes.
II. It may be congenital or acquired.
  A. Defective gonadal differentiation
  B. Defective gamete maturation

Pathophysiology

I. Defective gonadal differentiation occurs with intersex disorders (see Chap. 58).
  A. Errors in testicular differentiation have been described in female dogs with 78-XX, 79-XXY, or 78-XX/78-XY chromosome complements and true hermaphroditism.
  B. Errors in ovarian differentiation have been described in animals with X-chromosome monosomy and trisomy as well as X-chromosome mosaicism.
II. Lymphocytic oophoritis may result in ovarian failure.
  A. The inciting event or cause is unknown, but it is suspected to be immune mediated.
  B. Ovarian pathology includes degenerating follicles with infiltration of perifollicular lymphocytes, oocyte degeneration, and necrosis of follicle cells (Johnston, 1989).
  C. It can result in persistent anestrus (Johnston, 1989) or an abnormal estrous cycle (Nickel et al., 1991).
III. Defective gamete maturation may also arise from an insufficiency of thyroid hormone and its effects on the developing ovary.

Clinical Signs

I. In defective ovarian differentiation, there is failure to show signs of pubertal estrus by 24 months of age, i.e., primary anestrus.

II. Hypothyroidism may be associated with primary anestrus, prolonged anestrus, and extended proestrus (Manning, 1979).

Diagnosis

I. Measure plasma concentrations of pituitary gonadotropins (luteinizing hormone and follicle-stimulating hormone) to check for hypergonadotrophic states (Olson et al., 1992).
   A. Gonadal agenesis and lack of negative feedback inhibition may cause increased serum concentrations of gonadotropins (a hypergonadotrophic state).
   B. Assays for canine luteinizing hormone (LH) are commercially available.
      1. Normal levels depend on the phase of the estrous cycle.
      2. Repetitive sampling may be necessary to document persistently elevated levels.

II. Perform karyotyping to rule out an intersex disorder.

III. Thyroid function testing is also indicated in any case of anestrus or abnormal estrus.

Differential Diagnosis

I. Silent heat

II. Systemic disease, e.g., hyperadrenocorticism

III. Concurrent drug administration that suppresses cyclicity, e.g., corticosteroids

Treatment and Monitoring

I. No treatment is available for defective gonadal differentiation.

II. See Chap. 41 for treatment of hypothyroidism.

III. With thyroid supplementation, estrus will reappear but may take several months. Hypothyroid animals should not be part of a breeding program, however.

OVARIAN REMNANT SYNDROME

Definition and Causes

I. Ovarian remnant syndrome is the presence of functional ovarian tissue in a previously ovariohysterectomized bitch or queen (Wallace, 1991).

II. It develops from failure to remove all ovarian tissue.
   A. Improper placement of clamps or ligatures
   B. Poor visualization of surgical field
   C. Inadvertent dropping of a piece of ovarian tissue into the abdomen

III. The development of a granulosa cell tumor was reported in an ovariohysterectomized bitch at the site of a probable remnant (Pluhar et al., 1995).

Clinical Signs

I. Signs of proestrus and estrus occur.
   A. Bitch
      1. Vulvar swelling and/or bloody vaginal discharge
      2. Exhibition of flagging or standing behavior
      3. Attraction and/or acceptance of a male
      4. Pseudocyesis with or without signs of estrus
   B. Queen
      1. Vocalization, rolling, treading, or lordosis
      2. May attract or accept a tom

II. Signs may develop months to years after the ovariohysterectomy.

Diagnosis

I. Vaginal cytology reveals progressive cornification of vaginal epithelial cells, which is evidence of estrogen secretion.

II. Reproductive hormones may be assayed but have several disadvantages and may be costly.
   A. Single samples can be misleading if not taken at the appropriate time.
   B. Progesterone assays are more useful in the bitch than are estradiol levels.
      1. Progesterone concentrations of >2 ng/ml confirm the presence of functional corpora lutea.
      2. The queen is an induced ovulator, so evaluation of serum progesterone levels alone is not helpful.
   C. Hormone stimulation tests are more reliable than resting levels in both the bitch and the queen.
      1. Give HCG (500–1000 IU in the dog, 250 IU in the cat) or GnRH (2 μg/kg in the dog, 25 μg in the cat) IM during estrus.
      2. 2–3 weeks later, serum progesterone concentration is >2 ng/ml if functional tissue is present.

III. Surgical exploration of the abdomen is both diagnostic and therapeutic.

Differential Diagnosis

I. Vaginal neoplasia

II. Vaginitis

III. Uterine stump pyometra

IV. Trauma

Treatment and Monitoring

I. The treatment of choice is exploratory laparotomy and excision of remnant tissue.

II. The remnant tissue may be more easily identified if the animal is in estrus at the time of surgery.

III. Clinical signs resolve within days following corrective surgery.

OVARIAN NEOPLASIA

Definition

Ovarian neoplasms in the dog and cat are comparatively rare. They may be of several cell types.

I. Ovarian adenocarcinoma
   A. Tumor of the surface epithelial tubules
   B. May be cystic or papillary
   C. Occurs in older dogs
   D. Although the most commonly diagnosed ovarian tumor, overall incidence low
II. Ovarian cystadenoma
   A. It may be cystic or papillary.
   B. Hyperplastic, poorly organized nodules of epithelial tubules suggestive of adenoma are often found in the ovaries of aging dogs (Andersen and Simpson, 1973).
III. Tumors of gonadal stromal origin
   A. These tumors are composed of granulosa or thecal cells.
   B. They are the functional counterpart of Sertoli's cell tumors in the male patient.
   C. Granulosa cell tumors are probably the most common ovarian tumor in both the dog (Dow, 1960) and the cat (Norris et al., 1969).
   D. The English bulldog appears to be at extraordinary risk for the development of these tumors (Hayes and Young, 1978).
   E. Most granulosa cell tumors in the dog are benign, but malignancy with metastasis is commonly reported in the cat (Norris et al., 1969; Aliakbrai and Ivoghli, 1979).
   F. The development of a granulosa cell tumor was reported in an ovariohysterectomized bitch at the site of a probable remnant (Pluhar et al., 1995).
IV. Tumors of germ cell origin
   A. Dysgerminomas
      1. They are tumors of the primordial germ cells of the ovary.
      2. Metastasis of these tumors is rare but does occur.
   B. Teratomas
      1. They can be benign, well-differentiated neoplasms containing mature tissue elements such as hair, squamous epithelium, bone, cartilage, lymphoid follicles, and nervous tissue.
      2. Malignant teratomas also occur and contain both mature and embryonal anaplastic elements.
      3. The ovary is the most common location for the development of teratomas in the dog; approximately 5% of canine ovarian tumors are teratomas (Hayes and Young, 1978).
      4. The tumor has also been reported in the cat (Dehner et al., 1970).
V. Other tumors
   A. Primary: leiomyomas, fibromas
   B. Metastatic: lymphosarcoma and mammary carcinoma

Causes

I. The cause of most ovarian tumors is unknown.
II. Malignant ovarian adenocarcinomas have been produced by experimental administration of diethylstilbestrol in dogs as young as 8 months old (O'Shea and Jabara, 1967).

Clinical Signs

I. Most benign epithelial ovarian neoplasms produce no clinical signs unless they are very large.
II. Certain changes are associated with specific tumors.
   A. Ovarian adenocarcinoma
      1. Dogs may present because of vaginal bleeding unrelated to the estrous cycle.
      2. These tumors commonly rupture as they enlarge, spilling tumor cells into the abdomen.
         a) Ascites with abdominal enlargement follows growth of these tiny tumor nodules.
         b) Common abdominal sites for implantation or metastasis are the diaphragm, para-aortic lymph nodes, omentum, and mesentery.
   B. Teratomas and dysgerminomas
      1. They generally produce no clinical signs until the tumor mass is large enough to palpate.
      2. Affected animals with large tumors may show lethargy, anorexia, a bloody vaginal discharge, and signs of intermittent intestinal obstruction.
   C. Granulosa/theca cell tumors
      1. Because they may produce estrogen and progesterone, clinical signs of endocrine disease are sometimes found.
      2. Persistent or irregular signs of estrus, alopecia, and enlargement of the nipples and vulva may be present.
      3. Changes in the uterus range from cystic endometrial hyperplasia to pyometra.
      4. In one report, bone marrow hypoplasia with a bleeding diathesis resulted from high levels of estrogen produced by a granulosa cell tumor (McCandlish et al., 1979).

Diagnosis

I. Cytologic evaluation of ascitic fluid
   A. Sample is obtained by paracentesis.
   B. It may be difficult to distinguish malignant adenocarcinoma cell clusters from normal mesothelial cells.
II. Abdominal radiography, ultrasonography
   A. They may reveal a mass caudal to the kidney.
   B. Intravenous urography may be necessary to rule out renal enlargement.
III. Circulating estradiol levels: sometimes high (>15 pg/ml) in bitches with functional granulosa cell tumors
IV. Vaginal cytology: in dogs with estradiol-secreting tumors, reveals an abundance of superficial epithelial cells typical of a bitch in heat
V. Definitive diagnosis usually made by exploratory laparotomy and histopathologic examination of the excised ovary

Differential Diagnosis

I. Renal and adrenal tumors
II. Large renal and ovarian cysts

III. Other causes of a midabdominal mass
IV. Other causes of ascites, neoplastic effusion

Treatment and Monitoring

I. Ovariohysterectomy is the primary treatment for all types of ovarian neoplasia.
II. Ovarian adenocarcinoma also requires the following.
   A. The tumor is treated by radical resection of the primary and as many of the metastatic lesions as possible.
      1. If implantation of the tumor over the mesothelial surfaces has not occurred, it is important to avoid rupture of the tumor capsule and spillage of tumor cells during surgery.
      2. Surgical debulking improves survival but is not usually curative.
   B. Chemotherapy using melphalan, chlorambucil, or cyclophosphamide has been reported to induce remission in the dog (Greene et al., 1979).
   C. There are anecdotal reports of response to carboplatin and paclitaxel.
III. Germ cell and gonadal stromal tumors are treated as follows.
   A. Ovariohysterectomy is the primary therapy, as most of these tumors are localized to the ovary.
   B. Successful treatment of malignant teratoma has been reported in one dog with ovariohysterectomy, but approximately 33% of reported cases develop metastases (Jergens et al., 1987).
   C. Radiation therapy should be considered in the rare case of metastasis of a dysgerminoma, because they are exquisitely radiosensitive tumors.

Bibliography

Aliakbrai S, Ivoghli B: Granulosa cell tumor in a cat. J Am Vet Med Assoc 174:1306, 1979

Andersen AC, Simpson ME: The Ovary and Reproductive Cycle of the Dog (Beagle). Geron-X, Los Altos, CA, 1973

Andrews EJ, Stookey JL, Helland DR, et al: A histopathological study of canine and feline ovarian dysgerminomas. Can J Comp Med 38:85, 1974

Dehner LP, Norris HJ, Garner FM, et al: Comparative pathology of ovarian neoplasms. III. Germ cell tumours of canine, bovine, feline, rodent, and human species. J Comp Pathol 80:299, 1970

Dow C: Ovarian abnormalities in the bitch. J Comp Pathol 70:59, 1960

Feldman EC, Nelson RW: Canine and Feline Endocrinology and Reproduction. 2nd Ed. WB Saunders, Philadelphia, 1996

Gelberg HB, McEntee K, Heath EH: Feline cystic rete ovarii. Vet Pathol 21:304, 1984

Greene JA, Richardson RC, Thornhill JA, et al: Ovarian papillary cystadenocarcinoma in a bitch: case report and literature review. J Am Anim Hosp Assoc 15:351, 1979

Greenlee PG, Patnaik AK: Canine ovarian tumors of germ cell origin. Vet Pathol 22:117, 1985

Hayes HM, Young JL: Epidemiologic features of canine ovarian neoplasms. Gynecol Oncol 6:348, 1978

Jergens AE, Knapp DW, Shaw DP: Ovarian teratoma in a bitch. J Am Vet Med Assoc 191:81, 1987

Johnston SD: Premature gonadal failure in female dogs and cats. J Reprod Fertil 39:65, 1989

Manning PJ: Thyroid gland and arterial lesions of beagles with familial hypothyroidism and hyperlipoproteinemia. Am J Vet Res 40:820, 1979

McCandlish IAP, Munro CD, Breeze RG, et al: Hormone producing ovarian tumours in the dog. Vet Rec 105:9, 1979

Nickel RF, Okkens AC, van der Gaag I, van Haaften B: Oophoritis in a dog with abnormal corpus luteum function. Vet Rec 128:333, 1991

Norris HJ, Garner FM, Taylor HB: Pathology of feline ovarian neoplasms. J Pathol 97:138, 1969

Olson PN, Mulnix JA, Neff TM: Concentrations of luteinizing hormone and follicle-stimulating hormone in the serum of sexually intact and neutered dogs. Am J Vet Res 53:762, 1992

Olson PN, Wrigley RH, Husted PW, et al: Persistent estrus in the bitch. p. 1792. In Ettinger SJ (ed): Textbook of Veterinary Internal Medicine. 3rd Ed. WB Saunders, Philadelphia, 1989

O'Shea JD, Jabara AG: The histogenesis of canine ovarian tumours induced by stilboestrol administration. Pathol Vet 4:137, 1967

Pluhar GE, Memon MA, Wheaton LG: Granulosa cell tumor in an ovariohysterectomized dog. J Am Vet Med Assoc 207:1063, 1995

Rowley J: Cystic ovary in a dog: a case report. Vet Med Small Anim Clin 75:1888, 1980

Schille VM, Calderwood-Mays MB, Thatcher M: Infertility in a bitch associated with short interestrous intervals and cystic follicles: a case report. J Am Anim Hosp Assoc 20:171, 1984

Stabenfeldt GH, Pedersen NC: Reproduction and reproduction disorders. p. 144. In Pedersen NC (ed): Feline Husbandry. American Veterinary Publishers, Goleta, CA, 1991

Vaden P: Surgical treatment of polycystic ovaries in the dog. Vet Med Small Anim Clin 73:1160, 1978

Wallace MS: The ovarian remnant syndrome. Vet Clin North Am [Small Anim Pract] 21:501, 1991

55

Diseases of the Testes and Epididymides

Joni L. Freshman

CRYPTORCHIDISM

Definition

I. Cryptorchidism is a condition in which the testicle does not descend to its normal scrotal position.

II. It most commonly is unilateral.

III. The undescended testicle may be retained in the abdomen or may have descended through the inguinal ring.

IV. Controversy exists over which testicle is most likely to be retained.

V. With bilateral cryptorchidism, the affected dog is sterile, apparently owing to the effect of the higher abdominal temperature on spermatogenesis.

VI. The unilaterally cryptorchid male patient is often less fertile than one with both testicles normally descended.

Causes

I. It is usually a hereditary condition.
  A. It involves multiple gene influences.
  B. Likely breeds include the Yorkshire terrier, Pomeranian, miniature and toy poodle, Siberian husky, miniature schnauzer, Shetland sheepdog, and Chihuahua.
  C. Within closely related breeds (e.g., toy, miniature, and standard poodles), smaller breeds are at greater risk (Hayes et al., 1985).
  D. Degree of inbreeding is higher in bilateral than in unilateral cases (Cox et al., 1978).

II. Apparently, hereditary influences are not always involved in cryptorchidism, as some unilaterally cryptorchid male patients have been used as sires repeatedly with no evidence of the defect in their offspring (Whitney, 1961).

III. Insufficient gonadotropin stimulation during early gonadal development may be a cause.
  A. It occurs rarely.

B. Early administration of gonadotropins may allow the testis to descend and develop properly (Christiansen, 1984).

IV. Environmental contamination with endocrine-disrupting chemicals may be a cause (Colborn et al., 1993).
  A. Pesticides, especially organochlorines, may mimic diethylstilbestrol and act as estrogen agonists.
  B. Potential exposure of the affected dog or its dam should be considered.

Pathophysiology

I. The developing testicle is attached to the inguinal region by a mesenchymal structure called the gubernaculum.

II. During the first 2 weeks after birth, the distal part of the gubernaculum begins to increase enormously in length and volume and extends through the inguinal ring into the scrotal sac.

III. As the gubernaculum grows, traction is exerted on the testis, which is also drawn into the inguinal canal.

IV. The gubernaculum then regresses, becoming the proper ligament of the testis and causing the testis to descend further to its scrotal position.

V. In the dog this process is complete by 3 weeks after birth.

VI. This two-phase process appears to be controlled by a combination of testosterone and an unidentified nonandrogenic factor of testicular origin (Baumans et al., 1983).

Diagnosis/Differential Diagnosis

I. Although it is possible to diagnose cryptorchidism at about 3 weeks of age, the testicles are very small at this time and may be missed.

II. Puppies have a highly effective cremaster reflex, and palpation of the testicle may cause retraction of the testis toward the inguinal ring.

A. These animals may be mistakenly diagnosed as cryptorchid.

B. Generally, the testis can be manipulated down into the scrotum in the normal puppy; this maneuver is not possible in the cryptorchid patient.

III. Disparity in size of the inguinal ring and testis makes descent unlikely after 4 months of age, but it can occasionally occur later, e.g., 7–8 months of age.

Treatment and Monitoring

I. Castration is advisable for two reasons.

A. Cryptorchid animals should not be used for breeding because of the possible hereditary nature of the condition.

B. The risk of neoplasia in the undescended testicle of the cryptorchid dog is reported to be 13.6 times higher than in the normal testicle (Hayes and Pendergrass, 1976).

C. Remove both the descended and the retained testicles.

II. Descent of inguinal testicles has been reported with the use of human chorionic gonadotropin (HCG) 100–1000 IU every 5 days for 4 treatments or gonadotropin-releasing hormone 50–100 μg IV or SQ for 2 treatments, 7 days apart (Feldman and Nelson, 1996).

A. Success is higher with inguinal testes and in dogs <16 weeks of age.

B. Because no controlled study has been performed, it is possible that the reported descent was coincidental and would have occurred without treatment.

C. Purebred dog registries would consider these dogs ineligible for showing.

SENILE ATROPHY

Definition

I. Senile atrophy is an age-related change of the testicles associated with a gradual decline in and cessation of sperm production.

II. It may occur at a comparatively early age in some dogs, especially the giant breeds.

III. It is also referred to as idiopathic testicular degeneration.

Causes

I. The cause is unknown.

II. Serum levels of follicle-stimulating and/or luteinizing hormone or pituitary function may change with age.

III. Infection or inflammation leading to immune-mediated destruction of spermatogonia is more likely to occur in the aged male dog, ultimately resulting in testicular atrophy.

Clinical Signs and Diagnosis

I. Semen evaluation of the dog with senile testicular atrophy initially reveals oligospermia; later in the process, no spermatozoa are found in the ejaculate. See Semen Analysis in Chap. 60.

II. Affected testicles are small and soft, which is not surprising, as 85% of the testis is involved in sperm production; when the germinal epithelium atrophies, loss of testicular size occurs.

III. Testicular biopsy confirms the diagnosis.

A. Fix tissue in Bouin's or Zenker's solution to evaluate seminiferous tubules.

B. It is not often performed clinically because of the poor prognosis associated with prolonged azoospermia.

Differential Diagnosis

I. Testicular atrophy secondary to trauma or infection

II. Testicular atrophy associated with nonreproductive endocrinopathies (e.g., hypothyroidism, hyperadrenocorticism)

Treatment and Monitoring

I. There is no effective treatment of senile testicular atrophy at present because the loss of spermatogonia accompanying the disorder is irreversible.

II. Although fertility is diminished, the condition does not predispose the dog to other testicular diseases.

ORCHITIS/EPIDIDYMITIS

Definition

I. Orchitis and epididymitis are inflammatory conditions of the testis and epididymis, respectively.

II. Because they are closely related, inflammation of one organ often results in involvement of the other.

III. The inflammation may be unilateral or bilateral.

Causes

I. The most common cause of acute epididymitis in the canine is *Brucella canis*.

A. Palpable enlargement of the epididymis occurs within 15 weeks after infection, and an infiltration of plasma cells, lymphocytes, and macrophages is seen (George et al., 1979).

B. Semen may be affected as early as 5 weeks after infection, with numerous primary and secondary abnormalities of spermatozoa.

II. Some fungal diseases (e.g., blastomycosis and coccidioidomycosis) may produce granulomatous orchitis and epididymitis.

III. In the dog, septicemia may rarely result in bacterial infection of the male genital tract.

IV. Trauma to the testicle or epididymis sometimes produces inflammation and subsequent infection.

A. In dogs with scrotal pyoderma, constant licking of the scrotum may lead to bacterial infection of the underlying testicle and epididymis.

B. Bite wounds and abscesses of the testicles are particularly common in cats.

V. Canine distemper virus may produce both testicular and epididymal inflammation (Larsen, 1980).

Clinical Signs

I. Symptoms of acute testicular inflammation include the following.
   A. There may be heat, pain, and swelling.
   B. The testicle is usually firm in consistency, and fluid may accumulate between the tunics.
   C. The animal often aggravates the condition by licking at the testicle and epididymis, sometimes mutilating the organs.
   D. Generalized malaise, fever, and anorexia can be present.
II. An enlarged, firm, nonpainful testicle is seen in chronic granulomatous orchitis.
III. As the inflammatory process becomes more chronic, the testicle becomes atrophied, fibrotic, and irregular. Adhesions between the testicle and overlying scrotum are common.
IV. Careful palpation can detect a normal testis and enlarged epididymis in cases of primary epididymitis.

Diagnosis

I. Culture and evaluation of semen are useful tests, but pain may limit the animal's ability to have an erection and ejaculate.
II. Cytology of a testicular or epididymal aspirate may allow differentiation between purulent and granulomatous inflammation and can be used to culture for bacteria and mycoplasma.
III. Obtain a laboratory database.
   A. Serology for *B. canis* (see Chaps. 2 and 111)
   B. Complete blood count (CBC)
   C. Urinalysis and urine culture
   D. ± Biochemical profile
   E. ± Fungal titers
IV. Castration and histopathology of the involved testicles may be necessary to delineate the cause.

Differential Diagnosis

I. Testicular trauma
II. Testicular neoplasia
III. Immune-mediated orchitis
IV. Testicular torsion
V. Other lower urinary tract infections (e.g., urethritis, prostatitis)

Treatment

I. Appropriate antibiotic or antifungal therapy
   A. Brucellosis (see also Chap. 111)
      1. Give minocycline HCl 12 mg/kg PO BID for 14 days combined with streptomycin 5–10 mg/kg IM BID for 7 days.
      2. Tetracycline HCl 10 mg/kg PO TID for 28 days is less expensive but not as effective.
      3. Cure is unlikely in the male animal, so castration is advised, followed by antibiotic therapy.

B. Systemic mycoses (see Chap. 109)
   C. Other bacterial infections
      1. Antibiotics based on culture and sensitivity
      2. May require 2–4 weeks of therapy
II. Castration
   A. *Brucella*-positive dogs
   B. Severe testicular abscesses and/or necrosis
III. Removal of affected unilateral testis and epididymis may allow remaining testis to regain fertility.

Patient Monitoring

I. Sperm granulomas and obstruction of the ejaculatory duct may occur.
II. Immune-mediated infertility may develop (see later).

SPERMATOCELE AND SPERM GRANULOMA

Definition and Causes

I. Spermatocele: sperm-filled cystic dilatation within the epididymis at the level proximal to a ductal occulsion
II. Sperm granuloma: granulomatous inflammatory reaction to spermatocele caused by leakage of sperm across a degenerated tubular wall
III. Causes of the epididymal ductal occlusion
   A. Congenital aplasia
   B. Acquired occlusion from trauma, infectious epididymitis, or *B. canis* infection
IV. Can be unilateral

Clinical Signs and Diagnosis

I. Palpable nodule within epididymal structure
II. Decreased sperm output: azoospermia or oligospermia
III. Decrease seminal alkaline phosphatase concentration if lesions are complete and bilateral (see Chap. 60)
IV. Diagnosis confirmed with histopathology

Differential Diagnosis

I. Epididymitis
II. Neoplasia
III. *B. canis* infection

Treatment and Monitoring

I. There is no effective treatment.
II. The lesions may lead to production of autoantibody to sperm if granuloma forms.
III. Castration is recommended if bilateral abnormalities with azoospermia are present.

IMMUNE-MEDIATED ORCHITIS

Definition

I. Autoimmune orchitis results from invasion of lymphocytic cells into the testis.

II. This can result in acquired infertility.

Causes

I. Genetic influences may be a cause.
  A. Beagle dogs have a familial incidence of lymphocytic orchitis/thyroiditis (Fritz et al., 1976).
  B. A group of affected Scottish terriers were highly inbred over the past 20 generations (Olson, 1991).
II. Other potential causes have not yet been determined.

Pathophysiology

I. Spermatozoal antigens are anatomically separated from the immune system.
II. Anything that breaks down the blood-testis barrier (e.g., infection or trauma) may allow sensitization to sperm antigens and resultant antibody formation.
III. Sperm agglutination and sperm head phagocytosis by neutrophils are abnormalities suggesting the presence of antibodies on the surfaces of sperm.

Clinical Signs

I. Acute inflammation is not usually present.
II. The animal is often presented for acquired infertility and azoospermia.
III. Testes may be normal on palpation.

Diagnosis

I. Pedigree review for degree of inbreeding and evaluation of male relatives may be suggestive.
II. Definitive diagnosis requires histopathologic examination; the area of the rete testis is the most commonly affected.

Differential Diagnosis

I. Chronic orchitis (e.g., brucellosis)
II. Other causes of male infertility (see Chap. 60)
III. Testicular atrophy

Treatment and Monitoring

I. No treatment is available at this time.
II. Evaluate related dogs for a potentially heritable condition.

TESTICULAR TORSION

Definition

I. Testicular torsion is a condition of the dog in which the spermatic cord undergoes rotation, leading to infarction of the testicle.
II. It is commonly seen in retained, abdominal testes that have undergone neoplastic transformation but may occur in non-neoplastic, intrascrotal testes as well.

III. Age incidence ranges from 5 months to 10 years.
IV. Although there is no breed predilection, the condition is most commonly seen in breeds with a predilection for cryptorchidism.

Causes and Pathophysiology

I. In the neoplastic abdominal testicle, increased weight of the testicular mass may predispose to torsion of the spermatic cord.
II. Rotation of the spermatic cord in the fully descended testicle probably requires either previous traumatic rupture of the scrotal ligament or an anatomic lack of its development.
  A. Because the testicle and epididymis are attached to the spermatic fascia at the ventral border of the testicle by the scrotal ligament, partial rupture of the ligament allows limited rotation of the tunica vaginalis and testicle together.
  B. Complete rupture of the scrotal ligament allows a full range of torsion of the testis; rotations of 180°, 360°, 540°, and 720° have been described.

Clinical Signs

I. Acute torsion of an intrascrotal testicle
  A. Mild fever, severe vomiting, unwillingness to move, and a stiff gait are generally seen.
  B. With 180° torsions of the testicle, an abnormal location of the tail of the epididymis may be noted.
  C. Enlargement of the testicle and spermatic cord is not a constant finding.
  D. The twisted testicle is painful in the acute stages; after 24 hours or so, pain may disappear.
II. Acute torsion of an abdominal testicle
  A. Anorexia, fever, and vomiting may be present.
  B. There is a painful posterior abdominal mass.
III. Chronic or partial torsions
  A. They may be clinically silent for long periods of time.
  B. An incidental abdominal mass may be discovered.

Diagnosis

I. Rapid onset of an acutely painful scrotal testis, accompanied by systemic signs is suggestive.
II. Differentiation of a twisted abdominal testis is more difficult.
  A. Hemogram may reveal a leukocytosis with or without a left shift.
  B. Biochemical organ profile usually rules out other organ involvement.
  C. Ultrasonography may be helpful in delineating masses associated with other organs.
III. Diagnosis is sometimes confirmed only at surgery.

Differential Diagnosis

I. Scrotal torsion: acute orchitis, blunt testicular trauma, necrosis of testicular neoplasm (rare)

II. Abdominal torsion: other causes of acute abdomen syndrome (see Chap. 37)

III. Partial or chronic torsion: testicular neoplasia

Treatment and Monitoring

I. Intra-abdominal testicular torsion
   A. Stabilize the patient with preoperative intravenous fluids and supportive care.
   B. Perform immediate exploratory laparotomy with castration.
II. Intrascrotal testicular torsion
   A. Castration is the treatment of choice.
   B. In torsions of <180°, rotation of the testicle and repair of the scrotal ligament may be performed, avoiding orchiectomy (Young, 1979).
III. Surgery usually curative

CANINE TESTICULAR NEOPLASIA

Definition

I. Testicular neoplasia may develop from the following cells.
   A. Spermatogonia (germ cells): seminoma
   B. Leydig's (interstitial) cells: interstitial cell tumor (ICT)
   C. Sertoli's cells: Sertoli's cell tumor (SCT)
II. Testicular tumors are more common in the dog than any other domestic animal.
   A. The testicle is second in frequency only to skin as a site of neoplasia in the male dog.
   B. The incidence of neoplasia in the undescended testicle is 13.6 times higher than in the scrotal testicle (Hayes and Pendergrass, 1976).
      1. SCT is the most frequently found tumor in the cryptorchid testicle, with seminomas next most common.
      2. ICTs are generally found in normally descended testicles.
      3. Lymphosarcoma has also been diagnosed in the canine testis.
      4. Up to 35% of affected dogs have more than one tumor type present (Mattheeuws and Comhaire, 1977).
III. Age incidence is as follows.
   A. Dogs <6 years old are at low risk for the development of testicular neoplasia (Reif et al., 1979), but tumors may develop in dogs as young as 3 years old.
   B. The mean age for development of testicular tumors is 10.2 years (Lipowitz et al., 1973).
IV. The incidence of tumors developing in both testicles is very high.
V. Breeds with a high incidence of cryptorchidism are more likely to be affected with testicular neoplasia.
   A. Boxers
      1. High risk for all three types of testicular tumor
      2. Occurs independently of cryptorchidism

3. May occur at an earlier age
B. Weimaraners, Shetland sheepdogs: increased risk of SCT
C. German shepherd dogs: increased risk of seminomas

Causes

I. Neither the etiologic factors leading to the development of testicular tumors nor the reasons for the increased risk of neoplasia in the cryptorchid testicle are understood (Pearson, 1981).
II. Increased temperature of intra-abdominal testes may predispose to development of SCT (Wallace and Cox, 1980).
III. Scrotally located tumors are equally divided among the three cell types.

Clinical Signs

I. Because of the high incidence of testicular neoplasia, the physical examination of middle-aged and older dogs should always include a thorough palpation of the testicles.
   A. Enlargement in size, change in shape, or increased firmness in part or all of the testicle should lead to suspicion of a tumor.
   B. Palpation of a caudal abdominal mass in a cryptorchid animal may indicate testicular neoplasia.
II. Feminization may be present.
   A. May occur with any type of testicular tumor but is most common with SCT
   B. Signs
      1. Gynecomastia
      2. Pendulous prepuce
      3. Alopecia and hyperpigmentation of the skin
      4. Decreased libido, infertility
      5. Atrophy of the contralateral testicle
      6. Squamous metaplasia of the prostate
   C. May be associated with either high serum estrogen levels or increased estrogen/testosterone ratios (Pearson, 1981)
III. Signs of estrogen toxicity can occur with hyperestrogenism in any of the three tumor types.
   A. Infection, septicemia: leukopenia, pancytopenia
   B. Bleeding diatheses: thrombocytopenia
   C. Anemia, usually aplastic
IV. Other signs may also occur.
   A. Torsion of the spermatic cord and testicle (see earlier)
   B. Scrotal swelling due to obstruction of lymphatics with tumor

Diagnosis

I. Suspicious clinical signs and physical findings
II. Cytologic examination of testicular aspirate
   A. Seminoma
      1. Cells are fragile, and often only stripped nuclei are present on the slide.
      2. The cells have large nuclei with prominent nucleoli and scanty cytoplasm.

3. Giant nuclei, multinucleation, and mitotic figures are common.
B. SCT or ICT
1. Cells are cuboidal to columnar with a large amount of vacuolated cytoplasm.
2. SCT cells contain numerous small vacuoles of uniform size.
3. ICT cells contain fewer vacuoles of varying size.
III. Examination of stained preputial swab: epithelial cells influenced by estrogen (cornified)
IV. Examination of excised testicle
A. Gross appearance
1. The SCT is typically irregularly lobulated, brownish-yellow or white, and firm to hard; cystic areas may be present.
2. The ICT is bright yellow, orange, or brown, is firm in consistency, and often contains cysts.
3. The seminoma is usually soft, white to light yellow, and bulges on the cut surface. Slight lobulation is sometimes noted.
B. Histopathology
Definitive diagnosis of testicular neoplasia is made by histopathologic examination.

Differential Diagnosis

I. Chronic or previous orchitis
II. Partial or chronic testicular torsion

Treatment

I. Orchiectomy
A. Perform a CBC and platelet count preoperatively to rule out secondary effects of hyperestrogenism, and survey chest and abdominal radiographs to search for metastasis.
B. Because of the high incidence of tumors in both testes, the contralateral testicle is also removed.
II. Treatment of metastasis
A. Low incidence
1. SCT, seminoma: approximately 10%
2. ICT: very rare
B. SCT
Partial regression has been reported using methotrexate, vinblastine, and cyclophosphamide (Theilen and Madewell, 1979).
C. Seminoma
Metastatic seminomas in humans are extremely sensitive to both radiotherapy and chemotherapy (Javadpour, 1980; Drasga et al., 1982), but there is limited experience with these modalities in dogs.

Patient Monitoring

I. Watch for symptoms or hematologic changes that occur following excision of an estrogen-producing tumor.
A. CBC, platelet count
B. Signs of bleeding at surgical site
C. Onset of fever

II. Recovery of the bone marrow from hyperestrogenism is variable, depending on the cell types involved (see also Chaps. 63 and 64).
III. Successful excision of benign tumors should be followed by resolution of feminizing signs within 60 days.
IV. Monitor for evidence of metastasis.
A. Follow-up examinations at 3, 6, and 12 months
B. Common sites of metastasis
1. Sublumbar lymphatics and lymph nodes
2. Liver, lungs, eyes

Bibliography

Badinand F, Szumowski P, Breton A: Etude morphobiologique et biochimique du sperme de chien cryptorchide. Rec Med Vet 148:655, 1972

Baumans V, Dijkstra G, Wensing CJG: The role of a non-androgenic testicular factor in the process of testicular descent in the dog. Int J Androl 6:541, 1983

Carmichael LE: Canine brucellosis. p. 633. In Morrow DA (ed): Current Therapy in Theriogenology. WB Saunders, Philadelphia, 1980

Christiansen IJ: Reproduction in the Dog and Cat. Baillière Tindall, London, 1984

Colborn T, vom Saal FS, Soto AM: Developmental effects of endocrine-disrupting chemicals in wildlife and humans. Environ Health Perspect 101:378, 1993

Cox VS, Wallace LJ, Jessen CR: An anatomic and genetic study of canine cryptorchidism. Teratology 18:233, 1978

Drasga RE, Einhorn LH, Williams SD: The chemotherapy of testicular cancer. CA 32:66, 1982

Feldman EC, Nelson RW: Canine and Feline Endocrinology and Reproduction. 2nd Ed. WB Saunders, Philadelphia, 1996

Fritz TE, Lombard LS, Tyler SA, et al: Pathology and familial incidence of orchitis and its relation to thyroiditis in a closed beagle colony. Exp Mol Pathol 24:142, 1976

George LW, Duncan JR, Carmichael LE: Semen examination in dogs with canine brucellosis. Am J Vet Res 40:1590, 1979

Hayes HM, Pendergrass TW: Canine testicular tumors: epidemiologic features of 410 dogs. Int J Cancer 18:482, 1976

Hayes HM, Wilson GP, Pendergrass TW, Cox VS: Canine cryptorchidism and subsequent testicular neoplasia: case-control study with epidemiologic update. Teratology 32:51, 1985

Hulse DA: Intrascrotal torsion of the testicle in a dog. Vet Med Small Anim Clin 68:658, 1973

Javadpour N: Germ cell tumor of the testis. CA 30:242, 1980

Kawakami E, Tsatsui T, Yamada Y, Yamauchi M: Cryptorchidism in the dog: occurrence of cryptorchidism and semen quality in the dog. Jpn J Vet Sci 46:303, 1984

Larsen RE: Infertility in the male dog. p. 646. In Morrow DA (ed): Current Therapy in Theriogenology. WB Saunders, Philadelphia, 1980

Lipowitz AJ, Schwartz A, Wilson GP, et al: Testicular neoplasms and concomitant clinical changes in the dog. J Am Vet Med Assoc 163:1364, 1973

Lipshultz LI, Cunningham GR, Howards SS: Differential diagnosis of male infertility. p. 249. In Lipshultz LI, Howards SS (eds): Infertility in the Male. Churchill Livingstone, New York, 1983

Mattheeuws DRG, Comhaire MD: Tumors of the testes, p. 1054. In Kirk RW (ed): Current Veterinary Therapy VI. WB Saunders, Philadelphia, 1977

McNeil PE, Weaver AD: Massive scrotal swelling in two unusual cases of canine Sertoli-cell tumor. Vet Rec 106:144, 1980

Moore JA, Kakuk TJ: Male dogs naturally infected with *Brucella canis*. J Am Vet Med Assoc 155:1352, 1969

Morgan RV: Blood dyscrasias associated with testicular tumors in the dog. J Am Anim Hosp Assoc 18:970, 1982

Moulton JE: Tumors of the genital system. p. 309. In Moulton JE (ed): Tumors in Domestic Animals. University of California Press, Berkeley, 1978

Mumford DM, Warner MR: Male infertility and immunity. p. 265. In Lipshultz LI, Howards SS (eds): Infertility in the Male. Churchill Livingstone, New York, 1983

Olson PN: Clinical approach for evaluating dogs with azoospermia. Proc Soc Theriogenol 202, 1991

Pearson H, Kelly DF: Testicular torsion in the dog: a review of 13 cases. Vet Rec 97:200, 1975

Pearson JC: Endocrinology of testicular neoplasms. Urology 17:119, 1981

Pendergrass TW, Hayes HM: Cryptorchidism and related defects in dogs: epidemiologic comparisons with man. Teratology 12:51, 1975

Reif JS, Maguire TG, Kenney RM, et al: A cohort study of canine testicular neoplasia. J Am Vet Med Assoc 175:719, 1979

Theilen GH, Madewell BR: Tumors of the urogenital system. p. 357. In: Veterinary Cancer Medicine. Lea & Febiger, Philadelphia, 1979

Wallace LJ, Cox VS: Canine cryptorchidism. p. 1244. In Kirk RW (ed): Current Veterinary Therapy VII. WB Saunders, Philadelphia, 1980

Wensing CJG: Developmental anomalies, including cryptorchidism. p. 583. In Morrow DA (ed): Current Therapy in Theriogenology. WB Saunders, Philadelphia, 1980

Whitney LF: Non-inherited monorchidism. Vet Med 56:204, 1961

Young ACB: Two cases of intrascrotal torsion of a normal testicle. J Small Anim Pract 20:229, 1979

56

Diseases of the Uterus

Claudia L. Barton
Janice L. Cain

CYSTIC ENDOMETRIAL HYPERPLASIA/PYOMETRA COMPLEX

Definition

I. Cystic endometrial hyperplasia (CEH) is a continuum of proliferative and degenerative changes of the endometrium associated with aging.
   A. As the condition progresses, a diffuse chronic inflammatory infiltrate of lymphocytes and plasma cells is present within the endometrium.
   B. Mucometra or hydrometra may be seen occasionally in the dog or cat with advanced CEH.
      1. These conditions are characterized by variable amounts of thin to viscid mucus within the uterine lumen.
      2. In hydrometra, the mucin present is a watery fluid.
      3. In mucometra, the mucin may be thick or even a semisolid mass.
      4. No infection is present in these cases unless introduced by breeding or trauma.
II. Pyometra is a uterine inflammation/infection of the dog and cat, often from secondary bacterial infection of an abnormal uterus.
III. "Stump pyometra" is a bacterial infection of the remnant of the uterine body in the neutered animal.

Causes and Pathophysiology

I. Progesterone, produced during diestrus, promotes the accumulation of uterine secretions and stimulates endometrial hyperplasia.
   A. Repeated non-gravid cycles can increase the risk of CEH development as the bitch ages.
   B. Progesterone also inhibits local leukocyte responses to infection in the uterus.
II. Estrogen produces cervical dilatation during estrus.
   A. This allows bacteria (especially *Escherichia coli*) to ascend into the uterus.
   B. Estrogen also enhances the stimulatory effects of progesterone on the uterus.
III. The combination of pathogenic bacteria and an abnormal endometrium leads to pyometra.
IV. Estrogen compounds given for mismating can produce an acute pyometra or endometritis in young bitches 1–10 weeks following treatment.
V. Progesterone and synthetic progestins such as megestrol acetate have been incriminated as causes of cystic endometrial hyperplasia, mucometra and subsequent pyometra, and uterine stump infections in neutered cats.
VI. The development of CEH/pyometra in the queen can be due to progesterone or estrogen influence.
   A. Pseudopregnancy and the continuous influence of progesterone on the uterus may be a cause.
   B. Queens with follicular phase ovaries and basal (low) serum progesterone concentrations have also been diagnosed with CEH/pyometra (Lawler et al., 1991).
VII. Intrauterine foreign material (e.g., nonabsorbable sutures) or obstruction to drainage through the cervix may lead to mucometra.

Classification

I. Although the Dow classification of pyometra requires uterine biopsy and is therefore not very useful clinically, it does explain the progression of disease (Dow, 1957).
II. Stages of disease are as follows.
   A. Dow type I pyometra: uncomplicated cystic endometrial hyperplasia with no clinical signs of disease
   B. Dow type II pyometra
      1. Thickened endometrium with cystic, irregular elevations, mucus within the uterine lumen, and a diffuse chronic inflammatory infiltrate consisting of lymphocytes and plasma cells
      2. Mucoid vaginal discharge or infertility
   C. Dow type III pyometra

1. Cystic endometrial hyperplasia is present with a superimposed acute endometritis.
2. The uterus is somewhat enlarged radiographically, and purulent vaginal discharge, anorexia, and depression are presenting clinical signs.
3. Bacteria can be cultured from the vulvar discharge.

D. Dow type IV pyometra
1. Chronic endometritis is so extensive that cystic endometrial hyperplasia is no longer evident.
2. Marked myometrial damage is present.
3. If the cervix is closed, the uterus enlarges and the wall becomes extremely friable.
4. Clinical signs are directly proportional to the degree of cervical patency; the dog with a closed cervix rapidly becomes toxic, and peripheral leukocyte counts of $\geq 70,000/\mu l$ are possible.

Clinical Signs

I. Clinical signs of uncomplicated CEH may be limited to infertility due to impaired implantation of fertilized ova.
II. Signs of pyometra are generally manifested in older animals, 4–10 weeks following estrus.
III. Open-cervix pyometra is characterized by a purulent or sanguinopurulent vaginal discharge.
    A. Some bitches have systemic signs, such as lethargy, pyrexia, depression, anorexia, polyuria, and polydipsia.
    B. Signs of chronic immune-complex deposition (i.e., immune-mediated polyarthritis) can occur but are uncommon.
    C. Other animals appear normal except for a vaginal discharge.
IV. With closed-cervix pyometra, vaginal discharge is not present.
    A. Abdominal enlargement may occur as a result of material in the uterus.
    B. These animals often become severely ill from toxemia, with vomiting, dehydration, and azotemia progressing to shock, collapse, and coma.

Diagnosis

I. History
    A. Aged bitch in diestrus
    B. Young bitch recently given a mismating drug
    C. Prior treatment with megestrol acetate or another progestin
    D. Pseudopregnant queen
II. Physical examination
    A. Purulent vulvar discharge
    B. Palpably enlarged, soft, doughy uterus
III. Hematologic findings
    A. Depending on cervical patency, the white blood cell (WBC) count may be mildly to markedly elevated.

B. A nonregenerative anemia (packed cell volume = 25–35%) may be present.
IV. Urinary tract parameters
    A. Azotemia and hyperphosphatemia may be marked, especially if the animal becomes dehydrated.
    B. Urine specific gravity is variable.
        1. Some animals with pyometra have impaired ability to concentrate urine from *E. coli* endotoxemia.
        2. Polyuria and polydipsia result, with worsening of dehydration.
    C. Pyuria and bacteriuria may be present and are difficult to differentiate from urinary tract infection because voided urine is likely to be contaminated with uterine discharge. Cystocentesis is not recommended because of the risk of rupturing the friable uterus.
V. Other laboratory tests
    A. In most cases, hyperproteinemia with elevation of the globulin fraction is found.
    B. Hypoalbuminemia may be present from reduced protein intake and protein loss into the uterus.
    C. Cytology of the vaginal discharge reveals degenerated neutrophils and a few macrophages, with or without bacteria.
VI. Diagnostic imaging
    A. Radiographically, pyometra is a fluid-dense tubular structure in the ventrocaudal abdomen. Uterine size is variable; a dog with an open-cervix pyometra may not have a radiographically enlarged uterus.
    B. Ultrasonography allows determination of the size of the uterus and the thickness of the uterine wall and confirms that the intrauterine material is of fluid density.
VII. Endoscopy
    A. With an open-cervix pyometra, vaginoscopy may be necessary to determine whether the vulvar discharge is from the uterus or from the vagina.
    B. With pyometra, the vaginal mucosa usually appears normal.
    C. While the cervix is visualized, the uterus may be palpated abdominally, and material for cytology or culture can often be expressed through the cervix.
VIII. Exploratory laparotomy
    A. May be necessary to confirm the diagnosis of stump pyometra
    B. Allows differentiation of mucometra from pyometra in cats

Differential Diagnosis

I. Pregnancy
II. Neoplasia of the uterus and of other caudal abdominal organs
III. Vaginitis
IV. Mucometra or hydrometra

Treatment

I. Treatment is planned based on the following.
    A. In a dog with a closed-cervix pyometra, toxicity

develops extremely rapidly, so immediate ovario-hysterectomy is generally the treatment of choice.

B. Medical treatment is generally reserved only for the bitch with an open-cervix pyometra, with few signs of systemic illness, or with a pyometra that develops after treatment for mismating.

C. If the animal's principal value is as a breeding animal, medical treatment may be considered even in animals with closed-cervix or advanced pyometras. However, the owner should be warned of the potential dangers of delaying definitive surgical treatment.

II. Adequate fluid therapy before, during, and after surgical therapy is a necessity.

III. Broad-spectrum antibiotics are administered before surgery and are continued for 7–10 days afterwards. Prior to receiving culture and sensitivity data, trimethoprim-sulfamethoxazole or enrofloxacin would be appropriate choices.

IV. If the owner wishes to attempt to salvage the dog for breeding, medical therapy with prostaglandin $F_{2\alpha}$ (PGF$_{2\alpha}$) may be attempted.

A. PGF$_{2\alpha}$ causes contraction of the myometrium and inhibits steroidogenesis by the corpora lutea, leading to expulsion of the uterine exudate and a decreased plasma progesterone concentration.

B. Factors to consider before beginning PGF$_{2\alpha}$ therapy include the following.
1. It is not recommended in animals older than 8 years, with concurrent geriatric diseases, or with preexisting uterine pathology.
2. It should not be the treatment of choice in animals that are critically ill, because it may take up to 48 hours before a therapeutic effect is seen.
3. If the uterus is friable or the cervix is closed, there is potential for rupture of the uterus or retrograde expulsion of the uterine exudate into the abdominal cavity.

C. Because synthetic prostaglandins are more potent than the natural product, their use may be fatal. Use only the natural product (Lutalyse)!
1. An effective protocol for the dog is 0.25 mg/kg SQ SID for 5–7 days, with concurrent bactericidal antibiotics (Feldman and Nelson, 1996).
   a) A lower dose (0.1 mg/kg on day 1; 0.2 mg/kg on day 2) may be given to encourage the bitch to acclimate to the drug.
   b) Treat to effect using ultrasonography to evaluate resolution of luminal fluid.
2. A dosage of 0.1 mg/kg SQ SID has been shown to be effective in the cat (Davidson et al., 1992).

D. Common side effects include restlessness, hypersalivation, vomiting, panting, defecation, abdominal cramping, tachycardia, and fever.
1. These effects begin within 5–60 minutes and last 20–30 minutes.
2. Cats often show vocalization and intense grooming.
3. Bronchospasm may occur in cats with feline bronchial asthma.

E. Overdosage may result in severe hemorrhagic shock in the dog.

F. Clinical evidence that prostaglandins are producing the desired effects is as follows.
1. Resolution of systemic signs
2. Change of sanguineous or purulent vulvar discharge to serous discharge
3. Decrease in uterine diameter
4. Return of normal leukogram

G. Efficacy in *selected* animals with open-cervix pyometra is good.
1. Many dogs and cats have complete resolution of their uterine infection, but some animals require two courses of treatment (Feldman and Nelson, 1996).
2. Many PGF$_{2\alpha}$-treated bitches and queens subsequently whelp healthy litters.

H. Efficacy in closed-cervix pyometra is not as good and has greater risks than surgery.
1. In one study, only 34% of bitches had resolution of their uterine infection, but 100% of those who responded whelped healthy litters later (Feldman and Nelson, 1996).
2. Peritonitis may occur from retrograde flow of exudate into the abdominal cavity.
3. There is also an increased possibility of uterine rupture with the strong contractions induced by prostaglandins.

V. As long as the cervix is open, cranial vaginal infusions of soluble antibiotics may aid in controlling the pathogenic bacteria. Any attempt to cannulate a closed cervix in order to administer these solutions is generally futile, traumatic, and potentially dangerous because the infected uterus is friable.

Patient Monitoring

I. After successful treatment with PGF$_{2\alpha}$, the owner should be informed that clinical signs of pyometra may recur after subsequent periods of estrus.

II. Because future reproductive potential of a bitch successfully treated for pyometra is likely to be limited, the bitch should be bred during her next estrus.

III. A urine sample obtained by cystocentesis is cultured 3 weeks after treatment of the uterine infection to be sure that any concurrent cystitis has been effectively cured.

IV. In bitches treated surgically, the leukocyte count often increases dramatically for a few days after removal of the uterus.

UTERINE TORSION

Definition

I. Uterine torsion is a twisting of one of the uterine horns or the entire uterus perpendicular to its long axis.

II. It occurs rarely in the dog but more commonly in the cat.

III. Torsion can involve only a part of a horn containing one or more fetuses, which are generally found to be dead.
IV. Torsions of 180°–1080° have been described (Shull et al., 1978).

Causes

I. Because a heavy, pendulous uterus suspended by only the ovarian pedicle and broad ligament is more likely to undergo torsion, uterine torsion usually occurs in animals that are pregnant and near parturition.
II. Because tearing or stretching of the broad ligament of the uterus may occur with multiple pregnancies or large litters, multiparous animals are at higher risk.
III. Excessive fetal weight or movement may also contribute.
IV. Other uterine pathologic conditions causing increased uterine weight, such as uterine tumors and pyo-, muco-, or hematometra, may also predispose to torsion.

Clinical Signs

I. A history of prolonged unproductive labor is common.
II. Because uterine torsion may involve only one horn, there may be normal delivery of some offspring 24–48 hours earlier.
III. Torsions of 180° may persist for days or weeks without clinical signs until labor ensues.
IV. Other signs include anorexia, depression, lethargy, vomiting, and bloody or mucoid vulvar discharge.
V. A palpable caudal abdominal mass may be found on physical examination.
VI. The abdomen may be distended with serosanguineous fluid if uterine rupture with effusion has occurred.
VII. Fatal hemorrhage with shock occurs if the uterine artery ruptures.

Diagnosis

I. Abdominal radiography reveals an enlarged fluid-filled uterus or calcified fetal skeletons if the animal is near term. If fetal death has occurred in a horn that has undergone torsion, radiographic signs of fetal death are noted, such as fetal and intrauterine gas formation, collapse of the cranial bones, and decomposition.
II. Ultrasound examination of the abdomen may confirm the presence of hyperechoic material in the uterus, and helps determine whether remaining fetuses are dead or alive.
III. Definitive diagnosis of uterine torsion is possible only by exploratory surgery.

Differential Diagnosis

I. Pregnancy with dystocia
II. Pyo-, muco-, or hematometra

III. Uterine neoplasia or neoplasia of other caudal abdominal organs, such as the bladder

Treatment and Monitoring

I. Start supportive therapy, including treatment for shock or hemorrhage.
II. Ovariohysterectomy is generally recommended. With partial torsion, removal of only the affected horn is possible if the animal is valuable for breeding.
III. Although uterine torsion is not generally complicated by bacterial infection, pre- and postoperative antibiotics are indicated if fetal death, purulent discharge, or fever is noted.

UTERINE PROLAPSE

Definition

I. Uterine prolapse is the protrusion of the uterine body and/or one or both uterine horns through the cervix.
II. It is a rare condition but occurs more commonly in the queen than the bitch.
III. Prolapse of the uterus generally occurs during or after parturition or abortion, when the cervix is dilated.

Causes

I. Excessive traction on retained fetal membranes or forced fetal extraction
II. Excessive straining by the bitch or queen due to metritis or a retained placenta
III. Idiopathic causes following apparently normal parturition, especially in the cat

Clinical Signs

I. Partial prolapse of the uterus into the vagina: vaginal discharge, abdominal pain, straining, restlessness, or abnormal posture without an obvious external uterine mass
II. Mass protruding from the vulva in the postpartum or postabortion period
   A. Depending on the size and duration of the prolapse, the tissue may be ischemic or necrotic.
   B. Mutilation of ischemic or necrotic tissue by the animal is likely.
III. Hemorrhagic shock from rupture of an ovarian or uterine artery

Diagnosis

I. Complete prolapse of both horns can be determined visually during physical examination.
II. A partial prolapse into the vagina requires digital evaluation and/or vaginoscopic examination.

Differential Diagnosis

I. Vaginal prolapse: occurs during estrus rather than during the postpartum period

II. Neoplasia: transmissible venereal tumor, vaginal squamous cell carcinoma, vaginal leiomyoma

Treatment

I. Ovariohysterectomy is recommended if the animal's future reproductive capability is not important or if the prolapsed tissue is damaged and necrotic.
II. Epidural or general anesthesia is required before the uterine prolapse can be replaced.
III. Clean the prolapsed tissue with an antiseptic solution and débride or suture necrotic and lacerated areas.
IV. With partial prolapse, the perineum is elevated and digital pressure is applied to the prolapsed uterus.
V. Insert a sterile test tube or syringe case into the uterine horn or infuse a sterile solution under pressure to assist in completely reducing the prolapse. An episiotomy incision may allow for easier placement of the syringe case into the vagina.
VI. If external reduction is impossible, consider an exploratory laparotomy with internal reduction. Hysteropexy is not generally required, as the prolapse is not reported to recur.
VII. If the prolapsed tissue is damaged or necrotic, amputation of the uterine horn or an ovariohysterectomy may be required.

Patient Monitoring

I. Systemic antibiotics are administered both pre- and postoperatively.
II. After replacement of the prolapse, 5–10 units of oxytocin are given to assist in uterine involution.
III. Within 24 hours, the cervix should have closed tightly enough to prevent recurrence.
IV. Pregnancy and parturition have been reported following correction of uterine prolapse in the cat (Wallace et al., 1970), but the prognosis for future pregnancy in the dog is questionable.

NEOPLASIA

Definition

I. Lesions that mimic neoplasia
A. Hyperplastic endometrial polyps are pedunculated growths that project into the uterine lumen, appearing to arise from focal areas of cystic endometrial hyperplasia. They occur in both the dog and cat and are not known to be preneoplastic.
B. Adenomyosis is diffuse hyperplasia of the endometrial glands in the uterus and has been noted in the cat and dog.
II. Neoplastic lesions
A. Uterine leiomyoma and leiomyosarcoma are tumors of the smooth muscle cells of the uterine myometrium.
1. They appear as firm, white to tan-colored masses of the uterine wall.
2. Leiomyoma is the most common tumor of the

uterus of the dog and has been rarely reported in the cat.
B. Endometrial adenocarcinoma is a tumor of the endometrial glands that is principally found in the dog or cat >8 years of age.
1. The neoplasm appears to be rare in the dog.
2. It is the most common feline uterine neoplasm.
3. Grossly, the uterus of an animal with adenocarcinoma is thickened and nodular, with firm white masses filling the lumen. Solid and cystic areas are often present.
4. Because the endometrium is usually disrupted when an adenocarcinoma is present, the mucosal surface of the tumor may have a hemorrhagic appearance.
5. Metastasis is common and has been reported to occur in the lungs, abdominal viscera, heart, regional and bronchial lymph nodes, adrenal and thyroid glands, and the brain (Baldwin et al., 1992).
C. Chorionepithelioma is a very rare tumor of both the dog and the cat.
1. It arises from the placenta in the pregnant animal; neoplastic chorionic epithelial tumor cells invade the muscle and blood vessels of the uterus.
2. It is possible that subinvolution of the placental sites was misdiagnosed as chorionepithelioma in some older reports in the veterinary literature.
D. Hydatidiform mole is a rare proliferation of trophoblasts within the uterus that has been reported in both the dog and cat.
1. It appears grossly as multiple cysts within the uterine lumen and resembles a bunch of grapes.
2. The cysts are lined by chorionic epithelium and are filled with serous fluid.
E. Other reported primary uterine tumors include adenoma, fibroma/fibrosarcoma, and lymphosarcoma. Lipomas have been described in the broad ligament of the dog.

Causes

I. In rabbits, rats, and humans, there is a proven relationship between endometrial hyperplasia and adenocarcinoma that appears to be mediated by estrogen.
II. Such a relationship has *not* been proved in the dog or cat, however.

Clinical Signs and Diagnosis

I. A mass may be palpable in the caudal abdomen of an intact bitch or queen.
A. Uterine neoplasia may also occur in remnants of uterine tissue near the cervix of the neutered female.
B. A large mass may cause signs of stranguria and tenesmus (Baldwin et al., 1992).
II. A neoplasm located near the cervix may cause sec-

ondary mucometra or pyometra due to uterine obstruction.

III. A large intrauterine tumor may cause infertility, although it is not uncommon to find pregnancy coexisting with a benign uterine tumor. Alternatively, the tumor may produce a maternal obstructive dystocia in a whelping animal.

IV. Uterine tumors (especially leiomyomas and adenomas) are often clinically "silent" and may be found incidentally during ovariohysterectomy of an older bitch or queen.

V. With carcinoma, a vaginal discharge is commonly noted and may vary from purulent to mucoid to darkly hemorrhagic.

VI. Plain radiography is often inconclusive except to verify the presence of a caudal abdominal mass.

VII. Ultrasonography can be used to localize the abdominal mass to the uterus, to define the thickness of the uterine wall, and to rule out pyometra or pregnancy.

VIII. Surgical intervention with gross and histologic examination of the uterus is usually required for a definitive diagnosis.

IX. An animal with diffuse metastasis may present with a wide spectrum of clinical signs depending on the organs involved.

Differential Diagnosis

I. Vulvar discharge associated with uterine neoplasia must be differentiated from that associated with endometritis, subinvolution of the placental sites, uterine torsion, and vaginitis.

II. Rule out other causes of uterine enlargement, including subinvolution of the placental sites, pyometra, mucometra, and normal pregnancy.

Treatment

I. If no obvious metastases are present, complete ovariohysterectomy is the treatment of choice. For determining prognosis with endometrial adenocarci-

noma, biopsies of the sublumbar lymph nodes may be taken at the same time.

II. With no evidence of metastasis, ovariohysterectomy is potentially curative in some cases.

III. There are currently no reports in the veterinary literature assessing the efficacy of radiation therapy or chemotherapy for uterine tumors.

Patient Monitoring

I. After ovariohysterectomy for a malignant tumor, abdominal and thoracic radiography is repeated at 3–6 month intervals to check for metastasis.

II. Endometrial adenocarcinoma commonly spreads to the iliac and sublumbar lymph nodes, and lymphadenopathy may be visible on abdominal radiography.

A. The tumor may also locally extend to the ovary, broad ligament, and vagina.

B. Metastasis has also been reported to the lung, liver, kidneys, diaphragm, cerebrum, eyes, and adrenal gland.

III. Leiomyosarcoma apparently metastasizes late and most commonly to the lungs.

Bibliography

Baldwin CJ, Roszel JF, Clark TP: Uterine adenocarcinoma in dogs. Compend Contin Educ Pract Vet 14:731, 1992

Davidson AP, Feldman ED, Nelson RW: Treatment of feline pyometra in cats, using prostaglandin F2 alpha: 21 cases (1982–1990). J Am Vet Med Assoc 200:825, 1992

Dow C: The cystic hyperplasia-pyometra complex in the bitch. Vet Rec 69:1409, 1957

Feldman EC, Nelson RW: Canine and Feline Endocrinology and Reproduction. 2nd Ed. WB Saunders, Philadelphia, 1996

Lawler DF, Evans RH, Reimers TJ et al: Histopathologic features, environmental factors, and serum estrogen, progesterone, and prolactin values associated with ovarian phase and inflammatory uterine disease in cats. Am J Vet Res 52:1747, 1991

Shull RM, Johnston SD, Johnston GR et al: Bilateral torsion of uterine horns in a nongravid bitch. J Am Vet Med Assoc 172:601, 1978

Wallace LJ, Henry JD, Clifford JH: Manual reduction of uterine prolapse in a domestic cat. VM/SAC 65:595, 1970

57

Disorders of the Canine Vagina

Peggy M. Wykes
Susan F. Soderberg

CONGENITAL AND DEVELOPMENTAL DISORDERS

Peggy M. Wykes

Intersex Disorders

See Chap. 58.

Congenital Anomalies

Definition and Causes

I. Types of developmental vaginal defects identified (Wykes and Soderberg, 1983)
   A. Hymen membrane remnants located at vaginovestibular junction
      1. Bisecting vertical bands or septa
      2. Annular fibrous strictures
   B. Hypoplasia of the vaginal body or the vaginovestibular junction
   C. Elongated vertical septa bisecting the vagina and sometimes forming a double vagina
II. Causes and heritability: unknown

Pathophysiology

I. Normal embryologic development is as follows (Wykes and Soderberg, 1983).
   A. The paired paramesonephric ducts (mesonephric ducts) form the uterine horns and join caudally to form the body of the uterus, cervix, and vagina.
   B. The vestibule, urethra, and urinary bladder develop from the urogenital sinus.
   C. The hymen forms after fusion of the caudal portion of the paramesonephric ducts with the urogenital sinus and normally disappears by birth.
II. Anomalies result from either developmental inhibition of portions of the paramesonephric ducts or alterations in the pattern of their fusion to each other or to the urogenital sinus.
   A. Stenosis results from incomplete perforation of the hymenal membrane or hypoplasia of the genital canal at the vaginovestibular junction during development.
   B. Incomplete fusion of the two paramesonephric ducts and retention of part of the medial wall(s) result in a residual vertical vaginal band at the vaginovestibular margin, or a double vagina, with one portion usually ending as a blind pouch.
   C. Segmental aplasia from incomplete development of the caudal sections of the paramesonephric ducts clinically presents with compartmentalization of the vagina.
   D. Abnormal joining of the genital folds and genital swelling cause a stricture in the region of the vestibulovulvar junction, at the level of the vulvar labia.

Clinical Signs

I. Segmental aplasia or hypoplasia
   A. Can be seen anywhere along the length of the vagina
   B. Results in difficult breeding (dyspareunia) and/or dystocia, from reduced luminal diameter of the vagina
   C. Retention of uterine fluids during estrus in cases of complete vaginal aplasia resulting in signs similar to pyometra
II. Incomplete perforation of the hymen
   A. Pain during copulation: male refuses further advances
   B. Prevention of normal "tie" during breeding
   C. Urine pooling and retention of vaginal fluids in the vagina
      1. Secondary vaginitis with excessive licking at the vulva may occur.

601

2. A positional urinary incontinence may be observed clinically.
   D. Dystocia
   E. Normal estrous cycles and normal mating behavior
III. Vulvar stenosis
   A. Most commonly seen at the cranial boundary of the vulva
   B. May be more prevalent in collies and shelties
   C. Presents because of dyspareunia

Diagnosis

I. Signalment, history, and clinical signs as described are suggestive.
II. Visual inspection of the caudal reproductive tract is performed.
   A. Examine vulvar conformation for size and positioning.
   B. Vulvar mucosa and clitoris are examined for presence of inflammation, discharge, os penis (suggestive of intersex disorder), or clitoritis.
III. Digital vaginal examination is the best method for diagnosing abnormalities at the vaginovestibular and vulvar region, because a scope may inadvertently bypass the defect.
   A. Vaginal bands, elongated septa, or double vagina is considered when a small opening is palpated on either side of a central partition, just cranial to the urethral tubercle.
   B. Annular strictures and/or hypoplastic defects have a single small opening that prevents normal digital penetration of the ostium vaginum.
IV. Examination of the vestibule and caudal vagina can be performed with an otoscope or vaginal speculum.
V. A proctoscope or fiberoptic endoscope is necessary to examine the cranial vagina and cervical os.
   A. Adequate visualization may require insufflation of the vagina with air because the mucosal folds tend to collapse around the scope.
   B. The vaginal mucosa is normally smooth and pink but appears more thickened and edematous during estrus.
VI. A positive contrast vaginogram may demonstrate the location and expandability of a vaginal or vaginovestibular stricture, confirm the presence of a double vagina or vaginal mass, and outline any urethral or pelvic masses impinging on the vagina.
VII. Vaginal cultures obtained from the cranial vagina with a guarded swab, for isolation of aerobic and anaerobic bacteria, mycoplasma, and ureaplasma, are suggested if secondary vaginitis is evident.

Differential Diagnosis

I. Complete vaginal segmental aplasia must be differentiated from closed pyometra via radiography or ultrasonography.
II. Normal contraction of the vestibularis muscle during vaginal palpation may falsely suggest a stenosis at the vaginovestibular junction.
   A. Sedation may be necessary to relax the vestibularis muscle.
   B. A stenosis detected during anestrus may not be significant when the dog is examined during estrus because the tissues are relaxed owing to hormonal influences.
III. Rule out vaginitis or vestibulitis from other causes.
   A. Vaginal/vestibular foreign body
   B. Bacterial, immunologic, or allergic condition
   C. Primary cystitis resulting in secondary vestibulitis
IV. An annular fibrous stricture of the vaginovestibular junction must be differentiated from hypoplasia of the genital canal at the vaginal entrance, which also has a reduced lumen but lacks the fibrous ring that occurs with hymenal remnants.

Treatment

I. Congenital abnormalities of the vagina are frequently observed, but few are actually associated with clinical disease.
II. No treatment is necessary for nonbreeding, asymptomatic female dogs with partial obstructions.
III. Surgery is indicated if the anomaly will interfere with breeding and parturition, or if urogenital signs persist despite proper medical therapy.
   A. Vulvar stenosis: permanent episiotomy
   B. Annular strictures and hypoplasia at the vaginovestibular junction
      1. Respond poorly to bougienage alone because of subsequent cicatrix and stricture formation.
      2. Cicatrix formation is minimized if rotational mucosal flaps are used to cover mucosal defects after surgically enlarging the vaginal opening.
   C. Small thin vertical bands: visualized with speculum and digitally resected
   D. Large thick vaginal septum that resists digital breakdown
      1. Perform an episiotomy to assist visualization.
      2. Remove the band and oversew the origin and insertion.
   E. Caudal and midvaginal strictures in breeding bitches: resected followed by anastomosis of the vaginal segments (Wykes and Olson, 1985)
IV. Vaginectomy is indicated for cranial vaginal strictures, if urine pooling persists, or when surgical removal of the occlusive tissue at the vaginovestibular junction is unsuccessful.

Patient Monitoring

I. Animals may possess both types of imperforate hymen (annular stricture and vertical bands), so the diameter of the vaginal opening should be carefully evaluated at the time of septum removal.
II. Short vertical bands may "flatten" the vaginal opening to suggest a concurrent stricture, but the vaginal opening expands normally after band excision.
III. Prognosis is guarded after removal of severe annular strictures but excellent after band removal.

ACQUIRED VAGINAL DISEASES

Vaginal Edema
Peggy M. Wykes

Definition

I. Excessive vaginal tissue that develops during estrogenic stimulation (Johnson, 1989)
II. Formerly called vaginal hyperplasia or hypertrophy
III. Marked edema on histologic examination

Causes

I. It occurs during proestrus or estrus and is thought to be an exaggerated vaginal response to the presence of estradiol.
II. Some breeds of dogs are considered to be predisposed, but the condition is not proved to be hereditary.

Pathophysiology

I. Affected tissue arises initially from the floor of the vagina, just cranial to the urethral tubercle.
II. With time, increasing amounts of vaginal tissue become enlarged and everted.
  A. Type I
    1. There is slight to moderate eversion of the vaginal floor.
    2. No vaginal mucosa protrudes through the vulvar cleft, but the perineum may bulge.
  B. Type II: Prolapsing vaginal tissue protrudes through the vulvar cleft.
  C. Type III
    1. Vaginal prolapse is a donut-shaped eversion of the entire circumference of the vaginal wall, including the urethral orifice, which is visualized on the ventral aspect of the prolapsed tissue.
    2. With a partial vaginal prolapse, the cervix is not visible.
    3. With a complete prolapse, the cervix is exteriorized.

Clinical Signs

I. Signalment
  A. Age: occurs primarily in young bitches
  B. Breed: boxers, English bulldogs, mastiffs, German shepherd dogs, St. Bernards, Labrador and Chesapeake Bay retrievers, Airedale terriers, and Weimaraners
II. Clinical presentation
  A. Presence of a protruding mass from the vulvar cleft in an otherwise clinically asymptomatic animal
  B. Failure to mate normally
  C. Excessive licking of the vulvar area and bulging of the perineum
  D. Dysuria, stranguria
  E. Edematous tissue protruding before parturition

Diagnosis

I. Signalment, history, and a compatible stage in the estrous cycle are suggestive.
II. A pedunculated vaginal mass is detected by digital or vaginoscopic examination and found to originate just cranial to the urethral tubercle.
III. The hemogram, chemistry profile, and plasma hormone concentrations are usually normal.

Differential Diagnosis

I. Benign (inflammatory) vaginal polyps
II. Vaginal tumors: fibromas, leiomyomas, leiomyosarcomas

Treatment

I. Edematous tissue typically resolves spontaneously at the end of estrus.
  A. Keep exposed mucosa clean and moist with saline or topical antibiotic ointments.
  B. Prevent self-trauma with use of an Elizabethan collar.
  C. Consider placing temporary retention sutures in the vulva for 7–10 days to protect the mucosa.
  D. Ensure normal urination; place an indwelling catheter only if necessary.
II. The duration of estrogenic stimulation can be reduced by inducing ovulation.
  A. Ovulation can be induced during the follicular phase of the estrous cycle with a single dose of gonadotropin-releasing hormone (50 μg GnRH IV) or human chorionic gonadotropin (1000 U IM).
  B. These medications will not alter the course of the vaginal edema if they are given after the bitch has already ovulated.
III. Ovariohysterectomy is recommended as the primary treatment for bitches not intended for breeding.
  A. It will prevent recurrence.
  B. Recurrence rate is 66% without ovariohysterectomy.
IV. Indications to surgically resect prolapsed tissue include the following.
  A. With long-standing vaginal edema/prolapse, fibrous tissue may prevent resolution of the mass.
  B. The prolapsed tissue is devitalized or traumatized.
  C. Normal urination is prevented.
  D. The patient becomes systemically ill.

Vaginitis
Susan F. Soderberg

Definition

I. Vaginitis is an inflammation of the vaginal mucosa.
II. It frequently arises from a noninfectious cause, followed by overgrowth of resident microorganisms.

Causes and Pathophysiology

I. Bacterial infections are as follows.
- A. The normal vaginal flora contains a mixed population with a predominance of aerobic organisms.
- B. An overgrowth of normal organisms is generally identified with vaginitis.
  1. *Escherichia coli*
  2. *Staphylococcus* spp.
  3. *Streptococcus* spp.
  4. *Proteus* spp.
  5. *Pasteurella* spp.
  6. *Corynebacterium* spp.
- C. *Brucella canis*, although an uncommon cause, should also be considered.

II. *Mycoplasma* and *Ureaplasma* spp. have been identified both as normal flora and as causes of vaginitis.

III. Herpesvirus infection can cause chronic, intermittent inflammation.

IV. Predisposing factors may allow normal vaginal flora to proliferate.
- A. These factors cause chronic irritation to the vaginal mucosa or allow pooling of fluid in the vaginal vault.
- B. Potential predisposing factors include the following.
  1. Abnormal conformation of the vulva, vestibule, or vagina
     - a) Small vulva in a perivulvar fat roll causing perivulvar dermatitis
     - b) Vestibulovulvar strictures or septae
     - c) Compartmentalization of the vagina from segmental aplasia
     - d) Blind pouch or double vagina from incomplete fusion of two paramesonephric ducts
  2. Clitoral hypertrophy
     - a) Androgenic stimulation
     - b) Chronic inflammation
  3. Foreign bodies
  4. Vaginal tumors
  5. Vaginal immaturity (juvenile vaginitis)
     - a) Under 6 months of age
     - b) Resolves as puppy ages
     - c) If clinical signs other than vaginal discharge (discomfort, pain, licking), further evaluation indicated
  6. Urine pooling from abnormalities of the urethra or ureters (ectopia)

V. Urinary tract infections (UTIs) may cause or occur as the result of vaginitis.

Clinical Signs

I. Signs may develop in prepuberal, spayed, or intact females.

II. Vaginal licking or scooting is the most common sign, often accompanied by a mucoid or purulent discharge.

III. Discomfort after urination may be observed and may be associated with cystitis.

IV. Male dogs may show sexual interest in a spayed, anestrus, or juvenile female.

V. Systemic signs of illness are not usually present.

Diagnosis

I. Physical examination
- A. Evaluate the vulva, clitoris, and vaginal mucosa visually with a proctoscope, endoscope, or, in small breeds, otoscope.
  1. The mucosa of the vestibule is consistently congested and hyperemic.
  2. Erosions, ulcerations, and vesicles should be identified when present.
  3. Nodular lymphoid hyperplasia may be observed in the mucosa of the vulva, vestibule, or caudal vagina.
- B. Digitally examine the vaginal vault.

II. Laboratory evaluation
- A. Vaginal cytology
  1. Large numbers of neutrophils: healthy to degenerative
  2. Bacteria, possibly engulfed by the neutrophils
  3. Macrophages and lymphocytes: chronic vaginitis
  4. Intracytoplasmic inclusions: *Mycoplasma, Ureaplasma, Chlamydia*
- B. Bacterial culture of the vaginal vault
  1. Caudal vaginal cultures are difficult to interpret because of contamination and greater concentrations of normal bacterial flora.
  2. A guarded culture swab is preferred to obtain culture samples from the cranial vagina but may also be difficult to interpret because of overgrowth of normal flora.
  3. Isolation of *Mycoplasma* and *Ureaplasma* requires specialized media and laboratories.
- C. Urinalysis and culture are performed on samples collected by antepubic cystocentesis to rule out UTI.
- D. Hemogram and serum biochemistries are usually normal.
- E. Obtain titers for *B. canis* and herpesvirus.
- F. Obtain a biopsy of the vaginal mucosa to evaluate for the following.
  1. Lymphoplasmacytic infiltration
  2. Erosive ulceration
  3. Neoplasia

III. Radiography
- A. Abdominal radiographs and ultrasonography are normal.
- B. Positive-contrast vaginography can be used to rule out tumors or congenital anomalies not detected by physical examination.

Differential Diagnosis

I. Open-cervix pyometra (see also Chap. 56)
- A. History of estrus within the last 10 weeks
- B. Clinical signs of illness

C. Uterine enlargement detected on physical examination or abdominal radiography or ultrasonography
D. Systemic leukocytosis
II. Metritis (see also Chap. 56)
  A. History of whelping
  B. Clinical signs of illness
  C. Uterine discharge passing through cervix into vagina
III. Increased levels of androgens from endogenous or exogenous sources
IV. Congenital anomalies of the vagina
V. Foreign body within the vagina
VI. Vaginal neoplasia or hyperplasia

Treatment

I. Correct predisposing factors if possible.
II. Prepuberal vaginitis usually resolves with the first estrus or with ovariohysterectomy.
III. Eradicate infections.
  A. Systemic antibiotics
    1. Antibiotic selection is based on sensitivity results.
    2. If a culture cannot be performed, select an antibiotic effective against *E. coli*.
    3. Tetracycline, chloramphenicol, and enrofloxacin are the most effective agents against *Mycoplasma* or *Ureaplasma*.
    4. Administer for 14 days and at least 1 week beyond resolution of the vaginal discharge.
  B. Vaginal douches may be used as adjunct therapy BID until discharge resolves but should be discontinued 1 week prior to breeding because they may decrease fertility.
    1. Chlorhexidine 0.05% solution
    2. Povidone-iodine 0.5% solution
    3. Nitrofurazone 0.2% solution

Patient Monitoring

I. If clinical signs persist despite appropriate therapy or recur after therapy is discontinued, reevaluation is necessary.
II. Pursue additional diagnostic tests as outlined earlier to identify predisposing factors.
III. Reculture the anterior vaginal vault and urine to determine if bacteria present are resistant to previously administered antibiotics.
IV. Rule out infection in the uterus, e.g., pyometra (see Chap. 56).
V. Biopsy affected vaginal mucosa for histologic examination.

VAGINAL NEOPLASIA

Peggy M. Wykes

Definition and Causes

I. Benign tumors are much more common than malignant tumors (Thacher and Bradley, 1983).
  A. Benign tumors: leiomyomas (most common), fibromas, polyps, lipomas
  B. Malignant tumors: leimyosarcoma, squamous cell carcinoma, mast cell, transmissible venereal tumors (TVTs)
II. Vaginal tumors occur most often in older intact females, suggesting hormonal influences.
III. Etiology is unknown for most tumors.

Pathophysiology

I. Tumors may develop anywhere in the wall of the vagina or vestibule.
II. Benign tumors tend to be more pedunculated than malignant masses.
III. Metastasis is uncommon but may occur with TVT, leiomyosarcoma, or carcinoma.
IV. TVTs develop by transplantation of tumor cells through intercourse as well as by hematogenous or lymphatic spread (see Chap. 58).

Clinical Signs

I. Bulging of the perineal region or prolapse of tissue from the vulva
II. Dysuria and pollakiuria
III. Serosanguineous or bloody vaginal discharge
IV. Tenesmus, constipation
V. Difficulty mating

Diagnosis

I. Signalment, history, and clinical signs as described
II. Detection of a vaginal mass
  A. Vaginal and rectal palpation
  B. Vaginoscopy
  C. Positive contrast vaginogram
III. Exfoliative cytology and histopathology for definitive diagnosis
IV. Thoracic and abdominal radiographs to detect metastasis

Differential Diagnosis

I. Primary vaginitis/vestibulitis
II. Vaginal trauma: lacerations
III. Tumors originating from the distal urethra: squamous cell, transitional cell carcinoma
IV. Vaginal edema and prolapse, which occur in the young bitch during estrus

Treatment

I. The treatment of choice for most vaginal tumors (other than TVT) is surgical removal if no metastasis is noted.
  A. The need for an episiotomy depends on the tumor size and location within the vagina.
  B. An ovariohysterectomy is performed to eliminate hormonal influences.
II. Successful treatment of metastatic disease is difficult, and prognosis is poor.

III. TVT may be treated with surgery and chemotherapy (see Chap. 58).

Patient Monitoring

I. Periodic physical examination and thoracic radiographs are suggested at 1, 3, and 6 months after completion of treatment.

II. Prognosis is poor for malignant tumors, excellent for benign tumors and TVT.

Bibliography

Johnson SD: Vaginal prolapse. p. 1302. In Kirk RW (ed): Current Veterinary Therapy X: Small Animal Practice. WB Saunders, Philadelphia, 1989

Thacher C, Bradley RL: Vulvar and vaginal tumors in the dog: a retrospective study. J Am Vet Med Assoc 183:690, 1983

Wykes PM, Olson PO: The vagina. p. 1672. In Slatter DH (ed): Textbook of Small Animal Surgery. WB Saunders, Philadelphia, 1985

Wykes PM, Soderberg SF: Congenital abnormalities of the canine vagina and vulva. J Am Anim Hosp Assoc 19:995, 1983

58

Diseases of the External Genitalia

Jean-Pierre Held
Philip E. Prater

CONGENITAL DISORDERS

Intersex Disorders

Definition

I. An abnormal sexual phenotype can result from a defect in any step in the sequence of sexual development (Fig. 58–1).
II. Intersexuality, a condition in which the sex of the animal is ambiguous, can occur whenever any part of this complex sequence of events is disturbed.
   A. A hermaphrodite is an animal with gonads of both sexes represented either as one testis and one ovary or as ovotestes. The external genitalia are generally female in appearance.
   B. A pseudohermaphrodite is an animal with the gonads of one sex and external genitalia resembling those of the opposite sex or appearing ambiguous.
      1. Male pseudohermaphroditism: Gonads are histologically testicles.
      2. Female pseudohermaphroditism: Gonads are histologically ovaries.
III. Breeds with high reported incidence of intersex organs include the cocker spaniel, miniature schnauzer, pug, Kerry blue terrier, beagle, German shepherd dog, Alsatian blue terrier, German shorthaired pointer.

Causes and Pathophysiology

I. True hermaphroditism
   A. True hermaphrodite chimeras have XX/XY or XX/XXY chromosome combinations.
      1. The external appearance is that of female except for an enlarged clitoris. The presence of an os clitoris has been described.
      2. Internally, testicular and ovarian tissue is present in all cases.
   B. True hermaphrodites have an XX chromosome complement with the external appearance of females, often with an enlarged clitoris containing an os clitoris.
      1. Gonadal tissue usually consists of an ovotestis.
      2. Studies in American cocker spaniels and beagles show the trait to be inherited (Sommer and Meyers-Wallen, 1991).
   C. The XX male syndrome is a predominantly male phenotype with XX chromosome complement. These dogs are positive for the H-Y antigen.
      1. There are often bilateral varying degrees of masculinization of the external genitalia.
      2. Abnormal curvature and hypoplasia of the penis are common.
      3. It is reported in cocker spaniels, pugs, and Kerry blue terriers.
II. Male pseudohermaphroditism
   A. Inadequate synthesis of fetal testosterone
   B. Androgenic receptor defect at target organ
   C. Ineffective response to müllerian inhibiting factor leading to the persistent müllerian duct syndrome described in miniature schnauzers
III. Female pseudohermaphroditism
   A. Most are induced by exposure to exogenous androgens in utero (Olson et al., 1989).
   B. Metabolic errors causing decreased cortisol production or administration of progestational compounds during pregnancy can also result in the masculinization of female fetuses.

Clinical Signs

I. True hermaphrodite: clitoral enlargement, os clitoris, rudimentary penis and prepuce, internal testicular and ovarian tissue
II. Male pseudohermaphrodite: varying degree of masculinization, penile hypoplasia

607

GENETIC SEX: <u>XX</u>

GONADAL SEX: | OVARY |

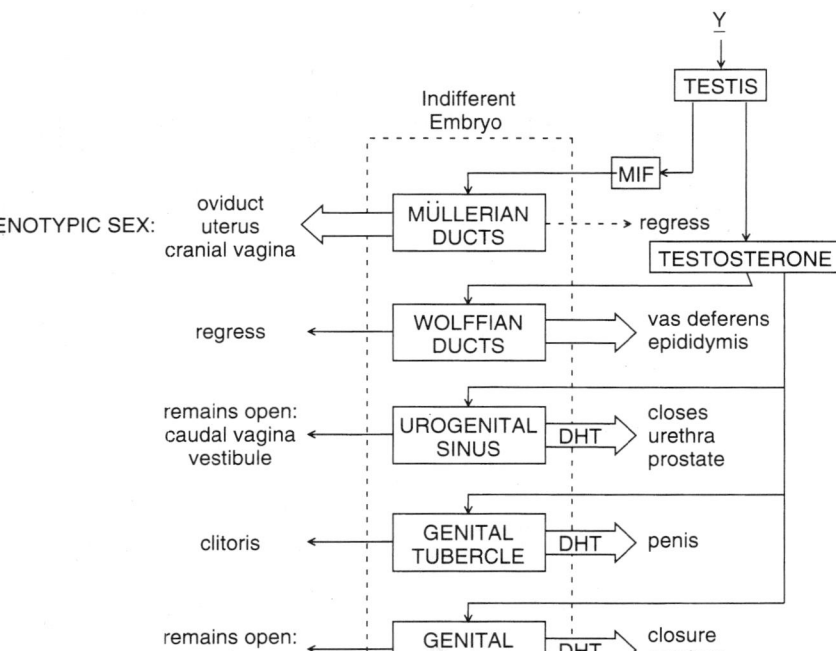

Figure 58–1. Differentiation of the internal and external genitalia after the gonad develops into a testicle or an ovary. MIF = müllerian inhibiting factor; DHT = dihydrotestosterone. (From Meyers-Wallen and Patterson, 1986, with permission.)

III. Female pseudohermaphrodite: varying degree of masculinization of female genitalia following exposure to exogenous androgens
IV. Other signs
  A. Cryptorchidism
  B. Infertility and/or irregular or absent estrous cycles due to segmental aplasia of the reproductive tract
  C. Hypospadias
  D. Penile hypoplasia
  E. Urinary incontinence, urethral abnormalities
  F. Cystic endometrial hyperplasia and pyometra

Diagnosis

  I. Thorough inspection of abnormal external genitalia
  II. Gross examination of gonads and secondary sex organs via laparotomy or laparoscopy
  III. Histologic examination of the gonads matched against karyotyping
  IV. History of administration of exogenous androgens or progestogens during pregnancy

Differential Diagnosis

  I. Abnormalities of chromosomal sex and phenotypic sex may have many of the same clinical signs.
  II. Differentiation among the numerous intersex syndromes can be made only through karyotype determination and/or histopathologic evaluation.

III. Other causes of infertility must also be ruled out.

Treatment

  I. Intersex disorders are compatible with a comfortable, functional life.
  II. Neutering is recommended to prevent reproductive tract disease such as pyometra or testicular tumors and to terminate any objectionable behavior.

Penile Hypoplasia

Definition

Penile hypoplasia is a congenital anomaly that is normally associated with the intersex condition of male pseudohermaphroditism (see also Intersex Disorders).

Causes and Pathophysiology

  I. Reported in 78-chromosome individuals with an XX karyotype
  II. Masculinization of a prenatal XX fetus by exogenous androgen administration

Clinical Signs

  I. May be asymptomatic
  II. Dysuria, hematuria
  III. Urinary incontinence, secondary to preputial urine pooling and infection

IV. May have bilateral cryptorchidism

Diagnosis

I. Thorough examination of external genitalia
II. Cytogenetic evaluation of the karyotype to differentiate from intersex disorders
III. Histopathology of gonadal tissue
IV. Serum H-Y antigen assay: not generally available at this time

Treatment

I. Treatment may not be necessary in the absence of clinical signs.
II. Surgical enlargement of the preputial orifice may prevent urine pooling and recurrent preputial infections in symptomatic dogs.

Hypospadias

Definition

Congenital anomaly of male external genitalia in which the urethral orifice opens on the ventral aspect of the penis or in the perineal area rather than at the tip of the penis (see also Intersex Disorders).

Causes

I. Induced by administration of exogenous progesterone or estrogens during pregnancy (Wensing, 1980)
II. Inadequate androgenic stimulation during fetal development

Clinical Signs

I. Mild deformity
   A. May be asymptomatic
   B. Abnormal location of urethral orifice on the cranial ventral penis
   C. Abnormal shape of preputial opening
   D. Infection and urine scalding of mucocutaneous surfaces
II. Severe deformity
   A. Urethral opening on the ventral midline in the perineal, scrotal, or caudal preputial area
   B. Urinary incontinence, urine scalding with adjacent mucocutaneous infection
   C. Other associated defects
      1. Cryptorchidism
      2. Incomplete scrotum and prepuce
      3. Persistent müllerian structures
      4. Unilateral renal agenesis (McFarland and Deniz, 1961)

Diagnosis

I. Thorough inspection of external genitalia
II. Catheterization of the urethra

Differential Diagnosis

Congenital hypospadias may be differentiated from traumatic urethral and preputial defects by the presence of associated preputial, scrotal, and perineal defects.

Treatment

I. Mild glandular hypospadias may be corrected by surgical reconstruction of the urethra.
II. Severe deformities require urethrostomy and castration with excision of the rudimentary penis, prepuce, and scrotum.

Persistent Penile Frenulum

Definition and Cause

I. Persistent penile frenulum is a congenital anomaly in which a thin sheet of fibrous connective tissue attaches the ventral aspect of the glans penis to the prepuce, resulting in ventral or lateral deviation of the penile tip (Johnston, 1986).
II. It is an uncommon condition but has been reported in several breeds.

Clinical Signs

I. Affected animals may be asymptomatic.
II. Discomfort can occur during urination or at erection.
III. The penis deviates ventrally during erection, resulting in inability to breed.
IV. Dermatitis may develop from urination onto the medial aspect of the hind legs.

Diagnosis

Diagnosis is made by thorough inspection of the penis.

Treatment and Monitoring

I. Surgically remove the frenulum.
II. After postoperative recovery, prognosis for natural copulation is good.

ACQUIRED DISORDERS

Urethral Prolapse

Definition

Prolapse of the urethra is an eversion of the urethral mucosa at the tip of the penis.

Causes

I. Trauma
II. Genitourinary tract infection with stranguria
III. Sexual excitement
IV. Primarily reported in the English bulldog and Boston terrier

Clinical Signs

I. Presence of a small, red, rounded tissue mass at the urethral opening
II. Hemorrhage from the everted urethral mucosa
III. Excessive licking of the penis and prepuce

Diagnosis

I. Observation of tissue mass at urethral opening
II. Observation of blood in urine or in prepuce

Differential Diagnosis

Other forms of urethral diseases such as calculi should be ruled out through both plain and contrast radiography.

Treatment

I. Treat any underlying cause such as cystitis.
II. Prolapse reduction is attempted only if the prolapsed tissue is not severely damaged.
   A. Reduction is accomplished by insertion of a urethral catheter and placement of a pursestring suture around the external urethral orifice.
   B. Remove suture in 5 days.
III. Amputation of prolapsed tissue may be needed (Sinibaldi and Green, 1973).
   A. A circular incision is made in the penile mucosa peripheral to the prolapsed tissue.
   B. To prevent retraction of the urethra, one half of the urethral mucosa is incised at a time and sutured to the penile mucosa.

Patient Monitoring

I. Administer antibiotics based on culture and sensitivity results for 5–7 days.
II. Prevent licking of the penis and self-mutilation with an Elizabethan collar.
III. Observe for urethral strictures postoperatively.

Paraphimosis

Definition

Paraphimosis is a condition in which the extruded penis cannot be withdrawn back into the preputial cavity.

Causes and Pathophysiology

I. Congenital or traumatic reduction in the size of the preputial opening, often aggravated by secondary inflammation (Elkins, 1984)
II. Laceration or malformation with enlargement of the preputial opening, causing chronic exposure of the tip of the penis
III. Strangulation of the penis by rubber bands, string, or hair
IV. Chronic balanoposthitis
V. Swelling of penile soft tissue from trauma or fracture of the os penis

Clinical Signs

I. Engorged penis protruding from the prepuce
II. Excessive licking of the exposed penis
III. Drying or necrosis of the exposed penis
IV. Stranguria, hematuria, and anuria

Diagnosis/Differential Diagnosis

I. Observation of a persistently exposed penis with an abnormally small or abnormally large preputial opening
II. Must be differentiated from priapism, which is sustained penile erection

Treatment

I. Treatment of exposed penis
   A. Cleanse edematous penile tissue.
   B. Reduce edema with cold soaks, massage, or application of hyperosmolar saline solutions.
   C. Penile amputation and perineal urethrostomy may be necessary if necrosis is severe.
II. Replacement of penis
   A. Lubricate exposed penis.
   B. Surgical enlargement of a small preputial opening may be performed.
      1. Make an incision along the dorsocranial aspect of preputial orifice, then suture the preputial mucosa to the skin edge along the margin of the incision.
      2. A ventrocranial approach to the preputial opening is not recommended because it may result in chronic exposure of the glans penis.
   C. Paraphimosis caused by an abnormally large preputial opening may be repaired by surgically narrowing the orifice.
III. Daily flushing of the prepuce with a dilute antiseptic solution combined with an antibiotic-steroid ointment is indicated to reduce accumulation of bacteria.
IV. If stranguria is apparent, insert a urethral catheter to evacuate the bladder.

Patient Monitoring

I. Adhesions may be prevented by daily extrusion of the penis for 5–7 days.
II. In cases of preputial alteration, reevaluation of the size of the preputial opening may be necessary.
III. Prevention of penile erection may be accomplished by the use of tranquilizers or castration.

Phimosis

Definition

Phimosis is a condition in which the preputial opening is too small to allow extrusion of the penis.

Causes

I. Trauma from lacerations or sucking of the prepuce by litter mates may reduce the size of the preputial opening.

II. Congenital preputial stenosis occurs in German shepherd dogs and golden retrievers.

Clinical Signs

I. If the preputial opening is large enough to allow urination, puppies may be asymptomatic.
II. Inability to protrude the penis and urine retention in the prepuce are noted.
III. Chronic balanoposthitis can develop and may result in septicemia in affected puppies.

Diagnosis

Diagnosis is made by observation of an anatomically small preputial opening.

Treatment and Monitoring

I. The preputial opening is surgically enlarged using a dorsocranial approach (see Paraphimosis).
II. Examine the preputial opening postoperatively to ensure adequate room for penile extrusion.

Priapism

Definition

Priapism is a persistent penile erection not associated with sexual excitement.

Causes and Pathophysiology

I. Injury or irritation of the innervation of the penis
II. Following amphetamine administration for narcolepsy (Johnston, 1986)
III. Thromboembolism of the cavernous venous supply at the base of the penis

Clinical Signs

I. Persistent erection
II. Variable tissue irritation depending on duration of penile exposure
III. Licking of the penis
IV. Neurologic signs associated with a nervous system injury

Diagnosis

Observation of persistent erection in the absence of sexual stimulation is definitive.

Differential Diagnosis

I. Priapism must be differentiated from paraphimosis.
II. The penis can be manually replaced in the prepuce with priapism, but manual replacement is usually not possible with paraphimosis.

Treatment

I. If possible, treat the underlying causes.
II. Spontaneous remission of priapism may occur.
III. Provide supportive care for persistent priapism.
   A. Keep the exposed penis clean and lubricated.
   B. Prevent licking and self-trauma.

Patient Monitoring

I. Neurogenic priapism may reverse, depending on the location and treatment of the neurologic injury.
II. Priapism from thromboembolism of the venous supply is usually permanent.

Balanoposthitis

Definition

Balanoposthitis is an inflammation of the penile and preputial mucosa.

Causes and Pathophysiology

I. It arises primarily from bacterial overgrowth of normal flora in the preputial mucosa, possibly following compromise of normal defense mechanisms.
II. Herpesvirus and blastomycosis infections have also been reported (Johnston, 1986).
III. Inflammation may also be secondary to trauma, foreign body, or penile lymphoid hyperplasia.

Clinical Signs

I. Many dogs are asymptomatic.
II. Purulent preputial discharge is found.
III. Irritation and licking of affected area occur.

Diagnosis

I. Diagnosis is based on gross appearance of the penis and prepuce.
II. Exfoliative cytology of the inflammatory lesions may reveal purulent exudate with degenerate neutrophils.
III. Penile lymphoid hyperplasia is definitively diagnosed by histopathology.
IV. Bacterial culture and sensitivity testing are advised for persistent or refractive lesions.

Differential Diagnosis

I. Urethritis
II. Early penile or preputial neoplasia, e.g., transmissible venereal tumor
III. Preputial trauma

Treatment

I. Perform daily preputial lavage with a 5% chlorhexidine solution in symptomatic dogs.
II. Apply an antibiotic ointment daily into the prepuce and administer systemic antimicrobials.

III. Give systemic antifungal agents for blastomycosis (see Chap. 109).
IV. Lymphoid hyperplasia requires more rigorous treatment.
   A. Scarification, cauterization of lymphoid papules with 5% silver nitrate solution
   B. Application of an antibiotic/corticosteroid ointment daily

Patient Monitoring

I. Extrude penis daily for 5–7 days to prevent adhesions.
II. Watch for recurrences once treatment has stopped.

Scrotal Dermatitis

Definition and Causes

I. Inflammation of scrotal epidermis/dermis
II. Can occur secondary to generalized dermatologic disease
   A. Pyoderma
   B. Flea-allergic dermatitis
III. Can occur as a primary disease
   A. Contact irritation from cleansers, insecticides, or fertilizers
   B. An allergic reaction to any substance
IV. May result in secondary orchitis/epididymitis
   A. May result in direct bacterial infiltration of testes/epididymides (uncommon)
   B. Can cause adhesions of testicular tunics to scrotum
V. May increase testicular temperature, resulting in decreased spermatogenesis

Clinical Signs

I. Ulcerated, crusted scrotal epidermis
II. Excessive grooming of scrotum
III. Other concurrent dermatologic signs
IV. Scrotal skin thickened if chronic

Diagnosis

I. Visual examination
II. Palpation for adhesions
III. Evaluation of underlying cause of dermatopathy (see Section XII)
IV. History of exposure to chemical irritants

Differential Diagnosis

I. Cutaneous neoplasia: mast cell tumor, squamous cell carcinoma
II. Trauma

Treatment

I. It is dependent on the underlying cause if part of a generalized dermatopathy.
II. Eliminate environmental exposure to chemical irritants or allergens.

III. Antibiotic and anti-inflammatory therapy is usually needed.
   A. Palliation of the irritation/infection can be achieved with topical antibiotic/corticosteroid ointment.
   B. Systemic antibiotic therapy with products directed against staphyloccocal organisms may be instituted.
   C. Short-term systemic corticosteroid therapy may be helpful.
IV. Prevent self-mutilation with an Elizabethan collar.

Patient Monitoring

I. Recurrent episodes can occur.
II. Associated infertility is usually transient, depending on the extent of adhesions or secondary orchitis/epididymitis.
III. Once lesions have resolved, allow 2–3 months for return to fertility (the time required to complete spermatogenesis).

NEOPLASIA

Transmissible Venereal Tumor

Definition

I. Transmissible venereal tumor (TVT) is a naturally occurring tumor of dogs that affects the external genitalia and other mucous membranes.
II. It has a worldwide distribution.
III. It has been documented in the literature for 150 years.
IV. Incidence is increased in areas with crowded canine populations and many unconfined, sexually active dogs.
V. Outbreaks are more common in temperate climates.

Cause

I. The TVT is a naturally occurring allograft.
   A. The cells are easily transplanted experimentally by subcutaneous injection.
   B. Exfoliated neoplastic cells are transmitted from tumor-bearing animals to new hosts during sexual or social contact.
   C. During natural transmission, neoplastic cells invade small abrasions of the mucosa.
II. The origin of the TVT cell is unknown. The tumor cells have a chromosome complement of 59 ± 5, which is distinctly different from the normal canine chromosome number of 78.

Pathophysiology

I. Biologic behavior
   A. The tumor characteristically grows rapidly during the first few weeks. Subsequent tumor growth is slower, and spontaneous regression may occur within 6 months.

B. Metastasis is uncommon, but the actual incidence of spread is unknown.
   1. Regional lymph nodes are the most common site.
   2. Other reported locations are brain, eye, testicle, and thoracic and abdominal viscera.
   3. Metastasis is most likely to occur in dogs that are unable to mount an immune response.
II. Immunology
   A. The immune system plays a significant role in tumor growth and metastasis.
   B. Humoral antibodies have been demonstrated in tumor-bearing dogs and are correlated with tumor regression.
      1. Antibodies persist after regression.
      2. Antibodies are of the immunoglobulin G (IgG) classification.
   C. A cellular immune response has also been demonstrated.
      1. A strong lymphoblastogenic response to TVT is demonstrated in dogs in which the TVT eventually regresses.
      2. A higher incidence of metastasis is seen in dogs with a weak lymphoblastogenic response.

Clinical Signs

I. Appearance
   A. The tumor is usually a lobulated, cauliflower-like, sessile mass; it is occasionally papillary or pedunculated.
   B. The exposed surface is friable and red early in the course of growth and pink or gray in later stages.
   C. Hemorrhage and necrosis are often present.
II. Location
   A. The most common sites are the external genitalia.
      1. Prepuce or penis
      2. Vulva, vestibule, or vagina
   B. It may also be located extragenitally, with or without genital involvement.
      1. Lips, oral cavity, nasal cavity
      2. Rarely in the integument, reportedly the result of transplantation of tumor cells to bite wounds
   C. Clinical signs associated with extragenital or metastatic tumors are related to the organs and sites involved.
III. Sometimes large tumors produce mechanical discomfort.
IV. Serosanguineous genital discharge and licking of the affected area are common.
V. Foul odor may be detected owing to tumor necrosis.

Diagnosis

I. The typical lobulated, cauliflower-like, bleeding mass is present.
II. Cytologic aspiration or impression smear is a reliable and inexpensive diagnostic tool.

A. Stain the sample with Diff-Quik or another hematology stain.
B. The smear is populated with large round to oval cells of relatively uniform size (Herron, 1988).
   1. Each cell has a large round nucleus and a prominent nucleolus.
   2. The cells have a moderate amount of cytoplasm containing vacuoles of varying numbers and sizes.
   3. Mitotic figures are common in some tumors.
III. Histopathology is helpful but may not differentiate the TVT from other tumors.
   A. Histiocytoma
   B. Lymphosarcoma
   C. Agranular (anaplastic) mast cell tumor
IV. Karyotyping is the most precise diagnostic test, as the tumor cells characteristically have 59 ± 5 chromosomes.

Differential Diagnosis

I. Until the neoplastic mass is found, the serosanguineous discharge may be confused with the following.
   A. Estrus
   B. Urethritis/cystitis
   C. Prostatitis
II. Other tumors of the genital mucosa must be ruled out, especially squamous cell carcinoma.

Treatment

I. Surgical resection may be curative, but recurrence after surgery is common. It is proposed that neoplastic cells might be transplanted to the incision site and account for recurrences.
II. Electrosurgery and cryosurgery may be combined with or substituted for surgery, depending on the size and location of the mass.
III. Radiotherapy alone or in combination with surgery is curative.
   A. A total dose of 1500–2000 rads is usually recommended (Theilen and Madewell, 1979).
   B. A 100% cure can be expected with localized disease.
IV. Chemotherapy is highly successful in treating TVT.
   A. Vincristine is the drug of choice.
      1. Dosage is 0.5 mg/m² IV weekly.
      2. Length of treatment depends on the rate of regression; 4–6 weeks of therapy is usually sufficient.
      3. Visible tumor regression should be noted within 2 weeks of the first treatment.
   B. Single-drug trials with other chemotherapeutic agents have not been successful (Amber et al., 1990).
V. Spontaneous regression after several months is reported in experimentally transplanted tumors.
   A. The regression is probably related to the immune response.
   B. The incidence of spontaneous recovery in naturally occurring tumors is not known.

Patient Monitoring

I. Limit exposure to other dogs until the tumor has regressed.
II. If chemotherapy is being used, observe the animal for vomiting and perform periodic white blood cell counts for leukopenia during treatment.
III. Monitor for recurrence, especially if surgical removal was the only form of treatment.
IV. Metastasis has been observed as late as 2 years after treatment of the primary tumor. Periodic physical examinations and radiography may be advisable.

TRAUMATIC DISORDERS

Penile Trauma

Definition and Causes

I. Traumatic injuries to the penis occur from accidents or fight wounds or from masturbation.
II. Contusions, lacerations, or puncture wounds may result.
III. Fracture of the os penis may also occur in any size or breed of dog, often when the animal attempts to jump a fence.

Clinical Signs

I. Hemorrhage, which may be profuse and recurrent
II. Local pain or irritation
III. Variable urethral signs: dysuria, hematuria, stranguria, anuria
IV. Systemic depression

Diagnosis

I. Diagnosis of soft tissue trauma is made from a history of trauma and thorough examination of the external genitalia.
II. Diagnosis of os penis fracture is made by radiography.
III. Urethral involvement is determined by urinary catheterization and/or retrograde urethrography.

Differential Diagnosis

I. Rule out other causes of urinary tract hemorrhage.
II. Rule out urethritis and urethral obstruction from calculi.

Treatment

I. Apply local pressure to control hemorrhage.

II. Clean, débride, and suture affected soft tissue as needed.
III. For fracture of os penis, surgical intervention may not be indicated in the absence of any bony displacement resulting in a urethral obstruction.
IV. A fractured os penis with displacement may be stabilized with stainless steel surgical wires or via bone plating.
V. In cases of masturbation, remove or prevent access to objects used for sexual stimulation. If the behavior is the manifestation of a compulsion, fluoxetine (Prozac) at a dose of 1 mg/kg once daily may be helpful. The male may have to be medicated for at least 1 month before any improvement can be noted.

Patient Monitoring

I. Manually extrude the penis daily and apply antibiotic ointment as needed to prevent adhesions.
II. Urethral stricture may occur postoperatively and may be prevented with urethral catheterization and lavage.

Bibliography

Amber EI, Henderson RA, Adeyanju JB, et al: Single-drug chemotherapy of canine transmissible venereal tumor with cyclophosphamide, methotrexate, or vincristine. J Vet Intern Med 4:144, 1990

Elkins AD: Canine paraphimosis of unknown etiology: a case report. Vet Med 79:638, 1984

Herron MA: Diseases of the external genitalia. p. 673. In Morgan RV (ed): Handbook of Small Animal Practice. Churchill Livingstone, New York, 1988

Johnston SD: Disorders of the canine penis and prepuce. p. 549. In Morrow DA (ed): Current Therapy in Theriogenology. WB Saunders, Philadelphia, 1986

McFarland LZ, Deniz E: Unilateral renal agenesis with ipsilateral cryptorchidism and perineal hypospadia in a dog. J Am Vet Assoc 139:1099, 1961

Meyers-Wallen VN, Patterson DF: Disorders of sexual development in the dog. p. 567. In Morrow DA (ed): Current Therapy in Theriogenology. WB Saunders, Philadelphia, 1986

Olson PN, Seim HB, Park RD: Female pseudohermaphroditism in three sibling greyhounds. J Am Vet Med Assoc 194:1747, 1989

Richardson R: Canine transmissible venereal tumor. Compend Contin Educ Pract Vet 3:951, 1981

Sinibaldi KR, Green RW: Surgical correction of prolapse of the male urethra in three English bulldogs. J Am Anim Hosp Assoc 9:450, 1973

Sommer MM, Meyers-Wallen VN: XX true hermaphroditism in a dog. J Am Vet Med Assoc 198:435, 1991

Theilen GH, Madewell BR: Tumors of the skin and subcutaneous tissues. p. 123. In: Veterinary Cancer Medicine. Lea & Febiger, Philadelphia, 1979

Wensing CJG: Developmental anomalies including cryporchidism. p. 583. In Morrow DA (ed): Current Therapy in Theriogenology. WB Saunders, Philadelphia, 1980

59

Diseases of the Mammary Glands

Barbara E. Kitchell
Andrew S. Loar

MASTITIS

Definition

I. Inflammation of the mammary glands is a condition primarily restricted to the postpartum or pseudopregnant animal (bitch or queen).
II. Mastitis may occur in acute, gangrenous, or chronic forms.
III. The incidence or significance of subclinical mastitis is not known.

Causes

I. Ascending bacterial infection, via the teat orifices, and hematogenous spread are the most likely causes.
II. Coliforms (especially *Escherichia coli*), staphylococci, and streptococci are most commonly isolated from infected milk (Johnston and Hayden, 1980).
III. Trauma from nursing pups or kittens as well as poor hygiene may contribute to mastitis.

Clinical Signs

I. Acute mastitis
   A. One or more warm, painful, reddened, and swollen glands are present; the caudal glands are more often affected.
   B. Pyrexia and malaise may be present.
   C. Dams may be presented owing to neonate morbidity or mortality.
   D. There may be secretions from affected gland(s).
      1. Not all portions of the gland may be inflamed; thus, not all teat orifices may yield an abnormal discharge.
      2. Brownish, hemorrhagic, or purulent secretions may be expressed.
II. Abscesses or gangrenous changes
   A. Affected glands may be dark, cool, and/or ulcerated.
   B. Signs of systemic sepsis may be present.
III. Chronic and subclinical mastitis
   A. Chronic bacterial mastitis may be an incidental finding in older, nonlactating queens (Colby and Stein, 1983).
      1. Inflammatory changes are usually minimal.
      2. Affected glands may appear thickened, and nodules may be palpable.
      3. Grossly these changes are indistinguishable from mammary neoplasia.
   B. Subclinical bacterial mastitis should be suspected in asymptomatic lactating dams whose young are presented for poor weight gain or other unexplained septic illness (Wheeler et al., 1984).
      1. Bacteria, leukocytes, and macrophages are found in the milk.
      2. It is unclear if this form of mastitis is a cause or effect of bacterial disease in the nursing neonate.

Diagnosis

I. Hemograms from dams with acute bacterial mastitis generally have a neutrophilic leukocytosis.
II. Fluid analysis and culture of milk from abnormal glands are useful.
   A. Estimated white blood cell (WBC) counts $>3000/\mu l$ are considered abnormal.
   B. Degenerate neutrophils are the predominant cell type noted.
   C. Phagocytized bacteria within degenerative neutrophils and macrophages are commonly found in mastitic milk.
   D. Elevated WBC counts in milk are occasionally noted in normal dams as well as in those with galactostasis.
   E. Bacterial culture and sensitivity and evaluation

of the pH of infected milk aid in antimicrobial selection.

Differential Diagnosis

I. Mastitis in a lactating dam must be considered in the differential diagnosis associated with illness or death in nursing neonates.
   A. Bitches and queens with acute mastitis may provide inadequate passive immunity, nutrition, and hydration to their young.
   B. Ingestion of infected milk is a suggested, although unproven, cause of neonatal septicemia.
   C. Theoretically, pups or kittens with bacterial diseases may cause ascending mastitis in the dam via suckling (Wheeler et al., 1984).
II. Many of the clinical signs of galactostasis are similar to those of bacterial mastitis.

Treatment and Monitoring

I. Give broad-spectrum antibiotics, based on culture results.
II. Evaluation of milk pH may be important in antibiotic selection.
   A. If milk is more acidic than normal plasma pH (dogs <7.3; cats <7.2), antibiotics that are weak bases are indicated.
      1. Trimethoprim-sulfadiazine 15–30 mg/kg PO BID × 21 days
      2. Erythromycin 10 mg/kg PO TID × 21 days
      3. Lincomycin 15 mg/kg PO TID × 21 days
   B. If milk is more alkaline than normal plasma (pH >7.4), antibiotics that are weak acids are indicated.
      1. Ampicillin 20 mg/kg PO TID × 21 days
      2. Cephalexin 30 mg/kg PO BID × 21 days
   C. Tetracycline HCl, doxycycline, and chloramphenicol appear in the milk in reasonable concentrations independent of pH.
      1. Tetracycline may cause yellow staining of tooth enamel in nursing pups and kittens.
      2. Because these antibiotics may cause adverse effects in nursing neonates, they are not recommended unless weaning occurs.
III. Aminoglycosides are not recommended owing to poor penetration of the blood–mammary gland barrier.
IV. These considerations may be less significant in the acutely inflamed mammary gland because of breakdown of the milk–plasma barriers.
V. With chronic or relapsing infections, culture and sensitivity and milk pH evaluations are critical for effective therapy.
VI. Keeping the affected gland(s) empty of abnormal secretions is important.
   A. Milking can be manually performed by the owner but is difficult to do effectively.
   B. It is controversial whether the young should be allowed to nurse from the mastitic gland(s).
      1. Most authors suggest continuation of nursing in the absence of abscessation or gangrene.

2. Ingestion of either infected secretions or milk containing antibiotics is rarely a problem to the young (Johnston and Hayden, 1980).
3. Affected milk does have a poor nutritional content, however.
VII. Gangrenous or abscessed mammary glands require further therapy.
   A. They may be a sequela to progressive, fulminant acute mastitis.
   B. Anaerobic organisms may play a role.
   C. Treat with surgical drainage and warm antiseptic compresses.
   D. Strip milk secretions from affected glands manually BID and prevent offspring from nursing.
   E. Infuse affected gland(s) with antibiotics or antiseptic solutions (0.5–1% povidone-iodine) BID × 2–5 days, using a lacrimal duct cannula or small-gauge polyethylene catheter.
   F. Chronic, persistently infected glands may ultimately require mastectomy.
VIII. Signs of septicemia demand aggressive support with intravenous fluids, appropriate antibiotic therapy, and intensive nursing care.
IX. If offspring are prevented from nursing, owners are offered advice regarding hand-rearing techniques.

GALACTOSTASIS

Definition and Causes

I. Excessive accumulation of milk in the mammary gland(s) concurrent with a lack of excretion
II. May be associated with sterile or septic mastitis
III. May also be noted after weaning or during pseudopregnancy

Pathophysiology and Clinical Signs

I. The engorgement of the gland(s) with residual milk causes mild to moderate inflammation, edema, and discomfort.
II. Insufficient nursing or inadequate removal of the secretions aggravates the condition.
III. In lactating queens the cranial glands are more commonly affected (Colby and Stein, 1983).
IV. Unless the condition is secondary to acute septic mastitis, the animal shows no signs of systemic illness.
V. If the condition persists, milk may become inspissated.

Diagnosis

I. Galactostasis is most likely to occur in the pseudopregnant animal or when nursing young are abruptly weaned.
II. In lactating dams an inverted, nonfunctional teat may be noted on the affected gland.
III. It is a likely sequela to mastitis.
IV. Cytology of milk from affected gland(s) shows the following.

A. Elevated WBC count (>3000/μl) is not uncommon (Wheeler et al., 1984).
B. Nondegenerated neutrophils, macrophages, and occasionally eosinophils occur in the absence of sepsis.
C. Increased relative numbers of macrophages suggest a more chronic reaction.
D. Phagocytized fat droplets are frequently noted.

Treatment and Monitoring

I. Treat underlying septic mastitis when present.
II. When secondary to abrupt weaning or pseudopregnancy, treat as follows.
  A. Any stimulus may increase milk production. Apply cool compresses 10–15 minutes infrequently if dam's comfort appears increased by the procedure.
  B. Do not encourage manual milking of glands, as it may cause additional milk production/letdown.
  C. In severe cases, mild diuretics and glucocorticoids for 2–5 days may be beneficial.
  D. It is best prevented by gradual weaning of offspring simultaneous with a modest reduction in food intake.
III. Involvement of a single gland during lactation calls for the following.
  A. Attempt to evert inverted nipple.
  B. Encourage nursing or massage of affected gland.
  C. Apply cool compresses.

AGALACTIA

Definition

I. True agalactia is the arrest of milk production and excretion (letdown).
II. This condition is extremely uncommon in small animals and is probably secondary to congenital abnormalities in mammary gland development and/or insufficient hormonal interactions.

Causes

I. Poor nutrition is an uncommon cause of decreased milk production
II. Young (primiparous) or anxious dams may psychologically impair milk letdown or be unwilling to allow nursing.
III. The cause and management of true agalactia in small animals are not well documented and reported.

Diagnosis

I. Diagnosis is based on the absence of milk in the mammary glands and the physical condition of the dam.
II. Mammae generally appear normal on physical examination.

Treatment and Monitoring

I. Severe debilitation from poor nutrition or systemic disease is managed accordingly.
II. Calm nervous dams with reassurance and a quiet environment.
  A. Acepromazine (0.125 mg/kg PO BID-TID) can be used.
  B. Acepromazine can also increase milk production because it antagonizes dopamine, which is a prolactin inhibition factor.

GALACTORRHEA

Definition

Galactorrhea is an excessive or inappropriate production and release of milk.

Causes and Pathophysiology

I. The hormonal basis for milk production is complex.
II. In the pregnant bitch approaching parturition, an abrupt decrease in serum progesterone levels with concurrent elevation of serum prolactin precedes lactation (Concannon, 1983).
III. Inappropriate lactation is probably most dependent on an abrupt decrease in serum progesterone levels.
  A. Luteal regression in the pseudopregnant (diestral) bitch is often associated with galactorrhea.
  B. Pseudopregnancy in the queen, although less common than in the bitch, may also be associated with lactation.
  C. Ovariohysterectomy during diestrus simulates luteal regression, sometimes producing lactation.
  D. Cessation of progestogen treatment has been reported to cause galactorrhea (Johnston and Hayden, 1980).
    1. Dogs and cats, of either sex
    2. Examples: megestrol acetate and methylprogesterone

Diagnosis

Inappropriate mammary development and lactation in the diestral or progestogen-treated animal suggest the diagnosis and cause of galactorrhea.

Treatment and Monitoring

I. It generally resolves in several days with no treatment.
II. Decrease food and water for 24–48 hours.
III. Androgen therapy has been recommended for persistent galactorrhea in bitches (Johnston and Hayden, 1980).
  A. Mibolerone 16 μg/kg PO SID × 5 days in bitches.
  B. Methyltestosterone 1–2 mg/kg PO (up to 25 mg) SID × 5–7 days (Johnston and Hayden, 1980).
  C. Androgens are not approved and are not recommended for use in cats.

MAMMARY FIBROEPITHELIAL HYPERPLASIA

Definition

   I. It is a benign proliferation of cellular elements of either the fibroglandular or ductular epithelial components of mammary tissues.
  II. The condition occurs most frequently in young queens after estrus and occasionally in animals of either sex receiving progestogens.
 III. Synonyms are benign fibroadenomatous hyperplasia, juvenile mammary hypertrophy, mammary fibroadenomatosis, and fibroglandular hypertrophy.

Causes

   I. An elevation in endogenous progesterone levels is a cause.
      A. Associated with pregnancy or the postestrous period in the pubescent queen
      B. Noted rarely in the young diestral bitch
  II. Elevated serum estrogen levels in the queen may also be a contributing factor (Colby and Stein, 1983).
 III. Long-term administration of progestogen compounds (e.g., megestrol acetate and methylprogesterone) to cats of either sex may be a cause.
  IV. The exact mechanism for development of the hyperplasia is not understood.

Pathophysiology

   I. Lesions are generally well circumscribed or encapsulated.
  II. The term "hypertrophy" is not really applicable to this condition.
 III. There are two distinct histologic forms.
      A. Diffuse fibroepithelial hyperplasia
         1. Proliferation of fibroglandular elements within the affected gland(s)
         2. Reported to be typical of the lesion found in young, postestral queens (Johnston and Hayden, 1980)
      B. Intraductular papillary hyperplasia
         1. Proliferation of mammary ductular epithelium
         2. Reported to be characteristic of lesions induced by progestogen therapy (Johnston and Hayden, 1980)
         3. May also be described as preneoplastic or adenomatous lesion
  IV. The two histologic forms appear to have a similar biologic behavior and response to treatment.

Clinical Signs

   I. There is a nonpainful, firm swelling in one or more mammary glands.
      A. It may be diffuse or nodular within the affected gland(s).
      B. Multiple nodules in multiple glands and/or chains may be noted.
      C. Glandular enlargement is often dramatic and bilateral.
  II. When gland enlargement is profound, gross evidence of inflammatory changes and discomfort may occur.
 III. Occasionally, brownish fluid is expressed from affected gland(s); it is aseptic with low cellularity.
  IV. Swelling generally lasts from days to weeks and may be progressive.
   V. Fluid-filled cysts have been noted in mammary tissues from young bitches.
      A. The surface of the gland may have a blue or brown tinge owing to the fluid-containing cysts.
      B. The condition generally resolves spontaneously or after ovariohysterectomy.
      C. In chronic cases, the affected glands contain a considerable amount of fibrous connective tissue.

Diagnosis

   I. Signalment, history, and clinical features are usually sufficient for a tentative diagnosis.
  II. Excisional biopsy may be indicated in selected cases.
      A. In older animals (>5 years)
      B. If inflammatory changes predominate
      C. If appropriate therapy does not result in regression within 3–4 weeks

Differential Diagnosis

   I. Galactorrhea
  II. Mammary neoplasia
 III. Mastitis

Treatment and Monitoring

   I. The condition generally regresses spontaneously without specific therapy.
      A. As ovarian hormone concentrations return to baseline levels
      B. After cessation of progestogen therapy
      C. Usually occurs within several weeks
  II. Ovariohysterectomy is usually helpful and may be the treatment of choice in severely affected cats.
      A. May hasten remission
      B. May be technically more difficult owing to mammary chain swelling, unless flank incision is used (cats)
 III. Testosterone administration is sometimes effective (Colby and Stein, 1983).
  IV. Surgical excision and biopsy may be indicated.
      A. When other therapies fail
      B. When the glands become traumatized, infected, or gangrenous
   V. Palliative therapy for inflammatory changes includes cool compresses, corticosteroids, and diuretics.

MAMMARY NEOPLASIA

Definition

   I. Mammary gland tumors arise primarily in the female animal from secretory epithelial, myoepithelial, or,

Table 59–1. *Morphologic Forms of Canine Mammary Tumors*

Benign mammary tumors
  Benign mixed tumor
  Complex adenoma
  Fibroadenoma
    Intracanalicular type
    Pericanalicular type
  Duct papilloma
  Simple adenoma
Malignant mammary tumors
  Tubular adenocarcinoma, simple and complex types
  Papillary adenocarcinoma, simple and complex types
  Papillary cystic adenocarcinoma, simple and complex types
  Solid carcinoma, simple and complex types
  Anaplastic carcinoma
  Other carcinomas: mucinous, squamous cell, spindle cell
  Sarcomas: osteosarcoma, fibrosarcoma, combined forms
  Malignant mixed tumor (carcinosarcoma)

less frequently, mesenchymal elements of the mammary tissues.

II. Table 59–1 lists the most commonly described histologic forms of mammary tumors.

III. Incidence is as follows.
  A. Dogs: most common tumor in the bitch; second most common tumor in dogs of either sex after skin neoplasms (Brodey et al., 1983)
    1. Incidence is approximately 2/1000 female dogs at risk (Dorn et al., 1968).
    2. Approximately 50% of mammary masses are malignant in the dog (Gilbertson et al., 1983).
  B. Cats: third most common site of cancer, after hematopoietic tissues and skin (Dorn et al., 1968)
    1. Incidence is approximately half that in humans and dogs (Hayes et al., 1981).
    2. 80–90% of mammary tumors in cats are malignant (Dorn et al., 1968).
  C. No clear breed predilection in either species
    1. Some studies suggest a higher incidence in spaniels, poodles, and terriers.
    2. Chihuahuas, boxers, greyhounds, and beagles may be at decreased risk.
    3. Siamese cat breeds may have up to twice the risk of tumor development as compared with other cats (Hayes et al., 1981).
    4. Spaying practices of breeders and veterinarians in different countries may confound the breed predisposition statistics (Kitchell, 1995).

IV. The median age is 10–12 years for both species (Else and Hannant, 1979; Hayes et al., 1981).
  A. Age ranges are 2–17 years in dogs and 9 months to 19 years in cats.
  B. Mammary tumors are extremely uncommon in animals <2 years of age.
  C. Siamese cats appear to develop tumors at a younger age than other cat breeds.
  D. Tumor development at a young age does not appear to correlate with a poorer prognosis.

  V. The posterior glands are most often affected because they are larger glands and thus have more cells at risk for malignant transformation (Bostock, 1975).
VI. Mammary tumors in male animals are extremely rare (1% of malignant mammary tumors seen in male dogs) and are generally aggressive in behavior.

Causes

I. Tumor development is profoundly hormone dependent.
  A. Unspayed cats and dogs have a sevenfold increased risk of mammary tumors than spayed animals (Dorn et al., 1968).
  B. Ovariohysterectomy (OHE) in the dog done prior to the first estrus is protective against the development of mammary carcinoma.
    1. OHE between the first and fourth heat cycle results in a gradually increasing risk of tumor development.
    2. After 2.5 years of age, OHE provides no protective effect.
  C. Intact cats are more likely to develop mammary tumors than ovariectomized cats (Hayes et al., 1981).
  D. The administration of progestogen compounds has also been associated with mammary neoplasia in cats and dogs.
    1. Progesterone, including progestins used for estrus control, induce benign nodules in mammary glands (Kwapein et al., 1980; Misdorp, 1991).
    2. Nortestosterone induced a high rate of mammary carcinomas in intact dogs in a high-dose, long-term study (Misdorp, 1991).
    3. Progestational drugs are strongly associated with mammary tumor development in cats (Hernandez et al., 1975).
  E. Presence of hormone receptors on mammary tumors may be important.
    1. Estrogen receptors and progesterone receptors have been detected on canine mammary tumor cells (Parodi et al., 1984).
      a) Approximately 40–60% of all tumors tested are positive for receptors (Hamilton et al., 1977; MacEwen et al., 1982).
      b) Receptors are present in approximately 70% of benign tumors, and tumors with high levels of receptors tend to be better differentiated (Sartin et al., 1992).
    2. Progesterone effects may be mediated through expression of growth hormone within the mammary tissue (Theilen and Madewell, 1987).
    3. Glucocorticoid and progesterone receptors have been found on feline mammary tumor cells (Johnston et al., 1984; Parodi et al., 1984).
    4. Only 10% of cat mammary tumors are positive for estrogen receptors (Hamilton et al., 1976).
    5. Some canine mammary tumors are positive

for prolactin receptors, and lower levels of prolactin receptor expression are seen with malignant tumors (Rutteman et al., 1986).
  F. Reproductive history is not usually a factor, because none of the following influences the risk of mammary tumor development in the bitch.
    1. Number of size of previous litters
    2. Previous episodes of pseudopregnancy
    3. Irregular or unpredictable estrous cycles
    4. Fertility problems
II. High fat diets are associated with an increased incidence of mammary carcinoma in humans and potentially in dogs. Dogs that are thin at 9 to 12 months of age have a reduced risk as compared with other spayed dogs (Sonnenschein et al., 1991).

Pathophysiology

I. Clinically and histologically, mammary neoplasia is an extremely heterogeneous disease.
II. The most significant clinical features of animals with mammary neoplasia are those that correlate with a specific prognosis.
  A. A mammary tumor that exhibits malignant behavior is one that has a high probability for local aggressiveness and/or postoperative recurrence.
  B. Histologic evidence of malignancy does not correlate invariably with malignant behavior in canine and feline mammary tumors (Withrow and MacEwen, 1996).
    1. Histologic criteria of malignancy are not uniformly interpreted by pathologists.
    2. Marked histologic variation may exist within a mass.
III. Gross physical examination findings can be indicative of malignant behavior.
  A. History of rapid tumor growth is a poor prognostic finding.
    1. Tumors whose appearance and growth are associated with estrus develop rapidly.
    2. Benign tumors may occasionally transform to rapidly progressive cancers.
    3. Occasionally, benign tumors exhibit sudden enlargement.
  B. Poorly circumscribed lesions suggest infiltration into the normal tissues and are difficult to excise with complete surgical margins.
  C. Gross evidence of infiltration into skin, abdominal muscle, or other adjacent tissues is a poor prognostic sign.
    1. Skin ulceration
    2. Fixation to skin or underlying tissues
  D. Evidence of inflammatory changes in the skin and adjacent tissues often indicates tumor invasion into dermal lymphatics and is an extremely unfavorable prognostic sign in the dog.
  E. Evidence of regional or distant metastatic lesions confirms malignancy.
    1. Tumor invasion into lymph nodes or vessels is correlated with a 95% postsurgery recurrence rate (Gilbertson et al., 1983).

    2. Other causes of lymphadenopathy must be considered.
    3. Common systemic sites of metastatic mammary cancer include lungs, liver, bone, kidneys, eyes, and regional or distant lymph nodes.
IV. Some clinical features have neither positive nor negative prognostic significance.
  A. The location of the primary tumor(s) within the mammary chain (e.g., anterior vs. posterior glands, right vs. left chain) (Theilen and Madewell, 1987)
  B. Whether tumors are located in single (75% of cases) vs. multiple glands
  C. The presence of abnormal glandular secretions (unless cytologic evidence of anaplasia)

Clinical Signs

I. Animals may present with solitary or multiple masses; tumor size varies considerably.
II. Lesions may appear as distinct nodules or as a diffuse swelling of the involved gland(s), with or without inflammation.
III. Multiple glands in one or both mammary chains may be affected.
IV. Cystic ducts associated with the tumor may cause fluid secretion through the nipple.
V. Regional or distant metastatic spread of mammary cancers may result in certain clinical signs.
  A. Lymphatic involvement may cause local swelling (lymphedema) and discomfort, especially of the hindlegs.
  B. Respiratory or other organ metastases may result in systemic problems (e.g., dyspnea, anorexia, vomiting, diarrhea).
  C. Paraneoplastic sequelae may cause signs of hypercalcemia or cancer cachexia.

Diagnosis

I. Preoperative work-up
  A. History: rate of growth, reproductive history, medication history, other systemic disorders
  B. Documentation and measurement of all mammary gland lesions
  C. Presurgical hematologic and biochemical profile, as for the geriatric patient
  D. Thoracic radiography, including two lateral and one dorsoventral view for metastasis
    1. The presence of metastatic disease generally contraindicates surgery.
    2. Mastectomy may be offered as a palliative treatment if metastatic lesions are small or if the primary tumor is causing the animal discomfort or other clinical problems.
  E. Cytology
    1. Abnormal teat secretions
      a) Rarely diagnostic for neoplasia
      b) May rule out septic mastitis
    2. Fine-needle aspiration from lesion(s)

a) Positive for carcinoma: consider more radical initial surgery
b) Negative: does not rule out malignancy

II. Incisional biopsy
   A. It is not therapeutic and is rarely indicated unless inflammatory carcinoma is suspected.
   B. Changes suggestive of inflammatory carcinoma preclude surgical intervention (Susaneck et al., 1983).
      1. Inflammatory carcinoma is uniformly unresectable and generally is systemic at initial presentation.
      2. Many of these animals have subclinical coagulopathies and are poor anesthetic risks.

III. Excisional biopsy
   A. Eliminates all gross evidence of disease.
   B. Provides an adequate tissue specimen for histopathology.
   C. Surgical options for obtaining a biopsy, as well as for therapeutic intervention, include the following.
      1. Nodulectomy (lumpectomy): isolated removal of small (<0.5 cm) tumor(s) from each affected gland
      2. Simple mastectomy: removal of the affected gland(s)
      3. En bloc resection (modified radical mastectomy): removal of tumor and its adjacent glands dependent on their lymphatic drainage
         a) Glands 1–3 drain to axillary and cranial sternal lymph nodes (Sautet et al., 1992).
         b) Glands 4 and 5 drain to the superficial inguinal nodes.
         c) Lymphatic drainage may cross midline to contralateral glands in the cat.
      4. Radical mastectomy (uni- or bilateral): removal of all mammary glands ipsilateral to the tumor(s) as well as the intervening tissues and regional lymphatic structures

IV. Histopathology of canine tumors
   A. Biopsy specimens must be adequate.
      1. They should allow the pathologist at least two, preferably three or four, sections for examination.
      2. A lumpectomy may provide insufficient tissue for evaluation of local invasiveness and lymphatic and blood vessel infiltration.
      3. Lymph node involvement is best confirmed by histologic examination (vs. cytology).
   B. The morphology and distribution of the various canine mammary tumors are far more variable than those of feline mammary tumors.
   C. There are several histologic classification systems.
      1. They are designed to provide morphologically descriptive names for each type of mammary tumor.
      2. These systems are not uniformly accepted.
      3. Histologic type, lymphoid reactivity in the tumor, and degree of anaplasia are correlated with prognosis.
      4. Gilbertson's classification scheme (Gilbertson et al., 1983) is based on morphologic criteria

*Table 59–2. **Histologic Stage Correlated with Disease-Free Interval after Mastectomy in 233 Dogs with Mammary Cancer***

Histologic Stage	Definition	Recurrence 2 Years After Mastectomy
0	Carcinoma in situ	19%
I	Invasive carcinoma without lymphatic or venous invasion	60%
II	Invasive carcinoma with vascular or lymphatic invasion or metastasis to regional nodes	97%
III	Evidence of distant metastasis	100%

From Kurzman ID and Gilbertson SP, 1986, with permission.

used in the classification of human breast cancers.
   a) Different categories of tumors show distinct, predictable biologic behavior.
   b) Distribution for several thousand mammary tumors in dogs using this scheme is as follows (Greenlee and Tappe, unpublished data, 1991).
      (1) Benign adenoma, 50%
      (2) Benign with atypia, 30%
      (3) Carcinoma in situ, 5%
      (4) Invasive, no infiltration, 10%
      (5) Invasive, with infiltration, 5%
   D. Prognosis may be based on histologic diagnosis (Tables 59–2 and 59–3).
      1. Pathologists using most histologic systems (except Gilbertson's) render a diagnosis of malignancy in about 50% of all mammary neoplasms evaluated.
      2. The percentage of malignant tumors that recur and/or cause the dog's death within 2 years of initial surgery varies between 20 and 95%, depending on the degree of malignancy.
      3. To aid the clinician in evaluating a biopsy report, the following characteristics are correlated with an unfavorable prognosis.

*Table 59–3. **Histologic Grading System and Correlates with Survival in 320 Dogs with Mammary Carcinoma***

Histologic Description	Median Survival Time (Weeks)	
	Invasive	*Noninvasive*
Papillary carcinoma	65	128
Tubular carcinoma	38	110
Solid carcinoma	26	82
Anaplastic carcinoma	11	Not applicable

Reprinted from European Journal of Cancer, Vol. II, Bostock BE, The prognosis following the surgical excision of canine mammary neoplasms, p. 389, © 1975, with kind permission from Elsevier Science Ltd., The Boulevard, Langford Lane, Kidlington 0X5 1GB, UK.

a) Evidence of microscopic invasion into tissues past the boundaries of tumor stroma

b) Tumor invasion into lymph nodes, lymph vessels, or blood vessels

c) Features indicative of mammary sarcoma

d) Features indicative of cellular anaplasia

e) Relatively few lymphocytes within the tumor stroma (Kurzman and Gilbertson, 1986)

V. Histology and behavior of feline mammary neoplasms

A. About 80–90% are malignant (Hayes and Mooney, 1985).

1. Most are adenocarcinomas.

2. Carcinoma in situ, as well as tubular, papillary, and solid types, has been reported.

3. Tumors diagnosed as carcinoma in situ generally do not recur after surgery (MacEwen et al., 1984).

4. No correlation has been shown between the other types of carcinoma and the survival time or recurrence rate.

B. Most feline mammary cancers show local invasion or lymphatic infiltration.

C. Most cats with large mammary carcinomas develop tumor recurrence and die within 1 year after surgery (Weijer et al., 1972).

D. The volume of the tumor appears to be a significant factor determining the survival time (MacEwen et al., 1984).

E. The type of surgical therapy offered also appears to influence the prognosis (see Treatment, later).

VI. Clinical staging of mammary neoplasms

A. See Table 59–4: tumor-node-metastasis (TNM) system

Table 59–4. Staging of Canine Mammary Carcinoma

T	T1—Less than 3 cm diameter
	T2—3–5 cm diameter
	T3—Greater than 5 cm in diameter
	Subgroups: a) not fixed to other tissues
	b) fixed to skin
	c) fixed to underlying muscle
	T4—Any size, but inflammatory carcinoma (dermal infiltrates)
N	N0—No nodal involvement
	N1a—Ipsilateral node, nonfixed
	N1b—Ipsilateral node, fixed
	N2a—Bilateral nodes, nonfixed
	N2b—Bilateral nodes, fixed
M	M0–No distant metastasis
	M1—Metastatic
Stage I	T0, T1 a, b, or c, N0, M0
Stage II	T0, T1 or T2, a, b, or c, N0 or N1a, M0
Stage III	Any T3 tumor, with any N, and M0 status or any T with Nb and M0 status
Stage IV	Any T, with any N and M1 status

T = tumor; N = node; M = metastasis
Staging classification of the World Health Organization.

B. Requires a thorough work-up

1. Mammary/node palpation

2. Thoracic and abdominal radiographs (or abdominal ultrasound)

3. Histologic examination of primary tumor(s) and nodes

C. Designed to predict postsurgical biologic behavior

1. It is useful only with malignant tumors.

2. It indicates the total body tumor burden and potential for metastasis and postoperative recurrence.

3. Dogs with stage III disease (primary tumors >5 cm in diameter) that have histologically invasive carcinomas have a significantly higher risk of tumor recurrence than dogs with less advanced invasive cancers (Loar, 1986).

4. Cats with small primary adenocarcinomas (<8 cm^3) have longer disease-free intervals and survival times than those with larger cancers (MacEwen et al., 1984).

Differential Diagnosis

I. Mastitis

II. Galactostasis

III. Mammary hyperplasia

Treatment

I. The simplest surgical procedure that removes known cancer in the mammary gland should be performed (Withrow and MacEwen, 1996).

A. Nodulectomy (lumpectomy)

1. Appropriate for tumors <0.5 cm diameter (Withrow and MacEwen, 1996)

2. Does not provide adjacent or lymphatic tissues for histopathology

3. May not be practical for dogs with multiple gland involvement

4. Does not eliminate the risk of de novo (new primary) lesions in remaining mammary tissues

B. Simple mastectomy

1. Provides histologic examination of tumor invasiveness

2. May be more difficult than en bloc resection because mammary glands are intimately associated with one another

3. Does not offer easy surgical access to adjacent lymph nodes

4. Lumpectomy with 2 cm margins equally effective as other surgical procedures (Allen and Mahaffey, 1989)

C. En bloc resection

1. Designed to remove regional metastatic sites

2. Based on lymphatic drainage patterns

a) Metastatic cells from glands 1, 2, and 3 traverse cranial to the ipsilateral axillary lymph node.

b) Tumor cells from glands 3, 4, and 5 drain toward the inguinal node.

c) Variation in lymph drainage probably occurs.
3. Technique (Withrow and MacEwen, 1996)
a) Tumor in gland 1 and/or 2: Remove three anterior glands, interposing tissues, and axillary node (if node is obviously enlarged).
b) Tumor in gland 4 and/or 5: Remove two most posterior glands, interposing tissues, and inguinal node.
D. Unilateral or bilateral mastectomy (''radical'' mastectomy)
1. Has the highest morbidity of all techniques
a) Wound closure and elimination of dead space may cause significant problems.
b) Excessive tension occurs at the incision site, especially if bilateral procedures are necessary.
2. Provides adequate tissue for histopathology
3. Indicated when both anterior and posterior glands are affected
E. Choice of technique
1. No study has confirmed the advantage of one surgical technique over any other in the dog.
2. The advantages of radical vs. local resection are still debated in the dog.
a) Less extensive surgery is associated with less morbidity and more rapid recovery.
b) More extensive surgery may prevent onset of de novo tumors and may be associated with better sample acquisition for histologic prognostication.
3. In the cat, radical mastectomy has been shown to provide a longer disease-free interval (remission duration) than simple mastectomy (MacEwen et al., 1984); however, overall survival times were not signficantly different.
II. Radiation therapy
A. No studies are available on the use of radiotherapy in treatment of dog and cat mammary carcinoma.
B. Inoperable or inflamed tumors have been treated with minimal success in animals.
C. Prospective trials are needed to establish the place of radiation therapy in veterinary medicine.
III. Chemotherapy
A. Indicated for animals whose biopsies suggest a high probability for postoperative recurrence or metastasis
1. Those whose biopsies indicate invasiveness or infiltration into lymph, lymphatic vessels, or blood vessels (i.e., stage II and III tumors)
2. Animals with distant metastatic disease (stage IV)
3. Any cat with mammary cancer, because of the aggressive nature of the tumors
B. Cytotoxic chemotherapy
1. Partial responses have occurred in dogs using doxorubicin at 30 mg/m^2 IV q 3 weeks up to four to eight treatments (Ogilvie et al., 1989).
2. Early reports utilizing various dosages of mi-

toxantrone have not been as promising (Ogilvie et al., 1991).
3. Cisplatin has been reported to have some efficacy in dogs (Withrow and MacEwen, 1996).
4. A report of combination therapy showed responses in cats with advanced carcinoma (Jeglum et al., 1985).
a) Doxorubicin (see previous dosage)
b) Cyclophosphamide 50 mg/m^2 PO SID on days 3, 4, 5, and 6 after doxorubicin
C. Hormone ablation
1. Use of antiestrogen drugs, e.g., tamoxifen and clomiphene, theoretically decreases growth stimulus in hormone-dependent tumors.
2. Estrogen-receptor assays are performed on biopsy specimens first.
3. Tamoxifen (median dose 0.42 mg/kg) was administered to seven dogs with inoperable or metastatic tumors in one study (Kitchell and Fidel, 1992).
a) Objective evidence of tumor shrinkage was seen in five of seven dogs.
b) Mean survival times were 4 months from start of tamoxifen therapy.
c) Adverse effects seen were related to antiestrogen effects (urinary incontinence), estrogen agonist effects (signs of estrus, vaginal discharge), and development of pyometra or cervical stump pyometra.
4. In another study, 10 of 18 dogs treated with tamoxifen had significant estrogen-like signs, and no dogs had evidence of antitumor activity (Morris et al., 1993).
5. No study has shown a decreased recurrence rate or improved survival time secondary to OHE at the time of tumor resection.
D. Biologic response modifiers
1. They are designed to augment the immune-mediated removal of residual tumor cells after surgical resection.
2. Nonspecific immunostimulants, i.e., levamisole, *Corynebacterium parvum,* and bacillus Calmette-Guérin (BCG), have been used most often (Brodey et al., 1983; MacEwen et al., 1985).
3. No consistent benefits have been documented.
4. Removal of circulating tumor antigen-antibody complexes has been used to initiate antitumor responses in dogs (Terman et al., 1980; Matus, 1983).
E. Palliative therapy
1. Symptomatic therapy for large, painful tumors may be of short-term benefit.
a) Antibiotics for secondary infections
b) Hot packs and other forms of physical therapy
c) Judicious débridement of ulcerated, draining lesions
2. Corticosteroids
a) May decrease tumor-associated inflam-

mation at the primary tumor or at distant metastatic sites

b) May improve attitude and appetite of debilitated animals

3. Metastatic pulmonary disease

a) Consider antitussives or bronchodilators.

b) Pulmonary nodules may grow slowly and need not necessitate euthanasia unless clinical signs are manifested.

Patient Monitoring

I. Prognosis is based on histologic diagnosis and clinical stage.

II. Animals with high potential for recurrence are examined at 1- to 3-month intervals, with thoracic radiographs being obtained every 2–4 months. High-risk cases include the following.

A. Animals with histologic evidence of invasiveness or lymphatic or vascular infiltration

B. Animals with primary tumors >5 cm in diameter (stage III)

C. Any cat with an adenocarcinoma

D. Animals with postoperative evidence of residual disease

III. If the histologic diagnosis was carcinoma in situ, re-examinations are scheduled at 3- to 6-month intervals, with thoracic radiographs every 6 months.

IV. Animals remaining free of disease for more than 24 months have a remote chance for subsequent relapse.

V. Any female animal with remaining mammary tissue is at risk for developing mammary tumors.

A. De novo tumors may develop.

B. New nodules are no less likely to be malignant than their predecessors and thus are managed accordingly.

Bibliography

Allen SW, Mahaffey EA: Canine mammary neoplasia: prognostic indicators and response to surgical therapy. J Am Anim Hosp Assoc 25:540, 1989

Bostock BE: The prognosis following the surgical excision of canine mammary neoplasms. Eur J Cancer 11:389, 1975

Brodey RS, Goldschmidt MH, Roszel JR: Canine mammary neoplasms. J Am Anim Hosp Assoc 19:61, 1983

Center SA, Randolph JF: Lactation and spontaneous remission of feline mammary hyperplasia following pregnancy. J Am Anim Hosp Assoc 21:56, 1985

Colby ED, Stein BS: Reproductive system. p. 511. In Pratt PW (ed): Feline Medicine. American Veterinary Publications, Santa Barbara, California, 1983

Concannon PW: Reproductive physiology and endocrine patterns of the bitch. p. 886. In Kirk RW (ed): Current Veterinary Therapy VIII. WB Saunders, Philadelphia, 1983

Dorn AS, Legendre AM, McGavin MD: Mammary hyperplasia in a male cat receiving progesterone. J Am Vet Med Assoc 182:621, 1983

Dorn DR, Taylor DON, Schneider R et al: Survey of animal neoplasms in Alameda and Contra Costa counties. II. Cancer morbidity in dogs and cats in Alameda county. J Natl Cancer Inst 40:307, 1968

Else RH, Hannant D: Some epidemiological aspects of mammary neoplasia in the bitch. Vet Rec 104:296, 1979

Ferguson RH: Canine mammary gland tumors. Vet Clin North Am [Small Anim Pract] 15:501, 1985

Gilbertson SR, Kurzman ID, Zachrau RE et al: Canine mammary epithelial neoplasm: biologic implications of morphologic characteristics assessed in 232 dogs. Vet Pathol 20:127, 1983

Hahn KA, Richardson RC, Knapp DW: Canine malignant mammary neoplasia: biological behavior, diagnosis and treatment alternatives. J Am Anim Hosp Assoc 28:251, 1992

Hamilton JM, Else RW, Forshaw P: Oestrogen receptors in feline mammary tumors. Vet Rec 99:477, 1976

Hamilton JM, Else RW, Forshaw P: Oestrogen receptors in canine mammary tumors. Vet Rec 101:258, 1977

Hampe AF, Misdorp W: Tumours and dysplasias of the mammary gland. Bull WHO 50:111, 1974

Harvey HJ, Gilbertson SR: Canine mammary gland tumors. Vet Clin North Am 7:213, 1977

Hayes AA, Mooney S: Feline mammary tumors. Vet Clin North Am 15:513, 1985

Hayes HM, Milne KL, Mandell CP: Epidemiologic features of feline mammary carcinoma. Vet Rec 108:476, 1981

Hernandez FZ, Fernandez BB, Chertach M et al: Feline mammary carcinoma and progestogens. Feline Pract 5:45, 1975

Jeglum KA, deGuzman E, Young KM: Chemotherapy of advanced mammary adenocarcinoma in 14 cats. J Am Vet Med Assoc 187:157, 1985

Johnston SD, Hayden DW: Non-neoplastic disorders of the mammary glands. p. 1224. In Kirk RW (ed): Current Veterinary Therapy VII. WB Saunders, Philadelphia, 1980

Johnston SD, Hayden DW, Kiang DT et al: Progesterone receptors in feline mammary adenocarcinomas. Am J Vet Res 45:379, 1984

Kitchell BE: Mammary tumors p. 1098. In Kirk RW (ed): Current Veterinary Therapy XII: Small Animal Practice. WB Saunders, Philadelphia, 1995

Kitchell BE, Fidel JL: Tamoxifen as a potential therapy for canine mammary carcinoma. Proc Vet Cancer Soc 12:91, 1992

Kurzman ID, Gilbertson SP: Prognostic factors in canine mammary tumors. Semin Vet Med Surg 1:25, 1986

Kwapein RP, Giles RC, Geil RC et al: Malignant mammary tumors in beagle dogs dosed with investigational oral contraceptive steroids. J Natl Cancer Inst 65:137, 1980

Loar AS: The management of canine mammary tumors. p. 480. In Kirk RW (ed): Current Veterinary Therapy IX. WB Saunders, Philadelphia, 1986

Loar AS, Susaneck SJ: Doxorubicin-induced cardiotoxicity in five dogs. Semin Vet Med Surg 1:68, 1986

MacEwen EG, Patnaik AK, Harvey HJ et al: Estrogen receptors in canine mammary tumors. Cancer Res 42:2255, 1982

MacEwen EG, Hayes AA, Harvey HJ et al: Prognostic factors for feline mammary tumors. J Am Vet Med Assoc 185:201, 1984

MacEwen EG, Hayes AA, Mooney S et al: Evaluation of effect of levamisole on feline mammary cancer. J Biol Response Mod 5:541, 1985

Matus RE: Intensive therapeutic plasmapheresis in veterinary medicine. p. 442. In Kirk RW (ed): Current Veterinary Therapy VIII. WB Saunders, Philadelphia, 1983

Misdorp W: Progestogens and mammary tumors in dogs and cats. Acta Endocrinol 125(suppl):27, 1991

Misdorp W, Hart AAM: Prognostic factors in canine mammary cancer. J Natl Cancer Inst 56:779, 1976

Morris JS, Dobson JM, Bostock DE: Use of tamoxifen in the control of canine mammary neoplasia. Vet Rec 133:539, 1993

Nelson LW, Weikel LH, Reno FE: Mammary nodules in dogs during four years treatment with megestrol acetate or chlormadinone acetate. J Natl Cancer Inst 51:1303, 1973

Ogilvie GK, Reynolds HA, Richardson RC et al: Phase II evaluation of doxorubicin for treatment of various canine neoplasms. J Am Vet Med Assoc 195:1580, 1989

Ogilvie GK, Obradovich JE, Elmslie RE et al: Efficacy of mitox-antrone against various neoplasms in dogs. J Am Vet Med Assoc 198:1618, 1991

Owen LN (ed): The TNM Classification of Tumours in Domestic Animals. WHO, Geneva, 1980

Parodi AL, Mialot JP, Martin PM et al: Canine and feline mammary cancers as animal models for hormone-dependent human breast tumors: relationships between steroid receptor profiles and survival rates. Prog Cancer Res Ther 31:357, 1984

Rutteman GR, Willekes-Koolschijn N, Bevers MM et al: Prolactin binding in benign and malignant mammary tissue of female dogs. Anticancer Res 6:829, 1986

Sartin EA, Barnes S, Kwapien RP et al: Estrogen and progesterone receptor status of mammary carcinomas and correlation with clinical outcome. Am J Vet Res 53:2196, 1992

Sautet JY, Ruberte J, Lopez C et al: Lymphatic system of the mammary glands in the dog: an approach to the surgical treatment of malignant mammary tumors. Canine Pract 17:30, 1992

Sonnenschein EG, Glickman LT, Goldschmidt MH, McKee LJ: Body conformation, diet and risk of breast cancer in pet dogs: a case-control study. Am J Epidemiol 133:694, 1991

Susaneck SJ, Allen TA, Hoopes J et al: Inflammatory mammary carcinoma in the dog. J Am Anim Hosp Assoc 19:971, 1983

Terman DS, Yamamoto T, Mattioli M et al: Extensive necrosis of spontaneous canine mammary adenocarcinoma after extracorporeal perfusion over Staph A. J Immunol 124:795, 1980

Theilen G, Madewell BR: Tumors of the mammary gland. p. 327. In Theilen G, Madewell BR (eds): Veterinary Cancer Medicine. 2nd Ed. Lea & Febiger, Philadelphia, 1987

Weijer K, Head KW, Misdorp W et al: Malignant mammary tumors. 1. Morphology and biology: some comparisons with human and canine mammary carcinomas. J Natl Cancer Inst 49:1697, 1972

Wheeler SL, Magne ML, Kaufman J et al: Postpartum disorders in the bitch. Compend Contin Educ Pract Vet 6:493, 1984

Withrow SJ, MacEwen EG: Tumors of the mammary gland. p. 356. In Withrow SJ, MacEwen EG (eds): Small Animal Clinical Oncology. 2nd Ed. WB Saunders, Philadelphia, 1996

60

Disorders of Canine Reproduction

Janice L. Cain
Autumn P. Davidson
Melissa S. Wallace
Melissa F. Goodman

INFERTILITY IN THE BITCH

Janice L. Cain

Definition

I. A diminution or absence of ability to produce off-spring
II. Includes bitches that fail to breed, conceive, or carry a litter to term
III. Classified based on reproductive history
   A. Failure to breed
   B. Normal estrous cycle
   C. Abnormal estrous cycle

Causes and Clinical Signs

I. Failure to breed
   A. Breeding management error
      1. Owners often believe that breeding should occur on predetermined dates relative to the day of the estrous cycle, e.g., days 9 and 11 or 11 and 13.
      2. If proestrus is either short or long, predetermined breeding dates may not correspond with behavioral estrus (see Chap. 53).
   B. Vaginal abnormality that prevents copulation (see Chap. 57)
   C. Decreased libido
      1. Bitches that dominate the stud dog
      2. Bitches that have had a prior traumatic breeding experience
   D. Abnormal stature or conformation making breeding physically difficult, e.g., English bulldog
II. Normal estrous cycle
   Consider the following in a bitch with normal interestrous intervals and duration of proestrus and estrus, that breeds naturally, and yet apparently fails to conceive or carry a litter to term.
   A. Breeding management error
      1. If a limited number of breedings occur prior to ovulation, sperm may not be viable when the bitch has mature ova available for fertilization.
      2. If a bitch is bred after the cytologic diestral shift (as determined by vaginal cytology), the fertile period may be missed.
   B. Stud dog infertility (see later discussion)
   C. Ovulatory failure
      1. Evaluation of progesterone concentration during diestrus can be used to retrospectively determine that a bitch has ovulated and has functional corpora lutea.
      2. Serum progesterone concentration ranges from 5–80 ng/ml during diestrus if the bitch has normal ovarian function, whether or not she is pregnant (Concannon et al., 1975).
   D. Occult illness
      1. Clinical signs such as polyuria, polydipsia, poor coat quality, weight loss or gain, and change in appetite warrant investigation.
      2. Endocrinologic diseases such as hyper- or hypoadrenocorticism, diabetes mellitus, and hypothyroidism can cause reproductive failure.
      3. Occult neoplasia is another cause of reproductive failure.
      4. Any underlying disease can cause reproductive failure.
   E. Infectious diseases
      1. All breeding bitches are screened for *Brucella canis* prior to breeding.
      2. Infection with canine herpesvirus can cause

failure to conceive, fetal loss in utero, still-born fetuses, and early neonatal death (Hashimoto and Hirai, 1986).

3. Low-grade, occult bacterial infection of the uterus may cause conception and/or implantation failure.
4. Bacteria of the normal vaginal flora do not cause infertility.
   a) Overgrowth of vaginal mycoplasma has been suspected as a cause of conception failure (Lein, 1986).
   b) More investigation is warranted in the interpretation of vaginal cultures for *Mycoplasma* sp. and the possible relationship of vaginal mycoplasmosis and infertility.
F. Cystic endometrial hyperplasia: conception and/or implantation failure (see Chap. 56)
G. Fetal resorption or abortion
   1. Fetuses that die in utero during the first two thirds of gestation may degenerate and be resorbed without outward signs.
   2. Some bitches may exhibit malaise, fever, inappetence, and a sanguineous or purulent vaginal discharge.
   3. Fetuses that die later in gestation will usually be aborted.
   4. Causes of fetal death include maternal infectious disease, endometrial disease, developmental defects in the fetuses, and progesterone insufficiency.
      a) Luteal insufficiency is a failure of corpora lutea to secrete adequate progesterone.
      b) Decrease in progesterone may be secondary to other factors such as fetal abnormalities, placentitis, and exogenous glucocorticoid therapy (Feldman and Nelson, 1996).
   5. A bitch can partially resorb or abort a litter and the remaining healthy fetuses may go to term (Feldman and Nelson, 1996).
   6. An incorrect diagnosis of pregnancy by palpation may cause an owner to inaccurately believe that resorption has occurred when the bitch fails to whelp a litter.
H. Stress from shipping
   1. Stress is a suspected, but difficult to prove, cause of conception failure or early fetal resorption.
   2. Some bitches have a split heat after shipping that may be stress related.
III. Abnormal estrous cycle
   A. Short interestrous interval
      1. Bitches that cycle as frequently as every 4 months or less are abnormal.
      2. A short interestrous interval may occur if a bitch fails to ovulate.
      3. If a bitch ovulates with each cycle, it is possible that the uterus has insufficient time to recover from the trophic effects of progesterone before the next cycle occurs (Al-Bassam et al., 1981).
      4. Cystic endometrial hyperplasia may develop

as a result of repeated diestral progesterone influence.
      5. Split heats may be occurring.
         a) There is an abrupt end to proestrus/estrus followed by 2–4 weeks of anestrus before beginning a new estrous cycle.
         b) Ovulation may eventually occur with the new cycle; fertility would be normal at that point.
         c) It is more common in pubertal bitches and may spontaneously resolve with maturity.
   B. Long interestrous interval
      1. An interestrous interval >10 months is abnormal for most breeds.
      2. Some breeds, such as the basenji, normally cycle only once per year.
      3. Some bitches cycle sporadically but are fertile.
      4. If the interestrous interval is sporadic or prolonged in a bitch that fails to conceive, consider the following.
         a) Underlying illness, including endocrinologic disease or neoplasia
         b) Drug administration such as glucocorticoids and antineoplastic agents
         c) Older bitches (>6–8 years)
            (1) There is a significant decrease in conception rate, number of puppies whelped, and puppy viability after 8 years of age.
            (2) Aged bitches have a high incidence of cystic endometrial hyperplasia and decreased frequency of ovulation.
      5. Silent, ovulatory estrus may be occurring.
         a) Outward signs of proestrus/estrus inapparent to the owner
         b) Possibly more common in bitches housed alone
   C. Persistent anestrus should be evaluated in a bitch over 2 years of age that has not had a pubertal estrus or in bitches that apparently cease estrous cyclicity.
      1. Estrous cycles may occur without outward signs of proestrus or estrus (silent estrus).
      2. Underlying systemic disease may cause persistent anestrus.
      3. If a bitch fails to show pubertal estrus, an intersex condition may exist (see Chap. 58).
      4. Premature ovarian failure may be a cause of persistent anestrus (see Chap. 54).
      5. Oophoritis or ovarian cysts may also be a cause.
   D. Abnormally long proestrus or estrus may also occur.
      1. Either phase lasting longer than 21 days is considered abnormal.
      2. Pubertal cycles may be abnormal but spontaneously normalize with maturity.
      3. Follicular cysts or ovarian neoplasms producing estrogen (± progesterone) may be a cause.

4. Idiopathic oophoritis may also cause estrous cycle abnormalities.

Diagnosis

I. Obtain a complete medical and reproductive history.
II. Perform a thorough physical examination with vaginal and rectal palpation.
III. Perform a vaginoscopic examination.
   A. Specialized equipment is necessary to insufflate and visualize the entire length of the canine vagina.
   B. An otoscope is insufficient in all but toy breeds.
IV. Rule out brucellosis.
   A. All bitches should be screened for *B. canis* prior to each breeding.
   B. Stud dogs should be screened every 6 months and bred only to tested bitches.
V. Determine ovulation timing to detect management errors (see Chap. 53).
VI. Screen for underlying illness with a hemogram, biochemistry profile, and urinalysis.
   A. Additional diagnostic tests to evaluate for hyper- or hypoadrenocorticism or hypothyroidism are performed when indicated by clinical signs.
   B. Bitches with confirmed endocrinologic diseases should not be used for breeding because of possible heritability.
VII. Consider hormonal assays.
   A. Progesterone determination is the most useful.
      1. When determined in diestrus, serum progesterone concentration >5 ng/ml indicates that the bitch ovulated and has functional corpora lutea.
      2. If luteal insufficiency is suspected, serum progesterone concentration should be monitored weekly during gestation.
      3. Gestational serum progesterone concentration <2 ng/ml is inadequate to support pregnancy (Concannon et al., 1977).
      4. A silent, ovulatory estrus can be documented (see Causes).
   B. Evaluation of serum estrogen concentration is generally unhelpful unless signs of prolonged proestrus/estrus are seen.
   C. Serum gonadotropins may be evaluated in cases of persistent anestrus.
      1. A luteinizing hormone (LH) assay is commercially available, but one for follicle-stimulating hormone (FSH) is not.
      2. Significant, repeatable elevation of LH concentration is consistent with ovariectomy or ovarian degeneration (see Chap. 54).
VIII. Ultrasonography helps characterize uterine changes.
   A. Detects pregnancy (approximately 20–23 days after last breeding), which is important in differentiating conception failure from fetal resorption
   B. Provides indication of fetal viability and estimation of litter size
   C. Allows differentiation of pyometra from pregnancy

D. May detect other uterine or ovarian disease, e.g., neoplasia
IX. A guarded swab may be used to culture the cranial vagina (see Chap. 57).
   A. Isolation of aerobic bacteria is difficult to interpret, because normal flora are often recovered (Bjurström and Linde-Forsberg, 1992).
   B. *Mycoplasma* spp. can be isolated with special handling, but positive growth may represent normal flora.
X. In a bitch with resorption of fetuses or abortion, test for canine herpesvirus (CHV).
   A. Viral isolation can be achieved from swab samples (Viral culturettes, Marion Scientific, Kansas City, MO) of vaginal discharge.
   B. Aborted fetal tissues and placentae should be chilled (not frozen) and submitted for CHV isolation.
   C. Serum antibody titers to CHV are relatively low (i.e., 1:2 up to 1:32) and generally persist only 4–8 weeks after exposure. Paired titers are suggested, but any positive titer, coincident with clinical signs, is significant.
XI. Karyotyping is recommended to evaluate for intersex conditions or other abnormalities in cases of primary anestrus or prolonged proestrus.
XII. Exploratory laparotomy is an aggressive but helpful diagnostic step.
   A. The uterus, ovaries, and areas of the oviducts can be directly palpated.
   B. Obtain uterine biopsies for evaluation of endometrial disease.
   C. Obtain cultures from the uterine lumen for aerobic bacteria and *Mycoplasma* spp.; positive growth from the uterus is significant.

Treatment

I. The key to treatment is finding the cause of apparent infertility and correcting the problem.
II. In a bitch that fails to breed, consider the following.
   A. Correct a vaginal stricture or other anomaly.
   B. Time ovulation to determine if the breeding is managed correctly (see Chap. 53).
   C. Change the environment.
      1. If either animal is apprehensive, provide an alternative setting.
      2. The stud dog may overcome an aggressive bitch if she is brought into his environment.
   D. Artificial insemination may be necessary if a cause cannot be found.
III. For bitches with normal estrous cycles, try the following.
   A. A test breeding should be conducted during the next estrus.
      1. Attempt natural matings with an aggressive stud dog that has recently sired litters.
      2. Ovulation timing is performed so that breedings occur during the period of optimum fertility.
      3. Do not ship the bitch for breeding.

B. If a bitch has ovulation failure, ovulation can be hormonally induced.
1. Give human chorionic gonadotropin (HCG) 500–1000 IU IM, SQ.
2. The HCG is injected at the point of maximal vaginal cornification.
3. Inappropriate administration of HCG can cause premature follicular luteinization and thereby prevent ovulation of viable ova.
C. If a large number of *Mycoplasma* spp. are recovered with a cranial vaginal culture, systemic antibiotics (chloramphenicol, tetracycline, or enrofloxacin) are given for 2–3 weeks.
1. The ideal time for such treatment is just preceding the next estrous cycle.
2. Antibiotic therapy is discontinued when behavioral estrus begins.
3. No studies have been published to prove that this regimen is effective.
D. For concerns during pregnancy when luteal insufficiency has been documented during a prior gestation and serum progesterone concentration is low (2–5 ng/ml), consider progesterone supplementation.
1. Inappropriate supplementation may induce masculinization of female fetuses, causing anomalous urogenital system development.
2. To maintain serum progesterone concentration >10 ng/ml, inject progesterone in oil 3 mg/kg IM daily (Scott-Moncrieff et al., 1990).
3. If progesterone supplementation is continued beyond days 50–55 of gestation, spontaneous parturition may be inhibited.
IV. For bitches with short interestrous intervals that ovulate with each cycle, try estrus suppression with mibolerone.
A. Give the usual dosage for 6–9 months.
B. No studies have been published to prove the efficacy of this protocol.
V. For bitches with primary anestrus for which an underlying cause cannot be determined, estrus induction has been suggested.
A. No published estrus induction protocols using commercially available hormones will reliably induce fertile estrus in bitches with normal estrous cycles, however.
B. A variety of protocols have been suggested, including the use of gonadotropin-releasing hormone (GnRH), GnRH analogues, gonadotropins, estrogens, and ergot derivatives (Cain, 1995; Feldman and Nelson, 1996).

Patient Monitoring

I. When a cause for the apparent infertility can be found and corrected, the prognosis for fertility is favorable.
II. Breeding management error is the most common cause of apparent infertility, and the easiest to correct.
III. Owners may not wish to pursue a thorough diagnos-

tic evaluation of a bitch that is of marginal breeding quality, and ovariohysterectomy may be considered.

PSEUDOCYESIS

Definition

A physical and behavioral condition simulating pregnancy that occurs in the nonpregnant bitch.

Causes and Pathophysiology

I. During diestrus, nonpregnant bitches with normal ovarian function have serum progesterone concentrations indistinguishable from pregnant bitches.
II. The reason that clinical manifestations of pseudocyesis occur in some bitches and not in others is unknown.
III. Decreasing serum progesterone concentrations and subsequent increases in prolactin secretion at the end of diestrus cause overt manifestations of periparturient behavior.
IV. Signs may be observed in bitches after ovariohysterectomy in diestrus because removal of the ovaries simulates parturition with a rapid drop in progesterone and a consequent rise in prolactin.

Clinical Signs

I. Mid-diestrus signs may be similar to signs of midgestation.
A. Mammary gland development
B. Behavioral changes such as aggression and lethargy
C. Possible weight gain in bitches from overfeeding because owners believe the bitch is pregnant
II. Toward the end of diestrus (60–80 days postestrus), overt periparturient signs appear.
A. Nesting, restlessness, aggression, anorexia
B. ''Mothering'' of inanimate objects
C. Lactation
1. Mammary glands may produce normal milk or a brownish watery fluid.
2. Mastitis in engorged mammary glands is a possible sequela.

Differential Diagnosis

I. Normal pregnancy must be ruled out.
II. The administration of progestogens may cause signs of pseudocyesis, and milk production may occur when the drug is discontinued.

Treatment

I. Therapy is generally necessary only in those bitches showing marked behavioral changes.
II. Signs of pseudocyesis can be abbreviated with mibolerone 16 µg/kg PO daily for 3–5 days (Brown, 1984).
III. Also consider abruptly decreasing the bitch's food

and water consumption for 24–48 hours to decrease lactation.

Patient Monitoring

I. Recurrence is common with subsequent estrous cycles.
II. There is no association with diminished fertility in future estrous cycles.

INFERTILITY IN THE MALE DOG

Melissa S. Wallace

Definition

I. The infertile male dog is unable to breed or to produce a pregnancy when bred to fertile bitches in estrus.
II. The subfertile dog has reduced ability to produce a pregnancy or produces pregnancies of small litter size.
III. There are several requirements for male dog fertility.
   A. The dog must be capable of erection, intromission, and ejaculation.
   B. The testes of the dog must produce sufficient numbers of normal, motile spermatozoa.
   C. The reproductive duct system must be patent to deliver the spermatozoa.
   D. The spermatozoa must be capable of capacitation, penetration of the zona pellucida of the ovum, and fertilization.

Causes and Pathophysiology

I. Failure to breed is one cause of male infertility.
   A. Breeding management errors
      1. Attempting to breed when the bitch is not in behavioral estrus
      2. Breeding inexperienced dogs to inexperienced bitches
      3. Attempting to breed dogs with behavioral problems such as excessive submission or aggression
   B. Physical inability of the dog to mount and achieve intromission
      1. Congenital or acquired defects of the penis or prepuce may prevent normal copulation (see Chap. 58).
      2. Disorders of the vulva or vagina may prevent normal intromission (see Chap. 57).
      3. Failure to achieve an "inside tie" during breeding is usually caused by engorgement of the bulbus glandis prior to penetration of the penis into the vagina.
         a) From overexcitement or inexperience
         b) Ejaculation unlikely to result in pregnancy
      4. Conformational characteristics acquired through selective breeding may result in dogs that cannot breed naturally.
      5. An orthopedic injury may cause temporary or permanent disability preventing natural breeding.
   C. Poor libido
      1. Behavioral disorders
      2. Congenital or acquired defects of the hypothalamic-pituitary-gonadal axis with hypotestosteronism
         a) Hypopituitarism (see Chap. 40)
         b) Acquired endocrine diseases: hypothyroidism, hyperestrogenism, hyperadrenocorticism
         c) Drugs: direct or indirect effects (Freshman, 1989)
      3. Any underlying illness
II. Infertility may occur in dogs with normal libido and ability to breed but that have ejaculatory failure or yield an incomplete ejaculation.
   A. Incomplete ejaculation
      1. Ejaculation without production of sperm-rich fraction (see Canine Semen Collection and Analysis)
      2. Fright, stress, or inexperience
      3. Pain or anticipation of pain
         a) Prostatic inflammation
         b) Failure of collector to retract the prepuce behind the bulbus glandis (Olson, 1991)
      4. During manual semen collection without a teaser bitch
   B. Retrograde ejaculation
      1. The spermatozoa are found in the urinary bladder after ejaculation.
      2. Abnormality of the internal urethral sphincter and/or sympathetic nervous system may allow retrograde ejaculation.
   C. Ejaculatory dysfunction
      1. Dogs have an erection but fail to produce any ejaculate (aspermia).
      2. Disorders of the sympathetic nervous system may be a cause.
III. Infertility and subfertility may occur in dogs with normal libido and breeding behavior that have abnormal sperm production and/or output.
   A. Abnormalities (see also Canine Semen Collection and Analysis)
      1. Azoospermia: essentially no sperm in the ejaculate
      2. Oligospermia: decreased amount of sperm in the ejaculate
         a) Relative to normal amount expected for age and breed
         b) Temporary decrease in sperm quantity from repeated daily ejaculation
      3. Teratozoospermia: high percentage of morphologically abnormal sperm
      4. Asthenozoospermia: high percentage of sperm without normal motility
      5. Seminal fluid changes: blood, urine, leukocytes, proteins, or antibodies
   B. Congenital causes
      1. Azoospermia may be caused by aspermatogenesis (Meyers-Wallen and Patterson, 1989).
         a) XXY syndrome

b) XX male syndrome

c) Testicular hypoplasia

2. Oligospermia may have a congenital cause (Meyers-Wallen, 1991).

   a) Unilateral segmental aplasia of the ductule system

   b) Unilateral cryptorchidism

   c) Testicular hypoplasia

3. Sperm motility or morphologic defects may occur with congenital problems, such as Kartagener's syndrome, which results in immotile cilia.

C. Acquired causes

1. Senile atrophy (see Chap. 55)

   a) Also referred to as idiopathic testicular degeneration

   b) Usually associated with advancing age

   c) May spontaneously occur at young ages, however

   d) Arrested spermatogenesis; seminiferous tubules degenerate, eventually atrophy

   e) An irreversible condition

2. Drugs

   a) Affect the germinal epithelium within the seminiferous tubules: antineoplastic, cytotoxic agents

   b) Interfere with the normal hypothalamic-pituitary-gonadal axis (Freshman, 1989)

     (1) Methyltestosterone

     (2) Estradiol

     (3) Diethylstilbestrol

     (4) Tamoxifen citrate

     (5) Glucocorticoids

     (6) Anabolic steroids

     (7) Anti-gonadotropin-releasing hormone (Anti-GnRH) analogues

     (8) GnRH agonists

   c) Inhibit androgen synthesis

     (1) Spironolactone

     (2) Ketoconazole

     (3) Cimetidine

3. Environmental toxins and radiation

4. Elevated environmental temperature, febrile episodes, or scrotal inflammation

5. Infectious orchiepididymitis

   a) Bacterial infections

   b) *Brucella canis*

   c) *Mycoplasma*

6. Immune-mediated orchiepididymitis; destruction of spermatogonia, inflammation and obstruction of the duct system

7. Testicular tumors

   a) Local invasion of testicular tissue

   b) May secrete steroidal hormones, which cause negative feedback to the hypothalamus and pituitary, resulting in aspermatogenesis (Feldman and Nelson, 1996)

8. Tumors of the hypothalamus or pituitary

D. Bilateral obstruction of the male duct system

1. Congenital segmental aplasia

2. Acquired obstruction from sperm granulomas or scar tissue

Clinical Signs

I. Signalment

  A. Geriatric dogs may have reduced sperm output (Lowseth et al., 1990).

  B. Pubertal dogs may have abnormal spermatozoa (Amann, 1986).

  C. Specific breeds of dogs are predisposed to hypothyroidism (see Chap. 41).

  D. Breed conformation may preclude natural breeding.

II. There are often no clinical signs in the infertile male dog.

III. Dogs with acute orchiepididymitis or prostatitis are symptomatic (see Chaps. 52 and 55).

Diagnosis

I. Perform a thorough physical examination, paying particular attention to the reproductive system.

  A. Examine the prepuce and penis for tumors, trauma, congenital abnormalities, or abnormal urethral discharge.

  B. Palpate the scrotum for abnormalities such as dermatitis, tumors, or adhesions of the scrotum to the testes.

  C. Palpate the testes for size, texture, and symmetry.

  D. Palpate the epididymides along the dorsolateral surface of each testis and follow each spermatic cord to the inguinal ring.

    1. Areas of thickening or nodules indicate granulomas or neoplasia.

    2. Absent areas in the tubular tract indicate segmental aplasia.

  E. Palpate the prostate gland abdominally and rectally.

II. A complete semen evaluation is undertaken as described later. Abnormalities in semen dictate further diagnostics.

III. Obtain a minimum laboratory database.

  A. Complete blood count, serum biochemical profile, urinalysis

  B. Screening test for brucellosis

  C. Thyroid evaluation in some cases

IV. Karyotyping is recommended if congenital infertility is suspected.

V. Cytology of the ejaculate is useful if the semen evaluation is abnormal.

  A. Elevated numbers of white blood cells (WBC) suggest inflammatory disease.

    1. Neutrophils may be contaminants from the urethra, but macrophages indicate chronic infection.

    2. Toxic neutrophils or phagocytosis of bacteria implies infection.

  B. Abnormal epithelial cells may be associated with prostatic neoplasia.

  C. Fractionating the ejaculate during collection into sperm-rich versus prostatic fluid, and comparing the two fractions, may help localize the site of disease.

VI. Culture and sensitivity of the ejaculate are indicated

in cases of oligozoospermia, poor sperm motility or morphology, increased inflammatory cells, or palpable abnormalities of the prostate, testes, or epididymides.

  A. Aerobic bacterial culture and sensitivity
  B. Isolation of *Mycoplasma* and *Ureaplasma*
    1. The semen should arrive chilled at the laboratory within 24 hours, or be placed in appropriate media, such as Amies without charcoal.
    2. Because these organisms can be part of the normal urethral flora, interpretation of their significance in cases of infertility is difficult.
  C. ± Anaerobic bacterial culture

VII. Consider assaying epididymal markers, i.e., substances found in high concentration in the epididymis but not in other areas of the reproductive tract (Olson, 1991).
  A. There are two uses for epididymal markers.
    1. Incomplete ejaculation is associated with low concentrations of an epididymal marker in the ejaculatory fluid.
    2. In cases of azoospermia, the concentration of an epididymal marker in the seminal plasma will be low with bilateral obstruction of the excretory ducts, but high with failure of spermatogenesis.
  B. Carnitine is an epididymal marker, but assays for it are not routinely available.
  C. Alkaline phosphatase is found in high concentrations in seminal plasma.
    1. It can be measured with the same techniques as for measuring serum alkaline phosphatase.
    2. Normal seminal plasma alkaline phosphatase is >5000 IU/L (Johnston, 1991).

VIII. Endocrinologic evaluation may be helpful.
  A. Assay serum testosterone concentrations in dogs with impaired libido and decreased sperm production.
    1. Normal resting serum testosterone concentration in intact male dogs is 0.5–5 ng/ml.
    2. Owing to fluctuations in secretion of testosterone, challenge testing is better than assaying resting values (Shille and Olson, 1989).
  B. Serum testosterone in normal dogs will rise following administration of HCG or GnRH.
    1. Give HCG 44 IU/kg IM.
      a) Measure testosterone at 0 and 4 hours.
      b) Normal post-HCG values = 4.6–7.5 ng/ml.
    2. Give GnRH 2.2 μg/kg IM.
      a) Measure testosterone before and 1 hour after administration.
      b) Normal values at 1 hour = 3.7–6.2 ng/ml.
      c) Remember that in using GnRH, the pituitary must be capable of gonadotropin release (Shille and Olson, 1989).
  C. Evaluation of serum gonadotropins may be useful in azoospermic dogs.
    1. Resting serum LH concentration must be interpreted cautiously.
      a) Because of episodic secretion, LH concentrations in normal and castrated dogs may overlap (Olson et al., 1992).
      b) At least three samples at 20- to 30-minute intervals are analyzed (Shille and Olson, 1989).
      c) If testosterone and LH are decreased, the cause of azoospermia is hypothalamic or pituitary.
      d) When testosterone is decreased and LH is increased, suspect a primary failure of Leydig's cells (Feldman and Nelson, 1996).
    2. Repetitive sampling of FSH may be helpful.
      a) Elevated FSH concentrations are indicative of testicular pathology (Freshman et al., 1988).
      b) As spermatogenesis fails, decreased secretion of inhibin by Sertoli's cells may occur, resulting in diminished negative feedback and secondary elevation of FSH concentration (Shille and Olson, 1989).
      c) Currently a canine-specific assay for FSH is not commercially available.
    3. Evaluation of plasma LH before and 10 minutes after administration of GnRH 250 ng/kg IV may be useful in localizing the cause of azoospermia (Shille and Olson, 1989).
      a) If testosterone response to challenge testing (described earlier) is abnormal, finding normal LH response to GnRH supports the diagnosis of primary testicular dysfunction.
      b) If the LH response to GnRH is abnormally low, azoospermia may be pituitary in origin.

IX. Radiography and ultrasonography are useful to evaluate dogs with infertility associated with testicular or prostatic disease or neoplasia.

X. Testicular biopsy is indicated in the persistently azoospermic or oligozoospermic dog.
  A. It is not a benign procedure, as it disrupts the blood-testis barrier.
  B. A wedge biopsy is obtained to provide enough seminiferous tubules for evaluation (Feldman and Nelson, 1996).
    1. The tissue must be fixed in Bouin's or Zenker's solution rather than formalin.
    2. Testicular tissue may be cultured at the time of biopsy.

XI. Epididymal aspiration is used for suspected epididymal disease or ductule obstruction.
  A. Consider whether the information gained will outweigh the risk of inducing a sperm granuloma.
  B. The technique involves the insertion of a fine needle into the caudal epididymis and gently aspirating fluid for cytologic evaluation.

Differential Diagnosis

I. Rule out infertility in the bitch.
II. Poor breeding management, particularly with respect to ovulation timing, must also be ruled out.

Treatment

I. General principles of therapy
  A. Treatment should be based on a specific diagnosis.
  B. Empirical hormonal therapies are mostly unhelpful and may be deleterious.
    1. Reserve hormonal therapies for cases that have persistent or worsening infertility.
    2. Use hormonal therapies only after a complete diagnostic evaluation.
    3. Testosterone administration decreases gonadotropin secretion and results in decreased spermatogenesis.

II. Therapy of systemic diseases
  A. Infertility associated with systemic diseases is often reversible if the drugs used to treat the diseases do not damage fertility further.
  B. When systemic endocrinopathies are controlled, fertility may improve.
    1. Breeding animals that have an endocrinologic disease is a questionable practice.
    2. A genetic tendency may be the underlying cause of many diseases.

III. Treatment of primary reproductive disorders
  A. Bacterial orchitis and epididymitis (see Chap. 55)
  B. Mycoplasmal infection of the prostate, epididymides, and testes
    1. Tetracycline 15–22 mg/kg PO TID for 3 weeks
    2. Doxycycline loading dose of 5 mg/kg, then 2.5 mg/kg PO SID for 10 days; repeated in 10 days
    3. Enrofloxacin 5 mg/kg PO BID or ciprofloxacin 5–10 mg/kg PO BID for 2–3 weeks
    4. Reinfection common, requiring repeated therapy
  C. Immune-mediated orchitis and/or epididymitis (see Chap. 55)
    1. Consider prednisone 2 mg/kg/day PO.
    2. Glucocorticoids impair spermatogenesis, making a return to fertility unlikely (Feldman and Nelson, 1996).
  D. Chronic bacterial prostatitis (see Chap. 52)
  E. Endocrine disorders of the reproductive system
    1. Dogs with low testosterone and elevated FSH and normal or elevated LH have primary testicular degeneration or atrophy.
      a) There is no known treatment.
      b) Administration of androgens is unsuccessful (Feldman and Nelson, 1996).
    2. Dogs with normal testosterone and LH but with elevated FSH usually have failure of spermatogenesis.
      a) No practical effective treatment is available.
      b) Possible future therapy in oligozoospermic dogs is pulsatile administration of GnRH using an implantable pump (Meyers-Wallen, 1991).
    3. Dogs with normal gonadotropin levels and infertility may have a variety of disorders.

      a) Because hormone levels are normal, hormonal therapy is unlikely to be successful.
      b) Therapy with antiestrogen agents such as tamoxifen and clomoxifen citrate has been suggested, but data are lacking for the dog.
    4. Dogs with decreased testosterone, LH, and FSH have hypogonadotropic hypogonadism, which is most likely acquired.
      a) Rule out a pituitary tumor prior to attempting treatment for infertility.
      b) The general well-being of the dog may outweigh reproductive capability.
      c) Various drugs with FSH and LH effects may be tried (Feldman and Nelson, 1996).
        (1) HCG 500 IU SQ twice weekly is used to stimulate Leydig's cell function.
        (2) FSH at 25 mg SQ once weekly or 1 mg/kg IM every other day may be used to stimulate spermatogenesis.
        (3) Oral methyltestosterone or the synthetic androgen mesterolone can be used to stimulate libido.
        (4) Therapy must be continued for at least 3 months, but once spermatogenesis is achieved, it may be maintained with HCG alone.

IV. Treatment of retrograde ejaculation and failure of ejaculation (aspermia)
  A. Alpha-adrenergic drugs may improve internal urethral sphincter tone, improving antegrade ejaculation (see Chap. 50).
  B. Alpha-adrenergic drugs may increase the response to stimulation from the sympathetic nervous system, which is required for ejaculation.

Patient Monitoring

I. Prognosis for a return to fertility varies with the cause.
  A. Some insults to the testes are potentially reversible.
    1. Drugs and toxins
    2. High environmental temperature and fever
  B. Infectious causes of infertility are treatable, but prognosis varies with the site and degree of damage.
  C. Many cases of male infertility have a poor to guarded prognosis in spite of appropriate diagnosis and therapy.

II. Repeat semen evaluations every 2–3 months.
  A. Spermatogenesis requires 62 days in the dog (Amann, 1986).
  B. Epididymal transit requires about 15 days.

III. Monitor semen quality for 6–12 months.
  A. Production of multiple generations of spermatozoa may be needed to raise the sperm count to normal.
  B. An insult to the spermatogonia may take 2 months to be fully reflected in the semen evaluation.

IV. Repeated diagnostic testing is based on the original diagnosis.
   A. Culture and cytology of the ejaculate
   B. Ultrasonography of prostate or testes
   C. Aspiration of persistent prostatic lesions for culture and cytology
   D. Frequency of repeated testing proportional to the severity of the disorder

CANINE SEMEN COLLECTION AND ANALYSIS

Melissa F. Goodman

Definition

I. Indications
   A. Breeding soundness examination
   B. Infertility investigation
   C. Artificial insemination
   D. Semen freezing
   E. Shipping chilled semen
II. Requirements for success
   A. Proper collection technique
   B. Good libido in stud dog

Preparation of Equipment

I. Materials coming in contact with the ejaculate *must* be free of any spermicidal residues from cleaning and/or sterilization procedures.
   A. Wash artificial vagina (AV) and collection tubes.
      1. Soak AV in boiling water for 20 minutes 2–3 times.
      2. Then wash AV and tubes in a mild dishwashing liquid, rinse 3 times in tap water and 3 times in distilled water before initial use.
   B. Reusable items are soaked in a disinfectant solution, then washed and rinsed as described earlier.
   C. Alternatively, use a disposable AV and tubes.
II. Collection equipment should be at room temperature or slightly warmer.
III. Attach a 15-ml polystyrene collection tube, with a small vent hole at the top, to the latex AV.
   A. Stretch the AV tip to cover the top of the collection tube so that it will not fall off during the collection procedure.
   B. Do not cover the vent hole, or the semen will not flow freely into the tube during collection.
IV. If using a disposable plastic AV, the collection tube does not need to be vented, but can be attached to the AV with a rubber ring.
V. Fold down the open end of the AV to form a cuff.
   A. The cuff should be 1 in. for large or giant breeds and 2–3 in. for small or medium dogs.
   B. The cuff allows ease in handling the AV when it is placed over the erect penis.
VI. Lubricants are not used because most are spermicidal and are rarely necessary.

Preparation of Dogs and Environment

I. Perform collections in a quiet area.
   A. Use a rubber-backed mat to provide secure footing.
   B. Be patient and nonthreatening.
II. One or two assistants should be available for restraint and to help separate collected fractions.
III. Allow stud dog to urinate completely before the collection to minimize urine contamination of ejaculate.
IV. Always use a teaser bitch.
   A. Increased libido of stud dog will significantly increase sperm count and motility quality.
   B. If libido is poor or the dog is reluctant to ejaculate, he can refrain from ejaculating sperm, even though presperm and prostatic fluids are ejaculated.
   C. Ideally, use a teaser bitch in estrus that is of the same approximate size as the stud dog.
   D. Alternatively, a placid bitch with estrus scent applied to her vulva can be used.
      1. Estrus secretions can be collected on a cotton swab, kept frozen, and thawed in 2–3 ml warm water, when needed.
      2. Stimulating chemicals may also be used but are not as effective as actual estrus secretions.
         a) *P*-Hydroxybenzoic acid methyl ester by Sigma Chemical Co., St. Louis, MO
         b) Eau d'Estrus by International Canine Genetics, Malvern, PA

Collection Technique

I. Allow the stud dog to mount the bitch; as he starts to thrust, slide the prepuce behind the bulbus glandis. Manual stimulation may be necessary if libido is poor.
   A. If 50% erection occurs before the prepuce is pulled back, do not force it over the enlarged bulbus glandis.
      1. Allow the dog to dismount, walk him away from the bitch, and allow his erection to subside.
      2. Then bring him back to the bitch, and this time slide the prepuce behind the bulbus glandis earlier.
   B. If full erection occurs within the prepuce, it is usually painful and may result in incomplete ejaculation.
II. Slip the AV, with the attached collection tube, over the exposed glans penis and the bulbus glandis.
III. The collector forms a ring with a thumb and forefinger proximal to the bulbus glandis to simulate the bitch's vaginal opening. Gently grasp the bulbus glandis, maintaining a gentle but constant pressure throughout the collection.
IV. Allow the dog to step over the collector's arm, redirecting the penis 180 degrees backwards between his legs; this approximates the position of the coital lock during a natural tie.
V. Separate the fractions during collection, which allows better evaluation and identification of the source of any problems present in the ejaculate.

A. Dogs ejaculate in three fractions.
  1. First fraction (presperm)
    a) Produced by the prostate and urethral glands
    b) Clear to slightly cloudy
    c) Released during the period of vigorous thrusting
    d) Contains few sperm cells
  2. Second fraction (sperm-rich)
    a) Made up almost entirely of spermatozoa
    b) White, opaque, thick
    c) Released just after vigorous thrusting ends and intromission is complete
  3. Third fraction (prostatic fluid)
    a) Produced by the prostate
    b) Clear to slightly cloudy
    c) Contains few sperm cells but contributes a major portion of the total volume of the ejaculate
B. Seminal plasma (nonsperm portion of the ejaculate) contributes volume and decreases the concentration of the semen, allowing motility.
  1. It is, however, detrimental to the longevity of sperm in vitro.
  2. This effect may be so dramatic that motility decreases within minutes after collection unless the fractions are separated.
  3. This effect is usually nonexistent with natural breeding.
C. There are two techniques for separation of the ejaculate.
  1. Switch collection tubes as the ejaculate changes.
    a) Fractions may be visualized as the semen flows into the clear collection tubes.
    b) In addition, most dogs have a detectable brief pause between fractions.
    c) It is easiest to have one person perform the collection and another switch the tubes.
      (1) After the first tube is removed from the AV, use additional tubes to collect the different fractions.
      (2) The AV tip is pinched and placed inside the additional tubes, as it is difficult to stretch the AV around the outside of a tube during the ejaculation process.
  2. If unable to switch tubes, the sample may be centrifuged.
    a) Centrifuge at 2000 g for 10–15 minutes.
    b) It is more traumatic to sperm than separating fractions during collection.
    c) A commercial product may protect the sperm during centrifugation (Semen Separating Solution by International Canine Genetics, Malvern, PA).
VI. Gently remove the AV from the penis by grasping the cuffed portion of the AV and pulling down.
  A. Apply lubricant to the engorged penis if needed.
  B. Be sure that the penis is fully retracted into the prepuce before returning the dog to the kennel.

Semen Analysis

I. Volume
  A. May be read directly from the calibrated collection tube
  B. Expected normal volume
    1. First fraction: 0.5–10 ml
    2. Second fraction: 0.25–3 ml
    3. Third fraction: 2–40 ml
  C. Results
    1. Variable from dog to dog
    2. Not an actual measure of sperm quality or quantity
II. Color
  A. Normal is white, ranging from opalescent to thick, depending on concentration of sperm cells.
  B. Yellow indicates urine contamination, which is toxic to sperm.
  C. Red/brown color indicates the presence of blood; blood is not spermicidal.
    1. Often the result of abrasions of the tip of the penis and/or stimulation of the highly vascular penis and prostate
    2. May reflect inflammation or infection anywhere along the reproductive tract
  D. Clear ejaculate indicates azoospermia.
    1. May be the result of poor libido and lack of release of the sperm-rich fraction
    2. May reflect infertility
III. Motility
  A. Place 1 drop of sperm-rich fraction on a pre-warmed slide, cover with a coverslip.
    1. Try to obtain a standard-sized drop.
    2. Examine under low magnification ($10\times$).
    3. Examine several fields, choosing an area near the center that does not contain air bubbles.
  B. If the sample is too concentrated to evaluate, mix one drop of semen with 1 drop of physiologic saline at 37°C and re-examine.
  C. Record percent motility, speed (slow, moderate, fast) of movement, and quality of forward progression.
    1. Excellent quality motility: smooth, straight, linear forward progression
    2. Good: minor degree of deviation from linear, yet still good forward progression
    3. Average: more deviation from linear, but overall still progressing forward
    4. Poor: sperm cells moving, but little or no forward progression; only jiggling in place or spinning
  D. Criteria for normal fertility is >70% progressively motile sperm; however, most normal healthy stud dogs produce semen with 90% motility, moderate to fast speed, and good to excellent quality of forward progression.
  E. It is important to use a slide warmer, because motility is greater at physiologic temperature (37°C) than at room temperature (25°C).
IV. Sperm count
  A. Owing to variability in ejaculate volume, sperm quantity per ejaculate rather than sperm concentration per ml is evaluated.

1. Normal sperm counts range from 200 million to 2–3 billion per ejaculate (depending on the breed).
2. Larger breeds have higher counts, reflecting higher seminiferous tubular volume.

B. Gently agitate the semen sample, because sperm cells settle at the bottom of the tube.

C. Use a Unopette #5853 (designed for WBC ± platelet counts) and hemocytometer.
   1. Fill the Unopette and let it sit at room temperature for 15 minutes.
   2. Charge the hemocytometer and allow it to sit for 5 minutes.
   3. Count three of the nine large hemocytometer squares.
      a) Add the three values together, multiply by 3, add 10% of the total, and divide by 10 to give the sperm concentration per ml.
      b) Multiply this result by the volume in the tube from which the Unopette sample was taken to determine the sperm count per ejaculate.

V. Morphology

A. Prepare the slide using eosin/nigrosin or Diff-Quik stain.

B. Examine under oil immersion and evaluate 100 sperm, noting number of abnormalities seen.
   1. Primary abnormalities associated with abnormal spermatogenesis are head defects and midpiece and tail deformities.
   2. Secondary abnormalities associated with maturation and transport through the epididymis, or caused by trauma to the sperm during the collection process, are detached normal heads, retained cytoplasmic droplets, and bent tails.

C. Decreased fertility has been reported when the number of morphologically normal sperm falls below 60% (Oettlé, 1993).

D. A morphology-specific stain has been recommended (Oettlé, 1995), but its reliability has not been established.

VI. Cytology

A. Centrifuge sample to concentrate the cells.

B. Examine Diff-Quik stained smear.

C. Subjectively note quantity of WBC, red blood cells (RBC), bacteria, and cellular debris.

VII. Semen pH

A. Place one drop of the sperm-rich and/or third fraction on test tape pH paper.

B. Normal canine semen pH is 6.3–7; that of prostatic fluid alone is 6.0–7.4.

C. There is no known correlation between pH and semen quality or fertility.

DYSTOCIA

Autumn P. Davidson

Definition

I. Normal parturition

A. Vaginal delivery of a litter at full term without difficulty

B. Consists of three stages
   1. First-stage labor
      a) It is preceded by a decline in plasma progesterone concentration to <2ng/ml and a subsequent drop in body temperature to <99°F.
      b) Onset occurs within 24 hours of the drop in body temperature. Owners should monitor body temperature twice daily for the last 7 days of gestation.
      c) Uterine contractions occur (not visible externally), with eventual cervical dilatation.
      d) Nesting, restlessness, panting, trembling, and inappetence or vomiting can occur.
      e) It averages 12–24 hours in duration.
   2. Second-stage labor
      a) There are visible contractions, with fetal expulsion occuring within 1 hour.
      b) Puppy delivery alternates between both uterine horns.
      c) The normal interval between puppies varies from minutes to several hours but does not normally exceed 1 hour with continuous contractions.
   3. Third-stage labor
      a) Expulsion of the placental membranes
      b) Alternates with stage II
      c) Placentae possibly eaten by the bitch and not detected

II. Dystocia

A. A bitch's inability or failure to expel fetus(es) through the birth canal at term

B. Can result in fetal or maternal morbidity or mortality without intervention
   1. Maternal death can occur from peritonitis, septic or hypovolemic shock, or disseminated intravascular coagulation.
   2. Fetal or neonatal death can occur from umbilical cord compression, premature placental separation, ineffective or compressive myometrial contractions, or incompatible fetal and maternal anatomy.

Causes and Pathophysiology

I. Prolonged gestation

A. Gestation of >70 days from the first breeding, >66 days from the LH surge, or >60 days of diestrus (Feldman and Nelson, 1996)

B. Occurs secondary to a small litter size, with failure of the fetus(es) to initiate labor

C. Also occurs secondary to primary uterine inertia, with failure to enter stage II labor

II. Maternal factors

A. Excessive nervousness

B. Primary uterine inertia
   1. No stage II labor occurs.
   2. Stage I occurs normally.

C. Secondary uterine inertia
   1. Stage II labor ceases often after prolonged efforts to deliver fetuses.

2. Myometrial exhaustion and subclinical hypocalcemia/hypoglycemia can be present.
   D. Anatomic abnormalities
      1. Uterine torsion or entrapment in hernias
      2. Vaginal masses, hyperplasia, strictures, or bands
      3. Pelvic stenosis, malalignment
   E. Metabolic disturbances
      1. Hypoglycemia
      2. Hypocalcemia
III. Fetal factors
   A. Oversize, often secondary to prolonged gestation or small litter size
   B. Malpresentation
      1. Normal presentations are anterior dorsal or posterior dorsal.
      2. Anterior ventral presentation, anterior presentation with abnormal positioning of the head or forelimbs, and transverse presentation are the most common malpresentations.
   C. Lack of lubricating fetal fluids or membranes
   D. Oversized fetal heads, with prevention of normal passage in the pelvic canal
   E. Fetal anomalies such as anasarca, hydrocephalus (uncommon)

Clinical Signs

I. Prolonged gestation of >70 days from the first breeding date may be detected.
II. Dystocia can be characterized by the following.
   A. Stage I labor for >24 hours without progression to stage II
   B. Stage II labor for >1 hour without fetal expulsion
   C. Stage III labor for >4 hours without resumption of visible contractions, with fetus(es) remaining
   D. An abnormal degree of pain or depression associated with labor
   E. Excessive hemorrhagic or malodorous vaginal discharge
   F. Uteroverdin (green-black vaginal discharge)

Diagnosis

I. Successful management of dystocia depends on differentiation of the contributing factors.
II. An accurate history is important.
   A. Accurately calculate the actual gestational length.
   B. The preovulatory LH rise can be estimated by serial serum progesterone concentrations evaluated every 48 hours (see Chap. 53); whelping should occur 65 ± 1 days later.
   C. The preovulatory LH surge can be identified using a daily assay (see Chap. 53).
   D. The first day of diestrus can be determined by serial vaginal cytologies and vaginoscopic examination of mucosal folds (see Chap. 53); whelping should occur 57 ± 2 days later.
   E. Estimation of whelping dates from breeding dates is inherently inaccurate because of the long period of sexual receptivity in the bitch.

III. Perform a careful physical examination of the bitch.
   A. Vital signs
   B. Abdominal palpation to determine uterine tone, presence of fetus(es)
   C. Digital vaginal examination for the presence of a fetus in the vaginal vault and to determine the nature of vaginal/pelvic ligament tone and vaginal discharge
   D. Direct visualization of the cervix using vaginoscopic equipment (difficult in the bitch because of vaginal anatomy)
   E. Evaluation of the mammary glands for colostrum
IV. Perform additional diagnostics as indicated.
   A. Abdominal ultrasonography to evaluate fetal viability
   B. Abdominal radiography to evaluate litter size and the presence of remaining fetuses or to rule out obstruction of the birth canal
   C. Plasma progesterone concentration of the bitch at term of <2 ng/ml (Feldman and Nelson, 1996)
   D. Serum ionized calcium and glucose measurements

Treatment and Monitoring

I. Successful induction of parturition in the bitch with prolonged gestation is not well documented.
   A. Elective cesarean section is advised.
   B. Documentation of adequate gestational age is made to avoid prematurity. This can be accomplished by radiographic evaluation of skeletal development and plasma progesterone measurement, especially if breeding dates are not well documented.

II. Treatment of dystocia varies according to the contributing factors.
   A. The presence of obstruction, either maternal or fetal in origin, is an absolute indication for cesarean section, unless it can be readily corrected (e.g., vaginal septum).
   B. Metabolic abnormalities may respond to medical intervention once obstruction has been ruled out.
      1. Give oxytocin 1–20 U IM, observe for 10–30 minutes.
      2. Digitally feather the dorsal vaginal wall to stimulate reflex contractions.
      3. Encourage the bitch to urinate and defecate if necessary; offer water and food.
      4. Give an IV infusion 10% calcium gluconate 2–10 ml in 5% dextrose/water over a 10-minute interval.
      5. Oxytocin can be repeated twice.
         a) Ineffective uterine contractions can compromise fetuses by compressing placental blood supply.
         b) Repeated oxytocin injections can cause this.
      6. Alternatively, an IV infusion of oxytocin 10 U in 5% dextrose/water, delivered over a 30-minute period, can be substituted with caution. Ineffective, tetanic uterine contractions can occur with too rapid an infusion (Feldman and Nelson, 1996).

C. Failure of medical management to stimulate vaginal delivery within 1–4 hours should be followed by a cesarean section.

III. Resuscitate the neonates when the bitch fails or is unable to do so.
   A. Establish an airway free of fluid, placental membranes, and meconium within 1–3 minutes of birth.
      1. Tear and remove placental membranes if present.
      2. Gently suction or swab the oral cavity and trachea; avoid aspiration of meconium.
      3. Expel fluids from the airway by swinging pup gently headfirst in a downward path while supporting head and trunk in a towel.
   B. Stimulate initiation of respiration by thoracic/facial massage with a dry, warm towel, using positive pressure ventilation if necessary.
   C. Provide oxygen by face mask if cyanosis persists.
   D. Monitor heartbeat by thoracic palpation/auscultation; perform external cardiac massage if none is detected.
   E. Consider pharmacologic intervention in poorly responsive neonates.
      1. For drug dosages, canine neonates range from 100–700 g body weight at birth (0.1–0.7 kg).
      2. If born by cesarean section, reverse any narcotic or barbiturate anesthetic agents used in the bitch with 1–2 drops of naloxone or doxapram.
         a) Administer IM or IV (i.e., use the umbilical vein).
         b) Analeptic agents such as doxapram are not absorbed across mucous membranes.
         c) Narcotic antagonists are 50-fold more potent when administered parenterally than when given orally.
      3. Prolonged asphyxiation (>5 minutes) can warrant correction of acidosis. Give sodium bicarbonate 4–5 mEq/kg body weight, diluted 1:1 with 5% dextrose/water, administered via the umbilical vein over 2–4 minutes.
      4. Prolonged bradycardia may be treated with the following.
         a) Epinephrine (1:10,000):0.1 ml/kg IV
         b) Atropine: 0.03 mg/kg IM, IV
   F. Completely dry the neonate, maintaining warmth (ambient temperature of 29.4–30°C).
   G. Encourage immediate suckling to provide calories, glucose, and colostrum, sparing limited glycogen stores.
      1. If nursing does not occur immediately, provide glucose (see also Chap. 119).
      2. Oral administration (Karo syrup), 2–5 drops

POSTPARTUM DISORDERS

Autumn P. Davidson

Puerperal Tetany (Eclampsia)
Definition
I. Periparturient hypocalcemia
II. Generally occurs within the first 2 weeks postpartum, but can also occur in the prepartum period

Causes
I. Improper perinatal nutrition of the bitch
II. Calcium supplementation of the bitch during gestation
III. Heavy lactational demands from large neonates or a large litter
IV. Increased incidence in toy breeds of dogs

Pathophysiology
I. Altered membrane potentials from hypocalcemia allow spontaneous discharge of nerve fibers and tonic contractions of skeletal muscle.
II. Hypoglycemia can occur concurrently.
III. It is exacerbated by metabolic conditions favoring protein binding of serum calcium (e.g., alkalosis).
IV. Prolonged seizure activity may cause cerebral edema.

Clinical Signs
I. Initial signs include behavioral changes (irritability and restlessness), salivation, limb pain, and facial pruritus.
II. Signs progress to ataxia and muscle spasms.
III. Tonoclonic muscle contractions or seizures occur and may be associated with hyperthermia and tachycardia.
IV. The bitch may remain obtunded or nonresponsive after correction of hypocalcemia if cerebral edema has developed.

Diagnosis
I. Clinical signs and history allow a presumptive diagnosis.
II. A pretreatment serum sample is collected for confirmation of hypocalcemia, but treatment is often required prior to laboratory confirmation.
III. Total serum calcium in affected dogs generally ranges from 4–7.5 mg/dl; ionized calcium is <1.0 mg/dl.
IV. Evaluate serum glucose concentration for evidence of concurrent hypoglycemia.

Differential Diagnosis
I. Rule out other causes of seizures such as hypoglycemia, toxicoses, and primary neurologic disorders, e.g., epilepsy (see Chap. 22).
II. Consider other causes of irritability and hyperthermia such as metritis or mastitis.

Treatment
I. Administer 10% calcium gluconate IV slowly to effect over 3–5 minutes.
   A. A total dose of 1–20 ml is generally required.
   B. Monitor heart rate with auscultation or electrocardiogram (ECG).
   C. If an arrhythmia develops, discontinue administration until rhythm and rate are normal and

resume administration at half the original infusion rate.

D. Muscle relaxation should be immediate.

II. If calcium infusion is ineffective, consider administering diazepam 1–15 mg IV.

III. Treat cerebral edema if indicated (see Chap. 23).

IV. Correct hyperthermia and hypoglycemia if present.

V. Once stable, repeat the total required dose of calcium gluconate SQ, diluted in an equal volume of normal saline, and repeat as needed TID to control clinical signs.

VI. Oral supplementation with calcium lactate, carbonate, or gluconate 30–100 mg/kg/day is begun and continued until lactation ceases.

VII. Consider weaning or providing pups with supplemental nutrition to decrease lactational demands.

VIII. Provide a balanced diet for the bitch with a commercial food designed for use during lactation or growth.

Patient Monitoring

I. Monitor calcium levels every several days and adjust calcium dosages accordingly.

II. Warn owners that this condition is likely to recur with future pregnancies.

III. Calcium supplementation during gestation will not prevent, and may contribute to, the development of eclampsia.

IV. Postpartum calcium supplementation in bitches with a history of eclampsia may be helpful.

Postpartum Endometritis

Definition and Causes

I. Acute and severe bacterial infection of the uterus occurring in the postpartum period

II. Several potential causes

A. Retained fetuses or placental membranes

B. Obstetric contamination of the cranial vagina, cervix, or uterus

C. Dystocia

D. No underlying cause may be found.

III. There is no association between this condition and a lack of oxytocin administration postpartum.

Pathophysiology

I. Though clinically similar to pyometra that occurs in the nongravid uterus, postpartum metritis is not caused by underlying uterine pathology and is not associated with elevated serum progesterone concentration (see also Chap. 56).

II. Uterine discharge is generally less purulent than that which occurs with the cystic endometrial hyperplasia/pyometra complex.

III. The relaxed postpartum cervix allows discharge of uterine contents.

Clinical Signs

I. Normal lochia is generally reddish-brown and persists 2–6 weeks.

II. Vaginal discharge with endometritis differs from normal lochia.

A. Usually sanguinopurulent or frankly hemorrhagic

B. May be copious

C. Often quite odorous

III. Systemic signs of illness are common.

A. Fever, inappetence, dehydration, and malaise

B. Inattention to pups

C. Decreased milk production

Diagnosis

I. Suspicious systemic and local signs are noted on physical examination.

II. Vaginal cytology is indicated to characterize the nature of the discharge.

A. Degenerated neutrophils

B. Epithelial cells and neutrophils with intracellular bacteria

III. Obtain a guarded cranial vaginal culture to determine pathogen(s) involved and their antibiotic sensitivity.

IV. Vaginoscopy can aid in localizing the source of vaginal discharge.

A. Determine if the origin is cranial to the cervix by evaluating the postcervical area for discharge.

B. Determine if vaginal trauma associated with parturition has caused the abnormal discharge.

V. A hemogram may reveal a moderate neutrophilia and left shift.

VI. Ultrasonography is performed.

A. Note any retained fetuses.

B. The finding of an enlarged uterus is expected in the postpartum period.

C. Ultrasonography determines whether the uterine lumen is fluid-filled.

VII. Abdominal radiography is not helpful because the postpartum uterus normally appears enlarged.

Differential Diagnosis

I. Lochia and mild fever: normal in the postpartum period

II. Vaginitis

III. Coagulopathy

IV. Other systemic disease, including mastitis

Treatment

I. Begin broad-spectrum antibiotic therapy (e.g., cephalosporins) while awaiting culture and sensitivity results.

II. Begin supportive care such as parenteral fluid therapy.

III. Ovariohysterectomy is curative if the bitch is not intended for future breeding.

IV. Prostaglandin F_2-alpha can be used to promote uterine evacuation as an alternative to ovariohysterectomy (see Chap. 56).

A. A dose of 0.1–0.25 mg/kg SQ SID–BID for 5–7 days is recommended.

B. Use ultrasonography to determine response to

treatment and end point of therapy; it may be necessary to treat to effect.

V. The bitch may be unable to care for pups during acute illness, and temporary orphan care may be necessary.

Patient Monitoring

I. Most bitches respond well to aggressive medical management.

II. Subsequent fertility is expected to be normal following prompt and successful resolution of the disease, but studies to document future fertility are lacking.

Subinvolution of Placental Sites (SIPS)

Definition

I. A delay in the process of placental degeneration and endometrial reconstruction that normally takes place after whelping

II. Source of chronic hemorrhage into the uterine lumen

Causes

I. The cause of this condition is unknown.

II. It is unlikely to be caused by bacterial infection or a failure to administer oxytocin in the immediate postpartum period.

Pathophysiology

I. Affected placental sites grossly appear as large ellipsoidal swellings with a thick, rough, gray to brown endometrial surface with areas of hemorrhage.

II. Not all placental sites in a uterus are affected (Al-Bassam et al., 1981).

III. Histologically, fetal trophoblastic cells persist in the myometrium.

A. They produce thinning and herniation of the subinvoluted endometrium through the muscle layer (Glenn, 1968).

B. Trophoblastic cells usually die promptly and spontaneously in the postpartum endometrium, and the reason for their persistence in SIPS is unknown.

Clinical Signs

I. Young (<3 years) bitches are most commonly affected.

II. Serosanguineous discharge persists beyond 6 weeks postpartum.

III. Bitch is otherwise normal.

Diagnosis

I. Physical examination reveals sanguineous vaginal discharge as the only abnormality.

II. Exfoliative vaginal cytology is indicative of anestrus.

A. Parabasal cells predominate; cellular debris and RBCs may be seen.

B. Syncytial trophoblast-like cells may be found (Wheeler, 1986).

III. Culture of the vaginal vault reveals normal flora.

IV. Laboratory parameters (hemogram, serum biochemistry profile, urinalysis, coagulation profile) are usually normal, but anemia as a result of blood loss may be present if hemorrhage is copious.

V. Ultrasonography may reveal echogenic foci in the endometrium, but often no abnormalities are detected.

VI. Vaginoscopy is performed to rule out vaginal causes of hemorrhage.

VII. Any bitch with an abnormal vaginal discharge should be tested for *Brucella canis*.

Differential Diagnosis

I. Vaginal origin of hemorrhage, or proestrus
II. Endometritis
III. Coagulopathy
IV. Neoplasia of the uterus, vagina, or urethra

Treatment

I. Specific treatment is not indicated if the bitch is intended for future breeding, because the lesions resolve spontaneously.

II. Ovariohysterectomy is curative, but only indicated if hemorrhage is copious.

Patient Monitoring

I. Vaginal hemorrhagic discharge can persist until the next proestrus.

II. Tendency for recurrence following future pregnancy is unknown but appears to be uncommon.

III. SIPS does not appear to diminish future fertility.

ESTRUS SUPPRESSION

Janice L. Cain

Mibolerone

Indications

I. Treatment of infertility in a bitch with naturally short, ovulatory interestrus intervals (see Infertility in the Bitch)

II. Owner or handler convenience

III. Only androgen approved for estrus suppression in the United States

Mechanism of Action

I. Androgenic, anabolic, and antigonadotropic

II. Prevents estrus by negative feedback mechanisms that inhibit synthesis and release of pituitary gonadotropins

Administration

I. Dosage of Cheque (Upjohn, Kalamazoo, MI) is based on body weight as per label instructions (see Appendix IV).
II. Administration is begun during anestrus and at least 30 days prior to the expected onset of proestrus.
III. It can be prescribed for 24 consecutive months.
IV. Return to estrus is normally within 7–200 days upon withdrawal.

Adverse Effects

I. Hepatocellular pathologic changes and possible increased serum concentrations of alanine aminotransferase and bilirubin
II. Masculinization of female fetuses if administered during pregnancy (Olson and Nett, 1983)
III. Premature epiphyseal closure if administered prior to maturity
IV. Mild clitoral hypertrophy and white-colored vaginal discharge
V. Interference with lactation (Olson and Nett, 1983)
VI. Deepening of voice, musky breath, epiphora, and worsening of preexisting seborrhea

General Considerations

I. Not recommended for bitches intended to be used for breeding (as per label instructions)
II. Contraindicated during pregnancy
   Note: Bitches should not be bred if estrus occurs during mibolerone administration (breakthrough estrus).
III. Contraindicated prior to pubertal estrus or in bitches with open physes

Megestrol Acetate

Indications

I. Only approved progestational compound for canine contraception in the United States
II. Can be used to prevent ovulation or delay the onset of estrus

Mechanism of Action

I. May cause negative feedback inhibition of the anterior pituitary and/or hypothalamus with decreased production and release of gonadotropins
II. A synthetic hormone that exerts a progesterone influence on the reproductive tract and other organs

Administration

I. To prevent ovulation and abbreviate estrus (Ovaban by Schering, Kenilworth, NJ)
   A. It must be commenced during the first 3 days of proestrus.
   B. Treat for 8 consecutive days at 2.2 mg/kg/day PO.

   C. If proestrus is short for a particular bitch, this treatment may not be successful.
II. To suppress or delay the onset of estrus
   A. Begin administering the drug at least 7 days prior to the expected onset of proestrus.
   B. Dose is 0.55 mg/kg/day PO for 32 consecutive days.
   C. If estrus occurs during therapy, continue treatment to inhibit ovulation at 2.2 mg/kg/day PO for 8 days, then discontinue the drug.

Adverse Effects

I. Reproductive tract effects
   A. Inhibition of local uterine immunity and endometrial gland proliferation, both of which increase the incidence of pyometra (Concannon, 1983)
   B. Possible development of cystic endometrial hyperplasia and subsequent infertility
   C. Exacerbated by the presence of naturally secreted estrogen during proestrus, therefore increased risk of endometrial disease with high-dose regimen during proestrus
II. Systemic effects (Concannon et al., 1980)
   A. Insulin resistance and diabetes mellitus
   B. Mammary gland proliferation and neoplasia
   C. Acromegaly
   D. Liver enlargement
   E. Polyphagia, lethargy, weight gain

General Considerations

I. The drug should not be used on known diabetics or in bitches with a history of liver or mammary gland disease.
II. It is not recommended for bitches that are intended for breeding purposes because of adverse effects on the reproductive tract.
III. It can be used to suppress estrus prior to elective ovariohysterectomy.

PREGNANCY TERMINATION

Autumn P. Davidson

Indications

I. Unplanned mating to unacceptable male or at an undesirable time or age (immature bitch)
II. Form of medical abortion to avoid unwanted puppies

Mismating Options

I. Determine the chance of conception based on the phase of the estrous cycle, i.e., a bitch may be bred but is unlikely to be fertile after the cytologic diestral shift.
II. Estrogenic compounds (orally or parenterally) have been advocated in the past as an effective mismating treatment but are no longer recommended (Jackson and Johnston, 1980; Soderberg and Olson, 1983; Bowen et al., 1985).

A. Poor efficacy unless relatively high doses of the more toxic compounds are used
B. Potential for irreversible aplastic anemia and other transient blood dyscrasias
C. Association with later development of the cystic endometrial hyperplasia–pyometra complex

Early Pregnancy Termination

I. Immunocontraceptive agents using zona pellucida antigens, isoquinoline anti-implantation compounds, or steroid synthesis inhibitors have been proposed (Galliani and Omodei-sale, 1982; Lerner, 1989; Keister et al., 1989).
   A. Problems with application of these methods include poor efficacy, narrow range of safety, and wide variety of side effects.
   B. Other methods are under investigation and are currently unavailable (e.g., epostane, a steroid synthesis inhibitor).
II. Administration of nonsynthetic prostaglandin F$_2$-alpha (Lutalyse) between days 5 and 10 of diestrus has been advised (Romagnoli et al., 1993).
   A. The dose used was 0.25 mg/kg SQ BID for at least 4 days.
   B. It caused luteolysis in 12 of 15 mated bitches.
   C. Pregnancy termination was attempted before pregnancy diagnosis could be confirmed.

Midgestation Abortion

I. Prostaglandin F$_2$-alpha administered after approximately day 30 of gestation can cause abortion (Feldman et al., 1993).
   A. Dosage is 0.1–0.25 mg/kg SQ TID to effect.
   B. End point of therapy is determined by ultrasonographic confirmation that all fetuses are expelled.
   C. Duration of therapy can range from 4–11 days.
II. Prior to medical abortion, pregnancy should be confirmed with ultrasonography 21–30 days after breeding.
III. Side effects of prostaglandin F$_2$-alpha include emesis, diarrhea, salivation, tachypnea, trembling, and urination after injection.
   A. These effects are often well tolerated and diminish in severity and duration as treatment progresses.
   B. Restlessness, hypothermia, nesting, and lochia may be observed prior to aborting.
   C. Bitches return to normal reproductive cycling after treatment, but because diestrus is shortened by the prostaglandin, the next estrous cycle can occur sooner than expected.

Other Abortifacients

I. Bromocriptine, a prolactin inhibitor, has been evaluated as an abortifacient (Concannon et al., 1987).
   A. Gastrointestinal side effects can occur.
   B. Efficacy is questionable.
II. Dexamethasone has been reported to cause fetal death during the latter half of gestation (Wanke et al., 1996).
   A. Dosage ranged from 0.1–0.2 mg/kg BID.
   B. Duration of therapy ranged from 7–13 days.
III. Misoprostol may be useful as a cervical softening agent given vaginally at 1–3 μg/kg/day to hasten midgestation abortion with prostaglandin F$_2$-alpha.

Bibliography

Al-Bassam MA, Thampson RG, O'Donnell L: Normal post-partum involution of the uterus in the dog. Can J Comp Med 45:217, 1981

Amann RP: Reproductive physiology and endocrinology of the dog. p. 532. In Morrow DA (ed): Current Therapy in Theriogenology. WB Saunders, Philadelphia, 1986

Bjurström L, Linde-Forsberg C: Long-term study of aerobic bacteria of the genital tract in breeding bitches. Am J Vet Res 53:665, 1992

Bowen RA, Olson PN, Behrendt MD, et al: Efficacy and toxicity of estrogens commonly used to terminate canine pregnancy. J Am Vet Med Assoc 186:783, 1985

Brown J: Efficacy and dose titration study of mibolerone for treatment of pseudopregnancy in the bitch. J Am Vet Med Assoc 184:1467, 1984

Cain JL: The use and misuse of reproductive hormones in canine reproduction. p. 1069. In Bonagura JD (ed): Current Veterinary Therapy XII: Small Animal Practice. WB Saunders, Philadelphia, 1995

Chandler ML: Canine neonatal mortality. Proc Soc Theriogenol 243, 1990

Concannon PW: Fertility regulation in the bitch: contraception, sterilization, and pregnancy termination. p. 901. In Kirk RW (ed): Current Veterinary Therapy VIII. WB Saunders, Philadelphia, 1983

Concannon PW, Altszuler N, Hampshire J, et al: Growth hormone, prolactin and cortisol in dogs developing mammary nodules and an acromegaly-like appearance during treatment with medroxyprogesterone acetate. Endocrinology 106:1173, 1980

Concannon PW, Hansel W, Visek WJ: The ovarian cycle of the bitch: plasma estrogen, LH, and progesterone. Biol Reprod 13:112, 1975

Concannon PW, Powers ME, Holder W, Hansel W: Pregnancy and parturition in the bitch. Biol Reprod 16:317, 1977

Concannon PW, Weinstein P, Whaley S, et al: Suppression of luteal function in dogs by luteinizing hormone antiserum and bromocryptine. J Reprod Fertil 81:175, 1987

Evermann JF: Diagnosis of canine herpetic infections. p. 1313. In Kirk RW (ed): Current Veterinary Therapy X: Small Animal Practice. WB Saunders, Philadelphia, 1989

Feldman EC, Davidson AP, Nelson RW, et al: Prostaglandin induction of abortion in pregnant bitches after misalliance. J Am Vet Med Assoc 202:1855, 1993

Feldman EC, Nelson RW: Canine and Feline Endocrinology and Reproduction. 2nd Ed. WB Saunders, Philadelphia, 1996

Freshman JL: Drugs affecting infertility in the male dog. p. 1224. In Kirk RW (ed): Current Veterinary Therapy X: Small Animal Practice. WB Saunders, Philadelphia, 1989

Freshman JL, Amann RP, Bowen RA, et al: Clinical evaluation of infertility in dogs. Compend Contin Educ Pract Vet 10:443, 1988

Galliani G, Omodei-sale A: Pregnancy termination in dogs with non-hormonal compounds: evaluation of selected derivatives. J Small Anim Pract 23:295, 1982

Gilroy BA, DeYoung DJ: Cesarean section. Vet Clin North Am [Small Anim Pract] 16:483, 1986

Glenn BL: Subinvolution of placental sites in the bitch. Gaines Vet Symp 18:7, 1968

Hashimoto A, Hirai K: Canine herpesvirus infection. p. 516. In Morrow DA (ed): Current Therapy in Theriogenology. WB Saunders, Philadelphia, 1986

Jackson WF, Johnston SD: Pregnancy prevention and termination. p. 1239. In Kirk RW (ed): Current Veterinary Therapy VII. WB Saunders, Philadelphia, 1980

Jezyk PF: Metabolic diseases: an emerging area of veterinary pediatrics. Compend Contin Educ Pract Vet 5:1026, 1983

Johnston SD: Performing a complete canine semen evaluation in a small animal hospital. Vet Clin North Am [Small Anim Pract] 21:545, 1991

Keister RF, Gutheil LD, Kaiser LD, et al: Efficacy of oral epostane administration to terminate pregnancy in mated laboratory bitches. J Reprod Fertil 39:241, 1989

Lein DH: Canine mycoplasma, ureaplasma, and bacterial infertility. p. 1240. In Kirk RW (ed): Current Veterinary Therapy IX. WB Saunders, Philadelphia, 1986

Lerner LJ: Development of novel embryotoxic compounds for interceptive fertility control in the dog. J Reprod Fertil 39:251, 1989

Lowseth LA, Gerlach RF, Gillet NA, et al: Age-related changes in the prostate and testes of the beagle dog. Vet Pathol 27:347, 1990

Meyers-Wallen VN: Clinical approach to infertile male dogs with sperm in the ejaculate. Vet Clin North Am [Small Anim Pract] 21:609, 1991

Meyers-Wallen VN, Patterson DF: Disorders of sexual development in dogs and cats. p. 1261. In Kirk RW (ed): Current Veterinary Therapy X: Small Animal Practice. WB Saunders, Philadelphia, 1989

Oettlé EE: Sperm morphology and fertility in the dog. J Reprod Fertil Suppl 47:257, 1993

Oettlé EE: Sperm abnormalities and fertility in the dog. In Bonagura JD (ed): Current Veterinary Therapy XII: Small Animal Practice. WB Saunders, Philadelphia, 1995

Olson PN: Clinical approach to evaluating dogs with azoospermia or aspermia. Vet Clin North Am [Small Anim Pract] 21:591, 1991

Olson PN, Mulnix JA, Nett TM: Concentrations of luteinizing hormone and follicle-stimulating hormone in the serum of sexually intact and neutered dogs. Am J Vet Res 53:762, 1992

Olson PNS, Nett TM: Small animal contraceptives. p. 1725. In Ettinger SJ (ed): Textbook of Veterinary Internal Medicine. 2nd Ed. WB Saunders, Philadelphia, 1983

Padgett GA, Bell TG, Patterson WR: Genetic disorders affecting reproduction and periparturient care. Vet Clin North Am [Small Anim Pract] 16:577, 1986

Romagnoli SE, Camillo F, Cele M, et al: Clinical use of prostaglandin F2α to induce early abortion in bitches: serum progesterone, treatment outcome and interval to subsequent oestrus. J Reprod Fertil Suppl 47:425, 1993

Scott-Moncrieff JC, Nelson RW, Bill RL, et al: Serum deposition of exogenous progesterone after intramuscular administration in bitches. Am J Vet Res 51:893, 1990

Sheffy BE: Nutrition and nutritional disorders. Vet Clin North Am 8:7, 1978

Shille VM, Olson PN: Dynamic testing in reproductive endocrinology. p. 1282. In Kirk RW (ed): Current Veterinary Therapy X: Small Animal Practice. WB Saunders, Philadelphia, 1989

Soderberg SF: Infertility in the male dog. p. 544. In Morrow DA (ed): Current Therapy in Theriogenology. WB Saunders, Philadelphia, 1986

Soderberg SF, Olson PN: Abortifacients. p. 945. In Kirk RW (ed): Current Veterinary Therapy VIII: Small Animal Practice. WB Saunders, Philadelphia, 1983

Wanke M, Loza ME, Monachesi N, Concannon PW: Clinical use of oral dexamethasone for termination of unwanted pregnancy in dogs [abstract]. Proc Internat Symp Reproduc Dogs, Cats, Exotic Carnivores. University of Utrecht, 3:1996

Wheeler SL: Subinvolution of placental sites in the bitch. p. 513. In Morrow DA (ed): Current Therapy in Theriogenology. WB Saunders, Philadelphia, 1986

61

Disorders of Feline Reproduction

Janice L. Cain

INFERTILITY IN THE QUEEN

Definition

I. Failure of the queen to breed, conceive, or carry a litter to term
II. Includes queens with abnormal ovarian cycles and uterine disease

Causes and Pathophysiology

I. Persistent seasonal estrus
  A. It may be caused by abnormal ovarian follicle growth patterns.
    1. The normal ovarian cycle is composed of repeated follicular phases of 6–7 days duration, with intervening interfollicular phases that are 8–9 days in duration (Shille et al., 1979).
      a) Sexual receptivity (estrus) normally begins 1–2 days after the onset of follicle growth and terminates at the end of the follicular phase.
      b) During the interfollicular phase the queen is normally not sexually receptive; this phase is also termed interestrus.
    2. If follicles form in overlapping cycles, estrus behavior may be continuous.
  B. Some queens have persistent estrus owing to a behavioral rather than a physiologic basis.
II. Persistent nonseasonal estrus
  A. Can occur as a result of cystic follicular degeneration of the ovaries
  B. More common in older, nulliparous queens
III. Unexpressed estrus
  A. Queens may fail to show estrus behavior even though they have normal cyclic ovarian activity (Shille and Stabenfeldt, 1980).
  B. It may occur in queens in group housing with other cycling queens.

C. Unexpressed estrus most commonly occurs in queens low in the social order.
IV. Persistent anestrus (no ovarian activity)
  A. Age
    1. Onset of first estrus generally occurs between 7 and 9 months of age, although purebred queens may become sexually mature later (9–12 months) (Jemmett and Evans, 1977; Povey, 1978).
    2. Queens over 8 years of age have reduced reproductive capacity and may cycle irregularly.
  B. Insufficient photoperiod exposure
    1. Under natural light (United States), queens cease ovarian activity during midautumn and resume ovarian activity as early as 30 days after the winter solstice, i.e., December 21 (Hurni, 1981).
    2. Queens housed in inadequate artificial light situations may not cycle.
  C. Queens low in the social order that are housed with other cycling queens may have ovarian inactivity.
  D. Ovarian inactivity is normal during lactation.
  E. Queens may not cycle because of underlying illness.
V. Ovulatory failure
  A. When in conjunction with normal copulatory activity, it most commonly occurs because breeding was too late in the follicular cycle and follicles are undergoing regression (Shille et al., 1979).
  B. It may occur from inadequate stimulation as a result of poor male libido or too few breedings allowed.
  C. Spontaneous ovulation without coital stimulation has been reported (Lawlor et al., 1993).
VI. Cystic endometrial hyperplasia (CEH)–pyometra complex
  A. CEH develops in nonbred queens because of

intermittent exposure of the uterus to estrogens of ovarian origin (Lawlor et al., 1991).
B. It may occur from diestral phase progesterone stimulation in the pseudopregnant queen, as in the bitch.
C. Corpora lutea were present in 40% of queens with pyometra or endometritis in one study (Potter et al., 1991).
D. Correlation of CEH to reproductive history (i.e., nulliparous vs. multiparous) is debated (Potter et al., 1991; Lawlor et al., 1991).
VII. Fetal loss owing to resorption or abortion
A. Gestational age of the fetus determines whether a nonviable fetus will be resorbed or aborted.
  1. Normal gestation is 63–66 days after breeding; fetuses delivered sooner than 60 days of gestation are usually stillborn (Prescott, 1973).
  2. Abortion in the queen generally occurs between days 50 and 58 of gestation.
  3. Resorption occurs with loss of fetal viability in the first half of pregnancy.
B. Infectious disease is a likely cause.
  1. Feline leukemia virus (FeLV) is implicated most often (Pedersen, 1991).
  2. Other infectious disorders causing abortion include herpesvirus type 1, *Mycoplasma* spp., *Chlamydia psittaci* var. *felis* feline infectious peritonitis (FIP), feline panleukopenia virus, and toxoplasmosis.
  3. Uterine infections with coliform bacteria, streptococci, staphylococci, and salmonellae may be involved (Christiansen, 1984).
  4. As in the bitch, normal vaginal flora are difficult to differentiate from potential pathogens (Clemetson and Ward, 1990).
C. Taurine deficiency has been identified as a cause (Dieter et al., 1993).
D. Inadequate progesterone secretion to maintain pregnancy is very rare in the queen.

Clinical Signs

I. Abnormal estrous cycles
A. Queens with persistent estrus generally show no other abnormalities.
B. Some queens with ovarian degeneration have weight loss and rough, thin hair coats.
C. Queens with unexpressed or persistent anestrus may demonstrate behavior typical of a queen at the low end of the social order (i.e., poor weight gain, poor coat, failure to socialize, and failure to thrive).
II. Ovulation failure
A. Queens continue estrus cyclicity without a luteal phase.
B. If caused by inadequate copulatory stimulus, the copulatory cry of the queen may be absent after mating.
III. Cystic endometrial hyperplasia
A. Usually infertility is the only clinical sign (Lein, 1983; Johnson, 1989).

B. If a secondary pyometra develops, signs typical of that condition are noted (see Chap. 56).
IV. Resorption and abortion
A. Resorption can occur without clinical signs.
B. Sanguineous vaginal discharge occurring during gestation is suspicious.
C. Expulsion of fetuses occurs with abortion.
D. Queens rarely exhibit listlessness and inappetence.

Diagnosis and Differential Diagnosis

I. A thorough medical and reproductive history is essential.
A. Timing the interval between estrous cycles determines if ovulation is occurring in the mated queen.
  1. Sterile mating that induces ovulation results in a luteal phase (pseudopregnancy); estrus does not occur for 45–50 days (Paape et al., 1975).
  2. Investigate the male for infertility.
  3. Very early embryonic loss may be occurring, but it is difficult to document.
B. If the queen appears not to ovulate, question breeding practices as to frequency of mating, occurrence of the postcopulatory cry, and how soon the pair is brought together after the onset of estrus behavior.
C. Check for infectious diseases in the cattery.
II. A complete physical examination is necessary.
A. It is useful to detect an underlying systemic disease.
B. Vaginal palpation in the queen is usually not possible or recommended.
III. Vaginal cytology can give an estimate of ovarian activity.
A. Changes in the prevalent cell type are indicative of estrogen influence (Table 61-1).

Table 61-1. **Vaginal Cytology in the Queen**

Stage of Cycle	Cytologic Changes Expected[a]
Anestrus/ prepuberty	Small parabasal epithelial cells

Estrus	Clearing of cellular debris from the background of the slide
	Cell types:
	  Superficial, nucleated epithelial cells—50%
	  Anuclear superficial epithelial cells—40%
	  Intermediate epithelial cells—10%

Interestrus	Background of slide has cellular debris that takes up stain
	Cell types:
	  Superficial, nucleated epithelial cells—45–50%
	  Anuclear superficial epithelial cells—5%
	  Intermediate epithelial cells—45–50%
	  Parabasal epithelial cells—2%

[a]For a description of vaginal epithelial cell types, see Chap. 53.

B. Cytology can determine whether persistent estrus is caused by ovarian activity.

C. Accurate evaluation of vaginal cytology in the queen requires considerable experience.

IV. Vaginoscopy using an otoscope cone may detect vaginal discharge or vesicles but must be used with care during estrus, as vaginal stimulation can induce ovulation.

V. Hormone concentrations may be assayed.

A. Serum estrogen concentration can be used to differentiate a queen with persistent anestrus from one with unexpressed estrus (Shille et al., 1979).

1. During the follicular phase and estrus, plasma concentrations of estradiol are >20 pg/ml.

2. During anestrus and interestrus, plasma estradiol concentrations are <20 pg/ml.

3. Repeated sampling is necessary to establish a pattern, but the cost may be prohibitive.

B. Serum progesterone concentration can be used to differentiate pseudopregnancy from anestrus.

1. Luteal phase serum progesterone concentration is >2 ng/ml.

2. Serum progesterone concentration <1 ng/ml indicates lack of luteal tissue (Shille et al., 1979; Stabenfeldt and Pedersen, 1991).

3. During gestation, the serum progesterone concentration should remain >2 ng/ml to sustain pregnancy.

VI. Obtain a routine laboratory database to screen for underlying illness.

A. Evaluate a hemogram, serum biochemistry profile, and urinalysis.

B. Test for FeLV and feline immunodeficiency virus (FIV).

VII. Ultrasonographic examination of the abdomen may detect an enlarged, nongravid uterus in a queen with cystic endometrial hyperplasia.

A. Provides necessary proof of pregnancy in a queen with suspected resorption of prior litters

B. Is a good method to assess fetal viability

VIII. Exploratory laparotomy can be used to obtain uterine biopsies and cultures for detection of cystic endometrial hyperplasia or occult endometritis and to examine the ovaries for evidence of follicular cysts.

IX. Perform a necropsy in any stillborn or aborted fetuses to detect possible infectious agents.

Treatment and Monitoring

I. Persistent seasonal estrus

A. Allow queen and tom to breed on a daily basis.

B. Cessation of estrus may indicate that ovulation has occurred.

II. Persistent nonseasonal estrus

A. No specific treatment exists for cystic follicular degeneration.

B. Consider ovariohysterectomy in the older queen with this condition.

III. Unexpressed estrus

A. Change the housing situation of the queen.

B. House the queen alone or with either another cycling queen or an intact male.

IV. Persistent anestrus

A. Change photoperiod exposure.

1. Expose to 14 hours of light daily (Hurni, 1981).

2. If this is done year-round, the queen usually cycles in the off-season.

B. Attempt induction of estrus.

1. Follicle-stimulating hormone (FSH-P) 2 mg IM once daily for 5 days (Wildt et al., 1978)

2. Generally induces estrus behavior by the fourth or fifth day of therapy

V. Ovulatory failure

A. Allow the queen and tom to breed repeatedly.

1. Place them together no later than the fourth day of behavioral estrus.

2. Allow them to breed repeatedly.

a) It is not unusual for the pair to copulate four times within the first hour.

b) If not too late in the cycle (i.e., after day 4) this activity should cause ovulation.

c) If in doubt, allow breeding at the first sign of estrus behavior and place the pair together daily for 1–2 hours until the termination of estrus.

B. Alternatively, try to induce ovulation.

1. Induction can often be accomplished by vaginal insertion of a metal or glass probe; success is indicated on elicitation of the copulatory cry by the queen.

2. Administer either of the following protocols.

a) Human chorionic gonadotropin (HCG) 250 IU IM on days 1 and 2 of estrus (Wildt and Seager, 1978)

b) Gonadotropin-releasing hormone 25 μg IM on day 2 of estrus (Chakraborty et al., 1979)

VI. CEH–pyometra complex: see Chap. 56

VII. Resorption or abortion

A. Treat the underlying cause when possible.

B. Impending abortion can rarely be prevented.

C. Prevention of infectious diseases should be emphasized. Consider vaccination schedules, husbandry practices, and isolation procedures for newly acquired cats and those taken to shows.

INFERTILITY IN THE TOM CAT

Definition

I. The lack of ability to cause conception

II. Includes failure to breed and failure to produce semen capable of fertilization

Causes and Clinical Signs

I. Poor libido

A. Physical causes

1. Any chronic illness may cause poor libido.

2. Adhesions of penis to prepuce owing to a congenital lesion or prior inflammation may cause the tom to be reluctant to mate.
3. Formation of hair rings at the base of the penis makes it difficult to achieve an erection or causes persistent erection (priapism).

B. Behavioral causes
1. Incompatability between queen and tom may cause the tom to appear uninterested.
2. The queen may dominate the tom and intimidate him, especially if they are housed together.
3. Serum testosterone concentration in the tom is often normal, hence inadequate testosterone production is not usually the cause.

II. Abnormal semen
A. Age may be a factor.
1. Spermatogenesis begins at 5 months of age, and sexual maturity is complete by 9 months.
2. Sperm quality decreases with age.
B. Causes of inadequate sperm quantity or quality have not been extensively evaluated in the tom.

III. Reproductive tract infections
A. They are considered an uncommon cause of infertility in the tom.
B. Effusive FIP can cause scrotal enlargement and associated testicular infection.

IV. Cryptorchidism
A. One or both testicles are retained in the abdomen or inguinal canal; the unilateral condition is more common (Millis et al., 1992).
B. Unilateral cryptorchid males may be fertile but should not be used for breeding because the trait is likely to be inherited.
C. Persians had a significantly higher incidence in one study (Millis et al., 1992).

V. Intersex condition
A. Tortoiseshell male cats have an abnormal genotype.
1. The tortoiseshell-calico pattern (i.e., black and orange coat) requires the presence of two X chromosomes.
   a) Normal male cats have 38 chromosomes with an XY sex chromosome combination.
   b) Tortoiseshell-calico males commonly have a 39, XXY karyotype.
   c) The estimated incidence in the feline population is 1 in 3000 (Chastain et al., 1988).
   d) The XXY karyotype in cats serves as a model for Klinefelter's syndrome in people.
2. Other sex chromosome combinations (e.g., mosaicism) can cause the tortoiseshell pattern but are less common.
B. Most males with this condition are sterile owing to seminiferous tubule dysgenesis. A fertile male tortoiseshell cat is rare but not necessarily valuable.

Diagnosis

I. As in the queen, a detailed medical and reproductive history is essential.

II. Perform a complete physical examination, including examination of the penis, which may require sedation.

III. Semen evaluation may be performed.
A. Semen collection
1. Tom cats can be trained (may take 3 weeks of training) to ejaculate into an artificial vagina.
2. Electroejaculation procedures can be done (Platz and Seager, 1978; Christiansen, 1984).
3. A postcoital vaginal wash may be used to determine if any sperm are present, but it is a poor technique to evaluate semen quality.
4. Retrograde ejaculation into the urinary bladder may be a significant element in the ejaculation process of tom cats (Dooley et al., 1991).

B. Semen analysis
1. Evaluation techniques are similar to those recommended for dogs (see Chap. 60).
2. The volume of semen released at each ejaculation ranges from 0.03–0.3 ml (Lein, 1989).
3. Normal sperm count ranges from 6×10^7 to 1.5×10^9 per ml of ejaculate.
4. Motility ranges from 65–90%.
5. Structurally abnormal spermatozoa should be <30%.

IV. Serum testosterone concentration can be helpful in certain circumstances.
A. Can differentiate castrated state from cryptorchidism
B. Approximate expected values
1. Scrotal testes: >1000 pg/ml
2. Cryptorchidism: 200-1000 pg/ml
3. Bilateral castrate: 25 pg/ml

V. Screen for underlying diseases
A. Evaluate a hemogram, serum biochemistry profile, and urinalysis.
B. Test for FeLV and FIV.
C. Evaluate serum thyroxine (T_4) concentration to rule out hyperthyroidism in an older tom.

Treatment and Monitoring

I. Poor libido
A. Change housing situation.
1. House males separately.
2. Bring the queen and tom together only for breeding.
3. Consider artificial insemination.
   a) It is possible if the male can be trained to ejaculate.
   b) The queen must also be induced to ovulate as described earlier.
B. Supplementation with testosterone is not recommended.
1. Will not increase libido
2. Can cause decreased spermatogenesis owing to negative feedback inhibition of pituitary gonadotropin secretion

II. Cryptorchid cats should be bilaterally castrated.

DYSTOCIA

Definition

I. The inability of the queen to deliver fetuses once the delivery process has begun
II. Relatively rare in cats when compared with other domestic species

Causes and Pathophysiology

I. Fetal presentation or size
    A. Because the limbs of feline fetuses are relatively short in comparison to the body, malpositioning does not usually result in dystocia.
    B. Abnormalities may occur with a small litter size and resultant fetuses that are too large for the pelvic canal.
II. Maternal factors causing obstruction
    A. Congenitally narrowed pelvis
    B. Previously fractured pelvis with a narrowed birth canal
III. Uterine inertia
    A. Primary uterine inertia occurs when the uterus is unable to respond to normal hormonal and physical stimuli at the onset of delivery. This is most common in overweight, sedentary queens and rarely in queens with large litters (Laliberte, 1986).
    B. Secondary uterine inertia occurs with prolonged, often difficult, deliveries.
IV. Uterine torsion, tear, or rupture
    A. Uterine torsion is relatively uncommon in cats.
        1. It tends to occur near or at the time of parturition.
        2. It can prevent the delivery of fetuses in the affected horn(s).
    B. A uterine tear involves the endometrium and possibly part of the myometrium without extending through the serosal surface.
    C. Uterine rupture is a tear in the uterus that extends through the serosal surface and can allow the passage of fetuses and placentas into the abdominal cavity.
V. Prolonged gestation
    A. The length of gestation in domestic shorthair cats has been reported to be 65.8 ± 2.5 days (Munday and Davidson, 1993).
    B. Some queens may fail to initiate labor by 66 days, causing concern for fetal well-being.
    C. It is difficult to decide how long to allow gestation to continue beyond 66 days before recommending cesarean section.

Clinical Signs

I. Suspect dystocia if there is failure to deliver a fetus after 30–60 minutes of straining.
II. Straining for >20 minutes to pass a fetus that is exposed at the vulva or is within the pelvic canal is also abnormal.
III. Greenish vaginal discharge indicates placental separation from the uterus.
IV. Evidence of hemorrhagic vaginal discharge that persists more than several minutes may indicate a uterine tear.
V. Hypovolemic shock can develop if prolonged, severe hemorrhage occurs.
VI. Evidence of abdominal pain and mental depression in the queen may develop with uterine torsion, tear, or rupture.

Diagnosis

I. Suspicious clinical signs
II. Abdominal radiography
    A. To determine number, size, and position of remaining fetuses
    B. To assess conformation of pelvic canal to rule out maternal cause for obstruction
    C. To identify fetus(es) located in abdominal cavity as evidence of a uterine rupture
III. Abdominal ultrasonography to assess fetal viability
IV. Exploratory laparotomy to detect uterine torsion

Treatment

I. For uterine inertia, try the following (Laliberte, 1986).
    A. Digital stimulation of the dorsal vaginal wall may stimulate uterine contractions.
    B. Administer oxytocin 2–5 U SQ or IM, which

Table 61–2. **Postparturient Disorders in the Queen**

Disorder	Clinical Significance	Diagnosis	Treatment
Vulvar discharge	Normal if red-brown or green-black for <3 weeks	If copious or purulent, may indicate metritis	See Chap. 56
Endometritis	Although unusual, may be severe in queens	As for bitches; see Chap. 60	See Chaps. 56 and 60
Septicemia	Occurs 2–10 days postpartum Origin of sepsis often not identified—may be from uterus or mammary glands	Signs of acute depression, anorexia, fever, agalactia, dehydration, and hypovolemic shock	Antibiotics based on culture and sensitivity, supportive care
Eclampsia	Uncommon in queens; may occur during early lactation, as in the bitch	Signs as in bitch; see Chap. 60	See Chap. 60

may be repeated after 45 minutes if no effect is seen.

   C. Slow IV infusion of 1–3 ml of 10% calcium gluconate solution may be beneficial to sensitize the uterus before the second oxytocin dose.

   D. Cesarean section may be necessary if medical management fails to cause delivery of fetuses.

  II. For uterine torsion, see Chap. 56.

 III. For uterine tear or rupture, ovariohysterectomy is advised after stabilization.

Patient Monitoring

Postpartum conditions are outlined in Table 61–2.

Bibliography

Chakraborty PK, Wildt DE, Seager SWJ: Serum luteinizing hormone and ovulatory response to luteinizing hormone-releasing hormone in the estrous and anestrous domestic cat. Lab Anim Sci 29:338, 1979

Chastain CB, Guilford WG, Schmidt D: The 38,XX/39,XXY genotype in cats. Compend Contin Educ Small Anim Pract 10:18, 1988

Christiansen IJ: Reproduction the Dog and Cat. Bailliere Tindall, London, 1984

Clemetson LL, Ward ACS: Bacterial flora of the vagina and uterus of healthy cats. J Am Vet Med Assoc 196:902, 1990

Dieter JA, Stewart DR, Haggarty MA, et al: Pregnancy failure in cats associated with long-term dietary taurine insufficiency. J Reprod Fertil Suppl 47:457, 1993

Dooley MP, Pineda MH, Hopper JG, Hsu WH: Retrograde flow of spermatozoa into the urinary bladder of cats during electroejaculation, collection of semen with an artificial vagina, and mating. Am J Vet Res 52:687, 1991

Herron MA: Feline vaginal cytologic examination. Feline Pract 1(7):36, 1977

Hurni H: Day length and breeding in the domestic cat. J Lab Anim 15:229, 1981

Jemmett JE, Evans JS: A survey of sexual behaviour in reproduction of female cats. J Small Anim Pract 18:31, 1977

Johnson CA: Uterine diseases. p. 1797. In Ettinger SJ (ed): Textbook of Veterinary Internal Medicine. 3rd Ed. WB Saunders, Philadelphia, 1989

Laliberte L: Pregnancy, obstetrics and postpartum management of the queen. p. 818. In Morrow DA (ed): Current Therapy in Theriogenology. WB Saunders, Philadelphia, 1986

Lawlor DF, Evans RH, Reimers TJ, et al: Histopathologic features, environmental factors, and serum estrogen, progesterone, and prolactin values associated with ovarian phase and inflammatory uterine disease in cats. Am J Vet Res 52:1747, 1991

Lawlor DF, Johnston SD, Hegstad RL, et al: Ovulation without cervical stimulation in domestic cats. J Reprod Fertil Suppl 47:63, 1993

Lein DH: Pyometritis in the bitch and queen. p. 942. In Kirk RW (ed): Current Veterinary Therapy VIII. WB Saunders, Philadelphia, 1983

Lein DH: Male reproduction. p. 1475. In Sherding RG (ed): The Cat: Diseases and Clinical Management. Churchill Livingstone, New York, 1989

Millis DL, Hauptman JG, Johnson CA: Cryptorchidism and monorchism in cats: 25 cases (1980–1989). J Am Vet Med Assoc 200:1128, 1992

Mills JN, Valli VE, Lumsden JH: Cyclical changes of vaginal cytology of the cat. Can Vet J 20:95, 1979

Mowrer RT, Conti PA, Rassow AF: Vaginal cytology: an approach to improvement of cat breeding. Vet Med Small Anim Clin 70:691, 1975

Munday HS, Davidson HPB: Normal gestation lengths in the domestic shorthair cat (Felis domesticus). J Reprod Fertil Suppl 47:559, 1993

Paape SR, Shille VM, Seto H, Stabenfeldt GH: Luteal activity in the pseudopregnant cat. Biol Reprod 13:470, 1975

Pedersen NC: Common infectious diseases of multiple cat environments. p. 163. In Pederson NC (ed): Feline Husbandry: Diseases and Management in the Multiple Cat Environment. American Veterinary Publications, Goleta, CA, 1991

Platz CC Jr, Seager SWJ: Semen collection by electroejaculation in the domestic cat. J Am Vet Med Assoc 173:1353, 1978

Potter K, Hancock DH, Gallina AM: Clinical and pathologic features of endometrial hyperplasia, pyometra, and endometritis in cats: 79 cases (1980–1985). J Am Vet Med Assoc 198:1427, 1991

Povey RC: Reproduction in the pedigree female cat. A survey of breeders. Can Vet J 19:207, 1978

Prescott CW: Reproduction patterns in the domestic cat. Aust Vet J 49:126, 1973

Shille VM, Lundstrom KG, Stabenfeldt GH: Follicular function in the domestic cat as determined by estradiol-17B concentrations in plasma: relation to estrous behavior and cornification of exfoliated vaginal epithelium. Biol Reprod 21:953, 1979

Shille VM, Stabenfeldt GH: Current concepts in reproduction of the dog and cat. Adv Vet Sci Comp Med 24:211, 1980

Stabenfeldt GH, Pedersen NC: Reproduction and reproductive disorders. p. 129. In Pedersen NC (ed): Feline Husbandry: Diseases and Management in the Multiple Cat Environment. American Veterinary Publications, Goleta, CA, 1991

Wildt DE, Kinney GM, Seager SWJ: Gonadotropin-induced reproductive cyclicity in the domestic cat. Lab Anim Sci 28:301, 1978

Wildt DE, Seager SWJ: Ovarian response in the estrual cat receiving varying dosages of HCG. Horm Res 9:130, 1978

Hemolymphatic System

62

Introduction

Karen M. Young

COMPONENTS AND FUNCTIONS

I. Blood cells are produced in the bone marrow from stem cells, acquire functional characteristics, are delivered to circulation, and are surveyed in the spleen.

II. Blood travels throughout the body delivering needed cells and plasma components.
   A. Erythrocytes: transport oxygen to tissues and carbon dioxide to lungs
   B. Leukocytes
      1. Neutrophils protect against bacterial infections.
      2. Eosinophils defend against parasites, abrogate hypersensitivity reactions, and participate in allergic reactions.
      3. Basophils play a role in defense against parasites and in hypersensitivity reactions.
      4. Monocytes/macrophages present antigens to lymphocytes, produce hematopoietic regulatory factors, modulate inflammation, and have antitumor effects.
      5. Lymphocytes play the major role in humoral and cell-mediated immunity; they also produce hematopoietic regulatory factors.
   C. Platelets and coagulation factors: critical to hemostasis and important in inflammation

III. Lymphoid tissue comprising bone marrow, thymus, lymph nodes, and spleen is central to development and maintenance of immune response to foreign antigens.

IV. Spleen also functions in blood filtration, removal of damaged or senescent blood cells, storage of blood cells, and extramedullary hematopoiesis.

ASSESSMENT

I. Blood analysis
   A. Blood is easy to obtain and analyze for cell counts, cell morphology, and quantitation and function of plasma constituents.
   B. Analysis of blood provides "window" to many body systems, often reflecting abnormalities or pathologic changes in diseased organs.

II. Bone marrow aspiration or biopsy
   A. Analysis provides useful information about production and maturation of hematopoietic cell lines.
   B. Aspirates are best for analysis of individual cell morphology.
   C. Biopsy is essential for detection of hypoplasia, aplasia, and fibrosis.
   D. Indications for bone marrow examination are the following.
      1. Nonregenerative anemia without identifiable extramarrow cause
      2. Pancytopenia
      3. Unexplained neutropenia or thrombocytopenia
      4. Presence of circulating abnormal or "atypical" cells
      5. Diagnosis of leukemia, plasma cell myeloma, or metastatic tumor
      6. Staging of certain neoplasms (e.g., lymphoma)
      7. Detection of hemotropic infectious organisms
      8. Determination of marrow iron stores

III. Lymph nodes and spleen
   A. Size and physical characteristics: palpation, imaging studies
   B. Cellular constituents, tissue architecture: biopsy, cytology

DISORDERS OF RED BLOOD CELLS

I. Anemia is a laboratory finding, not a disease, and may result from a primary red blood cell (RBC) abnormality or be secondary to an underlying disease process.
   A. Classification of anemia as regenerative or nonregenerative is essential to diagnosis and proper therapeutic management.

1. Regenerative anemias result from hemolysis or hemorrhage.
    2. Nonregenerative anemias can have both extramarrow and intramarrow causes.
  B. Hematologic data (RBC quantitation, indices, morphology, hemoglobin concentration, reticulocyte count) indicate the severity of the anemia, the presence or absence of a regenerative response, and sometimes the cause.
II. Polycythemia may be relative or absolute, with the latter category including primary (neoplastic) or secondary causes that are either physiologically appropriate or inappropriate.

DISORDERS OF WHITE BLOOD CELLS

  I. Quantitative and qualitative assessment of white blood cells (WBC) can give valuable information about the presence, progression, or resolution of a disease process.
 II. Neutrophils are critical to survival, with quantitation providing information on the balance between their production by bone marrow and utilization by tissues.
  A. Neutrophilia may be physiologic, stress-induced, or a response to inflammation.
  B. Neutropenia may indicate excessive tissue demand for neutrophils, decreased production, or immune-mediated destruction.
  C. Morphologic changes associated with disease include immaturity (left shift), toxic change, abnormalities of nuclear segmentation, and inclusions of infectious agents.
  D. Because neutrophils have a short life span, neutropenia may be the first reflection of damage to rapidly dividing cells caused by infectious agents (e.g., parvovirus) or by cytotoxic drugs.

LEUKEMIAS

  I. Both lymphoid and nonlymphoid leukemias are well documented in dogs and cats.
 II. Leukemias are classified as acute or chronic based on the degree of cellular differentiation.
III. A new subclassification system for acute non-lymphoid leukemias will permit acquisition of useful information about prognosis and treatment.

DISORDERS OF HEMOSTASIS

  I. Adequate hemostasis requires coordinated function of the vascular wall, platelets, and coagulation factors and a balance between clot formation and fibrinolysis.
 II. Hemostatic disorders may be acquired or inherited, with acquired disorders being more common.
III. Bleeding may result from quantitative or qualitative abnormalities in platelets or coagulation factors and from defects in the vessel wall.
  A. Pattern of bleeding (e.g., mucosal bleeding vs. bleeding into a body cavity) may indicate a defect in platelets or coagulation factors, respectively.
  B. Knowledge and appropriate use of laboratory tests for hemostatic components are essential to diagnosis and effective management of disorders of platelets and coagulation factors.
  C. Be aware that certain drugs and modified live virus vaccines can alter platelet number and function and further compromise hemostasis.
  D. Before surgical procedures, anticipate and be prepared for any bleeding complications.
IV. Thrombocytosis is usually secondary to another disease process and rarely causes clinical signs.

DISORDERS OF LYMPH NODES, LYMPHATICS, AND SPLEEN

  I. An intact immune system is essential for health and survival.
 II. Congenital disorders may result in aplasia or hypoplasia of lymph nodes or lymphatics.
III. Lymphadenopathy may signify lymphoid hyperplasia, inflammation, or neoplasia.
IV. Diseases affecting the spleen can disrupt splenic functions and can be diffuse or focal.

ONCOLOGY AND PARANEOPLASTIC SYNDROMES

  I. To provide accurate information to owners regarding prognosis and available therapy, understanding the principles of oncology is essential.
 II. Hypercalcemia, hypoglycemia, hyperhistaminemia, anorexia/cachexia, fever of unknown origin, inappropriate secretion of antidiuretic hormone, and hyperviscosity syndrome may be associated with and caused by various neoplasms.

ADVANCES IN TREATMENT

Many advances have been made in the treatment of neoplasia and disorders of the hemolymphatic system. These include the use of monoclonal antibodies, cytokines such as interferon, and immunoregulatory peptides such as liposome-encapsulated muramyl tripeptides. Others include the following.
  I. Transfusion medicine: safe and effective replacement of blood or blood components
  A. Transfusions are used to treat anemia, coagulopathies, and, less commonly, thrombocytopenia, thrombopathia, and hypoproteinemia.

B. Indications for transfusion with fresh whole blood, stored whole blood, or specific blood components, such as packed red cells, platelet-rich plasma, fresh-frozen plasma, or cryoprecipitate, vary.

C. Blood typing and cross-matching are important aspects of transfusion medicine.

D. Transfusion reactions may be mediated by immunologic or non-immunologic mechanisms.

II. Recombinant hematopoietic growth factors

A. Recombinant human erythropoietin (rh-EPO)

1. Its availability is a major advance in the treatment of anemia of renal disease.

2. Be aware of side effects and the potential for animals to develop antierythropoietin antibodies.

B. Recombinant canine granulocyte colony-stimulating factor (G-CSF) helps reduce morbidity and mortality in dogs receiving chemotherapy or total body irradiation.

III. Bone marrow transplantation

This technique has great promise in correcting inherited abnormalities, such as RBC enzyme deficiencies or mucopolysaccharidosis, and in treating certain disseminated neoplasms, such as lymphoma.

Bibliography

Beutler E, Lichtman MA, Coller BS, Kipps TJ (eds): Williams Hematology. 5th Ed. McGraw-Hill, New York, 1995

Weiss L (ed): Cell and Tissue Biology. A Textbook of Histology. 6th Ed. Urban & Schwarzenberg, Baltimore, 1988

63

Disorders of Red Blood Cells

David J. Fisher

LABORATORY ASSESSMENT OF RED BLOOD CELL ABNORMALITIES

Definitions and Causes

I. Red blood cells (erythrocytes, RBCs) are the cellular component responsible for transporting oxygen.

II. Anemia is defined as a decrease in the RBC mass. This decrease results in decreased oxygen delivery to the tissues.
   A. Anemias are classified as either regenerative or nonregenerative.
      1. Regenerative anemias are characterized by increased production and delivery of RBCs.
      2. Conversely, nonregenerative anemias are characterized by decreased production and delivery of RBCs.
   B. Functional anemia may also occur as a result of decreased oxygen-carrying capacity of hemoglobin, such as with methemoglobinemia or carbon monoxide poisoning.
   C. Anemia is not a disease, but a laboratory finding, and the underlying disease must be identified to allow for appropriate therapy.

III. Polycythemia is an increase in RBC mass (see Polycythemia later).

IV. Other abnormalities of RBCs may not cause anemia or polycythemia, but they do result in altered cell shape, cell size, and cytoplasmic constituents.
   A. Microcytosis and increased intracellular potassium in Akitas
   B. Macrocytosis in poodles
   C. RBC morphologic changes secondary to hepatic, splenic, or neoplastic diseases or to toxin or drug exposure

Clinical Signs

I. Anemia is typified by pallor and weakness.
   A. Development of other signs depending on severity and rate of progression
   B. Tachycardia, dyspnea, reduced exercise tolerance, and collapse (severe anemia)
   C. Occasional: heart murmur, jaundice, evidence of hemorrhage

II. Polycythemia is typified by mucous membrane congestion and cyanosis.

Diagnosis

I. The measurement of red blood cell mass is estimated based on the RBC count, hemoglobin concentration, and hematocrit (or packed cell volume). Packed cell volume is the easiest and quickest method for detecting anemia or polycythemia. Other laboratory values help further classify the pathologic process.
   A. RBC count may be obtained in two ways.
      1. Automated cell counters are the most accurate way to measure RBC numbers.
      2. Manual counts are inaccurate and time consuming and are not recommended.
   B. Hemoglobin (Hb) concentration usually is measured by colorimetric methods.
      1. The cyanmethemoglobin method is most common, but some automated instruments measure oxyhemoglobin spectrophotometrically.
      2. Artificially high values may be measured in the presence of lipemia, hemolysis, or large numbers of Heinz bodies.
   C. Packed cell volume (PCV) and hematocrit (HCT) are similar but not identical.
      1. HCT is calculated on automated counters by multiplying the RBC count and mean cell volume (MCV).
      2. PCV is measured using a microhematocrit tube and a microcentrifuge. The height of the RBC column divided by the height of the whole blood column is the PCV.
      3. HCT and PCV should be roughly the same, although the PCV can be 2–3% higher because of the space trapped between erythrocytes after centrifuging.

*Table 63–1. **Erythrocyte Parameters in Regenerative vs. Nonregenerative Anemias***

	Regenerative	Nonregenerative
Reticulocytes	Absolute: >60,000/µl Relative: >1%	Absolute: <60,000/µl Relative: <1%
Morphology	Increased anisocytosis and polychromasia Shape changes indicative of hemolysis (see Table 63–2)	Lack of or minimal anisocytosis and polychromasia Variable shape changes Hypochromasia: late iron deficiency
Indices	Macrocytic, hypochromic (usually) Normocytic, normochromic (<3 days duration; immune destruction of precursors)	Normocytic, normochromic (usually) Macrocytic, normochromic: FeLV related; dyserythropoiesis, B₁₂/folate deficiency, myelodysplasia or myeloproliferative disease Microcytic, normochromic: iron deficiency, dyserythropoiesis, liver disease Microcytic, hypochromic: late iron deficiency
Inclusions	Nucleated RBCs increased Howell-Jolly bodies ± Heinz bodies ± RBC parasites ± Basophilic stippling	Nucleated RBCs without appropriate reticulocytosis: dyserythropoiesis, lead toxicity, myelodysplasia, myeloproliferative disease, splenic or marrow disease
Bone marrow	Erythroid hyperplasia	Erythroid hypoplasia

II. Laboratory parameters used to assess the underlying cause of changes in RBC mass, in particular, whether an anemia is regenerative or not (Table 63–1), are as follows.
  A. RBC indices
    1. Mean cell volume (MCV)
      a) Average size of RBCs, typically expressed in femtoliters (fl)
      b) Either measured by a cell counter or calculated by the formula MCV (fl) = PCV × 10/RBC count (×10⁶)
      c) Increased MCV = macrocytic; normal MCV = normocytic; decreased MCV = microcytic
      d) Artifact: high MCV due to RBC clumping; low MCV if platelets counted as RBCs with automated counters
    2. Mean corpuscular hemoglobin concentration (MCHC)
      a) Average amount of hemoglobin concentration per RBC
      b) Calculated by the formula MCHC (g/dl) = [Hb] × 100/PCV
      c) Increased MCHC = hyperchromic (high MCHC is almost always an artifact caused by hemolysis, lipemia, Heinz bodies); normal MCHC = normochromic; decreased MCHC = hypochromic
    3. Red blood cell distribution width (RDW)
      a) Describes the variability in the size of RBCs
      b) Increased RDW = increased variation in RBC size, such as with regenerative anemias or iron deficiency
  B. Erythrocyte morphology on the blood smear (Table 63–2)
  C. Reticulocyte count

  1. Reticulocytes are immature, anucleated RBCs that are not fully hemoglobinized and still retain remnant RNA.
  2. Because of the retained RNA, they have a bluish color when stained with Wright's stain (i.e., reticulocytes = polychromatophils).
  3. Reticulocyte numbers are the most important factor in determining whether a regenerative response is present.
  4. They are counted by staining blood with new methylene blue dye, then counting the number of reticulocytes per 500–1000 RBCs to give the reticulocyte percentage.
    a) Cats have two types of reticulocytes: aggregate and punctate.
      (1) The aggregate reticulocytes are counted to assess for an active regenerative response.
      (2) The aggregate reticulocyte count closely corresponds to the degree of polychromasia.
      (3) Punctate reticulocytes circulate longer than aggregate reticulocytes and are indicative of the cumulative regenerative response rather than the active response.
    b) Normal count for both dogs and cats is less than 1% (i.e., counts greater than 1% are indicative of regeneration), but the percentage must be interpreted with respect to the degree of anemia (see discussion of corrected reticulocyte percentage and reticulocyte production index later).
    c) Usually, the degree of reticulocytosis for the degree of anemia is lower in cats than in dogs. A marked reticulocyte count in dogs is 20–50% reticulocytes; in cats, it is greater than 5%.

Table 63–2. **Morphologic Assessment of RBCs on a Blood Smear**

	Morphology	Description and Clinical Significance
Size	Anisocytosis	Variably sized RBCs; increased anisocytosis generally secondary to regeneration
	Macrocytosis	Large RBCs; usually reticulocytes, but occasionally fully hemoglobinized cells in some nonregenerative anemias (see Megaloblasts later)
	Microcytosis	Small RBCs; usually iron deficiency, also liver disease and fragmentation
Color	Polychromasia	Blue-colored RBCs; increased polychromasia is seen with reticulocytosis
	Hypochromasia	Hypochromic cells appear to have only a thin rim of hemoglobinized cytoplasm; microcytic, hypochromic cells are due to iron deficiency
Shape	Spherocytes	Dense, spherical, lack central pallor; usually seen with IMHA, occasionally with Heinz body and fragmentation anemias
	Eccentrocytes	RBCs with densely hemoglobinized area of cytoplasm leaving a pale cytoplasmic area to one side; oxidant exposure
	Schistocytes	RBC fragments; fragmentation hemolysis, iron deficiency
	Acanthocytes	RBCs with irregularly sized blunt projections from the surface; seen with hemangiosarcoma and liver disease
	Target cells	RBCs with dense central area separated by a clear area encircled by peripheral hemoglobinized region; associated with liver disease, also with regenerative anemia
	Stomatocytes	RBCs with a slit-like clear area in center of the cell; unusual, described in some breeds as a congenital RBC abnormality
	Autoagglutination	Diagnostic for IMHA, but must be distinguished from rouleaux formation; microscopically, agglutination looks like grape clusters, rouleaux look like stacked coins; rouleaux are dispersed with saline dilution
Inclusions	Nucleated RBCs	RBCs with retained nucleus, most mature form is the metarubricyte; increased numbers with regeneration but should be proportionate to reticulocytes; also can be increased with splenic or bone marrow disease, hemangiosarcoma, lead toxicity, splenic contraction
	Megaloblasts	Large RBCs with immature nuclear features but cytoplasm that is more fully hemoglobinized than expected for the degree of nuclear maturity and cell size; indicative of asynchronous maturation of the cytoplasm and nucleus, seen with myelodysplasia, myeloproliferative disease, FeLV, rarely folate/cobalamin deficiency
	Howell-Jolly bodies	Small, round nuclear fragments; increased with regeneration
	Heinz bodies	Pale, spherical projections from RBC surface; oxidant exposure, systemic disease in cats
	Basophilic stippling	Faint, punctate aggregations of residual RNA; may be seen with regeneration, also reported with lead toxicity
	Hemoparasites	*Hemobartonella* spp., *Babesia* spp., *Cytauxzoon felis*

IMHA = immune-mediated hemolytic anemia.

5. Absolute reticulocytes are calculated by multiplying reticulocyte percentage by the RBC count.
   a) Normal count for dogs is less than 60,000/μl; for cats, less than 50,000/μl.
   b) Determining absolute reticulocyte numbers is the most reliable way to assess regeneration in the peripheral blood, but it requires an RBC count.
6. If an RBC count is not done, then a corrected reticulocyte percentage (CR%) may be useful.
   a) CR% = reticulocyte % × HCT/normal HCT (45, dog; 37, cat)
   b) More accurate assessment of the regenerative response
   c) CR% >1% = evidence of regeneration
7. Reticulocyte production index (RPI) can be calculated in dogs if an absolute reticulocyte count is not done.
   a) The RPI is calculated by the following formula: RPI = reticulocyte percentage × (HCT/45) × (1/maturation time),

where maturation time of reticulocytes varies depending on HCT (45% = 1.0 day, 35% = 1.5 days, 25% = 2.0 days, 15% = 2.5 days).
   b) An RPI >2.0 indicates a good regenerative response.
D. Bone marrow examination
   1. Aspiration and/or biopsy is performed from sites such as the iliac crest, trochanteric fossa of femur, and craniodorsal humerus (see Chap. 3).
   2. Examination is indicated for nonregenerative anemias and to detect underlying dysplasia or neoplasia.
   3. Normal marrow has a myeloid to erythroid (M:E) ratio of approximately 1:1 to 2:1, with complete and orderly maturation in all hematopoietic lines. The M:E ratio may increase with age.
E. Plasma protein (refractometry)
   1. Protein generally decreases with external hemorrhage and increases with hemolysis.

Table 63–3. Reference Values in the Dog and Cat

	Canine	Feline
RBC ($\times 10^6/\mu$l)	5.5–8.5	5–10
Hemoglobin concentration (g/dl)	12–18	8–15
PCV (%)	37–55	24–45
MCV (fl)	60–77	39–55
MCHC (g/dl)	32–36	30–36

Values are ranges in normal dogs and cats.
From Jain NC (ed): Essentials of Veterinary Hematology. Lea & Febiger, Philadelphia, 1993.

2. Increased protein and PCV are indicative of dehydration.
III. Reference values are given in Table 63–3.

Differential Diagnosis

See Table 63–4.

REGENERATIVE ANEMIAS

Congenital or Hereditary Anemias

I. Most congenital RBC disorders of clinical significance cause hemolytic anemia.
II. See Table 63–5.

Erythrocytic Parasites

Definition

I. Hemolytic anemia is directly related to infection of the erythrocyte by a hemotropic rickettsial or protozoal organism.
II. Other infectious agents may cause anemias in a manner separate from actual RBC infection.

Causes

I. Hemobartonellosis: *Hemobartonella felis* (cats), *H. canis* (dogs; rare cause of anemia)
II. Babesiosis: *Babesia canis* (dogs), *B. gibsoni* (dogs)
III. Cytauxzoonosis: *Cytauxzoon felis* (cats)

Pathophysiology

I. *Hemobartonella* organisms are epicellular rickettsial parasites in the family Anaplasmataceae (Carney and England, 1993).
  A. The organism is transmitted by blood transfer, including by blood-sucking insects and by needles.
  B. Transplacental transmission may also occur.
  C. Infection causes RBC surface invagination, loss of RBC deformability, and antibody response to the parasite, all of which lead to increased RBC phagocytosis by macrophages.
    1. Many infected cats are also Coombs-positive and may have secondary immune-mediated hemolytic anemia.
    2. Cold agglutinins may be partially responsible for hemolysis, but this is controversial.
  D. Parasitemia develops 2–17 days after experimental infection and lasts 3–8 weeks.
  E. Cats that recover become carriers and may have relapses when exposed to stressful conditions.
  F. Risk factors include feline leukemia virus (FeLV) or feline immunodeficiency virus (FIV) infection, outdoor roaming, and stress from unrelated disease.
  G. Canine hemobartonellosis rarely causes clinical disease except in splenectomized dogs.
II. *Babesia* spp. are intracellular protozoal parasites (Taboada, 1995).
  A. Transmitted by ticks, primarily *Rhipicephalus sanguineus,* also *Dermacentor* spp. and *Haemaphysalis* spp.
  B. Transplacental or blood transfer also
  C. Incubation period: 10–21 days after exposure
  D. Mostly a problem in dogs, rare in cats
  E. Greyhounds: possibly greater risk of infection
  F. Frequently Coombs-positive (see Immune-Mediated Hemolytic Anemia later)
  G. Intra- or extravascular hemolysis
III. Cytauxzoonosis is almost always a fatal protozoal infection in cats (Hoover et al., 1994).
  A. The domestic cat is a dead-end host.
    1. The reservoir host is probably the bobcat. Infected cats are found in southern states from Oklahoma and Texas to Florida.
    2. The mode of transmission is uncertain, possibly ixodid ticks.

Table 63–4. Differential Diagnosis of Anemia: Regenerative vs. Nonregenerative Causes

Regenerative		Nonregenerative	
Hemorrhage	Hemolysis	Extramarrow	Intramarrow
Trauma	Immune-mediated	Chronic disease	Drug/toxic agent
Coagulopathy	Heinz body	Chronic renal or liver failure	Hypoplastic/aplastic
Ectoparasitism	Fragmentation	Endocrine disease	Myelofibrosis or necrosis
Gastrointestinal loss	Erythrocytic parasites	Nutrient/mineral deficiency	Myelodysplastic disease
Urinary loss	Intrinsic RBC defect		Hematopoietic malignancy
Neoplasia			Metastatic neoplasia

Table 63–5. **Congenital Red Blood Cell Diseases in Dogs and Cats**

Defect	Breed	Clinical and Laboratory Features	References
Pyruvate kinase (PK) deficiency	Basenji Beagle West Highland white terrier Cairn terrier Abyssinian cat	Moderate to severe hemolytic anemia with marked reticulocytosis, myelofibrosis, and osteosclerosis. Osteosclerosis not reported in Abyssinians. Abnormal PK kinetics and glycolytic intermediates. Genetic testing may be available for basenjis.	Giger and Noble, 1991 Giger and Kohn, 1995
Phosphofructokinase (PFK) deficiency	English springer spaniel American cocker spaniel	Chronic hemolytic disorder with acute hemolytic crisis precipitated by prolonged exercise, panting. Mild myopathy and pigmenturia found during acute exacerbation. Abnormal PFK activity, genetic testing available for English springer spaniel.	Giger and Harvey, 1987 Giger et al., 1992
Feline congenital porphyria	Domestic shorthair (DSH) Siamese	Variable anemia, brown/red discoloration of teeth and bones that fluoresce with ultraviolet light; partial deficiency of uroporphyrinogen III cosynthetase.	Weiser, 1995
Methemoglobin reductase deficiency	Several breeds of dogs DSH	Brown or muddy mucous membranes, weakness, lethargy, polycythemia; methemoglobin reductase activity is decreased and methemoglobin concentration is persistently increased (18–40% dogs, 50% cats).	Harvey et al., 1991, 1994
Hereditary or familial nonspherocytic hemolytic anemia	Beagles Poodles	Mild chronic hemolytic anemia, normal glycolytic enzymes, unknown defect Moderate hemolytic anemia with marked reticulocytosis, hemosiderosis, myelofibrosis, hepatosplenomegaly, possible membrane defect	Maggio-Price et al., 1988 Randolph, 1986
Hereditary elliptocytosis	Mixed breed dog	Elliptocytes, very mild anemia, erythrocyte membrane abnormality (protein 4.1)	Conboy et al., 1991
Stomatocytosis, macrocytosis	Alaskan malamute Miniature schnauzer Drentse patrijshond	Macrocytosis, normal PCV, mild reticulocytosis, chondrodysplasia in malamutes, membrane defect? Macrocytosis, hypertrophic gastritis	Brown et al., 1994 Slappendel et al., 1991
Familial macrocytosis and dyshematopoiesis	Poodles (miniature and toy)	Macrocytosis, normal PCV, hypersegmented neutrophils, impaired DNA synthesis?	Canfield and Watson, 1989
Dyserythropoiesis	English springer spaniel	Mild to moderate anemia, metarubricytosis, reticulocytosis absent, microcytosis, polymyopathy, cardiac disease, impaired DNA synthesis?	Holland et al., 1991
Selective cobalamin malabsorption	Giant schnauzer	Mild to moderate nonregenerative anemia, megaloblastic RBCs, low serum cobalamin, cachexia, dementia	Fyfe et al., 1989

3. The incubation period in experimental infections is 5–20 days.
B. The extraerythrocytic form proliferates in perivascular macrophages.
　1. Schizonts and macroschizonts are found in macrophages. These cells rupture and release merozoites that infect RBCs.
　2. RBC parasitemia is a late feature of infection.
　3. Blood stasis and death are typically rapid.
　4. Anemia is not well characterized, because death is usually rapid but may be caused by a combination of hemorrhage and hemolysis.

Clinical Signs

I. Hemobartonellosis: moderate to severe regenerative anemia, icterus, lethargy, depression, weight loss, pallor, ± fever
II. Babesiosis
　A. Young dogs (<6 months) are most susceptible.
　B. Clinical disease occurs in three forms.
　　1. Hyperacute disease: shock, disseminated intravascular coagulation (DIC), metabolic acidosis, rapid death
　　2. Acute disease: severe intravascular hemolysis

with hemoglobinuria and hemoglobinemia, icterus, lymphadenopathy, splenomegaly
   3. Subacute to chronic disease: fever, anorexia, depression, mild anemia
III. Cytauxzoonosis
   A. Depression, fever, hepatosplenomegaly, anorexia, ± icterus, rapid death
   B. Cats from southern states; no breed, age, or sex predilection; ± tick exposure

Diagnosis

I. In all cases, demonstration of the organism provides a definitive diagnosis.
   A. Parasitemia with *Hemobartonella* is transient or cyclic, and absence of the organism does not rule out infection.
      1. Small bacillary, coccoid, or ring forms are found on the surface or periphery of RBCs.
      2. Some anticoagulants (ethylenediaminetetraacetic acid [EDTA] may cause elution of the parasite from RBCs, and immediate preparation of blood smears may maximize the identification of organisms.
      3. If organisms are found in cats with a nonregenerative anemia, other causes of anemia should be investigated.
      4. Infected dogs generally are not anemic, and organisms are not found unless the dog is immunocompromised (splenectomized).
   B. *Babesia* organisms are most easily demonstrated in early infection.
      1. *B. canis*: usually paired piriform trophozoites in RBC
      2. *B. gibsoni*: smaller, single, annular, and pleomorphic
      3. Capillary blood probably best; infected cells at feathered edge of blood smear
   C. *Cytauxzoon* erythrocytic form is 1–2 μm in diameter and has the shape of a signet ring or safety pin, or tiny dots. Splenic or bone marrow aspirate is best suited to demonstrate extraerythrocytic form.
II. Serologic tests are available for *Babesia* infection.
   A. Serologic test does not distinguish between *B. canis* and *B. gibsoni*.
   B. Immunofluorescent antibody (IFA) titer >1:40 is considered positive for babesiosis.

Differential Diagnosis

I. Stain artifact or precipitate needs to be distinguished from *Hemobartonella* organisms.
II. *Hemobartonella* infections may occur concurrently with other disorders that also cause anemia, e.g., FeLV infection, immune-mediated hemolytic anemia.
III. Other causes of regenerative anemia must be ruled out if reticulocytosis is present.

Treatment

I. Hemobartonellosis: tetracycline 22 mg/kg PO TID for 2–3 weeks
II. Babesiosis (Taboada, 1995)
   A. Supportive therapy (intravenous fluids, transfusion) may be all that is required for treating acute disease caused by *B. canis*.
   B. The most effective babesicidal drugs are not available or approved for use in the United States except on a limited basis.
      1. Diminazene acetate (Berenil) 3.5 mg/kg IM
      2. Imidocarb dipropionate (Imizol) 5 mg/kg IM repeated in 14 days
   C. Infection due to *B. gibsoni* is less responsive to supportive therapy as well as to babesicidal therapy.
   D. There are anecdotal reports of successful treatment with clindamycin at 25 mg/kg PO divided BID.
III. Cytauxzoonosis: frequently fatal within a few days, no treatment

Patient Monitoring

I. *Hemobartonella*: carriers may re-express disease
II. *Babesia*: recovered dogs become inapparent carriers
III. Previously infected animals: not to be used as blood donors

Oxidant-Induced Anemia

Definitions

I. Oxidant damage of hemoglobin or cell membrane causes Heinz body or eccentrocyte formation with resultant decreased RBC life span.
   A. Heinz bodies are aggregates of precipitated hemoglobin.
   B. Eccentrocytes most likely result from oxidative injury to the RBC membrane.
II. Oxidation of heme iron results in methemoglobin.
III. Different oxidants may lead to the formation of Heinz bodies or eccentrocytes, or to methemoglobinemia, singly or in combination.

Causes

I. Various agents have been cited as causes of oxidative damage in dogs and cats.
   A. Onions
      1. Fresh, cooked, and dehydrated onions can cause Heinz body hemolytic anemia, mostly reported in dogs.
      2. Soup mixes and baby foods with onion powder have been implicated in clinical cases.
      3. Dogs appear to vary considerably in their susceptibility to onions.
   B. Acetaminophen
      1. In cats, methemoglobin values increase within 2–4 hours, followed by Heinz body formation (Harvey, 1995).
      2. In dogs, toxicity usually is associated with

a hepatopathy, but methemoglobinemia and anemia have also been described.

  C. Zinc toxicity
  1. The mechanism of hemolytic toxicity is unclear, but some animals with exposure to zinc have increased numbers of Heinz bodies.
  2. Zinc sources include pennies minted after 1982, zinc bolts, and zinc oxide ointment.

  D. Methylene blue
  The use of this agent as a urinary antiseptic has resulted in Heinz body hemolytic anemia, and it is no longer approved for such use.

  E. Phenazopyridine
  Used as a urinary analgesic, it has caused marked methemoglobinemia and Heinz body hemolytic anemia in cats.

  F. Benzocaine
  1. Over-the-counter topical preparations have caused primarily methemoglobinemia.
  2. Experimental use of benzocaine-containing spray on the larynx of cats caused marked methemoglobinemia.

  G. Vitamin K
  Vitamin K_3 can cause Heinz body hemolytic anemia in dogs and should not be used.

  H. DL-Methionine
  Used for urinary acidification, it produces Heinz body hemolytic anemia in cats.

  I. Propylene glycol
  This was used as a food additive in moist, soft cat food, but it was found to cause prominent Heinz body formation.

  J. Phenolic compounds (e.g., moth balls)

II. In cats, many types of systemic disease are reported to result in increased Heinz body formation, including diabetes mellitus, hyperthyroidism, lymphoma, and other nonhemic cancers (Christopher, 1989).

III. Hemolytic anemia has been described in five cats with diabetes mellitus and one cat with hepatic lipidosis, all of which had severe hypophosphatemia (<1.6 mg/dl) at the onset of the anemia. The pathogenesis of the anemia is uncertain but is possibly related to depletion of erythrocyte adenosine triphosphate (ATP) or increased susceptibility to oxidative damage (Adams et al., 1993).

Pathophysiology

  I. Heinz bodies (Christopher et al., 1990; Harvey, 1995)
  A. Oxidative damage to hemoglobin results in denaturation and Heinz body formation.
  B. Reduced RBC deformability causes decreased RBC life span.
  C. In dogs, pitting function of spleen (removal of Heinz bodies) may result in spherocyte formation. Clearance of Heinz bodies is independent of the spleen in the cat.
  D. Cats are more susceptible to Heinz body formation (Christopher et al., 1990).
    1. Decreased RBC reductive capacity compared with dogs

    2. More sulfhydryl groups on hemoglobin, easily oxidized to form irreversible disulfide bonds
    3. Heinz bodies of questionable significance in non-anemic cats

II. Methemoglobin
  A. It is formed by the oxidation of heme iron from the ferrous (2+) to ferric (3+) state.
  B. Only the ferrous state is able to reversibly bind oxygen.
  C. Formation of methemoglobin is normal to a degree (normal is 1–3%), but it is kept from accumulating by the reductive capacity of the cell.
  D. Drug toxicity (e.g., acetaminophen, benzocaine, phenazopyridine) may cause increased production.
  E. Decreased enzymatic reduction of methemoglobin occurs in animals with methemoglobin reductase deficiency (see Table 63–5).

Clinical Signs

  I. No age or sex predilection
  II. Heinz body hemolytic anemia
  A. Signs vary depending on the amount of oxidant exposure and the time elapsed since exposure.
  B. Pallor, ± icterus, weakness, depression, tachycardia, and hyperpnea occur if severe anemia is present.
  C. Vomiting, diarrhea, and anorexia may also occur.
  III. Methemoglobinemia
  A. Brown or muddy mucous membranes
  B. Tachycardia, hyperpnea, weakness, and lethargy
  C. With acetaminophen toxicity in cats, subcutaneous swelling, particularly of the face

Diagnosis

  I. Exposure to known oxidants
  II. Regenerative anemia with presence of Heinz bodies, eccentrocytes, ± spherocytes
  A. Heinz bodies may be seen with Wright's stain, but they are easiest to visualize with new methylene blue (NMB).
    1. With a NMB wet preparation, they are seen as dark refractile inclusions.
    2. With NMB used as a reticulocyte stain, they are seen as small to large, pale blue round projections or inclusions.
  B. Eccentrocytes are RBCs with hemoglobin that appears dense and constricted to one side of the cell, leaving a pale area that still contains a small amount of hemoglobin.
  III. Methemoglobinemia
  A. If methemoglobin concentration is greater than 10%, a drop of blood on filter paper appears brown compared with normal blood.
  B. Some referral laboratories are able to measure methemoglobin concentration.
  C. Methemoglobin reductase activity may be measured, but this typically requires a research laboratory.

Differential Diagnosis

I. Rule out other causes of regenerative anemia.
II. In cats with numerous Heinz bodies, the presence of systemic disease should be investigated.

Treatment

I. Heinz body hemolytic anemia
   A. Remove any oxidative substances and institute supportive care.
   B. Transfusions are usually not necessary.
II. Methemoglobinemia
   A. Removal of any oxidative substances
   B. In cats with acetaminophen ingestion
      1. Give *N*-acetylcysteine (Mucomyst) 140 mg/kg PO followed by 70 mg/kg PO QID for seven treatments (Harvey, 1995).
      2. Absorption of *N*-acetylcysteine is impaired by charcoal administration.
   C. Methylene blue (1% solution) 1 mg/kg IV slowly
      1. It should only be used in severe cases, and overuse must be avoided because too much methylene blue may result in increased oxidative damage.
      2. If used, PCV is monitored for 3 days afterward to detect development of a hemolytic anemia.

Patient Monitoring

I. Assess for good regenerative response, as blood repopulation is rapid with an intact marrow response.
II. Anemia nadir may not be reached for several days after exposure.

Immune-Mediated Hemolytic Anemia (IMHA)

Definition

I. This disorder arises from coating of the RBC surface with immunoglobulin and/or complement resulting in decreased RBC life span.
II. It is one of the most common immunohematologic disorders in dogs (Klag et al., 1993).

Causes

I. Idiopathic (primary or autoimmune)
   A. In dogs, it may constitute up to 60–75% of IMHA cases (Dodds, 1977; Jackson and Kruth, 1985).
   B. Recent review of 35 dogs with IMHA suggested a smaller percentage are idiopathic: 42.9% primary, 57.1% secondary (Jones and Gruffydd-Jones, 1991).
II. Secondary
   A. Neoplasia: most frequent cause of secondary IMHA
   B. Infectious or parasitic agents: FeLV, *H. felis, Ehrlichia canis,* dirofilariasis
   C. Drug-related
      1. Not well documented in animals
      2. Drugs suspected of causing IMHA: cephalosporins, penicillins, trimethoprim-sulfadiazine (Cotter, 1992)
   D. Neonatal isoerythrolysis: rare in cats and dogs; kittens born to type B queen mated to type A tom may be at greatest risk
   E. Vaccine-related (Dodds, 1977)
   F. Systemic immune-mediated disease (e.g., systemic lupus erythematosus)

Pathophysiology

I. Antigen is recognized on RBC membrane.
   A. May be self-antigen (autoimmune)
   B. Hidden or cryptic antigen exposed owing to membrane damage
   C. Drug, microorganism, or immune complexes bound to RBC membrane
   D. Infectious agents sharing antigenic determinants with RBC membrane proteins leading to cross-reacting antibodies
II. Immunoglobulin and/or complement coats the erythrocyte surface.
   A. IgG, IgM, and complement (C′) are most frequently involved.
   B. In dogs, IgG or both IgG and C′ are probably responsible for 50–70% of cases (Klag et al., 1993).
   C. Some classification schemes evaluate warm reactive (usually IgG) vs. cold reactive (usually IgM) antibodies. The diagnostic and therapeutic value of this is controversial (Cotter, 1992).
III. Coated RBCs are removed from circulation.
   A. If complement mediated (complete IgG or IgM both fix complement efficiently), then intravascular hemolysis may result.
   B. Removal by the mononuclear-phagocytic system (primarily in spleen and liver) results in extravascular hemolysis.
      1. Macrophages have receptors for complement and the Fc portion of antibody. They either completely phagocytize the coated RBC or phagocytize a portion of the RBC membrane, resulting in spherocyte formation.
      2. Extravascular hemolysis generally leads to hepatosplenomegaly.
IV. Cold agglutinating antibody is uncommon but may cause intravascular agglutination in small peripheral vessels during cold exposure and result in necrosis of extremities.

Clinical Signs

I. Signalment
   A. It may occur at any age, but it is most common in young and middle-aged animals (Dodds, 1977; Jackson and Kruth, 1985).
   B. Autoimmune hemolytic anemia is most common in female dogs. With secondary IMHA, there is

no sex predilection (Dodds, 1977; Jackson and Kruth, 1985).
  C. Commonly affected dog breeds include American cocker spaniels, poodles, Irish setters, and Old English sheepdogs, but there are no breed predilections in cats (Dodds, 1977; Stewart and Feldman, 1993).
 II. Seasonal incidence: most cases occur in spring (Klag et al., 1993)
III. Physical examination
  A. Animals are generally lethargic, weak, depressed, and anorectic.
  B. Physical examination reveals pale mucous membranes, tachycardia, hepatosplenomegaly, lymphadenopathy, icterus, fever, and ± heart murmur.
  C. Signs usually have insidious onset as a result of incomplete antibodies that cause a more slowly developing anemia, but onset may be acute with complete antibodies.

Diagnosis

  I. CBC and reticulocyte count
  A. Most commonly a regenerative, macrocytic, hypochromic anemia is present, but a significant portion of IMHA cases may be nonregenerative, as a result of peracute disease (<3 days) or antibody directed at reticulocytes or earlier precursors.
    1. Reticulocytes are usually more numerous than 60,000/μl (>1%).
    2. The percentage of cases with reticulocytosis at presentation varies from 59–69% (Jones and Gruffydd-Jones, 1991; Klag et al., 1993).
  B. RBC morphology reveals polychromasia and anisocytosis.
    1. Presence of autoagglutination is diagnostic for IMHA but must be distinguished from rouleaux formation (see Table 63–2).
    2. The presence of large numbers of spherocytes suggests IMHA, but they may also form as a result of other types of erythrocyte damage, e.g., removal of Heinz bodies.
    3. Spherocytes are difficult to identify in cats because of poor central pallor and small cell size normally.
  C. Neutrophilia with a left shift and monocytosis may occur.
 II. Biochemical profile and urinalysis: ± hyperbilirubinemia, hyperproteinemia, increased liver enzymes, bilirubinuria, hemoglobinuria (with intravascular hemolysis)
III. Direct antiglobulin test (DAT, also known as Coombs' test)
  A. A positive test result is consistent with the diagnosis of IMHA; however, the significance of a positive test in the absence of anemia is questionable.
  B. Reagents are species-specific and in most cases test for IgG, IgM, and complement together, although reagents can be used to detect these separately.
  C. It is routinely done at 37°C. It is not routinely run at 4°C because most positive results at this temperature are nonspecific (Cotter, 1992).
  D. The test is positive in about 60–70% of cases of IMHA (Cotter, 1992).
    1. False-positive results are not common, but it should be remembered that the test detects only the presence of immunoglobulin or complement on the surface of the RBC, and this occurs normally to some extent.
    2. False-negative results may be due to inadequate antibody or complement on RBCs, prozone effect, or previous corticosteroid therapy.
  E. No correlation exists between strength of reaction and the severity of clinical disease (Cotter, 1992).
  F. It is not necessary to do a Coombs' test in a patient with autoagglutination, because the presence of autoagglutination is already diagnostic for IMHA.
 IV. Bone marrow examination
  A. Generally, this procedure is not indicated for a regenerative anemia.
  B. If a nonregenerative anemia is present, but IMHA is suspected, bone marrow examination may be helpful to demonstrate erythroid hyperplasia, maturation arrest, increased iron stores, and/or increased erythrophagocytosis.
  V. Direct enzyme-linked antiglobulin test
  A. This test has shown correlation between severity of anemia and the amount of IgG bound to the RBC surface.
  B. It is not routinely available.

Differential Diagnosis

  I. Other causes of hemolytic anemia, including Heinz body anemia, microangiopathic hemolytic anemia, enzymopathies, and infectious agents, must be ruled out.
 II. Icterus may be caused by hemolysis or cholestatic disease.
  A. It is usually not necessary to determine the indirect and direct (unconjugated and conjugated) fractions of bilirubin to distinguish hemolytic icterus from hepatic icterus.
  B. Assessing other laboratory data (PCV, RBC morphology, liver enzymes) usually is sufficient to distinguish the two.
    1. Hemolytic icterus: anemia (usually regenerative), normal to mildly increased liver enzymes, ± spherocytes, Heinz bodies, parasites, or autoagglutination
    2. Hepatic icterus: PCV normal or mild nonregenerative anemia, increased liver enzymes, ± acanthocytes and/or target cells
III. In humans, hemophagocytic syndrome is a well-recognized cause of regenerative to nonregenerative anemias, as well as other cytopenias.
  A. This neoplastic or inflammatory proliferative disorder of histiocytes or monocytes that phagocy-

tize erythrocytes and other hemic cells results from pathogenic mechanisms that are not well understood.

B. Although this disorder is not well characterized in animals, four dogs and one cat with presumptive hemophagocytic histiocytosis have been described (Walton et al., 1996).

Treatment

I. Prednisone is the drug of choice and is given at 1–2 mg/kg PO BID (Cotter, 1992; Stewart and Feldman, 1993).
   A. This dose is continued until the PCV begins to rise, generally at 2–4 weeks.
   B. If PCV improves, reduce to SID for another 1–2 weeks, then reduce dosage by ½ and continue SID for another 1–2 weeks. Continue to taper accordingly.
   C. Other glucocorticoids may be used as alternatives, but adjust dosage according to relative potency.

II. Other immunosuppressive drugs in combination with prednisone are considered if there is fulminant hemolysis, autoagglutination, or lack of response to glucocorticoids (Cotter, 1992).
   A. Cyclophosphamide is administered at 50 mg/m² (2 mg/kg) PO or IV SID the first 4 days of a week or every other day. If possible, the drug is administered in the morning, and its use is limited to 4–6 weeks (Stewart and Feldman, 1993).
   B. Azathioprine is administered at 2 mg/kg PO SID initially, then reduced to 1 mg/kg PO SID after 7–10 days.
   C. There is no experimental evidence for which drug is more effective (Cotter, 1992).
   D. Response is not expected with these agents for 1–3 weeks, and drugs are tapered slowly over several months in recovering animals (Cotter, 1992).

III. Other drugs that may be effective include the following.
   A. Danazol 2–5 mg/kg PO TID in the dog (Stewart and Feldman, 1993)
   B. Human gammaglobulin 0.5–1.5 g/kg IV as a 12-hour infusion (Scott-Moncrieff et al., 1995)
   C. Cyclosporine 10 mg/kg/day PO or IM for 5 days, then skip 2 days

IV. If there is evidence of fulminant hemolysis or DIC, then heparin 100 U/kg SQ QID is administered.

V. Intravenous fluids are administered at 1–1.5 times the maintenance dose at initial presentation.

VI. Other therapeutic options include the following.
   A. Splenectomy is considered in cases of IMHA that have not responded to medical therapy or in recurring cases.
   B. Transfusions of whole blood or whole packed cells can be therapeutic and supportive and are used in animals with life-threatening anemia.

Patient Monitoring

I. PCV is measured at least SID initially to determine whether it is continuing to drop, leveling off, or beginning to increase.

II. Once the PCV is increasing, PCV measurement need be done only once a week to assess how therapy should be altered or tapered. Reduction of steroid therapy may take months.

III. Absent or poor reticulocyte response, leukopenia, and serum bilirubin concentration >10 mg/dl all have been associated with a worse prognosis (Klag et al., 1993).

IV. Use of cytotoxic drugs warrants monitoring of white blood cell and platelet counts, because neutropenia or thrombocytopenia may develop.

Fragmentation Hemolysis

Definition

I. Mechanical fragmentation of erythrocytes may lead to decreased RBC life span.

II. When caused by intravascular trauma, it is referred to as microangiopathic hemolytic anemia (Rebar et al., 1981).

Causes

I. Disseminated intravascular coagulation (DIC)
II. Cardiac or liver disease
III. Heartworm disease, vena cava syndrome
IV. Neoplasia, such as hemangiosarcoma
V. Splenic torsion
VI. Vasculitis
VII. Hemolytic-uremic syndrome (HUS)

Pathophysiology

I. Endothelial damage or coagulation system activation ultimately results in fibrin strands deposited in blood vessels, and as RBCs flow through the area, they are damaged by shearing.
   A. HUS is similar to DIC in that it occurs secondary to another pathologic process, ultimately resulting in thrombosis and coagulation factor depletion.
   B. In HUS, endothelial injury and platelet aggregation are initial events, whereas with DIC, widespread triggering of the coagulation system occurs first (Holloway et al., 1993).
   C. The occurrence of HUS is rare relative to DIC.

II. Turbulent blood flow or tissues with tortuous microvasculature, e.g., heart disease or neoplastic masses, may cause RBC fragmentation.

III. RBC fragments are cleared from the blood by the mononuclear-phagocytic system, resulting in decreased RBC life span.

Clinical Signs

I. Clinical signs of the inciting disorder predominate.

II. The rate of hemolysis may be subclinical, but occasionally acute hemolysis develops.

Diagnosis

I. Recognition of schistocytes, blister cells, keratocytes, or acanthocytes on blood smears
II. Coagulation panel to detect DIC: increased prothrombin time (PT) and activated partial thromboplastin time (aPTT), decreased platelet numbers, decreased fibrinogen concentration, increased fibrin split products, decreased antithrombin III concentration (see Chap. 66)
III. May have intravascular hemolysis with hemoglobinemia, hemoglobinuria
IV. HUS: microangiopathic hemolytic anemia, thrombocytopenia, acute renal failure
   A. Characterized by thrombosis on arterial side of circulation as opposed to venous side (DIC)
   B. Difficult to distinguish from DIC ante mortem

Differential Diagnosis

Other causes of hemolytic anemia

Treatment and Monitoring

I. Treatment must be directed at the underlying cause.
II. If DIC is present, heparin therapy and plasma transfusion should be considered (see Chap. 66).
III. Prognosis is generally guarded to poor.

Hemorrhagic Anemia

Definition

I. It results from the loss of RBCs from the vascular space.
II. Hemorrhage may occur internally (body cavities) or externally (lacerations, surgical blood loss, gastrointestinal bleeding, urinary loss).

Causes

I. Acute hemorrhage
   A. Trauma, surgery
   B. Hemostatic defect: acquired or hereditary coagulopathy, severe thrombocytopenia, or platelet dysfunction
   C. Neoplasia
II. Chronic hemorrhage
   A. Parasites: fleas, hookworms
   B. Gastrointestinal tumors, ulcers
   C. Renal hemorrhage (e.g., telangiectasia)

Pathophysiology

I. Within a few hours of blood loss, compensatory fluid shift to the vascular space results in decreased PCV and plasma protein concentration (Weiser, 1995).
II. If 30–50% of circulating volume is lost, shock may result.
III. Three to 4 days are required to see a regenerative response.
IV. If blood loss is low grade but chronic, anemia may or may not appear regenerative (see Nutritional or Mineral Deficiency later).

Clinical Signs

I. Hemorrhage from lacerations, surgery, other trauma
II. Epistaxis, petechiation, ecchymoses, melena, hematochezia, hemoptysis, hematuria
III. Pallor, lethargy, weakness

Diagnosis

I. Anemia is regenerative if blood loss occurred more than 3–4 days previously.
II. Plasma protein may be decreased.
III. Hemorrhage is evident.
   A. If from multiple sites: suggestive of hemostasis problem
   B. Radiography, ultrasonography, and body cavity centesis useful in detecting internal bleeding
IV. Occult blood is documented in feces.
   A. Two to 4 ml of blood in a 30 kg dog can result in a positive occult blood test, which is 20–50 times less than that required to cause melena.
   B. Diet may affect the results of occult blood testing, and diet modification (meat-free diet fed for 3 days prior to testing) is advisable.

Differential Diagnosis

Other causes of regenerative anemia

Treatment

I. Transfusion and fluid therapy with acute hemorrhage (see Chap. 69)
II. Chronic hemorrhage
   A. Correction of cause of hemorrhage
   B. Iron supplementation (see Nutritional or Mineral Deficiency)

Patient Monitoring

I. Acute hemorrhage: monitor for shock
II. Chronic hemorrhage: 60–120 days possibly required for normalization of RBC values

EXTRAMARROW NONREGENERATIVE ANEMIAS

Nutritional or Mineral Deficiency

Definitions

I. Iron is necessary for production of hemoglobin; deficiency results in decreased hemoglobin production and anemia.
II. Vitamin B_{12} (cobalamin) and folate both are necessary for DNA synthesis. Deficiency of either is a well-described cause of anemia in humans (e.g., pernicious anemia) but is reported infrequently in dogs or cats.

Causes

I. Iron deficiency
    A. In dogs and cats, almost always related to chronic blood loss rather than inadequate intake
        1. Young animals: severe flea infestation, hookworms
        2. Older animals: gastrointestinal disease (tumors, ulcers)
        3. Blood donors: overuse
    B. Weaning kittens with inadequate intake
II. Other deficiencies: cobalamin/folate deficiency, acquired or congenital

Pathophysiology

I. Iron deficiency
    A. Chronic external blood loss results in loss of iron. Deficiency can develop within 60–70 days in a medium-sized dog losing just 10 ml of blood per day (Weiser, 1995).
    B. Chronic blood loss results in nonregenerative anemia as animal becomes iron deficient.
        1. RBC size decreases in attempt to maintain cellular hemoglobin concentration (MCHC) at approximately 33%.
        2. As severity increases, hemoglobin concentration cannot be maintained and hypochromasia develops.
        3. Ultimately, a population of microcytic, hypochromic RBCs is created.
II. Folate or cobalamin deficiency
    A. Rare in both dogs and cats
    B. Dietary insufficiency, malabsorption, chronic folate inhibitor drug therapy (methotrexate, sulfas, anticonvulsants), congenital defect
        1. Cobalamin malabsorption in giant schnauzers has been reported as a congenital defect (see Table 63–5).
        2. Folate deficiency with macrocytic anemia was described in a Persian cat, probably from a folate-deficient diet and selective malabsorption.
    C. Defective DNA synthesis causing asynchronous maturation of nucleus and cytoplasm
        1. In humans, classically a macrocytic, normochromic anemia
        2. When recognized in dogs or cats, more often normocytic, normochromic
        3. Other cell lines possibly affected, e.g., hypersegmented neutrophils

Clinical Signs

I. Pallor, lethargy, weakness, exercise intolerance
II. Severe flea infestation, melena, hematochezia, diarrhea, emaciation

Diagnosis

I. Iron deficiency
    A. Microcytosis and hypochromia are late features.
    B. Serum iron (SI) is decreased.
        1. Total iron-binding capacity (TIBC) is normal to increased.
        2. Percent saturation (SI × 100/TIBC) is decreased (normal, approx. 33%).
    C. Bone marrow iron is absent.
    D. Perform occult blood test on fecal sample if melena or hematochezia is not evident.
II. Folate/cobalamin deficiency
    A. History of gastrointestinal disease or chronic folate inhibitor drug therapy
    B. Mild to moderate anemia, usually normocytic, normochromic, but may be macrocytic, normochromic; hypersegmented neutrophils
    C. Low serum cobalamin and/or folate concentration
    D. Correction of anemia with supplementation

Differential Diagnosis

I. Microcytosis
    A. Artifact from low RBC count and high platelet count with platelets counted as RBCs
    B. Occurs with liver disease (particularly portosystemic shunts), severe fragmentation anemias
II. Macrocytosis
    A. Artifact from RBC clumping
    B. Occurs with FeLV infection, dyserythropoiesis, reticulocytosis, myeloproliferative or myelodysplastic disease

Treatment and Monitoring

I. Correction of underlying cause of blood loss
II. Iron supplementation
    A. Administer ferrous sulfate 100–300 mg/day PO to dogs or 50–100 mg/day PO to cats.
    B. After PCV normalizes, reduce dosage by one half and continue supplementation.
    C. Injectable iron (iron dextran, 10–20 mg/kg) is considered if blood loss is gastrointestinal.
III. Cobalamin supplementation: 100–200 μg/day PO (dog); 50–100 μg/day PO (cat)
IV. Folic acid supplementation: 0.004–0.01 mg/kg/day (4–10 μg/kg/day)
V. May take weeks to months for anemia and RBC indices to correct

Anemia of Chronic Disease

Definition and Causes

I. Previously called anemia of chronic inflammatory disease, it consistently accompanies a variety of chronic disease problems, such as gingivitis, abscesses, dermatologic disease, and neoplasia.
II. It is probably the most common form of nonregenerative anemia.

Pathophysiology

I. Impaired marrow response to anemia (Weiss et al., 1983)

II. Sequestering of iron in mononuclear-phagocytic system

III. Shortened RBC life span

   A. Erythrocyte survival in cats with experimental sterile abscesses was significantly reduced.

   B. The decreased life span is a major factor in early stages of anemia in cats (Weiss and Krehbiel, 1983).

Clinical Signs and Diagnosis

I. Signs attributable to primary disease, not anemia

II. Mild to moderate nonregenerative anemia with evidence of other primary disease

III. Other causes of nonregenerative anemia ruled out

IV. Serum iron decreased, TIBC normal to decreased, percent saturation normal (approx. 33%)

Differential Diagnosis

I. Other causes of mild nonregenerative anemia

II. Decreased serum iron present in both chronic disease and iron deficiency

   A. TIBC should be measured in conjunction with serum iron to help distinguish it (see earlier).

   B. With chronic disease, bone marrow iron is increased as a result of increased iron sequestration; with iron deficiency, marrow iron is absent.

Treatment and Monitoring

I. Because anemia is generally mild, there is rarely a need to treat it directly.

II. Correction of the inciting cause typically corrects the anemia.

III. Monitoring is based on the primary disease process.

Anemia of Chronic Renal or Liver Failure

Definition

Both dogs and cats with chronic renal failure or chronic hepatic disease frequently develop a nonregenerative, normocytic, normochromic anemia of mild to moderate severity.

Causes and Pathophysiology

I. Chronic renal failure (King et al., 1992)

   A. Failure to produce adequate erythropoietin for the degree of anemia

   B. Impaired hematopoietic response to erythropoietin

   C. Shortened RBC life span

   D. Uremic toxins contributing to impaired response and shortened RBC life span

II. Chronic liver disease

   A. Altered RBC membrane lipid and cholesterol content results in RBC morphologic changes (acanthocytes, target cells) and possibly decreased life span.

   B. Other factors include RBC fragmentation and blood loss secondary to hepatic coagulopathies and gastrointestinal disease.

Clinical Signs

I. Clinical signs related to chronic renal failure or liver disease

II. Pallor, weakness, lethargy related to anemia

Diagnosis

I. Documentation of organ insufficiency/failure

   A. Renal failure: creatinine concentration roughly correlating to the degree of anemia (King et al., 1992)

   B. Liver disease: elevated liver enzymes, increased bile acids, hyperbilirubinemia, hypoalbuminemia, hypoglycemia, decreased BUN

II. Nonregenerative anemia

Differential Diagnosis

Rule out other causes of nonregenerative anemia.

Treatment and Monitoring

I. Anemia is not often severe enough to require transfusion, yet it may be serious and unremitting enough to worsen the quality of life.

II. In chronic renal failure, erythropoietin administered at 50–150 U/kg SQ 2–3 times weekly usually corrects the anemia (see Chap. 47).

III. With erythropoietin therapy, 20–30% of dogs and cats may develop anti-erythropoietin antibodies.

Anemia Related to Endocrine Disease

Definition

Endocrine disorders commonly result in a nonregenerative anemia of mild to moderate severity.

Causes

I. Hypothyroidism

II. Hypoadrenocorticism

Pathophysiology and Clinical Signs

I. Cortisol and thyroid hormones have stimulatory effects on RBC production, including facilitating the effect of erythropoietin on marrow.

II. Clinical signs are associated with the endocrine disorder.

Diagnosis

I. Mild nonregenerative anemia (dehydration with hemoconcentration may mask anemia)

II. Documentation of endocrine disease

Differential Diagnosis

Rule out other causes of nonregenerative anemia.

Treatment and Monitoring

I. Anemia is generally mild and is not treated.
II. Correction of the underlying endocrine disorder usually corrects the anemia.
III. In most cases, weeks to months may be required for complete resolution of anemia.

INTRAMARROW NONREGENERATIVE ANEMIAS

Drug/Toxin-Induced Anemia

Definition and Causes

I. Altered hematopoiesis from various drugs and/or toxic agents
II. Drug toxicity, e.g., phenylbutazone, estrogen, chloramphenicol, meclofenamic acid, trimethoprim-sulfadiazine, chemotherapeutic agents (Weiss and Klausner, 1990)
III. Neoplasia, e.g., estrogen-producing testicular tumors (Sertoli cell and interstitial cell)

Pathophysiology

I. Direct destruction of early to late precursors by drug or toxin, interference with cytokine and growth factor effects, and altered marrow microenvironment all may contribute to the development of cytopenias.
II. Estrogen may block the effect of erythropoietin on stem cells.
    A. Initial 2–3 weeks: thrombocytopenia, neutrophilia
    B. Neutropenia usually within 4 weeks, anemia slower to develop
III. Phenylbutazone causes a dose-independent, idiosyncratic reaction with neutropenia, thrombocytopenia, and slow-onset anemia.
IV. Chloramphenicol causes a reversible anemia and thrombocytopenia in some cats.
V. Trimethoprim-sulfadiazine induces both dose-dependent and idiosyncratic reactions.
    A. High doses reduce serum folate levels and may result in anemia (Weiss and Klausner, 1990).
    B. Pancytopenia associated with a polysystemic reaction has been described in Doberman pinschers.
VI. Meclofenamic acid has caused bone marrow failure in one reported case (Weiss and Klausner, 1990).
VII. Chemotherapeutic agents usually induce neutropenia and thrombocytopenia because of the shorter life spans of these cells.

Clinical Signs

I. Clinical signs: related to the degree of cytopenia
II. Neutropenia and thrombocytopenia usually more se-
vere, leading to opportunistic infections and bleeding, respectively
III. Estrogen: feminization, endocrine alopecia
IV. Chloramphenicol: central nervous system depression, anorexia, weight loss
V. Trimethoprim-sulfadiazine (in Doberman pinschers): shifting leg lameness, polyuria/polydipsia, skin rash, fever
VI. Other drugs: no specific clinical signs

Diagnosis

I. History of drug exposure, testicular tumor, cryptorchidism
II. Bone marrow evaluation generally revealing a hypoplastic marrow

Differential Diagnosis

Rule out other causes of multiple cytopenias.

Treatment

I. Removal of offending drug or toxin
II. Transfusions and antibiotics as indicated

Patient Monitoring

I. Monitor CBC weekly to detect recovering marrow.
II. If recovery is to occur, increasing cell counts are often seen within 1–3 weeks.
III. Estrogen-induced aplastic anemia is usually fatal, although recovery has been reported.

Hypoplastic Anemias

Definitions and Causes

I. Aplastic anemia and pure red cell aplasia (PRCA) are characterized by cytopenias in all cell lines or limited to the erythroid series, respectively; they are both manifested by severe nonregenerative anemias.
II. The cause of these anemias may either be primary or secondary.
    A. Primary: no causes are identified (idiopathic)
    B. Secondary
        1. Infectious agents: FeLV, *Ehrlichia*
        2. Drug toxicity (see earlier)
        3. Immune-mediated disease directed at early to late precursors
III. One case of presumptive congenital PRCA was described in a 3-month-old Samoyed dog that was similar to a syndrome in humans resulting from an intrinsic bone marrow defect.

Pathophysiology and Clinical Signs

I. Direct or indirect injury to pluripotent stem cells or early erythroid precursors or alterations in the marrow microenvironment may contribute to the pathogenesis.
II. Signs are related to the severity of cytopenias and

which cell lines are affected. Problems include opportunistic infections, weakness, lethargy, pallor, hemorrhage, and petechiation.

Diagnosis

I. Bone marrow aspiration and/or biopsy
   A. Marrow examination reveals hypoplasia or aplasia of at least the erythroid series.
   B. If there is severe hypoplasia, marrow core biopsy is better suited to demonstrate this rather than aspiration alone.
   C. Increased erythrophagocytosis and/or cytophagia may be observed in the marrow, as well as increased iron stores.
II. History of exposure to drugs, toxins, and ticks
   A. FeLV and *Ehrlichia canis* testing
   B. Coombs' test

Differential Diagnosis

Rule out other causes of severe nonregenerative anemia.

Treatment

I. Correction of preexisting problem if possible
II. Symptomatic and supportive care, including transfusions and broad-spectrum antibiotics
III. Immunosuppressive therapy: if aplasia is from immune disease (Weiss, 1992)
IV. Bone marrow stimulation
   A. Controlled studies in animals have not been done.
   B. Treatment with oxymetholone 2 mg/kg PO divided BID was successful in one dog with aplastic anemia (Weiss, 1992).
V. Bone marrow transplantation (not routinely available)

Patient Monitoring

I. Prognosis is generally guarded to poor.
II. In some instances, RBC suppression is transient with complete recovery of the marrow (Weiss, 1992).

Myelofibrosis and Marrow Necrosis

Definition and Causes

I. Myelofibrosis by definition is the replacement of marrow hemic tissue with fibrous tissue.
II. Marrow necrosis occurs as a result of degeneration of marrow elements secondary to infectious agents, toxins, drugs, or neoplasia.

Pathophysiology

I. Myelofibrosis is characterized by fibroblastic proliferation in the marrow cavity (Reagan, 1993).
   A. Primary disease is thought to be a myeloproliferative disorder, but in dogs and cats, it is possible that myelofibrosis is always secondary (Reagan, 1993).
   B. Secondary disease is a nonspecific attempt at marrow repair after damage such as radiation, congenital hemolytic anemia, marrow necrosis, myeloproliferative disease, myelodysplasia, and marrow inflammation.
II. The pathogenesis of marrow necrosis is poorly understood, but two mechanisms have been proposed (Weiss et al., 1985).
   A. Direct toxic damage to hematopoietic tissue by bacterial and viral infections, irradiation, myelotoxic chemicals
   B. Failure of the marrow microcirculation

Clinical Signs and Diagnosis

I. Signs are related to the severity of cytopenias and which cell lines are affected. Problems include opportunistic infections, weakness, lethargy, pallor, hemorrhage, and petechiation.
II. Fibrosis is better demonstrated on bone marrow core biopsy than on an aspirate.
III. Anemia, thrombocytopenia, and neutropenia are present. Dacryocytes (tear-shaped RBCs) may be found with fibrosis, but they are not a common feature.

Treatment

I. Supportive care including transfusions and antibiotics
II. Anti-fibrotic drugs: not evaluated in dogs or cats with myelofibrosis

Patient Monitoring

I. Monitor CBC weekly to evaluate need for supportive care.
II. Cases of marrow necrosis with prolonged survival have been reported (Weiss et al., 1985).

Myelodysplasia or Hematopoietic Neoplasia

See Chap. 65.

POLYCYTHEMIA

Definition

I. Relative: RBC mass not actually increased; plasma volume decreased as reflected by increased PCV, RBC count, Hb concentration, and plasma protein concentration
II. Absolute: RBC mass increased, resulting in increased PCV, RBC count, and Hb concentration
   A. Primary (polycythemia vera)
   B. Secondary
      1. Physiologically appropriate
      2. Physiologically inappropriate

Causes

I. Dehydration is the most common cause of polycythemia.

II. Physiologic causes include problems that result in decreased PaO_2, such as right-to-left heart shunt, high altitude, chronic pulmonary disease, massive obesity (pickwickian syndrome), and defective oxygen transport (chronic methemoglobinemia).

III. Physiologically inappropriate causes include the following.
   A. Tumors producing erythropoietin-like substance, including renal cell carcinoma, renal lymphoma, cerebellar hemangioblastoma, hepatoma, uterine leiomyoma, ovarian carcinoma, pheochromocytoma, adrenocortical adenoma (Campbell, 1990)
   B. Renal disease: cysts, hydronephrosis, pyelonephritis, localized renal hypoxia (Waters and Prueter, 1988)

IV. Polycythemia vera is a myeloproliferative disorder.

Pathophysiology

I. Relative polycythemia: dehydration results in a loss of intravascular fluid

II. Physiologic secondary polycythemia
   A. It is mediated by increased production of erythropoietin.
   B. Increased production is a compensatory physiologic response to increased tissue hypoxia.

III. Nonphysiologic secondary polycythemia
   A. It occurs secondary to production of erythropoietin or erythropoietin-like compounds.
   B. Increased production is not regulated by tissue oxygen concentration.

IV. Primary polycythemia
   A. Clonal disorder of the pluripotential stem cell
   B. Expansion of committed stem cells, primarily of erythroid line
   C. Erythropoietin independent

Clinical Signs

I. Relative polycythemia: fluid loss due to vomiting, diarrhea

II. Absolute polycythemia
   A. Generally older animals
   B. Congestion and cyanosis of mucous membranes
   C. Neurologic disturbances
   D. Hemorrhagic tendencies, retinal vascular tortuosity and hemorrhage, retinal detachment

Diagnosis

I. PCV >60% is indicative of polycythemia; PCV >70% suggests primary polycythemia.

II. Assess plasma protein, skin turgor, and mucous membranes to detect dehydration.

III. Decreased PaO_2 is suggestive of physiologic secondary polycythemia, although increased blood viscosity can decrease oxygen delivery with primary polycythemia.
   A. Normal PaO_2 is >97%.
   B. Polycythemia is physiologically appropriate when PaO_2 <92% (Campbell, 1990).

IV. Evaluate animal for history of cardiovascular or pulmonary disease to support decreased oxygen delivery.

V. Perform radiography, ultrasonography, and/or intravenous pyelogram to identify renal disease.

VI. Erythropoietin measurement does not always distinguish the cause of polycythemia, although in dogs the median erythropoietin concentration may be significantly decreased with polycythemia vera as compared with secondary polycythemia (Cook and Lothrop, 1994).

Differential Diagnosis

I. Differentiate relative from absolute polycythemia.

II. Differentiate secondary from primary polycythemia and physiologically appropriate from inappropriate responses.

Treatment

I. Fluid therapy to correct dehydration, treatment of underlying disease, and removal of contributing causes are the major therapies except for polycythemia vera.

II. Phlebotomy is used for patients with polycythemia vera but is contraindicated with physiologic secondary polycythemia (i.e., systemic hypoxia) unless it is severe.
   A. Removal of 20 ml/kg blood results in a decrease of approximately 15% in PCV.
   B. Replace blood with equal volume of saline or plasma expanders.
   C. Goal is to reach high normal PCV, although PCV of 50–60% is acceptable.

III. Hydroxyurea is an alternative therapeutic choice for treating polycythemia vera and is indicated if phlebotomy is needed more often than every 4–8 weeks (Campbell, 1990).
   A. Give 15 mg/kg PO SID until PCV normalizes (monitor PCV every 7–14 days).
   B. After PCV normalizes, recheck every 3–4 months.
   C. If cytopenias develop, discontinue drug, then restart at lower maintenance dose.

Patient Monitoring

I. Increased risk for thrombosis occurs with polycythemia and frequent phlebotomy.

II. Monitor PCV every 1–4 weeks depending on therapy.

III. Frequent phlebotomy may result in iron deficiency.

Bibliography

Adams LG, Hardy RM, Weiss DJ et al: Hypophosphatemia and hemolytic anemia associated with diabetes mellitus and hepatic lipidosis in cats. J Vet Intern Med 7:266, 1993

Brown DE, Weiser MG, Thrall MA: Erythrocyte indices and volume distribution in a dog with stomatocytosis. Vet Pathol 31:247, 1994

Campbell KL: Diagnosis and management of polycythemia in dogs. Compend Contin Educ Pract Vet 12:543, 1990

Canfield PJ, Watson ADJ: Investigations of bone marrow dyscrasia in a poodle with macrocytosis. J Comp Pathol 101:269, 1989

Carney HC, England JJ: Feline hemobartonellosis. Vet Clin North Am [Small Anim Pract] 23:79, 1993

Christopher MM: Relation of endogenous Heinz bodies to disease and anemia in cats: 120 cases (1978–1987). J Am Vet Med Assoc 194:1089, 1989

Christopher MM, White JG, Eaton JW: Erythrocyte pathology and mechanisms of Heinz body-mediated hemolysis in cats. Vet Pathol 27:299, 1990

Conboy JG, Shitamoto R, Parra M et al: Hereditary elliptocytosis due to both qualitative and quantitative defects in membrane skeletal protein 4.1. Blood 78:2438, 1991

Cook SM, Lothrop CD Jr: Serum erythropoietin concentrations measured by radioimmunoassay in normal, polycythemic, and anemic dogs and cats. J Vet Intern Med 8:18, 1994

Cotter SM: Autoimmune hemolytic anemia in dogs. Compend Contin Educ Pract Vet 14:53, 1992

Dodds JW: Autoimmune hemolytic disease and other causes of immune-mediated anemia. An overview. J Am Anim Hosp Assoc 13:437, 1977

Fyfe JC, Jesyk PF, Giger U et al: Inherited selective malabsorption of vitamin B_{12} in giant schnauzers. J Am Anim Hosp Assoc 25:533, 1989

Giger U, Harvey JW: Hemolysis caused by phosphofructokinase deficiency in English springer spaniels. J Am Vet Med Assoc, 191:453, 1987

Giger U, Kohn B: Feline hemolytic anemias. Proc Am Coll Vet Intern Med 13:230, 1995

Giger U, Noble NA: Determination of erythrocyte pyruvate kinase deficiency in Basenjis with chronic hemolytic anemia. J Am Vet Med Assoc 198:1755, 1991

Giger U, Smith BF, Woods CB et al: Inherited phosphofructokinase deficiency in an American cocker spaniel. J Am Vet Med Assoc 201:1569, 1992

Harvey JW: Methemoglobinemia and Heinz-body hemolytic anemia. p. 443. In Bonagura JD (ed): Kirk's Current Veterinary Therapy XII: Small Animal Practice. WB Saunders, Philadelphia, 1995

Harvey JW, King RR, Barry CR et al: Methemoglobin reductase deficiency in dogs. Comp Haematol Int 1:55, 1991

Harvey JW, Dahl M, High ME: Methemoglobin reductase deficiency in a cat. J Am Vet Med Assoc 205:1290, 1994

Holland CT, Canfield PJ, Watson ADJ et al: Dyserythropoiesis, polymyopathy, and cardiac disease in three related English springer spaniels. J Vet Intern Med 5:151, 1991

Holloway S, Senior D, Roth L et al: Hemolytic uremic syndrome in dogs. J Vet Intern Med 7:220, 1993

Hoover JP, Walker DB, Hedges JD: Cytauxzoonosis in cats: eight cases (1985–1992). J Am Vet Med Assoc 205:455, 1994

Jackson ML, Kruth SA: Immune-mediated hemolytic anemia and thrombocytopenia in the dog. A retrospective study of 55 cases diagnosed from 1969 through 1983 at the Western College of Veterinary Medicine. Can Vet J 26:245, 1985

Jones DRE, Gruffydd-Jones TJ: The haematological consequences of immune-mediated anemia in the dog. Comp Haematol Int 1:83, 1991

King LG, Giger U, Disereris D: Anemia of chronic renal failure in dogs. J Vet Intern Med 6:264, 1992

Klag AR, Giger U, Shofer FS: Idiopathic immune-mediated hemolytic anemia in dogs: 42 cases (1986–1990). J Am Vet Med Assoc 202:783, 1993

Maggio-Price L, Emerson CL, Hinds TR et al: Hereditary nonspherocytic hemolytic anemia in beagles. Am J Vet Res 49:1020, 1988

Randolph JF, Center SA, Kallfelz FA et al: Familial nonspherocytic hemolytic anemia in poodles. Am J Vet Res 47:687, 1986

Reagan WJ: A review of myelofibrosis in dogs. Toxicol Pathol 21:164, 1993

Rebar AH, Lewis HB, DeNicola DB: Red cell fragmentation in the dog: an editorial review. Vet Pathol 18:415, 1981

Scott-Moncrieff JL, Reagan WJ, Glickman LT et al: Treatment of nonregenerative anemia with human gamma-globulin in dogs. J Am Vet Med Assoc 206:1895, 1995

Slappendel RJ, van der Gaag I, Van Nes JJ et al: Familial stomatocytosis-hypertrophic gastritis (FSHG): a newly recognised disease in the dog (Drentse patrijshond). Vet Q 13:30, 1991

Stewart AF, Feldman BF: Immune-mediated hemolytic anemia. Part II. Clinical entity, diagnosis, and treatment theory. Compend Contin Educ Pract Vet 15:1479, 1993

Taboada J: Canine babesiosis. p. 315. In Bonagura JD (ed): Kirk's Current Veterinary Therapy XII: Small Animal Practice. WB Saunders, Philadelphia, 1995

Walton RM, Modiano JF, Thrall MA et al: Bone marrow cytological findings in 4 dogs and a cat with hemophagocytic syndrome. J Vet Intern Med 10:7, 1996

Waters DJ, Prueter JC: Secondary polycythemia associated with renal disease in the dog: two case reports and review of literature. J Am Anim Hosp Assoc 24:109, 1988

Weiser MG: Erythrocyte responses and disorders. p. 1864. In Ettinger SJ, Feldman EC (eds): Textbook of Veterinary Internal Medicine. 4th Ed. WB Saunders, Philadelphia, 1995

Weiss DJ: Aplastic anemia. p. 479. In Kirk RW, Bonagura JD (eds): Current Veterinary Therapy XI: Small Animal Practice. WB Saunders, Philadelphia, 1992

Weiss DJ, Klausner JS: Drug-associated aplastic anemia in dogs: eight cases (1984–1988). J Am Vet Med Assoc 196:472, 1990

Weiss DJ, Krehbiel JD: Studies of the pathogenesis of anemia of inflammation: erythrocyte survival. Am J Vet Res 44:1830, 1983

Weiss DJ, Krehbiel JD, Lund JE: Studies of the pathogenesis of anemia of inflammation: mechanisms of impaired erythropoiesis. Am J Vet Res 44:1832, 1983

Weiss DJ, Armstrong PJ, Reimann K: Bone marrow necrosis in the dog. J Am Vet Med Assoc 187:54, 1985

64

Disorders of White Blood Cells

Joyce S. Knoll

CONGENITAL DISORDERS

Canine Cyclic Hematopoiesis

Definition and Causes

I. In cyclic hematopoiesis there is periodic production and shutdown of all hematopoietic lines in the marrow at 10- to 14-day intervals (Jones et al., 1975).

II. It is characterized in the peripheral blood by cycles of neutropenia, monocytosis, thrombocytosis, and reticulocytosis.

III. All silver gray (not blue merle) collies are affected.

IV. It is inherited as an autosomal recessive trait, with one gene believed to be responsible for both hair coat color and the hematologic disorder.

V. Cause of the cyclic change is unknown, but it appears to be the result of a defect in the pluripotential stem cell (Abkowitz et al., 1988).

Pathophysiology

I. The cycles begin at birth and are continuous.

II. All cell lines are affected, but severe neutropenia is the most prominent finding because of the longer life span of other cells.

III. Neutrophils have a slightly decreased killing function; platelets have a defect in aggregation (Boney et al., 1985).

Clinical Signs

I. Periodic bacterial infections begin as early as 6–8 weeks of age.

II. Growth and sexual development are retarded.

III. Severity and number of infections are variable from dog to dog and are independent of granulocyte numbers. Most infections begin shortly after neutropenia and may persist beyond the period of neutropenia.

IV. Infections usually involve skin, lungs, gastrointestinal tract, kidneys, joints, and heart valves.

V. Acute infections are most common in young pups; chronic continuous infections are more common in older dogs.

Diagnosis

I. Suspicious breed and phenotype

II. Rare disorder in clinical practice; used as a model for abnormal hematopoiesis

III. Laboratory findings

A. Each blood cell type cycles independently, with the cycle length averaging 12 days.

1. Neutropenia lasts about 4 days, followed by a rebound neutrophilia.

2. Monocytosis is the first sign of recovery and occurs 2–4 days before neutrophilia.

3. Lymphocyte counts are highest during neutropenic episodes, and large, immature lymphocytes with basophilic cytoplasm (atypical lymphocytes) may be present.

4. Eosinophils are highest during neutropenic episodes.

5. Reticulocyte numbers are highest 3–6 days after neutrophilia.

B. Microcytic normochromic anemia is usually present because of either a stem cell defect or chronic infections.

C. Dogs may have increased circulating immunoglobulins.

D. Secondary amyloidosis may occur with time and is found on biopsy of affected organs.

Treatment

I. Bactericidal antibiotic therapy is indicated during febrile episodes.

II. Lithium carbonate 21–26 mg/kg/day PO stabilizes neutrophil numbers, reducing the severity of the cycling.

III. Administration of recombinant granulocyte colony-

stimulating factor prevents neutropenic episodes but does not correct cellular defects (Pratt et al., 1990).
IV. Bone marrow transplants from normal animals are curative.
V. Animals should be housed separately in a protected environment.

Patient Monitoring

I. Owner observation is important, with prompt institution of antibiotics as needed.
II. Prognosis is grave, as many animals are dead by 6 months, and few survive beyond 3 years of age.

Inherited Malabsorption of Vitamin B₁₂

Definition and Causes

I. The condition is caused by a selective malabsorption of cobalamin (vitamin B_{12}).
II. It is reported in giant schnauzers (Fyfe et al., 1989).
III. The inheritance pattern appears to be autosomal recessive.

Pathophysiology

I. Ileal enterocytes lack the receptor for the vitamin B_{12}–intrinsic factor complex (Fyfe et al., 1991).
II. Cobalamin is important for synthesis of nucleic acids, which are essential for growth and normal hematopoiesis.
   A. Deficiency causes failure to gain weight in spite of near normal linear growth.
   B. Abnormal maturation of hematopoietic cells results.
III. Cobalamin is also a cofactor in a common amino acid catabolic pathway; deficiency results in accumulation of the organic acid methylmalonic acid, which can be detected in urine.

Clinical Signs

I. Affected dogs show inappetence, lethargy, cachexia, and failure to thrive.
II. Clinical signs can usually be noted between 6 and 12 weeks of age, after body stores developed in utero are depleted.

Diagnosis

I. Laboratory findings are suggestive.
   A. Neutropenia with formation of hypersegmented neutrophils
   B. Nonregenerative anemia, marked anisocytosis and poikilocytosis of red blood cells (RBCs)
   C. Bone marrow hypocellular, with evidence of erythroid and granulocytic dysplasia
   D. Chronic proteinuria
II. Document decreased serum vitamin B_{12} levels in the face of a normal diet.
III. Document methylmalonic aciduria.

IV. Generalized intestinal malabsorption, exocrine pancreatic insufficiency, and bacterial overgrowth are ruled out, as these can also cause low serum cobalamin levels (see Chap. 32).

Treatment

The syndrome can be mitigated by administering parenteral (but not oral) vitamin B_{12} 0.5–1 mg IM weekly to every few months as needed.

Pelger-Huët Anomaly

Definition and Causes

I. This is a congenital disorder of leukocyte development resulting in hyposegmentation of granulocyte nuclei.
II. It is reported in a variety of species, including coonhounds, redbone hounds, foxhounds, basenjis, Boston terriers, cocker spaniels, Australian shepherds, Australian blueheelers, border collies, German shepherd dogs, Samoyeds, crossbred dogs, and domestic shorthair cats.
III. The inheritance pattern is unknown but is presumably autosomal dominant.

Pathophysiology

I. Neutrophils fail to undergo normal nuclear segmentation, resulting in granulocytes that resemble bands, metamyelocytes, and myelocytes.
II. The chromatin pattern remains mature and tightly condensed, and the cytoplasm is normal.
III. Neutrophil adherence, chemotaxis, phagocytosis, and bactericidal activity remain unimpaired (Latimer et al., 1989).
IV. Eosinophils, monocytes, and megakaryocytes (Latimer et al., 1987) show similar nuclear hyposegmentation.
V. The homozygous anomaly is associated with skeletal defects in cats and rabbits and is usually lethal in utero (Latimer et al., 1988).

Clinical Signs

Generally not associated with signs of illness

Differential Diagnosis

I. It must be differentiated from the severe left shift seen with some infections.
II. Pseudo–Pelger-Huët anomaly is an acquired condition that is identical in appearance to Pelger-Huët anomaly.
   A. It is seen with chronic inflammation, drug administration, or marrow neoplasia and resolves when the inciting condition is eliminated.
   B. The acquired condition usually affects fewer neutrophils than the true congenital anomaly.

Treatment

None is required.

Mucopolysaccharidosis

Definition and Causes

I. This syndrome is characterized by deficiency in one of several enzymes required for catabolism of mucopolysaccharides.
II. Skeletal, neurologic, and granulocyte abnormalities result.
III. Metachromatic granules are noted in granulocytes (Romanowsky-stained blood smears).
IV. Various manifestations of this condition are seen in Siamese and domestic shorthaired cats, dachshunds, plothounds, and English springer spaniels.
V. It is generally transmitted as an autosomal recessive trait.

Pathophysiology

I. Abnormal catabolism of mucopolysaccharides leads to accumulation in various tissues.
II. Mucopolysaccharidosis VI (Maroteaux-Lamy syndrome) occurs in Siamese cats from a deficiency in arylsulfatase B activity.
III. Mucopolysaccharidosis I (Hurler's syndrome) occurs in domestic shorthaired cats and plothounds from diminished α-L-iduronidase activity.
IV. Mucopolysaccharidosis VII in dogs (Haskins et al., 1984) and cats (Gitzelmann et al., 1994) occurs from a deficiency in β-glucuronidase activity.

Clinical Signs

See Chaps. 79 and 101.

Diagnosis

I. Presumptive diagnosis: clinical signs and presence of characteristic inclusions in leukocytes
   A. Neutrophils contain a few to numerous coarse metachromatic (pinkish-purple) granules.
   B. Eosinophil and basophil granules are enlarged and also metachromatic.
   C. Lymphocytes contain granules or are vacuolated.
II. Urine toluidine blue spot test
   A. This test detects increased amounts of mucopolysaccharide metabolic products in urine.
   B. It is measured as chondroitin sulfuric acid on paper chromatograms.
III. Enzymatic analysis of leukocytes or tissue biopsy for arylsulfatase B, α-L-iduronidase, or β-glucuronidase activity

Treatment and Monitoring

I. None is currently available; the disease is usually progressive.
II. Treatment with bone marrow transplantation has been attempted experimentally with some success (Gasper et al., 1984).
III. Prognosis is poor; euthanasia is indicated for progressive disease.

GM$_1$ Gangliosidosis

Definition and Causes

I. This syndrome is characterized by deficiency in one of several enzymes required for catabolism of gangliosides and related glycoproteins and glycolipids (Barker et al., 1986; Shell et al., 1989).
II. Neurologic, skeletal, and leukocyte abnormalities result.
III. This condition has been seen in Portuguese water dogs, English springer spaniels, mixed breed dogs, beagles, Siamese cats, a Korat cat, and a domestic shorthaired cat.
IV. It is generally transmitted as an autosomal recessive trait.

Pathophysiology

I. GM$_1$ gangliosidosis results from a deficiency of acid β-galactosidase.
II. Incomplete catabolism and intralysosomal accumulation of gangliosides occur in various tissues.
III. Lymphocytes are often vacuolated.

Clinical Signs

Signs of cerebellar dysfunction (e.g., ataxia) and/or lameness due to progressive skeletal dysplasia begin early in life (see Chap. 23).

Diagnosis

I. Documentation of reduced β-galactosidase activity in leukocytes, serum, and/or brain
II. Documentation of increased GM$_1$ ganglioside in brain or liver tissues

Treatment

None is available; the disease is rapidly progressive.

Carbohydrate Metabolism Disorders

Definition and Causes

These conditions are caused by deficiency in one of several enzymes required for lysosomal degradation of N- and O-linked oligosaccharides.

Pathophysiology

I. Neurologic, skeletal, and leukocyte abnormalities result owing to accumulation of partially degraded carbohydrates within various tissues.
II. Alpha-mannosidosis is caused by a deficiency in the

enzyme α-mannosidase (Jezyk et al., 1986; Cummings et al., 1988), with intralysosomal accumulation of mannose-rich oligosaccharides. This deficiency has been reported in Persian, domestic shorthaired, and domestic longhaired cats.

III. Fucosidosis is caused by a deficiency in the lysosomal enzyme α-L-fucosidase (Taylor et al., 1987), with intralysosomal accumulation of fucose-containing glycans. It has been reported in English springer spaniels, is transmitted as an autosomal recessive trait, and is prevalent in several pedigree lines in the United Kingdom (Barker et al., 1988).

IV. Vacuolated leukocytes, especially lymphocytes and monocytes, can be found in blood, bone marrow, and sometimes cerebrospinal fluid.

Clinical Signs

I. Alpha-mannosidosis causes neurologic signs, skeletal deformities, ocular abnormalities, and hepatomegaly, which develop early in life. The severity of the condition can vary (see also Chap. 23).

II. Fucosidosis causes multifocal neurologic signs that are generally evident by 2 years of age, with progressive motor and neurologic deterioration. No affected dogs have survived beyond 4 years of age.

Diagnosis

I. Alpha-mannosidosis is diagnosed by documenting reduced α-mannosidase activity in serum, brain, liver, and/or kidney. Increased amounts of oligosaccharides are present in urine.

II. Canine fucosidosis is diagnosed by documenting reduced α-L-fucosidase activity in plasma or leukocytes.

Treatment

None is available.

Abnormal Granulation Syndrome in Birman Cats

I. Fine acidophilic (pinkish-purple) granules appear in neutrophils of highly inbred Birman cats with this disorder (Hirsch and Cunningham, 1984).

II. The disease is not associated with abnormal function of granulocytes or clinical disease.

III. It is inherited as an autosomal recessive trait and must be distinguished from mucopolysaccharidosis VI.

Granulocytopathy Syndrome in Irish Setters

Definition and Causes

I. A syndrome characterized by decreased capacity of granulocytes to kill phagocytosed bacteria (Renshaw et al., 1975)

II. Autosomal recessive trait in Irish setters

III. Increased susceptibility to pyogenic infections

Pathophysiology

I. Hexose monophosphate shunt activity is defective.

II. Phagocytosis of bacteria is normal.

III. Biochemical oxidative burst does not occur, resulting in decreased oxygen-dependent bactericidal activity of neutrophils.

Clinical Signs

I. Recurring bacterial infections beginning in puppyhood
   A. Omphalophlebitis
   B. Dermatitis
   C. Gingivitis
   D. Osteomyelitis

II. Pyrexia and neutrophilia with a left shift

III. Lymphadenopathy

IV. Nonregenerative anemia of chronic disease

V. Hypergammaglobulinemia

Diagnosis and Treatment

I. It is difficult to confirm because neutrophils are morphologically normal.

II. Definitive diagnosis requires a bacterial killing assay available in specialized laboratories.

III. Continuous antibiotic therapy may be necessary to prevent severe bacterial infections.

IV. Bacteria may become resistant to treatment over time, and most of these dogs die at a few months of age.

Defective Neutrophil Function in Dobermans

Definition and Cause

I. Syndrome characterized by an impaired capacity of neutrophils to kill phagocytosed bacteria

II. Reported in eight closely related Doberman pinschers (Breitschwerdt et al., 1987)

III. Increased susceptibility to bacterial infection of the respiratory tract

Pathophysiology

I. Phagocytosis of bacteria is normal.

II. Bacterial killing is impaired from incapacity of neutrophils to generate oxygen radicals after stimulation.

III. Lymphocyte blastogenesis in response to mitogens is normal.

IV. Serum concentrations of immunoglobulins and complement are normal or increased.

Clinical Signs

I. Recurring respiratory infections, especially chronic rhinitis and pneumonia, occur beginning in puppyhood.

II. Neutrophils appear morphologically normal and are present in normal or increased numbers.

Diagnosis and Treatment

I. Neutrophils have a decreased capacity to reduce nitroblue tetrazolium.
II. Definitive diagnosis requires bacterial killing assay available in specialized laboratories.
III. Most bacterial infections are responsive to bactericidal antibiotics.
IV. Continuous antibiotic therapy may be necessary to prevent severe bacterial infections. Bacteria may become resistant to treatment over time.

Defective Neutrophil Function in a Weimaraner

I. A single 5-month-old Weimaraner was noted to have defective neutrophil phagocytosis (Hansen et al., 1995).
II. Neutrophil dysfunction resulted in recurrent bacterial infections.

RESPONSES OF WHITE BLOOD CELLS IN INFLAMMATION AND OTHER CONDITIONS

Neutrophils—Morphologic Changes Associated with Disease

Toxic Change

I. Toxic change is a combination of cytoplasmic changes caused by disturbances in neutrophil maturation in the bone marrow (Jain, 1986).
   A. Cytoplasmic basophilia and a foamy, moth-eaten pattern of vacuolation are common toxic changes.
   B. Döhle bodies are small blue-gray aggregates of rough endoplasmic reticulum. They occur more frequently in feline neutrophils than in those from other species.
   C. Toxic granulation, with prominent pink primary granules visible in mature neutrophils, is an infrequent toxic change in canine and feline neutrophils. This abnormality must be distinguished from storage diseases in cats and hereditary granulation anomaly in Birman cats (see earlier).
II. These changes usually occur as a result of septicemia or endotoxemia but can also occur with acute sterile inflammation or drug toxicity. A septic process should be suspected when most of the neutrophils appear "toxic."
III. Several hours of exposure to ethylenediaminetetra-

acetic acid (EDTA) can result in neutrophil vacuolation resembling toxic change.
IV. Toxic bands may be difficult to distinguish from monocytes. It often helps to find a recognizable neutrophil and monocyte on the same smear and compare them with the cell(s) in question.
   A. Monocytes tend to have greater cytoplasmic basophilia. Monocyte cytoplasm has a homogeneous, grainy texture as compared with the mottled texture of toxic neutrophil cytoplasm.
   B. Monocyte vacuoles are discrete and well-defined, rather than foamy and coalescing as they are in toxic neutrophils.
   C. Döhle bodies only occur in neutrophils.

Degenerate Neutrophils

I. Neutrophils become degenerate in the tissues because of local release of bacterial toxins.
II. These products alter cell membrane permeability, allowing water to enter the cell and the nucleus, by way of the nuclear pores.
III. Resulting nuclei are swollen, with decreased segmentation and loose, homogeneous, eosinophilic nuclear chromatin.
   A. The presence of degenerate neutrophils in a cytology sample (e.g., a thoracic or abdominal effusion) suggests a septic process.
   B. The presence of nondegenerate neutrophils does not rule out a septic process, because some bacteria are not toxin producers.

Nuclear Hyposegmentation

I. Nuclear hyposegmentation can occur as a result of neutrophil immaturity. The presence of >300 bands/μl is referred to as a left shift.
   A. A left shift is most commonly associated with neutrophilia but can also occur in conjunction with either neutropenia or a normal neutrophil count.
      1. Typically, there is an orderly pyramidal distribution of immature neutrophils with mature cells predominating.
      2. A severe left shift, in which the number of immature cells equals or exceeds the number of segmented neutrophils, is a poor prognostic sign.
   B. A left shift can be associated with any of the following conditions.
      1. Increased tissue consumption of neutrophils, from inflammatory disease
      2. Maturation arrest of the granulocytic series in the marrow
      3. Neutrophilia associated with the marked regenerative erythrocyte response resulting from hemolytic anemias
II. Nuclear hyposegmentation can also result from failure of mature neutrophils to undergo normal nuclear segmentation.
   A. Pelger-Huët anomaly is a congenital disorder of

leukocyte development resulting in hyposegmented leukocyte nuclei (see earlier).
B. Pseudo–Pelger-Huët anomaly is a poorly documented, acquired disorder associated with chronic inflammation, drug administration, and neoplasia. Some neutrophils have a band-shaped, indented, or round nucleus with mature, tightly condensed chromatin.

Nuclear Hypersegmentation

I. Canine and feline neutrophils are considered to be hypersegmented if a significant number of neutrophils have five or more nuclear lobes (Jain, 1986).
II. Neutrophil hypersegmentation occurs most typically as a senescent change in neutrophils with a prolonged circulation time secondary to the effects of endogenous (prolonged stress, hyperadrenocorticism) or exogenous corticosteroids.
III. Other less common conditions associated with hypersegmented neutrophils include granulocytic leukemia, myelodysplastic syndrome, vitamin B_{12}/folate deficiency, and congenital bone marrow dysplasia in miniature and toy poodles.

Cytoplasmic Inclusions

I. *Ehrlichia* inclusions are occasionally observed in circulating canine leukocytes.
A. Morulae are 0.5–2 μm, tightly packed clusters of deep blue to purple coccoid bodies.
B. *Ehrlichia* species can be distinguished by their host cell tropism.
1. *Ehrlichia canis, Ehrlichia risticii,* and *Ehrlichia chaffeensis* infect mononuclear cells, with infected cells rarely seen.
2. *Ehrlichia equi, Ehrlichia ewingii* (Anderson et al., 1992), *Ehrlichia phagocytophilia,* and a related but as yet unidentified species (Greig et al., 1994) have a predilection for neutrophils and occasionally eosinophils. Infected granulocytes can be found in the circulation of dogs early in the course of infection.
II. Canine distemper inclusions can be found in circulating leukocytes and erythrocytes during the early stages of disease and occasionally shortly after vaccination.
A. These are large (up to 3 μm), homogeneous, and circumscribed structures that stain from pale blue to reddish purple with Romanowsky stains.
B. They tend to occur more frequently in lymphocytes than in neutrophils or erythrocytes.
III. In disseminated histoplasmosis, *Histoplasma capsulatum* organisms can sometimes be found in circulating leukocytes.
A. Yeast forms are 2–4 μm and oval, with a thin cell wall. The central area of the organisms is basophilic and is frequently surrounded by an unstained halo.
B. Often, several yeast are clustered within a single cell.

C. Examination of a buffy coat preparation may facilitate discovery of infected leukocytes.
IV. Gametocytes of the protozoan *Hepatozoon canis* can occasionally be found in canine neutrophils and monocytes.
A. These are oval structures, measuring approximately 5 × 10 μm, staining ice-blue with Romanowsky stains.
B. If blood is allowed to sit before preparation of smears, the organism may escape from the leukocyte, leaving an easily overlooked, unstained capsule (Craig, 1984).
V. Abnormal granules may also be found (see Congenital Disorders, earlier).

Neutrophilia

Definition

An increase in circulating mature neutrophils to >12,000/ μl

Causes and Pathophysiology

I. Physiologic neutrophilia
A. This change occurs in response to epinephrine release from fear, excitement, or strenuous exercise. It commonly occurs after prolonged struggling during venipuncture.
1. Epinephrine causes a transient shift of marginated neutrophils into the circulating pool. Release of cells from the marrow remains unchanged, so there is no associated left shift. It occurs within minutes and persists for about 10–20 minutes.
2. This effect occurs more often in young animals than in adults and is more pronounced in cats than in dogs. The neutrophilia rarely exceeds 15,000/μl.
B. It can be accompanied by a lymphocytosis that may be of greater magnitude than the neutrophilia, especially in cats. Monocyte and eosinophil counts are usually unaffected.
II. Glucocorticoid-induced neutrophilia (stress neutrophilia)
A. This change occurs with increased levels of either endogenous cortisol or exogenous corticosteroid administration.
1. Corticosteroids increase neutrophil release from the marrow while also decreasing neutrophil adhesion to vessel walls, causing their shift into the circulating pool. A left shift is usually absent unless the marrow storage pool of mature neutrophils has been depleted.
2. A two- to threefold increase in neutrophil counts can be observed within 4–6 hours after steroid administration. The magnitude of neutrophilia is diminished with long-term corticosteroid exposure. Cell counts return to normal by 24 hours (Jain, 1986).
B. Corticosteroid-induced neutrophilia is typically associated with lymphopenia, eosinopenia, and monocytosis.

III. Neutrophilia in response to inflammatory disease
   A. The bone marrow responds to the presence of inflammatory disease by accelerating release of neutrophils. Neutrophilia occurs if the rate of neutrophil release from the marrow exceeds the rate of neutrophil migration into the tissues.
   B. Disorders associated with neutrophilia are varied.
      1. Any type of inflammation
         a) Infection: bacterial or fungal
         b) Tissue necrosis
         c) Trauma
      2. Hemolysis
      3. Neoplasia
   C. Marked neutrophilic leukocytosis with neutrophil counts >100,000/μl may occur with the following.
      1. Localized purulent inflammation: pyometra, peritonitis, pyothorax, or severe abscesses
      2. Certain systemic diseases: autoimmune hemolytic anemia, endocarditis, mycoses
      3. *Hepatozoon canis* infection (Craig, 1984)
      4. Certain neoplasms
         a) Renal tubular carcinoma (Lappin and Latimer, 1988)
         b) Fibrosarcoma (Chinn et al., 1985)
         c) Rectal adenomatous polyp (Thompson et al., 1992)
   D. Neutrophilia is accompanied by a left shift if the marrow storage pool of mature neutrophils has been depleted and neutrophils are released at a rate exceeding the capacity of the marrow to replenish it.
      1. Significant left shifts (>1000 bands/μl) are commonly associated with severe exudative processes involving pyogenic bacteria, fungi, foreign bodies, or tissue necrosis.
         a) The left shift diminishes as the marrow undergoes granulocytic hyperplasia and replenishes the storage pool.
         b) A decreasing left shift in the face of a persistent neutrophilia indicates the presence of a chronic suppurative process.
      2. A white blood cell (WBC) count >50,000/μl with a left shift including myelocytes and more immature forms is referred to as a leukemoid reaction because of its resemblance to leukemia (see Chap. 65).
         a) This benign process is most often caused by internal suppurative inflammation associated with pyometra, pyothorax, peritonitis, or acute necrosis of certain tissues or neoplasms. It is much more common than chronic granulocytic leukemia (CGL) but can be difficult to distinguish from CGL.
            (1) Leukemoid reactions show orderly cell maturation, with immature forms being less numerous than mature forms.
            (2) The presence of toxic vacuolation and Döhle bodies suggests a leukemoid reaction in response to infection.
         b) Leukemoid reactions are frequently associated with monocytosis and may or may not be accompanied by eosinophilia, depending on the cause.

Neutropenia

Definition

A decrease in circulating neutrophils to <3000/μl

Causes

I. Utilization of neutrophils beyond the rate of production
   A. Endotoxemia caused by gram-negative bacteria
      1. Endotoxin causes a rapid but transient neutropenia that develops during the first 1–2 hours after exposure and persists for 2–3 hours. This is caused by enhanced neutrophil margination and migration into the tissues.
      2. Within 6–8 hours after exposure to endotoxin, a rebound neutrophilia, about two to three times normal, occurs because of increased release of neutrophils from the marrow.
   B. Other infectious agents (e.g., other types of bacteria and some fungi)
   C. Other causes of severe inflammation
II. Decreased production
   A. Neutrophils have a circulating half-life of about 6 hours. Because of this short life span, neutropenia may be the first indication of marrow hypoplasia.
   B. Decreased production of neutrophils can occur from damage to stem cells or rapidly dividing cells in the bone marrow.
      1. Drugs and toxins
         a) Numerous therapeutic agents (Table 64–1)
         b) Myelosuppressive chemotherapeutic drugs (see Chap. 70)
            (1) These include cyclophosphamide, daunomycin, dimethylmyleran, doxorubicin, mitoxantrone, azathioprine, and 6-thioguanine.
            (2) Neutropenia occurs within 4–7 days, followed by thrombocytopenia and rarely anemia.
         c) Benzene-containing compounds such as eucalyptus oil, menthol, and camphor
         d) Other potential drugs: gold salts, thiacetarsamide, meclofenamic acid, quinidine gluconate, captopril, penicillamine
      2. Infectious diseases (Table 64–2)
         a) Feline immunodeficiency virus (FIV)
         b) Canine and feline parvovirus
         c) Feline leukemia virus (FeLV)
         d) Canine ehrlichiosis
      3. Bone marrow necrosis
   C. Decreased production of neutrophils (or other hematopoietic cells) can also occur from infiltrative bone marrow diseases.

Table 64–1. **Drug- and Hormone-Associated Neutropenia**

Drug	Sources/Uses	Hematologic Findings	Recovery	Associated Clinical Signs
Estrogen Estradiol (ECP) is more toxic than diethylstilbestrol (DES)	Endogenous hyperestrogenism: estrogen-secreting testicular or ovarian tumors, especially Sertoli cell tumors (McCandlish et al., 1979; Sherding et al., 1981; Morgan, 1982) Administration of ECP or DES: treatment of bitches for mismating and urinary incontinence; treatment of males for prostatic hyperplasia or perianal adenomas	Peripheral blood leukocytosis and thrombocytopenia are seen within 1–2 wk, along with granulocytic hyperplasia of the marrow and depletion of erythroid cells and megakaryocytes (Jain, 1986). Leukocytosis peaks at about 20 days, followed by neutropenia. Generalized marrow hypoplasia occurs in some dogs by day 10. Anemia can occur late.	Changes may or may not be reversible. Recovery, if possible, occurs within 3 mo. Young animals tend to recover more rapidly.	Endocrine alopecia, feminization, and signs of pancytopenia
Phenylbutazone	Nonsteroidal anti-inflammatory	Prolonged treatment can cause severe leukopenia or pancytopenia; this may be associated with toxic change or a left shift. The bone marrow appears hypoplastic.	Recovery, after drug withdrawal, is usually rapid but may take several months.	Anorexia, lethargy, vomiting (sometimes containing blood), signs of pancytopenia
Chloramphenicol	Antibiotic	Low doses (50 mg/kg) in cats can cause leukopenia and bone marrow hypoplasia within 2–3 wk (Penny et al., 1967; Watson and Middleton, 1978). Neutrophils may contain Döhle bodies and show evidence of defective maturation (vacuolation, giant bands, and metamyelocytes).	Recovery occurs within 1–2 wk after discontinuation of drug.	Anorexia, lethargy, soft feces or diarrhea, vomiting
Trimethoprim-sulfadiazine	Antibiotic	Dogs, especially Doberman pinschers, can develop leukopenia or pancytopenia within 10–21 days of treatment.	Recovery occurs within 1–2 wk after discontinuation of therapy.	Dobermans may show retinitis, nonseptic polyarthritis, glomerulonephropathy, polymyositis, and/or skin rash (Giger et al., 1985).
Cephalosporins	Antibiotic	Neutropenia occurs and is associated with toxic neutrophil morphology and granulocytic hypoplasia in the marrow (Bloom et al., 1987). Nonregenerative anemia can occur, with circulating spherocytes, erythroblastemia, and erythroid hypoplasia in the marrow.	Cytopenias are completely reversible on discontinuation of therapy.	
Methimazole	Treatment of hyperthyroidism	It most often causes mild eosinophilia, lymphocytosis, and leukopenia with a normal differential count. A small percentage of cats develop severe granulocytopenia and/or thrombocytopenia (Peterson et al., 1988).	Hematologic changes usually occur within the first 2 mo of treatment and resolve within 1–2 wk after cessation of treatment.	
Griseofulvin	Treatment of mycotic disease	Cats can develop leukopenia and bone marrow hypoplasia within 7–11 wk of treatment (Helton et al., 1986). Anemia can also occur but is uncommon.	Recovery occurs within 1–2 wk after discontinuation of therapy.	Anorexia, vomiting, diarrhea, depression, pruritus, ataxia, and disorientation Elevation of bilirubin and liver enzymes may occur.

Table 64–2. Infectious Diseases Affecting WBCs

Infectious Agent	Leukocyte Abnormalities
Feline leukemia virus	Neutropenia Granulocytic hypoplasia or aplasia, previously referred to as "panleukopenia-like syndrome" Hematopoietic dysplasia: severe neutropenia associated with marrow granulocytic hyperplasia but with disturbed granulocyte maturation and dysplastic granulocyte and/or erythroid or megakaryocyte precursors (see Chap. 65) Cyclic neutropenia (Gabbert, 1984; Swenson et al., 1987): recurrent neutropenia every 8–16 days associated with concurrent cyclic fluctuations in other cell lines Pancytopenia from bone marrow hypoplasia or aplasia Lymphopenia Leukemia: lymphoid and nonlymphoid (see Chap. 65)
Feline immunodeficiency virus	Neutropenia is common during the initial stages of disease. Neutrophilia and monocytosis are seen in response to opportunistic infections (Sparkes et al., 1993). Intermittent leukopenias are seen later as a result of neutropenia and/or lymphopenia (Shelton et al., 1995). Multiple cytopenias (lymphopenia, neutropenia, anemia) are more common in cats with advanced clinical disease. FeLV-negative leukemia, both lymphoid and nonlymphoid, may occur.
Parvovirus (canine and feline)	Neutropenia and lymphopenia are most severe during the first 3–4 days and may be accompanied by a left shift and toxic change. Leukopenia is more consistent and severe in cats than in dogs. Degree of leukopenia corresponds to the severity of the infection. Recovery often results in rebound leukocytosis with a left shift and atypical lymphocytes.
Canine ehrlichiosis	WBC counts vary; either transient leukopenia or occasionally leukocytosis can occur with acute disease (Kuehn and Gaunt, 1985). Neutropenia is sometimes seen with chronic disease, presumably because of marrow hypoplasia; an underlying immune-mediated mechanism has been proposed. Lymphocytosis involving large granular lymphocytes has been reported (Weiser et al., 1991). *Ehrlichia canis* organisms are infrequently observed in monocytes; *E. equi* and *E. ewingii* can be found in neutrophils in circulation and occasionally within synovial fluid. Inclusions consist of 1–2 μm deep purple to gray mulberry-like structures (morulae) composed of tightly packed organisms. Examination of a buffy coat preparation may increase the chance of observing infected leukocytes.

1. Leukemia
2. Nonhematopoietic neoplasm metastatic to the marrow cavity
3. Myelofibrosis or osteosclerosis
   a) Myelofibrosis is usually secondary to marrow necrosis or neoplasia.
   b) The presence of cytopenias and abnormally shaped erythrocytes in the circulation (e.g., dacrocytes [teardrops], keratocytes, and schistocytes [fragments]) may suggest myelofibrosis.
4. Disseminated granulomatous disease
D. Leukopenia or pancytopenia may be caused by ineffective hematopoiesis.
   1. Myelodysplasia (see Chap. 65)
   2. Inherited malabsorption of vitamin B_{12} in giant schnauzers (see Congenital Disorders, earlier)
E. Recurrent intermittent neutropenia can occur secondary to cyclic stem cell proliferation.
   1. Canine cyclic hematopoiesis of gray collie dogs (see Congenital Disorders, earlier)
   2. Associated with FeLV infection
   3. Cyclic fluctuation in hematopoietic cells reported in one cocker spaniel and a Pomeranian.

III. Neutropenia can also occur secondary to immune-mediated processes, resulting in either destruction of circulating neutrophils or suppression of granulopoiesis in the marrow.
   A. This cause requires confirmation by leukoagglutination or immunofluorescent techniques.
   B. Clinical cases of neutropenia without accompanying bone marrow hypoplasia have not been well documented in dogs and cats, although there have been anecdotal reports of steroid-responsive neutropenias.

Clinical Signs

I. The major clinical consequence of neutropenia is bacterial infection, which may occur when the neutrophil count is <1000/μl.
II. Infections often affect skin or mucous membranes.
III. Minimal exudate makes finding the site of infection difficult.
   A. May have pneumonia without radiographic changes
   B. May have urinary tract infection without pyuria
   C. Culture of any suspicious site indicated
IV. Animals usually present with fever, anorexia, and lethargy.

Diagnosis

I. There may be a history of acute or chronic infection.
   A. Acute infection may be either the cause or the result of neutropenia.
   B. Chronic or recurrent infection is more likely to be secondary to neutropenia or another immune deficiency.
II. Look for other evidence of a primary marrow disorder.
   A. Nonregenerative anemia, inappropriate numbers of nucleated erythrocytes (RBC), or other abnormalities of RBC morphology such as dacrocytes (teardrops)
   B. Abnormalities of WBCs such as blasts, giant bands or metamyelocytes, or other atypical cells
   C. Thrombocytopenia
III. A bone marrow aspirate may differentiate decreased production from increased utilization.
   A. Inflammation, with increased neutrophil consumption, should be associated with granulocytic hyperplasia.
   B. A core bone marrow biopsy may be needed to diagnose marrow hypoplasia, aplasia, or myelofibrosis.

Treatment

I. No treatment is indicated if neutropenia is not accompanied by fever or signs of illness.
II. Neutropenia from drugs/toxins abates without treatment if the cause is removed, unless permanent stem cell damage has occurred.
III. With neutropenia and sepsis, antibiotics are started as soon as appropriate culture specimens have been taken. *Note:* Delay could be life-threatening. Blood and urine are the most appropriate samples to submit for culture.
   A. Bacterial infection
      1. The most frequent pathogens are *Staphylococcus* or gram-negative organisms such as *Escherichia coli* or *Klebsiella.*
      2. Endogenous flora are often involved.
   B. Intravenous bactericidal antibiotics (e.g., gentamicin combined with a cephalosporin) may be the best initial choice.
   C. Antibiotic choice can be modified, depending on culture results.
   D. Infections usually improve rapidly as the neutrophil count rises.
   E. Antibiotics may be stopped soon after recovery of normal neutrophil numbers and abatement of fever.
   F. Antibiotics should be continued for at least 2 weeks if the neutrophil number remains low after defervescence.
IV. Recombinant canine granulocyte colony-stimulating factor (rcG-CSF; Amgen, Thousand Oaks, CA) at 5 μg/kg/day SQ may be useful in both dogs and cats for the treatment of transient neutropenia (Obradovich et al., 1991; Mishu et al., 1992; Ogilvie et al., 1992; Obradovich et al., 1993).
   A. G-CSF causes a dose-dependent increase in neutrophil and monocyte counts, as well as enhancing neutrophil function.
   B. Neutrophil counts increase significantly 24 hours after the first injection.
   C. Monocyte counts, in dogs, increase more slowly.
   D. Neutrophil counts return to pretreatment levels within 5 days after discontinuation of treatment.
   E. Mild irritation at the injection site is the only side effect noted.
   F. In dogs (Lothrop et al., 1988) and cats (Fulton et al., 1991), recombinant human granulocyte colony-stimulating factor (rhG-CSF) has been reported to cause a similar response that is more short-lived because of the development of neutralizing antibodies to rhG-CSF.
V. Lithium carbonate at 11 mg/kg BID PO may help stimulate granulopoiesis (Hall, 1992).

Patient Monitoring

I. Serial WBC counts and WBC differentials are indicated to follow progression of the problem.
   A. With recovery from myelosuppression, monocytes return before granulocytes; therefore, monocytosis is a favorable sign.
   B. Neutrophilia with a left shift signals recovery from neutropenia.
II. Prolonged neutropenia is more likely to indicate a primary marrow problem.

Lymphocytosis

Definition

Lymphocyte count of >5000/μl in the dog and >7000/μl in the cat

Causes

I. Young animals <6 months of age have slightly higher numbers of circulating lymphocytes.
   A. Puppies have 5700–6100 lymphocytes/μl.
   B. Young cats may have even higher lymphocyte counts.
II. It most often occurs in response to antigenic stimulation after vaccination or from chronic inflammation or infection.
   A. It may be associated with immunoblasts ("atypical lymphocytes") undergoing blastogenesis.
      1. These cells are large and have increased cytoplasm that is a deep royal blue. They may have an immature nucleus with fine chromatin, with or without nucleoli.
      2. Atypical lymphocytes may also be seen in animals with lymphoblastic leukemia or lymphoma. Morphologically, neoplastic lymphocytes cannot be distinguished from reactive lymphocytes responding to antigenic stimulation.
   B. Lymphocytosis involving large granular lymphocytes can also occur.

1. These lymphocytes have a cluster of large, dark pink granules adjacent to the nucleus.
2. In people, these lymphocytes have been demonstrated to have natural killer cell activity.
   C. A concurrent hypergammaglobulinemia, usually from a polyclonal gammopathy, may be present.
III. Lymphocytosis associated with epinephrine release occurs in young healthy animals similar to physiologic neutrophilia. This response can be pronounced in young cats with lymphocyte counts ≥24,000/μl.
IV. Lymphoid neoplasia also causes lymphocytosis.
   A. Lymphoma, especially if disseminated (see Chap. 67)
   B. Lymphoblastic or lymphocytic leukemia (see later)

Lymphopenia

Definition

Lymphocyte count of <1500/μl in cats and <1000/μl in dogs (consult reference intervals established by laboratory performing counts)

Causes

I. Stress, hyperadrenocorticism, corticosteroid administration: absence of lymphopenia in a stressed animal suggests glucocorticoid deficiency
II. Infectious agents causing lymph node atrophy/destruction or depletion of lymphocyte subpopulations: FeLV, FIV, canine distemper virus, canine parvovirus, infectious canine hepatitis, and feline panleukopenia virus (parvovirus)
III. Loss of lymphocyte-rich lymph from chylothorax or intestinal lymphangiectasia

Monocytosis

Definition

An increase in circulating monocytes to >1350/μl in dogs and >850/μl in cats

Causes

I. Monocytosis commonly occurs secondary to antigenic stimulation and hyperplasia of the mononuclear phagocytic system.
   A. Certain diseases are associated with monocytosis.
   1. Acute or chronic inflammation secondary to tissue necrosis or other causes of inflammation
   2. Neoplasia
   3. Pyogranulomatous inflammation
   4. Immune-mediated disease
   5. Internal hemorrhage or hemolytic anemia
   6. Chronic granulomatous infections, especially involving fungi or intracellular bacteria such as *Mycobacterium* or *Brucella* spp.
   B. Monocytosis is typically accompanied by neutrophilia.
   C. Occasionally with bacteremia or bacterial endo-

carditis, monocytosis may be the only hematologic abnormality (Calvert, 1982; Calvert and Greene, 1986).
II. Glucocorticoid therapy, hyperadrenocorticism, or acute stress resulting in release of cortisol may produce a monocytosis associated with neutrophilia, lymphopenia, and eosinopenia.
III. Monocytosis can be the first evidence of marrow recovery after neutropenia.

Eosinophilia

Definition

An increase in circulating eosinophils to >1000/μl

Causes

I. Parasitic disease, especially if associated with tissue invasion
II. Allergic disorders such as feline asthma, allergic dermatitis, eosinophilic pneumonitis, eosinophilic gastroenteritis
III. Eosinophilic granuloma complex of cats and Siberian huskies
IV. Mast cell tumor
   A. Eosinophilia is more common with visceral or disseminated mastocytosis.
   B. Peripheral eosinophilia is uncommon in association with cutaneous mast cell tumors.
   C. Eosinophilia is thought to result from mast cell degranulation and release of eosinophilic chemotactic factors (Jain, 1986).
V. Chronic inflammation of the skin, gastrointestinal tract, respiratory tract, or urogenital tract
   A. These tissues are rich in mast cells.
   B. Eosinophilic infiltrate can occur in these or other tissues in the absence of a circulating eosinophilia.
VI. Hypoadrenocorticism (occasionally)
VII. Paraneoplastic syndrome
   A. Fibrosarcoma (Couto, 1984) and mammary carcinoma (Losco, 1986) in dogs
   B. Lymphoma, myeloproliferative disease, pilomatrixoma, osteosarcoma, myxosarcoma, and basal cell tumor, as well as transitional cell, gastric, salivary, and renal carcinoma in cats (Center et al., 1990; Sellon et al., 1992)
   C. May be caused by production of either eosinophilopoietic or eosinophil chemotactic factors by tumor cells or by products of macrophages or T lymphocytes infiltrating the tumor
VIII. Hypereosinophilic syndrome of cats (Hendrick, 1981; Neer, 1991)
   A. This is an uncommon syndrome characterized by persistent eosinophilia of unknown etiology and eosinophilic infiltration of various tissues.
   1. Tissues most commonly infiltrated are small intestine, spleen, mesenteric lymph nodes, and liver.
   2. The most common clinical complaints are diarrhea, weight loss, vomiting, and anorexia.

3. Mean eosinophil counts are about 40,000/μl, with counts ranging from 3000–130,000/μl.
B. The cause of this syndrome is unknown.
C. This syndrome has responded poorly to chemotherapeutic agents and is usually fatal. Corticosteroids are useful in some cases, but other cats are refractory to this treatment.

Differential Diagnosis

I. Eosinophilia is mild in most of these conditions and rarely exceeds 5000/μl.
  A. The highest eosinophil counts have been reported in association with hypereosinophilic syndrome.
  B. Disseminated mast cell tumors, flea-allergy dermatitis, feline asthma, and eosinophilic granulomas occasionally result in eosinophil counts as high as 20,000–50,000/μl.
II. Extremely high eosinophil counts are commonly mistaken for eosinophilic leukemia (see Chap. 65).

Eosinopenia

Definition

I. Eosinophil count of <100/μl is demonstrated.
  A. This is best documented by obtaining absolute eosinophil counts using a hemocytometer and an eosin-based diluent.
  B. The Unopette system (Becton Dickinson) provides a convenient diluent for this purpose.
II. Occasional absence of eosinophils on the differential WBC count is not significant.

Causes

I. Eosinopenia is most commonly present as a component of a stress leukogram in response to acute infection or severe disease.
II. Persistent eosinopenia is seen with hyperadrenocorticism or during corticosteroid therapy.

Basophilia

Definition

A persistent elevation in the basophil count exceeding 2% of the leukocyte differential or >200 basophils/μl

Causes

I. Any conditions that cause eosinophilia: most common cause, in both dogs and cats, is heartworm infection
II. Myeloproliferative disorders (see Chap. 65)
III. Occasionally occurs in the absence of eosinophilia, in conditions associated with persistent lipemia (Jain, 1986)
  A. Conditions include diabetes mellitus, chronic liver disease, nephrotic syndrome, and hyperadrenocorticism.
  B. Basophils are a major source of heparin, which

enhances the activity of endothelial cell lipoprotein lipase in clearing fat from the circulation.
C. Basophilia, when it occurs, is usually mild.

LEUKEMIA

Acute Lymphoblastic Leukemia (ALL)

Definition and Cause

I. This lymphoid neoplasm arises from and primarily involves bone marrow.
II. Neoplastic cells are lymphoblasts, usually T cells in cats and most often B cells in dogs.
III. It is a rapidly progressive disease of young adult or middle-aged cats and dogs.

Clinical Signs

I. Lethargy, anorexia, weight loss
II. ± Bleeding
III. Nonspecific signs, including vomiting, polyuria/polydipsia, and shifting lameness
IV. Central nervous system (CNS) signs if meningeal invasion occurs
V. Physical examination
  A. Pale mucous membranes
  B. Splenomegaly ± hepatomegaly
  C. ± Lymphadenopathy, generally milder than with lymphoma
  D. Occasionally fever or other signs of bacterial infection

Diagnosis

I. WBC counts are usually elevated. Peripheral blood examination is sometimes diagnostic if the absolute number of lymphoblasts is markedly increased (≥20,000/μl).
II. Animals may be "aleukemic" (neoplastic cells absent from the circulation) and pancytopenic owing to myelophthisis; anemia and thrombocytopenia are common. Examination of a bone marrow aspirate is required in these cases and is strongly recommended even if large numbers of lymphoblasts are circulating.
III. Bone marrow is usually replaced by lymphoblasts, but early in the disease, focal infiltration of the marrow may not be detected by an aspirate, so a core bone marrow biopsy is preferred. Multiple biopsies may be required.
IV. Special cytochemical stains are sometimes necessary to distinguish lymphoblasts from myeloblasts or monocytoblasts.
V. Unlike lymphoma, sarcomatous (solid) masses are not present with true ALL. A small percentage of dogs and cats with lymphoma present with a leukemic blood picture.
VI. Pretreatment work-up includes the following.
  A. Complete blood count (CBC), platelet count, bone marrow aspirate

B. FeLV test for cats
C. Chemistry profile, urinalysis
D. Thoracic and abdominal radiography
E. A search for any preexisting infection
  1. Perform a careful physical examination.
  2. Culture the urine if indicated by the urinalysis.
  3. Perform other cultures as indicated.
  4. Treatment of any infection must be concurrent with chemotherapy.
  5. Chemotherapy cannot be delayed, as lymphoblastic leukemia progresses rapidly.
F. Fecal examination, heartworm test in dogs

Differential Diagnosis

I. Acute myeloproliferative disorder (see Chap. 65)
II. Chronic lymphocytic leukemia (CLL)—involves small, well-differentiated lymphocytes (see later)
III. Chronic antigenic stimulation-induced lymphocytosis (e.g., chronic canine ehrlichiosis)
IV. Other causes of pancytopenia ruled out in aleukemic animals

Treatment

I. General considerations include the following.
  A. If neutrophil count is >3000/μl, use a protocol for lymphoma employing myelosuppressive drugs (see Chaps. 67 and 70).
  B. If neutrophil count is <3000/μl or if platelet count is <75,000/μl, myelosuppressive drugs carry a high risk of causing infection or bleeding. Consider the following.
    1. Marrow-sparing drugs used in lymphoblastic leukemia in dogs include vincristine, prednisone, and L-asparaginase.
    2. L-Asparaginase has been less effective in cats than in dogs.
    3. Note that vincristine and L-asparaginase used concurrently can be myelosuppressive.
II. Various protocols are available; two chemotherapeutic protocols are outlined in Table 64–3.

Patient Monitoring

I. Monitor CBC 5–7 days after each dose of cyclophosphamide.
  A. If the granulocyte count is <1000/μl, discontinue cyclophosphamide until neutrophil count recovers.
  B. Subsequent doses are then reduced by 25%.
  C. Anemia and thrombocytopenia are common but are usually not serious.
II. Monitor urine for evidence of hemorrhagic cystitis and, if present, replace cyclophosphamide with chlorambucil (Leukeran) 15 mg/m² PO daily for 4 days of each week.
III. There are several potential complications of treatment.
  A. Infection is the most serious problem; if fever develops at the nadir of the granulocyte count, it is considered an emergency.
  B. Lack of marrow recovery, with persistent aplasia, may develop. If normal cells do not return to the blood by the fourth week, rebiopsy the marrow.
    1. May find persistent leukemia
    2. May find beginning of normal recovery
  C. For drug side effects, see Chap. 70.
  D. Leukemia may recur.
    1. Attempts can be made to reinduce remission with L-asparaginase or doxorubicin (Adriamycin; see Chap. 70).
    2. Second remissions are more difficult to achieve and are usually of shorter duration than first remissions.
IV. Length of treatment is as follows.

Table 64–3. ACOP Protocol for Treatment of Canine Acute Lymphoblastic Leukemia

| Drug | Weeks | | | | | | | | | | | | | | | |
	1	2	3	4	5	6	7	8	9	10	11	12	13	14	15	16etc.
L-Asparaginase (10,000 units/m² IM)	X	X	X	X												
Vincristine (0.75 mg/m² IV)	X	X	X	X			X			X			X			X
Cyclophosphamide (250 mg/m² PO)				X			X			X			X			X
Prednisone (1 mg/kg/day PO)	[--- daily ----]			[--------------------- alternate day ---------------------]												

Cyclophosphamide is given if the neutrophil count is >3000/μl. The initial dose is rounded off to the nearest whole tablet below 250 mg/m². Subsequent doses are decreased by 25% if the granulocyte count is <1000/μl 7 days after the previous administration.
An alternative protocol (COP) can be used in cats and some dogs: Give vincristine as above. Give prednisone as above in dogs, but at a dose of 2 mg/kg in cats. L-Asparaginase is eliminated. Cyclophosphamide is given on week 1 and then every 3 weeks, as above. In cats, cyclophosphamide can be given at 300 mg/m² (rounded off to the nearest 25 mg on the low side of the dose).
There is growing evidence that doxorubicin (Adriamycin) is efficacious in treating lymphoma and ALL. For a sample protocol, see Stone et al., 1991 and Chap. 67.

ACOP = L-asparaginase, cyclophosphamide, oncovin (vincristine), prednisone.

A. If there is no relapse after 1 year (cats) or 1.5 years (dogs), consider stopping therapy.
B. Continue to monitor the animal via physical examination and hemograms periodically after stopping chemotherapy.
V. Prognosis is generally grave and is dependent on several factors.
   A. Response rate to vincristine/prednisone combination is 27% in cats (Cotter, 1983). Response rate to prednisone alone is much lower.
   B. Remission duration is similar to that for lymphoma, except that leukemia has a higher risk of recurrence in the CNS.
      1. Response to vincristine, prednisone, L-asparaginase combination was 46% in dogs, with a median survival time of 150 days in responders and only 15 days in nonresponders (Matus et al., 1987).
      2. Response to vincristine and prednisone alone was only 19% in dogs, with a median survival of 19 days (Matus et al., 1983).
   C. Prognosis is worse if leukemia is accompanied by severe neutropenia, anemia, or thrombocytopenia.
      1. RBCs can be replaced by transfusion during therapy.
      2. Recovery of neutrophils and platelets may take 2–3 weeks, as blasts must be destroyed before normal cells repopulate.
   D. Prognosis is worse with any underlying organ failure or extreme debility.
   E. Prognosis is worse with preexisting infection, as infections may become worse with immunosuppressive and myelosuppressive therapy.

Chronic Lymphocytic Leukemia (CLL)

Definition

I. Slowly progressive disease of older dogs and cats; uncommon
II. Characterized by lymphocytosis with small lymphocytes

Clinical Signs and Diagnosis

I. Signs are minimal or absent initially; some cases are found when CBC is performed for another reason.
II. Lethargy is the most common complaint.
III. Splenomegaly and/or hepatomegaly may be present and may be mild to dramatic.
IV. There may be slight lymphadenopathy.
V. Chronic vomiting, diarrhea, and weight loss may be noted with infiltration of the gastrointestinal tract.
VI. Laboratory findings are the following.
   A. CBC shows a persistent, unexplained lymphocytosis ranging from 6000 to >100,000/µl (Leifer and Matus, 1986).
   B. Lymphocytes appear normal or have increased cytoplasm.
   C. Later, anemia, neutropenia, or thrombocytopenia

may occur; cytopenias tend to be less severe than with ALL.
   D. Marrow is infiltrated with small lymphocytes (>15%); replacement is usually not total as in ALL.
   E. Monoclonal gammopathy is seen in some dogs (Leifer and Matus, 1986).
VII. Some cats are also hyperthyroid.

Differential Diagnosis

I. Physiologic lymphocytosis, especially in cats
   This is a transient abnormality, whereas CLL is associated with a persistent lymphocytosis.
II. Antigenic stimulation-induced lymphocytosis (e.g., chronic canine ehrlichiosis)

Treatment

I. Pretreatment work-up is similar to that for lymphoblastic leukemia.
II. If an animal is asymptomatic with a total WBC count of <75,000/µl and not anemic, neutropenic, or thrombocytopenic, no treatment is needed; just monitor the CBC.
III. When clinical signs develop or a CBC indicates anemia, neutropenia, thrombocytopenia, or a lymphocyte count >75,000/µl, therapy is begun.
IV. Treatment need not establish immediate complete remission.
   A. CLL cells have a slow turnover rate compared with ALL cells.
   B. Remission in CLL may take longer to achieve than in ALL.
V. For treatment protocols, see Table 64–4.

Patient Monitoring

I. Prognosis for remission is good, and survival of 2–3 years is common. Survival data are not available for protocols I and II (see Table 64–4), but median survival for dogs treated with protocol III is 348 days (Leifer and Matus, 1986).
II. Monitor CBC weekly for the first month and then monthly.
III. Decrease chlorambucil if neutropenia occurs. Restart at a lower dose after neutrophil recovery.
IV. Consider stopping therapy after 1 year of remission. Monitor CBC every 1–2 months for signs of relapse.

Mastocythemia

Definition

I. Presence of mast cells in peripheral blood and/or bone marrow
II. May be an indication of a disseminated mast cell neoplasm (systemic mastocytosis)
III. Has been reported in dogs with acute inflammatory disease, including parvovirus enteritis (Stockham et al., 1984)
IV. Mild mastocythemia occasionally an incidental finding

Table 64–4. **Treatment of Chronic Lymphocytic Leukemia in the Dog**

Protocol	Drug	Dosage
I	Chlorambucil	15 mg/m² PO SID for 5 days; repeat every 3 wk
	Prednisone	1 mg/kg PO QOD
II	Chlorambucil	2–8 mg/m² (cat: 1.5 mg/m²) PO SID for 3 wk beyond remission, then 1.5 mg/m² PO SID for 15 days, then every third day
	Prednisone	1 mg/kg PO QOD
III	Vincristine	0.75 mg/m² IV weekly for 3 wk
	Chlorambucil	Administer after 3 wk of vincristine at 6 mg/m² PO SID for 7 days, then 3 mg/m² PO SID as maintenance therapy
	Prednisone	30 mg/m² PO SID for 7 days, then 20 mg/m² PO SID for 7 days, then 10 mg/m² PO SID for 7 days, then QOD

Chlorambucil is given if the neutrophil count is >3000/μl at the start of therapy. It is discontinued if the neutrophil count falls below 1000/μl.

Pathophysiology

I. Mast cells in blood or marrow may arise elsewhere, such as from tumors of the spleen, skin, or other organs.
II. Systemic mastocytosis, with significant mastocythemia, is much more common in the cat. It is not associated with FeLV infection.
III. Signs of illness are caused by several mechanisms.
  A. The marrow is invaded, causing suppression of hematopoiesis.
  B. Histamine release from mast cell granules causes increased hydrochloric acid production in the stomach, with secondary ulcers.
  C. Heparin release may cause increased bleeding tendencies.

Clinical Signs

I. Bone marrow involvement may be the primary problem, with resulting anemia or pancytopenia.
II. Other signs depend on organ involvement and are as follows.
  A. Enlarging abdomen from splenomegaly
  B. Skin nodules
  C. Acute collapse from perforated gastrointestinal ulcers or ruptured spleen
  D. Icterus from liver involvement
  E. Petechiation, bruising, melena

Diagnosis

I. Evaluate the hemogram.
  A. Mast cells are seen in the blood, especially along the feathered edge of the blood smears.
    1. Mild mastocythemia can be caused by either acute inflammation or a disseminated mast cell tumor.
    2. Significant mastocythemia (>10/blood smear) is typically associated with systemic mastocytosis.
  B. Eosinophilia may also occur.
  C. Poorly differentiated mast cells have fewer granules.

  D. Mast cell granules do not stain well with Diff-Quik stain.
II. Buffy coat preparations of peripheral blood can be examined for evidence of mastocythemia.
III. A bone marrow aspirate is useful for staging purposes; >10 mast cells/1000 nucleated cells is consistent with systemic mastocytosis.
IV. Aspirate of cutaneous nodules or spleen reveals mast cells.

Differential Diagnosis

The major differential is basophilic leukemia (see Chap. 65).
I. Basophils have lobular nuclei and few large granules; immature basophils, however, have round to indented nuclei.
II. Mast cells have round nuclei, and most have small granules.
III. Mast cells are usually larger than basophils.

Treatment

I. Some cases (about 50%) respond to corticosteroids.
  A. Give prednisone 40 mg/m² PO for 2–3 weeks.
  B. If tumor completely disappears, maintain on 30 mg/m² PO QOD for 1 year.
  C. If there is no response in 2–3 weeks, continuing treatment may not be of value.
II. Other chemotherapeutic agents have not been effective in the treatment of systemic mastocytosis in cats. L-asparaginase and vincristine may have some success in treating mast cell tumors in dogs (Ogilvie and Moore, 1995).
III. Localized tumors may respond to wide excision and radiation therapy.
IV. Splenectomy is indicated if splenomegaly is present (see Chap. 68).
V. Supportive care is indicated for secondary symptoms.
  A. Cimetidine 2–5 mg/kg PO BID helps prevent gastric ulceration.
  B. Consider sucralfate 0.5–1 g PO TID for gastrointestinal bleeding.

Patient Monitoring

I. Monitor hemogram and possibly the bone marrow during corticosteroid therapy. Avoid the temptation to stop steroids after a good response is seen.

II. Prognosis for mast cell leukemia varies from good to poor.
   A. Good prognosis is expected after splenectomy in cats with minimal residual tumor; the cat may live several years.
   B. Poor prognosis is indicated in animals not responsive to steroids.

Bibliography

Abkowitz JL, Holly RD, Hammond WP: Cyclic hematopoiesis in dogs: studies of erythroid burst-forming cells confirm an early stem cell defect. Exp Hematol 16:941, 1988

Anderson BE, Green CE, Jones DC et al: *Ehrlichia ewingii* sp. nov., the etiologic agent of canine granulocytic ehrlichiosis. Int J Syst Bacteriol 42:299, 1992

Barker WG, Blakemore WF, Dell A et al: GM_1 gangliosidosis (type 1) in a cat. Biochem J 235:151, 1986

Barker CG, Herrtage ME, Shanahan F et al: Fucosidosis in English springer spaniels: results of a trial screening programme. J Small Anim Pract 29:623, 1988

Bloom JC, Lewis HB, Sellers TS, Deldar A: The hematologic effects of cefonicid and cefazedone in the dog: a potential model of cephalosporin hematotoxicity in man. Toxicol Appl Pharmacol 90:135, 1987

Boney CM, McDonald TP, Jones JB: Abnormal function and thromboxane release from platelets of dogs with cyclic hematopoiesis. Exp Hematol 13:586, 1985

Breitschwerdt EB, Brown TT, DeBuysscher EV et al: Rhinitis, pneumonia, and defective neutrophil function in the Doberman pinscher. Am J Vet Res 48:1054, 1987

Calvert CA: Valvular bacterial endocarditis in the dog. J Am Vet Med Assoc 180:1080, 1982

Calvert CA, Greene CE: Bacteremia in dogs: diagnosis, treatment and prognosis. Compend Contin Educ Pract Vet 8:179, 1986

Center SA, Randolph JF, Erb HN, Reiter S: Eosinophilia in the cat: a retrospective study of 312 cases (1975–1986). J Am Anim Hosp Assoc 26:349, 1990

Chinn DR, Myers RK, Matthews JA: Neutrophilic leukocytosis associated with metastatic fibrosarcoma in a dog. J Am Vet Med Assoc 186:806, 1985

Cotter SM: Treatment of lymphoma and leukemia with cyclophosphamide, vincristine, and prednisone I and II: treatment of dogs and cats. J Am Anim Hosp Assoc 19:159, 1983

Cotter SM: Feline viral neoplasia. p. 490. In Greene CE (ed): Clinical Microbiology and Infectious Diseases of the Dog and Cat. WB Saunders, Philadelphia, 1984

Couto CG: Tumor-associated eosinophilia in a dog. J Am Vet Med Assoc 184:837, 1984

Cowell KR, Jezyk PF, Haskins ME, Patterson DF: Mucopolysaccharidosis in a cat. J Am Vet Med Assoc 169:334, 1976

Craig TM: Hepatozoonosis. p. 771. In Greene CE (ed): Clinical Microbiology and Infectious Diseases of the Dog and Cat. WB Saunders, Philadelphia, 1984

Cummings JF, Wood PA, deLahunta A et al: The clinical and pathologic heterogeneity of feline alpha-mannosidosis. J Vet Intern Med 2:163, 1988

Fulton R, Gasper W, Ogilvie GK et al: Effect of recombinant human granulocyte colony-stimulating factor on hematopoiesis in normal cats. Exp Hematol 19:759, 1991

Fyfe JC, Giger U, Hall CA et al: Inherited selective intestinal cobalamin malabsorption and cobalamin deficiency in dogs. Pediatr Res 29:24, 1991

Fyfe JC, Jezyk PF, Giger U et al: Inherited selective malabsorption of vitamin B_{12} in giant schnauzers. J Am Anim Hosp Assoc 25:533, 1989

Gabbert NH: Cyclic neutropenia in a feline leukemia-positive cat: a case report. J Am Anim Hosp Assoc 20:343, 1984

Gasper PW, Thrall MA, Wenger DA et al: Correction of feline arylsulphatase B deficiency (mucopolysaccharidosis VI) by bone marrow transplantation. Nature 312:467, 1984

Giger U, Werner LL, Millichamp NJ, Gorman NT: Sulfadiazine-induced allergy in six Doberman pinschers. J Am Vet Med Assoc 186:479, 1985

Gitzelmann R, Bosshard NU, Superti-Furga A et al: Feline mucopolysaccharidosis VII due to beta-glucuronidase deficiency. Vet Pathol 31:435, 1994

Greig B, Armstrong J, Dumler S: Granulocytic ehrlichiosis in Minnesota and Wisconsin dogs—a potential zoonotic disease (abstract). Vet Pathol 31:575, 1994

Hall EJ: Use of lithium for treatment of estrogen-induced bone marrow hypoplasia in a dog. J Am Vet Med Assoc 200:814, 1992

Hansen P, Clercx C, Henroteaux M et al: Neutrophil phagocyte dysfunction in a Weimaraner with recurrent infections. J Small Anim Pract 36:128, 1995

Haskins ME, Desnick RJ, DiFerrante N et al: β-Glucuronidase deficiency in a dog: a model of human mucopolysaccharidosis VII. Pediatr Res 18:980, 1984

Helton KA, Nesbitt GH, Caciolo PL: Griseofulvin toxicity in cats: literature review and report of seven cases. J Am Anim Hosp Assoc 22:453, 1986

Hendrick M: A spectrum of hypereosinophilic syndromes exemplified by six cats with eosinophilic enteritis. Vet Pathol 18:188, 1981

Hirsch VN, Cunningham TA: Hereditary anomaly of neutrophil granulation in Birman cats. Am J Vet Res 45:2170, 1984

Jain NC (ed): Schalm's Veterinary Hematology. 4th Ed. Lea & Febiger, Philadelphia, 1986

Jezyk PF, Haskins ME, Newman LR: α-mannosidosis in a Persian cat. J Am Vet Med Assoc 189:1483, 1986

Jones JB, Lange RD, Jones ES: Cyclic hematopoiesis in a colony of dogs. J Am Vet Med Assoc 166:365, 1975

Kuehn NF, Gaunt SD: Clinical and hematologic findings in canine ehrlichiosis. J Am Vet Med Assoc 186:355, 1985

Lappin MR, Latimer KS: Hematuria and extreme neutrophilic leukocytosis in a dog with renal tubular carcinoma. J Am Vet Med Assoc 192:1289, 1988

Latimer KS, Duncan JR, Kircher IM: Nuclear segmentation, ultrastructure, and cytochemistry of blood cells from dogs with Pelger-Huet anomaly. J Comp Pathol 97:61, 1987

Latimer KS, Kircher IM, Lindl PA et al: Leukocyte function in Pelger-Huet anomaly of dogs. J Leukocyte Biol 45:301, 1989

Latimer KS, Rowland GN, Mahaffey MB: Homozygous Pelger-Huet anomaly and chondrodysplasia in a stillborn kitten. Vet Pathol 25:325, 1988

Leifer CE, Matus RE: Chronic lymphocytic leukemia in the dog: 22 cases (1974–1984). J Am Vet Med Assoc 189:214, 1986

Losco PE: Local and peripheral eosinophilia in a dog with anaplastic mammary carcinoma. Vet Pathol 23:536, 1986

Lothrop CD, Warren DJ, Souza LM: Correction of canine cyclic hematopoiesis with recombinant human granulocyte colony-stimulating factor. Blood 72:5624, 1988

Madewell BR, Gribble DH: Infection in two dogs with an agent resembling *Ehrlichia equi*. J Am Vet Med Assoc 180:512, 1982

Matus RE, Leifer CE, McEwen EG: Acute lymphoblastic leukemia in the dog: a review of 30 cases. J Am Vet Med Assoc 183:859, 1983

Matus RE, Peterson PG, Greenlee PG et al: Acute lymphoblastic leukemia in 13 dogs: pathologic and immunologic studies and response to chemotherapy. Proc Vet Cancer Soc 7:30, 1987

McCandlish IAP, Munro CD, Breeze RG, Nash AS: Hormone producing ovarian tumours in the dog. Vet Rec 105:9, 1979

Mishu L, Callahan G, Allebban Z et al: Effects of recombinant canine granulocyte colony-stimulating factor on white blood cell production in clinically normal and neutropenic dogs. J Am Vet Med Assoc 200:1957, 1992

Morgan RV: Blood dyscrasias associated with testicular tumors. J Am Anim Hosp Assoc 18:970, 1982

Neer TM: Hypereosinophilic syndrome in cats. Compend Contin Educ Pract Vet 13:549, 1991

Obradovich JE, Ogilvie GK, Powers BE, Boone T: Evaluation of recombinant canine granulocyte colony-stimulating factor as an inducer of granulopoiesis. J Vet Intern Med 5:75, 1991

Obradovich JE, Ogilvie GK, Stadler-Morris S et al: Effect of recombinant canine granulocyte colony-stimulating factor on peripheral blood neutrophil counts in normal cats. J Vet Intern Med 7:65, 1993

Ogilvie GK, Moore AS: Managing the Veterinary Cancer Patient. Veterinary Learning Systems, Trenton, 1995

Ogilvie GK, Obradovich JE, Cooper MF et al: Use of recombinant canine granulocyte colony-stimulating factor to decrease myelosuppression associated with the administration of mitoxantrone in the dog. J Vet Intern Med 6:44, 1992

Penny RHC, Carlisle CH, Prescott CW, Davidson HA: Effects of chloramphenicol on the haemopoietic system of the cat. Br Vet J 123:145, 1967

Peterson ME, Kintzer PP, Hurvitz AL: Methimazole treatment of 262 cats with hyperthyroidism. J Vet Intern Med 2:150, 1988

Pratt HL, Carroll RC, McClendons S et al: Effects of recombinant granulocyte colony-stimulating factor treatment on hematopoietic cycles and cellular defects associated with canine cyclic hematopoiesis. Exp Hematol 18:1199, 1990

Renshaw HW, Chatburn C, Bryan GM et al: Canine granulocyto-pathy syndrome: neutrophil dysfunction in a dog with recurrent infections. J Am Vet Med Assoc 166:443, 1975

Sellon RK, Rottman JB, Jordan HL et al: Hypereosinophilia associated with transitional cell carcinoma in a cat. J Am Vet Med Assoc 201:591, 1992

Shell LG, Potthoff A, Carithers R et al: Neuronal–visceral GM_1 gangliosidosis in Portuguese water dogs. J Vet Intern Med 3:1, 1989

Shelton GH, Linenberger ML, Persik MT et al: Prospective hematologic and clinicopathologic study of asymptomatic cats with naturally acquired feline immunodeficiency virus infection. J Vet Intern Med 9:133, 1995

Sherding RG, Wilson GP, Kociba GJ: Bone marrow hypoplasia in eight dogs with Sertoli cell tumor. J Am Vet Med Assoc 178:497, 1981

Sparkes AH, Hopper CD, Millard WG et al: Feline immunodeficiency virus infection; clinicopathologic findings in 90 naturally occurring cases. J Vet Intern Med 7:85, 1993

Stockham SL, Basel DL, Schmidt DA: Idiopathic mastocytemia in dogs. Vet Clin Pathol 13:33, 1984

Stone MS, Goldstein MA, Cotter SM: Comparison of two protocols for induction of remission in dogs with lymphoma. J Am Anim Hosp Assoc 27:315, 1991

Swenson CL, Kociba GJ, O'Keefe DA et al: Cyclic hematopoiesis associated with feline leukemia virus infection in two cats. J Am Vet Med Assoc 191:93, 1987

Taylor RM, Farrow BRH, Healy PJ: Canine fucosidosis: clinical findings. J Small Anim Pract 28:291, 1987

Thompson JP, Christopher MM, Ellison GW et al: Paraneoplastic leukocytosis associated with a rectal adenomatous polyp in a dog. J Am Vet Med Assoc 201:737, 1992

Watson ADJ, Middleton DJ: Chloramphenicol toxicosis in cats. Am J Vet Res 39:1199, 1978

Weiser MG, Thrall MA, Fulton R et al: Granular lymphocytosis and hyperproteinemia in dogs with chronic ehrlichiosis. J Am Anim Hosp Assoc 27:84, 1991

65

Myeloproliferative Disorders

Karen M. Young

GENERAL CONSIDERATIONS

Definition and Classification

I. Myeloproliferative disorders (MPDs) are a group of primary diseases of bone marrow resulting from unregulated clonal proliferation of one or more hematopoietic (nonlymphoid) cell lines.
II. MPDs are uncommon in dogs but are more common in cats owing to feline leukemia virus (FeLV) infection.
III. Most MPDs can be classified as acute or chronic, depending on the degree of cellular differentiation.
  A. In acute MPD, proliferation of hematopoietic cells occurs with no or minimal cellular differentiation.
    1. Neoplastic cells have a blastic appearance.
    2. Cytochemical stains for the presence of cytoplasmic enzymes or other cellular constituents, identification of cell surface markers by flow cytometry, and ultrastructural analysis by electron microscopy are often required to identify the cell lineage.
    3. Acute MPDs are subclassified based on newly defined criteria (see later).
  B. In chronic MPD, proliferation is accompanied by some degree of differentiation, permitting recognition of the cell line involved.
    1. Chronic MPDs include polycythemia vera, chronic granulocytic leukemia and its variants, and essential thrombocythemia.
    2. Myelofibrosis, with excessive proliferation of marrow fibroblasts, is also considered an MPD in certain cases.
IV. Erythroleukemia complex in cats comprises chronic erythremic myelosis, erythroleukemia, and acute erythremic myelosis.
V. In occult MPD, leukemic blasts are present in bone marrow but are not yet manifested in peripheral blood.

Causes

I. In dogs, there is no known cause for spontaneously occurring MPD.
  A. Possible factors: genetic, environmental (drugs, irradiation, toxins), aberrant functioning of immune system
  B. Experimentally produced by irradiation (Dungworth et al., 1969; Seed et al., 1977)
II. In cats, FeLV is the most common cause.
  A. Strain of FeLV may be important (Theilen and Madewell, 1979).
  B. Combination of FeLV infection and increased marrow proliferation during recovery from viral panleukopenia or during hemobartonellosis may be important in development of neoplastic clone (Schalm et al., 1975).
  C. MPD can occur in FeLV-negative cats.

Pathophysiology

I. Defective proliferation and maturation of a clone of cells result from disturbances in the hematopoietic stem cell pool. Despite manifestation in a single lineage, MPDs affect all cell lines, and transitions from one form to another can occur.
II. Quantitative and qualitative abnormalities occur.
  A. Impaired production of normal hematopoietic cells leads to anemia, neutropenia, and/or thrombocytopenia.
  B. Leukemic cells, such as neutrophils in chronic granulocytic anemia, have impaired function.
  C. There are severe complications (e.g., hemorrhage and sepsis).
III. Organ dysfunction, especially involving the liver and spleen, results from infiltration by leukemic cells.
IV. MPD may be preceded by a myelodysplastic syndrome (MDS), sometimes termed "preleukemia." Distinction between MDS and MPD can be difficult.

Clinical Signs

I. There is no age, breed, or sex predilection.
II. Clinical signs common to all forms of MPD include the following.
   A. Anorexia, lethargy, weight loss, emaciation
   B. Fever, recurrent infections
   C. Splenomegaly, from neoplastic infiltration and extramedullary hematopoiesis
   D. Hepatomegaly, less commonly lymphadenopathy
   E. Pallor from anemia, petechiation from thrombocytopenia

Diagnosis

I. Definitive diagnosis of MPD requires examination of peripheral blood and bone marrow to identify leukemic cells and hypoplasia of other cell lines.
II. Diagnosis may be made by analysis of peripheral blood alone if abnormal cells are present in high enough frequency.
III. Bone marrow aspirates are usually hypercellular and easy to obtain. Aspirates are superior to core biopsy specimens for evaluation of individual cellular morphology by standard Romanowsky or special cytochemical stains.
IV. If aspirates are difficult to obtain, core bone marrow biopsies can be evaluated histopathologically.
   A. They usually reveal hypercellularity, associated with accumulation of leukemic cells, as well as hypoplasia of other lines.
   B. Individual cellular morphology is not well defined, and distinguishing nonlymphoid and lymphoid neoplasms can be difficult.
V. Other common laboratory findings include the following.
   A. Nonregenerative anemia, sometimes with modest reticulocytosis
   B. In cats, macrocytic erythrocytes and metarubricytosis
   C. Platelet numbers: low, normal, or high in chronic MPD; usually low in acute MPD
   D. Serum biochemical abnormalities and signs (e.g., icterus) associated with organ dysfunction secondary to infiltration by leukemic cells
   E. Cats usually FeLV-positive

Treatment

I. Cytoreductive drugs are required to control aberrant proliferation of leukemic cells and permit return of normal hematopoiesis.
II. Experimental modalities that may be available in the future include biologic response modifiers, total body irradiation and bone marrow transplantation, terminal differentiators, and cytokines (see Chap. 70; Grant and Shelton, 1989; Kurzman and MacEwen, 1989).
III. Transfusions may be required to treat severe anemia or thrombocytopenia (see Chap. 69).
IV. Antibiotics to treat bacterial infections are used most effectively after culture of the infected site to identify specific organism(s).

MYELODYSPLASTIC SYNDROME

Definition

I. Aberrant development of one or more hematopoietic cell lines, resulting in refractory cytopenias with no obvious neoplasm
II. Identified most commonly in FeLV-positive cats

Clinical Signs

I. Abnormalities in two or three cell lines in peripheral blood
   A. Normochromic anemia, sometimes macrocytic, and metarubricytosis out of proportion to reticulocyte response
   B. Neutropenia ± left shift or hypersegmented neutrophils
   C. Thrombocytopenia
II. ± Anorexia, lethargy, fever, pallor, hepatosplenomegaly

Diagnosis

I. Bone marrow cellularity is normal or increased.
   A. M:E (myeloid:erythroid) ratio is increased, and blast cells constitute <30% of nucleated cells.
   B. A form with erythroid predominance may be present (Jain et al., 1991).
II. There are dysplastic changes such as megaloblastic changes in erythroid precursors, giant forms and abnormal nuclei and granules in neutrophil precursors, or micromegakaryocytes.
III. Cats recovering from viral panleukopenia may have similar changes.

Treatment

I. No specific therapy: transfusions to improve degree of anemia
II. Antibiotics for specific bacterial infections in neutropenic animals
III. Agents with future potential: colony-stimulating factors, terminal differentiators

Patient Monitoring

This condition may progress to overt leukemia, stabilize with persistence of cytopenia(s), or, less frequently, resolve.

ACUTE MYELOPROLIFERATIVE DISORDERS

Definition and Classification

I. Group of rapidly progressive bone marrow diseases resulting in accumulation of immature blast cells of one or more hematopoietic cell lines in bone marrow, blood, and other organs

II. Subclassified by the Animal Leukemia Study Group based on cytochemical staining (see later)
   A. Acute undifferentiated leukemia (AUL), formerly reticuloendotheliosis
   B. Subtypes M1–M7
      1. M1: myeloblastic leukemia without differentiation
      2. M2: myeloblastic leukemia with some neutrophilic differentiation
      3. M3: promyelocytic leukemia, not reported in animals
      4. M4: myelomonocytic leukemia
      5. M5
         a) M5a: monocytic leukemia without differentiation
         b) M5b: monocytic leukemia with some differentiation
      6. M6
         a) M6: erythroleukemia
         b) M6Er: M6 variant with rubriblasts
      7. M7: megakaryoblastic leukemia

Clinical Signs and Diagnosis

I. Anemia, metarubricytosis, neutropenia, and thrombocytopenia are common. White blood cell (WBC) count is variable, ranging from leukopenia to >150,000/μl.

II. Blast cells are large mononuclear cells with high nuclear to cytoplasmic ratios and prominent nucleoli. They are usually present in high numbers in blood and bone marrow, as well as in other organs (e.g., spleen, liver, and lymph nodes).

III. In occult MPD, blast cells are increased in bone marrow but are in low numbers (subleukemic) or absent (aleukemic) in peripheral blood. Hematologic abnormalities (e.g., nonregenerative anemia, neutropenia, and/or thrombocytopenia) are present and are indications for bone marrow evaluation.

IV. Occasionally blast cells are found in cerebrospinal fluid of animals with central nervous system (CNS) involvement.

V. Definitive identification of the lineage of blast cells usually requires cytochemical staining (Table 65–1).
   A. Techniques are species-specific and can be performed according to described methods (Jain, 1986) or by veterinary hematology laboratories.
   B. In M4, blast cells originate from bipotent stem cells and have characteristics of both neutrophils and monocytes. In some cases, morphologic evaluation without special stains permits detection of monocytic features such as nuclear pleomorphism and cytoplasmic vacuolization.
   C. Differentiating among acute MPDs is often not essential, because the prognosis is uniformly poor. Distinguishing acute MPD from lymphoid leukemia, however, is important (see later).

VI. Electron microscopy may help identify blast cells (e.g., megakaryoblasts may contain demarcation membranes and alpha granules).

VII. Once the blast cell lineage is identified, a standardized scheme based on the percentage of bone marrow erythroid cells and blast cells is used to classify the disorder (Jain et al., 1991).

VIII. Serum lysozyme activity may be increased in dogs with acute granulocytic or myelomonocytic leukemia (Shifrine et al., 1973).

Differential Diagnosis

I. The main differentials for acute MPDs are the lymphoid leukemias (acute lymphoblastic leukemia, lymphocytic leukemia).

II. In dogs, lymphoid leukemias are more common, are more responsive to therapy, and have a better prognosis than nonlymphoid leukemias (acute MPD); distinction is critical when advising the owner about therapy and prognosis.

III. Sometimes definitive diagnosis can be made based on morphology: lymphoid cells have more condensed chromatin, fewer nucleoli, and less cytoplasm than myeloblasts; often, however, cytochemical stains are required to positively identify cells (see Table 65–1).

Treatment and Monitoring

I. Therapy for acute MPD has not been successful in most cases. Palliative supportive care (e.g., blood transfusions, antibiotics for bacterial infections) may be indicated.

II. If attempted, therapy is aimed at ablating the leukemic clone and then allowing recovery of normal

Table 65–1. **Acute Myeloproliferative Disorders**

Acute Leukemia	Lineage	Positive Cytochemical Staining/Immunostaining
Myelogenous (M1–3)	Neutrophil (myeloblast)	Sudan black B, peroxidase, periodic acid–Schiff, chloracetate esterase
Monocytic (M5)	Monocyte (monoblast)	Nonspecific esterases (with inhibition by sodium fluoride)
Myelomonocytic (M4)	Neutrophil and monocyte	Sudan black B, chloracetate esterase, nonspecific esterases
Megakaryoblastic (M7)	Megakaryocyte	Periodic acid–Schiff, platelet peroxidase, acetylcholinesterase, and immunostaining for von Willebrand factor and GPIIb/IIIa
Undifferentiated (AUL)	Unknown	No positive staining

Note: Lymphoid cells are negative in most of these reactions but may contain focal positivity for nonspecific esterase (NSE) activity, compared with diffuse positivity present in monocytic cells. NSE activity in lymphoid cells is not inhibited by sodium fluoride.

hematopoiesis. Veterinarians are advised to contact a veterinary oncologist about new protocols.

   A. Because of the rapidly progressive course of acute MPD, therapy must begin immediately.

   B. Aggressive therapy with cytosine arabinoside, 6-thioguanine, and doxorubicin in dogs (Theilen et al., 1987) and cyclophosphamide, vincristine, cytosine arabinoside, and prednisone in cats (Hardy and MacEwen, 1989) has been tried, but recovery of normal hematopoiesis rarely occurs before return of the leukemic clone or before death from hemorrhage or infection.

   C. Supportive therapy (e.g., blood transfusions, antibiotics) is usually required to treat myelosuppressive effects of chemotherapeutic drugs.

  III. The prognosis is grave; death from hemorrhage and infection is common.

  IV. Treatment modalities under investigation include total body irradiation with bone marrow transplantation, biologic response modifiers, terminal differentiators, serum factors, and cytokines (see Chap. 70).

Erythroleukemia Complex in Cats

Definition

   I. This complex comprises chronic erythremic myelosis, erythroleukemia, and acute erythremic myelosis.

  II. These disorders fall within the M6 and M6Er subtypes in the new classification system (see earlier).

Clinical Signs and Diagnosis

   I. Chronic erythremic myelosis: predominance of mature nucleated erythroid cells
    A. Peripheral blood: severe nonregenerative anemia with macrocytic mature erythrocytes and numerous nucleated red blood cells
    B. Bone marrow: erythroid hyperplasia with occasional abnormal forms

  II. Erythroleukemia: both erythroid forms and myeloblasts in blood and bone marrow

  III. Acute erythremic myelosis: predominance of large blastic erythroid cells with clumped chromatin, basophilic cytoplasm, and sometimes reddish cytoplasmic granules

Treatment and Monitoring

There is no known effective treatment, and the prognosis is grave (see earlier for future treatment modalities).

CHRONIC MYELOPROLIFERATIVE DISORDERS

Polycythemia Vera

See Chap. 63.

Chronic Granulocytic Leukemia (CGL)

Definition

   I. Neoplastic proliferation of neutrophil series with all stages of development present

  II. Variants: chronic myelomonocytic leukemia and chronic monocytic leukemia (defined by percentage of monocytes)

  III. Reported in dogs, but rarely

  IV. May terminate in "blast crisis" with transition to an acute MPD (Leifer et al., 1983)

Diagnosis

   I. Peripheral blood abnormalities
    A. High neutrophil count (can be >100,000/μl)
    B. Left shift, possibly disorderly, with presence of bands, metamyelocytes, and myelocytes and only small number of promyelocytes and myeloblasts
    C. ± Abnormal neutrophil morphology (e.g., giant bands)
    D. ± Monocytosis, eosinophilia with left shift, basophilia

  II. Bone marrow
    A. Granulocytic hyperplasia with or without morphologic abnormalities, such as maturation arrest or giant forms
    B. Erythroid hypoplasia common
    C. ± Micromegakaryocytes (dwarf forms), megakaryocytic hyperplasia

  III. Often difficult to differentiate from leukemoid reaction: requires careful search to rule out inflammation and sometimes biopsy to demonstrate infiltration of organs (e.g., the liver) by leukemic cells

Differential Diagnosis

CGL must be distinguished from the more common leukemoid reactions (high neutrophil count ± left shift) caused by inflammatory diseases.

   I. Conditions such as pyometra, abscesses (e.g., prostatic), and endocarditis, especially involving pyogenic bacteria

  II. Certain neoplasms (e.g., lymphoma or those accompanied by necrosis, sepsis, or production of hematopoietic growth factor)

  III. Immune-mediated diseases (e.g., autoimmune hemolytic anemia)

Treatment

   I. Administer hydroxyurea 20–25 mg/kg PO BID (Young and MacEwen, 1996).
    A. Use this dose for 4–6 weeks initially.
    B. When neutrophil count falls to 15,000–20,000/μl, continue therapy at half the dose, or administer 50 mg/kg two or three times weekly.
    C. Gradual reduction in the leukemic cell population is usually permissible.

  II. No successful therapy has been found for CGL with blast crisis.

Patient Monitoring

I. Prognosis for CGL is guarded; with therapy, animals may live several years.
II. Try to maintain neutrophil count in the range of 15,000–20,000/μl.
III. Monitor blood counts weekly and then monthly after remission is attained.
  A. Discontinue therapy if count falls below desired range.
  B. Reinstitute therapy if count climbs above desired range.
IV. Repeat bone marrow evaluation every few months initially and then at longer intervals.
V. Death usually results from complications of infection or hemorrhage.
VI. Prognosis for blast crisis is poor.

Eosinophilic Leukemia

Definition

I. Very rare form of leukemia with predominance of eosinophils
II. Reported primarily in cats, not associated with FeLV infection
III. Controversial as true entity (see Hypereosinophilic Syndrome, Chaps. 32, 64, and 85)

Clinical Signs

In cats, marked eosinophilia occurs with eosinophilic infiltrates in intestines, mesenteric lymph nodes, liver, spleen, and other organs (Hendrick, 1981).

Diagnosis

I. High numbers of circulating eosinophils, sometimes with left shift, and eosinophilic hyperplasia of bone marrow
II. Criteria for definitive diagnosis not established

Differential Diagnosis

I. Hypereosinophilic syndrome
II. Parasitic infection
III. Hypersensitivity disorders
IV. Mast cell tumor
V. Other neoplasms (e.g., lymphoma and carcinomas) rarely associated with eosinophilic infiltrates (Center and Randolph, 1991)

Treatment and Monitoring

As this disease has not been documented as a true entity, therapy is ill-defined and is similar to immunosuppressive therapy for hypereosinophilic syndrome, which is often refractory to treatment.
I. High-dose corticosteroids
  A. Administer prednisolone 1–2 mg/kg/day PO.
  B. If unsuccessful at reducing eosinophil count, try other preparations (e.g., triamcinolone).

II. Other agents with unproven efficacy: hydroxyurea, cyclosporine (Gregory, 1989)
III. Prognosis: grave unless primary antigenic stimulus can be identified and eliminated

Basophilic Leukemia

Definition

Very rare form of leukemia with basophilic predominance

Clinical Signs and Diagnosis

I. High numbers of circulating basophils without predisposing cause
II. Basophils differentiated from mast cells by segmented nucleus in the former and pale granules in feline basophils
III. ± Hepatosplenomegaly, lymphadenopathy, thrombocytosis

Differential Diagnosis

I. Basophilia in association with eosinophilic disorders
II. Occult dirofilariasis

Treatment and Monitoring

See Chronic Granulocytic Leukemia, earlier.

Essential Thrombocythemia

Definition

I. Persistent thrombocytosis from autonomous production of platelets
II. Rarely reported in animals
  A. In cats, thrombocytosis occurs as a component of other MPDs and rarely as a primary entity (Hammer et al., 1990).
  B. In dogs, thrombocytosis may accompany other MPDs or be a primary entity (Hopper et al., 1989; Simpson et al., 1990).

Clinical Signs and Diagnosis

I. Persistent and excessive thrombocytosis (platelet count >600,000/μl), bizarre platelets, and bone marrow megakaryocytic hyperplasia with abnormal forms
II. Absence of detectable causes of reactive thrombocytosis, blast cells, other MPDs
III. ± Splenomegaly
IV. Potential sequelae; bleeding, thrombosis

Differential Diagnosis

Reactive thrombocytosis, which is much more common (see Chap. 66)

Treatment and Monitoring

I. Asymptomatic animals may not benefit from therapy.
II. One dog was successfully treated with vincristine,

cytosine arabinoside, cyclophosphamide, and prednisone (Simpson et al., 1990).
III. Hydroxyurea may be used to control thrombocytosis
(see Chronic Granulocytic Leukemia, earlier).

Myelofibrosis

Definition and Causes

I. Myelofibrosis is marrow fibrosis with abnormal development of all hematopoietic cell lines.
II. FeLV can cause myelofibrosis or osteosclerosis in
cats.
III. Myelofibrosis and osteosclerosis can develop secondary to MPD.
IV. In most dogs, myelofibrosis occurs secondary to marrow damage or necrosis from ehrlichiosis, septicemia, drug toxicity (estrogens, cephalosporins), radiation damage, or congenital hemolytic anemias. In
some cases it is idiopathic.
V. There is one reported case similar to the human
syndrome of primary myelofibrosis with myeloid
metaplasia in a dog with megakaryocytic leukemia
(Rudolph and Hubner, 1972).

Clinical Signs

I. Anemia with metarubricytosis, anisocytosis, poikilocytosis
II. Neutropenia with left shift
III. ± Pancytopenia
IV. Myeloid metaplasia reported in liver, spleen, and
lung (Thompson and Johnstone, 1983); ineffective in
preventing or correcting cytopenias

Diagnosis/Differential Diagnosis

I. Diagnosis requires core biopsy of bone marrow for
histologic demonstration of myelofibrosis ± osteo-
sclerosis.
II. Rule out myelofibrosis secondary to marrow damage.
A. Pyruvate kinase deficiency (see Chap. 63)
B. Myelotoxic drugs and radiation therapy (see
Chaps. 64 and 70)
C. Ehrlichiosis, septicemia (see Chap. 113)

Treatment

I. No successful treatment has been described.
II. The following treatments have been tried, with limited success, in people: androgens, glucocorticoids,
busulfan, interferons, collagen synthetase inhibitors,
vitamin D congeners, and bone marrow transplantation (Lichtman, 1995).

Bibliography

Center SA, Randolph JF: Eosinophilia. p. 349. In August JR
(ed): Consultations in Feline Internal Medicine. WB Saunders,
Philadelphia, 1991
Dungworth DL, Goldman M, Switzer JW, McKelvie DH: Devel-
opment of a myeloproliferative disorder in beagles continu-
ously exposed to ^{90}Sr. Blood 34:610, 1969
Grant CK, Shelton GH: Biological response modifiers. p. 507. In
Kirk RW (ed): Current Veterinary Therapy X: Small Animal
Practice. WB Saunders, Philadelphia, 1989
Gregory CR: Cyclosporine. p. 513. In Kirk RW (ed): Current
Veterinary Therapy X: Small Animal Practice. WB Saunders,
Philadelphia, 1989
Hammer AS, Couto CG, Getzy D et al: Essential thrombocy-
themia in a cat. J Vet Intern Med 4:87, 1990
Hardy WD, MacEwen EG: Feline retroviruses. p. 362. In
Withrow SJ, MacEwen EG (eds): Clinical Veterinary Oncology.
JB Lippincott, Philadelphia, 1989
Harvey JW: Myeloproliferative disorders in dogs and cats. Vet
Clin North Am 11:349, 1981
Hendrick M: A spectrum of hypereosinophilic syndromes exem-
plified by six cats with eosinophilic enteritis. Vet Pathol
18:188, 1981
Hopper PE, Mandell CP, Turrel JM et al: Probable essential
thrombocythemia in a dog. J Vet Intern Med 3:79, 1989
Jain NC: Cytochemistry of normal and leukemic leukocytes. p.
909. In: Schalm's Veterinary Hematology. 4th Ed. Lea & Febiger, Philadelphia, 1986
Jain NC, Blue JT, Grindem CB et al: A report of the animal
leukemia study group. Proposed criteria for classification of
acute myeloid leukemia in dogs and cats. Vet Clin Pathol
20:63, 1991
Kurzman I, MacEwen EG: New developments in cancer therapy.
p. 128. In Withrow SJ, MacEwen EG (eds): Clinical Veterinary
Oncology. JB Lippincott, Philadelphia, 1989
Leifer CE, Matus RE, Patnaik AK, MacEwen EG: Chronic myelogenous leukemia in the dog. J Am Vet Med Assoc
183:686, 1983
Lichtman MA: Idiopathic myelofibrosis (agnogenic myeloid
metaplasia). p. 331. In Beutler E, Lichtman MA, Coller BS
et al (eds): Williams Hematology. McGraw-Hill, New York,
1995
MacEwen EG: Feline lymphoma and leukemias. p. 479. In
Withrow SJ, MacEwen EG (eds): Small Animal Clinical Oncology. 2nd Ed. WB Saunders, Philadelphia, 1996
MacEwen EG, Drazner FH, McClelland AJ, Wilkins RJ: Treatment of basophilic leukemia in a dog. J Am Vet Med Assoc
166:376, 1975
Madewell BR, Jain NC, Weller RE: Hematologic abnormalities
preceding myeloid leukemia in three cats. Vet Pathol 16:510,
1979
Maggio L, Hoffman R, Cotter SM et al: Feline preleukemia: an
animal model of human disease. Yale J Biol Med 51:469, 1978
Messick J, Carothers M, Wellman M: Identification and characterization of megakaryoblasts in acute megakaryoblastic leukemia
in a dog. Vet Pathol 27:212, 1990
Moulton JE, Harvey JW: Tumors of the lymphoid and hematopoi-
etic tissues. p. 231. In Moulton JE (ed): Tumors in Domestic
Animals. 3rd Ed. University of California Press, Berkeley, 1990
Raskin RE, Krehbiel JD: Myelodysplastic changes in a cat with
myelomonocytic leukemia. J Am Vet Med Assoc 187:171,
1985
Regan WJ: A review of myelofibrosis in dogs. Toxicol Pathol
21:164, 1993
Rudolph R, Hubner C: Megakaryozytenleukose beim hund.
Kleintier Prax 17:9, 1972
Schalm OW, Jain NC, Carroll EJ: The leukemia complex. p. 565.
In: Veterinary Hematology. 3rd Ed. Lea & Febiger, Philadel-
phia, 1975
Seed TM, Tolle DV, Fritz TE et al: Irradiation-induced erythroleu-
kemia and myelogenous leukemia in the dog. Hematology and
ultrastructure. Blood 50:1061, 1977
Shifrine M, Chrisp CE, Wilson FD, Heffernon U: Lysozyme
(muramidase) activity in canine myelogenous leukemia. Am J
Vet Res 34:695, 1973

Simpson JW, Else RW, Honeyman P: Successful treatment of suspected essential thrombocythemia in a dog. J Small Anim Pract 31:345, 1990

Theilen GH, Madewell BR: Leukemia–sarcoma disease complex. p. 204. In: Veterinary Cancer Medicine. 1st Ed. Lea & Febiger, Philadelphia, 1979

Theilen GH, Madewell BR, Gardner MB: Hematopoietic neoplasms, sarcomas and related conditions. p. 392. In Theilen GH, Madewell BR (eds): Veterinary Cancer Medicine. 2nd Ed. Lea & Febiger, Philadelphia, 1987

Thompson JC, Johnstone AC: Myelofibrosis in the dog: three case reports. J Small Anim Pract 24:589, 1983

Young KM, MacEwen EG: Canine myeloproliferative disorders. p. 495. In Withrow SJ, MacEwen EG (eds): Small Animal Clinical Oncology. 2nd Ed. WB Saunders, Philadelphia, 1996

66

Platelet and Coagulation Disorders

Mary K. Boudreaux

QUANTITATIVE PLATELET DISORDERS

Immune-Mediated Thrombocytopenia

Definition

I. Circulating platelets and/or megakaryocytes are destroyed by immune-mediated mechanisms.
II. Platelet number declines to <150,000/μl. Although platelet number alone cannot be used as a predictor of bleeding, numbers <50,000/μl are usually clinically significant.

Causes

I. Primary or autoimmune, idiopathic
II. Secondary to immune-complex absorption or neoantigen expression
 A. Vaccine induced
 B. Drug induced
 C. Rickettsia induced
 D. Virus induced
III. Incompatible transfusion
IV. Spurious thrombocytopenia

Pathophysiology

I. Primary or immune-mediated thrombocytopenia (IMT)
 A. The most common target antigen on platelets is the glycoprotein IIb-IIIa complex (also known as the fibrinogen receptor or as the integrin $\alpha_{IIb}\beta_3$). The second most common target antigen is the glycoprotein Ib-IX complex.
 B. Antibody may be against circulating platelets and/or bone marrow megakaryocytes.
 C. Antibody production is usually secondary to another event (see later); when seemingly "unprovoked," it is termed idiopathic.

II. Secondary IMT
 A. Vaccine-induced thrombocytopenia occurs 3–10 days after vaccination with modified live virus vaccines. Binding of viral particles or antigen-antibody complexes to the platelet surface results in immune clearance of platelets from the circulation.
 B. Drug-induced thrombocytopenia may be drug dependent or drug independent.
  1. Drug-dependent antiplatelet antibody binding requires the simultaneous presence of drug, suggesting that antibody-drug complexes bind to the platelet surface.
  2. Drug-independent antiplatelet antibody binding does not require the simultaneous presence of drug and persists after the removal of drug.
  3. Drugs most commonly associated with drug-induced thrombocytopenia include quinine/quinidine, acetaminophen, trimethoprim-sulfamethoxazole, gold compounds, and penicillin.
  4. Potentially any drug is capable of inducing drug-dependent or drug-independent antibodies.
 C. Rickettsia-induced thrombocytopenia can occur secondary to infection with *Ehrlichia canis, Ehrlichia platys*, or *Rickettsia rickettsii* (Rocky Mountain spotted fever).
  1. Although rickettsia-induced vasculitis with secondary platelet activation and consumption is a major cause of thrombocytopenia in acute *E. canis* and *R. rickettsii* infections, immune-mediated platelet clearance likely plays a role.
  2. Shortened platelet life span and accumulation of platelets within the spleen have been demonstrated in *E. canis* infection.
  3. Shortened platelet life span and thrombocytopenia in *E. platys* infections initially may result from direct platelet destruction by the rickettsial agent.

D. Virus-induced thrombocytopenias may be caused by direct platelet/megakaryocyte destruction or may be secondary to immune-mediated events similar to those described for modified live virus vaccines.

III. Incompatible transfusion
A. The platelet integrin $\alpha_{IIb}\beta_3$ is highly immunogenic and is the most frequent target antigen in IMTs.
B. Polymorphisms in the genes for the $\alpha_{IIb}\beta_3$ subunits result in changes in amino acids within the subunits that can be recognized by the immune system.
C. In human beings, PL^{A1} on β_3 is the most frequently implicated alloantigen in neonatal alloimmune thrombocytopenic purpura (NATP) and post-transfusion purpura (PTP).
D. PL^{A1} has been demonstrated on canine platelets.

IV. Spurious thrombocytopenia
A. Ethylenediaminetetraacetic acid (EDTA)–dependent pseudothrombocytopenia has been recognized in the dog. The sera of affected animals probably contain antibodies to platelet antigens that are not exposed on the platelet surface except in the presence of EDTA.
B. Heparin can cause sporadic spurious thrombocytopenia when used as an anticoagulant. Although both immune and nonimmune mechanisms have been established in humans, the mechanism is not known in domestic animals.

Clinical Signs

I. Mucosal bleeding, including epistaxis, gingival, gastrointestinal, and urinary tract hemorrhage, and petechial hemorrhages on the abdomen, ear pinnae, or gingiva, are common manifestations.
II. Vaccine-induced thrombocytopenia is usually not accompanied by clinical bleeding unless an underlying defect (e.g., von Willebrand's disease) is present as well.
III. IMTs may accompany immune-mediated anemias.
A. Anemias are generally spherocytic and markedly regenerative.
B. A neutrophilic leukocytosis is often present.
IV. NATP should be suspected in newly nursing puppies or kittens with mucosal-type bleeding and thrombocytopenia.
V. PTP should be suspected in recently transfused animals with mucosal bleeding and acute thrombocytopenia.
VI. Spurious thrombocytopenia is not accompanied by a bleeding diathesis.

Diagnosis

I. Platelet counts are usually <50,000/μl before bleeding is evident. Hemorrhage can occur with higher platelet counts if platelet function is also affected or if there is an accompanying qualitative defect such as von Willebrand's disease (vWD).
II. Low mean platelet volume (MPV) accompanying

severe thrombocytopenia (<20,000 platelets/μl) is a strong indicator of acute IMT in dogs.
A. This combination may be observed only very early in the disease.
B. Collection of blood into citrate for determination of MPV is advisable, because EDTA causes platelet swelling and spurious increases in MPV.
C. As the bone marrow responds, MPV increases above the reference range.
D. Lack of an increase in MPV with time may indicate antimegakaryocyte antibodies.
E. Thrombocytopenia is likely to persist if MPV does not increase.
F. Enzyme-linked immunosorbent assay (ELISA) and flow cytometric techniques for detecting increased immunoglobulin on the surface of platelets have been described (Kristensen et al., 1994b; Lewis et al., 1995).
III. Bone marrow megakaryocytes may be decreased or increased, depending on whether platelet destruction is acute and whether antibodies are present against megakaryocytes.
IV. Animals with autoimmune thrombocytopenia may also have high antinuclear antibody (ANA) titers or be lupus erythematosus (LE) cell positive.
V. History of recent vaccination aids in discriminating vaccine-induced thrombocytopenia. Lack of clinical bleeding and rapid return of platelet numbers to the reference range are also useful indicators.
VI. Drug-induced thrombocytopenia that is drug dependent should resolve with drug withdrawal.
A. Mixing of an animal's plasma in the presence of normal platelets and drug may result in platelet clumping with drug-dependent thrombocytopenia.
B. Antibody against the parent drug and not a metabolite is necessary for this test to be positive.
C. Drug-independent antibodies persist in the absence of drug, and this condition is difficult to specifically diagnose.
VII. Rickettsia-induced thrombocytopenias can be verified by titer analysis and also by response to treatment with tetracycline.
VIII. Virus-induced thrombocytopenia is difficult to diagnose definitively, but high antibody titers to suspected viral agents are supportive evidence.
IX. Spurious thrombocytopenia related to collection of blood into EDTA or heparin corrects when blood is collected in citrate.

Differential Diagnosis

I. IMT must be differentiated from bone marrow suppression, enhanced platelet consumption, and virus- or rickettsia-induced thrombocytopenia.
II. Usually myeloid and erythroid cell lines are affected as well as megakaryocytes with bone marrow suppression owing to drugs. Mean platelet volume is usually within the reference range.
III. Coagulation screening assays such as the activated partial thromboplastin time (aPTT), prothrombin time (PT), and thrombin time are prolonged with

enhanced platelet consumption owing to disseminated intravascular coagulation (DIC).

IV. Parasite-induced thrombocytopenia is supported by the finding of parasites within blood, but numbers may be too low to detect. Antibody or antigen tests may aid in diagnosing such parasites.

Treatment

I. Primary IMT may be treated with prednisolone alone or in combination with cyclophosphamide, azathioprine, vincristine, or danazol (Table 66–1). Severely thrombocytopenic animals may be treated with platelet-rich plasma or platelet concentrate (Table 66–2).

II. Vaccine-induced thrombocytopenia spontaneously resolves. Plasma or cryoprecipitate transfusion (Tables 66–2 and 66–3) may be required to arrest bleeding in a vWD dog after vaccination.

III. Treat drug-dependent thrombocytopenia by removing the drug; drug-independent thrombocytopenia is treated as primary IMT.

IV. Rickettsia-induced thrombocytopenia is treated with tetracycline 22 mg/kg PO TID for 2 weeks or doxycycline 5 mg/kg PO SID-BID for 2 weeks (acute disease) or doxycycline 10 mg/kg PO SID-BID for 3 weeks (chronic disease).

V. Incompatible transfusions are generally not preventable with steroids, but they may alleviate some of the acute inflammatory signs.

VI. EDTA-induced thrombocytopenia does not require treatment.

Patient Monitoring

I. Thrombocytopenia secondary to drugs, rickettsial agents, viruses, or incompatible transfusions is monitored with platelet counts until platelet number is >200,000/μl.

II. Animals with a history of drug-induced thrombocytopenia should be treated cautiously in the future, even if different medications are used. Platelet counts are performed periodically, and the owners are taught to examine the animal for petechial hemorrhages on the mucosa or abdomen at least once daily.

Drug-Induced Thrombocytopenia

Definition

I. Circulating platelets are directly destroyed by drug interaction or by immune-mediated mechanisms, or bone marrow megakaryocytes are suppressed or destroyed.

II. Platelet number can be profoundly decreased, particularly with bone marrow suppression.

Table 66–1. *Various Treatment Approaches for Immune-Mediated Thrombocytopenia*

1. Administer prednisolone 2 mg/kg PO BID for 2 wk (administer GI protectants such as H_2 blockers during treatment).
2. Check platelet counts every 1–2 days until count >75,000/μl. May discharge the animal at this time, with platelet counts every week.
3. When platelet count exceeds 200,000/μl, begin tapering sequentially as follows:

    1 mg/kg PO SID for 2–4 wk, then
    1 mg/kg PO QOD for 4–8 wk, then
    0.5 mg/kg PO QOD for 4–8 wk

4. If initial response is not good, combine prednisolone with azathioprine 50 mg/m² PO SID for 10–14 days, then 50 mg/m² PO QOD for 14 days, then 25 mg/m² PO QOD.

    OR

5. Combine prednisolone with cyclophosphamide at 2 mg/kg or 50 mg/m² PO SID for 4 days or administer vincristine 0.02 mg/kg or 0.25–0.3 mg/m² IV once.

    OR

6. Try combining prednisolone (1 mg/kg PO BID) with danazol (5 mg/kg PO BID). Taper prednisolone while maintaining danazol treatment as platelet numbers rise above 200,000/μl.

Table 66–2. *Transfusion Products for Treatment of Bleeding Disorders*

Intrinsic Platelet Disorders or Severe Thrombocytopenia

Platelet-rich plasma

CPDA₁ whole blood is centrifuged at 2000 × g for 3 min at room temperature.
Platelet-rich plasma is expressed from the surface of the red cells into a satellite bag.
Keep platelet-rich plasma at room temperature until use, which should be within 24 h.

Platelet concentrates

Platelet-rich plasma is centrifuged at 2000 × g for 10 min at room temperature.
Platelet-poor plasma is expressed from the surface of the platelet layer into a satellite bag, leaving about 50 ml of plasma for resuspension of platelets.
Leave platelets at room temperature, gently rocking if possible, for about 30 min prior to use.
Do not transfuse platelets that have visibly aggregated/clumped during isolation procedures.

Coagulation Disorders

Fresh frozen plasma (ffp)

CPDA₁ plasma is separated from whole blood by centrifuging at 2000 × g for 20 min at 4°C.
Plasma is quickly frozen at −80°C and stored at −30°C for up to 1 yr.

Cryoprecipitate (cryo)

Slowly thaw ffp at 4°C (refrigerator) for several hours until only few ice crystals remain (appears slushy).
Centrifuge at 2000 × g for 15 min at 4°C.
Decant plasma supernatant (good for treatment of vitamin K antagonism) and leave whitish sediment (cryo) in a volume of about 20 ml of plasma.
Warm and infuse into animal or further dilute with warm, sterile saline (0.15 M) and infuse.
May be refrozen and stored as cryoprecipitate, but this should not be done if cryo was prepared from 1-yr-old ffp.
Cryoprecipitate is a rich source of factor VIII coagulant, factor VIII–vWF, fibrinogen, and factor XIII.

Table 66–3. **Platelet Disorders, Diagnostic Tests, and Appropriate Transfusion Products**

Platelet Disorder	Tests	Bleeding Diathesis	Transfusion Product
Severe thrombocytopenia	Platelets <10,000/μl	Yes/No[a]	Platelet-rich plasma, platelet concentrate[b]
Von Willebrand's disease	vWF antigen <40%	Yes/No[a]	Cryoprecipitate, plasma, whole blood
Intrinsic disorder	Platelet reactivity absent or reduced[c]	Yes/No[a]	Platelet-rich plasma, platelet concentrate[b]

[a]Platelet disorders tend to result in sporadic bleeding, and tendency for spontaneous bleeding diathesis usually does not correlate well with platelet number or in vitro function. Bleeding is usually mucosal in nature.

[b]Whole blood should be administered to animals with packed cell volumes <20%; however, whole blood may not contain a sufficient number of platelets to curtail bleeding associated with thrombocytopenia or a platelet function disorder.

[c]Diagnosis of intrinsic platelet function disorders requires specialized testing (platelet aggregometry, flow cytometry, protein electrophoresis, etc.), and a definitive diagnosis usually requires that the affected animal be near or on the premises of the testing facility.

Causes

I. Primary: directly drug induced
II. Secondary: bone marrow suppression
   A. Hormones
   B. Anticancer drugs
   C. Antibiotics
   D. Other drugs
III. Secondary: immune mediated (see earlier)

Pathophysiology

I. Primary drug-induced thrombocytopenia
   A. The drug most notable is the antibiotic ristocetin.
   B. Ristocetin induces direct platelet agglutination/ aggregation, resulting in clearance of platelets from the circulation.
II. Bone marrow suppression and secondary thrombocytopenia
   A. Hormones
      1. Estrogen causes suppression of bone marrow stem cells, resulting in pancytopenia.
      2. Thrombocytopenia usually occurs prior to anemia or leukopenia.
      3. Estrogen may be administered pharmacologically or be secreted in excess from testicular or ovarian tumors.
   B. Anticancer drugs
      1. Cyclophosphamide, chlorambucil, triethylenethiophosphoramide, busulfan, melphalan, dacarbazine, and lomustine can cause thrombocytopenia, leukopenia, and, less commonly, anemia.
      2. Cisplatin can also cause myelosuppression, but it does so less frequently.
      3. Other drugs that can cause pancytopenia include methotrexate, 5-fluorouracil, and cytosine arabinoside.
   C. Antibiotics
      1. Chloramphenicol can cause pancytopenia in dogs and cats.
      2. Trimethoprim-sulfadiazine has caused reversible aplastic anemia in dogs.
   D. Other drugs

      1. Griseofulvin may cause idiosyncratic pancytopenia in cats.
      2. Ribavirin induces a dose-related toxic effect on bone marrow megakaryocytes in cats.
      3. Meclofenamic acid and phenylbutazone have been associated with idiosyncratic, apparently irreversible, bone marrow failure in dogs.

Clinical Signs

I. Mucosal-type bleeding may be present, depending on the degree of thrombocytopenia.
II. Animals may be leukopenic and anemic, depending on the duration of bone marrow suppression.
   A. Leukopenic animals are susceptible to infection and may have respiratory, gastrointestinal, and/ or urinary tract dysfunction.
   B. Anemic animals may be weak, lethargic, or even dyspneic.
III. Male dogs with testicular tumors may have feminizing changes.

Diagnosis

I. Physical examination, ultrasonography, radiography, biopsy, and/or exploratory surgery aid in the detection of ovarian or testicular tumors.
II. When administering anticancer medications, repeatedly evaluate for hematologic evidence of developing thrombocytopenia, leukopenia, or anemia.
   A. Bone marrow aspirates are helpful to determine the severity of cytopenia.
   B. Platelet MPV is often within the normal range even with coexisting thrombocytopenia.
III. Routine analysis of blood, including platelet counts, is performed in any animal receiving hormone or fungistatic drugs.
IV. Blood and bone marrow aspirates should be evaluated in animals receiving antibiotics or anti-inflammatory drugs that develop signs of mucosal bleeding.

Differential Diagnosis

I. Drug-induced thrombocytopenia must be differentiated from enhanced platelet consumption as seen in DIC.

II. DIC may also be observed in animals treated with anticancer, fungistatic, or antibacterial drugs (see later).

Treatment

I. Withdraw any offending drug.
II. Consider platelet-rich plasma or platelet concentrates to prevent catastrophic hemorrhage.
III. Whole blood transfusion may be necessary in severely anemic animals, but platelet numbers may not be adequate in whole blood transfusions to prevent thrombocytopenia-related hemorrhage.
IV. Lithium treatment (11 mg/kg PO BID) may be effective in treating estrogen-induced bone marrow hypoplasia.

Patient Monitoring

I. Continue monitoring platelet and white cell numbers, preferably every other day to twice weekly in severely affected animals. Erythrocyte numbers are evaluated once or twice weekly.
II. Perform bone marrow aspirates once weekly.

Enhanced Platelet Consumption

Definition

I. Platelets are removed from circulation secondary to activation at a rate faster than megakaryocytes can compensate.
II. Platelet number may be very low or marginally low, depending on the degree of platelet activation, chronicity of the event, and capacity of megakaryocytes to respond.

Causes

I. Parasites
II. Vasculitis
III. Viruses

Pathophysiology

I. Parasites
   A. Intravascular parasites, including *Plasmodium* and *Dirofilaria* spp., are capable of enhancing platelet reactivity, resulting in enhanced platelet consumption.
   B. Platelets have been demonstrated to kill intravascular parasites via an IgE-mediated mechanism.
II. Vasculitis
   A. Agents such as *E. canis* and *R. rickettsii* and feline infectious peritonitis (FIP) virus cause severe endothelial damage and vasculitis, resulting in enhanced platelet activation and consumption.
   B. Platelet activation/adherence may be caused by exposure of subendothelial components or upregulation of endothelial cell adhesive ligands.
III. Viruses
   A. FIP virus potentiates platelet responses in vitro.

B. It is possible that direct viral effects may contribute to the thrombocytopenia seen in this disease.

Clinical Signs

I. Mucosal-type bleeding may be present, depending on the severity of the thrombocytopenia.
II. Dogs or cats with heartworm disease may have respiratory signs, lethargy, or exercise intolerance.
III. Cats with FIP may have a distended abdomen and/or may be cachectic and anorexic.
IV. Animals with DIC may be in shock, be hyper- or hypothermic, or display a variety of abnormal signs referable to the gastrointestinal, nervous, urinary, or respiratory/cardiac system.

Diagnosis

I. Parasite infections may be diagnosed by detecting parasites and/or their antigens in blood.
II. Uncompensated DIC is usually accompanied by prolongation in routine coagulation screening tests such as the aPTT, PT, and thrombin time.
   A. Fibrinogen is usually <100 mg/dl.
   B. Fibrin/fibrinogen degradation products (FDPs) are usually >40 μg/ml.
   C. Platelet number is usually <100,000/μl, and MPV is usually above the reference range.
III. Rickettsial infection is best diagnosed by demonstrating a rise in titer to suspect agents (see Chap. 113).
IV. FIP infection is most reliably diagnosed post mortem (see Chap. 110).

Differential Diagnosis

I. Enhanced platelet consumption must be differentiated from immune-mediated platelet destruction and bone marrow suppression.
II. Immune-mediated platelet destruction is usually suspected when other causes have been ruled out.
III. Bone marrow aspirates demonstrate marked reduction in cellular elements with bone marrow suppression; megakaryocytes are hyperplastic with enhanced platelet consumption.

Treatment

I. Treat filarial and other parasite infections accordingly (see Chap. 12).
II. Determine the underlying cause of DIC and eliminate or alleviate the cause. Supportive care in the form of fluids or blood transfusions is important to maintain blood flow and prevent thrombosis.

Patient Monitoring

I. Platelet counts are performed until platelet number exceeds 200,000/μl.
II. The presence of filarial antigens or microfilaria is monitored every 6–12 months, and animals are placed on heartworm preventative.

Virus-Induced Thrombocytopenia

Definition

I. Platelets and/or megakaryocytes are destroyed directly by viruses or indirectly by immune-mediated mechanisms (see earlier).
II. Platelet production is suppressed owing to viral effects on megakaryocytes.

Causes

I. Feline leukemia virus (FeLV), feline immunodeficiency virus (FIV)
II. Parvovirus/panleukopenia virus
III. Canine distemper virus

Pathophysiology

I. FeLV-associated thrombocytopenia results from aplasia or atrophy of bone marrow stem cells or immune-mediated clearance of infected cells.
II. FIV-induced thrombocytopenia mechanisms are uncertain.
III. Parvovirus and panleukopenia virus are radiomimetic viruses and can cause profound pancytopenia.
IV. Canine distemper virus causes thrombocytopenia via immune-mediated events; later in the course of disease, direct infection and destruction of megakaryocytes may contribute to the thrombocytopenia observed.

Clinical Signs

I. Mucosal-type bleeding
II. FeLV-associated thrombocytopenia
   A. Other hematopoietic cell dyscrasias, anemia, and/or leukopenia
   B. Lethargy, anorexia, weakness, cachexia, or even dyspnea
III. Profuse bloody diarrhea in dogs infected with parvovirus
IV. Respiratory, gastrointestinal, and/or central nervous system dysfunction in dogs with canine distemper

Diagnosis

I. FeLV and FIV infections are best diagnosed using assays that demonstrate the presence of viral antigens (FeLV) or antiviral antibodies (FIV).
II. Parvoviral infections and canine distemper can be diagnosed by demonstrating a rise in antibody titer associated with signs of disease. Characteristic pathologic lesions associated with these diseases provide supportive evidence post mortem.

Differential Diagnosis

I. Virus-induced thrombocytopenia must be differentiated from bone marrow suppression caused by hormones or drugs and from immune-mediated megakaryocyte destruction.

II. Rising antibody titers or the presence of viral antigens provides supportive evidence of virus-induced thrombocytopenia.
III. Systemic signs referable to viral infection also provide supportive evidence.
IV. Lymphocytes of canine distemper–infected dogs may have viral inclusions.
V. Rule out the use of drugs and hormones and the presence of gonadal tumors.

Treatment

I. Treatment is supportive and includes fluids, antibiotics, and anti-inflammatory agents.
II. Whole blood transfusion (20 ml/kg) may be necessary for profound hemorrhage, particularly if the packed cell volume (PCV) is ≤20%.
III. Whole blood may not provide platelets in sufficient numbers to curtail platelet-related hemorrhage.

Patient Monitoring

I. Cats with FeLV or FIV that are responsive to treatment are reevaluated approximately every 6 months.
II. Dogs and cats responsive to treatment for canine distemper or parvovirus/panleukopenia infection should be vaccinated at least yearly (see Chap. 110).

Decreased Platelet Production

Definition

I. Platelet production is markedly decreased or absent.
II. Mean platelet volume is usually within the normal range in spite of coexisting severe thrombocytopenia.
III. Bone marrow megakaryocytes and other hematopoietic cells are markedly diminished or absent.
IV. Bone marrow space is occupied by neoplastic or fibroblastic cells and collagen.

Causes

I. Myelophthisis
II. Myelofibrosis

Pathophysiology

I. Metastatic or primary neoplasm replaces the existing normal hematopoietic environment.
   A. Primary neoplastic disorders include lymphoproliferative and myeloproliferative disorders.
   B. Metastatic disorders may include carcinomas, sarcomas, or other poorly differentiated tumors.
II. Myelofibrosis occurs from overpopulation of the bone marrow with fibroblasts and their collagenous by-product matrix.
   A. Myelofibrosis is a common sequela in nonspherocytic hemolytic anemia of poodles and may potentially occur with any severe chronic anemia.
   B. It may also occur secondary to myeloproliferative disease.

C. Myelofibrosis secondary to hemolytic anemia may be transitory and reversible, unlike myelofibrosis associated with myeloproliferative disease or severe congenital anemias.

Clinical Signs

I. Mucosal bleeding, weakness, lethargy, anorexia, lameness, dyspnea, and/or fever may occur as bone marrow platelet, leukocyte, and erythrocyte production declines.
II. Initial presenting signs may be related to the primary neoplasm if bone marrow failure has not yet occurred.

Diagnosis

I. Bone marrow and peripheral blood cytologic evaluation are needed for a diagnosis.
II. Bone marrow particle aspiration is difficult in advanced myelofibrosis; bone marrow core biopsy may be required for a diagnosis.

Differential Diagnosis

I. Decreased platelet production must be differentiated from other causes of thrombocytopenia.
II. Bone marrow and peripheral blood evaluation help differentiate myelofibrosis/myelophthisis from enhanced platelet destruction.
III. Drug-induced marrow suppression, especially secondary to estrogen toxicity, may eventually result in myelofibrosis.

Treatment and Monitoring

I. Treatments are aimed at the primary cause.
    A. Bone marrow transplantation has been shown to effectively reverse myelofibrosis associated with chronic congenital anemias.
    B. Unfortunately, bone marrow transplantation is not readily available, and most poodles with non-spherocytic hemolytic anemia develop profound marrow failure secondary to myelofibrosis before 4 years of age (Randolph et al., 1986).
II. Successful treatment of myeloproliferative or metastatic disease may be accompanied by regression of myelofibrosis.
III. Repeat bone marrow evaluations and peripheral blood cytology at least weekly to determine the progress of treatment.

Platelet Sequestration

See Splenomegaly in Chap. 68.

Thrombocytosis

Definition

I. Platelet numbers are increased above the normal reference range.

II. Mean platelet volume may be increased, normal, or decreased.

Causes

I. Myeloproliferative disorders (see Chap. 65)
II. Inflammatory disorders/neoplasia; reactive thrombocytosis
III. Splenic disorders

Pathophysiology

I. Myeloproliferative disorders may be associated with thrombocytosis, but thrombocytosis is rare even in megakaryoblastic leukemias.
    A. Platelet function may be impaired or enhanced, with the animal at risk for either hemorrhage or thrombosis.
    B. Mean platelet volume is variable.
    C. Myelofibrosis is a common finding with megakaryoblastic leukemias.
II. Inflammatory disorders or neoplasia may be accompanied by thrombocytosis.
    A. Interleukin-6 can induce thrombocytosis in dogs by enhancing megakaryocyte maturation.
    B. Other cytokines capable of enhancing megakaryocyte maturation or proliferation include leukemia inhibitory factor (LIF), interleukin-3, interleukin-11, granulocyte-macrophage colony-stimulating factor (GM-CSF), and thrombopoietin.
    C. Approximately 30% of cases of iron-deficiency anemia are accompanied by thrombocytosis. Inflammatory mediators, as mentioned earlier, are likely causes.
III. Splenic disorders and splenic removal generally result in a moderately increased platelet count.

Clinical Signs

I. Signs are usually referable to the primary disorder.
II. Thrombocytosis does not usually result in clinical signs, but affected animals may be susceptible to hemorrhage or thrombosis.

Diagnosis

I. Peripheral blood and bone marrow cytologic evaluation aids in the diagnosis of myeloproliferative disease or megakaryoblastic leukemia.
II. Normal platelet and megakaryocyte morphology is suggestive of a reactive thrombocytosis, with an underlying inflammatory or neoplastic disease suspected.

Differential Diagnosis

I. Reactive thrombocytosis must be differentiated from thrombocytosis associated with myeloproliferative disease.
II. Normal morphology of platelets and megakaryocytes

and the coexistence of inflammation or neoplasia help support a diagnosis of reactive thrombocytosis.

Treatment

I. Treatment of the underlying cause generally alleviates the thrombocytosis.
II. Anagrelide (induction at 1–1.5 mg PO QID, with maintenance at 1.5–4 mg PO SID) has successfully controlled the thrombocytosis associated with human myeloproliferative disease.

INHERITED/CONGENITAL QUALITATIVE PLATELET DISORDERS

Intrinsic Platelet Disorders

See Tables 66–3 and 66–4.

Extrinsic Platelet Disorders

Definition

I. Platelets are normal.
II. Plasma factors exterior to the platelet and necessary for normal platelet function are absent, reduced, or dysfunctional.

Causes

I. von Willebrand's disease
II. Afibrinogenemia

Pathophysiology

I. von Willebrand's disease
    A. Type I: reduced von Willebrand factor (vWF) levels
        1. The inheritance pattern is autosomal dominant, with variable expression in the dog.
        2. As a result of reduced vWF levels, factor VIII coagulant levels are also reduced, but usually not enough to affect the aPTT or to result in coagulopathy-like bleeding.
        3. This is the most common inherited bleeding disorder of dogs, and it has been described in the cat.
    B. Type II
        1. vWF high-molecular-weight multimers are reduced or qualitatively altered.
        2. It has been described in only three German shorthaired pointers.
    C. Type III
        1. vWF multimers of all sizes are not detectable.
        2. It is autosomal recessive, or affected individuals are doubly heterozygous.
II. Afibrinogenemia (see Factor I [Fibrinogen] Deficiency, later)

Clinical Signs

I. Mucosal bleeding is an intermittent finding. Platelet numbers are normal, however.
II. Spontaneous mucosal bleeding may not occur unless the animal is vaccinated or receives aspirin.
III. Bleeding is prolonged during and after surgical procedures and following trauma.
IV. The buccal mucosal bleeding time is prolonged (>5 minutes).

*Table 66–4. **Inherited/Congenital Qualitative Platelet Disorders***

Disorder	Dense Granule Content	Membrane Glycoproteins	Platelet Aggregation	Platelet Morphology
Great Pyrenees Glanzmann's thrombasthenia	Normal	IIb-IIIa ↓	Impaired	Normal
Otterhound thrombasthenic thrombopathia	Normal	IIb variably ↓ IIIa ↓ Ib ↑	Impaired	Bizarre giant forms
Chédiak-Higashi syndrome	Reduced	Normal	Impaired	Normal, large granules may be present
American cocker spaniel dense granule defect	Reduced	Normal	Impaired	Normal
Grey collie cyclic hematopoiesis	Reduced	Normal	Impaired	Normal
Basset hound thrombopathia	Normal	Normal[a]	Impaired	Normal
Spitz thrombopathia	Normal	Normal[a]	Impaired	Normal

[a]Basset hound thrombopathia and spitz thrombopathia may represent variant forms of Glanzmann's thrombasthenia. Variant Glanzmann's thrombasthenia is characterized by the presence of normal quantities of glycoproteins IIb and IIIa but an impaired ability to express ligand binding function. Gingival bleeding can be controlled by topically applying thrombin at areas of hemorrhage in dogs affected with spitz thrombopathia and basset hound thrombopathia. Topical thrombin is not effective in dogs with Glanzmann's thrombasthenia or thrombasthenic thrombopathia.

Diagnosis

I. vWD is best diagnosed by evaluating antigen levels (ELISA), although antigen levels often do not directly correlate with bleeding severity and cannot be used to predict the likelihood of a bleeding diathesis.

II. A qualitative botrocetin or coagglutinin cofactor assay, which evaluates the capacity of vWF to agglutinate platelets in the presence of venom from *Bothrops jararaca,* is available in few research laboratories.

III. Animals requiring surgery and suspected of having vWD should have a mucosal bleeding time performed prior to surgery.
   A. Although not diagnostic for vWD, the bleeding time provides useful information.
   B. Bleeding times ≥5 minutes are abnormal.

Differential Diagnosis

I. Extrinsic platelet function disorders must be distinguished from intrinsic platelet disorders and acquired qualitative disorders (see later).

II. Platelet function, evaluated in an aggregometer in response to various agonists such as adenosine diphosphate (ADP), collagen, and platelet activating factor (PAF), is normal in vWD.

III. Obtain a thorough history for prior drug treatment, particularly with aspirin. (Normal-dosage aspirin treatment alone does not induce spontaneous mucosal bleeding, and an underlying defect such as vWD should be suspected in these situations.)

IV. Evaluate affected animals for the existence of renal or hepatic disorders, leukemia, or infection.

Treatment

I. For vWD, a bleeding episode can be curtailed with IV transfusion of fresh plasma, fresh frozen plasma (6–10 ml/kg), or cryoprecipitate (1–1.5 ml/kg).
   A. Whole blood (20 ml/kg) may be required in an anemic animal (PCV <20%).
   B. DDAVP may be administered to the blood-donor dog at a dosage of 1 µg/kg SQ, 30–120 minutes before collecting blood for transfusion.

II. Administration of DDAVP to the affected dog just before a surgical procedure may be considered, but this is not totally effective in preventing excessive bleeding.

III. Animals documented to have excessive hemorrhage associated with vWD are transfused just prior to surgery (preferably with cryoprecipitate) and possibly during and after surgery as well.

Patient Monitoring

I. Periodic hemograms (complete blood count [CBC]) and iron determinations are performed to monitor for insidious blood loss.

II. Aspirin treatment is strongly discouraged.

III. Elective surgical procedures should be avoided; if performed, appropriate transfusion procedures must be available.

IV. vWD is a common inherited disorder, so dogs with vWD and a documented bleeding diathesis should not be bred.

V. Doberman pinschers have a particularly high incidence of vWD, and hypothyroidism may exacerbate coexisting vWD.
   A. Thyroid supplementation is recommended only in dogs documented to be hypothyroid.
   B. Thyroid supplementation is not recommended for euthyroid dogs, even if they do have clinically evident vWD.

Acquired Qualitative Platelet Disorders

Definition

I. Platelets develop an impairment in their ability to function.

II. Acquired platelet function defects tend to be reversible, unlike inherited defects.

Causes

I. Immune mediated
II. Drug induced
III. Infectious agent associated
IV. Myeloproliferative/lymphoproliferative disease associated
V. Renal failure and liver failure associated

Pathophysiology

I. Immune-mediated
   A. Antiplatelet antibodies may affect platelet reactivity with or without inducing concomitant thrombocytopenia.
   B. Platelet reactivity may be diminished or enhanced.

II. Drug-induced
   A. Binding of drugs to membrane receptors, altering their ability to recognize or respond to platelet activating agents
      1. β-Lactam antibiotics: penicillins and cephalosporins
      2. Aminoglycoside antibiotics: neomycin
      3. Anesthetics: cocaine, procaine, lidocaine, and dibucaine
      4. Others: ticlopidine
   B. Impairment of signal transduction via effects on cyclic adenosine monophosphate (cAMP)
      1. Inhibit cAMP phosphodiesterase: papaverine, dipyridamole, caffeine, theophylline, aminophylline
      2. Activate adenylate cyclase: iloprost
   C. Impairment of execution via effects on prostaglandin/thromboxane generation
      1. Nonsteroidal anti-inflammatory drugs (irreversible): aspirin
      2. Nonsteroidal anti-inflammatory drugs (reversible): phenylbutazone, acetaminophen, indomethacin, ibuprofen

D. Calcium channel blockers
 1. Barbiturates: pentobarbital, barbital
 2. Cardiovascular drugs: verapamil, diltiazem
III. Infectious agent–associated
 A. *E. canis* infection is often accompanied by platelet-type bleeding before or without the onset of thrombocytopenia, suggesting a rickettsial agent–associated platelet function disorder.
 B. *Yersinia pestis* outer membrane proteins inhibit thrombin- and ristocetin-induced human platelet aggregation, and prevention of platelet activation may be important during the initial stages of plague infection.
 C. FeLV can inhibit platelet reactivity with or without affecting platelet number.
IV. Myeloproliferative/lymphoproliferative disease–associated
 A. Myeloproliferative disease often results in abnormal function and morphology of one or more hematopoietic cells owing to defective stem cells.
 B. Hyperproteinemia associated with lymphoproliferative disease can inhibit platelet reactivity, possibly by interfering with platelet-platelet interactions.
V. Renal failure and liver failure–associated
 A. Although the mechanism is not fully understood, studies suggest that low-molecular-weight degradation products with amino acid sequences similar to ligand protein binding sites accumulate in uremia, resulting in inhibition of platelet aggregation.
 B. The liver is the clearing site for intermediate and end products of fibrinolysis, including FDPs. FDPs can bind to the fibrinogen receptor of platelets and competitively interfere with fibrinogen binding, thus impairing platelet aggregation.

Clinical Signs and Diagnosis

I. Mucosal bleeding is often present.
 A. Bleeding is acute and associated with disease or drug treatment, usually in an animal not previously documented to have a bleeding diathesis.
 B. Platelet numbers are within the reference range.
II. Biochemical tests for liver and/or renal function may be abnormal, and animals may display a variety of systemic signs, including icterus, polyuria/polydipsia, seizures, and vomiting.
III. Mucosal bleeding subsides with drug withdrawal (drug-related disorders) or response to treatment (infectious agent–associated platelet function disorders).
IV. Plasma protein levels are high in lymphoproliferative disorders affecting platelet reactivity.
 A. CBC and bone marrow analyses are abnormal with myeloproliferative disorders (see Chap. 65).
 B. Megakaryocyte and platelet morphology may be abnormal as assessed by light and electron microscopy.
V. Rising titers to infectious agents and the presence of viral antigens are supportive evidence for an infectious agent–induced platelet dysfunction.

Differential Diagnosis

I. Immune-mediated platelet dysfunction may be differentiated from an intrinsic platelet disorder by suspending normal platelets with plasma from the affected animal and vice versa.
 A. Intrinsic platelet disorders persist, as assessed by platelet aggregometry techniques, in the presence of normal plasma.
 B. Immune-mediated platelet dysfunction may normalize in the presence of normal plasma.
 C. More importantly, plasma from an affected animal with immune-mediated platelet dysfunction usually inhibits normal platelet reactivity.
II. Acquired qualitative platelet function disorders often resolve with response to treatment of the primary disease, removal of drugs, improved renal or hepatic function, or correction of plasma protein concentration.

Treatment

I. Treatment is aimed at the primary disease, whether it be infectious agent–associated, organ dysfunction–related, immune-mediated, or secondary to lympho- or myeloproliferative disease.
II. Drug-induced platelet function disorders are best treated by discontinuing drug treatment whenever possible.
III. Immune-mediated platelet function disorders are treated similarly to immune-mediated thrombocytopenias.

Patient Monitoring

I. Alleviation of mucosal bleeding occurs as the animal responds to treatment for the primary disease.
II. A buccal mucosal bleeding time may be performed to monitor the status of platelet function.

INHERITED/CONGENITAL QUANTITATIVE DISORDERS OF COAGULATION

Prekallikrein Deficiency

Definition and Causes

I. It is an autosomal recessive disorder, rarely diagnosed in domestic animals.
II. One reported case exists in a 14-year-old male poodle (Chinn et al., 1986).

Clinical Signs and Diagnosis

I. A bleeding diathesis is rare with prekallikrein deficiency in animals.
II. The aPTT is prolonged, and the PT and thrombin time are normal (Table 66–5).
III. Usually bleeding is not evident, and detection is fortuitous.

*Table 66–5. **Coagulation and Antithrombotic Protein Disorders, Diagnostic Tests, and Appropriate Transfusion Products***

Coagulation Factor Deficiency	Prolonged Tests	Bleeding Diathesis	Transfusion Product
Prekallikrein	aPTT, aCT	No	None
XII	aPTT, aCT	No	None
XI	aPTT, aCT	Mild, with trauma	Plasma, whole blood[c]
IX	aPTT, aCT	Yes[a]	Plasma, whole blood
VIII-C	aPTT, aCT	Yes[a]	Cryo, plasma, whole blood
VII	PT	Yes/No[b]	Plasma, whole blood
X	aPTT, aCT, PT	Yes	Plasma, whole blood
II	aPTT, aCT, PT	Yes	Plasma, whole blood
Fibrinogen	aPTT, aCT, PT, TT	Yes	Cryo, plasma, whole blood
Vitamin K antagonism	aPTT, aCT, PT	Yes	Plasma, whole blood
Antithrombin III	Activity < 70%	No (thrombosis)	Plasma

aPTT = activated partial thromboplastin time; aCT = activated coagulation time; PT = prothrombin time; TT = thrombin time; cryo = cryoprecipitate, administered at 1–1.5 ml/kg.
[a]Bleeding tendency correlates strongly with factor activity present and size/weight of the animal.
[b]There are sporadic reports of bleeding episodes in affected beagles.
[c]Whole blood (20 ml/kg) should be administered to animals with PCV < 20%. Plasma is administered at 6–10 ml/kg.

IV. Specific analysis of kallikrein activity is necessary for a diagnosis.

Differential Diagnosis

I. Prekallikrein deficiency must be differentiated from the presence of an inhibitor or deficiency of other factors within the intrinsic pathway above factor X.
II. Specific factor analysis determines which factor(s) are deficient and requires submission of citrated plasma to a specialized laboratory.

Treatment and Monitoring

I. Treatment is usually not necessary.
II. Bleeding should resolve with transfusion of autologous plasma.
III. Usually monitoring is not necessary.

Factor XII Deficiency (Hageman's Disease)

Definition and Causes

I. Autosomal recessive inheritance pattern in cats
II. Autosomal dominant inheritance pattern in one family of miniature poodles

Clinical Signs

I. Factor XII deficiency is not associated with a bleeding diathesis and did not enhance a coinciding factor IX deficiency in cats (Dillon and Boudreaux, 1988).
II. A predisposition to thrombosis and infection has been suspected in human beings, but this predisposition has never been documented in animals with Hageman's disease.

Diagnosis

I. The aPTT is prolonged, but the PT and thrombin time are normal (see Table 66–5).
II. Specific analysis of factor XII activity is necessary for a diagnosis.

Differential Diagnosis

I. Specific analysis of other factor activities within the intrinsic pathway rules out other factor deficiencies or the coexistence of other factor deficiencies.
II. A factor XII inhibitor may be present, but this has not yet been described in domestic animals.

Treatment and Monitoring

I. Treatment is not necessary.
II. Factor XII deficiency does not exacerbate a coexisting bleeding diathesis.

Factor XI Deficiency

Definition and Causes

I. Rare in domestic animals, factor XI deficiency has been diagnosed in only a few breeds of dogs.
II. The inheritance pattern in dogs is unknown, but there is an autosomal dominant inheritance pattern in human beings and an autosomal recessive inheritance pattern in cattle.

Clinical Signs

I. A spontaneous bleeding diathesis is rare in affected individuals.
II. Factor XI–deficient animals may bleed excessively after surgery or trauma.

Diagnosis

I. The aPTT is prolonged, and the PT and thrombin time are normal (see Table 66–5).
II. Specific analysis of factor XI activity is necessary for a diagnosis.
III. Antigen assay, if available, determines whether a quantitative or qualitative defect is present.

Differential Diagnosis

I. Other factor deficiencies within the intrinsic pathway must be ruled out.
II. The presence of an inhibitor to factor XI must be ruled out.
   A. Incubation of normal plasma with affected plasma (50:50 mixture) should correct the aPTT.
   B. If correction does not occur, an inhibitor should be suspected.

Treatment and Monitoring

I. Give plasma transfusion (6–10 ml/kg IV BID-TID or until bleeding stops) or whole blood transfusion (20 ml/kg) if PCV <20%.
II. Inhibitors of coagulation factors are usually produced secondary to underlying immunologic disease such as systemic lupus erythematosus (SLE), so identification and treatment of primary disease should eliminate the production of factor inhibitor.
III. Periodic CBC or PCV is monitored to assess for continued blood loss after transfusion.

Factor IX Deficiency (Hemophilia B)

Definition and Causes

I. It is a sex-linked recessive disease and the second most common inherited coagulopathy of domestic animals.
II. The incidence in dogs and cats is not known.
III. In the dog, two mutations for factor IX deficiency have been characterized at the gene level.

Clinical Signs

I. Because of factor IX's vital role in the intrinsic factor X activation complex, factor IX activity <3% of normal may be associated with profound spontaneous hemorrhage, particularly within body cavities such as joints, the thorax, or the abdomen or between muscle groups.
   A. Factor IX–deficient cats with recent internal hemorrhage may present with depression, anorexia, and fever as the only clinical signs.
   B. Lameness owing to hemorrhage into a joint cavity may be the only presenting complaint in small dogs or cats.
II. Small cats and dogs tolerate low factor levels better than larger animals, presumably because of their light weight.

A. Factor IX activities <1% of normal are probably not compatible with life.
B. Factor IX activities between 5 and 10% of normal are usually well tolerated.

Diagnosis

I. The aPTT is prolonged, and the PT and thrombin time are normal (see Table 66–5).
II. Specific analysis of factor IX activity is necessary for a diagnosis.
III. Antigen assay determines whether a quantitative or qualitative defect is present.

Differential Diagnosis

I. Factor IX deficiency must be differentiated from other factor deficiencies within the intrinsic pathway. Factor VIII coagulant deficiency is identical to factor IX deficiency in clinical presentation.
II. Rule out the presence of a factor IX inhibitor.
III. Factor IX is a vitamin K–dependent factor; therefore, rule out vitamin K antagonism by examining activities of other vitamin K–dependent factors (II, VII, and X).

Treatment and Monitoring

I. Plasma (6–10 ml/kg IV BID-TID or until bleeding stops) or whole blood transfusion (20 ml/kg if PCV <20%) curtails bleeding if an inhibitor is not present.
II. The presence of an inhibitor may require co-treatment with steroids. Acquisition of inhibitors by a hemophiliac is most likely to occur in animals treated with recombinant human products; therefore, these products are not recommended.
III. Cage rest may be the only treatment required in animals presenting with joint lameness and no evidence of continued bleeding.
IV. Euthanasia may be recommended in large-breed dogs with repeated hemorrhagic episodes, particularly if they result in crippling joint disease.
V. Do not perform thoracocentesis or abdominocentesis to remove blood from body cavities unless hemorrhage is impairing breathing.
VI. It is imperative to monitor PCV and/or CBC for evidence of continued blood loss into a body cavity such as the abdomen.

Factor VIII Deficiency (Hemophilia A)

Definition and Causes

I. It is a sex-linked recessive disease and the most common inherited coagulopathy of domestic animals.
II. The actual incidence of factor VIII deficiency in domestic animals is unknown.
III. Factor VIII coagulant is complexed with vWF in circulation.
   A. This relationship is vital to the stabilization and activity of factor VIII coagulant.

B. In severe vWD, factor VIII coagulant activity may decrease; however, in dogs, the decrease is rarely enough to affect the aPTT test or result in coagulopathy-type bleeding.

Clinical Signs

I. Because of factor VIII's cofactor role in the intrinsic factor X activation complex, factor VIII activity <3% of normal may result in profound hemorrhage similar to that described for factor IX deficiency (factor VIII and factor IX deficiencies are indistinguishable based on clinical signs).
II. Factor VIII activity <1% has not been reported and may be lethal.
III. Factor VIII activities between 5 and 10% of normal are well tolerated; prolonged bleeding may occur only following surgery or trauma.
IV. Cats or small dogs may present only with acute onset of lameness, depression, anorexia, and/or lethargy.

Diagnosis

I. The aPTT is prolonged, and the PT and thrombin time are normal (see Table 66–5).
II. Specific analysis of factor VIII coagulant activity is necessary for a diagnosis.
III. Antigen assay determines whether a quantitative or qualitative defect is present.

Differential Diagnosis

I. Factor VIII coagulant deficiency must be differentiated from other intrinsic pathway factor deficiencies, particularly factor IX deficiency.
II. An inhibitor of factor VIII coagulant may be present.

Treatment and Monitoring

I. Plasma (6–10 ml/kg IV BID-TID or until bleeding stops) or cryoprecipitate (1–1.5 ml/kg IV BID-TID or until bleeding stops) curtails a bleeding episode.
II. Whole blood transfusion (20 ml/kg) is given to animals with PCV <20%.
III. Mild bleeding into a joint may be treated with cage rest if the actual bleeding episode seems to have been arrested.
IV. Abdominocentesis or thoracocentesis is avoided in known hemophiliacs, and blood should not be removed from the thorax unless breathing is impaired.
V. Euthanasia may be recommended in large-breed dogs with repeated hemorrhagic episodes, particularly if they result in crippling joint disease.
VI. Periodic CBCs and/or PCVs are performed to assess response to treatment and to monitor for continued blood loss into body cavities.

Factor VII Deficiency

Definition and Causes

I. It is an autosomal recessive disease.
II. It is not common in animals but has been identified in beagles, miniature schnauzers, boxers, bulldogs, and Alaskan malamutes.
III. Factor VII, in complex with tissue factor (factor III), is an important enzyme in the extrinsic factor X activation complex.
IV. The factor VII–tissue factor complex is also an important activator of factor IX.

Clinical Signs

I. It is not associated with clinical signs and is discovered fortuitously, much like factor XII deficiency.
   A. There have been sporadic reports of bleeding diatheses in affected beagles.
   B. Bleeding is sometimes observed post partum in factor VII–deficient bitches.
II. Factor VII activity <1% of normal has not been reported and may be lethal. Activities between 1 and 3% of normal may be sufficient to prevent excessive hemorrhage in most situations.

Diagnosis

I. The PT is prolonged, and the aPTT and thrombin time are normal (see Table 66–5).
II. Specific analysis of factor VII activity is necessary for a diagnosis.
III. Antigen assay determines whether a quantitative or qualitative defect is present.

Differential Diagnosis

I. Factor VII is a vitamin K–dependent factor; therefore, factor VII deficiency may be a component of any vitamin K antagonism. Vitamin K antagonism would have to be very acute (<12 hours) for other vitamin K–dependent factors not to be affected and for the aPTT not to be prolonged.
II. Factor VII inhibitor may be present.

Treatment and Monitoring

I. It is usually discovered fortuitously, and treatment is not necessary.
II. Plasma (6–10 ml/kg IV) curtails a bleeding episode.
III. Pregnant animals with factor VII deficiency are monitored carefully.

Factor X Deficiency

Definition and Causes

I. It is an autosomal dominant disease with variable penetrance in dogs.
II. Factor X deficiency is rare and has been reported only in the American cocker spaniel and Jack Russell terrier breeds.
III. Factor X is important to both the extrinsic and the intrinsic pathways of coagulation.

Clinical Signs

I. Stillbirths and early deaths are common in puppies born to affected parents.

II. Bleeding diatheses range from mild to severe in dogs with factor X activities 3–68% of normal.
III. Factor X activities <1% of normal are likely lethal.
IV. Factor X activities of 1–3% are likely to be associated with serious hemorrhagic tendencies.
V. Even factor X activities as high as 50% of normal may still be associated with abnormal hemorrhage, particularly in association with trauma or surgery.

Diagnosis

I. The aPTT and PT are prolonged, and the thrombin time is normal (see Table 66–5).
II. Specific analysis of factor X activity is necessary for a diagnosis.
III. Antigen assay determines whether a quantitative or qualitative defect is present.

Differential Diagnosis

I. Factor X is a vitamin K–dependent factor; therefore, vitamin K antagonism must be ruled out.
II. Specific analysis of the activities of factors II, IX, and VII is necessary to rule in or out vitamin K antagonism.
III. Inherited vitamin K–dependent multifactor coagulopathy is also possible and is ruled out by documenting normal activities of other vitamin K–dependent factors.
IV. Levels of proteins induced by vitamin K absence or antagonists (PIVKA) are normal in congenital factor X deficiency.

Treatment and Monitoring

I. Plasma (6–10 ml/kg IV BID-TID or until bleeding stops) or whole blood transfusion (20 ml/kg if PCV <20%) curtails bleeding.
II. Factor X–deficient animals are susceptible to catastrophic hemorrhage and must be kept in protected environments.
III. Do not breed affected animals.

Factor II (Prothrombin) Deficiency

Definition and Pathophysiology

I. Factor II deficiency is extremely rare and has been diagnosed in only one 5-month-old female English cocker spaniel (Hill et al., 1982).
  A. Factor II activity in the affected dog was between 6 and 8% of normal.
  B. Antigen studies were not performed, so a dysprothrombinemia could not be ruled out in this case.
II. Deficiency of prothrombin is not very compatible with life, and reduced activities of the enzyme (<10% of normal) are not well tolerated.
III. Mucosal bleeding (gingival bleeding, epistaxis, petechial and ecchymotic hemorrhages) suggestive of a platelet disorder may also occur with severe prothrombin deficiency because thrombin is a platelet agonist.

Clinical Signs

I. In the one reported case, epistaxis and gingival hemorrhage were the presenting signs.
II. Coagulopathy-type bleeding into body cavities such as the thorax, abdomen, and joints is also possible.

Diagnosis

I. The aPTT and PT are prolonged, and the thrombin time is normal (see Table 66–5).
II. Specific analysis of factor II activity is necessary for a diagnosis.
III. Antigen assays determine whether a quantitative or qualitative defect is present.

Differential Diagnosis

I. Factor II is vitamin K dependent; therefore, vitamin K antagonism and vitamin K–dependent multifactor coagulopathy must be ruled out as described earlier under Factor X Deficiency.
II. An inhibitor of factor II may be present.

Treatment and Monitoring

I. Plasma (6–10 ml/kg IV BID–TID or until bleeding stops) or whole blood transfusions (20 ml/kg if PCV <20%) stop hemorrhage.
II. Affected animals should be kept in a protected environment.
III. Elective surgery is avoided unless transfusion products and procedures are readily available.

Factor I (Fibrinogen) Deficiency

Definition and Causes

I. Congenital afibrinogenemia has not been reported in dogs or cats.
II. Hypofibrinogenemia was reported in a St. Bernard in Switzerland in 1971 (Spurling, 1980).

Clinical Signs

I. Afibrinogenemia or severe hypofibrinogenemia is associated with severe hemorrhagic diatheses, not only from the inability to form clots but also from reduced to absent platelet aggregation.
II. A combination of mucosal bleeding and hemorrhage into body cavities is expected with severe hypofibrinogenemia.

Diagnosis

I. The aPTT, PT, and thrombin time are all prolonged (see Table 66–5).
II. The heat precipitation technique for fibrinogen and fibrinogen analysis by electrophoresis help diagnose quantitative and qualitative defects.

Differential Diagnosis

I. Specific analysis of the activity of other coagulation proteins is necessary to rule out other factor deficiencies in the intrinsic, extrinsic, and common pathways.
II. If coagulation protein consumption (DIC) is suspected, platelet counts and FDP analysis are appropriate. Thrombocytopenia and increased FDPs are expected in DIC.
III. Liver disease may result in profound decreases in many of the coagulation proteins.

Treatment and Monitoring

I. Plasma (6–10 ml/kg IV BID-TID or until bleeding stops), cryoprecipitate (1–1.5 ml/kg IV), or whole blood transfusion (20 ml/kg if PCV <20%) decreases bleeding.
II. Animals are kept in protected environments, and elective surgery is avoided.

Vitamin K–Dependent Multifactor Coagulopathy

Definition and Causes

I. An autosomal inheritance pattern is described in Devon rex cats (Soute et al., 1992).
  A. Vitamin K–dependent coagulation factors II, VII, IX, and X are reduced in activity.
  B. Factor deficiencies are caused by a defective gamma-glutamylcarboxylase enzyme that has a decreased affinity for both vitamin K hydroquinone and propeptide.
II. The vitamin K–dependent factors are vital to the intrinsic and extrinsic factor X activation complexes and the prothrombinase complex.

Clinical Signs

I. Deficiency of vitamin K–dependent factors results in severe hemorrhagic disease.
II. Several of the cats described with this disorder had major hemorrhage into body cavities, including the thorax and abdomen.

Diagnosis

I. The aPTT and PT are prolonged, and the thrombin time is normal.
II. Activities of the vitamin K–dependent coagulation factors (II, VII, IX, X) are reduced.
III. Animals respond to treatment with vitamin K_1.

Differential Diagnosis

I. Vitamin K antagonism must be ruled out.
  A. Obtain a thorough history to determine whether rodenticide exposure is possible.
  B. Affected animals may have to be isolated for several weeks to rule out rodenticide toxicity.

II. Vitamin K deficiency is possible in animals with chronic fat malabsorption/maldigestion.
III. Liver disease may cause coagulation factor deficiency, but other coagulation factors besides vitamin K–dependent factors would also be decreased.

Treatment

I. Affected cats respond to oral vitamin K_1 at 10 mg twice weekly or 5 mg daily.
II. Plasma or whole blood transfusion (PCV <20%) may be required to arrest acute hemorrhage.

Patient Monitoring

I. These animals are at continual risk for catastrophic hemorrhage.
  A. Provide a protective environment.
  B. Educate the owners to be alert for changes in behavior such as depression, lethargy, lameness, dyspnea, or anorexia.
II. Continued maintenance on oral vitamin K_1 may be required, but high doses have been associated with Heinz body hemolytic anemia.

ACQUIRED QUANTITATIVE DISORDERS OF COAGULATION FACTORS

Aquired Coagulation Factor Deficiencies

Definition

I. Usually, multiple coagulation factors are diminished to <40% of normal, but single factors may be affected.
II. Coagulation factor deficiencies are secondary to another disorder.
III. Most acquired coagulation factor deficiencies are associated with a bleeding diathesis.

Causes

I. Liver disease
II. Inhibitors
III. DIC
IV. Renal disease

Pathophysiology

I. Liver disease
  A. The liver is the major site of synthesis for the coagulation, fibrinolytic, and antithrombotic proteins.
    1. Exceptions include vWF, tissue plasminogen activator (TPA), and urokinase-type plasminogen activator (u-PA), which are synthesized by endothelials cells (vWF and TPA) and within the kidney (u-PA).

2. The liver also clears activated factors and both intermediate and end products of fibrinolysis.

B. Most coagulation factors have half-lives of <2 days; therefore, hepatic disease may result in a fairly rapid change in factor activity.
   1. Factor activities generally must decline to <10% of normal before spontaneous bleeding occurs.
   2. This requires widespread hepatic dysfunction secondary to inflammation, neoplasia, or fibrosis.

II. Inhibitors
   A. Production of antibodies recognizing one or more coagulation factors usually occurs secondary or in association with autoimmune diseases such as SLE.
      1. Such inhibitors often cause qualitative alterations in coagulation or antithrombotic protein function (see Acquired Qualitative Disorders of Coagulation Factors, later).
      2. Inhibitors, however, have been recognized in dogs without other evidence of autoimmune disease.
   B. Hemophiliacs may produce antibodies against factor VIII coagulant or factor IX with repeated transfusions.

III. DIC
   A. Overwhelming activation of the coagulation, fibrinolytic, and antithrombotic mechanisms can occur secondary to a wide variety of events, including septicemia, heat stroke, neoplasia, electric shock, burns, and hypothermia.
   B. Consumption of coagulation, fibrinolytic, and antithrombotic proteins is a dynamic process that occurs to varying extents and at varying rates, depending on the health of the animal at the onset, the underlying cause, and the ability of the animal to respond.
   C. Animals with DIC generally present with a hemorrhagic diathesis, but thrombosis may also occur, particularly in small vessels.

IV. Renal disease
   A. Antithrombin III is a potent inhibitor of activated coagulation proteins, particularly factors II and X.
   B. Antithrombin III activities of <70% place the animal at risk for thrombosis.
   C. The most common causes of antithrombin III deficiency include protein-losing renal disease, protein-losing enteropathy, and DIC.
   D. Antithrombin III has a molecular weight similar to that of albumin, so antithrombin III loss tends to parallel albumin loss.

Clinical Signs

I. With severe liver disease, the bleeding pattern may be platelet type owing to inhibition of platelet function and/or coagulopathy type owing to diminished production of coagulation proteins.

II. With DIC, the bleeding pattern is a combined platelet type and coagulopathy type owing to consumption of platelets and coagulation proteins. Breathing may be labored because of pulmonary thrombosis.

III. Animals with inhibitor development experience a coagulopathy-type bleeding that responds minimally to transfusion of blood or plasma.

IV. If the urinalysis reveals proteinuria, antithrombin III activity is monitored.

Diagnosis

I. Inhibitors should be suspected in animals not responsive to plasma transfusion.
   A. Mixing of normal plasma with affected plasma does not correct prolongations in the aPTT if inhibitors are present.
   B. Animals with SLE may have a positive ANA or LE test.

II. Uncompensated DIC is accompanied by prolongations in the aPTT, PT, and thrombin time; elevations in FDPs; and thrombocytopenia.

III. Compensated DIC is more difficult to diagnose, because varying combinations of normal and abnormal tests may be present as the animal begins to respond by increasing factor production, clearing FDPs, and increasing platelet production.

IV. FDP tubes using *Bothrops atrox* venom should not be used to measure FDPs in dogs.

V. D-dimer assays are of little to no value in domestic animals.

VI. Specific assays for antithrombin III are available, and antithrombin III activity is monitored in animals with protein-losing enteropathies or nephropathies.

Differential Diagnosis

I. Acquired quantitative disorders must be differentiated from inherited quantitative disorders.

II. Inherited disorders rarely involve more than one coagulation factor. Multifactor coagulopathy is one exception, and this defect involves only vitamin K–dependent factors.

Treatment

I. Liver disease widespread enough to cause coagulation factor deficiency and hemorrhage is a dire situation. Treatment is supportive, including blood transfusions to control hemorrhage.

II. Inhibitor effects often cannot be controlled with steroids, but steroid treatment coinciding with plasma transfusion may be attempted.
   A. Research is presently under way to determine the effectiveness of antibodies against tissue factor pathway inhibitor (TFPI) as a treatment for hemophilia.
   B. If effective, this treatment would be especially attractive for animals with inhibitor development.

III. Inhibitors secondary to SLE may resolve spontaneously with successful treatment or control of autoimmune disease.

IV. The underlying cause for DIC must be determined and treated or eliminated, if possible. Supportive care is vital and includes fluids, plasma, or blood transfusions (if PCV <20%) to maintain tissue perfusion and prevent thrombosis.

V. Animals with transient protein-losing conditions can be transfused with plasma to maintain antithrombin III activities above 70%. This is important not only to prevent thrombosis but also to enhance the effectiveness of heparin treatment during DIC.

Patient Monitoring

I. Serum liver enzyme and bilirubin analyses are performed on a weekly basis to determine whether hepatocellular necrosis is progressing or diminishing.

II. Coagulation screening tests are evaluated at least twice weekly to monitor for compensation and recovery from DIC.

III. Antithrombin III activity is monitored at least once or twice weekly in animals with protein-losing conditions or as part of the coagulation screening profile in animals with DIC.

INHERITED/CONGENITAL QUALITATIVE DISORDERS OF COAGULATION FACTORS

Dysfibrinogenemia

Definition and Causes

I. An autosomal disease is recognized in a family of Russian wolfhounds (Dodds, 1981).

II. Functional assays for fibrinogen were abnormal, but fibrinogen antigen levels were normal.

Clinical Signs

I. Affected Russian wolfhounds had a mild bleeding disorder until after trauma or surgery.

II. Dysfibrinogenemia, depending on the region of fibrinogen affected, may result in bleeding, thrombosis, or no clinical signs.

Diagnosis

I. The PT, aPTT, and thrombin time are prolonged (see Table 66–5).

II. The heat precipitation technique for fibrinogen does not correlate with functional activity.

III. Fibrinogen isolation and protein electrophoresis may aid in detecting gross qualitative changes in the fibrinogen molecule.

Differential Diagnosis

I. Dysfibrinogenemia must be differentiated from hypofibrinogenemia; DIC; vitamin K antagonism; liver disease; and factor V, II, or X deficiency.

II. Hypofibrinogenemia is ruled out with antigenic or physical assays for fibrinogen.

III. DIC is usually accompanied by thrombocytopenia and an increase in FDPs.

IV. Vitamin K antagonism can be ruled out with a careful history, lack of response to vitamin K therapy, specific analysis of vitamin K–dependent factor activities, and/or PIVKA analysis. The thrombin time is not prolonged with vitamin K antagonism.

V. Liver disease is ruled out by evaluating liver enzymes, dye clearance studies, radiography, ultrasonography, and/or biopsy.

VI. Other common pathway factor deficiencies are ruled out by evaluating specific factor activities.

Treatment

I. Bleeding as a result of dysfibrinogenemia is decreased with plasma (6–10 ml/kg) or cryoprecipitate (1–1.5 ml/kg) transfusion.

II. Whole blood (20 ml/kg IV) can be administered if the PCV is <20%.

Patient Monitoring

I. Animals are kept in a relatively protected environment.

II. Periodic CBCs are performed to evaluate for insidious blood loss.

III. Affected animals should not be bred.

Dysprothrombinemia

Definition and Causes

I. An autosomal inheritance pattern has been described in one boxer family (Dodds, 1979; Hill et al., 1982).

II. Functional assays for prothrombin were abnormal, but antigen assays were normal.

Clinical Signs

I. Affected adult boxer dogs had mild bleeding tendencies; bleeding was more severe in puppies.

II. Depending on the location of the prothrombin defect, animals may have major, minor, or no clinical bleeding.

Diagnosis

I. The PT and aPTT are prolonged, and the thrombin time is normal.

II. Factor II activity should be compared with antigenic assays for factor II.

Differential Diagnosis

I. Dysprothrombinemia must be differentiated from hypoprothrombinemia, vitamin K antagonism, DIC, liver disease, and factor X or V deficiency.

II. Hypoprothrombinemia is ruled out with antigenic assays.

III. Vitamin K antagonism is ruled out with a careful history, lack of response to vitamin K therapy, analysis of activities of other vitamin K–dependent factors, and/or PIVKA analysis.

IV. Uncompensated DIC is usually accompanied by thrombocytopenia, hypofibrinogenemia, and an increase in FDPs.

V. Liver disease is evaluated with liver enzyme activities, clearance of dyes, radiography, ultrasonography, and/or biopsy.

VI. Factor X and factor V activities are evaluated to rule out deficiencies of these factors.

Treatment and Monitoring

I. Bleeding as a result of dysprothrombinemia is decreased by plasma (6–10 mg/kg) or whole blood (20 ml/kg if PCV <20%) transfusion.

II. Keep animals in a relatively protected environment.

III. Do not breed affected animals.

ACQUIRED QUALITATIVE DISORDERS OF COAGULATION FACTORS

Vitamin K Antagonism/Deficiency

Definition and Pathophysiology

I. Vitamin K–dependent factors are vital players in the intrinsic and extrinsic factor X activation complexes and in the prothrombinase complex.

A. Vitamin K–dependent factors are synthesized by the liver and undergo post-translational modification that is vitamin K dependent.

B. As a result of this modification, functional coagulation factors become negatively charged.

II. Vitamin K antagonists inhibit the activity of the epoxide enzyme necessary for recycling of vitamin K. As a result of this antagonism, functional vitamin K–dependent factors are rapidly depleted while non-functional precursors (PIVKA) increase.

III. Vitamin K is a fat-soluble vitamin, so vitamin K deficiency may develop in animals with fat malabsorption/maldigestion.

Clinical Signs

I. Animals with vitamin K antagonism are at risk for profound hemorrhage.

II. Presenting signs can be quite variable and include depression, anorexia, dyspnea, lameness, weakness, seizures, and/or bloody diarrhea.

Diagnosis

I. The PT, aPTT, and activated clotting time (aCT) are prolonged in animals demonstrating excessive bleeding secondary to vitamin K antagonism or deficiency. The thrombin time is normal.

II. In early vitamin K antagonism, the PT may be the only abnormal screening test, because factor VII has the shortest half-life. This is most likely to occur

if samples are taken within 8 hours of rodenticide ingestion.

III. A careful history is imperative.

A. Owners may not be aware of rodenticide exposure if animals are free-roaming.

B. Secondary exposure by eating poisoned rodents is possible in cats.

C. Coprophagy is also a means of secondary exposure, particularly in dogs. Dogs being treated with vitamin K_1 after documented rodenticide ingestion must not be kenneled with other dogs who are coprophagic.

IV. A positive response to treatment with vitamin K_1 provides supportive evidence, as does specific analysis of vitamin K–dependent factor activities or PIVKA analysis.

Differential Diagnosis

I. Vitamin K antagonism must be differentiated from vitamin K deficiency, liver disease, and inherited vitamin K–dependent multifactor coagulopathy.

II. Vitamin K antagonism may be documented with a careful history, response to treatment with vitamin K_1, and cure without further treatment (provided re-exposure does not occur).

III. Vitamin K deficiency responds rapidly to one treatment, but a relapse is likely after several weeks to months if malabsorption/maldigestion is not corrected.

IV. Liver disease is evaluated with appropriate liver function tests, radiography, ultrasonography, and/or biopsy.

V. Inherited vitamin K–dependent multifactor coagulopathy is suspected if multiple siblings are affected, the animals are young, and there is no history of rodenticide exposure. Long-term vitamin K therapy may also be necessary for inherited multifactor coagulopathy.

Treatment

I. Vitamin K_1 0.25–2.5 mg/kg/day PO for 7 days is the recommended treatment for relatively short-acting coumarin compounds (see also Chap. 123).

A. These include warfarin and coumafuryl.

B. When compounds with moderately long half-lives, including brodifacoum and bromadiolone, are ingested, treatment may take as long as 3–4 weeks.

C. Indanedione compounds, including pindone, valone, diphacinone, and chlorophacinone, have half-lives as long as 15–20 days, and treatment may take 4–6 weeks.

D. Vitamin K_1 can be administered SQ, but IV administration may result in anaphylaxis.

II. Indanedione toxicity may not respond to lower doses of vitamin K_1 and may require higher dosages. (Vitamin K_1 dosages as high as 5 mg/kg have been associated with Heinz body anemia in dogs.)

III. Supportive care with oxygen, blood transfusions (20

ml/kg if PCV <20%), and steroids may also be required.

IV. Paracentesis to remove blood from body cavities is
not attempted unless breathing is impaired because
of massive thoracic hemorrhage.

V. Vitamin K_3 is not effective in treating vitamin K
antagonism.

VI. Malabsorption/maldigestion causes of vitamin K deficiency require SQ or IM administration of vitamin
K_1. Because the body can readily recycle vitamin K,
monthly injections are adequate if malabsorption/
maldigestion persists.

Patient Monitoring

I. Animals poisoned with shorter-acting coumarin- or
warfarin-type compounds have a much better prognosis than those poisoned with indanedione compounds.
  A. Most animals with warfarin toxicity can be managed at home with oral vitamin K_1.
  B. Indanedione-poisoned animals are more likely to
  require hospitalization and supportive or intensive care.

II. The PT is evaluated at the end of a treatment regimen
for vitamin K antagonism caused by coumarin compounds and is evaluated at least once weekly for
indanedione toxicity.

Coagulation/Antithrombotic Protein Inhibitors

Definition and Pathophysiology

I. Antibodies to one or more coagulation proteins may
result in altered function of those proteins.

II. Inhibitors may enhance or inhibit functional activity.

III. Inhibitors have been suspected to occur with autoimmune diseases such as SLE.

IV. Autoantibodies that inhibit in vitro phospholipid-de-
pendent coagulation reactions are termed lupus anticoagulants.

Clinical Signs

I. Depending on whether antibodies are inhibitory or
enhancing in their effect, animals may present with
bleeding or thrombosis.

II. Antibodies inhibiting coagulation protein activity
likely cause a bleeding pattern suggestive of a coagulopathy.

III. Antibodies inhibiting antithrombotic proteins such as
protein C or protein S may result in thrombosis.

Diagnosis

I. The aPTT and/or the PT may be prolonged, even in
animals presenting with thrombosis.

II. Animals with SLE may have positive ANA and/or
LE tests, anemia, and/or thrombocytopenia.

III. Measurement of soluble coagulation proteins in
blood, even suspect target antigens, likely yields nor-

mal antigen levels, because autoantibodies often do
not bind to soluble protein.

IV. Addition of suspect plasma to normal plasma pro-
longs the aPTT and/or PT. Normal plasma does not
correct the aPTT and/or PT of affected plasma.

V. Animals must not be heparinized when evaluating
the possibility of inhibitors.

VI. Inhibitors are most likely when animals present with
thrombosis yet coagulation screening tests are prolonged.

Differential Diagnosis

I. Inhibitor development must be differentiated from
DIC or other acquired or inherited disorders of coagulation.

II. Non-immunologic-related quantitative disorders of
coagulation proteins are corrected by addition of
normal plasma or missing factor. Addition of affected plasma does not affect normal plasma coagulation screening tests.

III. Uncompensated DIC is usually accompanied by prolongations in the aPTT, PT, and thrombin time and
by thrombocytopenia and an increase in FDPs.

IV. Compensated DIC is more difficult to differentiate,
but addition of normal plasma should correct coagulation screening test results.

Treatment and Monitoring

I. Treatment of the underlying autoimmune disease is
imperative; signs of thrombosis and/or bleeding resolve with successful control or cure.

II. Platelet concentrates, platelet-rich plasma, whole
blood, or plasma may be required to arrest hemorrhage, particularly if the PCV drops below 20%.

III. Animals in remission are monitored with a minimum
of a CBC and physical exam every 6 months.

Bibliography

Authement JM: Preparation of components. Adv Vet Sci Comp
Med 36:171, 1991

Axthelm MK, Krakowka S: Canine distemper virus–induced
thrombocytopenia. Am J Vet Res 48:1269, 1987

Bloom JC, Blackmer SA, Bugelski PJ et al: Gold-induced immune thrombocytopenia in the dog. Vet Pathol 22:492, 1985

Bloom JC, Meunier LD, Thiem PA, Sellers TS: Use of danazol
for treatment of corticosteroid-resistant immune-mediated
thrombocytopenia in a dog. J Am Vet Med Assoc 194:76, 1989

Blue TJ: Myelofibrosis in cats with myelodysplastic syndrome
and acute myelogenous leukemia. Vet Pathol 25:154, 1988

Boudreaux MK, Crager C, Dillon AR et al: Identification of an
intrinsic platelet function defect in spitz dogs. J Vet Intern Med
8:93, 1994

Boudreaux MK, Kvam K, Dillon AR et al: Type I Glanzmann's
thrombasthenia in a Great Pyrenees dog. Vet Pathol 33:503,
1996

Burstein SA, Downs T, Friese P et al: Thrombocytopoiesis in
normal and sublethally irradiated dogs: response to human
interleukin-6. Blood 80:420, 1992

Callan MB, Bennett JS, Phillips DK et al: Inherited platelet δ-
storage pool disease in dogs causing severe bleeding: an animal

model for a specific ADP deficiency. Thromb Haemost 74:949, 1995

Catalfamo JL, Dodds WJ: Hereditary and acquired thrombopathies. Vet Clin North Am [Small Anim Pract] 18:185, 1988

Cesbron JY, Capron A, Vargaftig BB et al: Platelets mediate the action of diethylcarbamazine on microfilariae. Nature 325:533, 1987

Cesbron JY, Hayasaki M, Joseph M et al: Monoclonal anti-idiotype antibody as antigen signal for the microfilaricidal cytotoxicity of diethylcarbamazine-treated platelets. J Immunol 141:279, 1988

Chinn DR, Dodds WJ, Selcer BA: Prekallikrein deficiency in a dog. J Am Vet Med Assoc 188:69, 1986

Cotter SM: Clinical transfusion medicine. Adv Vet Sci Comp Med 36:187, 1991

Davi G, Giammarresi C, Vigneri S et al: Demonstration of *Rickettsia conorii*–induced coagulative and platelet activation in vivo in patients with Mediterranean spotted fever. Thromb Haemost 74:631, 1995

Davidson MG, Breitschwerdt EB, Walker DH et al: Vascular permeability and coagulation during *Rickettsia rickettsii* infection in dogs. Am J Vet Res 51:165, 1990

Davie EW: Biochemical and molecular aspects of the coagulation cascade. Thromb Haemost 74:1, 1995

Dillon AR, Boudreaux MK: Combined factors IX and XII deficiencies in a family of cats. J Am Vet Med Assoc 193:833, 1988

Dodds WJ: Inherited bleeding disorders. Canine Pract 5:49, 1978

Dodds WJ: Prothrombin (factor II) deficiencies. p. 267. In Andrews EJ, Ward BC, Altman NH (eds): Spontaneous Animal Models of Human Disease. Academic Press, New York, 1979

Dodds WJ: Second international registry of animal models of thrombosis and hemorrhagic diseases. ILAR News 24:R16, 1981

Fernandez FR, Teachout DJ, Christopher MM: Vitamin K–induced Heinz body formation in dogs. J Am Anim Hosp Assoc 20:711, 1984

Gaunt SD, Baker DC, Babin SS: Platelet aggregation studies in dogs with acute *Ehrlichia platys* infection. Am J Vet Res 51:290, 1990

George JN, Shattil SJ: The clinical importance of acquired abnormalities of platelet function. N Engl J Med 324:27, 1991

Green RA: Clinical implications of antithrombin III deficiency in animal diseases. Compend Contin Educ Pract Vet 6:537, 1984

Green RA, Kabel AL: Hypercoagulable state in three dogs with nephrotic syndrome: role of acquired antithrombin III deficiency. J Am Vet Med Assoc 181:914, 1982

Grindem CB, Corbett WT, Levy MG et al: Platelet aggregation in dogs experimentally infected with *Rickettsia rickettsii*. Vet Clin Pathol 19:25, 1990

Hackett T, Kelton JG, Powers P: Drug-induced platelet destruction. Semin Thromb Hemost 8:116, 1982

Hall EJ: Use of lithium for treatment of estrogen-induced bone marrow hypoplasia in a dog. J Am Vet Med Assoc 200:814, 1992

Henderson WR, Rashed M, Yong EC et al: *Toxoplasma gondii* stimulates the release of 13- and 9-hydroxyoctadecadienoic acids by human platelets. Biochemistry 31:5356, 1992

Hill BL, Zenoble RD, WJ Dodds: Prothrombin deficiency in a cocker spaniel. J Am Vet Med Assoc 181:262, 1982

Holloway SA, Meyer DJ, Mannella C: Prednisolone and danazol for treatment of immune-mediated anemia, thrombocytopenia, and ineffective erythroid regeneration in a dog. J Am Vet Med Assoc 197:1045, 1990

Jans HE, Armstrong PJ, Price GS: Therapy of immune mediated thrombocytopenia: a retrospective study of 15 dogs. J Vet Intern Med 4:4, 1990

Jones BEV: Platelet aggregation in dogs after live-virus vaccination. Acta Vet Scand 25:504, 1984

Joseph M, Auriault C, Capron A et al: A new function for platelets: IgE-dependent killing of schistosomes. Nature 303:810, 1983

Kiefel V, Santoso S, Mueller-Eckhardt C: Serological, biochemical, and molecular aspects of platelet autoantigens. Semin Hematol 29:26, 1992

Kramer JW, Davis WC, Prieur DJ: The Chediak-Higashi syndrome in cats. Lab Invest 36:554, 1977

Kristensen AT, Weiss DJ, Klausner JS: Platelet dysfunction associated with immune-mediated thrombocytopenia in dogs. J Vet Intern Med 8:323, 1994a

Kristensen AT, Weiss DJ, Klausner JS et al: Comparison of microscopic and flow cytometric detection of platelet antibody in dogs suspected of having immune-mediated thrombocytopenia. Am J Vet Res 55:1111, 1994b

Lerner W, Caruso R, Faig D, Karpatkin S: Drug-dependent and non-drug-dependent antiplatelet antibody in drug-induced immunologic thrombocytopenic purpura. Blood 66:306, 1985

Leung KY, Reisner BS, Straley SC: YopM inhibits platelet aggregation and is necessary for virulence of *Yersinia pestis* in mice. Infect Immun 58:3262, 1990

Lewis DC, McVey DS, Shuman WS, Muller WB: Development and characterization of a flow cytometric assay for detection of platelet-bound immunoglobulin G in dogs. Am J Vet Res 56:1555, 1995

Mount ME, Feldman BF, Buffington T: Vitamin K and its therapeutic importance. J Am Vet Med Assoc 180:1354, 1982

Northern J, Tvedten HW: Diagnosis of microthrombocytosis and immune-mediated thrombocytopenia in dogs with thrombocytopenia: 68 cases (1987–1989). J Am Vet Med Assoc 200:368, 1992

Pancre V, Cesbron JY, Auriault C et al: IgE-dependent killing of *Brugia malayi* microfilariae by human platelets and its modulation by T cell products. Int Arch Allergy Appl Immunol 85:483, 1988

Randolph JF, Center SA, Kallfelz FA et al: Familial nonspherocytic hemolytic anemia in poodles. Am J Vet Res 47:687, 1986

Roubey RAS: Autoantibodies to phospholipid-binding plasma proteins: a new view of lupus anticoagulants and other "antiphospholipid" autoantibodies. Blood 84:2854, 1994

Sadler JE, Matsushita T, Dong Z et al: Molecular mechanism and classification of von Willebrand disease. Thromb Haemost 74:161, 1995

Silverstein MN, Petitt RM, Solberg LA Jr et al: Anagrelide: a new drug for treating thrombocytosis. N Engl J Med 318:1292, 1988

Soute BAM, Ulrich MMW, Watson ADJ et al: Congenital deficiency of all vitamin K–dependent blood coagulation factors due to a defective vitamin K–dependent carboxylase in Devon rex cats. Thromb Haemost 68:521, 1992

Spurling NW: Hereditary disorders of haemostasis in dogs: a critical review of the literature. Vet Bull 50:151, 1980

Sullivan PS, Arrington K, West R, McDonald TP: Thrombocytopenia associated with administration of trimethoprim/sulfadiazine in a dog. J Am Vet Med Assoc 201:1741, 1992

Umekita LF, Piazza RMF, Mota I: Role of platelets and complement in the clearance of epimastigote forms of *Trypanosoma cruzi*. Brazil J Med Biol Res 27:2391, 1994

Weiss DJ, Armstrong PJ: Secondary myelofibrosis in three dogs. J Am Vet Med Assoc 187:423, 1985

Weiss DJ, Klausner JS: Drug-associated aplastic anemia in dogs: eight cases (1984–1988). J Am Vet Med Assoc 196:472, 1990

Weiss RC, Cox NR, Boudreaux MK: Toxicologic effects of ribavirin in cats. J Vet Pharmacol 16:301, 1993

67

Diseases of Lymph Nodes and Lymphatics

David M. Vail

CONGENITAL DISORDERS

Primary Lymphedema

Definition

Edematous swelling of part of the body resulting from a developmental abnormality within the lymphatic system

Causes

I. Often idiopathic, occurring in many breeds
II. Two distinct genetic forms
   A. Congenital form in English bulldogs
      1. Lethal generalized lymphedema
      2. Exact mode of inheritance unknown
   B. Autosomal dominant with variable expression: absent or hypoplastic lymph nodes and lymphatics
III. May be precipitated by mild trauma, superficial skin infection, or both

Pathophysiology

I. Three morphologic types
   A. Aplastic form: lymph channels and/or lymph nodes absent
      1. Mechanical insufficiency in removing lymph
      2. Example: congenital lymphedema of English bulldogs
   B. Hypoplastic form: number and size of lymphatics reduced, with mechanical insufficiency in removing lymph
   C. Hyperplastic form: number and size of lymphatics greatly increased
      1. Lymphatic vessels are dilated (lymphangiectasia).
      2. Interendothelial lymphatic valves become incompetent.
      3. Lymph passes distally instead of proximally.
II. Further perpetuation of tissue edema from accumulation of macromolecules (i.e., protein) in the tissues, with subsequent increase in oncotic pressure
III. Long-term effects of lymphedema
   A. Susceptibility to secondary infection and cellulitis
   B. Progressive interstitial fibrosis resulting from high protein content and secondary infections

Clinical Signs

I. Signalment
   A. Present at birth or develops within the first months of life
   B. Occurs in many breeds, familial form in English bulldogs
   C. No sex predilection known
II. Transient or prolonged pitting edema present at birth or within the first months of life
   A. Anatomic sites vary.
      1. Hindlimbs more commonly affected than forelimbs
      2. Can be generalized in more severe cases: all limbs, head, trunk, and tail
   B. Edema is painless, with no associated lameness initially.
   C. Skin is soft and intact.
   D. Secondary inflammation can result in local pain, heat, seepage, and ulceration.
III. Regional lymph nodes: normal, small, or absent
IV. ± Dilated lymphatics (lymphangiectasia)
V. Death soon after birth with severe generalized form
VI. Spontaneous regression reported

Diagnosis

I. History and clinical signs are described earlier.
II. Consider the following tests (minimum database) to eliminate secondary causes of peripheral edema and secondary lymphedema.
   A. Complete blood count (CBC), biochemistry profile, urinalysis

B. Microfilaria test
C. Abdominal (hindlimb edema) or thoracic (forelimb edema) plain radiography
III. Fine-needle aspiration of edematous tissue reveals either nonspecific transudate or inflammatory cells if there is secondary infection.
IV. Lymphangiography is often diagnostic.
   A. Technique (Takahashi et al., 1984)
      1. Inject patent blue IV dye (1 ml) SQ distal to lesion (i.e., toe web) and allow time (5–10 minutes) for uptake.
      2. Incise skin and locate and cannulate dyed lymphatics.
      3. Infuse contrast material (roughly 4 ml of Lipiodol) intralymphatically.
   B. Distinguishes three morphologic forms
   C. May not be possible to cannulate lymphatics in aplastic form
V. Deep dermal cultures and biopsies may be beneficial in eliminating other causes of edema.

Differential Diagnosis

I. Age, absence of pain, history of affected littermates, and minimum laboratory database help eliminate other causes of peripheral edema.
   A. Venous stasis, arteriovenous fistula
   B. Hypoproteinemia
   C. Right heart failure
   D. Cellulitis, vasculitis
   E. Secondary lymphedema: obstructive, inflammatory, and neoplastic disease
II. Also rule out primary lymphangiectasia, a rare congenital dilatation of the lymphatic vessels.
   A. Signs may not appear until early adulthood.
   B. Concurrent primary lymphedema may also occur with congenital malformation of the lymphatics.
   C. The greatest clinical significance occurs with involvement of the intestinal lacteals (see Chap. 32).
   D. It may be a form of lymphangioma (see later).

Treatment

I. Conservative management
   A. Prolonged use of pressure wraps
      1. Robert-Jones bandages or elastic wraps
      2. Weeks to months, with frequent bandage changes
   B. Warm water massage
   C. Antibiotics for secondary infections
   D. No therapy for some mild cases; advise owner about the possibility of secondary infections and fibrosis
II. Medical therapy
   A. Benzo-pyrones have been used in dogs to decrease high protein edema (Casley-Smith and Casley-Smith, 1988; Fossum et al., 1992).
   B. These drugs include coumarin (no anticoagulative effects) and the rutosides.
      1. Coumarin 400 mg/day PO
      2. Rutin 3 g/day PO

3. Diosmin 3 g/day PO
   C. Such medications may be found in nutritional and health food stores.
III. Surgical management
   A. Goals
      1. Remove accumulated fluid
      2. Eliminate space for accumulation
      3. Encourage alternative routes of drainage
      4. Increase tissue tension (to decrease filtration)
   B. Techniques
      1. Excision of involved skin and subcutis
      2. Thompson's procedure: unites superficial and deep lymphatics
      3. Lymphatico-venous shunts
      4. Omental transpositions

Patient Monitoring

I. With conservative therapy, educate the owner about the potential for bandage complications.
II. Prognosis is variable.
   A. It is guarded with respect to reversibility.
   B. Mild cases may recover spontaneously.
   C. Generalized forms are usually lethal.
   D. Disorder is usually not life-threatening in animals surviving the neonatal period.
   E. Although no controlled clinical trials using the benzo-pyrones have been performed in dogs in the United States, the drugs appear to be safe.

Lymph Node Hypoplasia

Definition

I. Decreased lymphoreticular tissue in the lymph node, resulting in impaired immune and/or phagocytic function
II. Subclassifications
   A. Congenital or primary: rare
   B. Acquired or secondary
   C. Iatrogenic: most common

Causes

I. Congenital hypoplasia
   A. Feline leukemia virus (FeLV)
   B. Aplastic or hypoplastic forms of primary lymphedema
II. Acquired hypoplasia
   A. Advanced age
   B. FeLV and/or feline immunodeficiency virus (FIV)
   C. Neoplasia
   D. Malnutrition
   E. Hyperadrenocorticism
III. Iatrogenic hypoplasia
   A. Corticosteroid therapy
   B. Cytotoxic drug therapy (cancer chemotherapy)
   C. Radiation therapy

Pathophysiology

I. FeLV infection results in T-cell depletion in the thymus and other lymphoid tissues.

II. With age, germinal centers tend to disappear.
III. Corticosteroids, cytotoxic drugs, and radiation therapy may cause lymph node hypoplasia by their cytotoxic effects.
IV. Lymphoid depletion may result in immunosuppression and increased susceptibility to infection.

Clinical Signs

I. Associated with secondary disease sequelae
II. Includes fever of unknown origin, weight loss, poor development and weight gain, and chronic or recurrent infections

Diagnosis

I. Clinical signs and history are helpful.
II. Lymph node biopsy with histologic examination is diagnostic.
III. Determine FeLV and FIV status.
IV. Search for infectious nidus elsewhere in the body.
V. Perform lymphangiography if primary lymphedema is suspected.

Differential Diagnosis

I. Any cause of fever of unknown origin (see also Chap. 71)
   A. Infectious agents
   B. Immune-mediated disorders
   C. Neoplasia
II. Any cause of chronic or recurrent infections
   A. Insufficient or inappropriate antimicrobial therapy
   B. Malnutrition
   C. Stress
   D. Hyperadrenocorticism
   E. Diabetes mellitus

Treatment

I. None is available for congenital forms.
II. Treat the underlying cause and any secondary infections.
III. Specific and nonspecific immune stimulants may be available for trial in the future.

Patient Monitoring

I. Vigilance is required to detect early secondary infections.
   A. Body temperature monitoring by owner
   B. Body weight measurements
   C. CBCs
   D. Bacterial cultures (urine, blood, etc.)
II. Prognosis varies with the degree of immunocompromise.

ACQUIRED DISORDERS

Secondary Lymphedema

Definition

I. Edematous swelling of part of the body, resulting from acquired loss of lymphatic function
II. Occurs secondary to lymphatic occlusion, hypoplasia, or loss of lymphatic channels
III. Concomitant lymph node hypoplasia

Causes

I. Secondary to lymphatic obstruction with chronic lymph stasis
II. Disorders resulting in secondary lymphedema
   A. Surgical excision of lymphatics (e.g., after castration)
   B. Trauma
   C. Infection and inflammation: lymphangitis, lymphadenitis
   D. Neoplasia: pressure, embolization, or infiltration of lymphatics
   E. Radiation therapy

Pathophysiology

I. Acquired occlusion leads to the following.
   A. Gradual thinning and loss of lymphatics
   B. Lymphatic atrophy with progressive interstitial fibrosis from lymph stasis
   C. Development of interlymphatic and lymphaticovenous anastomoses
   D. Rerouting of lymph flow
II. Affected animals are predisposed to other problems such as bacterial or fungal infections and fibrosis.

Clinical Signs

I. Pitting edema of affected limb
II. Enlargement of local or regional lymph nodes
III. Regional or focal swellings with lymphedema secondary to neoplasia
   A. Sublumbar or inguinal node involvement: hindlimb edema
   B. Cranial mediastinal or cervical node involvement: head, neck, and forelimb edema
IV. Signs specific to the primary disease

Diagnosis

I. Confirm the presence of lymphedema as described for primary lymphedema, earlier.
II. Rule out other causes of subcutaneous swelling via aspiration cytology, cultures, etc.
III. Determine the underlying cause of lymphedema.
   A. Note any previous trauma or surgery.
   B. Obtain a minimum database as described for primary lymphedema, earlier.
   C. Search for site of neoplasia or source of infection.

1. Palpation of regional lymph nodes and abdomen
2. Digital rectal exam
3. Thoracic radiographs for head or forelimb edema: rule out mediastinal mass
4. Abdominal radiographs for hindlimb edema: rule out intra-abdominal or pelvic mass

IV. Perform lymphangiography as described earlier.
   A. Peripheral lymphatics are often dilated, tortuous, and increased in number.
   B. Bidirectional flow or stasis is present.
   C. Lymph nodes with metastatic or inflammatory foci may appear enlarged and have filling defects.

V. Surgically biopsy affected subcutaneous tissue, suspicious masses, or affected lymph nodes to confirm lymphedema and determine a possible etiology.

Differential Diagnosis

I. Primary lymphedema
II. Other causes of peripheral edema or swelling
   A. Venous stasis, arteriovenous fistula
   B. Hypoproteinemia
   C. Right heart failure
   D. Cellulitis, vasculitis
   E. Subcutaneous hematomas or contusions

Treatment

I. Treat the underlying cause, if possible.
II. If the underlying cause is unknown or unresolvable, consider the following.
   A. Conservative therapy as described for primary lymphedema.
   B. Postsurgical lymphedema may respond to anti-inflammatory drugs (e.g., prednisone), physical therapy, or diuretics.
   C. Surgical excision of affected lymphatics is sometimes curative for focal post-traumatic cases.
   D. Lymphatico-venous shunts
   E. Medical therapy as for primary lymphedema, earlier

Patient Monitoring

I. Prognosis depends on the reversibility of the underlying cause.
II. Some cases of focal lymphedema may be well tolerated without therapy.

Lymphangitis

Definition and Causes

I. Inflammation of any lymph vessel
II. Usually secondary to disease processes occurring within the tissues drained by involved lymphatics
   A. Infections: bacterial/mycoplasmal, fungal, and viral

   B. Neoplasia
   C. Trauma
   D. Immune-mediated disorders: dermatopathy, vasculitis, polyarthritis
   E. Chronic irritation (e.g., lick granuloma)
   F. Foreign body

Pathophysiology

I. Inflammation may be a direct extension of a regional disease.
II. Edema of surrounding tissue contributes to lymphatic obstruction, slowing lymph flow and ultimately exacerbating the lymphangitis.
III. Regional lymph nodes may enlarge in response to lymphangitis.
IV. It may result in secondary lymphedema.

Clinical Signs

I. If infectious or inflammatory in nature, systemic signs of fever, depression, and anorexia may occur.
II. Affected limb may be lame, swollen, warm, and painful.
III. Overlying skin can be ulcerated.
IV. Regional nodes are sometimes enlarged.
V. Lymphangitis can also be subclinical.

Diagnosis

I. Suspicious clinical signs as outlined earlier
II. No evidence of primary lymphedema
III. Cytologic/histologic assessment of suspicious area
IV. Microbial culture to diagnose an infectious component
V. Exploratory surgery to search for a foreign body or to obtain a biopsy

Differential Diagnosis

I. Primary or secondary lymphedema
II. Subcutaneous swelling or edema from venous stasis, arteriovenous fistula, hypoproteinemia, or right heart failure
III. Inflammation of subcutaneous tissues such as cellulitis, vasculitis
IV. Subcutaneous hematomas or contusions

Treatment

I. Treat any underlying problem.
II. Institute appropriate antimicrobial therapy based on culture and sensitivities.
III. Begin warm compresses, medicated soaks, and physical therapy.
IV. Surgical incision and drainage are indicated for foreign bodies, fistulous tracts, and abscesses.

Patient Monitoring

I. Monitor for appropriate response to antibiotic therapy; recurrence may be suggestive of foreign body.

II. Frequently reevaluate for progression or metastasis if lymphangitis is secondary to neoplasia.

III. Reevaluate if the animal is on immunosuppressive therapy for an immune-mediated etiology (see Chap. 74).

Lymph Node Hyperplasia

Definition

I. Hyperplasia is reactive or inflammatory enlargement of one or more lymph nodes.

II. Inflammation within lymph nodes is also known as lymphadenitis.

III. Lymphadenopathy refers to lymph node enlargement regardless of etiology (neoplastic or non-neoplastic).

Causes and Pathophysiology

I. Infectious etiologies: bacterial, viral, fungal, rickettsial, parasitic, and algal agents

II. Noninfectious etiologies
   A. Immune mediated (see Chap. 74)
      1. Systemic lupus erythematosus
      2. Vasculitis
      3. Polyarthritis
      4. Dermatopathies
   B. Trauma
   C. Postvaccination
   D. Aluminosilicate and polyurethane-induced granulomatous lymphadenopathy of dogs
   E. Drugs (e.g., diphenylhydantoin)
   F. Any generalized antigenic stimulus

III. Causes or syndromes unique to cats
   A. Generalized lymphadenopathy resembling lymphoma (GLRL) (Mooney et al., 1987)
      1. Some histologic changes are suspicious of lymphoma; however, lesions regress without therapy in 1–6 months.
      2. Maine coon cats may be predisposed.
      3. It is probably associated with some sort of host immune response, as it often follows either urinary tract or upper respiratory tract infections.
      4. Some of these cats were exposed to FeLV-positive cats but were not viremic.
   B. Distinctive peripheral lymph node hyperplasia (DPLH) (Moore et al., 1986)
      1. Lymphadenopathy characterized by distortion of lymph node architecture and proliferation of histiocytes, lymphocytes, immunoblasts, and plasma cells
      2. Age: 5 months to 2 years
      3. Idiopathic; however, two thirds of affected cats were positive for FeLV neutralizing antibodies
      4. Majority regressed spontaneously (one cat developed lymphoma)
      5. Half clinically normal; half had fever, lethargy, anorexia, hepatosplenomegaly
   C. Argyrophilic intracellular bacteria with idiopathic peripheral lymphadenopathy (Kirkpatrick et al., 1989)

1. Recently, biopsy specimens from some cats with GLRL and DPLH were re-examined with a silver-impregnation stain and found to contain argyrophilic coccobacilli.
      2. These bacteria may represent another cause of chronic lymph node hyperplasia in the cat.
   D. Plexiform vascularization of lymph nodes
      1. Vascular proliferation of lymph nodes with accompanying lymphoid atrophy
      2. Cats clinically healthy but have lymphadenopathy
      3. Etiology unknown: possibly related to ischemia
   E. FeLV- and FIV-associated lymphadenopathy
   F. Eosinophilic granuloma complex and hypereosinophilic syndrome (see Chap. 85)

Clinical Signs

I. Local, regional, or generalized lymphadenopathy
   A. ± Pain on palpation
   B. ± Fever

II. ± Evidence of source or site of antigenic stimulation or inflammation

III. Possible signs attributable to physical presence of the lymphadenopathy
   A. Mandibular or cervical nodes, tonsils: dysphagia or stertor
   B. Secondary lymphedema or vascular obstruction: limb edema
   C. Cranial mediastinal or cervical nodes: precaval syndrome
   D. Sublumbar node: tenesmus
   E. Thoracic node: dyspnea, cough, or pleural effusion

Diagnosis

I. Thorough physical exam to determine extent of disease and identify other abnormalities

II. Radiography to identify thoracic and abdominal node involvement

III. Lymph node cytology
   A. Reactive hyperplasia
      1. There are increased numbers of medium-sized lymphocytes, lymphoblasts, plasma cells, and macrophages.
      2. Small lymphocytes still predominate.
      3. Mitotic figures may be prominent.
   B. Inflammation
      1. Bacterial: increased neutrophils
      2. Fungal, algal: granulomatous or pyogranulomatous inflammation with presence of multinucleated giant cells and epithelioid cells (macrophages), sometimes neutrophils
      3. Inflammation of skin, respiratory tract, or gastrointestinal tract: increased eosinophils
      4. ± Features of reactive hyperplasia

IV. Lymph node biopsy
   A. Cutting needle biopsy: may not provide enough tissue to assess changes in architecture and presence of capsular invasion

B. Wedge biopsy
C. Excisional biopsy
  1. Preferred method: architecture and capsule preserved
  2. Especially important in lymphadenopathy syndromes of cats, which may mimic lymphoma
D. Microbial stains and cultures
V. Identify possible infectious etiology
  A. Serology
  B. Cytology and cultures from aspirates, fluids, biopsy material, blood, or urine
VI. Tests for immune-mediated disorders (see Chap. 74)

Differential Diagnosis

I. Lymphoma
II. Metastatic neoplasia

Treatment

I. Medical management: treat underlying cause
II. Surgical management
  A. Excision of affected lymph nodes for therapeutic reasons is rarely indicated.
  B. Abscessed or fistulated nodes may require surgical drainage or excision.

Patient Monitoring

I. Prognosis is dependent on responsiveness of underlying cause to therapy: removal of antigenic stimulus or infectious agent typically resolves the condition.
II. Consider repeat biopsy if lymphadenopathy persists or more nodes become involved.

NEOPLASTIC DISORDERS

Lymphangioma

Definition and Causes

I. A rare benign tumor characterized by proliferating lymph vessels
II. May be either a benign congenital tumor or a congenital malformation of the lymphatic system (i.e., hyperplastic form of primary lymphedema or lymphangiectasia)
III. Cause unknown

Pathophysiology

Lymphedema and lymphangiectasia occur secondary to the proliferation of lymph vessels.

Clinical Signs

I. In half the reported cases, dogs are 1 year of age, and the rest are middle-aged to older.
II. Smooth, soft, fluctuant masses are observed in the subcutis.

A. In dogs, lesions are on the limbs, on the head, retroperitoneally, in the axillae, and in the nasopharynx.
B. Clinical signs depend on the location of the mass.
III. Skin lesions may leak milky white fluid or have draining tracts.
IV. It may present as a cystic mass compressing or obstructing an organ.
V. Typically the course is protracted (months to years).

Diagnosis

I. Definitive diagnosis requires surgical biopsy and histopathologic examination.
II. Analysis of draining or compartmentalized fluid reveals proteinaceous chyle.

Differential Diagnosis

I. Other subcutaneous tumors
II. Lymphatics containing metastatic tumors
III. Non-neoplastic conditions
  A. Primary/secondary lymphedema
  B. Non-neoplastic cysts
  C. Fistulous tracts
  D. Lymphangitis

Treatment and Monitoring

I. Surgery
  A. Surgical excision: recurrence rates approach 50%
  B. Marsupialization to allow drainage of lymph to external surface or abdomen
II. Radiation therapy: only one report exists of a dog with a complete response for at least 2 years (Turrel et al., 1988)
III. Chemotherapy: no data available
IV. Prognosis: few data available; favorable outcome likely with complete excision

Lymphangiosarcoma

Definition and Cause

I. Rare malignant neoplasm arising from the endothelium of lymphatic spaces
II. Signalment
  A. Only five cases have been reported in dogs and three cases in cats.
  B. Ages range from 7.5 months to 13 years.
III. Cause unknown

Pathophysiology

I. Reported primary sites include the inguinal area, axilla, prepuce, limbs, chin, and skin of the abdominal wall and thigh in a cat.
II. They are locally invasive.
III. Metastasis appears to occur in approximately 25% of cases in dogs and rarely in cats. Metastasis occurs in regional lymph nodes or distantly in lungs, spleen, and kidney.

Clinical Signs

I. Firm mass is present subcutaneously.
II. Clinical signs depend on location of primary disease and presence of metastasis.

Diagnosis

I. Histologic diagnosis is essential.
  A. Fine-needle aspirate is only suggestive of mesenchymal tumor.
  B. Cutting needle or surgical wedge biopsy is diagnostic.
II. Stage the clinical disease.
  A. Regional lymph node assessment
  B. Thoracic radiography
  C. Abdominal imaging if hindlimb involvement

Differential Diagnosis

I. Mesenchymal tumors of the soft tissue sarcoma group: hemangiopericytoma, fibrosarcoma, neurofibrosarcoma, and hemangiosarcoma
II. Nonmesenchymal neoplasia
III. Benign mass lesions

Treatment

I. Surgical excision is the treatment of choice.
II. Radiotherapy may be attempted and is likely to be more efficacious following surgical cytoreduction or to downstage disease presurgically.
III. Consider chemotherapy with VAC protocol (vincristine, doxorubicin, cyclophosphamide) if surgery or radiotherapy is not an option.

Patient Monitoring

I. Prognosis is dependent on ability to control local disease with either surgery alone or surgery and radiotherapy in combination.
II. Frequent rechecks (every 3 months) for local recurrence and thoracic metastasis are recommended.

Lymphoma

Definition

I. Lymphoma (lymphosarcoma) is a lymphoid neoplasm primarily affecting lymph nodes or other solid visceral organs such as liver or spleen.
II. It is the most common neoplastic disorder of lymph nodes.

Causes

I. Retroviral etiology
  A. Demonstrated in a variety of species, including cats, chickens, cattle, and human beings
  B. Direct evidence for FeLV-induced lymphoma in cats
  C. Indirect evidence for FIV-induced lymphoma in cats

  D. No conclusive evidence for a viral etiology in dogs
II. Possible genetic predispositions
III. Possible role of exposure to carcinogenic agents, in particular, 2,4-D herbicide

Classification Systems

I. Classification is based on anatomic site in dogs.
  A. Multicentric lymphoma: most common form (84%)
  B. Alimentary lymphoma (6.9%)
  C. Cutaneous lymphoma (6.3%)
  D. Mediastinal lymphoma (2.2%)
  E. Miscellaneous extranodal sites (0.6%): central nervous system (CNS), bone, heart, nasal cavity, ocular structures
II. Prevalence of anatomic forms in cats varies with geographic location and appears to have changed concomitant with the widespread use of FeLV vaccines.
  A. Prior to FeLV vaccination, mediastinal and multicentric forms were the most prevalent (usually FeLV-positive cats).
  B. Now, gastrointestinal forms (FeLV-negative) appear more prevalent.
  C. Renal and other extranodal forms are also seen.
III. World Health Organization (WHO) clinical staging is also used to classify the extent of disease (Table 67–1).
IV. Histologic classification schemes also exist.

Clinical Signs

I. Dogs: middle-aged to older, many breeds
II. Cats: median age of 3 years for FeLV-positive and 7 years for FeLV-negative cats
III. Vary with anatomic site involved
  A. Multicentric lymphoma
    1. Generalized lymphadenopathy
    2. Inappetence, lethargy, and weight loss
    3. Polyuria/polydipsia: secondary to paraneoplastic hypercalcemia in dogs (see Chap. 71)
    4. ± Hepatosplenomegaly
    5. Ophthalmic abnormalities (33%): uveitis, ocular hemorrhage

Table 67–1. **Clinical Staging of Canine and Feline Lymphoma**

Stage[a]	Criterion
I	Involvement limited to a single node or lymphoid tissue in a single organ (excluding bone marrow)
II	Involvement of many lymph nodes in a regional area
III	Generalized lymph node involvement
IV	Liver and/or spleen involvement (± stage III)
V	Manifestation in the blood and involvement of bone marrow and/or other organ systems (± stages I–IV)

[a]Each stage is subclassified into (a) systemic signs absent or (b) systemic signs present.

B. Alimentary lymphoma
  1. Weight loss and lethargy
  2. Vomiting and diarrhea, with or without blood
C. Cutaneous lymphoma
  1. Single or multiple skin lesions with wide variation in appearance
  2. Begin as mild eczematous pruritic plaques and progress to nodular tumors
  3. Often pruritic
D. Mediastinal lymphoma
  1. Respiratory signs
  2. Precaval syndrome (i.e., facial and forelimb edema) from tumor compression or invasion of vena cava
  3. Polyuria/polydipsia, anorexia and weakness if hypercalcemic
E. Bone marrow involvement
  1. May result in clinically significant cytopenias
  2. Hemorrhage secondary to thrombocytopenia
  3. Immunosuppressed states secondary to neutropenia
  4. Anemia
F. Spinal lymphoma in cats: present as hindlimb paresis
G. Miscellaneous extranodal forms of lymphoma: highly variable signs

Diagnosis

I. Physical examination
  A. Palpate all lymph nodes (include rectal and abdominal palpation).
  B. Examine mucous membranes for pallor or petechia indicating anemia or thrombocytopenia from possible bone marrow involvement.
  C. Examine for evidence of visceral (liver or kidney) involvement, including icterus, uremic ulcers, and organomegaly.
  D. In cats, thoracic compression is performed to discern mediastinal masses.
II. Hematologic abnormalities
  A. ± Atypical circulating lymphocytes
  B. Thrombocytopenia, eosinopenia, lymphopenia, nucleated erythrocytes
  C. Anemia
    1. Anemia of chronic disease: normocytic, normochromic, and nonregenerative
    2. Regenerative anemia with blood loss or hemolysis
    3. Myelophthisic anemia
    4. Common in FeLV-positive cats
  D. Bone marrow aspirate/core biopsy
    1. ± Increased myeloid–erythroid ratio
    2. ± Infiltration with neoplastic lymphocytes
    3. Important for clinical staging
III. Biochemical abnormalities
  A. Hypercalcemia occurs in 15–20% of dogs with multicentric and in nearly half with mediastinal lymphoma.
  B. Elevations in blood urea nitrogen and serum creatinine occur from renal infiltration with tumor,

hypercalcemic nephrosis, or prerenal causes (e.g., dehydration).
  C. Liver-specific enzyme elevations result from hepatic parenchymal infiltration.
  D. Elevated serum globulins (usually monoclonal) occur with some B-cell lymphomas.
IV. Frequency of FeLV infection
  A. Mediastinal, multicentric, and spinal lymphoma: 80%
  B. Renal forms: 50%
  C. Alimentary forms: 5%
  D. A minority of cutaneous forms
V. Radiographic abnormalities
  A. Half of all dogs with lymphoma have radiographic evidence of sternal and sublumbar lymph node, spleen, and liver enlargement.
  B. Thoracic radiography is important to rule out mediastinal lymphoma.
VI. Histopathologic and cytologic diagnosis
  A. Fine-needle aspirates of enlarged lymph nodes, visceral organs, or other involved sites
    1. Predominance of a homogenous population of immature lymphoid cells suggests neoplastic disease; however, conclusive histologic diagnosis is recommended.
    2. Feline lymphoma is often difficult to distinguish cytologically from reactive hyperplasia.
    3. Granulated round cell tumors of cats or intestinal globule leukocyte tumors and large granular lymphocyte tumors appear as large mononuclear cells with prominent eosinophilic granules.
    4. Immunophenotypic analysis can be performed on fine-needle aspirate samples (see prognostic indicators under Treatment).
  B. Whole lymph node excision is preferred, as the orientation, invasiveness, and architecture are all better illustrated.
  C. Avoid sampling nodes draining reactive areas (e.g., submandibular lymph nodes in the presence of periodontal disease), because reactive hyperplasia may mask (or mimic) the true neoplastic condition.
  D. Immunophenotypic analysis can be performed on histologic samples (see prognostic indicators under Treatment).
  E. Pleural fluid analysis often reveals abnormal lymphoid cells with mediastinal forms.

Differential Diagnosis

I. Generalized lymphadenopathy
  A. Infectious diseases: bacterial, viral, rickettsial, parasitic, fungal
  B. Immune-mediated diseases: systemic lupus, polyarthritis, vasculitis, dermatopathy
  C. Other hematopoietic tumors: leukemia, multiple myeloma, mast cell neoplasia, malignant histiocytosis
  D. Tumors metastatic to lymph nodes (common ones listed here)
    1. Malignant melanoma

2. Mammary adenocarcinoma
3. Osteosarcoma
4. Perirectal adenocarcinoma
5. Prostatic adenocarcinoma
6. Soft tissue sarcomas
7. Squamous cell carcinoma

II. Alimentary lymphoma
  A. Lymphocytic–plasmacytic enteritis
  B. Granulated round cell tumors in cats
    1. Include globule leukocyte tumors and large granular lymphocyte lymphomas (may be variations of the same disease)
    2. Involve small intestine; may result in widespread metastasis
    3. Usually FeLV-negative
    4. Nonspecific gastrointestinal signs that may include intestinal obstruction
    5. Usually palpable intestinal mass; diagnosed via fine-needle aspirate or surgical biopsy
    6. Varied response to systemic chemotherapy
  C. Other intestinal neoplasms
  D. Granulomatous enteritis

III. Cutaneous lymphoma
  A. Infectious dermatitis
  B. Immune-mediated dermatitis (e.g., pemphigus)
  C. External parasitic infestations
  D. Other cutaneous neoplasms

IV. Mediastinal lymphoma (see Chap. 20)
  A. Ectopic thyroid tumors
  B. Heart base tumor (chemodectoma)
  C. Thymoma
  D. Pulmonary lymphomatoid granulomatosis
  E. Granulomatous disease (e.g., hilar lymphadenopathy with blastomycosis)

Treatment

I. Prognostic indicators
  A. Age, body weight, and breed do not affect duration of remission or overall survival for lymphoma.
  B. Most studies fail to reveal a relationship between WHO clinical stage and prognosis in the dog; however, bone marrow involvement and related cytopenias are associated with decreased long-term survival.
  C. Substage b (i.e., systemic signs) is associated with significantly poorer prognosis.
  D. Immunophenotype strongly predicts response and remission and survival duration in the dog.
    1. T-cell (CD3-positive) tumors respond poorly to therapy.
    2. CD3 analysis can be performed on fine-needle aspirate or biopsy specimens.
  E. Prolonged steroid therapy prior to initiation of combination chemotherapy is associated with poor prognosis.
  F. High tumor proliferation rates are associated with superior initial response to chemotherapy.
  G. Female dogs enjoy significantly longer remission and survival times when compared with similarly treated males (median survival of 375 days for females vs. 214 days for males).
  H. Cutaneous and leukemic forms have a poorer prognosis than multicentric forms.
  I. In cats, the higher the clinical stage, the poorer the remission rates and survival lengths (Mooney et al., 1989).
    1. Complete remission rates of 90% for stage I disease
    2. Remission rates of 50% for stage III or higher
  J. Other factors in the cat known to have a negative prognostic impact include the presence of leukemia, anemia, neutropenia, and sepsis.
  K. FeLV status does not affect remission rates but significantly shortens survival times.

II. Systemic chemotherapeutic protocols
  A. These are the mainstay of therapy for multicentric or systemic lymphoma.
  B. Without treatment, most animals die in 4–6 weeks.
  C. Examples of protocols for canine lymphoma are presented in Table 67–2.
  D. In the cat, protocols based on COP (cyclophosphamide, vincristine, and prednisone) are the gold standard with which future protocols are compared.
  E. The addition of doxorubicin to COP protocols has significantly increased duration of remission and survival times in cats with lymphoma.

III. Modification of chemotherapeutic protocols
  A. Therapy may need to be altered in the presence of thrombocytopenia ($<75,000/\mu l$) and neutropenia ($<2500/\mu l$).
  B. Use chemotherapeutic drugs that tend to spare the bone marrow (e.g., prednisone, L-asparaginase, and vincristine).
  C. If myelosuppression from chemotherapy occurs, discontinue those drugs known to affect bone marrow for 5–7 days.
    1. Then repeat a CBC and platelet count.
    2. When the counts have improved, reinstitute therapy at either a decreased dose or a decreased frequency.
    3. Recombinant canine granulocyte colony-stimulating factor (rcG-CSF) can be used long term in cats and dogs to alleviate neutropenias.
    4. Recombinant human G-CSF loses its effectiveness owing to antibody production after approximately 3 weeks.

IV. Therapy unique to extranodal lymphoma
  A. Extranodal lymphoma determined to be a local disease after thorough clinical staging can be treated locally without systemic therapy by either surgical excision or local radiotherapy.
  B. CNS lymphoma
    1. Therapy depends on location and the capabilities of drugs to cross the blood-brain barrier.
    2. Chemotherapeutic drugs that consistently cross the blood-brain barrier in therapeutic concentrations are prednisone and cytosine arabinoside.

Table 67–2. **Published Chemotherapeutic Protocols for Canine Lymphoma**

Protocol	Complete Remission Rate (%)	Median (Mean) Remission Time (Days)	Median (Mean) Survival Time (Days)	Reference
1. CTX 50 mg/m² PO 4 days/wk × 8 wk ARAC 100 mg/m² IV daily × 4 days VCR 0.5 mg/m²/wk IV × 8 wk Prednisone 40 mg/m² PO × 7 days, then 20 mg/m² PO QOD thereafter **Maintenance:** CTX 50 mg/m²/day PO × 4 days/wk Prednisone 10 mg/m² PO BID QOD *or* 6-MP 50 mg/m²/day PO *or* MTX 2.5 mg/m² PO BID weekly	65	66	186	Madewell, 1975
2. CTX 300 mg/m² PO every 3 wk VCR 0.75 mg/m²/wk IV × 4 wk, then every 3 wk Prednisone 1 mg/kg/day PO × 21 days, then QOD	75	180	N/R	Cotter, 1983
3. Protocol 2 above for 7 wk, then doxorubicin 30 mg/m² IV replaces every third CTX treatment; all therapy stops at 78 wk	83	210	N/R	Cotter and Goldstein, 1987
4. VCR 0.7 mg/m² IV on days 1 and 14 L-ASP 400 IU/kg IM on day 1 CTX 200–250 mg/m² IV on day 7 MTX 0.6–0.8 mg/kg IV on day 7 Repeat above every 21 days, except use L-ASP only for rescue and substitute chlorambucil 1.4 mg/kg PO for CTX if dog is in remission	77	140	265	MacEwen et al., 1981
5. Doxorubicin 30 mg/m² IV every 21 days × 5 treatments. Rescue with CTX, VCR, prednisone, L-ASP	76	206 (189)	270 (265)	Carter et al., 1987
6. L-ASP 400 IU/kg IM on day 1 VCR 0.7 mg/m² IV on days 1, 14, 35, and 49 CTX 200 mg/m² IV on days 7 and 42 Doxorubicin 30 mg/m² IV on days 21 and 56 See reference for maintenance schedule.	84	252	357	Keller et al., 1993

CTX = cyclophosphamide; ARAC = cytosine arabinoside; VCR = vincristine; 6-MP = 6-mercaptopurine; MTX = methotrexate; L-ASP = L-asparaginase; N/R = not reported.
Modified from MacEwen and Young, 1989, with permission.

3. Surgical intervention for diagnosis or removal of accessible tumors may be required.
4. More commonly, surgery is combined with adjuvant chemotherapy or radiotherapy.
5. Radiotherapy is also used successfully for the treatment of CNS lymphoma.
V. Rescue therapy
  A. It is defined as an attempt to reestablish remission once the lymphoma recurs.
  B. If the disease returns while the animal is on chemotherapy, those drugs should be discontinued in favor of alternative choices.
  C. If a drug used in the past is not currently being used when the disease recurs, it may still be an effective choice and can be reinstated if superior alternatives do not exist.
  D. Drugs with preliminary promise as rescue agents are actinomycin D, mitoxantrone, ifosfamide, and doxorubicin alone or in combination with dacarbazine.

E. The length of subsequent remissions is usually half that of the previous remission.
VI. Experimental therapies
  A. Immunotherapy in combination with traditional chemotherapy
    1. Nonspecific immunostimulants (e.g., levamisole) and various bacterial extracts: unproven efficacy
    2. Autochthonous tumor cell vaccines
    3. Tumor-specific monoclonal antibodies (MAb 231)
  B. Total body irradiation in combination with bone marrow transplant
VII. Therapy for paraneoplastic hypercalcemia (see Chap. 71)

Patient Monitoring

I. Animals receiving chemotherapy
  A. Monitor hemograms (CBC, platelet count) before

administering drugs known to suppress bone marrow.
  B. Monitor function of organs known to be adversely affected by chemotherapeutic drugs (e.g., cardiac function with doxorubicin).
  C. Recheck monthly to ensure completeness of remission.
 II. Extranodal lymphomas treated with local therapy
  A. Recheck 1 month after therapy and every 3 months thereafter to detect local recurrence or systemic spread.
  B. Thoroughly recheck local site and perform a CBC and biochemistry profile.
  C. Assess the bone marrow if the hemogram is abnormal.
 III. Prognosis
  A. Remission rates for feline lymphoma are roughly 65% with a 7-month median survival (Mooney et al., 1989).
  B. Median survival can approach 18 months in FeLV-negative stage I or II cats.
  C. Most dogs with lymphoma attain complete and lengthy remissions (see Table 67–2) and enjoy a good quality of life; however, cures are still rare.

Bibliography

Carmichael NG, Watson ADJ, Rothwell TLW: Secondary lymphoedema in a dog. J Small Anim Pract 27:335, 1986

Carter RF, Harris CK, Withrow SJ et al: Chemotherapy of canine lymphoma with histopathologic correlation: doxorubicin alone compared to COP as first treatment regimen. J Am Anim Hosp Assoc 23:587, 1987

Casley-Smith JR, Casley-Smith JR: The pathophysiology of lymphedema and the action of benzo-pyrones in reducing it. Lymphology 21:190, 1988

Cotter SM: Treatment of lymphoma and leukemia with cyclophosphamide, vincristine, and prednisone: II. Treatment of cats. J Am Anim Hosp Assoc 19:166, 1983

Cotter SM, Goldstein MA: Comparison of two protocols for maintenance of remission in dogs with lymphoma. J Am Anim Hosp Assoc 23:495, 1987

Drobatz KJ, Fred R, Waddle J: Globule leukocyte tumor in six cats. J Am Anim Hosp Assoc 29:391, 1993

Fossum TW, Miller MW: Lymphedema—etiopathogenesis. J Vet Intern Med 6:283, 1992

Fossum TW, King LA, Miller MW, Butler LM: Lymphedema—clinical signs, diagnosis and treatment. J Vet Intern Med 6:312, 1992

Jeglum KA: Chemoimmunotherapy of canine lymphoma with adjuvant canine monoclonal antibody 231. Vet Clin North Am [Small Anim Pract] 26:73, 1996

Keller ET, MacEwen EG, Rosenthal RC et al: Evaluation of prognostic factors and sequential combination chemotherapy with doxorubicin for canine lymphoma. J Vet Intern Med 7:289, 1993

Kirkpatrick CE, Moore FM, Patnaik AK, Whiteley HE: Argyro-philic intracellular bacteria in some cats with idiopathic peripheral lymphadenopathy. J Comp Pathol 101:341, 1989

Lucke VM, Davies JD, Wood CM, Whitbread TJ: Plexiform vascularization of lymph nodes: an unusual but distinctive lymphadenopathy in cats. J Comp Pathol 97:111, 1987

MacEwen EG, Brown NO, Patnaik AK et al: Cyclic combination chemotherapy of canine lymphosarcoma. J Am Vet Med Assoc 178:1178, 1981

MacEwen EG, Young KM: Canine lymphoma and lymphoid leukemia. p. 380. In Withrow SJ, MacEwen EG (eds): Clinical Veterinary Oncology. JB Lippincott, Philadelphia, 1989

Madewell BR: Chemotherapy of canine lymphosarcoma. Am J Vet Res 36:1525, 1975

Madewell BR: Hematological and bone marrow cytological abnormalities in 75 dogs with malignant lymphoma. J Am Anim Hosp Assoc 22:235, 1986

McEntee MF, Blue SH, Meuten DJ: Granulated round cell tumor of cats. Vet Pathol 30:195, 1993

Mills JN: Lymph node cytology. Vet Clin North Am [Small Anim Pract] 19:697, 1989

Mooney SC, Hayes AA, Matus RE et al: Treatment and prognostic factors in lymphoma in cats: 103 cases (1977–1981). J Am Vet Med Assoc 194:696, 1989

Mooney SC, Patnaik AK, Hayes AA, MacEwen EG: Generalized lymphadenopathy resembling lymphoma in cats: 6 cases. J Am Vet Med Assoc 190:897, 1987

Moore FM, Emerson WE, Cotter SM, DeLellis RA: Distinctive peripheral lymph node hyperplasia of young cats. Vet Pathol 23:386, 1986

Obradovich JE, Ogilvie GK, Powers BE et al: Evaluation of recombinant canine granulocyte colony-stimulating factor as an inducer of granulopoiesis. J Vet Intern Med 5:75, 1991

Obradovich JE, Ogilvie GK, Stadler-Morris S et al: Effect of recombinant canine granulocyte colony-stimulating factor on peripheral blood neutrophil counts in normal cats. J Vet Intern Med 7:65, 1993

Rudd RG, Veatch JK, Whitehair JG et al: Lymphangiosarcoma in dogs. J Am Anim Hosp Assoc 25:695, 1989

Takahashi JL, Farrow CS, Presnell KR: Primary lymphedema in a dog: a case report. J Am Anim Hosp Assoc 20:849, 1984

Teske E, Heerde P, Rutteman GR et al: Prognostic factors for treatment of malignant lymphoma in dogs. J Am Vet Med Assoc 205:1722, 1994

Theilen GH, Madewell BR (eds): Veterinary Cancer Medicine. 2nd Ed. Lea & Febiger, Philadelphia, 1987

Turrel JM, Lowenstine LJ, Cowgill LD: Response to radiation therapy of recurrent lymphangioma in a dog. J Am Vet Med Assoc 193:1432, 1988

Vail DM: Recent advances in chemotherapy for lymphoma of dogs and cats. Compend Contin Educ Pract Vet 15:1031, 1993

Vail DM, Kisseberth WC, Obradovich JE et al: Assessment of potential doubling time, argyrophilic nucleolar organizer regions, and proliferating cell nuclear antigen as predictors of therapy response in canine non-Hodgkin's lymphoma. Exp Hematol 24:807, 1996

Wellman ML, Hammer AS, DiBartola SP et al: Lymphoma involving large granular lymphocytes in cats: 11 cases (1982–1991). J Am Vet Med Assoc 201:1265, 1992

Zahm SH, Blair A: Pesticides and non-Hodgkin's lymphoma. Cancer Res 52(Suppl):5485(s), 1992

68

Disorders of the Spleen

Julia T. Blue

SPLENOMEGALY

Definition

Splenomegaly is diffuse, usually symmetrical enlargement of the spleen.

Causes and Pathophysiology

I. Non-neoplastic causes
   A. Congestive splenomegaly is produced by conditions that impede the flow of blood through the red pulp reticulum and venous vessels.
      1. Splenic torsion, which can occur alone or in association with gastric dilatation–volvulus complex, is a life-threatening cause of splenomegaly that requires rapid diagnosis and correction.
      2. Barbiturates, tranquilizers, and inhalant anesthetics cause relaxation of smooth muscle in the splenic capsule and trabeculae, which produces increased pooling of blood in the red pulp. The hematocrit of peripheral blood from an anesthetized dog or cat is spuriously lowered.
      3. Portal hypertension resulting from conditions such as right-sided congestive heart failure, obstruction of the caudal vena cava or portal vein, and increased intrahepatic vascular resistance (cirrhosis, hepatitis, lipidosis) can cause congestive splenomegaly in some dogs and cats (Johnson, 1987).
      4. Splenic infarction unrelated to splenic torsion is an uncommon cause of splenomegaly (Hardie et al., 1995). Occlusion of splenic vessels by thrombi or emboli can occur secondary to conditions leading to a hypercoagulable state (e.g., protein-losing nephropathy, hypercortisolemia, sepsis, and cancer), cardiac disease, and concurrent causes of splenomegaly.
   B. Hyperplastic splenomegaly results from increased white pulp volume with accumulation of lymphocytes and plasma cells in red pulp secondary to immunologic stimulation and/or from increased numbers of macrophages throughout the red pulp in response to particles to be phagocytized (work hyperplasia). Concurrent congestion often contributes to the enlargement. Diseases commonly accompanied by hyperplastic splenomegaly are as follows.
      1. Systemic immune-mediated diseases: systemic lupus erythematosus
      2. Chronic bacteremia: canine brucellosis, bacterial endocarditis
      3. Hemolytic anemias: immune mediated, Heinz body, hemobartonellosis, babesiosis, pyruvate kinase deficiency
      4. Canine ehrlichiosis
      5. Protozoal infections: leishmaniasis, trypanosomiasis, cytauxzoonosis
      6. Histoplasmosis
   C. Inflammatory cell infiltration is a relatively uncommon cause of splenomegaly.
      1. Suppurative splenitis can occur as an extension of septic, suppurative peritonitis or as the result of septicemia.
      2. Pyogranulomatous inflammation can be caused by feline infectious peritonitis, some systemic mycoses, toxoplasmosis, and mycobacterial infections.
      3. Eosinophilic infiltration associated with hypereosinophilic syndrome is a rare cause of splenic enlargement in cats.
   D. Extramedullary hematopoiesis can also cause splenic enlargement.
      1. Disorders associated with marked splenic hematopoiesis include severe chronic hemolytic anemias and chronic inflammatory diseases with intense stimulation of neutrophil production.
      2. In most cases, hematopoiesis in marrow is concurrently increased, but in rare cases marrow function is compromised and the spleen is the major hematopoietic site.
II. Neoplastic causes
   A. Lymphoma (see also Chap. 67)
      1. Lymphoma usually produces diffuse enlarge-

ment, but focal masses are formed in some animals.
   2. Concurrent enlargement of other abdominal organs is present in many cases.
B. Acute leukemias (see also Chaps. 64 and 65)
   1. Acute myeloid leukemia (AML) and acute lymphoblastic leukemia (ALL) arise in marrow and secondarily infiltrate spleen, liver, and lymph nodes.
   2. Splenomegaly is often present at the time of diagnosis.
C. Systemic mastocytosis
   1. Massive splenomegaly, caused by mast cell infiltration, and mastocythemia are consistent findings in affected cats.
   2. Bone marrow, liver, and lymph nodes usually are infiltrated with mast cells.
D. Chronic lymphocytic leukemia (CLL) (see also Chap. 64)
   1. CLL is an uncommon disease that affects dogs more often than cats.
   2. Splenomegaly is present in most animals with symptomatic CLL.
E. Multiple myeloma (see also Chap. 75)
   1. Marked infiltration of spleen by neoplastic plasma cells causes splenomegaly in some dogs and cats.
   2. Rarely, the spleen is the site of focal extramedullary plasmacytomas.
F. Malignant histiocytosis
   1. Splenomegaly is a consistent finding in this rare syndrome, which is characterized by proliferation of atypical, presumably neoplastic macrophages.
   2. Malignant histiocytosis has a familial occurrence in Bernese mountain dogs (Rosin et al., 1986) and sporadic occurrence in cats and other dog breeds, especially golden retrievers, rottweilers, and Doberman pinschers.
G. Chronic myeloid leukemia (CML) (see also Chap. 65)
   1. CML is a very rare disease in dogs and cats.
   2. Splenomegaly results from expansion of red pulp by neoplastic granulocytopoiesis.
H. Hypersplenism
   1. Primary hypersplenism was once thought to exist as a syndrome consisting of splenomegaly, cytopenias in blood, normal bone marrow, correction of cytopenias by splenectomy, and absence of other factors accounting for cytopenias. The concept of unprovoked splenic hyperfunction is obsolete, and use of the term is discouraged.
   2. Secondary hypersplenism refers to splenomegaly and cytopenias attributed to blood cell destruction or sequestration in the spleen secondary to other factors, such as antibody coating of blood cells, acquired or inherited red cell abnormalities, and enhanced macrophage function in inflammatory and infectious diseases.

Clinical Signs

I. Nonspecific signs attributable to splenomegaly include the following.
   A. Abdominal distention and pain
   B. Decreased appetite
   C. Lethargy and depression
   D. Vomiting and diarrhea
   E. Weight loss
   F. Polyuria and polydipsia
II. Clinical signs suggestive of some specific disorders include the following.
   A. Splenic torsion
      1. Predilection for large, deep-chested breeds of dogs
      2. Collapse, shock, anorexia, vomiting, depression, marked splenomegaly, abdominal pain, and hemoglobinemia/hemoglobinuria from lysis of red cells trapped in the spleen
   B. Systemic mastocytosis
      1. Affected cats typically show vomiting, diarrhea, and gastrointestinal bleeding caused by histamine released from mast cells.
      2. In affected cats, the spleen may be dramatically enlarged, filling the cranial ventral abdomen.
   C. Malignant histiocytosis
      1. Nonspecific signs of fever, lethargy, inappetence, and weight loss are common.
      2. Lymphadenopathy and hepatomegaly are concurrent with splenomegaly.
      3. Many affected Bernese mountain dogs have respiratory signs, including cough, dyspnea, and abnormal lung sounds (Rosin et al., 1986), but respiratory involvement is unusual in other breeds.

Diagnosis

I. History
   A. Signs associated with splenic torsion are usually of sudden onset, but some cases have a history of vague and intermittent abdominal distress for several weeks' duration (Stevenson et al., 1981).
   B. Most other causes of splenomegaly are associated with signs lasting days to weeks.
II. Physical examination findings
   A. Splenomegaly usually can be detected by abdominal palpation.
   B. Dogs with splenic torsion usually have the following.
      1. Pale mucous membranes
      2. Tense, painful abdomen
      3. Palpable mass in cranial abdomen, sometimes identifiable as spleen
   C. Splenomegaly caused by neoplastic infiltrate is often accompanied by palpable hepatomegaly, abdominal lymphadenopathy, or other intra-abdominal masses.
III. Hemogram
   A. Anemia, thrombocytopenia, leukopenia, or any combination of cytopenias in an animal with

splenomegaly may result from several mechanisms.
1. Sequestration or destruction of blood cells in the spleen
2. Myelophthisis and concurrent enlargement of the spleen by neoplastic lymphoid or hematopoietic cells
3. Disseminated intravascular coagulation (DIC)
4. Histamine-induced gastrointestinal bleeding secondary to systemic mastocytosis
B. Red cell morphologic abnormalities reflecting blood flow through an abnormal spleen include acanthocytes, fragmented red cells, normocytic target cells, nucleated red cells, and increased numbers of Howell-Jolly bodies.
C. The presence of spherocytes, Heinz bodies, or erythroparasites indicates causes of hemolysis that may result in splenic congestion and hyperplasia.
D. Circulating neoplastic leukocytes from lymphoma, acute leukemia, chronic leukemia, or systemic mastocytosis may be seen.
IV. Serum chemistry tests
A. Hypercalcemia is suggestive of lymphoma or multiple myeloma.
B. Hyperglobulinemia may be associated with chronic inflammatory diseases or lymphoid neoplasia, including multiple myeloma.
C. Hypoproteinemia and hypoalbuminemia are found in many dogs with malignant histiocytosis.
V. Bone marrow examination
A. Examination of marrow may show evidence of hemolymphatic neoplasms.
B. Erythroid hyperplasia is usually found in animals with hemolytic anemia.
C. Granulocytic hyperplasia suggests an inflammatory disorder.
VI. Immunologic tests
A. Direct Coombs' test
B. Antinuclear antibody (ANA) titer
C. Rheumatoid factor (RF) test
VII. Imaging procedures
A. Plain radiography
1. The size and location of the spleen can be assessed in radiographs unless abdominal effusion obscures detail.
2. Some enlargement of the spleen by congestion can be expected in anesthetized or sedated animals.
3. Patterns suggestive of splenic torsion include identification of the spleen in an abnormal location, displacement of other organs, C-shaped spleen in abnormal position, and gas bubbles in the spleen resulting from seeding of ischemic areas by gas-forming bacteria (Stickle, 1989).
B. Ultrasonography
1. Ultrasonic imaging provides information on soft tissue architecture not available in radiographs and information on size, location, and shape in the presence of poor abdominal radiographic contrast (Feeney et al., 1984).

2. Congestion and diffuse infiltration appear as enlargement with normal to decreased echogenicity.
3. Diffuse anechoic areas separated by small linear echoes, splenomegaly, and enlarged splenic veins form a pattern suggestive of splenic torsion (Konde et al., 1989).
4. Nonhomogeneous echoic patterns and poorly marginated hypoechoic to anechoic nodules have been reported for splenic lymphoma in dogs (Wrigley et al., 1988a).
5. Splenic infarction without splenic torsion appears as rounded hypoechoic to isoechoic foci or as a diffuse hypoechoic or heterogeneous lacy pattern (Hardie et al., 1995).
C. Radionuclide studies
1. Not widely available yet for dogs and cats
2. Measure capacity to clear particulate matter from blood
VIII. Cytology
A. Indications for percutaneous fine-needle aspiration of the spleen
1. Determination of causes of splenomegaly that are not identified by physical diagnostic procedures and other laboratory tests
2. High probability of collecting diagnostic material with the following
a) Good collection and smear preparation techniques are used (O'Keefe and Couto, 1987; MacWilliams, 1989).
b) Spleen is diffusely affected.
B. Contraindications for percutaneous aspiration of the spleen
1. If hemangiosarcoma is suspected, the risk of rupture and hemorrhage is high.
2. Clotting abnormalities are present.
3. The spleen cannot be immobilized.
4. Splenic enlargement is so great that manipulation may cause rupture.
C. Cytologic patterns of splenic aspirates: see Table 68–1
D. Complications of splenic aspiration: hemorrhage, seeding of tumor cells in abdomen
IX. Exploratory laparotomy
A. Indicated if less invasive procedures have failed to produce a diagnosis
B. Should be preceded by correction of severe anemia or coagulopathy, if present
C. Allows visual assessment of other organs for evidence of involvement
D. Allows collection of splenic tissue for cytologic and histologic examination
1. Examination of impression smears is a useful adjunct to histologic examination.
2. Cytology can provide immediate diagnosis in some cases.
3. Cells of hemolymphatic neoplasms are more easily differentiated in smears than in tissue sections.

Differential Diagnosis

I. Transient splenomegaly
A. Splenomegaly detected during routine physical

Table 68–1. **Cytologic Patterns in Splenic Aspirates**

Condition	Cytologic Pattern
Normal spleen	Blood (red cells, platelets, and granulocytes); heterogeneous lymphoid population (predominantly small lymphocytes with fewer large lymphocytes, lymphoblasts, and plasma cells); macrophages; ± clusters of connective tissue cells (reticular cells and endothelial cells); ± megakaryocytes and erythroid cells
Congested spleen	Same cells as normal spleen, but larger component of blood and relatively fewer lymphoid cells
Inflammation	Increased percentage of neutrophils, macrophages, and/or eosinophils compared with normal spleen; ± infectious agents; normal to reactive lymphoid population
Hemolytic anemia	Increased density of morphologically normal macrophages containing ingested red cells and hemosiderin; variable number of normal spleen cells
Hematoma or infarction	Aged blood cells
Extramedullary hematopoiesis	Spectrum of differentiating granulocytes, erythroid cells, and/or megakaryocytes; variable number of normal spleen cells
Sarcomas	Clusters of pleomorphic spindle-shaped cells and/or large numbers of spindle cells; variable number of normal spleen cells
Lymphoma, acute leukemias	High density of blast cells (discrete round cells with high nucleus-to-cytoplasm ratio, blue cytoplasm, fine chromatin, ± visible nucleoli)
Chronic lymphocytic leukemia	High density of small lymphocytes, morphologically homogeneous
Chronic myeloid leukemia	Very high density of differentiating neutrophils
Systemic mastocytosis	Very high density of mast cells
Malignant histiocytosis	High density of morphologically atypical macrophages—marked anisocytosis and anisokaryosis, round nuclei, nucleoli, multiple nuclei, many ingested red cells
Multiple myeloma or solitary plasmacytoma	High density of plasma cells, usually some morphologic atypia

examination of an apparently healthy animal may reflect a transient change (e.g., congestion) rather than a significant pathologic process.
  B. Reevaluation of splenic size at a later date may show return to normal size.
  C. A search for the cause of splenomegaly is indicated if clinical signs of illness are present.
II. Splenic masses (see later)
  A. In some cases, neoplasms that form splenic masses are extensive enough to produce generalized enlargement of the spleen.
  B. Focal enlargements (e.g., hematoma or abscess) may develop secondary to the cause of splenomegaly.
III. Enlargement of other abdominal organs
  A. Cranial abdominal masses arising in other organs
  B. Hepatomegaly and abdominal lymphadenopathy

Treatment

I. Medical therapy of underlying disease
  A. Chemotherapy for hemolymphatic neoplasms
  B. Appropriate antimicrobial therapy for splenomegaly secondary to infectious diseases
  C. Immunosuppressive therapy for immune-mediated diseases
II. Indications for splenectomy
  A. Splenic torsion
  B. Systemic mastocytosis

    1. Splenectomy is palliative, not curative, but is beneficial because it removes a large portion of the tumor cell burden.
    2. Survival times of months to years after splenectomy have been reported in both cats and dogs (Liska et al., 1979; O'Keefe et al., 1987).
  C. Splenic rupture caused by massive splenomegaly regardless of the underlying disease
  D. Immune-mediated hemolytic anemia or thrombocytopenia refractory to drug therapy (Feldman et al., 1985)
  E. Adjunct to chemotherapy for lymphoma (Brooks et al., 1987)
    1. Alleviation of signs of massive splenomegaly before initiation of chemotherapy
    2. Progressive splenomegaly despite chemotherapy
III. Supportive care
  A. Stabilize animals in shock before splenectomy, if possible.
    1. IV fluids, ± corticosteroids
    2. ± Sodium bicarbonate for correction of metabolic acidosis commonly present in dogs with splenic torsion
  B. Transfuse severely anemic animals with whole blood or packed red cells from a compatible donor.
  C. Before splenectomizing animals with mastocytosis, minimize the effects of mast cell degran-

ulation with antihistamines and H$_2$-receptor antagonists.

IV. Treatment not available
   A. No effective treatment has been described for malignant histiocytosis.
   B. Chemotherapy for acute myeloid leukemia in dogs and cats rarely produces remission.

Patient Monitoring

I. Postsplenectomy care
   A. Administer antibiotics perioperatively.
   B. Continue IV fluids as necessary for correction of hypovolemia in dogs with splenic torsion.
   C. Monitor for hemorrhage.
      1. Hemogram to assess hematocrit and indications of DIC
      2. Coagulation testing if development of DIC is suspected
      3. Peritoneal fluid analysis if effusion occurs
      4. Exploratory laparotomy and re-ligation of vessels if necessary
   D. Monitor dogs for cardiac arrhythmias for 3–4 days after surgery.
   E. Once the surgical site is healed, treat cats with systemic mastocytosis with prednisone 40 mg/m^2 PO SID for a week, then 20 mg/m^2 PO QOD (Couto, 1989b).
II. Potential consequences of splenectomy
   A. Increased platelet counts in some animals (not clinically significant)
   B. Decreased resistance to erythroparasite infections
   C. Increased susceptibility to septicemia, especially if immunosuppressed (Couto, 1989a)
III. Monitoring of medical therapy
   A. Effective treatment of underlying disorder should result in reduction of splenic size.
   B. Resolution of clinical signs and abnormal laboratory parameters also indicates a positive response.

SPLENIC MASSES

Definition

Splenic masses are focal areas of splenic enlargement.

Causes and Pathophysiology

I. Non-neoplastic causes
   A. Hematomas (common)
      1. Not associated with known traumatic event in most cases
      2. Often associated with nodular hyperplasia and may be caused by disruption of normal blood flow in the region of the hyperplastic tissue (Spangler and Culbertson, 1992)
   B. Nodular hyperplasia (common)
      1. Composed of hyperplastic lymphoid tissue or mixed lymphoid and hematopoietic foci
      2. Hemorrhagic areas and hematomas within or around many hyperplastic nodules

   C. Abscesses (rare)
      1. Caused by blood-borne bacteria
      2. Other splenic disease (e.g., lymphoma or torsion) usually concurrent
   D. Myelolipoma (very rare)
      1. Tumor-like mass composed of adipose tissue and hematopoietic cells resembling normal bone marrow
      2. Probably not neoplastic
II. Neoplastic causes
   A. Hemangioma/hemangiosarcoma
      1. Hemangiosarcoma is the most common splenic neoplasm in dogs, whereas hemangioma is rare (Spangler and Culbertson, 1992).
      2. Both types of tumors arise from vascular endothelium.
         a) The proliferation of endothelial cells results in the formation of irregular, sometimes cavernous, vascular spaces that are filled with blood and thrombi.
         b) Large areas of the mass may consist of hemorrhage, necrosis, and inflammation.
      3. The spleen is the primary site in many dogs.
   B. Nonangiogenic sarcomas: leiomyosarcoma, fibrosarcoma, liposarcoma, malignant fibrous histiocytoma, osteosarcoma, chondrosarcoma, rhabdomyosarcoma, myxosarcoma, and undifferentiated sarcoma
      1. Much less common than hemangiosarcoma
      2. Primary to the spleen in many instances
   C. Metastatic melanoma and carcinoma
      1. Metastatic tumors of the spleen result from hematogenous spread or by seeding of the capsule by tumor cells, because the spleen has no afferent lymphatic vessels.
      2. Splenic involvement by metastatic tumors is rare.
   D. Lymphoid neoplasms
      1. Lymphoma appears as splenic mass rather than splenomegaly in some cases.
      2. Plasmacytomas occasionally originate in the spleen.

Clinical Signs

I. Splenic masses, especially small or benign ones, may be clinically silent and detected incidentally.
II. Nonspecific signs attributable to large splenic masses are those described earlier for splenomegaly.
III. Abdominal effusion is present in some animals.
   A. Hemoperitoneum is commonly found in dogs with hemangiosarcoma.
   B. Effusion caused by nonangiogenic tumors is probably secondary to interference with blood or lymph circulation or inflammation resulting from tumor dissemination in the abdomen (Weinstein et al., 1989).
IV. Signs associated with splenic hemangiosarcoma are as follows.
   A. Progressive lethargy, weakness, inappetence
   B. Intermittent episodes of weakness with spontaneous recovery

C. Acute collapse and shock
D. Distended abdomen
E. Dyspnea caused by hemothorax from rupture of metastatic tumor

V. Age and breed predilections are similar for hematoma, hemangiosarcoma, nodular hyperplasia, and nonangiogenic sarcomas in dogs (Brown et al., 1985; Prymak et al., 1988; Spangler and Culbertson, 1992).
   A. Middle-aged or old dogs
   B. Medium- to large-size breeds, especially German shepherd dogs

Diagnosis

I. Physical examination findings
   A. Palpable mass in cranial to mid-abdomen
   B. Findings suggestive of hemangiosarcoma
      1. Pale, sometimes icteric, mucous membranes
      2. Hemoperitoneum, hemothorax, or hemopericardium detected by aspirating bloody, nonclotting fluid

II. Hemogram
   A. Animals with any cause of splenic mass can be anemic, but hemangiosarcoma is more likely if anemia is moderate to severe.
   B. Hemogram findings typical of hemangiosarcoma are as follows.
      1. Normocytic or macrocytic anemia
      2. Reticulocytosis
      3. Acanthocytes, schistocytes, keratocytes, nucleated red cells
      4. Neutrophilic leukocytosis, ± left shift, lymphopenia
      5. Thrombocytopenia

III. Coagulation tests
   A. DIC is common in animals with hemangiosarcoma but is only rarely associated with benign splenic masses.
   B. DIC is recognized by finding at least three of the following.
      1. Prolongation of prothrombin time (PT) and/or activated partial thromboplastin time (aPTT)
      2. Thrombocytopenia
      3. Hypofibrinogenemia
      4. Increased fibrin/fibrinogen degradation products (FDPs)

IV. Imaging procedures
   A. Plain radiography can confirm the presence of a splenic mass in many cases unless abdominal detail is obscured by fluid.
   B. Ultrasonography is more reliable than plain radiography for detection of splenic masses, especially if abdominal effusion is present (Wrigley et al., 1988b).
   C. Hemangiosarcoma usually produces a nonhomogeneous complex echo pattern because of the presence of hypoechoic blood-filled spaces and hyperechoic solid tissue (Wrigley et al., 1988b).
   D. Thoracic radiography is indicated to look for metastases and pleural effusion. Metastatic pulmonary hemangiosarcoma is most likely to appear as poorly defined, diffuse, nodular, and linear lung opacities (Hammer et al., 1993).

V. Cytology
   A. Fluid analysis
      1. If fluid collected from a serous cavity looks like blood, place some in a tube with EDTA and some in a tube without anticoagulant to assess for ability to clot.
      2. Hemorrhagic effusion is suggestive of hemangiosarcoma and has the following characteristics.
         a) Fluid looks like blood but does not clot.
         b) Macrophages containing red cells and hemosiderin are numerous.
         c) Reactive mesothelial cells are numerous.
      3. Modified transudates or exudates secondary to nonsarcomatous neoplasms may contain exfoliated tumor cells.
   B. Cytologic examination of splenic aspirate
      1. Percutaneous fine-needle aspiration of splenic masses is done with caution because of the risk of rupture and is guided by ultrasound localization of the mass.
      2. Cytologic patterns are shown in Table 68–1.

VI. Exploratory laparotomy and splenectomy
   A. Gross appearance of a splenic mass does not reliably distinguish splenic hematoma from hemangiosarcoma (Spangler and Culbertson, 1992).
   B. Histologic evaluation of splenic tissue is the most reliable method for specific identification.
      1. Differentiation of hematoma, hemangioma, and hemangiosarcoma can be difficult in some cases.
      2. Several pieces of the splenic mass or the entire spleen should be submitted for histologic examination to increase the probability of finding evidence of neoplasia.
   C. Cytologic examination of intraoperative aspirate or imprint can be helpful.
   D. Suspected metastatic masses in other abdominal organs should be biopsied.

Differential Diagnosis

I. Causes of splenomegaly (see earlier)
II. Masses in other abdominal organs

Treatment

I. Splenectomy
   A. Splenectomy for a splenic mass should be complete rather than partial to avoid leaving residual tumor tissue.
   B. Splenectomy is curative for hematoma, nodular hyperplasia, hemangioma, and myelolipoma.
   C. Splenectomy is palliative, rather than curative, for most sarcomas because metastases are present, especially in the following areas (Patnaik and Liu, 1977; Brown et al., 1985; Weinstein et al., 1989).
      1. Liver
      2. Omentum, peritoneum

Table 68–2. *Miscellaneous Splenic Disorders*

Disorder	Definition	Cause	Signs	Treatment
Accessory spleens	Congenital ectopic foci of splenic tissue supplied by branches of the splenic artery	Unknown	None	None
Splenosis	Ectopic foci of regenerated autotransplanted splenic tissue	Traumatic fragmentation of spleen	None	None
Splenic rupture	Interruption of normal splenic architecture	Traumatic or spontaneous caused by an underlying disease	1. Hemorrhagic shock after traumatic event, either immediate or delayed 2. Vague signs of abdominal discomfort caused by subcapsular hematoma 3. None	1. Medical therapy for hypovolemic shock 2. Splenectomy 3. Surgical repair

  3. Lymph nodes in the abdominal and thoracic cavities
  4. Lungs
  5. Kidneys, heart
II. Supportive care
  A. Stabilize animals with DIC or with severe abdominal hemorrhage before splenectomy.
    1. IV fluids, corticosteroids
    2. Whole blood transfusions
  B. Antibiotics are administered if there is evidence of septic peritonitis or splenic abscessation.
  C. Dogs with splenic masses are apt to have ventricular arrhythmias that require antiarrhythmic drugs (Knapp et al., 1993).

Patient Monitoring

  I. Postsplenectomy care
    A. Continue supportive care as necessary.
    B. Monitor for hemorrhage (see Splenomegaly, earlier).
    C. Medical therapy following surgical removal or reduction of hemangiosarcoma can have a beneficial effect.
      1. Dogs treated with combination chemotherapy consisting of vincristine, doxorubicin, and cyclophosphamide (Hammer et al., 1991) or doxorubicin and cyclophosphamide (Sorenmo et al., 1993) have prolonged survival compared with dogs treated by surgery alone.
      2. Immunotherapy in addition to splenectomy and chemotherapy with doxorubicin and cyclophosphamide further improves survival and metastasis-free interval (Vail et al., 1995).
  II. Potential consequences of splenectomy (see Splenomegaly, earlier)
  III. Monitoring for metastases in animals with sarcoma
    A. Death caused by metastatic tumors is common with hemangiosarcoma and nonangiogenic sarcomas, even if metastases are not evident at the time of initial diagnosis.
    B. Very few animals survive for longer than 1 year, and most die within a few months.
    C. Metastatic disease can be detected by the following methods.
      1. Periodic radiography or ultrasonography of the thorax and abdomen
      2. Periodic hemograms to look for recurrence of anemia or evidence of DIC
      3. Recurrence of clinical signs

MISCELLANEOUS SPLENIC DISORDERS

See Table 68–2.

Bibliography

Brooks MB, Matus RE, Leifert CE, Patnaik AK: Use of splenectomy in the management of lymphoma in dogs: 16 cases (1979–1985). J Am Vet Med Assoc 191:1008, 1987
Brown NO, Patnaik AK, MacEwen EG: Canine hemangiosarcoma: retrospective analysis of 104 cases. J Am Vet Med Assoc 186:56, 1985
Couto CG: Diseases of the lymph nodes and spleen. p. 2225. In Ettinger SJ (ed): Textbook of Veterinary Internal Medicine. 3rd Ed. WB Saunders, Philadelphia, 1989a
Couto CG: Oncology. p. 589. In Sherding RG (ed): The Cat: Diseases and Clinical Management. Churchill Livingstone, New York, 1989b
Feeney DA, Johnston GR, Hardy RM: Two-dimensional, gray-scale ultrasonography for assessment of hepatic and splenic neoplasia in the dog and cat. J Am Vet Med Assoc 184:68, 1984
Feldman BF, Handagama P, Lubberink AAME: Splenectomy as adjunctive therapy for immune-mediated thrombocytopenia and hemolytic anemia in the dog. J Am Vet Med Assoc 187:617, 1985

Hammer AS, Bailey MQ, Sagartz JE: Retrospective assessment of radiographic findings in metastatic canine hemangiosarcoma. Vet Radiol Ultrasound 34:235, 1993

Hammer AS, Couto CG, Filippi J et al: Efficacy and toxicity of VAC chemotherapy (vincristine, doxorubicin, and cyclophosphamide) in dogs with hemangiosarcoma. J Vet Intern Med 5:160, 1991

Hardie EM, Vaden SL, Spaulding K, Malarkey DE: Splenic infarction in 16 dogs: a retrospective study. J Vet Intern Med 9:141, 1995

Johnson SE: Portal hypertension. Part I. Pathophysiology and clinical consequences. Compend Contin Educ Pract Vet 9:741, 1987

Knapp DW, Aronsohn MG, Harpster NK: Cardiac arrhythmias associated with mass lesions of the canine spleen. J Am Anim Hosp Assoc 29:122, 1993

Konde LJ, Wrigley RH, Lebel JL et al: Sonographic and radiographic changes associated with splenic torsion in the dog. Vet Radiol 30:41, 1989

Liska WD, MacEwen EG, Zaki FA, Garvey M: Feline systemic mastocytosis: a review and results of splenectomy in seven cases. J Am Anim Hosp Assoc 15:589, 1979

MacWilliams PS: The splenic parenchyma. p. 199. In Cowell RL, Tyler RD (eds): Diagnostic Cytology of the Dog and Cat. American Veterinary Publications, Goleta, 1989

O'Keefe DA, Couto CG: Fine-needle aspiration of the spleen as an aid in the diagnosis of splenomegaly. J Vet Intern Med 1:102, 1987

O'Keefe DA, Couto CG, Burke-Schwartz C, Jacobs RM: Systemic mastocytosis in 16 dogs. J Vet Intern Med 1:75, 1987

Patnaik AK, Liu S-K: Angiosarcoma in cats. J Small Anim Pract 18:191, 1977

Prymak C, McKee LJ, Goldschmidt MH, Glickman LT: Epidemiologic, clinical, pathologic, and prognostic characteristics of splenic hemangiosarcoma and splenic hematoma in dogs: 217 cases (1985). J Am Vet Med Assoc 193:706, 1988

Rosin A, Moore P, Dubielzig R: Malignant histiocytosis in Bernese mountain dogs. J Am Vet Med Assoc 188:1041, 1986

Sorenmo KU, Jeglum KA, Helfand SC: Chemotherapy of canine hemangiosarcoma with doxorubicin and cyclophosphamide. J Vet Intern Med 7:370, 1993

Spangler WL, Culbertson MR: The prevalence, type and importance of canine splenic diseases (a diagnostic survey). J Am Vet Med Assoc 200:829, 1992

Stevenson S, Chew DJ, Kociba GJ: Torsion of the splenic pedicle in the dog: a review. J Am Anim Hosp Assoc 17:239, 1981

Stickle RL: Radiographic signs of isolated splenic torsion in dogs: eight cases (1980–1987). J Am Vet Med Assoc 194:103, 1989

Vail DM, MacEwen EG, Kurzman ID et al: Liposome-encapsulated muramyl tripeptide phosphatidylethanolamine adjuvant immunotherapy for splenic hemangiosarcoma in the dog: a randomized multi-institutional clinical trial. Clin Cancer Res 1:1165, 1995

Weinstein MJ, Carpenter JL, Mehlhaff Schunk CJ: Nonangiogenic and nonlymphomatous sarcomas of the canine spleen: 57 cases (1975–1987). J Am Vet Med Assoc 195:784, 1989

Wrigley RH, Konde LJ, Park RD, Lebel JL: Ultrasonographic features of splenic lymphosarcoma in dogs: 12 cases (1980–1986). J Am Vet Med Assoc 193:1565, 1988a

Wrigley RH, Park RD, Konde LJ, Lebel JL: Ultrasonographic features of splenic hemangiosarcoma in dogs: 18 cases (1980–1986). J Am Vet Med Assoc 192:1113, 1988b

69

Transfusion Medicine

Urs Giger

Definition

I. Transfusion therapy is the safe and effective replacement of blood or one of its components.
II. Transfusions are indicated for anemia, coagulopathy, and rarely for the correction of thrombocytopenia/thrombocytopathia and hypoproteinemia (Table 69–1). Fresh whole blood, packed red cells, and fresh frozen plasma are the most commonly used transfusion components in veterinary practice.
III. Specific blood component replacement provides the most effective and safest therapy and allows optimal use of every blood donation (Callan et al., 1996).
  A. Blood components are prepared from a single donation of blood by simple physical separation methods such as centrifugation.
  B. Fresh whole blood can be separated into packed red cells, platelet-rich plasma or concentrate, fresh frozen plasma, and cryoprecipitate.
IV. There are several books on veterinary transfusion medicine (Cotter, 1991; Hohenhaus, 1992; Kristensen and Feldman, 1995).

Blood Types

I. Blood types are genetic markers on erythrocyte surfaces that are antigenic and specific for each species. A set of blood types (two to several alleles) makes up a blood group system.
  A. Naturally occurring alloantibodies are found in the sera of unimmunized animals, whereas other alloantibodies occur only after sensitization by a transfusion.
  B. These alloantibodies may be responsible for hemolytic transfusion reactions and neonatal isoerythrolysis (NI).
  C. Alloantibodies can be detected by a blood cross-match or a blood back-typing test. In the latter, typed erythrocytes are incubated with the animal's plasma. Agglutination or hemolysis indicates the presence of alloantibodies (Callan et al., 1995).
II. Canine blood types are as follows.
  A. Dogs have at least 13 blood group systems known as dog erythrocyte antigens (DEA) (Giger et al., 1995; Hale, 1995).
    1. For all blood group systems other than the DEA 1 system, red blood cells from a dog can be positive or negative for that blood type (e.g., for the DEA 7 system, a dog's cells can be DEA 7 positive or DEA 7 negative).
    2. The DEA 1 system has three subtypes: DEA 1.1 (A_1), DEA 1.2 (A_2), and possibly A_3 (described in Australia).
     a) A dog's red blood cells can be DEA 1.1 positive or negative.
     b) DEA 1.1 negative cells can be DEA 1.2 positive or negative.
     c) Dogs that are DEA 1.1 negative are considered universal donors.

Table 69–1. **Indications for Blood Component Therapy**

Condition	Fresh Whole Blood	Stored Whole Blood	Packed Red Cells	Platelet-Rich Plasma[a]	Fresh Frozen Plasma	Cryo-precipitate
Anemia	X	X	⊗			
Thrombocytopenia/thrombocytopathia	X			⊗		
Coagulopathies	X				⊗	
von Willebrand's disease/hemophilia A	X				X	⊗
Hypoproteinemia	X				⊗	

[a]Also indicates platelet concentrate.
Circle indicates best component.

Table 69–2. **Canine Blood Type Frequencies**

Blood Type	Positive (%)	Negative (%)
DEA 1		
DEA 1.1 (A₁)	33–45	55–67
DEA 1.2 (A₂)	7–20	35–60[a]
DEA 3 B	5–10	90–95
DEA 4 C	87–98	2–13
DEA 5 D	12–22	78–88
DEA 7 Tr	8–45	55–92

[a]DEA 1.1 and 1.2 negative dogs.
Data from Giger et al., 1995.

   3. These blood types are codominantly inherited.
   4. The frequency of each blood type may vary geographically and among breeds (Table 69–2).
  B. Blood types that are strongly antigenic are of great clinical importance in dogs.
   1. Before sensitization (transfusion) of a dog, no clinically significant alloantibodies have been reported, although a small number of dogs may have antibodies against DEA 3, 5, and 7.
   2. Transfusion of DEA 1.1 positive cells to a DEA 1.1 negative dog elicits a strong alloantibody response.
     a) Anti-DEA 1.1 antibodies develop after >4 days and may cause a delayed transfusion reaction.
     b) Previously sensitized DEA 1.1 negative dogs develop an acute hemolytic reaction after transfusion of DEA 1.1 positive blood.
     c) NI has been documented only after sensitizing a bitch with a mismatched transfusion.
  C. Canine blood typing is recommended for blood donors and, if possible, for animals receiving transfusions.
   1. Because of the strong antigenicity of DEA 1.1, typing of donors (and recipients) for DEA 1.1 is strongly recommended.
     a) DEA 1.1 negative dogs should receive only DEA 1.1 negative blood.
     b) DEA 1.1 positive dogs may be transfused with DEA 1.1 positive or negative blood.
   2. A blood typing card to classify dogs as DEA 1.1 positive or negative is now available as a simple in-practice kit from DMS Laboratories, Inc. (2 Darts Mill Road, Flemington, NJ 08822; 800-567-4367).
     a) The assay requires a small amount of anticoagulated blood and is based on the agglutination reaction that occurs within 2 minutes when erythrocytes that are DEA 1.1 positive interact with a murine monoclonal antibody specific to DEA 1.1 (Andrews et al., 1992).
     b) Autoagglutination precludes typing and crossmatching.

   3. Some clinicians also recommend typing for other blood types, although their clinical importance has not been documented (Hale, 1995).
     a) Typing service and polyclonal antisera are available for DEA 1.1, 1.2, 3, 4, 5, and 7 from Dr. Robert Bull, B228 Life Sciences Building, Michigan State University, East Lansing, MI 48824; 517-355-4616.
     b) These typing procedures require some expertise and experience.
     c) Recent advice to use exclusively canine donors that are negative for all testable DEA except DEA 4 would unnecessarily eliminate many active and potential donors, would be cost prohibitive, and is not supported by any published clinical reports.
III. There are three feline blood types: A, B, and AB (Callan and Giger, 1994; Griot-Wenk and Giger, 1995).
  A. A is dominant over B.
   1. Cats with type A blood have a genotype A/A or A/B.
   2. Only homozygous B/B cats express the type B antigen on their erythrocytes.
   3. AB is inherited separately as a third allele that is recessive to A and dominant to B.
  B. The frequency of feline A and B blood types varies geographically and among breeds (Table 69–3).
   1. Type A is the most common blood type.
   2. Most domestic shorthair cats have type A, but this may vary regionally.

Table 69–3. **Blood Type Frequencies in Cats of the United States**

Breed	Type A (%)	Type B (%)
Abyssinian	86	14
Birman	84	16
British shorthair	60	40
Burmese	100	0
Cornish rex	66	34
Devon rex	59	41
Domestic shorthair		
Northeast	99.7	0.3
North central	99.6	0.4
Southeast	98.5	1.5
Southwest	97.5	2.5
West Coast	95.3	4.7
Himalayan	93	7
Japanese bobtail	84	16
Maine coon	98	2
Norwegian forest	93	7
Persian	86	14
Scottish fold	82	18
Siamese	100	0
Sphinx	81	19
Somali	83	17
Tonkinese	100	0

Data from Giger et al., 1991a, 1991b, including >10,000 cats.

3. Depending on the breed, the type B frequency may reach 40%.
4. Type AB cats are very rare (Griot-Wenk et al., 1996).

C. Cats have important naturally occurring alloantibodies (Bücheler and Giger, 1993).
1. All type B cats have very strong naturally occurring alloantibodies.
   a) Kittens receive alloantibodies through the colostrum from type B queens. Type A and AB kittens born to type B queens are at risk for NI.
   b) All type B kittens develop anti-A antibodies with high hemolysin and agglutinin titers ($>1{:}32$) after a few weeks of age.
   c) Type B cats receiving a mismatched transfusion with type A blood will have a very serious acute hemolytic transfusion reaction (Giger and Bücheler, 1991).
2. Type A cats have weak anti-B alloantibodies.
   a) The alloantibody titer is usually very low ($1{:}2$).
   b) These antibodies cause shortened survival of transfused B cells in type A cats but have not been associated with NI.

D. Feline blood typing is recommended to give matched transfusions and to breed blood-compatible mates.
1. There are no universal donor cats.
2. Donor and recipient cats should both be blood typed.
3. Feline blood typing cards to classify cats as type A, B, or AB are available as a simple in-practice test kit from DMS Laboratories, Inc. (2 Darts Mill Road, Flemington, NJ 08822; 800-567-4367).
4. The author's laboratory has typed over 10,000 cats (0.5 ml EDTA blood shipped by regular mail to Dr. Giger, Typing, Veterinary Hospital, University of Pennsylvania, 3900 Delancey Street, Philadelphia, PA 19104-6010), and commercial veterinary laboratories are now routinely blood typing cats.

Blood Crossmatch

I. A blood crossmatch test detects the serologic compatibility or incompatibility between the anemic recipient and the potential donor.
A. This test checks for the presence or absence of alloantibodies without determining the blood type (Table 69–4).
B. The major crossmatch tests for alloantibodies in the recipient's plasma against donor cells.
C. The minor crossmatch tests for alloantibodies in the donor's plasma against recipient's red blood cells and is of lesser importance, because the donor's plasma is diluted.

II. Because dogs do not have naturally occurring alloantibodies, the initial crossmatch of a dog that has not previously been transfused should show compatibility.

Table 69–4. *Instructions for Crossmatching Blood*

1. Collect blood from the recipient and possible donor(s) into EDTA tubes (or take one segment from the donor blood bag).
2. After centrifugation, remove plasma from each sample into labeled tubes.
3. Wash red blood cells (RBCs) 3 times with (phosphate buffered) saline; resuspend to make a 3–5% RBC suspension.
4. Prepare 3 tubes labeled major, minor, and recipient control. Add 2 drops (50 µl) of plasma and 1 drop (25 µl) of RBC suspension to each tube as follows:
   Major crossmatch: recipient plasma + donor RBCs
   Minor crossmatch: donor plasma + recipient RBCs
   Recipient control: recipient plasma + recipient RBCs
5. Mix gently and incubate for 15–30 minutes at 37°C.
6. After centrifugation, examine supernatant for hemolysis.
7. Gently resuspend button of cells by tapping tube with a finger and examine for macroscopic and microscopic agglutination.
8. Any hemolysis or agglutination in the major crossmatch is considered an incompatibility. Slight hemolysis or agglutination in a minor crossmatch does not preclude transfusion in an emergency situation, but careful monitoring is mandatory.
9. Autoagglutination or severe hemoglobinemia precludes testing.

A. A compatible crossmatch in a dog does not prevent sensitization against donor cells within 1–2 weeks.
B. Previously transfused dogs should always be crossmatched, even when receiving blood from the same donor.

III. Because cats have naturally occurring alloantibodies, a crossmatch test can detect A-B mismatches (Griot-Wenk et al., 1996).
A. If the major crossmatch is incompatible, the recipient is type B and the donor has type A blood.
B. If the minor crossmatch is incompatible, the recipient is type A and the donor has type B blood.
C. If the crossmatch is compatible, donor and recipient have the same blood type.

Blood Sources

I. Sources of blood
A. In-house blood donors kept on premises (expensive)
B. Voluntary blood donor programs, often relying on client- or staff-owned dogs and cats
C. Commercial animal blood banks
1. Animal Blood Bank, Vacaville, CA, 916-678-3009
2. Eastern Veterinary Blood Bank, Annapolis, MD, 800-949-3822 (only blood bank for canine and feline blood)
3. Hemopet, Irvine, CA, 714-252-8455
4. Midwest Animal Blood Bank Services, Inc, Stockbridge, MI, 517-851-8244
5. Penn Animal Blood Bank, Philadelphia, PA, 215-573-7222

D. Exsanguination of healthy animals that are to be euthanized

E. Autologous (self) transfusion
   1. Blood donated by an animal 4 weeks to 1 day before surgery is transfused back to the animal during or after surgery.
   2. Autotransfusion of shed blood salvaged intraoperatively can be reinfused after careful filtering. Do not reinfuse blood from long-standing, contaminated, or malignant hemorrhagic effusions.

II. Donor selection criteria
   A. Adequate packed cell volume (dogs >40%; cats >35%) or hemoglobin concentration (dogs >13 g/dl; cats >11 g/dl)
   B. Compatible blood type based on blood typing and crossmatching as outlined earlier
      1. Canine blood donor should be DEA 1.1 negative unless the recipient is known to be positive.
      2. All feline donors and recipients should be either blood typed to ensure an A-B matched transfusion or at least crossmatched.
      3. All previously transfused animals should be crossmatched.
   C. Healthy young adult animals weighing at least 25 kg (dogs) or 4 kg (cats) and with current vaccinations
   D. Prior pregnancy not an exclusion
   E. Free of infectious diseases
      1. Dogs are screened for *Dirofilaria*, *Babesia*, and *Ehrlichia*.
      2. Cats are screened for feline leukemia virus (FeLV), feline immunodeficiency virus (FIV), feline infectious peritonitis (FIP), and *Hemobartonella*.
   F. Splenectomy generally not recommended for donors
   G. Detailed records kept for each donor animal regarding blood type, dates of and data regarding health checks, and dates of blood withdrawal and amount of blood drawn

Blood Collection and Storage

I. Blood is collected aseptically by gravity or vacuum pump from the jugular vein.

II. Feline donors commonly are sedated with a combination of ketamine 10 mg, diazepam 0.5 mg, and atropine 0.04 mg by IV injection.

III. A closed collection system is preferred to avoid bacterial contamination.
   A. Plastic bags containing citrate-phosphate-dextrose-adenine (CPD-A) with or without satellite bags for blood component separation are optimal.
   B. A large plastic syringe containing 1 ml CPD-A or 3.8% citrate (if not for storage) per 7–9 ml blood connected to a three-way stopcock and 19-gauge butterfly needle is used commonly for cats (open system).
   C. Vacuum glass bottles are not recommended.

IV. Several anticoagulants and preservatives are available, but heparin is not recommended.

V. Donor animals are treated as follows.
   A. The maximal volume of blood to be donated is different for dogs and cats.
      1. Canine donors: 20 mg/kg or one regular blood unit (450 ml blood plus 63 ml CPD-A) per 25-kg dog
      2. Feline donors: 10 ml/kg or one feline unit of 50 ml for cats weighing >5 kg
   B. In-house blood donors are usually bled no more than every 6 weeks.
   C. Crystalloid fluids (2–3 times blood volume collected) may be administered to donor cats.
   D. Because iron supply may become limited for erythropoiesis, regularly used blood donors are supplemented with ferrous sulfate (10 mg/kg PO twice weekly).

VI. The separation and storage of blood components from a single donation of blood are performed according to the Technical Manual of the American Association of Blood Banking. Blood components are prepared within 8 hours from the time of collection (Price et al., 1988; Wardrop, 1995).
   A. Fresh whole blood with functional platelets is kept at room temperature with gentle agitation for <8 hours before transfusion.
   B. Stored whole blood can be maintained at 4°C for 1 month when collected by a closed system in CPD-A or a similar preservative.
   C. Packed red cells can be stored at 4°C for 1 month. Before transfusing packed red cells, physiologic saline may be added to decrease the viscosity (packed cell volume [PCV]).
   D. Platelet-rich plasma and platelet concentrate can be stored for only 24 hours at room temperature under constant agitation.
   E. Fresh frozen plasma (as well as stored frozen plasma and cryoprecipitate) can be stored at < −20°C for up to 1 year.
   F. Blood components that have been warmed, opened, and/or partially used should not be re-cooled and stored again.

Administration of Blood

I. Stored blood components may be prewarmed to temperatures of 22–37°C immediately or up to half an hour before transfusion in a water bath.

II. Blood bags are connected to blood infusion sets that have an in-line microfilter.

III. Blood components are best administered intravenously through an indwelling catheter (16–22 gauge).

IV. If intravenous access cannot be obtained, red blood cells and plasma may be infused via the intraosseous route through the trochanteric fossa of the femur using a standard needle, a spinal needle in young animals, or a bone marrow needle (Otto and Crowe, 1992).

V. Concurrent administration of drugs or fluids other than physiologic saline through the same catheter is avoided to minimize blood coagulation or lysis of erythrocytes.

VI. Rate of transfusion depends on the hydration status, degree of anemia, and general health of the animal.

   A. Start with 1–3 ml over the first 5 minutes and observe for any transfusion reactions, even with typed and crossmatched blood.

   B. Maximum rate in normovolemic animals is 10–20 ml/kg/h.

   C. In animals with cardiac failure, do not exceed 4 ml/kg/h.

   D. Transfusion of a single bag is completed within 4 hours to prevent functional loss of blood elements or bacterial growth.

VII. Volume of blood component to be administered depends on the degree of anemia, platelet defect or coagulopathy, and size of the animal.

   A. Consider the following when treating severe anemia.

      1. Administration of 2 ml whole blood/kg elevates the PCV by 1%.

         a) This formula assumes that the PCV of the blood bag is 40%.

         b) If packed red cells are used, administer half the volume, because packed red cells have a PCV of 70–80%.

      2. Increase the PCV to 15–20% in animals with major signs of anemia or to ≥20% in animals that require anesthesia and surgery.

   B. When treating bleeding disorders, see dosages given in Chap. 66.

Complications: Transfusion Reactions

I. Adverse reactions usually occur during or shortly after the transfusion and can be caused by any component of whole blood.

II. Most transfusion reactions can be avoided by carefully selecting only healthy donors; using appropriate collection, storage, and administration techniques; performing blood typing and crossmatching tests; and administering only needed blood components.

III. The most common sign of a transfusion reaction is fever, followed by vomiting and hemolysis.

   A. Hemolytic transfusion reactions can be fatal.

   B. Fever and vomiting are usually self-limited.

IV. Adverse effects of transfusions can be divided into nonimmunologic and immunologic reactions (Table 69–5).

   A. Fever is a rise in temperature of >1.5°F or 1°C.

      1. Stop transfusion, but keep IV line open.

      2. Consider giving antipyretics if temperature is >105°F (>40°C).

      3. Correct underlying cause.

      4. When acute hemolytic reactions and sepsis have been ruled out and fever is controlled, the transfusion may be continued slowly.

   B. Hemolytic transfusion reactions may be caused by alloantibodies or by improper collection, storage, or administration of blood (Giger and Bücheler, 1991; Giger et al., 1995; Callan et al.,

*Table 69–5. **Adverse Reactions to Transfusions***

Nonimmunologic	Immunologic
Fever (pyrogens)	Hemolysis
Transmission of infection	Acute: intra-/extravascular
Hemolysis (physical)	hemolysis, disseminated
Vomiting	intravascular coagulation,
Congestive heart failure	renal failure
Hypothermia	Delayed: extravascular
Citrate toxicity	hemolysis with gradual
Coagulopathy	packed cell volume
	decrease
	Fever (with or without
	hemolysis)
	Urticaria, anaphylaxis

1995). The former reactions are separated into two phases (Auer et al., 1982).

1. Phase I reactions (anaphylaxis) result from complement activation and typically occur in type B cats receiving type A blood within seconds to minutes of starting the transfusion.

   a) Hypotension (weak pulses), bradycardia

   b) Hypopnea, apnea

   c) Urination, defecation, vomiting

   d) Neurologic signs: lethargy, lateral recumbency, seizures, nystagmus

   e) Death

2. Phase II reactions (hemolytic) occur in DEA 1.1 negative dogs as well as type B, and sometimes type A, cats receiving mismatched blood and are seen within a few minutes to hours.

   a) Hemolysis, hemoglobinemia, hemoglobinuria, bilirubinuria, and icterus after 1 day

   b) Tachycardia, lethargy, disseminated intravascular coagulation, death

3. Stop the transfusion immediately and see treatment of anaphylaxis in Chap. 74.

4. Recheck red cell compatibility of donor and recipient.

5. Delayed hemolytic reactions occur 1–2 weeks after the blood transfusion and may not cause clinical signs except for rapid recurrence of anemia.

C. Transmission of infection must be minimized.

   1. Viral diseases (e.g., FeLV, FIV, and FIP) are of particular importance in cats.

   2. Blood donors should be screened by careful examination of peripheral blood smears and by available serologic techniques for *Babesia, Hemobartonella,* and *Dirofilaria.*

   3. Avoid bacterial contamination during collection, storage, or administration (Hohenhaus and Drusin, 1996).

D. Congestive heart failure may be induced in animals with preexisting heart disease and normovolemia by transfusing them too rapidly.

E. Vomiting may occur during or shortly after transfusion and may be associated with an infusion rate that is too rapid, or it may be facilitated by allowing an animal to eat immediately before or during a transfusion.

    F. Hypothermia may be caused by administering large volumes of cold blood components.

    G. With massive transfusions (>100 ml/kg), coagulation factors may be diluted and lead to bleeding, and the large quantity of citrate infused may cause hypocalcemia-related cardiovascular and neurologic signs.

Bibliography

Andrews GA, Chavey PS, Smith JE: Production, characterization, and applications of a murine monoclonal antibody to dog erythrocyte antigen 1.1. J Am Vet Med Assoc 201:1549, 1992

Auer L, Bell K: The AB blood group system in cats. Anim Genet 12:287, 1981

Auer L, Bell K, Coates S: Blood transfusion reactions in the cat. J Am Vet Med Assoc 180:729, 1982

Bücheler J, Giger U: Alloantibodies against A and B blood types in cats. Vet Immunol Immunopathol 38:283, 1993

Callan MB, Giger U: Transfusion medicine. p. 525. In August JR (ed): Consultations in Feline Internal Medicine. WB Saunders, Philadelphia, 1994

Callan MB, Jones LT, Giger U: Hemolytic transfusion reactions in a dog with an alloantibody to a common antigen. J Vet Intern Med 9:277, 1995

Callan MB, Oakley DA, Shofer FS, Giger U: Canine red blood cell transfusion practice. J Am Anim Hosp Assoc 32:303, 1996

Cotter SM: Comparative Transfusion Medicine. Academic Press, San Diego, 1991

Giger U: Feline transfusion medicine. p. 600. In Hohenhaus AE (ed): Problems in Veterinary Medicine. JB Lippincott, Philadelphia, 1992

Giger U, Bücheler J: Transfusion of type-A and type-B blood to cats. J Am Vet Med Assoc 198:411, 1991

Giger U, Bücheler J, Patterson DF: Frequency and inheritance of A and B blood types in feline breeds of the United States. J Hered 82:15, 1991a

Giger U, Griot-Wenk ME, Bücheler J, et al: Geographical variation of the feline blood type frequencies in the United States. Feline Pract 19:21, 1991b

Giger U, Gelens CJ, Callan MB, Oakley DA: An acute hemolytic transfusion reaction caused by dog erythrocyte antigen 1.1 incompatibility in a previously sensitized dog. J Am Vet Med Assoc 206:1358, 1995

Giger U, Oakley DA, Callan MB, Kohn B: Advances in canine blood typing, cross-matching, and donor programs. Proc Am Coll Vet Intern Med 14:22, 1996a

Giger U, Oakley D, Callan MB, et al: Current transfusion therapy for anemic cats. Proc Am Coll Vet Intern Med 14:24, 1996b

Griot-Wenk ME, Giger U: Feline transfusion medicine: feline blood types and their clinical importance. Vet Clin North Am [Small Anim Pract] 25:1305, 1995

Griot-Wenk M, Casal ML, Chisholm-Chait A, et al: Blood type AB in the feline blood group system. Am J Vet Res 57:1438, 1996

Hale AS: Canine blood groups and their importance in veterinary transfusion medicine. Vet Clin North Am [Small Anim Pract] 25:1323, 1995

Hohenhaus AE: Transfusion medicine. Problems Vet Med 4, 1992

Hohenhaus AE, Drusin LM: *Serratia marcescens* contamination of whole blood from a large feline blood donor colony. Proc Am Coll Vet Intern Med 14:760, 1996

Kristensen AT, Feldman BF (eds): Canine and feline transfusion medicine. Vet Clin North Am [Small Anim Pract] 25(6), 1995

Otto CM, Crowe DT: Intraosseous resuscitation techniques and applications. p. 107. In Kirk RW, Bonagura JD (eds): Current Veterinary Therapy XI: Small Animal Practice. WB Saunders, Philadelphia, 1992

Price CS, Armstrong PJ, McLeod DA, et al: Evaluation of citrate-phosphate-dextrose-adenine as a storage medium for packed canine erythrocytes. J Vet Intern Med 2:126, 1988

Schneider A: Blood components: collection, processing, and storage. Vet Clin North Am [Small Anim Pract] 25:1245, 1995

Wardrop KJ: Selection of anticoagulant-preservatives for canine and feline blood storage. Vet Clin North Am [Small Anim Pract] 25:1263, 1995

70

Principles of Oncology

Cheryl A. London
Angela E. Frimberger

Definition

I. A tumor (or neoplasm) is a tissue growth composed of abnormal cells that proliferate in an uncontrolled manner.
   A. Benign
      1. The abnormal cells remain clustered together in a single mass.
      2. Benign tumors often compress the surrounding tissues but do not possess the property of invasiveness.
      3. They are often curable by simple surgical excision.
   B. Malignant
      1. The cells have the ability to invade adjacent tissues.
      2. This property allows malignant cells to break loose, enter the blood stream or lymphatic vessels, and form secondary tumors (metastases).
      3. "Cancer" refers to a malignant tumor.
II. Tumors are classified according to the tissue and cell type they most resemble.
   A. Benign (examples)
      1. Epithelial, glandular: adenoma
      2. Smooth muscle: leiomyoma
   B. Malignant
      1. Epithelial: carcinoma
      2. Connective tissue or muscle: sarcoma
      3. Others: leukemias and some cancers of the nervous system

Causes

I. Carcinogenesis (the development of cancer)
   A. In general, a tumor arises from a single cell that has undergone a series of genetic mutations, affecting genes that regulate the growth and differentiation of cells.
   B. At least two, and as many as five, mutations may be required for malignant transformation (the development of malignant potential).
   C. Mutations may be inherited (leading to a predisposition to tumor development), spontaneous during the aging process, or the result of environmental agents.
II. Genetics of cancer
   A. Proto-oncogenes
      1. These are normal genes that regulate cellular responses to external signals that stimulate growth and differentiation.
      2. Gene products include growth factors (sis, int-2), growth factor receptors (kit, trk), cytoplasmic protein kinases (src, abl), and nuclear proteins (myc, jun).
      3. Oncogenes are altered forms of proto-oncogenes in which the level of expression or the gene product is changed (through a mutation), giving the cell malignant potential.
   B. Tumor suppressor genes
      1. These genes code for proteins that restrict or inhibit cellular proliferation.
      2. When gene function is lost, cells may grow in an uncontrolled manner, leading to development of a tumor.
      3. Examples include *p53* (mutated in up to 60% of human tumors) and *Rb*.
   C. Other genes
      1. Those coding for DNA repair enzymes
      2. Proteins important in cell adhesion
III. Environmental carcinogens
   A. Viruses
      1. Carcinogenic RNA viruses often carry an oncogene that is introduced into an infected cell and can rapidly induce transformation. Examples include feline leukemia virus (FeLV) and feline sarcoma virus.
      2. DNA viruses can cause cancer by making viral proteins that alter cell growth and differentiation. An example is papovavirus (papillomavirus).
   B. Chemicals
      1. Pesticides have been shown to increase the cancer risk for humans and animals. Examples

include chlordane, toxaphene, and 2,4-D, a lawn herbicide that has been implicated in canine lymphoma.

2. Food preservatives such as nitrite, nitrate, and polyvinyl chloride (a contaminant from packaging material) have carcinogenic activity in laboratory animals.

C. Radiation
  1. Ultraviolet radiation produces tumors in animals and humans. Lack of pigmentation and prolonged sunlight exposure predispose to the development of squamous cell carcinoma.
  2. Ionizing radiation includes x-rays and gamma rays.
    a) Radiation exposure in humans is linked to the development of leukemia and thyroid tumors.
    b) In humans and animals, second primary tumors occasionally have been found to develop after therapeutic radiation.

D. Others
  1. Hormones have been implicated in tumor development.
    a) Female dogs allowed to experience at least two estrous cycles develop mammary tumors seven times more frequently than dogs spayed before 2 years of age.
    b) Perianal gland tumors occur almost exclusively in intact male dogs.
  2. Parasitic infection with *Spirocerca lupi* has been associated with esophageal fibrosarcoma and osteosarcoma.

Pathophysiology

I. Tumor growth
  A. Cell cycle
    1. Tumor cell growth involves several mechanisms to increase cell number (Fig. 70–1).
    2. A population of cells can increase in number by the following means.
      a) Shortening the duration of the cell cycle
      b) Moving resting cells (in G_0) into the cell cycle
  B. Tumor kinetics
    1. Theoretically, tumors undergo Gompertzian growth.
      a) As the tumor grows, the blood supply may become inadequate.
      b) Poor perfusion results in a decrease in growth fraction and an increase in cell death.
      c) These two changes result in an increase in the tumor doubling time.
    2. A tumor is not detectable until it is approximately 1 g or 1 cm³. By this time, it has undergone 20 or more doublings and contains over several million cells.

II. Angiogenesis
  A. Tumor cells release substances into their environment that cause proliferation of vascular endothelium and growth of blood vessels into the tumor,

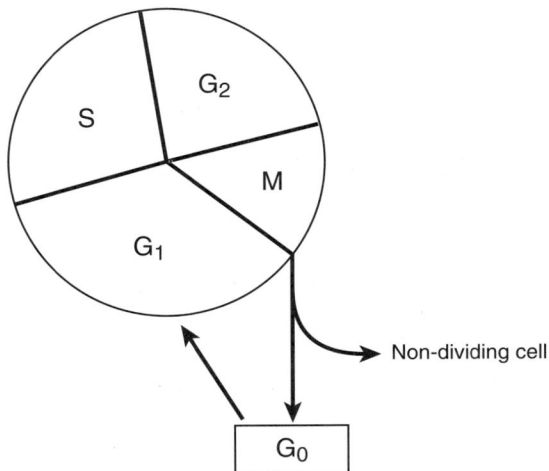

Figure 70–1. Cell cycle. A cell in mitosis (M) proceeds into a growth phase (G_1) in which new proteins are made. This is followed by a period of DNA synthesis (S) and another growth phase (G_2) before the next mitosis. Some cells may temporarily leave the cell cycle and enter a resting state (G_0) from which they can be rescued by appropriate stimuli to re-enter the cycle. Other cells may leave the cycle permanently after terminal differentiation.

processes essential for continued tumor development.
  B. The tumor vasculature is often "leaky," which may aid in metastasis.

III. Metastasis
  A. Fewer than 1 in 10,000 cells that leave the primary tumor survive.
  B. To succeed, the tumor cell must complete all the necessary steps.
    1. Detachment from the primary tumor mass
    2. Invasion into the vascular or lymphatic system
    3. Evasion of host defenses
    4. Arrest and attachment in vascular or lymphatic vessels
    5. Extravasation into the surrounding tissue
    6. Establishment of new tumor growth

Clinical Signs

I. Because tumors are not usually detectable until they have reached approximately 1 g in size, they may have already metastasized. Therefore, clinical signs may be related to the primary tumor or to metastatic disease in other locations.
II. Clinical signs of cancer are diverse and can mimic many infectious or autoimmune disorders.
  A. Pain
    1. Tumors invading bone and other tissues may be painful to the animal, especially osteosarcoma and multiple myeloma that cause osteolysis.
    2. Such pain may be manifested by chronic lameness.
  B. Fever

1. Tumor cells or the body's response to a tumor may generate pyrogenic factors.
    2. Tumor-associated fever is often intermittent.
  C. Nonhealing wound
    1. Any mass or wound that is chronically non-healing could be a tumor.
    2. Many skin neoplasms may be mistaken for simple skin infections.
  D. Other signs
    1. Anorexia, weight loss
    2. Vomiting, diarrhea
    3. Coughing, dyspnea
    4. Glaucoma, sudden blindness, seizures
    5. Clotting abnormalities
    6. Polyuria, polydipsia
III. Some tumors exhibit no clinical signs until they are quite large, e.g., hemangiosarcoma.

Diagnosis

  I. History
  A. Acquiring a complete history from the pet owner aids the clinician in the diagnostic process and provides information concerning the biologic behavior of the tumor.
  B. The duration of clinical signs gives clues as to both the nature of the disease and its potential aggressiveness.
    1. It is extremely useful to know how long any masses have been present and whether they have been growing.
    2. Rapid growth may indicate a biologically aggressive tumor.
  C. Knowledge of previous illness is particularly relevant.
    1. If the animal has had other tumors, the current problem may be a recurrence.
    2. Any other serious medical condition may influence the prognosis, course of treatment chosen, and diagnostic procedures performed.
 II. Physical examination
  A. A complete physical examination is essential in the evaluation of any tumor-bearing animal to help determine the extent of disease, as well as any underlying conditions that may affect the health of the animal.
  B. Determine whether any obvious mass is located within the skin or subcutaneous tissue and whether it is fixed to any underlying structures.
    1. A tumor that is infiltrating adjacent structures may be more difficult to remove.
    2. Be sure to search carefully for any other masses.
  C. Carefully palpate both local and distant lymph nodes for enlargement, as this may indicate metastatic disease.
  D. Rectal examination is important in the assessment of sublumbar lymph nodes, the prostate gland, and the urethra.
  E. Abdominal palpation may reveal organomegaly, which could represent the primary disease or be a manifestation of metastatic/systemic disease.
  F. Thoracic auscultation is important to assess lung and cardiac function (see Chap. 1).
    1. Metastatic disease in the lungs is usually not detectable by auscultation.
    2. Pleural effusion secondary to thoracic disease may be noted.
  G. The oral cavity should be examined thoroughly, as many tumors go unnoticed in this location until they become quite large.
  H. Anterior uveitis, chorioretinitis, and other ocular changes may occur with neoplastic disease.
III. Diagnostic procedures
  A. Complete blood count (CBC), serum biochemical profile, and urinalysis
    1. May aid in the primary diagnosis
    2. May demonstrate the existence of a paraneoplastic syndrome
    3. May reveal potentially complicating conditions unrelated to the neoplasm
  B. Fine-needle aspirate
    1. Any palpable mass on the animal is evaluated by fine-needle aspiration.
    2. This simple procedure often yields a diagnosis.
  C. Biopsy
    1. If fine-needle aspiration is not possible or does not provide a definitive diagnosis, it may be necessary to perform a surgical biopsy.
    2. It is important to remember that a properly performed surgical biopsy does not cause metastasis or negatively influence survival.
      a) Needle/incisional biopsy
        (1) It is performed using a punch biopsy needle (Tru-Cut) or a blade to obtain a wedge of tissue, often under local anesthesia.
        (2) The junction of normal and abnormal tissue is the best area for the pathologist to assess invasiveness.
        (3) Because the biopsy tract may be seeded with tumor cells, it is important to position the biopsy tract so that it can be easily removed upon subsequent excision of the tumor.
        (4) Indications for needle/incisional biopsy include any tumor too large for excisional biopsy, any tumor suspected of being malignant, and any tumor that may not be able to be entirely removed.
      b) Excisional biopsy
        (1) Every effort is made to obtain wide margins.
        (2) It is indicated when the tumor is very small and not amenable to needle aspiration (small dermal nodule) or if the treatment would not be changed by knowledge of the histologic type (splenic mass, testicular mass).
IV. Diagnostic imaging
  A. Radiography
    1. Abdominal radiography is useful for evaluat-

ing the size of organs; severe organomegaly is readily detected, but marginal organomegaly or a mass within a normal-sized organ may not be detected.
   2. Thoracic radiography is useful for detecting lesions in lungs, cardiomegaly, pleural effusion, or a cranial mediastinal mass.
   3. Contrast studies can be used to evaluate the morphology or function of a specific organ system (e.g., barium GI studies, contrast cystogram).
B. Special radiographic procedures
   1. Angiography can give an indication of the vascular organization of a tumor and whether a tumor may be invading an adjacent blood vessel.
   2. Scintigraphy can be used to evaluate bone, liver, and lung for tumors.
C. Ultrasonography
   1. It is an extremely useful noninvasive technique for evaluating both the abdomen and the thorax.
   2. It provides better evaluation of organ structure, including the presence of diffuse organ infiltration or the presence of small masses not detectable on radiographs.
   3. Structures not adequately visualized on radiographs, such as the pancreas, mesenteric lymph nodes, cranial mediastinal structures, and large blood vessels, can often be found by ultrasonography.
   4. Because it cannot penetrate air or bone, it is not useful for evaluating the lungs or the central nervous system (CNS).
D. Computed tomography (CT), magnetic resonance imaging (MRI)
   1. CT and MRI are more sensitive for detecting metastatic disease or small lesions than standard radiography or ultrasonography.
   2. MRI is particularly useful for delineating structures within the CNS.
V. Endoscopy/bronchoscopy
A. Endoscopy is excellent for assessing upper and lower gastrointestinal tracts.
B. Rhinoscopy and bronchoscopy are used to visualize the nasal cavity and large airway structures.
C. Bronchoscopy is also used for bronchoalveolar lavage, which can sometimes provide a cytologic diagnosis of pulmonary neoplasia.
VI. Bone marrow evaluation
A. Indications include the presence of hematologic abnormalities or suspicion of a hematologic malignancy.
B. Bone marrow aspiration is usually sufficient, but if an inadequate sample is obtained, a bone core biopsy using a Jamshidi needle may be necessary (see Chap. 3).
C. Significant hemorrhage is uncommon, so it can be done in the presence of severe thrombocytopenia.

Differential Diagnosis

I. The potential differential diagnoses are numerous, including infectious (especially fungal) disease, trauma, and autoimmune conditions.

II. Tumors sometimes generate secondary conditions such as autoimmune hemolytic anemia, clotting disorders, or renal failure that may mask the primary disorder.

Staging

I. It is extremely important to determine the extent of disease to arrive at an accurate prognosis and design an appropriate therapeutic regimen. The process of staging involves systematic determination of the extent of disease.

II. Staging is most commonly done using the TNM classification scheme of the World Health Organization (see Table 59–4). The exact criteria for the different stages vary with each tumor but follow a general pattern.
   A. T represents the extent of the primary tumor, with T0 denoting no evidence of primary tumor, and T1, T2, T3, and T4 indicating increasing size of the primary tumor.
      1. In general, the higher the number, the larger the tumor and, in most cases, the worse the prognosis.
      2. For example, an oral melanoma that is less than 2 cm in size is classified as T1.
   B. N refers to the extent of lymph node involvement, with N0 indicating no lymph node abnormalities, and N1, N2, and N3 referring to the specific characteristics of affected lymph nodes, including size and movability. For example, an oral melanoma with bilateral lymph node involvement is classified as N2.
   C. M represents the extent of distant metastases, with M0 indicating no metastatic disease and M1 indicating distant metastases.
   D. For T, N, and M, a designation of X means that it is impossible to assess the extent of the disease in that area.

III. The staging procedure is as follows.
   A. Primary tumor
      1. Carefully assess the size of the primary tumor and whether it is freely movable or fixed to adjacent tissues, while also noting other characteristics, such as ulceration, erythema, and so forth.
      2. Determine whether bony invasion is present (best evaluated by CT), as this will change the T classification.
   B. Lymph nodes
      1. Examine both local and distant nodes.
      2. Palpation often yields important information concerning lymph node size and consistency.
      3. Lymph nodes not amenable to palpation may be assessed by radiography, ultrasonography, CT, or MRI.
      4. Perform a fine-needle aspiration of any suspicious lymph node, but a negative finding does not rule out metastasis.
   C. Metastatic disease
      1. Thoracic radiographs are essential to determine whether obvious metastatic disease is present in the lungs.

a) Three views (both laterals and ventral/dorsal) are necessary to thoroughly examine the lungs.

b) Tumors smaller than 0.5–1 cm are not detectable by radiography; therefore, negative thoracic radiographs do not completely rule out the presence of microscopic metastatic disease.

  2. Ultrasonography is often important in evaluating abdominal organs for metastatic disease.

  3. Other useful modalities are scintigraphy, CT, and MRI.

IV. The importance of staging cannot be overemphasized, as the therapeutic regimen is based on the extent of disease.

General Therapeutic Approach

I. To appropriately select a treatment course as well as to choose a goal of treatment (see later), it is imperative to have a correct histologic diagnosis and to be aware of the extent of disease (stage).

II. The clinician should be compassionate, but communication must be clear and honest. A full range of treatment options is presented to the client.

III. Before undergoing cancer treatment, the animal is carefully evaluated for other medical problems that may affect the prognosis or that need to be considered in cancer treatment planning.

IV. It is important to determine from the beginning whether the goal of treatment is cure or palliation.

  A. Cure (the complete eradication of all tumor cells with proliferative potential) is an ideal outcome but is not always a realistic goal. If treatment is undertaken with curative intent, the approach must be aggressive from the start, and a higher level of short-term toxicity must be expected.

  B. If the intent is palliation, the primary goal is to improve the quality of life rather than to influence the disease course.

  C. It is rarely effective to start treatment with a palliative intent and then later attempt a cure, but it is common to attempt a cure and then switch to palliative treatment.

V. Tumors are measured before starting treatment and at each recheck.

  A. Whenever possible, the tumor is measured in three dimensions, and the product calculated to give a tumor volume.

  B. If multiple tumors are present, they are each noted and measured.

VI. The response to treatment is described using terms that have specific meanings.

  A. Clinical remission: no evidence of tumor detected using physical examination or routine imaging techniques, but not necessarily the same as a cure

  B. Complete response (CR): in response to a particular treatment, tumor regression to the point of clinical remission, but not necessarily a cure

  C. Partial response/remission (PR): a decrease in tumor volume of >50% and no new tumors

  D. Stable disease (SD): <50% decrease or <10% increase in tumor volume

  E. Progressive disease (PD): an increase in tumor volume >10% or the appearance of new tumors

VII. The clinician must be familiar with any treatment modality used, including the usual dosage, toxicities to be expected (and their management), drug mechanisms of action, and storage requirements.

VIII. Many of the therapeutic modalities are best employed in combination rather than singly, particularly if they have different mechanisms of action, because this allows additive efficacy without overlapping toxicity.

  A. Adjuvant therapy refers to the use of another modality, such as chemotherapy or ionizing radiation, following surgery.

  B. Neoadjuvant therapy refers to the use of another modality prior to surgery.

  C. Chemoradiotherapy refers to the use of chemotherapeutic drugs primarily as radiation sensitizers rather than for their direct cytotoxicity.

Chemotherapy

I. Chemotherapy is the only major treatment modality that is distributed through the entire body, so it remains the primary treatment for systemic diseases such as hematologic malignancies and metastatic disease.

  A. Chemotherapy is most effective against the smallest tumors and is rarely curative for large tumors (exception: transmissible venereal tumor).

    1. Chemotherapy is most active against dividing cells, and a greater proportion of cells in large tumors are quiescent owing to poor nutrition.

    2. Because of poor perfusion in large tumors, chemotherapeutic drugs may not reach all tumor cells.

    3. The larger the tumor, the greater the likelihood that a mutation for drug resistance has occurred.

  B. Chemotherapy can be used in combination with other modalities.

  C. Most chemotherapeutic drugs have a small therapeutic margin (i.e., the toxic dose is close to the therapeutic dose).

    1. It is important to be as accurate as possible when calculating and administering these drugs.

    2. To improve accuracy, dosages of many chemotherapeutic drugs are based on body surface area (BSA), derived from a table or calculation (Table 70–1); for some drugs, BSA is thought to be a better reflection of metabolic body size than is body weight.

II. A good understanding of the cell cycle is important, because many chemotherapeutic drugs are more effective against cells that are actively dividing or are more effective in a particular phase of the cell cycle (see Fig. 70–1).

III. Most chemotherapeutic drugs are highly toxic, and many are also mutagenic, so precautions must be taken when handling, administering, and disposing

Table 70–1. **Weight (kg) to Body Surface Area (m²) Conversion Chart**

Dogs						Cats		
kg	lb	m²	kg	lb	m²	kg	lb	m²
0.50	1.1	0.06	33	72.6	1.03	2.0	4.4	0.159
1	2.2	0.10	34	74.8	1.05	2.5	5.5	0.184
2	4.4	0.15	35	77.0	1.07	3.0	6.6	0.208
3	6.6	0.20	36	79.2	1.09	3.5	7.7	0.231
4	8.8	0.25	37	81.4	1.11	4.0	8.8	0.252
5	11.0	0.29	38	83.6	1.13	4.5	9.9	0.273
6	13.2	0.33	39	85.8	1.15	5.0	11.0	0.292
7	15.4	0.36	40	88.0	1.17	5.5	12.1	0.311
8	17.6	0.40	41	90.2	1.19	6.0	13.2	0.330
9	19.8	0.43	42	92.4	1.21	6.5	14.3	0.348
10	22.0	0.46	43	94.6	1.23	7.0	15.4	0.366
11	24.2	0.49	44	96.8	1.25	7.5	16.5	0.383
12	26.4	0.52	45	99.0	1.26	8.0	17.6	0.400
13	28.6	0.55	46	101.2	1.28	8.5	18.7	0.416
14	30.8	0.58	47	103.4	1.30	9.0	19.8	0.432
15	33.0	0.60	48	105.6	1.32	9.5	20.9	0.449
16	35.2	0.63	49	107.8	1.34	10.0	22.0	0.464
17	37.4	0.66	50	110.0	1.36			
18	39.6	0.69	52	112.2	1.41			
19	41.8	0.71	54	114.4	1.44			
20	44.0	0.74	56	116.6	1.48			
21	46.2	0.76	58	118.8	1.51			
22	48.4	0.78	60	121.0	1.55			
23	50.6	0.81	62	123.2	1.58			
24	52.8	0.83	64	125.4	1.62			
25	55.0	0.85	66	127.6	1.65			
26	57.2	0.88	68	129.8	1.68			
27	59.4	0.90	70	132.0	1.72			
28	61.6	0.92	72	134.2	1.75			
29	63.8	0.94	74	136.4	1.78			
30	66.0	0.96	76	138.6	1.81			
31	68.2	0.99	78	140.8	1.84			
32	70.4	1.01	80	143.0	1.88			

The values in the table are derived from the equation m² = 10.0 (10.1 in cats) × (weight in grams)$^{2/3}$/10,000.

From Hahn KA, Richardson RC: Cancer Chemotherapy: A Veterinary Handbook. Williams & Wilkins, Baltimore, 1995, p. 237, with permission.

of the drugs to ensure the safety of staff, clients, and the community.

A. Ideally, a fume hood is used to prepare all chemotherapeutic drugs, but most practices do not have access to one.
　1. Always use protective eyewear and a respirator mask when preparing drugs.
　2. The drugs are prepared in an area where drafts do not occur and other personnel will not be exposed.
B. Wear a gown with long sleeves and closed cuffs and heavy latex (not vinyl) gloves.
C. Hydrophobic filters (Chemo-Pins) are available to be placed between the drug vial and the syringe to equalize the pressure, reducing the risk of aerosolization.
　1. Use Luer-Lok syringes.
　2. If a Chemo-Pin is not used, gauze is wrapped around the vial top and the needle while the

needle is withdrawn to prevent aerosolization of the drug.
D. Drug-contaminated waste is kept separately in sealed bags and disposed of according to local requirements.
E. When oral chemotherapeutic drugs are dispensed for use at home, the owner is also given a supply of heavy latex gloves and a disposal bag.
　1. The bag is used to return any contaminated items, including the gloves and vials, to the clinician for disposal.
　2. Breaking and crushing of pills must be stringently avoided.
F. Cisplatin is excreted in the urine of treated dogs for up to 48 hours, so gloves are worn when cleaning up urine or contaminated areas.
G. After any drug handling, wash hands well even if gloves were worn.
IV. Major classes of chemotherapy drugs are as follows (Table 70–2).
A. Alkylating agents
　1. Mechanism of action: alkylation of DNA, causing cross-linkage and strand breaks
　2. Cell cycle specificity: nonspecific
　3. Major indications: primarily hematopoietic neoplasms
　4. Cautions
　　a) The main toxicity is myelosuppression.
　　b) Hemorrhagic cystitis is a unique toxicity of cyclophosphamide.
　5. Examples: cyclophosphamide, chlorambucil, melphalan, busulfan, nitrosoureas
B. Antimetabolites
　1. Mechanism of action: analogues of normal metabolites incorporated into DNA that interfere with enzyme activity or with transcription and translation
　2. Cell cycle specificity: S phase
　3. Major indications: not often indicated in veterinary medicine because of toxicity (especially 5-fluorouracil) and lack of concomitant efficacy
　4. Cautions
　　a) The main toxicity is myelosuppression.
　　b) An exception is 5-fluorouracil, which is neurotoxic; *do not give to cats.*
　5. Examples: cytosine arabinoside, 5-fluorouracil, methotrexate
C. Antibiotics
　1. Mechanism of action: topoisomerase II inhibition, free radical production, intercalation
　2. Cell cycle specificity: S phase/nonspecific
　3. Major indications: hematopoietic neoplasms, some carcinomas and sarcomas
　4. Cautions
　　a) Most drugs cause myelosuppression and gastrointestinal disturbances.
　　b) Many are cardiotoxic to varying degrees.
　　c) Extravasation causes severe sloughing.
　5. Examples: doxorubicin, mitoxantrone, actinomycin D
D. Mitotic inhibitors

Table 70–2. *Administration and Dosing Information for Selected Chemotherapy Drugs*

Drug (Brand Name, Supplier)[a]	Drug Class	Major Indications	Dosage,[b] Route, Frequency	Relative Cost[a]	Cautions/Major Toxicities[c]
Actinomycin D (Cosmegen, Merck)	Anthracycline antibiotic	Low-cost alternative for canine LSA	0.5–0.9 mg/m² IV *slowly* through a catheter every 3 wk	Low	MyS, V/D, extravasation-induced skin slough
L-Asparaginase (Elspar, Merck)	Enzyme	In combination protocols for canine and feline LSA	Dogs and cats: 10,000 IU/m² or 400 IU/kg IM up to weekly	Moderate	Anaphylaxis is rare when given IM; if anaphylaxis occurs, treat as shock and do not give any more drug; rarely causes pancreatitis; delays clearance of vincristine
Carboplatin (Paraplatin, Bristol-Myers-Squibb)	Platinum compound	Like cisplatin but *safe for cats;* some efficacy in melanoma	Dilute in 5% dextrose Large dogs: 350 mg/m² IV every 3 wk Small dogs: 300 mg/m² IV every 3 wk Cats: 210 mg/m² IV every 3 wk	Very high, but moderate for cats	MyS, thrombocytopenia; reduce dose if azotemia is present owing to reduced clearance
Chlorambucil (Leukeran, Burroughs Wellcome)	Alkylating agent	DOC for canine CLL in combination protocol; possible efficacy in MCT; substitute when cyclophosphamide not tolerated	Dosage varies with different protocols; generally 0.2 mg/kg PO daily for induction, then 0.1 mg/kg PO daily for maintenance	Low–moderate	MyS can occur; monitor CBC frequently and reduce dose as needed
Cisplatin (Platinol, Bristol-Myers-Squibb)	Platinum compound	DOC for canine OSA, TCC, malignant effusions; various carcinomas	Large dogs 60–70 mg/m² IV, small dogs 50–60 mg/m² IV, *in a 4–6 h saline diuresis protocol;* to reduce vomiting, give butorphanol 0.4 mg/kg IM at end of cisplatin Intracavitary: 50 mg/m² in 1 L/m² of 0.9% saline, with *saline diuresis*	High	Do not give to cats! Severely nephrotoxic in dogs (small dogs more sensitive) unless given in a diuresis protocol; vomiting is common during and shortly after treatment; eliminated in urine for 48 h
Cyclophosphamide (Cytoxan, Bristol-Myers-Squibb)	Alkylating agent	In combination protocols for canine and feline LSA; some carcinomas	50 mg/m² PO SID for 4 days per wk; or 250 mg/m² PO or 200 mg/m² IV once every 3 wk	Low	MyS, minor vomiting; severe sterile hemorrhagic cystitis may be prevented by giving with prednisone and in the morning
Cytosine arabinoside (Cytosar-U, Upjohn)	Antimetabolite	Few indications; possibly feline renal or CNS LSA	100 mg/m² per day continuous infusion for 4 days; or 300 mg/m² SQ BID for 2 days	Low	MyS, anorexia, vomiting
Dacarbazine (DTIC-Dome, Miles)	Unclassified	In combination protocols for canine LSA rescue; some efficacy in melanoma	200 mg/m² IV slowly daily for 5 days every 3 wk	High–Moderate	MyS, V/D, extravasation-induced skin slough
Doxorubicin (Adriamycin, Adria; generics and others)	Anthracycline antibiotic	DOC for canine and possibly feline LSA, especially in combination protocols; also for mammary gland tumors, other solid tumors	Dogs: 25–30 mg/m² IV at 1 ml/min through a catheter every 3 wk; at cumulative doses greater than 180 mg/m² precede each dose with echocardiogram Cats: 20–30 mg/m² IV at 1 ml/min every 3 wk	Moderate	Do not use with heparin—causes precipitation MyS, V/D, occasional severe hemorrhagic colitis; occasional allergic reaction can be prevented by giving slowly; cardiotoxic in dogs; caution in Dobermans or if preexisting cardiac disease; extravasation-induced skin slough; alopecia can occur; rare chronic renal toxicity reported
Etretinate (Tegison, Roche)	Retinoid	Cutaneous SCC, especially premalignant	2–3 mg/kg PO TID	High	Hepatotoxicity, nephrotoxicity reported
Hydroxyurea (Hydrea, Immunex)	Unclassified	DOC for polycythemia vera and CML	Dogs: 80 mg/kg PO every 3 days Cats: 25 mg/kg PO 3 times per wk	Low	MyS or anemia can occur; monitor CBC and reduce dose as needed
Ifosfamide (Ifex, Bristol-Myers-Squibb)	Alkylating agent	Canine LSA rescue, various sarcomas	350–375 mg/m² IV, with mesna, in a diuresis protocol, every 2–3 wk	Moderate	Give in diuresis protocol with mesna to prevent urotoxicosis; MyS, thrombocytopenia can occur
Lomustine (CeeNu, Bristol-Myers-Squibb)	Nitrosoureas, nitrogen mustard, alkylating agent	Canine CNS neoplasms (crosses BBB), possibly canine LSA rescue	90 mg/m² PO every 3–4 wk	Low–Moderate	Occasional nausea 24 h after administration; MyS 1–6 wk after, cumulative MyS with thrombocytopenia
Melphalan (Alkeran, Burroughs Wellcome)	Alkylating agent	DOC for canine multiple myeloma in combination protocols	0.1 mg/kg PO (or IV) daily for 10 days, then 0.05 mg/kg PO daily for maintenance	Low–Moderate	MyS can occur, especially cumulative—monitor CBC and adjust dose as needed; extravasation-induced skin slough
Methotrexate (Rheumatrex, Lederle; generics and others)	Antimetabolite	Few indications; possible role in LSA combination protocols	Dogs: 0.6–0.8 mg/kg IV every 3 wk or 2.5 mg/m² PO daily Cats: 0.8 mg/kg IV or PO every 4 wk	Low	MyS, V/D

Table continued on following page

Table 70–2. **Administration and Dosing Information for Selected Chemotherapy Drugs** (Continued)

Drug (Brand Name, Supplier)[a]	Drug Class	Major Indications	Dosage,[b] Route, Frequency	Relative Cost[a]	Cautions/Major Toxicities[c]
Mitotane (Lysodren, Bristol-Myers-Squibb)	Unclassified	Adrenal cortical tumors	50 mg/kg PO per day divided into 2 doses; when ACTH stimulation is normal, then 50 mg/kg per wk divided into 2–3 doses	Low–Moderate	Iatrogenic hypoadrenocorticism—adjust dose, give corticosteroids; can disrupt insulin regulation in diabetes
Mitoxantrone (Novantrone, Lederle)	Anthracycline antibiotic	Some efficacy in various canine and feline LSA, sarcomas, carcinomas; DOC for feline oral SCC in combination with radiation	Dogs: 5.5–6 mg/m² IV every 3 wk Cats: 6.5 mg/m² IV every 3 wk over at least 3 min	High	Heparin causes precipitation MyS, V/D; cardiotoxic but less than doxorubicin
Piroxicam (Feldene, Pfizer; generics and others)	Nonsteroidal anti-inflammatory	Canine TCC and SCC; additional good palliation for many dogs	0.3 mg/kg PO daily	Moderate	Occasional gastric upset; give with food; give with misoprostol if needed
Prednisone (generics, many)	Corticosteroid	In combination protocols for canine and feline LSA, CLL, MCT, other hematopoietic malignancies; palliative for CNS tumors	Dosage varies; for LSA, usually 30–40 mg/m² daily for 4 wk, then every other day; for MCT, 2.2 mg/kg BID for 2 wk, then SID for 2 wk, then QOD for 6 mo	Low	Iatrogenic hyperadrenocorticism; may accelerate the development of multiple drug resistance—do not give alone if combination chemotherapy is being considered
Vinblastine (Velban, Lilly, others)	Mitotic inhibitor	In combination protocols for canine and feline LSA when vincristine is not tolerated	Dogs and cats: 2.0 mg/m² IV slowly through a catheter, up to weekly	Low	Heparin in syringes causes precipitation MyS, nausea, vomiting, extravasation-induced skin slough
Vincristine (Oncovin, Lilly, others)	Mitotic inhibitor	In combination protocols for canine and feline LSA; DOC for TVT; causes platelet release from marrow	Dogs and cats: LSA: 0.7–0.75 mg/m² IV up to weekly TVT: 0.5 mg/m² IV weekly until resolution, usually less than 6 wk	Low	Heparin causes precipitation Neuropathy—peripheral, paralytic ileus; extravasation-induced skin slough

BBB = blood-brain barrier; CBC = complete blood count; CLL = chronic lymphocytic leukemia; CML = chronic myelogenous (granulocytic) leukemia; CNS = central nervous system; DOC = drug of choice; LSA = lymphoma; MCT = mast cell tumor; MyS = myelosuppression; OSA = osteosarcoma; SCC = squamous cell carcinoma; TCC = transitional cell carcinoma; V/D = vomiting and diarrhea.

[a]Before ordering a drug for the first time, check the most recent *Physicians' Desk Reference* or consult a pharmacist about suppliers and cost, because pharmaceutical companies may merge or change names, and the cost of a drug may decrease dramatically when generics become available.

[b]The dosages listed here are guidelines only. Dosages vary, particularly in combination protocols. Select a protocol appropriate to the case and use the dosages recommended therein. Also, if toxicity occurs, dose reduction is always an option.

[c]Always consult the package insert before giving a drug for the first time for the full details of toxicities and side effects.

1. Mechanism of action: interference with tubulin function to prevent normal spindle apparatus formation and mitosis
2. Cell cycle specificity: M phase
3. Major indications: hematopoietic neoplasms, transmissible venereal tumor (vincristine), possibly other tumors (paclitaxel)
4. Cautions: major toxicities vary
5. Examples: vincristine, vinblastine, paclitaxel

E. Platinum compounds
1. Mechanism of action: platinum complex binding of DNA, causing interstrand and intrastrand cross-links
2. Cell cycle specificity: nonspecific
3. Major indications: osteosarcoma, transitional cell and squamous cell carcinomas
4. Cautions
   a) Cisplatin is uniformly fatal to cats.
   b) In dogs, cisplatin is nephrotoxic unless given with saline diuresis.
   c) Carboplatin is myelosuppressive but safe for cats.
5. Examples: cisplatin, carboplatin

F. Others
1. L-Asparaginase
   a) Hydrolyzes serum asparagine; cytotoxicity relies on tumor cell's lack of asparagine synthetase, whereas normal cells are able to synthesize new asparagine.
   b) Main indication is lymphoma.
   c) Major toxicity is anaphylaxis, which is rare when the drug is given intramuscularly or when the PEGylated form is used (polyethylene glycol blocks immune recognition).
2. Prednisone
   a) It possesses cytotoxic activity against some lymphomas and some mast cell tumors; mechanism is unclear.
   b) It may also have palliative effects in some terminal cases.
   c) Major toxicity is iatrogenic Cushing's syndrome.
   d) It may accelerate the development of multiple drug resistance, so its use alone to treat lymphoma when combination chemotherapy is being considered is not recommended.
3. Hydroxyurea
   a) Inhibits ribonucleoside reductase, inhibiting DNA synthesis
   b) S-phase specific

c) Main indications: polycythemia vera and chronic myelogenous leukemia

d) Possible severe myelosuppression

V. Resistance to chemotherapy may be either inherent or acquired.

A. Inherent resistance

1. Drug may be physically unable to reach tumor cells.
   a) Blood-brain barrier
   b) Poor perfusion in tumors
2. Cell may not have receptors or activating enzymes for drug.
3. Cell may not be sensitive to mechanism of action of drug. For example, a cell that has asparagine synthetase will be resistant to L-asparaginase.

B. Acquired resistance

1. Spontaneous mutation
   a) Rate is higher in tumors than in normal tissues because of genetic instability and high rate of mitosis.
   b) The larger the tumor, the higher the likelihood that mutation has occurred.
2. Gene amplification of detoxifying protein (usually enzyme) is enhanced by the presence of a sublethal concentration of drug.

C. Multiple drug resistance

1. It is caused by a membrane pump that removes foreign substances from cells.
   a) Present on many normal cells, especially hepatocytes, intestinal mucosa, kidney
   b) Recognizes many natural chemotherapy drugs, especially anthracyclines and mitotic inhibitors, as well as other xenobiotics
   c) Alkylating agents not affected
2. It can be inherent (e.g., hepatocellular carcinoma) or acquired.
   a) Low levels of expression increase with exposure to chemotherapy.
   b) Gradually increasing intensity of chemotherapy encourages development.
3. It is a common cause of relapse in lymphoma.

VI. Toxicity of chemotherapy is reflected in a number of organ systems.

A. Myelosuppression

1. The nadir is the lowest point of the cell count.
   a) The white cell nadir usually occurs at 7–10 days.
   b) A platelet nadir may occur later.
   c) Nadirs vary with the drug used.
2. Although many animals have decreased white blood cell or platelet counts without showing clinical signs, when signs do occur, they range from fever and lethargy to septic shock.
   a) Clinical deterioration can be rapid, so animals must be watched closely, and these signs are considered a potential emergency.
   b) Owners are instructed to take the animal's temperature if they suspect a fever.
   c) Thrombocytopenia rarely causes clinical signs, but petechiae, ecchymoses, and mucosal bleeding may be noted.
3. Management of myelosuppression involves several considerations.
   a) The risk of life-threatening complications is small but real, and emergencies may require an aggressive response. If the clinician is not prepared to provide 24-hour emergency care, contact with a reliable local emergency/critical care clinic is established in advance.
   b) Do not give a myelosuppressive drug unless the starting neutrophil count is >2500/μl and the platelet count is >100,000/μl.
   c) If the neutrophil count is <1500/μl at the nadir, the dose of the myelosuppressive drug is reduced by 25% for future treatments, even if clinical signs do not occur.
   d) If the neutrophil count is <1500/μl, the risk of sepsis is significant. Even if there are no clinical signs, oral antibiotics are given at home with close monitoring.
   e) If mild clinical signs occur (i.e., mild fever without other complaints), oral antibiotics can be given at home with careful monitoring.
   f) If gastrointestinal signs, particularly hemorrhagic colitis, also occur, the risk of sepsis is increased considerably. Animals that have both myelosuppression and gastrointestinal toxicosis are admitted to the hospital for intravenous fluids (nonlactated if the patient has lymphoma) and broad-spectrum antibiotics.
   g) If sepsis occurs, high-rate intravenous fluids and intravenous broad-spectrum antibiotic therapy are started without delay.
   h) See Chap. 66 for therapy of severe thrombocytopenia.
4. Prognosis
   a) With nonclinical myelosuppression or a mild febrile episode, the prognosis is good.
   b) Sepsis is potentially life-threatening, but with aggressive management, most animals have a fair to good prognosis.

B. Gastrointestinal toxicity

1. Clinical signs range from inappetence to vomiting and diarrhea; doxorubicin can cause hemorrhagic colitis.
2. Management is related to severity (see Chaps. 30, 32, 33).
3. Prognosis is good in most cases, particularly if signs are mild and managed appropriately.
   a) Hemorrhagic diarrhea can potentiate sepsis when myelosuppression occurs concurrently.
   b) Extra caution is indicated after cisplatin therapy, when dehydration may potentiate nephrotoxicity.

C. Cardiac toxicity

1. It occurs mainly with long-term anthracycline therapy in dogs.
2. Anthracyclines may cause histologic cardiac changes in cats, but clinical cardiotoxicity has yet to be reported.
3. Acute cardiotoxicity consists of arrhythmias that occur during administration of the drug and are related to peak plasma level and histamine release.
   a) Occurrence is prevented by slow administration.
   b) Arrhythmias occasionally can cause collapse but are self-limited if administration is slowed.
4. Chronic cardiotoxicity resembles dilated cardiomyopathy.
   a) Echocardiographic changes are seen before clinical signs are evident.
   b) Clinical signs are those of congestive heart failure (see Chap. 10).
5. Total cumulative dose of doxorubicin should not exceed 240 mg/m^2.
   a) Breeds susceptible to dilated cardiomyopathy, particularly Dobermans, appear to be more sensitive to this toxicosis.
   b) Each dose of doxorubicin is preceded by careful cardiac auscultation, and a murmur warrants further investigation.
   c) At a cumulative dose of 180 mg/m^2 or greater, each doxorubicin treatment is preceded by echocardiography.
   d) Any evidence of dilatative changes warrants discontinuation of anthracyclines, because the changes can continue to progress after stopping the drug.
   e) When cardiotoxicity occurs, it is managed as dilated cardiomyopathy with congestive heart failure (see Chap. 10).
   f) Liposome-encapsulated doxorubicin may be less cardiotoxic.
6. Prognosis is generally poor to grave; therefore, every effort must be made to prevent this toxicosis.

D. Nephrotoxicity: mainly associated with cisplatin
1. Clinical signs are those of acute or chronic renal failure, azotemia, and uremia.
2. Management is as for acute or chronic renal failure, with dietary management and fluid therapy as needed (see Chap. 47).
3. Prognosis is generally poor to grave. Administration of cisplatin in a saline diuresis protocol significantly reduces the risk of nephrotoxicity.

E. Urothelial toxicity: usually associated with cyclophosphamide and ifosfamide
1. Clinical signs are those of hemorrhagic cystitis, with significant blood loss in severe cases.
2. To prevent cystitis, cyclophosphamide is given in the morning, and the animal is given free access to water and allowed to urinate often, particularly before bedtime.

3. If the animal is also receiving prednisone, both drugs are given on the same day to take advantage of the polyuria caused by prednisone.
4. Ifosfamide causes severe hemorrhagic cystitis so often that it must never be given without the uroprotective thiol drug mesna, which is packaged with ifosfamide.
5. Infectious cystitis is always ruled out by performing a urine culture.
6. Sterile hemorrhagic cystitis may resolve on its own with time, and anti-inflammatories (steroids, piroxicam, methyl sulfonyl methane [MSM]) may make the animal more comfortable.
7. If cystitis persists, intravesicular instillation of 20 ml of 1% formalin or 25% DMSO solution for 20 minutes may help reduce signs.
8. If hemorrhage persists, surgical débridement may be tried.
9. In all cases, cyclophosphamide must be discontinued and another alkylating agent such as chlorambucil substituted.
10. Prognosis is fair to good in most cases.

F. Extravasation reactions
1. Many chemotherapeutic agents are vesicants. Extravasation may cause tissue necrosis severe enough to result in loss of a limb.
   a) The animal may or may not show discomfort at the time of extravasation.
   b) After the incident, there is pain and swelling at the site, followed by a nonhealing lesion in 1–4 weeks.
2. When extravasation occurs, as much drug as possible is withdrawn through the catheter, and then the catheter is removed.
3. Ice or cold compresses are applied for 6–12 hours.
4. Prevent self-trauma and consider surgical intervention.
5. Prognosis is poor, so every effort must be made to avoid this occurrence.
   a) Any chemotherapeutic agent that is potentially caustic, if it requires slow administration, is given through a fresh, patent, "one-stick" catheter.
   b) The catheter is tested with a saline flush before the drug is administered and is flushed again with saline before it is removed.
   c) A butterfly catheter can be used for volumes less than 1 ml.

G. Allergic reactions
1. These are most often associated with L-asparaginase.
2. The risk increases with increased exposure to the drug, so occurrence is unlikely on the first treatment.
3. Doxorubicin may cause hypersensitivity reactions, but this is rarely a problem if the drug is given slowly.

4. Clinical signs may be immediate or slightly delayed but will occur within a few hours. They include general discomfort, erythema of the face and ears, pruritus, head shaking, crying, vomiting, collapse, and cardiovascular shock.
5. Management is as for other causes of anaphylaxis (see Chap. 74).
6. Reaction is uncommon if L-asparaginase is given intramuscularly.
7. Prognosis is good once the immediate episode is controlled, but the animal should not receive L-asparaginase again.

VII. Routes of administration
   A. Most chemotherapeutic drugs are given either orally or intravenously, occasionally intramuscularly or subcutaneously.
   B. Other routes of administration are sometimes used.
      1. Topical: 5-fluorouracil (dogs only)
      2. Intracavitary: particularly for malignant effusions
      3. Intralesional: in a colloid suspension to prevent systemic absorption
      4. Other routes: intrathecal, intra-arterial, intravesicular

VIII. Protocol design
   A. Most chemotherapeutic drugs are best used in combinations called protocols.
   B. Every drug in a protocol should have efficacy as a single agent.
   C. Benefit is greatest when drugs with different mechanisms of action or pathways of resistance are combined to complement one another in terms of antitumor efficacy.

Surgery

I. Indications
   A. Surgery remains the primary form of therapy for localized tumors and is more likely to provide a cure than any other form of therapy.
   B. Surgical aims may include the following.
      1. Cure
         a) A cure depends on the histologic diagnosis and stage.
         b) Benign tumors and well-localized malignant tumors are often cured by surgical removal alone.
         c) Depending on the tumor type, surgical removal followed by radiation (e.g., mast cell tumor) or chemotherapy (e.g., plasmacytoma) may result in a cure.
      2. Local control
         a) Some animals may benefit from local excision even though microscopic metastatic disease is present (e.g., anal sac adenocarcinoma).
         b) Some tumors grow so slowly that local excision may provide long-term tumor control (e.g., hemangiopericytoma).
      3. Debulking
         a) When a tumor is sufficiently large that it is unlikely to be affected by chemotherapy or radiation, the tumor may be debulked (cytoreduced) before using the other modality.
         b) This often reduces the tumor to microscopic disease, which is usually more susceptible to additional treatment modalities (such as radiation or chemotherapy).
      4. Metastatectomy
         a) It is sometimes performed in animals with osteosarcoma metastatic to the lungs. Extremely stringent criteria must be met before such a surgery is undertaken.
         b) Occasionally, lymph nodes containing metastatic disease are removed if they are generating a paraneoplastic syndrome or if they are significantly impairing the animal's quality of life.

II. Principles
   A. Preoperative work-up: staging, CBC, serum biochemical profile
   B. Surgical technique
      1. The first surgery has the best chance of cure; therefore, every effort is made to follow the guidelines described here.
      2. Wide excision of any tumor (1- to 3-cm margin of normal tissue around the tumor) is indicated unless it is known to be benign.
      3. Include needle aspirate or biopsy tracts within the surgical margins to remove any tumor cells that may have seeded these areas.
      4. During excision, the tumor tissue is not incised unless absolutely necessary.
      5. Once the tumor has been removed, clean instruments are used for closure to prevent seeding of tumor cells into the surgical site.
   C. Histopathology
      1. Every mass that has been removed from an animal is submitted for histopathologic evaluation.
      2. To aid in orienting the pathologist during examination of tumor margins, sutures or surgical clips can be used to mark the edges of the tumor (left, right, lateral, dorsal, ventral, and so forth).

III. Cryosurgery
   A. Involves the use of liquid nitrogen or nitrous oxide to induce a controlled rapid freezing and slow thawing of tissues
   B. Mechanisms of cell death after freezing
      1. Direct cellular death occurs immediately after freezing and is caused by ice crystal formation and subsequent damage to cell membranes and proteins.
      2. Vascular collapse secondary to thermal damage to small blood vessels leads to hypoxia and infarction of frozen tissues.
   C. Advantages
      1. Surgical time is short.
      2. Treatment is relatively easy to perform.

3. Multiple treatments and anesthesia are often not necessary.
D. Disadvantages
  1. Equipment can be expensive.
  2. Freezing causes tissue necrosis, so the margins of tumor destruction cannot be easily assessed.
  3. Postoperative care may be more involved than with surgery, as the necrotic tissue must be cleaned and periodically débrided.
E. Indications
  1. Small tumors, especially ones that are benign
  2. May have no advantage over standard surgery, which permits histopathologic identification and evaluation of tumor margins

Radiation Therapy

I. Types of radiotherapy
  A. Systemic therapy involves the systemic administration of the radioactive source (e.g., iodine 131 therapy for thyroid tumors); the animal must be quarantined.
  B. Brachytherapy involves the implantation of a radioactive source; the animal must be quarantined.
  C. Teletherapy involves the delivery of a beam of radiation from a source outside the body.
    1. Orthovoltage radiation is relatively low energy and is used only when megavoltage is not available.
      a) Almost completely absorbed by bone
      b) Poor penetration of soft tissues and uneven, unpredictable deposition relative to megavoltage
      c) More severe side effects to skin and superficial tissues and greater likelihood of serious late effects than with megavoltage
    2. Megavoltage radiation is produced by either a cobalt 60 source machine or a linear accelerator.
      a) High-energy radiation has greater penetration and a more even deposition in tissues.
      b) The predictability of deposition of the radiation allows the use of computer-assisted treatment planning.
      c) Energy does not build to a therapeutic level until it has passed through 5–10 mm of tissue or tissue-equivalent material (bolus), so side effects to skin are minimal.
      d) A linear accelerator can produce photons of different energies, as well as electrons, so flexibility is greater than with cobalt 60.
II. Indications
  A. In most cases it is useful only for diseases that are not systemic or metastatic (although in selected cases it may still be useful for palliation).
  B. Radiation may be used as the primary modality for small and superficial tumors that are radioresponsive (e.g., facial squamous cell carcinoma in cats, acanthomatous epulis).
  C. It is usually most effective when used in combination with other modalities.
    1. Preoperative (neoadjuvant) radiation may be used when a solid tumor is not operable, in the hope of achieving enough shrinkage to permit a surgical approach and to sterilize the edges of the tumor so that it is less likely to be disrupted in surgery.
    2. Postoperative radiation is used in an attempt to eradicate residual tumor when complete surgical excision is not possible.
    3. Intraoperative therapy delivers radiation directly to the surgically opened tumor bed.
    4. Chemotherapeutic drugs may be used to improve the efficacy of radiation by sensitizing the tumor cells (chemoradiotherapy). When drugs are used for this purpose, they may be given by a different schedule than when they are used for their direct cytotoxic effect.
    5. Radiation, surgery, and chemotherapy may be used together, e.g., for soft tissue sarcoma, feline oral squamous cell carcinoma.
  D. Palliative radiation is used when systemic or metastatic disease is present but the animal's quality of life can be improved by shrinking the primary tumor.
    1. When radiotherapy is done with palliative intent, the fractions are often large and infrequent to minimize the stress and time commitment of the animal and owner.
    2. Examples of palliative radiation include the following:
      a) Rapid shrinkage of lymphoma lesions (e.g., submandibular lymph nodes)
      b) Shrinkage of oral tumors, providing relief of pain and dysphagia (e.g., oral melanoma)
      c) Relief of pain associated with bone tumors (e.g., osteosarcoma)
III. Limitations of radiotherapy
  A. Tumor bulk inhibits the efficacy of radiotherapy.
    1. Large tumors have a higher proportion of hypoxic cells (see later).
    2. Large tumors have a higher proportion of cells in a quiescent phase of the cell cycle (G_0), and actively dividing cells are more sensitive.
    3. In most cases, large bulky tumors are surgically debulked before radiotherapy; the radiation oncologist should be consulted prior to surgery.
  B. Molecular oxygen is needed for the production of the free radicals that cause DNA damage, so hypoxic cells are relatively resistant to radiotherapy.
  C. Certain cell types and tumors are intrinsically more radiosensitive or resistant than others, or have better or worse repair capacity.
  D. Because of the sensitivity of certain normal tissues to radiation side effects, tumors in some locations require special consideration.
    1. Treatment of periocular tumors may cause serious ocular side effects (keratitis, cataracts).
    2. Treatment of spinal tumors may induce myelopathy.

3. Treatment of bladder tumors may produce bladder fibrosis.

4. Treatment of thoracic tumors may result in cardiac damage and pulmonary fibrosis.

IV. Treatment protocols

A. The preferred term for units of radiation therapy is the international unit gray (Gy), which equals 100 rad.

B. Total dose of radiation varies with the tumor to be treated, generally ranging from 48–60 Gy. Total dose is administered in individual fractions over the treatment interval.

   1. Frequency of treatment in veterinary medicine is 3–5 times per week.

   2. Time between fractions allows tumor cells to reoxygenate and to redistribute into the proliferative phase of the cell cycle (good) and allows normal and tumor cells to repair and repopulate (good and bad).

   3. Fraction size generally ranges from 2–4 Gy.

   4. Fraction size is the most important determinant of late radiation reactions, so smaller, more frequent fractions (finer fractionation) allow a higher total dose.

V. Complications

A. Early or acute

   1. Common, especially with orthovoltage

   2. Discomfort ranging from mild to severe

   3. Rarely serious, usually heal rapidly

   4. Tissues affected

      a) Skin: hair loss, erythema, dry desquamation, moist desquamation

      b) Oral mucosa: mucositis

      c) Eyes: radiation keratitis, keratoconjunctivitis sicca

   5. Management of complications

      a) To prevent self-trauma, use an Elizabethan collar, padded foot bandages, and so forth.

      b) Clean areas of moist desquamation with warm water, dry them, then apply nongreasy dressing such as aloe vera gel.

      c) For oral mucositis, rinse mouth with cool tea or dilute saline and feed soft, low-salt, aromatic foods.

      d) Enteral feeding tubes are used for animals that are anorexic secondary to radiation complications.

      e) Use artificial tears and antibiotic ointment as needed for keratoconjunctivitis sicca and monitor carefully for signs of corneal ulceration.

      f) Use analgesics as needed and corticosteroids only if discomfort is severe.

B. Late or chronic

   1. These are rare but can be severe.

   2. Organs affected include skin (nonhealing ulcers from loss of perfusion), joints/tendons (fibrosis), lungs (fibrosis), and eyes (cataracts, retinal degeneration).

   3. Secondary tumors, although rare, sometimes develop.

Biologic Response Modifiers

I. Biologic response modifiers are natural or synthetic substances that act to alter the host's response to a tumor, with a subsequent therapeutic benefit.

II. Evidence of the immune system's ability to recognize and eliminate cancer cells comes from several observations.

A. Spontaneous remissions

B. Increased incidence of tumors in immunosuppressed patients

C. Historic reports of tumor regression following treatment with immunomodulators

III. Recent advances in understanding the basis for immune responses have led to the development of new, more effective therapies.

IV. Nonspecific immunomodulators act to generate an antitumor response in an unrestricted fashion.

A. Cytokines

   1. Cytokines are glycoproteins that stimulate growth, differentiation, and effector functions of hematopoietic cells.

   2. Interleukin-2 (IL-2) is a pleiotropic cytokine that activates lymphocytes and natural killer cells, increasing their capacity to kill cancer cells.

      a) Although initially promising as a therapy for malignant melanoma and renal tumors in humans, its use has been limited owing to significant side effects when given systemically.

      b) Efforts are now under way to modify the delivery of IL-2 to limit toxicity (such as encapsulation in liposomes).

   3. IL-12 is another cytokine that activates lymphocytes and natural killer cells but exhibits less systemic toxicity. It is also more effective at directly stimulating cell-mediated immunity (cytotoxic T cells).

   4. Interferons are glycoproteins produced by cells in response to viral infections and other mitogens.

      a) They exhibit cytotoxic, cytostatic, immunomodulatory, and antiangiogenic properties.

      b) Interferons are probably best used in combination with other agents.

B. Hematopoietic growth factors (HGFs)

   1. HGFs are cytokines that promote the differentiation and effector functions of bone marrow–derived cells.

   2. Granulocyte-macrophage colony-stimulating factor (GM-CSF) stimulates the proliferation and maturation of neutrophils and monocytes in the marrow. It also enhances the function of granulocytes, monocytes, and macrophages, improving their ability to kill tumor cells.

   3. Granulocyte colony-stimulating factor (G-CSF) promotes the differentiation of immature neutrophils in the bone marrow. G-CSF is used primarily to decrease the extent and duration of neutropenia associated with some chemotherapy agents.

C. Bacterial agents
1. Bacillus Calmette-Guérin (BCG) is an attenuated mycobacterium shown to have activity in the treatment of some tumors.
2. Muramyl-tripeptide, a derivative of muramyl-dipeptide (a component of bacterial cell walls), nonspecifically activates monocytes and macrophages to kill tumor cells when encapsulated in liposomes. When used in the treatment of canine osteosarcoma and hemangiosarcoma in combination with chemotherapy, this agent produced significant increases in survival times when compared with animals given chemotherapy alone.
3. Other agents include *Corynebacterium parvum* and *Serratia marcescens*.
D. Other agents
1. Acemannan is a mannan polymer derived from the aloe vera plant that has been shown to enhance macrophage and lymphocyte function, primarily through the release of various cytokines. It has been reported to have activity against fibrosarcomas in dogs and cats.
2. Piroxicam (Feldene) is a nonsteroidal anti-inflammatory drug that inhibits the production of prostaglandin E_2, which is an inhibitor of several lymphocyte functions, including cytotoxic activity and cytokine production.
a) Piroxicam administration to dogs with transitional cell carcinoma of the bladder resulted in a 17% response rate.
b) This drug may be useful for other tumors, including squamous cell carcinoma.
3. Differentiating agents promote the maturation of neoplastic cells into a more differentiated, or mature, phenotype.
a) The retinoids are derivatives of vitamin A that have demonstrated some efficacy against epithelial neoplasms, such as squamous cell carcinoma and keratoacanthomas, and some forms of lymphoma (mycosis fungoides) and leukemia (acute promyelocytic leukemia in humans).
b) Etretinate and isotretinoin (Accutane) are two agents that have been used with some success.
V. Specific immunomodulators take advantage of the fact that tumor cells often produce abnormal proteins or embryonic proteins not made in normal cells. These altered or abnormal products can often be distinguished by immune cells, leading to a tumor-specific immune response.
A. Monoclonal antibodies are antibodies of a single specificity that can be engineered to recognize particular tumor-specific antigens. When administered systemically, often with another immunomodulator, they have the potential to recognize and bind to tumor cells, thereby permitting tumor cell destruction through antibody-dependent killing mechanisms.
B. Tumor vaccines are engineered using antigens that are considered unique to the tumor cells.

VI. Delivery of immunomodulators can be achieved in several ways.
A. Liposomes are lipid vesicles that are used to encapsulate various agents for systemic delivery.
1. In addition to limiting the toxicities of these agents, liposomes can be engineered to target specific cell populations.
2. Some forms of liposomes have been designed for oral administration.
B. Transfection of tumor cells with DNA-encoding cytokines or HGFs either in vitro or in vivo is now being used to deliver these agents directly to the tumor. This permits local production of the agent, thereby limiting toxicity.

Photodynamic Therapy

I. Photodynamic therapy (PDT) is a local therapy based on the interaction of a drug (the photosensitizer) with light of a specific wavelength.
II. Mechanism of action of PDT is as follows.
A. The photosensitizer is normally inert unless activated by light. It usually is given systemically and preferentially accumulates in the tumor (mechanism unknown).
B. When exposed to light of the specific wavelength, the drug becomes activated and interacts with molecular oxygen to produce cytotoxic oxygen radicals.
C. Oxygen radicals damage membrane organelles, causing cell death.
III. PDT has been used in veterinary medicine for feline cutaneous squamous cell carcinoma, canine transitional cell carcinoma, soft tissue sarcoma, and mast cell tumors.
IV. There are several considerations regarding administration.
A. Light sources
1. A laser is not absolutely necessary but greatly facilitates PDT. Examples include argon pumped dye, gold vapor, and diode lasers.
2. Wavelength-filtered halogen lamps may also be used.
B. Light administration
1. Fiberoptics allow light distribution to any cavity or lumen by endoscopy, laparoscopy, and so forth.
2. Fiberoptics are more compatible with lasers than with other light sources.
C. Photosensitizers
1. Classic examples are hematoporphyrin derivative (HPD) and Photofrin II.
2. Newer photosensitizers include the phthalocyanines, benzoporphyrin derivatives, chlorins, and others.
V. PDT has several advantages over other modalities.
A. Often only a one-time treatment
B. Can be repeated
C. Minimal toxicity to surrounding normal tissues, well tolerated
VI. Complications and limitations include the following.
A. Light penetration is 5 mm at best.

1. Avoid large tumors; debulking surgery may help.
2. Interstitial PDT buries fiberoptic tips in the tumor to improve penetration.
B. Photosensitizers can accumulate in normal tissues, and the clearance time varies with the photosensitizer used.
C. Rare hypersensitivity reactions have been reported.

Hyperthermia

I. Hyperthermia causes cell death by heating tissues to greater than 42°C.
II. It is most effective in combination with other modalities.
III. Hyperthermia can be applied regionally or to the whole body.
A. Whole body hyperthermia by radiant heat
1. It produces more even tissue heating and is more effective.
2. It is difficult to manage and monitor, so it is limited to institutional research settings.
B. Regional hyperthermia by microwave, radiofrequency, or ultrasound
1. Feasible in practice
2. Limited to lesions <1 cm in diameter
3. Destroys tissue
4. No advantage over traditional surgery

Palliation

I. Palliation is designed to improve the animal's quality of life rather than to affect the course of disease. It is often used in the face of a grave prognosis to ease discomfort.
II. It involves using drugs (analgesics) to manage pain.
A. For all drugs, analgesia is more effective if it is instituted *before* the onset of pain.
1. Anticipate pain whenever possible to prevent it.
2. During postoperative recovery, give analgesia as scheduled rather than postponing a dose because the animal appears comfortable.
B. Nonsteroidal anti-inflammatories provide good analgesia. Their main side effect is gastric upset and ulceration; therefore, give with food or use misoprostol concurrently.
1. Buffered aspirin 10 mg/kg PO BID–TID for dogs, QOD for cats
2. Piroxicam 0.3 mg/kg PO SID for dogs
C. Corticosteroids provide fair analgesia and may also stimulate appetite and a general sense of well-being. Do not over-rely on steroids to the exclusion of nonsteroidals.
D. Injectable narcotics may have a more profound analgesic effect than oral forms.
1. Butorphanol is usually well tolerated but may cause sedation.
a) Dose in dogs: 0.2–0.6 mg/kg IV, IM, or SQ q 1–4 h

b) Dose in cats: 0.1–0.4 mg/kg IV, IM, or SQ q 1–4 h
2. Buprenorphine may be a more potent analgesic than butorphanol.
a) Dose in dogs: 0.005–0.02 mg/kg IV, IM, or SQ q 4–12 h
b) Dose in cats: 0.005–0.01 mg/kg IV, IM, or SQ q 4–12 h
3. Fentanyl transdermal patch is a new analgesic option able to deliver long-term (up to 72 hours), steady-state blood levels of a potent analgesic narcotic at home.
a) Its main disadvantage is that it takes 12–24 hours to become effective; therefore, if pain can be anticipated, the patch should be applied the day before the painful event.
b) A patch can be applied and other analgesia added for the first 12–24 hours to keep the animal comfortable.
c) As the patch begins to lose effect, another can be applied before the first is removed.
d) The dose is 3–5 µg/kg.
III. Palliative radiation may improve the quality of life dramatically in some cases in which the disease is systemic or metastatic, by shrinking the primary tumor or decreasing the discomfort associated with it (see Radiation Therapy, earlier).
IV. Management of other symptoms is also important.
A. Loss of appetite associated with disease or chemotherapy often can be improved with cyproheptadine (Periactin). For dogs and cats the dose is 3 mg/kg PO BID–TID.
B. Corticosteroids often can improve overall sense of well-being, decrease mild pain, and improve appetite.

Bibliography

Abbas AK, Lichtman AH, Pober JS (eds): Cellular and Molecular Immunology. 2nd Ed. WB Saunders, Philadelphia, 1994

Cantley LC, Auger KR, Carpenter C et al: Oncogenes and signal transduction. Cell 64:281, 1991

Cross M, Dexter TM: Growth factors in development, transformation, and tumorigenesis. Cell 64:271, 1991

De Vita VT: Principles of chemotherapy. p. 276. In De Vita VT, Hellman S, Rosenberg SA (eds): Cancer, Principles and Practice. 4th Ed. JB Lippincott, Philadelphia, 1993

De Vita VT, Hellman S, Rosenberg SA (eds): Biologic Therapy of Cancer. JB Lippincott, Philadelphia, 1991

Dickinson KL, Ogilvie GK: Safe handling and administration of chemotherapeutic agents in veterinary medicine. p. 475. In Bonagura JD, Kirk RW (eds): Current Veterinary Therapy XII: Small Animal Practice. WB Saunders, Philadelphia, 1995

Dobson JM, Gorman NT (eds): Cancer Chemotherapy in Small Animal Practice. Blackwell Scientific Publications, Oxford, 1993

Frazier DL, Hahn KA: Commonly used drugs. p. 79. In Hahn KA, Richardson RC (eds): Cancer Chemotherapy, a Veterinary Handbook. Williams & Wilkins, Malvern, PA, 1995

Hellman S: Principles of radiation therapy. p. 248. In De Vita VT, Hellman S, Rosenberg SA (eds): Cancer, Principles and Practice. 4th Ed. JB Lippincott, Philadelphia, 1993

Henry CJ, Brewer WG: Drug interactions with antineoplastic

agents. p. 482. In Bonagura JD, Kirk RW (eds): Current Veterinary Therapy XII: Small Animal Practice. WB Saunders, Philadelphia, 1995

Klein MK: Anticancer drugs: dose schedule and guidelines. p. 478. In Bonagura JD, Kirk RW (eds): Current Veterinary Therapy XII: Small Animal Practice. WB Saunders, Philadelphia, 1995

Knapp DW, Richardson RC, Chan TCK et al: Piroxicam therapy in 34 dogs with transitional cell carcinoma of the urinary bladder. J Vet Intern Med 8:273, 1994

Levine AJ, Perry ME, Chang A et al: The 1993 Walter Hubert lecture: the role of the p53 tumor-suppressor gene in tumorigenesis. Br J Cancer 69:409, 1994

London CA, Vail DM: Tumor biology. p. 16. In Withrow SJ, MacEwen EG (eds): Small Animal Clinical Oncology. 2nd Ed. WB Saunders, Philadelphia, 1996

MacEwen EG, Kurzman ID, Helfand S et al: Current studies of liposome muramyl tripeptide (CGP 19835A Lipid) therapy for metastasis in spontaneous tumors: a progress review. J Drug Targeting 2:391, 1994

Moulton JE: Tumors in Domestic Animals. 3rd Ed. University of California Press, Berkeley, 1990

Ogilvie GK, Moore AS (eds): Managing the Veterinary Cancer Patient. Veterinary Learning Systems, Trenton, NJ, 1995

Tannock IF, Hill RP (eds): The Basic Science of Oncology. 2nd Ed. McGraw-Hill, New York, 1992

Théon AP: Indications and applications of radiation therapy. p. 467. In Bonagura JD, Kirk RW (eds): Current Veterinary Therapy XII: Small Animal Practice. WB Saunders, Philadelphia, 1995

Vail DM, MacEwen EG, Kurzman ID et al: Liposome encapsulated muramyl tripeptide phosphatidylethanolamine (L-MTP-PE) adjuvant immunotherapy for splenic hemangiosarcoma in the dog: a randomized multi-institutional clinical trial. Clin Cancer Res 1:1165, 1995

Weinberg RA: Finding the anti-oncogene. Sci Am 259:44, 1988

Weinberg RA: Oncogenes, anti-oncogenes, and the molecular basis of multistep carcinogenesis. Cancer Res 49:3713, 1989

Withrow SJ: Surgical oncology. p. 58. In Withrow SJ, MacEwen EG (eds): Small Animal Clinical Oncology. 2nd Ed. WB Saunders, Philadelphia, 1996

71

Paraneoplastic Syndromes

Philip J. Bergman

GENERAL CONSIDERATIONS

I. Paraneoplastic syndromes (PNS) are neoplasm-associated alterations in bodily structure and/or function that occur distant to the tumor.
II. Most PNS are systemic with an unknown cause.
III. PNS often result in more morbidity than the malignancy itself and are generally underestimated in importance.
IV. PNS may be the first sign of a malignancy.
V. Persistence of PNS after therapy may signify metastasis or ineffective therapy.

HUMORAL HYPERCALCEMIA OF MALIGNANCY

Definition

I. Synonyms include malignant hypercalcemia, malignancy-associated hypercalcemia, cancer-associated hypercalcemia, and pseudohyperparathyroidism.
II. Humoral hypercalcemia of malignancy (HHM) is characterized by a persistent elevation of serum calcium ($\geq$12 mg/dl) and ionized calcium ($\geq$5.5 mg/dl) in the presence of a non-parathyroid malignancy.
  A. HHM causes clinically important dysfunctions in many organ systems distant from the primary malignancy.
  B. HHM often causes more short-term morbidity and potentially more mortality than the malignancy itself; therefore, proper diagnosis and treatment are imperative for a good clinical outcome.
III. HHM has been reported in the dog and cat in association with a variety of malignancies, predominantly hematopoietic tumors and carcinomas.

Causes

I. The pathogenesis is unclear in some cases, but several pathways seem to operate separately or in tandem.

  A. Ectopic production of peptide similar to parathyroid hormone (PTH), called PTH-related protein (PTH-rP), or of PTH itself
  B. Osteolysis by prostaglandin E (PGE) series, e.g., PGE_{2M}
  C. Ectopic production of osteoclast activating factor (OAF) or OAF-like substances
  D. Direct tumor osteolysis
  E. Others: calcitriol (1,25-dihydroxyvitamin D)
II. Lymphoma is the most common cause of HHM in dogs. See Table 71–1 for neoplasms associated with HHM in domestic animals.

Pathophysiology

I. True humorally mediated bone resorption may produce the hypercalcemia.
  A. PTH-rP or PTH directly stimulates osteoclastic bone resorption.
    1. Parathyroid cancer or skeletal metastases are not present.
    2. PTH-rP is distinct from native PTH.
  B. Prostaglandins of the E series are produced.
    1. Potent local mediators of bone resorption
    2. Explains why some PGE blockers are effective therapeutically
  C. OAF and OAF-like substances are produced.
II. Bone resorption occurs by direct contact of tumor with bone.
  A. Resorbing bone itself increases the rate of osteolysis.
  B. Localization of tumor cells and/or mononuclear phagocytes in bone results in the release of aforementioned bone-resorbing factors.
III. The following sequence is essentially similar in all cases of HHM, but the severity can vary dramatically among cases and malignancies.
  A. Accumulation of calcium continues, despite ongoing homeostatic mechanisms to lower the calcium level.

Table 71–1. **Neoplasms Associated with Humoral Hypercalcemia of Malignancy in Domestic Animals**

Site	Neoplasm
Lymphoid tissue	Lymphoma (lymphosarcoma)
	Lymphocytic leukemia: acute, chronic
	Thymoma (epithelial malignancy)
	Multiple myeloma
Adbominal cavity	Exocrine pancreatic carcinoma
	Gastric carcinoma
Respiratory system	Nasal carcinoma/adenocarcinoma
	Epidermoid carcinoma
Skeletal tissue	Primary bone tumors
	Secondary (metastatic) bone tumors
Reproductive system	Mammary gland tumors
	Interstitial cell tumor
	Seminoma
Skin/soft tissue	Anal sac apocrine adenocarcinoma
	Fibrosarcoma

1. Increased calcitonin secretion, inhibiting bone resorption and antagonizing PTH actions
2. Reduced PTH secretion by parathyroids
3. Increased renal excretion of calcium
4. Decreased intestinal absorption of calcium

B. Continuing hypercalcemia leads to decreased neuromuscular function.
  1. Decreased Q–T intervals on the electrocardiogram
  2. Bradycardia and poor contractility
  3. Gastrointestinal hypomotility
  4. Weakness and sluggish response of muscles
  5. Central nervous system depression and possibly coma and/or seizures

C. Severe, potentially permanent damage to the kidney can occur.
  1. Decreased renal blood flow and glomerular filtration rate from vasoconstrictive properties of calcium
  2. Decreased sensitivity of distal convoluted tubules and collecting ducts to pH
  3. Degeneration of renal epithelial cells
  4. Decreased tubular reabsorption of electrolytes
  5. Decreased ability to concentrate urine, leading to necrosis and calcification of the renal epithelial cells, hypercalcemic nephropathy, and renal failure

Clinical Signs

  I. Anorexia, weight loss
 II. Vomiting
III. Constipation
 IV. Generalized muscle weakness
  V. Lethargy, dehydration
 VI. Polyuria, polydipsia
VII. Bradycardia or other cardiac dysrhythmias
VIII. Hypertension
 IX. Coma or seizures (rarely)

Diagnosis

  I. It is *not* based on clinical signs and physical findings alone; laboratory findings are crucial.
 II. If electrolyte imbalances are suspected from physical findings of neoplasia, perform calcium analysis.
   A. Calcium values must be interpreted in relation to serum albumin or total protein and pH.
   B. The preferred formula uses the albumin level, as it is more accurate than using the total protein corrective formula. The formula is valid only for adult dogs.
     1. Adjusted calcium (mg/dl) = calcium (mg/dl) − albumin (g/dl) + 3.5
     2. Adjusted calcium (mg/dl) = calcium (mg/dl) − 0.4 (total serum protein [g/dl]) + 3.5
   C. Remeasure calcium within 8–12 hours to document persistence of hypercalcemia and to rule out a spurious test result.
   D. Measure ionized calcium, because it is a better determination of true hypercalcemia and obviates the need to use corrective formulas.
   E. Moderate to severe persistent hypercalcemia ($>$14 mg/dl) or evidence of concurrent azotemia is an emergency situation requiring immediate treatment.
III. Other tests useful in the diagnosis of hypercalcemia include the following.
   A. Serum phosphorus
     1. Subnormal or normal concentrations suggest HHM or primary hyperparathyroidism.
     2. HHM-induced severe renal failure can induce hyperphosphatemia.
   B. Serum urea nitrogen and creatinine
     1. Normal early in the course of hypercalcemic nephropathy
     2. Elevated with widespread hypercalcemic nephropathy or primary renal disease
   C. Serum alkaline phosphatase
     1. Normal with cancer-associated hypercalcemia
     2. Elevated with primary hyperparathyroidism, neoplastic invasion of liver, or neoplastic osteolysis
     3. Tissue-specific isoenzyme analysis possibly helpful
   D. Hematologic and immunologic tests
     1. Complete blood count (CBC) may reveal atypical lymphocytes with lymphoma or lymphocytic leukemias.
     2. Serum protein electrophoresis may reveal a monoclonal spike in the gamma (or less likely the beta) region, indicating a possible lymphoproliferative disorder.
   E. Thorough radiographic exam
     1. Findings on skeletal films
       a) Neoplastic osteolysis: diffuse or focal, fractures possible
       b) Skeletal demineralization
         (1) Mild to none with HHM and primary hyperparathyroidism
         (2) Present with chronic renal disease and nutritional hyperparathyroidism

2. Thoracic abnormalities
   a) Mediastinal mass suggestive of lymphoma or thymoma
   b) Enlarged thoracic nodes
   c) Pulmonary metastasis
3. Possible abdominal findings
   a) Hepatosplenomegaly
   b) Enlarged abdominal lymph nodes
   c) Abdominal mass

F. Urinalysis
   1. Low urine specific gravity (usually <1.012)
   2. Hypercalciuria
   3. ± Bence Jones proteinuria
G. Biopsy for identifying neoplasia
   1. Fine-needle aspiration cytology
   2. Excisional or incisional biopsy
   3. Bone marrow aspiration or biopsy
H. Electrocardiogram
I. Rectal palpation/examination

IV. If the preceding diagnostic procedures fail to identify the cause of hypercalcemia, the following procedures may be attempted.
   A. Determination of PTH concentration and ionized calcium simultaneously (see Chaps. 2 and 42)
   B. Determination of prostaglandin concentrations
   C. Exploratory laparotomy and biopsy of any suspicious lesions
   D. Surgical exploration of neck
   E. Corticosteroid challenge test only as a last resort: hampers the diagnosis and potentially the prognosis of some malignancies

Differential Diagnosis

I. Primary hyperparathyroidism
II. Hypervitaminosis D
III. Primary renal disease
IV. Hyperproteinemia
V. Hypoadrenocorticism
VI. Septic osteomyelitis
VII. Normal growth in a young animal (rare)
VIII. Granulomatous disorders
IX. Laboratory error

Treatment

I. Treatment is directed at both the underlying malignancy and the hypercalcemia.
   A. Mild hypercalcemia (12–14 mg/dl): 0.9% NaCl at 50 ml/kg/day to rehydrate the animal and induce diuresis
   B. Moderate hypercalcemia (14–16 mg/dl)
      1. 0.9% NaCl at 50–70 ml/kg/day IV (supplemented with KCl if hypokalemic)
      2. Furosemide 1–3 mg/kg IV SID-BID after rehydration
      3. Prednisone 2 mg/kg PO SID-BID after reaching definitive diagnosis
   C. Hypercalcemic crisis (>16 mg/dl) with oliguric renal failure
      1. Institute more aggressive saline diuresis with ≥80 ml/kg/day IV.

2. Closely monitor urine output and keep output ≥2 ml/kg/hour.
3. Administer sodium bicarbonate only for *severe* acidosis, because acidosis increases the free ionized calcium fraction.
D. Additional treatments to consider in dogs
   1. Calcitonin 4–8 U/kg IM, SQ SID-BID
   2. Mithramycin 0.1–0.2 μg/kg IV for 1–2 doses
   3. Diphosphonates (Didronel) 10–30 mg/kg PO or IV for 1–2 doses
   4. Gallium nitrate 2.5 μg/kg IV SID for 5 days
II. See also therapy of renal failure in Chap. 47.

Patient Monitoring

I. Major complications of HHM include the following.
   A. Oliguric renal failure
   B. Reaction to anticancer therapy
   C. Acid–base and electrolyte disorders
   D. Muscle weakness, coma, and bradycardia
   E. Sepsis
II. Monitor serum calcium, urea nitrogen, and creatinine, as well as urine specific gravity, daily in animals with moderate to severe renal disease.
III. Broad-spectrum antibiotic coverage is usually useful, as many affected animals are immunocompromised.
IV. Serial measurements of calcium are recommended at least monthly during cancer therapy, as recurrence of hypercalcemia may precede clinical recurrence of the malignancy.
V. Warn owners that HHM worsens the prognosis in most instances.

HYPOGLYCEMIA

Definition and Causes

I. Pancreatic tumor hypoglycemia (PTHG) and extrapancreatic tumor hypoglycemia (EPTHG) are characterized by fasting hypoglycemia (<60 mg/dl) in the presence of a neoplasm.
II. PTHG is attributable to a functional pancreatic islet beta-cell tumor.
III. EPTHG may be caused by several malignant conditions in the dog and cat, with hematologic malignancies and carcinomas predominating.
   A. Lymphoma (lymphosarcoma)
   B. Lymphocytic leukemias
   C. Primary lung tumor
   D. Metastatic mammary tumor
   E. Hepatoma
   F. Hemangiosarcoma
   G. Leiomyosarcoma

Pathophysiology

I. PTHG is associated with hyperinsulinemia.
II. The pathogenesis of EPTHG is unclear, but several processes may be involved.
   A. Secretion of insulin or insulin-like substances such as insulin-like growth factor I (IGF-I) and IGF-II (''big'' IGF)

1. Ectopic insulin immunologically similar to native insulin
    2. Nonsuppressible insulin-like activity
  B. Upregulation of insulin receptors
  C. Failure of homeostatic mechanisms
    1. Inhibition of gluconeogenesis or glycogenolysis
    2. Destruction of liver by metastatic disease
    3. Decreased counterregulatory hormone release
  D. Excessive glucose utilization by tumor
III. Neuroglycopenic signs of cerebral dysfunction occur at blood glucose levels <40–45 mg/dl and mimic a wide variety of metabolic and neurologic disorders.
  A. Neuroglycopenic signs are related to the rate of blood glucose decrease and not necessarily to the severity of hypoglycemia.
  B. Onset, severity, and duration of neuroglycopenic signs can vary with external stimuli such as excitement, exercise, fasting, and eating.
  C. Prolonged and severe hypoglycemia can lead to persistent seizure activity and hypoxic damage to the cerebral cortex and lower centers, irreversible damage and significant neuronal degeneration, respiratory center depression, and possibly death.

Clinical Signs

  I. Disorientation and weakness
 II. Hunger or anorexia
III. Nervousness, collapse
 IV. Focal neurologic abnormalities
  V. Seizures, coma
 VI. Signs attributable to compensatory adrenergic effects: tachycardia, vomiting, restlessness

Diagnosis

  I. History may be suggestive of neuroglycopenic signs.
 II. Perform a biochemical panel to document fasting hypoglycemia.
  A. Repeat glucose if it is initially <60 mg/dl.
  B. Submit serum for concomitant insulin assay.
    1. Some animals need 24–48 hours of fasting to demonstrate reproducible hypoglycemia with hyperinsulinemia.
    2. Lengthy fasts require extremely careful monitoring to ensure that severe hypoglycemia does not occur.
  C. Determine amended insulin/glucose ratio (AIGR).
    1. Helps discriminate between insulinoma and other possible causes of hypoglycemia
    2. AIGR formula: serum insulin (μU/ml $\times$ 100) $\div$ [serum glucose (mg/dl) $-$ 30]
    3. AIGR >30: very suggestive of insulinoma
    4. AIGR $\leq$30: insulinoma *not* completely ruled out
III. Tumors associated with EPTHG are often large and may produce signs of a space-occupying lesion.
  A. Radiograph the chest and abdomen.
  B. Biopsy the mass, if present.
  C. Consider exploratory laparotomy to search for neoplasia.

IV. Provocative testing is useful when the diagnosis is uncertain.
  A. Glucagon tolerance test
  B. Glucose tolerance testing (IV or oral)
 V. Amelioration of neuroglycopenia upon treatment with glucose-containing solutions is supportive of the diagnosis but is not pathognomonic for EPTHG or PTHG.

Differential Diagnosis

EPTHG and PTHG must be differentiated from the other etiologies of hypoglycemia as reviewed in Chap. 45.

Treatment

  I. Nonspecific therapy for hypoglycemia
  A. Frequent small feedings
  B. Glucose-containing solutions IV or PO
  C. Hyperglycemic agents for dogs
    1. Prednisone 0.5–1 mg/kg PO BID
    2. Propranolol 10–40 mg PO TID
    3. Diazoxide 5–13 mg/kg PO BID-TID
    4. Hydrochlorothiazide 2–4 mg PO BID
    5. Glucagon 0.03 mg/kg IV
 II. Specific therapy directed at tumor
  A. Surgical excision of primary mass may lead to transient improvement of hypoglycemia, but insulinomas may be multiple or may have metastasized by the time of surgery.
  B. Somatostatin and somatostatin analogues may be useful in dogs, but dosages are presently not well characterized.
  C. Chemotherapy typically is not useful unless the etiology of the EPTHG is known to be responsive to chemotherapy.
  D. Radiation therapy is often of limited use for PTHG and abdominal EPTHG, but it may be of benefit in some cases of thoracic or peripheral EPTHG.

Patient Monitoring

  I. Monitor blood glucose at least every 2 weeks after initial tumor-specific therapy. Once stabilized, monitoring every 4–6 weeks is warranted, as recurrence of hypoglycemia typically precedes clinical recurrence of tumor by weeks to months.
 II. Watch closely for recurrence of neuroglycopenic signs.
III. Warn owner of likelihood of recurrence of tumor and the associated hypoglycemia.
 IV. Postsurgical PTHG cases are monitored for pancreatitis and transient diabetes mellitus.
  A. Owing to long-term endogenous beta-cell suppression, mild hyperglycemia is possible postoperatively in animals with PTHG.
  B. With time, the hyperglycemia abates and is not treated with insulin unless the animal becomes ketotic and/or has persistent blood glucoses >400 mg/dl.

HYPERHISTAMINEMIA

Definition and Causes

I. Increased release of histamine and other mast cell granule constituents from mast cell tumors has been reported primarily in the dog and less commonly in the cat.

II. Mast cell degranulation can occur with any of the following.
   A. Trauma to tumor site
   B. Rapid temperature changes
   C. Surgical manipulation of the tumor
   D. Chemotherapy-induced mast cell lysis

Pathophysiology

I. Mast cell granules and their components, particularly histamine, heparin, and proteolytic enzymes, are released.

II. Histamine binding to ubiquitous H_1 and H_2 receptors results in hypotension, arrhythmias, bronchospasm, and subcutaneous or dermal erythema and pruritus.

III. Histamine binding to gastric mucosal parietal cell H_2 receptors results in hyperacidity in gastric environment, hypergastrinemia, increased mucosal blood flow, gastric epithelial edema, and subsequent ulceration.

Clinical Signs

I. Animal possibly asymptomatic
II. Poor hemostasis, melena and hematemesis
III. Abdominal pain
IV. Subcutaneous or dermal erythema and potential hemorrhage
V. Pruritus
VI. Hypotension with collapse or weakness
VII. Arrhythmias
VIII. Bronchospasm with dyspnea
IX. Poor healing of traumatic or surgical sites

Diagnosis

I. Perform a fine-needle aspiration (FNA) of peripheral mass and examine cytologically to identify mast cells.
   A. Thirty seconds of fixation (step 1) in Diff-Quik system promotes identification of granules in mast cells.
   B. The preferred stains for identification of mast cell granules that do not stain with Diff-Quik are Wright's stain and toluidine blue.

II. Nonperipheral mast cell tumors may require additional diagnostic tests.
   A. Abdominal radiography
   B. Abdominal ultrasonography and guided biopsy or FNA
   C. Thoracic radiography
   D. Bone marrow aspiration and/or biopsy

III. Gastrin assays are rarely available.

Differential Diagnosis

I. See Chap. 91 for other causes of skin tumors.
II. See Chap. 68 for other causes of splenomegaly.
III. See Chap. 32 for other causes of melena.

Treatment

I. Minimize manipulation of or temperature changes to the primary mast cell tumor to decrease the chances of iatrogenic degranulation.

II. Perform a wide surgical excision of the mast cell tumor (3-cm margins laterally and at least one fascial plane deep).

III. Pretreat with the following agents if significant surgical manipulation and, therefore, degranulation are anticipated.
   A. Diphenhydramine (H_1 blocker) 1 mg/kg IM
   B. H_2 blockers
      1. Cimetidine 4–6 mg/kg PO, SQ, or IV BID-QID
      2. Ranitidine 1–2 mg/kg PO, SQ, or IV BID
   C. Corticosteroids: prednisone 1–2 mg/kg PO SID-BID

IV. H_1 and H_2 blockers may be useful until suture removal to promote healing at the surgical site, but no conclusive studies have been performed.

Patient Monitoring

I. Serial rechecks of the incision are recommended every 7 days to evaluate healing.

II. If the resection was incomplete, degranulation with subsequent poor healing and pruritus may result, necessitating measures (Elizabethan collars, side bars, neck rings, protective coverings, sedation, etc.) to ensure that the animal does not scratch or lick at the incision site.

III. Monitor for development of additional mast cell tumors.

CACHEXIA/ANOREXIA COMPLEX

Definition

I. It is a phenomenon characterized by severely reduced body weight leading to emaciation and debility associated with a decreased, unchanged, or increased appetite.

II. Cachexia can occur in the absence of anorexia from profound alterations in host metabolism.

III. This complex is a common finding in many animals with cancer at some time during the course of their illness.

Causes

I. Anorexia
   A. Altered odor or taste perception
   B. Substances associated with anorexia

1. Lactate
2. Ketones
3. Tumor-derived or tumor-induced circulating factors
   a) Tumor necrosis factor
   b) Interleukin-1 alpha
C. Direct effects of tumor on the appetite center
D. Modification of eating behavior by an aberrant metabolic compound
E. Physical impingement by tumor on upper gastrointestinal tract
II. Cachexia
   A. Imbalance between caloric intake and expenditure
      1. Hypophagia
      2. Poor digestion and absorption
      3. Tumor and host competing for nutrients
      4. External nutrient loss
      5. Increased host energy expenditure
   B. Altered metabolism of glucose and other fuel sources
      1. Increased basal metabolic rate in face of caloric deficit
      2. Increased Cori cycle (lactate breakdown) activity, resulting in increased inefficient energy expenditure
      3. Glucose intolerance
      4. Marked insulin resistance
      5. Abnormal insulin production
      6. Altered protein synthesis and catabolism
      7. Altered fat catabolism and synthesis
      8. Decreased anabolic enzymes
      9. Increased catabolic enzymes
   C. Factors implicated in altering metabolism
      1. Interferons (IFN-γ)
      2. Interleukins (IL-1 and IL-6)
      3. Altered thyroid homeostasis
      4. Adrenocorticotropic hormone (ACTH)–like hormone
      5. Tumor necrosis factor (TNF)
      6. Prostaglandin E_2
      7. D-factor

Pathophysiology

I. Syndrome often begins with anorexia and decreased absorption of nutrients.
II. Substantially increased metabolism, subsequent host depletion of stored carbohydrates and fats, and muscle breakdown occur early in the complex.
III. Organ structure and function begin to deteriorate, resulting in cachexia and increased morbidity.
IV. No direct relationship exists between the degree of cachexia and caloric intake, tumor burden, tumor cell type, or anatomic site of involvement, although gastrointestinal tumors compound the problems of anorexia and cachexia owing to sheer space limitations.

Clinical Signs

I. Early satiety
II. Anorexia, hypophagia
III. Weight loss, marked debilitation
IV. Anemia

Diagnosis

I. History of change in appetite concomitant with weight loss
II. Neoplastic condition(s) discovered on physical examination
III. Thoracic and abdominal radiographs, or abdominal ultrasonographic findings of masses with or without metastatic disease

Differential Diagnosis

I. Starvation
II. Extreme parasitic infestation
III. Endocrine disorders
   A. Hyperthyroidism
   B. Hypopituitarism
   C. Hypoadrenocorticism
   D. Diabetes mellitus
IV. Central nervous system lesions
V. Chronic infectious diseases
   A. Feline infectious peritonitis (FIP)
   B. Systemic mycoses
VI. Malabsorption/maldigestion syndromes

Treatment

I. Criteria for dietary supplementation
   A. Oral intake $\leq$80% of recommended protein and calories
   B. Presence of stomatitis or gastrointestinal problems
   C. Weight loss >10% of normal weight
   D. Fever or sepsis
   E. Albumin <2.5 g/dl
II. Dietary guidelines
   A. Special oral diets and nutrients
      1. Protein 4–7 g/kg/day (high biologic value: eggs, meat)
      2. Fat 1.3–1.5 g/kg
      3. Calories 75–120 kcal/kg/day
      4. Vitamin supplementation
      5. Carbohydrates 10–10.5 g/kg/day
   B. Tube feeding, e.g., percutaneous endoscopic gastrostomy (PEG) tube
   C. Total parenteral nutrition (TPN)
III. Enhanced palatability
   A. Warm food slightly.
   B. Flavor with meat or animal fat.
   C. Give multiple smaller feedings throughout the day.
   D. Flavor slightly with onion or garlic.
IV. Anabolic agents
   A. Questionable efficacy and can be hepatotoxic
   B. Stanozolol 1–4 mg PO BID
   C. Nandrolone decanoate 1–5 mg/kg IM weekly (maximum 200 mg/week)
V. Appetite stimulants
   A. Cyproheptadine (cats) 1–2 mg PO SID-BID

B. Diazepam (cats) 0.05–0.15 mg/kg IV SID-QOD or 1 mg PO SID

C. Megestrol acetate (questionable efficacy and potentially toxic) 0.5 mg/kg PO SID for 4–7 days, then weekly to every 2 weeks

D. Prednisone 1–2 mg/kg PO SID-BID

VI. Specific anticancer therapy

VII. Erythropoietin for severe anemia (see Chap. 47)

Patient Monitoring

I. Weigh the animal weekly.

II. Have the owner weigh food portions at home and keep a diary of intake.

III. Monitor for progressive emaciation.

IV. Perform CBC every 2 weeks, monitoring for anemia.

V. Perform biochemical profile monthly to monitor for changes in albumin, total protein, and other organ functions.

VI. Warn the owner that marked cachexia typically portends a poor prognosis and may be the most important prognostic factor in clinical outcome for a wide variety of tumor types.

VII. Consider these precautions.

A. Anticancer therapies can potentially worsen existing anorexia/cachexia.

B. Parenteral dietary manipulation may have significant adverse metabolic consequences; therefore, gastrostomy and/or jejunostomy tubes are preferred.

HYPERTROPHIC OSTEOPATHY

See Chap. 79.

FEVER OF UNKNOWN ORIGIN

Definition

I. Fever of unknown origin (FUO) is characterized by an intermittent or continuous body temperature of ≥103°F (39.7°C) that lasts ≥2 weeks and remains undiagnosed after multiple days of in-hospital diagnostic tests and evaluation.

II. Fever can be a common presenting sign in dogs and cats with neoplastic diseases.

Causes and Pathophysiology

I. Neoplasms associated with FUO in dogs and cats are as follows.

A. Lymphoma, especially hepatic

B. Various leukemias, myeloproliferative disorders (MPDs)

C. Multiple myeloma

D. Mast cell tumor (mastocytoma)

E. Hepatic neoplasms

F. Intracranial tumors

G. Can occur with any neoplasm, especially if undergoing active necrosis and/or secondary infection

II. Neoplasms may produce endogenous pyrogens, especially IL-1 and IL-6.

III. Interaction of sensitized host lymphocytes with tumor-related or tumor-specific antigens may result in release of various lymphokines that stimulate production of endogenous pyrogens by host macrophages and/or neutrophils.

Clinical Signs

I. Persistent fever

II. Weight loss

III. Anorexia

IV. Lethargy, dehydration

Diagnosis/Differential Diagnosis

I. Obtain a complete history and physical exam pursuing a diagnosis of neoplasia.

II. Measure body temperature every 8–12 hours to document persistence of fever.

III. Perform routine diagnostic tests.

A. CBC

B. Serum biochemical profile

C. Urinalysis

D. Thoracic and abdominal radiography

IV. Rule out other potential causes of FUO by performing the following.

A. Electrocardiogram and echocardiogram

B. Aerobic and anaerobic blood cultures

C. Arthrocentesis of multiple joints

D. Serologic testing

1. Rickettsial diseases

2. Immune-mediated diseases

3. Systemic mycoses

4. Bacterial and viral diseases

E. Abdominal ultrasonography

F. Upper and lower gastrointestinal contrast studies

G. Skeletal radiographic study

H. Excretory urography

V. If fever persists and the preceding tests suggest a potential disease process that cannot otherwise be adequately evaluated, consider invasive diagnostic tests.

A. FNA and cytology of any abnormal area

B. Bone marrow aspiration and/or biopsy

C. Lymph node aspiration and/or biopsy

D. Liver, spleen, bowel, or bone biopsy

E. Exploratory laparotomy

Treatment

I. Prophylactic antibiotic therapy is appropriate only for animals with concurrent leukopenia and/or inflamed, necrotic, or secondarily infected neoplasms.

II. Primary therapy against tumor involves surgery, chemotherapy, and/or radiation therapy.

III. Consider nonspecific antiprostaglandin therapy if fever persists.

A. Aspirin

1. Dogs: 5–10 mg/kg PO SID-BID

2. Cats: 3–6 mg/kg PO q 54 h (not routinely recommended, but may be tried)
   B. Gastrointestinal protectants in addition

Patient Monitoring

I. Record body temperature SID–QID.
II. Obtain a CBC every 2–4 weeks, monitoring for leukopenia and/or evidence of sepsis.
III. Watch for complications of existing leukopenia or infection, if present.
IV. Watch for evidence of tumor recurrence.
V. Weigh the animal every 1–2 weeks and manage nutrition appropriately.

INAPPROPRIATE SECRETION OF ANTIDIURETIC HORMONE

Definition

I. Syndrome of ectopic production and continued secretion of antidiuretic hormone (ADH) in the face of hyponatremia, low plasma osmolality, and high urine osmolality
II. Also known as ectopic ADH production syndrome, ectopic vasopressin syndrome, and syndrome of inappropriate ADH (SIADH)
III. Documented in dogs with lymphoma, undifferentiated carcinoma, and meningeal sarcoma

Causes

I. Neoplastic diseases
   A. Lymphoma
   B. Intracranial tumors (especially meningioma)
   C. Bronchogenic carcinoma
   D. Mesothelioma
   E. Pancreatic adenocarcinoma
   F. Leiomyosarcoma
   G. Thymoma
   H. Undifferentiated carcinomas
   I. Possibly associated with any tumor
II. Chemotherapeutic agents
   A. Cyclophosphamide
   B. Vincristine and vinblastine
III. Non-chemotherapeutic agents
   A. Opiates
   B. Barbiturates
   C. Histamine
   D. Isoproterenol
   E. Chlorpropamide

Pathophysiology

I. ADH causes increased permeability to water at the distal nephron and collecting ducts.
II. Marked expansion of extracellular fluid volume occurs.
III. Progressively worsening hyponatremia develops.
   A. Increased reabsorption of water
   B. Increased urinary sodium excretion

C. Shifting of sodium from extracellular to intracellular compartment
IV. Overall, plasma osmolality is reduced.
V. Increased urine osmolality arises from hypernatriuresis concurrent with reduced plasma osmolality.

Clinical Signs

I. Clinical signs may be absent in the initial phases.
II. Signs begin to occur when sodium level reaches a critical value (usually <125 mEq/L).
   A. Anorexia
   B. Nausea, vomiting
   C. Weakness, confusion, and stupor
   D. Seizures and coma
III. Increases in body weight may be noted from water retention.

Diagnosis

I. Suspicious laboratory test results
   A. Severe hyponatremia
   B. High urine osmolality
   C. Increased fractional excretion of sodium
   D. Normal renal function
II. Evidence of neoplastic disease in history and on physical examination
III. History of chemotherapeutic or other drug use as listed earlier
IV. Assay for ADH (bioassay or radioimmunoassay and reference ranges dependent on the laboratory performing the assay)

Differential Diagnosis

I. Excessive hypothalamic-pituitary release of ADH
   A. Head trauma
   B. Cerebrovascular accidents
   C. Infectious agents: bacterial, viral, mycotic, and mycobacterial
   D. Intracranial tumors
   E. Severe pulmonary infections
   F. Granulomatous inflammation
II. Chronic diuretic administration
III. Osmoregulatory system malfunction
   A. ADH release occurs at lower levels of plasma osmolality and sodium concentration than is normal.
   B. Sodium level is usually 125–135 mEq/L.
IV. Iatrogenic hypoadrenocorticism
V. Severe sodium depletion from variety of causes
VI. Chronic renal failure
VII. Severe hypothyroidism

Treatment

I. Treatment of the underlying malignancy is the primary objective.
II. Discontinue chemotherapeutics if they are thought to be causing the SIADH.
III. Mild hyponatremia is treated with the following.

A. Moderate water restriction (gradual and progressive)

B. 0.9% saline 50–60 ml/kg/day

C. Demeclocycline 3–6 mg/kg PO SID-BID to counteract action of ADH on renal tubules

D. In refractory cases, lithium carbonate 25 mg/kg PO SID to antagonize renal action of ADH

IV. Severe hyponatremia with onset of seizures and/or coma is treated with the following.

A. Hypertonic saline 5–20 ml/kg IV PRN

B. Aggressive furosemide diuresis at 1–4 mg/kg IV or IM SID-QID

C. Demeclocycline as earlier, once stabilized

Patient Monitoring

I. Adjust water intake and/or medication levels to attempt to keep sodium levels at 135–150 mEq/L or the urine:plasma osmolality ratio at 2.5–5.

II. Weigh the animal every 2–3 days; weight should slowly decrease on appropriate therapy as extracellular fluid volume returns to normal.

III. Measure serum sodium every 4 weeks once normalized.

IV. Begin monitoring plasma and urine osmolality with any recurrence of hyponatremia.

HYPERVISCOSITY SYNDROME

Definition and Causes

I. Hyperviscosity syndrome (HVS) is characterized by poor circulatory flow from an increased viscosity, or sludging, within the blood vascular system.

II. HVS disorders include blood sludging syndrome, M component disorder, hyperglobulinemia-hyperviscosity syndrome, and bleeding diathesis–associated HVS.

III. The pathogenesis of HVS is associated with either an increased protein level or a hypercellular state that impedes vascular movement owing to simple increased viscosity properties.

IV. The most common etiology of HVS in clinical practice is multiple myeloma.

V. Occasionally, infection-associated hyperglobulinemias (e.g., FIP, rickettsial diseases) reach a protein level consistent with the genesis of HVS.

VI. Other malignancies associated with HVS include the following.

A. Polycythemia

B. Hyperleukocytic acute or chronic leukemias

C. Lymphoma (lymphosarcoma)

D. Various dysproteinemias

E. Variety of solid tumors

F. Primary macroglobulinemia

Pathophysiology

I. Excessive secretion of immunoglobulin by a monoclonal line of immunoglobulin-producing cells occurs.

II. An excessive number of cells (either red cells or leukocytes) occurs, causing sludging within the vascular system and microvascular collapse owing to lodging of cells in small capillaries.

III. Hyperviscosity causes an increased demand on the heart, leading to a hypertrophic cardiomyopathy–like state.

IV. Decreased renal perfusion from increased viscosity leads to poor concentrating ability and potential renal epithelial damage from a partial hypoxic state.

V. HVS from elevated proteins interferes with normal platelet function, and the paraproteins act as coagulation factor inhibitors (and potentially bind coagulation factors), causing abnormally prolonged coagulation times.

VI. Severe sludging in the central nervous system can lead to weakness, disorientation, and potentially seizures in severe cases.

VII. Sludging in microcapillaries of bone and eye can lead to bone pain and to retinal hemorrhages and blindness, respectively.

Clinical Signs

I. Ecchymoses, petechiae, epistaxis, melena, and gingival bleeding

II. Blindness

III. Weakness, disorientation, and seizures

IV. Polydipsia/polyuria

V. Exercise intolerance

VI. Shifting limb lameness

VII. Anorexia, lethargy

Diagnosis

I. HVS is suspected when clinical signs are present with the following.

A. Increased protein concentration on biochemical profile

B. Increased cell count on CBC

II. Hyperviscosity is confirmed by the following.

A. Serum and urine protein electrophoresis

B. Serum (or urine) immunoelectrophoresis

C. Bence Jones protein test on urine

III. To determine the cause of HVS, consider the following tests.

A. Bone marrow aspiration and cytology

B. FNA or biopsy of any suspicious lesions

C. Chest and abdominal radiography

D. Retinal examination

E. Survey skeletal radiography

F. Coagulation profile

G. *Ehrlichia* titer and other rickettsial titers

H. Erythropoietin levels (see Chap. 63)

Treatment

I. Best therapy is to treat the inciting cause.

A. Multiple myeloma (see Chap. 75)

B. Lymphoma (see Chap. 67)

II. Administer IV fluids (0.45% NaCl or 5% dextrose

in water at 30–60 ml/kg/day) for dehydration and renal disease.
III. Consider broad-spectrum antibiotics, as many HVS animals are also immunocompromised.
IV. Plasmapheresis is indicated in severe cases that are not responsive to the preceding therapeutics.
  A. Blood is collected in plastic collection bags.
  B. The plasma is siphoned off, and the remaining red blood cells are resuspended in an equivalent volume of sterile normosaline for transfusion back to the animal.

Patient Monitoring

I. Gradual decreases in globulin can be expected over 4–8 weeks with proper treatment for multiple myeloma.
  A. A CBC and globulin level test are performed every 14 days until normal and then every 8 weeks.
  B. Monitor for recurrence and chemotherapy-associated leukopenia every 3–4 weeks.
II. Continue monitoring for bleeding problems until protein level returns to normal.
III. Prognosis is dependent on the etiology of HVS.

OTHER PARANEOPLASTIC SYNDROMES

See Table 71–2.

Bibliography

Bergman PJ, Bruyette DS, Coyne BE et al: Canine clinical peripheral neuropathy associated with pancreatic islet cell carcinoma. Prog Vet Neurol 5:57, 1994
Bick RL: Coagulation abnormalities in malignancy: a review. Semin Thromb Hemost 18:353, 1992
Braund KG: Remote effects of cancer on the nervous system. Semin Vet Med Surg (Small Anim) 5:262, 1990
Braund KG, McGuire JA, Henderson RA: Peripheral neuropathy associated with malignant neoplasms in dogs. Vet Pathol 24:16, 1987
Bunn PA, Ridgway EC: Paraneoplastic syndromes. p. 2026. In DeVita VT, Hellman S, Rosenberg SA (eds): Cancer: Principles and Practice of Oncology. JB Lippincott, Philadelphia, 1993
Center SA, Randolph JF, Erb HN, Reiter S: Eosinophilia in the cat: a retrospective study of 312 cases (1985–1986). J Am Anim Hosp Assoc 26:349, 1990
Chew DJ, Carothers M: Hypercalcemia. Vet Clin North Am [Small Anim Pract] 19:265, 1989
Chew DJ, Nagode LA, Carothers M: Disorders of calcium: hypercalcemia and hypocalcemia. p. 116. In DiBartola SP (ed): Fluid Therapy in Small Animal Practice. WB Saunders, Philadelphia, 1992
Comer KM: Anemia as a feature of primary gastrointestinal neoplasia. Compend Contin Educ Pract Vet 12:13, 1990
Couto CG: Tumor-associated eosinophilia in the dog. J Am Vet Med Assoc 184:837, 1984
Duncan ID: Peripheral neuropathy in the dog and cat. Prog Vet Neurol 2:111, 1990
Hammer AS, Couto CG, Swardsen C et al: Hemostatic abnormalities in dogs with hemangiosarcoma. J Vet Intern Med 5:11, 1991
Hargis AM, Feldman BF: Evaluation of hemostatic defects secondary to vascular tumors in dogs: 11 cases (1983–1988). J Am Vet Med Assoc 198:891, 1991
Helfand SC, Couto CG, Madewell BR: Immune-mediated thrombocytopenia associated with solid tumors in dogs. J Am Anim Hosp Assoc 21:787, 1985
Keller ET: Immune-mediated disease as a risk factor for canine lymphoma. Cancer 70:2334, 1992
Klebanow ER: Thymoma and acquired myasthenia gravis in the dog: a case report and review of 13 additional cases. J Am Anim Hosp Assoc 28:63, 1992
Leifer CE, Peterson ME: Hypoglycemia. Vet Clin North Am [Small Anim Pract] 14:873, 1984
Lennon VA, Kryzer TJ, Griesmann GE et al: Calcium-channel antibodies in the Lambert-Eaton syndrome and other paraneoplastic syndromes. N Engl J Med 332:1467, 1995
MacEwen EG, Hurvitz AI: Diagnosis and management of monoclonal gammopathies. Vet Clin North Am [Small Anim Pract] 7:119, 1977
Madewell BR, Feldman BF: Characterization of anemias associated with neoplasia in small animals. J Am Vet Med Assoc 176:419, 1980
Matus RE, Leifer CE: Immunoglobulin-producing tumors. Vet Clin North Am [Small Anim Pract] 15:741, 1985
Meuten DJ, Capen CC, Kociba GJ et al: Ultrastructural evaluation of adenocarcinomas derived from apocrine glands of the anal sac associated with hypercalcemia in dogs. Am J Pathol 107:167, 1982a
Meuten DJ, Chew DJ, Capen CC et al: Relationship of serum total calcium to albumin and total protein in dogs. J Am Vet Med Assoc 180:63, 1982b
Ogilvie GK: Alterations in metabolism and nutritional support for veterinary cancer patients: recent advances. Compend Contin Educ Pract Vet 15:925, 1993
Ogilvie GK, Walters LM, Fettman MJ et al: Energy expenditure in dogs with lymphoma fed two specialized diets. Cancer 71:3146, 1993
O'Keefe DA, Couto CG: Coagulation abnormalities associated with neoplasia. Vet Clin North Am [Small Anim Pract] 18:157, 1988
Rosol TJ, Capen CC: Biology of disease—mechanisms of cancer-induced hypercalcemia. Lab Invest 67:690, 1992
Ruslander D, Page R: Perioperative management of paraneoplastic syndromes. Vet Clin North Am [Small Anim Pract] 25:47, 1995
Silverman P, Distelhorst CW: Metabolic emergencies in clinical oncology. Semin Oncol 16:504, 1989
Tashjian AH: Prostaglandins, hypercalcemia and cancer. N Engl J Med 293:1317, 1975
Vail DM, Ogilvie GK, Wheeler SL: Metabolic alterations in patients with cancer cachexia. Compend Contin Educ Pract Vet 12:381, 1990a

Vail DM, Ogilvie GK, Wheeler SL et al: Alterations in carbohydrate metabolism in canine lymphoma. J Vet Intern Med 4:8, 1990b

Weir EC, Burtis WJ, Morris CA et al: Isolation of a 16,000-dalton parathyroid hormone–like protein from two animal tumors causing humoral hypercalcemia of malignancy. Endocrinology 123:2744, 1988a

Weir EC, Nordin RW, Matus RE et al: Humoral hypercalcemia of malignancy in canine lymphosarcoma. Endocrinology 122:602, 1988b

SECTION **X**

Immune System

72

Introduction

Kevin T. Schultz

GENERAL CONSIDERATIONS

Role and Components

I. The fundamental role of the immune system is to provide protection against invasion by microorganisms, chemical agents, and other foreign substances.
   A. The immune system accomplishes this by responding to molecules called antigens.
   B. The immune system has developed many means of reacting to and eliminating antigens, including neutralization of infectious organisms and biologically active molecules and lysis of foreign or altered cells (e.g., tumor cells or virus-infected cells, transplanted cells). This removal can be nonspecific or specific for a given antigen.

II. The host immune response is multicellular and can be divided into two main components.
   A. The nonspecific immune response (also called innate resistance) is one component and includes such barriers as skin, secretions, and the phagocytic and complement systems.
   B. The specific immune responses, which involve the humoral and cellular immune systems, are the other component.

IMMUNE SYSTEM

General Features

I. Specific: Cells of the immune system are genetically programmed for a particular antigen but respond to this antigen only after encountering it or a very similar (cross-reactive) antigen.

II. Heterogeneous: The immune system can respond to a wide variety of antigens.

III. Memory or learning: The immune system is capable of responding more rapidly on subsequent exposure to an antigen. This feature is important in immunization programs.

IV. Can distinguish self and nonself: Under normal circumstances the immune system does not respond to self-antigens (antigens of host origin).

A. The immune cells bind to structures (antigens) on self-cells. These structures are called major histocompatibility antigens (MHC).
B. The immune cells react only if a foreign antigen is on these same self-cells.

Anatomy

I. Primary lymphoid tissue
   A. Site of origin of lymphoid stem cells: fetal liver, bone marrow in the adult
   B. Sites of maturation and differentiation of lymphoid cells
      1. Bone marrow: probably the site of maturation and differentiation of B lymphocytes in mammals
      2. Thymus: site of maturation and differentiation of T lymphocytes

II. Secondary lymphoid tissue
   A. Once the lymphocytes reach functional maturity, they migrate from the primary lymphoid tissues and populate the secondary lymphoid structures located throughout the body.
   B. These secondary structures are the sites where antigen and lymphocytes interact to produce a specific immune response.
   C. The various secondary lymphoid structures include the following.
      1. Lymph nodes: filter and trap antigen from both tissue lymphatics and the bloodstream
      2. Spleen: filters and traps antigen directly from the bloodstream
      3. Mucosa-associated lymphoid tissue: responsible for initiating a specialized secretory immune response that acts to protect the various mucosal organs of the body

III. Cell types
   A. B lymphocytes (B cells)
      1. These cells mediate the humoral immune response.
      2. They produce antibody.
   B. T lymphocytes (T cells)
      1. These cells mediate the cellular immune response.

2. They are further divided into T-cytotoxic cells, which kill cells such as virus-infected cells, and T-helper cells, which produce substances called lymphokines that help other specific and nonspecific immune system cells to proliferate and/or differentiate.
C. Natural effector cells (NEC) and killer (K) cells
1. Both of these are naturally occurring, nonspecific, cytotoxic effector cells that do not require antigenic stimulation for function.
2. They lyse or "kill" virus-infected cells, tumor cells, or other foreign cells such as transplants.
3. Killer cells require an antibody-coated target cell to function.

Function

I. Humoral immune system
A. The function of the humoral immune system is the production of immunoglobulin (antibody) against specific antigens following antigenic challenge.
B. The immunoglobulins (Igs) found in the circulation are IgG, IgM, IgA, and IgE.
C. IgG and IgM are the major immunoglobulin classes involved in a systemic immune response.
1. Primary antibody response
a) Antigen is transported to the regional lymph node, where it is processed by macrophages.
b) The processed antigen is presented to T-helper cells, and these T-helper cells produce lymphokines called interleukins (ILs), such as IL-4, IL-5, and IL-6, which are involved in B-cell differentiation.
c) The B cell is activated to undergo division (clonal expansion) to form a large population of B cells with specificity to that particular antigen.
d) After clonal expansion, two populations of cells emerge—plasma cells producing antibody and memory cells.
e) The first antibody produced is of the IgM class.
f) As the response continues, the antibody class switches to IgG.
g) As the antibody removes antigen from the circulation, clonal expansion stops and the amount of antibody slowly decreases.
2. Secondary antibody response
a) There is a shorter period before antibody is detected.
b) Antibody is produced at a faster rate, the amounts are greater, and it persists longer.
c) The predominant class of antibody is IgG.
D. IgE is primarily involved in allergic reactions.
E. A special type of antibody, secretory IgA, is produced by plasma cells of the mucosa-associated lymphoid tissue. Secretory IgA is secreted into the lumen of the mucosal organ and bathes the epithelial cells to provide protection of the mucosal surface.

II. Cellular immune system
A. After activation of antigen-specific T cells, clonal expansion results in a large population of antigen-specific T cells as well as memory cells.
B. Two major types of effector mechanisms are operable in a cellular immune response.
1. Direct effect: T cells may lyse target cells directly and are called T-cytotoxic cells.
2. Indirect effect: Activated T cells (T-helper cells) release soluble factors called lymphokines that can act on cells of the nonspecific immune system such as macrophages. These macrophages may then eliminate the antigen. Alternatively, the lymphokines may kill a target cell directly.
C. Regulatory T cells regulate the immune response.
1. T-helper cells aid in the activation of B cells during an antibody response to an antigen.
2. Other T-helper cells act to "turn off" or suppress a humoral (antibody) or cellular immune response.

PHAGOCYTIC SYSTEM

General Features

I. Nonspecific
II. Lacks memory
III. Can distinguish self and nonself

Cell Types

I. Neutrophils: phagocytic cells that function primarily in bacterial infections
II. Monocytes: mononuclear phagocytic cells found in the peripheral blood
III. Macrophages
A. They are the tissue form of mononuclear phagocytes located primarily in the liver, spleen, lymph nodes, lungs, and connective tissue.
B. These cells act primarily as nonspecific barriers to antigens by filtering them out of the bloodstream. Those antigens that escape this barrier are exposed to the specific components of the immune system.

Function

I. Phagocytic cells have surface receptors for the Fc portion of immunoglobulin and a number of complement components, especially C3b. These receptors enhance phagocytosis of antibody- and complement-coated (opsonized) antigens.
II. Following phagocytosis, the antigen is degraded and eliminated from the body.
III. Macrophages can be "activated" by lymphokines secreted by T cells to become more efficient phagocytes, and are also involved in antigen processing.

COMPLEMENT SYSTEM

Components

I. This system consists of at least 20 chemically and immunologically distinct serum proteins. These proteins interact with each other, with antibody, and with cell membranes.

II. These interactions lead to the generation of various biologic activities.

    A. Inflammation: the most important biologic activity of complement activation

    B. Chemotaxis or directional migration of neutrophils

    C. Promotion of phagocytosis

    D. Lysis of bacteria, virus, virus-infected cells, tumor cells, and so forth

Bibliography

Benjamini E, Leskowitz S: Immunology: A Short Course. 2nd Ed. Wiley-Liss, New York, 1992

Tizzard I: An Introduction to Veterinary Immunology. 4th Ed. WB Saunders, Philadelphia, 1992

73

Immunodeficiency Disorders

Urs Giger
Peter J. Felsburg

GENERAL INFORMATION

Definition

I. Immunodeficiency disorders are caused by defects in the host defense and immune response against microorganisms, resulting in increased susceptibility to infectious diseases (Felsburg, 1994).

II. Key clinical features are seen with immunodeficiencies.
   A. Recurrent and chronic protracted course of infection
   B. Infection with common non-pathogenic or unusual infectious agents
   C. Most severe and often atypical infectious disease presentation
   D. Delayed, incomplete, or lack of response of antimicrobial therapy
   E. Adverse reactions to modified live virus vaccines

III. Immunodeficiency disorders represent a large heterogeneous group of diseases. Evaluation of immune function usually discloses the presence of one or more abnormalities of the immune system involving lymphocytes, phagocytes, and mechanical barriers.

IV. Immunodeficiencies can be divided into two major forms depending on whether they are inherited or acquired.
   A. Primary immunodeficiencies are also known as hereditary or congenital immunodeficiencies (Giger et al., 1988; Felsburg, 1994; Giger, 1994).
   B. Secondary immunodeficiencies are also known as acquired immunodeficiencies.

Primary Immunodeficiencies

I. They are genetically determined abnormalities in morphology, maturation, and/or function of leukocytes or the barrier system. Broadly, they can be classified into defects of the specific or nonspecific immune response.
   A. Deficiencies of the B-cell or humoral immune system affect the production of immunoglobulins and lead to an increased susceptibility to bacterial infections.
   B. Deficiencies of the T-cell or cell-mediated immune system are associated with viral, fungal, and protozoal infections, but bacterial infections can also occur.
   C. Disorders of the phagocytic system involve defects of neutrophils and monocytes and complement system and lead to pyogenic infections.
   D. Defects in the barrier system such as skin and mucosal surfaces result in specific organ infections, e.g., ciliary dyskinesia causing rhinosinusitis and bronchopneumonia with bronchiectasis (Edwards et al., 1992). Disorders of the barrier system are covered under the appropriate organ system (see Chaps. 17 and 82).

II. Although there is an increased susceptibility to opportunistic infections, the type of infection varies depending on the immunodeficiency. Only a few disorders predispose animals to a restricted group of infectious agents.
   A. Basset hounds have increased susceptibility to systemic avian mycobacteriosis, toxoplasmosis, and neosporidiosis (Carpenter et al., 1988).
   B. Male dachshunds appear predisposed to pneumocystis pneumonia.
   C. German shepherd dogs may be prone to develop systemic aspergillosis (Day et al., 1985).
   D. A genetic predisposition to demodicosis has been proposed in various canine breeds or families (see Chap. 87).

III. Infections may be systemic or restricted to a particular organ system.
   A. Respiratory infections with ciliary dyskinesia
   B. Skin and mucosal surface infections with IgA deficiency

C. Pyoderma with hereditary skin disorders
D. Skin infections with lethal acrodermatitis in bull terriers (Jezyk et al., 1986)
IV. In addition to the previously mentioned features of infections in immunocompromised hosts, primary immunodeficiencies may have other common manifestations.
A. Neonatal to juvenile, non–colostrum-deprived animals with overwhelming and recurrent infections
B. Tendency toward allergies
C. Increased bleeding tendencies
D. Growth failure
E. Characteristic coat color dilutions
V. Some morphologic leukocyte changes are not associated with any noticeable immunodeficiencies.
A. Chédiak-Higashi syndrome in smoke-colored Persian cats characterized by abnormally large eosinophilic granules in polymorphonuclear leukocytes (Kramer et al., 1977)
B. Pelger-Huët anomaly in dogs and cats with hyposegmented granulocytes (Bowles et al., 1979; Latimer et al., 1985)
C. Mucopolysaccharidosis in dogs and cats with lysosomal granules in white blood cells
D. Acidophilic granulation of neutrophils in Birman cats (Hirsch and Cunningham, 1984)
VI. The mode of inheritance of primary immunodeficiencies, where determined, is usually autosomal recessive.
A. Autosomal dominant trait for Pelger-Huët anomaly
B. X-Chromosomal recessive trait for severe combined immune deficiency due to common gamma chain interleukin-2 (IL-2) receptor defects

Secondary Immunodeficiencies

I. The immune system of animals with secondary immunodeficiencies is initially functional but becomes transiently or permanently impaired during or following an underlying primary disease condition.
II. They occur more commonly than primary immunodeficiencies.
III. They are associated with many organ disorders or exposure to different agents.
IV. Causes of immunosuppression include the following.
A. Colostrum deprivation with vulnerability to infection during the neonatal period
1. The susceptibility to infection is relatively low.
2. A transient hypoglobulinemia occurs between 2 and 6 months following the decline of maternal antibodies.
B. Viral infections suppressing the immune system
1. Feline leukemia virus
2. Feline immunodeficiency virus
3. Feline and canine parvovirus
4. Canine distemper virus
C. Chemicals and drugs
1. Cytotoxic agents
2. Estrogens (dog)

3. Glucocorticosteroids
4. Other immunosuppressive agents
D. Whole body irradiation
E. Organ diseases
1. Hyperadrenocorticism
2. Diabetes mellitus
3. Lymphangiectasia
4. Systemic lupus erythematosus, immune-mediated hemolytic anemia, and other immune-mediated diseases
5. Dysproteinemias
6. Cancer
F. Nutritional deficiencies
1. Vitamin A
2. Vitamin E and selenium
3. Zinc
4. General malnutrition
G. Aged animals
H. Barrier damage
1. Burns
2. Invasive catheters
3. Splenectomy

Treatment

I. The successful control of infections in immunodeficient animals depends on the underlying disease and which part of and how severely the immune system is affected.
II. There are currently no practical treatments for primary immunodeficiencies.
A. Some leukocyte defects cause overwhelming infections and death before 1 year of age, whereas others may not lead to a markedly increased predisposition to infection.
B. Early and aggressive antibiotic therapy is indicated even for mild infections with usually nonpathogenic agents.
C. Bone marrow transplantation has experimentally corrected several leukocyte defects.
D. Fresh whole blood may be transfused to animals with overwhelming infections, but the effect is very transient and limited.
E. Plasma transfusion or gamma globulin injection may be used to support humoral immunodeficiencies.
1. These products should not be used in animals with IgA deficiency, because they may cause anaphylactic reactions.
2. There is no commercial canine gamma globulin, and the human gamma globulin is exorbitantly expensive and may cause allergic reactions. There are no data to support their use in small animal practice.
F. Nonspecific immunostimulators have not been documented to be beneficial in animals with cell-mediated immunodeficiencies.
G. Modified live virus vaccines are not used in animals with T-cell deficiencies because they may develop clinical disease from the vaccine virus.

III. If the underlying disease causing a secondary immunodeficiency can be corrected, the infection is often easily controlled.
   A. Use bactericidal antibiotics until the bacterial infections are controlled.
   B. Treat underlying disease and remove triggering agents.
IV. Consider the potential zoonotic risks involved in keeping an immunodeficient animal with infections that may be contagious to humans, particularly immunosuppressed patients.

SPECIFIC PRIMARY IMMUNODEFICIENCIES

Cyclic Hematopoiesis

Definition and Cause

I. Cyclic hematopoiesis is characterized by a periodic production and maturation defect of hematopoietic cells in the bone marrow (Jones et al., 1975; Lothrop et al., 1988).
   A. All blood cell counts cycle at a 12–14 day interval.
   B. During periods of severe neutropenia, also known as cyclic neutropenia, dogs are highly susceptible to bacterial infections.
II. It is inherited as an autosomal recessive trait in the collie breed.
   A. No clinical case has been observed since the 1970s.
   B. Affected collies have hypopigmentation, and their coat appears silvery gray or light tan, thus the term ''gray collie syndrome.''

Clinical Signs

I. Clinical features start at 6–8 weeks of age (see Chap. 63).
   A. Regularly recurring bacterial infections
   B. Severe neutropenia ($<1000/\mu l$) every 12–14 days lasting for 3–4 days
   C. Cycling of all other blood cell counts at an interval of 12–14 days
II. Gingival bleeding may occur from platelet storage pool defect.
III. Death may arise from sepsis and organ failure before 1 year of age.

Diagnosis

I. Silver gray collies
II. Cyclic hematopoiesis
III. Systemic amyloidosis associated with secondary organ failures (e.g., azotemia)

Treatment and Prognosis

I. Antibiotics are indicated during episodes of infection.
II. Experimental bone marrow transplantation completely corrects the defect.

III. Experimental lithium carbonate only corrects the cycling at extremely high and toxic doses.
IV. Prognosis is poor.

Leukocyte Adhesion Deficiency

Definition and Cause

I. Leukocyte adhesion deficiency (LAD) is caused by a lack of family of three leukocyte integrins, also known as CD11a-c/CD18 heterodimers, which are essential for normal leukocyte-endothelial cell adherence and migration (Giger et al., 1987; Trowald-Wigh et al., 1992).
   A. A deficiency in the common β-subunit of the dimers results in the dysfunction of all three integrins.
   B. The lack of CD11b/18 is most important, as this is the CR3 receptor and binds C3bi and ICAM-1 (binds to a complement split product and endothelial surface protein).
   C. LAD has previously been described as canine granulopathy syndrome (Renshaw and Davis, 1979).
II. LAD is a rare autosomal recessive disorder in Irish setters and has recently been reported in the United States and Sweden.

Clinical Signs

I. Clinical features of severely increased susceptibility to infection begin at a few weeks of age.
   A. Recurrent pyogenic infections
   B. Poor wound healing
   C. Impaired inflammatory response with minimal pus formation
II. Death occurs at a young age unless the condition is aggressively treated with antibiotics.

Diagnosis

I. Deficiency of leukocyte-surface glycoproteins CD11a-c/CD18 by FACS analysis
II. Lack of neutrophil and monocyte adhesion
III. Asymptomatic carriers (heterozygotes): intermediate adhesion function and expression of CD11/CD18
IV. Persistent severe leukocytosis of $25,000-500,000/\mu l$
   A. Mature neutrophilia with hypersegmentation
   B. Variable lymphocytosis, eosinophilia, and monocytosis

Treatment and Prognosis

I. Antimicrobial therapy
II. Prognosis guarded to poor

Complement Component 3 (C3) Deficiency

Definition and Cause

I. Complement component 3, a key factor in the complement system, is required in opsonizing bacteria.

A. Affected dogs have a complete deficiency of C3 (0.1%) and markedly reduced plasma complement activity (<1%) (Winkelstein et al., 1982).

B. Phagocytosis by neutrophils is impaired wherever bacterial opsonization is required.

II. C3 deficiency has been reported in a colony of Brittany spaniels with a spinoneuromuscular disease and is inherited as an autosomal recessive trait (Blum et al., 1985).

Clinical Signs

I. Affected dogs have a moderately increased susceptibility to bacterial infections.

A. Occasional bacterial infections with protracted course

B. Renal failure with amyloidosis

II. Diagnosis is made by serum complement C3 determination.

Treatment

I. Antibiotics

II. Prognosis guarded

Neutrophil Bactericidal Defect Associated with Respiratory Infection

Definition and Cause

I. This neutrophil dysfunction is associated with partially reduced oxygen radical formation and bactericidal activity, despite normal phagocytosis of bacteria, resulting in an increased susceptibility to respiratory tract infection (Breitschwerdt et al., 1987).

A. The specific defect has not yet been identified.

B. Primary ciliary dyskinesia has not been completely ruled out. The cilia morphology appears normal, but no functional studies have been done.

II. The disease has only been described in closely related Doberman pinschers, and an autosomal recessive mode of inheritance is suggested.

Clinical Signs

I. Chronic intermittent respiratory tract infection starting at a few weeks of age

II. Coughing, sneezing, and mucopurulent nasal discharge

III. Seborrhea sicca

IV. Ancylostomiasis and trichinosis

V. Leukocytosis with neutrophilia and eosinophilia

Diagnosis and Treatment

I. No specific diagnostic tests are available.

II. Antibiotics are given during periods of infection.

III. Prognosis is guarded.

Susceptibility to Suppurative and Granulomatous Disease

Definition and Cause

I. An unidentified defect that affects phagocytic and humoral immune systems leads to suppurative and pyogranulomatous infections in Weimaraners (Studdert, 1984; Couto et al., 1989).

A. Decreased neutrophil chemiluminescence, low serum IgG and IgM concentrations, and increased levels of circulating immune complexes have been documented, but they may be secondary to inflammation and infection.

B. Causative infections are only rarely recognized.

II. This immunodeficiency appears to occur commonly in Weimaraners, but the mode of inheritance has not been determined.

Clinical Signs and Diagnosis

I. Clinical signs occur between a few months and several years of age.

A. Intermittent high fever (40–42°C)

B. Pyogranulomatous disease (cellulitis)

C. Large abscesses in muscle

D. Surface bleeding

E. Coat color dilution

F. Profound depression

II. The diagnosis is based on the breed predilection and characteristic clinical signs. No specific tests are available.

Treatment

I. Antibiotics

II. Supportive care

III. Prognosis guarded

X-Linked Severe Combined Immunodeficiency (XSCID)

Definition and Cause

I. This severe combined immunodeficiency is characterized by a failure in humoral and cell-mediated immunity with increased susceptibility to viral, bacterial, fungal, and protozoal infections (Jezyk et al., 1989; Felsburg, 1994; Felsburg et al., 1992).

A. The X-linked form of SCID is caused by different mutations in the common gamma (γc) chain gene that encodes for an essential component for the cytokine receptors for IL-2, IL-4, IL-7, IL-9, and IL-15.

1. Bassets with XSCID have a four base pair deletion that produces a frameshift and subsequent premature stop codon in exon 1 (Henthorn et al., 1994).

2. Cardigan Welsh corgis with XSCID have an insertion of cytosine resulting in a premature stop codon (Somberg et al., 1995).

B. The shared usage of the γc chain by several other cytokine receptors explains the profound

immunologic abnormalities (Jezyk et al., 1989; Somberg et al., 1994, 1996).
1. The ability of lymphocytes to bind and proliferate to IL-2 is severely impaired.
2. The development of thymocytes is drastically reduced with an increased proportion of immature CD4$^-$CD8$^-$ thymocytes.
II. The inheritance of XSCID is X-linked recessive.
   A. XSCID has been reported in an isolated family of basset hounds and Cardigan Welsh corgis.
   B. Male dogs are affected, whereas females can be carriers. The dams of affected dogs are carriers, and the sires are normal.

Clinical Signs and Diagnosis

I. Clinical signs occur after the decline of maternal immunity.
   A. Bacterial infections usually involving the skin and gastrointestinal and respiratory systems
   B. Thymus and lymph nodes absent or hypoplastic
   C. Failure to thrive
   D. Growth failure
   E. Adverse, and often fatal, reactions to modified live virus vaccines
   F. Death within a few months from systemic bacterial or severe viral infection
II. Diagnosis is reached by histopathology and immunologic testing.
   A. Low serum IgG and IgA levels, but normal IgM levels
   B. Marked hypoglobulinemia
   C. Impaired lymphocyte blastogenic response
   D. Thymic and lymphoid hypoplasia
   E. Polymerase chain reaction–based tests to identify the specific mutation in bassets and corgis

Treatment

I. Reconstitution of immunologic function has been achieved following experimental bone marrow transplantation.
II. Prognosis without transplantation is grave.

Hypotrichosis Congenita and Thymic Aplasia (Nude Athymic Kittens)

Definition and Cause

I. Hypotrichosis is lack of hair growth and thymic development.
   A. This defect is characterized by the birth of nude kittens with severe immunodeficiency.
   B. This is a homologue to the nude mice.
II. This syndrome is inherited by an autosomal recessive trait and is seen in the Birman breed (Casal et al., 1994).

Clinical Signs

I. Nude kittens born
II. Failure to thrive

III. No thymus and lymph nodes
IV. Death within a few days

Treatment

None available

Selective IgA Deficiency

Definition and Cause

I. Absent or markedly reduced and slowly developing serum IgA concentrations predispose to two types of immune diseases (Whitbread et al., 1984; Felsburg et al., 1985; Glickman et al., 1988).
   A. Young animals are predisposed to mucocutaneous infections.
   B. Adult animals may develop allergies and autoimmune disease.
II. Selective IgA deficiency has been reported in various canine breeds, including beagles, Shar peis, and German shepherd dogs, but the mode of inheritance has not been elucidated.

Clinical Signs and Diagnosis

I. Clinical signs of immunodeficiency occur in young dogs, whereas adult dogs may be normal.
   A. Chronic recurrent upper respiratory infections involving parainfluenza and *Bordetella bronchiseptica*
   B. Gastroenteritis with vomiting, diarrhea, and ulcerative colitis
   C. Pyoderma
   D. Recurrent or chronic otitis
   E. Atopic dermatitis and possibly other immune-mediated diseases
   F. Seizures
II. Diagnosis is made based on low serum IgA levels.
   A. Serum IgA concentrations need to be compared with age-matched controls.
   B. Serum IgG and IgM concentrations are normal.
   C. Some IgA-deficient dogs have a positive rheumatoid factor or anti-IgA antibodies.

Treatment

I. Antibiotics
II. Prognosis guarded

Immunodeficiency Syndrome in Shar Peis

Definition and Cause

I. This syndrome appears to be caused by T- and B-cell abnormalities with varied abnormal parameters.
   A. Variably low serum IgG, IgA, and IgM concentrations
   B. Decreased in vitro lymphocyte proliferative response after pokeweed mitogen stimulation
   C. Reduced IL-6 synthesis in vitro by mononuclear cells (Rivas et al., 1995)

II. It is possible that the previously described selective IgA deficiency is part of the syndrome in this breed (Moroff et al., 1986).
III. This immunodeficiency has been described in Shar peis, but the mode of inheritance remains unknown.

Clinical Signs and Diagnosis

I. Clinical signs occur between a few months and several years of age.
   A. Intermittent fever
   B. Recurrent gastrointestinal signs (ulcerative colitis)
   C. Recurrent pyoderma
   D. Adult onset demodicosis in some cases
   E. Intestinal adenocarcinoma and lymphoma
II. Diagnosis
   A. Breed predilection and characteristic signs
   B. Defective IL-6 synthesis in vitro

Treatment

I. Supportive
II. Prognosis guarded

Thymic Abnormalities and Dwarfism

Definition and Cause

I. This immunodeficiency is characterized by thymic cortex hypoplasia and dwarfism, but the cause has not been identified.
II. This syndrome has been described in one family of Weimaraners (Roth et al., 1980, 1984).

Clinical Signs and Diagnosis

I. Clinical signs occur early in life.
   A. Failure to thrive
   B. Growth retardation
   C. Recurrent infections
II. No definitive diagnostic tests are available.
   A. Reduced lymphocyte blastogenic response to phytohemagglutinin
   B. Low serum growth hormone concentrations after clonidine stimulation

Treatment

Bovine growth hormone therapy resulted in clinical improvement and marked increase in cortical thymus thickness.

Lethal Acrodermatitis

See Chap. 82.

Increased Susceptibility to Avian Mycobacteriosis in Basset Hounds

Definition and Cause

I. Dogs and cats are generally resistant to avian mycobacteria, an ubiquitous agent.

A. Increased susceptibility to avian mycobacteriosis and also to toxoplasmosis and neosporidiosis has been reported in several basset hounds of both genders (Carpenter et al., 1988).
B. An interleukin or RAMP protein deficiency is suspected.
II. Affected basset hounds have been found throughout the United States, but the mode of inheritance is unknown.

Clinical Signs and Diagnosis

I. Clinical signs of systemic avian mycobacteriosis are seen in juvenile to adult basset hounds.
   A. Diarrhea
   B. Weight loss
   C. Generalized lymphadenopathy
   D. Nasal and ocular mucopurulent discharge
   E. No response to antimicrobial therapy
II. Diagnosis is based on identifying *Mycobacterium avium.*
   A. Many acid-fast staining bacteria in tissue
   B. Bacterial culture
   C. Bacille Calmette-Guérin (BCG) tuberculin skin test

Treatment

I. None
II. Prognosis grave

Pneumocystis in Dachshunds

Definition and Cause

I. Pneumocystis occurs as a respiratory infection in dogs.
II. Several male dachshunds have been affected, but the mode of inheritance has not been determined (Farrow et al., 1972; Copeland, 1974; Botha and Van Rensburg, 1979).

Clinical Signs and Diagnosis

I. Clinical signs of respiratory infections are apparent.
II. Pneumocystis is found on exudates (transtracheal lavage) or at necropsy.

Treatment

I. None
II. Prognosis grave

Bibliography

Barta O, Turnwald GH: Demodicosis, pyoderma, and other skin diseases of young dogs, and their associations with immunologic dysfunctions. Compend Contin Educ Pract Vet 5:995, 1983

Blum JR, Cork LC, Morris JM et al: The clinical manifestations of a genetically-determined deficiency in the third component of complement in the dog. Clin Immunol Immunopathol 24:304, 1985

Botha WS, Van Rensburg IBJ: Pneumocystosis: a chronic respiratory distress syndrome in the dog. J S Afr Vet Assoc 50:173, 1979

Bowles CA, Alsaker RD, Wolfle TL: Studies of the Pelger-Huët anomaly in Foxhounds. Am J Pathol 96:237, 1979

Breitschwerdt EB, Brown TT, DeBuyssher EV et al: Rhinitis, pneumonia, and defective neutrophil function in the Doberman pinscher. Am J Vet Res 48:1054, 1987

Carpenter JL, Myers AM, Conner MW et al: Tuberculosis in five Basset hounds. J Am Vet Med Assoc 192:1563, 1988

Casal ML, Strauman U, Sigg C et al: Congenital hypotrichosis with thymic aplasia in nine Birman kittens. J Am Anim Hosp Assoc 30:600, 1994

Copeland JW: Canine pneumonia caused by *Pneumocystis carinii*. Aust Vet J 50:515, 1974

Couto CG, Giger U: Congenital and acquired neutrophil function abnormalities in the dog. p. 521. In Kirk RW (ed): Current Veterinary Therapy X: Small Animal Practice. WB Saunders, Philadelphia, 1989

Couto CG, Krakowa S, Johnson G et al: In vivo immunologic features of Weimaraner dogs with neutrophil abnormalities and recurrent infections. Vet Immunol Immunopathol 23:103, 1989

Daniel GB, Edwards DF, Harvey RC et al: Communicating hydrocephalus in dogs with congenital ciliary dysfunction. Dev Neurosci 17:230, 1995

Day MJ, Eger CE, Shaw SE et al: Immunologic study of systemic aspergillosis in German shepherd dogs. Vet Immunol Immunopathol 9:335, 1985

Edwards DF, Patton CS, Kennedy JR: Primary ciliary dyskinesia in the dog. Prob Vet Med 4:291, 1992

Farrow BRH, Watson ADJ, Hartley WJ: Pneumocystis pneumonia in the dog. J Comp Pathol 82:447, 1972

Felsburg PJ: Overview of the immune system and immunodeficiency disease. Vet Clin North Am [Small Anim Pract] 24:629, 1994

Felsburg PJ, Glickman LT, Jezyk PF: Selective IgA deficiency in the dog. Clin Immunol Immunopathol 36:297, 1985

Felsburg PJ, Somberg RL, Perryman LE: Domestic animal models of severe combined immunodeficiency: X-linked severe combined immunodeficiency in the dog and severe combined immunodeficiency in the horse. Immunodeficiency Rev 3:277, 1992

Giger U: Primäre Immundefekte beim Kleintier. Kleintierpraxis 39:433, 1994

Giger U, Boxer LA, Simpson PJ et al: Deficiency of leukocyte surface glycoproteins Mo1, LFA-1, and LeuMS in a dog with recurrent bacterial infections: an animal model. Blood 69:1622, 1987

Giger U, Fyfe JC, Haskins ME et al: Inherited leukocyte defects in dogs. Proc Am Coll Vet Intern Med 8:311, 1988

Glickman LT, Shofer FS, Payton AJ et al: Survey of serum IgA, IgG, and IgM concentrations in a large beagle population in which IgA deficiency had been identified. Am J Vet Res 49:1240, 1988

Healy MC, Gaafar SM: Immunodeficiency in canine demodectic mange. II. Skin reactions to phytohemagglutinin and concanavalin A. Vet Parasitol 3:133, 1977

Hirsch VN, Cunningham TA: Hereditary anomaly of neutrophil granulation in Birman cats. Am J Vet Res 45:2170, 1984

Jezyk PF, Felsburg PJ, Haskins ME, Patterson DF: X-linked severe combined immunodeficiency in the dog. Clin Immunol Immunopathol 52:173, 1989

Jezyk PF, Haskins ME, MacKay-Smith WE, Patterson DF: Lethal acrodermatitis in bull terriers. J Am Vet Med Assoc 188:833, 1986

Jones JB, Lange RD, Jones ES: Cyclic hematopoiesis in a colony of dogs. J Am Vet Med Assoc 166:365, 1975

Kramer JW, Davis WC, Prieur DJ: The Chédiak-Higashi syndrome in cats. Lab Invest 36:554, 1977

Latimer KS, Rakich PM, Thompson DF: Pelger-Huët anomaly in cats. Vet Pathol 22:370, 1985

Lothrop CD, Warren DJ, Souza LM: Correction of canine cyclic hematopoiesis with recombinant human granulocyte colony-stimulating factor. Blood 72:5624, 1988

Moroff SD, Hurvitz AI, Peterson ME et al: IgA deficiency in shar pei dogs. Vet Immunol Immunopathol 13:181, 1986

Renshaw HW, Davis WC: Canine granulopathy syndrome: an inherited disorder of leukocyte function. Am J Pathol 95:731, 1979

Rivas AL, Tintle L, Argentieri D et al: A primary immunodeficiency syndrome in Shar pei dogs. Clin Immunol Immunopathol 74:243, 1995

Roth JA, Lomax LG, Altszuler N et al: Thymic abnormalities and growth hormone deficiency in dogs. Am J Vet Res 41:1256, 1980

Roth JA, Kaeberle ML, Grier RL et al: Improvement in clinical condition and thymus morphologic features associated with growth hormone treatment of immunodeficient dwarf dogs. Am J Vet Res 45:1151, 1984

Somberg RL, Robinson JP, Felsburg PJ: T lymphocyte development and function in dogs with X-linked severe combined immunodeficiency. J Immunol 153:4006, 1994

Somberg RL, Pullen RP, Casal ML et al: A single neucleotide insertion in the canine interleukin-2 receptor gamma chain results in X-linked severe combined immunodeficiency disease. Vet Immunol Immunopathol 47:203, 1995

Somberg RL, Tripold A, Hartnett BJ et al: Postnatal development of T cells in dogs with X-linked severe combined immunodeficiency. J Immunol 156:1431, 1996

Studdert VP, Phillips WA, Studdert MJ et al: Recurrent and persistent infections in related Weimaraner dogs. Aust Vet J 61:261, 1984

Trowald-Wigh G, Hakansson L, Johannisson A et al: Leucocyte adhesion protein deficiency in Irish setter dogs. Vet Immunol Immunopathol 32:261, 1992

Whitbread TJ, Batt RM, Garthwaite G: Relative deficiency of serum IgA in the German shepherd dog: a breed abnormality. Res Vet Sci 37:350, 1984

Winkelstein JA, Johnson JP, Swift AJ et al: Genetically determined deficiency of the third component of complement in the dog: in vitro studies of the complement system and complement-mediated serum activities. J Immunol 129:2598, 1982

74

Immune-Mediated Diseases

Kristen A. Bernard

ANAPHYLAXIS

Definition

I. Anaphylaxis is an acute, systemic, severe manifestation of type I hypersensitivity reaction.
  A. It occurs immediately after introduction of an allergen (antigen) into the blood circulation of a sensitized animal.
  B. The binding of antigens to mast cells or basophilfixed IgE antibodies causes release of chemical mediators from these cells, resulting in anaphylactic shock or an urticarial reaction.
II. Anaphylactoid reactions are clinically similar to anaphylaxis but are not mediated through an antibody reaction.
  A. Certain substances act directly on mast cells, causing the release of mediators, or act via the formation of anaphylatoxins (C3a, C5a) through complement activation.
  B. Immediate therapeutic measures are the same as with true anaphylaxis.
III. Anaphylaxis is uncommon in the dog and extremely rare in the cat.

Causes

I. A variety of agents can cause anaphylactic reactions.
  A. Venoms from stinging and biting insects of the order Hymenoptera, including bees, wasps, hornets, ants
  B. Blood products, e.g., whole blood, plasma, cryoprecipitate
  C. Tetanus and venom antitoxins, vaccines, allergenic extracts
  D. Various drugs: antibiotics, iron dextran, hormones, local anesthetics, vitamin K, asparaginase, radiopaque dyes, sulfobromophthalein, opiate analgesics, nonsteroidal anti-inflammatory drugs, vaccines (especially leptospirosis bacterin)

II. The implicated agent is usually introduced parenterally, rarely orally.

Pathophysiology

I. On first exposure to an antigen, an antigen-specific IgE antibody is produced by B cells. The antibody then binds to the surface membrane of mast cells and basophils in tissues and blood, respectively. The animal is then sensitized.
II. Following a subsequent exposure, the antigen binds to the cell-fixed IgE antibodies; this triggers the release of chemical substances from the mast cells and basophils.
III. Major biologically active mediators released or generated by mast cells and basophils include histamine, leukotrienes, eosinophilic chemotactic factor, platelet-activating factor, kinins, serotonin, and proteolytic enzymes.
IV. These substances trigger numerous reactions, including vasodilation, increased vascular permeability, smooth muscle contraction, cellular infiltration, and complement activation.
V. The severity of the anaphylactic reaction depends on the type of antigen, degree of sensitization, and amount and route of antigen on re-exposure.

Clinical Signs

I. They usually occur within minutes after the exposure to the offending agent and can be mild to severe, with the severity directly related to the rapidity of onset.
II. The following signs may be seen alone or in combination, and progression is often rapid.
  A. Restlessness and excitement
  B. Pruritus around the head and/or antigen injection site
  C. Facial urticaria and angioedema
  D. Salivation and lacrimation
  E. Stridor from angioedema of the head
  F. Vomiting, abdominal pain, diarrhea

G. Hepatosplenomegaly in the dog

H. Dyspnea and cyanosis in the cat

I. Shock

J. Incoordination, collapse, convulsions, death

III. Facial urticaria and angioedema are more common than actual anaphylactic shock.

IV. Dogs differ from other domestic animals in that the major organ involved in acute anaphylaxis is not the lung but the liver. Therefore, signs in the dog are caused mainly by constriction of hepatic veins, which results in portal hypertension and visceral pooling. On necropsy, the liver and intestines are engorged with blood.

V. In cats the anaphylactic shock organs are the respiratory and intestinal tracts. Therefore, respiratory distress is often observed, and bronchoconstriction, emphysema, pulmonary hemorrhage, and edema are seen on necropsy.

Diagnosis

I. Suspicious clinical findings

A. History may reveal prior exposure to an offending agent.

B. Clinical signs, especially skin reactions, are suggestive.

II. Laboratory tests

A. Results are nonspecific and usually normal during the acute phase.

B. Later, changes result from hypovolemia, hypotension, and shock.

III. Pulmonary edema may be evident on radiography of the cat.

IV. *Do not* attempt to challenge the animal with the agent that is suspected to have caused the anaphylactic reaction.

Differential Diagnosis

I. Other types of shock

II. Certain toxicoses (see Chaps. 123, 124, 126)

III. Feline asthma

IV. Canine hemorrhagic gastroenteritis

V. Urticaria and angioedema of nonimmunologic causes

Treatment

I. Systemic anaphylaxis is a true emergency that requires immediate therapeutic intervention based on counteracting the effects of mediators, supporting vital organ function, and preventing further release of mediators.

II. Stop administration of the allergenic agent (drug, blood transfusion).

III. For animals in shock, consider the following.

A. If the animal is in respiratory distress, ensure a patent airway and administer oxygen.

B. Immediately administer epinephrine HCl (1:10,000) 0.2–1 ml IV. If unable to administer IV, then give 0.2–2 ml SQ and continue attempts to give IV.

C. Administer shock doses of IV fluids such as 5% dextrose/water (D5W) or lactated Ringer's solution (LRS) 50–100 ml/kg/hour for 1–2 hours. Alternatively, administer dextran at 5 ml/kg as an IV bolus, not to exceed a daily dose of 20 ml/kg.

D. Administer fast-acting corticosteroids such as dexamethasone 2–4 mg/kg IV.

E. Administer diphenhydramine (Benadryl) 2 mg/kg IM or slowly IV, or administer other antihistamines (Table 74–1).

F. Inject 0.2–0.5 ml epinephrine HCl 1:10,000 at the entrance site of the allergen (e.g., insect bite, parenteral medication) and apply cold to the site.

G. After 20–30 minutes, if clinical signs continue or worsen, repeat IV epinephrine injection.

IV. For animals manifesting less severe signs, do the following.

A. Administer 0.2–2 ml SQ epinephrine HCl 1:10,000.

B. Administer antihistamines (see Table 74–1).

C. If the animal is exhibiting stridor or dyspnea, monitor closely for airway patency.

D. Inject epinephrine HCl (1:10,000) 0.2–0.5 ml at the entrance site of the allergen, and apply cold to the site.

E. If shock develops, initiate the therapy outlined earlier.

Patient Monitoring

I. During the initial therapy, monitor airway patency, pulse strength, capillary refill time, blood pressure, central venous pressure, and urine production.

II. If the animal responds immediately (i.e., within 20–30 minutes) to intensive therapy, the prognosis is good.

III. Avoid or prevent future exposure to the allergenic agent and any related compounds.

URTICARIA AND ANGIOEDEMA

Definition

I. Urticaria, or hives, is an acute erythematous and edematous allergic skin disease usually associated with pruritus.

II. Angioedema is similar to urticaria but involves the deeper subcutaneous tissues around the head and/or extremities and is usually not painful or pruritic.

III. Both are uncommon in dogs and rare in cats.

Causes

I. Immunologic causes

A. Type I hypersensitivity reaction: the most common mechanism

1. Anaphylactic antigen induces a more localized anaphylactic reaction.

*Table 74–1. **Antihistamines for Use in Dogs and Cats**[a]*

Drug	Dose for Dogs	Dose for Cats
Chlorpheniramine	4–8 mg total IV, IM, SQ, PO BID	1–2 mg total PO BID
Cyproheptadine	1.1 mg/kg PO BID–TID	1.1 mg/kg PO BID–TID
Dimenhydrinate	4–8 mg/kg IV, IM, PO, TID	12.5 mg total IV, IM, PO TID
Diphenhydramine	2–4 mg/kg IV, IM, PO, TID–BID	2–4 mg/kg IV, IM, PO TID–QID
Hydroxyzine	2 mg/kg IM, PO BID–TID	Safety unknown
Meclizine	25 mg total PO SID	12.5 mg total PO SID
Promethazine	0.2–0.4 mg/kg IV, IM, PO TID–QID	0.2–0.4 mg/kg IV, IM, PO TID–QID
Terfenadine	2.5–5 mg/kg PO BID	2.5–5 mg/kg PO BID
Trimeprazine	0.5 mg/kg PO BID	0.5 mg/kg PO BID
Tripelennamine	1 mg/kg PO BID	1 mg/kg PO BID

[a]Side effects include sedation, central nervous system (CNS) stimulation, and possible teratogenesis. Use antihistamines with caution in cats, because severe CNS depression can occur with resulting apnea.

2. Food and inhalant allergens have also been incriminated (see Chap. 89)
B. Type II hypersensitivity: cytotoxic antibodies that activate the complement cascade and thereby produce C3a and C5a anaphylatoxins, e.g., transfusion reactions (see Chap. 69)
C. Type III hypersensitivity: immune complexes such as occur in serum sickness
D. Vaccine reactions: type I, II, III, or IV hypersensitivity reaction
II. Nonimmunologic causes
A. Agents that cause direct release of histamine
B. Agents that activate the complement pathway directly
C. Skin exposure to cold, heat, and pressure
D. Mast cell tumor or mastocytosis with release of histamine
E. Genetic Clq inhibitor deficiency

Pathophysiology

I. Mechanisms are similar to those described under Anaphylaxis earlier.
II. Increased vascular permeability is the most important pathophysiologic factor.
III. Initial redness is caused by dilation of capillaries.
IV. Wheal formation is caused by extravasation of fluid.

Clinical Signs

I. Localized or generalized wheals, with or without serum leakage
II. Marked edematous swelling of soft tissues of the head, particularly around the eyes, mouth, and ears
III. Isolated swelling of an extremity
IV. Variable pruritis and self-mutilation
V. Upper airway stridor, dyspnea secondary to laryngeal edema

Diagnosis

I. Clinical signs are diagnostic.
II. A careful history may reveal an etiologic factor.
III. Histopathologic changes are nonspecific.

Differential Diagnosis

I. Vasculitis, phlebitis, thromboembolism
II. Cellulitis
III. Diffuse cutaneous lymphoreticular and mast cell tumors
IV. Cranial vena cava syndrome
V. Lymphedema
VI. Contact dermatitis

Treatment

I. Remove the causative agent.
II. Many acute urticarial reactions regress spontaneously within hours.
III. Severe cases require medical treatment.
A. Epinephrine (1:10,000): 0.5–2 ml SQ
B. Corticosteroids: prednisone 2 mg/kg PO, IM BID
C. Antihistamines: diphenhydramine 2 mg/kg IM BID PRN, or others (see Table 74–1)

Patient Monitoring

I. The prognosis is usually good; however, massive pharyngeal and laryngeal swelling can be fatal, and airway patency must be carefully monitored.
II. Attempt to ascertain the cause to avoid the etiologic factor in the future.

DRUG ALLERGY

Definition

Drug allergy or hypersensitivity refers to an immune-mediated adverse drug reaction from the production of specific antibodies and/or sensitized T lymphocytes directed against the drug or its metabolites.

Causes

I. Proteinaceous substances such as sera, vaccines, and biologic and allergenic extracts are inherently antigenic and carry a high risk of evoking allergic reactions. This reaction is exemplified by serum sickness.

II. Most drugs are not antigenic per se but function immunologically as haptens. Haptens must covalently bind in vivo to a host protein molecule, forming the hapten–carrier complex that can induce an immune response. The development of allergy to a particular drug greatly depends on the ease with which the drug or its metabolite binds to the carrier.

III. Any drug or biologic product has the potential to cause an allergic reaction. The following drugs do not represent a complete list.

   A. Sulfonamides
      1. Doberman pinschers are suspected to have a genetic predisposition for trimethoprim-sulfa allergies.
      2. Polyarthritis and other signs have been described.
   B. Penicillins
   C. Cephalosporins
   D. Propylthiouracil (cats)
   E. Levamisole (dogs)
   F. Gold salts (dogs)
   G. Asparaginase
   H. Doxorubicin
   I. Phenothiazines
   J. Oxytetracycline
   K. Lincomycin
   L. Progesterone analogues
   M. Vaccines

IV. Some drugs cross-react antigenically and therefore cause cross-sensitivity in an animal, e.g., beta-lactam antibiotics or penicillins and first- or second-generation cephalosporins.

V. Drug dosage, drug formulation, route of administration, and length and interval of therapy can influence the development of a drug allergy.

VI. Genetic factors also influence individual susceptibility.

VII. Underlying metabolic and immunologic diseases can predispose to drug allergy.

VIII. Some drug reactions may mimic an allergy but are not immunologically mediated.

Pathophysiology

I. All four types of immunologic hypersensitivity reactions can occur, but the type of reaction to a particular drug has not been documented in small animals.

II. Type I reactions
   A. The drug–carrier complex binds to reagenic antibodies (usually IgE) fixed to mast cells and basophils, resulting in anaphylaxis, urticaria, or angioedema.
   B. See Anaphylaxis and Urticaria and Angioedema.

III. Type II reactions
   A. An antibody binds to a drug that has previously fixed to a cell membrane, and this complex then activates the complement pathway, causing cell lysis.
   B. The drug–antibody–complement complex is formed first in the plasma and fixes nonspecifically to cell membranes, after which lysis occurs.

   C. The drug may also affect the cell membrane so that hidden autoantigens are exposed, enabling the production of autoantibodies.

IV. Type III reactions
   A. Circulating drug–carrier antibody (immune) complexes are deposited along the endothelial surfaces of blood vessels, stimulating directly and via the complement pathway a neutrophilic inflammatory response and vascular damage.
   B. This action results in a multisystemic vasculitis most commonly affecting the joints, skin, and kidneys.

V. Type IV reactions
   A. Tissue-fixed drug–carrier complexes attract sensitized T lymphocytes, which on reaction with the complex produce tissue inflammation through the action of lymphokines.
   B. Lymphocytes and macrophages are the predominant cell type involved.

VI. Certain drug allergies may be expressions of more than one type of reaction.

Clinical Signs

I. The general features of drug allergy include the following.
   A. Reactions occur only after an induction period during which the animal becomes sensitized.
      1. None occurs on initial exposure.
      2. They occur at least 5 days following first exposure to the drug.
   B. It is seen only in a small percentage of animals.
   C. Clinical manifestations do not resemble known pharmacologic actions of the drug or the disease being treated.
   D. It often mimics signs of other immune-mediated diseases.
   E. Clinical signs induced by one drug can vary greatly among individuals.
   F. Clinical signs usually subside within days (to weeks) after withdrawal of the drug.
   G. On readministration, clinical signs recur either immediately or after a latent period of a few days.

II. The four types of hypersensitivity reactions can cause a variety of clinical manifestations.
   A. Fever
   B. Cutaneous manifestations
      1. Urticaria and angioedema
      2. Pruritus
      3. Erythema multiforme and/or papular rash
      4. Allergic contact dermatitis
      5. Toxic epidermal necrolysis
   C. Polyarthritis
      1. Shifting leg lameness
      2. Pain on joint manipulation
      3. Joint swelling (particularly distal joints)
   D. Myositis
   E. Ataxia
   F. Glomerulonephritis
      1. Proteinuria and isosthenuria
      2. Acute renal failure

G. Hematologic manifestations
   1. Hemolytic anemia
   2. Thrombocytopenia
   3. Neutropenia or neutrophilia
   4. Lymphadenopathy
H. Vomiting, diarrhea, and/or abdominal pain

Diagnosis

I. Clinical diagnosis
   A. A temporal relation is established between drug exposure and signs. All drugs given to an animal should be considered.
   B. Clinical signs are typical of immune-mediated disorders and subside promptly on withdrawal of the drug.
II. Laboratory tests
   A. Occasionally serologic tests (Coombs', antinuclear antibody [ANA], platelet factor 3 test) are positive.
   B. For suspicious findings of joint fluid analysis and radiography, see Nonerosive Polyarthritis in Chap. 78.
   C. Increased urinary protein excretion is compatible with glomerulonephropathy (see also Chap. 47).
   D. Histopathology and immunofluorescence results of biopsies are often diagnostic for antigen–antibody complex deposition.
   E. Positive delayed skin test occurs with contact allergy. However, skin tests for immediate hypersensitivity reactions may cause systemic signs.
   F. Serum complement and circulating immune complex levels, as well as the presence of antibodies to a drug, may be detected, but these assays are not widely available.
III. Drug challenge studies
   These studies are usually not recommended to confirm a suspected drug allergy because of the risk of fatal systemic reactions.

Differential Diagnosis

I. The differential diagnosis of drug allergy is complex and must be considered for each organ system affected.
II. If multiple organ systems are involved, the following differential diagnoses should be considered.
   A. Systemic infections with bacterial, rickettsial, viral, and fungal agents
   B. Other systemic immune-mediated diseases such as systemic lupus erythematosus (SLE) or other vasculitides
III. Nonimmunologic adverse drug reactions such as vasculitis of nonimmune origin must be ruled out.

Treatment and Monitoring

I. Withdraw the drug(s) suspected to be responsible.
   A. Discontinue all drugs that are not absolutely essential for the animal's well-being.
   B. If a substitute drug must be given, it should be one that is unlikely to cross-react antigenically.

C. In most cases clinical signs subside within hours to a few days after the drug has been withdrawn.
II. Give supportive treatment for life-threatening conditions.
   A. Epinephrine, antihistamines, and IV fluids for anaphylactic shock
   B. Aspirin in case of high fever
   C. Blood transfusions and corticosteroids for severe thrombocytopenia-related bleeding or severe hemolytic anemia
III. Corticosteroids are usually not required but may be used to decrease cell destruction and inflammation and to hasten the recovery from vasculitic reactions.
IV. The prognosis for fast and complete recovery is good.
V. Avoid future use of a suspected or proved allergenic drug (and related drugs).

SPECIFIC CELLULAR AND ORGAN IMMUNE-MEDIATED DISORDERS

Definition

I. The immunologic injury caused by a specific antibody–antigen interaction may be localized, affecting only one (or two) cell type(s) in one organ, or it may be systemic.
II. Most of these disorders are classified according to their etiology as idiopathic (primary) or secondary disorders.
III. Secondary immune-mediated injuries are induced by infections, neoplasms, and chemicals and are therefore more common than the true idiopathic or primary immunologic disorders.
IV. They occur in both dogs and cats.

Classification

I. Almost any organ or body system can be affected (Table 74–2).
II. For further discussion of the clinical signs, diagnosis, treatment, and monitoring of these disorders, see the section on immune disorders within each chapter.

SLE AND OTHER MULTISYSTEMIC IMMUNE-MEDIATED DISEASES (VASCULITIDES)

Definition

I. Systemic lupus erythematosus (SLE)
   A. SLE is a rare systemic inflammatory disease associated with the formation of autoantibodies and immune complex deposition in many organs caused by a failure in immunoregulation.
   B. Autoantibodies are directed against nuclear constituents (DNA, RNA, nonhistone components)

Table 74–2. *Disorders That Are Primarily or Partially Immune Mediated*

Type of Disorder	Specific Disease
Blood	Hemolytic anemia Thrombocytopenia Aplastic anemia Systemic lupus erythematosus (SLE) Neutropenia
Endocrine	Hypothyroidism (dogs) secondary to lymphocytic thyroiditis Diabetes mellitus secondary to autoantibodies Hypoadrenocorticism (dogs) Hypoparathyroidism (dogs) Male infertility secondary to autoantibodies (dogs) Polyendocrine disorders, e.g., Schmidt's disease: hypothyroidism, hypoadrenocorticism, and diabetes mellitus
Respiratory	Allergic rhinitis Allergic bronchitis Feline asthma Occult heartworm pneumonitis
Gastrointestinal	Plasmacytic-lymphocytic gingivitis/stomatitis Plasmacytic-lymphocytic enteritis Eosinophilic enterocolitis Chronic colitis Immunoproliferative small intestinal disease of basenjis Food allergy, gluten enteropathy Chronic active hepatitis (dog) Cholangiohepatitis (cat)
Renal	Immune complex glomerulonephritis Antiglomerular basement membrane glomerulonephritis
Ocular	Keratoconjunctivitis sicca (KCS) Uveitis, especially that caused by canine adenovirus type I Chorioretinitis Sjögren's syndrome: xerostomia, KCS, and arthritis or thrombocytopenia Granulomatous panuveitis and dermal depigmentation (dogs) Optic neuritis
Neurology	Distemper and rabies postvaccinal encephalomyelitis Acute polyradiculoneuritis (coonhound paralysis) Myasthenia gravis
Musculoskeletal	Masticatory myositis (dogs) Polymyositis Idiopathic polyarthritis Rheumatoid arthritis (dogs) Plasmacytic-lymphocytic arthritis SLE Chronic progressive and erosive polyarthritis (cats) Enteropathic arthritis
Dermatologic	Pemphigus complex Bullous pemphigoid Discoid lupus erythematosus SLE Dermatomyositis of collies and shelties

and/or mitochondrial and ribosomal structures, resulting in a positive ANA test.

  C. Although antinuclear antibodies are important features of SLE, a variety of other antibodies are also produced, e.g., rheumatoid factor and antibodies against blood cells and clotting factors.

  D. Depending on the site and extent of immune complex deposition, a variety of clinical features develop, including polyarthritis, dermatitis, glomerulonephritis, cytopenias, and fever.

  E. Classic SLE has a slight female predominance.

II. Immune vasculitis/polyarteritis

  A. It is a type III hypersensitivity reaction characterized by localization of antigen–antibody immune complexes.

  B. It can be associated with connective tissue disorders such as SLE and rheumatoid arthritis, or it may occur secondary to infectious diseases.

  C. It can be classified according to the type of vessel involved.

    1. Leukocytoclastic or hypersensitivity vasculitis

a) It affects small blood vessels (arterioles, capillaries, venules) of many organs, especially the skin.

b) Beagles and Doberman pinschers may be predisposed.

c) It is often induced by chemicals or infectious agents.

2. Polyarteritis nodosa

It is a rare multisystemic necrotizing vasculitis that affects small and medium-sized muscular arteries in kidneys, heart, skeletal muscle, and gastrointestinal tract but usually not in the skin.

Causes

I. The initiating cause of SLE usually remains unknown.

   A. Genetic, environmental, and viral factors probably contribute to a failure in immunoregulation.

   B. When immunologic control mechanisms are rendered ineffective, antibodies to self-antigens may be produced.

II. Almost any foreign substance that elicits a detectable antibody response can lead to the development of immune complex disease.

   A. Infections (usually chronic)

     1. Viral infections: feline infectious peritonitis, feline leukemia virus (FeLV) infection, canine adenovirus I

     2. Bacterial infections: endocarditis, prostatitis, pyometra, diskospondylitis, chronic abscess

     3. Rickettsial and protozoal infections

     4. Systemic fungal infections

     5. Parasitic infections: dirofilariasis

   B. Chemicals such as sulfonamides in dogs and propylthiouracil in cats

   C. Neoplasia, particularly hemolymphatic tumors

Pathophysiology

I. The major cause of the immunologic injury in SLE is a type III hypersensitivity reaction involving precipitating and nonprecipitating antibodies of the IgG and IgM classes.

   A. Low-affinity antibodies in the presence of slight antigen excess are more likely to form antigen–antibody complexes.

   B. On entrapment of the complex in the tissue, complement activation occurs, releasing mediators of inflammation that increase vascular permeability and attract neutrophils and other phagocytes, resulting in severe tissue damage.

   C. Immune complexes can directly stimulate macrophages and neutrophils as well as sensitize cytotoxic T cells, which also amplify the inflammatory response.

II. SLE and other multisystemic diseases can result from or be associated with type II and IV hypersensitivity reactions.

Clinical Signs

I. It often has a waxing and waning course.

II. Clinical signs of SLE are not truly specific and may mimic many other systemic diseases; they vary greatly depending on the extent and site of immune complex deposition.

III. Major signs (characteristic and common)

   A. Polyarthritis, usually nonerosive

   B. Glomerulonephritis

   C. Dermatitis

   D. Coombs-positive anemia

   E. Thrombocytopenia, leukopenia

IV. Minor signs (less specific, uncommon)

   A. Fever (common but fluctuant)

   B. Pleuritis

   C. Peripheral and central neuropathy

   D. Myocarditis/pericarditis

   E. Myositis (muscle weakness)

V. Other possible signs: lymphadenopathy, leukocytosis, hepatosplenomegaly, lethargy, anorexia

Diagnosis

I. Multisystemic immune-mediated diseases require numerous diagnostics to define the extent and severity of the disease.

II. Routine diagnostics include the following.

   A. Hemogram with reticulocyte and platelet counts

   B. Serum chemistry profile, including creatine phosphokinase

   C. Urinalysis with bacterial culture

   D. If polyarthritis is suspected

     1. Radiography of affected joints

     2. Joint fluid analysis with cytology, culture

     3. Synovial biopsy

   E. If glomerulonephritis is suspected

     1. Total urinary protein excretion, urine electrophoresis, urinary protein/creatinine ratio

     2. Creatinine clearance

     3. Renal biopsy for histopathology and direct immunofluorescence

   F. If skin lesions are present

     1. Scrapings of skin to rule out parasites

     2. Bacterial and fungal cultures

     3. Skin biopsy for histopathology and direct immunofluorescence examination

III. Tests for autoantibodies are as follows.

   A. ANA test

     1. Results are usually expressed as a titer of the highest serum dilution that causes a positive ANA test.

     2. Antibodies to double-stranded nucleic acid in dogs do not appear to be as specific for SLE as they are reported to be in people.

     3. A positive ANA test is not specific for SLE.

   B. LE cell test

     1. An LE cell is a phagocytic cell containing a large homogeneous eosinophilic inclusion that is ingested and degraded nuclear material.

     2. LE cells can form when leukocytes are incubated with serum from affected animals. LE

cells may be found in joint fluids of SLE patients with polyarthritis.

    3. It is less sensitive for SLE than the ANA test.

C. Rheumatoid factor (RF) test

    1. RF is defined as an IgG or IgM autoantibody against native IgG.

    2. A positive RF test is not specific for rheumatoid arthritis.

    3. Positive RF tests have been reported in SLE patients and probably reflect overlap between these diseases.

D. Direct immunofluorescence for immune complexes

    1. The test can be run on biopsies of skin, kidney, bone marrow, synovia, and so forth.

    2. With SLE, deposition of IgG at the dermo-epidermal junction is found in both affected and normal skin.

    3. A positive test supports a diagnosis of immune-mediated disease, but it is not diagnostic by itself.

E. Hematologic parameters

    1. Coombs' test at both 37° and 4°C

    2. Platelet factor 3 test

    3. Antimegakaryocyte and antiplatelet antibody tests

    4. Measurement of serum complement

    5. Detection of circulating immune complexes

IV. The definitive diagnosis of SLE requires a positive ANA titer in combination with at least two major or one major and two minor signs.

A. Probable SLE refers to cases with one major sign and positive serology.

B. Positive serology alone is not sufficient to reach a diagnosis of SLE because the ANA test can be positive in other diseases.

C. There are also many systemic disorders with clinical signs suggestive of SLE but with a negative ANA test.

V. All attempts should be made to define an underlying disease (infection, neoplasia) or cause (drug administration).

Differential Diagnosis

I. The list of differential diagnoses of multisystemic immune-mediated disorders is extremely long.

II. Many infectious diseases may induce a polysystemic disease by immunologic injury, so infections should be considered a potential cause.

III. Neoplastic diseases and exposure to chemicals (e.g., sulfadiazine, propylthiouracil, levamisole) may also induce an immune complex disease.

Treatment

I. Remove the causative agent and treat any underlying disorder.

A. Appropriate antibiotics for bacterial infections (weeks to months)

B. Surgical drainage of abscesses or infected tissues

C. Therapy for heartworm disease

D. Withdrawal of drugs

II. Immunosuppression and anti-inflammatory therapy may be given.

A. Indicated for autoimmune diseases in which no exogenous cause can be identified (SLE) or in which the underlying disease cannot be treated (e.g., viral infection)

B. Prednisone 1.1–2.2 mg/kg PO BID, gradually decreasing to QOD over several weeks

C. Azathioprine (Imuran) 2.2 mg/kg PO SID–QOD

    1. Use alone or in combination with corticosteroids.

    2. On remission, decrease dose to 1–2 mg/kg PO QOD.

D. Cyclophosphamide (Cytoxan) 50 mg/m² PO QOD or for 4 consecutive days of each week

    1. It may be used as an alternative to or rarely with azathioprine.

    2. Withdraw drug if side effects occur (chemical cystitis, leukopenia).

E. Cyclosporine 5 mg/kg PO SID (use with caution)

    1. Use alone or in combination with corticosteroids.

    2. Withdraw if side effects occur, such as gastritis, gingival hyperplasia, papillomatosis, lymphocytoid dermatitis, anorexia, vomiting, weight loss, or involuntary shaking.

III. Plasmapheresis may be tried for the removal of autoantibodies and immune complexes from plasma.

IV. Buffered aspirin may be used in severely painful and febrile patients, but it does not directly influence the disease process.

V. During active joint inflammation, enforced rest is also important.

VI. Correct any hormonal imbalances, in particular hypothyroidism.

Patient Monitoring

I. Monitor the progression of the disease, the response to therapy, and the potential development of drug side effects.

A. Perform weekly physical examinations.

B. Repeat routine blood tests and urinalyses initially on a weekly basis to monitor effects of cyclophosphamide and azathioprine.

C. Results of ANA, LE cell, RF, Coombs', and platelet tests are influenced by immunosuppressive therapy, thus they are not reliable indicators of response to treatment.

II. The prognosis for SLE and other systemic immune complex diseases is guarded to fair. If the cause can be identified and treated or removed, the prognosis is good after an initial response to therapy. In these cases, immunosuppressive therapy can be tapered more quickly.

III. Animals with autoimmune diseases treated with high-dose immunosuppressive therapy are prone to fatal systemic infections.

IV. Relapses occur commonly.

A. Repeat laboratory tests as on initial examination.

B. Reinstitute the therapy at the original dosages or begin one of the alternative therapies in conjunction with corticosteroids as described earlier.

C. Relapses are usually less responsive to therapy; therefore, treatments are tapered more gradually than before.

Bibliography

Cohen RD: Systemic anaphylaxis. p. 150. In Bonagura JD, Kirk RW (eds): Kirk's Current Veterinary Therapy XII: Small Animal Practice. WB Saunders, Philadelphia, 1995

Cronin ME, Leair DW, Jaronski S et al: Simultaneous use of multiple serologic tests in assessing clinical activity in systemic lupus erythematosus. Clin Immunol Immunopathol 51:99, 1989

Curtis R, Bell WJ, Laing PW: Polyarteritis in a cat. Vet Rec 105:354, 1979

Davis LE: Hypersensitivity reactions induced by antimicrobial drugs. J Am Vet Med Assoc 185:1131, 1984

Easley JR: Necrotizing vasculitis: an overview. J Am Anim Hosp Assoc 15:207, 1979

Felson DT, Anderson JJ, Meenan RF: The comparative efficacy and toxicity of second-line drugs in rheumatoid arthritis. Arthritis Rheum 33:1449, 1990

Garlepp M, Farrow B, Kay P et al: Antibodies to the acetylcholine receptor in myasthenic dogs. Immunology 37:807, 1979

George L, Carmichael L: Antisperm responses in male dogs with chronic *Brucella canis* infections. J Am Vet Res 45:274, 1983

Giger U, Werner LL, Millichamp NJ, Gorman NT: Sulfadiazine-induced allergy in six Doberman pinschers. J Am Vet Med Assoc 186:479, 1985

Gordon BR, Moroff S, Hurvitz AI et al: Circulating immune complexes in sera of dogs with benign and malignant breast disease. Cancer Res 40:3627, 1980

Gosselin SJ, Capen CC, Martin SL et al: Autoimmune lymphocytic thyroiditis in dogs. Vet Immunol Immunopathol 3:185, 1982

Grauer GF, Culham CS, Dubielzig RR et al: Effects of specific thromboxane synthetase inhibitor on development of experimental *Dirofilaria immitis* immune complex glomerulonephritis in the dog. J Vet Intern Med 2:192, 1988

Gray A, Evans C, Kidd A: Suspected adverse reactions to medicines during 1989. Vet Rec 126:376, 1990

Grinden CB, Johnson KH: Systemic lupus erythematosus: literature review and report of 42 new canine cases. J Am Anim Hosp Assoc 19:489, 1983

Haines DM, Penhale WJ: Autoantibodies to pancreatic islet cells in canine diabetes mellitus. Vet Immunol Immunopathol 8:149, 1985

Halliwell REW: Autoimmune diseases in domestic animals. J Am Vet Med Assoc 181:1088, 1982

Harcourt RA: Polyarteritis in a colony of beagles. Vet Rec 102:519, 1978

Hurvitz AI: Mechanisms of immune injury. J Am Vet Med Assoc 181:1080, 1982

Jordan SC: Intravenous gamma-globulin therapy in systemic lupus erythematosus and immune complex disease. Clin Immunol Immunopathol 53:5164, 1989

Kaswan RL, Martin CL, Dawe DL: Rheumatoid factor determination in 50 dogs with keratoconjunctivitis sicca. J Am Vet Med Assoc 183:1073, 1983

Kern TJ, Walton DK, Riis RC et al: Uveitis associated with poliosis and vitiligo in six dogs. J Am Vet Med Assoc 187:408, 1985

Lachman PJ, Peters DK (eds): Clinical Aspects of Immunology. Blackwell, Oxford, 1982

Longhofer SL, Frisbie DD, Johnson HC: Effects of thromboxane synthetase inhibition on immune complex glomerulonephritis. Am J Vet Res 52:40, 1991

Medleau L, Miller WH: Immunodiagnostic tests for small-animal practice. Compend Contin Educ Pract Vet 5:705, 1983

Miller WH: Nonsteroidal anti-inflammatory agents in the management of canine and feline pruritus. p. 566. In Kirk RW, Bonagura JD (eds): Current Veterinary Therapy XI: Small Animal Practice. WB Saunders, Philadelphia, 1992

Moise NS, Spaulding GL: Feline bronchial asthma: pathogenesis, pathophysiology, diagnostics and therapeutic considerations. Compend Contin Educ Pract Vet 3:1091, 1981

Osborne CA: Special therapy. p. 58. In Kirk RW, Bonagura JD (eds): Current Veterinary Therapy XI: Small Animal Practice. WB Saunders, Philadelphia, 1992

Pedersen NC, Boyle JF: Immunologic phenomena in the effuse form of feline infectious peritonitis. Am J Vet Res 41:868, 1980

Pedersen NC, Pool RR, Morgan JP: Joint diseases of dogs and cats. p. 2187. In Ettinger SJ (ed): Textbook of Veterinary Internal Medicine. 2nd Ed. WB Saunders, Philadelphia, 1983

Pedersen NC, Pool RR, O'Brien TR: Feline chronic progressive polyarthritis. Am J Vet Res 41:522, 1980

Peterson ME, Hurvitz AI, Leib MS et al: Propylthiouracil-associated hemolytic anemia, thrombocytopenia antinuclear antibodies in cats with hyperthyroidism. J Am Vet Med Assoc 184:806, 1984

Rahman MA, Emancipator SS, Sedor JR: Hydroxyl radical scavenger ameliorates proteinuria in rat immune complex glomerulonephritis. J Lab Clin Med 112:619, 1988

Randell MG, Hurvitz AI: Immune-mediated vasculitis in five dogs. J Am Vet Med Assoc 183:207, 1983

Schaer M, Riley WJ, Buergelt CD et al: Autoimmunity and Addison's disease in the dog. J Am Anim Hosp Assoc 22:789, 1986

Schrader LE, Hurvitz AI: Cold agglutinin disease in a cat. J Am Vet Med Assoc 183:121, 1983

Scott DW: Autoimmune dermatoses. p. 467. In Kirk RW (ed): Current Veterinary Therapy VIII: Small Animal Practice. WB Saunders, Philadelphia, 1983

Scott DW, Walton DK, Manning TO et al: Canine lupus erythematosus. J Am Anim Hosp Assoc 19:461, 1983

Shelton GD, Cardinet GH, Bandman E, Cuddon P: Fiber type-specific autoantibodies in a dog with eosinophilic myositis. Muscle Nerve 8:783, 1985

Stites DP, Stobo JD, Fudenberg HH, Wells JV (eds): Basic and Clinical Immunology. 5th Ed. Lange, Los Altos, CA, 1984

Tizard IR (ed): An Introduction to Veterinary Immunology. 3rd Ed. WB Saunders, Philadelphia, 1987

Van Hess J, Mason KV, Gross TL, Burren VS: Levamisole-induced drug eruptions in the dog. J Am Anim Hosp Assoc 21:255, 1985

Volz MA, Nelson HS: Drug allergy. Best diagnostic and treatment approaches. Postgrad Med 87:137, 1990

Werner LL: Immunologic diseases affecting internal organ systems. p. 2161. In Ettinger SJ (ed): Textbook of Veterinary Internal Medicine. 2nd Ed. WB Saunders, Philadelphia, 1983

Werner LL, Bright JM: Drug induced immune hypersensitivity disorders in two dogs treated with trimethoprim-sulfadiazine. J Am Anim Hosp Assoc 19:783, 1983

Werner LL, Gorman NT: Immune-mediated disorders of cats. Vet Clin North Am 14:1039, 1984

Werner LL, Halliwell REW, Jackson RF et al: An investigation of the role of immunologic factors in anemia associated with canine heartworm disease. Vet Immunol Immunopathol 7:285, 1984

75

Immunoproliferative Diseases

Jaime F. Modiano
Stuart C. Helfand

REACTIVE CONDITIONS

Definition

I. Reactive immunoproliferative conditions are characterized by proliferative expansion of cells as a result of either appropriate or excessive (inappropriate) responses to antigen by normal cells of the immune system.

II. The antigen can be infectious (e.g., viral, bacterial, protozoal) or noninfectious (e.g., metabolic or neoplastic disease).

III. Reactive immunoproliferative conditions are different from autoimmune disease, but these two entities can occur simultaneously.

Causes

I. Ehrlichiosis
  A. *Ehrlichia canis* generally stimulates polyclonal, oligoclonal, or occasional monoclonal B-cell activation and differentiation.
  B. Active disease associated with *E. canis* infection usually includes hematopoietic abnormalities (any combination of anemia, thrombocytopenia, and leukopenia or leukocytosis), bone marrow and splenic plasmacytosis, monoclonal to polyclonal hyperglobulinemia, and a positive test for anti–*E. canis* antibody. The titer to *E. canis* may not correlate with the presence or severity of the disease.
  C. *E. platys* (predominantly found in platelets and platelet precursors) and canine granulocytic ehrlichiosis can also be a cause.

II. Heartworm disease

III. Reactive histiocytosis
  A. Histiocytosis is characterized by a benign proliferation of histiocytes or macrophages secondary to infectious, neoplastic, or metabolic diseases.

  B. This condition can progress to hemophagocytic syndrome, resulting in blood cytopenias.
  C. The histiocytic proliferation occurs in the organs of the reticuloendothelial system, including the bone marrow, liver, spleen, and lymph nodes.

IV. Disseminated or chronic neoplasia of a non–immune cell origin

V. Feline infectious peritonitis (FIP)

VI. Lymphoid hyperplasia in cats with retrovirus infections

Pathophysiology

I. Reactive conditions generally involve polyclonal or oligoclonal immune cell activation.

II. These conditions frequently resolve, ameliorate, or subside if the primary or inciting mechanism is removed.

Clinical Signs

I. These conditions have similar signs as for any other chronic or active inflammatory disease.

II. It is often difficult to differentiate those clinical signs attributable to the pathogen or the primary disease and those that arise from an immune-mediated condition (e.g., *E. canis*–associated thrombocytopenia).

Diagnosis

I. Hematology results are variable and can include mild to moderate normocytic, normochromic, nonregenerative anemia (anemia of inflammatory or chronic disease), with or without leukocytosis, with or without thrombocytopenia.
  A. The leukemoid reaction is a response to an inflammatory condition where there is a pronounced leukocytosis with a marked left shift (often including progranulocytes).

B. This type of reaction can be seen as a response to overwhelming bacterial sepsis (e.g., pyometra) or other infectious organisms such as *Hepatozoon canis.*

C. The leukemoid reaction mimics chronic myelogenous leukemia (CML).

D. Unlike CML, leukemoid reactions include an orderly, pyramidal differentiation sequence.

E. Anemia and thrombocytopenia are not prominent features, except in cases where there is a mild, nonregenerative anemia consistent with anemia of chronic or inflammatory disease.

II. Hyperglobulinemia can occur, but hyperviscosity is uncommon.

A. Hyperglobulinemia is a useful indicator to identify some types of immunoproliferative disease, such as those that involve B cells.

B. The presence and type of hyperglobulinemia should be confirmed and classified further into monoclonal, oligoclonal, or polyclonal by serum protein electrophoresis (Fig. 75–1).

C. The globulin region where the proteins localize (α, β, γ) and the specific isotype for monoclonal gammopathies (immunoelectrophoresis) can be used to rule out other differential diagnoses.

D. It is imperative to differentiate hyperglobulinemias that are caused by increased immunoglobulin production from those that may represent the possible extreme of an acute phase reaction (α and β globulins such as α-macroglobulins, C-reactive protein, ceruloplasmin, fibrinogen, haptoglobins, transferrin, etc.).

III. Serum biochemistries are variable and reflect systemic condition and organ involvement.

IV. Urinalysis results are variable, although some cases may present with proteinuria.

A. Identify the source of the proteinuria.

B. Immunoglobulin light chains in the urine (Bence Jones proteins) are not detectable using routine procedures to quantify urine protein (see discussion of multiple myeloma later).

C. Proteinuria generally suggests some facet of renal involvement (see Chap. 47).

D. Urine protein:urine creatinine ratios are of value in assessing the relative severity of proteinuria.

V. Reactive conditions often mimic neoplasia based on their patterns of cellular infiltration, but generally these can be differentiated by microscopic examination of biopsies or fine-needle aspirates.

Differential Diagnosis

I. All of the causes listed previously must be ruled out.

II. See other sections for diagnostic advice.

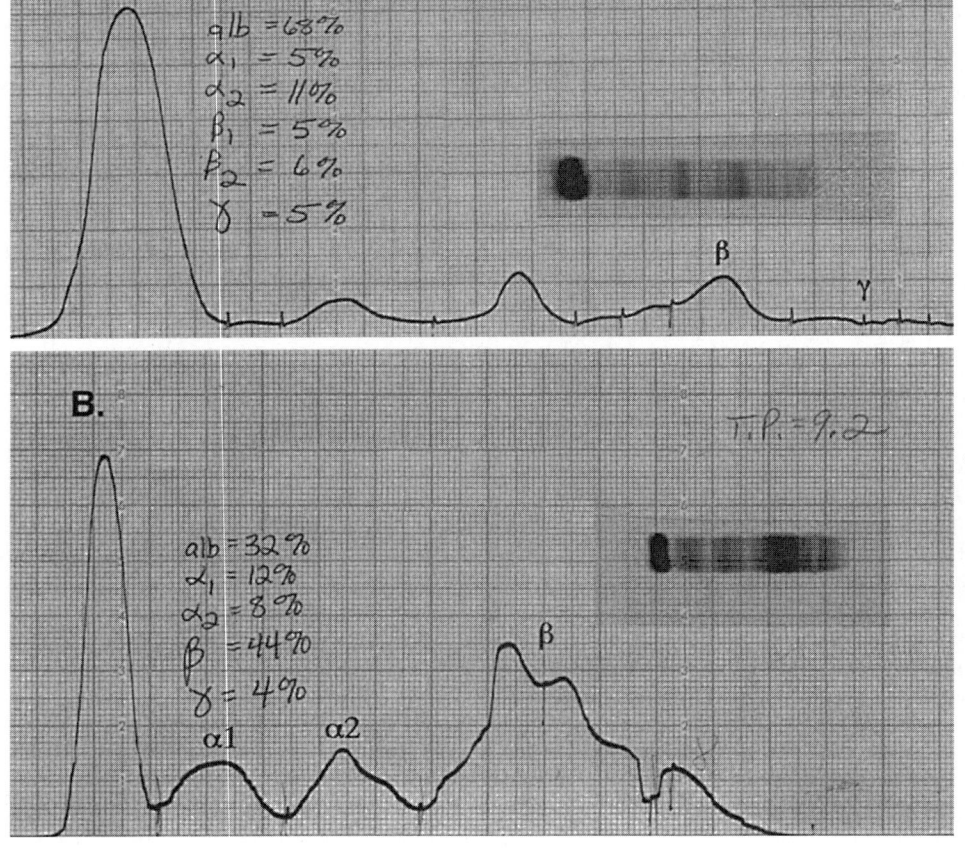

Figure 75–1. A. Normal canine serum protein electrophoresis. The tallest peak is albumin (left), and the immunoglobulins migrate to the β and γ regions (right). The bands on the acetate membrane in which the serum proteins were separated and stained (right) were analyzed with a densitometer to produce the graph. B. Serum protein electrophoresis from a dog with chronic thyroid neoplasia. There are marked elevations in the α and β regions, corresponding to increases of acute phase proteins and some immunoglobulins, respectively.

Treatment and Monitoring

I. Reactive immunoproliferative conditions may or may not respond to symptomatic treatment.
   A. Ideally, the inciting cause is found and appropriate treatment is instituted for the underlying disease.
   B. Immunosuppressive therapy may be counterproductive, although it is sometimes used for specific conditions such as the immune-mediated thrombocytopenia (IMT) associated with *E. canis* infection.
II. In FIP, clinical disease arises from an inappropriate humoral immune response to a pathogen, so immunosuppressive therapy is warranted.
III. The immunosuppressive agents that can be used when warranted include the following.
   A. Prednisone 2–4 mg/kg PO SID-BID
   B. Melphalan (numerous therapeutic protocols described)
      1. 7 mg/m² PO SID × 5 days every 3 weeks
      2. 1.5 mg/m² PO SID × 7–10 days, repeated every 3 weeks
      3. 0.1 mg/kg PO SID × 10 days, then 0.05 mg/kg PO SID until a clinical response or myelosuppression occurs

C. Cyclophosphamide
   1. 50 mg/m² PO SID × 4 days per week until clinical response or adverse effects
   2. 200 mg/m² IV weekly until clinical response or adverse effects
   3. *Caution:* side effects of cyclophosphamide well known and dose limiting

NEOPLASTIC DISEASES

Definition

I. Neoplastic immunoproliferative conditions are characterized by uncontrolled proliferation of a transformed population of clonal immune cells.
II. Excessive production of a monoclonal immunoglobulin called paraprotein or M component is a frequent characteristic of some of these malignancies, especially those arising from plasma cells or B lymphocytes.

Causes

I. Cell division is tightly regulated by the balanced action of gene products that promote or suppress growth (proto-oncogenes and tumor suppressor

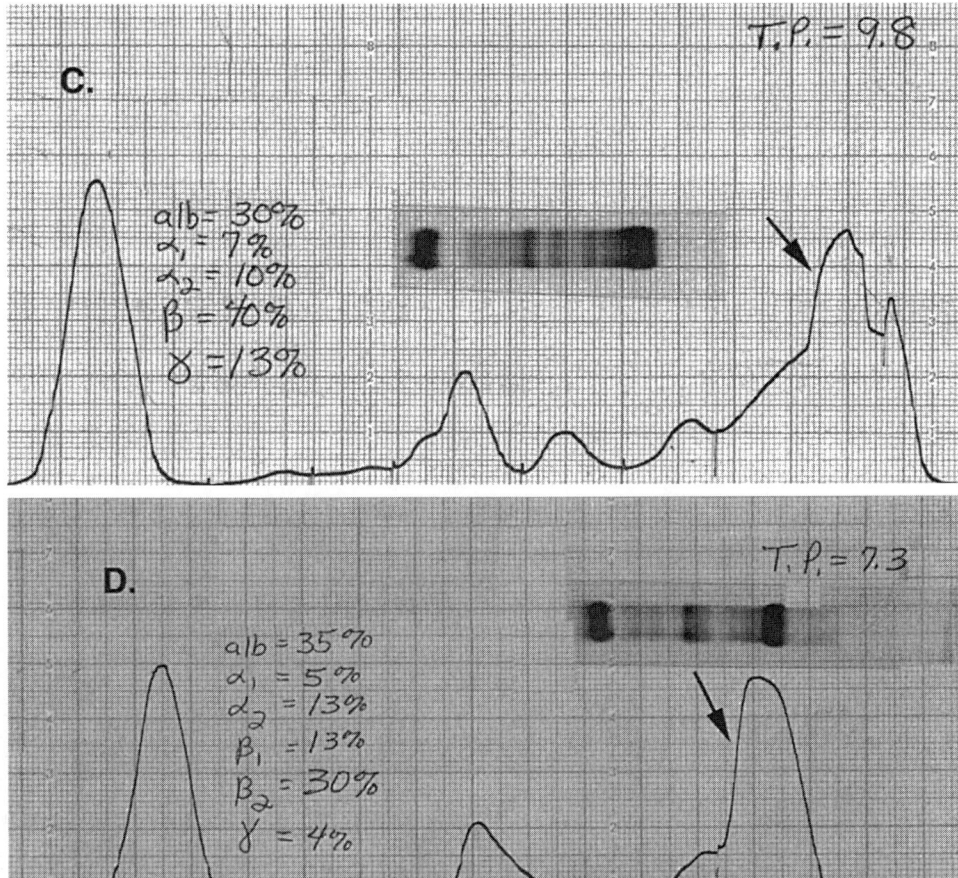

Figure 75–1 *Continued.* C. Serum protein electrophoresis from a cat with feline infectious peritonitis. Polyclonal gammopathy (arrow) is commonly associated with this illness as a result of an inappropriate humoral response induced by the virus. D. Serum protein electrophoresis from a dog with multiple myeloma. Monoclonal gammopathy (IgA type) is present (arrow) in the β₂ region.

genes, respectively). Mutations that affect the temporal expression or function of one of these regulatory genes may incite neoplastic transformation.

II. The cellular proliferation seen in neoplastic immunoproliferative conditions is not driven by antigen or normal environmental signals.

III. Some specific genetic events have been associated with neoplastic immunoproliferative disease.

  A. Chromosomal translocations and mutations involving the c-myc gene and the bcl-2 gene have been the most frequently described genetic defects in human and murine multiple myeloma.

    1. Rearrangements have been identified in canine and feline lymphohematopoietic malignancies.

    2. The prevalence of these rearrangements is unknown.

  B. The establishment of autocrine growth loops, where a cell makes excessive quantities of a factor that in turn promotes its own growth, has been defined in various species.

    1. Most involve abnormalities in the growth pathways regulated by interleukin-2.

    2. They include cutaneous lymphoma/leukemia involving natural killer cells in dogs.

  C. Viral insertions that disrupt the normal function of growth regulatory genes can also cause immunoproliferative disease, and this is known to occur in some feline leukemia virus (FeLV)–infected cats.

Pathophysiology

I. Multiple myeloma (including macroglobulinemia)

  A. Malignant plasma cells in bone marrow impair normal hematopoiesis, resulting in anemia, leukopenia, and thrombocytopenia.

  B. Plasma cell dysfunction results in immune deficiency and increased susceptibility to infection.

  C. Increased paraprotein can cause plasma hyperviscosity, hemostatic abnormalities, amyloidosis, and cryoglobulinemia.

  D. Increased antibody subunits (light chains) contribute to renal failure.

    1. Light chains filtered by glomerulus

    2. Overloading of tubule reabsorptive ability

    3. Tubular degeneration with cast formation

II. Solitary plasmacytoma

  A. Skin and oral mucous membranes

    1. Behave as space-occupying lesions and can interfere with tissue function locally

    2. Can ulcerate and bleed

    3. Not associated with immunoglobulin production or systemic pathology

  B. Gastrointestinal (GI) tract

    1. Can be solitary in the canine rectum, intestine, stomach

    2. Usually secrete clonal immunoglobulin, most often IgG

    3. Metastasize within the abdomen

    4. Interfere with normal GI function

  C. Osseous forms

    1. Rarely, solitary osseous plasmacytoma may precede recognition of systemic multiple myeloma.

    2. They should probably be considered a variant of multiple myeloma.

III. Tumors of the monocyte/macrophage or reticuloendothelial (RE) system

  A. Canine cutaneous histiocytoma

    1. Arises from Langerhans cells in the skin

    2. Most often seen in young dogs as a solitary nodule in an extremity, but can occur in dogs of any age and at any site in the skin

    3. Generally regress spontaneously

    4. Very rarely are locally invasive

  B. Systemic histiocytosis

    1. Familial disease of Bernese mountain dogs

    2. Characterized by infiltration of the skin and lymphoid organs by benign histiocytes

  C. Malignant histiocytosis

    1. Occurs in many breeds of dogs and rarely in cats

    2. Bernese mountain dogs and golden retrievers affected most often

    3. Characterized by infiltration of numerous organs or tissues by malignant histiocytes or macrophages

    4. Lung, lymph nodes, central nervous system, eye, spleen, bone marrow, skin/subcutis frequently affected

  D. Monocytic leukemia

    1. It is the most common canine myeloproliferative disease.

    2. Acute monocytic or monoblastic leukemia may present with an elevated white blood cell (WBC) count and circulating blasts, with a normal WBC count and circulating blasts (subleukemic), or with a decreased WBC count with no circulating blasts (aleukemic).

    3. It frequently results in anemia and thrombocytopenia from space-occupying effects in the bone marrow (myelophthisic lesion).

  E. Malignant fibrous histiocytoma

    1. It is also known as giant cell tumor of soft tissues.

    2. It is locally invasive, and the giant cell variant is highly metastatic (often to lymphoid organs).

    3. It is reported in dogs and cats; the genesis and biologic behavior may be different for each species.

    4. It most often arises in the subcutis.

  F. Pulmonary lymphomatoid granulomatosis

    1. It is an invasive, proliferative disease that affects the lungs and mediastinum of dogs.

    2. Cellular populations are mixed and include mononuclear cells (histiocytes and lymphocytes), granulocytic cells (neutrophils and eosinophils), and rarely multinucleated giant cells.

    3. Lesions may be malignant or premalignant.

    4. It is unknown whether the proliferative, invasive cells are lymphoid or histiocytic in origin.

Clinical Signs

I. Multiple myeloma
  A. Signs related to proliferation of malignant plasma cells
    1. Skeletal lesions resulting in pain and increased osteoclast activity
       a) Osteolytic lesions, pathologic fractures, osteoporosis
       b) Order of involvement: vertebrae, long bones, ribs, pelvis
       c) In 75% of dogs, rare in cats
    2. Neurologic signs in 40% of affected dogs
       a) Spinal cord compression: pain, weakness, paralysis, urinary incontinence
       b) Brain/meningeal infiltration
    3. Hepatosplenomegaly most common
    4. Lymphadenopathy (rare)
    5. Anemia in 50% of dogs
  B. Signs related to products of malignant plasma cells
    1. Bleeding diathesis in 30% of cases with epistaxis and petechia of mucous membranes
       a) Decreased platelet adhesiveness and platelet factor 3 (PF3) release
       b) Interference with coagulation factors
       c) Thrombocytopenia secondary to myelophthisis
    2. Hyperviscosity syndrome (HVS) in 10–20% of dogs and occasionally in cats from high molecular weight immunoglobulin (IgM), polymers of IgA, or high concentrations of IgG paraproteinemia
       a) Retinopathy: vessel tortuosity and hemorrhages
       b) Dementia, depression, coma
       c) Congestive heart failure from hypervolemia
    3. Renal dysfunction with proteinuria composed of Ig light chains (Bence Jones protein)
       a) Protein precipitation in tubules and glomerular damage
       b) Deleterious effects of hypercalcemia
       c) Poor renal circulation from HVS
    4. Life-threatening infections from depressed levels of normal immunoglobulins, granulocytopenia secondary to myelophthisis or impaired neutrophil function
    5. Hypercalcemia from osteoclast activating factor (OAF) secreted by plasma cells
       a) Polyuria, polydipsia
       b) Weakness, inappetence
II. Solitary plasmacytoma
  A. Skin and oral mucous membranes
    1. Smooth, dome-shaped, sessile mass
    2. Pink to bright red
    3. Millimeters to centimeters in size
    4. Found anywhere on the skin
    5. Not usually invasive of underlying bone when in the mouth
    6. Benign behavior
  B. Gastrointestinal tract
    1. Vomiting when located in the stomach or esophagus
    2. Anorexia
    3. Diarrhea, melena, tenesmus, and hematochezia associated with intestinal and rectal plasmacytomas
    4. Also secondary signs associated with monoclonal gammopathy
III. Macroglobulinemia
  A. Neoplastic infiltrates occur primarily in soft tissues and cause organomegaly, especially of the spleen, liver, and lymph nodes.
  B. Bony lysis is uncommon.
  C. Clinical signs are primarily related to hyperviscosity.
    1. Hemorrhages of the microcirculation of numerous organs including skin
    2. Neurologic signs
    3. Retinal vein distention and hemorrhage
    4. Anemia
IV. Tumors of the monocyte/macrophage or RE system
  A. Canine cutaneous histiocytoma: usually solitary nodule with no systemic effects
  B. Systemic histiocytosis
    1. Anorexia and weight loss
    2. Lethargy or depression
    3. Increased lung sounds
    4. Cutaneous nodular masses
    5. Lymphadenopathy
  C. Malignant histiocytosis
    1. Signs are generally nonspecific.
    2. It can result in anemia, thrombocytopenia, or leukopenia as a result of myelophthisis or hemophagocytosis.
    3. Many animals die of fulminant organ failure.
  D. Monocytic leukemia
    1. Signs are generally nonspecific and include lethargy, fever, weight loss, and inappetence.
    2. It can result in anemia, thrombocytopenia, or leukopenia as a result of myelophthisis.
  E. Malignant fibrous histiocytoma
    1. Generally a single skin mass
    2. Enlarged lymph nodes or splenomegaly from metastasis
  F. Pulmonary lymphomatoid granulomatosis
    1. Dyspnea or increased respiratory effort
    2. Nonproductive coughing
    3. Exercise intolerance

Diagnosis

I. Multiple myeloma
  A. Hemogram
    1. Normocytic, normochromic anemia
    2. Leukopenia in 30% of cases
    3. Occasional plasma cells at feathered edge
    4. Rouleaux formation
    5. Elevated plasma protein up to 16 g/dl
  B. Platelet count: thrombocytopenia (usually mild to moderate, but can be marked)
  C. Serum protein electrophoresis

1. Monoclonal gammopathy with protein peak in α, β, or γ regions (see Fig. 75–1)
   a) IgG, IgM, or IgA production, usually of a single immunoglobulin class
   b) Decreased concentrations of the uninvolved immunoglobulins
   c) Immunoelectrophoresis or Ig quantitation required to characterize abnormal Ig type
2. "Silent myeloma" characterized by proliferation of neoplastic plasma cells that do not secrete paraprotein

D. Biochemical profile
1. Elevated serum total protein (usually >9 g/dl)
2. Possibly normal serum protein if large protein loss occurring through kidneys
3. Hypercalcemia (10% of cases)
4. Elevated creatinine with advanced renal dysfunction
5. Elevated liver enzymes with hepatic plasma cell infiltration

E. Urinalysis
1. Bence Jones proteinuria may be detected via classical method utilizing heat precipitation.
2. Urine electrophoresis is more sensitive for detection of globulins and is the test of choice (Fig. 75–2).
3. Urine dipsticks are not sensitive to globulins or Bence Jones proteins.

F. Bone marrow aspirate or core biopsy
1. Essential to the diagnosis
2. Increased numbers of clustered primitive plasma cells (>10% of nucleated cells)
3. Decreased numbers of other marrow cells
4. Patchy marrow infiltration

G. Skeletal radiographic survey
1. 75% of dogs have skeletal lesions.
2. Most commonly these are punched out osteolytic lesions.

H. Serum viscosity >7 relative to water (normal serum viscosity = 1.6)

I. Definitive diagnosis of multiple myeloma of the following lesions

1. Demonstrate at least two of four of the following.
   a) Radiographic bony lesions
   b) Bone marrow infiltration with plasma cells
   c) Monoclonal gammopathy
   d) Bence Jones proteinuria or paraproteinuria
2. Preferably three of these four lesions are found, in order to avoid confusion with ehrlichiosis.

II. Solitary plasmacytoma
A. Skin and oral mucous membranes
1. Excisional biopsy is the preferred diagnostic procedure.
2. Intraoral tumors are radiographed to ascertain adjacent bone destruction prior to tumor excision.
3. A systemic work-up, as described for multiple myeloma, is usually not performed once the diagnosis of skin/oral mucous membrane plasmacytoma has been obtained because these tumors are not progressive.

B. Gastrointestinal tract lesions
1. If GI signs and/or abdominal masses are present, an abdominal work-up including radiography and ultrasonography is indicated.
2. If upper GI signs are present, endoscopic exam may be useful to obtain tissue for diagnosis.
3. If the animal is hyperproteinemic, conduct a systemic work-up as described for multiple myeloma to rule out bone marrow disease.
4. Absence of skeletal lesions may make the diagnosis elusive.

III. Macroglobulinemia
A. Serum protein electrophoresis usually shows elevated β peak.
B. Macroglobulinemia can be seen in conjunction with other B-cell malignancies, such as lymphoma and chronic lymphocytic leukemia.

IV. Tumors of the monocyte/macrophage or RE system
A. These diseases are often presumptive in certain

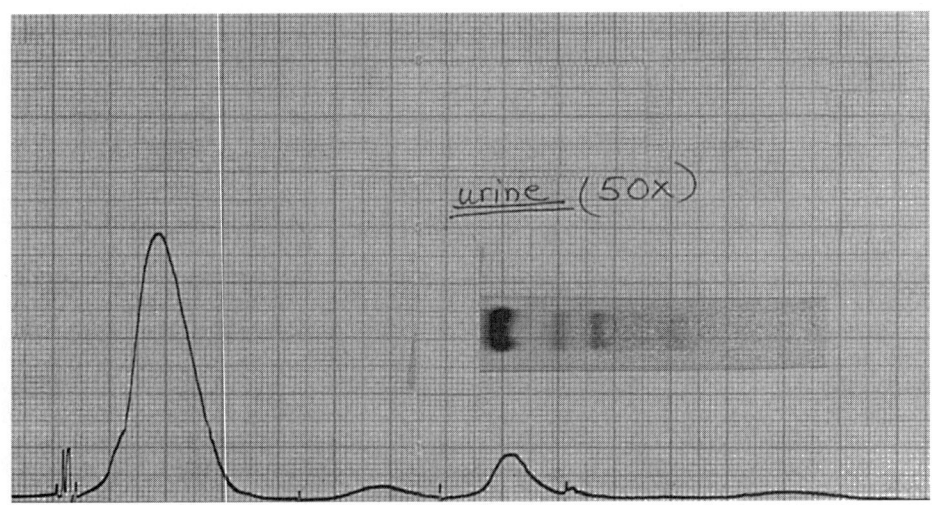

urine (50x)

Figure 75–2. Urine electrophoresis from a dog with multiple myeloma. The large peak on the left represents albuminuria; the smaller peak on the right represents paraprotein.

breeds such as Bernese mountain dogs and golden retrievers that show a predilection for histiocytic malignancies.
B. Cytologic examination of fine-needle aspirates is a useful diagnostic aid for most histiocytic disorders.
C. The diagnosis is always confirmed by histologic evaluation of affected tissues.
D. Cytochemistry or immunohistochemistry of cytologic or histopathologic samples provides a definitive diagnosis.

Treatment

I. Multiple myeloma
  A. Goals of therapy
    1. Reduce tumor cell mass, which will reduce quantity of paraprotein and specific syndromes
    2. Provide supportive care
  B. Criteria of objective response
    1. Decrease in abnormal serum protein by 50%
    2. Decrease in Bence Jones proteinuria by 50%
    3. Size and number of lytic bone lesions static or reduced
    4. Clinical reduction in the presenting signs (e.g., lameness, bone pain, lethargy, etc.)
  C. Chemotherapy
    1. Melphalan plus prednisone (most common protocol)
     a) Melphalan (Alkeran) 0.1 mg/kg PO SID × 10 days, then 0.05 mg/kg PO SID continuously (or 7 mg/m² PO SID × 5 days every 3 weeks, or 1.5 mg/m² PO SID on 3 alternate days per week)
     b) Prednisone 0.5 mg/kg PO SID × 10 days, then 0.5 mg/kg PO every other day
     c) Cyclophosphamide possibly used in place of melphalan, but more toxic
    2. Combination chemotherapy
     a) Multiagent chemotherapy as used in lymphoma
     b) Combinations of cyclophosphamide, doxorubicin, vincristine, and prednisone
     c) Dosages as for lymphoma
    3. Liposome-encapsulated doxorubicin: recently reported to induce remission in a dog with IgA myeloma refractory to conventional chemotherapy
    4. May be tried in cats
  D. Radiation therapy with ⁶⁰Co or linear accelerator
    1. To palliate bone pain
    2. For treatment of spinal cord compression
    3. For extramedullary plasmacytoma
  E. Surgical excision
    1. It is the treatment of choice for extramedullary plasmacytoma of skin and oral cavity.
    2. It is the initial therapy for gastrointestinal plasmacytoma.
  F. Supportive therapy
    1. Infections
     a) Maintain on antibiotics until remission is noted.
     b) Give trimethoprim/sulfa orally or gentamicin plus cephalosporin parenterally if life-threatening sepsis is present.
     c) Use clean technique for all venipunctures.
     d) Avoid intravenous catheters if possible.
    2. Hypercalcemia (see also Chaps. 47 and 71)
     a) Saline diuresis plus chemotherapy if Ca²⁺ <13.5 mg/dl
     b) Saline diuresis, furosemide, plus chemotherapy if Ca²⁺ >13.5 mg/dl
     c) If refractory, mithramycin at 1.25 μg/m² IV once weekly (decreases Ca²⁺ in 12 hours, but very expensive and rarely used)
     d) May normalize with tumor-specific chemotherapy only
    3. Plasmapheresis
     a) To remove immunoglobulins present in plasma
     b) Used as emergency treatment for HVS
II. Tumors of the monocyte/macrophage or RE system
  A. Surgical excision is the primary treatment for histiocytoma.
    1. For difficult surgical sites, cryotherapy and radiotherapy are alternatives.
    2. L-Asparaginase (400 IU/kg every 1–2 weeks × 4 treatments) has been used successfully to treat dogs with multiple cutaneous histiocytomas.
  B. Aggressive chemotherapy has been used for malignant histiocytosis.
    1. Combination chemotherapy with doxorubicin, cyclophosphamide, vincristine, and prednisone may be tried.
    2. Single agents provide minimal benefit, although prednisone alone may induce minimal short-lived responses.
  C. Adjuvant chemotherapy or radiation therapy has been used following surgical excision of malignant fibrous histiocytoma.
  D. Prednisone or combination chemotherapy (cytoxan, vincristine, prednisone) is reported to result in partial to complete responses for pulmonary lymphomatoid granulomatosis.

Patient Monitoring

I. Multiple myeloma shows the following trends.
  A. Response to therapy
    1. Melphalan can cause thrombocytopenia after 3–6 months of therapy, so monitor hemograms and platelet counts every month.
    2. A positive response to therapy is usually seen in 3–6 weeks.
    3. Perform serum protein electrophoresis or measure Ig levels every 3–4 weeks initially.
     a) Normal or improved results are usually seen in 6–8 weeks.
     b) Periodically (every 2 months) measure serum paraprotein concentrations during maintenance therapy.

4. Bone marrow aspiration is routinely repeated periodically to further assess remission.

B. Prognosis
1. Animals with Bence Jones proteinuria and hypercalcemia have a poorer prognosis.
2. Animals with pancytopenia or plasma cell leukemia have a very poor prognosis.
3. Irreversible renal function carries the worst prognosis.
4. Animals that respond early to therapy have a better prognosis.
5. If early sepsis and renal dysfunction are successfully managed, most dogs respond well to chemotherapy.
6. Prolongation of life up to 2 years is possible; median survival of 540 days is reported in dogs (Matus et al., 1986).
7. Limited reports of therapy in cats suggest the results to be inferior to that in dogs.

II. Extramedullary plasmacytoma of skin and oral mucous membranes have excellent prognosis with complete surgical excision.

III. Gastrointestinal extramedullary plasmacytomas are usually malignant and metastatic and carry a guarded to poor prognosis.

IV. Tumors of the monocyte/macrophage or RE system have a variable course.
A. Routine blood counts are done as for any patient receiving chemotherapy.
B. If possible, organ-specific exams (e.g., lung radiographs, abdominal ultrasonography/aspiration) are performed every 2 months to assess responses to chemotherapy.
C. Despite therapy, systemic histiocytosis, malignant histiocytosis, and giant cell variant of malignant fibrous histiocytoma are almost always progressive and fatal.
D. Stable disease can sometimes be maintained for 3–6 months with chemotherapy.
E. Histiocytoma is benign, nonprogressive, and curative with surgery, and spontaneous remissions can also occur.
F. Complete remissions are reported for pulmonary lymphomatoid granulomatosis, but prognosis is guarded.

Bibliography

Berry CR, Moore PF, Thomas WP et al: Pulmonary lymphomatoid granulomatosis in seven dogs (1976–1987). J Vet Intern Med 4:157, 1990

Breitschwerdt EB, Woody BJ, Zerbe CA et al: Monoclonal gammopathy associated with naturally occurring canine ehrlichiosis. J Vet Intern Med 1:2, 1987

Eastman CA: Plasma cell tumors in a cat. Feline Pract 24:26, 1996

Helfand SC, Modiano JF, Moore PF et al: Functional interleukin-2 receptors are expressed on natural killer-like leukemic cells from a dog with cutaneous lymphoma. Blood 86:636, 1995

Jackson MW, Helfand SC, Smedes SL et al: Primary IgG secreting plasma cell tumor in the gastrointestinal tract of a dog. J Am Vet Med Assoc 204:404, 1994

Kisseberth WC, MacEwen EG, Helfand SC et al: Response to liposome-encapsulated doxorubicin (TLC D-99) in a dog with myeloma. J Vet Intern Med 9:425, 1995

Matus RE, Leifer CE, Gordon BR et al: Plasmapheresis and chemotherapy of hyperviscosity syndrome associated with monoclonal gammopathy in the dog. J Am Vet Med Assoc 1883:215, 1983

Matus RE, Leifer CE, MacEwen EG, Hurvitz AI: Prognostic factors for multiple myeloma in the dog. J Am Vet Med Assoc 188:1288, 1986

Moore PF, Rosin A: Malignant histiocytosis of Bernese mountain dogs. Vet Pathol 23:1, 1986

Moriello KA, MacEwen G, Schultz KT: PEG-L-asparaginase in the treatment of canine epitheliotrophic lymphoma and histiocytic proliferative dermatitis. p. 293. In Ihrke PJ, Mason IS, White SD (eds): Advances in Veterinary Dermatology. Pergamon Press, New York, 1992

Pieden MM, Shen S: Immunoglobulin light chains and the kidney: an overview. Ultrastruct Pathol 18:105, 1994

Walton RM, Modiano JF, Thrall MA, Wheeler SL: Bone marrow cytological findings in 4 dogs and a cat with hemophagocytic syndrome. J Vet Intern Med 10:7, 1996

Waters CB, Morrison WB, DeNicola DB et al: Giant cell variant of malignant fibrous histiocytoma in dogs: 10 cases (1986–1993). J Am Vet Med Assoc 205:1420, 1994

Weinberg RA: The molecular basis of oncogenes and tumor suppressor genes. Ann N Y Acad Sci 758:331, 1995

Woody BJ, Hoskins JD: Ehrlichial diseases of dogs. Vet Clin North Am [Small Anim Pract] 21:75, 1991

76

Diseases of the Thymus

Jaime F. Modiano
Stuart C. Helfand

DISEASES OF REDUCED THYMIC MASS

Thymic Hypoplasia

Definition

I. It grossly appears as only a rudimentary thymus.
II. Decreased size may be from reduced numbers of thymic lymphocytes, decreased epithelial framework, or both.

Causes

I. Genetic disorders (see also Chap. 73)
 A. X-linked severe combined immunodeficiency (XSCID)
  1. Found in a colony of basset hounds established from a single affected female
  2. Arises from a defect in the gene encoding the common gamma chain of the interleukin-2 receptor (IL-2Rγ)
  3. Histologic dysplasia of the thymic epithelial component with severe lymphoid hypoplasia
 B. Growth hormone deficiency: immunodeficient dwarfism in a family of Weimaraners
  1. Growth hormone is thymotrophic.
  2. The condition is partially responsive to treatment with bovine growth hormone or thymosin fraction 5.
 C. Thymic atrophy of Mexican hairless dogs
  1. Pups are born with an apparently normal thymus.
  2. Thymus undergoes severe atrophy by the age of 2 months.
  3. T cell function is reduced in adults.
 D. Acrodermatitis with immunodeficiency: described in bull terriers
  1. Growth retardation
  2. Skin lesions and immunodeficiency
 E. Thymic aplasia in cats: syndrome of hairlessness in Birman kittens

II. Acquired disorders
 A. Infectious diseases
  1. Morbilliviruses: canine distemper virus
  2. Picornaviruses
   a) Canine parvovirus and feline panleukopenia virus
   b) Lympholytic and cause thymic necrosis
  3. Retroviruses
   a) Immunosuppressive C-type viruses
    (1) Feline leukemia virus (FeLV)
     i) FeLV subgroup C virus (replication deficient)
     ii) Requires helper virus (usually FeLV subgroup A)
     iii) Induces thymocyte apoptosis
    (2) Canine immunosuppressive retrovirus
     i) Lympholytic in peripheral lymphoid organs
     ii) Impairs T-cell function
     iii) Effect on thymic development unknown
   b) Lentiviruses
    (1) Feline immunodeficiency virus (FIV)
     i) Replication occurs primarily in T cells and monocytes or macrophages.
     ii) Thymic hypoplasia does not always occur with FIV infection.
     iii) It can be lympholytic; loss of infected and uninfected CD4 T cells may occur through apoptosis similar to that in human immunodeficiency virus.
    (2) Canine immunodeficiency virus (CIV)
     i) Isolated from a dog with myeloproliferative disease
     ii) Effects on thymocyte or T cell function, or on thymic development, unknown
 B. Environmental conditions
  1. Radiation
  2. Thymic hematomas

a) Idiopathic thymic hemorrhage
b) Traumatic thymic hemorrhage
C. Physiologic changes
  1. Corticosteroid administration
  2. Can be reversible

Pathophysiology

I. Thymic aplasia arises from failure of thymic elements to differentiate during development.
II. Thymic hypoplasia may arise from involution from gradual to acute loss of thymocytes.
  A. Lympholysis: necrosis of lymphocytes
  B. Apoptosis: programmed cell death or "cell suicide"

Clinical Signs

I. Other than viral-induced disease, thymic hypoplasia is extremely rare.
II. Immunosuppression (failure to thrive, recurrent infections) is a hallmark feature of thymic hypoplasia.

Diagnosis

I. Inspection of the thymus
II. Laboratory testing for viral causes
III. Especially warranted in "fading" puppies or kittens

Differential Diagnosis

I. Immunodeficiency of non-thymic origin
II. Reduced cellular immunity without loss of thymocyte mass

Treatment and Monitoring

I. If the cause is known, specific therapies are instituted.
  A. Aggressive antimicrobial therapy with supportive care for canine parvovirus and feline panleukopenia
  B. Surgery and supportive therapy for thymic hematomas
II. The usefulness of some commercially available immune modulators and biologic response modifiers (e.g., interferons, interleukins, or colony-stimulating factors) in the treatment of immunosuppression has not been rigorously confirmed and is controversial.
III. Severe immunosuppression is generally fatal.

NEOPLASTIC DISEASES OF INCREASED THYMIC MASS

Thymoma

Definition

I. The tumor originates from a transformed thymic epithelial cell (see also Chap. 20).
II. It is common in dogs, and the incidence in German shepherd dogs may be higher than in other breeds.
III. It is very rare in cats.

Classification and Pathophysiology

I. Benign thymoma
  A. It is generally well encapsulated.
  B. Epithelial cells promote T-cell proliferation with full differentiation (T cells account for most of the increased thymic mass).
II. Malignant thymoma: locally invasive to metastatic
  A. It may displace lymphoid tissue entirely.
  B. Angioinvasive thymomas may result in mediastinal or pleural hemorrhage or chylous effusion.

Clinical Signs

I. Dyspnea, dysphagia
II. Muffled heart sounds (especially if pleural effusion present)
III. Facial edema from impaired venous return via the cranial vena cava
IV. Non-compressible thorax in cats
V. Evidence of paraneoplastic syndromes
  A. Myasthenia gravis
  B. Polymyositis

Diagnosis

I. Benign thymoma
  A. It can usually be visualized radiographically or by ultrasonography
  B. Fine-needle aspirates usually yield samples that consist almost entirely of small lymphocytes.
    1. Occasionally mast cells are seen, but these may also be present in normal thymic tissue.
    2. Epithelial cells may be present in small numbers.
    3. Diagnosis should be confirmed histologically via ultrasound-guided biopsy or exploratory surgery.
II. Malignant thymoma
  A. Epithelial cells are a more prominent component.
  B. Small lymphocytes are still often the predominant cells seen on fine-needle aspirates.

Differential Diagnosis

I. Thymic hyperplasia
  A. Thymic nodular hyperplasia may occur in animals.
  B. It is usually an incidental finding at necropsy with no clinical significance.
II. Thymic cysts
  A. Congenital defect with thymic enlargement into cystic, multilobulated masses
  B. Clinically insignificant

Treatment

I. Surgery can be curative for benign thymoma.
II. Radiation is palliative for benign and malignant thymoma.
III. Chemotherapy may be tried.
  A. Prednisone may induce partial remission of the lymphoid component.

B. Multiagent chemotherapy as used in lymphoma (e.g., cyclophosphamide, doxorubicin, vincristine, prednisone) is minimally effective at inducing remission.

Patient Monitoring

I. Prognosis is favorable for benign thymoma.
II. Paraneoplastic diseases worsen the prognosis significantly.
III. Prognosis is guarded to poor for malignant thymoma.

Thymic Lymphoma

Definiton

I. It is a tumor of lymphoid origin.
II. It frequently involves mediastinal lymph nodes.
III. Malignant lymphoblasts can efface the thymus gland.
IV. It may occur alone or as part of multicentric disease.

Causes and Pathophysiology

I. It is commonly associated with FeLV infection in very young or aged cats.
II. Etiology is uncertain in dogs; a retroviral etiology has not been demonstrated.

Clinical Signs

I. Dyspnea, dysphagia
II. Muffled heart sounds, especially if pleural effusion present
III. Non-compressible thorax in cats

Diagnosis

I. It can often be visualized radiographically or ultrasonographically (see Chap. 20).
II. Pleural effusion is commonly present, and fluid analysis is usually helpful (see Chap. 19).
    A. Fine-needle aspirates yield large numbers of large lymphocytes and lymphoblasts.
    B. Neutrophils may be present from any associated inflammation.
    C. Fluid may be a transudate, modified transudate, or exudate.
        1. Neutrophils, vacuolated macrophages, and mesothelial cells invariably are present as a result of associated irritation or inflammation.
        2. Histopathology is used to confirm diagnosis and aid in establishing prognosis.

Treatment

I. Multiagent chemotherapy as used in lymphoma (see Chap. 67)
II. Usually induces complete remission in cats; less effective in dogs

Patient Monitoring

I. Prognosis is guarded with chemotherapy.
    A. Median survival of 17.5 months has been reported for FeLV-negative cats with thymic lymphoma (Mooney et al., 1989).
    B. Thymic lymphoma in dogs is often associated with hypercalcemia, and survival times are shorter.
II. FeLV-positive cats often develop additional lymphohematopoietic tumors, usually within 1 year of diagnosis.

Bibliography

Aronsohn M: Canine thymoma. Vet Clin North Am [Small Anim Pract] 15:755, 1985

Beebe AM, Dua N, Faith TG et al: Primary stage of feline immunodeficiency virus infection: viral dissemination and cellular targets. J Virol 68:3080, 1994

Bellah JR, Stiff ME, Russell RG: Thymoma in the dog: two case reports and review of 20 additional cases. J Am Vet Med Assoc 183:306, 1983

Coolman BR, Brewer WG, D'Andrea GH, Lenz SD: Idiopathic thymic hemorrhage in two littermate dogs. J Am Vet Med Assoc 206:156, 1995

Fukuta K, Koizumi N, Imamura K et al: Microscopic observations of skin and lymphoid organs in the hairless dog derived from the Mexican hairless. Jikken Dobutsu (Jap J Vet Res) 40:69, 1991

Macartney L, McCandlish IA, Thompson H, Cornwell HJ: Canine parvovirus enteritis 1: clinical, haematological and pathological features of experimental infection. Vet Rec 115:201, 1984

Modiano JF, Getzy DM, Akol KG et al: Retrovirus-like activity in an immunosuppressed dog: pathological and immunological findings. J Comp Pathol 112:165, 1995

Mooney SC, Hayes AA, MacEwen EG et al: Treatment and prognostic factors in lymphoma in cats: 103 cases (1977–1981). J Am Vet Med Assoc 194:696, 1989

Rojko JL, Fulton RM, Rezanka LJ et al: Lymphocytotoxic strains of feline leukemia virus induce apoptosis in feline T4-thymic lymphoma cells. Lab Invest 66:418, 1992

Roth JA: Possible association of thymus dysfunction with fading syndromes in puppies and kittens. Vet Clin North Am [Small Anim Pract] 17:603, 1987

Roth JA, Kaeberle ML, Grier RL et al: Improvement in clinical condition and thymus morphologic features associated with growth hormone treatment of immunodeficient dwarf dogs. Am J Vet Res 45:1151, 1984

Snyder PW, Kazacos EA, Felsburg PJ: Histologic characterization of the thymus in canine X-linked severe combined immunodeficiency. Clin Immunol Immunopathol 67:55, 1993

Somberg RL, Robinson JP, Felsburg PJ: T lymphocyte development and function in dogs with X-linked severe combined immunodeficiency. J Immunol 153:4006, 1994

Terry A, Fulton R, Stewart M et al: Pathogenesis of feline leukemia virus T17: contrasting fates of helper, v-myc, and v-tcr proviruses in secondary tumors. J Virol 66:3538, 1992

Tizzard IR: Veterinary Immunology: An Introduction. 5th Ed. WB Saunders Philadelphia, 1996

van der Linde-Sipman JS, van Dijk JE: Hematomas in the thymus in dogs. Vet Pathol 24:59, 1987

Musculoskeletal System

77

Introduction

Joseph Harari

GENERAL CONSIDERATIONS

I. The musculoskeletal system is composed of muscles, bones, cartilage, ligaments, and tendons.
  A. Bones of the skeletal system are classified into axial (vertebrae, skull, hyoid, ribs, and sternum), appendicular (pectoral and pelvic limbs), and heterotopic (os penis) divisions.
    1. Long, short, and sesamoid bones are found in limbs.
      a) Long bones are composed of a shaft (diaphysis) and two ends (epiphyses) covered by hyaline cartilage.
      b) The growth plate (physis) in growing bones separates the metaphyseal portion of the bone from the epiphyseal cartilage.
      c) Short bones have irregular shapes and are located in the carpus and tarsus.
      d) Sesamoid bones develop in tendons and serve as protection from friction.
    2. Flat and irregular bones constitute the skull and vertebral column.
  B. Skeletal muscles are attached to bone by connective tissue such as cord-like tendons or flat, sheet-like aponeuroses.
  C. Ligaments are bands of collagenous tissue that unite two or more bone ends at a joint.
II. The functions of the musculoskeletal system include structural support, protection, locomotion, respiration, mastication, and metabolism involving hormones, minerals, and vitamins.

SIGNS OF DYSFUNCTION

I. Abnormalities of the musculoskeletal system may cause focal, multifocal, or systemic disease and may involve other organs of the neurologic, endocrine, urologic, digestive, hemolymphatic, respiratory, and cardiovascular systems.
II. Classic clinical signs of musculoskeletal disorders include weakness, lameness, limb swelling, and joint dysfunction.
III. Motor or sensory neurologic dysfunction may occur secondary to traumatic, developmental, or neoplastic musculoskeletal lesions affecting central or peripheral nerves.
IV. Compromise of respiratory, cardiovascular, urologic, and digestive functions often occurs secondary to severe traumatic injuries.

EXAMINATION PROCEDURES

I. The goals of examination are to define and localize any musculoskeletal lesion(s).
  A. Diagnosis requires accurate evaluation of the signalment, medical history, and physical status of the animal.
  B. Ancillary diagnostic tests (see later) and multiple physical examinations may be required to completely assess the animal and the disease process.
II. Knowledge of the animal's signalment (age, weight, breed, and gender) helps delineate congenital, developmental, and acquired conditions.
III. The pertinent medical history (anamnesis) is reviewed with regard to onset, duration, previous treatments, and course of illness, as well as environmental conditions, diet, and pedigree of the animal.
IV. Lameness examination is critical for accurate evaluation of the musculoskeletal system and follows assessment of concurrent life-threatening injuries or multisystemic lesions.
V. Lameness evaluation is performed (if possible) not only while the animal is at rest but also while it is standing and rising and during locomotion.
  A. Characteristics of the lameness, such as single or multiple limb involvement, weight-bearing pattern, and increase or decrease in severity with exercise, are noted.
  B. Limb assessment includes evaluation of muscle mass, limb conformation, external wounds, and nail length and palpation of bones, joints, muscles, tendons, and ligaments in a distal to proximal manner (including spine and skull).
    1. Palpation of limb structures will reveal abnormal swelling; crepitation; craniocaudal, medi-

811

olateral, or rotational instability; luxation; decreased range of motion; and patient discomfort.

2. In the evaluation of a subtle or obscure lameness, serial palpations may be required, including examinations before and after exercise.

3. For the evaluation of fractious animals or those with extremely painful lesions, sedation or anesthesia may be necessary to permit limb palpation; the examination can be performed immediately before or after radiography.

USEFUL DIAGNOSTIC TESTS

I. Survey radiographs are useful in identifying soft tissue and osseous abnormalities.

  A. Two standard views are necessary and include mediolateral, craniocaudal, oblique, or tangential projections.

  B. Radiography of a contralateral unaffected limb is often useful in interpreting the clinical significance of malformations.

  C. Sedation or anesthesia is often required for proper positioning, and high-detail screen and film combinations are useful for optimum resolution and lesion identification.

  D. Use of a horizontally directed x-ray beam is helpful for evaluating peripheral limb injuries in recumbent animals that are in pain.

  E. Joints can be evaluated radiographically by stressing adjacent bones to detect instability or placing the joints in flexion and extension.

  F. Nuclear scintigraphy is used at referral centers to evaluate osseous lesions not easily identified by survey radiography.

II. Arthrocentesis is useful in identifying arthritides with septic, degenerative, immune-mediated, or traumatic causes (see Chap. 3).

III. Arthrography using aqueous iodinated solutions is useful in evaluating traumatic or development lesions of the humeral head and biceps tendon sheath (see Chap. 4).

IV. Electromyographic testing of muscular electrical activity and peripheral nerve conduction velocity is useful in identifying neuromuscular disorders that can cause lameness or weakness.

V. Muscle biopsy can provide diagnostic information about lameness caused by a degenerative, inflammatory, or metabolic myopathy.

Bibliography

Brinker WO, Piermattei DL, Flo GL: Physical examination for lameness. p. 267. In Brinker WO, Piermattei DL, Flo GL (eds): Handbook of Small Animal Orthopedics. 2nd Ed. WB Saunders, Philadelphia, 1990

Hazewinkel HA, Meutstege FJ: Locomotor system. p. 17. In Rijnberk A, deVries HW (eds): Medical History and Physical Examination in Companion Animals. Kluwer Academic Publishers, Boston, 1995

Schrader SC, Prieur WD, Bruse S: Diagnosis: historical, physical and ancillary examinations. p. 3. In Olmstead ML (ed): Small Animal Orthopedics. Mosby–Year Book, St. Louis, 1995

78

Diseases of Joints and Ligaments

James K. Roush

DEVELOPMENTAL DISORDERS

Aseptic Femoral Head Necrosis (Legg-Calvé-Perthes Disease)

Definition and Causes

I. Aseptic femoral head necrosis (AFHN) is a congenital deterioration and collapse of the proximal femoral articular surface.

II. Femoral head necrosis occurs in miniature- and small-breed dogs during late phases of growth. The cause of AFHN is unknown, although a recessive mode of inheritance is suspected in Manchester terriers (Vasseur et al., 1989).

Pathophysiology

I. Infarction of proximal epiphyseal and metaphyseal bone occurs from an unknown cause.

II. Infarction results in necrosis of the proximal femoral bone, but the proximal femoral articular cartilage remains normal.

III. Revascularization, resorption, and remodeling of infarcted bone occur.

IV. During remodeling, normal biomechanical stresses on the porotic resorbing subchondral bone cause collapse of the femoral head and neck.

V. Growth plate architecture is lost as fibrovascular tissue bridges the growth plate.

Clinical Signs

I. Onset of unilateral or bilateral hindlimb lameness in a miniature- or toy-breed dog between 4 and 11 months of age

II. Pain elicited on coxofemoral manipulation; reduced range of motion

III. Atrophy of thigh musculature in the affected limb

Diagnosis

I. Early radiographic lesions of affected hips include irregular densities within the metaphysis and discrete radiolucent areas within the proximal femoral epiphysis.

II. Late radiographic lesions include deformity of the epiphysis, thickening of the femoral neck, and increased joint space.

III. Severe cases demonstrate collapse and fragmentation of the femoral head with radiographic signs of secondary degenerative joint disease.

Differential Diagnosis

I. Proximal femoral physeal fracture

II. Traumatic hip luxation

III. Medial patella luxation

Treatment

I. Femoral head and neck excision is the treatment of choice.

II. Bilateral surgeries can be staged 4–6 weeks apart or performed simultaneously.

Patient Monitoring

I. Postoperatively, animals are allowed physical activity to encourage early use of the limb.

II. Animals are radiographed for signs of the disease in the opposite hindlimb.

III. Neutering is recommended because of the probable heritable nature of the disease.

Congenital Patella Luxation

Definition and Causes

I. The patella is an ossification in the tendon of insertion of the quadriceps muscle group and articulates with the trochlear groove of the femur.

II. Congenital patella luxation is hereditary in origin, but phenotypic expression is influenced by poorly understood environmental and nutritional factors.

Pathophysiology

I. Patella luxation has been characterized as an anatomic anomaly of the entire pelvic limb.
  A. Young dogs develop angular and torsional abnormalities secondary to limb conformation.
  B. Patella luxation gradually increases in severity as angular deformities worsen during growth.
  C. Secondary changes associated with patella luxation (shallow femoral trochlea, formation of a pseudotrochlea, coxa vara, genu varum, and medial rotation of the tibia) occur as a result of patellar-femoral malarticulation.
  D. Secondary degenerative joint disease develops because of abnormal biomechanical forces and cartilage damage on the articular surfaces of the patella and the femoral trochlea.
II. Medial luxation of the patella occurs most commonly in small- or miniature-breed dogs at a young age and may increase in severity during growth and adult life.
III. Lateral luxation is more common than medial luxation in large-breed dogs, but the pathogenesis is similar.
IV. In cats, patella luxation is usually medial, and a breed disposition has been described in the Devon rex (Houlton and Meynink, 1989).

Clinical Signs

I. Intermittent or chronic hindlimb lameness occurs in animals from 2 months to 10 years of age, associated with visible hindlimb conformational defects.
II. Often a ''skipping'' or ''hopping'' gait is described by clients, with spontaneous recovery a few steps later.

Diagnosis

I. Chronic hindlimb lameness and absence of pain during palpation of the stifle joint in a small-breed dog are highly suggestive of patella luxation.
II. Palpation of the stifle and patella confirms the abnormal position of the patella and allows determination of the accompanying femoral or tibial conformational defects.
III. Patella luxation is graded for surgical and prognostic purposes.
  A. Grade 1: patella can be manually luxated but returns to normal position when released
  B. Grade 2: patella luxates with stifle flexion or on manual manipulation and remains luxated until stifle extension or manual replacement occurs
  C. Grade 3: patella is luxated continually but can be manually reduced
  D. Grade 4: patella is luxated continually and cannot be manually reduced
IV. Stifle radiography demonstrates the abnormal position of the patella and the extent of secondary degenerative and conformational changes.

Differential Diagnosis

I. Legg-Calvé-Perthes diseases
II. Coxofemoral luxation
III. Torn cranial cruciate ligament
IV. Distal femoral physeal fracture

Treatment

I. Animals with grade 1 patella luxation often exhibit only temporary or occasional lameness, do not commonly develop secondary degenerative joint disease, and do not require surgical correction.
II. Animals with grade 2 patella luxation require surgical intervention with any or a combination of the following procedures (Roush, 1993).
  A. Joint capsule imbrication (on the side opposite the luxation)
  B. Fascial releasing incision (on the same side as the luxation)
  C. Trochleoplasty, chondroplasty, or trochlear wedge recession
  D. Tibial crest transposition
  E. Fabella to tibial tuberosity derotation sutures (on the side opposite the luxation)
III. Animals with grade 3 patella luxation require a combination of some or all of the previously listed procedures.
IV. Animals with grade 4 patella luxation often require femoral or tibial derotation osteotomy and multiple surgeries to correct patella luxation.
  A. Animals with grade 4 patella luxation during growth have a grave prognosis for long-term function.
  B. Limb amputation or stifle joint arthrodesis may be necessary.

Patient Monitoring

I. Postoperatively, limited exercise is allowed to provide for limited joint motion and to improve return to function.
II. Growing animals are monitored via radiography and palpation for progressive development or return of patella luxation after surgery.

Shoulder and Elbow Luxation

Definition and Causes

I. Congenital shoulder and elbow luxations are probably hereditary in origin but may occur secondary to trauma during growth.
II. Congenital elbow luxations have been reported in most small breeds, including the Yorkshire terrier, Boston terrier, miniature poodle, English bulldog, Pomeranian, and pug.

Pathophysiology

I. Luxation results from an embryonic failure in formation of intra-articular ligaments.

II. Congenital elbow luxation is characterized by lateral rotation of the ulna and internal rotation of the antebrachium.

Clinical Signs

I. Partial or non–weight-bearing lameness of one or both limbs and pain on palpation or movement of the affected joint(s)

II. Abnormal conformation of one or both forelimbs in young animals

III. Often bilateral, although only one side may be clinically affected at initial presentation

Diagnosis

I. Clinical signs and signalment

II. Physical examination and identification of malarticulation

III. Radiographic lesions such as malformations, particularly flattening of the joint surfaces, and torsional or angular deformities in adjacent bones

Differential Diagnosis

I. Traumatic joint luxation

II. Physeal injuries

Treatment

I. Congenital scapulohumeral or elbow luxation carries an extremely poor prognosis.

   A. Closed reduction and splint stabilization are unsuccessful.

   B. Surgical interventions have been described but carry a guarded prognosis.

II. Closed reduction and percutaneous fixation have been successful for congenital elbow luxation in dogs 4 months of age (Komtebedde and Vasseur, 1993).

III. Arthrodesis (see Traumatic Joint Luxation, later) is indicated for chronic luxation or severe secondary degenerative joint disease, but success is limited because of the often bilateral nature of the luxation.

Patient Monitoring

I. After surgical reduction, exercise is restricted for 4 weeks.

II. Radiography is performed 4 and 8 weeks after surgery to evaluate joint anatomy.

III. Prognosis is poor for long-term function.

Fragmented Medial Coronoid Process

Definition and Causes

I. The coronoid process is the cranial medial articular process of the ulna distal to the trochlear notch.

II. Fragmented medial coronoid process (FMCP), osteochondrosis, and ununited anconeal process fall into a syndrome known as elbow dysplasia (Wind, 1993).

III. FMCP is a congenital disease of dogs that has been shown to be related to osteochondrosis or to asynchronous growth of the radius and ulna.

IV. The disease may have a heritable component.

Pathophysiology

I. Elbow joint congruency is based on uniform growth of the humeral, radial, and ulnar joint components.

II. Asynchronous growth of the radius and ulna may lead to FMCP through biomechanical pressure on the coronoid process by the humerus during growth.

III. Cases of traumatically induced FMCP have been reported, primarily in racing greyhounds and other working breeds.

Clinical Signs

I. Forelimb lameness in large-breed dogs, with onset usually between 4 and 12 months of age

II. Pain during flexion of the elbow

III. Pain on palpation of the medial elbow joint compartment

IV. Elbow joint effusion

Diagnosis

I. Flexed lateral radiographs demonstrate periosteal proliferation on the dorsal anconeal process; occasionally, the separate coronoid fragment may be observed.

II. Cranial-caudal radiographs show the fragment in the medial joint compartment, often associated with an osteochondral defect of the distal medial humeral condyle.

III. The opposite elbow should be radiographed, because the disease is often bilateral.

IV. Older dogs may exhibit radiographic signs of degenerative joint disease, including periarticular osteophyte formation, decreased joint space, and increased periarticular soft tissue swelling or fibrosis.

Treatment

I. Removal of the coronoid process is undertaken through a medial arthrotomy.

II. Bilateral lesions may be treated by staged procedures performed 6 weeks apart or simultaneously.

Patient Monitoring

I. Soft padded bandaging and leash walking are instituted for 10–14 days.

II. Lameness in affected dogs often resolves within 1 month.

III. Lameness may recur owing to progressive secondary degenerative joint disease.

IV. Aspirin 10–25 mg/kg PO BID-TID may be given to reduce inflammation and joint pain.

V. Joint fluid modifiers (polysulfated glycosaminogly-can, hyaluronic acid) and oral nutraceuticals may be useful in ameliorating signs of degenerative joint disease, although objective clinical data are not yet available.

Hip Dysplasia

Definition and Causes

I. Hip dysplasia is characterized by faulty development of the coxofemoral joint that initially presents as varying degrees of joint laxity and later is characterized by femoral and acetabular remodeling and degenerative joint disease.
II. Hip dysplasia is a multifactorial disease of genetic origin.
III. Environmental factors, particularly overall increased energy level and increased percentage of calcium in the diet, also contribute to its development.

Pathophysiology

I. Hip dysplasia is initiated as a disparity between primary muscle mass and disproportionately rapid skeletal growth.
II. Coxofemoral joint instability leads to subluxation of the acetabulum and femoral head.
III. Bony changes such as a thickened femoral neck, osteophytosis, and sclerosis of the acetabulum occur secondarily to coxofemoral discongruity and subluxation.

Clinical Signs

I. Lameness of the hindlimb varies from barely detectable gait abnormalities to non-weight-bearing lameness. Lameness is especially evident after exercise periods.
    A. A "bunny-hopping" gait is often seen in affected young dogs and is characterized by simultaneous advancement of both hindlimbs while running.
    B. Young dogs often lie in ventral recumbency with limbs outstretched behind them.
II. Pain is elicited during full extension of the joint, and joint laxity is noted.

Diagnosis

I. Ortolani's sign is a muted pop elicited when dorsal pressure is applied to the femur by a hand placed on the knee while moving the limb from an adducted to an abducted position.
    A. The pop refers to relocation of the femoral head in the acetabulum.
    B. Animals can be placed in dorsal or lateral recumbency during testing.
    C. Absence of Ortolani's sign indicates a normal hip or advanced degenerative joint disease precluding movement of the femoral head out of the acetabulum.
    D. Presence of Ortolani's sign indicates joint laxity in a young animal. The angle of the femur to the midsagittal plane of the body at the time Ortolani's sign occurs is roughly correlated with the amount of joint laxity.
II. Ventrodorsal radiographic changes associated with hip dysplasia range from subluxation of the femoral head to severe degenerative joint disease.
    A. Animals less than 10 months of age often exhibit only varying degrees of subluxation. Clinical significance of the degree of subluxation is based on the dog's breed, age, and clinical signs.
        1. Generally, subluxation in which <25% of the head of the femur is in the acetabulum on ventrodorsal radiographs is considered severe and leads to rapid development of secondary degenerative joint disease.
        2. Milder degrees of subluxation may also lead to degenerative joint disease.
    B. Animals older than 10 months of age develop radiographic changes of degenerative joint disease at varying rates, depending on the degree of subluxation.
        1. Flattening of the femoral head
        2. A shallow acetabulum
        3. Osteophytes on the femoral neck and femoral margin of the joint capsule
        4. Narrowing of the joint space
        5. Subchondral sclerosis of the femoral head and acetabulum
    C. Compression and distraction of the hips during radiography may be useful in documenting joint laxity (Smith et al., 1990).
III. A dorsal rim acetabular view is used by some surgeons to evaluate acetabular conformation.

Differential Diagnosis

I. Traumatic luxation
II. Infectious or immune-mediated arthritis
III. Cranial cruciate ligament rupture
IV. Degenerative myelopathy (older dogs)
V. Femoral head or neck fractures

Treatment

I. Nonsurgical therapy
    A. Restrict activity.
    B. Administer nonsteroidal anti-inflammatory drugs.
        1. Buffered aspirin is the drug of choice at 10–25 mg/kg PO BID-TID.
        2. Carprofen is effective and may have fewer side effects at 2.2 mg/kg PO BID.
    C. See other medical therapies under Degenerative Joint Disease.
II. Surgical therapy (Manley, 1993)
    A. Triple pelvic osteotomy (TPO)
        1. It is indicated in young (≤10 months of age) large-breed dogs with hip subluxation and no signs of degenerative joint disease.
            a) Candidates for TPO should have some

remaining coverage of the femoral head by the acetabulum.
   b) Animals with complete subluxation are not good candidates for TPO.
   c) There are sporadic reports of TPO being performed in older animals with early degenerative signs, but clinical follow-up of these animals is inconclusive.
2. The surgery involves osteotomies of the pubis, ischium, and ilium; dorsal rotation of the acetabulum; and stabilization of the ilial osteotomy with a bone plate.
   a) Osteotomies of the bones are performed with oscillating or reciprocal saws.
   b) Bone plates used for TPO are specially designed and pre-bent to permit dorsal rotation of the acetabulum at 20–40° angles.
3. TPO is usually performed unilaterally at 1-month intervals in bilaterally affected dogs, but simultaneous bilateral surgeries have been reported with good results.

B. Femoral head and neck excision
1. This procedure is indicated for dogs of all ages with subluxation or degenerative joint disease.
2. It relieves joint pain and allows nonanatomic ambulation.
3. Success may relate more to postoperative physical therapy than to patient size.
4. A femoral osteotomy is performed on a line from the lateral aspect of the trochanteric fossa to just proximal to the lesser trochanter, and the head and neck are removed.
   a) The joint capsule is sutured over the acetabulum, and the incision is closed in routine fashion.
   b) The use of interpositional muscle flaps remains controversial.

C. Total hip replacement (THR)
1. Involves replacement of the femoral head and acetabulum with artificial components
2. Demands advanced technical expertise and equipment and strict aseptic technique
3. Indicated in dogs after growth plate closure occurs
4. Surgical treatment of choice in adult dogs weighing >20 kg to obtain functional and anatomic coxofemoral joint function
5. High success rate (>90%), although complications (infection, dislocation, loosening of implants) may be catastrophic

D. Pectineal muscle or tendon resection
1. Soft tissue resections may alleviate pain from abnormal joint motions.
2. Efficacy in resolving long-term joint degeneration is questionable.

E. Other procedures
1. Femoral neck lengthening has been described in dogs with subluxation and a shortened femoral neck.
2. Subtrochanteric osteotomy has been described

for dogs with subluxation and an excessive joint angle (coxa valga).
3. Biocompatible orthopedic polymer (BOP) shelf arthroplasty has been performed to increase dorsal acetabular coverage, although scientific validity of the procedure has been questioned.

Patient Monitoring

I. Animals given medical therapy are evaluated monthly for relief of pain and assessment of limb function.
II. After surgery, animals are monitored for common postoperative complications, and exercise must be restricted.
   A. Incisions are examined daily for redness, swelling, heat, or pain during the first 2 weeks.
   B. Postoperative analgesia is used to improve animal comfort.
      1. Epidural or systemic administration of narcotic agonists is recommended for the first 12–72 hours.
      2. Oral narcotic agonist/antagonists (butorphanol) or nonsteroidal anti-inflammatories are started as necessary 12 hours after surgery.
   C. Exercise is restricted to an approximately 4 by 4 foot area with good footing and leash walking with towel support for the first 2 months.
      1. After TPO or THR
      2. Until there are radiographic signs of healing
   D. Exercise is beneficial after femoral head and neck excision. Passive motion of the surgical site is recommended, either twice daily by owner manipulation or by swimming or other non–weight-bearing exercise.
III. Animals are radiographed 2 months after THR or TPO. THR animals are also radiographed yearly to monitor for signs of cement or implant loosening.
IV. Neutering is recommended for all dogs with hip dysplasia.

Osteochondrosis

Definition and Causes

I. Osteochondrosis (OC) is a defect in articular cartilage development.
II. Osteochondritis dissecans (OCD) is the term used for the disease when a cartilage flap forms as a result of progression of the articular cartilage defect.
III. In the dog, the exact cause of OC is unknown.
IV. OC is heritable in horses, pigs, humans, and other species.

Pathophysiology

I. OC is a defect in endochondral ossification that results in abnormal subchondral bone development (Probst and Johnston, 1993).
II. Hyaline cartilage in the growing dog epiphysis does not mature into bone, and the joint cartilage thickens at selected areas.

III. Cartilage at the base of the defect is unable to obtain nutrients via diffusion and dies, creating a non-attached cartilage segment.

IV. Joint movement and/or minor trauma can disrupt the cartilage, turning the detached segment into a flap or joint mouse.

V. The cartilage defect is unable to heal owing to lack of blood supply and subsequent lack of an inflammatory response.

VI. Abnormal cartilage congruency or joint debris causes inflammation of the synovium and subsequent degeneration of the joint owing to release of inflammatory mediators.

Clinical Signs

I. Unilateral or bilateral lameness occurs in any limb.

II. The disease often affects the scapulohumeral joint, elbow, tarsus, and stifle in the dog.

III. Joint effusion is variable.

IV. Pain is often noted during palpation or range-of-motion manipulations.

Diagnosis

I. Lateral, medial, or craniocaudal radiographs of the affected joint demonstrate a flattened or concave subchondral defect.

II. Radiographic OC lesions may be present without clinical signs.

III. Radiographic signs (osteophytosis, subchondral bone sclerosis, joint mice) of secondary degenerative joint disease may be present.

IV. Contrast arthrography may be performed to delineate subtle dissecting lesions or cartilage flaps (see Chap. 4).

V. The opposite joint should be radiographed, because the disease is often bilateral.

Differential Diagnosis

I. Panosteitis

II. Traumatic joint injury

III. Septic arthritis

IV. Immune-mediated arthritis

V. Ununited anconeal process

VI. Fragmented coronoid process

Treatment

I. Arthrotomy, removal of the cartilage flap, and curettage of the OC lesion to stimulate fibrocartilage formation are performed.

A. Joint mice are removed if possible to decrease subsequent degenerative joint disease.

B. In animals with bilateral radiographic lesions, only joints with clinical signs of disease are curetted.

II. Experimental procedures using fibrin or cyanoacrylate glues to replace cartilage flaps, and efforts to stabilize the flap with absorbable pins, have been unsuccessful.

Patient Monitoring

I. The degree of degenerative joint disease and size of the subchondral defect determine clinical outcome.

II. Prognosis for OCD is generally best in the shoulder, followed by the stifle and elbow; it is poor for OCD in the tibiotarsal joint.

III. Radiography and physical examination are performed at 6- or 12-month intervals to monitor animals with clinically significant osteoarthritis.

Ununited Anconeal Process

Definition and Causes

I. The anconeal process is the hook-shaped portion of the olecranon at the proximal end of the ulna.

II. Ununited anconeal process (UAP) is a congenital disease of dogs that has been related to osteochondrosis or to unequal growth of the radius and ulna (Sjöström et al., 1995).

III. The disease may have a heritable component in German shepherd dogs.

Pathophysiology

I. The anconeal process develops as a separate center of ossification and normally unites with the proximal ulna at 20–24 weeks of age.

II. Failure of the anconeal process to unite results in mild to moderate elbow instability and development of secondary degenerative joint disease.

III. Recent evidence suggests that UAP may be the result of premature closure of the distal ulna or asynchronous growth of the radius and ulna, resulting in biomechanical stress on the anconeal process.

Clinical Signs

I. Forelimb lameness in large dogs beginning at 5 months of age

II. Pain elicited on extension of the elbow joint and palpation of the proximal ulna

III. ±Joint effusion in affected elbows

Diagnosis

I. Lateral elbow radiographs (straight or flexed) demonstrate the absence of union in dogs >6 months of age.

II. Radiographs of the contralateral elbow are obtained for comparison and to rule out bilateral disease.

III. Signs of secondary degenerative joint disease (effusion, osteophytosis) may also be evident on lateral radiographs.

IV. Elbow radiographs are assessed for additional lesions such as panosteitis, fragmented coronoid process, and osteochondritis dissecans.

Differential Diagnosis

I. Fragmented medial coronoid process

II. Panosteitis

III. Osteochondrosis
IV. Septic arthritis
V. Traumatic elbow injuries

Treatment

I. Surgical removal of the UAP following a lateral arthrotomy is most frequently performed.
II. An alternative surgical approach is lag screw fixation of the anconeal process to the ulna.
III. Reports indicate that midshaft ulnar osteotomy may provide effective relief of asynchronous growth and result in union of the anconeal process and ulna (Sjöström et al., 1995).

Patient Monitoring

I. Soft padded bandage and leash walking for 10–14 days to minimize swelling and seroma formation
II. Radiography 6 and 12 weeks after surgery to assess bone union following lag screw fixation or ulnar osteotomy

DEGENERATIVE DISORDERS

Degenerative Joint Disease

Definition and Causes

I. Degenerative joint disease is a progressive diarthrodial joint deterioration characterized by hyaline cartilage thinning, joint effusion, and periarticular osteophyte production.
II. It occurs with or after inciting joint injuries such as trauma, sepsis, prolonged immobilization, immune-mediated disease, congenital malarticulation (e.g., hip dysplasia), or developmental diseases (e.g., osteochondrosis).

Pathophysiology

I. The inciting cause stimulates the formation and release of degradative enzymes from chondrocytes, resulting in loss of cartilage matrix.
II. Matrix loss accelerates the rate of damage to cartilage under normal use and leads to further pathology, cartilage breakdown, and chondrocyte death.
III. Degradative enzymes and prostaglandins from cartilage breakdown irritate the synovial membrane and cause pain and continued inflammation.
IV. Cartilage destruction and abnormal joint biomechanics perpetuate the degradative processes, pain, and inflammation.

Clinical Signs

I. Episodic or persistent lameness along with periods of inactivity
   A. Lameness may improve during activity, leading to the observed phenomenon of ''warming-out'' of lameness.

B. Strenuous activity results in increased severity of lameness, particularly after a previous rest period.
   C. Noticeable pain and lameness on joint movement may increase in frequency and severity as the disease progresses.
II. Pain during joint palpation or joint movement
III. ± Joint effusion or swelling palpable on examination
IV. ± Crepitation from joint fragments or periarticular calcification during joint manipulation

Diagnosis

I. Clinical signs, history, and signalment may be suggestive.
II. Radiographic signs of degenerative joint disease include joint effusion, perceived narrowing of joint spaces (owing to cartilage thinning), osteophyte formation, and subchondral sclerosis.
III. Joint aspiration (see Chap. 3) indicates a nonseptic and noninflammatory process (Table 78–1).

Differential Diagnosis

I. Trauma
II. Developmental joint disease
III. Infectious or immune-mediated arthritis

Treatment

I. Prevention is the best treatment through prompt and aggressive attention to inciting causes (accurate fracture reduction in traumatized joints or joint lavage for septic joints).
II. Weight loss is important to reduce load bearing by cartilage and bones.
III. Limitation of exercise or exercise at regular intervals may modulate the clinical signs.
IV. Treatment with pharmaceuticals is directed at minimizing clinical signs (Table 78–2).
   A. Nonsteroidal anti-inflammatory drugs (NSAIDs)
      1. Buffered aspirin at 10–25 mg/kg PO BID-TID is the drug of choice. Side effects are usually limited to gastric irritation, which may be prevented by simultaneous administration of H_2 blockers.
      2. Carprofen has fewer side effects than aspirin and is given at a dosage of 2.2 mg/kg PO BID.
      3. Phenylbutazone at 13 mg/kg PO BID-TID (maximum 800 mg/day) provides similar control to aspirin in the dog. Its use is not recommended in cats.
      4. Ibuprofen and other NSAIDs (e.g., meclofenamic acid) may cause gastric ulcers and perforations in small animals and should not be used.
   B. Polysulfated glycosaminoglycans and hyaluronic acid may function as chondroprotective agents in

Table 78–1. **Synovial Fluid Analysis**

Condition	Color	Viscosity	RBCs	WBCs (μl)	PMNs (%)
Normal	Clear	Normal	None	250–3000	0–6
Degenerative arthritis	Pale yellow	Normal	Few	1000–5000	0–12
Hemarthrosis	Red	Reduced	Many	3000–10,000	60–75
Erosive arthritis	Yellow	Reduced	Few	8000–40,000	75–85
Nonerosive arthritis	Yellow	Reduced	Few	10,000–100,000	40–65
Septic arthritis	Gray/turbid	Reduced	Medium	80,000–300,000	90 +

RBCs = red blood cells; WBCs = white blood cells; PMNs = polymorphonuclear neutrophils.

small animals. The efficacy of these compounds is still being tested in objective clinical trials.
C. Corticosteroids are reserved as a last attempt to control clinical signs. The most common drug used is prednisone at 1–2 mg/kg PO BID initially, then gradually decreased to 0.25 mg/kg QOD as needed.
D. Dimethyl sulfoxide and other substances such as orgotein have been used to alleviate clinical signs of degenerative joint disease, but efficacy in controlled studies has not been established.
E. Cimetidine (5–10 mg/kg PO TID) and sucralfate (0.5–1 g PO BID) can be used in combination with NSAIDs to prevent gastric ulcers.
V. Surgical treatment is used to recover limb function.
A. Joint replacement alleviates clinical signs but is limited in clinical veterinary medicine to the canine coxofemoral joint.
B. Resection arthroplasty may effectively alleviate clinical signs in cats and dogs. Removal of the femoral head or glenoid has been reported to alleviate discomfort in the coxofemoral and scapulohumeral joints, respectively.
C. Arthrodesis is an effective method to eliminate discomfort from a degenerative joint, and arthrodesis of joints below the elbow and stifle (in the dog) allows acceptable function in most instances.

Patient Monitoring

I. Once initiated, low-dose NSAIDs may be necessary to control clinical signs.
II. Animals are monitored every 1–4 months, and medi-

cation and dosage are adjusted as necessary to maintain optimum quality of life.
III. Following arthrodesis or implant surgery, radiography is performed at 6 and 12 weeks to evaluate healing.

INFECTIONS

Bacterial Arthritis

Definition and Causes

I. Septic arthritis is a bacterial joint infection secondary to joint contamination from hematogenous or exogenous routes.
II. The most common bacteria isolated are staphylococci, streptococci, and coliforms.
III. Hematogenous spread occurs primarily in young, aged, or immunologically deficient animals.
IV. Rarely, infection by atypical fungal organisms occurs, usually in immune-deficient animals.

Pathophysiology

I. Contamination of the synovium results in hyperemia and edema of the synovium, followed by infiltration of polymorphonuclear leukocytes.
II. Extravasation of fibrin, clotting factors, polymorphonuclear leukocytes, and serum occurs into the joint.
III. Lysosomal enzymes from polymorphonuclear leukocytes are released and break down cartilage matrix and collagen.
IV. Synovial fluid dynamics and cartilage nutrition are altered.

Table 78–2. **Pharmacologic Management of Degenerative Joint Disease**

Drug	Dosage	Frequency	Route	Duration
Buffered aspirin	Dog: 10–25 mg/kg	BID-TID	PO	As needed
	Cat: 6 mg/kg	q 48–72 h	PO	As needed
Phenylbutazone[a]	Dog: 0.5–1 mg/kg	TID	PO	As needed
Carprofen	Dog: 2.2 mg/kg	BID	PO	As needed
Prednisone	1–2 mg/kg	BID	PO	Decrease dosage to QOD as needed
Meclofenamic acid	1.1 mg/kg	SID	PO	For 4–7 days, then 0.5 mg/kg
Polysulfated glycosaminoglycans	5 mg/kg	SID	IM	Once weekly for 6–8 wk

[a]Should not be used in cats.

V. The combination of continued enzymatic degradation, altered biomechanical stresses, and fibrin deposition on cartilage surfaces accelerates the process of cartilage destruction.

Clinical Signs

I. Erythema, swelling, hyperthermia, and pain in one or more joints
   A. Monoarticular signs occur in exogenously introduced (traumatic or iatrogenic) organisms.
   B. Polyarticular signs occur following hematogenous spread.
II. Marked lameness in one or more limbs
III. Pyrexia, lethargy, or anorexia

Diagnosis

I. Arthrocentesis and synovial fluid evaluation (see Table 78–1) confirm the diagnosis.
II. Radiographic lesions supportive of septic arthritis include bone lysis, joint surface irregularity, effusion, and soft tissue swelling.
III. Nuclear scintigraphy may be useful to assess relative joint inflammation and arthritis in multiple joints.
IV. Aerobic, anaerobic, and fungal culture and sensitivity tests are performed on joint fluid. Inoculation of blood culture medium is the most reliable method of culture (Montgomery et al., 1989).

Differential Diagnosis

I. Traumatic injuries: fractures, torn ligaments
II. Periarticular tumors: synovial sarcoma
III. Other infectious arthritides: mycoplasmosis, calicivirus (Dawson et al., 1994), coronavirus, bacterial L-forms

Treatment

I. Institute systemic broad-spectrum antibiotics (fluoroquinolones, cephalosporins) pending culture and sensitivity results.
II. Joint decompression and copious lavage via arthrotomy and surgical debridement are essential.
   A. The best initial lavage solution is sterile, warmed lactated Ringer's solution at volumes exceeding 5 L/joint.
   B. Addition of antibiotics and antiseptics to lavage solutions is controversial and may be detrimental to cartilage survival.
   C. All fibrin clots, purulent exudate, and foreign material within the joint are removed by debridement or lavage.
III. Joints are ideally managed as open wounds until second-intention healing occurs.
IV. Forced joint mobility (passive therapy, swimming, leash walks) during resolution of infection and healing minimizes the destructive changes of septic arthritis.

Patient Monitoring

I. Daily (or more frequent) aseptic bandage changes are necessary until the infection resolves and the wound heals.

II. Parenteral antibiotics based on bacterial culture and antimicrobial sensitivity testing are continued for a minimum of 4 weeks.

Borreliosis (Lyme Disease)

Definition and Causes

I. Borreliosis is an infectious zoonotic arthropathy endemic in the northern and eastern United States (see Chap. 111).
II. *Borrelia burgdorferi* is a spirochete carried by the deer tick (*Ixodes dammini* in the eastern and mid–United States, and *Ixodes pacificus* in California and other western states).

Pathophysiology

I. The white-footed mouse is the main reservoir for *B. burgdorferi* and is the preferred host of larval and nymphal forms of the ticks.
II. A bite from an infected tick initiates the disease.
III. In dogs, borreliosis is primarily a polyarthritis that may be septic in origin or immune-mediated because of the presence of the spirochete in the synovium.

Clinical Signs

I. Lameness may be either acute or chronic and is often progressive.
II. Anorexia, lethargy, and weight loss may be noted in the history.
III. Signs of systemic infection on physical examination may include pyrexia, anorexia, joint pain, lymphadenopathy, lethargy, and weight loss.
IV. Swelling and effusion of one or more joints are often evident.

Diagnosis

I. Radiographs commonly show little or no evidence of degenerative joint disease.
II. Laboratory evaluation is undertaken.
   A. Complete blood count (CBC) and serum chemistry profiles are often normal.
   B. Serum immunofluorescent antibody (IFA) or enzyme-linked immunosorbent assay (ELISA) titers of 1:128 or 1:256 for borreliosis indicate possible infection, and titers ≥1:512 are highly positive and indicative of chronic infection.
   C. Animals with high titers and no clinical signs may be recently infected and should be retested in 1 month.
III. Culture of the organism is seldom successful.
IV. Joint fluid analysis is usually consistent with degenerative joint disease (see Table 78–1).
V. Histologic findings from synovial biopsy include chronic lymphocytic infiltration, microvascular proliferation, and nonspecific villus hypertrophy.

Differential Diagnosis

I. Immune-mediated polyarthritis: rheumatoid arthritis or systemic lupus erythematosus
II. Septic arthritis, particularly *Mycoplasma* spp.

Treatment

I. Prevention
    A. A commercially licensed killed bacterin has been tested for efficacy on experimental animals challenged with *B. burgdorferi.* Protection against natural infection and disease has not been established, and the vaccine is not currently recommended.
    B. Limit exposure to tick-infested areas. Premise sprays may be used to reduce tick populations.
    C. Use of tick repellents in the form of dips, powders, collars, and sprays may reduce the incidence of Lyme disease.
II. Therapy for active borreliosis
    A. In endemic areas, low positive titers are usually incidental findings.
    B. Treat animals with clinical signs of borreliosis and positive titers with systemic antibiotics for 21 days.
        1. Tetracycline 15–20 mg/kg PO TID
        2. Doxycycline 10 mg/kg PO BID
        3. Cephalexin 22 mg/kg PO TID (best choice for chronic infection)
    C. Animals from endemic areas with clinical signs suggesting borreliosis and negative serum titers should be evaluated for other causes of polyarthritis and, in the absence of other etiologies, treated for borreliosis. Recheck serum titers in 1 month.
III. NSAIDs for secondary degenerative joint disease in chronic cases (see earlier).

Patient Monitoring

I. Animals are monitored every 1–4 months by physical examination for return of clinical signs after successful therapy.
II. Antibiotic therapy is continued for 2 weeks after resolution of clinical signs.

Ehrlichiosis

See Chap. 113.

Rocky Mountain Spotted Fever

See Chap. 113.

IMMUNE-MEDIATED DISEASES

Erosive Polyarthritis

Definition and Causes

I. Erosive arthritis is characterized by the destruction of articular cartilage and subchondral bone.
II. Rheumatoid arthritis is the most common cause in the dog.
III. Other erosive arthritides in small animals include erosive polyarthritis of greyhounds and feline chronic progressive polyarthritis.

IV. Specific etiologies for rheumatoid arthritis and other erosive polyarthritides have not been identified.

Pathophysiology

I. Instigating infectious systemic diseases such as staphylococci, mycoplasmas, *Corynebacteria*, bacterial L-forms, and viruses have been implicated.
II. Cellular and humoral immunopathogenic factors develop against collagen, cartilage proteoglycans, and synovial antigens.
III. Deposition of immune complexes in the joint and periarticular tissues leads to complement fixation, neutrophil chemotaxis, and release of chondrodestructive enzymes, including collagenases and proteases.
IV. Articular cartilage destruction occurs secondary to the synovial inflammatory process.

Clinical Signs

I. Clinical signs commonly involve multiple joints and most often affect distal limb joints such as the carpus, tarsus, and interphalangeal joints.
II. Lameness, pain, joint effusion, periarticular soft tissue swelling, and palpable joint hyperthermia may be present.
III. Joint-related signs may be accompanied by systemic signs such as fever, malaise, anorexia, and generalized muscle pain.
IV. Clinical signs may be intermittent or persistent over the course of the disease and may shift from limb to limb.
V. Dogs with rheumatoid arthritis are usually adult, small-breed dogs. Greyhounds with erosive polyarthritis are affected at 3–30 months of age.
VI. Cats with feline chronic progressive polyarthritis are most often male and 1–5 years of age.

Diagnosis

I. Survey radiography of affected joints demonstrates signs of degenerative joint disease, including collapse of the joint space, periarticular swelling, subchondral bone cysts, and periarticular osteophyte production. In chronic cases, joint subluxation may be evident, resulting in an appearance similar to that of nonerosive arthritides.
II. Arthrocentesis reveals synovial fluid of characteristic appearance and cellularity (Table 78–1).
III. Serologic testing is often positive for rheumatoid factor (RF) and should be negative for antinuclear antibody antigen (ANA).
    A. Only 25% of dogs test positive for RF.
    B. A negative ANA must be present to permit a diagnosis of rheumatoid arthritis.
    C. Animals with positive ANA titers are treated for systemic lupus erythematosus.
IV. Synovial fluid cultures for aerobic, anaerobic, and mycoplasmal organisms are negative.

V. Histologic evaluation of joint biopsy specimens is characterized by villous synovial hypertrophy and plasmacytic, lymphocytic infiltration of synovial tissue. Articular cartilage erosion may be noted at the joint margins.

Differential Diagnosis

I. Nonerosive polyarthritides
II. Septic arthritis
III. Degenerative joint disease of any etiology

Treatment

I. NSAIDs are the drugs of choice in mildly affected animals (Table 78–3).
II. Alternatively, systemic glucocorticoids are administered at anti-inflammatory doses.
III. If refractory disease occurs, therapy is expanded to include combinations of glucocorticoids and cytotoxic drugs such as cyclophosphamide, azathioprine, and methotrexate.
IV. Weekly injections of 1 mg/kg sodium aurothioglucose have been successful in the treatment of rheumatoid arthritis.
V. Surgical arthrodesis or synovectomy may be performed on selected severely affected joints, but surgery as an effective therapy is often limited by the number of joints affected.

Patient Monitoring

I. Resolution of erosive arthritis is rare, but remission may be achieved within 3–6 months.
II. Animals treated with cytotoxic drugs are monitored with CBCs and platelet counts every 1–3 weeks, depending on dosage.
III. After remission of clinical signs, therapy may be discontinued or continued at a decreased dosage and interval.
IV. The animal is monitored by physical examination at 1–6-month intervals for return of clinical signs.
V. Treatment regimens for greyhounds afflicted with erosive polyarthritis have been unrewarding, and the prognosis for this disease is poor.
VI. Cats are monitored at yearly intervals for feline leukemia virus if treated with cytotoxic drugs.

Nonerosive Polyarthritis

Definition and Causes

I. Nonerosive polyarthritis is characterized by periarticular inflammation with no radiographic or histopathologic evidence of joint destruction in early stages.
II. Systemic lupus erythematosus (SLE) and idiopathic nondeforming arthritis are the most common disease syndromes resulting in nonerosive polyarthritis.
III. Nonerosive polyarthritis has also been associated with various concurrent conditions, including diskospondylitis, enteropathy, and bacterial endocarditis, and with the administration of some pharmacologic agents.

Pathophysiology

I. A type III hypersensitivity reaction induces the formation and deposition of immune complexes in periarticular tissues.
II. An inflammatory response, including activation of the complement cascade, occurs.
III. Autoantibodies to nuclear material from various cells are produced (antinuclear antibody).
IV. Subsequent weakening of ligamentous periarticular structures occurs and leads to joint instability.
V. Chronic joint instability results in progressive degenerative changes and joint subluxation or luxation.

Clinical Signs

I. Clinical signs commonly involve multiple joints and most often affect distal limb joints such as the carpus, tarsus, and interphalangeal joints.
II. Lameness, pain, joint effusion, periarticular soft tissue swelling, and palpable joint hyperthermia may be present.
III. Joint-related signs may be accompanied by systemic signs such as fever, malaise, anorexia, and generalized muscle pain.
IV. Clinical signs may be intermittent or persistent over the course of the disease and may shift from limb to limb.
V. SLE is accompanied by signs of other organ disease such as renal, hepatic, dermatologic, or neuromuscular disease. Systemic signs of malaise, lethargy, anorexia, and pyrexia may occur early in the course of disease.

Table 78–3. *Drug Regimens for Control of Immune-Mediated Arthritis in the Dog*

Drug	Dosage	Frequency	Route	Duration
Acetylsalicylic acid	10–25 mg/kg	BID-TID	PO	As needed
Prednisone	1–2 mg/kg	BID	PO	Maintain at lowest effective dose
Cyclophosphamide	1.5–2.5 mg/kg	SID (4 days/wk)	PO	Maintain until regression
Azathioprine	2 mg/kg	SID	PO	Maintain until regression
Gold sodium thioglucose	1 mg/kg	Once weekly	IM	Maintain until regression

Diagnosis

 I. In early stages, survey radiographs demonstrate subluxation or luxation, joint effusion, and periarticular soft tissue swelling of affected joints.
   A. Destruction of cartilage is not often evident radiographically at this stage.
   B. Stress radiographs may be necessary to demonstrate joint instability.
 II. In later stages, survey radiographs may appear identical to those of erosive arthritides and advanced degenerative joint disease, and include collapse of the joint space, periarticular swelling, subchondral bone cysts, and periarticular osteophyte production.
 III. Arthrocentesis reveals synovial fluid of characteristic appearance and cellularity (see Table 78–1).
 IV. LE preparations may be positive (LE cells are polymorphonuclear phagocytes that have engulfed antibody-coated material from other cells).
 V. Serologic testing is positive for antinuclear antibody and negative for rheumatoid arthritis and infectious causes of arthritis.
 VI. Synovial fluid cultures for aerobic, anaerobic, and mycoplasmal organisms are negative.
 VII. SLE is accompanied by systemic signs of other organ disease.
 VIII. Histologic evaluation of joint biopsy specimens is characterized by mild synovitis and some polymorphonuclear neutrophil infiltration of synovium. Articular cartilage destruction is absent in early stages but may be evident in advanced disease.

Differential Diagnosis

 I. Erosive polyarthritides
 II. Septic arthritis
 III. Degenerative joint disease of any etiology
 IV. Infectious polyarthritis: calicivirus, coronavirus, mycoplasmosis

Treatment

 I. In early stages, systemic glucocorticoids are administered at anti-inflammatory doses (see Table 78–3).
 II. If refractory disease occurs, therapy is expanded to chemotherapy combinations of glucocorticoids and cytotoxic drugs such as cyclophosphamide, azathioprine, and methotrexate.
 III. Arthrodesis may be performed on selected severely affected joints, but the utility of arthrodesis is often limited by the number of affected joints.

Patient Monitoring

 I. After remission of clinical signs, therapy is continued at reduced dosages (prednisone 1 mg/kg PO QOD). If remission continues on reduced therapy, elimination of therapy may be tried after 1–3 months.
 II. The patient is monitored by physical examination at 1- to 6-month intervals for return of clinical signs.

NEOPLASTIC DISEASES

Synovial Sarcoma

Definition and Causes

 I. Synovial sarcoma is a malignant tumor arising from mesenchymal cells outside the synovial surface.
 II. The etiology of synovial sarcoma is unknown.

Clinical Signs

 I. Slowly progressive lameness of a single limb, most commonly in large-breed dogs
 II. Slowly progressive swelling near a joint, most commonly one of the large limb joints (elbow, stifle)
 III. Pain elicited during joint palpation and motion

Diagnosis

 I. Survey radiography reveals bone lysis in epiphyseal regions of both bones constituting the joint. Irregular periosteal reactions and soft tissue calcification may be evident in joint regions as well.
 II. Arthrotomy and synovial biopsy demonstrate characteristic histology of an epithelioid, fusiform, and spindle tumor mass with large, discrete cytoplasmic vacuolation.

Differential Diagnosis

 I. Bone tumors
 II. Septic arthritis
 III. Chronic luxation and fibrosis

Treatment

 I. Limb amputation is the therapy of choice.
   A. Local excision is not sufficient, and regrowth is inevitable.
   B. Median survival after amputation is 17 months (Vail et al., 1994).
 II. Efficacious adjunctive chemotherapeutic protocols have not been established.

Patient Monitoring

 I. Affected animals are monitored for signs of regional and distant metastasis.
 II. The long-term metastatic rate for synovial cell sarcoma is 40–50% (Vail et al., 1994).

TRAUMATIC DISORDERS

Cranial Cruciate Ligament Rupture

Definition and Causes

 I. The cranial cruciate ligament in the dog normally restricts cranial movement (cranial drawer) and internal rotation of the tibia in relation to the femur.

II. Excessive trauma of a weakened or degenerate ligament is the most frequent cause of cranial cruciate ligament rupture.

III. Some authors have suggested that an immune-mediated ligament degeneration precedes cranial cruciate ligament rupture.

IV. Abnormal conformation in straight-legged dogs (rottweilers, Dobermans) may also predispose the ligament to stress and rupture.

Pathophysiology

I. Two clinical syndromes are evident: acute traumatic rupture from catastrophic loading and twisting of the ligament, and chronic ligament degeneration leading to subsequent rupture.

II. Excessive instability and abnormal joint function lead to medial meniscal injury, joint effusion, and pericapsular fibrosis.

Clinical Signs

I. Acute hindlimb lameness is often noted.
  A. Obvious lameness within the first 72 hours of rupture, with partial to no weight-bearing, and gradual improvement over several weeks.
  B. After approximately 6 weeks, development of degenerative joint disease leads to gradually increased lameness.

II. Pain can usually be elicited on palpation of the stifle joint.

III. Stifle joint effusion is variable.

IV. Signs referable to secondary joint disease may be present in animals with chronically ruptured ligaments, such as stifle joint swelling, elicitation of pain on joint palpation, and pain and crepitation on joint movement.

V. Large-breed, obese dogs are prone to acute rupture.

Diagnosis

I. The diagnosis is based primarily on elicitation of a cranial drawer movement during physical examination.
  A. The distal femur is grasped in one hand from the caudal aspect by placing the thumb on the lateral femoral condyle and the fingers over the patella.
  B. The proximal tibia is grasped in the opposite hand from the caudal aspect by placing the thumb over the fibular head and the fingers over the tibial crest.
  C. Increased cranial movement (>3–5 mm) of the tibia in relation to the femur indicates rupture of the cranial cruciate ligament; joint laxity in flexion is usually associated with partial tears.
  D. An alternative method of physical diagnosis involves tensing the gastrocnemius muscle by flexion of the hock while the femur is held at 90° in relation to the tibia (tibial compression). Forward movement of the tibia is a positive diagnostic test for cranial cruciate ligament injury.

II. In chronic cases, radiographic signs of degenerative joint disease are present at 4–6 weeks after injury and progress rapidly.
  A. Impingement of or decrease in the cranial fat pad
  B. Peripatellar or peritrochlear osteophyte production
  C. Osteophyte presence on the proximal tibia
  D. Cranial subluxation of the tibia in relation to the femur

III. Medial joint fibrosis (medial buttress formation) on joint palpation is pathognomonic for joint instability, including medial meniscal injury.

IV. Arthroscopy has been advocated for diagnosis, but its utility is limited by the availability of suitable-sized arthroscopic equipment.

Differential Diagnosis

I. Caudal cruciate ligament rupture
II. Stifle joint sprain or meniscal injuries
III. Bilateral: hip dysplasia, myelopathies
IV. Patellar luxation

Treatment

I. In very small (<5 kg) dogs and in cats, exercise restriction and subsequent joint fibrosis for 2–4 weeks may result in alleviation of clinical signs.

II. In larger dogs or cats, surgical stabilization is recommended to limit development of secondary degenerative joint disease.
  A. Extracapsular suture stabilization is useful in small (5–10 kg) dogs or cats. This is accomplished by passing and tightening a nonabsorbable or slowly absorbable lateral suture (1-0) around the lateral fabella and through the tibial crest.
  B. In larger (>10 kg) dogs, extracapsular suture material is recommended and includes double-stranded monofilament nylon (#2) used laterally and possibly medially.
  C. Fibular head transposition uses the lateral collateral ligament to resist cranial movement and internal rotation of the tibia. The fibular head is transposed cranially and reattached with a Kirschner wire or bone screw.
  D. Intracapsular repair techniques are extremely popular for dogs >20 kg.
    1. The "under and over fascial technique" has gained widespread use and acceptance (Vasseur, 1993).
    2. In this procedure, a lateral tensor fascia lata strip is created and passed under the intermeniscal ligament and over the lateral femoral condyle and then attached to the femoral condyle.
    3. Similar procedures include medial, lateral, and middle patella tendon grafts.
  E. The lateral retinaculum is usually tightened during all surgical procedures.
  F. Some surgeons perform intra- *and* extracapsular procedures in large (>30 kg), active dogs.

III. When radiographic evidence of avulsion of the tibial insertion is present, the bone fragment may be re-attached with crossed Kirschner wires.

Patient Monitoring

I. Postoperative management includes bandage support and exercise restriction for 1 month, followed by controlled leash walks and physical therapy to maintain joint health.
II. Animals are rechecked between 6 and 12 weeks postoperatively to assess limb function and stifle stability.
III. Weight loss is important in obese animals to limit stress on the repair and to ease clinical signs related to existing degenerative joint disease.
IV. Owners should be informed of the frequent incidence of rupture of the opposite cruciate ligament in obese animals.
V. The dog is also monitored for the continued development of degenerative joint disease, and any appropriate pharmacologic control is initiated.
VI. Concurrent medial meniscal injuries increase morbidity.
VII. Most surgeons report an 80–90% success rate, regardless of surgical technique.

Caudal Cruciate Ligament Rupture

Definition and Causes

I. The caudal cruciate ligament in the dog restricts caudal movement (caudal drawer) of the tibia in relation to the femur.
II. Isolated rupture of the caudal cruciate ligament occurs infrequently.
III. Most lesions occur in conjunction with cranial cruciate and meniscal injury in a severely affected joint.

Clinical Signs

I. Acute hindlimb lameness from known or suspected traumatic incident
II. Mild stifle joint pain or effusion in isolated ruptures

Diagnosis

I. Presence of caudal drawer sign (see cranial drawer technique, earlier)
II. Radiographic evidence of avulsion of the caudal tibial insertion of the ligament
III. Joint effusion, hemarthrosis, pain elicited on palpation or movement of the joint

Differential Diagnosis

I. Cranial cruciate ligament rupture
II. Stifle joint sprain
III. Meniscal injury
IV. Patellar luxation

Treatment

I. Clinical signs in animals with isolated caudal cruciate ligament injuries often resolve after cage rest or other exercise restriction.

II. If lameness persists >1 month, extra-articular stabilization may be effective (Vasseur, 1993).

Patient Monitoring

I. Caudal drawer motion may persist in treated or untreated animals without evidence of lameness.
II. Radiography at yearly intervals may be useful in evaluating joint degeneration if lameness persists.

Stifle Meniscal Injury

Definition and Causes

I. The menisci are semilunar fibrocartilaginous pads interposed between the femoral condyles and tibia that provide energy transfer across the joint, joint lubrication, and joint stabilization.
II. Isolated meniscal injuries are rare in small animals.
III. Medial meniscal injuries are frequently associated with cranial cruciate ligament rupture.

Pathophysiology

I. Loss of the cranial cruciate ligament results in repeated cranial subluxation of the tibia.
II. The medial meniscus is bound to the tibial plateau by cranial and caudal ligaments, and the caudal portion of the meniscus becomes wedged between the femur and tibia during subluxation.
III. Tearing or folding of the medial meniscus occurs from compressive and shear forces during subluxation.

Clinical Signs

I. Lameness of the affected limb
II. Joint effusion or pain on palpation of the affected stifle
III. A palpable and sometimes audible "click" during stifle motion

Diagnosis

I. Diagnosis is based on clinical assessment and an associated cranial cruciate ligament injury.
II. Diagnosis may be aided in large dogs by magnetic resonance imaging of the affected stifle.
III. Arthroscopy and direct visualization of the affected meniscus is limited to large dogs.
IV. Arthrotomy confirms any meniscal injury.

Differential Diagnosis

I. Cranial cruciate ligament tear
II. Medial collateral ligament injury

Treatment

I. Vascular access channeling may be an effective method of repairing tears of the meniscal margins (Vasseur, 1993).

II. Partial meniscectomy of torn axial meniscal tissue is frequently performed because of lack of tissue healing response.

III. Complete meniscectomy results in secondary degenerative joint disease and should be avoided if possible.

IV. Local or systemic administration of polysulfated glycosaminoglycans may provide protection to articular surfaces of meniscectomized dogs.

Patient Monitoring

I. Postoperatively, institute controlled and limited exercise for 1–3 months during recovery from cranial cruciate ligament and meniscal injury.

II. Radiography and stifle joint palpation are indicated for persistently lame patients to reassess the diagnosis.

Collateral Ligament Rupture

Definition and Causes

I. Collateral ligaments (medial and lateral) are present in the stifle, elbow, hock, carpus, and metacarpal-phalangeal, metatarsal-phalangeal, and interphalangeal joints.

II. Trauma and excessive loading of the joint are the inciting causes of rupture of the collateral ligaments of diarthrodial joints

Clinical Signs

I. Lameness in one or more limbs
II. Pain on palpation of the affected joint
III. ± Joint effusion
IV. Periarticular soft tissue swelling of the affected joint
V. Laxity or instability on the side of the injured collateral ligament

Diagnosis

I. Joint laxity detected during palpation by medial or lateral stressing of the affected joint

II. Increased or asymmetrical joint space visible on stress radiographs of the affected joint

III. Bone avulsion fragments possibly visible at the origin or insertion of the ligaments

Differential Diagnosis

I. Other ligament or meniscal injuries
II. Joint sprains
III. Degenerative joint disease
IV. Infectious or immune-mediated arthritis

Treatment

I. Surgical repair is necessary to prevent continued joint instability and development of degenerative joint disease.

A. Splinting without surgical stabilization is often ineffective.

B. Primary suturing of ligamentous ruptures is possible but is often ineffective because of shredding or stretching of collateral ligaments during injury.

C. For most joints (e.g., stifle, elbow), prosthetic collateral ligaments can be constructed by placing screws at the origin and insertion of the ligament and applying orthopedic wire or monofilament nonabsorbable suture in a figure-eight fashion around the screws (DeCamp, 1995).

D. In the hock, long and short components of the collateral ligaments are replaced separately (DeCamp, 1995).

E. Postoperative splinting for 4 weeks may be used to supplement surgical repair.

II. Surgical arthrodesis is reserved for joint salvage in animals with chronic rupture and severe secondary degenerative joint disease.

Patient Monitoring

I. Monitor postoperative splints or support bandages at weekly intervals for proper application.

II. Assess ligament stability by palpation 4 and 8 weeks postoperatively.

Traumatic Joint Luxation

Definition and Causes

I. Joint luxation is the complete separation of two normally articulating bone surfaces.

II. Luxation occurs as a result of severe trauma such as motor vehicle or firearm accidents.

Clinical Signs

I. Lameness in affected limb, often with complete lack of weight-bearing
II. Pain elicited on palpation or motion of affected joint
III. Abnormal limb angulation originating at a joint
IV. Joint swelling or hyperthermia
V. Abnormal limb length: limb becomes shorter or longer than opposite normal limb as a result of bone displacement

Diagnosis

I. Clinical signs and history of trauma are suggestive.
II. Radiographs of affected joints reveal joint dislocation and direction of displacement.

Differential Diagnosis

I. Septic arthritis
II. Neoplasia
III. Bony fractures

Treatment

I. Most joint luxations occur subsequent to traumatic collateral or other ligamentous injury. In general, luxations are treated by joint reduction (either closed or open) and surgical repair of associated ligamentous injuries.

II. Coxofemoral luxations commonly displace in a craniolateral direction.
   A. Closed reduction is attempted first. If closed reduction is successful and the coxofemoral joint can be manually reluxated only with difficulty, an Ehmer sling or cage rest (4 weeks) will maintain reduction.
   B. Closed reductions that are not inherently stable can be supplemented with a flexible external fixator (McLaughlin and Tillson, 1994).
   C. Unsuccessful closed reductions or unstable reductions are further reduced and stabilized through a craniolateral approach. Successful methods of surgical stabilization include the following (DeCamp, 1995).
      1. Primary joint capsule repair
      2. Trochanteric transposition (caudal and distal)
      3. Extracapsular suture stabilization
      4. Transarticular pin stabilization
      5. Toggle pin fixation (Flynn et al., 1994)
      6. Ischioilial (Devita) pinning (Beale et al., 1991)
      7. Triple pelvic osteotomy
   D. Chronic coxofemoral luxations with severe secondary degenerative joint disease may be treated by femoral head and neck excision or total hip replacement.
III. Although some scapulohumeral luxations may be closed-reduced and stabilized with a Velpeau's bandage, many require surgical intervention for stabilization (DeCamp, 1995).
IV. Complete stifle luxations generally carry a poor prognosis because of the associated multiple ligamentous and meniscal injuries present.
V. Elbow luxations often are stable after closed reduction and may not require surgical stabilization.
VI. Although acute carpal and tarsal luxations may be closed-reduced, they often require surgical stabilization because of the routinely poor outcome of splint stabilization.
VII. Joint arthrodesis is reserved for animals with chronic luxation and severe secondary degenerative joint disease.
   A. Pancarpal or pantarsal arthrodesis results in near-normal limb function.
   B. Stifle and elbow arthrodesis severely restricts limb function but eliminates discomfort.
   C. Stabilization methods vary with the joint, but in general, principles for surgical joint arthrodesis include the following.
      1. Curettage of remaining cartilage from joint surfaces
      2. Cancellous bone graft applied to joint surfaces
      3. Reduction and rigid fixation of joint at a normal weight-bearing angle

Patient Monitoring

I. Bandages or slings are examined daily as part of routine care.

II. Exercise restriction for 4–8 weeks after reduction is necessary to allow repair of ligamentous structures.
III. Radiography is performed at 6 and 12 weeks to confirm joint reduction and stability of implants.

Physeal Fractures

See Chap. 79.

Bibliography

Alexander JW: Canine hip dysplasia. Vet Clin North Am [Small Anim Pract] 22:50, 1992
Beale BS, Lewis DD, Parker RB et al: Ischio-ilial pinning for stabilization of coxofemoral luxations in twenty-one dogs: a retrospective evaluation. Vet Comp Ortho Traum 4:28, 1991
Chauvet AE, Johnson AL: Evaluation of fibular head transposition, lateral fabellar suture and conservative treatment of CrCL rupture in large dogs. J Am Anim Hosp Assoc 32:247, 1996
Dawson S, Bennett D, Carter SD et al: Acute arthritis of cats associated with feline calicivirus infection. Res Vet Sci 56:133, 1994
DeCamp CE: Dislocations. p. 333. In Olmstead ML (ed): Small Animal Orthopedics. Mosby–Year Book, St. Louis, 1995
DeHaan J, Goring R, Beale B: Evaluation of polysulfated glycosaminoglycan for the treatment of hip dysplasia in dogs. Vet Surg 23:177, 1994
Flynn MF, Edmiston DN, Roe SC et al: Biomechanical evaluation of a toggle pin technique for management of coxofemoral luxation. Vet Surg 23:311, 1994
Harari J, Johnson AL, Stein LE et al: Evaluation of experimental transection and partial excision of the caudal cruciate ligament in dogs. Vet Surg 16:151, 1987
Houlton JF, Meynink SE: Medial patellar luxation in the cat. J Small Anim Pract 30:349, 1989
Huber ML, Bill RL: The use of polysulfate glycosaminoglycans in dogs. Compend Contin Educ Pract Vet 16:501, 1994
Komtebedde J, Vasseur PB: Elbow luxation. p. 1729. In Slatter DH (ed): Textbook of Small Animal Surgery. 2nd Ed. WB Saunders, Philadelphia, 1993
Korvick DL, Johnson AL: Surgeons' preferences in treating cranial cruciate ligament ruptures in dogs. J Am Vet Med Assoc 205:1318, 1994
Manley PA: The hip joint. p. 1786. In Slatter DH (ed): Textbook of Small Animal Surgery. 2nd Ed. WB Saunders, Philadelphia, 1993
McLaughlin RM, Tillson DM: Flexible external fixation for craniodorsal coxofemoral luxations in the dog. Vet Surg 23:21, 1994
Montgomery RD, Long IR, Milton JL et al: Comparison of aerobic culturette, synovial membrane biopsy and blood culture medium in detection of canine bacterial arthritis. Vet Surg 18:300, 1989
Probst CW, Johnston SA: Osteochondrosis. p. 1944. In Slatter DH (ed): Textbook of Small Animal Surgery. 2nd Ed. WB Saunders, Philadelphia, 1993
Roush JK: Canine patellar luxation. Vet Clin North Am [Small Anim Pract] 23:855, 1993
Sjöström L, Kasström H, Källberg M: Ununited anconeal process in the dog. Vet Comp Ortho Traum 8:170, 1995
Smith GK, Biery DN, Gregor TP: New concepts of coxofemoral joint stability and development of a clinical stress radiographic method for quantitating hip joint laxity in the dog. J Am Vet Med Assoc 196:59, 1990
Todhunter RJ, Lust G: Polysulfate glycosaminoglycan in the treatment of osteoarthritis. J Am Vet Med Assoc 204:1245, 1994
Tomlinson J, McLaughlin R: Medically managing canine hip dysplasia. Vet Med 91:48, 1996

Vail DM, Powers BE, Getzy DM et al: Evaluation of prognostic factors for dogs with synovial sarcoma: 36 cases (1986–1991). J Am Vet Med Assoc 205:1300, 1994

Vasseur PB: Stifle joint. p. 1817. In Slatter DH (ed): Textbook of Small Animal Surgery. 2nd Ed. WB Saunders, Philadelphia, 1993

Vasseur PB, Foley P, Stevenson S, Heitter D: Mode of inheritance of Perthe's disease in Manchester terriers. Clin Orthop Rel Res 244:281, 1989

Wind AP: Elbow dysplasia. p. 1966. In Slatter DH (ed): Textbook of Small Animal Surgery. 2nd Ed. WB Saunders, Philadelphia, 1993

79

Diseases of Bone

Joseph Harari

DEVELOPMENTAL DISORDERS

Craniomandibular Osteopathy

Definition and Causes

I. Craniomandibular osteopathy is a non-neoplastic, proliferative bone disease of growing animals affecting the mandible and tympanic bullae.
II. The cause of the condition is unknown, although a genetic basis has been suggested owing to disease occurrence in a few select breeds (Alexander, 1983).

Pathophysiology

I. Bilaterally symmetrical resorption of normal lamellar bone and replacement by deposition of woven (immature) bone occur along endosteal and periosteal surfaces.
II. Bone resorption and deposition occur in a cyclic fashion during growth of the animal.
III. Although the woven bone may eventually be replaced by mature bone, normal osseous architecture is rarely recovered.

Clinical Signs

I. Some patients may be asymptomatic.
II. It is frequently diagnosed in terrier breeds 3–10 months of age with a history of oral discomfort.
   A. Animals exhibit difficulty in mastication, with subsequent weight loss and dehydration.
   B. Intermittent fever may be present.
   C. Palpable and sometimes painful enlargement of the mandible may be detected.
III. The disease is infrequently seen in other breeds such as the Labrador retriever, Great Dane, English bulldog, Doberman pinscher, and boxer.

Diagnosis

I. Suspicious clinical signs, physical examination, signalment, and history
II. Classic radiographic changes in the skull, such as bilaterally symmetrical bony proliferation of the mandible and tympanic bulla
III. Histologic evaluation of biopsy specimen revealing noninflammatory changes characterized by haphazard bone deposition and resorption

Differential Diagnosis

I. Similar symptoms: myositis, temporomandibular joint malformations, or trauma
II. Similar radiographic findings: bone infection or neoplasia

Treatment

I. No specific therapy has been identified, and the bone growth usually stops by 12 months of age (skeletal maturity).
II. Therapy is symptomatic.
   A. Aspirin 10–22 mg/kg PO BID or corticosteroids (infrequently) to reduce discomfort
   B. Soft foods to reduce masticatory movement and pain
   C. Pharyngotomy or gastrostomy tubes to provide nutrition for animals unable to eat
   D. Surgical reduction of bone mass usually not successful
   E. Euthanasia in severely progressive cases

Patient Monitoring

I. Control or reduce discomfort and maintain adequate level of nutrition.
II. Repeat clinical and radiographic examinations every 6–8 weeks to monitor disease progression until remission.

Hypertrophic Osteodystrophy

Definition and Causes

I. Hypertrophic osteodystrophy is a developmental disorder of the metaphyses of long bones in young large- and giant-breed dogs.

830

II. The exact cause of the condition is unknown, although speculation has focused on vitamin C deficiency, excessive dietary supplementation, and infection.

Pathophysiology

I. Bilateral disturbance in metaphyseal blood supply develops, leading to a failure or delay in ossification, especially in the distal radius and ulna.
II. Metaphyseal bone trabeculae fracture; necrosis and inflammation may occur, as well as periosteal new bone formation.

Clinical Signs

I. Bilateral, symmetrical metaphyseal swelling, pain, and lameness in large or giant dogs 2–8 months of age
II. Possibly fever, anorexia, and depression
III. Clinical signs usually episodic
IV. Angular limb deformities in severely affected dogs

Diagnosis

I. Clinical signs, physical examination, signalment, and history
II. Radiographic examination revealing metaphyseal lucency, representing trabecular necrosis and circumferential metaphyseal periosteal bone formation
III. Hematologic changes: normal or mild leukocytosis

Differential Diagnosis

I. Panosteitis
II. Osteomyelitis
III. Hypertrophic osteopathy
IV. Trauma

Treatment

I. No primary treatment has been delineated.
II. Correct or avoid any dietary imbalances and oversupplementation.
III. Aspirin is used to reduce discomfort.
IV. Corticosteroids and vitamin C are not recommended (Bellah, 1993; Manley and Romich, 1993).
V. Padded kennels, supportive fluid, and nutritional care are required for severely affected animals.
VI. Correction of persistent angular limb deformities may be necessary in lame, mature dogs.

Patient Monitoring

I. The condition is episodic in nature, and complete remission can occur in mildly or moderately affected animals.
II. Severely affected animals may become moribund and require extensive supportive therapy.
III. In mature animals, physical deformities may persist owing to excessive periosteal proliferation or asynchronous bone growth in the radius and ulna.

Multiple Cartilaginous Exostoses (Osteochondromatosis)

Definition and Causes

I. Osteochondromatosis is a proliferative disease of young dogs and cats characterized by multiple ossified protuberances arising from the metaphyseal cortical surface of long bones, vertebrae, or ribs.
II. Although the exact etiopathogenesis of the condition is uncertain, it is suspected to have a familial tendency in dogs and possibly a viral-associated malignant transformation in cats (Poole, 1993; Jacobsen and Kirberger, 1996).

Pathophysiology

I. Displacement of chondrocytes from the growth plate occurs, followed by osseous differentiation along a juxtacortical position.
II. In dogs, these osseous nodules usually cease growth at skeletal maturity.
III. In cats, the lesions may continue to progress after skeletal maturity and resemble a sarcoma (Poole, 1993).

Clinical Signs

I. Animals are usually asymptomatic unless bone enlargements encroach on neurovascular, tendinous, or ligamentous structures.
II. Signs can range from discomfort and lameness to paralysis.
III. Most affected animals are young dogs (6–18 months) and mature cats (2–4 years).

Diagnosis

I. Palpation reveals firm swellings arising from long bones, ribs, or vertebrae.
II. Radiography reveals pedunculated or sessile excrescences with smooth or irregular surfaces arising from multiple cortical surfaces.
III. Biopsy reveals a cartilage cap overlying a trabecular base of bone.

Differential Diagnosis

I. Neoplasia
II. Trauma
III. Calcinosis circumscripta

Treatment

I. Neutering of affected dogs is recommended because of the possible heritable nature of the condition.
II. Surgical excision of masses may be performed in dogs if clinical signs (lameness, pain, paralysis) are present.
III. In cats, surgical excision may only be palliative because of the condition's association with malignant

transformation and feline leukemia virus (Poole, 1993).

Patient Monitoring

I. Clinical and radiographic evaluations are indicated every 6 months to monitor the progressive or static nature of the lesions.
II. Surgical treatment is undertaken if neurologic or locomotor dysfunction develops.
III. Prognosis is poor in cats because of malignant transformation.
IV. Prognosis in dogs depends on the extent of skeletal involvement.

Panosteitis

Definition and Causes

I. Panosteitis is a spontaneous, self-limiting disease of young, rapidly growing large or giant dogs involving the diaphyseal and metaphyseal regions of long bones.
II. The exact cause of the condition is unknown, although a hereditary predisposition in German shepherd dogs has been postulated.
III. Other factors such as stress, infection, metabolic or autoimmune conditions, and parasitism have been suggested but not proved.

Pathophysiology

I. Fatty degeneration of the bone marrow is followed by stromal cell proliferation and osteoid production.
II. Vascular congestion secondary to osteoid production leads to endosteal and periosteal reactions and subsequent resorption of new bone.
III. Resorption is followed by reestablishment of normal marrow vascularity and adipose tissue.

Clinical Signs

I. The most typical signs include an acute, cyclic, single or multiple limb lameness in large or giant dogs at 6–14 months of age.
II. Males are more commonly affected than females.
III. Palpation of the diaphyses and metaphyses of long bones reveals pain and discomfort.
IV. The ulna, radius, humerus, femur, and tibia are affected, in decreasing order of prevalence.
V. Affected animals may also have periodic episodes of pyrexia, anorexia, and depression.

Diagnosis

I. Signalment, clinical signs, and physical examination are highly suggestive.
II. Radiography reveals increased intramedullary multifocal densities and irregular endosteal surfaces in long bones.

Differential Diagnosis

I. Hypertrophic osteodystrophy
II. Osteochondroses

III. Hip dysplasia
IV. Trauma

Treatment

I. No specific treatment has been identified; therapy is supportive to alleviate pain and discomfort.
II. Anti-inflammatory and analgesic therapy with aspirin (10–22 mg/kg PO BID) during periods of illness is often recommended.
III. Short-term corticosteroids (0.25–0.50 mg/kg PO SID for 3–5 days) are less frequently recommended.

Patient Monitoring

I. The condition is cyclic in nature and characterized by waxing and waning episodes, with eventual complete remission.
II. Clinical recovery is usually permanent by 18 months of age.

Radial and Ulnar Dysplasia

Definition and Causes

I. Abnormal development of the radius and ulna can occur because of asynchronous growth rates associated with damage to the proximal and/or distal growth plates.
II. Physeal damage may result from direct trauma, improper development or ossification, restrictive implants, or fracture healing (synostosis of the radius/ulna).
III. Dysplasia of the bones leads to both angular and length deformities, as well as carpal and elbow joint subluxations and arthritides.
IV. Disproportionate ulnar and radial growth is common in achondroplastic (bulldog, pug, Boston terrier) and hypochondroplastic (dachshund, beagle, basset hound) breeds and is related to desired breed traits (Manley and Romich, 1993).

Pathophysiology

I. Synchronous growth of the radius and ulna is essential for development of a normal forelimb.
  A. Although the growth rate for each physis of the respective bones is variable, unrestricted growth is necessary for proper bone and joint alignments.
  B. Alteration of growth in either bone deleteriously affects development of the adjacent bone and proximal/distal joints.
II. The radius is the major weight-bearing bone of the forearm and receives approximately 60% of its length from the distal physis.
III. The ulna receives 85% of its length from the distal physis.
IV. In most dogs, physeal growth accelerates at 4–8 months of age and declines at 9–11 months of age.

Clinical Signs

I. Most animals present with varying degrees of lameness, joint pain, and limb deformation (length and angulation).

II. Signs are usually unilateral in cases involving trauma and bilateral in developmental lesions (retained ulnar cartilage cores).

Diagnosis/Differential Diagnosis

I. Suggestive clinical signs, physical examination, signalment, history, and radiography

II. Premature closure of the distal ulnar physis

   A. It is the most common of all growth disturbances caused by a crush injury of the germinal cells in the distal cone-shaped physis.

   B. A shortened ulna restrains the radius and causes several forelimb abnormalities.

   1. Increased humeroulnar articulation and elbow subluxation

   2. Cranial bowing, external rotation, and shortening of the radius

   3. Valgus deviation at the carpus

   4. Degenerative joint disease in the elbow and carpus in chronic cases

   C. Radiography reveals a premature closure of the distal ulnar physis and bone/joint changes as described earlier.

III. Premature closure of the distal radial physis (uncommon)

   A. Lesions can be partial (asymmetrical) or complete (symmetrical).

   1. Asymmetrical closure usually involves the caudolateral physeal region.

   a) Produces a valgus deformation at the carpus owing to continued medial radial physeal growth.

   b) Radial length and elbow incongruity may not be clinically significant.

   2. Symmetrical distal radial physeal closure produces a shortened radius, elbow and carpal joint malarticulations, and caudal bowing of the radius and ulna.

   B. Radiography reveals partial or complete premature physeal closure and bone/joint changes mentioned earlier.

   C. A fragmented medial coronoid process of the ulna has also been described in dogs with distal radial physeal closure (Macpherson et al., 1992).

IV. Premature closure of proximal radial physis (uncommon)

   A. It produces a shortened radius, increased humeroradial joint space, and humeroulnar malarticulation if there is continued ulnar growth.

   B. Radiography reveals a prematurely closed proximal radial physis and the bone/joint changes mentioned earlier.

Treatment

I. The goal of surgery is to realign the radius/ulna and elbow/carpus to maintain limb function and prevent degenerative arthritis.

II. The type of surgery performed depends on the location of the lesion, age of the animal, and degree of limb deformation.

   A. Immature animals with growth potential (usually <6–8 months)

   1. Closure of distal ulnar physis

   a) Normal elbow joint

   (1) Partial distal ulnar ostectomy and interposition of free fat graft to reduce constraint on growing radius

   (2) Postoperative bandage support

   b) Humeroulnar malarticulation

   (1) Proximal ulnar osteotomy for "dynamic" muscular reduction of elbow joint incongruity (Gilson et al., 1989)

   (2) Bone realignment with single intramedullary pin

   2. Asymmetrical closure of distal radial physis

   a) Resection of closed physis and interposition of free fat graft

   b) Radial osteotomy and distraction with external fixator to maintain limb length and elbow articulation (Yanoff et al., 1992)

   c) Partial distal ulnar ostectomy; may not correct angular deformity and may require distal radial epiphysiodesis (Henney and Gambardella, 1990)

   d) Dome osteotomy of distal radius and external coaptation to correct deformity and maintain limb length (MacDonald and Matthiesen, 1991)

   3. Symmetrical closure of distal radial physis

   a) Midshaft radial osteotomy and distraction with external fixator to maintain limb length and elbow articulation

   b) Partial distal ulnar ostectomy to correct humeroradial malarticulation (Henney and Gambardella, 1990)

   c) Midshaft radial ostectomy and fat graft interposition; may produce radioulnar synostosis (Vechten and Vasseur, 1993)

   d) Multiple midshaft radial osteotomies, distractions, and bone plating to maintain limb length

   4. Closure of proximal radial physis

   a) Transverse radial osteotomy and distraction with external fixator

   b) Multiple radial osteotomies and bone plate fixation

   c) Partial distal ulnar ostectomy and fat interposition

   d) Proximal ulnar ostectomy and intramedullary pinning for mild radial shortening, at or near maturity

   B. Mature patients with little or no growth potential (usually >8–10 months)

   1. Premature closure of distal ulnar physis

   a) Oblique or dome radial and transverse ulnar osteotomies; internal (plate or cross-pinning) or external skeletal fixation (Sikes et al., 1986)

b) Proximal dynamic ulnar osteotomy to correct humeroulnar malarticulation
2. Premature closure of proximal or distal radial physis
   a) Oblique or dome osteotomy and internal or external fixation to correct angular deformity
   b) Transverse osteotomy, distraction, and fixation to correct limb shortening
   c) Stair-step osteotomy and bone plate fixation to correct limb shortening
   d) Proximal ulnar ostectomy and intramedullary pinning to correct mild elbow malarticulation

Patient Monitoring

I. Traumatic limb injuries in immature animals should be monitored clinically and radiographically every 1–2 weeks.
   A. Limb conformation is examined for angulation or shortening.
   B. The elbow and carpal joints are palpated for range of motion and crepitation.
   C. Radiography of the bones and joints is performed.
II. Postoperatively, animals are evaluated clinically and radiographically every 2–4 weeks, depending on the lesion(s), type of surgery, and age of the animal. Examine carefully for the following.
   A. Healing of operative sites
   B. Stability of surgical devices
   C. Limb length and angulation
   D. Joint function

Retained Ulnar Cartilage Cores

Definition and Causes

I. Retained ulnar cartilage cores is a developmental disorder of the distal ulnar physis of young large or giant dogs.
II. Although the exact cause of the condition is unknown, suspected etiologies include excessive dietary supplementation, vascular impairment, or osteochondrosis.

Pathophysiology

I. Retarded endochondral ossification at the distal ulnar physis leads to slow growth and restraint on radial development, similar to premature traumatic physeal closure.
II. The matrix septa in the hypertrophic zone of the physis fails to calcify normally and delays bone production and remodeling.

Clinical Signs

I. Bilateral angular limb deformities in young large or giant dogs characterized by carpus valgus, external rotation, and cranial bowing of the radius

II. Forelimb lameness associated with elbow or carpal joint dysfunction

Diagnosis

I. A tentative diagnosis can be made from clinical signs, physical examination, signalment, medical history, and radiography.
II. Radiographs reveal a radiolucent cartilage core in the center of the distal ulnar physis and extending proximally into the metaphysis.

Differential Diagnosis

I. Premature closure of the distal ulnar physis
II. Hypertrophic osteodystrophy

Treatment

I. Cessation of dietary supplements; feeding of normal, nutritionally balanced maintenance diet
II. Partial distal ulnar ostectomy and fat graft interposition to reduce constraint on radial growth
III. Corrective radial osteotomy in mature patients with angular limb deformity

Patient Monitoring

I. Physical and radiographic examinations every 2 weeks to monitor limb development
II. Routine postoperative care to monitor healing and straightening of the limb following osteotomy or ostectomy

Scottish Fold Osteodystrophy

Definition and Cause

I. Scottish fold osteodystrophy is a heritable condition affecting homozygous cats of this breed.
II. It is characterized by skeletal deformations involving the coccygeal vertebrae, metacarpal/metatarsal bones, and phalanges (Matthews et al., 1995).
III. Osteodystrophic changes in the distal extremities of mature and immature cats cause lameness.

Pathophysiology

I. Disordered endochondral ossification in the physes of affected bones
II. Active secondary centers of ossification associated with plantar exostoses of the tarsal joint, entrapping nerve and muscle fibers

Clinical Signs

I. Thick, shortened, inflexible tail
II. Forelimb and hindlimb lameness
III. Shortened paws
IV. Osseous palmar and plantar swellings involving the carpus, tarsus, and digits

Diagnosis

I. Diagnosis is by signalment, clinical signs, and radiography.
II. Radiography reveals malformed coccygeal vertebrae, metacarpal/metatarsal bones, and phalanges; palmar and plantar exostosis along the distal aspect of forelimbs and hindlimbs; and tarsal and carpal joint degeneration.

Differential Diagnosis

I. Trauma
II. Infection (osteomyelitis)
III. Neoplasia

Treatment

I. Removal of exostoses affecting soft tissue structures
II. Arthrodesis of carpal or tarsal joints to reduce joint pain

Patient Monitoring

I. Because of the heritable nature of the condition, sexually intact cats should be bred only to straight-eared cats.
II. Exostectomy is evaluated with radiographs every 6 months to assess for bone regrowth.
III. Arthrodesis is evaluated at 6 and 12 weeks to confirm joint fusion.

INFECTION

Osteomyelitis

Definition and Causes

I. Osteomyelitis is inflammation of the medullary cavity, cortex, and periosteum of bone and is most commonly associated with bacterial infection.
II. Aerobic bacteria are most frequently identified as causative agents (Johnson, 1994).
   A. *Staphylococcus* spp.
   B. *Streptococcus* spp.
   C. *Escherichia coli*
   D. *Proteus* spp.
   E. *Pasteurella* spp.
   F. *Pseudomonas* spp.
   G. *Brucella canis*
III. Anaerobic bacteria are less frequently isolated and may be part of a polymicrobial infection.
   A. *Bacteroides* spp.
   B. *Fusobacterium* spp.
   C. *Clostridium* spp.
IV. Fungal infections may arise based on the geographic location of the animal.
   A. *Coccidioides immitis* (southwestern states)
   B. *Blastomyces dermatitidis* (southeastern, central states)
   C. *Histoplasma capsulatum* (central states)
   D. *Cryptococcus neoformans* (worldwide)

   E. *Aspergillus* spp. (worldwide)
V. Noninfectious primary sources of osteomyelitis include implant corrosion or loosening and foreign substances such as sponges or bone wax.

Pathophysiology

I. Osteomyelitis results from an imbalance between bacterial growth and host defense mechanisms.
II. Factors contributing to bone infection include bacterial invasion, vascular stasis (ischemia), focal accumulation of inflammatory cells, release of degradative enzymes, and subsequent bone necrosis.
III. Abscessation may produce dead segments of bone (sequestrum) surrounded by reactive, vascular bone (involucrum) attempting to prevent spread of the infection.
IV. Bacterial sources include open traumatic injuries, prolonged surgical exposures, extension from adjacent infected tissue, or hematogenous routes.
V. Fungal infections are often multicentric and disseminated hematogenously after pulmonary inoculation.

Clinical Signs

I. Acute osteomyelitis
   A. Signs developing within 2 weeks of surgery, injury, or previous illness
   B. Focal pain, swelling, excessive warmth, lameness
   C. Depression, anorexia, pyrexia
II. Chronic osteomyelitis
   A. Signs developing usually months to years after naturally occurring trauma, surgery, or exposure to pathogens
   B. Persistent or recurrent lameness
   C. Draining sinus tracts over affected site
   D. Waxing and waning episodes of pyrexia, anorexia, depression

Diagnosis

I. It is often based on a combination of clinical signs, radiography, and laboratory findings.
II. Radiographic changes include soft tissue swelling, bone lysis, irregular periosteal reaction, loose implants, bone sequestration, and involucrum formation.
III. Fistulography can be used to outline the location and source of draining tracts.
IV. Nuclear scintigraphy may reveal excessive uptake of the radioisotope from the effects of inflammation.
V. Deep fine-needle aspiration, biopsy, or cytology may accurately reveal the microbial source of infection and appropriate antimicrobial therapy.
   A. Samples are submitted for aerobic and anaerobic bacterial culturing.
   B. In animals with systemic illness, serial blood cultures may be obtained.
VI. Hematologic tests may reveal an acute leukocytosis or anemia resulting from chronic inflammation.

Differential Diagnosis

I. Trauma-induced periosteal reaction
II. Neoplasia
III. Implant failure

Treatment

I. Acute osteomyelitis
   A. Antibiotic therapy is based on known or expected bacterial pathogens (determined by bacterial culture, Gram's stain) and is administered for at least 2–4 weeks.
      1. Amoxicillin-clavulanic acid 22 mg/kg PO TID
      2. Cephalexin 30 mg/kg PO BID
      3. Cefazolin 20 mg/kg IV, IM, SQ QID
      4. Clindamycin 11 mg/kg IV, IM, PO BID-TID
      5. Enrofloxacin 15 mg/kg PO BID
      6. Ciprofloxacin 11 mg/kg PO BID
      7. Metronidazole 15 mg/kg PO, IV BID
      8. Amikacin 15 mg/kg IV, IM, SQ SID
      9. Gentamicin 6 mg/kg IV, IM, SQ SID
      10. Oxacillin 22 mg/kg IV, IM, SQ, PO TID-QID
   B. See Chap. 109 for treatment of specific fungal diseases.
   C. Other treatments include the following.
      1. Soft tissue wound debridement, lavage, and drainage
      2. Delayed wound closure (Bardet et al., 1983)
      3. Removal of loose implants, necrotic and infected bone
      4. Maintenance of fracture stability with new implants if necessary
II. Chronic osteomyelitis
   A. Long-term (4–6 weeks) antimicrobial therapy based on aspiration or biopsy results
   B. Soft tissue wound debridement and drainage
      1. Delayed wound closure
      2. Continuous or intermittent closed lavage with sterile saline solution
      3. Open wound packing with moistened sterile saline–soaked sponges, covered with bandages
   C. Sequestrectomy and curettage
   D. Removal, replacement of implants
   E. Antibiotic-impregnated methylmethacrylate beads for local sustained delivery (Tobias et al, 1996)
   F. Autogenous cancellous grafting to stimulate bone healing (Bardet et al., 1983)
   G. Myocutaneous grafts for closure of extensive wounds (Pavletic, 1992)
   H. Limb amputation in severely progressive, irreversible lesions

Patient Monitoring

I. Clinical, radiographic, and laboratory evaluations are indicated for 2–6 months to confirm osseous and soft tissue healing.
II. Clinical evaluations of limb function, overall health, external fixators, and open wounds are performed every 1–2 weeks as indicated by the severity of the infection.
III. Hematologic and microbiologic tests are repeated every 1–2 weeks as needed to assess focal or systemic bacterial infection.
IV. Radiographs of bones and implants are taken at 2- to 4-week intervals to assess fracture healing and stability of fixation devices.
V. Prognosis for recovery depends on the severity of the condition; appropriate antimicrobial therapy, along with timely wound and fracture therapies, can effectively reduce morbidity.

IDIOPATHIC CONDITIONS

Bone Cysts

Definition and Causes

I. Bone cysts are single or multilocular fluid-filled spaces found in the metaphyseal, epiphyseal, or diaphyseal regions of long bones in young animals.
II. The exact cause of the condition is unknown, although developmental trauma or hereditary causes (in Doberman pinschers) have been proposed (Halliwell, 1993).
III. Aneurysmal bone cysts are considered tumor-like and are associated with intraosseous arteriovenous shunting of blood.

Pathophysiology

I. Solitary bone cysts are lined by a thin layer of connective tissue and contain serosanguineous fluid.
II. Aneurysmal bone cysts are large, multilocular lesions filled with blood.

Clinical Signs

I. Pain and swelling localized to the affected region of bone
II. Lameness from pathologic bone fracture or expansive intramedullary swelling of bone
III. Some animals asymptomatic

Diagnosis

I. Diagnosis is based on physical examination, signalment, radiography, aspiration, and biopsy.
II. Radiography reveals single or multiple radiolucent defects within long bones; the surrounding cortex may be thin or fractured.
III. Aspiration reveals clear or serosanguineous acellular fluid or blood with cellular elements.
IV. Biopsy reveals a connective tissue lining of the cyst, along with mononuclear inflammatory cells; aneurysmal cysts are characterized by multinucleated cells and osteoid spicules.

Differential Diagnosis

I. Neoplasia
II. Trauma
III. Infection

Treatment

I. If clinical lameness is present, cyst drainage, curettage, and autogenous cancellous bone grafting are performed to stimulate osteogenesis in the bone defect.
II. External support may be useful to prevent bone fracture during healing.

Patient Monitoring

I. Clinical and radiographic evaluations are performed at 6 and 12 weeks to assess obliteration of the defect and osteosynthesis following grafting.
II. The prognosis is good for lesions located away from the physis or epiphysis.

Hypertrophic Osteopathy

Definition and Causes

I. Hypertrophic osteopathy is a diffuse periosteal proliferative condition of long bones in dogs and, rarely, in cats.
II. The cause of the periosteal reaction is excessive peripheral periosteal vascularization associated (inexplicably) with neoplastic or infectious masses in the thoracic or abdominal cavity.

Pathophysiology

I. The pathogenic mechanisms of hypertrophic osteopathy are not fully known.
II. Increased peripheral vascularity produces periosteal congestion and reduced oxygenation, which may lead to periosteal new bone formation in the phalanges and distal bones.

Clinical Signs

I. Diffuse progressive long bone pain, lameness, joint stiffness in mature animals
II. Signs referable to neoplastic or infectious diseases in the thorax or abdomen

Diagnosis

I. Diagnosis is by physical examination, medical history, radiography, and ultrasonography.
II. Physical examination reveals bilaterally symmetrical lameness, bone swelling, and increased warmth of affected peripheral extremities.
III. Radiography and ultrasonography of the thorax or abdomen may reveal masses. Radiography of the extremities reveals periosteal proliferation that is especially prominent in the phalanges and metacarpal/metatarsal bones.

Differential Diagnosis

I. Skeletal neoplasia
II. Osteomyelitis
III. Trauma
IV. Hypervitaminosis A (cats)
V. Hypertrophic osteodystrophy

Treatment

I. Surgical resection of primary thoracic or abdominal mass
II. Unilateral intrathoracic vagotomy in animals with nonresectable masses, to block a suspected neurovascular reflex associated with increased peripheral circulation
III. Anti-inflammatory analgesics (dog: aspirin 10–22 mg/kg PO BID; dog or cat: prednisolone 0.25–0.5 mg/kg PO SID) to reduce peripheral limb discomfort

Patient Monitoring

I. Clinical and radiographic examinations are performed 6 and 12 weeks after surgery to monitor regression of peripheral periosteal lesions following removal of primary thoracic or abdominal masses.
II. The prognosis is fair if the underlying cause of disease in the thorax or abdomen can be identified and treated properly.

NUTRITIONAL/METABOLIC DISEASES

Nutritional Secondary Hyperparathyroidism

Definition and Causes

I. Nutritional secondary hyperparathyroidism is a nutritional/metabolic disorder caused by elevation of parathyroid hormone (PTH), usually secondary to poor nutrition.
II. The condition is most common in young animals fed an all-meat or all-grain diet.

Pathophysiology

I. Inadequate diet with low elemental calcium, high phosphate, or low vitamin D produces hypocalcemia, which stimulates increased PTH release.
II. Intestinal malabsorption of normal diets may also cause hypocalcemia.
III. Increased PTH causes bone resorption and promotes calcium transfer into the extracellular fluid.
IV. Depletion of bone osteoid leads to deformities, fractures, and loss of structural support.

Clinical Signs

I. Young animals, especially kittens, with lameness or bone deformities
II. Spontaneous fractures of long bones or vertebrae

Diagnosis

I. Diagnosis is by clinical signs, signalment, dietary history, radiography, and laboratory findings.
II. Laboratory findings include increased serum phosphorus (PO_4), alkaline phosphatase (SAP), and PTH levels. Serum calcium (Ca) may be normal or decreased.
III. Radiography reveals systemic bone resorption, fractures, and increased linear metaphyseal densities.

Differential Diagnosis

I. Renal secondary hyperparathyroidism
II. Congenital bone deformities
III. Other primary causes of osteopenia: disuse atrophy, pseudohyperparathyroidism, hyperthyroidism, hyperadrenocorticism

Treatment

I. Dietary correction and calcium supplementation
II. Restriction of activity to prevent bone fractures
III. External splintage for support of bone fractures

Patient Monitoring

I. Laboratory (SAP, PO_4, PTH, Ca) and radiographic evaluations are indicated every 1–3 months following onset of treatment.
II. Animals without severe bone deformations have a good prognosis; bones often become normal in 2–3 months (Manley and Romich, 1993).
III. Fractures may have delayed healing (>3 months).

Renal Secondary Hyperparathyroidism

Definition and Causes

I. Renal secondary hyperparathyroidism is caused by increased PTH levels associated with congenital or acquired renal insufficiency.
II. The condition may be seen in young or old animals with progressive renal disease.

Pathophysiology

I. Impaired renal phosphorus excretion and diminished conversion of vitamin D to its active form result in hypocalcemia.
II. Hypocalcemia stimulates PTH release and subsequent bone resorption.
III. Impaired vitamin D metabolism leads to decreased osteoclastic activity and subsequent osteomalacia.

Clinical Signs

I. Metabolic disturbances associated with uremic syndrome include the following.
   A. Polydipsia/polyuria
   B. Vomiting, diarrhea
   C. Weight loss
   D. Anorexia
II. Locomotor lesions are not frequently seen.
III. Loosening of teeth and mastication problems ("rubber jaw") may occur.
IV. Soft tissue calcification in lungs, kidneys, stomach, and heart may also be found.

Diagnosis

I. Diagnosis is by clinical signs, medical history, laboratory findings, and radiography.
II. Laboratory findings include increased blood urea nitrogen (BUN), serum creatinine, phosphorus, alkaline phosphatase, and plasma PTH.
III. Radiography reveals bone resorption, especially in the skull.

Differential Diagnosis

I. Nutritional secondary hyperparathyroidism
II. Hypovitaminosis D
III. Primary hyperparathyroidism (see Chap. 42)

Treatment

I. Treat underlying cause of renal failure (see Chap. 47).
II. Institute medical therapies to reduce BUN, creatinine, and phosphorus elevations.
   A. Dietary protein restriction
   B. Fresh drinking water ad libitum
   C. Oral phosphate-binding gels (30–90 mg/kg/day)
   D. Vitamin D_3 (calcitriol) 0.025 µg/kg/day PO
III. Parathyroidectomy may be attempted when progressive disease is unresponsive to medical and surgical treatments for renal failure.

Patient Monitoring

I. Prognosis depends on identification and treatment of underlying renal disease (infection, neoplasia, and so forth).
II. Blood gases, serum electrolytes, BUN, and creatinine levels are evaluated at weekly or monthly intervals, depending on azotemia and urine concentration ability.

Hypovitaminosis D

Definition and Causes

I. Hypovitaminosis D is a metabolic bone disease that arises from a dietary deficiency or lack of sunlight.
II. The condition is termed rickets in young animals and osteomalacia in adults.

Pathophysiology

I. Vitamin D increases bone cellular activities and enchondral ossification.
II. In mature animals, bone osteoclastic resorption is impaired, leading to osteomalacia.

Clinical Signs

I. Lameness, bone deformations
II. Pathologic fractures

Diagnosis

I. Diagnosis is by clinical signs, signalment, and laboratory and radiographic evaluations.
II. Laboratory tests reveal hypocalcemia and decreased vitamin D metabolites.
III. Radiography reveals irregular physes, metaphyseal mushrooming, and thin cortices in young animals, and bone resorption in mature animals.

Differential Diagnosis

I. Nutritional secondary hyperparathyroidism
II. Congenital bone deformations

Treatment

I. Nutritionally balanced diets containing adequate amounts of calcium, phosphate, and vitamin D
II. Surgical correction of persistent angular limb deformities in mature patients

Patient Monitoring

I. Clinical, laboratory, and radiographic evaluations at monthly intervals to evaluate bone
II. Good prognosis for patients without severe deformations
III. Guarded for patients with pathologic fractures and delayed healing (>3 months)

Hypervitaminosis A

Definition and Causes

I. Hypervitaminosis A is a metabolic disorder of cats that are fed predominantly whole liver and milk diets, resulting in excessive intake of vitamin A.
II. The condition requires prolonged abnormal dietary intake and is not reported in cats fed commercial diets.

Pathophysiology

I. Hypervitaminosis A causes physeal degeneration, osteoporosis, and exostoses.
II. Exostoses may be periarticular along long bones and the cervicothoracic regions of the vertebrae.

Clinical Signs

I. Reluctance to move
II. Forelimb lameness
III. Muscle weakness
IV. Cervical pain and rigidity
V. Paresis

Diagnosis

I. Diagnosis is by clinical signs, signalment, dietary history, radiography, and laboratory evaluations.
II. Serum concentrations of vitamin A may be increased; normal serum vitamin A is 20–80 μg/dl (Goldman, 1992).
III. Radiography reveals periarticular exostoses and vertebral body fusions.

Differential Diagnosis

I. Mucopolysaccharidosis
II. Trauma
III. Cervical disk disease

Treatment

I. Nutritionally balanced diet
II. Elevated feeding bowls to reduce cervical discomfort
III. Oral analgesics: aspirin 6 mg/kg every 48–72 hours

Patient Monitoring

I. Clinical evaluations to monitor morbidity are indicated every 2–4 weeks.
II. Prognosis is guarded for animals with severe bone changes (Schrader and Sherding, 1994).
III. Ankylosis of the vertebrae is irreversible.

Mucopolysaccharidosis

Definition and Causes

I. Mucopolysaccharidosis is an inherited disorder affecting glycosaminoglycan metabolism in cats and, rarely, in dogs (Schrader and Sherding, 1994; Bennett and May, 1995).
II. Glycosaminoglycans are constituents of the ground substance in connective tissue.

Pathophysiology

I. The metabolic defect is related to specific lysosomal enzyme deficiencies that cause excessive urinary glycosaminoglycan excretion and musculoskeletal abnormalities (see Chap. 64).
II. Osseous changes include epiphyseal and metaphyseal long bone enlargement, exostoses, dysplastic joints, and fused vertebrae.

Clinical Signs

I. Most commonly affected breeds: Siamese cats, Plott hounds, and dachshunds
II. Lameness, gait changes: crouching gait, abducted stifles
III. Facial dysmorphia: broadening of the maxilla, enlarged head
IV. Neurologic deficits from spinal cord or nerve root compression
V. Chronic diarrhea, respiratory and ocular discharges

Diagnosis

I. Diagnosis is by clinical signs, signalment, and laboratory and radiographic evaluations.

II. Urinalysis reveals glycosaminoglycosuria; examination of blood smears reveals abnormal cytoplasmic granules in neutrophils.

III. Radiography reveals periarticular exostoses, joint and vertebral fusions, dysplastic hips, and pectus excavatum.

Differential Diagnosis

I. Hypervitaminosis A

II. Trauma

III. Neoplasia

IV. Other lysosomal storage diseases (sphingomyelinosis)

Treatment

I. There is no known treatment.

II. Supportive care, with SQ or IV fluids and analgesics, is provided as needed.

III. Experimental bone marrow transplantation from a normal sibling to an affected cat has produced clinical improvement (Beekman, 1993).

Patient Monitoring

I. Affected animals without neurologic disease may live for 4–5 years.

II. Prognosis is guarded for progressively deteriorating animals.

NEOPLASIA

Definition

I. Skeletal tumors can be primary, secondary (metastatic), or locally invasive from adjacent soft tissue structures.

II. Skeletal neoplasms are inherently malignant and produce severe bone destruction characterized by osteolytic and osteoproliferative reactions.

Causes and Classification

I. Primary bone tumors

  A. Osteosarcoma

    1. Most common (90%) of all skeletal tumors in dogs and cats

    2. Common sites: distal radius, proximal humerus, distal femur, and proximal tibia

    3. Mature large- and giant-breed dogs frequently affected

    4. Early metastatic spread to lungs

  B. Chondrosarcoma

    1. Second most common primary bone tumor in dogs; uncommon in cats

    2. Flat bones (skull, ribs) more frequently affected than long bones

    3. Medium to large breeds, middle-aged dogs affected

    4. Slower growing and more protracted clinical course than osteosarcoma

  C. Fibrosarcoma

    1. Occurs infrequently in dogs and cats

    2. Affects metaphyseal area of long bones or periosteal tumor of mandible/maxilla

    3. Variable growth rate

  D. Hemangiosarcoma

    1. Most commonly affects proximal humerus or femur in older dogs, particularly German shepherd dogs

    2. Early hematogenous dissemination common at time of diagnosis

  E. Multiple myeloma

    1. Rarely a multicentric tumor in dogs and cats

    2. Most commonly affects flat bones, vertebrae, and proximal femur or humerus

II. Secondary bone tumors

  A. Less frequently diagnosed than primary bone tumors

  B. Most common types: lymphosarcoma; adenocarcinoma from primary mammary, prostatic, or lung lesions

III. Contiguous bone tumors

  A. Oropharyngeal tumors invading underlying bone

    1. Malignant melanoma

    2. Acanthomatous epulis

    3. Squamous cell carcinoma

    4. Fibrosarcoma

  B. Tumors of the digits arising from the subungual epithelium: squamous cell carcinoma

Clinical Signs

I. Lameness, swelling, pain in affected limb or site

II. Acute pathologic fractures with minimal trauma

III. Anorexia, weight loss

IV. Dyspnea from metastatic lesions

Diagnosis

I. Diagnosis is by clinical history, signalment, physical examination, and radiographic and histologic evaluations.

II. Radiographic changes associated with skeletal neoplasia include osteolysis (''moth-eaten,'' ''punched-out'' lesions), osteoproliferation, periosteal reaction, soft tissue swelling, pathologic fractures, and metastatic lung lesions.

III. Skeletal survey radiography or nuclear scintigraphy is sometimes useful to determine multiple site involvement.

IV. Multiple biopsy samples of affected tissue should be obtained using a Michel bone trephine or Jamshidi bone biopsy needle (Straw, 1996).

  A. Samples can also be obtained for microbiologic cultures and antimicrobial sensitivity testing to rule out fungal or bacterial osteomyelitis.

  B. The extracellular matrix is examined for osteoid, cartilage, or fibrous tissue.

C. Accurate diagnosis is based on proper sample size (2-cm length) and location (central area of lesion) and experience of the pathologist in evaluating animal bone specimens.

Differential Diagnosis

I. Osteomyelitis
II. Trauma
III. Bone infarcts (emboli)
IV. Benign cystic lesions

Treatment

I. Osteosarcoma (Table 79–1)
  A. Limb amputation
    1. Median survival of 5 months in dogs (Spodnick et al., 1992)
    2. Median survival of 4 years in cats (Bitteto et al., 1987)
  B. Limb amputation and chemotherapy (carboplatin, cisplatin, doxorubicin)
    1. One-year survival rates range from 35–60%
    2. Median survival rate of approximately 10 months in dogs (Straw, 1996)
  C. Limb amputation and adjuvant immunotherapy
    1. Macrophage-stimulating agent: liposome-encapsulated analogue of *Mycobacterium* cell wall used to enhance tumor destruction (Straw, 1996)
    2. Prolongs survival after amputation by affecting metastatic lesions
    3. Used in combination with cisplatin
  D. Limb-sparing, cisplatin, and radiotherapy
    1. Involves en bloc resection of tumor (usually distal radius) and replacement with cortical allograft and a stabilizing bone plate (Straw et al., 1990)
    2. Provides a functional limb and similar survival rates as amputation and chemotherapy

  E. Metastectomy (O'Brien et al., 1993b; Straw, 1996)
    1. Controversial removal of lung masses
    2. May be useful for dogs with <3 metastatic nodules in one lung developing >300 days after diagnosis of the primary tumor
II. Chondrosarcoma
  A. Limb amputation
    1. Median survival of 1.5 years
    2. Adjuvant radiation and chemotherapy not effective
  B. Fair prognosis owing to slower growth than osteosarcoma (Davidson, 1995)
III. Fibrosarcoma
  A. Similar surgical treatments as osteosarcoma; chemotherapy may not be useful
  B. Guarded prognosis; metastasis to heart, skin, and other bones rather than lung (Ablin et al., 1991)
IV. Hemangiosarcoma
  A. Amputation and chemotherapy using doxorubicin and cyclophosphamide
  B. Poor prognosis owing to vascular dissemination and metastasis; most dogs are dead within 5 months of surgery (MacEwen, 1996)
V. Multiple myeloma
  A. Combination chemotherapy with melphalan and prednisolone (see Chap. 75)
  B. Good prognosis
VI. Metastatic bone tumors
  A. Therapy is palliative owing to multiple sites of disease.
  B. Amputation is reserved for solitary metastatic lesions.
  C. Radiation therapy for reduction of bone pain may produce relief for several months (Kisseberth and MacEwen, 1996).
VII. Contiguous lesions
  A. Partial or complete bone excision may be performed.
  B. Chemotherapy, irradiation, cryotherapy, and hy-

Table 79–1. Adjuvant Chemotherapy Agents Used with Amputation to Treat Osteosarcoma in Dogs

Drug	Dosage (mg/m²)	Survival	Comments
Cisplatin	70 IV every 21 days (2 times)	40% at 1 yr Median 272 days	Given before or after amputation
Cisplatin	50 IV every 28 days (up to 9 times)	62% at 1 yr Median 413 days	Longer survival with higher doses
Cisplatin	50 IV at 14 and 49 days after amputation	30% at 1 yr Median 290 days	Improved survival vs. amputation alone
Carboplatin	300 IV every 21 days (4 times)	35% at 1 yr Median 321 days	Maximum dosage not described
Doxorubicin	30 IV every 14 days (5 times)	50% at 1 yr	Tumor necrosis predicted survival
Doxorubicin and cisplatin	Doxorubicin at 30 IV day 1 and cisplatin at 60 IV day 21 (2 times)	37% at 1 yr Median 300 days	No difference compared with cisplatin alone
Cisplatin and biodegradable polymer (OPLA-Pt)	80 implanted at amputation	41% at 1 yr Median 278 days	New trials, results pending

From Straw RC, 1996, with permission.

perthermia may be useful, depending on the tumor and location.

Patient Monitoring

I. Usual cause of death following surgery for osteosarcoma is diffuse pulmonary metastasis.
II. Thoracic radiography is performed every 3–6 months to monitor metastatic disease, or earlier if there is respiratory compromise.
III. Laboratory evaluations (complete blood counts, platelet counts, serum chemistries) to monitor response to chemotherapy are performed according to the chemotherapeutic protocol.

TRAUMA

Fractures

Definition and Causes

I. A bone fracture is a break in the continuity of bone structure caused by external trauma, excessive muscular contractions, or an underlying disease that weakens the bone.
II. Fractures can be open or closed; complete or incomplete; simple, comminuted, or segmental.
III. Specific disruptive forces that produce fractures include compression, tension, bending, and rotation; clinically, they occur in a combined manner.

Pathophysiology

I. A bone fractures when localized stresses exceed bone strength and disrupt its stiffness.
II. Compressive forces can cause impacted metaphyseal fractures in young animals and collapse of vertebrae.
III. Tensile forces produce apophyseal distraction at the olecranon, calcaneus, and tibial tuberosity.
IV. Concentric compression of a curved bone (radius) or eccentric loading of a straight bone (femur) produces bending and subsequent transverse and oblique long bone fractures.
V. Torsion causes high internal shear and tensile stresses to produce spiral fractures.

Clinical Signs

I. Acute lameness, focal swelling, crepitation, shortness of limb, subcutaneous hemorrhage
II. Possibly neurologic deficits secondary to regional inflammation or direct bone trauma
III. Possibly compromised vital signs and bowel/bladder function
IV. External skin wounds; possible communication with underlying bone

Diagnosis

I. Diagnosis is based on clinical signs, physical examination, medical history, and radiography.

II. Radiography usually requires multiple views obtained in a sedated or anesthetized, stable animal.
  A. Obscure or subtle lesions may be identified by comparing views of the affected limb with the contralateral, normal leg.
  B. Radiographic examination provides detailed and accurate information regarding the nature and severity of the injury and the attendant osseous, soft tissue, and joint lesions.

Differential Diagnosis

I. Neoplasia
II. Congenital or developmental bone anomalies
III. Joint luxations

Treatment

I. Destabilizing forces at the fracture site(s) must be neutralized to permit primary (direct) or secondary (indirect, callus formation) bone union.
II. Treatments include external splints or casts, internal implants (pins, wires, plate, screws), or external fixators.
  A. Selection of operative or nonoperative treatment is based on the type of fracture and animal, expertise of the surgeon, availability of equipment, financial constraints of the owner, and environment for postoperative care.
  B. Circumferential casts are usually reserved for minimally displaced (or relatively stable) fractures below the elbow or stifle joint in young animals.
  C. Intramedullary pins are used to maintain axial alignment (prevent bending) and reduce rotational forces (multiple or stack pinning).
  D. Circumferential (cerclage) orthopedic wires and Kirschner wires are ancillary implants used for fragmentary apposition and some rotational support.
  E. A bone plate and screws can be used to counteract all distractive forces at the fracture site(s) and provide a rapid return of limb function. Screws can also be used as ancillary implants to provide interfragmentary compression and antirotational stability.
  F. External skeletal fixation (ESF) is a versatile stabilizing technique used to neutralize all fracture distractive forces.
    1. Percutaneous pins and connecting bars are used to design various ESF configurations based on the nature of the fracture.
    2. Application of ESF can be accomplished via open surgical techniques to obtain anatomic reduction (in conjunction with pins or wires) or via closed techniques to minimize soft tissue trauma and promote natural biologic healing (Aron et al., 1995).
    3. External bars and clamps of the fixator can be reused to reduce equipment costs.
    4. External configurations can be easily modified during the healing process to stress the bone

and enhance collagen remodeling and osteo-synthesis.
III. Autogenous cancellous grafts obtained from the greater tubercle of the humerus, wing of the ilium, or tibial tuberosity provide cellular constituents, a lattice, and biochemical stimulus to enhance fracture healing.
IV. Antibiotics are used perioperatively to reduce bacterial infection following fracture repair.
  A. Preoperatively, antibiotics are given intravenously to prevent infection (most commonly *Staphylococcus* spp., *E. coli*) in closed fractures when surgical repair is prolonged and/or infection would seriously endanger the animal or render the operation unsuccessful. Doses are repeated during surgery (Harari, 1993; Roush, 1996).
    1. Cefazolin sodium 22 mg/kg IV every 2 hours
    2. Oxacillin 22 mg/kg IV every 2 hours
  B. Therapeutic antibiotics (see drugs listed for Osteomyelitis) are used to treat open, contaminated fractures (preexisting infection) and are given postoperatively based on bacterial culture and antimicrobial sensitivity testing. Doses are given IV or IM initially and then PO.
V. Perioperative analgesia is useful in alleviating discomfort and enhancing biologic and psychologic recuperation (Keegan, 1996).
  A. Epidural narcotics
    1. Given preoperatively
    2. Morphine 0.1 mg/kg diluted with saline 0.25 ml/kg
  B. Systemic narcotics
    1. Morphine
      a) Dogs: 0.25–0.5 mg/kg, IM, SQ
      b) Cats: 0.05–0.1 mg/kg IM, SQ
    2. Oxymorphone
      a) Dogs: 0.025–0.05 mg/kg IV, IM, SQ
      b) Cats: 0.025–0.05 mg/kg IM, SQ
    3. Butorphanol 0.1–0.2 mg/kg IM, SQ
  C. Sedative given with opioid postoperatively Acepromazine 0.025 mg/kg IV, IM, SQ

Patient Monitoring

I. Physical examinations are performed daily after surgery, then at weekly and monthly intervals to assess limb function, wound healing, overall health, and the status of any external fixators or splints.
  A. Aspirin (10–22 mg/kg PO BID) can be used during the first postoperative week as an anti-inflammatory, antipyretic, analgesic agent to alleviate discomfort.
  B. Physical therapy is used to reduce morbidity and enhance recovery of functional limb usage (Hodges and Palmer, 1993).
    1. Local hypothermia (ice bags) is used in acute injuries to reduce vascular permeability, decrease nerve (pain) conduction, and produce muscle relaxation.
    2. Superficial hyperthermia (warm-water heating blankets) is used 48–72 hours after injury to improve circulation and reduce muscular tension and pain.
    3. Massage is useful in improving circulation and muscular activity.
    4. Passive and active exercises improve circulation, joint function, muscular activity, and coordination.
  C. Nutritional requirements are determined, and adequate intake of proteins, lipids, carbohydrates, fiber, and water must be maintained (Layton, 1996).
    1. Surgery and trauma increase the energy requirements (60–80 kcal/kg/day) of animals by 1.5-fold.
    2. Initial delivery of nutrients is by the simplest, least invasive, most physiologic route.
      a) Oral feedings
      b) Orogastric intubation
      c) Nasoesophageal feeding tube
      d) Pharyngostomy feeding tube
      e) Esophagostomy feeding tube
      f) Gastrostomy feeding tube
      g) Enterostomy feeding tubes or catheters
      h) Parenteral nutrition (IV)
  D. Naturally occurring external wounds are treated with sterile bandaging techniques, are permitted to close by second-intention healing, or are repaired by delayed wound closure (Lozier, 1993).
    1. Wound lavage with dilute antiseptic solutions (chlorhexidine, povidone-iodine) or saline is useful in reducing bacterial and foreign debris contamination.
    2. Delayed wound closure with sutures is performed 3–5 days after initiation of lavage and debridement, as wound contamination decreases and healing of tissues occurs.
II. Radiographs are taken at 3- to 6-week intervals to assess fracture healing and stability of implants.
  A. In general, pins and bone plates can be removed from long bone fractures following clinical and radiographic evidence of fracture healing and bone union.
  B. Normal fracture healing can be delayed, produce deformation (malunion), or be nonexistent (nonunion) and thus require a second surgery.
  C. Rates and type (primary or secondary bone union) of fracture healing depend on the nature of the injury, age of the animal, type of surgical repair, and postoperative care.
III. The prognosis for clinical recovery following fracture repair is good if surgical principles are followed and quality perioperative care (nutrition, physical therapy, wound care, antibiotics) is provided.
  A. Halstead's principles of surgery
    1. Gentle tissue handling
    2. Preservation of tissue vascularity
    3. Accurate hemostasis
    4. Strict aseptic technique
    5. Anatomic approximation of tissues without tension
    6. Obliteration of dead space
  B. Orthopedic guidelines

1. Rigid external or internal fixation
2. Preservation of periosseous neurovascular elements
3. Realignment of limb axis and maintenance of joint parallelism above/below fractured bones
4. Rapid return of limb usage to maintain functions of joints, muscles, and tendons

Bibliography

Ablin LW, Berg J, Schelling SH: Fibrosarcoma of the canine appendicular skeleton. J Am Anim Hosp Assoc 27:303, 1991

Alexander JW: Selected skeletal dysplasias: craniomandibular osteopathy, multiple cartilaginous exostoses, and hypertrophic osteodystrophy. Vet Clin North Am [Small Anim Pract] 13:55, 1983

Aron D, Palmer R, Johnson A: Biologic strategies and a balanced concept for repair of highly comminuted long bone fractures. Compend Contin Educ Pract Vet 17:35, 1995

Bardet JF, Hohn RB, Basinger R: Open drainage and delayed autogenous cancellous bone grafting for treatment of osteomyelitis in dogs and cats. J Am Vet Med Assoc 183:312, 1983

Beekman GK: Mucopolysaccharidosis VI in a kitten. Fel Pract 21:7, 1993

Bellah JR: Hypertrophic osteodystrophy. p. 858. In Bojrab MJ (ed): Disease Mechanisms in Small Animal Surgery. 2nd Ed. Lea & Febiger, Philadelphia, 1993

Bennett D, May C: Joint diseases of dogs and cats. p. 2032 In Ettinger SJ, Feldman EC (eds): Textbook of Veterinary Internal Medicine. 4th Ed. WB Saunders, Philadelphia, 1995

Bergman PJ, MacEwen EG, Kurzman ID et al: Amputation and carboplatin for treatment of dogs with osteosarcoma. J Vet Intern Med 10:76, 1996

Bitteto WV, Patnaik AK, Schrader SC et al: Osteosarcoma in cats: 22 cases (1974–1984). J Am Vet Med Assoc 190:91, 1987

Brinker WO, Piermattei DL, Flo GL: Disease conditions in small animals. p. 547. In Brinker WO, Piermattei DL, Flo GL (eds): Handbook of Small Animal Orthopedics and Fracture Treatment. WB Saunders, Philadelphia, 1990

Davidson JR: Canine and feline chrondrosarcoma. Compend Contin Educ Pract Vet 17:1109, 1995

Gilson SD, Piermattei DL, Schwarz PD: Treatment of humeroulnar subluxation with a dynamic proximal ulnar osteotomy: a review of 13 cases. Vet Surg 18:114, 1989

Goldman AL: Hypervitaminosis A in a cat. J Am Vet Med Assoc 200:1970, 1992

Halliwell WH: Tumorlike lesions of bone. p. 933. In Bojrab HJ (ed): Disease Mechanisms in Small Animal Surgery. 2nd Ed. Lea & Febiger, Philadelphia, 1993

Harari J (ed): External skeletal fixation. Vet Clin North Am [Small Anim Pract] 22:1, 1992

Harari J: Perioperative antibiotic therapy. p. 293. In Harari J (ed): Surgical Complications and Wound Healing in the Small Animal Practice. WB Saunders, Philadelphia, 1993

Henney LH, Gambardella PC: Partial ulnar ostectomy for treatment of premature closure of the proximal and distal radial physes in the dog. J Am Anim Hosp Assoc 26:183, 1990

Hodges CC, Palmer RH: Postoperative physical therapy. p. 389. In Harari J (ed): Surgical Complications and Wound Healing in the Small Animal Practice. WB Saunders, Philadelphia, 1993

Jacobsen LS, Kirberger RM: Canine multiple cartilaginous exostoses: unusual manifestations and a review of the literature. J Am Anim Hosp Assoc 32:45, 1996

Johnson KA: Osteomyelitis in dogs and cats. J Am Vet Med Assoc 205:1882, 1994

Keegan RD: Anesthesia. p. 11. In Harari J (ed): Small Animal Surgery. Williams & Wilkins, Baltimore, 1996

Kisseberth WC, MacEwen EG: Complications of cancer and its treatment. p. 129. In Withrow SJ, MacEwen EG (eds): Small Animal Clinical Oncology. 2nd Ed. WB Saunders, Philadelphia, 1996

Layton CE: Nutritional support of surgical patients. p. 39. In Harari J (ed): Small Animal Surgery. Williams & Wilkins, Baltimore, 1996

Lozier SM: Topical wound therapy. p. 63. In Harari J (ed): Surgical Complications and Wound Healing in the Small Animal Practice. WB Saunders, Philadelphia, 1993

MacDonald JM, Matthiesen D: Treatment of forelimb growth deformity in 11 dogs by radial dome osteotomy and external coaptation. Vet Surg 20:402, 1991

MacEwen EG: Miscellaneous tumors. p. 521. In Withrow SJ, MacEwen EG (eds): Small Animal Clinical Oncology. 2nd Ed. WB Saunders, Philadelphia, 1996

Macpherson GC, Lewis DD, Johnson KA: Fragmented coronoid process associated with premature distal radial physeal closure in four dogs. Vet Comp Ortho Traum 5:93, 1992

Manley PA, Romich JA: Miscellaneous orthopedic diseases. p. 1984. In Slatter D (ed): Textbook of Small Animal Surgery. 2nd Ed. WB Saunders, Philadelphia, 1993

Matthews KG, Koblik PD, Knoeckel MJ et al: Resolution of lameness associated with Scottish fold osteodystrophy following bilateral ostectomies and pantarsal arthrodesis. J Am Anim Hosp Assoc 31:280, 1995

Morgan JP, Leighton RL: Fracture description. p. 8. In Morgan JP, Leighton RL (eds): Radiology of Small Animal Fracture Management. WB Saunders, Philadelphia, 1995

O'Brien MG, Straw RC, Withrow SJ: Recent advances in the treatment of canine appendicular osteosarcoma. Compend Contin Educ Pract Vet 15:939, 1993a

O'Brien MG, Straw RG, Withrow SJ et al: Resection of pulmonary metastases in canine osteosarcoma: 36 cases (1983–1992). Vet Surg 22:105, 1993b

Olmstead ML, Egger EL, Johnson AL et al: Principles of fracture repair. p. 111. In Olmstead ML (ed): Small Animal Orthopedics. CV Mosby, St. Louis, 1995

Pavletic M: Myocutaneous flaps and muscle flaps. p. 309. In Pavletic M (ed): Atlas of Small Animal Reconstructive Surgery. JB Lippincott, Philadelphia, 1992

Poole RP: Osteochondromatosis. p. 821. In Bojab MJ (ed): Disease Mechanisms in Small Animal Surgery. 2nd Ed. Lea & Febiger, Philadelphia, 1993

Roush JK: Diseases affecting developing bone. p. 1073. In Birchard SJ, Sherding RG (eds): Saunders Manual of Small Animal Practice. WB Saunders, Philadelphia, 1994

Roush JK: Infection control. p. 23. In Harari J (ed): Small Animal Surgery. Williams & Wilkins, Baltimore, 1996

Schrader SC, Sherding RG: Disorders of the skeletal system. p. 1599. In Sherding RG (ed): The Cat—Diseases and Clinical Management. Churchill Livingstone, New York, 1994

Sikes RI, Olds RB, Renegar W: Dome osteotomy for the correction of long bone malunions: case reports and discussions of surgical technique. J Am Anim Hosp Assoc 22:221, 1986

Spodnick GJ, Berg J, Rand WH et al: Prognosis for dogs with appendicular osteosarcoma treated by amputation alone: 162 cases (1978–1988). J Am Vet Med Assoc 200:995, 1992

Straw RC: Tumors of the skeletal system. p. 287. In Withrow SJ, MacEwen EG (eds): Small Animal Clinical Oncology. 2nd Ed. WB Saunders, Philadelphia, 1996

Straw RC, Withrow SJ, Powers BE: Management of canine appendicular osteosarcoma. Vet Clin North Am [Small Anim Pract] 20:1141, 1990

Taylor R, McGehee R: Orthopedic procedures. p. 187. In Taylor R, McGehee R (eds): Manual of Small Animal Postoperative Care. Williams & Wilkins, Baltimore, 1995

Tobias KS, Schneider RK, Besser TE: Use of antibiotic-impregnated methylmethacrylate beads for treatment of infections. J Am Vet Med Assoc 208:841, 1996

Vechten VB, Vasseur PB: Complications of mid-diaphyseal radial ostectomy performed for treatment of premature closure of the distal radial physis in two dogs. J Am Vet Med Assoc 202:97, 1993

Watson ADJ: Diseases of muscles and bone. p. 657. In Whittick WG (ed): Canine Orthopedics. 2nd Ed. Lea & Febiger, Philadelphia, 1990

Yanoff SR, Hulse DA, Palmer RH: Distraction osteogenesis using modified external fixation devices in five dogs. Vet Surg 21:480, 1992

80

Diseases of Muscles and Tendons

Giselle Hosgood
Jacqueline R. Davidson

CONGENITAL/INHERITED MYOPATHIES

See Table 80–1.

INFECTIOUS MYOSITIS

Protozoal Polymyositis

Definition and Causes

I. Rarely, infectious agents may cause generalized myositis.
II. *Toxoplasma gondii* is the most common cause of infectious myositis.
III. *Neospora caninum* causes similar signs and may have been misdiagnosed as toxoplasmosis in the past.

Clinical Signs

I. Both organisms tend to cause more severe signs in very young animals and have an increased likelihood of causing signs in immunosuppressed animals.
II. Toxoplasmosis is often associated with canine distemper infection, whereas neosporosis is not associated with concurrent infection.
III. Gait abnormalities are present.
   A. Hopping gait
   B. Progressive hindlimb paresis
   C. Rigid extension of the hindlimbs
   D. Progressive ascending paralysis more common with neosporosis
   E. Severe muscle pain possible initially
   F. Gradual muscle atrophy as the disease progresses
IV. There is evidence of central nervous system (CNS) disease.
   A. Stupor
   B. Seizures
   C. Chorioretinitis
V. It has been reported to cause death within 48 hours of initial signs.

Diagnosis

I. Suspicious clinical signs are present.
II. Creatine kinase is elevated during the active phase of the disease.
III. Histopathologic findings in muscle biopsy are as follows.
   A. Pronounced fiber atrophy
   B. Severe multifocal or diffuse myonecrosis
   C. Mononuclear granulomatous inflammation
   D. Severe interstitial fibrosis in chronic cases
   E. Presence of organisms (free or in cysts) definitive, but not always found
IV. Serum with antibodies to *N. caninum* does not react with *T. gondii* organisms, and vice versa.
   A. Single titers may be unreliable.
   B. Rising titers support the diagnosis but require a long delay before results are obtained.
V. Cerebrospinal fluid (CSF) analysis reveals the following.
   A. Mixed pleocytosis
   B. High protein content
VI. Indirect fluorescent antibody test of serum, CSF, or tissue aids in distinguishing *N. caninum* from *T. gondii*.
VII. Definitive diagnosis of *N. caninum* may be made at necropsy using electron microscopy and immunohistochemical methods.

Differential Diagnosis

I. *Leptospira icterohaemorrhagiae*
   A. Diffuse myositis occurs in rare cases of leptospirosis.
   B. In addition to the renal and hepatic signs of

Table continued on following page

Table 80–1. *Congenital Myopathies*

Disorder and Definition	Breeds Affected	Cause and Inheritance	Clinical Signs	Diagnosis	Differential Diagnosis	Treatment and Prognosis	References
Type II muscle fiber deficiency Predominance of type I and deficiency of type II muscle fibers, causing gait disturbance	Labrador retriever	Cause unknown Simple autosomal recessive	<5 mo of age Initial gait abnormality progresses to generalized weakness, inability to hold head up Exacerbated by exercise Marked skeletal muscle atrophy Stunted growth Progressive signs until maturity, then signs stabilize Normal neurologic exam possible	Clinical signs in Labrador Creatinuria[a] up to 30× normal; CK[b] < normal Muscle biopsy: variable fiber diameter with increased endo- and perimysial connective tissue Deficiency of ATPase staining type II fibers EMG may reveal myotonic discharges.	Myasthenia gravis (older dogs; response to edrophonium chloride, EMG shows decremental response) Nutritional myodegeneration (history of abnormal diet, progressive) Congenital myotonia	None Diphenylhydantoin PO ineffective Diazepam PO may alleviate some signs. Poor prognosis since no treatment, but normal life span possible	Kramer et al., 1981 Sharp et al., 1989
Sex-linked myopathies Myopathies inherited via the X-gene	Alaskan malamute Golden retriever Groenendaeler shepherd Irish terrier Samoyed Male cats	Inability to produce dystrophin (cytoskeletal protein of muscle fibers) X-linked inheritance Males exhibit clinical signs. Carrier females may have mild elevations in muscle enzymes without clinical signs. Similar to Duchenne-type muscular dystrophy in humans	Dogs: Onset at 6–8 wk of age Rapid progression of signs Difficulty swallowing, drooling Stiff gait, rigid neck Hypertrophy of tongue and caudal thigh muscles Atrophy of other muscles, particularly truncal and temporal muscles Lumbar kyphosis Exercise intolerance Normal neurologic exam initially, with later proprioceptive deficits and hyporeflexia Cats: Onset at 12 mo of age Slow progression of signs Stiff, rigid neck Adduction of hocks Symmetrical muscular hypertrophy Lumbar kyphosis Reduced cardiac contractility and biventricular enlargement	Clinical signs in reported breeds Increased CK, aldolase, AST, ALT, and LDH Muscle biopsy variable: fiber necrosis and regeneration, hypertrophy (cat), fiber loss and fibrosis (dog), and myofiber mineralization (both) EMG: bizarre high-frequency discharges (golden retriever), diffuse, continuous myotonic discharge (Irish terrier) Normal nerve conduction velocity	Congenital myotonia of dogs (myotonic dimple) Hypokalemic myopathy of cats (elevated serum potassium) Inherited myopathy of Devon rex cats (normal CK, AST, characteristic head and neck ventroflexion, megaesophagus, generalized muscle weakness and fatigue) Immune-mediated polymyositis (characteristic cellular infiltrate in histologic specimens)	None Disease is progressive, less rapidly after 6 mo of age (dogs). Poor prognosis	Cardinet and Holliday, 1979 Kornegay, 1984 Malik, 1993 Presthues and Nordstoza, 1989 Robinson, 1992 van Ham et al., 1993 Vos et al., 1986 Wentworth et al., 1972

Table 80–1. Congenital Myopathies (Continued)

Disorder and Definition	Breeds Affected	Cause and Inheritance	Clinical Signs	Diagnosis	Differential Diagnosis	Treatment and Prognosis	References
Congenital myotonia Involuntary contraction of a muscle that persists after a voluntary effort or stimulation	Chow chow Cocker spaniel Labrador retriever Samoyed Staffordshire terrier West Highland white terrier	Cause unknown Low membrane chloride conductance and accumulation of potassium in the tubular system may cause postexcitement depolarization of the muscle membrane and continued contraction of the muscle. Autosomal recessive inheritance in chow chow, but considered to have multifactorial etiology	Abnormal stiff gait at 2–3 mo of age, lessens with exercise: Abduction of forelimbs "Bunny hop" Arched back Muscle hypertrophy of all skeletal muscles, especially proximal appendicular muscles, tongue, and anal sphincter Normal muscle tone at rest Characteristic myotonic dimple persists for 30–40 sec after direct muscle stimulation (tongue or shaved limb). Dysphagia often observed	Clinical signs in a reported breed with myotonic dimple EMG: high-frequency myotonic discharges with continuous insertional activity and possible decremental response Normal nerve conduction velocity CK may be elevated. Muscle biopsy variable: hypertrophy, atrophy, and degeneration	Nutritional myodegeneration Cerebellar dysmyelinogenesis: also reported in young chow chows Animals with cerebellar disease can potentially recover, are not stiff, and have a continuous tremor of the head, neck, and trunk; they typically "bounce" repetitively on the hindlimbs.	None Disease is not progressive. Procainamide and quinidine may lessen initial weakness. Diphenylhydantoin has no benefit. Avoid prolonged exercise. Fair to guarded prognosis	Averill, 1980 Duncan and Griffiths, 1983 Hill et al., 1995 Shires et al., 1983

a Creatinuria (normal = 0.1–1.6 mg/ml).
b CK = creatine kinase (normal = 45–125 IU/dl).
EMG = electromyography; AST = aspartate aminotransferase; ALT = alanine aminotransferase; LDH = lactate dehydrogenase.

leptospirosis, the animal has a stiff gait and muscle pain.
  C. Histopathology shows mononuclear cell infiltration, hemorrhage, and necrosis of muscle fibers.
II. Congenital myopathy
III. Nutritional myodegeneration
IV. Polymyositis
V. *Dirofilaria immitis*
  One case of myositis of the hindlimb has been reported as a result of a tissue reaction to aberrant adult heartworm (Cooley et al., 1987).
VI. Hepatozoonosis

Treatment and Monitoring

I. Clindamycin 10–40 mg/kg/day PO divided TID or QID is given.
II. Trimethoprim/sulfadiazine 30 mg/kg PO BID and pyrimethamine 0.5–1 mg/kg/day PO for 14–28 days (dogs) or 0.5 mg/kg/day PO for 7–10 days (cats) is the recommended treatment for systemic toxoplasmosis and can be used instead of clindamycin.
III. Animals with acute systemic disease may respond well, but long-term prognosis is guarded because of other immunosuppressive diseases or concomitant CNS lesions.

Localized Infectious Myositis

Definition and Causes

I. Bacterial infection may cause local myositis after infection through wounds or spread from osteomyelitis.
  A. *Staphylococcus intermedius* and *Clostridium perfringens* are most common.
  B. Other bacteria include *Salmonella typhimurium*, *Streptococcus* sp., *Corynebacterium* sp., *Mycobacterium* sp., and other species of *Clostridium.*
II. Parasites of muscle are usually not pathogenic in dogs and cats.
  A. *Sarcocystis* spp. have been reported as a pathogen in debilitated or immunosuppressed animals.
  B. *Trichinella* may cause signs with a heavy infection.
  C. *Dirofilaria* spp. may aberrantly migrate to muscle.

Clinical Signs

I. Bacterial myositis
  A. Lameness and localized swelling
  B. Fever
  C. May disseminate systemically and cause death within 24 hours of the onset of clinical signs
II. Parasitic myositis
  A. Muscle pain
  B. Fever

Diagnosis

I. Bacteria are identified by tissue cultures.
II. Parasites may be identified on muscle biopsy.

Treatment and Monitoring

I. Local bacterial myositis
  A. Wounds may require surgical drainage and lavage.
  B. Antibiotics, selected on the basis of culture and sensitivity testing results, are administered for at least 5–7 days.
II. Local parasitic myositis
  A. Symptomatic; alleviation of pain
  B. Treatment for *Dirofilaria* spp.
    1. Debride and lavage wound.
    2. Administer broad-spectrum antibiotics for severe infections.
    3. Consider systemic treatment with adulticide for *D. immitis.*

IDIOPATHIC MYOPATHIES

Fibrotic Myopathy

Definition

I. Fibrotic myopathies are chronic, progressive disorders that result in severe muscle contracture and fibrosis.
II. Fibrotic myopathy has been reported in the semitendinosus, quadriceps, supraspinatus, infraspinatus, rectus femoris, and gracilis muscles in dogs.
III. It has also been reported in the semitendinosus muscle in a cat.

Causes and Pathophysiology

I. The cause is unknown.
II. Fibrotic myopathy may be the result of primary neuropathy or myopathy, frequent intramuscular injections, exercise-induced trauma, or chronic trauma with tearing and stretching of muscle fibers, or it may be congenital.
III. Muscle is replaced by dense collagenous connective tissue, resulting in a taut fibrous band.

Clinical Signs

I. A nonpainful, mechanical lameness develops.
II. The limb involved and the severity of the lameness depend on which muscle is involved and the extent of the fibrosis.
  A. With fibrotic myopathy of the semitendinosus muscle in the dog, there is external rotation of the hock and internal rotation of the stifle as the leg is advanced. The anterior stride is shortened, and the leg is pulled backward several inches before the foot contacts the ground.
  B. In the cat, there is an exaggerated flexion of hip, stifle, and hock as the leg is advanced, with an abruptly shortened anterior stride and limited abduction (Lewis, 1988).

Diagnosis

I. Physical examination
  A. A thin fibrous band can be palpated, which replaces the muscle belly.
  B. Neurologic exam is normal.
II. Histopathology of affected muscles
  A. Muscle fibers are replaced with dense collagenous connective tissue.
  B. There is minimal inflammation.
III. Electromyography (EMG)
  A. No activity is detected from the fibrous band.
  B. Bizarre high-frequency discharges may occur with incomplete replacement of muscle fibers.

Treatment and Monitoring

I. Surgery is not recommended unless the lameness is disabling.
II. The goal of surgery is to release the fibrous band.
  A. This may involve tenotomy, myotenotomy, Z-plasty, or complete excision of the fibrotic tissue.
  B. Surgery usually resolves the lameness and restores range of motion.
III. Prognosis is guarded because of the likely recurrence of fibrous band and lameness within 3–8 months.

Infraspinatus Muscle Contracture

Definition

I. Infraspinatus muscle contracture consists of fibrosis of the infraspinatus muscle.
II. It occurs primarily in hunting or working breeds of dogs.
III. It is usually unilateral but may be bilateral.

Causes and Pathophysiology

I. The cause is unknown but is thought to be a primary muscle disorder rather than a neuropathy.
II. It may be associated with trauma, either self-induced or external.
III. It is theorized that trauma to the shoulder causes incomplete rupture of the muscle, which results in progressive fibrosis and contracture over 2–4 weeks.

Clinical Signs

I. Initially, the dog has an acute onset of pain in the shoulder during or soon after exercise. The lameness gradually subsides, but never resolves.
II. Two to 4 weeks after the initial injury, a nonpainful, mechanical lameness of the foreleg develops. The gait is characterized by adduction of the elbow and abduction of the foreleg, with outward rotation of the antebrachium and carpus. The limb is laterally circumducted with each stride, and the foot flips forward.

Diagnosis

I. Signalment and history are usually consistent with those described earlier.

II. Palpation of the forelimb helps confirm the diagnosis.
  A. The humerus rotates outward when the elbow is flexed.
  B. Range of motion in the shoulder joint is limited.
  C. Disuse atrophy of the infraspinatus, supraspinatus, and spinous deltoid muscles is evidenced by a prominent scapular spine.
  D. If the limb is forcefully pronated, the proximal border of the scapula abducts from the thorax.

Treatment and Monitoring

I. Treatment consists of a tenotomy of the tendon of insertion of the infraspinatus muscle.
  A. It may be necessary to dissect the tendon free from the shoulder joint capsule.
  B. The forelimb is immediately more easily adducted, and shoulder range of motion is improved.
  C. Activity should be limited for 1–2 weeks.
II. Prognosis for a full recovery is excellent.

Myositis Ossificans

Definition

I. Myositis ossificans is the heterotopic formation of bone in muscle. The term is probably inaccurate, as there is usually minimal inflammation, and muscle is not always involved.
II. Generalized and localized forms have been described based on clinical behavior.
  A. Localized myositis ossificans
    1. It is characterized by heterotopic, non-neoplastic bone formation in one muscle or a group of muscles.
    2. It has been reported in both dogs and cats.
    3. It has been well described in Doberman pinschers and involves the muscles of the hip. Some authors hypothesized this to be a separate disease entity and named it von Willebrand heterotopic osteochondrofibrosis in Doberman pinschers (Dueland et al., 1990).
  B. Progressive or generalized myositis ossificans
    1. Also known as progressive ossifying fibrodysplasia or progressive or generalized ossifying myositis
    2. Characterized by the development of excessive fibrous connective tissue, which results in widespread muscle degeneration and ultimately leads to dystrophic calcification and ossification
    3. Has been reported in young to middle-aged cats

Causes and Pathophysiology

I. Cause unknown
II. Localized form
  A. It may be associated with trauma.
  B. Other proposed etiologies include infection, ossifying hematoma, and metaplasia of muscle and connective tissue to cartilage and bone.

C. In Doberman pinschers, it is speculated that the combination of bleeding tendencies associated with von Willebrand's disease and trauma results in microvascular bleeding, with subsequent fibrosis or mineralization.

III. Progressive form
 A. Thought to be congenital and hereditary
 B. May be a defect of fibroblasts in collagenous connective tissue with secondary degeneration of muscle, rather than a primary muscular lesion

Clinical Signs

 I. Localized ossifying myositis
  A. Palpable firm enlargement in affected muscle
  B. Chronic lameness with muscle atrophy
  C. Pain after exercise
  D. In Doberman pinschers: hindlimb lameness associated with a caudal hip mass that limits extension
 II. Progresive ossifying fibrodysplasia
  A. Young to middle-aged cat
  B. Firm nodules anywhere on the body, but predominantly on the neck and back
  C. Mild gait stiffness progressing to difficulty walking
  D. Stiffness usually worse in hindlegs
  E. Proximal limb musculature enlarged and firm
  F. Painful when being handled or when walking
  G. Limited range of motion in the proximal leg joints
  H. May be severely disabled within 2 weeks to several months

Diagnosis

 I. Localized ossifying myositis
  A. Signalment, history, and clinical signs
  B. Radiography
   1. Soft tissue mineralization within 3–6 weeks of injury
   2. Mature bone in soft tissue after 2–6 months
   3. Parosteal or extraosseous mineralization
   4. Possible central radiolucent area in calcified mass
   5. ± Periosteal reaction
  C. Histopathology of lesion
   1. Zone phenomena occur, with progression of bone maturation centrally to peripherally.
    a) Central zone contains undifferentiated cells and fibroblasts and may resemble a sarcoma.
    b) Intermediate zone contains osteoid and some areas of immature bone.
    c) Peripheral zone contains mature bone and may exhibit resorption and remodeling.
   2. It does not invade surrounding soft tissue.
  D. Evaluation for coagulopathies
   1. Buccal mucosal bleeding time
   2. Von Willebrand's factor
   3. Thyroid function tests
 II. Progressive ossifying fibrodysplasia

A. Suspicious clinical signs are highly suggestive.
B. Radiographs show multiple mineralized densities within the affected musculature.
C. Serum creatine kinase may be elevated.
D. Histopathology of affected muscle reveals the following.
 1. Excessive connective tissue between muscle fibers
 2. Mononuclear infiltration and muscle atrophy
 3. Hyaline degeneration

Differential Diagnosis

 I. Localized ossifying myositis
  A. Dystrophic calcification or calcinosis circumscripta
  B. Callus formation secondary to bone healing
  C. Osteomyelitis
  D. Traumatic subperiosteal ossification
  E. Neoplasia of the bone or joint
  F. Mineralized or ossified soft tissue tumor
 II. Progressive ossifying fibrodysplasia
   Localized ossifying myositis

Treatment and Monitoring

 I. Localized ossifying myositis
  A. No treatment indicated if clinical signs are minimal
   1. Lesions sometimes regress or resorb in humans (Bone and McGavin, 1985).
   2. Rest, compression bandages, and aspirin may help relieve acute pain.
  B. Surgical excision of mineralized region
   1. Surgery is indicated to alleviate discomfort, restore normal limb function, or obtain a definitive diagnosis.
   2. In humans, if excision is performed within 6 months (when the lesion is immature), there is a high rate of recurrence.
   3. Postoperative physical therapy is important.
   4. Indomethacin or salicylates for 3–6 weeks postoperatively can inhibit ectopic bone formation, but beware of bleeding tendencies caused by these drugs.
 II. Progressive ossifying fibrodysplasia
  A. There is no effective treatment.
  B. Corticosteroids may help temporarily but will not prevent ectopic bone formation.
  C. Diphosphonate and dietary changes have been unsuccessful in preventing disease progression.

METABOLIC MYOPATHIES

Feline Hypokalemic Polymyopathy

Definition

 I. Feline hypokalemic polymyopathy is a manifestation of chronic potassium depletion, which usually presents as an acute onset of weakness.

II. It is thought to be one of the most common causes of generalized muscle weakness in cats.

III. A similar syndrome has been reported as a heritable disease of Burmese cats, which may be more sensitive to the effects of low potassium or may be afflicted with a variant of the syndrome.

Causes

I. The cause of the hypokalemia is unclear. It is thought to be a total body depletion of potassium rather than a redistribution between the intracellular and extracellular compartments.

II. A combination of low dietary intake of potassium and increased urinary potassium loss over a period of months may lead to depletion of body stores.

Pathophysiology

I. Hypokalemia may directly affect the muscle cell membrane.
   A. Extracellular potassium drops more rapidly than the intracellular concentration, inducing muscle cell membrane hyperpolarization.
   B. It is hypothesized that the sarcolemma then becomes more permeable to sodium, triggering hypopolarization.
   C. Hypopolarization of the muscle cell causes muscle weakness.

II. Hypokalemia may affect muscle blood flow. After potassium depletion, the normal increase in muscle blood flow in response to exercise is attenuated, which can lead to ischemic necrosis.

Clinical Signs

I. Acute onset of generalized weakness
II. Persistent ventroflexion of the neck
III. Reluctance to walk
IV. Stiff gait
V. Muscular pain when handled or palpated
VI. Muscle atrophy
VII. Anorexia, weight loss
VIII. Respiratory paralysis in severe cases

Diagnosis

I. Presence of typical clinical signs; neurologic exam normal
II. Serum chemistries
   A. Low potassium (<3.5 mEq/L)
   B. Elevated creatine kinase (500–10,000 IU/L)
   C. Elevated creatinine (2.5–5 mg/dl)
   D. Low-normal serum bicarbonate, indicating mild to moderate metabolic acidosis
III. Urinalysis
   A. Low specific gravity
   B. Increased fractional urinary excretion of potassium (normal = 4.7–14.3%)
IV. EMG abnormalities found in multiple muscle groups
   A. Frequent positive sharp waves
   B. Fibrillation potentials
   C. Occasional bizarre high-frequency discharges
   D. Normal nerve conduction velocities
V. Histopathology usually normal
   A. Mild myofiber necrosis and macrophage infiltration may be seen.
   B. Relative absence of inflammation is striking.
VI. Favorable response to potassium treatment

Differential Diagnosis

I. Polymyositis
II. Neuromuscular junction diseases
   A. Myasthenia gravis
   B. Organophosphate toxicosis
   C. Spider bite
III. Polyneuropathies
   A. Long-standing diabetes mellitus
   B. Prolonged treatment with vincristine
   C. Polyradiculoneuritis
IV. Electrolyte-induced muscle dysfunction
V. Ethylene glycol toxicosis
VI. Severe anemia
VII. Sepsis
VIII. Thiamine deficiency
IX. Thyrotoxicosis

Treatment

I. Potassium supplementation is instituted.
   A. Oral administration of potassium is the safest treatment and may be given as potassium-containing elixirs or potassium salts (KCl, $KHCO_3$).
      1. KCl has an objectionable taste and may potentiate any metabolic acidosis.
      2. Potassium gluconate elixir is more palatable and nonacidifying.
      3. Potassium gluconate powder is available for long-term supplementation.
      4. Oral dose is 5–8 mEq of potassium per day in two divided doses for cats with significant hypokalemia (<3 mEq/L).
   B. Parenteral KCl may be diluted in a balanced electrolyte solution such as lactated Ringer's solution (LRS) in cats with profound hypokalemia.
      1. High concentrations of KCl in LRS may be given as a constant IV infusion at rates of 0.4 mEq/kg/h in severely hypokalemic cats.
      2. IV fluid administration tends to lower serum potassium initially and can precipitate respiratory paralysis. This can occur even with fluids containing high concentrations of KCl.
II. Dopamine infusion can be used instead of parenteral potassium in a life-threatening situation.
   A. Dopamine at 0.5 μg/kg/minute IV can induce a transient increase in serum potassium by redistributing potassium from the intracellular to the extracellular compartment.
   B. Concurrent oral potassium must be started immediately.
III. Restrict activity.

Patient Monitoring

I. Oral potassium supplementation
   A. Monitor serum potassium daily until it is in the normal range (usually 1–3 days).
   B. Then monitor serum potassium weekly and adjust the dosage to maintain the concentration within the normal range.
   C. Most cats can be maintained on 2–4 mEq of potassium per day. In some cats with no renal dysfunction, feeding a diet with adequate potassium ($>0.6\%$) may be sufficient.
   D. Periodically monitor serum potassium to help prevent recurrence.
II. Parenteral KCl
   A. Monitor for phlebitis.
   B. Monitor the electrocardiogram (ECG) continuously for lethal arrhythmias.
   C. Monitor serum potassium every 3–6 hours, and slow the infusion once the potassium concentration reaches 3.5 mEq/L.
III. Prognosis
   A. Prognosis is excellent if the condition is diagnosed and treated early.
   B. Initial fluid administration, even when supplemented with potassium, may decrease serum potassium concentrations and precipitate complete paralysis.

Nutritional Myodegeneration

Definition

I. Nutritional myodegeneration is a generalized muscle weakness associated with low dietary levels of selenium, vitamin E, or both.
II. It is also known as white muscle disease, nutritional myopathy, and selenium-responsive myopathy.
III. It is very uncommon because commercially available diets are well balanced.

Causes

It may be seen in an animal that has been fed an unusual diet for a prolonged period, such as diets containing large amounts of unsaturated fats.

Pathophysiology

I. Vitamin E is a protective antioxidative agent for unsaturated fatty acids.
II. In the absence of vitamin E, the quantity of unsaturated fatty acids diminishes, which results in destabilization of lysosomes.
III. Continuous rupture of lysosomes leads to autodigestion of muscle.

Clinical Signs

I. Gait abnormalities
   A. Generalized weakness
   B. Stiff or stilted gait
   C. Difficulty rising from recumbent position
   D. Signs sometimes exacerbated with exercise
   E. Swollen, hot, painful muscles
II. Dysphagia
III. Sialosis
IV. Sudden death in newborn puppies

Diagnosis

I. History of an unusual diet consumed by the animal or by the dam of a newborn
II. Elevated serum muscle enzymes
III. EMG: abnormal electrical activity at rest
   A. Myopathic potentials
   B. Positive waves
   C. Fibrillation potentials
   D. Bizarre high-frequency discharges
IV. Gross pathology
   A. Skeletal muscle lesions are bilaterally symmetrical and affect individual muscles or muscle groups.
   B. The muscle is pale, with chalky longitudinal striations.
V. Histopathologic findings of muscle at necropsy
   A. Widespread myonecrosis
   B. Phagocytosis
   C. Intense granular calcification of fibers
   D. Proliferation of hypertrophic sarcoplasmic nuclei
   E. Reactive histiocytes and macrophages filling the interstitial spaces
   F. Loss of myofiber striations
   G. Fiber regeneration

Differential Diagnosis

I. Infectious myopathy
II. Congenital myopathy
III. Swimmer puppy syndrome

Treatment and Monitoring

I. Selenium and vitamin E replacement therapy
   A. Give vitamin E 100–400 IU PO BID until clinically normal.
   B. Institute diet containing adequate levels of selenium.
II. Possibly dramatic response to therapy if diagnosis is made early
III. Prognosis usually grave owing to involvement of cardiac, diaphragmatic, and intercostal muscles

Malignant Hyperthermia

Definition

I. Malignant hyperthermia is a hypermetabolic disorder of skeletal muscle.
II. It is characterized by the peracute development of skeletal muscle hypercatabolism and contracture.

Causes

I. It can be a response to certain inhalant anesthetics.
   A. Usually associated with halothane, but other anesthetics have also been implicated

B. May not be associated with the first exposure to the agent

II. It may also be associated with other drugs, such as succinylcholine and lidocaine.

III. It is thought to be inherited, with a polygenic mode of transmission.

IV. It may be induced by stress alone.

V. It is more common in male dogs and in heavily muscled breeds.

VI. Fever or high ambient temperature may also increase the risk.

Pathophysiology

I. Malignant hyperthermia is believed to be related to abnormal regulation of myoplasmic calcium, which leads to overstimulation of glycogenolysis and contractile protein activity.

II. This results in depletion of glycogen stores, hypoxia, heat production, and accumulation of CO_2 and lactic acid.

Clinical Signs

I. Insidious
   A. Tachycardia
   B. Tachypnea or hyperpnea
   C. Pyrexia

II. Fulminant
   A. Severe muscle rigidity: generalized or limited to the masseter muscles
   B. Heart failure
   C. Renal failure
   D. Pulmonary edema
   E. Disseminated intravascular coagulation
   F. Respiratory and cardiac arrest

Diagnosis

I. Characteristic clinical signs when the animal is anesthetized (between 30 minutes and 5 hours after exposure)

II. Extreme generalized muscle rigidity immediately after death

III. Gross pathology: muscles pale, soft, and exudative

IV. Histopathology of muscles
   A. Variable fiber size
   B. Fiber hypertrophy
   C. Increased number of internal nuclei in muscle cells

V. In vitro muscle contracture tests: done on viable muscle as a screening test for animals suspected to be susceptible (Kirmayer et al., 1984)

Differential Diagnosis

I. Exertional myopathy

II. Heat prostration

Treatment

I. Remove the triggering agent.
   A. Stop anesthesia and change the breathing circuit.
   B. Hyperventilate with 100% oxygen.

II. Begin symptomatic therapy.
   A. Chilled IV fluids: isotonic saline at 90 ml/kg/h IV
   B. Sodium bicarbonate based on blood gas analysis
   C. Total body cooling with ice packs
   D. Corticosteroids controversial but probably will not harm the animal

III. Dantrolene sodium may be administered once at 2–5 mg/kg IV.
   A. It is a skeletal muscle relaxant that may prevent the increase in myoplasmic calcium content.
   B. In humans, dantrolene is continued orally for 72 hours, but the appropriate dosage in dogs has not been documented.

Patient Monitoring

I. Measure urine output, especially if myoglobinuria develops.

II. Monitor serum potassium, because it may be elevated initially and decreased later in the syndrome.

III. Monitor the ECG for arrhythmias. Treat tachyarrhythmias with procainamide rather than lidocaine, because lidocaine may worsen the condition.

IV. Prognosis is poor, especially with the fulminant form.

Exertional Myopathy

Definition

I. Exertional myopathy is a syndrome of muscle damage caused by strenuous exercise.

II. It occurs most commonly in racing greyhounds and working dogs.

III. It is also known as exertional rhabdomyolysis, Monday morning disease, tying-up, azoturia, and paralytic myoglobinuria.

Causes

I. Acute muscle ischemia precipitated by the following
   A. Lack of fitness
   B. Excessive frequency of work
   C. Heat stress
   D. Excessive excitement

II. Also reported secondary to prolonged seizures

Pathophysiology

It is believed that local muscle ischemia and lactic acidosis cause lysis of muscle walls and resultant myoglobin release, which may result in nephropathy.

Clinical Signs

I. Mild cases: generalized muscle pain and swelling for 24–72 hours after a race

II. Severe cases
   A. Muscle swelling and pain, especially over the back and hindquarters
   B. Stiffness that is worse in hindlegs
   C. Hyperpnea
   D. Extreme distress
   E. Acute collapse

F. Severe myoglobinemia, leading to nephropathy, acute renal failure, and death within 48 hours

Diagnosis

I. Signalment, history, and clinical signs cause a high level of suspicion.
II. Urine produced during or shortly after exercise contains myoglobin.
III. Serum potassium and phosphorus may be elevated, depending on the extent of muscle and renal damage.
IV. Muscle enzymes become elevated.
V. Histopathology of muscle at necropsy reveals multifocal hemorrhage and myonecrosis.

Differential Diagnosis

I. Heat prostration
II. Malignant hyperthermia

Treatment and Monitoring

I. Supportive care includes the following.
  A. IV fluids to aid renal excretion of myoglobin, prevent acute renal failure, and combat shock
  B. Bicarbonate (if indicated by blood gases) to combat muscle acidosis and prevent precipitation of myoglobin in renal tubules
  C. Cooling of the body with tepid water baths
  D. Rest and massage of the muscles
  E. Muscle relaxants such as diazepam 0.5 mg/kg IV to effect
II. Monitor renal function and urine output.
III. Prognosis depends on severity of signs at presentation.

Polymyopathy Associated with Canine Hyperadrenocorticism

See Chap. 44.

IMMUNE-MEDIATED MYOPATHIES

Canine Polymyositis

Definition

I. Polymyositis is a generalized noninfectious disease that can affect any muscle group.
II. It can present as either an acute or a chronic problem.
III. It usually occurs in adult dogs with no gender predilection.

Causes

I. Usually, no underlying cause is identified.
II. It is thought to be a manifestation of an immune-mediated myositis.
III. It has been associated with systemic lupus erythematosus (Krum et al., 1977), myasthenia gravis, and thymoma.

Clinical Signs

I. May be chronic and progressive or episodic with acute attacks
II. General signs
  A. Depression, lethargy
  B. Fever
  C. Anorexia and weight loss
III. Gait abnormalities
  A. Weakness
  B. Rapid onset of fatigue; improvement with rest
  C. Stiffness
  D. Shifting lameness
IV. Muscular changes
  A. Myalgia
  B. Muscles either swollen or atrophied
V. Abnormalities of deglutition
  A. Dysphagia
  B. Muscles of mastication: swollen or atrophied
  C. Megaesophagus: regurgitation, aspiration pneumonia
VI. Dysphonia

Diagnosis

I. Physical examination is consistent with clinical signs listed earlier.
  A. Vague signs of weakness and muscle pain should create suspicion.
  B. Neurologic exam is normal.
II. Muscle enzymes such as creatine kinase may be elevated, but findings are inconsistent and not diagnostic.
III. EMG demonstrates generalized spontaneous electrical activity in many muscles, including those of mastication.
  A. Positive sharp waves
  B. Fibrillation potentials
  C. Polyphasic motor unit potentials
  D. Motor unit potentials of decreased duration
  E. Complex repetitive discharges
  F. Increased insertional activity
  G. Bizarre high-frequency discharges
IV. Muscle biopsy can confirm the diagnosis.
  A. Biopsy of a muscle group that is abnormal on EMG
    1. Since the disease is usually symmetrical, perform EMGs on one side and get the biopsy from the other side to avoid needle artifacts.
    2. If EMG is not available, biopsy a swollen or painful muscle.
  B. Histopathologic changes
    1. Focal, multifocal, or diffuse myonecrosis
    2. Phagocytosis
    3. Lymphoplasmacytic cellular infiltrates
    4. Fiber size variation
    5. Areas of fiber regeneration
V. Ancillary tests include the following.
  A. Radiographs may be helpful to screen for megaesophagus or pneumonia.
  B. Lupus erythematosus cell preparation and antinu-

clear antibody titer may be positive in dogs with concomitant systemic lupus erythematosus.
C. Serum titers may be performed to rule out leptospirosis and toxoplasmosis.

Differential Diagnosis

I. Polymyositis associated with other immune-mediated disorders
   A. Polyarthritis
   B. Polyarteritis
   C. Lupus erythematosus
   D. Dermatomyositis
   E. Myasthenia gravis
II. Polyneuropathy
III. Acute episodes: may resemble meningitis, peritonitis, or skeletal diseases
IV. Infectious myopathy
V. Masticatory myositis

Treatment

I. Corticosteroids are the treatment of choice.
   A. Administer immunosuppressive doses of prednisone at 1–2 mg/kg PO BID for 3–4 weeks.
   B. Taper the dose over 2–3 months, watching for recurrence of signs.
   C. Maintain on low-dose alternate-day therapy, if possible.
II. Other immunosuppressive agents may be added if the response to prednisone is poor or to allow a decrease in the dosage of prednisone.
   A. Azathioprine 2 mg/kg PO SID (dogs)
   B. Cyclophosphamide 1–2 mg/kg PO SID for 4 days on, 3 days off for up to 3 weeks

Patient Monitoring

I. Clinical signs should improve within the first 3 days of therapy.
II. Serial evaluations of muscle enzymes may be useful, if they were initially elevated.
III. If clinical signs or elevated muscle enzymes recur at any point during therapy, increase the prednisone to the previous dose and do not attempt further reductions for several weeks.
IV. Complete withdrawal of medications must be monitored carefully and may not be possible.
V. Relapses are not uncommon.
VI. Prognosis is favorable, provided megaesophagus and aspiration pneumonia do not develop.

Masticatory Myopathy

Definition

I. Masticatory myopathy or masticatory myositis is an acute or chronic myopathy that affects the muscles of mastication, primarily the temporal and masseter muscles.
II. It usually affects large-breed dogs, with no age or gender predilection.
III. It has also been described as eosinophilic myositis or atrophic masticatory myositis, but these are thought to be variants or stages of the same disease.

Causes

I. The actual cause is unknown.
II. It is thought to be an immune-mediated disease.
   A. Autoantibodies have been demonstrated that are specifically directed against fiber proteins found in the masticatory muscles.
   B. The masticatory muscles are antigenically different from other skeletal muscle.
   C. It generally responds to immunosuppressive doses of corticosteroids.
   D. It can occur simultaneously with other immune-mediated disorders.

Clinical Signs

I. Acute onset of swelling of the masticatory muscles
   A. Usually symmetrical, but may be asymmetrical
   B. Pain on opening the mouth or passive manipulation of the jaw
   C. Trismus (difficulty opening the mouth)
   D. Reluctance to chew: anorexia, weight loss
   E. Exophthalmos, which can cause blindness by compressing or stretching the optic nerve
   F. Possible enlargement of tonsils and mandibular lymph nodes
   G. ± Fever
   H. Acute signs lasting 2–3 weeks, peaking within 10–14 days
   I. Recurrent episodes
II. Progressive contracture and atrophy of the masticatory muscles herald the chronic stage of masticatory myopathy, which can occur without evidence of a preceding acute phase.
   A. Trismus: mouth cannot be opened, even under general anesthesia
   B. Atrophy of temporal and masseter muscles
   C. Enophthalmos

Diagnosis

I. Clinical signs of swelling or atrophy of masticatory muscles
II. Hemogram
   A. Usually normal
   B. Eosinophilia present occasionally
III. Serum chemistry
   A. Globulin levels may be elevated.
   B. Muscle enzymes may be normal or slightly elevated.
IV. EMG: spontaneous electrical activity in the masticatory muscles only
   A. Positive sharp waves
   B. Fibrillation potentials
   C. Polyphasic motor unit potentials
   D. Bizarre high-frequency discharges
   E. Electrical silence in areas of fibrosis
V. Muscle biopsy
   A. Biopsy is often diagnostic, although the affected area may be missed with a single biopsy.

B. Usually the temporalis muscle is biopsied.
C. Histopathologic changes can include the following.
  1. Lymphoplasmacytic cellular infiltrates with eosinophils seen less frequently
  2. Loss of muscle fibers and muscle fiber atrophy
  3. Increase in connective tissue and fibrosis
  4. No pathologic abnormalities
VI. Ancillary tests
  A. Radiographs may be helpful to rule out temporomandibular joint disease.
  B. Antinuclear antibody titer is usually negative but may help evaluate concurrent disease.
  C. Assays to demonstrate circulating serum autoantibodies against type 2M fiber proteins or immune complexes on muscle prepared by frozen section may be useful, but their diagnostic value has not been established.

Differential Diagnosis

I. Polymyositis
II. Infectious myopathy
III. Dermatomyositis
IV. Trigeminal neuropathy
V. Temporomandibular joint disease
VI. Retrobulbar abscess

Treatment

I. Spontaneous regression has been observed.
II. Corticosteroids are the treatment of choice.
  A. Administer immunosuppressive doses of prednisone at 1–2 mg/kg PO BID for 3–4 weeks.
  B. Taper the dose over 2–3 months, watching for recurrence of signs.
  C. Maintain on low-dose alternate-day therapy, if possible.
III. Other immunosuppressive agents (e.g., azathioprine 2 mg/kg PO SID [dogs]) may be added if the response to prednisone is poor or to allow a decrease in the dosage of prednisone.
IV. Long-term medication may be needed to maintain remission.

Patient Monitoring

I. Monitor response to therapy by the ability to open the jaw.
II. Serial evaluations of muscle enzymes may be useful, if they were initially elevated.
III. If clinical signs or elevated muscle enzymes recur at any point during therapy, increase the prednisone to the previous dose and do not attempt further reductions for another 2–4 weeks.
IV. Complete withdrawal of medications should be monitored carefully and may not be possible.
V. Relapses are common.
VI. Prognosis is favorable if the disease is treated early.
  A. In cases with muscle atrophy, the clinical response may be slow, with long term, low-dose therapy being required.
  B. If severe trismus is present, the prognosis may be more guarded, but corticosteroids may help even with fibrosis.

NEOPLASIA

Definition and Causes

I. Primary tumors originating from the skeletal muscle
  A. Rhabdomyoma (benign)
  B. Rhabdomyosarcoma (malignant)
II. Secondary tumors within the muscle that represent metastatic spread from tumors originating elsewhere
  A. Lymphosarcoma
  B. Adenocarcinomas of mammary, renal, and thyroid origin
  C. Hemangiosarcoma
  D. Malignant melanoma
III. Local invasion of tumors into the muscle from rapidly expanding cutaneous or bone tumors (Easton, 1994; Cook et al., 1995)
  A. Fibrosarcoma
  B. Osteosarcoma
  C. Mast cell tumor
  D. Hemangiopericytoma

Clinical Signs

I. The age of onset is variable.
  A. Primary muscle tumors can occur in young or old animals.
  B. Secondary muscle tumors usually occur in middle-aged animals.
II. Clinical signs depend on the muscle group affected.
III. Firm, nonpainful swelling, distortion of the area, and lameness are common.
IV. Common sites of primary neoplasia include the muscles of the head, appendicular skeleton, and heart.

Diagnosis

I. Diagnosis is confirmed by biopsy and histopathologic assessment.
II. Staging the disease with lymph node biopsy and thoracic radiographs is important.

Treatment and Monitoring

I. For primary neoplasia, surgical excision is preferred but may be ineffectual if the neoplasm is difficult to reach or invasive. Amputation of a limb may be indicated to attain adequate surgical margins.
II. For secondary neoplasia, treatment depends on the therapy indicated for the primary tumor.
III. Prognosis is generally poor in the presence of metastatic disease or inadequate surgical excision.
IV. Prognosis may be improved if the tumor is localized, easily excised, or benign.

MUSCLE AND TENDON TRAUMA

See Table 80–2.

Text continued on page 864

Table 80–2. *Traumatic Muscle Injuries*

Injury	Causes and Pathophysiology	Clinical Signs	Diagnosis	Treatment and Prognosis	References
Forelimb					
Rupture of the serratus ventralis	Acute trauma, although also presented as chronic injury Reported in the dog and cat	Upward displacement of the scapula with forelimb lameness Usually unilateral	History and clinical signs	Acute injuries treated conservatively with a shoulder sling or other non-weight bearing bandage for 3–4 wk Chronic injuries may require surgical repair of the muscle or fixation of the scapula to the ribs using wire. Very good prognosis	Bloomberg, 1995 Hoerlein et al., 1960
Disruption of the tendon of origin of the biceps brachii	Avulsion: acute trauma Avulsion of tendon of origin from the supraglenoid tubercle in young large-breed dogs (4–8 mo of age) Displacement: repetitive injury Medial displacement of the tendon of origin from the intertubercular groove in the racing greyhound; also reported in miniature poodle and border collie	Weight-bearing lameness (acute for avulsion; chronic for displacement) and pain on flexion and extension of the shoulder	Clinical signs and radiographs Avulsion: avulsed segment of bone (supraglenoid tubercle) may be present on radiographs Displacement: palpation of medial displacement of the tendon during flexion of the shoulder or during extension of the elbow with the shoulder held in partial flexion	Avulsion: surgical reattachment of the tendon (pin and tension band or screw) associated with a good prognosis Displacement in athletic animals: surgical reconstruction of the intertubercular ligament using screws and figure-of-eight suture across the tendon as it sits in the groove Displacement in sedentary animals: rest and administration of anti-inflammatory drugs may be successful Displacement with surgical stabilization has a good prognosis for return to function and fair prognosis for return to racing.	Goring et al., 1984
Tenosynovitis of the biceps brachii tendon	Unknown, but likely secondary to trauma, overuse, and repetitive injury Middle-aged or older medium- and large-breed dogs No breed or sex predilection	Usually unilateral, but may be bilateral Intermittent, chronic, or progressive weight-bearing forelimb lameness that worsens after exercise and improves with rest Resistance to flexion and extension of the shoulder	History, clinical signs, and physical exam findings Acute pain elicited when pressure is applied directly to the bicipital tendon during flexion and extension of the shoulder Atrophy of the infraspinatus and supraspinatus muscles Radiographs (including craniodistal-cranioproximal flexed view) may identify dystrophic calcification of the tendon, osteophytes in the intertubercular groove, or a mineralized joint mouse within the tendon sheath.	Acute cases: nonsteroidal anti-inflammatory medication (aspirin) with limited activity for 4–6 wk Severe or chronic cases: intra-synovial injection of 10–40 mg methylprednisolone acetate no more than every 2 wk; do not exceed 2 injections; rest for at least 2 wk after injection Surgery indicated for refractory cases (dogs that do not improve after 1 or 2 injections of corticosteroids), or for removal of joint mice if identified Prognosis for return to function is generally good.	Muir et al., 1992

Condition	Etiology / Description	Clinical signs	Diagnosis	Treatment / Prognosis	References
			Contrast arthrography may demonstrate filling defects along the tendon, adhesions between the tendon sheath and tendon, or joint mice. No radiographic changes may be apparent in acute cases. Cytology of synovial fluid consistent with degenerative joint disease, but may be normal Diagnosis confirmed by exploratory arthrotomy and microscopic examination of biopsied tissue		
Rupture of the origin of the long head of the triceps	Typically racing greyhounds Avulsion of the origin from the posterior edge of the scapula	A hollow depressed area posterior and distal to the scapula	Based on history and clinical signs	Conservative management with rest may be sufficient. Surgical reattachment of the muscle to the caudal scapula may be required. Prognosis for return to racing is fair; same level of racing may not be attained owing to decreased range of motion of the shoulder.	Anson and Betts, 1989 Davies and Clayton-Jones, 1982 Gilmore, 1984
Avulsion of the triceps tendon	Associated with trauma, local corticosteroid injection, or spontaneous avulsion Detachment of the triceps tendon occurs from its point of insertion on the olecranon. Immature animals may have avulsion of the proximal epiphysis of the olecranon.	Acute injury or chronic lameness Acute non-weight-bearing lameness with pain and reduced range of motion on flexion and extension of the elbow Chronic disruption associated with thickening and fibrosis over olecranon, muscle atrophy of affected forelimb	Based on clinical signs and radiographs Avulsed fragment of bone proximal to the olecranon may be seen on radiographs.	Surgical repair of tendon using tension-relieving tendon sutures or reattachment of the olecranon epiphysis using a pin and tension band or screw is indicated. Coaptation of the limb for 2 wk with physiotherapy and restricted exercise advised for a further 3–4 wk Prognosis after acute injury is good, but joint motion may be restricted. Prognosis after chronic injury is fair.	
Injury of the flexor carpi ulnaris	Chronic, repetitive injury in racing greyhounds Transverse tears may occur through the tendon of the humeral head. The insertion of the ulnar head and a bony fragment may avulse from the accessory carpal bone ("bowed tendon").	Poor performance Mild lameness After repeated injury, swelling and bruising are observed over the accessory carpal bone.	Based on history and clinical signs	Transverse tears and avulsions should be surgically repaired. Postoperative coaptation is required. Prognosis for return to racing after transverse tears of the humeral head is good. Prognosis for avulsion of the ulnar head is poor.	

Table continued on following page

Table 80–2. **Traumatic Muscle Injuries** *(Continued)*

Injury	Causes and Pathophysiology	Clinical Signs	Diagnosis	Treatment and Prognosis	References
Injury to the digital flexor and extensor tendons	Lacerations above or below the metacarpal and metatarsal pads. Digital extensor tendon injury is less critical owing to the many anastomoses of the tendon after they branch from the main tendon.	Laceration may be accompanied by profuse hemorrhage. Postural changes: superficial digital flexor injury alone may result in little change; deep digital flexor tendon injury results in flattening of one or more digits. Chronic injury may result in excoriation of the metacarpal or metatarsal pads owing to prolonged postural changes.	Based on clinical signs and surgical exploration of the laceration site. Pressure, using the palm of the hand, on the bottom of the pads may allow detection of any postural change in the digits.	Surgical repair is required if there are postural changes; coaptation is indicated if there are no postural changes. Prognosis for acute injuries is good. Prognosis for chronic injuries is poor owing to fibrosis and the inability to anastomose tendon if there are extensive deficits.	
Hindlimb					
Injury to the tensor fascia lata	Injury of racing greyhounds Tearing of the musculotendinous junction Most often the left rear leg of dogs racing in the United States	Weight-bearing lameness Palpable and visible depression in the proximal cranial area of the thigh	Based on clinical signs and palpation of thigh depression	Surgical repair is indicated. Prognosis for return to racing after primary repair is good.	Dee, 1989
Rupture of the gracilis muscle	Injury of the racing greyhound, but also seen in working dogs Exact cause is unknown; sudden exercise in an unfit animal may predispose to injury. Substantial hemorrhage can occur. Unilateral injury is more common.	Ventral displacement of the origin (or dorsal displacement of the insertion) is observed and palpated on the inside of the thigh. Significant bruising over the inside of the thigh Hindlimb lameness and difficulty rising, particularly 12–24 h after the injury	Based on clinical signs and palpation of the muscle avulsion	Surgical repair or reattachment of the avulsed tendon to the bone may be indicated if return to racing is desired. Prognosis for return to racing is fair. Fibrosis at the surgical site may restrict motion.	Eaton-Wells, 1992

| Quadriceps contracture | Associated with inadequate fracture repair, osteomyelitis, severe trauma, or overzealous tissue handling
Adhesions form between the quadriceps muscle and the femur.
Usually occurs in young animals
Prolonged immobilization of the hindleg in extension or failure to bear weight soon after internal fixation may also be factors.
Also reported as a congenital disorder and in association with toxoplasmosis
Disuse osteoporosis, irreversible degenerative joint disease of the stifle, and growth disturbances can occur (hip luxation, bone hypoplasia, increased femoral torsion, medial patellar luxation, and limb shortening). | Hindleg held with the stifle and hock stiff in extension
May be non-weight-bearing or use the leg as a peg leg
The affected leg is held cranial with respect to the other hindlimb.
Later clinical signs, if left untreated, include atrophy of the thigh muscles, bending of the stifle caudally in genu recurvatum with the hock extended, proximal positioning or medial luxation of the patella, and subluxation of the hip. | Based on history and clinical signs
In chronic cases, radiographs may reveal changes consistent with degenerative joint disease of the stifle, hip luxation, or disuse osteoporosis of the long bones. | Surgery is indicated to attempt to restore stifle joint mobility; adhesions between the quadriceps muscles and the femur are broken down and the stifle is flexed carefully to release any remaining fibrous tissue (excessive force could result in a Salter fracture of the distal femur or proximal tibia).
Sliding myoplasty or Z-myoplasty of the quadriceps may be indicated.
Postoperative maintenance of stifle flexion using a 90-90 flexion sling, a Robinson sling, or an external pin splint for 4-5 days is indicated.
Physical therapy is also required.
Results are unpredictable; surgery may result in 50-75% restoration of limb use.
If surgery is unsuccessful or there is advanced osteoarthritis of the stifle joint, stifle arthrodesis or amputation may be required.
Prevention of this condition is preferable; femoral fracture repair in young animals should be stable and allow early return to function.
Animals exhibiting signs of hyperextension following femoral fracture repair should have a flexion sling or external pin splint applied. | Bardet and Hohn, 1984
Drake and Hime, 1967
Stead et al., 1977 |

Table continued on following page

Table 80–2. Traumatic Muscle Injuries (Continued)

Injury	Causes and Pathophysiology	Clinical Signs	Diagnosis	Treatment and Prognosis	References
Disruption of the tendon of origin of the long digital extensor	Traumatic avulsion of the tendon of origin occurs in immature, large-breed dogs. Displacement of the tendon occurs in young dogs.	Avulsion causes mild weight-bearing lameness and pain on manipulation of the affected stifle. Lateral soft tissue swelling may be present. Displacement causes chronic, mild weight-bearing lameness.	Based on clinical signs and radiographs. Radiographs may show avulsed bone and cartilage near the extensor fossa of the lateral femoral condyle, best observed on the lateral projection. In a very young dog, the portion of bone may consist primarily of cartilage and not be visible on the radiograph. Diagnosis is confirmed by exploratory arthrotomy. Displacement can be palpated during extension and flexion of the stifle, which allows detection of the tendon moving in and out of the muscular groove.	Surgical reattachment of the avulsed segment using bone screws is the treatment of choice. Prognosis for return to function after acute injuries is good to excellent. For displacement, surgical stabilization of the tendon by reconstruction of the supporting retinacular tissue, use of a staple to make a roof over the tendon, or tenotomy and transplantation of the tendon to the craniolateral aspect of the proximal tibia (as a last resort) is indicated. Prognosis after surgery for displacement is variable.	
Avulsion of the lateral or medial head of the gastrocnemius muscle	Trauma Reported in the fox terrier, German shepherd dog, and Labrador retriever	Weight-bearing lameness and soft-tissue swelling over the caudal aspect of the stifle are apparent. Hyperflexion of the stifle and hock is present.	Based on clinical signs and radiographs revealing caudal and distal displacement of the fabella	Surgical reattachment of the tendon is indicated. Prognosis for acute injuries is good.	
Avulsion of the tendon of the popliteal muscle	Trauma	Weight-bearing lameness and soft tissue swelling over the lateral aspect of the stifle	Based on clinical signs and radiographs, which reveal displacement of the popliteal sesamoid bone and possibly a bony fragment from the lateral femoral condyle, positioned caudal to the point of attachment of the popliteal tendon	Surgical reattachment of the tendon Prognosis for acute injuries is good.	

| Disruption of the Achilles mechanism | Rupture occurs primarily in mature working or racing dogs. Injury has also been reported in cats. Result of an animal jumping and landing on its rear legs. May be bilateral. Rupture secondary to parasitic disease of the gastrocnemius muscle also reported. Disruption of the connective tissue over the superficial digital flexor tendon causes displacement of the tendon during weight bearing. | Tarsal hyperflexion (<90°) and stifle hyperextension owing to the inability to extend the tarsus. Degree of tarsal hyperflexion depends on the completeness of Achilles mechanism disruption. The animal walks on the plantar surface of the tarsus. Displacement of the superficial digital flexor tendon is associated with a mild, chronic weight-bearing lameness with the hock slightly hyperflexed but not to the degree as with complete calcaneal tendon disruption. Tissue thickening around the tuber calcanei may be apparent. | Clinical signs of tarsal hyperflexion and palpable flaccidity of the calcaneal tendon. If the superficial digital flexor tendon is intact, the digits will flex when the tarsus is flexed. Standing or stress radiographs may aid diagnosis, particularly in partial ruptures, because the entire tendon must be disrupted before excessive tarsal hyperflexion is present. Displacement of the superficial ditigal flexor tendon is diagnosed on clinical signs and palpation of the tendon and thickened tissue to one side of the tuber calcanei. | Acute damage requires tenorrhaphy, or apposition of the muscle-tendon or tendon-bone junction. Chronic rupture or injury can be treated by shortening the calcaneal tendon to reestablish function. Prognosis for acute rupture or severance of the Achilles mechanism in most animals is good. Prognosis in very large dogs, or in racing dogs for return to racing, is poor. Prognosis for chronic injuries with fibrosis is less favorable, although function may be improved after surgery. Arthrodesis of the tibiotarsal joint may be required if surgical repair is unsuccessful. Prognosis for normal function after surgical stabilization of the superficial digital flexor tendon is very good. | Mughannam and Reinke, 1994 Parker and Cardinet, 1984 |

(common calcaneal tendon)

Common calcaneal tendon composed of three major musculotendinous units
- gastrocnemius muscle
- superficial digital flexor
- common tendon of the biceps femoris, semitendinosus, and gracilis muscles

Bibliography

Anson LW, Betts CW: Triceps tendon avulsion in a dog: surgical management and xeroradiographic evaluation. J Am Anim Hosp Assoc 25:655, 1989

Averill DR Jr: Disease of the muscle. Vet Clin North Am [Small Anim Pract] 10:223, 1980

Bardet JF, Hohn RB: Subluxation of the hip joint and bone hypoplasia associated with quadriceps contracture in young dogs. J Am Anim Hosp Assoc 20:421, 1984

Basinger RR, Aron DN, Crowe DT et al: Osteofascial compartment syndrome in the dog. Vet Surg 16:427, 1987

Bennett RA: Contracture of the infraspinatus muscle in dogs: a review of 12 cases. J Am Anim Hosp Assoc 22:481, 1986

Bloomberg M: Tendon, muscles and ligament injuries and surgery. p. 1473. In Olmstead ML (ed): Small Animal Orthopedics. Mosby, St Louis, 1995

Bone DL, McGavin MD: Myositis ossificans in the dog: a case report and review. J Am Anim Hosp Assoc 21:135, 1985

Cardinet GH, Holliday TA: Neuromuscular disease of domestic animals: a summary of muscle biopsies from 159 cases. Ann NY Acad Sci 317:290, 1979

Coles LD, North C, Schillhorn van Veen TW: Special article—adult *Dirofilaria immitis* in hind leg abscesses of a dog. J Am Anim Hosp Assoc 24:363, 1988

Cook JL, Huss BT, Johnson GC: Periosteal osteosarcoma in the long head of the triceps in a dog. J Am Anim Hosp Assoc 31:317, 1995

Cooley AJ, Clemmons RM, Gross TL: Heartworm disease manifested by encephalomyelitis and myositis in a dog. J Am Vet Med Assoc 190:431, 1987

Davies JV, Clayton-Jones DG: Triceps tendon rupture in the dog following corticosteroid injection. J Small Anim Pract 23:779, 1982

de Haan JJ, Beale BS: Compartment syndrome in the dog: case report and literature review. J Am Anim Hosp Assoc 29:133, 1993

Dee JF: Soft tissue surgery in the racing greyhound. Proc Refresher Course on Greyhounds, University of Sydney, Australia 122:527, 1989

Dow SW, LeCouteur RA: Hypokalemic polymyopathy of cats. p. 812. In Kirk RW (ed): Current Veterinary Therapy X. WB Saunders, Philadelphia, 1989

Dow SW, LeCouteur RA, Fettman MJ et al: Potassium depletion in cats: hypokalemic polymyopathy. J Am Vet Med Assoc 191:1563, 1987

Drake JC, Hime JM: Two syndromes in young dogs caused by *Toxoplasma gondii*. J Small Anim Pract 8:621, 1967

Dubey JP: *Neospora caninum:* A look at a new *Toxoplasma*-like parasite of dogs and other animals. Compend Contin Educ Pract Vet 12:653, 1990

Dueland RT, Wagner SD, Parker RB: von Willebrand heterotopic osteochondrofibrosis in Doberman pinschers: five cases (1980–1987). J Am Vet Med Assoc 197:383, 1990

Duncan ID, Griffiths IR: Myotonia in the dog. p. 696. In Kirk RW (ed): Current Veterinary Therapy VIII. WB Saunders, Philadelphia, 1983

Easton CB: Extraskeletal osteosarcoma in a cat. J Am Anim Hosp Assoc 30:59, 1994

Eaton-Wells R: Surgical repair of acute gracilis muscle rupture in the racing greyhound. Vet Comp Orthop Traumatol 5:18, 1992

Farnbach GC: Myositis in the dog. Compend Contin Educ Pract Vet 1:183, 1979

Gannon JR: Exertional rhabdomyolysis (myoglobinuria) in the racing greyhound. p. 783. In Kirk RW (ed): Current Veterinary Therapy VII. WB Saunders, Philadelphia, 1980

Gilmore DR: Triceps tendon avulsion in the dog and cat. J Am Anim Hosp Assoc 20:239, 1984

Gilmour MA, Morgan RV, Moore FM: Masticatory myopathy in the dog: a retrospective study of 18 cases. J Am Anim Hosp Assoc 28:300, 1992

Goring RI, Parker RB, Dee L: Medial displacement of the tendon of origin of the biceps brachii muscle in the racing greyhound. J Am Anim Hosp Assoc 20:933, 1984

Hill SL, Shelton GD, Lenehan TM: Myotonia in a cocker spaniel. J Am Anim Hosp Assoc 31:506, 1995

Hoerlein BF, Evans LE, Davis JM: Upward luxation of the canine scapula: a case report. J Am Vet Med Assoc 136:258, 1960

Kirmayer AH, Klide AM, Purvance JE: Malignant hyperthermia in a dog: case report and review of the syndrome. J Am Vet Med Assoc 185:978, 1984

Kornegay JN: Golden retriever muscular dystrophy. Proc Am Coll Vet Intern Med 2:470, 1984

Kornegay JN, Gorgacz EJ, Dawe DL et al: Polymyositis in dogs. J Am Vet Med Assoc 176:431, 1980

Kramer JW, Hegreberg CA, Hamilton MJ: Inheritance of a neuromuscular disorder of Labrador retriever dogs. J Am Vet Med Assoc 179:380, 1981

Krum SH, Cardinet GH, Anderson BC et al: Polymyositis and polyarthritis associated with systemic lupus erythematosus in a dog. J Am Vet Med Assoc 170:61, 1977

Lewis DL: Fibrotic myopathy of the semitendinosus muscle in a cat. J Am Vet Med Assoc 193:240, 1988

Lincoln JD, Potter K: Tenosynovitis of the biceps brachii tendon in dogs. J Am Anim Hosp Assoc 20:385, 1984

Malik R: Hereditary myopathy of Devon rex cats. J Small Anim Pract 34:539, 1993

Matsen FA III, Winquist RA, Krugmire RB Jr: Diagnosis and management of compartment syndromes. J Bone Joint Surg [Am] 62:286, 1980

Moore RW, Rouse GP, Piermattei DL et al: Fibrotic myopathy of the semitendinosus muscle in four dogs. Vet Surg 10:169, 1981

Mughannam A, Reinke J: Avulsion of the gastrocnemius tendon in three cats. J Am Anim Hosp Assoc 30:550, 1994

Muir P, Goldsmid SE, Rothwell TLW et al: Calcifying tendinopathy of the biceps brachii in a dog. J Am Vet Med Assoc 201:1747, 1992

Norris AM, Pallett L, Wilcock B: Generalized myositis ossificans in a cat. J Am Anim Hosp Assoc 16:659, 1980

Parker RB, Cardinet GH: Myotendinous rupture of the Achilles mechanism associated with parasitic myositis. J Am Anim Hosp Assoc 20:115, 1984

Perry MO: Compartment syndromes and reperfusion injury. Surg Clin North Am 68:853, 1988

Pettit GD, Chatburn CC, Hegreberg GA et al: Studies on the pathophysiology of infraspinatus muscle contracture in the dog. Vet Surg 1:8, 1978

Poonacha KB, Donahue JM, Nightengale JR: Clostridial myositis in a dog. J Am Vet Med Assoc 194:69, 1989

Presthues J, Nordstoza K: Probable X-linked myopathy in a Samoyed litter. Proc Eur Soc Vet Neurol 10:52, 1989

Reinke JD, Mughannam AJ, Owens JM: Avulsion of the gastrocnemius tendon in 11 dogs. J Am Anim Hosp Assoc 29:410, 1993

Robinson R: Spasticity in the Devon rex cat. Vet Rec 132:302, 1992

Rorabeck CH, McGee HMJ: Acute compartment syndrome. Vet Comp Orthop Traumatol 3:117, 1990

Ruehlmann D, Podell M, Oglesbee M et al: Canine neosporosis: a case report and literature review. J Am Anim Hosp Assoc 31:174, 1995

Sharp NJH, Kornegay JN, Lane SB: The muscular dystrophies. Semin Vet Intern Med 4:133, 1989

Shelton GD, Cardinet GH, Bandman E: Canine masticatory muscle disorders: a clinicopathological and immunochemical study of 29 cases. Muscle Nerve 10:753, 1987

Shires PK, Nafe LA, Hulse DA: Myotonia in a Staffordshire terrier. J Am Vet Med Assoc 183:229, 1983

Stead AC, Camburn MA, Gunn HM et al: Congenital hindlimb rigidity in a dog. J Small Anim Pract 18:39, 1977

Stobie D, Wallace LJ, Lipowitz AJ et al: Chronic bicipital tenosynovitis in dogs: 29 cases (1985–1992). J Am Vet Med Assoc 207:201, 1995

Valentine BA, George C, Randolph JF et al: Fibrodysplasia ossificans progressiva in the cat. J Vet Intern Med 6:335, 1992

van Ham LML, Desmidt M, Tshamata M et al: Canine X-linked muscular dystrophy in Belgian Groenendaeler shepherds. J Am Anim Hosp Assoc 29:570, 1993

Van Vleet JF: Experimentally induced vitamin E-selenium deficiency in the growing dog. J Am Vet Med Assoc 166:769, 1975

Vaughan LC: Muscle and tendon injuries in dogs. J Small Anim Pract 20:711, 1979

Vos JH, van der Linde-Sipman JS, Goedegeburre SA: Dystrophy like myopathy in a cat. J Comp Pathol 96:335, 1986

Watt PR: Posttraumatic myositis ossificans and fibrotic myopathy in the rectus femoris muscle in a dog: a case report and literature review. J Am Anim Hosp Assoc 28:560, 1992

Wentworth GH, Van Der Unde SJ, Keijer AEFH et al: Myopathy with a possible recessive X-linked inheritance in a litter of Irish terriers. Vet Pathol 9:238, 1972

Dermatologic System

81

Introduction

Diane E. Bevier

Dermatologic History

I. Obtain a complete medical history.
   A. Note the age, sex, and breed of the animal.
   B. In addition, record both the general medical and dermatologic history.
II. Dermatologic history taking should be consistent from animal to animal (Table 81–1).

Examination of the Skin

I. Systematic examination is necessary to arrive at an appropriate differential diagnosis.
   A. Observe the entire animal at a distance of several feet.
   B. Observe for an impression of attitude and general health.
   C. Determine distribution pattern of dermatologic disease: generalized vs. localized; bilaterally symmetrical or unilaterally irregular.
II. Closely examine the skin.
   A. Palpate the skin and hair coat, evaluating texture, elasticity, and thickness of the skin.
      1. Note whether the hair is coarse, fine, dry, or oily and the ease of epilation.
      2. Determine whether the skin is unusually warm or cool to the touch.
   B. Examine every inch of the skin and mucous membranes.
      1. Pay close attention to sparsely haired areas.
      2. Clipping of hair and mild cleansing of lesions may aid in visualization.
      3. Determine whether the dermatosis is confined to a specific region of the body.
III. Identify primary and secondary lesions.
   A. Primary lesions are those that develop spontaneously as a direct result of the underlying disease and are often suggestive of a specific dermatosis or group of diseases.
      1. Macule-patch: A macule is a circumscribed, not raised, area of color change up to 1 cm in size. A patch is a macule >2 cm.
      2. Papule-plaque: A papule is a small, solid ele-

Table 81–1. Questions Pertinent to a Dermatologic History

1. What is the major complaint regarding the animal's skin condition: pruritus, odor, appearance, fear of contagious disease?
2. For what length of time has the current skin problem been present? Have there been prior episodes of dermatologic disease?
3. Was the onset of the dermatologic problem sudden or gradual?
4. Is the dermatologic problem continual or intermittent?
5. Is the problem seasonal, and is there any time of the year when the owner considers the pet to be normal?
6. What areas of the body are involved with the dermatologic problem?
7. Does the pet scratch, chew, bite, or lick itself? How many times an hour does this activity occur, and does the pet keep the owner awake at night?
8. Is there loss of hair, and if so, is the animal removing it or is it falling out?
9. Is there any change in the color of the hair or skin?
10. What other pets are in the household, and do they have any skin problems? Is there opportunity for this pet to be exposed to other animals (boarding, groomers, wild animals)?
11. Do any of the pet's relatives have any skin problems?
12. Do any members of the household have skin problems?
13. Describe the pet's diet over the last year.
14. What percentage of time does the pet stay indoors vs. outdoors?
15. What does the pet contact indoors in terms of rugs, bedding, and cleaning products?
16. What does the pet contact outdoors? Inquire whether the pet is leash walked, in a fenced yard, in fields, or swimming, and what is used for bedding or runs.
17. Does the pet ever have fleas or ticks?
18. Describe prior treatments, including specific drugs and length of treatment time.
19. Has there been a beneficial response to any of the treatments used?
20. Is the pet on treatment now? If so, what kind?
21. When did the pet last receive treatment, and what was it?
22. Does the pet have any other medical problems? Include allergies to medications.
23. Does the pet have other abnormal clinical signs?

vation of the skin up to 1 cm in diameter. A plaque is formed by the extension or coalition of papules and is a larger, flat-topped lesion.

3. Pustule: A pustule is a small, circumscribed elevation of the skin that contains pus. Pustules may be intraepidermal or follicular in location.

4. Nodule: A nodule is a small, circumscribed, solid elevation >1 cm in diameter that usually extends into the deeper layers of the skin.

5. Tumor-neoplasia: A neoplastic enlargement may involve any structure of the skin or subcutaneous tissue.

6. Vesicle-bulla: A vesicle is a sharply circumscribed elevation of the epidermis filled with clear fluid. A bulla is a vesicle >1 cm in diameter.

7. Wheal: A wheal is a sharply circumscribed, raised lesion consisting of edema.

B. Secondary lesions evolve from primary lesions or are artifacts induced by the patient or by external factors such as trauma, time, or medications.

1. Scale–epidermal collarette: Scale is an accumulation of loose fragments of the stratum corneum. An epidermal collarette is a special type of scale arranged in a circular rim of loose keratin flakes and is the remnant of the "roof" of a vesicle, bulla, or pustule.

2. Crust: A crust is formed when dried exudate, serum, pus, blood, cells, scales, or medications adhere to the surface and mingle with the hair.

3. Scar: A scar is an area of fibrous tissue that has replaced damaged dermis or subcutaneous tissue.

4. Erosion-ulcer: An ulcer is a break in the continuity of the epidermis with exposure of the underlying dermis. An erosion is a shallow ulcer that does not penetrate the basal laminar zone and, therefore, heals without scarring.

5. Comedo: A comedo is a dilated hair follicle

filled with cornified cells and sebaceous material.

6. Fissure: A fissure is a linear cleavage into the epidermis (at times extending into the dermis) caused by disease or injury.

7. Excoriation: Excoriation is an area of superficial loss of the epidermis, usually caused by scratching, biting, or rubbing.

8. Lichenification: Lichenification is a thickening and hardening of the skin characterized by an exaggeration of the superficial skin markings.

9. Hyperpigmentation-hypopigmentation: Hyperpigmentation is due to increased epidermal and occasionally dermal melanin. Hypopigmentation is loss of epidermal melanin.

10. Hyperkeratosis-callus: Hyperkeratosis is an increase in thickness of the stratum corneum. A callus is an area of hyperkeratosis over a pressure point.

IV. Characterize the specific type of dermatologic problem present.

A. Determine the configuration of lesions within an area: single, multiple, discrete, diffuse, grouped or confluent, linear or annular, polycyclic, serpiginous, with or without central healing.

B. Using palpation, delineate the depth (elevated, surface, or deep) and consistency (indurated, soft, fluctuant, atrophied, or rolled border) of the lesion.

C. Ascertain the quality of the lesions with respect to surface condition, i.e., dry, moist, greasy, oozing, bleeding, secondarily infected, and/or purulent.

D. Note the color: erythematous, violaceous, yellow, brown, white, gray, and/or black.

V. Proceed to diagnostic and laboratory tests.

A. Correlate the historical, physical examination, and laboratory data and arrive at a differential diagnosis.

B. Narrow the list of differential diagnoses by planning additional tests and instituting therapeutic trials.

82

Congenital/ Developmental Dermatoses

Robert G. Buerger

CONGENITAL DISORDERS

Alopecias

Definition

I. Alopecia, or hairlessness, can be total or partial.
II. It may be a desired or undesired trait and may or may not have a genetic basis.

Causes

I. In certain breeds, hairlessness is a desired trait.
  A. Dog breeds: Chinese crested, Mexican hairless, Abyssinian, African sand dog, Turkish naked dog, Peruvian hairless, Xoloitzcuintl
  B. Cat breed: sphinx, Canadian hairless
  C. Autosomal dominant in dogs and recessive in the sphinx cat and Birman cat
II. Congenital hypotrichosis and ectodermal defect have been reported in males, suggesting a sex-linked or sex-limited trait.
III. Degenerative or delayed (tardive) alopecias are discussed in Chap. 83.

Pathophysiology

I. The term *congenital hypotrichosis* implies abnormal or incomplete development of hair follicles.
II. The term *congenital ectodermal defect* implies abnormal development of multiple ectoderm-derived tissues (hair follicles, sebaceous glands, apocrine glands, claws, whiskers, teeth, etc.) and perhaps also arrector pili muscles.

Clinical Signs

I. Congenital hypotrichosis or congenital ectodermal defect has been reported in the following breeds.
  A. Dogs: cocker spaniel, Belgian shepherd, whippet, schipperke, Labrador retriever, beagle, basset hound, miniature poodle, bichon frise, rottweiler, and French bulldog
  B. Cats: Siamese, Devon Rex, and Birman cat
II. Alopecia may be present at birth or may become evident within several weeks after birth.
III. Alopecia may be total or partial.
  A. There is often an associated scaliness and/or greasiness.
  B. Hairs can be dry, rough, or shortened.
IV. Claws and/or dentition may be abnormal.
V. Alopecia is associated with thymic aplasia in Birman cats (lethal).

Diagnosis

I. It is based on clinical findings.
II. Biopsy reveals a variety of changes, including absence or decrease in the number of appendages, absence of hair follicles, decreased hair follicle density, empty follicles, dystrophic hairs, predominance of telogen hairs, follicular keratosis, surface hyperkeratosis, absence of arrector pili muscles, and hypermelanosis.

Differential Diagnosis

I. If the alopecia is present at birth, these syndromes are usually not confused with other dermatoses.
II. Causes of alopecia occurring shortly after birth include demodicosis, dermatophytosis, bacterial pyoderma, alopecia areata, traumatic alopecia (self-, littermate-, or dam-induced), and endocrinopathies.

Treatment

I. Usually none is required.
II. Greasiness and/or scaliness may require antiseborrheic shampoos.

III. Protection from cold and actinic damage can be provided by clothing and sunscreens.

Patient Monitoring

I. The alopecia usually does not progress with time.
II. Affected animals are not known to be prone to other problems.

Uncommon Disorders

See Table 82–1.

DEVELOPMENTAL DISORDERS

Lethal Acrodermatitis

Definition

An inherited syndrome of English bull terriers characterized by growth retardation, acrodermatitis, pyoderma, paronychia, diarrhea, pneumonia, and abnormal behavior that results in death usually before 15 months of age

Causes and Pathophysiology

I. It is inherited as an autosomal recessive trait.
II. It is thought to be similar to acrodermatitis enteropathica in people and lethal trait A46 in black pied Danish cattle, and it resembles experimentally induced zinc deficiency in dogs and other animals.
III. There is evidence to suggest that a zinc absorption defect is present in affected individuals.

Clinical Signs

I. General signs
   A. More lightly pigmented at birth than normal bull terriers
   B. Are weak, nurse poorly, and have difficulty chewing and swallowing
   C. High arch to hard palate
   D. Smaller than normal littermates
   E. Splayed feet
II. Cutaneous signs
   A. By 6–10 weeks of age, crusted lesions occur interdigitally and pyoderma is evident around the body orifices and on the ears and extremities.
   B. Pyoderma may become generalized.
   C. The footpads develop fissures.
   D. The nails are dystrophic and paronychia develops.
III. Systemic signs
   A. Diarrhea of varying severity occurs.
   B. Respiratory infections are common, and a hypoplastic trachea is found in some individuals.
   C. Behavioral abnormalities such as aggressiveness, poor responsiveness to external stimuli, or excessive sleeping may be noted.
   D. Light or mottled pigmentation around the pupillary border of the iris has been noted.

Diagnosis

I. Physical findings are suggestive.
   A. Affected breed
   B. Age of onset
   C. Suspicious clinical signs
II. Decreased serum zinc levels are found in affected dogs. The mean serum zinc concentration in affected dogs is 55.2 ± 9.04 μg/dl, whereas that of age- and breed-matched normal dogs is 70.4 ± 8.29 μg/dl (Mundell, 1988).
III. Serum chemistry abnormalities are nonspecific.
   A. Low serum alkaline phosphatase and alanine transaminase
   B. Hypercholesterolemia
IV. Hematology often reveals neutrophilia.
V. Documented immunologic abnormalities include decreased lymphocyte blastogenesis and dysgammaglobulinemia.
VI. Pathologic examination of affected animals helps confirm the diagnosis.
   A. Small or nonidentifiable thymus
   B. Small lymphoreticular organs, i.e., nodes, spleen
   C. Enlargement of lateral cerebral ventricles
   D. Parakeratosis, ulceration, superficial infection, and occasionally *Demodex* mites within hair follicles

Differential Diagnosis

I. Demodicosis
II. Dermatophytosis
III. Bacterial pyoderma
IV. Zinc-responsive dermatosis
V. Generic dog food dermatosis
VI. Zinc deficiency
VII. Pemphigus foliaceus
VIII. Lupus erythematosus

Treatment

I. None is known to be effective.
II. Oral zinc supplementation has not been beneficial.

Patient Monitoring

I. The median survival time is 7 months, and all affected dogs are dead by 15 months of age.
II. Siblings and parents of affected dogs are not to be used for breeding.

Acral Mutilation Syndrome

Definition

I. It is a rare, hereditary sensory neuropathy of German shorthaired and English pointers that results in a loss of nociception.
II. Clinically there is self-mutilation of the distal extremities.

*Table 82–1. **Uncommon Congenital Dermatoses***

Disorder	Definition	Causes	Breeds	Cutaneous Signs
Aplasia cutis	Localized or regionalized absence of skin at birth	Possible autosomal recessive, teratogens, trauma, amniotic adherences	—	Absence of skin resulting in ulceration
Chédiak-Higashi syndrome	A disease of partial oculocutaneous albinism and an increased susceptibility to infection and bleeding	Autosomal recessive	Persian cats	Light "blue smoke" coat color (see also Chap. 73)
Cyclic hematopoiesis	A lethal syndrome of collies characterized by a gray coat color, cyclic formation of blood cells (especially neutrophils), and increased susceptibility to infection	Autosomal recessive	Collie dogs	Silver or beige hair coat color (see also Chap. 64)
Dermoid sinus	A defect of development that results in an incomplete separation of the skin and the neural tube	Possibly inherited as a simple recessive	Rhodesian ridgebacks	Single or multiple indentations on dorsal midline (especially cervical)
Epidermolysis bullosa of cat	A disease of abnormal coherence at the dermoepidermal junction	Probably autosomal recessive	Siamese and Oriental cats	Beginning at 5 weeks of age claws shed with minimal trauma and regrow misshapen
Familial cutaneous vasculopathy	A disease characterized by vasculitis and collagenolysis affecting puppies 4–7 weeks of age	Autosomal recessive	German shepherd dogs	Swelling, crusting, ulceration, ± depigmentation of nose, ear margins, paw pads; fever; ± lameness; ± joint swelling
Footpad hyperkeratosis	A disease of paw pads usually noted before 6 months of age	Autosomal, exact mechanism unknown	Dogues de Bordeaux, Irish terriers	Paw pad hyperkeratosis, fissures, ± pain on ambulation
Ichthyosis	A disease of abnormal keratinization characterized by severe scaling and hyperkeratosis	Probably autosomal recessive	—	Thick, adherent, dry, tan-gray scales and keratinous "feathers"
Lupoid dermatosis	An exfoliative dermatosis of young adult dogs that has histopathologic similarities to lupus erythematosus	Unknown	German shorthaired pointers	Regionalized to generalized hyperkeratotic scaling and alopecia
Seborrhea oleosa of cats	A seborrheic skin disorder recognized in kittens days or weeks after their birth	Possibly recessive	Persian cats	Curly, unkempt, matted, dirty, greasy, and scaly coat with rancid odor
Tyrosinemia	A defect in tyrosinase metabolism that results in the accumulation of tyrosine crystals in tissues	Unknown	Reported in one 7 week old German shepherd dog (Kunkle et al., 1984)	Painful ulcerations on the planum nasale, tongue, footpads, and nail folds

Causes and Pathophysiology

I. The condition is inherited, probably as an autosomal recessive trait.
II. There is insufficient development of the primary sensory neuron with a significant decrease in the size of spinal ganglia and dorsal roots and in the number of ganglionic neurons.
III. A slowly progressive, postnatal degeneration of myelinated and unmyelinated sensory neurons occurs.
IV. There is evidence that substance P (thought to mediate pain perception) is deficient in affected dogs as well.

Clinical Signs

I. By 3–5 months of age, affected puppies of either sex begin chewing and licking their feet.
II. Self-inflicted ulceration and mutilation continue unabated, resulting in possible autoamputation.

Diagnosis

I. Affected animals are identifiable soon after birth because of their lack of response to painful stimuli, such as pin pricks or digital compression, or to extremes of temperature.
II. Gross and histopathologic findings at necropsy are distinctive.

Differential Diagnosis

I. Rule out dermatologic causes of foot licking or chewing.
   A. Hypersensitivities
      1. Atopy
      2. Food allergy
      3. Contact
   B. Irritant contact dermatitis
   C. Infectious pododermatitis
      1. Bacterial
      2. Fungal
   D. Parasitic pododermatitis
      1. Demodicosis
      2. *Pelodera* dermatitis
      3. Hookworm dermatitis
II. Rule out causes of stereotypic behavior with self-mutilation (i.e., boredom, psychosis).

Treatment

I. None is known to be effective.
II. Bandages, muzzles, or Elizabethan collars are not effective for long-term management.
III. Euthanasia is perhaps best for severe cases.

Patient Monitoring

I. The prognosis is poor.
II. Genetic counseling is necessary for owners of parents and siblings (even if clinically not affected), because these dogs are not to be used for breeding.

Acanthosis Nigricans

Definition

Acanthosis nigricans is a cutaneous reaction pattern characterized by symmetrical and often progressive axillary hyperpigmentation, lichenification, alopecia, greasiness, and odor.

Causes

I. Primary (rare): possibly inherited in dachshunds
II. Secondary (common)
   A. Hypersensitivities such as atopy, food, contact
   B. Friction from poor conformation and obesity
   C. Infectious agents, especially staphylococcal pyoderma and *Malassezia* dermatitis
   D. Endocrinopathies
      1. Hypothyroidism
      2. Hyperadrenocorticism
      3. Sex hormone–related
         a) Hyper- or hypoestrogenism
         b) Hyper- or hypoandrogenism
   E. Associated with internal malignancy, e.g., hepatic carcinoma, thyroid adenocarcinoma

Pathophysiology

I. The exact pathophysiology of primary acanthosis nigricans is obscure. Although abnormalities of pituitary or pineal hormones (i.e., thyrotropin, melanocyte-stimulating hormone [MSH], melatonin) and sex hormones have been incriminated, none of these have proven roles in the pathogenesis of lesions.
II. Secondary acanthosis nigricans due to hypersensitivities or friction results from chronic inflammation, repeated local trauma, or irritation.

Clinical Signs

I. Early symmetrical axillary hyperpigmentation occurs with or without inflammation and/or pruritus depending on the cause.
   A. Primary acanthosis nigricans begins in dogs younger than 1 year of age and is usually noninflammatory and nonpruritic.
   B. If inflammation or pruritus precedes the development of hyperpigmentation, secondary causes of acanthosis nigricans should be pursued.
II. Untreated, the hyperpigmentation is often progressive, with lichenification, alopecia, scales, greasiness, and seborrheic odor. The depths of the lichenified folds may be moist.
III. Lesions may ultimately involve the forelimbs, the ventral neck, chest, and abdomen; the pinnae; inner thighs; perineum; and hocks.

Diagnosis

I. An accurate history is critical to understanding the development of lesions and the underlying cause.
II. Skin scrapings and dermatophyte cultures are indicated to rule out demodicosis and fungal infections.

III. Thyroid and adrenal function test results are usually normal.
IV. Skin biopsy reveals the following.
   A. Irregular epidermal hyperplasia, focal spongiosis, melanosis of the stratum basale and superficial dermis, surface hyperkeratosis with focal para-keratosis, and superficial perivascular infiltrate of mononuclear cells, and lesser numbers of neutro-phils
   B. Variable follicular keratosis
V. Serologic evaluation of sex hormones often yields confusing and misleading results.

Differential Diagnosis

I. Rule out other inflammatory dermatoses.
II. Rule out generalized hyperpigmentation and licheni-fication associated with endocrinopathies.

Treatment

I. Any underlying disease or contributing factor must be resolved or controlled.
II. Melatonin (Rickards Research Foundation, Cleve-land, OH) may be tried for primary forms.
   A. It promotes melanosome aggregation with subse-quent blanching of skin.
   B. Give 1–2 mg SQ SID for 3–5 days, then weekly to monthly as needed.
   C. This treatment does not have wide acceptance among dermatologists, as most cases of acantho-sis nigricans are secondary in nature.
   D. Concurrent alternate-day prednisone therapy may be tried.
III. Corticosteroids may be effective because of their anti-inflammatory effects or because of an inhibition of MSH release from the pituitary gland.
   A. Give prednisone in anti-inflammatory doses (0.55–1.1 mg/kg PO QOD).
   B. A clinical response should be seen within 2–4 weeks.
IV. Vitamin E has been shown to be effective in improv-ing and controlling inflammation, lichenification, pruritus, greasiness, and odor, but not hyperpigmen-tation.
   A. Administer 200 IU PO BID (2 hours before or after a meal).
   B. Improvement should be seen in 60 days.
V. Antiseborrheic shampoos help control odor, greasi-ness, scales, and surface bacteria.
   A. Bathe twice weekly.
   B. Use shampoos containing sulfur and salicylic acid.
VI. Topical tretinoin (Retin-A) cream alone or in combi-nation with topical corticosteroid creams may be of value.
VII. Treatment with thyroid-stimulating hormone (TSH), antithyroid drugs (to promote TSH production by the pituitary), or thyroid hormone is not appropriate and is reserved for those cases in which thyroid disease has been documented.

Patient Monitoring

I. The disease is controllable but not curable.
II. Once pigmentation has stabilized, reevaluate every 3 months for exacerbation of lesions.

Dermatomyositis

Definition

I. Dermatomyositis is a group of hereditary mechano-bullous diseases characterized by dermatitis and/or myositis.
II. Dogs initially described as having epidermolysis bul-losa simplex probably had a mild form of dermato-myositis.

Causes and Pathophysiology

I. In collies, it is inherited as an autosomal dominant trait with variable expressivity.
II. It may be an immune-mediated disease.
III. Infectious and/or environmental factors, including temperature, trauma, and exposure to sunlight, may contribute to the formation of skin lesions.
IV. Mechanical trauma may result in activation of cyto-lytic enzymes within the epidermis and cause a sec-ondary disruption of the intact epithelium.

Clinical Signs

I. It has been reported in collies, shelties, Australian cattle dogs, Pembroke Welsh corgis, chow chows, German shepherd dogs, and other purebred dogs.
II. Onset of signs is usually between 3 and 6 months of age.
III. Affected puppies may be small, unthrifty, and weak.
IV. Skin lesions vary in severity, and occasional cases present with only muscle disease.
   A. Initially nonpruritic papules, pustules, vesicles, erosions, ulcers, crusts, erythema, and alopecia develop on the face, eyelids, muzzle, lips, ear tips, and tip of the tail and over bony promi-nences on the extremities.
   B. Lesions can remain mild and often spontaneously regress by 6–8 months of age, leaving alopecic scars.
   C. Lesions may wax and wane for the life of the ani-mal.
V. Muscle changes are often imperceptible or minimal.
   A. Dogs with severe skin lesions often develop se-vere atrophy of the muscles of mastication by 1 year of age, which may impair drinking and eating.
   B. In severe cases, generalized weakness, muscle atrophy, and megaesophagus may occur.

Diagnosis

I. Clinical signs are suggestive.
   A. Breed
   B. Age of onset

C. Appearance and distribution of lesions
II. Skin biopsy is often definitive.
  A. Follicular atrophy, dermal and perifollicular fibrosis, and perifolliculitis are the most common findings.
  B. Less commonly, hydropic degeneration, colloid bodies, and subepidermal or intrabasilar vesicles are found.
III. Muscle studies are helpful.
  A. Results of muscle enzyme assays for serum creatine phosphokinase and serum aspartate aminotransferase are usually normal.
  B. Electromyography often reveals positive sharp waves and fibrillation potentials, particularly in the masseter muscles, tongue, laryngeal muscles, and the muscles of the distal extremities and tail.
  C. Muscle biopsy reveals interstitial accumulation of mononuclear cells, fibrosis, and muscle fiber necrosis, atrophy, degeneration, and regeneration.
  D. Immunologic tests such as the direct Coombs, antinuclear antibody, lupus erythematosus prep, rheumatoid factor, and direct immunofluorescence are usually negative or nondiagnostic.

Differential Diagnosis

I. Demodicosis
II. Dermatophytosis
III. Bacterial folliculitis
IV. Lupus erythematosus

Treatment

I. Systemic corticosteroids
  A. Corticosteroid therapy is reserved for severely affected dogs.
  B. Prednisolone 1.1 mg/kg PO SID-BID may be helpful.
  C. With clinical remission, taper the dosage and frequency to QOD.
II. Oral vitamin E 100–400 IU/day may be helpful for skin lesions.
III. Pentoxifylline at 10 mg/kg PO SID-QOD (given with food) may result in improvement after 2–3 months of therapy.
IV. Provide a trauma-free environment because lesions occur at sites of trauma.

Patient Monitoring

I. Prognosis in all but the most severe cases is good, as most dogs undergo spontaneous remission. In severe cases, the skin and muscle changes may not be compatible with long-term existence.
II. Evaluate dogs receiving corticosteroids at 3-month intervals for level of control and for adverse effects from the therapy.
III. Affected dogs, their siblings, and their parents are not to be used for breeding.

Bibliography

Anderson RK: Canine acanthosis nigricans. Compend Contin Educ Pract Vet 1:466, 1979

August JR, Chickering WR, Rikihisa Y: Congenital ichthyosis in a dog: comparison with the human ichthyosiform dermatoses. Compend Contin Educ Pract Vet 10:40, 1988

Campbell KL: Canine cyclic hematopoiesis. Compend Contin Educ Pract Vet 7:57, 1985

Casal ML, Straumann U, Sigg C et al: Congenital hypotrichosis with thymic aplasia in nine Birman kittens. J Am Anim Hosp Assoc 30:600, 1994

Charach M: Dermatomyositis in a Shetland sheepdog with needle electromyographic abnormalities. Proc Am Coll Vet Dermatol 7:90, 1991

Chastain CB, Swayne DE: Congenital hypotrichosis in male Basset hound littermates. J Am Vet Med Assoc 187:845, 1985

Conroy JD, Rasmussen BA, Small E: Hypotrichosis in miniature poodle siblings. J Am Vet Med Assoc 166:697, 1975

Cummings JF, de Lahunta A, Winn SS: Acral mutilation and nociceptive loss in English pointer dogs. Acta Neuropathol 53:119, 1981

Cummings JF, de Lahunta A, Simpson ST et al: Reduced substance P-like immunoreactivity in hereditary sensory neuropathy of pointer dogs. Acta Neuropathol 63:33, 1984

Frieden IJ: Aplasia cutis congenita: a clinical review and proposal for classification. J Am Acad Dermatol 14:646, 1986

Grieshaber TL, Blakemore JC, Yaskulski S: Congenital alopecia in a Bichon Frise. J Am Vet Med Assoc 188:1053, 1986

Gross TL, Kunkle GA: The cutaneous histology of dermatomyositis in collie dogs. Vet Pathol 24:11, 1987

Hargis AM, Haupt KH, Hegreberg GA et al: Familial canine dermatomyositis. Am J Pathol 116:234, 1984

Hargis AM, Haupt KH, Prieur DJ, Moore MP: A skin disorder in three Shetland sheepdogs: comparison with familial canine dermatomyositis of collies. Compend Contin Educ Pract Vet 7:306, 1985

Hargis AM, Prieur DJ, Haupt KH, Collier LL: Post-mortem findings in a Shetland sheepdog with dermatomyositis. Vet Pathol 23:509, 1986

Ihrke PJ, Mueller RS, Stannard AA: Generalized congenital hypotrichosis in a female Rottweiler. Vet Dermatol 4:65, 1993

Jezyk PF, Haskins ME, MacKay-Smith MA, Patterson DF: Lethal acrodermatitis in bull terriers. J Am Vet Med Assoc 188:833, 1986

Johnstone I, Mason K, Sutton R: A hereditary junctional mechanobullous disease in the cat. Proc Am Coll Vet Dermatol 8:111, 1992

Kramer JW, Davis WC, Prieur DJ: The Chediak-Higashi syndrome of cats. Lab Invest 36:554, 1977

Kunkle GA: Congenital hypotrichosis in two dogs. J Am Vet Med Assoc 185:84, 1984

Kunkle GA, Jezyk PF, West CS: Tyrosinemia in a dog. J Am Anim Hosp Assoc 20:615, 1984

Kunkle GA, Gross TL, Fadok V: Dermatomyositis in collie dogs. Compend Contin Educ Pract Vet 7:185, 1985

Mann GE, Stratton J: Dermoid sinus in the Rhodesian ridgeback. J Small Anim Pract 7:631, 1966

Muller GH: Ichthyosis in two dogs. J Am Vet Med Assoc 169:1313, 1976

Muller GH, Kirk RW, Scott DW: Small Animal Dermatology. WB Saunders, Philadelphia, 1989

Mundell AC: Mineral analysis in bull terriers with lethal acrodermatitis. Proc Am Coll Vet Dermatol 4:22, 1988

O'Neill CS: Hereditary skin disease in the dog and the cat. Compend Contin Educ Pract Vet 3:791, 1981

Paradis M: Footpad hyperkeratosis in a family of Dogues de Bordeaux. Vet Dermatol 3:75, 1992

Paradis M, Scott DW: Hereditary primary seborrhea oleosa in Persian cats. Fel Pract 18:17, 1990

Prieur DJ, Collier LL, Bryan GM, Meyers KM: The diagnosis of feline Chediak-Higashi syndrome. Fel Pract 9:26, 1979

Robinson R: The Canadian hairless or sphinx cat. J Heredity 64:47, 1973

Schmeitzel LP, Laratta LJ, Braund KG, Patton CS: Dermatomyositis in an Australian cattle dog. Proc Am Coll Vet Dermatol 7:11, 1991

Scott DW, Walton DK: Clinical evaluation of oral vitamin E for the treatment of primary canine acanthosis nigricans. J Am Anim Hosp Assoc 21:345, 1985

Selcer EA, Helman RG, Selcer RR: Dermoid sinus in a shih tzu and a boxer. J Am Anim Hosp Assoc 20:634, 1984

Selmanowitz VJ, Kramer KM, Orentreich N: Congenital ectodermal defect in miniature poodles. J Heredity 61:196, 1970

Stogdale L, Botha WS, Saunders GN: Congenital hypotrichosis in a dog. J Am Anim Hosp Assoc 18:184, 1982

Vroom MW, Theaker MJ, Rest JR et al: Lupoid dermatosis in five German short-haired pointers. Vet Dermatol 6:93, 1995

Weir JA, Yeager JA: Familial cutaneous vasculopathy of German shepherd dogs. Proc Am Coll Vet Dermatol 9:95, 1993

White SD, Shelton GD, Sisson A et al: Dermatomyositis in an adult Pembroke Welsh corgi. J Am Anim Hosp Assoc 28:398, 1992

83

Degenerative Skin Diseases

Michele M. Brignac
Diane E. Bevier

FELINE SYMMETRICAL ALOPECIA

Definition

I. Feline symmetrical alopecia is a rare bilaterally symmetrical hypotrichosis that is not self-inflicted.
II. The name feline symmetrical alopecia is preferred to feline endocrine alopecia, because an endocrine cause has not been proved.
III. Most cats presented for bilaterally symmetrical hair loss are pulling their hair out and therefore do not have feline symmetrical alopecia.

Causes and Pathophysiology

I. Exact cause is unknown.
II. Sex hormone imbalance has not been documented. Therapy with sex hormones is often successful, but this may in part be the result of other factors, such as psychotropic effects.
III. Thyroid function has been studied, but hypothyroidism has not been proved. Thyroid hormone has been used with some success but can produce hair growth in various nonthyroidal illnesses.

Clinical Signs

I. Signalment
  A. Predominantly neutered male and female cats, males possibly predisposed
  B. Rarely affects purebreds
  C. Age: 2–12 years
II. Clinical picture
  A. Diffuse thinning of hair usually begins in the perineal and anogenital regions, progresses to involve the medial thighs, ventral abdomen, and proximal tail, and eventually may extend to the lateral thorax, flanks, and caudal forelimbs.

B. The hair loss is not self-inflicted.
C. Hair may epilate easily.
D. The underlying skin appears normal.
E. Pruritus is absent.
F. There are no signs or history of systemic disease or a stressful event.

Diagnosis

I. Rule out infectious disease.
  A. Skin scrapings
  B. Wood's lamp, fungal culture for dermatophytes
II. Rule out self-inflicted hair loss.
  A. Trichogram
    1. Pluck 10–20 hairs, mount in mineral oil, and examine microscopically on low power.
    2. Hair tips should be intact and pointed, indicating that hair loss is not self-inflicted.
    3. Fractured hair tips indicate excessive grooming or diseases that damage the hairshaft, such as psychogenic alopecia and dermatophytosis, and suggest the need to proceed with a workup for pruritic or psychogenic dermatoses.
  B. Elizabethan collar test
    1. An Elizabethan collar is applied 24 hours a day for a 30-day trial period.
    2. Hair regrowth during this period indicates a self-inflicted cause of alopecia.
    3. Cats with feline symmetrical alopecia do not show regrowth.
III. Biopsy shows a predominance of telogen hair follicles.
IV. Consider performing certain laboratory tests.
  A. Hemogram, serum chemistries, urinalysis, and adrenal function tests are normal.
  B. Thyroid function tests are variable.
    1. Serum total triiodothyronine (T_3) and thyroxine (T_4) are usually normal.
    2. Depressed response to stimulation with thyro-

tropin (TSH) was reported in one study (Thoday, 1986).
3. A true hypothyroid state has not been documented. Further investigation of thyroid function in cats with this disorder is needed.

Differential Diagnosis

I. Definite self-inflicted hair loss
   A. Psychogenic alopecia
   B. Flea bite hypersensitivity
   C. Other allergy (atopy, food)
II. Possible self-inflicted hair loss
   A. Dermatophytosis
   B. Demodicosis
III. Hair loss not self-inflicted
   A. Telogen or anagen defluxion
   B. Hypothyroidism (extremely rare)
   C. Hyperadrenocorticism (extremely rare)
   D. Megestrol acetate–induced alopecia
   E. Excessive shedding
   F. Hereditary hypotrichosis

Treatment

I. Combined androgen/estrogen therapy is the preferred initial treatment.
   A. Repositol testosterone (testosterone propionate in oil) 12.5 mg/cat IM and either repositol diethylstilbestrol (Stilphostrol) 0.625 mg/cat IM or repositol estradiol (ECP) 0.5 mg/cat IM are the hormones of choice.
   B. Give both hormones simultaneously, and repeat in 6 weeks if no new hair growth is evident.
   C. Side effects are possible with this treatment.
      1. Females may show signs of estrus.
      2. Males may exhibit urine spraying or aggressiveness.
      3. Overdosage can result in severe hepatobiliary disease or death.
      4. These drugs are not approved for use in cats in the United States.
II. Thyroid hormone therapy has been successful in some cases and can be tried if combined androgen/estrogen therapy is unsuccessful.
   A. Sodium levothyroxine 0.05–0.1 mg/cat PO BID is given initially.
   B. Sodium liothyronine 20 μg/cat PO BID, increased by 10 μg BID every third day to a maximum of 50 μg BID, can be tried if there is no response to sodium levothyroxine.
   C. Significant hair regrowth should be apparent after 3 months.
   D. Side effects are apparently rare with this therapy.
III. Progestagens are discouraged because of their serious and potentially life-threatening side effects.
   A. Injectable drugs
      1. Repositol progesterone (progesterone in oil) 2.2–22 mg/kg IM, SQ or medroxyprogesterone acetate (Depo-Provera) 50–175 mg/cat IM, SQ may be given.
      2. Repeat in 6 weeks if new hair growth is not evident.
      3. Do not use in unspayed females.
   B. Oral drug: megestrol acetate (Ovaban, Megace)
      1. Induction dose: 2.5–5 mg/cat PO QOD until hair regrowth is evident
      2. Maintenance dose: 2.5–5 mg/cat PO every 1–2 weeks
   C. Side effects
      1. Polyphagia and weight gain, polydipsia
      2. Personality changes
      3. Pyometra, mammary hyperplasia and neoplasia (both sexes)
      4. Diabetes mellitus, adrenocortical suppression
      5. Bilaterally symmetrical alopecia
      6. Not approved for use in cats in the United States

Patient Monitoring

I. Of patients treated with injectable compounds, 50% relapse within 6 months to 2 years, but retreatment is usually successful.
II. The disease is not life-threatening; therefore, the owner may choose not to treat the condition.

PINNAL ALOPECIA

Definition

Pinnal alopecia is a bilaterally symmetrical noninflammatory alopecia confined to the pinnae of dogs and cats.

Causes and Pathophysiology

I. Exact cause is unknown.
II. Hormonal imbalance is suspected in some cases.
   A. Hypothyroidism
   B. Sex hormone imbalances
III. May be hereditary in dachshunds.

Clinical Signs

I. Dogs
   A. Signalment
      1. Most common in dachshunds
      2. Other affected short-coated breeds
         a) Chihuahua
         b) Whippet
         c) Boston terrier
         d) Italian greyhound
         e) Basset hound
      3. Seldom noticed in dogs <1 year old
   B. Clinical picture
      1. Diffuse thinning of hair occurs and may progress to complete alopecia of the pinnae by 8–9 years of age.
      2. Underlying skin is normal.
      3. Pruritus is absent.
      4. Other areas of the body are not affected.
      5. Systemic signs are not present.

6. Hair loss is usually permanent.
II. Cats
   A. Signalment
      1. Siamese cats may develop a periodic alopecia of the pinnae.
      2. No age or sex predilection is reported.
   B. Clinical picture
      1. Onset may be sudden or slow.
      2. Hairs may epilate easily.
      3. Hair usually regrows in several months without treatment.

Diagnosis

I. History, physical examination, and absence of inflammatory skin lesions are suggestive.
II. Histopathology shows an overwhelming predominance of hair follicles in the inactive (telogen) phase.

Differential Diagnosis

I. Endocrinopathies
   A. Alopecia is usually not confined to the pinnae.
   B. Systemic signs are often present.
II. Inflammatory dermatoses
   A. These include ear margin seborrhea, contact dermatitis, pinnal vasculitis, and infectious and parasitic dermatoses.
   B. Erythema, scale, and crusts are usually present.
III. Periodic alopecia of miniature poodles
   A. Mature poodles suddenly lose large tufts of hair from the pinnae.
   B. Hair loss continues for several months, then hair regrows spontaneously over 3–4 months.
IV. Alopecia areata
   A. This rare disease of dogs and cats has a suspected immunologic basis and is characterized by well-circumscribed patches of alopecia as opposed to diffuse thinning of hair.
   B. Histopathology reveals a mononuclear infiltrate around the hair bulbs.

Treatment and Monitoring

I. In general, none is available.
II. Various hormonal therapies have been tried in dogs.
   A. Levothyroxine sodium 0.02–0.04 mg/kg PO divided BID may be tried.
   B. Methyltestosterone for male dogs 1 mg/kg PO QOD, to a maximum dose of 30 mg has had some success.
   C. If hair regrowth occurs, a low maintenance dose is instituted.
   D. If no hair growth occurs in 3 months, therapy should be discontinued.

PATTERN ALOPECIA

Definition

I. Pattern alopecia is a bilaterally symmetrical noninflammatory alopecia recognized in certain breeds of short-coated dogs.

II. In males, pinnal alopecia may be the only manifestation.

Causes and Pathophysiology

I. Exact cause is unknown.
II. A hereditary basis is suspected.

Clinical Signs

I. Signalment
   A. Most common in dachshunds
   B. Other affected short-coated breeds
      1. Manchester terrier
      2. Miniature pinscher
      3. Chihuahua
      4. Basset hound
   C. Begins <1 year of age
II. Clinical picture
   A. In males, hair loss on the pinnae progresses to complete pinnal alopecia by 8–9 years of age.
   B. Females develop ventral thinning of hair, which may progress to total baldness of the ventrum.
   C. Inflammatory lesions and pruritus are absent.
   D. There are no systemic signs.

Diagnosis

I. History and physical examination are normal except for the noninflammatory alopecia.
II. Rule out endocrinopathies, such as hypothyroidism and hyperadrenocorticism.
III. Biopsy shows a predominance of hair follicles in the inactive (telogen) phase.
IV. Diagnosis is usually based on clinical presentation and ruling out endocrine or hereditary conditions listed under Differential Diagnosis.

Differential Diagnosis

I. Female estrogen-responsive dermatosis (ovarian imbalance II)
   A. This disease may also present with a similar pattern of alopecia, but perineal alopecia and an infantile vulva are usually present.
   B. The condition responds to estrogen therapy.
II. Hypothyroidism
III. Hyperadrenocorticism
IV. Other sex hormone imbalances
V. Telogen or anagen defluxion
VI. Congenital or hereditary disorders, such as hereditary hypotrichosis
VII. Idiopathic pinnal alopecia (male dogs)

Treatment and Monitoring

I. No known treatment is effective.
II. Hair loss is permanent.

PREAURICULAR FELINE ALOPECIA

Definition and Cause

I. Preauricular feline alopecia is a physiologic sparseness of hair in the temporal region between the ear and eye of normal cats.
II. The cause is unknown.

Clinical Signs

I. Sparsity of hair confined to an area along the lateral forehead between the eye and ear
II. May be less noticeable in long-haired or densely coated animals
III. May be mistaken for disease by owners

Diagnosis

I. Clinical appearance is pathognomonic.
II. Underlying skin is normal.

Differential Diagnosis

Pruritus-induced self-inflicted hair loss

Treatment and Monitoring

I. None is required.
II. The degree of preauricular alopecia varies among breeds and individuals.

TRACTION ALOPECIA

Definition and Cause

I. It is transient or permanent alopecia in dogs that results from prolonged or too tight application of barrettes, rubber bands, or other methods to tie up the hair.
II. Mechanical trauma results in an inflammatory plaque that progresses to alopecia and an atrophic, scarred patch.

Clinical Signs

I. It is seen primarily in small, long-haired breeds such as the Yorkshire terrier, Maltese, Lhasa apso, and Shih Tzu.
II. It occurs at any age.
III. Initially an inflammatory plaque develops and progresses to alopecia on the top or lateral aspects of the head.

Diagnosis

I. Characteristic history and physical findings are suggestive.
II. Rule out other diagnoses.

A. Dermatophyte culture
B. Biopsy for histopathology: fairly characteristic

Differential Diagnosis

I. Alopecia areata
II. Dermatophytosis

Treatment

I. Instruct the owner in proper placement of hair-holding devices.
II. If scarring is present, cosmetic excision may be done.

SEASONAL ALOPECIAS

Definition

I. Cyclic follicular dysplasia (CFD) is seasonal thinning of the hair coat in a generalized or localized pattern. The generalized pattern is more common in Alaska, suggesting that duration of light exposure may be important.
II. Seasonal flank alopecia (SFA) is a localized follicular alopecia that occurs in spring or fall and appears to have some genetic basis.

Causes and Pathophysiology

I. The exact cause is unknown.
II. Photoperiod is extremely important in determining hair cycle changes in the dog.
III. Increased incidence in far northern climates and at times of the year when photoperiod is in flux implies involvement of photoperiod in the pathophysiology.
IV. A strong breed predilection exists for SFA, and affected families have been reported.

Clinical Signs

I. Signalment
A. CFD: Labrador retriever, mixed breed dogs, Yorkshire terrier, Airedale terrier
B. SFA: Airedale terrier, English bulldog, boxer, miniature schnauzer and poodle, Doberman pinscher, Bouvier des Flandres, Scottish terrier, French bulldog
C. Both conditions: adult dogs
D. SFA: possibly more common in spayed females
II. Clinical picture
A. Truncal alopecia or marked thinning of the hair coat is typically seen with CFD.
1. The flank area is often affected.
2. Scaling and inflammation are usually absent.
3. Some dogs have only 1–2 episodes, but others develop alopecia every year.
B. Dogs with SFA develop bilaterally symmetrical non-scarring alopecia confined to the thoracolumbar region.
1. Lesions are annular to polycyclic.
2. Lesions have a well-demarcated border.

3. Lesions are usually very hyperpigmented.
4. Scaling and bacterial folliculitis may occur in alopecic areas.
5. Hair regrowth occurs in 3–4 months and may be normal or a different color, texture, or both.
6. In more than half the cases, the hair loss occurs at least twice in successive years.

Diagnosis

I. Rule out the common endocrinopathies and sex hormone abnormalities with appropriate tests.
II. Rule out infectious diseases via skin scrapings and dermatophyte cultures.
III. Histopathology reveals follicular atrophy and infundibular hyperkeratosis and melanized sebaceous glands and is similar to that of other endocrinopathies.

Differential Diagnosis

I. Endocrinopathies: hypothyroidism, hyperadrenocorticism, sex hormone imbalance
II. Infectious diseases: demodicosis, dermatophytosis

Treatment and Monitoring

I. There is currently no treatment available.
II. Prognosis is unpredictable in any given dog.
   A. Some develop seasonal problems every year. Lesions may remain the same or worsen.
   B. Some dogs have an occasional year of involvement interspersed with normal years.
   C. In some dogs, alopecia is permanent.

TELOGEN AND ANAGEN DEFLUXION

Definition

I. Telogen defluxion and anagen defluxion are sudden hair losses induced by a variety of temporary stressful events that cause disruption of the hair cycle.
II. Anagen defluxion occurs when the active phase of hair growth (anagen) is temporarily interrupted.
III. Telogen defluxion occurs when the anagen phase of the hair cycle is shortened, and large numbers of hair follicles are simultaneously forced into the telogen (resting) phase.

Causes

I. Anagen defluxion
   A. Surgery
   B. High fever
   C. Metabolic and endocrine disorders
   D. Infectious diseases
   E. Antimitotic drugs: cyclophosphamide, methotrexate
II. Telogen defluxion

   A. Parturition, pregnancy
   B. Surgery, anesthesia
   C. High fever
   D. Shock
   E. Any severe illness
   F. Certain drugs: ampicillin, sulfonamides, hetacillin, heparin, thallium

Pathophysiology

I. In anagen defluxion, interruption in the growth process results in structural defects of the hair shaft and hair follicle. The hair resumes growth once the source of stress is removed, but the hair is weakened at these points and breaks easily.
II. In telogen defluxion, a large number of follicles are forced into the resting (telogen) phase at once. These synchronized follicles subsequently shed their hairs as a new hair cycle begins, resulting in alopecia.

Clinical Signs

I. Anagen defluxion
   A. Sudden onset of hair loss occurs several days to weeks following a stressful event.
   B. Because only the actively growing hairs are affected, some hair remains.
   C. The trunk may be the most severely affected area.
II. Telogen defluxion
   A. Sudden shedding of a large number of hairs occurs 2–3 months following a stressful event.
   B. By the time alopecia occurs, owners may have forgotten about the initial event.
   C. If the source of stress persists, as in an untreated endocrinopathy, alopecia may be persistent and progressive.
III. In both conditions, the hair regrows without treatment once the stressful insult is removed.

Diagnosis

I. A thorough history is necessary to determine the source of stress (i.e., illness, drug administration, surgery).
II. A careful physical examination should be performed; however, by the time the animal is presented for hair loss, the precipitating illness or stressful circumstance may have resolved.
III. A trichogram is helpful in determining whether anagen or telogen defluxion has occurred.
   A. 10–20 hairs are plucked, mounted in mineral oil, and examined microscopically.
   B. Anagen hairs are recognized by their larger root ends, which are surrounded by a root sheath. Telogen hairs have a club root with no root sheath.
   C. In anagen defluxion, a mixture of anagen and telogen hairs is present.
      1. The anagen hairs have structural abnormalities, including defects of the hair cortex and

irregular narrowing of the diameter of the hair shaft.
2. Hairs may be broken at the points of structural damage.
D. In telogen defluxion, all hairs are in the telogen phase, and the hair structure is normal.

Differential Diagnosis

I. Endocrinopathy
II. Pattern alopecia
III. Alopecia areata
IV. Feline symmetrical alopecia
V. Follicular dysplasias (for anagen defluxion)
VI. Excessive shedding

Treatment and Monitoring

I. Identify and eliminate the stressful insult.
II. A completely normal coat may not be evident for several months.

EXCESSIVE SHEDDING

Definition

Dogs and cats are occasionally presented to the veterinarian for shedding what the owner deems to be an inordinate amount of hair.

Causes

I. A number of factors influence the hair cycle and, therefore, the rate of shedding of the hair coat.
II. The diverse nature of dog and cat breeds and coat types results in differences in shedding.

Pathophysiology

I. Photoperiod is the predominant influencing factor. Seasonal changes in the amount of light exposure that the pet receives interact in a complex manner with numerous other factors to trigger shedding.
II. Other factors include ambient temperature, nutrition, hormones, general health, genetics, and certain poorly understood ''intrinsic factors.''

Clinical Signs

I. In temperate latitudes (northern United States and Canada), dogs and cats tend to shed more hair in the spring and fall.
II. Animals exposed to significant amounts of artificial light (those housed indoors) may shed throughout the year.

Differential Diagnosis

I. Anagen or telogen defluxion
II. Endocrinopathy

Treatment and Monitoring

I. Determine the general health and nutritional status to rule out illness, nutritional deficiencies, and anagen or telogen defluxion caused by various sources of physiologic stress.
II. Adjustment of light and temperature has been suggested as a method of altering shedding behavior, but it is not likely to be successful or practical for the dog or cat owner because of the complex interaction of factors that influence the hair cycle.
III. Provide regular grooming to remove dead telogen hairs.
IV. It is difficult to predict the degree and duration of shedding because of the highly variable nature of this process among different breeds and individuals.

POST-CLIPPING ALOPECIA

Definition

I. It is failure to regrow hair for up to 24 months following clipping and is relatively uncommon.
II. This syndrome occurs more frequently in breeds at increased risk for congenital adrenal hyperplasia-like syndrome.

Causes and Pathophysiology

I. The exact cause is unknown, although two theories have been proposed.
II. It may occur as the result of vascular perfusion changes in response to cutaneous temperature changes.
III. The hairs may also be in their catagen stage at the time of clipping.

Clinical Signs

I. Signalment
A. Commonly in Siberian husky and chow chow; possibly any dog
B. No age or sex predilection
II. Clinical picture
A. In the affected areas, the coat looks exactly as it did after clipping.
B. The remainder of the hair coat appears normal and does not epilate easily.

Diagnosis

I. History and clinical signs are strongly suggestive.
II. Rule out infectious skin diseases.
III. Rule out an endocrine disorder.

Differential Diagnosis

I. Infectious diseases: demodicosis, dermatophytosis
II. Endocrinopathies: hypothyroidism, hyperadrenocorticism, sex hormone abnormality
III. Other causes of localized alopecia: alopecia areata, sebaceous adenitis

Treatment

No therapy is necessary because most affected dogs regrow hair in the clipped areas after they go through a heavy shedding.

SHORT HAIR SYNDROME OF SILKY BREEDS

Definition

I. A rare condition of Yorkshire and silky terriers in which the long, silky hairs characteristic of these breeds are lost or fail to achieve full length.
II. Different forms affect juvenile and mature dogs.

Cause and Pathophysiology

I. The cause is unknown.
II. It is theorized that the hair cycle has been shortened by an unknown factor, resulting in the shedding of hairs before they reach their normal length.

Clinical Signs

I. Mature dogs
  A. The age of onset in these dogs is 1–5 years.
  B. The long hair coat is lost and replaced with hairs that never grow to full length.
  C. The new, shorter hairs appear structurally normal.
  D. The underlying skin is normal.
II. Juvenile dogs
  A. The abnormal coat becomes apparent at 5 months of age.
  B. The puppy coat is normal but is replaced with a permanent shorter coat, which never attains the correct length.

Diagnosis

I. Signalment, history, and physical examination are suggestive.
II. Perform a trichogram to ensure that hair is not being broken or chewed off. Hair tips should taper to a point.

Differential Diagnosis

I. Endocrinopathy
II. Congenital or hereditary disorders

Treatment and Monitoring

I. No treatment is available.
II. The abnormally short coat appears to be permanent.

Bibliography

Conroy JD: The etiology and pathogenesis of alopecia. Compend Contin Educ Pract Vet 1:806, 1979

Foil CS: Feline alopecia. Proc Am Coll Vet Dermatol 6:89, 1990

Griffin CE, Rosenkrantz WS, Tarvin G: Diseases of the external ear and pinna. p. 937. In Morgan RV (ed): Handbook of Small Animal Practice. Churchill Livingstone, New York, 1988

Miller WH: Symmetrical truncal hair loss in cats. Compend Contin Educ Pract Vet 12:461, 1990

Muller G, Kirk RW, Scott DW: Small Animal Dermatology III. WB Saunders, Philadelphia, 1983

Muller G, Kirk RW, Scott DW: Small Animal Dermatology IV. WB Saunders, Philadelphia, 1989

Reedy LM: Alopecia. p. 524. In Kirk RW (ed): Current Veterinary Therapy VIII. WB Saunders, Philadelphia, 1983

Scott DW: Feline dermatology 1900–1978: a monograph. J Am Anim Hosp Assoc 16:331, 1980

Scott DW: Feline dermatology 1979–1982: introspective retrospections. J Am Anim Hosp Assoc 20:537, 1984

Scott DW: Feline dermatology 1983–1985: "The secret sits." J Am Anim Hosp Assoc 23:255, 1987

Thoday KL: Differential diagnosis of symmetric alopecia in the cat. p. 545. In Kirk RW (ed): Current Veterinary Therapy IX. WB Saunders, Philadelphia, 1986

84

Infectious Skin Diseases

Karen L. Campbell
Carol S. Foil

BACTERIAL SKIN DISEASES

Karen L. Campbell

Surface Bacterial Infections

Acute Moist Dermatitis

Definition

Acute moist dermatitis (pyotraumatic dermatitis, "hot spots," moist eczema) is a rapidly developing, ulcerative inflammation of the skin resulting from self-inflicted trauma.

Causes

    I. Ectoparasites: fleas, *Sarcoptes, Demodex, Cheyletiella, Pelodera, Otodectes, Trombicula* (chiggers), etc.
   II. Allergies: parasitic, inhalant, dietary
  III. Localized irritations and inflammation
     A. Anal sac impactions/infections
     B. Otitis externa
     C. Foreign bodies
     D. Irritant contact substances
     E. Hair mats
     F. Musculoskeletal disorders, e.g., hip dysplasia, osteoarthritis, etc.
  IV. Behavioral disorders (see Chap. 116)

Pathophysiology

    I. The animal bites, rubs, or scratches at a part of its body in an attempt to alleviate an itch or painful stimulus.
   II. Self-induced trauma results in hair loss, excoriation, and serum exudation.
  III. Lesions rapidly progress in an itch-scratch cycle.
  IV. Secondary bacterial colonization is common; *Staphylococcus intermedius* is the most common isolate.

Clinical Signs

    I. Lesions develop rapidly.
   II. Typical lesions are red, moist, and weeping, with a coagulum of proteinaceous exudate in the center surrounded by a halo of erythematous skin.
  III. Hair loss is usually present in the center of the lesions.
  IV. The margins of the lesions are sharply demarcated from the surrounding normal skin and hair. "Satellite" papules or pustules are absent; when present, these are indicative of a deeper folliculitis, e.g., pyotraumatic folliculitis (Reinke and Stannard, 1987).
   V. Lesions are tender and painful to the animal.

Diagnosis

    I. History of acute onset
   II. Physical appearance of lesions
  III. Usually associated with an underlying painful or pruritic stimulus
  IV. Biopsy differentiation from pyotraumatic folliculitis

Differential Diagnosis

Rule out the following conditions with the test described.
    I. Dermatophytosis: fungal culture
   II. Demodicosis: skin scrapings, biopsy
  III. Candidiasis: cytology, culture
  IV. *Malassezia*: cytology
   V. Dermatophilosis: cytology, culture, biopsy
  VI. Pyotraumatic folliculitis: biopsy
 VII. Neoplasia: cytology, biopsy

Treatment

    I. Sedate animal to facilitate treatment, because lesions are extremely painful.
   II. Clip hair away.
  III. Cleanse affected area using a mild antiseptic, e.g., chlorhexidine-containing cleanser.
  IV. Topical antiseptics and/or astringents such as 5% aluminum acetate (Domeboro), 5% tannic acid with 5% salicylic acid and 70% alcohol (Tansal solution), and benzoyl peroxide gel (Pyoben gel, OxyDex gel) aid drying of the lesions.

V. Topical analgesic products may be helpful in breaking the scratch-itch cycle. Examples include topical diphenhydramine hydrochloride (Histacalm spray), lidocaine (Derma Cool), pramoxine hydrochloride (Relief Spray, Dermal-Soothe spray), and hydrocortisone (Cortisoothe).

VI. Dry, crusted lesions can be treated with topical antibiotic/corticosteroid creams or emollients (Panalog cream, Humilac).

VII. Break the scratch-itch cycle with an Elizabethan collar, a bucket, or tranquilization.

VIII. Short-term corticosteroids (prednisolone 1.1 mg/kg/day PO for 5 days) may be helpful in alleviating inflammation and breaking the itch-scratch cycle. *Caution: Do not* use in dogs with "satellite" papules and pustules surrounding the central lesions because these dogs have a deep suppurative folliculitis and require systemic antibiotic therapy.

IX. Systemic antibiotics are required only for cases with a deep suppurative folliculitis.

X. Eliminate or control the predisposing factors, including ectoparasites, allergies, otitis externa, etc.

Patient Monitoring

I. Recheck at 1 week.
  A. Topical therapy for lesions that are now dry is changed to softening creams or emollients (Panalog cream, Humilac).
  B. Nonresponding cases should be biopsied for histopathology and/or treated with systemic antibiotic therapy.

II. Institute appropriate prophylaxis.
  A. Control of ectoparasites
  B. Good dermal hygiene: baths, grooming, ear cleaning, anal sac evacuation
  C. Control of other predisposing factors

Skin Fold Dermatitis

Definition

I. Skin fold dermatitis (intertrigo, skin fold pyoderma) is produced by skin rubbing against skin.

II. Anatomic areas frequently involved include the following.
  A. Facial, nasal folds: brachycephalic breeds especially the Pekingese, English bulldog, and pug
  B. Lip folds: especially dogs with large lip flaps such as the spaniels and Saint Bernard
  C. Body folds: obese dogs, legs of achondrodysplastic dogs such as the dachshund and basset hound, necks of the Labrador retriever and Shar pei
  D. Vulvar fold: especially obese dogs with recessed vulvas
  E. Tail fold: under "corkscrew" tails of the English bulldog, pug, Boston terrier

Causes

I. Skin folds "trap" moisture from glandular secretions and excretions such as tears (facial folds), saliva (lip folds, any area being licked), or urine (vulvar fold).

II. "Trapped" moisture coupled with friction of skin rubbing against skin results in skin maceration and bacterial growth.

III. Bacteria acting on the secretions/excretions produce breakdown products with an unpleasant odor.

Clinical Signs

I. Facial folds may rub on the cornea and cause severe keratitis and ulceration.

II. Fetid odors are often a presenting complaint.

III. A seropurulent exudate is found in folds with bacterial colonization.

IV. Areas affected vary with the conformation of the dog with the skin usually being edematous and erythematous.

Diagnosis

I. Physical examination with the finding of a purulent exudate in the crevice of a body fold is diagnostic.

II. Swabs from the affected area can be smelled to prove that the odor is coming from the folds and not from halitosis.

Differential Diagnosis

I. Halitosis: vs. lip fold pyoderma

II. Neoplasia: vs. chronic skin fold pyodermas

III. Demodicosis: vs. facial fold pyoderma, body fold pyoderma

IV. Seborrheic skin diseases ("rancid fat odor"): vs. body fold pyoderma

Treatment

I. Weight reduction is beneficial for obese dogs.

II. Daily benzoyl peroxide washes (OxyDex shampoo, Pyoben shampoo) are palliative.

III. Surgical correction is curative in many cases.
  A. Removal of facial folds
  B. Cheiloplasty
  C. Episioplasty (vulvoplasty)
  D. Tail amputation

Patient Monitoring

I. If surgical correction is not possible, palliative treatment may be needed for the life of the dog.

II. Dogs with facial fold pyoderma should be started on ocular protective agents and monitored for irritation and pigmentation of the cornea.

Superficial Bacterial Infections
Impetigo
Definition and Causes

I. Impetigo is a superficial bacterial infection involving the nonhairy areas of the skin.

II. In dogs, the predominant organism is *S. intermedius,* with occasional isolation of *Pseudomonas* spp. or *Escherichia coli.*

III. In cats, the predominant organisms are *Pasteurella multocida* and beta-hemolytic streptococci.

Pathophysiology

I. Impetigo develops secondary to a variety of factors.
  A. Ectoparasites
  B. Viral infections, e.g., canine distemper
  C. Dirty environment
  D. Immunodeficiencies (see Chap. 73)
  E. Poor nutrition
  F. Endocrinopathies, e.g., hyperadrenocorticism, hypothyroidism, diabetes mellitus
  G. Overzealous "mouthing" of kittens by the queen
  H. Debilitation
II. Bacteria colonize skin damaged by ectoparasites, scratching, chewing, or adverse environmental factors.
III. Viral infections, poor nutrition, immunodeficiencies, and debilitation impair the skin's normal defense mechanisms, resulting in the establishment of a secondary pyoderma.

Clinical Signs

I. Small subcorneal pustules and yellowish crusts
II. Lesions not involving hair follicles
III. Minimal pruritus or discomfort
IV. Dogs: most common sites—the glabrous areas of the inguinal and axillary regions
V. Kittens: lesions usually on the back of the neck, head, and wither

Diagnosis

I. History and physical examination findings of nonfollicular subcorneal pustules are suggestive of the disorder.
II. Cytology from direct smears of the pustules reveals bacteria and neutrophils.
III. Cultures usually isolate bacteria from lesions.
IV. Biopsies with histopathology show nonfollicular subcorneal pustules.
V. Look for predisposing factors, such as ectoparasites, inadequate hygiene, poor nutrition, endocrine diseases, etc.

Differential Diagnosis

I. Superficial bacterial folliculitis
II. Subcorneal pustular dermatosis
III. Pemphigus foliaceus

Treatment

I. Correct any predisposing factors.
II. Begin daily antibacterial shampoos with benzoyl peroxide, chlorhexidine, or ethyl lactate.
III. Apply topical antiseptics, such as aluminum acetate wet dressings, benzoyl peroxide gel, povidone-iodine spray, or other antibacterial agents, e.g., mupirocin ointment (Bactoderm).
IV. Immunosupressed animals may require systemic antibiotics (see Treatment of Superficial Bacterial Folliculitis later).

Patient Monitoring

I. Recheck in 7–14 days.
II. Reevaluate cases that have not responded to topical treatment for other underlying disorders and start systemic antibiotics.
III. Watch for recurrences.

Superficial Bacterial Folliculitis

Definition and Causes

I. Superficial folliculitis is a very common bacterial infection involving hair follicles and the adjacent epidermis.
II. The primary organism involved is *S. intermedius*.
III. Predisposing conditions, especially in recurrent cases, are listed below.
  A. Ectoparasites: fleas, *Demodex*, etc.
  B. Allergies: fleas, dietary, inhalant, contact
  C. Endocrinopathies: hypothyroidism, hyperadrenocorticism
  D. Immunodeficiencies (see Chap. 73)
  E. Unsanitary environment
  F. Keratinization disorders (see Chap. 88)

Pathophysiology

I. The pathogenesis is not well understood.
II. Some dogs have depressed neutrophil function.
III. Some dogs have elevated levels of antistaphylococcal IgE with a possible type I hypersensitivity reaction to staphylococci resulting in pruritus and impairment of local defense mechanisms.
IV. Bacterial exotoxins or cell wall antigens may also elicit a type III hypersensitivity reaction.
V. Follicular inflammation stops the growth of hair and the hairs "fall out," resulting in circular areas of alopecia and a "moth-eaten" appearance to the hair coat.

Clinical Signs

I. The primary feature is a pustule with a hair shaft protruding from the center.
II. Secondary lesions include crusts, epidermal collarettes, hyperpigmentation, "bulls-eye" or "target" lesions with erythematous borders and clearing centers, excoriations, and alopecia.
III. Distribution patterns are variable.
  A. Truncal form with "moth-eaten" alopecia
  B. "Short-coated pyoderma," where follicular papules are common, resulting in a "lumpy bumpy" skin
  C. Less commonly superficial pustules in the axillary and groin regions

Diagnosis

I. Examine direct smears of pustules for staphylococcal organisms.

II. Obtain bacterial cultures for organism identification and antibiotic sensitivity.

III. Histopathologic findings from skin biopsies reveal a neutrophilic exudate within hair follicles.

IV. Look for any underlying, predisposing factors.

Differential Diagnosis

I. Rule out dermatophytosis with a fungal culture.

II. Rule out demodicosis with skin scrapings.

III. Rule out immune-mediated dermatoses with skin biopsies.

IV. If pruritus continues after resolution of the pyoderma, then consider ectoparasitism and allergies.

V. For recurrent cases, search for other predisposing diseases.

Treatment

I. Identify and correct any predisposing factors.

II. Systemic antibiotics are administered for a minimum of 7 days past complete resolution of clinical signs.
    A. Initial choices
       1. Erythromycin 10–15 mg/kg PO TID
       2. Lincomycin 20 mg/kg PO BID
       3. Clindamycin 5 mg/kg PO BID
       4. Ormetroprim-sulfadimethoxine 27 mg/kg PO SID
       5. Trimethoprim-sulfadiazine combinations 15–30 mg/kg PO BID
    B. Recurrent cases
       1. Amoxicillin–clavulanic acid 15–22 mg/kg PO TID
       2. Oxacillin 22 mg/kg PO TID
       3. Cephalexin 22–30 mg/kg PO BID

III. Bathe twice weekly with antimicrobial shampoos during episodes of pyoderma and as an aid in prophylaxis.
    A. Benzoyl peroxide is the most effective antimicrobial shampoo but may bleach hair and carpets and can be drying.
    B. Chlorhexidine is the second most effective antimicrobial shampoo.
    C. Ethyl lactate shampoos may also be useful.

IV. Immunomodulators may be considered for recurrent cases; few controlled studies have been done to document their efficacy.
    A. Staphage lysate 0.5 ml SQ twice weekly during initial treatment, then every 7–14 days for maintenance
    B. *Propionibacterium acnes* (ImmunoRegulin) 0.2–0.25 ml/7 kg IV q 3–4 days for 2 weeks, then weekly until condition is resolved
    C. Staphoid AB diluted 1:1 with saline and injected once weekly; dose is split with 0.1 ml ID and remainder SQ, starting with 0.25 ml total dose and increasing by 0.25 ml increments until reaching a dose of 2 ml (split 0.1 ml ID and 1.9 ml SQ)
    D. Autogenous bacterins (obtain from commercial or state laboratories, most require a liability release form to be signed by the owner)

E. Levamisole 2–3 mg/kg PO Monday, Wednesday, and Friday

F. Cimetidine 6–8 mg/kg PO TID

V. Extended antibiotic regimens may be indicated for animals that (1) have recurrences of pyoderma within days of finishing appropriate antibiotic therapy and (2) have failed to respond to adjuvant treatments including antibacterial shampoos, immunomodulators, and correction of predisposing factors.
   A. With pulse therapy, antibiotics are given at a full dosage every other week or at longer intervals.
   B. Low-dose continuous treatment is controversial because of the increased risk of developing drug resistance.

VI. *Do not* use corticosteroids because they will mask pruritus and dampen inflammation, which may increase the likelihood of relapses.

Patient Monitoring

I. Recheck at 7 days, and if no response has occurred, reevaluate the choice of antibiotics.

II. Recheck at the end of antibiotic therapy, making certain that antibiotics have been given a minimum of 7 days past complete remission of clinical signs.

III. Inform owner of the likelihood of recurrence, particularly if underlying diseases have not been detected and treated.

IV. Also monitor for evidence of adverse drug reactions.
    A. Evaluate tear production every 2–3 weeks while on sulfa-drug therapy.
    B. Instruct the owner to return the animal for reexamination if any new problems develop during therapy.

Dermatophilosis

Definition and Causes

I. Dermatophilosis (cutaneous streptothricosis) is an extremely rare, superficial, crusted dermatitis caused by *Dermatophilus congolensis*.

II. *D. congolensis* is a gram-positive actinomycetic coccus that is transmitted from carriers, usually farm animals.

Pathophysiology

I. Motile zoospores are released following contact with moisture.

II. The zoospores are chemotropically attracted toward carbon dioxide diffusing from the surface of skin that has been damaged by ectoparasites, minor trauma, maceration, inflammation, or infection.

III. The zoospores germinate to produce a filament that invades the epidermis.

Clinical Signs

I. The classic "paint brush" lesion is a crust with imbedded hairs. When the crust is pulled away, the skin underneath has an oval, bleeding, ulcerated surface caked with green purulent exudate.

II. Early lesions are erythematous papules and pustules with crusts that may expand to several centimeters in diameter.
III. Older lesions have dry crusts, scaling, hyperpigmentation, and alopecia.
IV. Lesions are usually located over the dorsal back, scapula, and lateral thighs.

Diagnosis

I. On direct smears of exudate and crusts, look for parallel rows of gram-positive cocci (''railroad tracks'').
II. To culture, grind crusts with sterile distilled water and incubate 30 minutes prior to inoculation of media.
III. Histopathology of skin biopsies shows a ''palisading'' crust with orthokeratotic-parakeratotic hyperkeratosis, neutrophils, and branching parallel chains of organisms.

Differential Diagnosis

I. Staphylococcal pyodermas: impetigo, superficial bacterial folliculitis
II. Acute moist dermatitis
III. Dermatophytosis
IV. Keratinization disorders
V. Zinc-responsive dermatitis
VI. Pemphigus foliaceus

Treatment

I. Start daily soaks with 10% povidone-iodine or 3% lime-sulfur solution.
II. Remove and destroy crusts by incineration or chemical disinfectants.
III. Institute systemic antibiotics for 7–10 days with tetracycline, ampicillin, or high doses of penicillin.
IV. Eliminate primary inciting factors such as moisture, ectoparasites, and trauma.

Patient Monitoring

I. Positive cultures may be obtained from the skin of healed cases for up to 15 months.
II. Instruct owners to return the animal for re-examination if new lesions develop.

Deep Bacterial Infections

Deep Folliculitis and Furunculosis

Definition

I. This is a follicular infection that breaks through the hair follicle to produce furunculosis and cellulitis.
II. Furunculosis occurs when hair follicles rupture and is frequently associated with tissue eosinophilia.
III. Folliculitis, furunculosis, and cellulitis are normally present as a pathologic continuum.
IV. They may be diffuse or may be localized to certain anatomic areas (e.g., nasal folliculitis and furunculosis, muzzle folliculitis and furunculosis, pododermatitis).

Causes

I. These conditions are secondary to other contributing factors.
  A. Demodicosis and other parasites
  B. Dermatophytes
  C. Hypothyroidism and hyperadrenocorticism
  D. Immunosuppression
    1. Inherited (see Chaps. 64, 73, and 82)
      a) Combined immunodeficiency: basset hounds
      b) Granulocytopathy: Irish setters, Doberman pinscher, Weimaraner
      c) Cyclic hematopoiesis: gray collies, Pomeranian, cocker spaniel
      d) Complement deficiency: Brittany spaniels
      e) Immunoglobulin deficiencies: many breeds
      f) Zinc deficiency: bull terriers
      g) Unknown type: German shepherd dogs
    2. Secondary to neoplasia
    3. Secondary to debilitation
    4. Iatrogenic from certain drugs: corticosteroids, azathioprine, methotrexate, and other chemotherapeutic drugs
  E. Foreign bodies
  F. Trauma
  G. Immune-mediated diseases
II. Many organisms have been isolated.
  A. *S. intermedius* (most common)
  B. *Proteus* spp.
  C. *Pseudomonas* spp.
  D. *E. coli*
  E. Hemolytic staphylococci

Pathophysiology

I. Folliculitis and furunculosis start as a surface or follicular infection.
II. Rupture of hair follicles results in a foreign body reaction to keratin and hair shafts. Initially tissue eosinophilia develops, and later a pyogranulomatous or granulomatous dermatitis occurs.
III. Muzzle folliculitis and furunculosis are most common in young short-coated breeds.
IV. In long-coated breeds, most lesions start as a pyotraumatic dermatitis that rapidly progresses to a deep folliculitis and furunculosis.

Clinical Signs

I. Lesions are usually follicular in origin.
  A. Early: clusters of papules and pustules
  B. Late: ulcers, fistulas, furunculosis, alopecia, and hyperpigmentation
II. In the short-coated breeds, they are most common over the abdomen, trunk, and pressure points.
III. Muzzle lesions (canine acne) involve the chin and lips.
IV. German shepherd dogs usually develop the disease during middle age.

A. Most are intensely pruritic with excoriation and crusts.
B. Lesions start on rump, back, ventral abdomen, and thighs.
C. Peripheral lymphadenopathy is common.

V. Long-coated breeds, such as the golden retriever, Irish setter, and Saint Bernard, have superficial ulceration with a moist exudate that becomes crusted with thickened skin and surrounded by satellite papules and pustules. These lesions are very pruritic and, in the early stages, resemble pyotraumatic dermatitis but rapidly progress to a suppurative folliculitis and furunculosis.

Diagnosis

I. History and physical examination findings are suggestive.
II. Cytology demonstrates degenerate neutrophils and phagocytized cocci in the exudate.
III. Bacterial culture and antibiotic sensitivity testing are indicated to document the presence of mixed bacterial infections (often *Staphylococcus* spp. plus a gram-negative bacterium) and select appropriate antibiotics for long-term therapy.
IV. Certain tests are needed to eliminate other cutaneous diseases.
  A. Skin scrapings to rule out *Demodex* cases
  B. Fungal cultures to rule out dermatophytes
  C. Skin cytology to rule out concurrent *Malassezia*
  D. Hemogram and serum chemistry panel to rule out systemic diseases
  E. Thyroid-stimulating hormone (TSH) response test (or thyroid hormone profiles if TSH not available) to rule out hypothyroidism
V. Immune function tests are necessary to identify the inherited immunodeficiency diseases.
  A. Immunoglobulin quantitation
  B. Lymphocyte transformation
  C. Bactericidal assay
  D. Chemotaxis assay
  E. Serum complement quantitation
VI. Skin biopsies help characterize the lesions, identify a cause, and rule out neoplasia.

Differential Diagnosis

I. Folliculitis, furunculosis, and cellulitis are almost always secondary to another clinical abnormality.
II. Differentiation of these lesions from superficial infections is made by the clinical findings of nodular lesions or fistulous lesions with satellite papules and pustules.
III. The diagnosis of a deep pyoderma with folliculitis, furunculosis, and cellulitis may be confirmed by skin biopsy and histopathology.

Treatment

I. Clip hair from the lesions.
II. Administer systemic antibiotics.
  A. Base choice on culture and sensitivity.

B. Continue for a minimum of 7 days beyond clinical resolution.
C. Total length of treatment is often 6–10 weeks.
III. Consider topical therapy to promote drainage and healing.
  A. Whirlpool baths
  B. Wet soaks several times daily with antiseptics (chlorhexidine, povidone-iodine, aluminum acetate)
IV. Localized lesions can be cleaned daily with benzoyl peroxide shampoos and topical benzoyl peroxide gel.
V. Correct all predisposing causes.

Patient Monitoring

I. Recheck at 7–10 days.
II. Discuss with owner the probability of relapse if the underlying cause is not identified and corrected.
III. Reevaluate every 3–4 weeks during therapy for side effects of medications and for 2–3 months following cessation of antibiotics for evidence of relapse.

Subcutaneous Cellulitis/Abscesses

Definition

I. Anaerobic cellulitis is a severe, deep, suppurative infection occurring in areas with low oxygen tension.
II. Subcutaneous abscesses are deep, suppurative infections and are most common in cats.

Causes

I. Cat fights: bite wounds, scratches
II. Dog bites
III. Other penetrating wounds and foreign bodies
IV. May also occur secondary to
  A. Diabetes mellitus
  B. Demodicosis
  C. Immunodeficiency: congenital or acquired
V. Aerobic organisms frequently found
  A. *Pasteurella multocida*
  B. Beta-hemolytic streptococci
  C. *Bacteroides* spp.
  D. Fusiform bacilli
  E. *Actinomyces* spp.
VI. Anaerobic organisms often originating from body fluids or feces
  A. *Clostridium* spp.
  B. *Bacteroides* spp.
  C. Peptostreptococci
  D. Enterobacteriaceae

Pathophysiology

I. Conditions that create a local decrease in oxygen tension predispose to anaerobic infections.
II. Contamination with body fluids (especially feces) provides bacterial inoculum.
III. Bacteria are often inoculated under the skin via a puncture wound, then the wound surface seals.
IV. Bacteria proliferate resulting in abscess formation, usually within 2–4 days after the injury.

V. Infection causes local pain.
VI. Gas may accumulate within the tissues.
VII. Bacterial toxins and tissue necrosis produce systemic toxicity.

Clinical Signs

I. Signs compatible with cellulitis
  A. Tissue edema and discoloration of overlying skin
  B. Depression, fever, malaise
II. Signs associated with subcutaneous abscesses
  A. Commonly located around tail base, neck, and shoulders
  B. May rupture and drain purulent material
III. Signs suggestive of anaerobic cellulitis
  A. Overlying skin is friable, darkly discolored, and often necrotic.
  B. Area of infection is poorly defined.
  C. Extensive edema and tissue gas accumulation may occur.
  D. Mixed anaerobic infections are often putrid.
  E. Animal may be systemically ill from toxins.

Diagnosis

I. History and physical examination
II. Cytology of exudate
  A. Degenerate neutrophils with phagocytosis of bacteria
  B. Gram's stain of exudate: often mixed infections with gram-negative rods, gram-positive rods, and gram-positive cocci
III. Aerobic and anaerobic culture and sensitivity testing

Differential Diagnosis

I. Cellulitis
  A. Sterile panniculitis
  B. Mycobacterial infections
  C. Neoplasia
II. Recurrent or nonhealing abscesses
  A. Feline leukemia or immunodeficiency viruses
  B. Sterile panniculitis
  C. Other less common infections capable of producing focal subcutaneous infections
    1. *Nocardia* spp.
    2. *Yersinia pestis*
    3. Mycobacteria
    4. Mycoplasma
    5. Cryptococcoses, blastomycoses, histoplasmosis
  D. Foreign bodies

Treatment

I. Surgically débride and remove any necrotic tissue.
II. Provide drainage for focal abscesses.
III. Use whirlpool therapy or wet dressings to improve drainage, increase circulation, and promote healing of both open and closed lesions.
IV. Institute antibiotics.
  A. *Clostridium* spp.: high dosages of penicillin
  B. Anaerobic infections (based on sensitivity testing)
    1. Clindamycin 5 mg/kg PO BID
    2. Amoxicillin 22 mg/kg PO, SQ BID
    3. Chloramphenicol 50 mg/kg PO, IV, SQ TID dog (BID cat)
    4. Metronidazole 25 mg/kg PO BID
  C. Aerobic infections
    1. Amoxicillin–clavulanic acid 15–22 mg/kg PO BID TID
    2. Oxacillin 22 mg/kg PO TID
    3. Cephalexin 22–30 mg/kg PO BID
V. Provide supportive care as needed.
  A. Nutritional intake sufficient to promote a positive nitrogen balance
  B. Antipyretics for fevers above 106°F (aspirin 10 mg/kg PO BID for dogs, 6 mg/kg PO QOD for cats)
VI. Correct predisposing factors.

Patient Monitoring

I. Recheck at 5–7 days.
  A. Swelling decreased, minimal drainage: remove drain, continue antibiotics for 2 additional weeks.
  B. No improvement: reopen sealed drainage holes, review antibiotic administration by owner, repeat culture and sensitivity, consider need for further débridement.
II. Castration is recommended for intact male cats to decrease roaming and fighting behavior.

Mycobacterial Infections
Definition

I. Mycobacteria are organisms of the genus *Mycobacterium.*
II. Atypical mycobacteria are acid-fast bacilli that normally exist as saprophytes in the environment and sporadically cause disease. They are subdivided based on their rate of growth and pigment production.
  A. Slow growing: more than 7 days
  B. Fast growing: less than 7 days
  C. Chromogens: pigment producing
    1. Photochromogens: produce yellow pigment in presence of light
    2. Scotochromogens: produce orange pigment independent of light
  D. Nonchromogens: do not produce pigment

Causes

I. Cutaneous tuberculosis
  A. *M. tuberculosis* (65–75% canine cases)
  B. *M. bovis* (25–35% canine cases)
  C. *M. avium* (very rare in dogs)
II. Feline leprosy
  A. Acid-fast tubercle
  B. Does not appear to be *M. lepraemurium* or *M. leprae*
III. Atypical mycobacteria species isolated from dogs and cats

A. *M. fortuitum, M. chelonei, M. phlei*
B. *M. xenopi, M. thermoresistibile, M. smegmatis*

Pathophysiology

I. Cutaneous tuberculosis
   A. Rare except in endemic areas
   B. Routes of exposure: close contact with infected owner or diet of contaminated meat or milk
II. Feline leprosy: natural mode of infection unknown
III. Atypical mycobacterial infections
   A. Organisms are ubiquitous in soil and water.
   B. Inoculation occurs through injury or injection.
   C. They cause chronic subcutaneous abscesses and fistulas.

Clinical Signs

I. Cutaneous tuberculosis
   A. Single or multiple ulcers, abscesses, plaques, and nodules
   B. Thick yellow-to-green purulent exudate
   C. Most common on the head, neck, and limbs
   D. Usually systemically ill with anorexia, weight loss, fever, and lymphadenopathy
II. Feline leprosy
   A. Single or multiple cutaneous nodules
   B. Ulcerative lesions or abscesses
   C. Usually involves young cats (1–3 years)
   D. Not systemically ill
III. Atypical mycobacterial infections
   A. Lesions develop slowly.
   B. Usual presentation is a chronic nonhealing wound.
   C. Soft tissue abscessation occurs with ulcers and draining fistulas.
   D. Common locations are often the groin, thorax, or abdomen.
   E. Animals are seldom systemically ill.

Diagnosis

I. Cutaneous tuberculosis
   A. History and physical examination
   B. Biopsy
      1. Pyogranulomatous inflammation
      2. Few-to-many acid-fast organisms
   C. Guinea pig inoculation with death in 6–8 weeks
   D. Calmette-Guérin bacillus test (dogs only)
      1. Inject 0.1 ml ID.
      2. Positive test is severe erythema with central necrosis and ulceration at 10–14 days.
      3. Normal dogs may ulcerate at the injection site around 18–21 days.
II. Feline leprosy
   A. History and physical examination
   B. Biopsy
      1. Epithelioid granulomas with sparse acid-fast organisms
      2. Lepromatous granulomas with abundant acid-fast organisms
   C. Guinea pig inoculation without death
III. Atypical mycobacterial infections

A. History and physical examination
B. Biopsy
   1. Nodular-to-diffuse dermatitis or panniculitis
   2. Acid-fast bacilli
C. Culture using blood agar, Löwenstein-Jensen medium, or Stonebrink's medium

Differential Diagnosis

I. Cutaneous tuberculosis
   A. Other mycobacterial infections
   B. Neoplasia
   C. Deep mycotic infections
   D. Foreign body abscesses
II. Feline leprosy
   A. Tuberculosis
   B. Atypical mycobacterial granulomas
   C. Deep mycotic infections
   D. Eosinophilic granuloma complex (see Table 85–2)
   E. Neoplasia
III. Atypical mycobacterial infections
   A. Tuberculosis
   B. Feline leprosy
   C. Panniculitis due to other causes
   D. Abscesses due to other causes

Treatment

I. Cutaneous tuberculosis
   A. Euthanasia of affected animal is recommended.
   B. Notify public health authorities.
II. Feline leprosy
   A. Surgical excision may be curative for solitary lesions.
   B. Medical therapy may be tried for multiple lesions or diffuse disease.
      1. Clofazimine 8 mg/kg/day PO × 6 weeks
      2. Dapsone 1 mg/kg PO BID × 4–6 weeks; may result in hemolytic anemia
III. Atypical mycobacterial infection
   A. Surgical excision may be curative for solitary lesions.
   B. Drainage with antiseptic lavages (chlorhexidine) is indicated for areas with cellulitis and/or panniculitis.
   C. Antibiotics are based on sensitivity testing. Continue treatment for a minimum of 6 weeks.
      1. Enrofloxacin 2.5 mg/kg PO BID
      2. Doxycycline 5 mg/kg PO BID
      3. Erythromycin 11 mg/kg PO TID
      4. Chloramphenicol 50 mg/kg PO TID dogs, BID cats
      5. Tetracycline 22 mg/kg PO TID
      6. Polymyxin 2 mg/kg IM BID

Patient Monitoring

I. Feline leprosy
   A. No known public health risk
   B. Best prognosis if lesions surgically removed
   C. Variable response to antibiotics
II. Atypical mycobacterial infections

A. Prognosis is guarded.
B. Lesions may spontaneously regress.
C. Recurrent fistulas are common.

VIRAL, RICKETTSIAL, AND PROTOZOAL SKIN DISEASES

Karen L. Campbell

See Table 84–1.

Feline Poxvirus Infection

Definition and Causes

I. Feline poxvirus is an orthopoxvirus similar in morphology to cowpox that produces skin lesions in cats, cows, and people.
II. The precise identity of feline poxvirus is controversial.
   A. Early reports of pox lesions in cats implicated the cowpox virus.
   B. More recent reports suggest the virus be named feline poxvirus or catpox.
III. The epizootiology of feline poxvirus is not known, but small wild mammals such as voles may be reservoirs.
IV. It has been reported in the United Kingdom and Europe.

Pathophysiology

I. Cases peak in autumn when the vole population is highest.
II. Pock lesions are first seen on the face and paws, often spread, and heal in 2–4 weeks leaving hairless skin.
III. Owners may also be affected, as it is a zoonotic disease.

Clinical Signs

I. May have history of a bite wound
II. Multiple circular 5–10 mm diameter skin lesions
III. Crusted papules, plaques, nodules, and crateriform ulcers
IV. Most common on face, limbs, paws, and dorsal lumbar area
V. Variable pruritus
VI. Systemic signs
   A. Anorexia, lethargy, pyrexia
   B. Vomiting, diarrhea
   C. Conjunctivitis
   D. Dyspnea, icterus

Diagnosis

I. History and physical examination
II. Skin biopsy
   A. Histopathology: epidermal hyperplasia, ballooning degeneration, reticular degeneration, microvesicle formation, necrosis of epidermis and outer root sheath of hair follicle; eosinophilic intracytoplasmic inclusion bodies within keratinocytes
   B. Electron microscopy of dried scabs for detection of viral particles within intracytoplasmic inclusions
   C. Virus isolation with hemorrhagic pocks on chorioallantoic membranes of chick embryos
III. Serology: single sample for virus neutralization titer (2–3 ml, refrigerated) sent to Liverpool University, Department of Clinical Pathology, P. O. Box 147, Liverpool L68 3BX England; 051-709-6022

Differential Diagnosis

I. Eosinophilic granuloma complex
II. Cutaneous bacterial infections
III. Cutaneous fungal infections
IV. Neoplasia

Treatment

I. Recovery is often spontaneous and occurs in 1–2 months.
II. Symptomatic treatment with broad-spectrum antibiotics can be administered to control secondary bacterial infections.

Table 84–1. **Skin Lesions Associated with Selected Viral, Rickettsial, and Protozoal Diseases**

Disease	Dermatologic Signs
Feline leukemia virus	Chronic or recurrent pyoderma, abscesses, and cellulitis Chronic paronychia Poor wound healing Seborrhea Generalized pruritus Lymphosarcoma
Feline immunodeficiency virus	Pustular dermatitis Chronic gingivitis Chronic stomatitis Chronic abscesses
Canine distemper virus	Nasal hyperkeratosis Digital hyperkeratosis ("hard pad") Pyoderma
Rocky Mountain spotted fever	Conjunctivitis Mucopurulent oculonasal discharge Lymphadenopathy Petechial and ecchymotic hemorrhages Edema of extremities and dependent areas
Leishmaniasis	Alopecia with silvery white scales Periorbital alopecia ("lunettes") Nasal depigmentation Long brittle nails Skin ulcerations (especially on limbs) Generalized nodular disease (boxers may be predisposed) Generalized skin pustules (trunk, abdomen, axillae, groin)

III. *Avoid* glucocorticoids because they have been associated with exacerbation of the condition.

Patient Monitoring

I. Evaluate for underlying immunosuppression.
  A. Feline leukemia virus (FeLV) and feline immunodeficiency virus (FIV) tests
  B. Biochemical profile
II. Have owners wear gloves when handling infected cats; cowpox virus is infectious to people, and cats have been implicated as a source of infection in several recent human outbreaks in Europe.

FUNGAL DISEASES

Carol S. Foil

Superficial Mycoses

Dermatophytosis

Definition

I. Dermatophytosis is an infection of keratinaceous structures (hair, claws, stratum corneum) by saprophytic or parasitic keratinophilic fungi.
II. Dermatophytosis of dogs and cats is a common (in cats) and underdiagnosed infection with zoonotic potential that is often confused with other common skin diseases.

Causes

I. A variety of free-living fungi, as well as dermatophyte species, may be isolated from the hair of normal dogs and cats.
  A. Both *Microsporum canis* and *M. gypseum* may be carried on dogs or cats following exposure to a contaminated environment.
  B. *M. canis* can cause an inapparent or subclinical infection in cats, especially those with long hair, and is of great epidemiologic significance in multicat households and as a potential source of zoonotic infections.
II. Most dermatophytosis in dogs and cats is caused by one of three species: *M. canis, M. gypseum,* or *Trichophyton mentagrophytes.*
  A. *M. gypseum* infections are more common in warm, humid climates and during warm seasons.
  B. *M. canis* causes 50–70% of dermatophytosis in dogs and 90–98% in cats.
  C. Other species isolated include both anthropophilic species, e.g., *Trichophyton rubrum,* and geophilic species, e.g., *M. cookei.*

Pathophysiology

I. In dogs and cats, dermatophytosis is largely an infection of the hair shaft and follicle structure (exception: *M. persicolor*).
II. Host responses to follicle infection vary and determine the clinical outcome of an infection.
  A. Young and immunosuppressed animals are more

likely to become infected and develop more severe infections, which may become widespread.
  B. Infections in healthy adult dogs are often self-limiting, because specific and nonspecific immunity and inflammation can eliminate the infection.
  C. Cats may fail to develop an effective response to infection and can develop persistent but relatively quiescent infections, which may be both widespread and subclinical.
  D. Infections with geophilic and unusual species of dermatophytes often cause highly inflamed lesions.
III. Transmission is via exposure of the surface of the skin to fungal arthrospores.

Clinical Signs

I. History usually of limited benefit
  A. Pruritus is variable.
  B. A history of immunosuppressive drugs or illness can occasionally be elicited when dermatophytosis is generalized.
II. Clinical findings in cats (highly variable)
  A. Irregular or circular alopecia with or without scale
  B. Miliary dermatitis
  C. Focal or multifocal pruritic dermatitis, especially concurrent with corticosteroid or megestrol acetate therapy
  D. Onychomycosis (rare)
  E. Granulomatous dermatitis
    1. Seen in Persian and Himalayan cats with generalized dermatophytosis
    2. One or more well-circumscribed, ulcerated or fistulated dermal nodules that have tissue grains apparent on cut surface
  F. Asymptomatic carrier
III. Clinical findings in dogs
  A. Classic ringworm: foci of alopecia with follicular papules at the periphery and scale admixed with crust
  B. Facial folliculitis and furunculosis: often associated with *T. mentagrophytes* infection
  C. Folliculitis/furunculosis localized to one limb or generalized
  D. Seborrheic syndrome with greasy scale
  E. Kerion
    1. Often from *M. gypseum* infection
    2. Exudative variably circumscribed nodule with either hyperkeratosis or crusting and ulceration on the surface
    3. Most often located on the face or limbs
  F. Onychomycosis (rare)
    1. Often associated with ungual fold inflammation, occasionally with footpad hyperkeratosis and crusting
    2. Brittle, misshapen, sloughing nails

Diagnosis

I. Fungal culture is necessary for definitive diagnosis.
  A. Collection of specimens

1. Choose new lesions or the progressing edges of active lesions and sample several sites.
2. Clip hair, pat with 70% alcohol, and dry.
3. Collect hair with hemostats and scale with a dull scalpel blade.
4. For onychomycosis, culture pieces of clipped nails or scale/hair from around affected claws.

B. Culturing technique
1. Use dermatophyte test medium (DTM) or other selective agar-containing bacterial and saprophytic fungal inhibitors and pH indicators to demonstrate the metabolic habits of dermatophytes.
2. Observe the specimens daily for a color change in the medium (red in DTM) that occurs simultaneously with fungal colony growth.

C. Culturing asymptomatic animals
1. Indications include culturing pets from households with an infected person, searching for asymptomatic carriers in catteries, or monitoring treatment.
2. A newly purchased or sterilized toothbrush is used to brush the entire coat for 1 minute, then the bristles are pressed directly into the surface of the culture medium.

II. Hair and scale can also be directly examined microscopically.
A. Specimens are mounted on a microscope slide in a drop of 10% KOH and inspected after 1 to several hours for fungal spores and hyphae.
B. The technique is time-consuming, requires practice, and is not as reliable as culturing.

III. Wood's light observation *cannot* be used alone to rule out the possibility of a dermatophyte infection.
A. *M. canis* infections often (50–80%) fluoresce.
B. A positive result is a *very* bright apple-green fluorescence within/along the hair shafts.
C. Greasy scale and medication can have a greenish hue under the light, giving a false-positive impression.
D. Always culture fluorescing hairs for confirmation.

IV. Biopsy is not as sensitive as culture results to diagnose dermatophytosis but can be used to confirm infection where the culture results are questionable.

Differential Diagnosis

I. Classic ringworm
A. Rule out staphylococcal folliculitis and demodicosis in the dog.
B. In the cat, any cause of alopecia can resemble dermatophytosis, so submit a fungal culture from all cats with skin disease.
II. Miliary dermatitis in the cat: allergies
III. Regional (facial or limb) or generalized folliculitis: staphylococcal folliculitis, demodicosis, autoimmune skin disease, especially pemphigus foliaceus
IV. Nodular dermatophytosis: other infectious and noninfectious granulomatous diseases, neoplasia
V. Onychomycosis: autoimmune disease, vasculitis, developmental claw defects, drug eruptions, bacterial and yeast infections

Treatment

I. Topical therapy
A. Clip lesions or entire body of long-haired cats and apply some form of topical therapy to reduce the spread of infectious organisms. (This may worsen the symptoms at first.)
B. Use antiseptic baths and rinses to remove scale, crusts, exudate, and infected hairs.
1. Useful shampoos: ketoconazole- or miconazole-containing formulations; used twice weekly
2. Medicated rinses: enilconazole (where available) or lime sulfur; applied twice weekly
C. For localized cases and single lesions, creams or lotions may hasten resolution.
1. Miconazole and clotrimazole are available in the United States; ketoconazole and enilconazole are also available in Europe.
2. Highly inflamed lesions may resolve faster if a combination of an imidazole and a topical corticosteroid is applied for a few days (Lotrisone or Tresaderm).

II. Systemic therapy: griseofulvin, ketoconazole, or itraconazole
A. Systemic therapy is not indicated in every case.
1. Localized dermatophytosis in healthy dogs is often self-limiting.
2. Highly inflamed localized dermatophytosis, such as in the kerion reaction, may not require systemic therapy.
B. Griseofulvin is not water soluble, and gastrointestinal absorption is variable and incomplete.
1. Absorption is enhanced by administration with a fat-containing meal and is affected by particle size.
2. Recommended dose for microsized griseofulvin in dogs and cats is 10–30 mg/kg PO BID for 4–6 weeks.
3. Recommended dose for ultramicrosized griseofulvin is 2.5–5 mg/kg PO SID-BID for 4–6 weeks.
4. Side effects are many and may be serious.
a) The most common are vomiting, diarrhea, and anorexia, which may be ameliorated by dividing the doses more frequently or lowering the dose.
b) The most serious side effect, generally seen in cats, is bone marrow suppression with neutropenia, anemia, or pancytopenia.
c) The hematologic side effects may be dose dependent or idiosyncratic; the latter are seen most often in FIV-infected cats (Shelton et al., 1990).
d) Griseofulvin is teratogenic; it should be avoided in the first two thirds of pregnancy.
C. Ketoconazole is a fungistatic agent that is moderately effective in dermatophytosis.

1. Recommended uses include animals that do not tolerate griseofulvine or in proven resistance to griseofulvin (rare).
2. It is also a useful agent in onychomycosis or chronic feline dermatophytosis, which may require months of therapy to clear.
3. Recommended dose is 10 mg/kg PO SID.
4. It should not be used in breeding animals.
5. Side effects include anorexia, hepatitis, pruritus, alopecia, and a lightening of the hair coat.

D. Itraconazole is a triazole antifungal agent that is secreted in sweat and sebum and binds to keratinocytes.
   1. It is the most efficacious antifungal agent. Side effects are minimal, but increased liver enzymes and/or icterus may be seen.
   2. It is renally excreted, so use with caution in animals with renal insufficiency.
   3. Recommended dose is 10 mg/kg PO SID for 3 weeks.

III. Environmental control
   A. Remove infected hair, scale, and debris from the environment via thorough vacuuming, washing with bleach, and discarding all bedding. Repeat for three cycles.
   B. Thoroughly disinfect or discard grooming implements.
   C. In affected catteries, identify infected cats by culturing lesions or brush-culturing asymptomatic individuals, and institute the following measures.
      1. Separation of infected cats from uninfected
      2. Thorough environmental decontamination
      3. Topical treatment of all cats
      4. Systemic treatment of infected cats
      5. Treatment of all kittens to eliminate sale of infected animals
      6. Follow-up brush cultures of all cats on a regular basis

Patient Monitoring

I. Patients should be treated for 1–2 weeks beyond a clinical cure as demonstrated by a negative brush culture.
II. Monitor animals on griseofulvin with a hemogram every 2 weeks and liver enzyme assays monthly.
III. Monitor liver enzymes initially, then every 4–6 weeks in animals on ketoconazole or itraconazole therapy.

Superficial Candidiasis

Definition

I. It is a rare local proliferation of *Candida* spp. on mucous membranes or on chronically traumatized or wet skin.
II. Because *Candida* spp. are normal flora of the oral, gastrointestinal, and genital mucosa, proliferation and disease would imply a predisposing injury or immunodeficiency.

Causes

I. *C. albicans* and *C. parapsilosis* are the most frequent isolates in clinical cases (Greene and Chandler, 1990).
II. *Candida* is a dimorphic fungus that usually exists as a small, thin-walled, oval yeast but can form blastoconidia, pseudohyphae, and branching septate hyphae in invasive disease.

Pathophysiology

I. When normal epithelial barriers are chronically disrupted or when normal microflora are disturbed by broad-spectrum antibiotic therapy, the yeast may proliferate.
II. Disease also develops in animals with profoundly disturbed cell-mediated immunity.
III. Infection may be superficial, invasive, or disseminated.

Clinical Signs

I. Lesions are most often found at mucocutaneous sites and ungual folds, but any chronically diseased skin such as skin fold dermatitis or burn sites may become infected.
II. Cutaneous and mucocutaneous lesions consist of erosions or shallow ulcers, with erythematous and slightly proliferative margins.
   A. Mucous membrane lesions may have whitish pseudomembranes.
   B. Skin and ungual fold lesions are exudative and covered with macerated crusts.

Diagnosis

I. Diagnosis is made with a combination of identification by culture and histopathologic or cytologic demonstration of epithelial invasion and colonization.
   A. Because *Candida* spp. are normal inhabitants, positive culture alone is not sufficient to establish a diagnosis.
   B. Submit tissue samples from skin or mucous membranes for fungal culture as well as pathologic examination.
   C. Cytology of scrapings or smears may reveal large numbers of yeasts.
   D. In disseminated disease, the organism can also be isolated from blood cultures.
II. Perform a systemic work-up to search for an underlying disease.

Differential Diagnosis

Note: Many of the diseases mentioned here can predispose to the development of superficial candidiasis, and thus the fungal infection may be a secondary complication.

I. Mucous membrane ulceration: autoimmune diseases (pemphigus vulgaris, bullous pemphigoid, systemic lupus erythematosus), drug eruption (erythema multiforme), toxic epidermal necrolysis, bacterial mucositis, vasculitis (including toxic and uremic vasculitis)

II. Mucocutaneous crusting and erosion: necrolytic migratory erythema (hepatocutaneous syndrome, diabetic dermatopathy), autoimmune diseases (pemphigus, bullous pemphigoid, systemic lupus erythematosus), drug eruption, cutaneous vasculitis

III. Cutaneous crusting erosions: *S. intermedius, Malassezia pachydermatis,* mixed bacterial infections, *Dermatophilus* infection (rare)

IV. Facial and ungual fold dermatitis: demodicosis, dermatophytosis, bacterial infection, and *Malassezia* dermatitis

Treatment

I. Identify and correct any predisposing causes.

II. Mucosal and cutaneous lesions can be treated with topical nystatin (BID-TID for 1–2 weeks) or ketoconazole (BID 1–2 weeks), or oral ketoconazole as described later.

III. In widespread or chronic disease, or when underlying problems cannot be corrected, systemic ketoconazole is the treatment of choice.
A. Dose is 5–10 mg/kg PO SID.
B. Extend treatment for several days beyond clinical resolution and repeat as needed if relapses occur.

Patient Monitoring

I. The prognosis varies with the underlying cause but is only fair in superficial candidiasis because relapses are common; systemic candidiasis carries a grave prognosis.

II. In superficial candidasis, response to treatment is usually rapid.

Malassezia (Pityrosporum) Dermatitis

Definition

I. It is a superficial seborrheic and/or pruritic dermatitis of dogs (and possibly cats) associated with overgrowth of *Malassezia (Pityrosporum) pachydermatis.*

II. An underlying keratinization and sebaceous gland dysfunction or immunodeficiency may also exist.

Causes

I. *M. pachydermatis* is a part of the normal flora of the external ear canal and moist fold areas of the skin in both dogs and cats.

II. The organism exists primarily as a yeast but can rarely develop hyphae and pseudohyphae.

Pathophysiology

I. Factors that may lead to yeast overgrowth and skin disease are incompletely defined.
A. In otitis externa, yeast overgrowth may be associated with ceruminous or allergic otitis or with antibiotic therapy.
B. In dogs, skin disease has been associated with a familial keratinization defect in West Highland white terriers (Scott and Miller, 1989).

C. The organism is frequently found at intertriginous sites in animals with other keratinization defects such as familial seborrhea oleosa of dogs or feline acne.

D. Other diseases that have been associated with overgrowth of *Malassezia* on the skin include hepatocutaneous syndrome (or liver disease), atopy, drug eruption, and antibiotic therapy (McNeil, 1991).

II. When organisms multiply in great numbers, a contact dermatitis-like inflammation seems to occur, which may involve irritant factors and/or specific hypersensitivity responses.

Clinical Signs

I. Canine dermatitis
A. It has features of both contact allergic dermatitis and seborrheic dermatitis: ventral distribution with marked, well-circumscribed erythema and pruritus, with greasy whitish or red-brown exudate.
B. Papular or pustular eruptions that resemble bacterial folliculitis may be found.
C. Chronic cases have marked seborrheic changes with lichenification, hyperkeratosis, and hyperpigmentation superimposed on erythematous skin.

II. Feline acne: poorly defined cause

III. Otitis externa (see Chap. 105)

Diagnosis

I. Diagnosis requires a combination of identification of the organism on affected skin and response to antifungal therapy.

II. Cytologic specimens may be collected in a variety of ways.
A. Very greasy or mucoid exudate may be scraped from the surface of the skin with a dull scalpel blade and smeared onto a slide for staining with Diff-Quik or Gram's stain.
B. Drier skin areas may be sampled with transparent tape or with slides prepared with transparent adhesive (Duro-Tak slides).
C. In feline acne, follicular material may be squashed and smeared on a glass slide.
D. In the author's opinion, more than five organisms per oil power field ($1000\times$) is abnormal.

III. The organism may be identified histopathologically in skin biopsy sections, but it is unusual to find organisms by this method when cytologic preparations have not revealed large yeast counts.

IV. The yeast may be cultured from skin surface swabs; however, it is difficult to quantify the numbers of organisms present by this method.

V. Response to antifungal therapy confirms the diagnosis.

Differential Diagnosis

I. The major differential considerations in the dog include the following.

Table 84–2. *Subcutaneous Mycoses of Dogs and Cats*

Disorder	Agents	Source	Clinical Findings	Diagnosis	Treatment

Sporotrichosis	*Sporothrix schenckii*	Moss, wood, bark, thorns	Nodules, ulcers: localized or widely disseminated	Pathology, fungal culture	Localized
					  Cat: Na iodide 0.5 ml 20%/5 kg/day PO
					  Dog: K iodide 0.4 ml SSKI/10 kg PO BID-TID
					Disseminated
					  Ketoconazole 10–20 mg/kg/day PO
					  Itraconazole 10 mg/kg/day PO

Zygomycosis	Mucorales[a] Entomophthorales[b]	Ubiquitous opportunists Saprophytes, insect bites?	Systemic disease possible Nodules and plaques and/or ulcers; infarction with Mucorales	Pathology *and* culture Cytology may be helpful	Based on in vitro sensitivity testing Amphotericin B and/or ketoconazole possibly useful Local hyperthermia may be useful in some. Response unpredictable
Hyalohyphomycosis	Nonpigmented fungi[c]	Soil saprophytes, opportunistic	Systemic or cutaneous disease Nodules, plaques, ulcers	Pathology *and* culture Fluorescent antibody tests for some agents	Based on in vitro sensitivity testing Ketoconazole for *Aspergillus* Response to therapy highly variable
Pheohyphomycosis	Pigmented fungi[d]	Saprophytes, opportunistic	Systemic or cutaneous disease Nodules, plaques, ulcers	As for hyalohyphomycosis	Cutaneous lesions: wide excision Medical treatment as for hyalohyphomycosis
Eumycotic mycetoma	Various fungi[e]	Saprophytes or plant pathogens Opportunistic, wound contamination	Nodules/swellings with tracts, tissue grains (black or white) Often on head or limbs	Cytologic examination of tissue grains Pathology and culture	Wide surgical excision/débridement Lesions on trunk often have visceral involvement Ketoconazole, itraconazole, or K iodide may be tried.
Pythiosis	*Pythium insidiosum* (a protozoan with fungal characteristics in tissue)	Exposure of (injured?) skin to contaminated swampy water Also gastrointestinal, disseminated forms	Plaque or erosion progressing to ulcerated nodule; possible cutaneous infarction	KOH exam of tissues Pathology and culture Fluorescent antibody test available	Wide surgical excision May try K iodide Does not respond to standard antifungal treatment

[a]Includes the genera *Rhizopus, Rhizomucor, Mucor, Mortierella,* and *Absidia.*
[b]Includes *Conidiobolus* (*Entomophthora*) and *Basidiobolus.*
[c]Agents that have been found in dogs or cats include *Aspergillus, Penicillium, Paecilomyces, Pseudoallescheria, Geotrichum,* and *Trichosporon.*
[d]Agents implicated in dogs and cats include *Xylohypha* (*Cladosporium*) *bantiana, Bipolaris* (*Drechslera*) *spicifera, X. emmonsii, Exophiala jeanselmei, Moniliella suaveolens, Phialomonium obovatum, Phialophora verrucosa, Alternaria alternata, Pseudomicrodochium suttonii, Scolecobasidium humicola,* and *Stemphyllium* spp.
[e]Black-grain mycetoma in dogs or cats: *Curvularia geniculata, Madurella grisea;* white-grain mycetoma: *Pseudoallescheria boydii, Acremonium hyalinum.*

898

Table 84–3. **Cutaneous Manifestations of Systemic Mycoses**

Disorder	Cutaneous Findings	Diagnosis	Differential Diagnosis

Cryptococcosis	± Associated with systemic disease
	Localized, multifocal, or disseminated
	Usually on face, especially near nares
	Nodules, ulcers with mucopurulent exudate
		Cytology
		  Aspiration or exudate
		    Wet mounts: KOH, new methylene blue
		    Dry smears: Diff-Quik, Gram's stain
		Biopsy for pathology, culture
		Latex agglutination
			Other granulomatous diseases: infectious and sterile
			Neoplasms: mast cell, basal cell, squamous cell
			Eosinophilic ulcer

Blastomycosis	Associated with disseminated disease[a]
	Common presenting sign (up to 40% of cases)
	Lesions variable: nodules, ulcers, tracts
	Hemorrhagic-purulent exudate
		Cytology
		  Aspiration, exudate, impression
		    Diff-Quik stain
		Biopsy for pathology, culture
		Serology, radiography
			Other pyogranulomatous diseases with systemic manifestations
			Other systemic mycoses, actinomycosis, nocardiosis, tuberculosis
			Metastatic or multicentric neoplasia: lymphosarcoma, multiple myeloma, mast cell tumor, systemic histiocytosis
			Toe lesions: trauma, neoplasia, foreign body
			Nasal lesions: other mycoses, neoplasia, autoimmune skin disease

Histoplasmosis	Uncommon manifestation of dissemination Nodules, ulcers, abscesses	As for blastomycosis	As for blastomycosis
Coccidioidomycosis	As for histoplasmosis	As for blastomycosis More difficult to diagnose cytologically from skin lesions	As for blastomycosis

[a]Inoculation blastomycosis is rare, results in localized cutaneous disease; may result from bite of infected dog.

A. Seborrheic dermatitis and contact dermatitis: most important
B. Allergic dermatitis
C. Sarcoptic mange
II. Feline acne is more commonly caused by bacterial follicle infections (see Table 88–3).

Treatment and Monitoring

I. Topical therapy is indicated when overgrowth is identified.
  A. Treat *Malassezia* dermatitis in dogs with selenium disulfide, chlorhexidine, or ketoconazole- or miconazole-containing shampoos every other day until resolution of clinical signs, then once or twice weekly for maintenance.
  B. Use benzoyl peroxide or chlorhexidine-containing preparations or antifungal lotions for feline acne.
II. Systemic therapy is warranted when topical therapy fails or when it is necessary to have a very rapid resolution of symptoms.
  A. Ketoconazole or itraconazole is given at 5–10 mg/kg PO SID-BID for at least a month beyond resolution of signs.
  B. Response to treatment is usually rapid and dramatic.
  C. Relapse after the cessation of therapy is common and may, in some cases, be prevented with topical shampoo therapy or intermittent ketoconazole (pulse) therapy.
  D. Concurrent bacterial pyoderma is common and is treated with appropriate antibiotics (e.g., cephalexin).

Subcutaneous Mycoses

See Table 84–2.

Systemic Mycoses

See Table 84–3.

Bibliography

Abramson JS, Dahl MV, Walsh D et al: Antistaphylococcal IgE in patients with atopic dermatitis. J Am Acad Dermatol 7:105, 1982

Becker AM, Janik TA, Smith EK et al: *Propionibacterium acnes* immunotherapy in chronic recurrent canine pyoderma. An adjunct to antibiotic therapy. J Vet Intern Med 3:26, 1989

Bennet M: The laboratory diagnosis of orthopoxvirus infection in the domestic cat. J Small Anim Pract 26:653, 1985

Bevier DE: Canine staphylococcal pyoderma. Choosing the appropriate antibiotic. Vet Med Report 2:288, 1990

Center SA: Multiple cutaneous horns on the footpads of a cat. Fel Pract 12:26, 1982

Chapman WL Jr, Hanson WL, Alving CR, Hendricks LD: Antileishmanial activity of liposome-encapsulated meglumine antimonate in the dog. Am J Vet Res 45:1028, 1984

Chong H: Oriental sore. A trend in and approaches to the treatment of leishmaniasis. Int J Dermatol 25:615, 1986

DeBoer DJ: Strategies for management of recurrent pyoderma in dogs. Vet Clin North Am [Small Anim Pract] 20:1509, 1990a

DeBoer DJ: Canine staphylococcal pyoderma. Newer knowledge and therapeutic advances. Vet Med Report 2:254, 1990b

DeBoer DJ, Moriello KA, Thomas CB et al: Evaluation of a commercial staphylococcal bacterin for management of idiopathic recurrent superficial pyoderma in dogs. Am J Vet Res 51:636, 1990

Donnelly TM, Jones MR: Diffuse cutaneous granulomatous lesions associated with acid-fast bacilli in a cat. J Small Anim Pract 23:99, 1982

Ferrer L, Rabanal R, Fonderila D et al: Skin lesions in canine leishmaniasis. J Small Anim Pract 29:381, 1988

Gardner SA: Current concepts of feline immunodeficiency virus infection. Vet Med 86:300, 1991

Greene CE, Chandler FW: Candidiasis. p. 723. In Green CE (ed): Infectious Diseases of the Dog and Cat. WB Saunders, Philadelphia, 1990

Ihrke PJ: The management of canine pyodermas. p. 505. In Kirk RW (ed): Current Veterinary Therapy VIII. WB Saunders, Philadelphia, 1983

Ihrke PJ: Therapeutic strategies involving antimicrobial treatment of the skin in small animals. J Am Vet Med Assoc 185:1165, 1984

Ihrke PJ: An overview of bacterial skin disease in the dog. Br Vet J 143:112, 1987

Keenan CM: Visceral leishmaniasis in the German shepherd dog. I. Infection, clinical disease, and clinical pathology. Vet Pathol 21:74, 1984a

Keenan CM: Visceral leishmaniasis in the German shepherd dog. II. Pathology. Vet Pathol 21:80, 1984b

Kirkpatrick CE: *Leishmania chagasi* and *L. donovani*: experimental infections in domestic cats. Exp Parasitol 58:125, 1984

Kunkle GA: Clinical management of canine pyoderma. Proc Annu Kal Kan Symp 11:55, 1987

Kwochka KW, Kowalski JJ: Prophylactic efficacy of four commercial antimicrobial shampoos against *Staphylococcus intermedius* in dogs. Am J Vet Res 52:115, 1991

Longstaffe JA, Guy MW: Canine leishmaniasis—United Kingdom update. J Small Anim Pract 27:663, 1986

Martin WB: Poxvirus infection of cats. Vet Rec 115:36, 1984

Mason KV, Evans AG: Dermatitis associated with *Malassezia pachydermatis* in 11 dogs. J Am Anim Hosp Assoc 27:13, 1991

McNeil PE: *Pityrosporum* in canine skin biopsies. Br Vet Derm Newsletter 13:17, 1991

Moriello KA: The cutaneous mycoses of dogs and cats. Vet Med Report 1:1, 1988

Moriello KA, DeBoer DJ: Fungal flora of the coat of pet cats. Am J Vet Res 52:602, 1991

Muller GH, Kirk RW, Scott DW: Small Animal Dermatology. 4th Ed. WB Saunders, Philadelphia, 1989

Mundell AC: Effectiveness of clofazimine in the treatment of feline leprosy. Proc Am Acad Vet Derm 4:44, 1988

Nelson DA: Clinical aspects of cutaneous leishmaniasis acquired in Texas. J Am Acad Dermatol 12:985, 1985

Quaife RA, Womar SM: *Microsporum canis* isolations from show cats. Vet Rec 110:333, 1982

Reinke SI, Stannard A: Histopathologic features of pyotraumatic dermatitis. J Am Vet Med Assoc 190:57, 1987

Scott DW, Miller WH: Epidermal dysplasia and *Malassezia pachydermatis* infection in West Highland white terriers. Vet Dermatol 1:25, 1989

Shelton GH, Grant CK, Linenberger ML et al: Severe neutropenia associated with griseofulvin therapy in cats with feline immunodeficiency virus infection. J Vet Intern Med 4:317, 1990

Snider WR: Tuberculosis in canine and feline populations. Review of the literature. Am Rev Respir Dis 104:877, 1971

Swango LJ, Bankemper KW, Kong LI: Bacterial, rickettsial, protozoal, and miscellaneous infections. p. 265. In Ettinger SJ (ed): Textbook of Veterinary Internal Medicine. 3rd Ed. WB Saunders, Philadelphia, 1989

Thomsett LR: Cowpox in cats. J Small Anim Pract 30:236, 1989

Ward JM: *M. fortuitum* and *M. chelonei*: fast growing mycobacteria. Br J Dermatol 92:453, 1975

White PD, Kowalski JJ: Enrofloxacin-responsive cutaneous atypical mycobacterial infection in two cats. Proc Am Acad Vet Derm 7:95, 1991

White SD, Caprille KA: Maintenance antibacterial agents in recurrent pyoderma. Vet Med Report 2:296, 1990

Willemse A, Egberink HF: Transmission of cowpox virus infection from domestic cat to man. Lancet 1:1515, 1985

Wisselink MA, Bernardina WE, Willemse A et al: Immunologic aspects of German shepherd dog pyoderma. Vet Immunol Immunopathol 19:67, 1988

85

Inflammatory Skin Diseases

Karen A. Moriello

EOSINOPHILIC INFLAMMATORY DISEASES

Feline Eosinophilic Ulcers, Plaques, and Granulomas

Definition

I. Feline eosinophilic ulcer (indolent ulcer, rodent ulcer) is a common painless unilateral or bilateral erosion on the upper lip of cats.

II. Eosinophilic plaques are raised, focal areas of intense pruritus occurring on haired skin; the intense pruritus results in self-mutilation, and the area becomes ulcerated, excoriated, and exudative.

III. Feline eosinophilic granuloma is predominantly an asymptomatic skin disease characterized by linear or nodular areas of dermal collagen necrosis that clinically appear as well-circumscribed raised, firm to hard, nodular or linear masses in the skin of cats, particularly in young cats.

IV. Feline eosinophilic ulcer, plaque, and granuloma are distinct clinical entities; however, one or more may be present at the same time on a cat.

V. These three entities appear to be related because they all are probably common manifestations of feline allergic skin disease.

Causes and Pathophysiology

I. The cause of ulcers, plaques, and granulomas is unknown but is hypothesized to be the result of type I hypersensitivity reactions.

II. The most commonly recognized hypersensitivity reactions include flea allergy dermatitis, atopy, and insect-bite hypersensitivity, and food allergy.

III. Eosinophilic ulcers develop as a result of the influx of inflammatory cells, particularly eosinophils and neutrophils, and not from self-trauma.

IV. Eosinophilic plaques are intensely pruritic, and le-

sions are most likely the result of self-trauma/self-mutilation.

V. Eosinophilic granulomas develop spontaneously and do not appear to be the result of self-trauma but may develop in response to chronic antigenic stimulation.

VI. Some cats may be genetically predisposed to develop lesions; lesions often spontaneously resolve (Power and Ihrke, 1995).

Clinical Signs

Differentiating features are summarized in Table 85–1.

Diagnosis

I. Presumptive diagnosis is often made by clinical appearance, especially with eosinophilic ulcers.

II. Skin biopsy is diagnostic for eosinophilic plaque and linear granuloma but not necessarily for eosinophilic ulcer (see Table 85–1).

III. Peripheral blood eosinophilia is unpredictable, does not accurately reflect tissue eosinophilia, and may occur in response to the underlying allergic disease, rather than the ulcer, plaque, or granuloma.

IV. Cytologic examination of a fine-needle aspirate of an ulcer or granuloma, or impression smear of exudate from a plaque, may show eosinophils, mast cells, and other inflammatory cells; this test is not diagnostic.

V. Search for underlying causes such as flea allergy dermatitis, food allergy, insect-bite hypersensitivity, atopy, or other unidentified allergic diseases.

VI. The presence or absence of seasonal occurrence, location on the body, and combination with other lesions may be suggestive of an underlying cause.

A. Food allergy should be suspected in the following cases.

1. Recurrent eosinophilic ulcers, particularly in young cats

2. Recurrent granulomas on the head, ears, lip, or chin

3. Nonseasonal eosinophilic plaques on the head

Table 85–1. Feline Eosinophilic Inflammatory Diseases

Condition	Most Common Locations	Clinical Appearance	Pain/Pruritus	Biopsy Findings
Indolent ulcer	Upper lips at border of lip and haired skin	Well-circumscribed, red-brown, hairless, glistening depression with a raised border. Lip and margins look as if they are "melting away." Unilateral or bilateral	Rare	Nonspecific superficial perivascular dermatitis with a hyperplastic ulcerated epidermis is found. Fibrosing dermatitis may be present.
Eosinophilic plaque	Haired skin: ventral abdomen, inner thigh, face, neck, base of tail	Round to oval, well-circumscribed raised areas. The surface is often bright red and ulcerated. Serum and exudate ooze from the area, matting surrounding hair. Old lesions may be yellow-brown as a result of dried blood and exudate.	Intense	Superficial and deep perivascular dermatitis with focal to diffuse eosinophilic dermatitis is present. Spongiosis of the epidermis and outer root sheath is a key diagnostic finding. Eosinophilic microvesicles and microabscesses, ulceration, serocellular crusts, and large numbers of mast cells in the dermis are common findings.
Eosinophilic granuloma	Caudal thigh, chin, lips, and ears	Raised, firm to hard, well-circumscribed nodules. Nonexudative, hair intact. Yellow to pink discoloration of the skin. Lesions on chin or lip make cat look as if the cat has a "fat lip" or is "pouting." Lesions may be single or multiple. Females may be predisposed.	Rare	Nodular to diffuse granulomatous dermatitis with multifocal areas of collagen degeneration is found. Eosinophils and multinucleated giant cells may be seen. Palisading granuloma formation around foci degenerating collagen is common.
Feline hypereosinophilic syndrome	Multisystemic disease: affects internal organs, rarely skin involvement	Skin: diffuse maculopapular eruption and erythema Systemic signs: vomiting, diarrhea, weight loss, anorexia, weakness	Intense	Marked to severe infiltrate of skin and other organs with eosinophils is the primary finding.
Feline insect hypersensitivity	Dorsal muzzle, ears, junction of pads and haired skin, and other thinly haired areas	Glistening ulcerative lesions with or without crusted papular lesions	Common and variable in intensity	Superficial and deep eosinophilic inflammation in a perivascular to diffuse pattern. Collagen degeneration is common.

and/or neck with or without concurrent ulcers or granulomas
B. Flea allergy dermatitis should be suspected in the following cases.
   1. In northern climates, seasonal eosinophilic plaques occurring on the neck, abdomen, base of tail, or inner thigh
   2. In southern climates, nonseasonal eosinophilic plaques occurring anywhere on the body, especially if miliary dermatitis is present concurrently
   3. Nodular eosinophilic granulomas occurring on the head and neck
C. Feline atopy should be suspected in the following cases.
   1. Recurrent ulcers that are not caused by food allergy
   2. Recurrent ulcers that are increasingly more refractory to antibiotic or glucocorticoid therapy
   3. Eosinophilic plaques that are not caused by food allergy or flea allergy
   4. Eosinophilic plaques that are initially responsive to glucocorticoid therapy but become recurrent and more difficult to treat
D. Insect-bite hypersensitivity should be suspected in the following cases.
   1. Cats that go outdoors, especially when mosquitoes, gnats, and other biting insects are prevalent
   2. Cats with ulcerative to papular lesions on the thinly haired areas of the dorsal muzzle, ear tips, and/or junction of the pad and haired skin
   3. Cats with onset of lesions during the spring or a history of seasonal dermatopathies

Differential Diagnosis

I. Eosinophilic ulcers
   A. Infectious ulcers: deep bacterial, systemic fungal, feline immunodeficiency virus (FIV) or feline leukemia virus (FeLV) associated
   B. Trauma
   C. In young cats, focal necrosis from electrical cord bite
   D. Neoplasia: squamous cell carcinoma, mast cell tumor, lymphosarcoma
   E. Chemical and thermal burns
II. Eosinophilic plaques
   A. Infectious cutaneous ulcers: bacteria, dermatophytes, sporotrichosis, FIV- or FeLV-associated nonhealing wounds
   B. Neoplasia: lymphosarcoma, mast cell tumor
   C. Feline eosinophilic syndrome (see Table 85–1)
III. Eosinophilic granuloma
   A. Infectious granulomas (see Table 85–2)
   B. Neoplasia

Treatment

I. Indolent ulcer
   A. Lesions in young cats may respond to antibiotic therapy for 21 days.
      1. Trimethoprim-sulfadiazine 30 mg/kg PO BID
      2. Cefadroxil 22 mg/kg PO BID
      3. Amoxicillin clavulanate 20 mg/kg PO TID
   B. Induce remission with glucocorticoids; injectable agents are often the treatment of choice.
   C. Give methylprednisolone acetate 20–40 mg/cat SQ or IM every 2 weeks until the ulcer is healed. In severe cases, this may require more than six treatments.
   D. Try prednisolone 4.4 mg/kg PO SID until the lesion is completely healed. For unknown reasons, oral prednisolone often is less efficacious than parenteral glucocorticoids in treatment of indolent ulcers.
   E. Lesions may require up to 8–12 weeks to heal.
   F. Idiopathic recurrent ulcers may be treated with long-term corticosteroids alone or in combination with chlorambucil (0.1–0.2 mg/kg PO QOD-SID) or chrysotherapy at 1 mg/kg IM q 7 days until lesion is in remission and then slowly tapered to every 30 days.
II. Eosinophilic plaques
   A. Severely exudative lesions may be secondarily infected and require antibiotic therapy.
      1. Clean with chlorhexidine shampoo or solution SID-BID.
      2. Administer ampicillin 20 mg/kg PO TID for 7–10 days.
   B. Use an Elizabethan collar, bandages on the hind feet, adhesive nail covers, and/or a cotton stockingette on the cat's body to prevent continued self-trauma.
   C. Alleviate pruritus with acepromazine 1–2 mg/kg PO BID or chlorpheniramine maleate 2–4 mg/cat PO BID or TID.
   D. The use of corticosteroids concurrently with antibiotics is best avoided.
      1. Many cats respond very well to the previous three treatment steps (A–C) and do not require exogenous corticosteroids.
      2. Identification of the underlying cause is often delayed significantly or complicated by the use of corticosteroids.
      3. Corticosteroids interfere with wound healing and the body's cellular response to bacterial infections.
   E. If the cat is still pruritic after the secondary bacterial infection has resolved, induce lesion remission as described earlier for indolent ulcer.
III. Eosinophilic granuloma
   A. Many lesions spontaneously regress without treatment, especially in young cats.
   B. Treatment is not necessary unless the lesion is of discomfort to the cat, disfiguring, or displeasing to the owner.
   C. If treatment is indicated, induce lesion remission as described earlier for indolent ulcer.
   D. Persistent or recurrent lesions are uncommon and warrant further diagnostic testing for allergic diseases.
IV. Specialized diagnostic testing/therapy
   A. Diet challenge

1. Begin the diet trial after the lesion has been treated successfully with glucocorticoids or after the lesion has healed. It is optimal to begin the diet trial 2 weeks prior to the anticipated recurrence of the ulcer, plaque, or granuloma.
2. A commercial or homemade diet consisting of rabbit, venison, or lamb mixed with cooked whole grain rice is fed exclusively for 10 weeks. Diets containing fish, chicken or turkey, or beef are not suitable because these are common ingredients in commercial cat foods.
3. At the end of the diet trial, the patient's response to the diet is noted and the former diet reinstituted. If a food allergy is present, the lesion will begin to recur within 1–3 weeks of reinstituting the former diet.

  B. Flea control (see Chap. 87)

  C. Intradermal skin testing

1. It is recommended that a food trial and flea control be prescribed before performing intradermal skin testing.
2. Glucocorticoids must be withdrawn for a minimum of 6 weeks prior to intradermal skin testing. Injectable or long-acting glucocorticoids may require a withdrawal period of more than 12 weeks before testing.

V. Alternative therapies

  A. Inadequate response to therapy is often caused by too short a duration of therapy, too small a dose of glucocorticoids, patient or owner noncompliance, or failure to recognize an underlying cause.

  B. Idiopathic recurrent lesions may become refractory to methylprednisolone, prednisone, or prednisolone.

1. If this therapy is ineffective, use alternative glucocorticoids, e.g., triamcinolone, dexamethasone, betamethasone, or flumethasone.
2. Intralesional injection of glucocorticoids is difficult to do without chemical restraint; in addition it is often painful. There is no objective evidence to suggest that this technique is superior to intramuscular or subcutaneous administration of glucocorticoids.
3. Megestrol acetate has been used successfully in the treatment of ulcers, plaques, and granulomas; however, it is not recommended because of potential for severe side effects (diabetes mellitus, adrenocortical suppression).
4. Surgical excision, cryotherapy, radiation, and laser therapy have been used in rare instances with occasional success (Manning, 1987).

Patient Monitoring

I. The ulcer, plaque, or granuloma is measured before and during the treatment period to determine whether therapy is effective.

II. In most cases, a noticeable decrease in the size or number of the ulcer, plaque, or granuloma(s) should be seen within 7–14 days of the initiation of therapy.

III. If the ulcer, plaque, or granuloma is recurrent, it is important to identify the pattern of recurrence because this will aid in evaluating the response to special diagnostic testing.

Canine Sterile Eosinophilic Pustulosis

Definition and Cause

I. This is a rare idiopathic skin disease of dogs.

II. This disease is characterized by a peripheral eosinophilia, sterile pustules, eosinophilic infiltration of pustules, and marked responsiveness to systemic glucocorticoids (Scott, 1984, 1987).

III. The cause is unknown.

Clinical Signs

I. There is no known age, sex, or breed predilection.

II. The disease manifests as an acute onset of multifocal or generalized pruritic, follicular, and nonfollicular papules and pustules that develop into epidermal collarettes and erosions.

III. Lesions may appear clinically identical to a superficial pyoderma.

IV. Affected dogs may be febrile, anorexic, or depressed, with a peripheral lymphadenopathy.

Diagnosis

I. Perform a touch preparation of a pustule.

  A. Bacteria should not be present.

  B. Direct smears reveal large numbers of eosinophils with lesser numbers of nondegenerative neutrophils and occasional acantholytic cells.

II. Bacterial culture of pustules shows no growth of bacteria.

III. Biopsy a representative pustule.

  A. Histopathology reveals intraepidermal eosinophilic pustular dermatitis, folliculosis, and/or furunculosis.

  B. Direct immunofluorescence of tissue is negative.

IV. Repeated hemograms show a persistent eosinophilia.

Differential Diagnosis

I. Bacterial pyoderma may be clinically indistinguishable, but bacterial culture, cytology of a pustule, and response to antibiotic therapy differentiate these two skin diseases.

II. Demodicosis may mimic any skin disease, but deep skin scrapings of suspect lesions should reveal mites.

III. Pemphigus foliaceus may be difficult to differentiate from sterile eosinophilic pustulosis.

  A. Skin biopsy of pemphigus foliaceus shows intragranular or subcorneal acantholysis with cleft or pustule formation. Eosinophils are less prominent, but they may be present in large numbers.

  B. Direct immunofluorescence of a pustule shows intercellular fluorescence; however, in many cases such testing is negative.

C. Bacterial culture of a pustule is negative.

D. Cytologic examination of pustule exudate shows neutrophils, no bacteria, and rafts of acanthocytes; acanthocytes are not a feature of canine eosinophilic pustulosis.

IV. Systemic lupus erythematosus (SLE) may mimic any skin disease.

A. Multisystemic organ involvement is present in SLE.

B. Antinuclear antibody assay ideally is positive.

C. Skin biopsy most commonly shows interface and or a lichenoid dermatitis involving both the basement membrane zone and outer root sheath of the hair follicles.

Treatment

I. Most dogs respond well to oral glucocorticoids.

II. Prednisolone 2.2–4.4 mg/kg PO daily for 5–10 days induces lesion remission, prevents development, or causes obvious healing of new lesions.

A. Alternate-day glucocorticoid therapy is instituted as soon as lesion remission is obvious.

B. Life-long therapy is almost always necessary, as cessation of therapy results in relapses.

C. The dose of oral glucocorticoids may be reduced by using concurrent azathioprine at 2.2 mg/kg PO SID-QOD.

Patient Monitoring

I. This disease is not life-threatening, but the pruritus is distressing to both the dog and owner.

II. After clinical normalcy has been established, animals should be rechecked bimonthly for evidence of relapses or adverse reactions to therapy.

A. Long-term glucocorticoid therapy eventually results in clinical and biochemical findings consistent with iatrogenic hyperadenocorticism and chronic glucocorticoid administration.

B. Silent urinary tract infections are common in dogs receiving long-term glucocorticoid therapy, so urinalysis and urine culture via cystocentesis is recommended every 4–6 months.

C. Patients are at risk for becoming unresponsive to prednisolone if used long term (steroid tachyphylaxis). Equivalent doses of triamcinolone, betamethasone, or flumethasone are recommended as alternatives.

GRANULOMATOUS INFLAMMATORY DISEASES

Granulomatous Dermatitis

Definition and Causes

I. A granuloma is a response to a foreign substance in the skin that has resisted routine destruction by acute inflammation.

II. Granulomatous dermatitis is the reaction of the host to a persistent foreign agent. The inciting cause may or may not be infectious.

III. Granulomatous dermatitis has many causes, including bacteria, fungi, algae, parasites, hypersensitivity reactions, metabolic diseases, foreign body reactions, and idiopathic etiologies (Table 85–2).

Pathophysiology

I. Foreign material or an antigenic stimulus elicits an acute inflammatory reaction, but it does not eliminate the foreign material or the antigenic stimulus persists.

II. Macrophages migrate to the area of inflammation and remain there producing and releasing interferon, plasminogen activators, collagenases, elastases, complement components, and endogenous pyrogens, which all contribute to the formation of a granuloma.

Clinical Signs

I. Granulomatous dermatitis is characterized by proliferative to nodular cutaneous reactions that may be focal or multifocal, exudative, ulcerative, painful, rapid or slow to develop.

II. Pruritus is variable.

III. Concurrent systemic signs of illness, such as fever, malaise, weight loss, lymphadenopathy, cough, and vomiting, are variable and depend on the causative agent.

Diagnosis

I. Definitive diagnosis often requires multiple, deep, wedge biopsies.

A. Special stains are required to identify infectious agents.

B. Tissue should also be examined with a polarized light to identify foreign material.

II. Cytologic examination of exudate for infectious agents is very useful.

III. Also submit wedges of tissue for bacterial and fungal culture.

Differential Diagnosis

See Table 85–2.

Treatment

I. Specific therapy is dependent on the underlying cause (see Table 85–2).

II. Sterile nodular granulomas/pyogranulomas are treated with glucocorticoids.

A. Prednisone 2.2–4.4 mg/kg PO daily until lesions regress (7–21 days), then slowly discontinued.

B. If lesions recur, repeat therapy and then administer alternate-day therapy. This may be long-term or life-long.

C. Animals unresponsive or intolerant of glucocorticoids may respond to other immunosuppressive drugs.

1. Azathioprine 2.2 mg/kg SID until remission

Table 85–2. **Differential Diagnosis of Granulomatous Dermatitis**

Disease or Syndrome	Clinical Signs	Recommended Diagnostic Tests	Treatment and Prognosis
Bacterial Infections			
Botryomycosis (*Staphylococcus, Pseudomonas, Proteus*)	Nodular mass with macro- or microscopic tissue grains, draining fistulas, single or multiple	Biopsy with special stains, tissue culture	Surgical excision. Relapses are common. Antibiotic therapy is usually ineffective.
Actinomyces, Nocardia	Ulcerated nodules and draining tracts, mycetomas, granules may or may not be present	Biopsy and bacterial culture results, cytology, and Gram's stain	Surgical débridement is most important, followed by antibiotic therapy. Actinomycetes infections are treated with penicillin G 100,000 U/kg PO BID or penicillin V 50 mg/kg PO BID. Nocardial infections are treated with sulfadiazine 80 mg/kg PO TID. Fair to guarded prognosis.
Atypical *Mycobacterium*	Nonhealing wounds	Deep wedge biopsy with special stains. See Chap. 84.	Antibiotic sensitivity testing recommended. Ciprofloxacin 10–15 mg/kg PO for 30 days after clinical cure. Clofazimine 8–12 mg/kg PO for 30 days after clinical cure
Feline leprosy	Single or multiple draining nodules on head and limbs	Biopsy, acid-fast stain	Surgical excision. Clofazimine 2–3 mg/kg PO for 30 days after clinical cure
Fungal Infections			
Mycetoma	Single or multiple swellings with draining tracts, and granules	Biopsy with special stains, bacterial and fungal cultures	Surgical excision, possible amputation
Pseudomycetoma due to *M. canis*	Affects cats with dermatophytosis. Nodular lesions in skin	Biopsy and tissue culture for fungi and bacteria	Surgical excision. Relapses are common. Topical antifungal treatment with lime sulfur. Griseofulvin 50–60 mg/kg PO SID, or itraconazole 10 mg/kg PO SID
Kerion reaction (any dermatophytic fungi)	Swollen, painful, draining lesion	Biopsy and tissue culture	None, will usually heal spontaneously
Pheohyphomycoses (pigmented or dematiaceous fungi)	Single or multiple nodules, ulcers, draining tracts, abscesses	Biopsy and tissue culture	Surgical excision and itraconazole 5–10 mg/kg PO SID–BID
Pythiosis	Nonhealing wound, swelling, fistulas, tracts, ulcers, exudation. Early lesions may resemble a hot spot or lick granuloma. Intense pruritus	Biopsy and culture on vegetable extract agar	Wide surgical excision, amputation. Nonresponsive to systemic antifungal drugs.
Blastomycosis Histoplasmosis Cryptococcosis Coccidioidomycosis	Multiple dermal or subcutaneous masses that may ulcerate, drain, and form fistulous tracts and abscesses. Systemic signs are common.	Cytologic examination of exudate. Biopsy of tissue with special stains. Culturing not recommended.	Systemic antifungal drugs: amphotericin B, ketoconazole, itraconazole

Table 85–2. **Differential Diagnosis of Granulomatous Dermatitis** (Continued)

Disease or Syndrome	Clinical Signs	Recommended Diagnostic Tests	Treatment and Prognosis
Infection with Algae			
Prototheca	Multiple draining lesions in subcutaneous tissue. Exudate is thick, mucoid, and yellow to pink.	Culture on Sabouraud's dextrose agar of exudate or tissue, or by specific fluorescent antibody reagents on formalin-fixed tissues	Poor to grave prognosis. Surgical excision of solitary nodules may be curative. Organism nonresponsive to systemic antifungal drugs.
Parasitic Infestations			
Heartworm infection	Granulomas on head and forelegs	Biopsy	Good if heartworm infection is treated
Leishmaniasis	Ulcerated nodules with patchy hair loss, erythema, scaling	Biopsy with Giemsa stain	Reportable disease. Euthanasia recommended because of human health risk. Organism sensitive to ketoconazole
Tick bites	Papular to small dermal nodules in areas of previous tick attachment	Biopsy	See Chap. 87.
Hypersensitivity Reactions			
Feline eosinophilic granuloma	Linear or nodular raised, pink to yellow lesions on hindlegs, chin, ears, lips	Biopsy	None, lesion often heals spontaneously. Will respond to glucocorticoids
Canine eosinophilic granuloma	Lesions on tongue, soft palate, fetid odor from mouth. Nodular reactions may occur on skin with or without skin lesions.	Biopsy	Prednisolone 0.5–2.2 mg/kg PO SID for 20 days or until lesions resolve. May be recurrent.
Idiopathic sterile pyogranuloma	Single or multiple nodules over body that ulcerate and drain	Biopsy	Prednisolone 2.2–4.4 mg PO SID BID for 7–21 days or until lesions resolve. Unresponsive lesions may be treated with azathioprine 2.2 mg/kg PO SID or asparaginase 10,000 IU IM weekly until lesions regress, and then as needed.
Miscellaneous Causes			
Xanthomas secondary to diabetes mellitus, chronic megestrol acetate, or hyperlipidemia	Pale to erythematous papules and nodules	Biopsy	Treat underlying cause
Foreign bodies (exogenous and endogenous, e.g., keratin, lipid, calcium, urates)	Nodules that ulcerate, nonhealing wounds, draining tracts	Biopsy and demonstration of foreign material	Removal of foreign material

is induced, then continued as alternate-day therapy

2. Asparaginase 10,000 IU IM, once weekly until lesions regress (1–2 weeks), then as needed

Patient Monitoring

I. The prognosis for patients with sterile/idiopathic granulomatous skin disease is good if lesions respond to therapy.

II. Hemograms and platelet counts are monitored for anemia and thrombocytopenia if azathioprine or asparaginase is used.

III. Prognosis and specifics for patient monitoring for other granulomatous skin diseases vary (see Table 85–2).

Panniculitis

Definition

I. Panniculitis is an inflammatory skin disease of the subcutaneous fat in dogs and cats.

II. The disease is characterized by multiple cutaneous draining tracts and subcutaneous nodules.

Causes

I. Trauma and secondary ischemia

II. Infectious agents
   A. Bacteria: *Pseudomonas, Proteus, Actinobacillus, Staphylococcus, Nocardia,* atypical *Mycobacterium*
   B. Fungi: dermatophytes and systemic fungal organisms

III. Immunologic abnormalities
   A. SLE
   B. Drug eruptions

IV. Nutritional disorders: vitamin E deficiency

V. Neoplasia: lymphosarcoma

VI. Vascular abnormalities: vasculitis, thromboembolism

VII. Sterile or idiopathic forms

Pathophysiology

I. Each cause of panniculitis results in damage to the lipocytes and liberation of lipids that undergo hydrolysis into glycerol and fatty acids.

II. Fatty acids are potent inflammatory agents, and further inflammation ensues.

Clinical Signs

I. Any breed may be affected, but dachshunds may be predisposed.

II. Clinical appearance of lesions varies.
   A. Lesions may be single or multiple and occur in clusters or groups. Cats often have solitary lesions.
   B. Size may vary from a few millimeters to a few centimeters.
   C. Nodules may be firm and well-localized or soft and ill-defined.
   D. Lesions begin in the subcutaneous tissue but often ulcerate and drain an oily, yellow-brown to bloody discharge.
   E. Nodules may or may not be painful, and they heal with scarring.

III. Affected animals may be systemically ill with fever, depression, and anorexia, especially cats with multiple lesions.

Diagnosis

I. Diagnosis can be made only by multiple deep *excisional biopsies* of subcutaneous nodules.

II. Tissue is submitted for aerobic and anaerobic bacterial, fungal, and mycobacterial cultures, and cultures of pythiosis, in addition to histopathology.

III. Biopsy shows lobular, septal, diffuse, or any combination of granulomatous, pyogranulomatous, suppurative panniculitis with or without fat necrosis or thrombosis of subcuticular blood vessels.

Differential Diagnosis

Panniculitis may be confused clinically with deep pyoderma, cutaneous cysts, or cutaneous neoplasia.

Treatment

I. Therapy is dependent on identifying a cause.

II. In sterile nodular panniculitis, careful surgical excision of solitary nodules may be curative.

III. Sterile multifocal panniculitis is treated with systemic glucocorticoids.
   A. Prednisolone is given to dogs 2 mg/kg PO daily and to cats 4 mg/kg PO daily.
   B. Administer steroids until lesions regress (3–12 weeks) and then on an alternate-day schedule for an additional 4–6 weeks.
   C. Gradually diminish and stop steroid therapy; recurrent cases may require long-term alternate-day therapy.
   D. Concurrent vitamin E 400 IU PO BID may also be useful and may replace steroids in the long-term management of some patients.

Patient Monitoring

I. Cutaneous signs improve within 7–10 days of the initiation of therapy, and systemic signs of illness may improve sooner.

II. If an underlying cause can be identified, glucocorticoid therapy may be discontinued permanently.

Injection Reactions

Definition

I. It is an increasingly common sequela to subcutaneous injections with secondary alopecia and, in some cases, inflammation.

II. Reactions occur in both dogs and cats.
   A. An inflammatory reaction that is either a panniculitis or vasculitis

B. No gross inflammation; hair simply falls out
III. There is a reported association with the administration of subcutaneous rabies vaccination in the cat and increased risk of developing sarcomas at the site of injection.

Causes and Pathophysiology

I. Lesions are usually associated with subcutaneous injections of rabies vaccine, although any vaccine, repositol steroid or progestin, or injectable praziquantel may produce lesions.
II. The pathogenesis is unclear, although histopathologic findings suggest an idiosyncratic hypersensitivity or immune-mediated process.
III. A strong breed predilection in dogs suggests a genetic role.
IV. Biopsies from some feline post-vaccinal sarcomas reveal a crystalline foreign material consistent with aluminum, a common adjuvant used in vaccines.

Clinical Signs

I. Signalment in dogs
  A. Age ranging from 5 months to 12 years
  B. No sex predilection
  C. Most common in miniature poodles, other small-breed dogs
II. Signalment in cats: no age, breed, or sex predilection
III. Clinical picture
  A. Lesions appear 2–4 months after an injection.
  B. Lesions are most commonly seen over the shoulders, back, and thighs at sites where injections are given.
  C. Inflammatory reactions appear as a circular to oval erythematous plaque that is firm on palpation.
    1. Some lesions are not inflamed and appear as an atrophic, hypopigmented circular area.
    2. Chronic lesions are alopecic, hyperpigmented, and shiny (with or without scaling).
    3. Cats may develop a pruritic ulcerative form that occurs secondary to infection.

Diagnosis

I. Rule out infectious skin diseases.
II. Histopathology is necessary to make the diagnosis.
  A. Excisional biopsies are preferred and are obtained with wide margins because of the propensity for sarcoma formation.
  B. Marked lymphoplasmacytic inflammatory infiltrates in the deep dermis and panniculitis with or without vasculitis may be seen.
  C. Lymphoid nodules may occur, followed by foci of necrosis and extensive fibroplasia.
  D. Immunofluorescence testing with antibodies to rabies antigen shows positive deposits in dermal blood vessel walls and hair follicle epithelium.

Differential Diagnosis

I. Infectious causes of alopecia: demodicosis, dermatophytosis, folliculitis, cellulitis
II. Noninfectious causes of alopecia: alopecia areata, localized scleroderma, feline ulcerative linear dermatosis

Treatment and Monitoring

I. Usually none required
II. Hair regrowth variable
  A. It may take months to years.
  B. New hairs may be a different color.
III. Surgical excision curative
  A. It is strongly advised in cats because of the risk of developing sarcomas.
  B. In the dog, observation and/or surgery may be chosen.
IV. Good vaccination records
  A. Record the vaccine type, lot number, and manufacturer.
  B. Record specific location and depth (IM, SQ) of vaccine.
  C. Use different injection sites when giving more than one vaccine.

Granulomatous Sebaceous Adenitis

Definition and Cause

I. Granulomatous sebaceous adenitis is an uncommon idiopathic skin disease primarily of dogs in which the sebaceous glands are the focus of granulomatous inflammation.
II. This disease is rare in cats.
III. Although the cause is unknown, occurrence in specific breeds suggests a genetic factor.

Clinical Signs

I. There is some evidence that males are more commonly affected than females.
II. Any breed may be affected but vizslas, Akitas, Samoyeds, and black and apricot standard poodles appear to be predisposed.
III. There is preliminary evidence for an autosomal recessive mode of inheritance (Dunstan and Hargis, 1995).
IV. Early lesions begin as mild scaling with or without hair loss.
V. Unless a secondary pyoderma or *Malassezia* colonization is concurrently present, pruritus is not a feature of this disease.
VI. Standard poodles may appear clinically normal and still have the disease, as marked hyperkeratosis (silver-white scales) may occur initially, followed by hair loss.
VII. Lesions may appear as annular rings of alopecia and scaling, as areas of superficial pyoderma, or as severe areas of hair loss and seborrhea in longer coated dogs.

Diagnosis

I. Diagnosis is made only by skin biopsy.
II. Skin biopsy reveals a marked granulomatous tissue

reaction at the level of the sebaceous glands; sebaceous glands are obliterated by macrophages.

III. Interstitial dermal inflammation is conspicuously absent.

Differential Diagnosis

I. Skin scrapings are negative for demodicosis.

II. Dermatophyte culture is negative, and lesions do not respond to oral antibacterial therapy for a superficial pyoderma.

III. Rule out endocrine hair loss (see Chap. 88).

IV. Also rule out idiopathic seborrhea (see Chap. 88).

Treatment

I. There is no cure, although lesion severity may wax and wane.

II. Topical therapy is the most beneficial in minimizing clinical signs.

   A. Antiseborrheic shampoos are used 2–3 times weekly or as needed to control scaling.

   B. Emollient rinses or humectant sprays may be useful in minimizing scaling or as an alternative to frequent baths in cold weather.

III. Response to systemic drug therapy is unpredictable.

   A. Prednisolone 2.2 mg/kg PO SID

   B. Isotretinoin 1 mg/kg PO SID

   C. Asparaginase 10,000 IU IM weekly for 2–3 weeks, then as needed to control clinical lesions of scaling

   D. Cyclosporine 5 mg/kg PO BID

Patient Monitoring

I. Prognosis is poor for resolution of clinical signs.

II. Lesions usually progress, and dogs often become refractory to previously successful therapies.

III. This disease is not life-threatening or discomforting to the dog. The disease is displeasing to the owner because of the unaesthetic appearance of the dog.

Juvenile Cellulitis

Definition

I. Juvenile cellulitis is an idiopathic skin disease of puppies 3–16 weeks of age.

II. The disease varies in severity from mild to severe and, if untreated, can cause severe cutaneous scarring and even death.

III. The disease has also been called puppy strangles and juvenile pyoderma.

Cause and Pathophysiology

I. An etiologic agent has not been identified.

II. Studies have suggested an infectious cause, but attempts at transmitting the disease to unaffected puppies or isolating an infectious agent were unsuccessful (Reiman et al., 1989).

III. Currently, this disease is considered to be an immune dysfunction.

Clinical Signs

I. Any breed may be affected, but golden retrievers, dachshunds, pointers, Labrador retrievers, and beagles are most commonly affected.

II. One or more puppies in a litter may be clinically affected.

III. Clinical signs may vary from mild to severe.

IV. Lesions are concentrated on the head and face and mucocutaneous areas of eyes and mouth.

   A. Skin is swollen, red, and glistening.

   B. Vesicles or pustules often ooze serum or pus from affected areas.

   C. Clinical signs of a deep pyoderma (pain, swelling, exudation of blood and/or pus) may be present.

   D. In mild cases, affected areas are concentrated around the lips or eyelid margins.

   E. The pinnae are often swollen and exudative, with intact pustules or vesicles often seen.

   F. Older puppies may also have truncal panniculitis.

   G. Dramatic regional or generalized lymphadenopathy is common and considered a hallmark of the disease, but it is not always found in mild cases.

   H. Signs of systemic illness are often present and include fever, anorexia, and depression.

   I. Death may result if the disease is left untreated. The cause of death is unknown.

Diagnosis

I. Diagnosis is usually based on the clinical appearance, especially in predisposed breeds.

II. Skin biopsy is diagnostic and reveals diffuse pyogranulomatous inflammation with no etiologic agents identified.

III. Skin scrapings are negative for *Demodex* mites.

IV. Lymph node aspirate reveals septic or granulomatous inflammation; bacterial cultures are usually negative.

V. Complete blood count reveals an inflammatory leukogram.

VI. Skin lesions are poorly responsive to antibiotic therapy alone.

Differential Diagnosis

I. Demodicosis with or without a concurrent deep pyoderma is the most important differential diagnosis.

II. Deep pyoderma should be ruled out via culture.

III. Severe systemic infections must also be ruled out.

Treatment

I. Begin topical therapy with antibacterial shampoos (chlorhexidine or benzoyl peroxide) or chlorhexidine solution (1:4 dilution) rinses (following a bath in a cleansing solution) SID-BID.

II. Cephalexin 30 mg/kg PO BID (or 20 mg/kg PO TID) is instituted, but it is important to remember that antibiotic therapy alone is ineffective.

III. Systemic glucocorticoids are indicated in all cases.

   A. Give prednisolone 2.2 mg/kg PO SID until all clinical signs resolve (7–28 days).

B. Alternate-day therapy is used for another 14–21 days after clinical signs subside.

C. Relapse is common if corticosteroids are withdrawn too soon.

Patient Monitoring

I. Rapid recognition of this disease is crucial because puppies may die or be permanently scarred as a result of intense inflammation.

II. Too rapid withdrawal of oral glucocorticoids often results in a fulminate exacerbation of clinical signs.

III. Monitor puppies carefully for secondary complications of glucocorticoid therapy, such as vomiting, diarrhea, and silent urinary tract infections.

IV. Prognosis is favorable if puppies respond to therapy in 4–5 days.

V. Evidence of scarring with failure to regrow hair and a leathery texture to the skin may not be apparent until several months after the episode.

Bibliography

Dunstan RW, Hargis AM: The diagnosis of sebaceous adenitis in standard poodle dogs. p. 619. In Bonagura JD (ed): Kirk's Current Veterinary Therapy XII. WB Saunders, Philadelphia, 1995

Fadok VA: Granulomatous dermatitis in dogs and cats. Semin Vet Derm 2:186, 1987

Hirsh BC, Johnson WC: Concepts of granulomatous inflammation. Int J Dermatol 23:90, 1984

Manning TO: Three cases of feline eosinophilic granuloma complex (eosinophilic ulcer) and observations on laser therapy. Semin Vet Med Surg 2:206, 1987

Muller GH, Kirk RW, Scott DW: Small Animal Dermatology. 4th Ed. WB Saunders, Philadelphia, 1989

Neer TM: Hypereosinophilic syndrome in cats. Compend Contin Educ Prac Vet 13:549, 1991

Power HT, Ihrke PJ: Selected feline eosinophilic skin diseases. Vet Clin North Am [Small Anim Pract] 25:833, 1995

Reedy LM: Results of allergy testing and hyposensitization in selected feline skin diseases. J Am Anim Hosp Assoc 18:618, 1982

Reiman KA, Evans LV, Turner S et al: Clinicopathologic characterization of canine juvenile cellulitis. Vet Pathol 26:499, 1989

Scott DW: Sterile eosinophilic pustulosis in the dog. J Am Anim Hosp Assoc 20:585, 1984

Scott DW: Sterile eosinophilic pustulosis in dog and man: comparative aspects. J Am Acad Dermatol 16:1022, 1987

Scott DW, Anderson WI: Panniculitis in dogs and cats: a retrospective analysis of 78 cases. J Am Anim Hosp Assoc 24:551, 1985

Stewart LJ, White SD, Carpenter JL: Isotretinoin in the treatment of sebaceous adenitis in two vizslas. J Am Anim Hosp Assoc 27:65, 1991

86

Idiopathic Dermatoses

W. Dunbar Gram
William H. Abbott

ACRAL LICK DERMATITIS

Definition

I. It is a syndrome in which the animal licks excessively at the distal anterior portion of a limb, resulting in an alopecic, thickened plaque or ulcer.
II. The condition is also known as a "lick granuloma."

Causes

I. Psychogenic disorders: boredom
II. Anatomic abnormalities
  A. Orthopedic: fracture, osteophyte, arthritis
  B. Neural injury: neural entrapment due to trauma
  C. Prior wound
  D. Foreign body

Pathophysiology

I. An underlying cause results in an abnormal sensation leading to excessive licking of affected area.
II. Persistent licking leads to alopecia, hyperpigmentation, or extensive ulcerative plaque formation.
III. Both the underlying cause and lesion formation perpetuate the abnormal sensation and persistent licking.

Clinical Signs

I. Signalment
  A. Large-breed dogs: Doberman pinscher, Labrador retriever, golden retriever, German shepherd dog, Great Dane, and Irish setter
  B. Sex: male:female ratio = 2:1
II. History of excessive licking of the dorsal aspect of the carpus or tarsus
III. Appearance of lesions: alopecia, hyperpigmentation, folliculitis, furunculosis, and ulcerative plaque formation

Diagnosis

I. Clinical signs as described
II. History of an active dog in an environment that lacks stimulation
III. No underlying primary anatomic abnormality on radiography
IV. No demonstrable neurologic disorder on neurologic examination or nerve conduction velocity tests
V. A skin biopsy exhibiting "characteristic" collagen and adnexal changes
  A. Evidence of chronic dermatitis
  B. An ulcerative epidermis bordered by epidermal hyperplasia
  C. Vertical orientation of dermal fibroblasts and collagen fibrils
  D. Sebaceous gland hyperplasia

Differential Diagnosis

I. Neoplasia: ruled out with histopathology
II. Demodicosis: identified on skin scrapings
III. Dermatophytosis: isolated by fungal culture or microscopic identification
IV. Trauma: compatible history
V. A focal manifestation of allergic dermatitis: ± other characteristic signs of atopy
VI. Acral mutilation syndrome (see Chap. 82)

Treatment

I. Initial therapies
  A. Identification and treatment of underlying cause (see Chap. 116)
  B. A minimum of 6 weeks of antibiotics based on culture and sensitivity to treat any secondary infection
  C. Topical fluocinolone and DMSO (Synotic) with flunixin meglumine (Banamine)
    1. Mix one bottle of Synotic with 3 ml of flunixin meglumine.
    2. Apply to the lesion BID-TID.

D. Chronic application of Elizabethan collar or bandages until the lesion is totally healed

II. Additional therapies for refractory lesions
  A. Intralesional steroid injections
  B. Cryosurgery: freeze-thaw cycle repeated 2–3 times
  C. Surgical excision: may heal poorly postoperatively
  D. Psychotherapeutic agents
    1. Naltrexone 1–2.2 mg/kg PO SID has been reported to be relatively effective.
    2. They are expensive, and recurrences after discontinuing treatment are common.
    3. Amitriptyline 0.5–1 mg/kg PO BID may also be helpful and is considerably less expensive.
  E. Acupuncture: positive anecdotal reports
  F. Radiation therapy: two doses of 900–1000 cGy, 1 week apart

Patient Monitoring

I. This dermatologic disorder can be quite refractory to treatment.
II. Monitor for potential sequelae.
  A. Periosteal reaction of bones underlying severe chronic lesions is often evident.
  B. Functional loss of the affected limb can occur in severe cases.

FELINE PSYCHOGENIC ALOPECIA AND DERMATITIS

Definition

A chronic inflammatory dermatitis resulting from incessant licking and scratching of focal areas of skin

Causes and Pathophysiology

I. Some underlying cause results in excessive grooming, licking, or scratching of affected areas, which may lead to alopecia, abrasions, ulcers, and secondary infection.
II. Examples of potential causes include any pruritic dermatitis, infected ears or anal sacs, or behavioral abnormalities such as ''excessive nervousness.''

Clinical Signs

I. Alopecia may affect any combination of the following sites: the inner thigh, lower abdomen, caudal dorsal midline, the limbs, or tail.
II. Initially, the underlying skin is often normal.
III. In chronic cases the skin may become lichenified and hyperpigmented.
IV. The hair in affected areas may be darker.

Diagnosis

I. Clinical signs as described are suggestive.
II. There may be a history of a potentially psychologi-cally disturbing incident or change in the animal's normal routine.
III. A history of excessive licking or chewing is not always present, because cats may not groom in the presence of the owner.
IV. Perform a thorough exam to determine any underlying causes.
V. The hair in affected areas may feel like broken stubble.
VI. Microscopic examination of hair reveals broken hair shafts as opposed to tapered ends.
VII. The hair regrows normally when an Elizabethan collar or protective clothing prevents the cat from licking or grooming.
VIII. A skin biopsy should be performed to rule out other causes of alopecia.

Differential Diagnosis

I. Allergic dermatitis: inhalant, flea, or food allergies
II. Ectoparasites: fleas, *Cheyletiella, Notoedres, Demodex,* and *Otodectes* mites
III. Dermatophytosis
IV. Endocrine alopecia: hyperadrenocorticism
V. Telogen effluvium
VI. Feline symmetrical alopecia (see Chap. 83)

Treatment

I. Eliminate the stressor or anxiety-producing situation, if possible (see Chap. 117).
II. Give diazepam 1–2 mg PO SID-BID as needed to control symptoms. (Idiopathic lethal hepatic necrosis has been associated with diazepam use in cats.)
III. If diazepam is not effective, try phenobarbital 4–8 mg PO BID as needed.
IV. Provide mechanical restraint with Elizabethan collars, or prevent licking by having the cat wear baby pajamas.

Patient Monitoring

I. Periods of stress or anxiety may lead to recurrences.
II. Recurrence of clinical signs is also common after treatment is discontinued.
III. Reinstitute medical therapy when clinical signs recur.

ACQUIRED CUTANEOUS LAXITY

Definition and Cause

I. A rare disease of the dermal collagen resulting in the rapid adult onset of large folds of pendulous skin overlying a focally extensive gelatinous subcutis
II. Cause unknown

Pathophysiology

I. It is theorized that vascular insufficiency compromises focal areas, resulting in necrosis of the subcutaneous fat, with loss of function and integrity of the dermis.

II. The accumulation of necrotic fat and loss of integrity of the dermal collagen result in the development of skin folds.

Clinical Signs

I. Signalment: reported in an English setter and a mixed breed dog
II. Clinical findings
   A. One or more areas of the trunk or head affected
   B. Rapid onset of large gelatinous folds of pendulous skin

Diagnosis

I. Clinical signs as already described are suggestive.
II. A biopsy reveals a thin dermis, loosely interspersed and small fragmented collagen bundles, normal elastin, and noninflammatory areas of necrotic subcutaneous fat and vessels.
III. Potential causes of a vasculopathy should be investigated.

Differential Diagnosis

I. Hematoma: In time, a hematoma will resolve.
II. Lipoma: Biopsy of the lesion is diagnostic.

Treatment and Patient Monitoring

I. Attempt to identify and treat possible causes of the underlying vasculopathy.
II. Corrective surgery to remove affected areas may be necessary.
III. The condition is usually nonprogressive and self-limiting.

ULCERATIVE DERMATOSIS OF SHETLAND SHEEPDOGS AND COLLIES

Definition and Cause

I. It is an ulcerative condition that may be a severe form or subgroup of familial dermatomyositis.
II. The cause is unknown, but a genetic predisposition is suspected.

Clinical Signs

I. Affected dogs are adult Shetland sheepdogs and collies of either sex.
II. Lesions are located primarily in intertriginous areas of the groin and axillae but may also occur on the mucocutaneous junctions of the mouth, ears, eyes, genitalia, and anus.
III. Bilateral partial symmetrical alopecia may also be present.

IV. Signs may be induced or aggravated by estrus and/or trauma.
V. Some dogs experience pain, especially if secondary bacterial pyoderma is present.
VI. Concomitant asymptomatic myositis may also occur.

Diagnosis

I. Suspicious breed and clinical signs
II. Negative anti-nuclear antibody and direct immunofluorescence assays
III. Biopsy findings
   A. Hydropic degeneration, vacuolation, and necrosis of individual basal cells that may include occasional individual keratinocytes of stratum spinosum
   B. Cleft and vesicle formation progressing to dermal-epidermal separation and ulceration
   C. No follicular atrophy
   D. Superficial perivascular to partially lichenoid mixed mononuclear dermal inflammation

Differential Diagnosis

I. Erythema multiforme
II. Systemic lupus erythematosus
III. Pemphigus vulgaris
IV. Discoid lupus erythematosus
V. Bullous pemphigoid

Treatment and Monitoring

I. Minimize trauma and self-trauma.
II. Start antibiotics for any secondary bacterial infection.
III. Additional therapy to consider includes corticosteroids, vitamin E, and pentoxifylline.
IV. The disease is difficult to control and often has a cyclical nature.

MUCINOSIS OF SHAR PEIS

Definition

A condition of young Shar peis characterized by severe pitting mucinous edema of the face and extremities

Causes and Pathophysiology

I. Based on the breed predisposition, the disease may have a genetic basis.
II. Because some cases respond to glucocorticoid therapy, the condition may have an inflammatory or immunologic etiology.
III. The pruritus seen in some cases is suggestive of an allergic etiology.
IV. For whatever reason, an excessive accumulation of subcutaneous mucin occurs.

Clinical Signs

I. Signalment: young Shar peis of either sex
II. Clinical findings

A. Generalized puffiness and pitting pockets of fluid-like material cause excessive wrinkling of the face and extremities and a cobblestone appearance of the skin.
B. Occasionally epidermal vesicles develop that contain a clear, viscous mucinous substance.
C. Pruritus is variable.

Diagnosis

I. Clinical signs are highly suggestive.
II. When a needle is inserted through a dependent area of epidermis into the dermis, a clear viscid mucinous substance may be squeezed out (positive "prick" test).
III. Skin biopsy reveals an increased amount of acid mucopolysaccharides when stained with Hale's iron or alcian blue stain. A nonspecific perivascular pattern of a mixed inflammatory cell population is also seen.

Differential Diagnosis

I. Severe myxedema associated with hypothyroidism
II. Transient angioedema associated with immune hypersensitivity

Treatment and Monitoring

I. Spontaneous resolution may occur with the passage of puberty.

II. Anti-inflammatory doses of prednisone (0.25 mg/kg PO QOD) may be helpful in cases with pruritus but should be used cautiously in young animals.
III. Secondary skin fold dermatitis and pyoderma may occur and should be managed with systemic antibiotics and/or topical antibacterial therapy (see Chap. 84).

Bibliography

Dodman NH, Shuster L, White SD et al: Use of narcotic antagonists to modify stereotypic self-licking, self-chewing, and scratching behavior in dogs. J Am Vet Med Assoc 193:815, 1988
Griffin C: Common dermatoses of the akita, shar pei and chow chow. Proc Am Coll Vet Derm 4:31, 1988
Gross TL, Ihrke PJ, Wilder EJ: Veterinary Dermatopathology: A Macroscopic and Microscopic Evaluation of Canine and Feline Skin Disease. Mosby–Year Book, St. Louis, 1992
Ihrke PJ, Gross TL: Ulcerative dermatosis of Shetland sheepdogs and collies. p. 639. In Bonagura JD (ed): Kirk's Current Veterinary Therapy XII. WB Saunders, Philadelphia, 1995
Lyman R: Dematopathies. p. 94. In Fenner WR (ed): Quick Reference to Veterinary Medicine. JB Lippincott, Philadelphia, 1982
Muller GH: Skin diseases of the Chinese shar pei. Vet Clin North Am [Small Anim Pract] 20:1665, 1990
Owen LN: Canine lick granuloma treated with radiotherapy. J Small Anim Pract 30:454, 1989
Scott DW, Miller WH, Griffin CE (eds): Muller & Kirks' Small Animal Dermatology. 5th Ed. WB Saunders, Philadelphia, 1995
Wilcock BP, Yager JA: Focal cutaneous vaculitis and alopecia at sites of rabies vaccination in dogs. J Am Vet Med Assoc 118:1174, 1986

87

Parasitic Skin Diseases

Linda Medleau

PARASITIC INFESTATION

Ancylostomiasis and Uncinariasis

Definition

I. Dermatitis caused by cutaneous penetration and migration of hookworm larvae
II. Also known as hookworm dermatitis

Causes

I. The three most common species are *Ancylostoma caninum, A. braziliense* (southern United States), and *Uncinaria stenocephala* (northern United States).
II. Eggs are shed in feces and mature in soil and grass of warm, moist climates.
III. Third-stage larvae invade areas of skin that frequently contact the ground.

Pathophysiology

I. The larvae enter areas of desquamation or, occasionally, through hair follicles and migrate into the dermis. From there they migrate to the lungs and small intestine to finish maturation.
II. Histopathology reveals hyperplastic, spongiotic, perivascular dermatitis with eosinophils and neutrophils. Larvae are rarely found.
III. Hypersensitivity has been implicated as a cause of the lesions.

Clinical Signs

I. Pruritic, papular eruptions
 A. Primarily on the feet
 B. Also affected: sternum, ventral abdomen, tail, pubic and preputial surfaces, lateral and posterior legs, and elbows, hocks, and ischial tuberosities
II. Uniform erythema, thickening of the skin, and alopecia
 A. Feet are often swollen, hot, and painful.
 B. Footpads may be spongy and soft, with erythema of interdigital webs and deformity of claws.

C. Arthritis of the interphalangeal joints may be present.

Diagnosis

I. History of poor sanitation and poor response to antibiotic therapy
II. Clinical signs as described earlier
III. Skin scrapings and biopsies rarely diagnostic
IV. Fecal examination positive for hookworm ova
V. Positive response to treatment

Differential Diagnosis

I. Pelodera dermatitis
II. Scabies
III. Other ectoparasites (Table 87–1)

Treatment

I. Institute anthelmintic treatment for all affected and in-contact dogs.
II. Improve sanitation, with frequent removal of feces, provision of dry or paved runs, and treatment of soil with 10 lbs. Borax per 100 square feet.
III. Improve foot hygiene; keep nails trimmed short and paws clean and dry.

Patient Monitoring

I. Recheck and retreat with anthelmintic at 3–4 weeks.
II. Signs usually resolve within 2–3 weeks.

Cheyletiellosis

Definition

I. A mild, nonsuppurative, transmissible dermatitis caused by a surface-dwelling mite of the family Cheyletidae
II. Also known as "walking dandruff"

Table 87–1. **Common Parasitic Infestations**

Infestation	Clinical Signs	Diagnosis	Treatment

Flea bite dermatitis
Ctenocephalides felis (cat flea)
C. canis (dog flea)
Pulex irritans (human flea)
Echidnophaga gallinacea (chicken sticktight flea)
	Mild irritation
	Pruritic papular eruptions
	Alopecia
	Acute moist dermatitis
	Miliary dermatitis
	"Psychogenic" alopecia (cat)
	Eosinophilic granuloma complex (cat)
	Anemia
	Tapeworms
	± Asymptomatic carriers
		History of exposure, inadequate flea control
		Identify fleas, flea dirt, or tapeworm segments on animal
		Fecal exam positive for *Dipylidium* segments
			Treat all affected and in-contact animals with insecticidal dip, solution, spray, foam, or powder
			Dogs: pyrethrin, rotenone, imidacloprid, permethrin, malathion, fipronil, phosmet, chlorpyrifos, carbamate, dichlorvos, supona, synthetic pyrethroid
			Cats: rotenone-pyrethrin, imidacloprid, pyrethrin, carbamate, fipronil, d-limonene, synthetic pyrethroid
			Treat all affected and in-contact animals with oral lufenuron once a month
			Environmental control
			  Vacuum regularly
			  Insecticidal products for premises containing pyrethrin, resmethrin, carbaryl, malathion, chlorpyrifos, diazenon, methoprene, and/or pyriproxyfen
			  Professional exterminator
			Prednisone 0.5 mg/kg (dogs), 1 mg/kg (cats) PO BID × 7 days, then SID × 7 days, then QOD × 7 days, then stop or use lowest effective dose to control pruritus
			Consider antibiotics for secondary pyoderma

Ear mites
Otodectes cynotis
	Prevalent in younger animals
	Intensely pruritic ears
	Thick, red-brown-black crusts in external ear canals
	± Miliary dermatitis
	± Mites on neck, rump, tail
	± Asymptomatic carrier
		History and physical findings suggestive
		Ear swab positive for mites and/or ova
		Direct visualization of moving white specks on otoscopic exam
		Positive pinnal-pedal reflex: cat scratches ipsilateral rear limb when ear is swabbed
			Treat all affected and in-contact animals
			Otic miticidal products
			  Mitox: 2–4 drops/ear SID × 3 days, then q 72 h × 21 days
			  Tresaderm 2–4 drops/ear SID × 7 days, stop × 7 days, then repeat treatment
			  Mitaban: 1 ml per 33 ml mineral oil, 2–4 drops/ear twice weekly; treat 2 wk beyond clinical cure. Not approved for this use in United States.
			  Canex: 1 part:3 parts mineral oil, 2–4 drops/ear twice weekly, later once weekly; treat 2 wk past clinical cure

Table continued on following page

Table 87–1. **Common Parasitic Infestations** (Continued)

Infestation	Clinical Signs	Diagnosis	Treatment
Ear mites *Otodectes cynotis (continued)*			Insecticidal dip, spray, powder, or shampoo (see Flea Allergy Dermatitis) once or twice each wk for 4 wk to treat mites outside ears Alternatively, consider ivermectin 0.2–0.3 mg/kg PO or SQ twice, 2 wk apart. Not labeled for this use in United States. Will kill heartworm microfilariae. Not safe at this dose in collies or shelties. Environmental cleaning and treatment (see Flea Allergy Dermatitis)
Pediculosis *Heterodoxus spiniger* (dogs) *Linognathus setosus* (dogs) *Trichodectes canis* (dogs) *Felicola subrostratus* (cats)	Lice accumulate in hair mats around ears and orifices Intense pruritus Papules, crusts, scales Anemia Weight loss Behavioral changes: anxiety, hostility ± Asymptomatic carriers ± Transient infestation of owner	History of exposure, crowding, poor nutrition, poor hygiene, or poor sanitation Direct visualization Scotch tape prep (see Cheyletiellosis) Microscopic exam of hair shaft positive for eggs attached along entire length and at one end	Correct predisposing factors: anemia, malnutrition, and debilitation Treat all affected and contact animals Clip hair mats and bathe in mild shampoo (Allergroom or HyLyt EFA) Insecticidal dip, shampoo, spray, or powder 1–2 times each wk for 4-wk minimum (see Flea Allergy Dermatitis) Clean and disinfect environment, bedding, and grooming implements (see Flea Allergy Dermatitis)
Ticks *Dermacentor variabilis* (American dog tick) *Otobius megnine* (spinous ear tick) *Rhipicephalus sanguineus* (brown dog tick)	Otitis externa Dermatitis, nodules at bite site Anemia Tick paralysis or systemic signs associated with diseases transmitted by ticks	History of exposure Direct visualization	Manual removal of ticks, including mouthparts: Soak tick in alcohol or ether, then remove with mosquito forceps Never apply gasoline, kerosene, or burning cigarette to ticks Treat animal with insecticidal dip, spray, powder, or foam (see Flea Allergy Dermatitis) Treat premises and outdoors with insecticidal products (see Flea Allergy Dermatitis) Professional extermination for severe infestation
Trombiculidiasis Chiggers Harvest mites	Lesions on skin-ground contact areas: legs, feet, head, ears, and ventrum Intensely pruritic, papulocrustous eruptions Nonpruritic pustules and crusts Secondary scaling and alopecia	History of exposure to moist woods or fields Seasonality (summer and fall) Identify red-orange mites in lesions; however, mites may not be present at time of exam	Parasiticidal dip one or twice (see Flea Allergy Dermatitis) Prednisone 0.5 mg/kg (dogs), 1 mg/kg (cats) PO SID–BID for 2–3 days for severe pruritus Avoid exposure to contaminated areas

Causes

I. The three most common mite species are *Cheyletiella blakei* (cats), *C. parasitovorax* (rabbits), and *C. yasguri* (dogs).

II. The mites are not strictly species specific and may affect humans as well.

Pathophysiology

I. The mites live in pseudotunnels in the keratin layers of the epidermis.

II. The mites are highly contagious, especially between young host animals, with transmission by direct contact or fomites.

III. *Cheyletiella* spp. are obligate parasites, but adult females can live for up to 10 days off the host and thus may serve as a source of reinfestation.

IV. Histopathology reveals superficial perivascular dermatitis with occasional mite segments in the stratum corneum and variable numbers of eosinophils.

Clinical Signs

I. Young animals are usually affected most severely.

II. The primary lesion is excessive scaling over the dorsal midline, with a slightly oily coat.

III. Pruritus is variable and may be present without any primary lesions.

IV. Adult dogs, rabbits, and cats may be asymptomatic carriers.

Diagnosis

I. History and physical examination are suggestive.

II. Demonstration of mites or mite eggs is accomplished by several methods.
  A. Superficial skin scrapings from over a large area
  B. Scotch tape prep
    1. Puppies are initially affected over the rump, spreading to the head and back.
    2. Cats tend to be affected over the back.
  C. Flea comb
  D. Vacuum technique
    1. Cover the mouth of a handheld vacuum with a clean white piece of tissue and vacuum widely over the animal's coat.
    2. Microscopically examine the debris collected.
  E. Fecal flotation for ova and mites
  F. Inspection of dandruff with a high-power magnifying loupe, looking for accessory mouthparts that terminate in prominent hooks
  G. Examination of hair shafts for eggs attached at one end

Treatment

I. Apply parasiticidal dip, powder, or shampoo once a week for 4 weeks.
  A. Dogs may be treated with lime sulfur, pyrethroids, carbamates, or organophosphates.
  B. Cats may be treated with lime sulfur, pyrethrins, or carbaryl.

II. Alternatively, give ivermectin 0.2–0.3 mg/kg SQ twice, 2–3 weeks apart.

III. Treat all in-contact animals.

IV. Clean and treat environment with flea insecticides.

Patient Monitoring

I. Recheck at 4 weeks. If mites persist, continue treatments, and recheck at 2-week intervals until no mites can be found.

II. Monitor for signs of insecticide toxicity. Treat as necessary.

III. Ivermectin kills heartworm microfilaria rapidly at this dose. Test all dogs for heartworm disease before treating with ivermectin.

IV. Monitor all dogs for signs of ivermectin toxicity, such as diarrhea, mydriasis, depression, ataxia, tremors, drooling, paresis, recumbency, excitability, stupor, coma, and death.

V. Ivermectin at this dosage is not to be used in collies or shelties.

Canine Demodicosis

Definition and Causes

I. Demodicosis is an inflammatory skin disease caused by the presence of excessive numbers of demodectic mites.

II. *Demodex canis* is a follicular mite of the family Demodicidae measuring 40 μm × 225 μm.

Pathophysiology

I. *D. canis,* in small numbers, is a normal inhabitant of canine skin.

II. Transmission occurs from mother to neonate during the first 2–3 days of life.

III. Immunosuppression from immune system deficiency, underlying disease, or immunosuppressive therapy allows the mite to overcolonize hair follicles and overpopulate the skin.

IV. Demodicosis occurs in three clinical forms.
  A. Localized demodicosis
    1. It is most common in dogs less than 1 year old.
    2. Most cases resolve spontaneously within 4–8 weeks.
    3. Minority of cases progress to generalized disease.
    4. Predisposing factors include adolescence, estrus, endoparasitism, growth, poor nutritional status, surgery, pregnancy, and other transient stresses.
  B. Generalized demodicosis (two types)
    1. Generalized juvenile-onset demodicosis
      a) Age at onset: 3–12 months
      b) 30–50% of cases spontaneously resolve; however, close monitoring of progress required
      c) Familial and breed predisposition: Afghan hound, beagle, Boston terrier, boxer, Chi-

huahua, Shar pei, chow chow, collie, dalmatian, dachshund, Doberman pinscher, English bulldog, German shepherd dog, Great Dane, Old English sheepdog, pointer, pit bull terrier, pug, Staffordshire bull terrier
2. Generalized adult-onset demodicosis
   a) Age at onset: >1 year
   b) No breed or sex predilection
   c) May be caused by underlying disease: endogenous or iatrogenic hyperadrenocorticism, immune deficiency, hypothyroidism, diabetes mellitus, neoplasia, immunosuppressive therapy
C. Pododemodicosis
   1. Chronic digital and interdigital disease
   2. May or may not have history of generalized demodicosis
   3. Secondary superficial or deep pyoderma
   4. Especially large breeds: Great Dane, Saint Bernard, Newfoundland, and Old English sheepdog

Clinical Signs

I. Localized demodicosis
   A. Lesions usually on muzzle, periocular skin, commissures of the mouth, head, ear canal, forelegs, and trunk
   B. One to five areas of alopecia
   C. Variable erythema, hyperpigmentation, and scaling
   D. Not pruritic unless secondary pyoderma present
II. Generalized demodicosis
   A. Begins as localized disease that spreads
   B. Patchy to diffuse alopecia
   C. Erythema, scaling, folliculitis
   D. Secondary pyoderma
   E. Pruritus, especially with pyoderma
   F. Peripheral lymphadenopathy
   G. ± Animal systemically ill
III. Pododemodicosis
   A. Digital and interdigital pain, erythema, and swelling
   B. Secondary superficial or deep pyoderma
   C. ± History of generalized demodicosis
   D. ± Lesions elsewhere on the body
   E. Often extremely resistant to therapy

Diagnosis

I. Localized, generalized juvenile-onset, and pododemodicosis
   A. Demonstration of mites may be accomplished by several methods.
      1. Multiple deep skin scrapings
      2. Fecal flotation
      3. Biopsy: especially for Shar pei and pododemodicosis/pododermatitis cases
      4. Ear swab
   B. Bacterial culture and sensitivity of pyogenic skin lesions are done to rule out associated pyoderma.

II. Generalized adult-onset demodicosis
   A. Demonstrate presence of mites as described earlier.
   B. Obtain routine database with a hemogram, chemistry profile, and urinalysis.
   C. Rule out underlying hypothyroidism, hyperadrenocorticism, and neoplasia.

Differential Diagnosis

I. Dermatophytosis
II. Superficial pyoderma
III. Atopy
IV. Food allergy
V. Flea allergy dermatitis
VI. Canine acne
VII. Pemphigus complex
VIII. Dermatomyositis

Treatment

I. Localized demodicosis
   A. Many lesions resolve without treatment.
   B. Improve local health of the skin with 2.5–3% benzoyl peroxide shampoo, lotion, or cream or 5% gel applied to lesions SID.
   C. Consider miticides.
      1. Rotenone in oil (Canex) applied to lesions SID
      2. Benzyl benzoate lotion SID
      3. Topical amitraz (Mitaban) 0.66 ml/8 oz water applied topically to lesions SID
   D. Repeat skin scrapings every 2–4 weeks, and treat until skin scrapings are negative and skin lesions have resolved.
II. Generalized demodicosis: standard therapy
   A. Total body clip for medium- and long-coated breeds prior to acaricidal dip
   B. Benzoyl peroxide shampoo prior to dip
   C. Amitraz (Mitaban) dip weekly (5.3 ml/gal water)
   D. Multiple deep skin scrapings every 2–4 weeks
   E. Continued treatment for 3–4 weeks following first negative skin scrapings
   F. Skin scraping 4–6 weeks following final acaricidal treatment
   G. Treatment of ear canals with 1 ml amitraz in 10–20 ml mineral oil QOD
   H. Antibiotics for pyoderma (4 weeks minimum)
   I. Corticosteroids: *contraindicated*
   J. Treatment of any underlying disease
III. Generalized demodicosis: alternative therapy
   A. These treatments are not approved for this use in the United States and are reserved for dogs that do not respond to standard therapy or those with unacceptable side effects to amitraz therapy.
   B. Ivermectin 0.4–0.6 mg/kg PO SID is continued for 1 month past negative skin scrapings or for at least 3 months, whichever is longer.
      1. Ivermectin toxicosis may occur acutely or after chronic use.
      2. Attempt to prevent acute toxicosis by giving 0.1 mg/kg on day 1, 0.2 mg/kg on day 2, 0.3

mg/kg on day 3, and so on, until delivering 0.6 mg/kg/day.

   3. It is contraindicated in purebred or mixbred collies, shelties, Old English sheepdogs, and Australian shepherds.

   4. Success rate with 0.6 mg/kg dose is about 85%; success rate with 0.4 mg/kg is only about 42%.

C. Milbemycin oxime 2 mg/kg PO SID is given for 4 weeks past negative skin scrapings.

   1. Milbemycin toxicosis is uncommon.

   2. Signs of toxicity include salivation, ataxia, tremors, and recumbency.

   3. Success rate is approximately 85%.

   4. Lower dosages have significantly lower success rates.

D. Daily amitraz therapy can be started after a total body clip for medium- and long-coated breeds.

   1. The dog is bathed with benzoyl peroxide shampoo once weekly.

   2. A 0.125% amitraz solution (1 ml Taktic or 0.6 ml Mitaban per 100 ml water) is applied to one half of the body each day, alternating halves.

   3. Continue treatments 4 weeks past negative skin scrapings.

   4. Success rate is about 75%.

   5. It is a messy therapy, with continual human exposure to a pesticide.

   6. It is less expensive than milbemycin and may be considered when ivermectin is not tolerated or is ineffective.

IV. Pododemodicosis: standard therapy

A. Total body hair coat clip and dips as for generalized juvenile-onset disease

B. Local foot treatment

   1. Mix 0.66 ml amitraz (Mitaban) in 100 ml water and apply to feet SID. Prepare a fresh solution daily.

   2. Alternatively, mix 0.5–1 ml amitraz (Mitaban) in 30 ml mineral oil or propylene glycol and apply to the feet every 1–3 days.

     a) Amitraz in propylene glycol or water is unstable and must be prepared fresh daily.

     b) Amitraz in mineral oil should be prepared fresh every 2 weeks.

C. Long-term antibiotics (6–8 weeks minimum)

D. Treatment of any underlying disease

V. Pododermatitis: alternative therapy

   Same as for alternative therapies for generalized demodicosis

Patient Monitoring

I. Monitor for side effects of acaricidal treatment, i.e., drowsiness, depression, bradycardia, anorexia, gastrointestinal upset.

A. Drowsiness can be minimized by feeding the dog prior to the dip.

B. Yohimbine 0.1 mg/kg IV has been reported to prevent or reverse side effects of IV amitraz. Its efficacy as an antidote for topically applied amitraz has not been established.

II. Generalized juvenile-onset demodicosis has a good to fair prognosis. However, it may recur and require either local treatments or lifelong maintenance therapy.

III. It is advisable to neuter any dog with generalized juvenile-onset demodicosis because of its hereditary predisposition.

IV. Generalized adult-onset demodicosis has a fair to guarded prognosis, depending on the underlying diseases present.

V. Pododemodicosis can become chronic and extremely resistant to treatment.

VI. Avoid systemic corticosteroids in all successfully treated animals, or relapses may occur.

Feline Demodicosis

Definition and Causes

I. It is an inflammatory skin disease caused by the presence of *Demodex cati,* a mite very similar to *D. canis,* which colonizes and overpopulates hair follicles.

II. A second, unnamed demodectic mite may be found only in the stratum corneum. This mite has a broad, blunt abdomen and is approximately half the length of *D. cati* or *D. canis.*

Pathophysiology

I. Disease occurs in two forms, localized or generalized.

II. Localized demodicosis is a rare condition.

III. Generalized demodicosis is very rare and is frequently associated with underlying diseases such as diabetes mellitus, feline leukemia virus (FeLV), feline immunodeficiency virus (FIV), systemic lupus erythematosus (SLE), toxoplasmosis, upper respiratory tract infections, or hyperadrenocorticism.

IV. Burmese and Siamese cats appear to be more susceptible to generalized demodicosis than other breeds.

Clinical Signs

I. Localized demodicosis

A. Lesions on eyelids, periocular area, head, and neck

B. Pruritus variable

C. Patchy alopecia, erythema, scaling, and crusting

D. ± Ceruminous otitis externa

E. May be self-limiting and spontaneously resolve

II. Generalized demodicosis

A. It may involve the head, neck, legs, trunk, flanks, and/or ventrum.

B. Lesions are not as severe as in canine demodicosis.

C. Patchy or symmetrical alopecia, erythema, scaling, crusts, circumscribed macules, and/or hyperpigmentation are common.

D. Pruritus is variable.

E. The unnamed demodectic mite can cause severe pruritus, leading to excoriations.
F. Ceruminous otitis externa and secondary pyoderma may also be present.

Diagnosis

I. Demonstration of mites
   A. Deep and superficial skin scrapings
   B. Ear swab
II. Eosinophilia on hemogram

Differential Diagnosis

I. Dermatophytosis
II. Notoedric mange
III. Atopy
IV. Food allergy
V. Flea allergy dermatitis
VI. ''Psychogenic'' alopecia
VII. Seborrheic dermatitis

Treatment

I. Localized demodicosis
   A. Spontaneous resolution possible
   B. Topical rotenone (Canex) applied to lesions SID
   C. Topical amitraz (Mitaban) applied to lesions SID (0.66 ml amitraz/8 oz water mixed fresh daily); not approved for use in cats
II. Generalized demodicosis
   A. Treat underlying disease.
   B. Dip weekly until skin scrapings are negative (usually 3–4 weeks).
      1. Lime sulfur 2%
      2. Amitraz 2.5–5 ml/gal water: not approved for use in cats

Patient Monitoring

I. Monitor for side effects of acaricidal treatment.
   A. Amitraz may produce transient sedation and salivation.
   B. If depression, anorexia, or diarrhea occurs, reduce amitraz concentration to 2.5 ml/gal water and treat every 2 weeks.
II. Diabetic cats should not be treated with amitraz, as human diabetes has been aggravated by use of the agent.
III. Prognosis is good to guarded, depending on the underlying cause.

Notoedric Mange

Definition

I. A highly contagious, intensely pruritic parasitic disease of cats caused by the sarcoptid mite *Notoedres cati*
II. Also known as feline scabies

Causes

I. *N. cati* belongs to the Sarcoptidae family.
II. *N. cati* is an obligate parasite of cats but may also infect foxes, dogs, rabbits, and people.

Pathophysiology

I. Transmission is by direct contact or fomites.
II. The mites prefer hairless skin, and as they spread, hair is lost.
III. Histopathology reveals varying degrees of superficial perivascular dermatitis with pronounced focal parakeratotic hyperkeratosis. Mite segments may be found in superficial epidermis. Eosinophils vary in number.

Clinical Signs

I. There is no age, sex, or breed predilection.
II. Lesions consist of erythematous papules on the edges of the pinnae that spread to the face and neck and may also spread to the feet and perineum.
III. Affected areas become thickened, wrinkled, and alopecic.
   A. Dense, tightly adhering yellow-gray crusts develop.
   B. Excoriated areas may become secondarily infected.
   C. Peripheral lymphadenopathy may also be present.
IV. If untreated, lesions may spread over large areas of the body.
V. Uncommon sequelae include toxemia, emaciation, anorexia, and death.

Diagnosis

I. Distribution of lesions in hairless regions
II. Intense pruritus
III. Skin scrapings revealing large numbers of mites
IV. Fecal flotation showing ova or mites
V. Demonstration of mites with the vacuum technique, as described for cheyletiellosis
VI. Poor response to steroid therapy; positive response to parasiticidal treatments

Differential Diagnosis

I. *Otodectes cynotis*
II. Dermatophytosis
III. Cheyletiellosis
IV. Pediculosis
V. Atopy
VI. Food allergy
VII. Pemphigus foliaceus or erythematosus
VIII. SLE
IX. Traumatic (fight) wounds

Treatment

I. Give ivermectin 0.2 mg/kg PO, SQ, twice, 2 weeks apart, or 0.4 mg/kg SQ once. Ivermectin is not labeled for use in the cat.

II. Dip with 2–3% lime sulfur once weekly for 4–8 weeks or until skin scrapings are negative. Clip hair and bathe first to loosen crusts.
III. Apply amitraz 5.3 ml/gal water topically once. Amitraz is not labeled for use in cats.
IV. Treat all in-contact animals as well.

Patient Monitoring

I. Recheck every 2 weeks. Treat until skin scrapings are negative and lesions have resolved.
II. Monitor for adverse reactions to parasiticidal therapy.
  A. Adverse reactions to ivermectin include diarrhea, mydriasis, depression, ataxia, tremors, drooling, paresis, recumbency, excitability, stupor, coma, and death. Treatment is symptomatic or supportive.
  B. Adverse reactions to organophosphates include depression, anorexia, salivation, vomiting, diarrhea, ataxia, tremors, and dyspnea. Immediate treatment is with atropine 0.1–0.2 mg/kg IV, repeated as needed based on signs such as respiratory distress, cyanosis, and heart rate.

Pelodera Dermatitis

Definition and Causes

I. Pelodera dermatitis is a nonseasonal dermatitis of dogs caused by cutaneous infestation of *Pelodera strongyloides* larvae.
II. It is also known as rhabditic dermatitis.
III. *P. strongyloides* is a free-living nematode that lives in damp soil, decaying organic debris, straw bedding, or marsh hay.

Pathophysiology

I. Transmission is by direct contact with larvae in organic material.
II. The nematode larvae invade the hair follicles, causing folliculitis.
III. Histopathology may reveal larvae and some parthenogenic females in the hair follicles, with varying degrees of perifolliculitis, folliculitis, and furunculosis and numerous eosinophils.

Clinical Signs

I. Skin lesions on areas that contact the ground: feet, legs, perineum, ventrum, and under the tail
II. Erythema, alopecia
III. Papules, crusts, and scales
IV. Mild to intense pruritus
V. Secondary pyoderma

Diagnosis

I. History of contact with damp organic material or straw bedding and intense pruritus
II. Deep skin scrapings revealing small, motile nematode larvae
III. Biopsy

Differential Diagnosis

I. Hookworm dermatitis
II. Dirofilariasis
III. Strongyloidiasis
IV. Scabies
V. Contact dermatitis
VI. Demodicosis
VII. Bacterial folliculitis
VIII. Dermatophytosis

Treatment and Monitoring

I. Identify and remove source of contamination.
  A. Remove and destroy all bedding material.
  B. Thoroughly wash and spray beds, kennels, and cages with malathion or diazinon.
II. Bathe dog with Oxydex, Sulfoxydex, or Pyoben to soften and remove crusts and flush follicles.
III. Administer parasiticidal dips once weekly for 2 weeks.
IV. If pruritus is severe, give prednisolone 0.5 mg/kg PO SID-BID for 2–5 days.
V. Consider antibiotics for secondary pyoderma.

Sarcoptic Mange

Definition

I. Sarcoptic mange is a nonseasonal, intensely pruritic, highly contagious dermatitis of dogs caused by infestation with *Sarcoptes scabiei* var. *canis*.
II. It is also known as scabies.

Causes

I. *S. scabiei* var. *canis* is a burrowing mite.
II. It primarily affects dogs but can also attack cats, foxes, and human beings transiently.
III. The mite is susceptible to desiccation and usually dies within 3–4 days off of the host; however, under certain conditions, it may survive long enough to be a source of reinfestation.

Pathophysiology

I. The mite burrows through the stratum corneum, laying eggs in the tunnels. The hatched larvae and nymphs live and feed on the skin surface.
II. The mites prefer glabrous areas but can affect large regions of the body.
III. Transmission is by direct contact or fomites.
IV. The mite causes intense pruritus by mechanical irritation, production of irritating by-products, and secretion of allergenic substances that produce a hypersensitivity reaction in sensitized individuals.
V. The hypersensitivity reaction can produce severe pruritus in response to very few mites. Pruritus may persist long after the mites have been destroyed.
VI. Histopathology is rarely conclusive unless mites are found in the biopsy.
  A. Biopsy of an active papule may reveal varying degrees of superficial perivascular dermatitis.

B. There may also be focal epidermal edema, exocytosis, degeneration, and necrosis, as well as pronounced focal parakeratotic hyperkeratosis.

Clinical Signs

I. Distribution of lesions in glabrous regions, i.e., hocks, elbows, pinnal margins, and ventrum
   A. Some animals have no ear margin lesions.
   B. Lesions spread quickly over large areas of the body.
II. Intense pruritus
   A. Most intense at night and in warm environments
   B. Nonseasonal
III. Alopecia
IV. Erythematous papular eruptions with thick yellow crusts
V. Secondary excoriations and pyoderma
VI. ± Peripheral lymphadenopathy
VII. Poor response to steroid treatment
VIII. Asymptomatic carrier state in some dogs

Diagnosis

I. History of prior exposure or suspicious lesions in human contacts
II. Distribution of lesions and intense pruritus
III. Positive pinnal-pedal reflex: rub the ear margin and the animal responds by rapidly kicking the ipsilateral rear limb
IV. Skin scrapings
   A. As many as 50–75% of scrapings are negative.
   B. Mites prefer noninflamed skin, so obtain wide superficial scrapings from 5–10 areas.
V. Fecal flotation revealing mites or ova
VI. Demonstration of mites using vacuum technique as described for cheyletiellosis
VII. Response to scabicidal treatment

Differential Diagnosis

I. Atopy
II. Flea allergy dermatitis
III. Food allergy
IV. Contact dermatitis
V. Ectoparasites: pediculosis, cheyletiellosis, pelodera dermatitis, otodectic acariasis, demodicosis
VI. Dermatophytosis
VII. Generalized pyoderma
VIII. Seborrheic dermatitis

Treatment

I. Topical therapy
   A. Consider clipping all medium- and long-haired dogs.
   B. Bathe in antiseborrheic shampoo to remove crusts.
   C. Administer acaricidal dips weekly for 2 weeks beyond remission or for a minimum of 5 weeks.
      1. Lime sulfur 2% (Lym Dyp): safe for young and debilitated animals

2. Malathion
3. Mercaptomethyl phtalimide (Paramite)
   D. Use amitraz (Mitaban) 5.3 ml/gal water three times at 2-week intervals.
   E. Keep animal dry between treatments.
II. Systemic therapy
   A. Ivermectin 0.2–0.3 mg/kg PO, SQ given twice, 2 weeks apart
      1. Inexpensive and nearly 100% effective, but not labeled for this use in the United States
      2. Not to be used in collies or shelties
      3. Kills heartworm microfilariae rapidly
   B. Milbemycin oxime 0.75 mg/kg PO SID for 30 days (not labeled for this use in the United States)
III. Additional therapy
   A. Treat all contact animals.
   B. Dispose of all bedding, vacuum thoroughly, and treat environment with parasiticidal sprays.
   C. Give antibiotics for secondary pyoderma.
   D. Consider prednisolone 0.5 mg/kg PO SID for 2–5 days for severe pruritus.

Patient Monitoring

I. Some mite species are resistant to various acaricidal dips, necessitating trials with alternative topical products or systemic ivermectin treatment.
II. Monitor for adverse reactions to ivermectin.

PARASITIC HYPERSENSITIVITY

Cutaneous Dirofilariasis

Definition and Cause

I. It is a cutaneous reaction to aberrant microfilarial migration.
II. Causal relationship has not been definitively proved; however, lesions resolve following treatment for heartworm infection.

Pathophysiology

I. Circulating microfilariae migrate out of blood vessels into subcutaneous tissues and stimulate a pyogranulomatous response.
II. Hypersensitivity to *Dirofilaria immitis* has been suggested.
III. Histopathology reveals angiocentric pyogranulomatous dermatitis.
   A. Microfilariae are present within granulomatous dermal nodules and within blood vessels central to the lesions.
   B. Eosinophil numbers vary.

Clinical Signs

I. Pruritic, ulcerative, nodular dermatitis of the head, trunk, and limbs

A. Papulocrustous dermatitis resembling canine scabies
B. Chronic ulcerative dermatitis
C. Pustular eruptions
II. Erythematous, alopecic dermatitis of the chest and limbs
III. Secondary seborrheic skin disease
IV. Cutaneous granuloma (cat)
V. No response to corticosteroids, antibiotics, antifungals, shampoos, ointments, or sedatives

Diagnosis

I. Positive heartworm test
II. Microfilariae in tissues on biopsy
III. Response to treatment for heartworm disease

Differential Diagnosis

I. Acral lick dermatitis
II. Sporotrichosis
III. Dermatophytosis
IV. Mycetoma
V. Actinomycosis
VI. Atypical mycobacterial granuloma
VII. Feline leprosy
VIII. Neoplasia

Treatment and Monitoring

I. Treat for heartworm disease (see Chap. 12).
II. Lesions should resolve 5–8 weeks following completion of treatment for heartworm disease

Flea Allergy Dermatitis (FAD)

Definition and Causes

I. Allergic reaction to bites inflicted by *Ctenocephalides felis, Ctenocephalides canis,* or *Pulex irritans.*
II. FAD is caused by hypersensitivity to allergens and haptens in flea saliva.

Pathophysiology

I. Hypersensitivity is believed to involve four types of immune reactions.
A. Type I: IgE and, perhaps, IgG
B. Type IV: cell-mediated immunity
C. Late-onset IgE response
D. Cutaneous basophil hypersensitivity
II. Most flea-allergic dogs develop both immediate and delayed hypersensitivity reactions on intradermal skin tests. A minority of individuals manifest only one of these reactions.
III. Only immediate hypersensitivity has been reported in the cat.
IV. Studies indicate that atopy may predispose animals to FAD.

Clinical Signs

I. Most common age of onset: 3–6 years
II. Distribution of lesions over posterior one third of body
III. Miliary dermatitis on head and neck of cats
IV. Eosinophilic granuloma complex of cats
V. Pruritus
VI. Papulocrustous eruptions
VII. Secondary alopecia, excoriations, pyoderma
VIII. Hyperpigmentation and lichenification in dogs

Diagnosis

I. History of exposure, age at onset, and physical examination demonstrating lesions and distribution patterns compatible with FAD
II. Presence of fleas or flea dirt on the animal
III. Fecal examination positive for *Dipylidium* spp.
IV. Intradermal skin testing: false-negatives possible because the extract is made from whole fleas rather than from purified antigen
V. Response to treatment for fleas

Differential Diagnosis

I. Atopy
II. Food allergy
III. Drug hypersensitivity
IV. Intestinal parasite hypersensitivity
V. Bacterial folliculitis
VI. Other ectoparasites
VII. Dermatophytosis
VIII. Eosinophilic complex in cats

Treatment

I. Administer insecticidal sprays, foams, solutions, or dips every 7–30 days as labeled.
II. Treat from spring to first snowfall, or treat year-round in warm climates.
III. Administer the insect development inhibitor lufenuron (Program) 10 mg/kg PO to dogs and 30 mg/kg PO to cats with food once a month.
IV. Administer the flea adulticide imidacloprid (Advantage) or fipronil (Frontline) topically to dogs and cats once a month.
V. Treat all in-contact animals.
VI. Prevent animals from roaming.
VII. Treat the premises.
A. Professional extermination with flea growth regulators (methoprene, pyriproxyfen) is preferred.
B. Exterminate quarterly in regions with year-round warm climate.
VIII. Treat outdoors with insecticidal or biologic products designed for such use, where animal spends most of its time.
IX. Administer decreasing doses of prednisone 0.5 mg/kg (dogs) or 1 mg/kg (cats) PO BID for 7 days, then SID for 7 days, then QOD for 7 days, then stop or continue at lowest effective dose to control pruritus.
X. Use antibiotics and antibacterial shampoos (Oxydex, SulfOxydex) as necessary for pyoderma.

XI. Hyposensitization therapy is controversial at best and is probably rarely effective (Muller et al., 1989).

Patient Monitoring

I. Strict flea eradication is the *only* effective treatment for FAD.
II. Once FAD has developed, it becomes more severe over time, requiring increasingly vigilant and stringent flea control measures.

Intestinal Parasite Hypersensitivity

Definition and Causes

I. It is a cutaneous reaction to intestinal parasite antigens.
II. Hypersensitivity reactions have been noted in response to infestation with roundworms, hookworms, whipworms, and tapeworms.

Pathophysiology

I. Ascarid antigen has been shown to stimulate a profound IgE response in dogs and cats.
II. Both respiratory and cutaneous allergic reactions to ascarid antigen have been demonstrated in dogs.
III. Migrating parasites seem to be more antigenic than those that do not migrate.

Clinical Signs

I. Generalized or multifocal pruritic, papulocrustous dermatitis
II. Pruritic seborrheic skin disease
III. Pruritic urticaria
IV. Pruritus without skin lesions
V. ± Other signs of intestinal parasitism

Diagnosis

I. History of exposure, poor sanitation, and lesions as described earlier
II. Fecal examination revealing parasite ova
III. Positive response to anthelmintic therapy
IV. Skin scrapings, Wood's lamp examination, fungal culture, and intradermal skin testing to rule out other diseases, especially if no response to anthelmintic treatment

Differential Diagnosis

I. Atopy
II. Flea allergy dermatitis
III. Food allergy
IV. Drug hypersensitivity
V. Scabies
VI. Demodicosis
VII. Other ectoparasites (see Table 87-1)
VIII. Bacterial folliculitis or pyoderma
IX. Dermatophytosis

Treatment

I. Anthelmintic therapy
II. Antibacterial or antiseborrheic shampoos for secondary pyoderma, seborrhea, or papulocrustous lesions
III. Soaks for crusted lesions
IV. Antibiotics for secondary pyoderma
V. Prednisone 0.5 mg/kg (dogs) or 1 mg/kg (cats) PO in decreasing doses for severe pruritus

Patient Monitoring

I. Signs resolve with anthelmintic treatment.
II. Signs recur with parasitic reinfestation.

Otodectic Acariasis

Definition and Causes

I. It is a widespread cutaneous reaction to otodectic infestation.
II. The cause is unknown, but hypersensitivity appears to be involved.

Pathophysiology

I. Experimentally infected cats showed immediate, but not delayed, reactions when skin tested with mite extract.
II. Over time these cats also showed Arthus-type reactions to skin testing with mite extract as well as serum-precipitating antibodies.

Clinical Signs

I. *Otodectes cynotis* infestation
II. Intense pruritus, with widespread pruritic, papulocrustous dermatitis

Diagnosis

I. Suspicious physical examination findings
II. Demonstration of mite on ear swab cytology or on skin scrapings
III. Positive response to treatment for ear mites

Treatment

I. See Table 87-1 for mite therapy.
II. Give decreasing doses of prednisone as described for FAD (earlier) to relieve pruritus.
III. Consider antibiotics for secondary pyoderma.

Tick Bite Hypersensitivity

Definition and Causes

I. It is an exaggerated cutaneous response to tick bites.
II. Hypersensitivity to tick bites has been demonstrated in dogs and people; it is also believed to occur in cats.

Pathophysiology

I. It is considered to be a combination of type III (immune complex) and type IV (cell-mediated) immune response to tick antigen.

II. Histopathology reveals leukocytoclastic vasculitis with hemorrhage, necrosis, and ulceration or nodular to diffuse dermatitis owing to granulomatous or pyogranulomatous inflammation. Tick mouth parts are rarely found.

Clinical Signs

I. Focal necrosis and ulceration at site of bite
II. Nodules with or without erythema, pruritus, and ulceration
III. Pruritic pododermatitis

Diagnosis

I. History and physical examination are suggestive.
II. Biopsy may be supportive.

Treatment and Monitoring

I. Removal of ticks
II. Prevention or control of ticks
III. Surgical excision of severe or persistent reactions
IV. Prednisone 1 mg/kg (dogs) or 2 mg/kg (cats) PO SID-BID for 7–10 days for severe or persistent reactions

Bibliography

Bussieras J, Chermette R: Amitraz and canine demodicosis. J Am Anim Hosp Assoc 22:779, 1986

Cullen LK, Reynoldson JA: Central and peripheral-adrenoceptor actions of amitraz in the dog. J Vet Pharmacol Ther 13:86, 1990

de Jaham C, Henry CJ: Treatment of canine sarcoptic mange using milbemycin oxime. Can Vet J 36:42, 1995

Foley RH: Parasitic mites of dogs and cats. Compend Contin Educ Pract Vet 13:783, 1991

Hsu WH, Hopper DL: Effect of yohimbine on amitraz-induced CNS depression and bradycardia in dogs. J Toxicol Environ Health 18:423, 1986

Hsu WH, Lu Z-X, Hembrough FB: Effect of amitraz on heart rate and aortic blood pressure in conscious dogs: influence of atropine, prazosin, tolazoline, and yohimbine. Toxicol Appl Pharmacol 84:418, 1986

Hsu WH, McNeel SV: Amitraz-induced prolongation of gastrointestinal transit and bradycardia in dogs and their antagonism by yohimbine: preliminary study. Drug Chem Toxicol 8:239, 1985

Kalkofen UP: Hookworms of dogs and cats. Vet Clin North Am [Small Anim Pract] 17:1341, 1987

Kwochka KW: Fleas and related diseases. Vet Clin North Am [Small Anim Pract] 17:1235, 1987a

Kwochka KW: Mites and related diseases. Vet Clin North Am [Small Anim Pract] 17:1263, 1987b

MacDonald JM: Parasiticidal therapy: Part II. Rational treatment of canine demodicosis and scabies. Proc Mich Vet Conf 15:1, 1990

Medleau L, Brown CA, Brown SA et al: Demodicosis in cats. J Am Anim Hosp Assoc 24:85, 1988

Medleau L, Willemse T: Efficacy of daily amitraz therapy for refractory generalized demodicosis in dogs: two independent studies. J Am Anim Hosp Assoc 31:246, 1995

Merchant SR: Zoonotic diseases with cutaneous manifestations—Part II. Compend Contin Educ Pract Vet 12:515, 1990

Miller WH, Scott DW, Cayatte SM et al: Clinical efficacy of increased dosages of milbemycin oxime for treatment of generalized demodicosis in adult dogs. J Am Vet Med Assoc 207:1581, 1995

Muller GH, Kirk RW, Scott DW: Small Animal Dermatology. 4th Ed. WB Saunders, Philadelphia, 1989

Paradis M, Scott D, Villeneuve A: Efficacy of ivermectin against *Cheyletiella blakei* infestation in cats. J Am Anim Hosp Assoc 26:125, 1990

Pukay BP: Cheyletiellosis. p. 137. In August JR (ed): Consultations in Feline Internal Medicine. WB Saunders, Philadelphia, 1990

Reedy LM: Common parasitic problems in small animal dermatology. J Am Vet Med Assoc 188:362, 1986

Reedy LM, Miller WH: Allergic Skin Disease of Dogs and Cats. WB Saunders, Philadelphia, 1989

Ristic Z, Medleau L, Paradis M et al: Ivermectin for treatment of generalized demodicosis in dogs. J Am Vet Med Assoc 207:1308, 1995

Schaffer DD, Hsu WH, Hopper DL: The effects of yohimbine and four other antagonists on amitraz-induced depression of shuttle avoidance responses in dogs. Toxicol Appl Pharmacol 104:543, 1990

Scheidt VJ: Flea allergy dermatitis. Vet Clin North Am [Small Anim Pract] 18:1023, 1989

Scheidt VJ, Medleau L, Seward RL et al: An evaluation of ivermectin in the treatment of sarcoptic mange in dogs. Am J Vet Res 45:1201, 1984

Schmeibel LP: Cheyletiellosis and scabies. Vet Clin North Am [Small Anim Pract] 18:1069, 1989

Schneck G: Use of ivermectin against ear mites in cats. Vet Rec 123:599, 1988

Scott DW: Feline dermatology 1900–1978: a monograph. J Am Anim Hosp Assoc 16:331, 1980

Scott DW: Feline dermatology 1979–1982: introspective retrospections. J Am Anim Hosp Assoc 20:537, 1984

Scott DW: Feline dermatology 1983–1985: "the secret sits." J Am Anim Hosp Assoc 23:255, 1987

Scott DW, Horn RT: Zoonotic dermatoses of dogs and cats. Vet Clin North Am [Small Anim Pract] 17:117, 1989

88

Endocrine/Metabolic Skin Diseases

Rodney A. W. Rosychuk
Margaret S. Swartout

KERATINIZATION DISORDERS

Margaret S. Swartout

Seborrhea

Definition

I. Seborrhea is an alteration in epidermal keratinization and sebum production, leading to excessive scale formation, skin and hair greasiness, and often secondary inflammation.
II. It affects primarily dogs and can occur as either a primary or a secondary condition; classification is important for therapeutic purposes.

Causes

I. Primary disorders of keratinization
  A. Primary canine seborrhea (Table 88–1)
    1. Familial disorder of epithelial hyperproliferation affecting certain breeds most often
      a) American cocker spaniel
      b) English springer spaniel
      c) West Highland white terrier
      d) Basset hound
      e) Irish setter
      f) German shepherd dog
      g) Dachshund
      h) Doberman pinscher
      i) Shar pei
      j) Labrador retriever
      k) Golden retriever
      l) Poodle
    2. Diagnosis made by exclusion of underlying causes of secondary seborrhea and by histopathology of skin biopsy
  B. Primary feline seborrhea: rare heritable disease reported in Persian cats
  C. Other primary disorders of keratinization (see later).

II. Secondary seborrhea: caused by underlying systemic or cutaneous disorder, the most common type
  A. Pyoderma
    1. Can cause secondary flaking and pruritus
    2. Often difficult to identify which process is primary and which is secondary
  B. Allergies
    1. Flea allergy: common cause
    2. Allergic inhalant dermatitis: common cause
    3. Food allergy: uncommon cause
  C. Endocrine disorders (common cause)
    1. Hypothyroidism: most common endocrine cause
    2. Adrenal disorders
      a) Hyperadrenocorticism: second most common endocrine cause
      b) Adrenal sex hormone imbalance, previously called "growth hormone–responsive dermatosis" (Schmeitzel et al., 1995)
    3. Estrogen imbalances (Schmeitzel, 1990)
      a) Hyper-, hypoestrogenism of female dogs
      b) Testicular neoplasia
    4. Androgen imbalances (Schmeitzel, 1990)
      a) Testicular neoplasia
      b) Testosterone-responsive dermatosis of male dogs
      c) Castration-responsive dermatosis of dogs
    5. Diabetes mellitus (seborrhea sicca)
    6. Hepatocutaneous syndrome in severe liver disease, glucagonoma, and other intestinal disorders (rare)
  D. Parasites
    1. Scabies
    2. Cheyletiellosis
    3. Demodicosis
    4. *Otodectes* spp.
    5. Pediculosis
  E. Dermatophytosis

Table 88–1. **Distinguishing Features of Seborrhea**

Disorder	Clinical Findings
Primary seborrhea of dogs	Onset 18–24 mo of age, progressing as dog ages
	Oiliness and scaliness in patches or generalized
	Ventral neck, dorsum of trunk, inguinal and interdigital areas, axillae, elbows, hocks, and ears most severely affected
	Clusters of fatty particles adhering to hair resembling louse nits
	Rarely papules and pustules
	Plaques with erythema and crusting
	Pruritus, rancid odor
	Ceruminous otitis common
Primary seborrhea of cats	Onset 2 days to 6 wk of age
	Scale and grease on whole body
	Alopecia, rancid odor
	Waxy debris in face folds and ears
Secondary seborrheas	
Flea allergy	Seborrhea in dorsal lumbosacral area, medial and caudal thighs, ventral abdomen
Atopy	Moderate to severe pruritus and variable scaliness of the axillae, abdomen, face, ears, and feet
	Also generalized dry scale
Food allergy	Pruritus and seborrhea, especially of ears, paws, and face
Hypothyroidism	Seborrhea sicca, symmetrical alopecia
Adrenal imbalances	Seborrhea sicca, symmetrical alopecia, and possible hyperpigmentation
Estrogen imbalances	Seborrhea, symmetrical alopecia, possible hyperpigmentation; thin skin in hypoestrogenism and gynecomastia in hyperestrogenism
Andogren imbalances	Seborrhea
	Tail gland and perianal tissue hyperplasia, with testicular neoplasia
	Thin skin in testosterone-responsive dogs
	Symmetrical alopecia in testosterone-responsive and castration-responsive dogs
	Hyperpigmentation in castration-responsive males
Malassezia dermatitis	Face, feet, abdomen, posterior thighs, and forelimbs affected
	Erythema, hyperpigmentation, alopecia, lichenification, and scale
Zinc-responsive skin disease	Moderate to severe adherent crusting and scaling of pinnae, pressure points, periocular and perioral areas, muzzle, and chin
	Hyperkeratotic footpads

F. *Malassezia* dermatitis (see Chap. 84)
G. Nutritional disorders (see Chap. 90)
  1. Essential fatty acid (EFA) deficiency
    a) Although infrequent, it is the most common nutritional deficiency resulting in seborrhea.
    b) Deficiency can cause dry or oily seborrhea.
  2. Vitamin A–responsive dermatosis
  3. Zinc-responsive skin disease
  4. Protein deficiencies (uncommon)
  5. Malabsorption/maldigestion
H. Autoimmune skin diseases
  1. Secondary seborrhea may be present from decreased cohesion of keratinocytes.

  2. Pemphigus foliaceus is the most common autoimmune disorder to cause seborrhea.
  3. Seborrhea may be present in one third of dogs with systemic lupus erythematosus (SLE).
I. Cutaneous lymphoma
  1. Infiltrative disease leads to scales that exfoliate in large sheets.
  2. It may present as a severe seborrhea sicca.
J. Abnormal skin surface drying
  1. Low ambient humidity
  2. Overshampooing
  3. Too-frequent dipping
  4. Forced-air heat
  5. Hot-air blow-dryers

Pathophysiology

I. Normally, epidermal keratinocytes are produced in the basal cell layer of the epidermis, move to the skin surface, and are shed from the stratum corneum. In seborrheic dogs, keratinocyte transit time (normally 22 days) is decreased to as little as 8 days, resulting in excessive scale (Kwochka, 1993a).
II. Surface lipids are also altered (Horwitz and Ihrke, 1977).
  A. Surface film contains smaller amounts of diester waxes and increased free fatty acids.
  B. Surface bacteria act on sebaceous secretions, resulting in the production of inflammatory fatty acids with secondary pruritus and odor.
III. Seborrheic skin also has a higher number of coagulase-positive *Staphylococcus* spp. than does normal skin, predisposing to pyodermas and pruritus (Muller et al., 1989).
IV. Any disorder affecting normal epidermal turnover rate, keratinization, sebum production, or scale cohesiveness can result in seborrhea.

Clinical Signs

I. Seborrhea presents as excessive scaliness, which can be accompanied by skin and coat greasiness.
II. Several different manifestations of seborrhea are possible, although overlap can make them difficult to differentiate.
III. Similar alterations are present in the lipid layer, desquamation characteristics, and bacterial flora of the different forms; manifestations may be affected by breed variations.
  A. Seborrhea sicca
    1. Dry skin, dry and dull hair coat
    2. Focal to diffuse scaling
    3. Accumulation of white to gray nonadherent scales
    4. Typically affected breeds: Irish setter, German shepherd dog, dachshund, Doberman pinscher
  B. Seborrhea oleosa
    1. Focal or diffuse scale
    2. Brownish-yellow clumped scales adhering to skin and hair
    3. ''Nit-like'' flakes on hairs

4. Odiferous and oily coat
5. Common breeds: American cocker spaniel, English springer spaniel, Shar pei, West Highland white terrier
C. Seborrheic dermatitis
1. Scaling with evidence of focal or diffuse inflammation
2. Often associated with folliculitis
3. Localized circular lesions with alopecia, erythema, marginal epidermal scaling, and central hyperpigmentation
4. Common breeds: American cocker spaniel, English springer spaniel, West Highland white terrier, basset hound
D. Ceruminous otitis
1. Oily yellow film or flakes in external canal
2. Dry adherent flakes and scales in or around the external ear canal
3. May have a rancid odor

Diagnosis/Differential Diagnosis

I. Initially search for an underlying cause.
II. Primary seborrhea is diagnosed only after all other possible causes have been excluded via an exhaustive search.
III. Obtain a thorough history, paying particular attention to the following.
A. Age, sex, breed
B. Presence of pruritus: allergies, parasites, pyoderma, some fungal infections
C. Presence of polyuria, polydipsia, polyphagia: hyperadrenocorticism
D. Heat-seeking: hypothyroidism, other illnesses
E. Seasonality or pattern to symptoms
F. Current diet
G. Response to previous therapy
IV. Perform a thorough physical examination, noting the distribution of cutaneous lesions and any evidence of other underlying disorders.
V. Undertake the following to identify underlying causes.
A. Detection of fleas
B. Skin scrapings for mites
C. Microscopic examination of epilated hairs for growth stage, whether broken or intact, presence of parasites
D. Microscopic examination of Scotch tape impressions of scale for small parasites, eggs, epidermal debris
E. Wood's lamp examination of plucked hair roots, microscopic examination of potassium hydroxide–digested hairs, dermatophyte culture
F. Cytology of stained dry skin scrapings for yeast, bacteria, and cells
G. Impression smears of pustules, masses
H. Bacterial culture and sensitivity testing
VI. Consider these measures, depending on history, clinical signs, signalment, and initial work-up.
A. Hemogram, serum biochemistry, urinalysis
B. Fecal flotation
C. Skin biopsy

1. Histopathology may elucidate an underlying cause; identify bacterial, parasitic, and fungal/yeast agents; or suggest primary seborrhea.
2. Perform immunofluorescence or immunoperoxidase testing for immune-mediated diseases.
D. Rule out allergic skin disease with intradermal skin testing or in vitro testing.
E. Begin endocrine assays.
F. Consider dietary changes, EFA supplementation.

Treatment

I. For secondary seborrhea, correct the underlying cause.
II. Objectives of antiseborrheic topical therapy include the following.
A. Remove scales and crust, reduce oiliness, control odor, relieve pruritus, decrease inflammation, and maintain/restore protective skin surface emulsion.
B. Decrease doses of systemic drugs needed.
C. Control recurrence of problem.
D. Topical therapies are a valuable adjunct to treatment but rarely resolve the problem as a sole therapy (Kwochka, 1993b, 1995).
III. Topical therapy involves the following.
A. Many dogs benefit from a close hair trim, facilitating bathing and skin aeration.
B. Begin a bathing program (Table 88–2).
1. For mild seborrhea, bathe once to twice weekly until control is attained, then once weekly as maintenance or until resolution.

Table 88–2. *Topical Shampoo Agents for Seborrheic Animals*

Class of Agent	Mechanism of Action	Specific Ingredients
Keratolytic	Damages cells in stratum corneum, resulting in sloughing of cells	Sulfur, salicylic acid, tar
Keratoplastic	Decreases basal cell mitosis with slowing of keratinocyte production	Sulfur, salicylic acid, tar, selenium sulfide
Degreasing	Removes greasy exudate	Benzoyl peroxide, tar, selenium sulfide
Antibacterial	Kills or retards growth of bacterial organisms	Chlorhexidine, sulfur, iodine, triclosan, ethyl lactate, benzoyl peroxide
Antifungal/ antiyeast	Kills or retards growth of fungal and yeast organisms	Chlorhexidine, sulfur, iodine, miconazole, ketoconazole, selenium sulfide
Emollient	Rehydrates skin, decreases transepidermal water loss	Emollient oils, lanolin, lactic acid, urea, glycerin, fatty acids
Antipruritic	Decreases itching	Sulfur, salicylic acid, tar, colloidal oatmeal, pramoxine HCl, diphenhydramine, hydrocortisone

Note: Tar and selenium products are contraindicated for use in cats.

2. Severely affected dogs require bathing every 48 hours until control is attained, then twice weekly as maintenance or until resolution.
3. Shampooing first with hypoallergenic shampoo removes dirt and scale, preparing the skin for medicated shampoos.
4. Shampoos work best if they are diluted 1:5 to 1:10 with water before application to the pet (Shanley, 1990).
5. Most medicated shampoos require 8–15 minutes of application on the pet for maximum efficacy.
6. Shampoo type is matched to clinical signs (Kwochka, 1993b, 1995; Scott et al., 1995).
   a) Seborrhea sicca
      (1) Emollient shampoos are used for dryness and mild flaking.
      (2) For intercurrent pyoderma, use emollient-based chlorhexidine or ethyl lactate products.
      (3) More severe flaking necessitates the use of sulfur–salicylic acid shampoos.
      (4) For very severe dry flaking, mild light tar products must be used with caution, as tar's degreasing action can increase transepidermal water loss and worsen seborrhea.
      (5) Strong coal tar products, benzoyl peroxide products, and selenium sulfide products are contraindicated because of associated transepidermal water loss.
   b) Seborrhea oleosa
      (1) Moderately greasy animals need sulfur–salicylic acid or mild tar shampoos.
      (2) Very greasy dogs require stronger coal tar shampoos.
      (3) For associated pyodermas, use a benzoyl peroxide shampoo.
      (4) It is important to shampoo initially to remove scales and grease or to use a combination of products to achieve management of different symptoms of oily seborrhea.
   c) Concurrent yeast infections
      (1) Remove scales and exudate first, using benzoyl peroxide, 1% selenium sulfide, or sulfur–salicylic acid shampoos.
      (2) Antifungal 2% ketoconazole or 2% miconazole/0.5% chlorhexidine shampoos kill yeast.
      (3) Treat systemically for severe generalized yeast dermatitis with ketoconazole 10 mg/kg PO BID or itraconazole 5–10 mg/kg/day PO for 3–4 weeks.
      (4) Topical application of 2% miconazole nitrate cream, powder, or spray powder or 1% clotrimazole cream BID

can be helpful (takes 20 minutes to penetrate).
7. After-bath rinses are applied while the skin and fur are still damp and are allowed to remain on the pet as it dries (Kwochka, 1993b, 1995; Scott et al., 1995).
   a) Emollient rinses and humectants aid cutaneous hydration.
      (1) Rinses with linoleic acid are most effective.
      (2) Apply via misting bottle between baths for comfort and to decrease number of baths needed.
   b) Antimicrobial after-bath rinses aid treatment of concurrent infections.
   c) Creme rinses are designed to be applied to fur and skin after bathing; some are rinsed out and some remain on the fur and skin.
C. Antiseborrheic ointments or gels decrease focal crust and scale and have follicular flushing action.
D. Dips are indicated to control underlying parasites.
   1. Lime-sulfur is also keratolytic, keratoplastic, antibacterial, and antifungal.
   2. They may prove to be drying to skin.
IV. Corticosteroid therapy may be tried to relieve erythema and pruritus.
A. Prednisone 0.5 mg/kg PO QOD
   1. Short-term use only to decrease inflammation
   2. Contraindicated long term because it may worsen seborrhea
      a) Can suppress sebum production and increase scale formation
      b) May predispose to bacterial infections
B. Topical corticosteroids: creams, ointments, sprays
   1. Sometimes useful locally
   2. May draw pet's attention to area and increase licking
   3. May be absorbed through owner's skin
V. Antibiotics are indicated to decrease surface bacteria and the production of inflammatory fatty acids and for concurrent pyoderma. Choice of antibiotics is based on culture and sensitivity.
VI. Synthetic retinoid therapy affects keratinocyte proliferation, differentiation, and desquamation and may have some immunomodulating effects (Power and Ihrke, 1995).
A. Etretinate (Power and Ihrke, 1995)
   1. May be beneficial for generalized primary seborrhea
   2. Dose: 1 mg/kg PO SID or divided BID
   3. Response expected in 2–6 months: decrease in scale, pruritus, and odor and softened seborrheic plaques
   4. Maintenance tailored to pet's needs: dosing 5 out of 7 days, alternating weeks on and off, or months on and off of medication
   5. No effect on ceruminous otitis

6. Side effects
   a) Keratoconjunctivitis sicca (KCS), anorexia with weight loss, vomiting, diarrhea, increased thirst, pruritus, conjunctivitis, chelitis, stiffness, and hyperactivity are uncommon.
   b) Minor to moderate changes in transaminases, cholesterol, and triglycerides have been noted in dogs.
   c) Teratogenicity is a major concern, as medication is stored in body fat for 2 years; do not use in intact females or breeding males.
   d) Serum biochemistries and Schirmer's tear test values are obtained before treatment and 30 days after beginning therapy. Tear testing is continued every 30 days thereafter for the first 6 months, and serum chemistries are repeated as clinically indicated.
   e) Discontinue retinoid therapy if KCS occurs. Tear production may return in some dogs or respond to cyclosporine ointment.
7. Lifetime use indicated if positive response to therapy
8. Effective in primary seborrhea in cocker spaniels, springer spaniels, golden retrievers, and Irish setters; ineffective in West Highland white terriers and basset hounds
9. Schnauzer comedo syndrome, ichthyosis: may benefit from etretinate or isotretinoin
B. Isotretinoin (Power and Ihrke, 1995)
   1. Ineffective in the treatment of primary seborrhea
   2. Effective in the treatment of schnauzer comedo syndrome, canine ichthyosis, and feline acne
   3. Dose: 1–2 mg/kg/day or divided BID PO in dogs; 10 mg/day PO in cats
   4. Side effects: teratogenicity
C. Topical tretinoin (Power and Ihrke, 1995)
   1. Reduces keratinocyte cohesion and increases epidermal turnover
   2. Useful in nasal/digital hyperkeratosis, canine and feline acne
   3. 0.025% topically every 24–72 hours in cats (use sparingly to avoid irritation) and 0.05% SID-QOD in dogs
   4. Hydrocortisone cream 1% on alternate days to decrease irritation
VII. Fatty acid supplementation
A. Fatty acid imbalances may occur in seborrheic dogs.
   1. A relative deficiency of linoleic acid increases transepidermal water loss.
   2. A balanced fatty acid supplement containing linoleic acid may normalize cutaneous fatty acids.
B. The modification of leukotriene and prostaglandin synthesis and activity may decrease inflammation.

Patient Monitoring

I. Warn the owner that for primary seborrhea, a cure is not possible, but signs can be managed with varying degrees of success, depending on disease severity and the frequency of treatments rendered.
II. Therapy usually provides short-term relief for secondary seborrhea until the cause can be diagnosed and treated, and it helps hasten recovery of hair and skin.
III. Prognosis for secondary seborrhea is generally good if the underlying cause is identified and treated.

Seborrheic Syndromes

See Table 88–3.

Hyperkeratotic Syndromes

See Table 88–4.

CUTANEOUS ENDOCRINOPATHIES

Rodney A. W. Rosychuk

Disorders of Thyroid Hormone

Definition and Causes

Skin changes are associated with both deficiencies and excesses of thyroid hormones.

Pathophysiology

I. In the hypothyroid state, several events occur.
   A. Anagen fails to be initiated, and hair follicles enter telogen or the resting stage of the hair cycle. There is abnormal shedding (decreased or excessive) and increased ease of epilation with poor or absent regrowth.
   B. Epidermal keratinization becomes disordered, producing superficial and follicular hyperkeratosis (scaling, skin thickening, comedones).
   C. Sebaceous glands atrophy, and sebaceous secretions are decreased and/or qualitatively abnormal.
   D. There are alterations of cutaneous fatty acid concentrations.
   E. The accumulation of abnormal and potentially irritating ceruminous secretions in ears can cause otitis externa.
   F. Hyperpigmentation often occurs, but the mechanism is unknown.
   G. Myxedema may develop, especially in more chronic, severe hypothyroidism.
      1. Decreased catabolism of dermal mucopolysaccharides
      2. Mucopolysaccharide binding of excessive water
   H. The skin may become cool to the touch from slowed metabolism or peripheral vasoconstriction.

Table 88–3. ***Characteristics and Management of Seborrheic Syndromes***

Disorder	Affected Breeds	Clinical Signs	Pathophysiology	Treatment
Tail gland hyperplasia of dogs	Any dog	1. Swelling dorsum of tail 1–2 in. from tailhead 2. Hyperpigmentation 3. Comedones 4. Occasional papules, pustules 5. Greasy, scaly skin	1. Hyperplasia of perianal and sebaceous tail glands crowds out hairs, leading to swelling and alopecia 2. Associated with sex hormone imbalances, testicular neoplasia, seborrhea 3. Idiopathic	1. Correct underlying causes. 2. Apply benzoyl peroxide gels. 3. Castration may be helpful. 4. Surgical resection is indicated if idiopathic. 5. Progestational compounds may help.
Tail gland hyperplasia of cats	Most often in confined cats, especially male cats	1. Scaliness, matting and crusting of hair diffusely along dorsum of tail 2. Focal alopecia 3. Hyperpigmentation 4. Rarely pyoderma	1. Accumulation of increased secretions from tail sebaceous and apocrine glands 2. Poor grooming	1. Provide more inside living space, or let cat outside. 2. Clip and clean area. 3. Apply benzoyl peroxide shampoo to area. 4. Clean daily or as needed with alcohol.
Canine acne	Short-coated breeds: Doberman pinschers, English bulldogs, boxers, Great Danes, any dog at puberty	1. Comedones, papules, and pustules worse around rostral mandible and lips 2. Furuncles and draining tracts in chronic cases	1. Increased androgen circulation at puberty (3–12 mo) leads to hypertrophy and hyperplasia of sebaceous glands. 2. Alteration of keratinization of follicular epithelium leads to comedone formation. 3. Bacterial infection occurs. 4. Foreign body granulomas (hair, keratin) may complicate chronic cases.	1. Mild cases heal spontaneously. 2. Clip and clean area. 3. Shampoo area with benzoyl peroxide daily. 4. Use benzoyl peroxide gel BID. 5. Give severe and chronic cases systemic antibiotics. 6. Topical fluocinolone acetate in DMSO may benefit chronic cases. 7. Apply tretinoin 0.05% daily, with decreased frequency for maintenance.
Feline acne	Any cat	1. Comedones, papules, and pustules on chin and lips 2. Folliculitis, furunculosis, and cellulitis in severe cases	1. Idiopathic keratinization disorder results in comedones, papules, and pustules; suppurative folliculitis and cellulitis can develop. 2. May be episodic or constant	1. Clip and clean chin; apply warm compresses. 2. Benzoyl peroxide shampoo may be beneficial. 3. Provide maintenance cleaning with alcohol or shampoo 3 times a week. 4. Systemic antibiotics are indicated for pyoderma. 5. Apply topical tretinoin 0.01–0.025% q 24–72 h. 6. Metronidazole 0.75% gel may prove useful. 7. Isotretinoin 10 mg/day for refractory or uncooperative cats.
Schnauzer comedo syndrome	Miniature schnauzers	1. Comedones along dorsal midline from neck to lumbosacral area 2. Secondary pyoderma or folliculitis	1. It is an inherited dysplasia of the hair follicle resulting in obstruction of the follicle, which becomes filled with sebum and keratin. 2. Contents of plugged follicle protrude above skin surface. 3. Rupture of follicle contents into dermis leads to inflammation.	1. Clip and clean if severe surface crusting exists. 2. Shampoo with benzoyl peroxide or keratolytic shampoo. 3. Apply benzoyl peroxide gel BID as needed. 4. Rub alcohol on back 2–3 times a week. 5. Isotretinoin 1–2 mg/kg/day PO or etretinate 1 mg/kg/day can be effective within 3–4 wk.

Table continued on following page

Table 88–3. **Characteristics and Management of Seborrheic Syndromes** (*Continued*)

Disorder	Affected Breeds	Clinical Signs	Pathophysiology	Treatment
Ear margin seborrhea	Dachshunds, Boston terriers, and breeds with pendulous ears	1. Greasy plugs adherent to pinnal margins 2. Partial alopecia of pinnae may be present in dachshunds. 3. Inflammation and necrosis of ear magins can occur.	1. Idiopathic 2. Possibly thrombosis of vessels of ears	1. Hot pack or warm-water soaks followed by keratolytic shampoo 2. Follow with moisturizing rinses. 3. Treat underlying dermatitis. 4. Topical steroids lessen inflammation. 5. Prednisone 1 mg/kg PO daily for 7–10 days for severe inflammation 6. Boston terriers: etretinate 1 mg/kg/day PO 7. Pentoxifylline 400 mg/dog/day (200 mg/dog/day if <10 kg body weight) may help increase microvascular blood flow.
Epidermal dysplasia	West Highland white terriers	1. Develops at 2–6 mo of age 2. Severe pruritus 3. Lichenification, scale, alopecia, hyperpigmentation, erythema, papules, crusting 4. Greasy skin and hair coat 5. Ceruminous otitis externa 6. Peripheral lymphadenopathy	1. Heritable alteration of epidermal development 2. Possible altered immune defense mechanisms 3. Overgrowth of *Malassezia pachydermatis* 4. Possible development of fungal hypersensitivity	1. Follow keratolytic shampoos with ketoconazole or miconazole shampoos and use a 0.5% chlorhexidine or povidone-iodine in water rinse. 2. Administer ketoconazole 10 mg/kg PO BID or itraconazole 5–10 mg/kg/day PO.

I. There is also a predisposition to superficial and deep bacterial pyodermas, *Malassezia* infections, and demodicosis.
   1. Increased bacterial colonization in abnormal cutaneous surface microenvironment

2. Acquired immunodeficiencies related to hypothyroidism
J. Poor healing and increased bruising can occur.
   1. Defects in fibroblast function and collagen metabolism

Table 88–4. **Characteristics and Management of Hyperkeratotic Syndromes**

Disorder	Signalment	Clinical Signs	Pathophysiology	Treatment
Nasal hyperkeratosis	Generally older dogs	1. Raised, firm, dry accumulations of horny tissue with occasional fissures developing on rostral planum nasale 2. Infrequent hypopigmentation	1. Age-related retention of statum corneum 2. Associated with other diseases: pemphigus erythematosus, discoid lupus erythematosus, pemphigus foliaceus, or canine distemper	1. Wet dressings followed by petroleum jelly rehydrate the nose 2. Topical steroids are beneficial. 3. Topical tretinoin may be effective when used with emollients.
Digital hyperkeratosis	Generally older dogs	1. Accumulation of horny tissue on peripheral aspects of pads 2. Often accompanies nasal hyperkeratosis	1. Keratin not worn on periphery of pads 2. Accompanies other diseases: pemphigus erythematosus, pemphigus foliaceus, distemper, zinc-responsive dermatosis, discoid or systemic lupus erythematosus, or hepatocutaneous syndrome	Usually none required
Canine ichthyosis	Genetically predisposed individuals affected at birth	1. Body covered with scales and keratinous projections 2. Thickened footpads	Caused by a genetic keratinization defect	1. Incurable 2. Management with keratolytic shampoos 3. Isotretinoin 1 mg/kg PO BID 4. Etretinate 1 mg/kg PO SID or divided BID

2. Increased bleeding tendencies from platelet defects
II. The hyperthyroid state produces two basic changes.
   A. Psychoactive effects result in lack of attention to proper grooming and/or hair pulling (cats).
   B. Hypermetabolic state produces increased skin temperature and vasodilatation, which may also be pruritogenic (cats).

Clinical Signs

I. Canine hypothyroidism
   A. Cutaneous signs develop slowly over several months.
   B. The hairs are dull, dry, coarse, and brittle and may become bleached out or discolored (e.g., black to reddish).
   C. The skin tends to be dry and scaly (seborrhea sicca).
   D. On occasion, abnormal sebaceous secretions may accumulate to produce an oily or greasy coat/skin (seborrhea oleosa).
   E. Alopecia is common.
      1. Poor or absent regrowth following clipping
      2. Abnormal shedding patterns, increased shedding, increased ease of epilation
      3. Initially, often patchy or asymmetrical, primarily affecting areas of wear, e.g., dorsum of tail
      4. May become more bilaterally symmetrical and truncal but spares the head and distal extremities
      5. Undercoat often preferentially lost, giving the coat a coarse appearance
      6. Initially, hair loss over extremities in giant breeds
   F. Comedones are common and most prevalent over the ventral abdomen.
   G. Hyperpigmentation is first noted in alopecic areas and then becomes more generalized and symmetrical.
   H. Myxedema is seen as thickening and folding of the skin and is most commonly noted over the head (tragic expression) and distal extremities.
   I. Skin changes are nonpruritic; when pruritus is present, it is attributed to secondary bacterial pyoderma and severe seborrhea.
   J. In congenital hypothyroidism, initially there is a retention of the puppy coat and poor growth of primary hairs.
   K. Secondary/tertiary hypothyroidism generally produces milder changes than primary acquired hypothyroidism.
II. Feline hypothyroidism
   A. Coat and skin are generally dull, dry, and scaly.
   B. Pinnal alopecia (medial and lateral) is common.
   C. There is variable regrowth after clipping.
   D. Symmetrical, truncal alopecia is uncommon.
III. Feline hyperthyroidism
   A. There is usually excessive shedding, matting, and scaling and a general unkempt appearance.
   B. The skin may be warm and moist.

C. Alopecia caused by self-trauma is most commonly noted over the caudal thighs, inguinal regions, back, and sides.
D. There is an increased rate of nail growth.

Diagnosis

I. See Chap. 41 for specific laboratory diagnostic tests.
II. Histologic changes may be helpful in supporting the diagnosis.
   A. Nonspecific changes of an endocrinopathy
      1. Orthokeratotic and occasionally parakeratotic hyperkeratosis, follicular keratosis
      2. Telogen hairs predominating; follicles devoid of hairs
      3. Follicular atrophy or dilatation
      4. Sebaceous gland atrophy
      5. Epidermal melanosis
   B. Changes more characteristic of hypothyroidism
      1. Dermal thickening
      2. Myxedema
      3. Hypertrophy and vacuolation of arrector pili muscles (controversial)
   C. Normal, thickened, or thinned epidermis
   D. May see inflammatory changes owing to secondary seborrheas and/or pyodermas

Differential Diagnosis

I. Hyperadrenocorticism
II. Sex hormone imbalance
III. Adult-onset hyposomatotropism (growth hormone–responsive dermatosis)
IV. Follicular dysplasia
V. Color mutant alopecia
VI. Cyclic flank alopecia
VII. Sebaceous adenitis
VIII. Follicular arrest
IX. Telogen defluxion
X. Pattern baldness

Treatment and Monitoring

I. Hypothyroid disorders
   A. Adequate thyroid hormone supplementation should resolve both clinical and histologic manifestations.
   B. First hair regrowth is usually within 3–4 weeks of starting therapy.
   C. Return to full coat may take 4–6 months.
   D. During the first 2–6 weeks of therapy, increased shedding, scaling, and pruritus can result from reactivation of cutaneous metabolism.
      1. Administer antiseborrheic shampoos and moisturizers.
      2. If the skin is pruritic, consider a short course of oral prednisolone, starting at 0.5–1 mg/kg/day and decreasing over 1–3 weeks.
II. Hyperthyroid disorders
   A. Institute grooming program and resolve hyperthyroidism.

B. Coat/skin condition usually takes 1–3 months to significantly improve.

Disorders of Glucocorticoids

Definition and Causes

I. Cutaneous manifestations of glucocorticoid insufficiencies are rare in the dog and cat.
II. Skin changes are most commonly associated with excess concentrations of exogenous or endogenous glucocorticoids.
  A. Canine hyperadrenocorticism
    1. Primary, spontaneous
    2. Iatrogenic
  B. Feline hyperadrenocorticism
    1. Cats are generally more resistant to the deleterious effects of glucocorticoids.
    2. Endogenous forms are rare.

Pathophysiology

I. Glucocorticoids in excess quantities produce the following.
  A. Antimitotic and depressive effects on the initiation of anagen, with telogenization of hair follicles
  B. Disordered keratinization (orthokeratotic hyperkeratosis), with excessive scaling and comedones
  C. General catabolic effects
    1. Depression of fibroblast proliferation and decreased production of dermal collagen and ground substance
    2. Epidermal and dermal atrophy, loss of elasticity, and vascular fragility
  D. Sebaceous gland atrophy and decreased production of sebaceous secretions, with drying of the coat and skin
  E. Immunosuppressive effects predisposing to bacterial or fungal infections or demodicosis
  F. Degenerative changes in skin proteins, which predispose to calcium deposition in collagen and elastin fibers (calcinosis cutis)
II. High levels of adrenocorticotropic hormone (ACTH) produced with pituitary-dependent hyperadrenocorticism and hypoadrenocorticism may have a melanocyte-stimulating hormone (MSH)–like effect, promoting hyperpigmentation.

Clinical Signs

I. Canine hyperadrenocorticism
  A. Cutaneous signs generally develop slowly over several months or years.
  B. Characteristic skin changes may not occur in animals with rapidly growing adrenal tumors.
  C. Alopecia is the most common finding.
    1. Starts as focal hair loss over points of wear
    2. Progresses to bilaterally symmetrical, truncal alopecia, usually sparing head and distal extremities
    3. Hairs more readily epilated
    4. Occasionally may see extensive facial alopecia
    5. Thin and patchy coat, with a moth-eaten appearance in short-coated breeds
  D. Coat color may lighten; black hairs may become reddish.
  E. The skin is usually dry, with variable degrees of scaling (seborrhea sicca); scaling may be very heavy.
  F. Comedones are common and most prevalent over the ventral abdomen and caudodorsal back.
  G. The skin is usually thin and lacks elasticity and tone.
    1. Wrinkles over abdomen, inguinal region
    2. Simulates dehydration
    3. Prominent subcutaneous vasculature
    4. Atrophy often first affecting old scars
  H. Increased bruising occurs with petechiation or ecchymoses, especially following venipuncture or trauma.
  I. Delayed wound healing may be noted.
  J. Hyperpigmentation usually begins in alopecic areas but tends to become generalized and bilaterally symmetrical.
  K. There may be marked atrophy (paper-thin) of old scars.
  L. Calcinosis cutis is most common over the ventral abdomen, inguinal regions, back, and dorsal cervical regions.
    1. Initially creamy colored papules and plaques
    2. May become inflamed, exudative, crusty, ulcerated
    3. Variably pruritic; may be severe
    4. Predisposes to secondary bacterial infections
    5. Most common with endogenous disease, but may occur with iatrogenic
  M. Phlebectasias are occasionally found.
    1. Small, 1–6 mm, slightly raised blood blister–like lesions
    2. Most consistently associated with excessive glucocorticoid exposure (exogenous or endogenous)
    3. Definitively diagnosed on histologic examination
    4. Do not resolve with resolution of hyperadrenocorticism
  N. Perianal adenomas may develop in neutered males or females from the overproduction of testosterone or other androgens from hyperplastic adrenal glands.
II. Feline hyperadrenocorticism
  A. Alopecia of trunk or ventral abdomen, distal extremities
  B. Readily epilated hairs
  C. Thin skin, prominent vasculature
  D. Recurrent superficial and deep infections
  E. Variable hyperpigmentation of skin
  F. ± Increased friability of skin
    1. Full-thickness tears following minimal trauma
    2. May occur before significant hair loss noted
  G. Calcinosis cutis not known to occur

H. Signs of iatrogenic hyperadrenocorticism generally milder
III. Canine hypoadrenocorticism
   A. Occasionally hyperpigmentation
   B. Nonspecific truncal alopecia and scaling, probably from debilitating nature of the disease

Diagnosis

I. Specific adrenal function diagnostic tests are described in Chap. 44.
II. Skin biopsies often reveal changes suspicious of hyperadrenocorticism.
   A. Nonspecific changes of an endocrinopathy (see Disorders of Thyroid Hormone, earlier)
   B. Changes more suggestive of hyperadrenocorticism
     1. Dystrophic mineralization
     2. Thin dermis
     3. Absence of arrector pili muscles

Differential Diagnosis

I. Hypothyroidism
II. Same differentials as for hypothyroidism in dogs (see earlier)
III. Megesterol acetate administration in cats
IV. Pancreatic paraneoplastic alopecia in cats
V. Alopecia as a result of self-trauma in cats
VI. Telogen defluxion in cats
VII. Diabetes mellitus in cats

Treatment and Monitoring

I. Continuous normalization of serum cortisols is required to totally resolve the dermatologic manifestations of endogenous hyperadrenocorticism.
   A. Hair regrowth begins within 3–6 weeks of cortisol normalization.
   B. Normalization of hair coat/skin may take 4–6 months.
   C. Within first 2–6 weeks, a transient increased scaling, hair loss, and pruritus may be noted and can be managed with antiseborrheic shampoos and moisturizers.
   D. New hair may be of a different color (usually darker) but often becomes more normal following the next hair cycle.
II. Calcinosis cutis is treated with antiseborrheic shampoos and astringents (e.g., aluminum acetate) if it is inflamed and exudative.
   A. Antistaphylococcal antibiotics are indicated when secondary infections are suspected.
     1. Cephalexin 11–22 mg/kg PO TID for 3–4 weeks
     2. Enrofloxacin 2.5 mg/kg PO BID for 3–4 weeks
   B. Resolution should occur in most cases but may take many months ($\geq$6–12).
III. Skin changes associated with iatrogenic hyperadrenocorticism are reversible with discontinuation of the administered steroid.

A. The time to resolution is dependent on the severity of the iatrogenic changes.
B. Times to improvement generally parallel those outlined for well-treated endogenous hyperadrenocorticism.
IV. In cats, skin tears may not be amenable to suturing because of friability and may require the use of special occlusive dressings (BioDres [DVM]) and body bandages.

Disorders of Growth Hormone

Definition and Causes

I. Both excesses and deficiencies of growth hormone can be associated with skin changes.
II. The following disorders may present with dermatologic abnormalities (see also Chap. 40).
   A. Pituitary dwarfism
   B. Adult-onset hyposomatotropism (growth hormone–responsive dermatosis)
   C. Acromegaly

Pathophysiology

Growth hormone has many effects on the skin.
I. Stimulates hair growth
II. Stimulates sebaceous gland growth and secretion
III. Stimulates dermal collagen and mucopolysaccharide production
IV. Normalizes dermal elastin and pigmentation

Clinical Signs

I. Pituitary dwarfism
   A. Skin/coat may appear normal at birth.
   B. By 2–3 months, primary hair growth is seen only over the face and distal extremities.
   C. Puppy coat is retained.
   D. Hairs are more readily epilated.
   E. Bilaterally symmetrical truncal alopecia develops, with the pericervical and caudal thighs more severely affected.
   F. Skin becomes thin, hypotonic, scaly, and hyperpigmented.
   G. Comedones are common.
   H. Concurrent hypothyroidism may accentuate skin changes.
II. Adult-onset hyposomatotropism
   A. Affected breeds: many, but especially chow chow, Pomeranian, miniature poodle, keeshond, Samoyed, American water spaniel
   B. Males predisposed 10:1
   C. Age of onset for alopecia
     1. 1–2 years for most
     2. Range of 9 months to 11 years
   D. Gradual development of bilaterally symmetrical, nonpruritic alopecia in one of three forms
     1. Pericervical, caudomedial thighs, pinnae, tail
     2. Truncal alopecia without hyperpigmentation
     3. Flank alopecia with or without hyperpigmentation

Table 88–5. **Cutaneous Manifestations of Sex Hormone Imbalances**

Disorder	Causes	Clinical Signs	Diagnosis	Treatment and Monitoring
Female dog				
Hyperestrogenism	Cystic ovaries (follicular) Ovarian tumors (rare) Exogenous estrogen overdose	Alopecia: perineum, perigenital, ventrum, flanks, thorax; symmetrical Seborrhea (sicca or oleosa) ± Hyperpigmentation, ceruminous otitis externa, pruritus, gynecomastia, vulvar enlargement	Skin biopsies: endocrinopathy Vaginal cytology Ultrasonography Laparotomy Elevated serum estradiol in 30% Response to therapy	Discontinuation of exogenous estrogen Ovariohysterectomy Rupture or removal of cyst HCG or GnRH therapy
Estrogen-responsive dermatosis	Hypoestrogenism (suspected) Following ovariohysterectomy In noncycling, intact females Occasionally during pseudopregnancy	Alopecia: perineum, perigenital, caudomedial thighs, ventrum, pericervical, truncal, ears; symmetrical; on occasion, only flanks involved Short-coated breeds: hair/skin very soft Occasionally increased scaling, pruritus	Skin biopsies: endocrinopathy; sebaceous glands relatively spared Serum estrogen concentrations poorly predictive Response to estrogen therapy	Ovariohysterectomized bitches: diethylstilbestrol 0.02 mg/kg (max = 1 mg) PO SID for 14 days, then QOD for 2 wk, then twice weekly for a 3-mo trial If estrus is induced, stop until it abates, then resume maintenance dose Regrowth may be transient If estrogen fails, try testosterone or mibolerone Intact females: FSH (Carlson, 1985) DES, LH, FSH protocol (Moses and Shille, 1988)
Male Dog				
Testicular feminizing tumors	Estrogen excess: Sertoli's cell tumor, seminoma, interstitial cell tumor (rare cause)	Boxers, Shetland sheepdogs, Weimaraners predisposed Associated with male pseudohermaphrodism in miniature schnauzers Alopecia: perineum, genitals, ventrum, flanks, neck, chest; symmetrical; may only be flanks Coat color change ± Seborrhea, hyperpigmentation Line of hyperpigmentation and/or erythema along ventral prepuce Gynecomastia, enlarged nipples	Skin biopsies: endocrinopathy Serum estradiol increased in 30–40% Preputial cytology: cornification as seen in estral bitch (in advanced disease) Abdominal radiography, ultrasonography, exploratory laparotomy	Castration: first hair regrowth within 3–6 wk; complete resolution of symptoms within 3–6 mo May see transient increases in hair loss, scaling, and pruritus during the first few weeks following castration
Castration-responsive dermatosis	Unknown: 30–40% may have elevated serum estradiol, testosterone, or progesterone	Chow chow, Samoyed, keeshond, Pomeranian, husky, malamute predisposed Intact; testicles normal Alopecia: onset 1–3 yr; caudomedial thighs, neck, shoulder, flank, dorsolumbar Hyperpigmentation common Variable degrees of seborrhea Hair regrowth at sites of trauma	Skin biopsies: endocrinopathy; flame follicles (catagen arrest) 30–40% have elevated serum estradiol, testosterone, or progesterone Response to therapy	Castration: hair regrowth starts within 3–6 wk; may take 6–8 mo for complete normalization Response may be transient (recurrence of hair loss)
Adrenal hyperprogesteronism/ hyperandrogenism (congenital adrenal hyperplasia–like syndrome)	Adrenal enzyme deficiency causes excessive adrenal androgen or progesterone secretion	Pomeranians, other breeds Males and females affected (neutered or intact) Alopecia: onset 1–5 yr; neck, trunk, caudomedial thighs; symmetrical Hyperpigmentation common	Skin biopsies: endocrinopathy Increased progesterone, 17-hydroxyprogesterone, and androgens after ACTH stimulation	Mitotane as for pituitary-dependent hyperadrenocorticism (see Chap. 44) Castration Methyltestosterone (see Testosterone-responsive dermatosis)

Table 88–5. **Cutaneous Manifestations of Sex Hormone Imbalances** (*Continued*)

Disorder	Causes	Clinical Signs	Diagnosis	Treatment and Monitoring
Male Dog (*Continued*)				
Hyperandrogenism	Androgen-producing testicular tumors (especially interstitial tumors)	Tail gland hyperplasia; perianal hyperplasia Seborrhea common Prostatomegaly	Response to castration	Resolution of signs within 3–4 mo
Idiopathic male feminizing syndrome	Unknown; unlikely to be an endocrinopathy	Middle-aged or older; intact Alopecia: perineum, ventrum, chest, flanks, face; symmetrical Hyperpigmentation, seborrhea, lichenification, pruritus, gynecomastia all common	Skin biopsies: superficial perivascular dermatitis Response to therapy	Castration Oral testosterone (see below for dosages) Antiseborrheic topical therapy Systemic glucocorticoids
Testosterone-responsive dermatosis	Hypoandrogenism (suspected) Older, neutered males Atrophied testicles Testicular neoplasia	Alopecia: perineum, genitals, ventrum, flanks, neck, chest; dorsolateral lumbar and flanks may be primarily affected Variable hyperpigmentation Seborrhea sicca common Skin may be thin, hypotonic (mimics dehydration)	Skin biopsies: endocrinopathy; relative sparing of sebaceous glands Response to therapy	Methyltestosterone or fluoxymesterone 0.5 mg/kg (max = 30 mg) PO QOD for 3-mo trial Initial regrowth in 4–8 wk Once complete regrowth, give above dose as maintenance 2–3 times/wk Complications: aggressive behavior (uncommon), hepatotoxicity (rare)
Cat				
Feline acquired symmetrical alopecia (feline endocrine alopecia)	Unknown Sex hormone imbalance related to premature neutering? Abnormal thyroid function?	Rare disease (see also Chap. 83) Most commonly neutered males and females Alopecia: perineum, inguinal region, caudal thighs; may extend to trunk, forelegs Nonpruritic	Skin biopsies: telogenization of hair follicles Response to therapy	Megestrol acetate: 2.5–5 mg PO QOD until regrowth, then PRN Repositol testosterone: 12.5 mg total IM; if no response in 6 wk, repeat 50% relapse in 6 mo to 2 yr; repeat as necessary May see transient aggression, urine spraying Trial thyroid hormone supplementation

HCG = human chorionic gonadotropin; GnRH = gonadotropin releasing hormone; FST = follicle-stimulating hormone; DES = diethylstilbestrol; LH = luteinizing hormone; ACTH = adrenocorticotropic hormone.

E. Readily epilated hairs in affected areas
F. Thin, hypotonic, inelastic skin with advanced disease
G. Hair regrowth in tufts at sites of skin trauma
III. Acromegaly
   A. Thickened, myxedematous skin with prominent folds
   B. Hypertrichosis (thick coat), hyperpigmentation
   C. Thick, hard nails

Diagnosis

I. For specific diagnostic tests, see Chap. 40.
II. Skin biopsies can reveal the following.
   A. Pituitary dwarfism and adult-onset hyposomatotropism
      1. Nonspecific changes of an endocrinopathy (see Disorders of Thyroid Hormone, earlier)
      2. Changes more consistent with growth hormone deficiency
        a) Thin dermis
        b) Decreased number and size and fragmentation of dermal elastin fibers

      (1) Present only if signs of adult-onset hyposomatotropism chronic (>2 years)
      (2) Flame follicles (catagen hair follicles)
   B. Acromegaly
      1. Orthokeratotic hyperkeratosis, hypergranulosis
      2. Epidermal, dermal hyperplasia
      3. Myxedema

Differential Diagnosis

I. Pituitary dwarfism: hypothyroidism
II. Adult-onset hyposomatotropism
   A. Hypothyroidism, hyperadrenocorticism
   B. Castration-responsive dermatosis
   C. Estrogen/testosterone–responsive dermatosis
   D. Follicular dysplasia
   E. Cyclic flank alopecia
   F. Congenital adrenal hyperplasia–like syndrome
III. Acromegaly: hypothyroidism

Treatment and Monitoring

I. Pituitary dwarfism
   A. Cutaneous signs respond to bovine, porcine, or synthetic human growth hormone. Give 0.1 IU/kg SQ three times weekly for 4–6 weeks.
   B. Hair regrowth often begins within 3–4 weeks of starting therapy.
   C. Duration of regrowth is variable (months to years).
II. Adult-onset hyposomatotropism
   A. Because changes are restricted to skin and are not discomforting/debilitating, no therapy may be needed.
   B. Bovine, porcine, or human synthetic growth hormone can be given.
      1. Dose: 0.1 IU/kg SQ QOD for 30 days
      2. Initial hair regrowth in 2–8 weeks
      3. Good overall response by 3 months
      4. Variable duration of regrowth (6 months to 3 years)
      5. Successful retreatment possible
   C. Potential side effects
      1. Diabetes mellitus (usually transient)
      2. Hypersensitivity reactions
III. Acromegaly
   A. Discontinue progesterone therapy, consider ovariohysterectomy.
   B. See Chap. 40 for further advice.

Disorders of Sex Hormones

See Table 88–5.

Bibliography

Campbell KL, Small E: Identifying and managing the cutaneous manifestations of various endocrine diseases. Vet Med Report 86:118, 1991

Carlson RA: Endocrine alopecia in a dog showing response to FSH administration. J Am Anim Hosp Assoc 21:735, 1985

Horwitz LN, Ihrke PJ: Canine seborrhea. p. 519. In Kirk RW (ed): Current Veterinary Therapy VI. WB Saunders, Philadelphia, 1977

Kwochka KW: Retinoids in dermatology. p. 553. In Kirk RW (ed): Current Veterinary Therapy X: Small Animal Practice. WB Saunders, Philadelphia, 1989

Kwochka KW: Primary keratinization disorders of dogs. p. 176. In Griffin CE, Kwochka KW, McDonald JA (eds): Current Veterinary Dermatology. Mosby–Year Book, St. Louis, 1993a

Kwochka KW: Symptomatic topical therapy of scaling disorders. p. 191. In Griffin CE, Kwochka KW, McDonald JA (eds): Current Veterinary Dermatology. Mosby–Year Book, St. Louis, 1993b

Kwochka KW: Shampoos and moisturizing rinses in veterinary dermatology. p. 590. In Bonagura JD (ed): Kirk's Current Veterinary Therapy XII: Small Animal Practice. WB Saunders, Philadelphia, 1995

Miller WH: Follicular dysplasia in adult black and red Doberman pinschers. Vet Dermatol 1:181, 1990

Moses DL, Shille VM: Induction of estrous in greyhound bitches with prolonged idiopathic anestrus or with suppression of estrus after testosterone administration. J Am Vet Med Assoc 192:1541, 1988

Muller GH, Kirk RW, Scott DW: Small Animal Dermatology. 4th Ed. WB Saunders, Philadelphia, 1989

Power HT, Ihrke PJ: The use of synthetic retinoids in veterinary medicine. p. 585. In Bonagura JD (ed): Kirk's Current Veterinary Therapy XII: Small Animal Practice. WB Saunders, Philadelphia, 1995

Rosychuk RAW: Endocrine alopecia in a chow chow. Vet Med Report 2:55, 1990

Schmeitzel LP: Sex hormone-related and growth hormone-related alopecias. Vet Clin North Am [Small Anim Pract] 20:1579, 1990

Schmeitzel LP, Lothrop CD: Sex hormones and skin disease. Vet Med Report 2:28, 1990

Schmeitzel LP, Lothrop CD, Rosenkrantz WS: Congenital adrenal hyperplasia–like syndrome. p. 600. In Bonagura JD (ed): Kirk's Current Veterinary Therapy XII: Small Animal Practice. WB Saunders, Philadelphia, 1995

Scott DW, Miller WH: Epidermal dysplasia and *Malassezia pachydermatis* infection in West Highland white terriers. Vet Dermatol 1:25, 1989

Scott DW, Miller WH, Griffin CE: Small Animal Dermatology. 5th Ed. WB Saunders, Philadelphia, 1995

Shanley KJ: The seborrheic disease complex—an approach to underlying causes and therapies. Vet Clin North Am [Small Anim Pract] 20:1557, 1990

White SD, Cerugoli KL, Bullock LP et al: Cutaneous markers of canine hyperadrenocorticism. Compend Contin Educ Pract Vet 11:4446, 1989

89

Immune-Mediated Skin Diseases

Lowell J. Ackerman

AUTOIMMUNE DISORDERS

Pemphigus Complex

Definition and Causes

I. The term pemphigus is used to describe a group of dermatoses characterized by autoantibody deposition within the intercellular spaces of the epidermis, which causes the separation of epidermal cells from one another (acantholysis).

II. This complex is subdivided into four disorders, based on clinical presentation, location of intraepidermal clefting, and immunopathologic findings.
  A. Pemphigus vulgaris is the most severe manifestation of pemphigus but not the most common.
  B. Pemphigus foliaceus is probably the most common form.
  C. Pemphigus erythematosus is relatively common in animals and is believed to be a more benign form of pemphigus foliaceus, or perhaps a crossover syndrome between pemphigus and lupus erythematosus.
  D. Pemphigus vegetans is the rarest form and appears to be a more benign variant of pemphigus vulgaris.

Pathophysiology

I. The lesions of pemphigus result from binding of an autoantibody to an antigen (or antigens) in or near the epidermal cell membrane.

II. This results in detachment of epidermal cells from one another, with clefting and the formation of vesicles, bullae, and ulcerative lesions.

Clinical Signs

I. Signalment
  A. No sex predisposition
  B. Breed predisposition

1. Pemphigus foliaceus has been more commonly reported in the Akita, bearded collie, chow chow, dachshund, Doberman pinscher, Finnish spitz, Newfoundland, and schipperke.
2. Pemphigus erythematosus has been more commonly reported in the collie, German shepherd dog, and Shetland sheepdog.
  C. Age predisposition: usually occurs in middle-aged to older animals

II. Specific clinical features
  A. Pemphigus vulgaris
    1. It is an ulcerating disease initially affecting the nonhaired mucous membranes (mouth, anus, conjunctiva, nasal mucosa, vagina, prepuce) and their junctions with the skin, before becoming generalized.
    2. Oral lesions are found in most cases.
      a) The lesions consist of erosions and ulcerations.
      b) Intact blisters rarely occur because of the fragility of the blister roof.
    3. Additional findings include a positive Nikolsky's sign (when lateral pressure is applied to skin near a lesion, extension of the lesion or the creation of a new lesion occurs).
    4. Secondary bacterial complications may develop, and severely affected individuals can be anorectic, depressed, and febrile.
  B. Pemphigus foliaceus
    1. It is characterized by a scaling, crusting, and/or pustular dermatitis that often originates on the head and ears before becoming generalized.
    2. Mucosal and mucocutaneous involvement is not prominent, but the footpads are frequently involved and are hyperkeratotic.
    3. In cats, mammary glands and nail beds are frequently affected.
    4. Intact vesicles can appear transiently, but they rapidly become purulent and are usually sterile on culture.

5. Secondary infection, lymphadenopathy, edema, depression, and lameness are less common than expected, and animals usually do not become systemically ill.

C. Pemphigus erythematosus
   1. Pemphigus erythematosus is clinically indistinguishable from pemphigus foliaceus but usually remains localized to the head and face.
   2. Occasionally the footpads are involved.

D. Pemphigus vegetans
   1. Groups of pustules evolve into eruptive papillomatous lesions and verrucous vegetative masses.
   2. These lesions often erode and exude serum.

Diagnosis

I. Biopsy
   A. Histopathology
      1. Hallmark findings are acantholysis and intraepidermal clefting. Clefting is suprabasilar in pemphigus vulgaris and vegetans, and subcorneal in pemphigus foliaceus and erythematosus.
      2. Surface crust may reveal acantholytic keratinocytes from ruptured vesicles or pustules.
   B. Immunopathology
      1. Biopsies of normal perilesional skin for immunopathology are occasionally helpful.
         a) Submit in Michel's fixative for immunofluorescent antibody assays.
         b) Submit in formalin for peroxidase-antiperoxidase assays.
      2. Most cases of pemphigus have positive staining in the intercellular spaces. Pemphigus erythematosus may demonstrate positive staining at the basement membrane zone in addition to intercellular spaces.
      3. This test is not very sensitive, because only 50–60% of confirmed cases have positive staining.
      4. Biopsies taken from normal footpads or nose often have positive staining for IgM.

II. Cytology
   A. Submit preparations from aspirates of intact pustules or from impression smears of crusts.
   B. Cytologic evaluation may include the presence of numerous acantholytic cells and neutrophils.

III. Laboratory tests
   A. Antinuclear antibody (ANA) is not a very useful test in pemphigus. Occasionally, ANA is weakly positive in pemphigus erythematosus.
   B. Serum protein electrophoresis may reveal elevations of gamma globulins but is not specific for pemphigus.
   C. Hematology and biochemical profiles rarely reveal significant abnormalities, although secondary bacterial infections may result in leukocytosis with a left shift.

Differential Diagnosis

I. Pemphigus vulgaris: bullous pemphigoid, systemic lupus erythematosus (SLE), toxic epidermal necrolysis, drug eruption, cutaneous T-cell–like lymphoma, lymphoreticular neoplasia, and ulcerative stomatitis

II. Pemphigus foliaceus: bacterial folliculitis, dermatophytosis, dermatophilosis, demodicosis, candidiasis, keratinization disorders, SLE, pemphigus erythematosus, subcorneal pustular dermatosis, drug eruption, zinc-responsive dermatitis, dermatomyositis, tyrosinemia, cutaneous T-cell–like lymphoma, and lymphoreticular malignancy

III. Pemphigus erythematosus: pemphigus foliaceus, SLE, cutaneous (discoid) lupus erythematosus, nasal pyoderma, demodicosis, dermatophytosis, actinic dermatosis, dermatomyositis, epidermolysis bullosa simplex, and uveodermatologic syndrome

IV. Pemphigus vegetans: pemphigus vulgaris, bacterial folliculitis, pemphigus foliaceus, lichenoid dermatoses, cutaneous neoplasms

Treatment

I. Pemphigus vulgaris and pemphigus foliaceus
   A. Corticosteroids are useful but are rarely effective on their own. Give prednisone 2.2–6.6 mg/kg/day PO to initiate control.
   B. Adjunctive therapy includes azathioprine, chlorambucil, cyclophosphamide, and gold salts (chrysotherapy).
      1. Azathioprine 50 mg/m² PO QOD with prednisone
      2. Chlorambucil 0.1–0.2 mg/kg PO QOD with prednisone
      3. Cyclophosphamide 50 mg/m² PO QOD with prednisone
   C. Gold salt injections of aurothioglucose (Solganal) are commenced with two test doses spaced a week apart.
      1. Cats and small dogs initially are given 1 mg IM, then 2 mg IM a week later.
      2. Larger dogs (>10 kg) are given 5 mg IM, then 10 mg IM a week later.
      3. If no adverse reactions are encountered, therapy is continued at 1 mg/kg IM weekly until the condition responds, then tapered to biweekly, then monthly.
      4. Prednisone 1.1 mg/kg PO BID is given concurrently until resolution is evident, then tapered if possible.
   D. Oral gold salt therapy with auranofin 0.1–0.2 mg/kg PO BID may be tried.
   E. Corticosteroid pulse therapy with methylprednisolone sodium succinate 11 mg/kg IV SID in 5% dextrose/water for 3 days has been tried in a few dogs, but clinical relapse was common (White et al., 1987).
   F. Cats failing to respond to oral prednisone may do better with dexamethasone (0.2–0.4 mg/kg PO) or triamcinolone (0.4–0.8 mg/kg PO) daily

until the condition is in remission, then every 2–3 days for maintenance.

II. Pemphigus erythematosus and pemphigus vegetans
  A. Both conditions are considered to be fairly benign and self-limiting, so they should not be overtreated.
  B. Topical corticosteroids may be sufficient in some cases.
  C. Anti-inflammatory to mild immunosuppressive doses of corticosteroids may be used for more involved cases.
    1. Administer prednisone 1.1 mg/kg/day PO daily for 14 days.
    2. Switch to alternate-day therapy for another 14 days.
    3. Continue to decrease to the lowest possible dosage that keeps clinical signs in remission.
  D. Combinations of tetracycline (2.5–5 mg/kg) and niacinamide (2.5–5 mg/kg) are beneficial in about 25% of cases.
    1. Each is given TID until remission is evident, then the dosage interval can be decreased to SID-BID.
    2. Gastrointestinal upsets are usually caused by the niacinamide, which can be reduced in dosage if problems occur.

Patient Monitoring

I. Monitoring of animals on cytotoxic drugs or chrysotherapy is important, because adverse effects can be anticipated at some point in the therapy.
  A. Animals receiving azathioprine or cyclophosphamide
    1. Monitor hemograms twice weekly initially to detect anemias, leukopenias, or thrombocytopenias.
    2. If no abnormalities are detected, taper the hemograms to weekly, biweekly, monthly, and eventually quarterly.
    3. Biochemical profiles are submitted biweekly at first, then quarterly later.
    4. It is not unusual for elevated liver enzymes to occur with azathioprine therapy.
  B. Animals receiving chrysotherapy
    1. Prior to each injection, a urinalysis and complete blood count are performed.
    2. Monitor for proteinuria, anemia, and eosinophilia.
II. Treatment for pemphigus vulgaris and foliaceus may need to be continued for the life of the animal.

Pemphigoid Complex

Definition and Causes

I. Pemphigoid refers to a complex of dermatoses characterized by autoantibody deposition at the junction of the epidermis and dermis, with blister formation occurring immediately below the epidermis.
II. Two varieties are apparent, bullous pemphigoid and cicatricial pemphigoid.

Pathophysiology

I. Bullous pemphigoid is an autoimmune inflammatory disorder in which autoantibodies are directed against an antigen found in the lamina lucida of the basement membrane zone of squamous epithelium.
II. Evidence indicates that circulating bullous pemphigoid autoantibodies alone are not very pathogenic, but that both antibody and complement must be present to initiate dermal-epidermal separation.

Clinical Signs

I. Signalment
  A. Apparent breed predilection for collies, Shetland sheepdogs, and perhaps Doberman pinschers
  B. No apparent age or sex predisposition
II. Cutaneous findings
  A. Bullous pemphigoid has a similar distribution to pemphigus vulgaris.
    1. The principal lesions are transient blisters, crusts, epidermal collarettes, and ulcerations.
    2. Mucous membranes, head, neck, axillae, ventral abdomen, and the footpads are particularly susceptible regions.
  B. Cicatricial pemphigoid is a rare, chronic blistering disease affecting primarily the mucous membranes of the mouth and eyes.
  C. Bullous pemphigoid and cicatricial pemphigoid are indistinguishable on the basis of histopathology and immunopathology but may be differentiated by their clinical presentation.

Diagnosis

I. Biopsies for histopathologic assessment are the best diagnostic tests.
  A. An inflammatory subepidermal vesiculating disorder is evident.
  B. Inflammatory infiltrates consisting of granulocytes and mononuclear cells are common.
  C. Acantholysis is not a feature of pemphigoid.
II. Immunopathology may support the diagnosis.
  A. Biopsies of normal perilesional skin are occasionally helpful.
  B. Most cases of pemphigoid have positive staining in the basement membrane zone of the dermal-epidermal junction.
    1. Only 50–60% of confirmed cases have positive staining.
    2. Other conditions that may also have positive linear staining in this region include lupus erythematosus, linear IgA disease, dermatitis herpetiformis, and epidermolysis bullosa acquisita.

Differential Diagnosis

I. Bullous pemphigoid: pemphigus vulgaris, SLE, toxic epidermal necrolysis, drug eruption, cutaneous T-cell–like lymphoma, lymphoreticular neoplasia, ulcerative stomatitis

II. Cicatricial pemphigoid: other causes of ulcerative stomatitis and blepharitis

Treatment

I. Treatment of pemphigoid is identical to that for pemphigus and includes corticosteroids, cytotoxic agents, and chrysotherapy (see earlier).
II. Cicatricial pemphigoid usually does not require immunosuppressive therapy and may respond to topical or intralesional corticosteroids.

Patient Monitoring

I. Some cases of bullous pemphigoid can be controlled on low-dose corticosteroids and go into complete remission.
II. Other cases can be quite resistant, requiring lifelong therapy. See monitoring advice for pemphigus complex, earlier.

Cutaneous (Discoid) Lupus Erythematosus

Definition

I. Cutaneous (discoid) lupus erythematosus is generally regarded as a less harmful variant of SLE, wherein systemic involvement is absent and autoantibodies are rarely found.
II. SLE is discussed in Chap. 74.

Causes and Pathophysiology

I. Cutaneous lupus erythematosus is characterized by circulating autoantibodies and immune complexes that participate in immune-mediated tissue injury against the basement membrane zone of cutaneous epithelium.
II. The lesions of discoid lupus are exacerbated by sunlight.

Clinical Signs

I. Signalment
   A. Breed predilections exist for the collie, German shepherd dog, Shetland sheepdog, Siberian husky, Brittany spaniel, and German shorthaired pointer.
   B. There may be a sex predisposition for female dogs.
II. Cutaneous findings
   A. The most common presenting sign is a red, scaling dermatitis of the face, often affecting the nose, ears, and nasal mucosa.
   B. Nasal and digital hyperkeratosis may also be noticed.
   C. Depigmentation, especially of the nasal mucosa, often accompanied by erosion and ulceration, is frequently noted and is an important feature.

Diagnosis

I. Histopathologic findings are often variable.
   A. Common inflammatory patterns include interface dermatitis, vasculitis, and panniculitis.
   B. Increased amounts of glycosaminoglycans are often noted.
II. Immunopathology of older, active, nonulcerated skin lesions may be beneficial. Immunofluorescent staining is at the dermal-epidermal junction.
III. Serum ANA titers and lupus erythematosus (LE) cell preparations are rarely positive.
IV. Hemograms, biochemical profiles, and other tests (urinalysis, rheumatoid factor, etc.) are usually normal, because there is no systemic involvement.

Differential Diagnosis

I. Rule out infectious diseases such as demodicosis, dermatophytosis, and nasal pyoderma.
II. Rule out other immune-mediated diseases that affect the nose, such as pemphigus erythematosus, zinc-responsive dermatosis, dermatomyositis, uveodermatologic syndrome.
III. Also consider nutritional disorders such as zinc-responsive dermatosis.

Treatment

I. The treatment of cutaneous lupus erythematosus differs from that of SLE in that immunosuppressive therapy may not be warranted.
II. Topical fluorinated corticosteroids (e.g., fluocinolone, betamethasone) may be used to achieve remission, then progressively safer products (e.g., triamcinolone), can be substituted. The goal is to manage with very safe products (e.g., 1% hydrocortisone).
III. Anti-inflammatory doses of prednisone 1–1.5 mg/kg/day PO, eventually tapered to QOD, will control the condition.
IV. Administer tetracycline and niacinamide to dogs.
   A. Dogs 5–15 kg: 250 mg each drug PO TID, then wean
   B. Dogs >15 kg: 500 mg each drug PO TID, then wean
V. Administer vitamin E 200–800 IU PO BID with prednisone.
VI. Limiting exposure to sunlight or the use of topical sunscreens may also benefit these animals.

Patient Monitoring

I. Treatment is usually lifelong, although there may be a waxing and waning pattern to the clinical course.
II. The overall prognosis is good if immunosuppressive therapy is not needed. Few cases ever become systemic, and those that do may reflect an inaccurate initial diagnosis.

IMMUNE-MEDIATED VASCULAR DISORDERS

Cutaneous Vasculitis

Definition and Causes

I. Cutaneous vasculitis is a collection of disorders in which the underlying problem includes destructive and inflammatory changes in the blood vessels.
II. It may occur secondary to a number of processes.
   A. Infections: bacterial, mycoplasmal, rickettsial, viral, fungal
   B. Drug reactions or eruptions caused by foods and food additives
   C. Immune-mediated disorders: SLE, scleroderma, dermatomyositis, rheumatoid arthritis
   D. Exposure to cold
   E. Trauma
   F. Reactions to injections: rabies vaccinations
   G. Chronic diseases: diabetes mellitus, chronic respiratory disease, cancer
   H. Arthropod bites
   I. Hypersensitivity reactions
   J. Idiopathic reasons

Pathophysiology

I. Cutaneous vasculitis is not a specific entity but rather a collection of disorders in which the underlying problem includes destructive and inflammatory changes in the blood vessels.
II. Most vasculitis syndromes are associated with immune complex deposition in the blood vessel walls.

Clinical Signs

I. Vasculitic lesions occur most frequently on the dependent parts of the body, feet, and ears.
II. The most common lesion is an elevated bruise or so-called palpable purpura.
III. In later stages, when the blood vessels have been thoroughly compromised, the tissue may die, leaving a visibly depressed area.
IV. An erosive-ulcerative process is inevitable at some stage of the disease.
V. Systemic involvement may also occur.

Diagnosis

I. A diagnosis is often suspected based on characteristic clinical signs.
II. Biopsies for histopathologic evaluation reveal damage to blood vessels and, depending on the cause, a variable inflammatory infiltrate with granulocytes, mononuclear cells, or a mixed cell population.
III. Numerous tests may be necessary to define the underlying etiology.
   A. Immune tests: ANA, circulating immune complexes (C1q assay), rheumatoid factor,
   B. Hypoallergenic food trial

C. Microbial cultures: aerobic, anaerobic
D. Serology for infectious diseases

Differential Diagnosis

I. Urticaria/angioedema
II. Cellulitis or septicemia
III. Focal trauma
IV. Disseminated intravascular coagulopathy or other clotting disorders

Treatment and Monitoring

I. Treatment is directed at the underlying cause if it is known.
II. If no cause has been determined, therapy is initiated with corticosteroids.
   A. Begin prednisone 1 mg/kg PO BID for 14 days.
   B. If the condition resolves, give prednisone 1 mg/kg PO QOD for another 14 days, and continue to taper.
   C. Decrease dosage to the lowest alternate-day dose that maintains remission. In some cases, prednisone can be discontinued.
III. Dapsone or sulfasalazine is often used in cases of leukocytoclastic vasculitis, a histopathologic diagnosis in which fragmentation of leukocytes is noted in the vicinity of damaged vessels.
   A. Dapsone 1 mg/kg PO TID for 14 days, then BID for 14 days, then SID for 14 days, then QOD indefinitely
   B. Sulfasalazine 10 mg/kg PO TID until remission, then BID for another 3 weeks
IV. Pentoxifylline is currently being evaluated as a treatment option.

Cold Agglutinin Disease

Definition

Cold agglutinin disease refers to cutaneous damage occurring from vascular insufficiency caused by the precipitation of cryoglobulins and cryofibrinogens in tissue.

Causes and Pathophysiology

I. It is a rare disease in dogs and cats associated with cold-reacting (usually IgM) autoantibodies.
II. It has also been associated with lead poisoning in dogs and with upper respiratory infection in cats.
III. Skin lesions are associated with intracapillary hemagglutination at cool temperatures.

Clinical Signs

I. Most affected tissues are in peripheral locations (ears, tail, paws, nose) and are made worse by exposure to cold.
II. Lesions include erythema, purpura, necrosis, hyperpigmentation, and ulceration.

Diagnosis

I. A definitive diagnosis requires demonstration of significant titers of cold agglutinins, also called cryoglobulins.
II. Occasionally, skin biopsies are supportive of the diagnosis if thrombotic vessels or vasculitis is seen.

Differential Diagnosis

I. Cutaneous vasculitis
II. Circulatory disorders of other origins
III. Frostbite

Treatment and Monitoring

I. Therapy is directed at correcting the underlying cause.
II. Avoidance of cold is helpful.
III. Immunosuppressive doses of corticosteroids or azathioprine may be indicated for long-term control if underlying causes are not identified and corrected.
A. Prednisone 2.2–6.6 mg/kg/day PO
B. Azathioprine 50 mg/m² PO QOD with prednisone

HYPERSENSITIVITY DISORDERS

Allergic Inhalant Dermatitis

Definition and Causes

I. Allergic inhalant dermatitis, or atopy, is one of the most common dermatologic problems seen in dogs and perhaps also in cats.
II. Animals react to a variety of inhaled substances, including tree, grass and weed pollens; molds; house dust; house dust mites; feathers; and dander.

Pathophysiology

I. Inhalant allergies may be mediated by IgE of IgG, which cause an immediate hypersensitivity reaction when allergen contacts antibody on the surface of a tissue mast cell or circulating basophil.
II. Allergens causing inhalant allergies must be present in significant quantities, be buoyant enough to become airborne, and also be of a certain size and weight (5000–60,000 daltons and 2–60 μm) to reach the terminal portions of the respiratory tract.

Clinical Signs

I. Signalment
A. Atopy may be a familial disorder, because signs usually become apparent between 6 months and 3 years of age.
B. Breeds predisposed to atopy include the terrier breeds (especially the West Highland white terrier, Skye terrier, Scottish terrier, and Boston

terrier), the golden retriever, poodle, dalmatian, German shepherd dog, Shar pei, Shih Tzu, pug, Irish setter, and miniature schnauzer.
II. Clinical findings
A. Signs may be seasonal or year-round, depending on the allergen.
B. Pruritus is often marked.
1. Licking and chewing at the feet are common.
2. The flanks, groin, and axillae are also commonly affected.
3. Many animals rub their faces on the carpet, furniture, or other convenient surfaces.
4. The pinnae are often erythematous and pruritic.
5. Periocular and perineal areas may also be involved.
C. The characteristic pattern of allergic inhalant dermatitis is erythema and pruritus without primary lesions.
D. Self-traumatized areas may develop secondary bacterial infections.
E. Thickening and hyperpigmentation are chronic secondary changes of the skin.

Diagnosis

I. A careful history and physical examination often suggest allergy.
II. Corroborative tests include hematology, skin scrapings, dermatophyte cultures, and hypoallergenic diet trials. These tests are invariably negative in cases of inhalant allergy.
III. Intradermal allergy testing is currently the best test available for evaluating sensitivity to inhaled substances.
A. It measures the ability of allergen-specific IgE antibody to bind to effector mast cells in the dermis and initiate mast cell degranulation with an associated inflammatory response (wheal).
B. Positive reactions on a skin test indicate only sensitivity to a particular allergen. It is then necessary to interpret whether the information is relevant to the particular animal tested.
C. Candidates for skin testing are chosen on the following basis.
1. The diagnosis of allergic inhalant dermatitis is fairly certain from the history and clinical signs.
2. Corticosteroid doses needed to control pruritus are unsafe, cause undesirable side effects, or are unacceptable to the owner.
3. Other forms of symptomatic therapy (e.g., soothing baths, antihistamines, omega-3/6 fatty acid supplements) are unsuccessful, too expensive, or unacceptable to the owner.
4. The owner thoroughly understands the concept of testing and immunotherapy and is prepared to invest the required time and money.
D. Allergy testing can have false-negative and false-positive reactions and can be difficult to interpret.
E. The disadvantages of skin testing are that it re-

quires some expertise to perform, results and reproducibility may be variable, the source of allergens is unstandardized, and interpretation is subjective, based on the examiner.

IV. In vitro allergy tests purportedly measure levels of free allergen-specific IgE in the bloodstream.
  A. Enzyme-linked immunosorbent assay (ELISA) and the radioallergosorbent test (RAST) are commercially available.
  B. The indications for using in vitro tests are as follows.
    1. Intradermal testing is not available.
    2. Intradermal allergy testing was performed but the results are not consistent with the history.
    3. The owner will not allow the coat to be clipped for intradermal testing.
    4. Successful withdrawal of corticosteroids or antihistamines is not possible or is insufficient to allow accurate intradermal testing.
  C. There are several disadvantages of in vitro allergy testing.
    1. Conditions other than allergy may cause elevations of serum IgE, and elevated levels of allergen-specific IgE do not necessarily mean that the animal is allergic.
    2. Most allergy-mediating antibodies are tissue- or cell-bound and are not easily harvested and measured.
    3. Blood tests appear to have about 50% agreement with skin test results.

Differential Diagnosis

  I. Adverse food reactions
  II. Parasite infestations or hypersensitivities
  III. Contact allergy or eruptions
  IV. Keratinization disorders

Treatment

  I. Immunotherapy
    A. This involves serial injections of progressively larger amounts of the offending allergen(s) to increase tolerance to agents that the animal has been deemed sensitive to.
    B. Many animals treated with the regimen respond and have a decreased need for other medications.
    C. It is a slow process, sometimes taking up to a year before improvement is noticed.
  II. Environmental control
    A. Unless the offending allergens are cats, furniture stuffing, houseplants, or other removable items, environmental control is aimed at limiting exposure.
    B. High-efficiency particulate air (HEPA) filters can clear over 95% of the pollens, molds, yeasts, bacteria, and viruses in the air, and when coupled with a charcoal filter, they can remove most of the dust. These filters may be the best choice for treating the household environment.
  III. Corticosteroids
    A. Corticosteroids are occasionally suitable treat-

ment alternatives, but side effects are often problematic.
  B. If the allergic season is short or the amount of prednisone required to control clinical signs is small (<0.5 mg/kg PO QOD), corticosteroids may be considered a reasonable choice.
  C. Repository forms of corticosteroids such as methylprednisolone acetate or triamcinolone acetonide have little or no place in the maintenance therapy of atopic dogs, but they may be used safely in some cats.
IV. Antihistamines
  A. Antihistamines may offer clinical relief in 20–35% of allergic dogs and cats.
  B. Antihistamines acceptable for use in the dog include the following.
    1. Clemastine (Tavist) 0.05–0.1 mg/kg PO BID
    2. Hydroxyzine (Atarax) 2.2 mg/kg PO BID-TID
    3. Diphenhydramine hydrochloride (Benadryl) 1–2 mg/kg PO BID-TID
    4. Terfenadine (Seldane) 2.5–5 mg/kg PO BID
    5. Chlorpheniramine maleate (Chlor-Trimeton) 0.5–1 mg/kg PO BID-TID
    6. Trimeprazine (Temaril) 1–2 mg/kg PO BID
    7. Amitriptyline 1 mg/kg PO BID
  C. Chlorpheniramine 1–2 mg PO BID is the antihistamine of choice in the cat. Second choice is clemastine 0.67 mg/cat PO BID.
V. Omega-3 and -6 fatty acids
  A. The omega-3 fatty acids include eicosapentanoic acid, docosapentanoic acid, and docosahexanoic acid. The omega-6 fatty acids include gamma linolenic acid.
  B. Their positive effects are likely the result of mild and very safe anti-inflammatory properties. They may be effective in 20% of atopic animals.
  C. Give DermCaps, EFA-Z Plus, etc. in standard dosages (see Chap. 90).

Patient Monitoring

  I. Allergic inhalant dermatitis is not a systemic disease, and the prognosis is excellent unless therapies cause adverse effects.
  II. Immunotherapy results in improvement of 50–75% of cases. On average, 6–8 months may be required before benefit is seen.
  III. Most animals (90%) respond to anti-inflammatory doses of corticosteroids but must be carefully monitored.
    A. Perform hemogram and biochemical profile every 3–12 months, depending on the dosage used.
    B. Long-term continuous administration of corticosteroids may result in iatrogenic Cushing's disease and should be discouraged.

Food Hypersensitivity

Definition

Food hypersensitivity refers to an immunologically mediated adverse reaction unrelated to any physiologic effect of the food or food additive.

Causes and Pathophysiology

I. This hypersensitivity reaction may be a type I (mediated by IgE), type III, or type IV hypersensitivity reaction.

II. Although IgE may be the principal immunoglobulin capable of sensitizing mast cells and basophils to food antigens, a short-term sensitizing IgG antibody has also been reported.

III. Animals react adversely to individual ingredients, *not* specific brands of food. Allergenic fractions of food are usually glycoproteins with a molecular weight of 18,000–36,000 daltons and are generally heat and acid stable.

IV. Hypersensitivity responses to ingested antigens are very specific. Any factors that alter the antigenicity of dietary components, such as cooking, processing, or digestion, can significantly alter a substance's ability to evoke a specific hypersensitivity response.

Clinical Signs

I. Many affected animals have been fed the offending antigen for 2 or more years before developing clinical signs.

II. The most consistent cutaneous manifestation is a nonseasonal pruritic maculopapular dermatitis, with associated erythema and/or exfoliation.
   A. The pruritus may be generalized or limited to the head, feet, axillae, inguinal region, or ears.
   B. In cats, this maculopapular eruption is often accompanied by erosions and ulcerations and most commonly involves the head and neck.
   C. Miliary dermatitis and eosinophilic plaque also occur in the cat.
   D. Urticaria and angioedema are seen in a small percentage of affected animals.
   E. Superficial recurrent pyoderma and/or pyotraumatic dermatitis may occur secondarily.

III. Noncutaneous manifestations in dogs are less common.
   A. Gastrointestinal signs: vomiting, diarrhea, pruritus ani, flatulence
   B. Respiratory abnormalities: sneezing, asthma-like conditions
   C. Possible neurologic conditions: behavioral changes and seizures

Diagnosis

I. Food hypersensitivity may be suspected on the basis of history and clinical signs.
   A. Nonseasonal pruritic dermatosis
   B. Variable response to corticosteroids
   C. Normal or negative results from skin scrapings, evaluation for internal parasites, hematologic and biochemical profiles
   D. ± Evidence of inhalant allergies on intradermal skin testing

II. Definitive diagnosis requires a hypoallergenic diet trial.
   A. No food source is nonallergenic, and foods are considered hypoallergenic based on circumstance, such as when the pet has never eaten them before.
      1. If the pet has not been exposed to lamb, it is considered hypoallergenic.
      2. Rabbit, venison, duck, and bear meat are other alternatives.
   B. A diet is prepared by mixing 1 part venison, duck, or rabbit to 2 parts rice and/or potatoes. All ingredients are served boiled and fed in the same total volume as the pet's previous diet.
   C. During the trial, hypoallergenic foods and fresh, preferably distilled water must be fed *exclusively*. No treats, snacks, vitamins, chew toys, or even flavored heartworm preventive tablets may be given.
   D. Access must be denied to the food of other pets, and any opportunity for coprophagia eliminated.
   E. Administer the trial diet for at least 8–12 weeks.

III. In vitro tests for food hypersensitivity using ELISA and RAST assays can be misleading and are of little value as a diagnostic tool.

IV. Gastroscopic food hypersensitivity testing requires further evaluation to determine its reliability and diagnostic value (Guilford et al., 1991).

Differential Diagnosis

I. Physiologic intolerance to food or food additives
II. Inhalant allergy
III. Parasite hypersensitivities or infestations
IV. Lupus erythematosus
V. Metabolic dermatopathies (see Chap. 88)

Treatment and Monitoring

I. Commercial hypoallergenic diets appear to be about 80% effective. Examples include Hill's d/d diets, NutroMax, Protocol, Nature's Recipe, Condition, Wysong, IVD, and Avoderm.

II. Balanced homemade hypoallergenic diets can also be formulated for both dogs and cats.
   A. A vitamin-mineral supplement may be added (including taurine for cats) if it does not affect the clinical signs.
   B. Check plasma taurine levels every 4–6 months in cats receiving a homemade diet.

III. Challenge feeding may identify the actual ingredients causing the problem so that they can be avoided.
   A. Add one new food item each week to the hypoallergenic diet.
   B. If the food substance fails to initiate an adverse reaction within a week, assume that it may be tolerated by the pet.

IV. The prognosis for food hypersensitivity is good if a hypoallergenic diet is accepted by the pet and can be fed exclusively.

Allergic Contact Dermatitis

Definition and Causes

I. Allergic contact dermatitis is a type IV (delayed) hypersensitivity reaction in the dog and cat.

II. Documented causes include plants such as *Tradescantia fluminensis* (wandering Jew), carpet deodorizers, plastics or rubber (toys, bowls), leather, detergents, floor waxes, wool and synthetic rugs, carpets, fertilizer, mulch, concrete, and fabrics or fabric cleansers.

Pathophysiology

I. Most antigens capable of causing allergic contact dermatitis have relatively low molecular weights and act as haptens. Once applied to the skin, these haptens are able to penetrate the epidermis, where they bind to carrier proteins and become immunogenic.
II. Factors that damage the integrity of the epithelial barrier may predispose animals to allergic contact dermatitis by allowing penetration of haptogenic substances through the epidermis.
III. The development of a true allergic contact dermatitis usually requires frequent contact with the offending agent over prolonged periods of time, although under certain ideal conditions, dogs may become sensitized in 3–5 weeks.

Clinical Signs

I. Areas that have a sparse covering of hair and are frequently in contact with the ground are predisposed to develop allergic contact dermatitis. These sites include the axillae, inguinal area, perineum, scrotum, pressure points, chin, muzzle, pinnae, and the palmar, plantar, and interdigital surfaces of the feet.
II. If the contact allergen is a liquid, haired regions may be equally involved.
III. Pruritus is the primary sign, which may be accompanied by erythema, macules, vesicles, papules, and pustules.
IV. With chronic disease, thickening, hyperpigmentation, lichenification, and crusting of the skin; hair loss; pyoderma; and keratinization abnormalities may also be found.

Diagnosis

I. History and physical findings may be suggestive.
II. The animal can be bathed, then boarded or hospitalized on stainless steel with no blankets or towels available for 3–5 days to determine the degree of improvement. Marked improvement strengthens but does not confirm the diagnosis.
III. Histopathologic changes are not diagnostic but may be helpful in some cases.
   A. Intercellular and intracellular edema
   B. Interface dermatitis with lichenoid band of mononuclear cells
   C. Serocellular crusting
IV. Patch testing can be performed to confirm allergic contact dermatitis.
   A. Suspect allergens and control agents are applied to a shaved area over the thoracic wall and an occlusive wrap applied.
      1. The wrap is removed after 48 hours, and test

sites are evaluated both 30 minutes and 24 hours later.
      2. Erythema, papules, macules, swelling, and possibly even vesicle formation are seen at positive sites.
   B. False-positive and false-negative results can occur.
   C. Standardization of the allergen is difficult (if not impossible) when using material brought from home. The concentration and dose of the allergen, the vehicle used, and the application time all influence the results of patch testing.

Differential Diagnosis

I. Irritant contact dermatitis
II. Allergic inhalant dermatitis
III. Adverse food reactions
IV. Lupus erythematosus
V. Dermatophytosis
VI. Demodicosis

Treatment

I. Removal or avoidance of the allergen is preferable but not always possible.
II. Corticosteroids are often helpful early in the course.
   A. Topical hydrocortisone combined with antipruritic agents (Dermacool HC)
   B. Topical triamcinolone for 7–14 days
   C. Prednisone 1 mg/kg PO SID for 7 days, then 0.5–1 mg/kg PO QOD
III. Frequent bathing with hypoallergenic shampoo (Episoothe, Allergroom, Dermacleanse) and mechanical barriers such as socks or T-shirts may also be helpful.

Patient Monitoring

I. Animals usually show dramatic improvement within 5 days of identifying and removing the allergen.
II. Prognosis is good if the allergen is identified and removed but is poor if the allergen is not identified.
III. The length of treatment can be as little as 5 days if the allergen is permanently removed from the environment, intermittent if the allergen recurs periodically, or lifelong if the allergen is not identified or impossible to remove from the environment.

IMMUNE-MEDIATED DISORDERS

Drug Eruptions

Definition

I. Drug eruption is a rare, pleomorphic cutaneous/mucocutaneous reaction to a drug or its metabolite.
II. It occurs only after an initial exposure that sensitizes the animal.
III. Clinical signs do not resemble the known pharmacologic actions of the drug and may vary greatly among individuals.

IV. Signs usually subside within days to weeks after withdrawal and recur upon readministration of the offending drug.

Causes

I. Any drug may cause an eruption, and no specific type of reaction results from any one drug (Table 89–1).
II. Inciting drugs may be administered orally, topically, by injection, or by inhalation.
III. The incidence of drug eruption is unknown in animals.

Pathophysiology

I. Mechanisms of most drug eruptions are unknown but are thought to include all four types of hypersensitivity.
II. Eruptions may occur at *any time* in the course of therapy.

Clinical Signs

I. Drug eruption can mimic many dermatoses.
II. Several clinical forms of cutaneous drug eruptions exist.
   A. Erythema multiforme: see later
   B. Erythroderma: erythematous nodules that are pruritic and sometimes painful
   C. Exfoliative dermatitis: scaling and peeling
   D. Fixed drug reaction: dermatitis confined to focal area only
   E. Papular dermatitis: papules, pustules, comedones
   F. Purpura: petechiae or ecchymoses that become confluent
   G. Toxic epidermal necrolysis: see later
   H. Urticaria/angioedema: see Chap. 74
   I. Vesicular/bullous disease with secondary erosions or ulcers
   J. Otitis externa: see Chap. 105
III. Some drug eruptions are accompanied by systemic signs such as lameness and joint effusion, polyuria with proteinuria, fever, and malaise.

Diagnosis

I. It is imperative to obtain accurate and temporal knowledge of the medications given to any animal with an undiagnosed dermatosis.

Table 89–1. *Drugs Reported to Cause Eruptions in Dogs and Cats*

Sulfonamides	Penicillin
Cephalosporins	Cyclosporine
Ampicillin	Griseofulvin
Levamisole	Primidone
Aurothioglucose	Prednisone
Asparaginase	Streptomycin
Doxorubicin	Tetracycline
Phenothiazines	Vaccines/bacterins

II. There are no specific characteristic findings to allow a presumptive diagnosis, although erythematous pruritic papules are suggestive.
III. Laboratory tests are indicated to rule out other diseases.
   A. Immunologic tests: ANA, Coombs' test, platelet factor
   B. Joint fluid analysis and radiography
   C. Renal function and excretion tests
   D. Dermatohistopathology and immunofluorescent studies
IV. Clinical signs subside on withdrawal of the drug.
V. Provocative tests are not usually recommended because of the risk of fatal systemic reaction.

Differential Diagnosis

I. The differential diagnosis is complex, as drug eruption may mimic virtually any dermatosis, especially other immune-mediated conditions.
II. A drug eruption is not a drug reaction (side effect). Drug reactions are divided into two groups (see Chap. 130).
   A. Predictable: usually dose dependent and related to pharmacologic actions of the drug
   B. Unpredictable: dose independent and related to the individual's immunologic response or genetic difference in susceptibility (idiosyncrasy)

Treatment and Monitoring

I. Discontinue the offending drug.
II. Start supportive care for any life-threatening conditions, such as shock or anaphylaxis.
III. Glucocorticoids are usually not required but may be used for persistent pruritus.
IV. Institute symptomatic therapy with topical and systemic medications for secondary pyoderma, excessive scaling, and otitis externa.
V. Avoid chemically related drugs.
VI. Drug eruptions usually resolve within 7–14 days of removal of the offending agent but can sometimes persist for several weeks.

Erythema Multiforme and Toxic Epidermal Necrolysis

Definition

I. Erythema multiforme (EM) is an acute, self-limited syndrome of distinctive skin lesions with or without mucosal involvement.
II. Toxic epidermal necrolysis (TEN) is an uncommon, peracute, painful, vesicular/bullous, and ulcerative disorder of the mucosa and skin.
III. It is not known whether TEN is a separate disease or simply the most severe clinical form of EM.

Causes

I. Both conditions are currently considered to be hypersensitivity reactions associated with drugs, neoplasia, infections, and connective tissue diseases.

A. Drug therapy: aurothioglucose, cephalexin, chloramphenicol, diethylcarbamazine, gentamicin, levamisole, L-thyroxine, trimethoprim-sulfadiazine, other sulfas

B. Neoplasia: myeloproliferative disorders, splenic tumors

C. Infections: staphylococcal folliculitis, anal gland sacculitis, bacterial endocarditis

II. Accumulated clinical evidence points to drugs as the most important, if not the only, cause of TEN.

Pathophysiology

I. Despite recognition of multiple underlying or precipitating causes, the pathophysiology of these diseases is not fully understood.

II. Histopathologic and immunopathologic studies suggest an epithelial lymphocyte/macrophage–mediated immunologic reaction.

III. Abnormalities associated with EM are limited to the skin, but the clinical sequelae from TEN are similar to those of a massive second-degree burn, with fluid, electrolyte, and colloid losses and increased risk of secondary infection.

Clinical Signs

I. Skin lesions of EM are variable but are usually characterized by the following.
   A. Erythematous maculas that spread peripherally and clear centrally (target)
   B. Urticarial plaques
   C. Vesicles or bullae
   D. Some combination of the preceding

II. Two clinical forms are recognized.
   A. Minor
      Animals have macular papular eruptions but are usually asymptomatic.
   B. Major: Stevens-Johnson syndrome or TEN
      1. Animals are systemically ill, with extensive blistering and ulcerative lesions involving mucocutaneous areas and skin.
      2. Fever, malaise, collapse, shock, and death may occur with TEN.

Diagnosis

I. Definitive diagnosis is based on history, physical examination, and skin biopsy.

II. Because of the high likelihood of drugs inducing EM and TEN, an extensive review of current or past medications is imperative.

III. Laboratory tests may reveal leukocytosis with either a neutropenia or neutrophilia, electrolyte abnormalities, hypoproteinemia, and altered renal function.

IV. Histopathologic changes are found predominantly in the epidermis and basement membrane.
   A. Ballooning degeneration of the epidermal cells with sparse lymphohistiocytic infiltration is noted early.
   B. Full-thickness epidermal necrosis with subepidermal bullae formation and infiltration of neu-

trophils eventually occurs in all but the mildest lesions.
   C. Tissue immunofluorescence is usually negative.
   D. Because of the wide variety of lesions, multiple histologic sections should be submitted.

Differential Diagnosis

I. Bacterial folliculitis
II. Dermatophytosis
III. Other vesicular and pustular disorders, especially the autoimmune diseases

Treatment

I. Remove any causative agents and, if possible, treat the primary cause.

II. Many cases of EM run a mild course and spontaneously regress in a few weeks.
   A. An underlying cause should be sought and removed whenever possible.
   B. Prednisone 0.5–1 mg/kg/day PO may be given for persistent pruritus.

III. Treatment of more severe forms, especially TEN, involves symptomatic and supportive measures.
   A. IV fluid therapy with electrolyte supplementation and plasma replacement
   B. Parenteral bactericidal antibiotics
   C. Topical care of skin lesions by the clipping of hair and gentle cleansing

IV. The use of systemic glucocorticoids for both diseases is controversial and may be detrimental.

Patient Monitoring

I. By definition, EM is a self-limiting disease with a good prognosis.

II. The prognosis for TEN is guarded to poor, with a 50% mortality rate.
   A. Mortality is greatest in idiopathic cases.
   B. Clinical findings associated with a poor prognosis are old age, consistent neutropenia, elevated renal function tests, and hyperkalemia.

Hormonal Sensitivity

Definition and Causes

I. Hormonal hypersensitivity is a rare, pruritic, crusting dermatitis of dogs, associated with hypersensitivity reactions to sex hormones.

II. Although the exact cause is unknown, results of intradermal skin testing suggest a type I and/or type IV immunologic reaction to endogenous progesterone, estrogen, or testosterone.

Clinical Signs

I. No age or breed predilections have been reported; over 90% of reported cases have occurred in intact female dogs.

II. Clinically affected dogs appear similar to chronic

atopic animals but have enlargement of the vulva and nipples.
  III. The dermatologic signs usually coincide with estrus (which may be irregular) or pseudopregnancy.

Diagnosis

  I. Presumptive diagnosis is made from a combination of suspicious history, physical examination findings, intradermal skin testing, and response to therapy.
  II. Histopathology is nondiagnostic.

Differential Diagnosis

  I. Parasite (flea bite) hypersensitivity
  II. Food hypersensitivity
  III. Atopy
  IV. Drug allergy
  V. Folliculitis

Treatment and Monitoring

  I. Ovariohysterectomy or castration is indicated. Response to neutering is dramatic, with marked improvement within 5–10 days.
  II. Response to systemic glucocorticoids is usually unsatisfactory.

Vogt-Koyanagi-Harada–Like Syndrome in Dogs

Definition and Causes

  I. Vogt-Koyanagi-Harada–like syndrome (VKH) is a term used to describe a triad of signs in the dog.
    A. Granulomatous panuveitis
    B. Poliosis: depigmentation of hair
    C. Vitiligo: depigmentation of skin
  II. The disease is suspected to be an immune-mediated disorder, with melanocytes as the target cell.

Pathophysiology

  I. Pigmented tissues or tissues heavily laden with melanocytes, such as the uveal tract, skin, and mucous membranes, are primarily involved.
  II. Ocular tissues appear to be affected early in the course, with diffuse infiltration of lymphocytes, plasma, and epithelioid cells.
  III. Later in the course, melanocytes of the skin and hair bulbs are affected.
  IV. Unlike VKH in people, auditory and meningeal abnormalities have not been documented in the dog.

Clinical Signs

  I. The disease has been reported only in dogs.
    A. Most common breeds: Akita, Irish setter, Siberian husky, Samoyed, Shetland sheepdog, and chow chow
    B. Age: usually 1.5–6 years
    C. Onset: often acute, but occasionally can be chronic
  II. The clinical syndrome is characterized by acute onset of uveitis, followed by depigmentation of the nose, lips, eyelids, and occasionally the footpads, and lightening of the hair (see also Chaps. 97 and 100).
  III. Dermatologic signs are usually symmetrical and have a predilection for the head.
    A. In chronic cases, there is no visible inflammation of the depigmented skin.
    B. In acute cases, mucocutaneous ulceration and crusting occur, similar to other immune-mediated diseases.
    C. Poliosis may be widespread, dramatically changing the appearance of the animal.

Diagnosis

  I. A presumptive diagnosis can often be made from the history and physical examination findings.
  II. Definitive diagnosis is based on histopathology.
    A. Dermatohistopathologic findings are characterized by a lichenoid interface dermatitis.
      1. Large histiocytes, small mononuclear cells, and multinuclear giant cells are a major cellular component.
      2. In some specimens, plasma cells and lymphocytes predominate.
      3. Melanin is decreased or absent in the epidermis and hair follicles.
    B. Direct and indirect immunofluorescence testing is usually negative.
  III. Laboratory data are often normal.
    A. Changes in the hemogram or biochemistries are rare.
    B. ANA assays have been negative.
    C. Serology and cultures have not revealed an infectious disease.

Treatment

  I. For a discussion on the treatment of ocular signs, see Chaps. 97 and 100.
  II. Cutaneous abnormalities require systemic immunosuppressive therapy.
    A. Prednisone 1–2 mg/kg/day PO, eventually tapering to 0.5 mg/kg PO QOD
    B. ± Azathioprine 2 mg/kg/day PO, tapering slowly to 0.5 mg/kg PO SID
    C. ± Cyclophosphamide 2 mg/kg PO SID × 4 days each week

Patient Monitoring

  I. If therapy is instituted early, cutaneous repigmentation may occur.
  II. Dogs usually require chronic alternate-day glucocorticoid therapy and/or prolonged azathioprine for months to years to prevent recurrence.
  III. The disease has a protracted course, and recurrences can be expected.

IV. Dermatologic manifestations are not life-threatening, but severe ocular changes may result in euthanasia.

Feline Plasma Cell Pododermatitis

Definition and Causes

I. Plasma cell pododermatitis is an uncommon cutaneous disorder affecting the footpads of cats.
II. The cause is unknown.

Pathophysiology

I. An immune-mediated pathogenesis is suspected based on the following findings.
  A. Tissue plasmacytosis
  B. Consistent hypergammaglobulinemia
  C. Beneficial response to immunomodulating drugs
II. Some cases have seasonal recurrences, suggesting an allergic disorder.

Clinical Signs

I. No age, breed, or sex predilection is apparent.
II. Plasma cell pododermatitis begins as a soft, nonpainful swelling of multiple footpads on multiple paws.
  A. Lesion are pink, smooth, and non-ulcerated initially.
  B. With time, the margins of the footpad may ulcerate and become painful.
III. Metacarpal and metatarsal pads are usually affected.
  A. If one or more pads become ulcerated, pain, lameness, and regional lymphadenopathy may occur.
  B. A few cats also have plasma cell stomatitis/pharyngitis.
  C. Occasionally, glomerulonephritis or renal amyloidosis is also documented.

Diagnosis

I. Definitive diagnosis is based on the following.
  A. Physical examination findings as described earlier
  B. Aspiration cytology: plasma cells predominate
  C. Sterile bacterial cultures
  D. Dermatohistopathology
    1. Subepidermal infiltration of plasma cells and some lymphocytes
    2. Numerous Mott cells (bright-pink staining plasma cells containing immunoglobulin)
II. Laboratory data
  A. Neutrophilia and lymphocytosis may be seen.
  B. Hypergammaglobulinemia is typical.
  C. ANA tests and direct immunofluorescence are usually nondiagnostic.

Differential Diagnosis

I. Contact irritant or allergy
II. Trauma or burns
III. Neoplasia, especially early squamous cell carcinoma

Treatment

I. Plasma cell pododermatitis may be asymptomatic and spontaneously regress without treatment in some cases.
II. Treatment is indicated for involvement of multiple paws, especially when accompanied by ulceration and pain.
  A. Systemic corticosteroids are given initially.
    1. Prednisone 1–2 mg/kg/day PO
    2. Methylprednisone acetate 10–20 mg IM biweekly for 1–3 treatments
    3. Triamcinolone 2–4 mg PO SID–QOD
  B. If systemic steroids cannot be tapered or lesions are resistant to glucocorticoids, chrysotherapy can be tried with aurothioglucose (Solganal).
    1. Test dose of 1 mg IM
    2. Then 1 mg/kg IM every 1–2 weeks until remission, then monthly

Patient Monitoring

I. Many cases respond to transient corticosteroid therapy within a few weeks.
II. Other lesions, especially those accompanied by plasmacytic pharyngitis, glomerulonephritis, or amyloidosis, are more refractive and often require prolonged continuous therapy.
III. In the complicated cases, prognosis is poor.

Bibliography

Ackerman LJ: Pemphigus and pemphigoid in the dog and cat. Part I: Pemphigus. Compend Contin Educ Pract Vet 7:89, 1985

Ackerman LJ: Pemphigus and pemphigoid in the dog and cat. Part II: Pemphigoid. Compend Contin Educ Pract Vet 7:281, 1985

Ackerman LJ: Recognizing the signs and sources of canine inhalant allergies. Vet Med 83:770, 1988

Ackerman LJ: Diagnosing inhalant allergies: intradermal or in vitro testing? Vet Med 83:779, 1988

Ackerman LJ: Medical and immunotherapeutic options for treating atopic dogs. Vet Med 83:790, 1988

Ackerman LJ: Food hypersensitivity: a rare, but manageable disorder. Vet Med 83:1142, 1988

Ackerman LJ: Adverse reactions to foods. Vet Focus 2:5, 1990

Bettenay S: Diagnosing and treating feline atopic dermatitis. Vet Med 86:488, 1991

Breitschwerdt EB: Immunoproliferative enteropathy of basenjis. Kal Kan Symp 8:111, 1984

Bronner AK, Hood AF: Cutaneous complications of chemotherapeutic agents. J Am Acad Dermatol 9:L645, 1983

Campbell KL, McLaughlin SA, Reynolds HA: Generalized leukoderma and poliosis following uveitis in a dog. J Am Anim Hosp Assoc 22:121, 1986

Crawford MA, Foil CS: Vasculitis: clinical syndromes in small animals. Compend Contin Educ Pract Vet 11:400, 1989

Daniel GB, Patterson JS: Toxic epidermal necrolysis: a case report. J Am Anim Hosp Assoc 21:631, 1985

De Swarte RD: Drug allergy—problems and strategies. J Allergy Clin Immunol 74:209, 1984

Fabries L: Syndrome "VKH" chez le chien: au sujet de deux cas cliniques. Prat Med Chirurg Anim Comp 19:393, 1984

Giger U, Werner LL, Millichamp NJ, Gorman NT: Sulfadiazine-induced allergy in six Doberman pinschers. J Am Vet Med Assoc 186:479, 1985

Goldberg GN: Erythema multiforme: controversies and recent advances. Adv Dermatol 2:73, 1987

Guilford WG, Olsen J, Riel D et al: Gastroscopic food sensitivity in the dog. J Vet Intern Med 5:132, 1991

Hendricks PM: Dermatitis associated with the use of primidone in a dog. J Am Vet Med Assoc 191:237, 1987

Jeffers JG, Shanley KJ, Meyer EK: Diagnostic testing of dogs for food hypersensitivity. J Am Vet Med Assoc 198:245, 1991

Kalaher KM, Scott DW: Discoid lupus erythematosus in a cat. Feline Pract 19:7, 1991

Kern TJ, Walton DK, Riis RC et al: Uveitis associated with poliosis and vitiligo in six dogs. J Am Vet Med Assoc 187:408, 1985

Kunkle GA: Contact dermatitis. Vet Clin North Am [Small Anim Pract] 18:1061, 1988

Mason KV: Subepidermal bullous drug eruption resembling bullous pemphigoid in a dog. J Am Vet Med Assoc 190:881, 1987

Medleau L: Linking chronic steroid-responsive pruritus to allergies. Vet Med 85:259, 1990

Merot Y, Saurat JH: Clues ot pathogenesis of toxic epidermal necrolysis. Int J Dermatol 24:165, 1985

Miller WH Jr, Griffin CE, Scott DW et al: Clinical trial of DVM Derm Caps in the treatment of allergic disease in dogs: a nonblinded study. J Am Anim Hosp Assoc 25:163, 1989

Miller WH, Scott DW: Efficacy of chlorpheniramine maleate for management of pruritus in cats. J Am Vet Med Assoc 197:67, 1990

Nesbitt GH, Kedam GS, Caciolo P: Canine atopy. Part I. Etiology and diagnosis. Compend Contin Educ Pract Vet 6:73, 1984

Panciera DL, Bevier D: Management of cryptococcosis and toxic epidermal necrolysis in a dog. J Am Vet Med Assoc 191:1125, 1987

Paradis M, Scott DW, Giroux D: Further investigations on the use of nonsteroidal and steroidal antiinflammatory agents in the management of canine pruritus. J Am Anim Hosp Assoc 27:44, 1991

Parsons JM: Management of toxic epidermal necrolysis. Cutis 38:305, 1985

Romatowski J: A uveodermatological syndrome in an Akita dog. J Am Anim Hosp Assoc 21:777, 1985

Rosenthal RC, Dworkis AS: Adverse reactions to Leukocell[R]. J Am Anim Hosp Assoc 23:515, 1987

Schmeitzel LP: Recognizing the cutaneous signs of immune-mediated diseases. Vet Med 86:138, 1991

Scott DW: Feline dermatology 1900–1978: a monograph. J Am Anim Hosp Assoc 16:331, 1980

Scott DW: Dermatologic use of glucocorticoids. Vet Clin North Am [Small Anim Pract] 12:19, 1983

Scott DW: Feline dermatology 1983–1985: "the secret sits." J Am Anim Hosp Assoc 23:255, 1987

Scott DW, Smith FWK, Smith CA: Erythema multiforme and pemphigus-like antibodies associated with sulfamethoxazole-trimethoprim administration in a dog with polycystic kidneys. Canine Pract 133:35, 1986

Scott DW, Walton DK, Manning TO et al: Canine lupus erythematosus. II. Discoid lupus erythematosus. J Am Anim Hosp 19:481, 1983

Van Hess J, Mason KV, Gross TL, Burren VS: Levamisole-induced drug eruptions in the dog. J Am Anim Hosp 21:255, 1985

Westly ED, Wechsler HL: Toxic epidermal necrolysis: granulocytic leukopenia as a prognostic indicator. Arch Dermatol 120:71, 1984

White JV: Cyclosporine prototype of a T-cell selective immunosuppressant. J Am Vet Med Assoc 189:566, 1986

White SD: Food hypersensitivity. Vet Clin North Am [Small Anim Pract] 18:1043, 1989

White SD, Stewart LJ, Bernstein M: Corticosteroid (methylprednisolone sodium succinate) pulse therapy in five dogs with autoimmune skin disease. J Am Vet Med Assoc 191:1121, 1987

Willemse A, van den Brom WE, Rijenberk A: Effect of hyposensitization on atopic dermatitis in dogs. J Am Vet Med Assoc 184:1277, 1984

Wintroub BU, Stern R: Cutaneous drug reactions: pathogenesis and clinical classification. J Am Acad Dermatol 13:167, 1985

90

Nutritional Disorders of the Skin

Richard K. Anderson

PROTEIN DEFICIENCY

Definition

I. Because the hair is 95% protein and the keratinization process going on in the normal skin consumes 25–30% of the animal's daily protein requirements, protein deficiencies are potential causes of dermatologic changes.

II. The nutritional value of proteins depends on their essential amino acid profiles as well as on the efficiency of digestion, absorption, and utilization by the body.

Causes

I. Decreased food intake
   A. Starvation
   B. Disease-induced inappetence
II. Diets inadequate in quality or quantity of protein
   A. Growing puppies and kittens, whose protein needs are higher
   B. Late gestation and lactation, when protein needs are higher
   C. Feeding cats commercial dog foods
   D. Feeding dogs very low protein diets
III. Protein loss
   A. Maldigestion/malabsorption syndromes
   B. Protein-losing enteropathy/nephropathies
   C. Intestinal parasitism
   D. Systemic disease, such as neoplasia, with increased protein catabolism

Pathophysiology

I. Dietary protein and essential amino acids are important precursors of the structural proteins of developing skin and hair.

II. Protein deficiency results in decreased hair diameter and atrophy of the skin, as the body tries to conserve protein synthesis for more vital structures.

Clinical Signs

I. Patchy alopecia in which hairs become dry, dull, and brittle
II. Slow hair growth and a prolonged shedding period
III. Skin that appears dry and thin and may have increased pigmentation
IV. Decubital ulcers and impaired healing
V. Edema of feet and legs

Diagnosis

I. Nutritional history suspicious of poor or inadequate protein intake
II. Physical examination findings, especially muscle wasting, alopecia, scales, and crusts
III. Investigation of systemic disease
   A. Hemogram, chemistry profile, plasma amino acids, and urinalysis
   B. Thyroid profile, adrenal function tests
IV. Response to therapy: see later

Differential Diagnosis

I. Any metabolic disease that may affect the intake, absorption, utilization, or excretion of various nutrients
II. Seborrheic skin disease (see Chap. 88)
III. Endocrinopathies, especially hypothyroidism, hyperadrenocorticism, diabetes mellitus

Treatment

I. Improve the diet by including adequate protein.
   A. On a dry-matter basis, 25% for the dog and 33% for the cat is therapeutic.
   B. Most commercial diets are actually extremely high in protein.
   C. High-quality protein from eggs, meat, or milk is important in supplementation.
II. Treat any existing systemic disease.

955

Patient Monitoring

I. Gradual improvement with decreased scaling and regrowth of a more normal hair coat should be seen within 1–3 months.

II. Be careful of oversupplementation.

A. Protein and calorie excess in the growing dog may result in skeletal abnormalities and, in adult dogs, results in obesity.

B. Monitor weight and adjust supplementation, depending on response.

FATTY ACID DEFICIENCY

Definition

I. From a dermatologic viewpoint, fat deficiency usually means essential fatty acid (linoleic, linolenic, arachidonic) deficiency.

II. Linoleic acid is an essential fatty acid required in the diet of all domestic animals.

A. The dog can synthesize both linolenic and arachidonic acid from linoleic acid.

B. The cat can convert only linolenic acid from linoleic acid and requires arachidonic acid in the diet.

III. Arachidonic acid is a constituent of animal fats and is not present in plant products.

Causes

I. Dietary deficiency

A. Commercial semi-moist dog foods, poorly supplemented table food diets, and unsupplemented low-fat dry dog foods are most frequently implicated.

B. Animals receiving special low-fat diets to help control hyperlipoproteinemia, hepatic or pancreatic disorders, or obesity are also at risk.

C. Improper packaging, prolonged storage, or inadequate antioxidants, such as vitamin E, may cause fats to become rancid.

II. Disease processes interfering with fat digestion or absorption

A. Pancreatic and liver disease

B. Intestinal malabsorption syndromes

Pathophysiology

I. Essential fatty acids are necessary for cell membrane structure and function and act as precursors for prostaglandins, leukotrienes, and other eicosanoids, which in turn act as pro- or anti-inflammatory agents.

II. Deficiency produces abnormal keratinization, resulting in epidermal hyperplasia, hypergranulosis, and orthokeratosis and/or parakeratotic hyperkeratosis.

III. Decreases in dietary fat lead to initial reduction in surface lipid production and then an overcompensatory increase in surface lipids using a different biochemical pathway.

IV. Changes in the lipid film of the skin surface lead to alterations in the microbial flora.

V. Animals must be fed a diet deficient in fatty acids for several months before skin problems become evident.

Clinical Signs

I. Initially, dry and lusterless hair and fine scaling of the skin

II. Later, greasy or waxy skin and hair from excess surface lipid production, especially affecting the ears and between the toes

III. Variable hair loss, erythema, pruritus, and secondary bacterial or *Malassezia* infections

Diagnosis

I. Determine the brand, type, and length of storage of the food used.

II. Physical examination findings are as described earlier.

III. Rule out other keratinization and scaling disorders.

A. Skin scrapings, fungal culture

B. Hormone assays

C. Fecal parasite and fat studies

D. Skin biopsy with compatible findings, including epidermal hyperplasia, hypergranulosis, and orthokeratotic and/or parakeratotic hyperkeratosis

IV. Diagnosis is based primarily on exclusion of other dermatologic conditions and response to appropriate supplementation.

Differential Diagnosis

I. Primary keratinization defects

A. Primary idiopathic seborrhea

B. Vitamin A–responsive dermatosis

C. Zinc-responsive dermatosis

D. Epidermal dysplasia of West Highland white terriers (Muller et al., 1989)

E. Sebaceous adenitis

F. Ichthyosis

II. Other diseases characterized by scaling and crusting

A. Ectoparasites

B. Pyoderma

C. *Malassezia* dermatitis

D. Dermatophytosis

E. Endocrinopathy, especially hypothyroidism

F. Autoimmune dermatoses, especially pemphigus foliaceus

G. Cutaneous neoplasia, especially mycosis fungoides

H. Environmental factors, especially dry heat

I. Other dietary deficiencies, such as protein deficiency

J. Allergic dermatoses

Treatment

I. Unintentional dietary abnormality

A. Change to a well-balanced diet containing a high fat content.

1. Dogs should be fed a canned food diet containing a minimum of 3% fat or a dry diet with 7–8% fat.
2. Cats usually need 30–40% of their calories provided by fat.
   B. Supplement with 1 teaspoonful of an equal mixture of an animal (pork or poultry) fat and a vegetable (safflower or corn oil) fat per cup or can of food.
   C. Because the clinical syndrome can be caused by several deficiencies, use of a balanced supplement ensures that the skin condition is being adequately treated.
   1. EFA-Z Plus (Allerderm/Virbac) 2.5 ml/5 kg PO SID
   2. Pet-Tabs/F.A. granules (Pfizer Animal Health) 1 tsp/5 kg PO SID
II. Animal on a low-fat diet for medical reasons
   A. Apply a fatty acid product such as HY-LYT efa (DVM Pharmaceuticals) as a spray on short-coated dogs or as an after-bath rinse for long-haired or densely coated animals.
   B. Use a balanced omega-6 and omega-3 fatty acid supplement such as DermCaps (DVM Pharmaceuticals) 1 ml/10 kg or 1 capsule/20 kg PO SID.

Patient Monitoring

I. If the dermatosis is an essential fatty acid deficiency, supplementation resolves the signs in 6–8 weeks.
II. Excessive supplementation must be avoided, because it causes obesity and unbalances the diet.
III. Use caution when supplementing fats in diets of dogs with pancreatitis or with maldigestion/malabsorption syndromes, as they may exacerbate the problem.
IV. If the underlying cause cannot be corrected, continue to supplement indefinitely.

ZINC-RESPONSIVE DERMATOSIS

Definition

I. It is a nutritionally responsive dermatosis affecting several breeds of dogs (Siberian huskies, Alaskan malamutes, bull terriers).
II. Primary and secondary zinc deficiencies, as well as nutrient-sensitive disease that responds to zinc, occur in dogs.

Causes

I. A genetically controlled abnormality in zinc absorption from the intestines, or zinc metabolism such that the dog's zinc requirement cannot be met by commercial foods
II. High-calcium diets and diets high in cereal phytates, binding zinc to produce a relative deficiency
III. Generic dog foods deficient in zinc
IV. Possibly precipitated by stress, estrus, and gastrointestinal disorders affecting absorption

Pathophysiology

I. Zinc is a component of over 70 metalloenzymes affecting carbohydrate, lipid, protein, and nucleic acid metabolism.
II. Zinc must be supplied continuously, because only small amounts of readily available zinc are stored in the body.
III. Zinc is important for the maintenance of normal epidermal integrity, taste acuity, and immunologic homeostasis.

Clinical Signs

I. Partial alopecia with erythematous, crusted plaques occurs around the eyes, mouth, ears, and pressure points such as the elbows and hocks.
II. Footpads may be hyperkeratotic and fissured.
III. In addition to scaling and crusting, these dogs may have secondary bacterial or *Malassezia* infection, lymphadenopathy, depression, and anorexia.

Diagnosis

I. Breed predilection: Siberian husky, Alaskan malamute, bullterrier
II. History including a complete record of diet
III. Compatible physical examination findings
IV. Skin biopsy
   A. The most suggestive feature is a marked surface and follicular parakeratotic hyperkeratosis.
   B. Intraepidermal pustular dermatitis and suppurative folliculitis reflect secondary bacterial infection.
V. Blood zinc analysis: unreliable because of the difficulty in avoiding contamination from glassware, rubber, and other containers
VI. Hair analysis: great variation in normal values, interpretation difficult
VII. Response to therapy

Differential Diagnosis

I. Pyoderma
II. Demodicosis
III. Dermatophytosis
IV. Autoimmune dermatoses, especially pemphigus foliaceus, systemic lupus erythematosus (SLE)
V. Seborrheic skin disease
VI. Necrolytic migratory erythema (superficial necrolytic dermatitis)

Treatment

I. Dietary imbalances are corrected, and zinc supplementation is given.
   A. Zinc sulfate 10 mg/kg PO SID crushed and mixed with food
   B. Zinc methionine, e.g., PALA-Z (Virbac), 1.7 mg/kg PO SID
   C. If oral treatment shows no benefit: zinc sulfate 15 mg/kg IV weekly for at least 4 weeks, then taper to a maintenance interval

II. Topical therapy daily or as often as necessary: wet dressings or whole body warm-water soakings for 5–10 minutes, then bathing with an antiseborrheic shampoo, e.g., Sebolux (Allerderm), followed by emollient rinses, e.g., Humilac (Allerderm)

Patient Monitoring

I. Response to therapy should be noted within 3 weeks.
II. Huskies and malamutes usually need lifetime therapy, with the dosage adjusted to maintenance levels (based on response) after remission is achieved.
III. Most bullterriers do not respond; almost all die before 15 months of age (see Chap. 82).
IV. The most significant side effects associated with zinc therapy are nausea, inappetence, and vomiting, which can be managed by dividing the daily dosage and administering the drug with food.

VITAMIN A–RESPONSIVE DERMATOSIS

Definition

I. It is a rare nutritionally responsive dermatosis primarily of American cocker spaniels and occasionally other breeds.
II. It does not represent a true dietary deficiency of vitamin A, in that plasma levels of vitamin A are within the normal range.

Causes

I. The cause is unknown.
II. Breed predisposition in the cocker spaniel suggests a genetic factor.

Pathophysiology

I. The histologic lesion reflects a severe disturbance in keratinization.
II. Vitamin A inhibits abnormal epithelial keratinization and proliferation.
III. Clinical response to vitamin A may represent one of the following.
  A. An increased need at the epidermal level
  B. A positive pharmacologic effect of high doses on the epidermis, overriding a metabolic impairment of the normal keratinization process

Clinical Signs

I. It usually develops within the first 2–3 years of life.
II. Marked follicular plugging (comedones) and hyperkeratotic plaques with frond-like keratinous plugs on their surfaces are typically seen.
III. The hyperkeratotic plaques are most prominent on the ventral and lateral aspect of the chest and abdomen.
IV. Generalized scaling, a dry hair coat with easy epila-

tion, and ceruminous otitis externa may also be present.

Diagnosis

I. Breed predilection: cocker spaniel
II. History of seborrheic skin disease and ceruminous otitis externa refractory to topical antiseborrheic medication, antibiotics, glucocorticoids, and thyroid hormone replacement therapy
III. Physical examination as described earlier
IV. Other keratinization disorders ruled out
  A. Skin scrapings, fungal culture
  B. Hemogram, serum chemistry profile, urinalysis
  C. Thyroid profile
V. Skin biopsy from follicular plugs and hyperkeratotic plaques
  A. Lesions are characterized by marked orthokeratotic hyperkeratosis of hair follicles, compared with mild orthokeratotic hyperkeratosis of the surface epidermis.
  B. Although these histologic changes are highly suggestive, the final diagnosis of vitamin A–responsive dermatosis can be confirmed only by response to therapy.

Table 90–1. Vitamin B Deficiencies

Deficient Vitamin	Clinical Signs
Biotin	1. Depigmentation and partial alopecia around the eyes (spectacle eye) 2. Generalized crusted lesions in advanced cases 3. Papulocrustous (miliary) dermatitis in cats
Riboflavin	1. Fissuring and dry scaling of the lips and commissures of the mouth (cheilosis) 2. Erythema and a dry, flaky dermatitis of the rear legs, chest, and abdomen 3. Alopecia about the head, chest, and forelegs in cats
Niacin	1. Reddening and ulceration of the oral mucosa, tongue, and lips (pellagra) 2. Rough hair coat and a scaly pruritic dermatitis of the rear legs and abdomen
Pyridoxine	1. Edema with swelling, hyperkeratosis, and necrosis of the ears, paws, nose, and lips in dogs 2. A dull waxy hair coat with generalized fine, white scales and multiple areas of alopecia in cats
Pantothenic acid	1. Depigmentation of hair (leukotrichia) 2. Inflammation of the skin and mucous membranes at mucocutaneous junctions

Differential Diagnosis

I. Primary idiopathic seborrhea
II. Fatty acid deficiency
III. Zinc-responsive dermatosis
IV. Endocrinopathy, especially hypothyroidism
V. Sebaceous adenitis

Treatment

I. Give vitamin A (retinol) 10,000 IU PO SID with a fatty meal.
II. Synthetic retinoids have been ineffective in the treatment of this disorder.
III. Keratolytic shampoos containing benzoyl peroxide, e.g., Oxydex (DVM Pharmaceuticals), hasten recovery.

Patient Monitoring

I. Improvement should be noted within 4–6 weeks.
II. Therapy should be continued for life, as attempts at lowering the dose usually result in relapse.
III. Signs of toxicosis include loss of appetite and weight, bone and joint pain, and possibly a worsening of the dry, scaly skin.

VITAMIN B DEFICIENCIES

See Table 90–1 and Chap. 120.

Bibliography

Fadok VA: Nutritional therapy in veterinary dermatology. p. 591. In Kirk RW (ed): Current Veterinary Therapy IX: Small Animal Practice. WB Saunders, Philadelphia, 1986

Ihrke PJ, Goldschmidt MH: Vitamin A–responsive dermatosis in the dog. J Am Vet Med Assoc 182:687, 1983

Kunkle GA: Zinc-responsive dermatosis in dogs. p. 472. In Kirk RW (ed): Current Veterinary Therapy VII. WB Saunders, Philadelphia, 1980

Lewis LD: Cutaneous manifestations of nutritional imbalances. Proc Am Anim Hosp Assoc 48:263, 1981

Lewis LD, Morris ML, Hand MS: Small Animal Clinical Nutrition III. Mark Morris Associates, Topeka, KS, 1987

Miller WH: Nutritional considerations in small animal dermatology. Vet Clin North Am [Small Anim Pract] 1:497, 1989

Miller WH, Scott DW, Buerger RG et al: Necrolytic migratory erythema in dogs: a hepatocutaneous syndrome. J Am Anim Hosp Assoc 26:573, 1990

Muller GH, Kirk RW, Scott DW: Small Animal Dermatology. 4th Ed. WB Saunders, Philadelphia, 1989

Norton A: Skin lesions seen in cats with vitamin B (pyridoxine deficiency). Proc Am Acad Vet Dermatol 3:24, 1987

Sousa CA: Nutritional dermatosis. p. 189. In Nesbitt GH (ed): Dermatology Contemporary Issues in Small Animal Practice. Churchill Livingstone, New York, 1987

Sousa CA, Stannard AA, Ihrke PJ et al: Dermatosis associated with feeding generic dog food: 13 cases (1981–1982). J Am Vet Med Assoc 192:676, 1988

91

Cutaneous Neoplasia

Michael H. Goldschmidt
Frances S. Shofer

Table 91–1. Skin Tumors of the Dog and Cat

Tumor	Species/Breed/Sex Affected	Age	Site Predilection	Gross Appearance	Treatment	Prognosis
Basal cell	Kerry blue terrier, cockapoo, Siberian husky, Shetland sheepdog, cocker spaniel, miniature poodle	Dog: 4–8 yr Cat: 7–13 yr	Head, neck	Elevated mass, varies in size from 1–5 cm in diameter; overlying epidermis alopecic, thin, hyperpigmented; may be ulcerated; on cut section often multilobulated, well demarcated from surrounding tissue; may be pigmented and/or cystic	Surgical excision	Excellent; seldom recur following surgical excision
Feline basal cell carcinoma		9–13 yr	May be multicentric	Cannot be distinguished from basal cell tumor on clinical evaluation; histopathology reveals the infiltrative nature of the tumor	Surgical excision	Good following wide excision; may recur, but metastasis not reported
Canine squamous cell carcinoma	a. Skin: bloodhound, basset hound, standard poodle, miniature poodle b. Digit: schnauzer, Gordon setter, dachshund, Scottish terrier, Labrador retriever	7–13 yr	a. Skin: head, perineum/abdomen, rear leg b. Digit: may involve multiple digits	Hyperemia; hyperplastic ulcerated or nodular skin lesion; lesions are expansile, often associated with ultraviolet irradiation in light-skinned dogs exposed to the sun. Digital lesions may present as paronychia or a markedly swollen and deformed digit with secondary infection	Surgical excision	A proportion of cases recur or show lymph node metastasis
Feline squamous cell carcinoma	White cats with blue eyes	9–14 yr	External ear (pinna), eyelid, planum nasale	Hyperemia, ulcerated skin lesion progressing to invasion; destructive, ulcerated, infiltrative tumor	Surgical excision, radiation therapy	Good at sites where wide excision possible (ear); often recur at other sites (eyelid, planum nasale)
Sebaceous adenoma	Cocker spaniel, Siberian husky, Samoyed, West Highland white terrier, dachshund, miniature poodle (common in the dog, uncommon in the cat)	Dog: 8–14 yr	Head, neck, forelimbs, hindlimbs	Elevated mass with an extensive intradermal component; vary in size from 0.5–5 cm in diameter, ulceration may occur; white or pigmented on cut section; often polypoid	Surgical excision	Good; usually do not recur following wide excision; small percentage (3%) are multicentric
Sebaceous carcinoma	Cavalier King Charles spaniel, Cairn terrier, cocker spaniel, Siberian husky (common in the dog, very uncommon in the cat)	Dog: 8–15 yr	Head, neck, hindleg	Intradermal mass, usually white/yellow; may show invasion of subcutaneous tissue; rapid growth rate. Regional lymph nodes may show metastatic disease	Surgical excision and lymph node evaluation for metastasis	Guarded; widespread metastatic disease uncommon
Canine hepatoid gland (perianal) adenoma	Siberian husky, Samoyed, Pekingese, cocker spaniel, Brittany spaniel, Shih Tzu, beagle, Lhasa apso, cockapoo 3:1 M:F ratio, primarily intact males	8–13 yr	Perianal area, tail, ventral abdomen (preputial), back. Many cases have more than one tumor in the perianal area	Elevated, intradermal masses, 0.5–10 cm in diameter, covered by hairless skin or often ulcerated and necrotic; cut sections are pale brown, multilobulated; may show extensive hemorrhage and necrosis; invade underlying muscle and soft tissue	Surgical excision and castration of intact male dogs. Radiation therapy for advanced cases	Good; additional tumors represent de novo tumors, not recurrence

Table continued on following page

Table 91–1. *Skin Tumors of the Dog and Cat* (Continued)

Tumor	Species/Breed/Sex Affected	Age	Site Predilection	Gross Appearance	Treatment	Prognosis
Canine hepatoid gland (perianal) carcinoma	Malamute, Siberian husky 9:1 M:F, primary intact males	9–14 yr	Perianal area, ventral abdomen	Cannot be differentiated from adenomas; identification of metastatic disease to sacral and sublumbar lymph nodes most useful	Surgical excision, radiation therapy	Guarded
Meibomian adenoma	Gordon setter, malamute, collie, Shih Tzu, Siberian husky (uncommon in cats)	Dog: 7–12 yr	Eyelid margin	Elevated, hyperpigmented mass, usually less than 0.5 cm in diameter Overlying skin may be ulcerated	Surgical excision	Good with wide excision Recurrence often owing to incomplete excision of large tumors
Meibomian carcinoma	Very rarely seen; older dogs	Dog: 7–12 yr	Eyelid margin	Cannot be differentiated from adenomas	Surgical excision	Guarded; may show lymphatic invasion with lymph node metastasis
Apocrine adenoma	Old English sheepdog, collie, German shepherd dog, English springer spaniel	Dog: 6–12 yr Cat: 7–14 yr	Head, neck, abdomen	Slightly elevated mass, varying from 1–4 cm in diameter; alopecia and hyperpigmentation of overlying epidermis; cut section solid or cystic, white, or slight brown discoloration of fluid	Surgical excision	Good; seldom recur following surgical excision
Apocrine carcinoma	Norwegian elkhound, German shepherd dog	Dog: 9–13 yr Cat: 8–13 yr	Axilla, inguinal, perineal areas	Variable, nodular intradermal mass infiltrating deeper tissue or erosive, ulcerated, hyperemic lesion that mimics an eczematous dermatitis	Surgical excision ± chemotherapy	Very guarded; often have lymph node and pulmonary metastasis
Ceruminous adenoma and carcinoma	Cocker spaniel, German shepherd dog, toy poodle	Dog: 7–13 yr Cat: 6–14 yr	External ear canal	Elevated mass, often ulcerated with secondary inflammation and infection; may be hyperpigmented Carcinoma is often infiltrative and invades underlying connective tissue stroma	Surgery ± chemotherapy	Good following wide surgical excision of adenomas; carcinomas may require surgical ablation of the ear and evaluation of regional lymph nodes for metastasis
Anal sac gland carcinoma	English cocker spaniel, dachshund, English springer spaniel, German shepherd dog, mix-breed dogs Increased incidence in spayed female and castrated male dogs	Dog: 8–13 yr	Anal sac	Vary in size from 0.5–8 cm in diameter; smallest tumors identified only on rectal digital palpation; large masses mimic gross appearance of hepatoid gland adenomas; may be ulcerated; metastasis to sacral and sublumbar lymph nodes may cause difficulty in urination and defecation, hypercalcemia secondary to pseudohyperparathyroidism presents as polyuria and polydipsia	Surgical excision ± lymph node resection, chemotherapy	Guarded, often metastatic to sacral and sublumbar lymph nodes

Tumor	Breed/Incidence	Age	Location	Clinical Appearance	Treatment	Prognosis/Comments
Canine intracutaneous cornifying epithelioma (keratoacanthoma)	Norwegian elkhound, Lhasa apso, Yorkshire terrier, German shepherd dog, standard poodle	4–11 yr	Multiple sites on back, tail (elkhound, Lhasa apso)	Intradermal masses, often exophytic, varying from 0.5–3 cm in size; often have a central pore through which a gray keratinous material may be expressed; intradermal and subcutaneous component well demarcated from surrounding tissue	Surgical excision	Good, except in dogs that have multiple tumors, as additional masses continue to develop over time
Trichoepithelioma	Basset hound, standard poodle, Irish setter, English springer spaniel, golden retriever, English setter, miniature schnauzer, Airdale terrier 3:2 F:M ratio (common in dogs, uncommon in cats)	Dog: 5.5–11.5 yr	Multicentric, back, neck, tail	Intradermal masses, often exophytic, ranging in size from 1–5 cm in diameter; many are ulcerated, on cut sections, multiple gray-white foci of keratinous material are separated by thin connective tissue trabeculae; others may be cystic, and infiltrative type associated with sclerotic change	Surgical excision	Infiltrative type often recurs at surgical site Remainder cured by surgery alone <1% malignant with metastasis to regional lymph nodes and lungs
Canine pilomatrixoma	Kerry blue terrier, standard poodle, Old English sheepdog, basset hound, miniature poodle (common in dogs, uncommon in cats)	Dog: 3.5–10 yr	Back, neck, tail	Elevated, intradermal skin mass from 1–6 cm in diameter; may ulcerate or show alopecia and hyperpigmentation; cut section white, chalky appearance, may be multilobulated; often difficult to transect owing to bone within the tumor	Surgical excision	Good; seldom recur following surgical excision; occasional cases of malignant pilomatrixoma with lymph node and lung metastasis may be found
Dermal melanoma	Miniature schnauzer, standard schnauzer, vizsla, Doberman pinscher, Brittany spaniel, Irish setter, golden retriever Higher incidence in males than females	Dog: 6–12 yr Cat: 8–14 yr	Multiple: Doberman pinscher, Irish setter Eyelid: vizsla, Brittany spaniel, Weimaraner Back: miniature schnauzer Head, ear: feline	Intradermal mass, usually covered by hyperpigmented epidermis; may extend through panniculus adiposus into the subcutis; black but degree of pigmentation is variable	Surgical excision ± chemotherapy	Good following surgical excision
Malignant melanoma	Irish setter, Scottish terrier, standard schnauzer, miniature schnauzer Higher incidence in males than females	Dog: 8–14 yr Cat: 8–14 yr	Less than 10% of cases in the dog occur in the skin; major predilection sites are oral cavity (55%), lip (25%), and digit (10%) Digit: Irish setter, Scottish terrier, standard and miniature schnauzer Skin of abdomen, scrotum: miniature schnauzer Nose: cat	a. Digit: Loss of nail, destruction of P3, lameness; on section, tumor may be pigmented b. Skin: intradermal and subcutaneous mass with variable degree of pigmentation	Surgical excision ± chemotherapy	Guarded; metastasis occurs via lymphatics in regional lymph nodes and lungs

Table continued on following page

Table 91–1. Skin Tumors of the Dog and Cat (Continued)

Tumor	Species/Breed/Sex Affected	Age	Site Predilection	Gross Appearance	Treatment	Prognosis
Canine dermal fibroma	German shepherd dog, Doberman pinscher, boxer, golden retriever	5.5–11 yr	Multiple: German shepherd dog; forelimb, hindlimb	Elevated, alopecic intradermal and subcutaneous mass; very firm on palpation; white and glistening on cut section, dermis lacks adnexal structures	Surgical excision	Good following excision; some German shepherd dogs may develop syndrome of multiple dermal fibromas, uterine leiomyosarcoma, and renal carcinomas; this is a heritable condition
Canine dermal fibrosarcoma	Gordon setter, Irish wolfhound, Brittany spaniel, golden retriever, Doberman pinscher	5–12 yr	Forelimb, hindlimb, abdomen	Infiltrative intradermal and subcutaneous mass; gray/white on cross section; rapidly growing tumors have central necrosis and hemorrhage	Surgical excision	Guarded; because of infiltrative nature, may require amputation of affected limb; young dogs more likely to show pulmonary metastasis
Feline dermal fibrosarcoma	Any cat	Any age Cats with single or multiple tumors <5 yr old: associated with FeSV Cats with multiple tumors >5 yr old: 25% FeSV positive Cats with single tumors >5 yr old: no association with FeSV	Limbs, head, neck; may arise at site of prior subcutaneous vaccination	Firm, intradermal mass often infiltrating subcutaneous tissue; may be covered by hairless skin or ulcerated; white on cut section; may see necrotic center	Surgical excision	Guarded
Canine hemangiopericytoma	German shepherd dog, Irish setter, Siberian husky, mixed-breed dogs Females have a higher incidence than males	7.5–13 yr	Hindlimb and forelimb (over joints); thorax	Infiltrative intradermal mass; overlying skin alopecic, may be ulcerated; white on cut section, may appear multilobulated	Surgical excision; may require limb amputation after multiple recurrences	Guarded; commonly recur at surgical site, especially when over joints or where wide excision is difficult; very few metastasize
Canine myxoma and myxosarcoma	Beagle, Labrador retriever, mixed breed	7–13 yr	Thorax, forelimb, hindlimb	Soft intradermal and subcutaneous mass; on excision has a very mucoid appearance; edges of tumor difficult to identify at surgery	Surgical excision, may require limb amputation after multiple recurrences	Guarded; often recur at surgical site because of difficulty in identifying borders of tumor
Neurofibroma and neurofibrosarcoma	Rare in both dogs and cats	Usually older	Head, trunk	May be difficult to differentiate from fibroma, fibrosarcoma, and hemangiopericytoma Diagnosis based on histiopathologic findings of neuroid differentiation	Surgical excision	Good for neurofibroma if excision is complete Guarded for neurofibrosarcoma; tend to recur locally

Tumor	Breed	Age	Location	Clinical Features	Treatment	Prognosis
Hemangioma	Airedale terrier, boxer, English springer spaniel, German shepherd dog, golden retriever, Old English sheepdog, fox terrier	Dog: 5.5–12 yr Cat: 8–14 yr	Hindlimb, tail	Intradermal and subcutaneous mass Small lesions may be papilliferous and hyperpigmented; larger lesions often dark red in appearance; may bleed if skin is ulcerated and traumatized; on cut section, multiple blood-filled channels subdivided by fine, white trabeculae	Surgical excision	Good; may be multicentric Some cases may develop from chronic sun exposure
Hemangiosarcoma	German shepherd dog, golden retriever	Dogs: 7–11 yr Cats: 8–14 yr	Variable	Similar to hemangioma: many cases present with multiple intradermal and subcutaneous masses	Surgical excision ± chemotherapy	Guarded: cutaneous lesions may represent metastasis from a primary tumor of liver, spleen, or right auricular appendage
Lymphangioma	Affects primary dogs	Young dogs Older dogs	Ventral abdomen (inguinal area) and axillae	May present as subepidermal vesicles or as large infiltrative intradermal and subcutaneous mass; very spongy in texture; clear fluid may exude onto skin surface or when incised	Surgical excision	Guarded; difficult to identify surgical borders, so recurrence is common
Lipoma	Doberman pinscher, Labrador retriever, miniature schnauzer, mixed-breed dogs Females, especially spayed overweight animals	Dog: 6–11 yr Cat: 8–13 yr	Thorax, abdomen	Soft mass, easily movable in subcutis; some, however, are infiltrative and involve surrounding tissue, especially muscle; cross section white and oily, may have a thin capsule; large tumors may show central necrosis, float in water and 10% formalin	Surgical excision	Good following wide excision, except for infiltrative type, which may recur
Liposarcoma	Shetland sheepdog, beagle	Dog: 8–13 yr	Thorax, hindlimb, forelimb	Intradermal and subcutaneous mass; white to yellow to yellow/green on cut section; may infiltrate locally; histopathology required to differentiate from lipoma	Surgical excision	Relatively good following wide surgical excision; 30% may recur at surgical site; very few show metastatic spread
Canine mast cell tumor	Boxer, pug, Boston terrier, Weimaraner, Labrador retriever, beagle, golden retriever	5–12 yr	Rear limbs, perineum, scrotum, abdomen 5% of cases present as multiple tumors	Many mimic other tumors; intradermal mass of varying size that may be soft or firm; locally infiltrative, thus precluding adequate evaluation of borders at time of surgery Cytology very useful in establishing original diagnosis, thus allowing wide excision of tumor	Surgical excision, corticosteroids, radiation therapy	Guarded; tumors may become multicentric; metastatic spread is to regional lymph nodes, spleen, and liver
Feline mast cell tumor	Siamese	6–12 yr Siamese <4 yr old	Head, neck	Elevated, intradermal alopecic nodules; solitary or multiple; pink to yellow or white, pruritic and may be ulcerated	Surgical excision, corticosteroids	Good for single lesions Guarded for recurrent or multiple lesions or if systemic involvement occurs

Table continued on following page

Table 91–1. **Skin Tumors of the Dog and Cat** (Continued)

Tumor	Species/Breed/Sex Affected	Age	Site Predilection	Gross Appearance	Treatment	Prognosis
Cutaneous lymphosarcoma	Briard, English bulldog, Scottish terrier, golden retriever	Dog: 6–18 yr Cat: 8–14 yr	Multicentric	Variable: tumor may present as alopecic, hyperemic, seborrheic skin disease that progresses to multiple elevated plaques, nodules, and ulcerated intradermal masses. Histopathology shows infiltration of neoplastic lymphoid cells with or without epidermotropism	Nitrogen mustard for superficial epidermotropic form. Standard lymphosarcoma protocol for more advanced disease not proved useful	Guarded; lesions are progressive, with metastasis to lymph nodes, liver, and spleen
Canine cutaneous histiocytoma	Scottish terrier, boxer, Boston terrier, rottweiler, Doberman pinscher, Labrador retriever, cocker spaniel	6 mo–3 yr	Head (ear)	Hyperemic, alopecic, elevated intradermal nodule, 0.5–1.5 cm in diameter; may show surface ulceration	Surgical excision	Excellent; many regress spontaneously
Cutaneous plasmacytoma (solitary plasmacytoma)	Cocker spaniel, Airedale terrier, Scottish terrier, standard poodle	8–14 yr	Lip, ear, digits; small percentage may be multiple	0.5–1 cm elevated, bright red, intradermal mass, devoid of hair; may extend into the subcutis; may resemble histiocytoma, but usually found in older dogs. Cytology reveals round cells with abundant cytoplasm, occasional multinucleated cells	Surgical excision	Good; respond well to surgical excision except those tumors producing amyloid (which may recur)

M = male; F = female; FeSV = feline sarcomavirus.

Table 91–2. Common Tumor-Like Lesions of the Skin

Lesion	Species/Breed Affected	Age	Site Predilection	Gross Appearance	Treatment	Prognosis
Canine adnexal nevus	Weimaraner, dalmation, Labrador retriever, Doberman pinscher	6–12 yr	Limbs, abdomen	Elevated, hyperpigmentation, firm skin, may be polypoid Cut section often reveals multiple, small, keratin-filled cysts	Surgical excision	Excellent
Cutaneous tag	Rottweiler, Great Dane, boxer, Doberman pinscher, Labrador retriever (common in the dog, uncommon in the cat)	4–11 yr	Limbs, abdomen, thorax	Elevated, hyperpigmented, alopecic, papilliferous lesion, often with narrow baase	Surgical excision	Excellent
Epidermal inclusion cyst	Common in dogs and cats	All ages	Back	Intradermal mass, 0.3–2 cm in diameter: cut section reveals central soft gray/brown material (keratin) with a thin wall at periphery	Surgical excision	Excellent; however, rupture of cyst wall releases keratin into dermis, where it evokes a pyogranulomatous inflammatory response
Follicular cyst	Common in dogs, uncommon in cats	Young dogs	Top of head, elbows, hip	Intradermal cysts filled with keratin and hair shafts Overlying skin may be hyperpigmented, thickened, and devoid of hair	Surgical excision	Good; lesions are usually post-traumatic in origin
Apocrine cyst	Old English sheepdog, Weimaraner, collie	6–12 yr	Head, neck, multiple	Exophytic, intradermal, fluid-filled cyst(s), often with a light-blue discoloration: on cut section, fluid is colorless, cysts collapse	Surgical excision	Single cysts good; multiple cysts are probably senile change and increase in number with advancing age
Sebaceous hyperplasia	Standard poodle, Manchester terrier, Kerry blue terrier, bichon frise, cocker spaniel, poodle, cocker spaniel, West Highland white terrier, Siberian husky (very common in dog, uncommon in cat)	≥8 yr	Multiple; head, forelimb, hindlimb	Small (0.3–0.7 cm), yellow/white, elevated, umbilical nodules covered by thin, hairless epidermis	Senile change of unknown etiology New lesions may occur with increasing age	Good
Ceruminous hyperplasia	Cocker spaniel, miniature poodle	6–12 yr	External ear canal	Hyperplastic, polypoid, often papilliferous masses; often occurs secondary to chronic otitis externa, may occlude ear canal	Surgical excision, may require ablation of ear if severe	Fair to good
Ceruminous cyst	Common in cat, uncommon in dogs	≥8 yr	External ear canal	0.1–0.2 cm elevated, dark brown nodules, may be multiple	Ear cleaning ± excision	Good, but may predispose to recurrent otitis exema

Bibliography

Bevier DE, Goldschmidt MH: Skin tumors in the dog. Part I. Epithelial tumors and tumor-like lesions. Compend Contin Educ Pract Vet 3:389, 1981

Bevier DE, Goldschmidt MH: Skin tumors in the dog. Part II. Tumors of the soft (mesenchymal) tissues. Compend Contin Educ Pract Vet 3:506, 1981

Carpenter JL, Andrews LK, Holzworth J: Tumors and tumor-like lesions. p. 406. In Holzworth J (ed): Diseases of the Cat. WB Saunders, Philadelphia, 1987

Conroy JD: Canine skin tumors. J Am Anim Hosp 19:91, 1983

Goldschmidt MH, Bevier DE: Skin tumors in the dog. Part III. Lymphohistiocytic and melanocytic tumors. Compend Contin Educ Pract Vet 3:588, 1981

Macy DW: Canine and feline mast cell tumors: biologic behaviour, diagnosis, and therapy. Semin Vet Med Surg 1:72, 1986

Pulley LT, Stannard AA: Tumors of the skin and soft tissue. p. 23. In Moulton JE (ed): Tumors in Domestic Animals. 3rd Ed. University of California Press, Berkeley, CA, 1990

Scott DW, Miller WH, Griffin CE: Neoplastic diseases. p. 990. In: Muller & Kirk's Small Animal Dermatology. 5th Ed. WB Saunders, Philadelphia, 1995

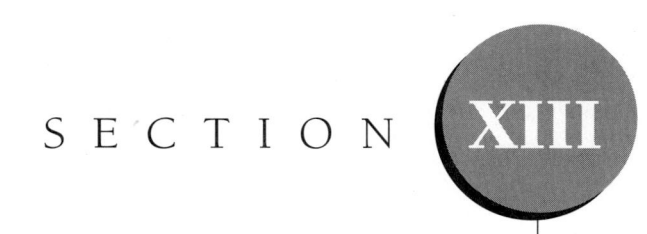

SECTION XIII

Diseases of the
Eye

92

Introduction

Cynthia S. Cook

Problems related to the eyes are a frequent reason for presentation of companion animals to the veterinary practitioner. Owners are particularly sensitive to the appearance of their pets' eyes and empathetic to any indication of discomfort or vision impairment. The initial owner observation usually falls into one of the following categories: (1) loss of vision, (2) change in appearance of the globe, (3) ocular discharge, and/or (4) ocular/orbital pain. In Table 92–1, reference is made to a condition as it occurs alone. For example, a lens luxation alone may not result in ocular pain, but if accompanied by secondary glaucoma (as is often the case), ocular pain results from the elevated intraocular pressure. "Change in appearance" refers to the changes likely to be observed by the owner; a plus sign = observed, a minus sign = not seen, and ± means may or may not be seen.

*Table 92–1. **Diseases of the Eye and Observed Signs***

	Loss of Vision	Change in Appearance	Ocular Discharge	Pain
Eyelids (see Chap. 93)				
Coloboma	−	+	+	±
Dermoid	−	+	±	±
Entropion	±	±	+	+
Ectropion	−	±	±	−
Trichiasis	±	−	±	±
Distichiasis	−	−	±	±
Ectopic cilia	−	−	+	+
Lagophthalmos	±	−	±	−
Hordeolum	−	+	±	−
Chalazion	−	+	±	−
Blepharitis	−	+	±	±
Dermatomyositis	−	+	±	−
Neoplasia	−	+	±	−
Trauma	−	+	±	+
Conjunctiva and Third Eyelid (see Chap. 94)				
Prolapse of third eyelid gland	−	+	±	−
Eversion of cartilage of third eyelid	−	+	−	−
Conjunctival cyst	−	+	−	−
Dermoid	−	+	+	±
Symblepharon	±	+	+	±
Conjunctivitis	−	+	+	±
Protrusion of third eyelid	±	+	−	−
Conjunctival neoplasia	−	+	±	−
Trauma	−	+	±	+
Lacrimal and Nasolacrimal System (see Chap. 95)				
Imperforate puncta	−	−	+	−
Keratoconjunctivitis sicca	±	+	+	±
Dacryocystitis	−	−	+	−
Dacryops	−	+	−	−
Neoplasia	−	+	±	−
Trauma	−	+	±	±

Table continued on following page

Table 92–1. *Diseases of the Eye and Observed Signs* (Continued)

	Loss of Vision	Change in Appearance	Ocular Discharge	Pain
Cornea and Sclera (see Chap. 96)				
Dermoid				
Corneal stromal dystrophy	±	+	+	±
Corneal pigmentation, vascularization, fibrosis	−	+	−	−
Eyelid abnormalities	±	+	+	±
Keratoconjunctivitis sicca	±	+	+	±
Chronic superficial keratitis	±	+	±	−
Eosinophilic keratitis	±	+	±	−
Corneal inflammatory infiltrate				
Infectious keratoconjunctivitis	±	±	+	±
Corneal abscess	±	±	±	±
Episclerokeratitis	−	+	−	−
Corneal edema				
Ulcerative keratitis	±	+	+	+
Persistent pupillary membranes	−	+	−	−
Endothelial dystrophy, degeneration	±	+	−	−
Uveitis	±	+	±	+
Infectious canine hepatitis	±	+	±	±
Glaucoma	+	+	−	±
Corneal sequestrum	±	+	+	+
Neoplasia	±	+	−	−
Anterior Uveal Tract (see Chap. 97)				
Persistent pupillary membranes, coloboma, anterior segment dysgenesis, cyst	±	+	−	−
Uveitis (all causes)	±	+	±	+
Iris atrophy	−	+	−	−
Iris melanosis	−	+	−	−
Hyphema	−	+	−	−
Lipid-laden aqueous	±	+	−	−
Anisocoria	−	+	−	−
Afferent deficit	+	+	−	−
Efferent deficit	−	+	−	−
Neoplasia	±	+	−	−
Lens (see Chap. 99)				
Cataract (all causes)	±	+	−	−
Nuclear sclerosis	−	±	−	−
Lens luxation	±	±	−	±
Vitreous (see Chap. 99)				
Persistent hyperplastic primary vitreous (PHPV)/persistent tunica vasculosa lentis (PTVL)	±	±	−	−
Vitritis	−	−	−	−
Asteroid hyalosis	−	−	−	−
Hemorrhage	±	±	−	−
Cholesterolosis bulbi	−	−	−	−
Syneresis	−	−	−	−
Posterior Segment (see Chap. 100)				
Retinal dysplasia				
Multifocal	±	−	−	−
Generalized	+	−	−	−
Collie eye anomaly	±	−	−	−
Congenital tapetal hypoplasia	−	−	−	−
Optic nerve hypoplasia	+	−	−	−
Optic nerve coloboma	±	−	−	−
Retinal degeneration (all causes)	+	−	−	−
Retinal detachment (all causes)	+	−	−	−
Chorioretinitis	±	−	−	±
Optic neuritis	+	−	−	−
Neoplasia	±	±	−	−
Orbit/Globe as a Whole (see Chap. 103)				
Microphthalmia	+	+	±	−
Phthisis bulbi	+	+	±	−
Orbital cellulitis	±	+	+	+
Eosinophilic myositis	±	+	−	+
Orbital cyst	−	+	−	−
Orbital neoplasia	±	+	±	±
Proptosis	±	+	±	+

93

Diseases of the Eyelids

Denise M. Lindley

CONGENITAL/ DEVELOPMENTAL DISORDERS

Eyelid Agenesis

Definition

I. Eyelid agenesis is a congenital defect of the eyelid margin resulting in absence of a focal area of eyelid skin, palpebral conjunctiva, and fornices.
II. Upper eyelid agenesis is most common and usually involves the lateral one third or two thirds of the eyelid margin.
III. Coloboma is a term that is often used to describe this condition.

Causes

I. The cause is unknown.
II. It is generally considered a sporadic, noninherited defect.
III. Some cases may be inherited, but the genetics are not defined.

Pathophysiology

I. Failure of eyelid folds to completely form during the first 3 weeks of development is proposed.
II. Failure of the optic fissure to close in cats is often associated with eyelid agenesis.
   A. As eyelid development is induced by contact of the early optic vessel with the surface ectoderm, microphthalmia may be primary to eyelid agenesis.
   B. Unilateral or bilateral iris, ciliary body, and posterior segment colobomas in the ventral globe at the site of the optic fissure are not uncommon (Bellhorn et al., 1971).
   C. Craniofacial abnormalities and hypoplasia/aplasia of the lacrimal gland may also be associated with eyelid agenesis.

Clinical Signs

I. Signalment
   A. Occurs infrequently in the cat, especially domestic shorthairs; even rarer in the dog
   B. Can be observed as early as eyelid opening at 14 days
   C. No sex predilection
II. Clinical presentation
   A. Usually bilateral, but not necessarily symmetrical
   B. Can be asymptomatic and presented for cosmetic repair
   C. Chronic blepharospasm
   D. Chronic epiphora
   E. Secondary changes
      1. Exposure keratitis
      2. Irritation to cornea and exposed conjunctiva from trichiasis
         a) Superficial corneal ulcers are fortunately infrequent.
         b) Corneal vascularization is common with chronic irritation.
         c) Corneal pigmentation very rarely occurs in the cat but can develop in the dog.
   F. With multiple ocular defects, occasionally visual deficits and/or abnormal behavior

Diagnosis

I. Definitive diagnosis is based on the presence of the eyelid defect during the ophthalmic examination.
II. A thorough ocular examination is performed to identify the presence of other ocular malformations.
   A. Ocular colobomas
   B. Lacrimal gland deficiency

Differential Diagnosis

I. Other causes of blepharospasm
   A. Entropion
   B. Ulcerative keratitis secondary to trauma or infection
   C. Foreign body

973

II. Other causes of corneal neovascularization
III. Acquired eyelid defects

Treatment

I. In the young animal, ophthalmic lubricant ointments (TID-QID) to decrease exposure keratitis and irritation
II. Cryoepilation of trichiasis
   A. Permanent removal of hairs that rub the cornea and conjunctiva
   B. Spray application of liquid nitrogen or application of nitrous oxide probe
      1. Ice ball should extend 2 mm past hair follicles that are being treated.
      2. Immediately repeat the freeze-thaw procedure.
   C. Advantages and disadvantages
      1. Effective at alleviating clinical signs of discomfort associated with trichiasis
      2. Less costly than reconstructive procedures
      3. Does not alleviate exposure keratoconjunctivitis
III. Surgical reconstruction of eyelid agenesis
   A. Surgical goals include coverage of globe with both conjunctiva and overlying skin.
   B. Several techniques are available (Peiffer, 1981; Dziezye et al., 1989).
   C. Preferred technique provides a conjunctival graft to line a skin flap (Dziezyc and Millichamp, 1989).
      1. The conjunctival graft is sutured to the edge of the freshened dorsal bulbar conjunctiva with 6-0 absorbable suture material so that epithelium faces epithelium.
      2. The anterior cut edges of the conjunctival graft and skin flap are sutured together with 6-0 absorbable suture material.
      3. 5-0 nonabsorbable skin sutures close the remainder of skin flap incisions.

D. The main disadvantage of all techniques using a pedicle skin flap from the lower eyelid is that trichiasis from the repositioned skin flap can occur.

Patient Monitoring

I. Postoperative care
   A. Apply topical antibiotic ophthalmic ointment to eye and suture lines TID until suture removal.
   B. Use an Elizabethan collar to decrease self-trauma.
   C. Restain the cornea with fluorescein 24 hours postoperatively and at time of suture removal (or sooner if ocular discharge and/or pain develop) to check for ulceration.
   D. Keep incision lines clean and remove sutures at 10–14 days.
   E. Monitor tear function and continue to treat as needed (see Chap. 95).
II. Reevaluate eyelid coverage of globe 6–8 weeks after surgery.
III. Cryoepilate any trichiasis associated with the pedicle flap 6–8 weeks after surgery.

Dermoid

See Chap. 94.

Entropion

Definition

I. Inversion of the eyelid margin toward the globe (Fig. 93–1)
II. Three classifications
   A. Heritable/conformational entropion
   B. Spastic entropion
   C. Cicatricial entropion

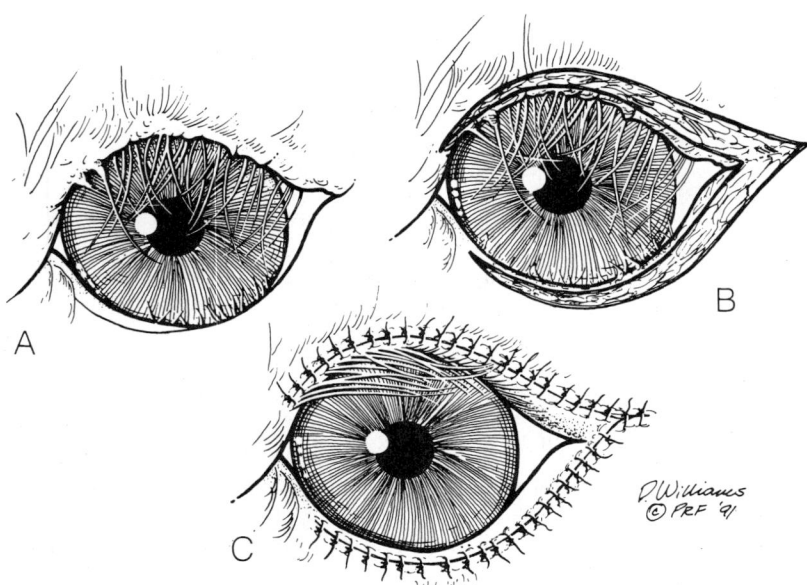

Figure 93–1. A. Upper and lower eyelid margins and lateral canthus are inverted, resulting in trichiasis. B. Sharp excision of eyelid skin adjacent to inverted eyelid margin has been performed. C. Closure of eyelid incision with numerous small sutures results in normal eyelid position. (From Purdue Research Foundation, with permission.)

Causes

I. Heritable/conformational entropion is a common anatomic defect that is considered to be a polygenic trait. Genes that influence skin, orbital contents, and skull conformation contribute to this problem.
  A. Medial canthal entropion
    1. Involves the medial eyelids
    2. Brachycephalic breeds: pug, Pekingese, Lhasa apso, Shih Tzu
    3. Mesocephalic breeds: poodle, bichon frisé
  B. Lateral canthal entropion
    1. Involves lateral upper and lower eyelid
    2. Common breeds: St. Bernard, chow chow, rottweiler, Shar pei, English bulldog, Newfoundland, bullmastiff
  C. Lower eyelid entropion: golden retriever, Labrador retriever, pointers, cats
II. Spastic entropion is acquired secondary to squinting caused by ocular irritation and may be transient.
  A. Foreign body, trichiasis
  B. Ulcerative keratitis, blepharitis
  C. Uveitis
III. Cicatricial entropion is eyelid scarring following trauma or chronic inflammatory disease that results in abnormal eyelid margin–globe conformation and trichiasis.

Pathophysiology

I. Heritable/conformational entropion is associated with poor canthal tension and excessive lid length.
  A. This results in "inward rolling" of the eyelids.
  B. It is advised that most affected dogs not be used for breeding.
II. With spastic entropion, ocular irritation increases tone in the orbicularis oculi muscle, causing blepharospasm and accentuating eyelid inversion.
  A. This accentuates eyelid margin inversion from severe blepharospasm.
  B. Eyelid margin inversion is worsened by enophthalmos.
III. Cicatricial entropion is uncommon and arises secondary to fibrosis and contraction from eyelid injury.

Clinical Signs

Clinical signs vary with severity, time of onset, and degree of trichiasis.
I. Epiphora, blepharospasm
II. Conjunctival injection, chemosis
III. Corneal scarring, vascularization, pigmentation
IV. Ulcerative keratitis, corneal perforation

Diagnosis

I. Evaluate the eyelid conformation at rest and while testing palpebral response.
II. Apply topical anesthetic or administer a palpebral nerve block to determine any spastic component of the entropion (spastic entropion resolves with local anesthesia).
III. Determine amount of required correction by digitally everting the eyelid margin to a normal position.

Differential Diagnosis

I. Other causes of epiphora and blepharospasm
  A. Distichiasis
  B. Trichiasis
  C. Ectopic cilia
  D. Ulcerative keratitis
II. Ectropion

Treatment

I. Medical therapy is addressed first.
  A. Lubricate cornea with ophthalmic antibiotic ointment TID-QID to decrease irritation before surgery.
  B. Treat corneal ulcers with topical antibiotics and cycloplegics.
  C. Correct underlying causes of spastic entropion.
II. Surgical therapy is indicated for any type of entropion when it causes persistent clinical signs.
  A. Surgical options
    1. Spastic entropion is surgically corrected when alleviation of the primary ocular irritation does not correct inversion of the eyelid.
    2. Choice of procedure depends on the cause of the entropion, the location, the amount of eyelid affected, and the age of the animal.
  B. Eyelid tacking using local anesthesia (Miller and Albert, 1988; Johnson, 1988)
    1. Eyelid tacking is used for temporary eyelid eversion in a young animal that has not reached adult head conformation (<4–6 months of age).
    2. This procedure is also good for an animal that is a poor anesthetic risk, because it can be done with the animal awake.
    3. Sedation may be necessary in an uncooperative animal.
    4. Two or three vertical mattress sutures of 4-0 nonabsorbable material on a cutting needle are used to evert the eyelid margin.
    5. The sutures are kept clean, treated with topical antibiotics TID, and allowed to remain in place as long as effective (up to 3 weeks).
    6. Alternatively, small surgical staples may be used to evert the eyelids.
  C. Permanent eyelid eversion (Miller and Albert, 1988) (see Fig. 93–1)
    1. Initial skin incision is made 2–3 mm from the eyelid margin, approximately 1 mm away from the haired-nonhaired margin of the eyelid skin.
    2. An ellipse of skin of predetermined width is excised, and the resulting defect is closed with 4-0 or 5-0 simple interrupted sutures.

Patient Monitoring

I. Apply topical antibiotics to eye and suture line TID and keep the eyelids clean.

II. Use an Elizabethan collar to help prevent traumatic dehiscence, and remove sutures in 7–14 days.
III. Ulcers from sutures rubbing the cornea are a potential postoperative complication. Fluorescein staining is indicated if blepharospasm or ocular discharge develops postoperatively.
IV. It is better to undercorrect and repeat the surgery at a later date than to overcorrect the entropion, thus causing ectropion.

Ectropion

Definition

I. Eversion of the eyelid
II. Most commonly affects the lower central eyelid
III. Can also affect the upper eyelid but with few clinical signs

Causes

I. Heritable/conformational
  A. Genetics undetermined: probably polygenic
  B. Predisposed breeds: English and American cocker spaniels, bloodhound, St. Bernard, mastiff, Newfoundland, English bulldog, basset hound
II. Cicatricial
  A. Caused by fibrosis secondary to trauma or chronic inflammatory eyelid disease
  B. May be more common than cicatricial entropion but less common than heritable ectropion

Pathophysiology

I. Heritable/conformational ectropion is associated with excessive eyelid length and poor eyelid tone.
II. The eyelid does not rest against the globe, so the conjunctiva and cornea are not well protected.
III. It may also be associated with medial or lateral entropion.

Clinical Signs

I. Signs vary with severity of ectropion.
  A. Some animals are asymptomatic.
  B. Other animals exhibit epiphora and chronic conjunctival injection.
II. Exposure keratoconjunctivitis occurs and can (rarely) result in corneal ulceration, vascularization, and pigmentation.

Diagnosis/Differential Diagnosis

I. Ancillary ophthalmic diagnostic tests such as fluorescein stain application and nasolacrimal flushing are usually normal.
II. Rule out other eyelid and corneal diseases that cause similar signs, such as conjunctivitis, entropion, distichiasis, trichiasis, and blepharitis.

Treatment

I. Medical therapy consists of treatment of exposed cornea and conjunctiva with antibiotic or antibiotic-corticosteroid ophthalmic ointment BID-TID.
II. Surgical therapy is indicated when chronic, persistent medical management is required, when secondary changes involving the cornea or conjunctiva are severe, or for cosmetic reasons to decrease conjunctival exposure.
  A. Wedge resection of the lateral lower eyelid is simple, effective, permanent, and the preferred technique (Slatter, 1990).
    1. Make full-thickness incision through the eyelid 1–2 mm from lateral canthus.
    2. Amount of lid margin removed corresponds to degree of shortening necessary to have eyelid margin cover the adjacent limbus.
    3. Conjunctiva is closed with 6-0 absorbable suture in a continuous pattern with buried knots.
    4. Meticulous closure of the eyelid margin is accomplished with a horizontal mattress or figure 8 suture, keeping the knot away from the eyelid margin.
    5. Close remaining skin incision with 5-0 nonabsorbable suture in a simple interrupted pattern.
  B. Other surgical techniques to correct ectropion are described elsewhere (Slatter, 1990).

Patient Monitoring

I. Use an Elizabethan collar postoperatively to prevent traumatic dehiscence.
II. Keep suture lines clean, apply antibiotic ophthalmic ointment TID, and remove sutures in 7–14 days.
III. With adequate correction, eyelid margins cover edge of adjacent limbus after healing has occurred.

Trichiasis

Definition

Trichiasis is a condition in which hair growing from normal sites contacts the cornea and/or conjunctiva.

Causes and Pathophysiology

I. Medial canthal entropion and aberrant dermis in brachycephalic breeds
  A. The condition is a heritable/conformational defect, but the genetics are unknown.
  B. Multiple genes probably contribute to head and adnexal conformation.
  C. The tarsal plate and eyelid tension are poorly developed in this area.
II. Upper eyelid agenesis
III. Prominent nasal folds in brachycephalic breeds
IV. Dermoids affecting eyelids, conjunctiva, and cornea
V. Long upper eyelashes (cocker spaniels) and facial hair
VI. Secondary to eyelid trauma or poorly performed eyelid surgeries

VII. Shar pei: eyelashes point ventrally and touch the dorsal cornea and ventral fornix

Clinical Signs

I. May be asymptomatic
II. Epiphora or increased seromucoid discharge, ± blepharospasm
III. Nasal keratoconjunctivitis with pigmentation and superficial vascularization
IV. Matting of periocular hair secondary to chronic moist dermatitis and excoriation of skin

Diagnosis/Differential Diagnosis

I. Diagnosis is based on observation of hair touching the cornea and/or conjunctiva.
II. It is necessary to rule out other causes of blepharospasm, ocular discharge, corneal vascularization, and pigmentation.
   A. Keratoconjunctivitis sicca
   B. Distichiasis
   C. Ectopic cilia
   D. Entropion
   E. Ulcerative keratitis

Treatment

I. Medical therapy
   A. It is indicated to relieve clinical signs on a temporary basis, or for asymptomatic animals.
   B. Trim any offending facial hair.
   C. Ophthalmic ointments (antibiotics or lubricants TID-QID) decrease ocular irritation until permanent removal of offending hairs is performed.
II. Surgical therapy
   A. It is indicated when clinical signs associated with trichiasis are present.
   B. See Table 93–1 for surgical options.

Patient Monitoring

I. Apply an Elizabethan collar and keep incision lines clean.
II. Topical antibiotic-corticosteroid ointments (TID for 7–10 days) decrease inflammation associated with cryoepilation.
III. Re-examine approximately 8 weeks after cryoepilation or electroepilation to determine whether any lashes are recurring.
IV. Monitor medial canthoplasties and entropion surgeries carefully for suture contact with the cornea and for dehiscence.

Distichiasis

Definition

Cilia originate from within dysplastic meibomian glands and emerge from the meibomian gland openings onto the eyelid margin.

Causes and Pathophysiology

I. Probably inherited in purebred dogs
   A. Predisposed breeds include the American cocker spaniel, miniature poodle, golden retriever, Shetland sheepdog, Chesapeake Bay retriever, Lhasa apso, and Shih Tzu.
   B. Genetics are undetermined.
II. May develop as an isolated incident in any dog or cat
III. May occur from incomplete differentiation of the meibomian glands, which are modified hair follicles

Clinical Signs

I. Variable, depending on number, size, position, and stiffness of cilia
II. May be asymptomatic
III. Epiphora, blepharospasm
IV. Conjunctival injection, chemosis
V. Corneal vascularization, scarring, ulceration

Diagnosis/Differential Diagnosis

I. Definitive diagnosis requires identification of cilia emerging from meibomian gland openings on adnexal examination.
II. Rule out other causes of secondary corneal changes.
   A. Schirmer's tear test is performed to rule out keratoconjunctivitis sicca.
   B. Fluorescein staining of the cornea is indicated to rule out ulcerative keratitis.
   C. Other considerations include trichiasis, ectopic cilia, entropion.

Treatment

I. Indications for treatment
   A. Some asymptomatic dogs with numerous fine distichia (cocker spaniels in particular) may require no treatment.
   B. Symptomatic animals usually require permanent removal of cilia to alleviate clinical signs.
II. Medical therapy
   A. Topical ointments (antibiotic or lubricant TID-QID) decrease ocular irritation until permanent removal of the cilia is performed.
   B. Manual epilation temporarily relieves clinical signs until cilia regrow.
III. Surgical therapy (see Table 93–1)
   A. It is the only effective way to alleviate the problem permanently.
   B. All procedures for removal of cilia require the use of magnification.

Patient Monitoring

I. Postoperatively, topical antibiotic-corticosteroid ointment is applied TID if fluorescein staining of the cornea is negative.
II. Reevaluate the animal at 2 weeks after surgery to remove loose dead lashes and determine the extent of any secondary lid damage.

Table 93–1. **Surgical Options for Trichiasis and Distichiasis**

Surgical Technique	Application/Advantages	Disadvantages/Sequelae	References
Cryoepilation	Good for trichiasis and distichiasis Can be used anywhere on eyelids Negligible regrowth of lashes No sutures required Can be performed with local anesthesia in the cooperative animal	Temporary eyelid swelling Depigmentation of eyelid margin for as long as 16 wk	Slatter, 1990 Chambers and Slatter, 1984
Eyelid eversion	Expensive equipment not needed; best for trichiasis, especially from the upper eyelid Same procedure as for correction of entropion	May not solve medial canthal trichiasis	Miller and Albert, 1988
Medial canthoplasty	Applicable for medical canthal trichiasis, prominent nasal folds	High incidence of dehiscence unless precautions taken May not correct epiphora	Gross, 1990
Eyelid splitting	Does not require cryosurgical equipment and cryogen Procedure is best used when many distichia are present	Incision of eyelid margin is difficult Eyelid scarring and cicatricial entropion can result Recurrence possible because of failure to completely remove hair follicle	Peiffer et al., 1981
Electroepilation	Electrolysis is a good method for permanent removal of single cilia	It is tedious for removal of many cilia Delivery of high-frequency current can cause severe tissue necrosis and scarring of eyelid margins	Slatter, 1990
Excision of aberrant dermis	Expensive equipment not necessary Can be combined with lower medial eyelid eversion in brachycephalic breeds	Nasolacrimal system must be identified and avoided	
Basal meibomian gland cautery	Easy to perform Requires only disposable ophthalmic cautery Does not affect the eyelid margin	Applicable only to distichiasis	Riis, 1982
Stades procedure	Good for upper eyelid trichiasis Involves excision of eyelashes Upper eyelid skin heals cosmetically without hair follicles	May need cryoepilation for recurrence of eyelashes	Stades, 1987

III. Reevaluate at 8 weeks postoperatively to identify regrowth of any cilia, and repeat the preceding procedures as necessary.

Ectopic Cilia

Definition

Ectopic cilia are hairs that emerge from the meibomian glands through the conjunctival surface of the eyelid, usually 2–6 mm from the eyelid margin, and lie perpendicular to the cornea.

Causes and Pathophysiology

I. The cause is unknown, although some breeds may be predisposed, such as the Shih Tzu, golden retriever, English bulldog, Boston terrier, and pug.
II. Aberrant meibomian gland follicles are usually present at birth, but the problem may not be evident until cilia grow through the conjunctival surface.

Clinical Signs

I. Young animals: usually <1 year of age
II. Epiphora, blepharospasm

III. Conjunctival injection
IV. Mild, focal corneal edema, scarring, vascularization, or pigmentation
V. Elevated or pigmented area of palpebral conjunctiva, usually at the 12 o'clock position
VI. Corneal ulceration
  A. Superficial, in dorsal half of cornea
  B. Slow or nonhealing with medical therapy
  C. Recurrent

Diagnosis

I. Evert the eyelid margin and examine the conjunctival surface of the eyelid using magnification.
  A. Check all palpebral conjunctiva, because more than one cilium can be present.
  B. Cilia can be very difficult to see and may require biomicroscopic examination or examination under anesthesia using an operating microscope.
II. Fluorescein stain uptake on adjacent corneal surface helps identify the position of the cilia.
III. Perform a complete ocular examination to rule out other causes of epiphora, blepharospasm, conjunctival injection, and corneal ulceration.

Differential Diagnosis

I. Trichiasis
II. Distichiasis
III. Conjunctival foreign body
IV. Corneal ulceration from other causes

Treatment

I. Preferred treatment is en bloc excision of affected conjunctiva (Slatter, 1990).
II. Cryosurgical ablation of ectopic cilia using liquid nitrogen may also be performed but is less reliable.

Patient Monitoring

I. Surgical treatment is usually curative.
II. Recurrences can occur at old or new sites at a later date.
III. If clinical signs return, re-examine for cilia regrowth.

Macropalpebral Fissure/ Lagophthalmos

Definition

I. Macropalpebral fissure is a term used to describe an enlarged, rounded eyelid fissure. This eyelid conformation typically allows the underlying sclera (which is normally not seen) to be visible.
II. Lagophthalmos is the inability to completely cover the globe with the eyelids because of an abnormal prominence or position of the eye.
III. Another term sometimes used to describe this condition is relative exophthalmos.

Causes and Pathophysiology

I. Present primarily in brachycephalics
  A. These breeds have shallow orbits and large palpebral fissures.
  B. Predisposed breeds include the pug, Lhasa apso, Boston terrier, and Shih Tzu.
II. Abnormal tear film dynamics and decreased corneal sensation
  A. Both may lead to corneal dryness and central corneal ulceration and pigmentation.
  B. Concurrent keratoconjunctivitis sicca further compromises corneal health.
III. Predisposition to proptosis owing to shallow orbit and facial conformation

Clinical Signs

I. Large, round palpebral fissure with up to 360° of visible sclera present
II. Central corneal ulceration and vascularization
III. Corneal pigmentation, often in a young dog
IV. Failure to completely close the eyelids during sleep or during normal blink cycle

Diagnosis

I. Diagnosis depends on signalment, history of corneal disease, and recognition of large palpebral fissures.
II. A complete external ophthalmic examination is indicated to rule out other causes of a prominent globe and corneal disease.
  A. Perform Schirmer's tear test to identify concurrent keratoconjunctivitis sicca.
  B. Stain the cornea with fluorescein to identify corneal ulceration.
  C. Rose bengal staining may identify a central area of corneal dryness and epithelial degeneration.
  D. Elicit blink to determine ability to actively close the eyelids.

Differential Diagnosis

I. Acquired lagophthalmos
  A. Following traumatic proptosis
  B. Secondary to buphthalmos
II. Seventh cranial nerve paralysis with ptosis and functional inability to close the eyelids (see Chap. 23)
III. Acquired exophthalmos
  A. Orbital neoplasia
  B. Eosinophilic myositis
  C. Orbital cellulitis or abscess
  D. Zygomatic mucocele

Treatment

I. Medical therapy
  A. Topical lubrication with ophthalmic ointments TID-QID provides temporary relief.
  B. It does not correct the primary problem of poor eyelid coverage of the globe.
II. Surgical therapy

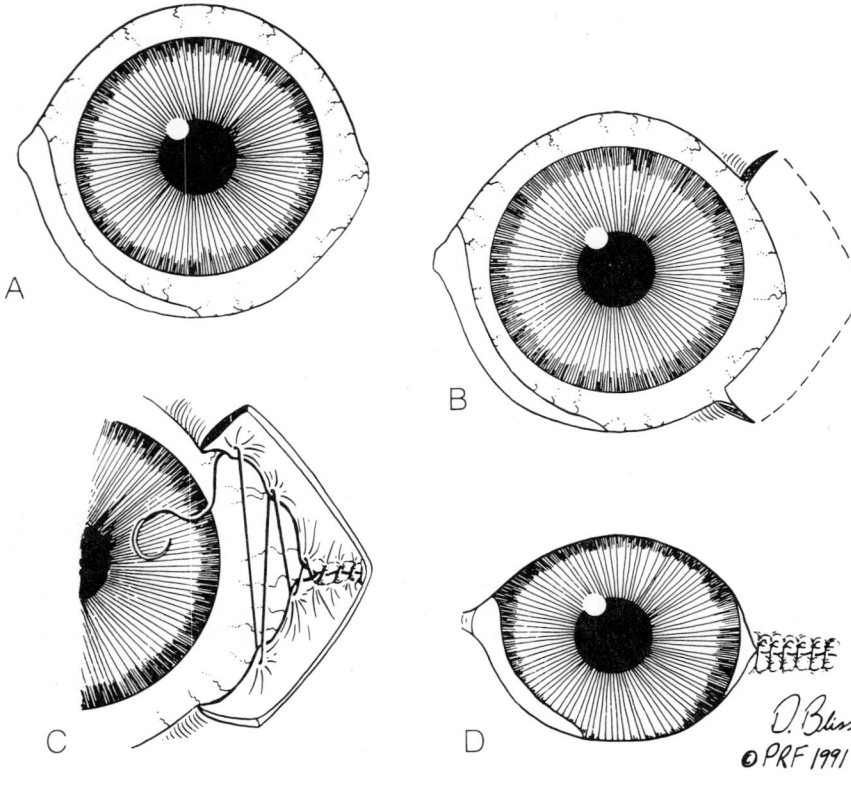

Figure 93–2. A. Macropalpebral fissure with exposure of perilimbal conjunctiva and underlying sclera. B. Lateral eyelid margin is excised so that new lateral canthus will approximate lateral limbus. C. Conjunctiva is closed with continuous absorbable suture with buried knots. D. Skin is closed with simple interrupted sutures. Note that the palpebral fissure size is reduced so that little or no conjunctiva is exposed. (From Purdue Research Foundation, with permission.)

A. Surgery is indicated when clinical signs of secondary corneal disease are present.

B. The goal of surgery is to shorten the palpebral fissure to permanently provide coverage of the globe by the eyelids.

C. Perform lateral canthoplasty or lateral permanent tarsorrhaphy (Slatter, 1990) (Fig. 93–2).
   1. This is the preferred technique because it is easy to perform and requires no special equipment.
   2. The lateral eyelid margin is excised, and the tissue is apposed in two layers: 6-0 absorbable suture in the conjunctiva and 5-0 nonabsorbable suture in the skin.
   3. The lateral canthus is closed until it is directly adjacent to the lateral limbus.
   4. The immediate postoperative result should appear slightly overcorrected, as the palpebral fissure will widen over the subsequent 4–6 weeks.

D. Perform medial canthoplasty or medial permanent tarsorrhaphy (Gross, 1990).
   1. It is indicated when corneal pathology affects the nasal quadrant. It also corrects medial canthal entropion and protects the cornea from prominent nasal folds.
   2. The lacrimal drainage system must be avoided, or chronic epiphora will result.

Patient Monitoring

I. Postoperative care includes the use of topical antibiotics TID and an Elizabethan collar and suture removal in 14 days.

II. The goals of surgery include resolution of active keratitis, increased corneal protection and cosmesis, and prevention of proptosis.

INFLAMMATORY DISORDERS

Neonatal Ophthalmia

Definition

Neonatal ophthalmia is infection that develops under the closed or partially closed eyelids in the early postnatal period (7–14 days old).

Causes and Pathophysiology

I. Infections are usually caused by *Staphylococcus* spp. or other normal adnexal flora.

II. Delayed eyelid opening may contribute by trapping organisms and accumulated secretions between eyelids and cornea.

III. It can be associated with upper respiratory infection (herpesvirus, chlamydia) in kittens.

Clinical Signs

I. Unilateral or bilateral
II. Protruding eyelids that are sometimes discolored
III. May have purulent exudate at the medial canthus
IV. ± Systemic signs: sneezing, fever, lethargy

Diagnosis/Differential Diagnosis

I. Diagnosis is made by ophthalmic examination demonstrating incomplete eyelid opening, swelling, and discharge.
II. Rule out other congenital conditions of the eyelids on examination.
III. Culture and sensitivity of exudate confirm bacterial and/or viral infection (cat).

Treatment

I. Apply warm, wet compresses to soften exudate adhered to eyelids.
II. Use gentle traction to separate eyelids.
III. If necessary, separate area of eyelid fusion (ankyloblepharon) with blunt scissors (Brightman, 1985).
IV. Flush fornices with saline to remove exudate.
V. Initially administer topical antibiotic ointment TID.
  A. Tetracycline for kittens
  B. Bacitracin-neomycin-polymixin for dogs
VI. Change topical antibiotics as needed on the basis of culture and sensitivity.

Patient Monitoring

I. Examine corneal integrity after eyelid opening using a focal light source and magnification.
II. Examine at weaning to evaluate tear production and to access corneal scarring via Schirmer's tear test and external ophthalmic examination.
III. Infrequently, animals develop symblepharon, panophthalmitis, rupture of the globe, orbital abscessation, and/or keratoconjunctivitis sicca if not treated quickly and aggressively.

Blepharitis

Definition

I. Blepharitis is an inflammation of the eyelids.
II. A hordeolum or stye is a focal infection of the sebaceous glands of the skin or meibomian glands.
III. A chalazion refers to a lipogranuloma of the meibomian glands.

Causes and Classification

I. Blepharitis can arise as a primary disease of only the eyelids or be a component of a dermatologic problem.
II. The causes of blepharitis are numerous (Table 93–2).

Clinical Signs

I. Nonspecific signs of blepharitis
  A. Erythema, swelling (focal or diffuse)
  B. Change in pigmentation
  C. Alopecia
  D. Pruritus
  E. Mucoid to mucopurulent discharge
II. Specific signs of underlying disorder (see Table 93–2)

III. ± Systemic signs: lymphadenopathy, fever, lethargy

Diagnosis/Differential Diagnosis

I. Skin scraping for parasites, Gram's stain, and cytology
II. Culture and sensitivity
  A. Assay for both bacteria and fungi.
  B. Submit meibomian gland contents, material from unopened pustules, or tissue specimens.
III. Biopsy and histopathology (see also Section XII)
  A. Especially for all mass lesions
  B. For all dermatoses not confined to eyelids
  C. For chronic, unresponsive blepharitis
IV. Direct immunohistopathology for all suspected immune-mediated cases
  A. Especially when bullae are present
  B. Requires separate tissue sample in Michel's fixative if fluorescent antibody testing is to be done
V. Skin or serum testing for allergic causes

Treatment

I. Supportive therapy for all forms of blepharitis
  A. Elizabethan collar to decrease self-trauma
  B. Hot, wet compresses to clean exudates and decrease tissue swelling
II. Bacterial blepharitis
  A. Topical antibiotic-steroid ophthalmic preparations (bacitracin-neomycin with prednisolone acetate, or gentamicin with dexamethasone) BID-TID
  B. Appropriate systemic antibiotics that are effective against *Staphylococcus* spp., such as oxacillin 10–20 mg/kg PO TID for a minimum of 3 weeks (see also Chap. 84)
  C. Careful application to eyelids (avoid ocular contact) of benzoyl peroxide SID until signs resolve
III. Juvenile cellulitis or pyoderma (see Chap. 85)
  A. Aggressive, systemic glucocorticoids
  B. Appropriate systemic antibiotics
IV. Staphylococcal hypersensitivity
  A. Topical antibiotic-steroid ophthalmic preparations as for bacterial blepharitis
  B. ± Systemic antibiotics that are effective against *Staphylococcus* spp.
  C. Careful topical application of benzoyl peroxide SID
  D. Systemic prednisone 0.5–1 mg/kg PO BID, tapering over several weeks
  E. Surgical curettage of meibomian glands to evacuate inspissated material
  F. ± Systemic bacterins and lysates (see Chap. 84)
V. Mycotic blepharitis
  A. Topical chlorhexidine solution TID for dermatophytes
  B. Intraconazole 5 mg/kg PO SID or ketoconazole 10 mg/kg PO SID-BID (see Chaps. 84 and 109)
VI. Parasitic blepharitis
  A. Topical chloramphenicol or eserine ophthalmic ointment SID
  B. Surgical removal of cuterebra larvae

Table 93–2. **Types of Blepharitis**

Causes	Characteristic Signs
Bacterial	
Staphylococcus spp.	Erythema, eyelid thickening, alopecia, crusts, pustules, moderate pruritus, ± cutaneous fistulas
Juvenile pyoderma, "strangles"	Animal usually < 6 mo old, fever, inappetence
	Facial edema, crusts, alopecia, erythema, and regional lymphadenopathy; eyelids, pinnae, and muzzle primarily involved
Staphylococcal hypersensitivity	Erythema, eyelid thickening, alopecia, crusts ± cutaneous fistulas, focal subconjunctival swelling
Mycotic	
Dermatomycoses (*Microsporum canis,* *Trichophyton mentagrophytes,* *Microsporum gypseum*)	Periocular alopecia and crusts
Systemic mycoses (histoplasmosis, blastomycosis, cryptococcosis)	Eyelid thickening, ulceration, and draining tracts ± focal eyelid masses
Parasitic	
Demodicosis	Periocular alopecia, crusts
Sarcoptic mange	Pruritus, alopecia, erythema
Cuterebra	Open hole in skin with surrounding associated eyelid swelling
Allergic	
Atopy	Erythema, eyelid thickening, pruritus
Food allergy	Erythema, eyelid thickening, pruritus
Contact allergy from neomycin or gentamicin	Alopecia, depigmentation of eyelids, dramatic conjunctival hyperemia
Insect bites	Focal, raised, erythematous masses
Immune-mediated	
Vogt-Koyanagi-Harada–like syndrome	Periocular and eyelid depigmentation, ulceration, blepharitis, poliosis
	Epiphora, corneal edema, aqueous flare, miosis
Pemphigus complex Pemphigus foliaceus Bullous pemphigoid Pemphigus vulgaris	Eyelid and muzzle depigmentation, alopecia, crusts, ulcer formation
Systemic lupus erythematosus and discoid lupus erythematosus	Eyelid and muzzle depigmentation, alopecia, crusts, ulcer formation
Dermatomyositis (epidermolysis bullosa simplex)	Familial in collie, Shetland sheepdog
	Other systemic signs
Drug-induced	
Sulfa drugs	Crusting, ulceration, alopecia of eyelids and ear pinnae with purulent discharge (McMurdy, 1990; Medleau et al., 1990)
Nutritional	
Zinc-responsive dermatosis	Affected breeds: Siberian husky, Alaskan malamute, Doberman pinscher, Great Dane
	Young, fast-growing dogs on high-calcium diet
	Erythema and crusts around mouth, eyes, ears, chin
	Nonpruritic scaling and hyperpigmentation
Vitamin A–responsive dermatosis	Alopecia, generalized scaling, hyperkeratosis, seborrhea of eyelids
Associated with generic dog foods	Similar to zinc-responsive dermatosis
Idiopathic	
Eosinophilic blepharitis of cats	Thickening, erythema, depigmentation of eyelids, focal masses
	Excoriation at medial canthus (Latimer and Dunstan, 1987)
Nodular granulomatous episclerokeratitis (NGE)	Focal, smooth, raised, pinkish mass involving palpebral conjunctiva and undelying tissues in eyelid
	Overlying skin usually normal
Periadnexal multinodular granulomatous dermatitis	Appearance same as NGE, but accompanied by numerous subcutaneous masses over trunk and sometimes anterior uveitis with focal iris granulomas (Carpenter et al., 1987)

VII. Allergic blepharitis
    A. Elimination of offensive allergen
    B. Topical ophthalmic corticosteroid or antihistamine preparations

    C. Desensitization techniques SID-BID (see Chap. 89)
VIII. Immune-mediated blepharitis
    A. Systemic prednisone 1–2 mg/kg PO SID to control signs, then tapered over several weeks

B. Azathioprine 2 mg/kg SID PO for resistant cases
C. No effective treatment for dermatomyositis

Patient Monitoring

I. Anti-inflammatory therapy may be required for weeks and is slowly decreased to effect.
II. Each individual disease component must be treated in complicated cases.
III. Depending on diagnosis, some require lifelong treatments, e.g., immune-mediated and allergic diseases.

NEOPLASIA

Definition

I. Neoplasms discussed here are tumors of the skin, glands, or conjunctiva of the eyelids.
II. Neoplasms can be classified as primary or secondary or as benign or malignant.
   A. Most neoplasms of the eyelid are benign in the dog.
   B. Neoplasms of the eyelid in the cat are less common than in the dog and tend to be malignant.

Classification

I. Benign
   A. Meibomian gland (sebaceous) adenoma
      1. It is the most common eyelid tumor in the dog.
      2. Even tumors with an aggressive histologic appearance usually have a benign behavior.
   B. Papilloma
   C. Melanocytoma
   D. Fibroma
   E. Histiocytoma
II. Malignant
   A. Squamous cell carcinoma: most common in the cat
   B. Sebaceous adenocarcinoma: rare
   C. Basal cell carcinoma: low malignant potential
   D. Mast cell tumor
   E. Fibrosarcoma: more common in cats than in dogs
   F. Lymphosarcoma
   G. Melanoma

Pathophysiology

I. Direct destruction and replacement of eyelid tissue
   A. Examples of neoplasms that are destructive and locally invasive include meibomian gland (sebaceous) adenoma, squamous cell carcinoma, malignant melanoma, mast cell tumor, and fibrosarcoma.
   B. Examples of neoplasms that are slowly expansile include papilloma and melanocytoma.
II. Secondary effects include corneal and conjunctival irritation, increased ocular discharge, and drainage or hemorrhage from the mass.

Clinical Signs

I. Mass identified on ophthalmic examination
II. Variable ocular discharge
III. Conjunctival injection
IV. Eyelid distortion resulting in poor protection of the globe

Diagnosis

I. Fine-needle aspirate, exfoliative cytology, or impression smears are helpful but may not be diagnostic.
II. Excisional biopsy with histopathology is diagnostic.
III. Systemic work-up is indicated for diagnoses of mast cell tumor and lymphosarcoma.
IV. Consider thoracic radiography with diagnosis of malignant lesions.

Differential Diagnosis

I. Non-neoplastic masses involving the eyelids
   A. Chalazion or hordeolum
   B. Fibrous histiocytoma (nodular granulomatous episclerokeratitis)
   C. Foreign body granuloma
   D. Mycotic or parasitic granuloma
   E. Eosinophilic granuloma complex of cats (Latimer and Dunstan, 1987)
II. Other ulcerative, destructive lesions of the eyelids
   A. Necrosis secondary to systemic vascular disease, cryosurgery, or cautery
   B. Trauma
   C. Causes of blepharitis that are ulcerative

Treatment

I. Full-thickness V-plasty eyelid resection (Slatter, 1990)
   A. Indicated when mass involves both skin and conjunctiva or suspected to be malignant
   B. Used when tumor affects less than one third of the eyelid margin
   C. Conjunctiva closed first using 6-0 absorbable suture with buried knots
   D. Skin closed with simple interrupted 5-0 nonabsorbable suture
II. H-plasty eyelid resection
   A. Excision of full-thickness masses affecting greater than one third of the eyelid margin may require a skin flap and conjunctival graft to close the defect (Fig. 93-3).
   B. Conjunctiva and skin are closed in two separate layers.
III. Cryosurgical ablation (Roberts, 1986)
   A. It is indicated for eyelid masses located near the lacrimal canaliculi (cryosurgery does not permanently damage the nasolacrimal passageway) or those too large for eyelid resection.
   B. Obtain a biopsy of the mass before application of the cryogen.
   C. Cryosurgery can be used as an adjunct to other therapies.
IV. Diode laser therapy

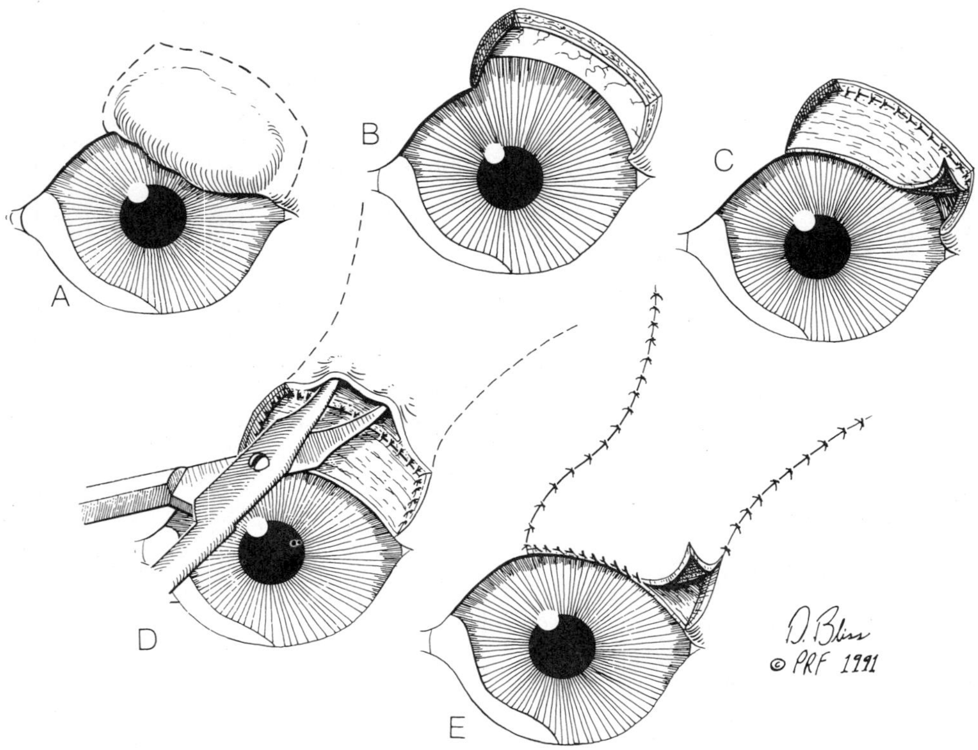

Figure 93–3. A. Eyelid mass involving more than one third of upper eyelid margin. B. En bloc full-thickness excision of the eyelid mass has been performed. C. Conjunctival graft is sutured into place covering underlying bulbar conjunctiva and dorsal cornea. D. Skin flap is undermined and released with tenotomy scissors. E. Skin flap is advanced and sutured to adjacent skin and anterior edge of conjunctival graft. (From Purdue Research Foundation, with permission.)

A. May be useful for small pigmented masses
B. Applied following biopsy of mass
V. Radiation therapy (especially effective for squamous cell carcinoma)
  A. Obtain a histopathologic diagnosis of the tumor before therapy.
  B. Surgically debulk the mass before radiation therapy to increase effectiveness.
  C. Both brachytherapy and teletherapy may be utilized.
VI. Chemotherapy
  A. Rarely used for eyelid tumors
  B. May help shrink a mass before surgical excision or radiation therapy
  C. Beneficial with mast cell tumors

Patient Monitoring

I. Complete local excision is curative for most canine eyelid tumors, especially for meibomian gland adenomas or papillomas (see also Table 91–1).
II. Some neoplasms such as malignant melanoma, squamous cell carcinoma, and fibrosarcoma are likely to recur locally.
  A. Re-examine at 1 and 6 months after surgery.
  B. Animals with no recurrence at 12 months are considered cured.
III. Monitor for distant metastasis with histologically malignant tumors.
  A. Physical examination
  B. Submandibular lymph node cytology
  C. Thoracic and abdominal radiography
  D. Serum chemistries

Bibliography

Barrie KP, Gelatt KN, Parshall CP: Eyelid squamous cell carcinoma in four dogs. J Am Anim Hosp Assoc 18:123, 1982

Bellhorn RW, Barnett KC, Hendkind P: Ocular coloboma in domestic cats. J Am Vet Med Assoc 159:1015, 1971

Brightman AH: Eyelid surgery. p. 1448. In Slatter DH (ed): Textbook of Small Animal Surgery. WB Saunders, Philadelphia, 1985

Carpenter JL, Thornton GW, Moore FM, King NW: Idiopathic periadnexal multinodular granulomatous dermatitis in 22 dogs. Vet Pathol 24:5, 1987

Chambers ED, Slatter DH: Cryotherapy of canine distichiasis: an experimental and clinical report. J Small Anim Pract 25:647, 1984

Dziezyc J, Millichamp NJ: Surgical correction of eyelid agenesis in a cat. J Am Anim Hosp Assoc 25:513, 1989

Gross SL: Lids. p. 68. In Bojrab MJ (ed): Current Techniques in Small Animal Surgery. Lea & Febiger, Philadelphia, 1990

Gwin RM, Gelatt KN, Williams LW: Ophthalmic neoplasms in the dog. J Am Anim Hosp Assoc 18:853, 1982

Johnson BW: Non-surgical correction of entropion in Shar pei puppies. Vet Med 83:482, 1988

Johnson BW, Campbell KL: Dermatoses of the canine eyelid. Compend Contin Educ Pract Vet 11:385, 1989

Krehbiel JD, Langham RF: Eyelid neoplasms of dogs. Am J Vet Res 36:115, 1975

Latimer C, Dunstan RW: Eosinophilic plaque involving eyelids of a cat. J Am Anim Hosp Assoc 23:649, 1987

McMurdy MA: A case resembling erythema multiforme major (Stevens-Johnson syndrome) in a dog. J Am Anim Hosp Assoc 26:297, 1990

Medleau L, Shanely KJ, Rakich PM, Goldschmidt MH: Trimethoprim-sulfonamide-associated drug eruptions in dogs. J Am Anim Hosp Assoc 26:305, 1990

Miller WW, Albert RA: Canine entropion. Compend Contin Educ Pract Vet 10:431, 1988

Nasisse MP: Disorders of the eyelids and conjunctiva. p. 624. In Kirk RW (ed): Current Veterinary Therapy IX: Small Animal Practice. WB Saunders, Philadelphia, 1986

Peiffer RL: Feline ophthalmology. p. 253. In Gelatt KN (ed): Textbook of Veterinary Ophthalmology. Lea & Febiger, Philadelphia, 1981

Peiffer RL, Gelatt KN, Karpinski LG: Canine eyelids. p. 277. In Gelatt KN (ed): Textbook of Veterinary Ophthalmology. Lea & Febiger, Philadelphia, 1981

Riis RC: Basal meibomian gland cautery, a surgical technique for distichiasis. Proc Am Soc Vet Ophthalmol 12:88, 1982

Roberts SM: Prevalence and treatment of palpebral neoplasms in the dog—200 cases (1975–1983). J Am Vet Med Assoc 189:1355, 1986

Slatter DH: Eyelids. p. 147. In: Fundamentals of Veterinary Ophthalmology. 2nd Ed. WB Saunders, Philadelphia, 1990

Stades FC: A new method for surgical correction of upper eyelid trichiasis-entropion: operation method. J Am Anim Hosp Assoc 23:603, 1987

Stades FC, Boeve MH: Surgical correction of upper eyelid trichiasis-entropion: results and followup in 55 eyes. J Am Anim Hosp Assoc 23:607, 1987

Williams LW, Gelatt KN, Gwin RM: Ophthalmic neoplasms in the cat. J Am Anim Hosp Assoc 17:999, 1981

94

Disorders of the Conjunctiva and Third Eyelid

Cecil P. Moore

CONGENITAL/ DEVELOPMENTAL DISORDERS

Prolapse of Third Eyelid Gland

Definition

I. Gland protrudes above the free border of the third eyelid.
II. Protrusion may be unilateral or bilateral and may have associated lymphoid hyperplasia or cartilage eversion.

Causes

I. Likely genetic predisposition
II. Secondary to inflammation (rare)
III. May be spontaneous without recognized inciting cause

Pathophysiology

I. There is a suspected anatomic abnormality in the fibrous attachment of the gland to periorbital fascia (endorbita) or other orbital tissues.
II. Swelling and enlargement of the gland and periglandular tissues may occur from persistent inflammation, e.g., chronic conjunctivitis and lymphoid hyperplasia.
III. Primary hyperplasia of the gland is not a factor.
IV. Chronic prolapse of the gland may result in loss of secretory activity and reduced tear production, with subsequent keratoconjunctivitis sicca (KCS).

Clinical Signs and Diagnosis

I. Signalment and history
   A. Breed predisposition
      1. Dogs: beagle, American cocker spaniel, poodle, Shar pei, basset hound, Boston terrier, Lhasa apso, English bulldog, and other brachycephalic breeds
      2. Cats: Burmese (Albert et al., 1982)
   B. Typical history: acute appearance of a pink mass in the medial canthus that may persist or periodically disappear
   C. Predominantly young animals: 6 weeks–12 months
II. Clinical picture
   A. Pink mass present at the medial canthus
   B. Mass typically smooth but occasionally has "cobble-stone" appearance (lymphoid hyperplasia)
   C. Mucoid or mucopurulent conjunctivitis often present
   D. Ocular discomfort minimal or absent

Differential Diagnosis

I. Third eyelid cartilage eversion
II. Third eyelid neoplasia
III. Third eyelid cysts
IV. Third eyelid protrusion (many causes)
V. Ocular trauma or orbital inflammation with third eyelid swelling

Treatment

I. Medical management usually provides only a temporary response.
   A. Manual replacement can be tried using a cotton-tipped applicator under topical anesthesia.
   B. Apply topical antibiotic-corticosteroids TID for 7 days, then BID for 7 days.
II. Surgical repair is the recommended treatment.
   A. Several techniques have been described for replacing the gland and securing it in position (Table 94–1; Figs. 94–1 to 94–3).

Table 94–1. **Techniques for Replacement of Third Eyelid (TE) Glands**

Type	Reference	Description
Anchoring or "tacking"	Blogg, 1979	Involves subconjunctival dissection over the gland on the posterior side of the TE and suturing the gland to the ventral epibulbar fascia
	Albert et al., 1982	Reported for repair of congenital TE gland prolapses in Burmese cats; differs from Blogg technique in that TE gland is anchored to the ventral oblique muscle
	Gross, 1983	Modification of Blogg's technique; involves securing TE gland to the ventral equatorial sclera
	Kaswan and Martin, 1985	Anchors TE gland to periosteum by incising the conjunctiva anterior to TE, placing suture through the orbital periosteum, the base of the TE, the prolapsed gland, and back through the base of the TE and tying the suture
	Stanley and Kaswan, 1994	Modification of Kaswan and Martin (1985) technique by using skin incision in addition to or in place of conjunctival fornix incision (Fig. 94–3)
Imbrication, pocket	Moore, 1983	Conjunctivectomy with Lembert imbrication used to stimulate fibrosis over the gland; an elliptical section of conjunctiva is removed over the prolapsed gland, and the remaining conjunctiva overlying the gland is freed by blunt dissection and undermining; the TE gland is secured with 2–3 preplaced subconjunctival Lembert sutures
	Morgan et al., 1992	A pocket technique, similar to Lembert imbrication technique; two parallel, 1-cm incisions are made on the posterior surface of the TE, one 2–3 mm from the free margin and the other 6–7 mm toward the base; the gland is replaced and fixed in position by suturing the two incisions together (Fig. 94–1)
Modified pursestring	Moore, 1990a	Technique advocated for repair of acute TE gland prolapses in puppies; following scarification of the conjunctiva overlying the gland, several bites of conjunctiva are taken around the gland in a modified pursestring fashion; the gland is replaced to its normal position and the suture is tied (Fig. 94–2)

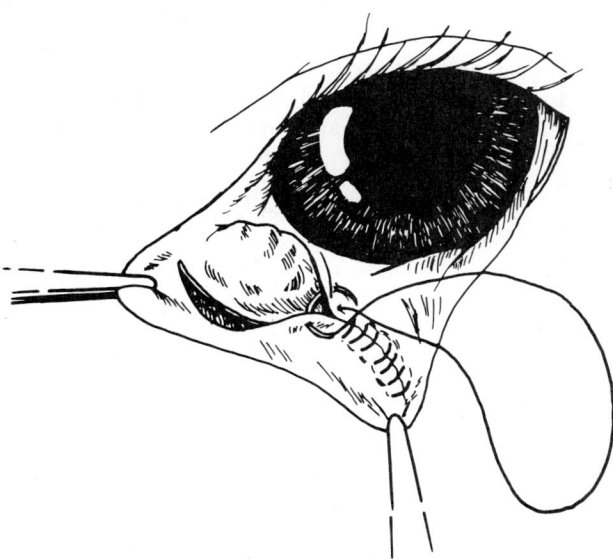

Figure 94–1. Repair of a prolapsed third eyelid gland using a pocket technique. One-centimeter incisions are made on the posterior surface of the third eyelid on either side of the prolapsed gland parallel to the free margin. The incisions are sutured together with 6-0 polyglactin 910 in a simple continuous, two-layered pattern without removing the conjunctiva. (From Morgan et al., 1992, with permission.)

B. In cases of unilateral gland prolapse, the opposite unaffected gland may be prophylactically sutured.
C. Administer triple antibiotic ointment postoperatively TID for 7 days or until signs of conjunctivitis abate.
III. Partial removal of gland involves debulking by removing only the exposed portion (approximately one third).
A. Less optimal than replacement procedures, which should be used as the primary method of gland prolapse repair
B. Performed after attempts at replacement have failed
C. May reduce aqueous tear secretion; check Schirmer's tear test (STT) before removing tissue and perform only if measurements are ≥20 mm/minute
IV. Total removal of gland is *not* recommended, as this may result in KCS at a later date.

Patient Monitoring

I. Recheck 2–3 days postoperatively for swelling, discomfort, and possible corneal irritation or erosion from the sutures.

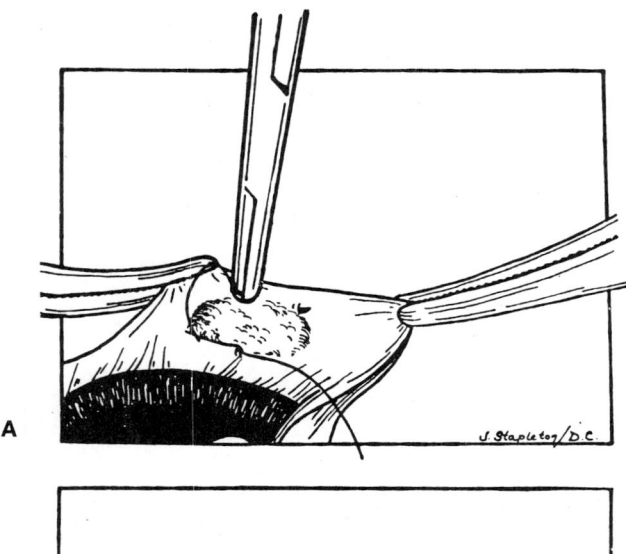

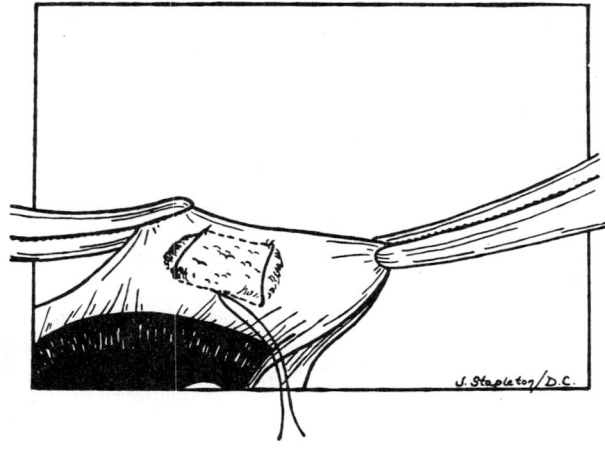

Figure 94–2. Placement of a modified pursestring suture around the prolapsed third eyelid gland. The initial bite is taken in the ventral fornix at the base of the third eyelid, and the second bite is taken between the body of the gland and the free margin of the third eyelid (A). The modified pursestring is completed when the final bite is placed back into the fornix to exit near the point of initial entry, drawn together, and tied (B). To stimulate adequate adhesion, the conjunctiva over the prolapsed gland is scarified prior to suture placement. (From Moore, 1990a, with permission.)

II. Check aqueous tear production with STT monthly for 3 months. If normal, recheck STT at 3- to 6-month intervals. If STT values are low, initiate medical treatment for KCS (see Chap. 95).
III. Alert owner to observe for recurrence; if it occurs, options include the following.
   A. Repeat surgical repair using techniques that maximize postoperative fibrosis, i.e., more extensive dissection and/or use of more reactive materials.
   B. Use modified orbital anchorage method (Stanley and Kaswan, 1994); this procedure results in immobility of the third eyelid.
   C. Examine for concurrent cartilage defect; repair if present (see Eversion of Third Eyelid Cartilage, later).
   D. Try partial removal of affected gland.
   E. Forgo any further attempts at surgical repair and medically manage any secondary conjunctivitis.

IV. There is a paucity of information on postoperative results of the various surgical techniques for repairing third eyelid gland prolapses. One retrospective study found a higher success rate using the pocket technique as compared with the modified Blogg technique (Morgan et al., 1992).

Eversion of Third Eyelid Cartilage

Definition

I. Defect in the cartilage that allows either an outward (more common) or inward scrolling of the third eyelid
II. Usually occurs as a single problem, although it is occasionally observed with gland prolapse

Causes and Pathophysiology

I. Large canine breeds, which tend to be enophthalmic, are primarily affected.
   A. An atypical spatial relationship may exist whereby the third eyelid does not lie properly against the globe, resulting in instability and abnormal positioning of the third eyelid.
   B. A primary defect of the stem of third eyelid cartilage may also be present.
II. In Burmese cats, cartilage eversion has been associated with gland prolapse (Albert et al., 1982).
III. It may occur with damage to the cartilage from bending or chronic tension.
   A. Chronic third eyelid gland prolapse results in displacement of the third eyelid and distortion of the cartilage.
   B. Placement of a third eyelid flap with sutures improperly inserted under the ''wings'' of the cartilage may bend the cartilage anteriorly.

Clinical Signs and Diagnosis

I. Signalment and history
   A. Juvenile large-breed dogs: Great Dane, St. Bernard, Newfoundland, German shorthaired pointer
   B. Usually acute, unilateral, and persistent
II. Clinical picture
   A. The third eyelid is more prominent and the normally tapered and pigmented free border is obscured because of displacement caused by the defective cartilage.
   B. Opaque, glistening cartilage may be seen through the exposed conjunctiva.
   C. Exposed tissue has a smooth, relatively flat appearance.
      1. Cartilage eversions do not have the fleshy appearance of a third eyelid gland prolapse.
      2. Lymphoid hyperplasia is usually not present.
   D. Mild conjunctivitis with mucoid ocular discharge is common.
   E. Affected animals appear oblivious to the presence of cartilage eversion.

Differential Diagnosis

I. Third eyelid gland prolapse
II. Third eyelid neoplasia

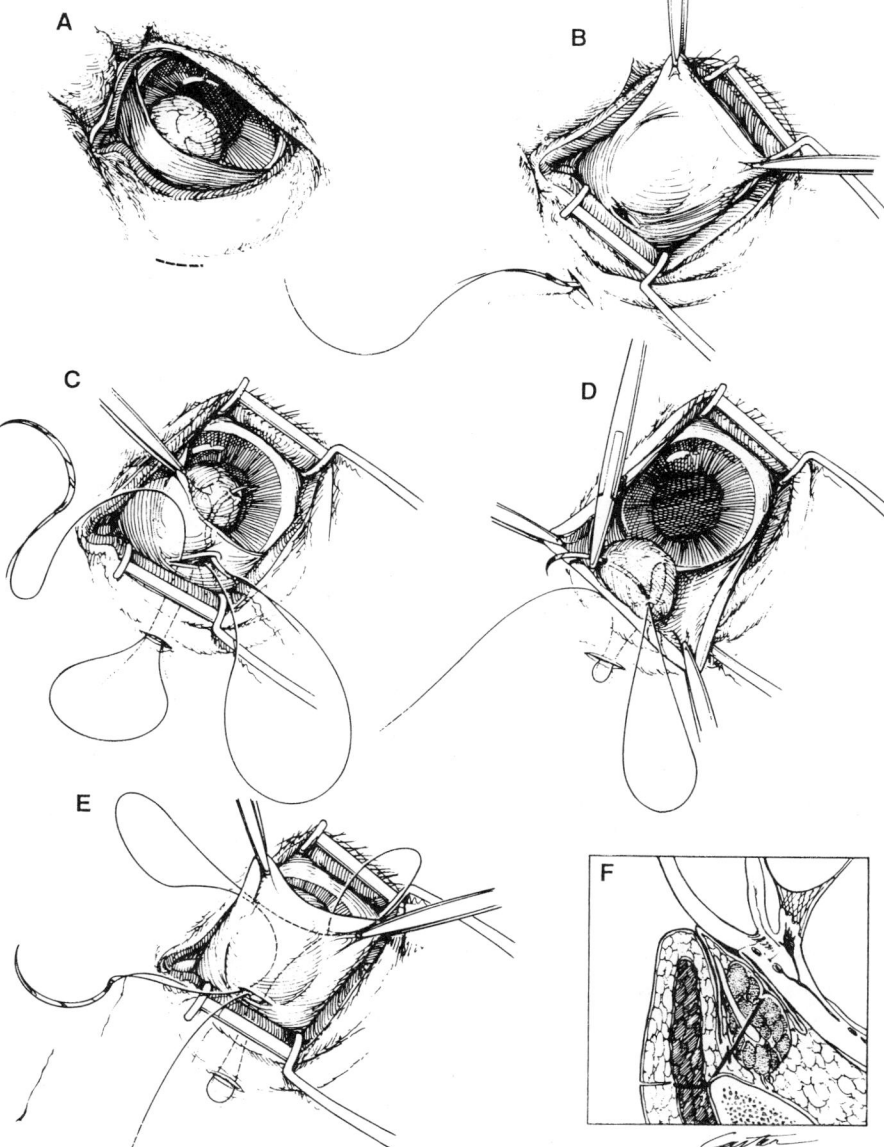

Figure 94–3. Diagram of a modification of the orbital rim anchorage method for surgical replacement of the gland of the third eyelid in dogs. A 5-mm skin incision is made parallel and subjacent to the ventral periorbital rim (A). A second incision is made parallel to the skin incision in the ventral conjunctival fornix. Nonabsorbable, monofilament suture (2-0 to 4-0 nylon, depending on the size of the dog) on a ⅜ circle cutting needle is passed through the skin, the periosteal rim, and the conjunctival incision (B). This is repeated with a second needle attached to the other end of the suture. The first needle is passed through the conjunctiva and emerges through the dorsal gland (C). The needle is passed back through the gland as shown in (D) and then back out the conjunctival incision (E). A knot is tied securing the repair (F). Neither conjunctiva nor skin is sutured. (From Stanley and Kaswan, 1994, with permission.)

III. Third eyelid cyst
IV. Third eyelid protrusion (many causes)
V. Ocular trauma with third eyelid swelling

Treatment

I. Treatment is indicated when conjunctivitis or persistent ocular irritation is present or when the owner is concerned about the abnormal appearance.
II. Treatment consists of surgical removal of the scrolled or defective portion of the cartilage.
   A. An incision is made in the posterior conjunctiva over the everted cartilage and the cartilage is dissected free of the conjunctiva.
   B. The cartilage is cut with scissors under the scrolled portion near its base and at the junction of the stem and wings.
   C. No conjunctival closure is necessary.

III. Apply topical antibiotics TID for 5 days, then BID for 5 days.

Patient Monitoring

I. Surgery results in an immediate resolution of the cartilage eversion; resolution of associated conjunctivitis is anticipated within 5–7 days.
II. Recurrences following cartilage resection are rare.
III. If recurrence is a problem, reevaluate the position of the third eyelid gland. Secondary prolapse of the gland is an uncommon complication of partial cartilage excision. If this occurs, stabilize the gland with one of the replacement procedures listed earlier.

Subconjunctival Cyst
Definition

I. Subconjunctival cysts, also referred to as conjunctival cysts, are congenital or acquired.

II. "Dermoid cyst" is a misnomer; dermoid refers to a congenital tumor in small animals and not a cyst (see Dermoid, later).

Causes and Pathophysiology

I. Congenital
   A. Displaced secretory tissue
   B. Anomalous formation of secretory ductules
II. Acquired (most common)
   A. Inversion/implantation of secretory epithelium: epithelial inclusion cyst
   B. Disruption of secretory ductules: ductal cyst
   C. Accumulation of nonseptic inflammatory fluids
   D. Trauma induced

Clinical Signs

I. Progressive subconjunctival swelling that results in displacement and bulging of the conjunctival surface
II. Fluctuant mass that may be translucent
III. Minimal associated conjunctivitis
IV. Negligible discomfort

Diagnosis

I. Compatible clinical signs
II. Centesis and aspiration of clear or amber viscous fluid
III. Imaging procedures to identify density of contents
   A. Ultrasonography: hypoechoic center
   B. Computed tomography: fluid density
IV. Excisional biopsy: allows definitive diagnosis

Differential Diagnosis

I. Local inflammation
   A. Subconjunctival abscess
   B. Dacryoadenitis
   C. Foreign body granuloma
II. Neoplasia (see Table 94–3, later)
III. Herniated periocular fat
IV. Zygomatic salivary mucocele

Treatment

I. Drain cyst by aspiration (usually provides only temporary relief).
II. Surgical excision is the treatment of choice.
   A. Incise conjunctiva over mass and bluntly dissect around mass to facilitate complete excision and avoid rupturing the cyst.
   B. Remove cyst completely, as well as all associated secretory tissue, then perform a two-layer closure using 6-0 polyglactin 910 (Vicryl) in a continuous pattern.
III. Postoperatively, apply topical triple antibiotic TID for 5 days, then BID for 5 days.
IV. Submit all excised tissue for histopathology.

Patient Monitoring

I. Examine for recurrence at 6- to 8-week intervals up to 6 months postoperatively.

II. Recurrence of a cystic lesion may indicate incomplete excision of secretory elements that requires further surgery or may necessitate a reassessment of the original diagnosis.

Dermoid

Definition

I. Congenital lesion (choristoma) containing tissue types not normally present at involved site
II. Contains surface ectoderm, with elements of normal skin, growing from the conjunctiva and/or cornea

Causes

I. Genetic predisposition
   A. Dogs: dachshund, St. Bernard, golden retriever, mastiff, German shepherd dog
   B. Cats: Burmese (Koch, 1979)
II. Occurs sporadically in other breeds

Pathophysiology

I. Embryologic sequestration of cutaneous ectoderm occurs on the epibulbar surface.
II. Induced irritation depends on its size and the presence of hairs.
III. Any effect on vision is related to the extent of corneal involvement.
IV. Additional congenital anomalies, e.g., persistent pupillary membranes, are occasionally seen in young dogs with ocular dermoid, but it is not known whether these are related or coincidental findings.

Clinical Signs

I. Appearance of lesion
   A. Elevated conjunctival mass most commonly present at or near the temporal limbus
   B. Usually pigmented and often has a tuft of hair arising from the surface
II. Other ocular signs: epiphora, interference with blink response, variable reduction in vision

Diagnosis

I. Clinical appearance is highly suggestive of dermoid.
II. Histopathologically, the lesion is composed of keratinizing, stratified squamous epithelium and other epidermal elements, such as hair follicles, sebaceous glands, and sweat glands.

Differential Diagnosis

I. Scarring and tissue displacement of palpebral and/or bulbar conjunctiva following eyelid lacerations or focal trauma
II. Inflammatory pseudotumors: nodular granulomatous episclerokeratitis
III. Neoplasia: epibulbar melanocytoma

Treatment

I. Conjunctivectomy
   A. An incision is made around the base of the dermoid leaving 2 mm of normal-appearing conjunctiva adjacent to the mass.
   B. Conjunctiva is undermined beneath the mass by blunt dissection, the mass is elevated and removed, and the defect is repaired by suturing the conjunctival wound with 6-0 polyglactin 910.
   C. Postoperatively, apply topical antibiotics TID-QID for 7 days.
II. Keratectomy (when the cornea is involved)
   A. Complete excision often necessitates performing a partial lamellar keratectomy.
   B. The iatrogenic corneal defect is treated with topical antibiotics TID-QID for 10 days or until the cornea heals, and topical 1% atropine SID for 3 days, then QOD for three additional treatments.

Patient Monitoring

I. Monitor healing of conjunctiva and cornea.
   A. Recheck at 5–7 days for infection, swelling, or pain.
   B. Instill fluorescein stain to assess corneal integrity.
II. Scarring is variable, depending on the extent of surgery.
   A. Conjunctival scarring is usually minimal.
   B. Corneal scarring may result in permanent opacities.
III. Discourage breeding, as the condition may be genetic.

INFLAMMATORY DISORDERS

Symblepharon

Definition

I. It involves adhesions of two apposing epithelial surfaces.
II. Scarring between palpebral and bulbar conjunctiva is most commonly seen, although adhesions may also involve the cornea and third eyelid.
III. It is more common in the cat than in the dog.

Causes

I. Severe infectious conjunctivitis, especially neonatal conjunctivitis of kittens from feline herpesvirus
II. Ocular surface trauma, e.g., abrasion or penetration
III. Chemical keratoconjunctivitis

Pathophysiology

I. Following extensive ulceration of apposing epithelial surfaces, fibrosis results in dense adhesions.
II. Adhesions are detrimental to normal ocular functions.
   A. Conjunctival fornices are obliterated or extensively altered, and this reduces mobility of the globe and interferes with aqueous tear dynamics.
   B. Scarring of the lacrimal puncta may result in chronic epiphora.
   C. Corneal involvement results in scarring and opacification, which reduces vision.
   D. Third eyelid adhesions may further immobilize the globe, creating varying degrees of enophthalmos.

Clinical Signs and Diagnosis

I. For some cats, a history of severe (ulcerative) keratoconjunctivitis weeks to months earlier is reported.
II. Corneal opacification occurs to varying degrees.
   A. Focal in area(s) of solitary adhesions
   B. Generalized with failure to visualize normal cornea in extensive cases
III. Multiple adhesions can occur with the eyelid(s) fixed to bulbar conjunctiva, cornea, or third eyelid, causing a reduced size of the palpebral fissure.
IV. Partial immobilization of the globe and enophthalmos are common in severe cases.
V. Epiphora is a frequent but variable finding.
VI. Mucopurulent discharge occurs in complicated cases, especially those with secondary bacterial conjunctivitis or concurrent KCS.

Differential Diagnosis

I. Developmental anomalies of the eyelids, conjunctiva, third eyelid, or cornea
II. Chronic keratoconjunctivitis
   A. Chronic infections: feline herpesvirus, chlamydial, and staphylococcal agents
   B. KCS
   C. Foreign body

Treatment

I. Consider surgical therapy, but understand the limitations and general expectations of surgery.
   A. Recurrent adhesions and additional corneal scarring may occur following attempts to correct symblepharon.
   B. In severe cases, the realistic goal of surgical correction is improvement of ocular function and return of some vision rather than total correction of all associated abnormalities.
II. Various surgical procedures can be tried for both focal and extensive adhesions (Table 94–2; Fig. 94–4).

Patient Monitoring

I. Recheck schedule depends on whether a conformer is used.
   A. If a conformer is not applied, re-examine at 5-day intervals over 3 weeks to inspect and to separate surfaces as necessary.
   B. If a conformer is used, weekly rechecks are rec-

Table 94–2. **Surgical Techniques for Symblepharon Repair**

Type of Adhesion	Surgial Technique	Reference	Postoperative Care
Focal adhesions	Manual separation	Munger, 1985	Antibiotic ointment TID-QID × 3 wk Use blunt instrument to maintain separation
	Surgical separation	Moore, 1993	Same as for manual separation
Extensive adhesions with corneal opacification	Grafting procedures: Arlt (local); Teale-Knapp (extensive)	Munger, 1985	Apply Elizabethan collar Ophthalmic ointment TID-QID × 3 wk Manually disrupt readhesions with blunt instrument
	Conjunctivectomy and lamellar keratectomy with soft contact lens and corneal-scleral conformer (Fig. 94–4)	Moore, 1990b	Instill topical antibiotic solution TID × 3 wk Systemic antibiotics × 10 days Remove tarsorrhaphy, contact lens, and conformer in 3 wk After corneal healing, an antibiotic-corticosteroid ointment is used TID × 2 wk, BID × 2 wk, then reevaluate

ommended to assess tolerance of the conformer and integrity of tarsorrhaphy sutures and to observe for signs of infection.

II. Monitor for corneal healing and readhesions 3 weeks following surgery or after conformer is removed.
  A. Negative fluorescein stain: use antibiotic-corticosteroid ointment TID for 2 weeks, then BID for 2 weeks and recheck again.
  B. Positive fluorescein stain: use *only* antibiotic ointment TID and restain in 1 week.
  C. Topical antiviral therapy may be instituted in cats with confirmed or suspected herpesvirus.
III. Reevaluate at 2 months for degree of improvement and to assess whether additional surgery is necessary.

Conjunctivitis

Definition

  I. Inflammation of ocular mucous membrane
  II. Most common cause of "red eye" in animals and humans

Causes

  I. Infectious agents
    A. Bacteria: gram-positive cocci, coliforms, mycoplasma
    B. Chlamydia: *Chlamydia psittaci*

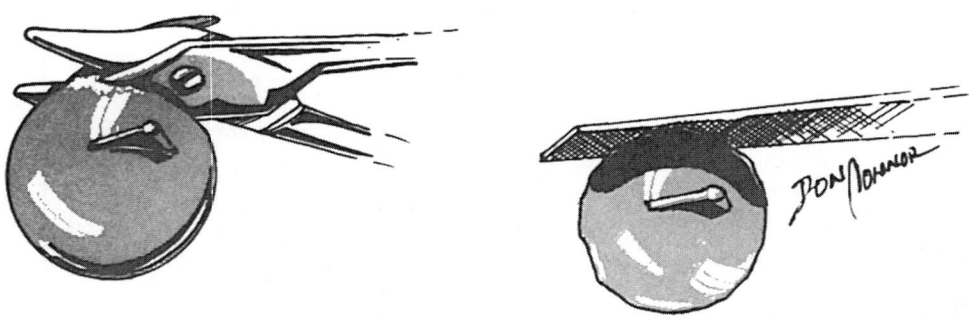

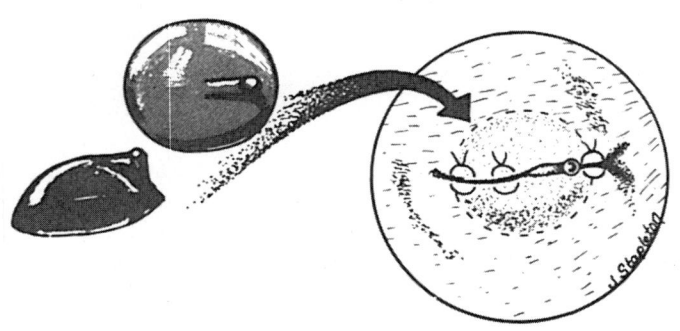

Figure 94–4. Formation of a corneoscleral overlay from a Crouch corneal protector (Storz, St. Louis) for use following extensive symblepharon correction. After conjunctival adhesions are freed by performing a keratoconjunctivectomy, a soft contact lens is placed on the cornea and the smoothed overlay is inserted under the eyelids. Three temporary tarsorrhaphy mattress sutures are placed in the eyelids to secure the overlay. (From Moore, 1990b, with permission.)

C. Viruses: feline herpesvirus, calicivirus, canine distemper virus
II. Foreign body: plant material most common
III. Parasites: *Thelazia, Cuterebra, Dirofilaria* larvae
IV. Immune-mediated causes
  A. Allergies
  B. Plasma cell infiltrate
  C. Eosinophilic conjunctivitis
  D. Ulcerative conjunctivitis of Doberman pinschers (Ramsey et al., 1996)
V. Irritants
  A. Contact irritants: topical medications, e.g., preservatives, aminoglycosides
  B. Environmental irritants: dust particles, plant material (including pollen)
  C. Eyelid diseases: trichiasis, distichiasis, ectopic cilia, eyelid masses, e.g., tumors and chalazia
VI. Surface drying
  A. Exposure
    1. Inadequate eyelid closure: ectropion, macropalpebral fissure with lagophthalmos, facial nerve paralysis, proptosis
    2. Neurogenic: loss of sensory innervation (cranial nerve V)
  B. KCS
VII. Trauma: bruises, abrasions, lacerations

Pathophysiology

I. Acute insults result in vasodilatation of conjunctival vessels, edema, neutrophilic/lymphocytic infiltrates, and, if severe, ulceration of conjunctival epithelium.
II. Prolonged insults cause chronic changes, including squamous metaplasia of epithelium, loss of conjunctival goblet cells, lymphocytic/plasmacytic infiltrates, and lymphoid follicle formation.

Clinical Signs

I. Hyperemia of conjunctival vessels (in contrast to injection of deeper episcleral vessels)
II. Ocular discharge: serous, mucoid, mucopurulent, hemorrhagic, or combination of these
III. Chemosis
IV. Discomfort: squinting, photophobia
V. Proliferative lesion(s)
  A. Focal masses: granulomas, tumors with local inflammation and secondary infection
  B. Multifocal or generalized proliferative lesions: follicles, papillary hypertrophy

Diagnosis

I. History
  Determine any previous trauma, chemical exposure, contact with other animals, past or present medical or surgical problems, concurrent treatments (either ophthalmic or systemic), and the particular use of the animal, e.g., hunting dogs.
II. Complete physical and ocular examinations
  A. Assess Schirmer's tear tests and fluorescein stain retention, examine for foreign bodies, measure intraocular pressure.
  B. Characterize nature of discharges, location and appearance of masses or proliferative lesions.
III. Cytology
  A. General considerations
    1. Evaluate conjunctival scrapings to characterize cellular response and to identify organisms.
    2. It is most informative in the early, active phase of disease.
    3. Remove exudates first and obtain samples before use of fluorescein stain.
  B. Method
    1. Use a metal or disposable spatula to collect the specimen; the Kimura platinum spatula is preferred because it can be flame sterilized.
    2. Following topical anesthesia, several scrapes are made in the same direction until a small droplet of material is collected.
    3. Transfer the cellular material to a glass slide and gently blot to form a thin layer.
    4. Prepare a minimum of three slides and allow them to air dry before staining.
    5. Unstained slides can also be submitted for indirect fluorescent antibody or polymerase chain reaction assays for feline herpesvirus and chlamydial species.
IV. Bacterial and special cultures
  A. They are indicated for nonresponsive, severe, or chronic infections.
  B. Take samples preferably before manipulating tissues.
  C. Viral culture and herpesvirus polymerase chain reaction (PCR) are the most sensitive diagnostic tests available; both require special test media and handling.
V. Conjunctival biopsy
  Consider histopathology to differentiate inflammatory from neoplastic diseases and in suspected cases of mucin deficiency (Moore et al., 1986).

Differential Diagnosis

Rule out other causes for a "red eye."
I. Scleritis: episcleral injection, thickened sclera, ± corneal involvement, variably painful, vision and intraocular pressure usually normal, ± concurrent uveitis
II. Uveitis: episcleral injection, miosis, decreased intraocular pressure, painful, cloudy aqueous, congested irides, ± poor vision
III. Glaucoma: episcleral injection, corneal edema, mydriasis, increased intraocular pressure, variably painful, poor vision
IV. Keratitis: either ulcerative or non-ulcerative (see Chap. 96)

Treatment

I. Treat primary disease(s) when identified.
  A. Remove irritants and foreign bodies or surgically correct eyelid disorders.

B. Treat KCS as needed (see Chap. 95).
C. Treat underlying infections.
1. Antiviral agents for herpesvirus: trifluridine, vidarabine, idoxuridine (sporadically unavailable)
2. Tetracyclines for chlamydia or mycoplasma; erythromycin an alternative topical agent
3. Triple antibiotics or chloramphenicol for gram-positive bacteria
4. Aminoglycosides or ciprofloxacin for gram-negative bacteria
5. Nystatin or miconazole for yeasts
6. Miconazole or natamycin for filamentous fungi
II. Remove discharges.
A. Initially clip periocular hairs and use moistened cotton to soak and remove exudates.
B. For maintenance, use an eyewash solution or sterile saline to cleanse the ocular surface and remove exudates SID-BID or as needed.
III. Anti-inflammatory agents are often helpful.
A. Indications
1. Allergic conjunctivitis: acute and chronic inhalant or contact allergies
2. Proliferative conjunctivitis: plasmacytic, eosinophilic, follicular, or granulomatous conjunctivitis
3. Ulcerative conjunctivitis of Doberman pinschers
4. Symptomatic therapy: irritant, foreign body, or trauma-induced conjunctivitis
B. Types of drugs
1. Corticosteroids
a) Topical (solutions, suspensions, ointments) or systemic (injectable, oral)
b) Topical corticosteroids contraindicated in cases of primary infectious conjunctivitis or when a corneal ulcer is present
2. Antihistamines
a) Antazoline 0.5% (H_1 antagonist) often combined with 0.05% naphazoline (sympathomimetic)
b) May be less effective in animals than humans
3. Cromolyn sodium 4% 4–6 doses daily
a) Inhibits degranulation of mast cells, therefore most effective when used before exposure to known allergens
b) Used less frequently in animals than humans
4. Nonsteroidal anti-inflammatory drugs (NSAIDs)
a) Flurbiprofen 0.03% (Ocufen), suprofen 1% (Profenal), diclofenac 0.1% (Voltaren), or ketorolac 0.5% (Acular) topical solutions: given BID-TID for 3–5 days to treat acute allergic chemosis
b) Flunixin meglumine 0.5–1 mg/kg IV
c) Aspirin 10 mg/kg PO BID
d) Not to be used in animals with clotting abnormalities or renal disease

5. Cyclosporine 0.2% (Optimmune)
a) Improves health of cornea and conjunctiva when used to treat KCS
b) Promising for treatment of ulcerative conjunctivitis of Doberman pinschers
C. Treatment frequency and duration
1. Acute inflammation
a) Give topical 0.1% or 1% prednisolone acetate, 1% hydrocortisone, or 0.1% dexamethasone drops 2–6 times daily, or ointments 1–4 times daily.
b) Reduce frequency every 3–4 days and discontinue at 7–10 days or a few days after signs subside.
c) Systemic corticosteroids and/or antihistamines may be indicated initially for acute severe chemosis with accompanying eyelid edema.
2. Chronic or recurring inflammation
a) Topical corticosteroids may be used intermittently or as needed to control inflammation.
b) Consider subconjunctival injections for refractory immune-mediated cases.
Note: Topical corticosteroids or NSAIDs should be used with caution in cats with conjunctivitis because of concerns about recrudescent feline herpesvirus.

Patient Monitoring

I. Monitor progress biweekly until conjunctivitis resolves or chronic conditions are effectively managed.
II. If nonresponsive, reassess the diagnosis and repeat STT, cytology, culture, or biopsy.

PROTRUSION OF THIRD EYELID(S)

Definition

I. Extension of the third eyelid over the globe without overt third eyelid pathology
II. Alters the appearance of the animal and may interfere with vision

Causes and Clinical Signs

I. Developmental
A. Conformational: breed-related enophthalmos, passive protrusion
B. Associated with microphthalmia: sporadic occurrence, genetic in some breeds, e.g., Australian shepherds, miniature schnauzers (Rubin, 1989)
C. Normal anatomy: nonpigmented third eyelids are more noticeable because they appear pink, which may give the impression that the third eyelid protrudes abnormally
II. Alteration of normal globe–orbit relationship
A. Anterior shift and protrusion of globe (exophthalmos)

Table 94–3. *Neoplasia of the Conjunctiva and Third Eyelid (TE)*

Type	Clinical Features	Treatment	Prognosis
Primary			
Epithelial			
Squamous cell carcinoma	Most common in white cats Often ulcerated Nonpigmented	Local excision ± grafting Cryosurgery Hyperthermia Radiation therapy	Focal mass: good Extensive: guarded to poor
Papilloma	Viral-induced Most often seen in young dogs Granular surface Pedunculated	Self-limiting Local excision Cryosurgery	Good
Melanocytic			
Limbal melanoma	Darkly pigmented Smooth surface Focal tension at limbus Slow growth	Local excision Cryosurgery Diode laser photocoagulation	Good
Conjunctival melanoma	± Heavy pigmentation Variable growth Focal lesion or broad-based Differentiate from epibulbar melanocytome (limbal melanoma)	Extensive excision Consider exenteration if broad-based Ancillary cryosurgery, radiation therapy, or chemotherapy	Guarded to poor
Vascular			
Hemangioma	Focal lesion Elevated Dark red	Local excision Ancillary radiation therapy	Good to guarded
Hemangiosarcoma	Focal or diffuse Dark red Tortuous vessels within mass	Wide excision Consider exenteration Ancillary oncotherapy	Guarded to poor
Angiokeratoma	Discrete Superficial Telangiectatic Elevated	Local excision	Good
Glandular			
Adenoma	Thickened TE Slow growth Smooth surface Minimal displacement of TE	Local excision	Good
Adenocarcinoma	Thickened TE Rapid growth Considerable displacement of TE Surface smooth or rough	Wide excision Consider TE amputation Consider ancillary oncotherapy	Guarded to poor
Free-ranging cells			
Histiocytoma	Smooth Elevated Solitary or multifocal Variant of nodular granulomatous episcleroconjunctivitis?	Excision Cryosurgery Local steroid therapy	Good
Mastocytoma	History of redness and swelling Broad-based or pedunculated Initial slow growth May exhibit aggressive behavior	Excision Local corticosteroids Consider systemic corticosteroids	Good to guarded
Secondary			
Lymphosarcoma	Diffuse infiltrates of TE or perilimbal conjunctiva Look for systemic signs May cause concurrent uveitis	Systemic chemotherapy (see Chap. 67) Local corticosteroids	Good if isolated to TE Guarded to poor if diffuse or multicentric
Adenoma/ adenocarcinoma			
Lacrimal	Orbital mass that affects conjunctiva secondarily Ventromedial displacement of globe	Excision via orbitotomy or exenteration	Guarded
Tarsal glands	Adenomas common in old dogs Secondarily involve tarsal conjunctiva Cauliflower appearance	Eyelid resection Cryosurgery Debulking and electroepilation See Chap. 93	Good

B. Posterior shift and recession of globe (enoph-
thalmos)
III. Systemic diseases
   A. Dehydration/emaciation with loss of orbital fluid
   or fat
   B. May accompany general malaise and lethargy of
   many systemic diseases
   C. Tetanus
IV. Neurologic disorders
   A. Horner's syndrome
      1. Accompanied by miosis, ptosis, and enoph-
      thalmos of affected eye
      2. Many causes (see Chap. 102)
   B. Bilateral sympathetic deficits (feline "Haw's
   syndrome")
      1. Occurs spontaneously; cause unknown, but a
      viral etiology has been proposed
      2. Otherwise healthy animal or mild gastrointestinal signs
      3. No other detectable autonomic deficits
      4. Responds to instillation of topical 2.5% phen-
      ylephrine or 0.1% epinephrine
V. Ocular pain: keratitis, uveitis, glaucoma
VI. Trauma with swelling or hemorrhage of third eyelid

Pathophysiology

I. Orbital disease causes changes in the spatial relationships between structures within the orbit, resulting in
displacement of the globe and third eyelid.
II. Neurogenic causes affect the position of the third
eyelid by compromising its sympathetic innervation
(Horner's and Haw's syndromes) or by producing
contraction of extraocular muscles with retraction of
the globe (tetanus toxin).
III. Pain causes reflex retraction of the globe with secondary third eyelid protrusion.

Diagnosis

I. Perform complete physical examination and appro-
priate diagnostic procedures to rule out systemic dis-
ease.
   A. Note evidence of weight loss, fever, anemia,
   masses, signs of tetanus.
   B. If systemic abnormalities are found, pursue diagnostic work-up with routine laboratory tests, radiography, and serology.
II. Examine both eyes carefully.
   A. Inspect for orbital/ocular symmetry.
   B. Palpate orbital margins and retropulse globe.
   C. Check pupillary light responses, note anisocoria.
   D. Rule out primary third eyelid disease by applying
   topical anesthesia and examining both sides of
   the third eyelid.
   E. Rule out other ocular diseases by examining all
   extraocular and intraocular structures and measuring the intraocular pressure.
III. Consider pharmacologic testing of both eyes for ab-
normal sympathetic innervation.
   A. Unilateral Horner's syndrome: see methodology
   and interpretation in Chap. 102.

B. Haw's syndrome: instill 1 drop of 2.5% phenylephrine or 0.1% epinephrine into each eye and
watch for affected third eyelids to almost completely retract within 20 minutes.

Treatment and Monitoring

I. Treat any underlying primary systemic or ocular disease.
II. For sympathetic "denervation" syndromes, consider
the following.
   A. One option is no treatment, as conditions usually
   improve with time.
   B. Empirical treatment with topical sympathomimetic agents (phenylephrine 1–5% or epinephrine 0.1–0.5% BID-TID) may be indicated when
   third eyelid protrusion reduces vision.
   C. Most cases of bilateral deficits in cats are self-
   limiting and subside in 4–6 weeks.
   D. Many cases of Horner's syndrome improve over
   7–8 weeks, although some persist indefinitely.
III. Conformational (breed-related) protrusions do not require treatment, and although shortening the third
eyelid has been reported, it is not generally recommended.
IV. Tattooing the free margin and anterior surface is a
nonsurgical option for cosmetic treatment of prominent nonpigmented third eyelids.

NEOPLASIA

See Table 94–3.

Bibliography

Albert RA, Garrett PD, Whitley RD: Surgical correction of
everted third eyelid in two cats. J Am Vet Med Assoc
180:763, 1982
Blogg JR: Surgical replacement of a prolapsed gland of the third
eyelid ("cherry eye"), a new technique. Aust Vet J 9:75, 1979
Bonney CH, Koch SA, Dice PF, Confer AW: Papillomatosis of
the conjunctiva and adnexa in dogs. J Am Vet Med Assoc
176:48, 1980
Buyukmihci N, Stannard AA: Canine conjunctival angiokerato-
mas (two cases). J Am Vet Med Assoc 178:1279, 1981
Collins BK, Collier LL, Miller MA et al: Biological behavior
and histologic characteristics of canine conjunctival melanoma.
Prog Vet Compar Ophthalmol 3:135, 1993
Cook CS, Rosenkrantz W, Peiffer RL, MacMillan A: Malignant
melanoma of the conjunctiva in a cat. J Am Vet Med Assoc
186:505, 1985
Dugan SJ, Severin GA, Hungerford LL et al: Clinical and histo-
logic evaluation of the prolapsed third eyelid gland in dogs. J
Am Vet Med Assoc 201:1861, 1992
Gross S: Effectiveness of a modification of the Blogg technique
for replacing the prolapsed gland of the canine third eyelid.
Proc Am Coll Vet Ophthalmol 14:28, 1983
Johnson BW, Brightman AH, Whiteley HE: Conjunctival mast
cell tumor in two dogs. J Am Anim Hosp Assoc 24:439, 1988
Kaswan RL, Martin CL: Surgical correction of third eyelid pro-
lapse in dogs. J Am Vet Med Assoc 186:83, 1985
Koch SA: Congenital ophthalmic abnormalities in the Burmese
cat. J Am Vet Med Assoc 174:90, 1979

Kuhns EL: Replacement of canine membrana nictitans with a lip graft. Mod Vet Pract 62:773, 1981

Martin CL: Canine epibulbar melanomas and their management. J Am Anim Hosp Assoc 17:83, 1981

Moore CP: Alternative technique for prolapsed gland of the third eyelid. p. 52. In Bojrab MJ (ed): Current Techniques in Veterinary Surgery. 2nd Ed. Lea & Febiger, Philadelphia, 1983

Moore CP: Imbrication technique for replacement of prolapsed third eyelid gland. p. 126. In Bojrab MJ (ed): Current Techniques in Veterinary Surgery. 3rd Ed. Lea & Febiger, Philadelphia, 1990a

Moore CP: Surgery of the conjunctiva. p. 76. In Bojrab MJ (ed): Current Techniques in Veterinary Surgery. 3rd Ed. Lea & Febiger, Philadelphia, 1990b

Moore CP: Diseases of the eyelids, conjunctiva, and third eyelid. p. 139. In Bojrab MJ (ed): Disease Mechanisms in Small Animal Surgery. 3rd Ed. Lea & Febiger, Philadelphia, 1993

Moore CP, Wilsman NJ, Nordheim EV et al: Selection of biopsy site for quantitation of canine conjunctival goblet cells. Proc Am Coll Vet Ophthalmol 17:272, 1986

Morgan RV, Duddy JM, McClurg K: Prolapse of the gland of the third eyelid in dogs: a retrospective study of 89 cases (1980–1990). J Am Anim Hosp Assoc 29:56, 1992

Munger RJ: The conjunctiva. p. 1469. In Slatter DH (ed): Textbook of Small Animal Surgery. WB Saunders, Philadelphia, 1985

Nasisse M: Feline herpesvirus ocular disease. Vet Clin North Am [Small Anim Pract] 20:667, 1990

Ramsey DT, Ketring KL, Glaze MB et al: Ligneus conjunctivitis in four doberman pinschers. J Am Anim Hosp Assoc 32:439, 1996

Rubin LF: Inherited Eye Diseases in Purebred Dogs. Williams & Wilkins, Baltimore, 1989

Stanley RG, Kaswan RL: Modification of the orbital rim anchorage method for surgical replacement of the gland of the third eyelid in dogs. J Am Vet Med Assoc 205:1412, 1994

Wheeler CA, Blanchard GL, Davidson H: Cryosurgery for treatment of recurrent proliferative keratoconjunctivitis in five dogs. J Am Vet Med Assoc 195:354, 1989

Wilcock B, Peiffer R: Adenocarcinoma of the gland of the third eyelid in seven dogs. J Am Vet Med Assoc 193:1549, 1988

Williams LW, Gelatt KN, Gwin RM: Ophthalmic neoplasms in the cat. J Am Anim Hosp Assoc 15:999, 1981

95

Disorders of the Lacrimal and Nasolacrimal System

Thomas J. Kern

CONGENITAL DISORDERS

Imperforate Punctum

Definition

The term imperforate punctum refers to the congenital absence of the opening of the upper and/or lower lacrimal canaliculi on the conjunctiva near the medial canthus.

Causes

I. Genetic factors are the primary cause.
II. Cocker spaniels and poodles, as well as other breeds, are commonly afflicted.

Pathophysiology

I. Epiphora is the predominant ocular clinical sign.
II. If only the upper punctum is imperforate, epiphora may be mild or absent.
III. In dogs with light coat color, reddish discoloration of the facial hair may result, and occasionally moist dermatitis may develop from chronic wetness.

Diagnosis

I. Fluorescein stain test
   A. Instillation of fluorescein into the conjunctival sac (*not* followed by irrigation with eyewash) allows determination of the structural and functional patency of the nasolacrimal system.
   B. Failure of fluorescein to appear at the distal naris suggests (but does not confirm) functional and/or structural obstruction.
II. Manual flushing
   A. Following topical anesthesia, the puncta are identified and cannulated with a 23-gauge (or smaller) nasolacrimal cannula and flushed with eyewash or normal saline solution.
   B. Apparent absence of one or both puncta suggests they are imperforate.
   C. If one punctum can be cannulated and flushed, the conjunctiva overlying the opposite imperforate punctum may appear to bulge or elevate from trapped fluid.

Differential Diagnosis

I. Other causes of punctal stenosis include cicatrization following these events.
   A. Trauma
   B. Inflammation of the conjunctiva, especially in cats from infection with feline herpesvirus or other agents
II. Other causes of epiphora include the following.
   A. Structural obstruction
      1. Nasolacrimal duct atresia or attenuation
      2. Dacryocystitis
      3. Acquired nasolacrimal duct obstruction from inflammation, infection, foreign body
   B. Functional obstruction
      1. Punctal malposition associated with medial canthal entropion or ectropion
      2. Trichiasis, resulting in wicking of tears onto facial hair
      3. Shallow lacrimal lake
         The potential space near the medial canthus where tears collect before drainage into the puncta may be smaller than normal from breed conformation, buphthalmos, or exophthalmos.
   C. Excessive lacrimation
      1. Extraocular causes
         a) Eyelid abnormalities such as entropion, ectopic cilium, distichiasis, trichiasis
         b) Ulcerative keratitis

c) Foreign bodies
d) Conjunctivitis
2. Intraocular causes
a) Uveitis
b) Glaucoma

Treatment and Monitoring

I. Surgical opening of puncta
A. Either general anesthesia or topical anesthesia with tranquilization can be used.
B. The conjunctiva overlying the single imperforate punctum is tented upward by irrigation from the patent punctum and then excised with iris or tenotomy scissors.
C. Alternatively, fine nylon suture material (2–0) is passed retrograde up the nasolacrimal duct from the orifice in the distal naris to tent the overlying conjunctiva, which is then excised.
II. Topical corticosteroids are instilled several times daily for 21 days to discourage re-epithelialization and scarring.
III. Postoperative closure may occur from conjunctiva overgrowing the surgically created punctal orifice (Gelatt, 1991).
IV. Indwelling nasolacrimal cannulation may be indicated following surgical opening of the puncta or, especially, after secondary repair following punctal cicatrization and closure (Slatter, 1990).
A. A monofilament nylon thread (2–0, with a smooth melted end) is passed through the surgically opened punctum to emerge through the distal naris.
B. Fine polyethylene tubing (PE90) or polyvinyl tubing with a beveled end is passed over the thread.
C. Halstead's forceps are clamped behind the tubing, which is pulled from the nasal end by forceps on the thread. The tubing is then pulled down the nasolacrimal duct and sutured to the skin near the medial canthus and distal nares.

Dacryops

Definition

I. Cystic disorders that represent dilatations of the canaliculi or nasolacrimal duct are termed dacryops.
II. Usually identified in young animals, they often but not invariably cause epiphora (Playter and Adams, 1977; Gerding, 1991; Grahn and Mason, 1995).

Causes

I. Embryonic malformation of the lacrimal excretory ducts or associated lacrimal glands is suspected.
II. Basset hounds are overrepresented in the few reported cases. If genetic, the mode of inheritance has not been established.

Pathophysiology

I. Epiphora usually associated with a painless facial or medial canthal swelling is the predominant sign.
II. Cysts are lined by epithelium.
III. The degree of nasolacrimal excretory obstruction is variable.

Clinical Signs

I. Fluctuant or fixed soft tissue swelling at or near the medial canthus
II. Variable epiphora

Diagnosis

I. Fluorescein stain test—as described for imperforate punctum
II. Manual flushing—as described for imperforate punctum
A. Obstruction may be absent, partial, or complete.
B. Rarely, flushing may cause increased soft tissue swelling.
III. Skull radiography
A. Plain films may show cysts or other abnormalities of the nasal cavity.
B. Positive contrast dacryocystorhinography may show only obstruction, with cystic dilatation of duct, or suggest external compression of duct by an adjoining cyst of presumed glandular origin.
IV. Ultrasonography
V. Magnetic resonance imaging

Differential Diagnosis

I. Other structural causes of epiphora
A. Imperforate puncta
B. Nasolacrimal duct atresia
C. Dacryocystitis
D. Acquired ductal stenosis caused by inflammation, infection, foreign body, trauma
II. Functional obstruction
A. Punctal malposition
B. Trichiasis
C. Shallow lacrimal lake
III. Excessive lacrimation (see Imperforate Punctum)
A. Extraocular causes
B. Intraocular causes
IV. Other causes of orbital masses or swelling (see Chap. 103)
A. Orbital cellulitis/abscess
B. Zygomatic salivary mucocele or adenitis
C. Masticatory muscle myositis
D. Orbital neoplasia

Treatment and Monitoring

I. Surgical excision or marsupialization of cyst is the treatment of choice.
A. Performed under general anesthesia
B. Incision over cyst followed by careful anatomic dissection from nasolacrimal duct.

1. Closure is performed to avoid ductal stenosis.
2. Curettage may be beneficial if complete excision is not possible.
II. Indwelling nasolacrimal cannulation may be indicated (see Imperforate Punctum; Slatter, 1990).
III. Incomplete removal may result in recurrence.
IV. Permanent obstruction and epiphora may result from postoperative cicatrization.

DEGENERATIVE DISORDERS

Keratoconjunctivitis Sicca

Definition

I. The inflammatory and degenerative changes of the cornea and conjunctiva that result from reduced aqueous tear secretion are defined as keratoconjunctivitis sicca (KCS).
II. KCS may be categorized as primary (lacrimal secretory failure) or secondary (failure of tear delivery).

Causes

I. Primary KCS
  A. Infection of the lacrimal glands by canine distemper virus
  B. Congenital absence of functional lacrimal tissue, especially in toy breeds of dogs
  C. Possible immune-mediated inflammation of the lacrimal glands
    1. Genetic predisposition suggested for many breeds, e.g., cocker spaniel, English bulldog, Lhasa apso, Shih Tzu, others
    2. Middle-aged and older dogs predisposed
    3. Sex predisposition uncertain in dogs; females perhaps at greater risk
  D. Drug toxicity
    1. Sulfa products: salicylazosulfapyridine (sulfasalazine), sulfadiazine, sulfisoxazole, sulfamethoxazole, trimethoprim/sulfas
    2. Phenazopyridine
    3. Atropine: parenteral or topical (Hollingsworth et al., 1992)
  E. Neurogenic secretory dysfunction resulting from parasympathetic denervation of lacrimal glands associated with facial neuropathy
  F. Excision of the prolapsed gland of the third eyelid, especially in breeds with an inherited predisposition for KCS
  G. Trauma
    1. Following severe orbital trauma, e.g., traumatic proptosis of the globe
    2. Following transient or permanent damage to the lacrimal glands, their innervation, or blood supply
II. Secondary KCS
  A. Conjunctival inflammation and/or scarring from infection (bacterial, viral), allergy, chemical and ulcerative/keratitis, exposure, etc. may occlude lacrimal gland ductules.
  B. If inflammation resolves quickly, KCS may be transient, but if scarring results, KCS is permanent.

Pathophysiology

I. Reduction or absence of lacrimal secretion results in corneal and conjunctival changes.
  A. Metabolic derangements: altered gas, nutrient exchange; hypertonicity of tear film
  B. Increased trauma from eyelid motion and contact and environmental insults
  C. Increased susceptibility to infection caused by reduction in antimicrobial properties of tears and increased epithelial trauma facilitating bacterial colonization
II. With chronicity, secondary effects of dryness such as bacterial infection, neovascularization, and inflammation promote goblet cell abnormalities and surface wettability changes.

Clinical Signs

I. Mucoid or mucopurulent ocular discharge is the hallmark sign of KCS.
II. Corneal changes include the following.
  A. Corneal ulceration
    1. Commonly complicates KCS
    2. Minor superficial ulceration from dryness
    3. Bacterial infection with deep ulceration, corneal melting, and/or perforation
  B. Superficial vascularization: focal or diffuse
  C. Corneal melanosis
III. Conjunctivitis and mucoid discharge may be the only signs in the early stages.
IV. Blepharospasm can occur from corneal irritation or ulceration.
V. Loss of vision follows chronic corneal vascularization, scarring, and melanosis.
VI. Primary KCS is likely to be a bilateral disorder, although initially it may be unilateral.
VII. Secondary KCS may either be uni- or bilateral, depending on the inciting cause.

Diagnosis

I. Schirmer's tear test (STT) is performed to estimate aqueous tear production.
  A. Normal values are >21 ± 4.2 SD mm/min for dogs and >16.2 ± 3.8 SD mm/min for cats.
  B. Low STT values in the presence of mucoid or mucopurulent discharge and conjunctivitis strongly suggest KCS.
  C. The test must be performed before instillation of any diagnostic solutions, topical anesthetics, or medications that would invalidate the result.
  D. If conjunctival inflammation and/or infection are present, STT should be repeated following appropriate treatment to discriminate permanent from transient KCS.
II. Consider bacterial culture of the conjunctiva.
III. A conjunctival scraping can be performed to assess

the type of cellular response (neutrophil vs. lymphocyte) and the presence of intracellular bacteria.

Differential Diagnosis

I. Primary conjunctivitis caused by infection, allergy, trauma
II. Dacryocystitis
   A. Mucoid or mucopurulent discharge is located over the medial canthus.
   B. The STT is normal.
   C. Conjunctivitis is absent.
III. Corneal/conjunctival hypesthesia from dysfunction of the ophthalmic branch of the trigeminal nerve (cranial nerve V)
   A. Corneal hypesthesia is suggested by absence of blink and globe retraction following corneal stimulation by a wisp of cotton.
   B. The STT is low, yet significant conjunctivitis or ocular discharge may be absent.
IV. Low STT values in the absence of signs suggestive of KCS or ocular hypesthesia are common findings in cats for unknown reasons and make evaluation of a single STT difficult in this species.

Treatment

I. Stimulate lacrimation.
   A. Topical cyclosporine
      1. A 2% solution in oil applied BID results in improvement in lacrimation and reduction in keratoconjunctivitis in approximately 66–75% of treated dogs.
      2. The exact mechanism is unknown, but a primary lacrimogenic effect as well as an anti-inflammatory effect have been postulated (Kaswan and Salisbury, 1990; Kaswan, 1992; Bounous et al., 1995).
      3. An effective 0.2% cyclosporine ointment is available (Optimmune, Schering-Plough) (Johnson et al., 1994).
      4. Reported side effects have been limited to blepharoconjunctivitis in some dogs, the specific cause of which is unclear.
      5. Indications for and safety of use in cats have not been reported.
   B. Oral ophthalmic pilocarpine
      1. One to 4 drops of 2% solution BID–TID was previously recommended to stimulate lacrimation. Its efficacy has been questioned (Smith et al., 1994) and may be of most value in rare cases of neurogenic KCS.
      2. Side effects include diarrhea, ptyalism, tachycardia, and pancreatitis.
      3. Because of its apparent safety and efficacy, topical cyclosporine has replaced pilocarpine administration.
II. Provide topical lubrication.
   A. Use a combination of aqueous and viscous artificial tear preparations.
      1. Aqueous solutions may contain methylcellu-

lose, polyvinyl alcohol, and/or prolonged contact polymers.
      a) They must be instilled frequently for significant benefit (6–12 times daily).
      b) Their use alone is both impractical and ineffective for management of most cases of KCS (Kern et al., 1988; Carrington et al., 1988).
         (1) Few owners can manage sufficiently frequent treatments.
         (2) Maximum contact time is only a few hours.
      2. Ophthalmic lubricating ointment containing petrolatum, mineral oil, or other agents is instilled 4–6 times daily, preceded by an aqueous solution.
   B. Parotid duct transposition may be considered if therapy with cyclosporine and tear replacement is unsatisfactory.
      1. Preoperative evaluation
         a) Eyelid function and structure must be normal. Animals with lagophthalmos, ectropion, or facial paralysis do not benefit, because normal blinking is required to distribute saliva over the cornea and conjunctiva.
         b) Salivary function must be present; therefore, rule out xerostomia.
         c) Corneal ulceration must be resolved before surgery is performed.
         d) Corneal scarring and pigment from chronic KCS may not resolve postoperatively.
         e) Animals need to receive food many times daily to stimulate salivation and subsequent ocular lubrication.
      2. Postoperative complications
         a) Precipitation of salivary secretions on the cornea, conjunctiva, and facial hair may cause irritation and reduction in vision.
            (1) Frequent irrigation with eyewash and meticulous removal of ocular discharge are helpful.
            (2) Topical 1% NaEDTA BID-QID may reduce mineral precipitation.
         b) If corneal ulceration develops, healing may be delayed because of stromal mineralization.
         c) The volume of saliva delivered to the eye is large, and overflow keeps the face wet, with possible secondary dermatitis.
III. Treat any secondary bacterial infections.
   A. For new infections (suggested by numerous polymorphonuclear neutrophil leukocytes [PMNs] on exfoliative conjunctival cytology), prescribe broad-spectrum antibiotic ointment (QID) or solution (q 3–4 h) for 14 days, then reevaluate with conjunctival cytology to assess success as judged by decreased PMN response.
   B. Improved lacrimation owing to cyclosporine therapy has been associated with reduced ocular surface bacterial populations (Salisbury et al., 1995).

C. Do *not* treat continuously with antibiotics, because this encourages overgrowth of resistant bacterial strains.

IV. Reduce conjunctivitis and nonulcerative corneal complications.
   A. Prescribe corticosteroid ointment (QID) or solutions (q 3–4 h) for specific short intervals (e.g., 14 days or 1 week of every 3–4 weeks) to discourage corneal melanosis and neovascularization.
      1. Use only *if* tear stimulants and replacement therapies fail to decrease these complications.
      2. Continuous corticosteroid therapy seems less efficacious than intermittent high-frequency, short-term (14-day) therapy.
   B. The corneal complications of KCS predictably result in blindness; therefore, their retardation is critical.
   C. Always rule out the presence of corneal ulceration *before* prescribing corticosteroids.
   D. Results of surgical keratectomy in cyclosporine-responsive dogs have been poor (Stiles et al., 1995).

Patient Monitoring

I. Primary KCS is usually bilateral and incurable, but prognosis for control of signs and retention of vision is fair to good with excellent owner compliance.
II. Secondary KCS usually resolves with resolution of the inciting cause.
III. Regular follow-up examinations are recommended every 2–4 months.
   A. These are necessary to identify corneal complications and assess adequacy of ongoing therapy.
   B. At each visit, repeat STT, stain cornea with fluorescein, and repeat conjunctival scraping for cytology. Consider bacterial culture submission if cytology shows numerous PMNs and/or intracellular bacteria.
IV. Recurrent bacterial conjunctivitis is suggested by purulent discharge and can be discouraged by optimal therapy.
   A. Diagnosis is by culture sensitivity and/or cytology, and therapy should be specific, adequate, and short term.
   B. Bacterial culture and sensitivity testing should be repeated for infections that persist despite adequate therapy.
V. Corneal changes resulting in blindness are a constant threat.
   A. The best insurance against them is adequate therapy.
   B. Animals that respond well to topical cyclosporine appear to have a better long-term prognosis for vision than nonresponders.
   C. Initial cyclosporine therapy should be continued for 12 weeks before treatment failure is certain.
      1. STT is performed every 2–3 weeks while initial response is being determined, about 3 hours following cyclosporine instillation.
      2. For some dogs responding with STT ≥20

mm/minute, treatment frequency may be reduced to SID-QOD.
      3. If treatment is stopped, ≥90% of responders have a decreased STT in 24–48 hours. For most dogs, QOD-BID treatment is necessary indefinitely.

IDIOPATHIC QUALITATIVE TEAR FILM ABNORMALITIES

Lipid Abnormalities

Definition

Abnormalities in volume or composition of the external lipid monolayer of the precorneal tear film produced by the meibomian (tarsal) glands (Moore, 1990)

Causes

I. Inflammation and/or infection of the eyelid margins and meibomian glands, most commonly by *Staphylococcus* spp.
II. Rupture of meibomian glands with release of lipid secretions into surrounding tissue.

Pathophysiology

I. Altered volume and/or composition of oil layer by tarsal gland inflammation is the primary defect.
II. Because the oil layer normally retards evaporation between blinks, increased evaporation of the aqueous tear layer occurs.
III. Altered distribution of tear film over the ocular surface also develops from tear viscosity alterations.
IV. Toxic products from inflamed meibomian glands may damage corneal epithelium.

Clinical Signs

I. Superficial keratitis (vascularization, edema, cellular infiltrate), especially involving the peripheral cornea
II. Epiphora with normal STT values.
III. Conjunctivitis
IV. Marginal blepharitis: hyperemia, swelling of tarsal glands, enhanced prominence of meibomian gland openings on lid margins, crusted exudate, cutaneous fistulization (see Chap. 93)

Diagnosis

I. Inspection of eyelid margins with magnifying loupe, looking for eyelid margin swelling, enlarged tarsal glands, with or without nodules, hyperemia of mucocutaneous junction, chalazia, dry and crusted marginal exudate
II. Assessment of expressed meibomian gland secretions
   A. Cytology: inflammatory cells, bacteria
   B. Culture: commonly *Staphylococcus* spp.
   C. Physical appearance: normal viscous oil appearance is replaced by thick, opaque, cheesy, or semi-solid secretion secondary to inflammation

Differential Diagnosis

  I. KCS
 II. Keratoconjunctivitis from infectious, inflammatory, traumatic causes
III. Mucin deficiency of tear film

Treatment

  I. Ocular lubricants containing petrolatum, mineral oil, or vegetable oil are used QID to reduce frictional trauma and retard evaporation of the aqueous tear component.
 II. Systemic and topical antibiotic therapy based on bacterial culture and sensitivity results may also be required for resolution of recurrent infections.
III. Surgical curettage of meibomian gland granulomas (chalazia) may be indicated if antibiotic therapy alone is ineffective.
 IV. Warm compresses are also applied to eyelids for 10 minutes TID-QID.

Patient Monitoring

  I. Not every animal with clinical marginal blepharitis has ocular surface disease.
 II. Prolonged therapy and repeated follow-up examinations may be necessary for several weeks.
III. Inspect lid margin and palpebral conjunctival surface for resolution of hyperemia, swelling, gland enlargment, and nodules.

IDIOPATHIC QUANTITATIVE TEAR FILM ABNORMALITIES

Mucin Deficiency

Definition

Insufficient production of mucous glycoprotein by the conjunctival goblet cells (Moore, 1990)

Causes

  I. Chronic conjunctivitis from many causes
   A. Aqueous tear deficiency (KCS) with alteration of goblet cell function
     1. Primary: secretory failure
     2. Secondary: obstruction of tear access from conjunctival inflammation or scarring
   B. Bacterial, viral infections
   C. Immune-mediated disorders
 II. Vitamin A deficiency (experimental)

Pathophysiology

  I. Reduced volume and/or composition of mucin alters the distribution and binding of the aqueous component of the tear film to the corneal and conjunctival epithelium.
 II. Chronic subconjunctival inflammation or hypovita-minosis A may alter the differentiation of conjunctival cells into goblet cells, with subsequent decrease in mucin production.

Clinical Signs

  I. Keratoconjunctivitis
 II. Relative absence of ocular discharge
III. Corneal ulceration of variable severity and duration
 IV. Normal STT values

Diagnosis

  I. Requires conjunctival biopsy to determine the relative prevalence of goblet cells, which are usually sparse or absent
   A. The specimen is taken under topical anesthesia from the ventral conjunctival fornix anterior to the base of the third eyelid (Moore, 1990).
   B. The ratio of goblet cells to all epithelial cells is determined (normal ratio, 0.3).
 II. Tear film breakup time measurement
   A. One to 2 drops of fluorescein stain are instilled while the eyelids are manually retracted to prevent blinking (Moore, 1990).
     1. Time is recorded from the last blink until appearance of the first dry spot on the cornea, which appears as a dark area in the yellow-green film.
     2. Normal breakup time in dogs is 19 ± 5 seconds.
   B. Test reliability is variable and is influenced by technical performance, preexisting ocular surface abnormalities, preservatives in the irrigating solution used, and other factors.

Differential Diagnosis

  I. KCS
 II. Keratoconjunctivitis caused by infection, nonseptic inflammation
III. Lipid abnormalities of the tear film

Treatment

  I. Topical artificial tear preparations containing mucinomimetic agents (Adsorbobase, Alcon Laboratories, Fort Worth) or viscoelastic substances such as hyaluronate or 2% methylcellulose are applied q 3–4 h.
 II. Infection is controlled with topical broad-spectrum antibiotics (ointment QID; drops q 4 h) for 7- to 14-day periods.
III. Conjunctivitis is treated with topical corticosteroids for short (7- to 14-day) periods.

Patient Monitoring

  I. Clinical signs may be difficult to prove.
 II. Careful owner compliance is required to sustain a beneficial result with topical therapy.
III. Progressive corneal disease usually causes blindness in inadequately treated animals.

IV. Frequent and regular rechecks are important.
   A. Weekly examinations are indicated during periods of active infection or keratitis, every 1–2 months during uneventful maintenance periods.
   B. Assess corneal wettability by instilling artificial tears; observe for even distribution over corneal surface.
   C. Repeat fluorescein staining of cornea.
   D. Repeat conjunctival cytology to document resolution of infection and/or inflammation.

INFECTIOUS/INFLAMMATORY DISORDERS

Dacryocystitis

Definition

Inflammation within the lacrimal sac and nasolacrimal duct (Slatter, 1990)

Causes

I. Infection, with or without antecedent nasolacrimal duct obstruction
   A. Bacterial infection most likely
      1. Primary
      2. Secondary to dental and nasal diseases
   B. Fungal infection possible but rare
II. Foreign body, e.g., weed awn
III. Trauma
IV. Dental abscess

Pathophysiology

I. Predisposing factors include congenital and acquired abnormalities of the puncta, canaliculi, or nasolacrimal duct that interefere with normal tear flow.
II. Absence of normal flushing action of tear drainage may allow microbial overgrowth.
III. Foreign bodies may cause septic or nonseptic inflammation.
IV. Even if nasolacrimal duct obstruction does not precede dacryocystitis, it is a frequent sequela.

Clinical Signs

I. Thick mucopurulent exudate centered at the medial canthus
II. Epiphora
III. Minimal to mild conjunctivitis; may be recurrent
IV. Expression of mucopurulent material from puncta following pressure applied to the medial canthus or during nasolacrimal irrigation
V. Variable local pain
VI. Medial canthus dermatitis
VII. Abscess formation at the medial canthus (rare)
VIII. May be unilateral or bilateral

Diagnosis

I. Presence of suggestive clinical signs
II. Established by demonstration of inflammatory exudate collected from puncta by nasolacrimal irrigation or by manual expression
III. ± Foreign body flushed out of opposite punctum
IV. Dacryocystorhinography
   A. May demonstrate foreign body or localize site of obstruction
   B. Types
      1. Positive contrast: aqueous or oil-based media
      2. Scintigraphy with technetium-99

Differential Diagnosis

I. KCS
II. Conjunctivitis caused by infection, nonseptic inflammation
III. Functional epiphora with secondary excoriation at medial canthus
IV. Cutaneous fistulization secondary to dental disease

Treatment

I. Flush nasolacrimal duct to reestablish and maintain duct patency and remove foreign bodies.
   A. Flush saline or eyewash through a 23-gauge lacrimal cannula introduced into upper or lower punctum. Occlude the opposite punctum, then flush with *moderate* pressure in an attempt to reduce obstruction.
   B. Short- and long-term cure rates are uncertain; failure results in permanent epiphora.
II. Prescribe topical broad-spectrum antibiotic therapy, based on bacterial culture and sensitivity results.
   A. Solutions (every 4 hours) may be preferable to ointments because of their presumed direct access to the affected area.
   B. Continue therapy for 2–3 weeks.
III. Indwelling nasolacrimal duct catheterization with 2-0 nylon or a fine polyethylene (PE90) or polyvinyl tubing may be indicated for recurrent dacryocystitis with obstruction.
   A. Stent is sutured to the skin of the face near the medial canthus and distally near the nares.
   B. Remove suture or tubing in 2–3 weeks.
IV. Dacryocystotomy is reserved for recurrent dacryocystitis not responsive to antibiotic therapy, to remove foreign bodies, or to explore swellings of the lacrimal sac.
   A. Entry is made into the lacrimal sac through an incision parallel to the lower lid near the medial canthus over the lacrimal bone.
   B. Inpissated material or foreign bodies are removed.
   C. Indwelling catheterization through the incision is used to establish and maintain patency of the nasolacrimal duct.
V. Systemic treatment may also be necessary.
   A. Systemic antibiotics are prescribed for nasolacrimal abscessation, severe dermatitis, or dental abscess.
   B. Systemic antifungal therapy may be indicated if mycotic infection is documented by culture or cytology.

VI. Treatment of primary causes is as follows.
 A. Treat dental abscess with systemic antibiotic and tooth extraction.
 B. Use multiple flushes, alternating through upper and lower puncta, to dislodge foreign bodies.

Patient Monitoring

 I. Follow-up evaluation is performed after 2–3 weeks of therapy.
 A. Nasolacrimal flush and cytologic examination of exudate are performed to determine presence or absence of inflammation or infection.
 B. Continue antibiotic therapy (topical ± systemic) for 1 week after resolution of clinical signs and normal flush cytology.
 C. Recurrences may develop immediately or weeks to months later.
 II. Dacryocystorhinography is recommended for recurrent dacryocystitis before surgical intervention.

NEOPLASIA

Definition

 I. Abnormal growth of cells derived from a tissue type native to the nasolacrimal system (primary)
 II. Mass affecting the system by distant metastasis from a primary site or local extension from the orbit, sinuses, cranium, or oral cavity (secondary)
 III. Types of neoplasia
 A. Lacrimal gland and nictitans gland adenocarcinomas are the primary neoplasms most commonly reported.
 B. Secondary neoplasms are usually malignant.

Causes

 I. Precise or specific causes are unknown.
 II. Incidence probably increases with age.

Pathophysiology

 I. Neoplasms of the lacrimal gland or gland of the third eyelid may result in reduced tear secretion and may displace the globe or change the position of the third eyelid.
 II. Neoplasms of the orbit or nasal cavity may secondarily involve the nasolacrimal secretory or excretory system.
 III. Primary neoplasms are rare.

Clinical Signs

 I. Space-occupying mass involving the superotemporal or inferomedial orbit or third eyelid
 II. Epiphora if the medial canthus is involved or the globe is exophthalmic
 III. KCS possible, but rare

 IV. Exophthalmos if neoplasma arises or extends behind globe
 V. Enophthalmos if neoplasm involves third eyelid or anterior orbit

Diagnosis

 I. Ocular and physical examinations
 A. Space-occupying mass within or around orbit suggests neoplasia if it is relatively painless and slow growing.
 B. Check submandibular and cervical lymph nodes for enlargement, suggestive of metastasis.
 C. Perform a careful oral examination, especially of the soft palate, to check for swelling or necrosis.
 II. Skull radiography
 A. For primary orbital or lacrimal system neoplasia, radiographs are usually normal.
 B. For neoplasia of nasal cavity or cranial bones, radiographs are usually diagnostic.
 III. Thoracic radiography to check for metastasis
 IV. Orbital imaging
 A. Ultrasonography
 1. B-scan more useful than A-scan
 2. Provides three-dimensional characterization of location, size, and extent of soft tissue masses
 3. Echogenicity characteristics of mass
 a) Cystic masses are hypoechoic.
 b) Solid masses (neoplastic or inflammatory) are usually hyperechoic.
 B. Computed tomography, magnetic resonance imaging
 1. Provide excellent cross-sectional imaging at many planes of view
 2. Best resolution for localization of orbital, nasal lesions
 3. Expensive and of limited availability
 V. Surgical biopsy specimen from mass
 A. Orbital exploration may be necessary to expose the mass.
 B. Before the third eyelid is removed completely for a nictitans mass, neoplasia should be documented by core biopsy.
 C. If available, ultrasound-guided percutaneous biopsy is recommended for masses not directly accessible, before conventional open surgical biopsy.

Differential Diagnosis

 I. Granulomatous inflammation of the orbit or third eyelid caused by infection, foreign body
 II. Zygomatic adenitis or mucocele (dog, ferret)
 III. Orbital cysts (see Chap. 103)
 IV. Primary or secondary orbital neoplasia
 V. Other causes of exophthalmos or prolapse of the third eyelid

Treatment

 I. Orbital lacrimal gland tumors
 A. Exenteration is usually the treatment of choice.

B. Local excision can rarely be performed.
II. Third eyelid gland neoplasms
 A. Wide excision of the third eyelid is indicated if the mass is confined to the nictitans.
 B. Exenteration is indicated if the mass extends beyond the third eyelid.
III. Cryotherapy
 A. Immediately following third eyelid removal if tumor extension is suspected or completeness of mass excision is uncertain
 B. For small localized lesions of third eyelid, medial canthus, anterior orbit
IV. Radiation therapy
 A. Radiosensitivity
  1. Sensitive: glandular, epithelial, lymphoid neoplasms
  2. Resistant: osseous, connective tissue, vascular neoplasms
 B. Modalities
  1. Teletherapy usually requires general anesthesia, fractionated dosages, and multiple treatments.
  2. Interstitial therapy usually requires general anesthesia and prolonged hospitalization with isolation, per radiation safety guidelines.

Patient Monitoring

 I. KCS may develop after removal of affected gland or teletherapy.
 II. Follow-up examinations include physical examinations 3–4 times per year and skull and thoracic radiography 3–4 times per year.
 III. Death from metastasis is variable.
 A. Malignant lacrimal, orbital, sinus, and nasal tumors have a poor prognosis, with survival times likely to be <1 year.
 B. The rare benign lacrimal neoplasm has a good long-term prognosis for survival.

Bibliography

Berger SL, Scagliotti RH, Lund EM: A quantitative study of the effects of Tribrissen on canine tear production. J Am Anim Hosp Assoc 31:236, 1995

Bounous DI, Carmichael KP, Kaswan RL et al: Effects of ophthalmic cyclosporine on lacrimal gland pathology and function in dogs with keratoconjunctivitis sicca. Vet Comp Ophthalmol 5:5, 1995

Carrington S, Bedford PGC, Guillon J-P et al: Biomicroscopy of the tear film: aqueous and lipid tear substitutes in the normal and abnormal eye. Vet Rec 123:329, 1988

Gelatt KN: Canine lacrimal and nasolacrimal system. p. 309. In Gelatt KN (ed): Veterinary Ophthalmology. 2nd Ed. Lea & Febiger, Philadelphia, 1991

Gerding PA Jr: Epiphora associated with *Canaliculops* in a dog. J Am Anim Hosp Assoc 27:424, 1991

Grahn BH, Mason RA: Epiphora associated with dacryops in a dog. J Am Anim Hosp Assoc 31:15, 1995

Hirsh SG, Kaswan RL: A comparative study of Schirmer tear test strips in dogs. Vet Comp Ophthalmol 5:215, 1995

Hollingsworth SR, Canton DD, Buyukmihci NC, Farver TB: Effect of topically administered atropine on tear production in dogs. J Am Vet Med Assoc 200:1481, 1992

Johnson CK, Lockwood PW, Weingarten AJ: US field of efficacy of a cyclosporine (CsA) ophthalmic ointment in the treatment of canine chronic idiopathic keratoconjunctivitis sicca (KCS). J Am Vet Med Assoc 8:158, 1994

Kaswan RL: Diagnosis and management of tear film disorders. p. 1092. In Kirk RW, Bonagura J (eds): Current Veterinary Therapy XI: Small Animal Practice. WB Saunders, Philadelphia, 1992

Kaswan RL, Salisbury MA: A new perspective on canine keratoconjunctivitis sicca: treatment with ophthalmic cyclosporine. Vet Clin North Am [Small Anim Pract] 20:583, 1990

Kaswan RL, Salisbury MA, Ward DA: Spontaneous canine keratoconjunctivitis sicca. A useful model for human keratoconjunctivitis sicca: treatment with cyclosporine eye drops. Arch Ophthalmol 107:1210, 1989

Kern TJ, Erb HN, Schaedler JM et al: Scanning electron microscopy of experimental keratoconjunctivitis sicca in dogs: cornea and bulbar conjunctiva. Vet Pathol 25:268, 1988

Laing EJ, Spiess B, Branington AG: Dacryocystotomy: a treatment for chronic dacryocystitis in the dog. J Am Anim Hosp Assoc 24:223, 1988

Lavach JD, Severin GA, Roberts SM: Dacryocystitis in dogs: a review of 22 cases. J Am Anim Hosp Assoc 20:463, 1984

Moore CP: Qualitative tear film disease. Vet Clin North Am [Small Anim Pract] 20:565, 1990

Moore CP, Collier LL: Ocular surface disease associated with loss of conjunctival goblet cells in dogs. J Am Anim Hosp Assoc 26:458, 1990

Moore CP, Wilsman NJ, Nordheim EP et al: Density and distribution of canine conjunctival goblet cells. Invest Ophthalmol Vis Sci 28:1925, 1987

Morgan RV, Abrams KL: Use of topical cyclosporine for keratoconjunctivitis sicca in dogs. J Am Vet Med Assoc 199:1043, 1991

Olivero DK, Davidson MG, English RV et al: Clinical evaluation of 1% cyclosporine for topical treatment of keratoconjunctivitis sicca in dogs. J Am Vet Med Assoc 199:1039, 1991

Playter RF, Adams LB: Lacrimal cyst (dacryops) in 2 dogs. J Am Vet Med Assoc 171:736, 1977

Rebhun WC, Edwards NJ: Two cases of orbital adenocarcinoma of probably lacrimal gland origin. J Am Anim Hosp Assoc 13:691, 1977

Salisbury MA, Kaswan RL, Brown J: Microorganisms isolated from the corneal surface before and during topical cyclosporine treatment in dogs with keratoconjunctivitis sicca. Am J Vet Res 56:880, 1995

Salisbury MA, Kaswan RL, Ward DA et al: Topical application of cyclosporine in the management of keratoconjunctivitis sicca in dogs. J Am Anim Hosp Assoc 26:269, 1990

Slatter D: Lacrimal system. p. 237. In Slatter D (ed): Fundamentals of Veterinary Ophthalmology. 2nd Ed. WB Saunders, Philadelphia, 1990

Smith EM, Buyukmihci NC, Farver TB: Effect of topical pilocarpine treatment on tear production in dogs. J Am Vet Med Assoc 205:1286, 1994

Stiles J, Carmichael P, Kaswan R et al: Keratectomy for corneal pigmentation in dogs with cyclosporine responsive chronic keratoconjunctivitis sicca. Vet Comp Ophthalmol 4:25, 1995

Wyman M, Gilger B, Mueller P, Norris K: Clinical evaluation of a new Schirmer tear test in the dog. Vet Comp Ophthalmol 5:211, 1995

96

Diseases of the Cornea and Sclera

Susan E. Kirschner

CONGENITAL DISORDERS

Dermoid

See Chap. 94.

Superficial Opacities

Definition and Causes

I. These opacities are confined to the epithelium and subepithelial stroma of the cornea and are first visualized on opening of the neonatal eyelids.
II. The exact cause is not known, but they may arise from incomplete development of the corneal epithelium at the time of lid opening, or subsequent to metabolic deficiencies of the early cornea.

Clinical Signs

I. Faint multifocal gray patches within the superficial cornea, usually in the interpalpebral space
II. No associated blepharospasm or ocular discharge

Diagnosis

I. Diagnosis is based on clinical appearance and the absence of any history or signs of prior infectious, inflammatory, or traumatic diseases.
II. Fluorescein dye tests are negative.

Differential Diagnosis

I. Deep corneal opacities such as endothelial dystrophies
   A. These also may be associated with anterior chamber or iris abnormalities.
   B. Slit-lamp biomicroscopy is helpful to define the location of the opacities.
II. Corneal scarring or keratitis from neonatal infections
   A. Usually associated with corneal vascularization

   B. History or signs of ocular discharge
III. Corneal ulceration
   A. Fluorescein dye tests are positive.
   B. Pain, redness, and discharge are present.

Treatment and Monitoring

I. No treatment is required; most lesions disappear by 3–6 months of age.
II. Periodic rechecks help confirm the diagnosis.

Deep Stromal and Endothelial Opacities

Definition

I. Usually occur from malformations of the corneal endothelium
II. Often seen as congenital bilateral focal or diffuse corneal opacities

Causes and Pathophysiology

I. Deep opacities may be related to persistent pupillary membranes.
   A. A persistent pupillary membrane may attach to the endothelial surface of the cornea, resulting in a gray or pigmented dense plaque.
   B. Persistent pupillary membranes are inherited in the basenji and are common in other breeds (Roberts and Bistner, 1968).
II. Deep corneal opacities also occur with the anterior chamber cleavage syndrome.
   A. This is a syndrome consisting of microphthalmia, absence of the anterior chamber, lens abnormalities, and retinal dysplasia or detachment.
   B. It has been described in the Doberman pinscher and the St. Bernard (Bergsjo et al., 1984).

Clinical Signs and Diagnosis

I. Opacities associated with persistent pupillary membranes

A. These are white, gray, or pigmented and do not usually involve >25% of the corneal surface.
B. The presence of a uveal strand originating from the collarette region of the iris and inserting into the cornea is diagnostic.
II. Anterior cleavage syndrome
A. The cornea is often diffusely opaque.
B. The anterior chamber and pupil are difficult to identify (see Table 97–1).
C. The eye is often microphthalmic.

Differential Diagnosis

I. Corneal edema
A. Usually associated with inflammation or glaucoma
B. Usually diffuse, not focal or multifocal
II. Corneal scarring
A. May have history of prior trauma or infection
B. Corneal vascularization common
III. Corneal ulceration
A. Fluorescein dye test positive
B. Associated with ocular discharge, pain, redness

Treatment and Monitoring

No effective treatment is available for either anterior cleavage syndrome or opacities caused by persistent pupillary membranes.

ACQUIRED NONINFLAMMATORY OPACITIES

Lipid Stromal Opacities

Definition

I. Lipid, cholesterol, and/or neutral fats accumulate within the cornea.

II. Often the location and appearance of the infiltrate are distinctive and allow classification of the lesion.
III. Although described as both dystrophic and degenerative in nature, this distinction is somewhat arbitrary.
A. Dystrophy implies a primary, spontaneous, bilateral, inherited condition.
B. Degeneration refers to a pathologic condition secondary to some inciting cause.

Causes and Pathophysiology

I. May be hereditary (Table 96–1)
II. Associated with hypercholesterolemia and diseases resulting in hypercholesterolemia, such as hypothyroidism and thyroid carcinoma
III. Following inflammation with vascularization of the cornea
A. Pannus
B. Trauma and ulceration
C. Episcleritis
D. Keratoconjunctivitis sicca (KCS)
IV. Possibly following long-term topical corticosteroid therapy
V. Idiopathic

Clinical Signs and Diagnosis

I. Most lipid opacities have a characteristic smooth, shiny, crystalline appearance commonly referred to as "ground glass."
II. They are slowly progressive or nonprogressive, nonpainful, and often bilateral in nature.
III. Inherited lesions vary in location and appearance (see Table 96–1).
IV. Lipid deposition associated with systemic hypercholesterolemia is most often seen as a dense yellow-white arc at the limbus.
A. It may also be found centrally, where it is usually

Table 96–1. *Canine Corneal Dystrophies*

Breed	Age	Location	Appearance	Other Data
Shetland sheepdog	>4 mo	Epithelial-subepithelial	Multiple small focal spots or rings	Recurrent erosions common
Rough collie, Cavalier King Charles spaniel	Any age	Central anterior stroma	Oval gray opacity with "ground-glass" appearance	Composed of lipids; no associated systemic disease
Beagle	>3 yr	Central anterior stroma	Solid oval or doughnut-shaped gray opacity	Composed of various lipids; no associated systemic disease
Siberian husky, Samoyed	>6 mo	Anterior, mid, and deep stroma	Gray/tan hazy oval opacity in anterior stroma, or refractile crystals in deep stroma; often clearer centrally	Recessive inheritance; composed of lipids
Airedale terrier	>6 mo	Starts centrally, progresses toward limbus	Dense milky infiltrative, usually clear at the limbus	Can cause blindness; composed of lipids; no associated systemic disease
American cocker spaniel	>1 yr	Endothelium, Descemet's membrane	Multifocal gray spots, patches, or streaks	May be dominantly inherited; no associated corneal edema
Boston terrier, Chihuahua	>5 yr	Starts temporally, progresses nasally	Gray reticulated opacity typical of corneal edema	Severe edema may result in corneal bullae and/or recurrent erosions

oval, with the typical gray ground-glass appearance.
  B. It is reported most often in the German shepherd dog, golden retriever, and rottweiler.
  C. See Chap. 41 for tests to confirm hypothyroidism.
V. Lipid deposition associated with corneal vascularization is usually found at the leading edge of the vessels.

Differential Diagnosis

  I. Corneal calcium infiltrate
 II. Corneal scarring
III. Endothelial or epithelial congenital opacities
 IV. Corneal edema

Treatment and Monitoring

  I. No effective therapy is known for inherited lipid infiltrates, and fortunately, most do not ever reach a size that threatens vision.
 II. If associated with corneal vascularization, the progression of the infiltrate may, in some cases, be slowed or halted with the use of topical corticosteroids.
III. For lipid infiltrates associated with hypercholesterolemia, lowering the blood cholesterol may halt the progression of disease and in some cases may improve it.
  A. Low-cholesterol diets
  B. Treatment of the hypothyroidism (see Chap. 41)
 IV. In some cases of idiopathic dystrophies, the opacity spontaneously resolves.

Calcium Infiltration

Definition

  I. Calcium accumulates within the subepithelial or superficial stromal cornea, often within the interpalpebral tissue.
 II. Dogs are more commonly affected than cats.

Causes

  I. Secondary to chronic keratitis
 II. Associated with systemic diseases
  A. Hyperadrenocorticism
  B. Chronic renal disease
III. Idiopathic

Pathophysiology

  I. It is not well understood why calcium becomes deposited in some corneas.
 II. Calcification is a common response to cellular injury in other tissues such as muscle.

Clinical Signs

  I. Dense, chalky-white appearance, often deposited in small clumps or spicules

 II. Commonly located in the central cornea, and usually oval in shape
III. May be associated with persistent or recurrent corneal ulceration, from disruption of the corneal epithelium over the deposits
 IV. May have a history of prior ulceration or trauma with corneal vascularization

Diagnosis

  I. It may occur at any age or in any breed if related to corneal trauma or inflammation.
 II. If it is associated with systemic disease, older dogs of smaller breeds are usually affected.
III. Diagnosis is based on typical clinical appearance on ocular examination.
 IV. The deposits may feel gritty when touched with a cotton swab or scalpel blade.

Differential Diagnosis

  I. Corneal lipid opacity
 II. Corneal scarring
III. Corneal ulceration
 IV. Corneal endothelial dystrophy

Treatment

  I. Diagnosis and treatment of the underlying cause, if possible, are of primary importance.
 II. Removal of the infiltrate is not necessary unless the animal experiences discomfort or secondary corneal erosions.
  A. Superficial keratectomy can be performed if lubricants are unsuccessful in relieving pain.
  B. The deposits will return unless the underlying cause is concurrently treated.
III. Lubricating ophthalmic ointments may be helpful in cases in which the overlying epithelium is fragile.
 IV. Disodium EDTA
  A. Remove the epithelium over the deposits and irrigate the deposits continuously for 15–20 minutes with 0.01 *M* or 0.37% disodium EDTA solution.
  B. Alternatively, administer a topical 1% solution BID-TID for several weeks.

Patient Monitoring

  I. Monitor affected animals for development of corneal erosions.
 II. If corneal calcification progressively worsens, reevaluate the animal for underlying systemic diseases.

Endothelial Dystrophies and Degenerations

Definition

  I. These include all abnormalities of Descemet's membrane or the corneal endothelium that may result in corneal edema or corneal ulceration.

II. The corneal endothelium is composed of nondividing cells, so if cell density decreases below a certain level, corneal edema develops.

Causes

I. Hereditary or familial forms
   A. Dogs: Boston terrier, Chihuahua, American cocker spaniel
   B. Cats: domestic shorthair, Manx
II. Senile degeneration

Pathophysiology

I. The corneal endothelium is a single layer of nonmitotic cells that functions to maintain the cornea in a relatively dehydrated state.
II. This is accomplished primarily via membrane-associated ATPase pumps found in the lateral cell membrane of endothelial cells.
III. If endothelial cells are lost through trauma or degeneration, a decrease in total corneal pump function occurs, and corneal overhydration, seen as corneal edema, develops.

Clinical Signs

I. Hereditary or familial forms
   A. Posterior polymorphous dystrophy in the American cocker spaniel (Gwin et al., 1983)
      1. Begins at 1–7 years of age
      2. Usually causes no clinical signs and is diagnosed as an incidental finding
      3. Dominant or incompletely dominant inheritance pattern
      4. Multifocal linear to vesicular corneal opacities corresponding to loss of endothelial cells and other endothelial cell abnormalities
   B. Endothelial dystrophy of the Boston terrier and Chihuahua (Martin and Dice, 1982)
      1. Begins in middle or old age, more common in females
      2. Edema first in the temporal cornea and progresses nasally
      3. May result in blindness
   C. Endothelial dystrophy in the cat
      1. Manx (Bistner et al., 1976)
         a) Edema begins at 4 months of age or later.
         b) Severe corneal edema develops, often resulting in bullous keratopathy and corneal ulceration.
      2. Domestic shorthair cat (Crispin, 1982)
         a) Edema begins at 3–4 weeks of age and is rapidly progressive.
         b) The central cornea becomes edematous initially, but eventually the entire cornea is involved.
II. Senile endothelial degeneration
   A. Usually seen in older dogs
   B. Corneal edema without any signs or history of inflammatory disease, trauma, or glaucoma
   C. Usually bilateral, although one eye may be less affected than the other
III. Bullous keratopathy
   A. Severe corneal edema may result in epithelial or subepithelial bullae.
   B. These may rupture, forming recurrent corneal ulcers.
   C. In addition, severely edematous corneas are particularly prone to rapid stromal melting once ulceration has occurred.
   D. Acute bullous keratopathy is a particular syndrome in the cat.
      1. Acute corneal edema begins focally but rapidly becomes diffuse.
      2. Corneal stromal melting followed by perforation is common (Glover et al., 1994).

Diagnosis

I. Breed, age, history, and typical clinical appearance are suggestive.
II. Rule out other causes of corneal edema with a thorough ocular exam, including measurement of intraocular pressure.

Differential Diagnosis

I. Other causes of focal or diffuse corneal edema
   A. Anterior uveitis
      1. Infectious canine hepatitis infection
      2. Hepatitis vaccine reaction
      3. Other causes of anterior uveitis (see Chap. 97)
   B. Glaucoma
   C. Acute anterior lens luxation
   D. Following intraocular surgery
   E. Drug toxicities: tocainide reaction in Doberman pinschers (Gratzek et al., 1993)
II. Other causes of corneal opacity
   A. Lipid deposition
   B. Ulceration
   C. Scarring

Treatment

I. Topical hyperosmotics may be helpful.
   A. Do not usually cause the cornea to appear clearer, but may help improve epithelial edema and decrease the incidence of corneal ulceration
   B. Sodium chloride 5% ointment or drops applied up to 6 times daily
   C. Glucose 40% ointment applied up to 6 times daily
II. Permanent conjunctival flap may be performed for cases with recurrent ulcerative disease.
III. Thermokeratoplasty using microcautery may slow progression of the edema and decrease recurrent ulcerative disease.
IV. Full-thickness keratoplasty may be considered for cases with bullous keratopathy or impending loss of vision.

Patient Monitoring

I. Animals with corneal edema but without corneal bullae are rechecked every 6 months.

II. Animals with edema and corneal bullae are rechecked at least every 2–4 months.

III. Watch cases with both corneal edema and ulcers extremely closely, as these may rapidly progress to perforation.

INFLAMMATORY DISORDERS

Ulcerative Keratitis

Definition

I. A superficial erosion is defined as loss of the corneal epithelium only.

II. A stromal ulcer involves loss of both the epithelium and some portion of stroma.

III. With a descemetocele, stroma is lost down to Descemet's membrane.

IV. A perforation is a wound in Descemet's membrane with leakage of aqueous humor and/or iris prolapse.

Causes

I. Trauma
  A. External sources: cat scratch, foreign body, etc.
  B. Eyelid disease: distichiasis, ectopic cilia, entropion

II. Tear film disease
  A. KCS
  B. Goblet cell deficiency

III. Lagophthalmos
  A. Macropalpebral fissure
  B. Exophthalmos: pathologic or conformational
  C. Buphthalmos
  D. Decreased blink frequency
  E. Palpebral nerve palsy

IV. Infection
  A. Bacterial
  B. Fungal: aspergillosis (Marlar et al., 1994)
  C. Viral: feline herpesvirus
    1. Infection may be primary or may be from recurrence of latent infection.
    2. Infection may be more common in immunodepressed or stressed cats.

V. Thermal or chemical burns
  A. Detergent agents
  B. Acids
  C. Alkaline agents

VI. Immune-mediated: marginal keratitis (Parshall and Kellum, 1987)

VII. Secondary to other corneal disease
  A. Neurotrophic keratitis (De Haas, 1962)
  B. Calcium infiltrate
  C. Edema (bullous keratopathy)
  D. Corneal epithelial basement membrane disorder

Pathophysiology

I. Minutes after an injury to the corneal epithelium, leukocytes enter the tear film and surrounding epithelial cells start to migrate over the wound.

A. Within 24 hours, the mitotic rate of the basal epithelial cells at the wound edge and at the limbus has increased.

B. Usually the wound is resurfaced within 1–4 days.

II. Tears supply many mediators of healing, so when the tear film is abnormal, as with KCS or lagophthalmos, healing may be delayed.

III. Chronic trauma such as entropion, ectopic cilia, or self-trauma may injure the migrating epithelium.

IV. Infections prevent healing through direct cytopathic effects and by inducing chemotaxis of neutrophils, which cause degradation of corneal constituents.

V. Herpesvirus keratitis involves the following.
  A. Most primary infections are seen in young cats and are associated with upper respiratory infection. Of these, about 80% will become latent (Gaskell and Povey, 1977).
  B. Latency is a condition in which the virus does not cause clinical signs of disease but continues to exist in the trigeminal ganglia and perhaps in corneal cells.
  C. From a state of latency, the virus can be reactivated spontaneously, by stress, or by topical steroids. Signs of upper respiratory infection are usually absent.

Clinical Signs

I. Superficial erosions
  A. Blepharospasm
  B. Epiphora (except in cases of KCS)
  C. Congestion of conjunctival vessels
  D. ± Miosis

II. Stromal ulcers
  A. All the signs of superficial erosions
  B. Visible pit or defect in the stroma
  C. Mucopurulent discharge
  D. ± Hypopyon, flare, or diffuse corneal edema
  E. Perilimbal vascularization ("brush border")

III. Descemetoceles
  A. All the signs of stromal ulcers are usually present.
  B. Bed of the ulcer is dark and smooth, not gray, and does not retain fluorescein stain.

IV. Perforated corneal ulcers
  A. All the signs of descemetoceles; blepharospasm very intense
  B. Fibrin or a pigmented mass (iris prolapse) in the ulcer bed
  C. ± Fluid leaking from the wound

V. Herpesvirus keratitis
  A. Young kittens
    1. Signs of upper respiratory infection
    2. Ocular discharge associated with corneal ulceration
  B. Adult cats
    1. Upper respiratory infection rarely seen
    2. May see very small epithelial linear or dendritic lesions, or erosions and ulcers of any shape and size
    3. Commonly secondary KCS

Diagnosis

I. Test palpebral nerve function and ability to blink. Normal dogs blink at least 4 times per minute.

II. Carefully examine the lids for adnexal disease and behind the nictitans and in the cornea for any foreign body.

III. Unless there is obvious epiphora, perform a Schirmer's tear test.

IV. Consider submitting a bacterial, fungal, or viral culture and scraping for cytology and Gram's stains.

    A. For feline herpesvirus keratitis, the most sensitive diagnostic test is polymerase chain reaction (PCR) assay.

    B. Immunologic testing of conjunctiva or cornea may be helpful in acute cases of herpesvirus; direct immunofluorescent testing is the most available test.

V. Stain the cornea with fluorescein dye to confirm the presence of an ulcer (except in some cases of descemetocele).

Differential Diagnosis

I. Anterior uveitis may also cause pain, epiphora, miosis, and congestion of episcleral vessels. However, a fluorescein dye test is negative.

II. Glaucoma may cause pain, epiphora, and episcleral vessel congestion, but the pupil is usually nonresponsive and there is often lack of normal menace reflex; the fluorescein dye test is negative.

III. Entropion, distichiasis, and ectopic cilia may cause pain, epiphora, and conjunctival hyperemia without a concurrent corneal erosion or ulcer.

Treatment

I. Topical antibiotics

    A. Apply them TID-QID for superficial erosions, 4–12 times a day for stromal ulcers.

    B. Stromal ulcers are treated with antibiotics that are bactericidal and broad spectrum.

    C. Gentamicin or tobramycin is the antibiotic of choice for rapidly progressive ulcers.

II. Topical atropine

    A. Give to effect—usually SID-QID is sufficient; some cases require increased frequency.

    B. It is also indicated for anterior uveal inflammation as manifested by miosis, flare, and hypopyon.

III. Topical antiviral medications

    A. Trifluorothymidine solution (Viroptic, Burroughs Wellcome)

        1. Five times more effective than the next best medication in vitro (Nasisse et al., 1989)

        2. Expensive

        3. Used 2–8 times daily

    B. Idoxuridine solution (Herplex, Allergan; Stoxil, SmithKline & French)

        1. Less effective than trifluorothymidine, more irritating

        2. Used 6–8 times daily

    C. Vidarabine ointment (Vira-A, Parke-Davis)

        1. Less effective than idoxuridine or trifluorothymidine

        2. Used 3–8 times daily

IV. Topical antifungal agents

    A. Natamycin is the only drug currently available for use in the eye and, although effective, is very expensive.

    B. Miconazole IV solution can also be used topically.

    C. Nystatin is fungistatic, not fungicidal, and is made by mixing 50,000 U soluble powder in 1 ml saline.

V. Subconjunctival antibiotics

    A. Indicated for septic stromal (deep) ulcers or perforations

    B. Gentamicin 4–10 mg every 24–48 hours

VI. Contact lenses

    A. Soft contact lenses are indicated for superficial nonhealing erosions and are contraindicated in infected corneal ulcers.

    B. Collagen contact lenses can be rehydrated in topical antibiotic solution and used in infected corneal ulcers (lasts 24–72 hours).

VII. Surgical therapy (Table 96–2)

    A. Nictitans flaps

        1. Useful to protect ulcers secondary to lagophthalmos, decreased blink frequency, poor lid conformation, and KCS

        2. Contraindicated in rapidly progressive ulcers, as they prevent monitoring of the condition

    B. Conjunctival flaps

        1. Indicated for descemetoceles or for deep stromal ulcers

        2. Act as a graft with an intact blood supply rather than a bandaging effect

    C. Primary closure

        1. Used for descemetoceles and for ruptured corneal ulcers <2–3 mm diameter

        2. If used in larger wounds, may distort the cornea excessively

    D. Corneoscleral transposition and lamellar grafts (Brightman et al., 1989)

        1. Used for closure of descemetoceles and perforated corneal ulcers too large to close primarily

        2. Require healthy adjacent cornea to transpose

Patient Monitoring

I. Recheck visits are important.

    A. Superficial erosions: in 5–7 days

    B. Stromal ulcers: every 2–3 days until re-epithelialized or until there is no purulent discharge

II. Watch for signs of infection (change from epiphora to purulent discharge, increased depth of the lesion).

    A. Culture the wound.

    B. Increase antibiotic frequency and/or change antibiotics.

    C. Consider surgical intervention.

III. If not healed in 1–2 weeks, a thorough ocular exam

Table 96–2. **Surgical Therapies for Corneal Ulcers**

Surgery	Indications	Contraindications	Technique	Reference
Nictitans flap	Ulcers associated with exposure keratitis or KCS	Rapidly progressive ulcers	Use mattress pattern to suture nictitans to superior bulbar conjunctiva or to upper lid.	Slatter, 1990
Conjunctival flap	Descemetoceles, deep stromal ulcers, rapidly progressive ulcers	Corneal perforations in which the anterior chamber is difficult to maintain (must use additional means of corneal support)	Use tenotomy scissors to dissect thin flap (pedicle, bridge, 180°, 360°) of conjunctiva from the limbus, based in the fornix. Suture to ulcer wall (pedicle flap), to normal cornea (bridge or 180° flap), or to conjunctiva (360°) using 6-0 to 8-0 suture. Reform anterior chamber if necessary.	Hakanson and Merideth, 1987
Corneoscleral transposition, corneal lamellar graft	Descemetoceles, deep stromal ulcers, perforated ulcers	No normal cornea exists	Make partial-thickness corneal flap, a free lamellar graft, or a corneal flap attached to a conjunctival pedicle flap, using a scalpel blade (cornea) and tenotomy scissors (conjunctiva). Slide the prepared graft over the defect and suture in place with 7-0 or 8-0 absorbable suture, thus sealing the wound. Reform anterior chamber if necessary.	Slatter, 1990 Brightman et al., 1989
Primary closure	Small descemetoceles and perforations (<3 mm)	Large defects	Close with simple interrupted or mattress sutures of 7-0 to 8-0 absorbable material. Reform anterior chamber if necessary.	Slatter, 1990

is repeated to rule out any previously undiagnosed etiology.

IV. Postoperative rechecks are scheduled every 2–3 days for a week, then every 1–2 weeks until the cornea is healed.

V. Herpesvirus keratitis is controllable but not curable.
  A. Periodic flare-ups are common.
  B. Testing for feline leukemia and immunodeficiency viruses is indicated in cats with refractory herpesvirus ulcers.

Persistent/Indolent Corneal Erosions

Definition

I. An erosion that persists beyond 2 weeks despite appropriate therapy
II. Characterized by lack of normal adhesion of epithelium to the underlying corneal stroma

Causes and Pathophysiology

I. The primary disorder is an abnormality of adhesion between the corneal epithelium and the stroma.
II. This condition has been associated with abnormal basement membrane and hemidesmosomes, with corneal edema presumably from endothelial degeneration, and with an abnormal layer of noncelluar material beneath the epithelium (Cook and Wilcock, 1995).
III. In basement membrane disorders, the basement

membrane is thickened and misshapen, and there is a decrease in hemidesmosome density, resulting in abnormal epithelial adhesion.

IV. In dogs with presumed endothelial disease, there is corneal epithelial cell and intercellular edema, as well as stromal edema; this is thought to prevent normal migration and adhesion of corneal epithelium.

Clinical Signs

I. Epiphora, conjunctival hyperemia, variable blepharospasm
II. Corneal defect not involving stroma
III. Loose or edematous epithelium that is easily removed with only gentle debridement
IV. ± Corneal vascularization
V. ± Corneal edema
  A. Focal in basement membrane disorders
  B. Diffuse in presumed endothelial disorders

Diagnosis

I. Based on characteristic clinical findings
II. Exclusion of other causes of corneal erosions

Differential Diagnosis

I. Rule out other causes of corneal ulcers, including trauma, bacterial or fungal infections, and entropion.
II. In young dogs, search for an underlying cause such as ectopic cilia.

Treatment

I. Initial treatment
   A. Debridement
      1. Under topical anesthesia, all loose epithelium is carefully removed with a cotton swab, spatula, or scalpel blade.
      2. This usually enlarges the denuded area of the erosion by 50–200%.
   B. Elizabethan collars
      1. Place on all affected animals.
      2. Even mild trauma from occasional rubbing may be enough to prevent healing.
   C. Topical antibiotics are used 2–4 times a day.
   D. Topical atropine is used to effect for anterior uveal signs (miosis, photophobia).
   E. Many heal within 3 weeks using this therapeutic regimen.
II. Ancillary therapies
   A. Indicated when initial treatment fails
   B. Soft contact lenses
      1. Used in combination with initial therapy
      2. Left in place for 2–6 weeks
   C. Superficial punctate keratotomy (Munger and Champagne, 1987)
      1. Create a series of shallow punctures in the anterior corneal stroma, using a 22- to 25-gauge needle.
      2. Perform the punctures after débridement, and place them not only in the bed of the erosion but also into the normal epithelium around the erosion.
   D. Superficial stromal keratectomy
   E. Hyperosmotic ophthalmic solutions and ointments
      1. 5% NaCl or 40% glucose SID-TID
      2. May be helpful in cases associated with epithelial or stromal edema
   F. Collagen shields
      1. Theoretically protect the cornea for 72 hours
      2. Efficacy for persistent erosions questionable
   G. Third eyelid flap
      1. Provides a bandage over the cornea
      2. May be combined with other therapies, e.g., punctate keratotomy, superficial keratectomy

Patient Monitoring

I. Recheck in 2–3 weeks, unless additional signs occur.
II. If not healed in 2 weeks, consider an additional therapy as outlined earlier.
III. It is the author's experience that many erosions associated with basement membrane disorders heal within 2–3 weeks with débridement, application of an Elizabethan collar, and contact lens placement, but cases associated with corneal edema are more refractory, requiring 3–6 weeks to heal.

Feline Corneal Sequestration

Definition and Causes

I. In this condition, a portion of corneal stroma turns brown or black from coagulative necrosis.

II. The cause is not definitively known, although it has been associated with feline herpesvirus infection.

Pathophysiology

I. Usually follows chronic keratitis or a nonhealing corneal erosion, especially those caused by herpesvirus
II. Can occur in any breed of cat, but may be more common in purebred cats, perhaps because of an increased incidence of herpesvirus in catteries
III. Cause of the characteristic brown/black color not definitively known

Clinical Signs

I. Round focal brown or black lesion in the cornea, often located centrally
II. Mild to moderate epiphora and blepharospasm
III. ± Corneal vascularization and edema
IV. ± Concurrent corneal ulceration

Diagnosis

I. Diagnosis is based on characteristic clinical appearance.
II. Submit cultures or scrapings for the detection of herpesvirus.
III. Assess tear function and eyelid conformation.

Differential Diagnosis

I. Corneal foreign body
II. Other types of corneal ulcers
III. Corneal melanosis (extremely rare in the cat)
IV. Chromophoric fungal keratitis

Treatment

I. Topical antibiotics are indicated for concurrent corneal ulceration.
II. Avoid corticosteroids, as they may activate herpesvirus.
III. Lubricating ointments may help decrease discomfort.
IV. Topical antivirals are indicated for active viral infections. (See treatment of Ulcerative Keratitis.)
V. Superficial keratectomy to remove the lesion may be useful for large, well-defined lesions, especially if they are causing pain.
VI. Correct any eyelid deformities and provide lubrication if tear production is reduced.

Patient Monitoring

I. If surgery is not performed, the necrotic area may eventually slough; periodic rechecks are indicated during this interval.
II. Once resolved, continue to monitor any underlying problems, consider long-term lubricants as a protective measure, and watch for recurrence.

Pigmentary Keratitis

Definition

I. This is a condition in which melanin pigment accumulates in the corneal stroma.
II. It may become severe enough to cause blindness.

Causes

I. Lagophthalmos
  A. Macropalpebral fissure
  B. Exophthalmos
  C. Buphthalmos
  D. Decreased blink frequency
  E. Palpebral nerve palsy
II. Chronic keratitis of any cause, especially KCS
III. Chronic trauma
  A. Distichiasis, trichiasis
  B. Medial canthal entropion

Pathophysiology

I. Corneal melanosis is most common in the Pekingese, pug, and other brachycephalic breeds.
II. It is a response to chronic tissue injury or inflammation.

Clinical Signs

I. Brown pigmentation in a portion or all of the cornea
II. ± Associated corneal neovascularization
III. Not associated with corneal ulceration

Diagnosis

I. Diagnosis is based on finding corneal pigmentation in association with other ocular surface abnormalities.
II. A thorough ocular exam is performed, with emphasis on the following.
  A. Blink frequency (normal, 4 blinks/min)
  B. Ability to completely close the lids
  C. Presence of entropion, trichiasis, distichiasis
  D. Schirmer's tear test
  E. Tear film breakup time (normal, 19 ± 5 seconds)

Differential Diagnosis

I. Corneal lamellar scarring and fibrosis
II. Corneal/scleral melanoma

Treatment

I. Treatment of the underlying disease is the first priority.
  A. Administer topical corticosteroids 2–6 times daily for active keratitis.
  B. Consider topical cyclosporine ointment BID.
  C. Protect the cornea with topical lubricant ointments BID indefinitely.
  D. Surgically correct any eyelid abnormalities (see Chap. 93).

II. Surgical removal is generally not indicated, because an exaggerated inflammatory response occurs postoperatively with the rapid return of pigment.

Patient Monitoring

I. Rechecks are scheduled every 3–6 months.
II. If pigmentation progresses, increase the frequency of medical treatment, switch to a more potent steroid, and reevaluate the underlying cause.
III. The eventual success of treatment is dependent on the correction of the underlying etiology; it is often not curable, only controllable.
IV. Because long-term topical corticosteroids suppress the adrenocortical axis, they should be used judiciously.
V. Warn the owners to watch for symptoms of corneal ulceration, because these breeds of dogs are prone to ulceration of the cornea, and topical steroid use may increase the risk of surface bacterial infections.

Pannus

Definition

I. Pannus is a bilateral nonulcerative condition that is manifested by pigmentation, vascularization, and inflammatory cell infiltration.
II. A variant of pannus affecting the nictitans independently of or concurrently with the cornea has been termed atypical pannus, or plasmoma.

Causes

I. The cause is poorly defined.
II. Exposure to ultraviolet radiation is thought to increase the severity of the condition.
III. Because pannus is commonly seen in German shepherd dogs and greyhounds, a familial basis for the disease has been proposed.

Pathophysiology

I. The cornea becomes vascularized, with infiltration of plasma cells and lymphocytes.
II. Superficial vascularization typically begins at the inferotemporal limbus and may be preceded by a gray haze.
III. The nictitans is often concurrently infiltrated with increased numbers of lymphocytes and plasma cells.

Clinical Signs

I. Bilateral vascularization of the cornea occurs, often associated with melanin pigment. In advanced cases, the cornea is thickened by a pink infiltrate that resembles granulation tissue.
II. Although it starts inferotemporally and progresses nasally, the whole cornea may become involved.
III. Pannus is usually nonulcerative and nonpainful.
IV. Rarely, a mild mucopurulent discharge or slight, patchy fluorescein uptake is associated with the condition.

V. In atypical pannus, the nictitans becomes hyperemic, thickened, bumpy, and depigmented.

Diagnosis

I. Diagnosis is based primarily on clinical signs.
II. Conjunctival or corneal scraping, or biopsy demonstrating plasmacytic/lymphocytic inflammation, is confirmatory.
III. Rule out the presence of other ocular diseases with a thorough ocular exam, including Schirmer's tear and fluorescein dye tests.

Differential Diagnosis

I. Corneal granulation tissue: unilateral, with history of prior ocular trauma, foreign body, or ulceration
II. Pigmentary keratitis: usually in brachycephalic dogs with underlying eyelid or tear film abnormalities
III. Squamous cell carcinoma of the cornea: unilateral, uncommon in dogs

Treatment

I. Corticosteroids are the mainstay of treatment.
  A. Topical 0.1% dexamethasone or 1% prednisolone acetate is used initially.
  B. Subconjunctival corticosteroids are given in severe or refractory cases.
    1. Betamethasone 1–2 mg
    2. Triamcinolone 4–8 mg
    3. Methylprednisolone 4–12 mg
  C. Frequency of topical treatment depends on the severity of disease and may range from QOD to 6–8 times daily.
II. Cyclosporine ointment BID may be helpful in some cases, especially those involving primarily the nictitans.
III. Other therapies that may be used include beta radiation and cryosurgery (Rickards, 1980; Whitley, 1991).
IV. Surgical removal of the lesion is not usually recommended unless the dog is blind despite aggressive medical therapy. Keratectomy does not cure the disease, and unless the cornea is aggressively treated postoperatively, blindness will recur.

Patient Monitoring

I. Treatment is lifelong; the condition is controllable but not curable.
II. Rechecks are scheduled every 4–6 months in mild cases, every 2–3 months in more severe cases.
III. At each recheck, a thorough ophthalmic examination is performed, including Schirmer's tear and fluorescein dye tests.
IV. Warn owners that the condition may worsen periodically, often in warm, sunny months.

Eosinophilic Keratitis

Definition

I. Infiltrative condition of the cornea of cats characterized by vascularization and infiltration with eosinophils, lymphocytes, plasma cells, and, occasionally, mast cells
II. May be unilateral or bilateral

Causes

I. A definitive cause has not been determined.
II. An allergic or immune-mediated basis has been proposed.
III. Herpesvirus has been isolated in some cases (Morgan et al., 1996).
IV. The relationship of eosinophilic keratitis with the feline dermatologic eosinophilic granuloma complex is unknown.

Clinical Signs

I. Elevated pink or white vascularized lesions are seen originating at the inferior nasal or dorsotemporal limbus and progressing centrally.
II. Often a yellow-white, cheesy exudate clings to the surface of the lesion.
III. It may be unilateral or bilateral.
IV. The condition may be nonpainful, but mild blepharospasm and mucoid ocular discharge may be seen.
V. Fluorescein dye tests may reveal patchy ulceration of the surface of the lesion or of the conjunctiva.

Diagnosis

I. Definitive diagnosis is based on the presence of eosinophils or mast cells in corneal or conjunctival scrapings.
II. In some cases, scrapings reveal only lymphocytes and plasma cells; these probably represent a variant of eosinophilic keratitis.
III. Test for feline herpesvirus infection by culture or immunocytology.

Differential Diagnosis

I. Feline herpesvirus stromal keratitis: usually vascularization and scarring, without proliferative infiltrate
II. Corneal granulation secondary to prior corneal disease: history of prior ocular injury or ulceration, more often central than limbal
III. Chronic corneal ulceration: positive fluorescein dye test, painful
IV. Squamous cell carcinoma: uncommon, usually seen in cats with unpigmented lids and conjunctiva

Treatment

I. Topical corticosteroids are the drugs of choice.
  A. Apply topical dexamethasone or prednisolone acetate.
  B. Use 2–6 times a day until the cornea becomes clear, then as needed to prevent recurrence.
  C. In severe cases, subconjunctival corticosteroids (see Pannus, earlier) are helpful.

II. Topical antivirals are indicated for concurrent herpesvirus infection.
III. In refractory cases, consider the following.
   A. Megestrol acetate 0.5 mg/kg PO SID for up to 2 weeks, then PRN; monitor for diabetes mellitus
   B. Prednisone 5–10 mg/day PO for 7–14 days

Patient Monitoring

I. This is often not a curable condition, but a controllable one.
II. Recheck the animal every 2 weeks until the cornea is clear, then every 2–6 months to monitor for recurrence.
III. If lesions return, reinitiate or increase the frequency of therapy as recommended earlier.

Blepharitis/Keratitis Complex

See Chap. 93.

Episcleritis

Definition

I. Inflammation of conjunctival and episcleral tissue, with infiltration of the perilimbal cornea
II. Known by a variety of names, including nodular fasciitis, nodular granulomatous episclerokeratitis, and fibrous histiocytoma

Causes and Pathophysiology

I. It is believed to be immune mediated in origin, but the specific etiology is unknown.
II. Histologic examination of the episcleral fascia reveals a mixture of fibrovascular tissue and plasma cells, lymphocytes, and neutrophils. Individual cases vary as to the predominant cell type involved in the inflammation and the amount of fibrous tissue present.

Clinical Signs

I. Focal episcleritis
   A. Usually seen in collies or collie-like dogs
   B. Raised, pink, smooth tumor-like lesion most commonly at the temporal limbus
   C. Usually bilateral, but may be unilateral
   D. Uncommonly found in nonlimbal conjunctiva, external eyelids, nictitans
II. Diffuse episcleritis
   A. There is no documented breed predisposition, but American cocker spaniels, Airedale terriers, and rottweilers seem overrepresented (Slatter, 1990).
   B. Thickening and hyperemia of conjunctival and episcleral tissues occur between the limbus and the equator of the globe.
   C. It often originates at the temporal limbus but may extend around the entire circumference and posteriorly to affect the retina and choroid.
   D. It is usually bilateral, but can be unilateral.

III. Both forms: nonpainful, minimal or no ocular discharge
IV. Secondary corneal changes adjacent to the episcleral lesion: edema, vascularization, and infiltration with stromal lipid deposits

Diagnosis

I. Signalment and clinical findings are suggestive.
II. Definitive diagnosis is based on biopsy with characteristic histopathologic findings.

Differential Diagnosis

I. Focal episcleritis
   A. Episcleral tumors: hemangioma, mast cell tumor, lymphoma, amelanotic melanoma, fibrosarcoma
   B. Granulomatous conjunctivitis: fungal, parasitic, foreign body, following subconjunctival injection
II. Diffuse episcleritis
   A. Conjunctivitis: allergic, bacterial
   B. Pannus
   C. Glaucoma
   D. Panophthalmitis

Treatment

I. Corticosteroids are the mainstay of treatment.
   A. Topical 1% prednisolone or 0.1% dexamethasone is used 4–6 times per day for several weeks beyond resolution of signs.
   B. Subconjunctival corticosteroids (see Pannus, earlier) are often required initially.
   C. Systemic prednisone (1–2 mg/kg/day PO) should be considered for refractory or recurrent cases.
II. Parenteral azathioprine may be indicated for severe, poorly responsive cases.
   A. Dosage is 2 mg/kg/day PO for 5–30 days, then tapered to three times a week until remission is assured.
   B. Monitor hemogram for decreases in total white blood cell and platelet counts.
   C. Gastrointestinal disturbances and elevation of liver enzymes are also potential side effects.
III. Surgical excision of focal episcleritis is not often curative but yields tissue for histopathology.
IV. Cryotherapy has been shown to be effective in resolving focal lesions (Wheeler et al., 1989).

Patient Monitoring

I. This is often a difficult and frustrating condition to treat.
   A. Some dogs require chronic or intermittent topical steroids to control the disease.
   B. Recurrences are common.
II. Rechecks are scheduled every 2–3 weeks until lesions resolve, then at 4- to 6-month intervals.

NEOPLASIA

Limbal Melanomas

Definition

I. Limbal or epibulbar melanomas probably originate from limbal melanocytes.
II. Their biologic behavior is relatively benign in the dog (Wilcock and Peiffer, 1986).
III. They are darkly pigmented, focal raised masses located near the limbus.

Causes and Pathophysiology

I. These tumors are composed of plump pigment-containing cells and small spindle cells.
II. They are characterized by local growth and extension into surrounding structures, including the anterior chamber.
III. They have not been reported to metastasize.

Clinical Signs

I. Age of onset is 1–10 years.
II. They may occur in any breed, but the German shepherd dog is overrepresented.
III. The lesion appears as a smooth, black, raised mass originating from near the limbus, with the superior limbus being the most common location.
IV. Mild anterior uveitis, localized corneal haziness, or stromal lipid infiltrates may also occur.

Diagnosis

I. The clinical appearance is highly suggestive.
II. Gonioscopy is indicated to rule out drainage angle involvement and to confirm the limbus as the site of origin.
III. Definitive diagnosis is based on biopsy.

Differential Diagnosis

I. Outward extension of an anterior uveal melanoma
II. Limbal staphyloma

Treatment

I. Excision by lamellar sclerokeratectomy is the treatment of choice for small lesions.
   A. Recurrence is common if excision is incomplete (Diters et al., 1983).
   B. Biologic behavior remains benign if the tumor should recur.
II. Cryosurgical therapy following tumor debulking may prevent recurrence (Harling et al., 1986).
III. Full-thickness sclerocorneal resection is indicated for large lesions (Wilkie and Wolf, 1991).
   A. Decreases chance of recurrence
   B. May use heterologous cornea, cartilage of third eyelid, or synthetic graft material to fill the defect created

IV. Photocoagulation by Nd:YAG or diode laser may be effective (Sullivan et al., 1996).

Patient Monitoring

I. If surgical removal is not performed because the lesion is very small and/or the animal is aged, recheck every 3–4 months.
   A. Perform a thorough ocular exam, including gonioscopy to watch for extension of tumor into the anterior chamber.
   B. Measure intraocular pressure if the drainage angle is affected.
II. If surgically removed, recheck every 1–3 weeks until healing is complete, then every 3–6 months to check for recurrence.
III. If the tumor recurs, a second surgical resection may be attempted, or if the globe is blind and painful, it may be removed.

Squamous Cell Carcinoma

Definition

I. It results from neoplastic transformation of the epithelium of the conjunctiva and/or the cornea.
II. Most commonly, neoplasia originates from the conjunctiva and extends into the cornea secondarily.
III. The tumor may be primary in the cornea.

Causes and Pathophysiology

I. In most species, squamous cell carcinoma (SCC) is associated with little or no ocular pigment.
II. Ultraviolet radiation damage to epithelium is thought to predispose to SCC.
III. In dogs, horses, and cattle, viral infection of epithelial cells (papillomavirus) is theorized to predispose to SCC, although this has not been shown in cats.
IV. It is thought to begin as a benign hyperplastic change, then progresses to carcinoma in situ, then to frank neoplasia.

Clinical Signs

I. SCC usually starts as thickening and hyperemia of the conjunctiva, nictitans, and/or lids.
II. It often becomes ulcerated, at which point there is usually an ocular discharge.
III. Corneal SCC is usually an extension of adnexal neoplasia.
   A. Pink, raised, roughened infiltrate in the cornea
   B. Conjunctival swelling, thickening, and hyperemia
   C. Usually unilateral, but occasionally bilateral

Diagnosis

I. Conjunctival or corneal biopsy is definitive.
II. Occasionally, scrapings for cytology are helpful; however, false-negatives are common.
III. With diffuse conjunctival and lid involvement, skull

radiography, computed tomography (CT) scans, or magnetic resonance images are indicated to rule out posterior orbital and optic nerve involvement.

Differential Diagnosis

I. Herpesvirus keratoconjunctivitis: can also cause conjunctival swelling and hyperemia; biopsy and culture may be necessary to differentiate
II. Eosinophilic keratitis: also unilateral, appears granulomatous; biopsy or cytology of conjunctival scrapings will differentiate

Treatment

I. Local excision
   A. Indicated for limited involvement of the conjunctiva and/or cornea
   B. Lamellar keratectomy in combination with conjunctivectomy
   C. Often recurs because conjunctival tumor margins are difficult to determine and disease is often diffuse
II. Enucleation, exenteration of orbit
   A. These are indicated for diffuse involvement of the conjunctiva or lids.
   B. Removal of the lids and all the conjunctiva, as well as the globe, is necessary (see Chap. 103).
III. Other treatments
   A. Radiation therapy: occasionally radiosensitive
   B. Cryosurgery: noninvasive technique, but recurrence likely if cryosurgery is the only therapeutic modality used
   C. Hyperthermia: efficacious in some cases of feline SCC

Patient Monitoring

I. Tumor often invades the surrounding bone and may extend into nasal cavities and the brain.
II. Recheck every 3 months in early cases, every few weeks in more advanced cases.
III. Skull radiographs and other imaging techniques are helpful if recurrence is suspected.
IV. Prognosis is guarded to grave for long-term survival with any therapeutic regimen.

Bibliography

Bergsjo T, Arnesen K, Heim P, Nes N: Congenital blindness with ocular developmental anomalies, including retinal dysplasia, in Doberman pinscher dogs. J Am Vet Med Assoc 184:1383, 1984

Bistner SI, Aguirre G, Shively JN: Hereditary corneal dystrophy in the Manx cat: a preliminary report. Invest Ophthalmol Vis Sci 15:15, 1976

Brightman AH, McLaughlin SA, Grogden JD: Autogenous lamellar corneal grafting in dogs. J Am Vet Med Assoc 195:469, 1989

Cook C, Wilcock B: A clinical and histologic study of canine persistent superficial corneal ulcers. Proc Am Coll Vet Ophthalmol 26:139, 1995

Crispin SM: Corneal dystrophies in small animals. Vet Annu 22:298, 1982

De Haas EBH: Desiccation of cornea and conjunctiva after sensory denervation. Arch Ophthalmol 67:79, 1962

Diters RW, Dubielzig RR, Aguirre GD, Acland GM: Primary ocular melanoma in dogs. Vet Pathol 20:379, 1983

Gaskell RM, Povey RC: Experimental induction of feline viral rhinotracheitis: re-excretion in FVR-recovered cats. Vet Rec 100:128, 1977

Glover TL, Nasisse MP, Davidson MG: Acute bullous keratopathy in the cat. Vet Comp Ophthalmol 4:66, 1994

Gratzek AT, Calvert CA, Martin KL, Kaswan RL: Corneal edema in dogs treated with tocainide. Vet Comp Ophthalmol 3:47, 1993

Gwin R, Cunningham DE, Shaver RP: Posterior polymorphous dystrophy of the cornea in cocker spaniels: preliminary clinical and specular microscopic finding. Proc Am Coll Vet Ophthalmol 14:154, 1983

Hakanson N, Merideth RE: Conjunctival pedicle grafting in the treatment of corneal ulcers in the dog and cat. J Am Anim Hosp Assoc 23:641, 1987

Harling DE, Peiffer RL, Cook CS, Belkin PV: Feline limbal melanomas: four cases. J Am Anim Hosp Assoc 22:795, 1986

Havener WH: Ocular Pharmacology. 5th Ed. CV Mosby, St. Louis, 1983

Kirschner SE, Niyo Y, Betts DM: Idiopathic persistent corneal erosion. Clinical and pathologic findings in 18 dogs. J Am Anim Hosp Assoc 25:84, 1989

Marlar AB, Miller PE, Canton DD et al: Canine keratomycosis: a report of eight cases and literature review. J Am Anim Hosp Assoc 30:331, 1994

Martin CL, Dice PF: Corneal endothelial dystrophy in the dog. J Am Anim Hosp Assoc 18:327, 1982

Morgan RV, Abrams KL, Kern TJ: Feline eosinophilic keratitis: a retrospective study of 54 cases (1989–1994). Vet Comp Ophthalmol 6:131, 1996

Munger RJ, Champagne ES: Multiple superficial punctate keratotomy for the treatment of recurrent erosions in dogs. Proc Am Coll Vet Ophthalmol 18:103, 1987

Nasisse MP, Guy JS, Davidson MG et al: In vitro susceptibility of feline herpesvirus 1 to vidarabine, idoxuridine, trifluridine, acyclovir or bromovinyldeoxyuridine. Am J Vet Res 50:158, 1989

Parshall CJ, Kellum KE: Canine progressive collagenolytic keratopathy. Proc Am Coll Vet Ophthalmol 18:addendum, 1987

Rickards DA: Cryosurgery in small animal ophthalmology. Vet Clin North Am 10:471, 1980

Roberts SR, Bistner SI: Persistent pupillary membranes in basenji dogs. J Am Vet Med Assoc 153:523, 1968

Slatter D: Fundamentals of Veterinary Ophthalmology. 2nd Ed. WB Saunders, Philadelphia, 1990

Sullivan TC, Nasisse MP, Davidson MG, Glover TL: Photocoagulation of limbal melanoma in dogs and cats: 15 cases (1989–1993). J Am Vet Med Assoc 208:891, 1996

Wheeler CA, Blanchard GL, Davidson H: Cryosurgery for treatment of recurrent proliferative keratoconjunctivitis in five dogs. J Am Vet Med Assoc 195:354, 1989

Whitley RD: Canine cornea. p. 322. In Gelatt KN (ed): Veterinary Ophthalmology. Lea & Febiger, Philadelphia, 1991

Wilcock BP, Peiffer RL: Morphology and behavior of primary ocular melanoma in 91 dogs. Vet Pathol 23:418, 1986

Wilkie DA, Wolf ED: Treatment of epibulbar melanocytoma in a dog, using full-thickness eyewall resection and synthetic graft. J Am Vet Med Assoc 198:1019, 1991

97

Diseases of the Anterior Uveal Tract

Michael G. Davidson

DEVELOPMENTAL/ CONGENITAL ANOMALIES

Persistent Pupillary Membranes

Definition

I. Persistent pupillary membranes (PPMs) are remnants of fetal anterior uveal tissue.
II. Several types of PPMs occur, including iris to iris, iris to lens, iris to cornea, and free-floating strands in the anterior chamber.

Causes

I. An inherited trait in basenji dogs, transmitted through an undefined mode of inheritance (Roberts and Bistner, 1968)
II. Unknown in other breeds of dogs and cats
III. Usually occurs as a sporadic, presumed noninherited event

Pathophysiology

I. The pupillary membrane is a sheet of fetal tissue arising from the iris collarette, which covers the pupil and provides a vascular supply to the developing lens.
II. Failure of normal involution by 4–5 weeks post partum (dogs) results in persistent strands of uveal tissue.
III. They may also be associated with multiple ocular defects such as microphthalmia, opacification of the cornea, dyscoria, cataract, and retinal dysplasia.

Clinical Signs

I. Affected breeds include the basenji, collie, chow chow, Pembroke Welsh corgi, and mastiff; it occurs sporadically in other breeds of dogs and is rare in cats.

II. In most instances, the animal is asymptomatic.
III. Large and numerous strands are more likely to cause lesions and vision impairment.
IV. Iris-to-cornea PPMs may result in defects in the endothelium, with stromal fibrosis and edema at or adjacent to the site of corneal attachment.
V. Iris-to-lens strands may cause a focal nonprogressive capsular and subcapsular cataract.
VI. They may also result in focal pigment deposition on the anterior lens capsule or corneal endothelium.

Diagnosis/Differential Diagnosis

I. Direct examination of the anterior segment
  A. Diagnosis involves visualization of strands of iridal tissue.
  B. Evaluate the eye for the presence of other congenital defects, particularly microphthalmia.
II. Characteristic clinical findings
  A. PPMs can be distinguished from senile iris sphincter muscle atrophy by origination of the strand on the iris collarette rather than the pupillary margin and by being congenital rather than acquired.
  B. Focal pigment from remnants of PPMs on the lens or corneal endothelium can usually be distinguished from postinflammatory synechiae pigment deposition by being punctate, often multiple, and axial (central).
III. Rule out other congenital abnormalities of the anterior uvea (Table 97–1).

Treatment and Monitoring

I. Usually none required
II. Penetrating keratoplasty and synechotomy
  A. May be indicated for extensive central corneal PPMs that interfere with vision
  B. Rarely performed
III. Cataract extraction and synechotomy

Table 97–1. Congenital/Developmental Anomalies of the Anterior Segment

Defect	Definition	Pathophysiology	Clinical Findings	Treatment/Advice
Iris coloboma	Absence of sector of the iris, usually "typical" at 6:00 position	Failure of complete closure of embryonic fissure (typical)	Variable-sized sectorial notch in iris, may also involve ciliary body and choroid	None necessary, with exception of Australian shepherd, not considered genetic event
Anterior segment dysgenesis	Number of congenital abnormalities resulting from improper embryogenesis of iris, ciliary body, iridocorneal angle, and cornea	Improper embryogenesis of neural crest cell derivatives, with abnormal development of lens and retina and faulty cleavage of structures forming anterior chamber and iridocorneal angle	Blindness, microphthalmia of varying degrees, opacification of the cornea, and occasionally congenital glaucoma and buphthalmia	No treatment. Affected animals should not be used for breeding
Aniridia	Near or complete congenital absence of iris	Presumed arrested differentiation of optic cup	Widely dilated pupil with rudimentary iris ± photophobia	No treatment. Affected animals should not be used for breeding
Polycoria	Congenital presence of more than one pupil (rare)	Abnormal embryogenesis of developing iris stroma	Two or more pupils present, both associated with pupillary light reflexes	No treatment
Dyscoria (congenital)	Abnormally shaped pupil	Developmental anomaly of iris stroma and/or iris intrinsic musculature	Abnormally shaped pupil. Minor degrees of congenital dyscoria are common.	No treatment
Heterochromia iridis	Congenital color difference between the two irides or difference in color in same iris	Hypopigmentation of iris generally correlated with hair coat color genetics	Blue-colored iris or portions of iris ± Iris stroma hypoplasia in affected area ± Associated deafness (Waardenburg's syndrome)	No treatment. Animals with deafness should not be used for breeding

A. May be indicated for PPMs causing complete cataracts and vision loss
B. Performed only if other ocular structures are normal, as determined by ultrasonography and electroretinography

IV. Breeding of affected basenji dogs discouraged

Anterior Uveal Cysts

Definition

Anterior uveal cysts arise from the pigmented epithelium of the posterior surface of the iris and occasionally from the ciliary body (Corcoran and Koch, 1993).

Causes

I. Congenital: often breed related, especially in the Boston terrier, golden retriever; uncommon in cats
II. Acquired
 A. Spontaneous
 B. Following uveal irritation, e.g., chronic anterior uveitis
 C. Secondary to uveal degeneration, e.g., iris atrophy

Clinical Signs

I. The animal is usually asymptomatic and presented for a dark-brown, circular structure within the eye.
II. Clinical appearance of the cysts may vary.
 A. Attached to pupillary margin

B. Freely floating in anterior chamber
C. Attached to ciliary body and difficult to visualize unless pupil is pharmacologically dilated

III. Collapsed cysts may cause focal pigment deposition on the corneal endothelium or anterior lens capsule.

Diagnosis

I. Anterior uveal cysts are fluid-filled, translucent structures, which usually can be transilluminated.
II. They have minimal or no attachment to the iris margin.
III. They do not usually alter or affect the structure or contour of the iris.

Differential Diagnosis

I. Anterior uveal neoplasia
 A. Dark-brown, opaque, cannot be transilluminated
 B. Altered structure and contour of anterior uveal tissues
II. Focal pigment deposition on cornea or lens from other causes
 A. Postinflammatory synechia: usually also other evidence of prior uveitis
 B. PPMs: congenital, present at birth

Treatment and Monitoring

I. Usually no treatment is necessary, because the cysts do not interfere with function of surrounding tissues or vision.

II. Surgical removal is indicated if cysts are large and interfere with vision.
   A. Aspiration of cysts may be performed with the animal under general anesthesia through a small limbal incision with a blunt 20-gauge needle or automated irrigation/aspiration unit.
   B. Q-switched neodymium:YAG or diode laser may be used to puncture the cyst wall in an unanesthetized animal.

DEGENERATIVE DISORDERS

Iris Atrophy

Definition and Causes

I. Iris atrophy is defined as a structural loss or thinning of iris stroma or muscle.
II. It is usually a senile, degenerative change.
III. Uncommonly, it may develop following inflammation (uveitis).

Clinical Signs

I. Mild forms near the pupillary margin
   A. Dyscoria
   B. Strands of tissue at pupillary margin
   C. Poor or incomplete pupillary light reflex (in older animals)
II. More severe forms with loss of central iridal tissue
   A. Large holes in central iris with isolated strands
   B. Large transillumination defects through which tapetal or fundic reflex can be visualized with coaxial illumination
   C. Normal pupillary margin
III. Usually subclinical, occasionally photophobia

Diagnosis

I. Clinical appearance and location of iridal strands at the pupillary margin allow a presumptive diagnosis.
II. Consider topical miotic challenge.
   A. Use a direct-acting parasympathomimetic agent, e.g., 2% pilocarpine.
   B. Failure to induce miosis distinguishes iris atrophy from neurologic mydriasis. With the latter, a functional pupillary sphincter muscle is present, which responds to direct pharmacologic stimulation.

Differential Diagnosis

I. PPMs
II. Neurologic lesions resulting in mydriasis and incomplete pupillary light reflexes

Treatment and Monitoring

I. None is available.
II. Keep animals exhibiting photophobia out of bright sunlight.

Iris Melanosis

Definition

I. Iris freckle
   A. Focal, flat accumulation of melanocytes
   B. Does not alter thickness of iris
II. Iris nevus
   A. Benign accumulation of melanocytic cells of a variety of sizes and shapes (Gelatt et al., 1979)
   B. May be slightly raised
III. Benign iris melanosis
   A. It is a benign, multifocal or diffuse, increased pigment in the iris.
   B. Potential for progression to iris melanoma in cats is incompletely defined.

Causes and Pathophysiology

I. Exact cause is unknown.
II. Melanocytes are normal components of iris stroma and posterior epithelium.
III. Preliminary information suggests that the condition represents a preneoplastic change in some cats (Dubielzig and Lindley, 1993).

Clinical Signs and Diagnosis

I. History: subclinical, iris color change noticed by owner
II. Signalment: usually older animal, most often unilateral
III. Ocular examination
   A. Single to multiple pigmented foci in iris
   B. Flat, nonraised surface to rounded, smooth mass-like lesions
   C. Normal pupil size and shape
   D. No involvement of iridocorneal angle on gonioscopy
   E. No detectable secondary uveitis or glaucoma

Differential Diagnosis

I. Early iris melanoma (especially in cats)
II. Iris color change from chronic anterior uveitis

Treatment and Monitoring

I. Re-examine every 3–6 months for progression to raised iridal lesion.
II. If mass-like lesions develop, consider possible iris biopsy or fine-needle aspiration for cytology.
III. If the growth rate changes rapidly, if the drainage angle becomes infiltrated, or if blindness from uveitis or glaucoma develops, consider a diagnosis of iris melanoma and enucleate the globe.
IV. Photocoagulation therapy with a diode laser may be of value in progressive lesions in dogs.

INFLAMMATORY CONDITIONS

Anterior Uveitis

Definition

Anterior uveitis refers to an inflammatory process affecting the iris and ciliary body that is caused by a heterogeneous group of endogenous and exogenous insults to the eye (Hankanson and Forrester, 1990).

Causes and Classification

I. Systemic infectious diseases
   A. Systemic mycoses
      1. Blastomycosis (Buyukmihci and Moore, 1987)
      2. Histoplasmosis
      3. Cryptococcosis
      4. Coccidioidomycosis (Angell et al., 1985)
   B. Bacterial infections
      1. Any condition associated with bacteremia, endotoxemia, or exotoxemia
      2. Certain infections in dogs
         a) Brucellosis
         b) Leptospirosis
         c) Borelliosis (suggested, but not proved)
      3. Cats: *Yersinia* infection (speculative)
   C. Viral infections
      1. Canine infectious hepatitis
      2. Feline leukemia virus (FeLV)
      3. Feline infectious peritonitis (FIP)
      4. Feline immunodeficiency virus (FIV) (English et al., 1990)
   D. Protozoal infections
      1. Toxoplasmosis: primarily cats (Lappin et al., 1989)
      2. Neosporosis: speculative in dogs
      3. Leishmaniasis: primarily dogs
   E. Rickettsial infections
      1. Rocky Mountain spotted fever (Davidson et al., 1989)
      2. Ehrlichiosis
         a) *Ehrlichia canis* (Swanson, 1990)
         b) *Ehrlichia platys* (Glaze and Gaunt, 1986)
   F. Algal infections: *Prototheca* spp. in dogs
   G. Parasitic agents
      1. Aberrant nematode larval migration
         a) Toxocariasis (ocular larva migrans)
         b) Dirofilariasis (L2 or L3 larvae)
         c) Ancylostomiasis
         d) Angiostrongylosis
      2. Ophthalmomyiasis interna with dipterous fly larvae (Gwin et al., 1984)
II. Lens-induced uveitis
   A. Phacolytic uveitis occurs with resorption of a hypermature cataract and is a common cause of uveitis in dogs.
   B. Phacoclastic uveitis is associated with disruption of the anterior lens capsule (Wilcock and Peiffer, 1986).
III. Immunologically mediated uveitis
   A. Canine adenovirus infection
      1. Associated with a vaccinal reaction to canine adenovirus-1 (CAV-1) or canine adenovirus-2 (CAV-2)
      2. Rarely, secondary to naturally occurring infection (see also Chap. 110)
   B. Uveodermatologic syndrome
      1. A presumed immune-mediated panuveitis (anterior and posterior uveitis) associated with skin and hair lesions (Kern et al., 1985; Morgan, 1989)
      2. Usually young dogs (1–4 years)
      3. Predominantly Arctic Circle or Asian breeds, including Akita, Samoyed, Siberian husky, Alaskan malamute, chow chow
   C. Idiopathic anterior uveitis
      1. Often, despite exhaustive clinical and clinicopathologic investigation, a specific etiologic agent cannot be identified.
      2. The likelihood of a specific diagnosis is inversely related to the duration of the uveitis.
      3. Idiopathic uveitis is common in older male cats (Davidson et al., 1991), and although it is less common in dogs, it may occur with increased frequency in the golden retriever.
IV. Ocular neoplasia: primary, secondary (metastatic)
V. Trauma
VI. Miscellaneous causes of disruption of the blood aqueous barrier
   A. Systemic hypertension (Morgan, 1986)
   B. Hyperviscosity syndromes: multiple myeloma, ehrlichiosis
   C. Therapeutic radiation therapy to the head (Jamieson et al., 1991)
   D. Secondary to ulcerative or inflammatory corneal/scleral diseases (reflex uveitis)

Pathophysiology

I. Infectious agents may cause anterior uveitis by direct replication or migration of organisms, by inciting an immune-mediated inflammation, or by allowing secondary opportunistic infections to occur.
II. Lens-induced uveitis results from exposure and release of lens proteins or other antigens through an intact lens capsule, inciting a complex immune-mediated, inflammatory response (phacolytic uveitis), or following massive and sudden release of lens proteins from a penetrating wound, leading to reversal of T-lymphocyte tolerance (phacoclastic uveitis).
III. Canine adenovirus infection
   A. Acute findings are related to viral replication causing a direct cytopathic effect.
   B. Subacute findings occur from anterior uveal and corneal endothelial immune complex deposition (type III hypersensitivity).
   C. Clinical signs occur more often with natural infections and the use of CAV-1 modified-live vaccine, although the condition may rarely be seen following use of the CAV-2 vaccine.
IV. Uveodermatologic syndrome
   A. This is suspected to be an immune-mediated re-

sponse to components of melanocytes of the eyes and skin.
B. Histopathologically, the disease is characterized by a granulomatous inflammatory reaction within ocular tissues and a lichenoid inflammatory cell infiltrate pattern in dermal tissues.
V. Idiopathic uveitis
A. Many cases of idiopathic anterior uveitis are presumed to be immunologically mediated, because intraocular tissues are immunologically privileged with unique immunologic responses to myriad insults.
B. Histopathologic findings often reveal lymphocytic/plasmacytic cellular infiltrates, and clinically, there is often at least partial response to anti-inflammatory or immunosuppressive therapies.

Clinical Signs

I. Ophthalmic findings (Table 97–2)
II. Uveitis associated with infectious diseases
A. Anterior uveal findings predominate with viral-induced uveitis.
B. Posterior segment findings predominate with fungal and algal infections and with secondary anterior uveitis.
C. Although they may be seen separately, anterior and posterior uveitis are often both present with bacterial, rickettsial, and protozoal infections.
III. Lens-induced uveitis
A. Phacolytic uveitis is associated with a hypermature or resorbing cataract (sometimes subtle resorption is difficult to detect), and older dogs tend to have more severe clinical signs than younger dogs.
B. Phacoclastic uveitis is generally a severe anterior uveitis following ocular injury.
1. Delay in onset of uveitis 1–14 days after injury
2. Visible rent in capsule, inflammatory cell infiltrate, or fibrin covering rent
3. Often unrelenting, with secondary glaucoma or phthisis bulbi as the outcome
IV. Canine adenovirus infection
A. Natural acute infection: mild anterior uveitis, conjunctivitis

Table 97–2. Clinical Signs of Anterior Uveitis

Acute findings	Chronic findings
Aqueous flare	Secondary cataract
Conjunctival and scleral vascular injection	Secondary glaucoma
Hypotony	Keratic precipitates
Posterior synechiae	Hyperpigmentation of iris (chronic)
Corneal edema	Vitreal cellular infiltrate
Photophobia	Vitreal syneresis
Miosis, resistance to pharmacologic mydriasis	
Iridal thickening and hyperemia	

B. Postvaccinal (subacute, 7–21 days after vaccination)
1. Usually more severe and unilateral
2. Moderate to severe anterior uveitis
3. Varying degrees of corneal edema, which is often diffuse and precludes visualization of anterior segment
4. Occasionally, secondary glaucoma
V. Uveodermatologic syndrome
A. Posterior uveitis may result in retinal detachment and acute blindness or focal chorioretinitis.
B. Secondary sequelae may include cataracts, glaucoma, and retinal degeneration.
C. For a description of dermal lesions, see Chap. 89.
VI. Idiopathic uveitis
A. Clinical findings of chronic uveitis
B. Secondary glaucoma a common sequela in cats

Diagnosis/Differential Diagnosis

I. Perform a thorough ocular examination and characterize ocular findings as acute or chronic.
II. Perform a complete physical examination, noting any systemic abnormalities.
III. A diagnostic database often consists of the following.
A. Complete blood count, serum chemistry profile, and urinalysis
B. Serology, viral assays
1. Appropriate clinicopathologic evaluation is dictated by the physical findings and incidence of common pathogens in specific areas.
2. Typical serologic tests in dogs include the following.
a) Blastomycosis and histoplasmosis in the southern and mideastern United States
b) Coccidioidomycosis in the southwestern United States
c) *Rickettsia rickettsii* and *Ehrlichia canis* titers in areas where tick-borne diseases are endemic
d) Brucellosis and borelliosis titers
3. Serologic tests for cats include the following.
a) *Toxoplasma gondii* (IgM and IgG titers)
b) FeLV
c) FIV
d) FIP
C. Plain thoracic radiography
1. Indicated in dogs with uveitis
2. Rarely diagnostic or necessary in cats with non-neoplastic uveitis
IV. Consider other tests.
A. Paracentesis of the anterior chamber or vitreous
1. Anterior chamber paracentesis
a) It is occasionally useful in supporting a diagnosis of ocular toxoplasmosis in cats by measuring aqueous and serum antibody levels to diagnose local antibody production.
b) Aqueocentesis is performed by stabilizing the globe with forceps at the limbus and directing a 25-gauge needle into the anterior chamber, taking care to direct the

needle parallel with the iris surface, avoiding damage to the cornea, iris, or lens.
  2. Vitreocentesis
    a) Occasionally useful for identifying fungal and algal agents
    b) Rarely necessary, as organism may be identified more readily and safely from other organ systems
    c) Performed by stabilizing the globe with forceps and directing a 22-gauge needle, 6 mm posterior to the temporal limbus, into the vitreal cavity
    d) Usually reserved for blind eyes owing to risks of hemorrhage or retinal detachment
  B. Skin biopsy for suspected uveodermatologic syndrome
V. Diagnosis of the following is often made by clinical findings, exclusion of other causes, or historic incidence.
  A. Lens-induced uveitis
  B. Canine adenovirus infection
  C. Idiopathic (immune-mediated) uveitis

Treatment

I. Treatment of the specific primary agent, if possible
II. Topical anti-inflammatory therapy
  A. Topical corticosteroids are indicated despite active organism replication within ocular tissues.
    1. Use a highly soluble topical corticosteroid, such as 1% prednisolone acetate, to facilitate delivery of the drug.
    2. Frequency is determined by the severity of uveitis.
      a) Mild uveitis: 2–4 times daily
      b) Moderate uveitis: 4–6 times daily
      c) Severe uveitis: 6–12 times daily
  B. Topical nonsteroidal agents (0.03% flurbiprofen, 0.1% suprofen, 0.1% diclofenac) may be used in conjunction with topical steroids.
    1. Synergistic but not additive with steroidal agents
    2. Generally used only for severe uveitis or before intraocular surgery
    3. Frequency: 2–6 times daily
    4. May increase intraocular pressure
III. Topical mydriatic/cycloplegic therapy
  A. Used to prevent posterior synechiae formation and painful ciliary or iridal muscle spasms
  B. Parasympatholytic agents
    1. Atropine 1%
      a) Most frequent agent used
      b) Given to effect, i.e., 1–6 times daily
    2. Atropine 4%
      a) Used for cases unresponsive to 1% atropine
      b) Frequency: 2–6 times daily
      c) Systemic toxicity possible in small dogs and cats with overusage
    3. Tropicamide 1%
      a) Very short acting (1–4 hours)

    b) Useful as an alternative if secondary glaucoma is possible
  C. Sympathomimetic agents
    1. Phenylephrine 2.5–10% may be used with atropine 2–6 times daily for recalcitrant cases.
    2. Overdosage in small animals may result in tachycardia or arrhythmias.
    3. It is a less powerful mydriatic than atropine.
IV. Subconjunctival corticosteroids
  A. Triamcinolone 4–8 mg
  B. Methylprednisolone acetate 4–8 mg
V. Systemic anti-inflammatory agents
  A. Corticosteroids
    1. Prednisone 0.25–0.5 mg/kg PO BID, then tapering dose for 21–28 days, is indicated for moderate to severe cases of anterior uveitis.
    2. Immunosuppressive dosages (1–2 mg/kg PO BID) of prednisone are indicated with certain forms of immune-mediated uveitis, for example, uveodermatologic syndrome.
    3. Do *not* use systemic steroids until after a thorough diagnostic evaluation has eliminated the possibility of an infectious systemic disease.
  B. Nonsteroidal agents
    1. Buffered aspirin 10 mg/kg PO BID for 7–21 days in dogs or 6 mg/kg PO every 48–72 hours in cats
    2. Less effective than steroids, but may be useful when systemic steroids are contraindicated (e.g., diabetes mellitus, certain infectious diseases).
VI. Surgical therapy
  A. Lentectomy
    1. Some cases of phacolytic uveitis fail to respond to a 3- to 4-week course of anti-inflammatory therapy, and uncommonly, early lentectomy may be indicated.
    2. Medical amelioration of mild cases of lens-induced uveitis with anti-inflammatory therapy is preferred prior to surgical lens extraction.
    3. In cases of phacoclastic uveitis, with capsular rents >1.5 mm, primary corneal or scleral laceration repair and early lentectomy are advised.
  B. Enucleation
    1. Enucleation may be necessary for unrelenting, severe, or chronic cases that have failed to respond to aggressive medical therapy or that present with irreversible blindness accompanied by pain from chronic inflammation and/or secondary glaucoma.
    2. It is indicated for blind eyes with large subretinal granulomas from systemic mycosis.
VII. Other specific therapy
  A. Systemic infectious disease: see Section XV
  B. Uveodermatologic syndrome
    1. If corticosteroids alone do not control disease or if treatment cannot be tapered, consider azathioprine 2 mg/kg/day PO, tapering slowly to 0.5 mg/kg/day PO.

2. Azathioprine can also be used in combination with systemic corticosteroids early in the course of treatment to decrease the dosage of steroids used.
   C. Systemic, broad-spectrum antibiotics: following any penetrating injury to the globe

Patient Monitoring

I. Timing and frequency of reevaluations depend on the severity and the underlying cause.
   A. Reevaluate 48–72 hours after initiation of therapy.
   B. Recheck weekly until improvement or resolution of clinical signs is evident.
   C. At each exam, also do the following.
      1. Measure intraocular pressure to monitor for secondary glaucoma.
      2. Scrutinize the lens, watching for secondary cataract formation.
      3. Examine the fundus to document posterior segment lesions.
II. Prognosis for anterior uveitis varies widely.
   A. Fungal uveitis
      1. Focal granulomatous chorioretinal lesions and mild anterior uveitis often resolve with systemic antimycotic therapy and topical anti-inflammatory therapy.
      2. Progression to panuveitis or endophthalmitis with blindness and retinal detachment requires enucleation.
   B. Bacterial uveitis: generally good prognosis with rapid resolution of clinical signs
   C. Toxoplasmic uveitis: prognosis often good
   D. Rickettsial uveitis
      1. Prognosis excellent with Rocky Mountain spotted fever.
      2. Prognosis fair with *E. canis*.
   E. Lens-induced uveitis
      1. Phacolytic uveitis, if diagnosed early, usually responds well to topical corticosteroid therapy.
      2. Phacoclastic uveitis responds less readily and is often unresponsive to medical therapy.
   F. Canine adenovirus–induced uveitis
      1. Prognosis is generally favorable.
      2. 10–15% of cases have permanent corneal edema.
      3. Animals receiving atropine should be monitored for the development of secondary glaucoma, and atropine should be discontinued if this occurs.
   G. Uveodermatologic syndrome
      1. Long-term therapy is often necessary to maintain remission, and recurrences are common.
      2. Long-term prognosis for vision is often poor.
   H. Idiopathic (immune-mediated) uveitis
      1. Recurrence of idiopathic, immune-mediated uveitis is common.
      2. Prognosis is only fair to good, as many cases respond incompletely to anti-inflammatory therapy.

3. Follow-up evaluation should include intraocular pressure measurements, because secondary glaucoma is a common sequela, particularly in cats.

NEOPLASIA

Definition

I. Primary ocular (anterior uveal) neoplasia arises from neuroectodermal and supporting tissues within the eye.
II. Secondary neoplasia refers to metastatic tumors or, less commonly, tumors invading from adjacent tissues.

Causes

I. Primary ocular neoplasia
   A. Melanoma
      1. Arises from melanocytes of the iris and/or ciliary body
      2. Nodular (dogs, cats) or diffuse (cats) forms
   B. Ciliary body neoplasia
      1. Ciliary epithelium: adenoma or adenocarcinoma
      2. Medulloepithelioma arising from undifferentiated neuroectoderm of ciliary body
   C. Undifferentiated intraocular sarcoma (cats)
      1. Cell origin unknown
      2. Occurs months to years following blunt or penetrating injury to the eye (Peiffer et al., 1983)
II. Secondary ocular neoplasia
   A. Lymphosarcoma
      1. Ocular involvement with multicentric forms of lymphosarcoma is common (Khrone et al., 1994).
      2. It is the only secondary neoplasm to commonly affect the iris and ciliary body.
   B. Other metastatic neoplasia: adenocarcinomas more common than sarcomas

Pathophysiology

Ocular neoplasia causes tissue damage by various means.
I. Direct invasion and subsequent dysfunction of ocular tissues
II. Secondary compressive and vascular (ischemic) effects
III. Disruption of the blood-ocular barrier
IV. Infiltration of aqueous outflow pathways, causing secondary glaucoma

Clinical Signs

I. Age
   A. Most tumors: older, aged animals
   B. Medulloepithelioma: young dogs (1–4 years)
   C. Lymphosarcoma
      1. Biphasic age distribution in dogs correlating with occurrence of multicentric forms

2. Any aged cat
 D. Ocular sarcoma: predominantly adult or older cats
II. Ophthalmic findings
 A. Nodule or mass on iris/ciliary body
  1. Brown mass is generally but not always indicative of a melanoma.
  2. Pinkish mass on ciliary body is often indicative of ciliary body adenoma/adenocarcinoma.
 B. Darkening of iris color
  1. Seen with diffuse iris melanoma in cats
  2. Can be difficult to distinguish from benign melanosis
   a) Melanomas are raised masses that change the contour of the iris surface.
   b) Iridocorneal angle involvement is common.
   c) Melanomas grow or progress at a steady rate over several months.
 C. Distortion of pupil size, shape, mobility
 D. Anterior uveitis: more severe with lymphosarcoma
 E. Secondary glaucoma
 F. Displacement of the lens
 G. Hyphema, blindness

Diagnosis

I. Direct visualization of the mass
II. Ultrasonography of the eye
 A. Useful when neoplasia suspected but cannot be visualized
 B. Potential findings
  1. A hyperechoic mass in the region of the iris or ciliary body
  2. Lens displacement, retinal detachment
  3. Organized, clotted blood producing a hyperechoic effect
III. Aqueocentesis (paracentesis of the anterior chamber)
 A. Usually most diagnostic for lymphosarcoma
  1. Rarely necessary for multicentric forms
  2. Variable cytologic findings
 B. Performed under general anesthesia using a 25-gauge needle with the globe stabilized at the limbus by a forceps
IV. Iris biopsy
 A. This may be necessary for cats with early diffuse iris melanoma, which may be confused with benign iris melanosis.
 B. Fine-needle aspirate with a 25-gauge needle may be of value; however, the absence of neoplastic melanocytes does not conclusively rule out melanoma.
 C. Sector iridectomy, with frozen histologic examination, and subsequent immediate enucleation for malignancy may be necessary.
V. Systemic evaluation
 A. Thorough physical examination
 B. Complete blood count, serum chemistries, urinalysis
 C. FeLV and FIV testing
 D. Thoracic and abdominal radiography

 E. Aspiration and/or biopsy of affected lymph nodes, other masses, or bone marrow

Differential Diagnosis

I. Rule out anterior uveitis from other causes.
II. Rule out hyphema from other causes.
III. Uveal cysts may be confused with melanomas.
IV. Differentiate benign iris melanosis from diffuse iris melanoma in cats.

Treatment

I. Primary neoplasia
 A. Anterior melanomas in cats are often malignant. Early enucleation may offer the greatest protection against metastasis (Duncan and Peiffer, 1991).
 B. In dogs, melanomas, adenomas, and adenocarcinomas have a low metastatic rate.
 C. Localized lesions (<6–8 mm) in dogs may be treated by photocoagulation with a diode laser.
 D. Larger lesions are generally enucleated when they cause discomfort from anterior uveitis or secondary glaucoma. Enucleation is usually curative (Peiffer, 1983; Wilcock and Peiffer, 1986).
II. Secondary neoplasia
 A. Lymphosarcoma
  1. Chemotherapy (see Chaps. 67 and 70)
  2. Topical corticosteroids
   a) Prednisolone acetate 1% 4–8 times daily initially
   b) Taper dosage, depending on response to chemotherapy
  3. Maintenance of mydriasis with 1% atropine BID-QID
 B. Other metastatic neoplasia
  1. Investigate and treat primary site if possible.
  2. Enucleate for palliative relief if globe is blind and painful.
III. Prophylaxis
 Early enucleation may be indicated in cats with severely traumatized, blind eyes or phthisical globes to prevent intraocular sarcoma formation.

Patient Monitoring

I. Prognosis variable with tumor type
 A. Canine uveal melanomas (Wilcock and Peiffer, 1986)
  1. Most (approximately 95%) are benign with no or low metastatic potential.
  2. Criteria for malignancy based on nuclear cytopathia and a mitotic index >4 per 10 high-power fields.
 B. Ciliary epithelial neoplasia
  1. Predominant type is benign adenoma.
  2. Adenocarcinomas also appear to have low metastatic potential.
 C. Feline uveal melanomas
  1. There is an estimated 60% metastatic rate

within 6–24 months (Patnaik and Mooney, 1988).
  2. Most reliable indicator of malignancy and metastasis appears to be a high mitotic index; however, relatively few cases have been studied.
  D. Intraocular sarcoma in cats
    1. Highly aggressive with local invasion, regional metastasis
    2. Usually lethal within 6 months of diagnosis
  E. Lymphosarcoma
    Prognosis and response to therapy generally correlate with response to systemic chemotherapy and stage of tumor at initiation of therapy.
II. Follow-up evaluation after enucleation
  A. Primary intraocular neoplasia in the dog
    1. Recheck 1–2 times per year.
    2. Perform plain thoracic radiography at 12-month recheck.
  B. Iris melanomas in cats
    1. Reevaluate every 3–4 months.
    2. Obtain biannual abdominal and thoracic radiographs and assay hepatic enzymes. Lung and liver are the most common sites of metastasis.
  C. Intraocular sarcoma in cats
    1. Monthly reevaluation is recommended.
    2. Carefully palpate the enucleation site and regional lymph nodes.
  D. Lymphosarcoma (see Chaps. 67 and 70)

HYPHEMA

Definition

Hyphema is the accumulation of blood in the anterior chamber.

Causes

  I. Trauma
  II. Severe anterior uveitis
  III. Coagulopathies
    A. Thrombocytopenia/thrombocytopathias
    B. Clotting factor deficiencies
    C. Disseminated intravascular coagulopathy
    D. Hyperviscosity syndromes
  IV. Ocular neoplasms
  V. Systemic hypertension
  VI. Chronic glaucoma
  VII. Secondary to retinal detachment
  VIII. Iatrogenic
    A. During diagnostic paracentesis of the eye
    B. During intravitreal gentamicin injection
    C. During intraocular surgery

Clinical Signs

  I. Fresh hemorrhage
    A. Bright red in color
    B. Often diffuse throughout anterior chamber

  II. Organized or old hemorrhage
    A. Clot generally forms within 24–48 hours with extensive hyphema.
    B. Clot may settle to ventral anterior chamber.
    C. Contraction of the blood clot may cause a rebleeding episode.

Diagnosis

  I. Rule out coagulopathies, especially if other (systemic) signs of bleeding are present.
    A. Complete blood and platelet counts
    B. Coagulation profile
  II. Consider serology for infectious causes of uveitis, especially any endemic rickettsial diseases.
  III. Ocular B-scan ultrasonography is useful to diagnose an intraocular tumor, retinal detachment, or movement of the lens.

Treatment

  I. Treat underlying condition if possible.
  II. Administer topical 1% prednisolone acetate 3–6 times daily until resolution.
  III. Consider topical 1% atropine therapy to maintain mydriasis.
    A. The use of atropine is controversial, because it may interfere with clot organization and resolution.
    B. However, hyphema is associated with or followed by uveal inflammation, making atropine therapy useful.
  IV. Consider topical phenylephrine 2.5–10% for its vasoconstrictor and mydriatic properties.
  V. Consider tissue plasminogen activator (TPA)
    A. Injection of 0.1 ml of 250 µg/ml solution of TPA into anterior chamber (Martin et al., 1993)
    B. Highly beneficial in resorbing blood or fibrin clots in anterior chamber that are less than 1 week old
    C. Useful in preventing damaging sequelae to hyphema
    D. Generally used only when underlying causes of hyphema have been corrected; contraindicated with bleeding disorders

Patient Monitoring

  I. Monitor for rebleeding at 48-hour intervals.
  II. Monitor for secondary glaucoma.
    A. During topical atropine therapy
    B. From posterior synechia and iris bombé several weeks to months later
  III. Prognosis for vision is dependent on amount of blood present and occurrence of rebleeding episodes.

Bibliography

Acland GM, McLean IW, Aguirre GD et al: Diffuse iris melanoma in cats. J Am Vet Med Assoc 176:52, 1980
Angell JA, Merideth RE, Shively JN, Sigler RL: Ocular lesions associated with coccidioidomycosis in dogs: 35 cases (1980–1985). J Am Vet Med Assoc 190:1319, 1987

Buyukmihci NC, Moore PF: Microscopic lesions of spontaneous ocular blastomycosis in dogs. J Comp Pathol 97:321, 1987

Corcoran KA, Koch SA: Uveal cysts in dogs: 28 cases (1984–1991). J Am Vet Med Assoc 203:545, 1993

Curtis R, Barnett KC: The ocular lesions of infectious canine hepatitis: 1. Clinical features. J Small Anim Pract 14:375, 1973

Davidson MG, Breitschwerdt EB, Nasisse MP et al: Ocular manifestations of Rocky Mountain spotted fever in dogs. J Am Vet Med Assoc 194:777, 1989

Davidson MG, Nasisse MP, English RV et al: Feline anterior uveitis: a study of 53 cases. J Am Anim Hosp Assoc 27:77, 1991

Dubielzig RR, Lindley DM: The transition from iris freckle to diffuse iris melanoma of cats: a histopathologic study. Proc Am Coll Vet Ophthalmol 24:56, 1993

Duncan DE, Peiffer RL: Morphology and prognostic indicators of anterior uveal melanoma in cats. Prog Vet Comp Ophthalmol 1:23, 1991

English RV, Davidson MG, Nasisse MP et al: Intraocular disease associated with feline immunodeficiency virus infection in cats. J Am Vet Med Assoc 196:1116, 1990

Gelatt KN, Johnson KA, Peiffer RL: Primary iridal pigmented masses in three dogs. J Am Anim Hosp Assoc 15:339, 1979

Glaze MB, Gaunt SD: Uveitis associated with *Ehrlichia platys* infection in a dog. J Am Vet Med Assoc 188:916, 1986

Gwin RM, Merideth R, Martin CL, Kaswan RL: Ophthalmomyiasis posteria interna in two dogs and a cat. J Am Anim Hosp Assoc 20:481, 1984

Hankanson N, Forrester SD: Uveitis in the dog and cat. Vet Clin North Am [Small Anim Pract] 20:715, 1990

Jamieson VE, Davidson MG, Nasisse MP et al: Ocular complications of radiotherapy to the head region. J Am Anim Hosp Assoc 27:51, 1991

Kern TJ, Walton Dk, Riis RC et al: Uveitis associated with poliosis and vitilgo in six dogs. J Am Vet Med Assoc 187:408, 1985

Krohne SDG, Henderson NM, Richardson RC et al: Prevalence of ocular involvement in dogs with lymphosarcoma: prospective evaluation of 94 cases. Vet Comp Ophthalmol 4:127, 1994

Lappin MR, Greene CE, Winston S et al: Clinical feline toxoplasmosis: serologic diagnosis and therapeutic management of 15 cases. J Vet Intern Med 3:139, 1989

Martin C, Kaswan R, Gratzek A et al: Ocular use of tissue plasminogen activator in companion animals. Prog Vet Comp Ophthalmol 3:29, 1993

Morgan RV: Systemic hypertension in four cats: ocular and medical findings. J Am Anim Hosp Assoc 22:615, 1986

Morgan RV: Vogt-Koyanagi-Harada syndrome in humans and dogs. Compend Contin Educ Pract Vet 11:1211, 1989

Patnaik AK, Mooney S: Feline melanoma: a cooperative study of ocular, oral and dermal neoplasms. Vet Pathol 25:105, 1988

Peiffer RL: Ciliary body epithelial tumors in the dog and cat; a report of 13 cases. J Small Anim Pract 24:374, 1983

Peiffer RL, Monticello T, Bouldin TW: Primary ocular sarcomas in the cat. J Small Anim Pract 24:105, 1983

Roberts SR, Bistner SI: Persistent pupillary membranes in basenji dogs. J Am Vet Med Assoc 153:533, 1968

Swanson JF: Ocular manifestations of systemic disease in the dog and cat: recent developments. Vet Clin North Am [Small Anim Pract] 20:849, 1990

Wilcock BP, Peiffer RL: Morphology and behavior of primary ocular melanomas in 91 dogs. Vet Pathol 23:418, 1986

Wilcock BP, Peiffer RL: The pathology of lens-induced uveitis in dogs. Vet Pathol 24:544, 1987

98

Glaucoma

Robert L. Peiffer, Jr.

Definition

I. Glaucoma is an elevation of intraocular pressure (IOP) beyond that compatible with normal ocular function.
   A. "Normal" IOP in the dog and cat is somewhat variable but usually lies within the range of 15–30 mmHg. IOP is the result of the relationship between intraocular fluid volume and the elasticity or rigidity of the cornea and sclera.
   B. IOP is dependent on several dynamic factors.
      1. Aqueous humor production by the ciliary epithelium
         a) Dog: 2 μl/min
         b) Cat: 14–20 μl/min
      2. Aqueous humor drainage through the outflow pathway, composed of pectinate ligament, ciliary cleft, trabecular meshwork, and scleral venous plexus (Fig. 98–1)
      3. The state of vitreous hydration
   C. Pathologic elevations of IOP may result from the obstruction of aqueous humor circulation through the pupil, at the iridocorneal angle, ciliary cleft, or trabecular meshwork.
II. Glaucoma is classified as either primary or secondary.
   A. Primary glaucoma may be genetically determined and occurs without antecedent or concurrent ocular disease (Table 98–1).
   B. Secondary glaucoma may arise from any ocular disease that results in obstruction of aqueous circulation or outflow.
III. Different types of glaucoma are described based on the appearance of the iridocorneal angle and ciliary cleft, using gonioscopy (Fig. 98–2).
   A. In an open angle, the usual anatomic relationships still exist between the iris and the peripheral cornea, and the angle appears clinically normal.
      1. The ciliary cleft may be open or collapsed.
      2. If the cleft is open, the pectinate fibers are well defined.
      3. If the cleft is collapsed, the pectinate fibers are not visible and the iris root is apposed to the outer pigment zone.
   B. In a closed angle, the iris base lies against the cornea, obliterating the ciliary cleft and obscuring the superficial pigment zone on gonioscopy.
   C. Goniodysgenesis refers to an embryologic malformation of the iridocorneal angle characterized by incomplete perforation of the pectinate ligament.
      1. The ciliary cleft and trabecular meshwork may be dysplastic.
      2. There is an anatomic predisposition to collapse of the ciliary cleft with resultant acute glaucoma.

Causes

I. The exact cause of primary glaucoma is unknown.
   A. The condition is inherited as an autosomal recessive trait in the beagle.

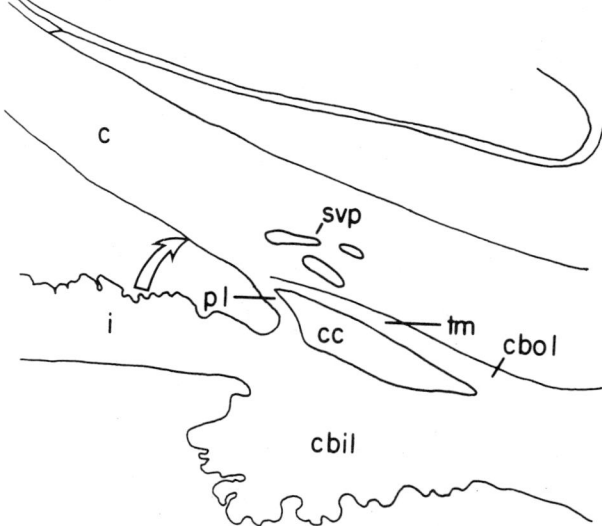

Figure 98–1. Schematic cross-sectional anatomy of the normal canine outflow pathway. c = cornea; i = iris; cbil = inner leaflet of ciliary body; cbol = outer leaflet of ciliary body; tm = trabecular meshwork; cc = ciliary cleft; pl = pectinate ligament; svp = scleral venous plexis; arrow = iridocorneal angle.

Table 98–1.
Breeds Predisposed to Primary Glaucoma

Breed	Age of Onset (years)	Anatomic Abnormality
Beagle	1–3	None initially
American cocker spaniel	3+	Goniodysgenesis
Basset hound	3+	Goniodysgenesis
English cocker spaniel	3+	Goniodysgenesis
Bouvier des Flandres	3+	Goniodysgenesis
Siberian husky	3+	Goniodysgenesis
Norwegian elkhound	?	Open
Cairn terrier	>5	Open, infiltrated by melanocytosis
West Highland white terrier	>5	Open, infiltrated by melanocytosis
Chow chow	3+	Goniodysgenesis
Miniature poodle	3+	Open
Sharpei	3+	Goniodysgenesis
Samoyed	3+	Narrow[a]
Domestic shorthair cat	3+	Narrow
Siamese cat	5+	Open

[a] Although the angle is narrow on gonioscopy, the primary defect is probably goniodysgenesis predisposing to collapse of the ciliary cleft.

B. In open-angle glaucoma in the beagle, the process likely involves a structural and/or biochemical defect that physically and/or metabolically limits outflow of aqueous through the trabecular meshwork into the trabecular veins.

C. The relationship between congenital goniodysgenesis and delayed-onset cleft collapse is not well understood; although the anatomic defect is congenital, glaucoma may not occur until middle age, or may not develop at all.

II. Secondary glaucoma occurs for a variety of reasons.
  A. Anterior uveitis

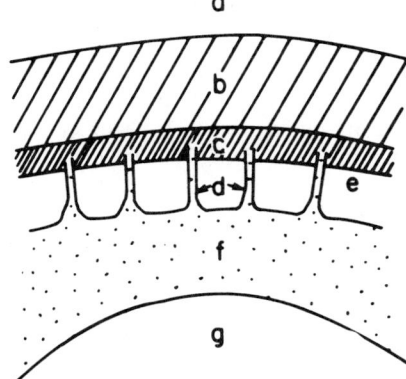

Figure 98–2. Schematic gonioscopic anatomy of the normal canine outflow pathway. Inner or deep pigment zone corresponds to outer leaflet of ciliary body; outer or superficial pigment zone corresponds to corneoscleral limbal pigment. a = corneal dome; b = superficial band of pigment zone (varies in density); c = deep band of pigment zone; d = individual fibers of the pectinate ligament; e = ciliary cleft (space of Fontana) containing the uveal trabecular meshwork; f = iris; g = pupil.

1. Exudation of protein (primarily fibrin) results in increased aqueous viscosity.
  a) Adjacent tissues tend to adhere to each other.
  b) Organization of fibrin forms permanent adhesions (synechiae) and/or membranes.
2. Infiltration of inflammatory cells may occlude the ciliary cleft.
3. Posterior synechiae may obstruct aqueous flow from the posterior to the anterior chamber.
4. Peripheral anterior synechiae between the iris root and inner cornea collapse the ciliary cleft and close the iridocorneal angle.
5. It is a common cause of glaucoma in cats.

B. Lens luxation
1. Lens luxation may occur because of a variety of causes (see Chap. 99).
2. Displacement of the lens causes obstruction of aqueous flow through the pupil.
3. Posterior subluxations and luxations usually do not cause glaucoma; anterior luxations frequently do.

C. Obstruction or infiltration of the angle
1. Tumors
  a) Anterior uveal melanomas
  b) Ciliary body adenoma/adenocarcinomas
  c) Metastatic neoplasia
2. Pre-iridal fibrovascular membranes (rubeosis iridis)
  a) Caused by angiogenic factors released by a hypoxic and/or chronically detached retina, intraocular neoplasms, or chronic uveitis
  b) May span and obstruct the iridocorneal angle or lead to angle closure
3. Pigment cells (melanocytosis)
  a) Proliferating melanocytes occlude the ciliary cleft and trabecular meshwork.
  b) This rare disorder occurs in elderly Cairn and West Highland white terriers.

Pathophysiology

I. Glaucoma is an abnormality of aqueous drainage; hypersecretion of aqueous has never been documented.
II. Glaucoma causes tissue damage through a variety of mechanisms (Table 98–2).
  A. Direct and indirect effects on cells
  B. Tissue hypoxia from IOP that exceeds ocular capillary pressure
  C. Deleterious metabolic effects from stagnation of aqueous

Clinical Signs

I. Signs of acute glaucoma
  A. Serous ocular discharge
  B. Pain: squinting or generalized depression
  C. Corneal edema, perilimbal vascularization (less common in the cat)

TABLE 98-2.
Pathophysiology of Ocular Changes in Glaucoma

Tissue	Effect	Result
Globe	Direct pressure	Globe enlargement, exposure keratitis
Conjunctiva/episclera	Indirect pressure (compression of vasculature with resultant increased venous pressure)	Vascular injection, hyperemia
Corneal endothelium	Hypoxia (aqueous stagnation)	Corneal edema
	Direct pressure	Breaks in Descemet's membrane (striae)
Uvea	Tissue hypoxia	Aqueous flare, fixed mid-size pupil
Lens	Hypoxia (aqueous stagnation)	Cataract
	Direct pressure	Luxation or subluxation
Vitreous	Direct pressure?	Syneresis (liquefaction)
Retina	Direct pressure	Retinal atrophy (especially ganglion cells)
	Indirect pressure	
	Tissue hypoxia	
Optic nerve	Direct pressure	
	Indirect pressure (compression of ganglion cell axons at the lamina cribrosa)	Optic atrophy, ± cupping, demyelination
	Tissue hypoxia	

  D. Episcleral vascular congestion (less common in the cat)
  E. Aqueous flare (variable)
  F. Fixed mid-sized to dilated pupil
  G. Blindness with lack of response to direct or indirect light stimulus
  H. Optic nerve and retinal edema
  I. Occasional focal retinal hemorrhages
  J. Acute globe enlargement in young animals (<1 year)
 II. Signs of chronic glaucoma
  A. Globe enlargement
  B. ± Secondary lagophthalmos and exposure keratitis
  C. Corneal edema and linear striae from breaks in Descemet's membrane
  D. Cataract (variable)
  E. Lens luxation
  F. Tapetal hyperreflectivity from retinal thinning
  G. Peripapillary hyperpigmentation, hyperreflectivity
  H. Optic nerve atrophy and cupping with loss of myelin
  I. Irreversible vision loss

Diagnosis

  I. Glaucoma can be suspected from the breed, history, and clinical signs.
 II. Quantification of IOP by tonometry is required to definitively diagnose glaucoma.
  A. Schiøtz (indentation) tonometry
   1. Inexpensive instrument available to all practitioners
   2. Based on the principle that there is an inverse relationship between IOP and the amount that the cornea is idented by a given force
   3. Best performed under topical anesthesia with the nose elevated and the instrument applied perpendicular to the central cornea

    a) Manually retract the lids without compressing the globe.
    b) Compression of the jugular veins during restraint results in artifactual elevation of IOP.
   4. Influenced by a number of variables, including corneal curvature and resiliency
    a) Obtain three consecutive readings and average them.
    b) Use species-specific tables to convert scale readings to actual IOP (see Appendix III).
    c) Clean the tonometer regularly so that the plunger is freely mobile.
    d) Accurate readings depend on a structurally intact cornea of adequate size to accommodate the instrument and on a cooperative patient.
  B. Applanation tonometry
   1. Based on the principle that the force necessary to flatten a given area of cornea is proportional to IOP
   2. More accurate and versatile, but expensive
   3. Types available: electronic, pneumatic
 III. Gonioscopy delineates the type of glaucoma present but often has little prognostic or therapeutic value.
  A. May be limited by corneal edema
  B. Should always also be performed on the fellow eye, as angle abnormalities are generally bilateral

Differential Diagnosis

  I. Exophthalmos secondary to a space-occupying orbital lesion
  A. With an orbital tumor, the history usually indicates a slowly progressive process.
  B. Unless the optic nerve is involved (uncommon), pupils are normal and the animal is usually sighted.
  C. IOP may be slightly elevated (30–35 mmHg) from compression of the globe.

II. Uveitis
   A. The pupil is usually miotic, and the IOP is low.
   B. The diagnosis of secondary glaucoma from uveitis is made by the presence of elevated IOP with signs indicative of chronic inflammation, such as peripheral anterior synechiae, iris bombé, rubeosis iridis, and keratic precipitates.
III. Other causes of conjunctival and episcleral injection: conjunctivitis, episcleritis, keratoconjunctivitis sicca
IV. Other causes of corneal edema: uveitis, endothelial dystrophy or degeneration
V. Other causes of blindness with anisocoria: retinal and/or optic nerve atrophy (see Chap. 100)

Treatment

I. Glaucomatous eyes can be segregated into two groups: those that are potentially visual (acute or mild glaucoma in dogs, most glaucoma in cats) and those that are irreversibly blind.
   A. In dogs with acute congestive glaucoma, the prognosis for vision is poor with pressures >50 mmHg after 48–72 hours.
   B. The presence of vision on functional testing, a consensual pupillary light reflex, and/or minimal funduscopic changes indicate the potential for preservation of vision.
   C. In dogs older than 6 months of age, globe enlargement (buphthalmos) is a poor prognostic sign.
II. The objective of treatment in eyes with visual potential is both prompt and prolonged maintenance of IOP at levels <25 mmHg.
III. Immediate control of IOP involves the following.
   A. Hyperosomotic agents (dehydrate the vitreous)
      1. Mannitol 1–2 g/kg IV over 30–45 minutes
      2. Glycerin 1–2 ml/kg PO
      3. May repeat both drugs once within 6 hours
   B. Carbonic anhydrase inhibitors (decrease aqueous production)
      1. Dichlorphenamide
         a) Dog: 2–4 mg/kg PO BID-TID
         b) Cat: 1 mg/kg PO BID-TID
      2. Methazolamide 1–2 mg/kg PO BID-TID
      3. Acetazolamide, dog: 2–5 mg/kg PO TID or 5–10 mg/kg IV; use with caution, toxic
   C. Topical autonomic agents
      1. Pilocarpine 2% may be administered, 1 drop q 15 min until effect or maximum of six treatments, then q 2–6 h; it is not effective if IOP is >40 mmHg.
      2. Timolol and levobunolol 0.5% (beta-adrenergic blockers) may be tried BID, but efficacy is unknown in concentrations <4%.
   D. Newer topical agents
      1. Of unknown efficacy in animals
      2. Alpha-blockers, e.g., apraclonidine
      3. Carbonic anhydrase inhibitors, e.g., dorzolamide
   E. Aqueous decompression
      1. It may be performed in an emergency to rapidly lower IOP by inserting a 30-gauge needle through the limbus.
      2. Its effect is transient (about 12–24 hours).
      3. Intraocular hemorrhage and lens trauma are potential sequelae.
IV. Long-term treatment of visual eyes usually requires surgery.
   A. Medical therapy
      1. Expensive and rarely effective for long-term control
      2. Indications
         a) Uveitis-induced glaucoma
         b) Certain infiltrative conditions (melanosis, pre-iridal membranes)
      3. Involves administration of both carbonic anhydrase inhibitors and topical autonomic agents (see earlier)
   B. Surgical therapy
      1. Options for primary glaucoma include filtering procedures, cyclocryotherapy, and laser cyclophotocoagulation
      2. Treatment for secondary glaucoma must address the primary condition.
         a) Lens luxation: lens removal and vitrectomy
         b) Secondary angle closure: filtering procedure, laser cyclophotocoagulation
         c) Intraocular tumor: laser therapy or enucleation
      3. Filtering procedures allow for external drainage of aqueous via a surgically created scleral defect or via silicone drainage devices placed into the anterior chamber (Bedford, 1989).
         a) Advantages: immediate lowering of IOP
         b) Disadvantages: poor long-term success for surgical filtering blebs, expense of drainage devices
      4. Transscleral cyclocryotherapy causes partial destruction of the ciliary body with a subsequent reduction in aqueous production.
         a) A cryoprobe (2–2.5 mm) is applied to the surface of the globe 5 mm posterior to the limbus (Vestre, 1984).
            (1) Two freeze/thaw cycles of 1–2 minutes' duration are used to cool the ciliary epithelium to −15°C.
            (2) Six different sites are treated, avoiding the 9 o'clock and 3 o'clock positions.
         b) The procedure is noninvasive and can be performed quickly and easily.
         c) The technique does cause intense chemosis for 24–72 hours postoperatively and has other potential side effects, such as uveitis, transient rise in IOP for 1–2 days, retinal detachment, and phthisis bulbi.
         d) The effects may not be permanent; additional applications may be needed within 6–12 months.
      5. Laser cyclophotocoagulation also destroys the ciliary body, thereby reducing aqueous production (Nasisse et al., 1988; Cook et al., 1996).

a) Using a hand-held neodymium:yttrium, aluminum, garnet (YAG) laser, 7–8 joules of energy are delivered across the sclera at a point 5 mm posterior to the limbus with a total of 230–250 joules delivered over 25–30 sites.

b) Using a diode laser, a total of 70–80 joules is delivered over 25–35 sites.

c) The procedure is easy to perform but requires expensive equipment that may not be readily available.

d) Potential side effects include postoperative elevations of IOP, cataract formation, mild corneal edema, and hyphema.

e) It may be performed prophylactically for the fellow eye.

V. The major goals when treating a blind eye are to achieve a comfortable eye that is cosmetically acceptable to the client.

A. Ocular hypotensive medications may be tried in an attempt to avoid surgery.

1. They are most efficacious for glaucoma secondary to uveitis or infiltrative conditions.

2. They are expensive and are not usually very effective in the long term.

B. Surgical intervention is indicated when the globe is painful or unsightly, when the IOP is consistently >50 mmHg, or if the cornea is diseased from lagophthalmos.

1. Enucleation is an effective, predictable procedure that provides acceptable cosmesis.

a) It is especially indicated in eyes with confirmed or suspected intraocular neoplasia.

b) Always submit enucleated eyes for histopathology.

2. Cyclocryotherapy may be tried but is not often effective permanently as a single treatment.

3. Laser photocoagulation is highly efficacious if available.

4. Evisceration with implantation of an intraocular prosthesis is a reasonable choice if retention of a cosmetic globe is important to the client.

a) It is contraindicated in the presence of intraocular neoplasia or infectious disease.

b) Examine all eviscerated intraocular tissue histopathologically.

c) Because of the propensity for cats to develop post-traumatic intraocular sarcomas, perform this procedure only on dogs.

5. Pharmacologic ablation of the ciliary body with intraocular gentamicin effectively lowers IOP but causes a transient uveitis and cataracts, and may lead to phthisis bulbis (Moller et al., 1986).

a) Vitreous (0.5–1 ml) is aspirated with a 22- to 23-gauge needle inserted 6 mm posterior to the dorsotemporal limbus and directed toward the optic nerve.

b) Gentamicin (25–50 mg) and dexamethasone (0.2–0.5 mg) are then injected into the vitreous cavity.

c) It is inexpensive and can be performed under light sedation.

d) The technique is contraindicated in cases with suspected intraocular neoplasia or infections, and in cats because of possible induction of post-traumatic sarcoma.

Patient Monitoring

I. Monitor IOP with tonometry frequently.

A. If there is no response to medical therapy within 48 hours, then surgery is indicated.

1. IOPs >40 mmHg cause irreversible retinal damage within 24–48 hours.

2. Early surgical intervention is indicated if there is the potential to save vision.

B. Animals managed medically are hospitalized until IOP is in the normal range, and then rechecked at 1-week, 1-month, and 3-month intervals as long as the IOP remains normal.

1. Monitor for side effects associated with carbonic anhydrase inhibitors, including restlessness, disorientation, nausea and vomiting, and panting from metabolic acidosis, as well as hypokalemia.

2. Some animals exhibit discomfort with application of topical miotics.

C. Surgical failures generally occur within the first 6 postoperative months.

1. Filtering procedures may close from fibrous scars and require reoperation.

2. Shunts and valves may plug with fibrin or cells and require flushing or replacement, and reservoirs may become encapsulated with dense scar tissue that requires excision.

3. Ciliary body epithelium may regenerate following cyclocryotherapy or laser ablation with recurrence of ocular hypertension within 6 weeks to 12 months.

II. Primary glaucoma or glaucoma secondary to primary lens luxation is a bilateral disease.

A. Examine fellow eyes with gonioscopy and tonometry at 3- to 6-month intervals.

B. Instruct owners to seek assistance at the first sign of any ocular problem (including discharge, hyperemia, cloudiness, pain, and/or visual impairment) in the unaffected eye.

III. Prophylactic treatment of ''normal'' fellow eyes may be considered.

A. There is no documented evidence that prophylactic treatment prevents the onset of glaucoma, but statistically it may increase the interval until the opposite eye is affected (Slater and Erb, 1986).

B. Topical therapy is preferred.

1. Pilocarpine 1–2% BID

2. Timolol maleate or levobunolol 0.5% SID-BID

IV. Prognosis for vision is always considered guarded at best. Success rate for control of IOP with long-term restoration or maintenance of vision is probably <50%.

Bibliography

Bedford PGC: The etiology of primary glaucoma in the dog. J Small Anim Pract 16:217, 1975

Bedford PGC: A gonioscopic study of the iridocorneal angle in the English and American breeds of cocker spaniel and the basset hound. J Small Anim Pract 18:631, 1977a

Bedford PGC: The surgical treatment of canine glaucoma. J Small Anim Pract 18:713, 1977b

Bedford PGC: The clinical and pathological features of canine glaucoma. Vet Rec 107:53, 1980a

Bedford PGC: The etiology of canine glaucoma. Vet Rec 107:76, 1980b

Bedford PGC: A clinical evaluation of a one-piece drainage system in the treatment of canine glaucoma. J Small Anim Pract 30:68, 1989

Brightman AN, Vestre WA, Helper RC, Jones JE: Cryosurgery for the treatment of canine glaucoma. J Am Anim Hosp Assoc 18:319, 1984

Cook CS, Davidson MG, Abrams KL et al: Diode laser cyclophotocoagulation for treatment of primary glaucoma in the dog: results of 6 and 12 month follow up. Vet Compar Ophthalmol (in press)

Corcoran K, Koch S, Peiffer RL: Glaucoma in the chow. Vet Compar Ophthalmol 4:193, 1994

Cottrell BD, Barnett KC: Primary glaucoma in the Welsh springer spaniel. J Small Anim Pract 29:185, 1988

Gelatt KN: Familial glaucoma in the beagle dog. J Am Vet Med Assoc 8:23, 1960

Gelatt KN, Gum GG, Samuelson DA et al: Evaluation of the Krupin-Denver valve implant in normotensive and glaucomatous beagles. J Am Vet Med Assoc 191:404, 1987

Lovelin LL, Belhorn RW: Clinicopathologic changes in primary glaucoma in the cocker spaniel. Am J Vet Res 29:379, 1968

Martin CL, Wyman M: Glaucoma in the basset hound. J Am Vet Med Assoc 153:1320, 1968

Martin CL, Wyman M: Controversial problems in veterinary practice. Primary glaucoma in the dog. Vet Clin North Am 8:257, 1978

Moller I, Cook CS, Peiffer RL et al: Indications for and complications of pharmacologic ablation of the ciliary body for the treatment of chronic glaucoma in the dog. J Am Anim Hosp Assoc 22:319, 1986

Nasisse MP, Davidson MG, MacLaughlin NJ et al: Neodymium: yttrium, aluminum, garnet laser energy delivered transclerally to the ciliary body of dogs. Am J Vet Res 49:1972, 1988

Peiffer RL, Gelatt KN, Jessen CR et al: Calibration of the Schiotz tonometer for the canine eye. Am J Vet Res 38:1881, 1977a

Peiffer RL, Gwin RM, Gelatt KN, Schenk M: Combined posterior sclerectomy, cyclodialysis, and trans-scleral iridencleisis in the management of primary glaucoma. Canine Pract 4:54, 1977b

Peiffer RL, Wilcock BP, Yin H: Pathogenesis and significance of preiridial fibrovascular membranes in domestic animals. Vet Pathol 27:41, 1990

Peterson-Jones SM: Abnormal ocular pigment deposition associated with glaucoma in the Cairn terrier. J Small Anim Pract 32:19, 1991

Slater MR, Erb HN: Effects of risk factors and prophylactic treatment on glaucoma. J Am Vet Med Assoc 88:1028, 1986

Smith RIE, Peiffer RL, Wilcock BP: Some aspects of the pathology of canine glaucoma. Vet Compar Ophthalmol 3:16, 1993

Van der Linde-Sipman JS: Dysplasia of the pectinate ligament and primary glaucoma in the Bouvier des Flandres dog. Vet Pathol 24:201, 1987

Vestre WA: Cryosurgical techniques in veterinary ophthalmology. Compend Contin Educ Pract Vet 6:481, 1984

Walde von I: Glaukom bein Hunde. Kleintier-Praxis 27:223, 1982

Watson P: Comparative aspects of glaucoma. J Small Anim Pract 11:129, 1970

Wilcock BP, Peiffer RL, Davidson MG: The causes of glaucoma in cats. Vet Pathol 27:35, 1990

99

Diseases of the Lens and Vitreous

Robert V. English

CONGENITAL MALFORMATIONS OF THE LENS

See Table 99–1.

CATARACTS

Definition

I. An opacity in the lens
II. Classification of cataracts
   A. Stage of development
      1. Cataracts are staged by judging the degree of lens opacification and the degree of lens liquefaction.
         a) The intensity of fundic reflex seen is an excellent way to evaluate the degree of lenticular opacification.
         b) The greater the loss of the fundic reflex, the more complete the cataract.
         c) Cataracts may undergo liquefaction resulting in the loss of lens fibers and a decrease in lens thickness.
      2. Stages are classified as follows (Playter, 1977).
         a) Incipient: cataract is focal or does not obscure retinal detail.
         b) Immature: the entire lens is not opaque.
         c) Mature: essentially the entire lens is opaque, and the fundic reflex is absent.
         d) Hypermature cataracts have the following characteristics.
            (1) Lens liquefaction has begun. The anterior chamber becomes deeper and the anterior lens capsule becomes wrinkled.
            (2) The fundic reflex may again be visible.
            (3) A morgagnian cataract is a hypermature cataract in which the nucleus has sunk to the bottom of the capsular bag because the surrounding lens cortex has liquefied.
            (4) Rarely does resorption progress to a point that functional vision is restored, except in young (<1 year) dogs.
   B. Location
      1. There are four general areas for lens opacities.
         a) Anterior or posterior capsule
         b) Anterior or posterior cortex
         c) Equator
         d) Nucleus
      2. Accurate localization requires slit lamp biomicroscopy (Gelatt, 1991a).
         a) Observing the direction of cataract movement during eye movement allows gross localization.
         b) Opacities in the anterior cortex or capsule move in the same direction as the eye, opacities in the posterior cortex or capsule move opposite the eye, and nuclear cataracts remain central.
         c) Equatorial cataracts are at the periphery of the lens and require full mydriasis to be seen.
      3. Localization is helpful in determining etiology and progression (Tables 99–2 and 99–3).
         a) Cortical and equatorial cataracts usually progress.
         b) Capsular and nuclear cataracts are less likely to progress.
   C. Age of onset
      1. Congenital or perinatal: cataract present when eyes open
      2. Juvenile and adult onset
         a) Classically, juvenile is <2 years old and adult is 2–6 years old, but these distinctions are arbitrary.
         b) Inherited cataracts can be congenital, juvenile, or adult in onset.

Table 99–1. **Congenital Malformations of the Lens**

Condition	Definition	Ophthalmic Findings	Comments and Associated Findings	Differential Diagnosis	Treatment and Patient Monitoring
Aphakia	Absence of lens	No evidence of a lens or lens capsule	Rare, usually associated with multiple ocular defects	Previous lentectomy Resorbed cataract Posterior lens luxation	No specific treatment indicated
Microphakia	Small lens	Decreased lens diameter, lens equator and elongated zonules visible in pupil	Lens luxation and/or glaucoma may occur.	Lens luxation	Frequent reevaluations of lens position and intraocular pressure recommended Lentectomy if lens luxation or associated complications occur
Lenticonus	Conical protrusion of lens	Conical extension of the lens, usually posteriorly into vitreous Cataract may be present.	Seen with congenital cataracts in miniature schnauzers	Persistent tunica vasculosa lentis	Lentectomy if cataract impairs clinical vision
Lens coloboma	Notch defect in lens	Notch defect in the lens, commonly at ventral lens equator	Coloboma of iris or optic nerve may be present. Large defects can cause lens luxation.		No specific treatment Lentectomy if lens luxation or associated complications occur
Cataract	Opacity in lens	See Cataract section in text	Multiple ocular defects including micro-ophthalmia and retinal dysplasia	See Cataract section in text	See Cataract section in text

3. Geriatric onset
   a) Senile cataracts
   b) Usually develop in dogs >10 years old

Causes

I. Inherited (most common)
II. Metabolic
   A. Hyperglycemia or galactosemia
   B. Hypocalcemia
   C. Storage diseases
   D. Tyrosinemia
III. Toxin-induced
   A. Disophenol and dimethyl sulfoxide (DMSO)
   B. Others (Grant, 1986; Gelatt, 1991b)
IV. Nutritional
   A. Cataracts have occurred in orphaned puppies and kittens fed milk replacer (Remillard, 1993).
      1. Arginine deficiency is the likely cause.
      2. Commercial milk replacement formulas claim to have corrected the deficiency, but orphaned pets should be monitored closely.
      3. Opacities at the equator, posterior capsule, and the Y sutures are seen most frequently.
      4. Opacities are mild and reversible when dietary deficiency is corrected early.
   B. Nutritional cataracts secondary to hyperparathyroidism and resultant hypocalcemia can result from all-meat diets (see also Chap. 120).

C. Deficiency of certain amino acids or vitamins can also cause cataracts but is rare in pets on quality commercial foods.
V. Traumatic
   A. Penetrating ocular injury
      1. Causes a severe lens-induced uveitis (phacoclastic uveitis)
      2. Prompt lentectomy recommended (Davidson et al., 1991b)
   B. Electrical shock
VI. Orthovoltage or megavoltage radiation (Roberts et al., 1987; Jamieson et al., 1991)
VII. Associated with retinal degeneration
VIII. Sequelae to intraocular inflammation (uveitis)
IX. Age-related (geriatric or senile cataracts)

Pathophysiology

I. Alterations in electrolyte and water balances (Quinn 1981; Gelatt 1991b)
   A. Maintenance of relative lens dehydration and precise lens fiber organization is required for optical clarity.
   B. Increased membrane permeability or altered osmotic gradients alter the ability of the lens to maintain water and electrolyte balance.
      1. For example, hyperglycemia/hypergalactosemia causes the saturation of hexose kinase

Table 99–2. *Characteristics of Selected Hereditary Cataracts in Dogs*

Breed[a]	Age of Onset	Mode of Inheritance	Location	Progression	Associated Findings[b]
Afghan	Juvenile	Not defined	Equatorial	Progressive	None
Akita	Congenital	Not defined	Nuclear and cortical	Variable progression	Microophthalmia, retinal dysplasia
Alaskan malamute	Juvenile	Not defined	Posterior subcapsular	Variable progression	None
American cocker spaniel	Juvenile or adult	Autosomal recessive	Cortical	Progressive	None
Australian shepherd	Congenital	Not defined	Nuclear and cortical	Nonprogressive	Microophthalmia, retinal dysplasia, colobomas
Basenji	Congenital	Not defined	Anterior capsular	Nonprogressive	Persistent pupillary membranes (PPM)
Beatle	Congenital	Not defined	Anterior capsular	Nonprogressive	PPM
Boston terrier	Congenital	Not defined	Nuclear and cortical	Progressive	None
	Adult	Not defined	Equatorial, subcapsular	Slow progressive	None
Cavalier King Charles spaniel	Congenital	Not defined	Nuclear and cortical	Progressive	Microophthalmia, lenticonus
Chesapeake Bay retriever	Juvenile or adult	Not defined	Posterior subcapsular	Variable progression	None
Chow chow	Congenital	Not defined	Nuclear and cortical	Variable progression	Microophthalmia, persistent pupillary membrane, retinal dysplasia, nystagmus
Collie	Congenital	Not defined	Nuclear and cortical	Unknown	Microophthalmia, retinal dysplasia, coloboma
Doberman pinscher	Congenital	Dominant with incomplete penetrance	Posterior subcapsular	Variable progression	Persistent hyperplastic primary vitreous or tunica vasculosa lentis
English cocker spaniel	Congenital	Not defined	Anterior capsular	Nonprogressive	PPM, microophthalmia, retinal dysplasia
Flat coat retriever	Juvenile or adult	Not defined	Posterior subcapsular	Nonprogressive	None
German shepherd dog	Congenital	Autosomal dominant	Nuclear	Nonprogressive	None
	Juvenile	Autosomal recessive	Posterior Y suture	Variable progression	None
Golden retriever	Juvenile or adult	Not defined	Perinuclear	Progressive	None
	Juvenile or adult	Not defined	Posterior subcapsular	Nonprogressive	None
Labrador retriever	Congenital	Incomplete dominance	Nuclear and cortical	Variable progression	Vitreoretinal dysplasia, skeletal chondrodysplasia
	Juvenile or adult	Not defined	Perinuclear	Progressive	None
	Juvenile or adult	Not defined	Posterior subcapsular	Nonprogressive	None
Miniature schnauzer	Congenital	Autosomal recessive	Nuclear and cortical	Variable progression	Posterior lenticonus, microophthalmia
Old English sheepdog	Congenital	Not defined	Nuclear and cortical	Progressive	PPM, microophthalmia, retinal dysplasia
Poodles					
Toy and miniature	Juvenile or adult	Not defined	Cortical	Progressive	None
Standard	Juvenile	Not defined	Equatorial	Progressive	None
Rottweiler	Juvenile or adult	Not defined	Posterior subcapsular and cortical	Nonprogressive	None
Samoyed	Congenital	Autosomal recessive	Nuclear and cortical	Variable progression	Retinal detachment, skeletal chondrodysplasia
Siberian husky	Juvenile	Not defined	Posterior subcapsular, equatorial	Variable progression	None
Staffordshire terrier	Congenital	Not defined	Nuclear and cortical	Progressive	None
	Congenital	Not defined	Posterior subcapsular	Nonprogressive	Persistent hyperplastic primary vitreous or tunica vasculosa lentis
Welsh springer spaniel	Juvenile	Autosomal recessive	Cortical	Progressive	None
West Highland white terrier	Congenital	Autosomal recessive	Nuclear and cortical	Progressive	Microophthalmia
	Juvenile	Not defined	Posterior Y suture	Nonprogressive	None

[a]All dogs with cataracts should be evaluated for retinal degeneration.
[b]These findings may or may not be present.

1038

Table 99–3. **Characteristics of Selected Nonhereditary Cataracts**

Etiology	Location and Description	Progression	Recommendations	Comments
Diabetes mellitus	Equatorial vacuoles	Progressive	Lentectomy once visual impairment occurs, providing diabetes is controlled	Common in diabetic dogs Not common in diabetic cats
Hypocalcemia	Punctate, cortical opacities	Slow, incomplete progression	Lentectomy not indicated because progression to visual impairment is rare	Severity and progression may relate to levels of hypocalcemia
Geriatric	Linear or triangular cortical opacities	Slowly progressive	Lentectomy rarely needed; indicated only if visual impairment present	Progression to visual impairment rare except in long-lived breeds
Secondary to retinal degeneration	Posterior cortical	Progressive	Lentectomy not indicated	Ophthalmoscopic retinal changes and visual impairment often present before cataracts
Secondary to uveitis	Subcapsular and cortical	Variable progression	Lentectomy indicated if retinal function is normal and uveitis resolved	Potential for recurrence of severe uveitis after lentectomy and therefore decreased prognosis for vision

with subsequent glucose-6-phosphate (G6P) buildup in lenticular cells.
2. Aldose reductase converts G6P to sorbitol, which osmotically pulls water into lens fibers.
3. Protein and electrolyte concentrations are therefore altered, resulting in a loss of lens fiber integrity and cell degeneration.
II. Free radical damage to lens fiber membranes and proteins
   A. Accumulation of oxidative damage with age
      1. Light- and metabolism-associated production of endogenous oxygen free radicals
      2. Decreased glutathione levels with age
   B. Chronic inflammation
III. Mechanical disruption of lens fibers
   A. Lens rupture from trauma
   B. Electrical current
IV. Disruption of normal lens embryogenesis
   A. Congenital cataracts
   B. Predominantly affects the lens nucleus and capsule
   C. Tunica vasculosa lentis abnormalities (see later)
V. Except for hyperglycemia/galactosemia, pathophysiology of cataract formation poorly understood

Clinical Signs

I. Signalment (see Table 99–2)
II. History
   A. Visual impairment
      1. Except in working dogs, vision loss associated with unilateral cataracts is rarely noted by owners.
      2. Pets with slow onset bilateral cataracts often navigate familiar environments with minimal difficulty.
   B. White to bluish-white appearance to eye
   C. History of
      1. Toxin exposure
      2. Chronic intraocular disease
      3. Trauma
      4. Metabolic disorders
      5. Orphaned neonate on milk replacer
      6. Cataracts in related animals
III. Ophthalmic findings (see Tables 99–2 and 99–3)
   A. Lens opacification
      1. Full mydriasis is essential.
      2. Retro-illumination using the tapetal/fundic reflex is helpful.
   B. Visual impairment
      1. It relates to the degree of lenticular opacification if the rest of visual pathway is normal.
      2. Cataracts do not inhibit normal pupillary light responses.
   C. Other potential ophthalmic changes
      1. Lens-induced uveitis: may occur with any stage of cataract, but seen most commonly with hypermature cataracts
      2. Lens luxation: primary or secondary
      3. Secondary glaucoma
         a) Associated with intumescent cataracts
            (1) A large swollen lens from a sudden increase in lens hydration
            (2) Seen in rapidly progressing cataracts
            (3) Results in shallow anterior chamber and collapse of the iridocorneal angle
         b) Associated with a luxated cataract
         c) Associated with lens- (cataract)-induced uveitis
      4. Retinal degeneration
      5. Vitreal abnormalities

6. Multiple congenital ocular anomalies
IV. Signs of systemic disease
  A. Cataracts may be the first clinical change recognized in diabetics.
  B. See also Chaps. 43 and 101.

Diagnosis

I. Presence of cataract on ophthalmic exam diagnostic
II. Determining cause
  A. Rule out metabolic disorders with physical and clinicopathologic exam.
  B. Diagnosis of inherited cataract is based on signalment, absence of other abnormalities, and localization.

Differential Diagnosis

I. Lenticular sclerosis associated with age
  A. Most dogs >6 years of age have lenticular sclerosis.
  B. The lens becomes denser with age, giving it a bluish appearance centrally, with a clear cortical zone peripherally.
  C. Lenticular sclerosis does not block the fundic reflex, as do cataracts, and has minimal effect on vision.
II. Other causes of ocular media opacification
  A. Corneal edema or scarring
  B. Aqueous humor opacification as seen in uveitis
  C. Intraocular tumors
  D. Vitreal inflammation or congenital vitreal abnormalities
  E. Retinal detachment
III. Other causes of visual impairment associated with cataracts
  A. Retinal degeneration: rule out with fundic exam or electroretinogram (ERG)
  B. Retinal detachment: rule out with ERG and ultrasonography
  C. Congenital vitreal abnormalities: rule out with biomicroscopy and detailed posterior segment examination

Treatment

I. Medical therapy
  A. No medical therapy has demonstrated clinical efficacy in reversing cataracts in dogs and cats.
  B. Diet-related lens opacities in orphaned puppies and kittens may be reversible with improved nutrition.
    1. Orphaned animals on milk replacer should be examined at 3–4 weeks of age for lens opacities.
    2. Wean these animals onto a high-quality commercial food as soon as possible if opacities are present.
II. Surgical cataract removal (lentectomy)
  A. Only clinically proven therapy for vision improvement in animals with cataracts
  B. Presurgical considerations

1. Owners should be informed of the time and financial commitment required.
2. When should cataract surgery be performed?
  a) Traditionally, cataracts were not removed until pets were functionally blind, because cataract surgery is not 100% successful and aphakic (no lens) vision is poor.
  b) However, recent improvements in cataract surgery, the availability of intraocular lenses, and higher reported success rates for immature cataracts support early lentectomy (Davidson et al., 1990).
3. Intraocular lenses (IOLs) are now available for dogs and cats.
  a) IOLs are plastic lenses placed inside the empty lens capsule after cataract extraction.
  b) Aphakic eyes are extremely far-sighted.
  c) Most animals with only aphakic vision are able to negotiate their environment without difficulty, but visual impairment is still functionally evident.
  d) Implantation of an IOL after lentectomy is recommended, as it is well tolerated and provides near-normal vision (Davidson et al., 1991a; Peiffer et al., 1991).
4. The presence of lens-induced uveitis before surgery may decrease the long-term success rate.
5. Preoperative medical therapy includes the following.
  a) Prophylactic control of inflammation
  b) Mydriasis to allow lens removal
  c) Perioperative antimicrobial therapy
  d) Preoperative medical regimen highly variable among surgeons (Gelatt, 1991b)
C. Three surgical techniques
1. Intracapsular cataract extraction: reserved for luxated lens
2. Standard extracapsular extraction
  a) Technique involves manual removal of lens from the capsule after making a large incision (15 mm) in the perilimbal cornea or sclera; the posterior lens capsule remains intact.
  b) Reported success rates vary, but approximately 70–85% of dogs have vision after surgery (Rooks et al., 1985; Paulsen et al., 1986, Davidson et al., 1990).
  c) Advantages include less equipment required compared with phacoemulsification and excellent exposure.
  d) Disadvantages include collapse of the eye during surgery, difficulty in removal of peripheral lens cortex, and large corneal incision.
3. Phacoemulsification cataract extraction
  a) This procedure involves aspiration of the lens after it is fragmented and emulsified with high-frequency sound waves. The anterior chamber is maintained by irriga-

tion of fluid into the eye throughout the procedure (Boldy, 1988; Nasisse et al., 1991)

    b) Reported success rate is 85–95% (Miller et al., 1987; Davidson et al., 1991a).

    c) Advantages include small corneal incision, maintenance of globe shape during surgery, subjectively less postoperative inflammation, and better ability to remove all lens material.

    d) Disadvantages include cost of equipment and potential for damage to intraocular structures by the phacoemulsification instruments.

D. Postoperative therapy
1. Control of intraocular inflammation
    a) Topical 1% prednisolone acetate q 4–6 h, decreasing the frequency over several weeks to months as inflammation subsides
    b) Aspirin 3–5 mg/kg PO BID and/or prednisolone 1 mg/kg PO SID for 7–10 days
2. Topical antimicrobials for 7–14 days
3. Mydriatic agents for postoperative miosis

E. Potential complications
1. Glaucoma secondary to surgically induced uveitis
2. Pupillary seclusion
    a) Extensive posterior synechia resulting in loss of the pupil
    b) Laser synechotomy or surgical iridectomy required to improve vision
3. Posterior capsular fibrosis
    a) It is one of the leading causes of decreased vision after cataract surgery.
    b) Surgical or laser capsulotomy improves vision.
4. Retinal detachment: mechanism incompletely understood, surgical correction or laser photocoagulation sometimes possible

III. Lens resorption
A. Cataractous lens fibers may liquefy and ''leak'' out of the lens capsule (see Hypermature cataracts, earlier).
B. Such lens resorption can result in the return of vision.
1. The amount of vision restored depends on the degree of lens resorption.
2. Lens resorption occurs more commonly in young (<1.5 years) animals.
3. Unfortunately, resorption is rarely complete and is often accompanied by lens-induced uveitis (Rubin and Gelatt, 1968).

Patient Monitoring

I. Monitoring of animals before cataract surgery
A. Monitor the degree of lens involvement and visual impairment every 3–6 months to determine when and if surgery is indicated.
B. Monitor for complications associated with cataracts, such as the development of ocular cloudiness, ocular redness, blepharospasm, or increased discharge.

II. Monitoring of animals after cataract surgery
A. The level of intraocular inflammation, intraocular pressure (IOP), and pupil position should be evaluated at 1–2 weeks and 4–6 weeks postoperatively, and then every 3–4 months during the first year after surgery.
B. Sudden increase in corneal edema, ocular discharge, or blepharospasm warrants immediate re-evaluation.

LENS LUXATION

Definition

I. Abnormal lens position
II. Subluxation
A. Malpositioned lens, but still in the posterior chamber
B. Some zonule attachment still present
III. Complete luxation
Complete loss of zonule attachment and displacement of the lens from the posterior chamber

Causes and Pathophysiology

I. Primary lens luxation (inherited)
A. Exact pathophysiology is not known.
B. Reports of inflammatory cells associated with the zonules suggest that subclinical ocular inflammation may be involved (Gwin et al., 1982).
C. Other reports have not found inflammatory cells and suggest a primary defect in the zonules (Martin, 1978; Curtis, 1983).
II. Secondary lens luxation
A. Globe enlargement secondary to glaucoma
1. Enlargement causes physical stretching and rupture of zonules; glaucoma occurs before lens luxation.
2. Primary lens luxation can also cause glaucoma, because of mechanical blockage of aqueous drainage.
3. Cataractous lenses may luxate, especially in older animals, probably secondary to chronic lens-induced uveitis.
B. Intraocular inflammation: zonule rupture from proteolytic and oxidative damage associated with chronic inflammation
C. Intraocular tumors of the ciliary body or posterior segment: mechanically displace the lens
D. Trauma
1. Blunt trauma to the orbit can potentially disrupt zonules.
2. There is little documentation of traumatic lens luxations in small animals.
E. Microphakia/lens coloboma: overextension of zonule attachments or absence of zonular attachment
F. Ehlers-Danlos syndrome (extremely rare in animals)

1. Hereditary defect in collagen synthesis
2. Results in weak zonules and subsequent lens luxations

Clinical Signs

I. Primary lens luxations
   A. Signalment
      1. Reported breeds
         a) Jack Russell terrier
         b) Fox terrier
         c) Sealyham terrier
         d) Miniature bull terrier
         e) Tibetan terrier
         f) Border collie
      2. Adults: 3–8 years of age
      3. Females more common than males
   B. History
      1. Sudden change in appearance of eye
      2. Blepharospasm, ocular redness, and cloudiness, especially if secondary glaucoma present
   C. Ophthalmic findings
      1. Subluxation
         a) Aphakic crescent
            (1) Fundic reflex visible around the edge of a subluxated lens
            (2) Usually dorsolateral
            (3) Mydriasis helpful: however, mydriasis contraindicated if IOP is elevated
         b) Increased lens motility when eye moves
         c) Iridodonesis: iris tremoring
         d) Subtle change in anterior chamber depth
         e) Vitreous or zonules in anterior chamber
      2. Complete luxation
         a) Anterior luxation (most common)
            (1) Loss of detectable anterior chamber
            (2) Lens equator visible anterior to iris
            (3) Corneal edema
         b) Posterior luxation
            (1) Very deep anterior chamber and vitreous within the pupil or anterior chamber
            (2) Marked iridodonesis
            (3) Lens fully displaced in posterior vitreous cavity
      3. Other potential ophthalmic changes
         a) Increased IOP
            May occur with any form of lens luxation, but is especially common with anterior lens luxations
         b) Anterior uveitis
         c) Corneal edema due to cornea–lens contact and/or elevated IOP
II. Secondary lens luxation
   A. Ocular signs of chronic anterior uveitis or vitritis
      Chronic uveitis is reported as the most common cause of lens luxation in cats, with feline immunodeficiency virus the most common cause identified (Olivero et al., 1991).
   B. Globe enlargement due to glaucoma

1. Breeds predisposed to primary glaucoma (see Chap. 98)
2. Ocular changes consistent with chronic glaucoma and a history of glaucoma before lens luxation
3. Lens most often posteriorly subluxated
   C. Cataracts
      1. History of cataracts before lens luxation
      2. Often hypermature cataract
      3. Ocular evidence of past or current uveitis
   D. Presence of a space-occupying mass of the iris or ciliary body and associated ophthalmic changes (see Chap. 97)
   E. Ehlers-Danlos syndrome
      1. Rare autosomal dominant disease
      2. Usually presented early in life, <1 year old
      3. Also cataracts, corneal edema, and hyperelastic skin and eyelids
   F. Trauma: history or physical evidence of serious head trauma
   G. Microphakia or lens coloboma

Diagnosis

I. Ocular examination confirms the diagnosis, but ultrasonography is helpful if ocular opacification precludes detailed ocular exam.
II. Determination of a cause may not be easy.
   A. Primary luxation: breed predisposition and lack of historical or exam findings to support secondary luxation
   B. Secondary luxation
      1. Diagnosis depends on detecting a known cause of secondary luxation on examination.
      2. With enlarged glaucomatous eyes, the temporal relationship between the onset of the glaucoma and the lens luxation, along with breed predisposition, is helpful in determining whether the luxation is primary or secondary. This is important in making a prediction for the fellow eye, because the presence of globe enlargement most likely indicates that irreversible vision loss has already occurred.

Differential Diagnosis

I. Subluxation or anterior luxation
   A. Microphakia
   B. Hypermature cataract (morgagnian cataract)
      1. Hypermature cataracts have a wrinkled anterior capsule, a reduced lens thickness, and a deep anterior chamber.
      2. See Cataract section, earlier.
II. Posterior luxation
   A. Previous lentectomy
   B. Congenital aphakia: rare
   C. Resorbed cataract: capsular bag is present in pupil

Treatment

I. Medical therapy for associated ocular changes
   A. Glaucoma

1. Control IOP as outlined in Chap. 98.
2. When lentectomy is desired for a subluxated or posterior luxated lens, miotic therapy (such as pilocarpine) for glaucoma is contraindicated because it makes lens removal difficult.
3. Although miotic therapy (topical 1% pilocarpine BID-TID) is beneficial in preventing posterior displacement of an anterior luxated lens before lentectomy, it may induce a significant increase in IOP and should be used for <24 hours preoperatively.
4. Miotic therapy is also beneficial in preventing anterior displacement of a posterior luxated lens when lentectomy is *not* desired.
5. Glaucoma may not be controllable without lentectomy.
B. Uveitis
1. Administer topical 1% prednisolone acetate TID-QID as needed if uveitis is present.
2. If lens extraction is planned, anti-inflammatory therapy is indicated as described for preoperative therapy of cataracts.
II. Intracapsular lens extraction
A. Indications
1. It is recommended for anterior luxated lenses and for subluxated lenses associated with increased IOP.
2. Any subluxated lens not associated with complications may be removed or simply monitored for the development of secondary ocular changes.
3. Necessity of surgery for posterior luxated lenses is controversial.
a) Lens may move from posterior to anterior segment, resulting in secondary complications.
b) Effect of the lens in the vitreous on retinal function is unknown.
c) Removal of posteriorly luxated lens is more difficult.
B. Advantages of lentectomy
1. To prevent or help control glaucoma and therefore preserve vision
a) Maintenance of normal IOP is often easier after removal of a luxated lens.
b) Chronic secondary glaucoma or the presence of iridocorneal angle changes may decrease the benefit of lentectomy.
c) Consequently, lens removal does not always result in control of glaucoma associated with lens luxation.
d) Removal of a lens luxated *secondary* to glaucoma is not indicated.
2. To prevent chronic uveitis, corneal endothelial damage, and other complications associated with lens luxations
3. To implant a ciliary sulcus-based intraocular lens to improve vision
C. Disadvantages of lentectomy
1. Complications associated with lentectomy (see Cataracts, earlier)
2. Potential worsening of any underlying uveitis

D. Pre- and postoperative considerations
1. Control of uveitis and prevention of ocular infection are accomplished as described for cataract lentectomy.
2. Medical control of glaucoma (if possible) before lentectomy is beneficial.
3. The use of miotics or mydriatics depends on the IOP and lens position.
a) Mydriatics are used for <24 hours preoperatively for posterior luxated and subluxated lenses.
b) The use of short-acting mydriatics such as tropicamide (BID-QID) instead of atropine is recommended in the event that mydriasis results in increased IOP.
c) Miotics may be beneficial preoperatively for an anteriorly luxated lens to prevent inadvertent movement behind the pupil; however, they may cause increased IOP.
III. Lens couching
A. It involves manual displacement of an anteriorly luxated lens into the vitreous as a salvage procedure in an attempt to control glaucoma, in animals who are already blind or who are not good candidates for surgery.
B. It is never performed in animals for whom lentectomy is ultimately desired.
C. See Gelatt (1991b) for technique.
D. Successful couching is followed with miotic therapy to keep the pupil aperture small enough to prevent recurrent anterior luxation of the lens.

Patient Monitoring

I. Monitor IOP and lens position in animals with subluxations or posterior luxations.
A. Monthly to bimonthly exams are advised.
B. The development of ocular cloudiness, ocular redness, blepharospasm, or increased ocular discharge warrants immediate evaluation.
II. Monitor fellow eye in cases of unilateral primary lens luxation.

CONGENITAL VITREAL DISORDERS

Persistent Primary Vitreous

Definition

I. Failure of the primary vitreous to regress
II. Non-patent remnants of the hyaloid artery or primary vitreous
A. Mittendorf's dot: a ring or dot on the anterior vitreous face, visible on biomicroscopy in most animals
B. Persistent, non-patent hyaloid remnant: extending a variable length from the axial posterior lens into the vitreous
C. Bergmeister's papilla

1. Small white tube extending from the optic disk into the vitreous
2. Occasional finding in dogs <6 months old
   D. Incidental findings: cause no clinical problems
III. Dysplastic remnants of the hyaloid artery or primary vitreous
   A. Persistent hyperplastic primary vitreous (PHPV): persistence of fibrovascular tissue extending from the optic disk, often to the anterior vitreal face or posterior lens capsule
   B. Persistent hyperplastic tunica vasculosa lentis (PHTVL): persistence of fibrovascular tissue around the lens

Causes

I. Unknown
II. Inherited trait in Doberman pinschers and Staffordshire bull terriers
   A. Multiple locus inheritance pattern has been postulated in Dobermans (Stades, 1983a, 1983b).
   B. Exact mode of inheritance in Staffordshire bull terriers is unknown (Leon et al., 1986).

Pathophysiology

I. The primary vitreous is a vascular tissue arising from mesenchymal tissue within the optic cup.
   A. Hyaloid artery of the primary vitreous branches to form the tunica vasculosa lentis, a vascular net surrounding the developing lens.
   B. These tissues atrophy during late gestation and early postpartum period.
      1. No patent remnants are normally present after 13–17 days post partum (Duddy et al., 1983).
      2. Small non-patent remnants may be present up to 6 months.
II. Reason for failure of regression or persistence is unknown.
   A. Retinal angiogenic factors and vitreal anti-angiogenic factors may control development and regression of hyaloid artery and tunica vasculosa lentis.
   B. Loss of the normal balance of these factors during development is postulated as a cause of PHPV/PHTVL.

Clinical Signs

I. Signalment
   A. Breed predilections
      1. Doberman pinscher
      2. Staffordshire bull terrier
      3. Single reports of PHPV: greyhound, German shepherd dog, miniature poodle, Irish setter, Border collie
   B. Usually presented in the first year of life
II. History
   A. Visual impairment
      Mild to functionally blind depending on the degree of primary vitreous persistence and lens changes

   B. Abnormal appearance of eye
III. Ophthalmic findings
   A. Leukocoria: white pupil
   B. Variable degrees of visual impairment
   C. Lenticular and perilenticular opacities
      1. Posterior lens capsule pigmentation
      2. Retrolental fibrovascular membranes
      3. Hyaloid artery remnants in the vitreous
      4. Posterior lenticonus: conical protrusion of the lens into vitreous
      5. Cataracts
   D. Persistent pupillary membranes
   E. Retinal dysplasia
      1. Hard to see clinically because of lenticular changes
      2. More frequent and severe in the Staffordshire bull terrier than in the Doberman pinscher
      3. Occasional retinal detachment reported
   F. Microphthalmia, lens coloboma, microphakia, and lens luxations (Doberman pinschers)

Diagnosis

I. Signalment
   The condition is present since birth, although cataracts and therefore the prominence of the ocular opacification may progress with age.
II. Diagnosis based on ocular findings
   A. Presence of posterior lens capsule pigmentation and/or a retrolental fibrovascular membrane
   B. Slit lamp biomicroscopy and indirect ophthalmoscopy essential for accurate assessment of changes
   C. Ultrasonography and electroretinography useful for evaluation of retinal changes when ocular opacities preclude posterior segment visualization

Differential Diagnosis

I. Leukocoria
   A. Cataract
   B. Retinal detachment
   C. Congenital intraocular neoplasia (rare)
   D. Endophthalmitis
   E. Differentiated with detailed ophthalmic exam, along with ultrasonography and electroretinography as needed
II. Vitreoretinal dysplasia
   A. Seen in Labrador retrievers, Siberian huskies, Samoyeds
   B. Usually associated with skeletal dwarfism
   C. May present with cataracts and retinal detachment
   D. Differentiated on basis of signalment, ophthalmic exam, and ultrasonography

Treatment

I. Lentectomy and anterior vitrectomy may be considered.
   A. Indicated only for eyes where lenticular and ante-

rior vitreous opacities are a major cause of visual impairment.
  B. Success rate (improvement in vision) is reported as 50% (Stades, 1983a).
  C. Thorough retinal evaluation including electroretinography and ultrasonography is important before considering surgery.
II. Mydriatics (topical 1% atropine every 2–3 days) may improve vision in animals with predominantly central opacities.

Patient Monitoring

  I. Cataract progression
    A. Cataracts are reported as slowly progressive.
    B. Progression appears to be related to the severity of the PHPV, with greater progression reported in Dobermans than in Staffordshire bull terriers (Leon et al., 1986).
    C. Histopathologically, the severity of lenticonus and cataract is related to the degree of posterior lens capsule thinning and retrolental fibrovascular plaque development (van der Linde-Sipman et al., 1983).
  II. Development of secondary ocular complications in eyes that do not undergo surgery
    A. None reported, but long-term follow-up not available
    B. Recurrent intraocular hemorrhages, glaucoma, and retinal detachment reported in humans

ACQUIRED VITREAL DISORDERS

Asteroid Hyalosis

Definition

  I. Crystals of phospholipids and calcium in the vitreous
  II. Not associated with other systemic or ocular disease

Causes

  I. Unknown
  II. Age-related degeneration suspected

Pathophysiology

  I. Electron microscopy of asteroid hyalosis in humans reveals phospholipid crystals and calcium.
  II. Products of degenerated retinal epithelial cells are proposed as a source of the phospholipids.

Clinical Signs and Diagnosis

  I. Signalment and history
    A. Primarily geriatric patients
    B. Usually no clinical evidence of visual impairment
    C. Occasionally ''fly-biting'' behavior reported
  II. Ophthalmic findings

    A. White refractile bodies scattered throughout the vitreous
    B. Minimal to no free movement and do not settle ventrally

Differential Diagnosis

  I. Cholesterolosis bulbi: settle ventrally in the vitreous
  II. Vitritis: inflammatory cells in the vitritis usually associated with uveitis and/or retinitis

Treatment and Monitoring

  I. Incidental finding
  II. No specific treatment warranted

Cholesterosis Bulbi

Definition

  I. Cholesterol crystals in the vitreous
  II. Associated with vitreal liquefaction

Causes and Pathophysiology

  I. Unknown
  II. May represent a secondary phenomenon after intraocular hemorrhage, inflammation, or retinal degeneration
  III. Also known as syneresis scintillans

Clinical Signs and Diagnosis

  I. Rare and usually bilateral
  II. Ophthalmic findings
    A. Angular, glittering, golden bodies in the vitreous
    B. Settle ventrally but will distribute throughout the vitreous with head or eye movement

Differential Diagnosis

  I. Asteroid hyalosis: ophthalmic appearance or history of previous ocular disease helps distinguish from asteroid hyalosis
  II. Vitritis: usually associated with uveitis or retinitis

Treatment and Monitoring

  I. It is considered an incidental finding, but always evaluate the eye for retinal hemorrhage or inflammation.
  II. No specific treatment is warranted.

Bibliography

Boldy KL: Current status of canine cataract surgery. Semin Vet Med Surg (Small Anim) 3:62, 1988
Curtis R: Clinical and pathological observations concerning the aetiology of primary lens luxation in the dog. Vet Rec 112:238, 1983
Davidson MG, Nasisse MP, Rusnak IM et al: Success rates of unilateral vs. bilateral cataract extraction in dogs. Vet Surg 19:232, 1990

Davidson MG, Nasisse MP, Jamieson VE et al: Phacoemulsification and IOL implantation in dogs: a study of surgical results in 182 dogs. Prog Vet Comp Ophthalmol 4:233, 1991a

Davidson MG, Nasisse MP, Jamieson VE et al: Traumatic anterior lens capsule disruption. J Am Anim Hosp Assoc 27:410, 1991b

Duddy JA, Wolodymyr PC, Rubin LF: Hyaloid artery patency in neonatal beagles. Am J Vet Res 44:2344, 1983

Dziezyc J, Brooks D: Canine cataracts. Compend Contin Educ Pract Vet 5:81, 1983

Gelatt KN: Ophthalmic examination and diagnostics. p. 224. In: Textbook of Veterinary Ophthalmology. 2nd Ed. Lea & Febiger Philadelphia, 1991a

Gelatt KN: The canine lens. p. 429. In: Textbook of Veterinary Ophthalmology. 2nd Ed. Lea & Febiger, Philadelphia, 1991b

Grant WM: Toxicology of the Eye. 3rd Ed. Charles C Thomas, Springfield, IL, 1986

Gwin RM, Samuelson DA, Powell NG et al: Primary lens luxation in the dog associated with lenticular zonule degeneration and its relationship to glaucoma. J Am Anim Hosp Assoc 18:485, 1982

Jamieson VE, Davidson MG, Nasisse MP, English RV: Ocular complications following cobalt-60 radiotherapy of neoplasms in the canine head region. J Am Anim Hosp Assoc 27:51, 1991

Leon A, Curtis R, Barnett KC: Hereditary persistent hyperplastic primary vitreous in the Staffordshire bull terrier. J Am Anim Hosp Assoc 22:765, 1986

Martin CL: Zonular defects in the dog: a clinical and scanning electron microscopic study. J Am Anim Hosp Assoc 14:571, 1978

Miller TR, Whitley RD, Meek LA, Garcia GA: Phacofragmentation and aspiration for cataract extraction in the dogs: 56 cases (1980–1984). J Am Vet Med Assoc 190:1577, 1987

Nasisse MP, Davidson MG, Jamieson VE et al: Phacoemulsification and IOL implantation: a study of surgical technique in 182 dogs. Prog Vet Comp Ophthalmol 4:225, 1991

Olivero DK, Riis RC, Dutton AG et al: Feline lens displacement. A retrospective analysis of 345 cases. Prog Vet Comp Ophthalmol 1:239, 1991

Paulsen ME, Lavach JD, Severin GA, Eichenbaum JD: The effect of lens induced uveitis on the success of extracapsular cataract extraction: a retrospective study of 65 lens removals in the dog. J Am Anim Hosp Assoc 22:49, 1986

Peiffer RL, Gaiddon J: Posterior chamber intraocular lens implantation in the dog: results of 65 implants in 61 patients. J Am Anim Hosp Assoc 27:453, 1991

Playter RF: The development and maturation of a cataract. J Am Anim Hosp Assoc 13:317, 1977

Quinn AJ: Embryology, anatomy, and physiology of the lens. Canine Pract 8:19, 1981

Remillard RL, Pickett JP, Thatcher CD, Davenport DJ: Comparison of kittens fed queens milk with those fed milk replacers. Am J Vet Res 54:901, 1993

Roberts SM, Lavach JD, Severin GA et al: Ophthalmic complications following megavoltage irradiation of the nasal and paranasal cavities in dogs. J Am Vet Med Assoc 190:43, 1987

Rooks RL, Brightman AH, Musselman EE et al: Extracapsular cataract extraction: an analysis of 240 operations in dogs. J Am Vet Med Assoc 187:1013, 1985

Rubin LF, Gelatt KN: Spontaneous resorption of the cataractous lens in dogs. J Am Vet Med Assoc 152:139, 1968

Stades FC: Persistent hyperplastic tunica vasculosa lentis and persistent hyperplastic primary vitreous (PHTVL/PHPV) in Doberman pinschers in 90 closely related Doberman pinschers: clinical aspects. J Am Anim Hosp Assoc 16:740, 1980

Stades FC: Persistent hyperplastic tunica vasculosa lentis and persistent hyperplastic primary vitreous in Doberman pinschers: techniques and results of surgery. J Am Anim Hosp Assoc 19:393, 1983a

Stades FC: Persistent hyperplastic tunica vasculosa lentis and persistent hyperplastic primary vitreous in Doberman pinschers: genetic aspects. J Am Anim Hosp Assoc 19:759, 1983b

van der Linde-Sipman JS, Stades FC, de Wolf-Rouendaal D: Persistent hyperplastic tunica vasculosa lentis and persistent hyperplastic primary vitreous in Doberman pinschers: pathological aspects. J Am Anim Hosp Assoc 19:791, 1983

100

Disorders of the Posterior Segment

Cynthia A. Wheeler

CONGENITAL/DEVELOPMENT DISORDERS

Retinal Dysplasia

Definition

I. Retinal dysplasia is an abnormal development (folds, rosettes, generalized disorganization) of the retina present at birth.
II. It can be localized (focal, multifocal, geographic) or generalized (severe, detachment).
III. When severe, it causes visual impairment or blindness.

Causes

I. In many breeds the condition is inherited as an autosomal recessive trait.
II. Certain external factors may cause retinal dysplasia during fetal development.
    A. Exposure to radiation
    B. Infectious diseases: feline leukemia virus, feline panleukopenia, canine herpesvirus, adenovirus, and parvovirus
    C. Toxins
    D. Nutritional disorders: vitamin A deficiency
    E. Intrauterine trauma

Pathophysiology

I. Invagination of the outer retinal layers occurs, which resembles rosettes.
II. The effect on retinal function and vision is dependent on the amount of retina involved.
    A. In mild cases (folds), no visual deficits are noted.
    B. With large geographic lesions, visual deficits may be observed, particularly in dogs marking game in the field.
    C. Animals with retinal detachments are blind.

Clinical Signs

I. Most dogs have good vision and behave normally.
II. Retinal detachments may occur soon after birth or before 1 year of age with subsequent blindness.
III. Some breeds of dogs also have skeletal achondrodysplasia.
    A. Labrador retrievers (Carrig et al., 1974, 1988)
    B. German shepherd dog
    C. Samoyed (Acland and Aguirre, 1991)

Diagnosis

I. The condition is congenital and can be seen on fundic examination as soon as the eyes are opened.
II. Best evaluation, particularly for small lesions, is made at 4–6 weeks and after 10 weeks.
III. The appearance of lesions varies (Table 100–1).
    A. Multifocal folds
        1. These are unilateral or bilateral, multiple round or linear lesions that have a blue-gray appearance before 16 weeks of age.
        2. When few in number, they are most commonly seen adjacent to the optic disk and may disappear as the dog matures.
        3. In the adult, tapetal lesions are dark and hyperreflective.
        4. In nontapetal areas, lesions are well demarcated and light in color.
    B. Geographic lesions
        1. These are larger areas of dysplasia in the tapetal retina dorsal to the optic disk.
        2. Lesions appear blue-white in young dogs and may be difficult to see.
        3. They degenerate into retinal scars that are hyperreflective and hyperpigmented, resembling postinflammatory lesions.
        4. They may result in retinal tears and detachments.
    C. Retinal detachment: may be seen floating behind a dilated pupil

Table 100–1. Funduscopic Appearance of Retinal Dysplasia in Different Breeds

Multifocal Folds	Geographic Lesions	Detachment
Akita	Akita	Afghan
American cocker spaniel	Bedlington terrier	Airedale terrier
Australian shepherd	Border collie	Akita
Beagle	Cavalier King Charles spaniel	Bearded collie
Bearded collie	English springer spaniel	Bedlington terrier
Bedlington terrier	Golden retriever	Border collie
Border collie	Labrador retriever	English springer spaniel
Bullmastiff	Samoyed[a]	Golden retriever
Cavalier King Charles spaniel	Sealyham terrier	Labrador retriever[a, b]
Clumber spaniel	Welsh corgi, Pembroke	Sealyham terrier
Collie	Yorkshire terrier	
Doberman pinscher		
English cocker spaniel		
English springer spaniel		
German shepherd dog[a]		
Golden retriever		
Labrador retriever[a]		
Mastiff		
Newfoundland		
Norwegian elkhound		
Old English sheepdog		
Petit Basset Griffon Veneen		
Puli		
Rottweiler		
Samoyed		
Sealyham terrier		
Soft-coated wheaten terrier		
Welsh corgi, Cardigan		
Welsh corgi, Pembroke		

[a]Skeletal changes.
[b]No skeletal changes.

D. Vitreous degeneration
  1. It may be a predisposing cause of retinal detachment and subsequent blindness.
  2. Viewed through the pupil, thin vitreous strands are seen moving when the eye moves.

Differential Diagnosis

I. Inherited retinal dysplasia cannot be distinguished funduscopically from acquired retinal disorganization and scarring.
II. The larger lesions of retinal dysplasia resemble post-inflammatory lesions.
III. Small physiologic folds or vermiform streaks are similar in appearance, but usually disappear by 6 months of age and are not considered clinically significant.

Treatment and Monitoring

I. There is no treatment available.
II. Except for the development of retinal detachment, the lesions of retinal dysplasia do not progress.
III. The breeding of animals with folds and multifocal dysplastic lesions is controversial.
  A. In most breeds of dog, the decision has been left to the discretion of the owner, although retinal dysplasia should be considered a genetic fault.

B. In the Labrador retriever, Samoyed, and English springer spaniel, breeding is discouraged.
IV. Animals with geographic lesions, retinal detachments, skeletal abnormalities, or concurrent vitreous degeneration should not be bred.

Collie Eye Anomaly (CEA)

Definition and Cause

I. A spectrum of malformations present at birth, ranging from inadequate development of the choroid (choroidal hypoplasia) to defects of the choroid, retina, or optic nerve (coloboma) and complete retinal detachment
II. Inheritance: autosomal recessive

Pathophysiology

I. It is believed to be a failure of induction of the choroid and sclera by a defective retinal pigmented epithelium resulting in choroidal and tapetal hypoplasia, hypopigmentation of the choroid, and neuroectodermal dysplasia at the optic disk.
II. Lesions near the optic disk can be detected in the embryo after the 28th day.

Clinical Signs

I. Affected breeds: rough and smooth collies, Border collie, Shetland sheep dog, Australian shepherd
II. Vision is normal except when there is retinal hemorrhage or detachment or a very large coloboma.

Diagnosis

I. It is recommended that puppies be examined at 6–10 weeks of age.
II. Diagnosis is based on characteristic funduscopic changes.
   A. Choroidal hypoplasia: a pale area temporal to the optic disk, consisting of localized absence of tapetum, loss of pigment in the retinal pigmented epithelium and underlying choroid, a decrease in and disorganization of choroidal vasculature, and exposure of the underlying sclera
   B. Coloboma: in or adjacent to the optic disk, accompanied by an area of choroidal hypoplasia
   C. Retinal detachment: partial or total
   D. Retinal vascular tortuosity: a subjective observation of uncertain significance
   E. Intraocular hemorrhage and microphthalmia: less common findings
III. Diagnosis of the anomaly in merle-colored animals may be difficult; look for a nonpigmented zone or distortion of the choroidal vascular pattern temporal to the optic disk.
IV. Some puppies demonstrate choroidal hypoplasia at an early age, but later the area becomes pigmented, creating a more normal appearance.

Differential Diagnosis

I. Coloboma resulting from failure of the fetal fissure to close properly
   A. Breeds: basenji, collie, Australian shepherd
   B. Typical coloboma: occurs at the ventral, 6 o'clock position and often affects the optic disk
   C. Atypical coloboma: occurs at locations other than the 6 o'clock position
   D. No associated areas of choroidal hypoplasia
II. Retinal dysplasia
III. Tapetal color variations
   A. Color-dilute animals (merles or merle-factored) may have irregular or no pigmentation in the fundus, mimicking choroidal hypoplasia.
   B. The normal tiger-striped choroidal vascular pattern should be intact (Table 100–2).

Patient Monitoring

I. It is believed that the incidence and severity of this entity have been decreased by breeding only "mildly affected" collies.
II. Phenotypically normal collies may carry the gene for CEA. These dogs produce CEA in some puppies when bred to an affected dog.
III. Genetically normal collies are increasing in availability for breeding.

Table 100–2. *Tapetal Variations and Abnormalities*

Normal juvenile tapetum
  Color first appears at 6 weeks
    1. 6 weeks: gray-magenta
    2. 8–12 weeks: blue-green
    3. 12–16 weeks: green-yellow/orange
Normal adult tapetum
  Possible colors
    1. Blue-green: thin tapetum over dark choroid pigment; dark-brown irises
    2. Yellow/orange: normal tapetum over brown choroid pigment; hazel-brown irises
    3. Yellow/white: normal tapetum over pigment-poor choroid; blue irises
    4. Hypoplasia: no or poorly visible tapetum; color-dilute animals
  Potential shapes
    1. Triangular: most dogs
    2. Semicircular: most cats
    3. Isolated patches: toy breeds, color-dilute animals
    4. Mosaic/mottled: color-dilute animals, yellow coat coloration
    5. Islets: toy breeds, color-dilute animals
  Types of margins
    1. Sharply delineated tapetal–nontapetal borders
    2. Irregular borders
    3. Dull muted coloration at margins (resembling early progressive retinal atrophy): golden retriever, yellow Labrador retriever, basenji, buff-colored cockers
Tapetal dysplasia of beagle
    1. Autosomal recessive trait
    2. Tapetal cells develop abnormally and later degenerate
    3. Fundus has no visible tapetum

IV. The only certain way to reduce or eliminate the problem is to avoid breeding affected animals.

Hypoplasia/Micropapilla of the Optic Nerve

Definition

I. Micropapilla is a small optic disk without apparent blindness.
II. Optic nerve hypoplasia (ONH) is a congenital underdevelopment of the optic nerve that causes blindness in the affected eye(s).
III. The two conditions may rarely occur in the same animal and are difficult to differentiate on ophthalmoscopic examination.
IV. Optic nerve aplasia is the absence of a visible optic nerve.

Causes

I. In the dog, ONH and aplasia appear to be inherited conditions.
II. They may also be associated with microphthalmos.

Pathophysiology

I. In micropapilla, the small optic disk probably is caused by abrupt cessation of myelination of retinal nerve fibers at the lamina cribrosa.
II. In ONH, there are reduced numbers of ganglion cells in the retina, resulting in a thin nerve fiber layer with a small optic disk and nerve.
III. In optic nerve aplasia, there is no clinical evidence of an optic nerve. Histologic evaluation may disclose some nerve or glial cell remnants.
IV. ONH and aplasia can be unilateral or bilateral.

Clinical Signs

I. Affected breeds
  A. Micropapilla: miniature and toy poodles, Belgian sheep dog and Tervuren, dachshund, Irish wolfhound
  B. ONH: collie, dachshund, English cocker spaniel, German shepherd dog, miniature and toy poodle
  C. Aplasia: miniature poodle, domestic shorthair cats (rare)
II. Vision
  A. Unilateral ONH does not affect functional vision and may go undetected until mydriasis is noted on clinical examination.
  B. Bilateral ONH causes visual deficits proportional to the degree of hypoplasia. Owners may note no vision dysfunction until the animal is tested.
  C. Animals with optic nerve aplasia are blind in the affected eyes.

Diagnosis and Differential Diagnosis

I. Micropapilla
  A. The optic disk is smaller than usual but normal in appearance.
  B. A dark ring of pigment or a thin hyperreflective crescent or circle may surround it.
  C. Pupillary light responses are normal.
II. Optic nerve hypoplasia
  A. Optic disk is small, discolored, or very dark.
  B. Abnormal, sluggish pupillary light responses are the only way to distinguish it from micropapilla.
  C. The electroretinogram (ERG) is of normal amplitude and waveform.
  D. The visual evoked response (VER) is reduced in severe cases.
III. Optic nerve aplasia
  A. There is no visible optic disk, and retinal vasculature may be abnormal.
  B. There are no pupillary light responses in the affected eye.
  C. The ERG and VER are absent in the affected eye(s).

Patient Monitoring

I. The diseases are not progressive.
II. Animals with optic nerve aplasia or severe hypoplasia should not be bred.

DEVELOPMENTAL AND DEGENERATIVE DISORDERS

Generalized Progressive Retinal Atrophy

Definition

I. In normal dogs, continued maturation of the retinal photoreceptors occurs from birth through 12 weeks.
II. Animals with progressive retinal atrophy (PRA) have either arrested development or early degeneration of the rods and/or cones.
III. The end result is blindness.

Causes and Pathophysiology

I. PRA is usually inherited as an autosomal recessive disease in most breeds of dogs.
  A. Siberian husky: X-linked from (Acland et al., 1993)
  B. Abyssinian cat: autosomal dominant
II. The actual triggering mechanism for photoreceptor degeneration varies but may involve altered enzyme function or abnormal protein synthesis.

Classification

I. Progressive retinal atrophy is a descriptive term that is applied to numerous types of photoreceptor abnormalities.
II. PRA can be classified by whether the rods and cones never develop properly (dysplasia) or degenerate early (degeneration).
  A. Rod-cone dysplasia: Irish setter (rcd-1), collie (rcd-2), miniature schnauzer
  B. Rod dysplasia: elkhounds; Abyssinian cats in England, mixed-breed cats
  C. Early rod degeneration: elkhounds
  D. Progressive rod-cone degeneration
    1. Prcd-1 (same genetic locus): miniature poodles, English cockers, American cockers, and Labrador retrievers
    2. Prcd-2 (different gene): Tibetan terrier
    3. Abyssinian cats of Sweden
    4. Unspecified types: numerous breeds
III. Photoreceptor dysplasias have an early onset (9–60 days) and progress to blindness rapidly (usually 1 year).
IV. Photoreceptor degenerations have a later onset (1–8 years) and progress more slowly to blindness (Table 100–3).

Clinical Signs

I. Night blindness occurs initially because rods (responsible for dim light vision) are affected first.
II. In most cases, cones are eventually affected, resulting in day blindness later.
III. The age of onset and rate of progression vary and are usually breed-specific (see Table 100–3).

Table 100–3. **Age of Onset for Generalized Progressive Retinal Atrophy**

Breed	Age (Years)	Breed	Age (Years)
Afghan	2	Irish water spaniel	ND
Airedale terrier	2	Italian greyhound	ND
Akita	1–3	Japanese chin	ND
Alaskan malamute	4	Keeshond	ND
American cocker spaniel	2–3; 5[a]	Kerry blue terrier	ND
American Staffordshire terrier	1.5	Labrador retriever	4
Australian cattle dog	3–5; 6[a]	Lhasa apso	ND
Australian shepherd	4	Lowchen	ND
Australian terrier	1	Maltese	ND
Basenji	ND	Manchester terrier (toy)	ND
Basset hound	3; 6–8[a]	Manchester terrier (standard)	ND
Beagle	3–5; 10–13[a]	Mastiff	ND
Bearded collie	1	Miniature pinscher	ND
Bedlington terrier	1.5	Miniature schnauzer	3–5; 10–13[a]
Belgian sheep dog	ND	Norwegian elkhound	0.5; 0.25[a]
Belgian Tervuren	ND	Nova Scotia duck tolling retriever	3–5
Bernese mountain dog	1	Old English sheepdog	ND
Black and tan coonhound	1.5	Papillon	ND
Border collie	2	Pekingese	ND
Border terrier	ND	Pit bull terrier	ND
Borzoi	ND	Pointer	ND
Boston terrier	5	Pomeranian	ND
Boxer	ND	Poodle, miniature	3–5
Briard	ND	Portuguese water dog	ND
Brittany spaniel	4	Puli	ND
Brussels griffon	4	Queensland blue heeler	ND
Bull terrier	ND	Rottweiler	ND
Cairn terrier	1	Saluki	ND
Cavalier King Charles spaniel	ND	Samoyed	3–5
Chesapeake Bay retriever	0.75–1	Schipperke	ND
Chihuahua	ND	Scottish terrier	ND
Chow chow	0.5	Sealyham terrier	ND
Collie	0.5; 5–7[a]	Shetland sheep dog	ND
Curly-coated retriever	3–5	Shih Tzu	ND
Dachshund	1, 4[a]	Siberian husky	ND
Dalmatian	ND	Silky terrier	ND
Doberman pinscher	1	Soft-coated wheaten terrier	ND
English cocker spaniel	4	Swiss hound	ND
English setter	1.5; 7–8[a]	Tibetan spaniel	ND
English springer spaniel	2; 5	Tibetan terrier	1–3
Field spaniel	4	Toy Havanese	ND
German shepherd dog	1.5	Vizsla	ND
German shorthaired pointer	ND	Welsh corgi, Cardigan	1
Giant schnauzer	3–4	Welsh corgi, Pembroke	ND
Golden retriever	2	Whippet	ND
Gordon setter	1	Wirehaired fox terrier	ND
Great Dane	ND	Yorkshire terrier	ND
Greyhound	1.5	Abyssinian cat	8–12 wks;
Irish setter	0.25; 4–5[a]		1.5–2 yr[a]
Irish terrier	ND		

[a]Two forms reported.
ND, Not documented.

IV. PRA affects only the eyes; the rest of the animal remains normal.

Diagnosis

I. A history of progressive vision loss, with bilateral clinical signs of sluggish pupil responses, retinal ves-sel atrophy, and tapetal hyperreflectivity are sugges-tive of PRA.

II. Maze testing in various types of ambient light may be helpful in assessing the loss of vision (see Table 102–1).

III. Ocular examination findings may include the follow-ing.

A. Dilated, poorly responsive pupils

B. Nystagmus in Abyssinian cats
C. Cataract
D. Funduscopic changes
1. Increased tapetal reflectivity and granularity
2. Depigmentation of the nontapetal region
3. Attenuation of retinal blood vessels
4. Pallor or graying of the optic disk
5. Early-stage variant: central strip of healthy retina near the optic disk and area centralis surrounded by dull, gray, degenerate retina
IV. Definitive diagnosis requires electroretinography.
A. The ERG is a quantitative measurement of retinal photoreceptor activity in response to light stimulation.
B. Different retinal degenerations have specific identifying ERG features, such as abnormal wave amplitudes and latencies (Acland, 1988).
C. The ERG is capable of detecting the photoreceptor abnormalities of PRA before they become apparent clinically.
V. The gene responsible for rcd-1 in the Irish setter has been isolated. Irish setters may be tested by submitting a blood sample in sodium citrate preservative (yellow top tube) to the Baker Institute at Cornell University, Ithaca, NY.

Differential Diagnosis

I. Nutritional retinal degeneration: central progressive retinal atrophy (CPRA)
II. Nyctalopia (night blindness)
A. Congenital nyctalopia of the briard
1. Associated with accumulations of arachodonic acid in neural cells and axons, including the retina and optic nerve (Riis and Aguirre, 1983)
2. May be a storage disease, with systemic signs
3. Congenital but does not progress to total blindness
4. Normal-appearing fundus
B. Congenital stationary night blindness of the Tibetan terrier
1. Also called retinal degeneration with inclusions (RDI)
2. Involves buildup of electron-dense inclusions resembling ceroid lipofuscin in all layers of the retina by 8 weeks
3. Night blind by 2 months
4. Funduscopic changes not evident until 3–4 years of age
C. Stationary night blindness of the collie
1. A reduction in the photoreceptor cell layer by as much as 50% (Lindley et al., 1990)
2. Onset by 12 months, progression unknown
III. Sudden acquired retinal degeneration (SARD)
IV. Postretinal causes of blindness (see Chap. 102)
A. Optic nerve disease
B. Central blindness

Treatment and Monitoring

I. No treatment is available.
II. Most animals go blind slowly. Dogs with a central

region of healthy retina may retain vision longer than those with total retinal involvement and may never go totally blind.
III. Most pets are able to adapt to their blindness with minimal difficulty.
IV. Secondary cataracts may result in vision impairment before the retinal degeneration causes blindness; therefore, evaluation of retinal function before lens removal is recommended.
V. Affected animals should not be bred.

Day Blindness

Definition and Causes

I. Day blindness (hemeralopia) is an inherited degeneration of the retinal cones.
II. It is believed to be a simple autosomal recessive trait in the Alaskan malamute and miniature poodle.

Pathophysiology

I. Cones begin to deteriorate at 6 weeks of age and are gone at 6 months.
II. Rods are not affected; the retina of affected adults is morphologically a pure rod retina.

Clinical Signs

I. Breeds affected and age of onset
A. Alaskan malamute: 8 weeks
B. Miniature poodle: 3 months
C. Standard poodle: 1 year
II. Blind in bright light but retain vision in dim or dark light

Diagnosis

I. The history and clinical signs may be suspicious.
II. On ocular examination, the pupillary light responses are normal and the fundus appears normal.
III. ERG confirms the diagnosis.

Differential Diagnosis

I. PRA
II. Central blindness
III. Congenital nyctalopia

Treatment and Monitoring

I. No treatment is available.
II. The disease is not progressive.
III. Affected animals should not be bred.

Central Progressive Retinal Atrophy

Definition

I. It is a progressive retinal degeneration in which photoreceptor degeneration occurs secondary to an abnormality of the underlying retinal pigmented epithelium.

II. Central progressive retinal atrophy (CPRA) is diagnosed frequently in Great Britain but is uncommon elsewhere and has only rarely been seen in dogs bred and raised in the United States.

Causes

I. This clinical entity appears to be caused by poor nutrition.

II. With changes in diet preparation in Europe, this disease has essentially disappeared.

Pathophysiology

I. Hypertrophy and clumping of retinal pigment epithelial cells occur followed by loss of photoreceptor cell outer segments and then photoreceptor cells.

II. Lesions are first seen in the area centralis, temporal to the disk, and progress to involve the peripheral tapetal areas then nontapetal retina.

Clinical Signs

I. In most breeds, lesions usually develop between 1.5 and 3.5 years of age.

II. Central (day) vision is altered early in the disease, leading to a typical history of poor working performance and an inability to mark or catch thrown objects.

III. With time, rods also begin to degenerate, leading to poor vision at any time of the day. Total blindness may not occur.

Diagnosis

I. History of poor working performance coupled with signs of pigment aggregation in the tapetal retina creates suspicion of CPRA.

II. Funduscopic changes are variable, depending on the stage.
   A. Early in the disease, retinal changes are pathognomonic.
   B. There are brown pigmented spots in the area centralis of the tapetal fundus, which are variable in size, shape, and density.

III. With maze testing under different light conditions, dogs have difficulty catching things or seeing stationary objects at a distance or at ground level.

IV. The ERG remains normal until the later stages of the disease.

Differential Diagnosis

I. Vitamin A or E or other antioxidant vitamin deficiency
   A. They usually present as night blindness and are associated with prolonged dietary deficiency.
   B. The ERG is extinguished early.

II. Generalized PRA

Treatment and Monitoring

I. Progression is slow, and some animals never lose vision.

II. Early in the disease, a change in diet may halt its progress.

INFLAMMATORY DISEASES

Chorioretinitis

Definition

I. Chorioretinitis is inflammation of the choroid and adjacent retina.

II. It is often a manifestation of a generalized or systemic illness (see Chap. 101).

Causes

I. Viruses: feline immunodeficiency virus (FIV), feline infectious peritonitis (FIP), canine and feline distemper, canine parvovirus, canine herpesvirus

II. Bacteria: brucellosis, colibacillosis, tuberculosis

III. Mycoses: cryptococcosis, coccidioidomycosis, blastomycosis, histoplasmosis, geotrichosis

IV. Protozoa: toxoplasmosis

V. Algae: prototothecosis

VI. Rickettsia: Rocky Mountain spotted fever, ehrlichiosis

VII. Toxins: lead, ethylene glycol, high levels of oxygen

VIII. Trauma: blunt trauma (proptosis), surgery, foreign body

IX. Immune-mediated diseases: uveodermatologic (VKH-like) syndrome, idiopathic thrombocytopenia, systemic lupus erythematosus, autoimmune hemolytic anemia

X. Parasites: toxocara larval migrans, dirofilariasis

XI. Metabolic disorders: diabetes mellitus, hypertension, uremia, lipemia, hyperviscosity syndrome, anemia

XII. Neoplasia: lymphosarcoma, monoclonal gammopathies, choroidal melanoma, reticulosis (pseudotumor), metastatic tumors, malignant histiocytosis

Pathophysiology

I. The retina has only a limited number of responses to inflammatory disease.

II. The destructive effects of inflammation and subsequent reparative processes in the eye may be more severe than that of the original infection or trauma.

III. Fibroplastic organization of the inflammatory exudates may obstruct vision, block aqueous outflow causing glaucoma, and/or produce detachment of the retina, all resulting in a nonvisual eye.

IV. Depending on the cause of the inflammation, different patterns of chorioretinitis may be seen, i.e., focal, diffuse, peripapillary, etc.

Clinical Signs

I. In many cases systemic signs overshadow ocular ones.

II. Ocular signs include defective vision or blindness, ocular pain, and evidence of secondary glaucoma or accompanying anterior uveitis.

Diagnosis

I. A thorough examination of both the anterior and posterior segments is indicated for every ill animal.
II. Funduscopic changes indicative of chorioretinitis include the following.
   A. Active lesions
      1. Cellular infiltrates
         a) Gray-white fluffy areas; cotton wool spots
         b) Raised granulomas
         c) Diffuse gray or brown discoloration of the tapetal retina
      2. Indistinct borders around lesions
      3. Perivascular cuffing: gray or white sheathing effect
      4. Tortuous retinal vessels, especially arterioles
      5. Edema or exudation within portions of the retina or around the optic disk
      6. Hemorrhage
         a) Intraretinal (deep): focal round spots or dots in the inner and outer plexiform layers
         b) Intraretinal (superficial): radiating, brush- or flame-shaped that follow the axon fiber layer; may be associated with retinal vessels
         c) Preretinal (along vitreal face): keel shaped, may overlay retinal vessels
         d) Subretinal (below the photoreceptor layer or in the choroid): large, dark, unassociated with retinal vessels
      7. Retinal detachment: focal or diffuse
      8. Vitreal haze: cellular or protein infiltrates
   B. Inactive (old) lesions
      1. Pigment epithelial hyperplasia and migration: discrete dark-brown ''cigarette burn'' spots
      2. Tapetal hyperreflectivity: focal, diffuse, or patchy
      3. Nontapetal depigmentation: gray to white foci, with clumping of pigment
      4. Distinct borders
      5. Vascular thinning and attenuation
      6. Choroidal atrophy revealing underlying deep choroidal vessels and white sclera
      7. Retinal atrophy: focal or generalized
III. Discovery of chorioretinitis necessitates a thorough medical work-up to differentiate the cause, including a hemogram, biochemical profile, urinalysis, survey radiography, serology for infectious diseases, and sometimes vitreal aspirate.

Differential Diagnosis

I. Bilateral lesions are more likely to represent systemic disease.
II. Differentiating trends in the appearance of lesions are as follows.

   A. Granulomatous (gray to white) lesions: systemic mycoses, tuberculosis, FIP, neoplasia
   B. Hemorrhagic lesions: toxoplasmosis, lymphosarcoma, FIP, hypertension, idiopathic thrombocytopenia, other bleeding disorders, diabetes mellitus, ehrlichiosis
   C. Perivascular cuffing: viral or bacterial septicemias, lymphosarcoma, FIP, uremia, hypertension, hyperviscosity syndrome
III. Rule out other causes of retinal hemorrhages such as blood dyscrasias, collie eye anomaly, persistent hyaloid remnants, anemia, and vascular anomalies.
IV. Differentiate from retinal dysplasia, CPRA, and PRA.
V. Rule out immune-mediated panuveitis (see Chap. 97).

Treatment

I. Where possible, treat the specific cause.
II. Where the causative agent is unknown, consider the following nonspecific treatments.
   A. Corticosteroids
      1. Use cautiously in areas with endemic infectious diseases
      2. Prednisolone 0.5–2 mg/kg PO BID, tapering the dose as the condition improves
      3. Methylprednisolone 0.2 mg/kg PO BID (fewer side effects)
      4. Subconjunctival steroids
         a) Dexamethasone sodium succinate 0.25–1.25 mg SID
         b) Betamethasone sodium succinate 0.25–0.5 mg once
         c) Flumethasone 0.125–1 mg SID
   B. Nonsteroidal anti-inflammatory drugs
      1. Flunixin meglumine
         a) For use in dogs; not recommended for cats
         b) Dose: 0.25–0.5 mg/kg IV SID-BID for only 1–3 doses
         c) Potential side effects, especially when used with corticosteroids: gastrointestinal bleeding and death
      2. Aspirin
         a) Dogs: 10 mg/kg PO BID
         b) Cats: 6–10 mg/kg PO QOD
   C. Broad-spectrum antibiotics
      1. Chloramphenicol 25–50 mg/kg PO TID
      2. Trimethoprim/sulfadiazine 15–30 mg/kg PO BID
      3. Ampicillin 11–22 mg/kg PO TID (has better blood-aqueous penetration than amoxicillin)

Patient Monitoring

I. Initial funduscopic evaluations are made at least SID-BID to assess treatment progress.
   A. Favorable signs
      1. Active lesions regressing, becoming inactive
      2. Stabilization of intraocular pressure to normal range

B. Unfavorable signs: increased size, type, or number of lesions
II. If chorioretinitis does not improve, reconsider the diagnosis and submit more diagnostic tests.
III. Monitor for secondary sequelae.
    A. Vitreal fibrovascular membranes
    B. Retinal detachment
    C. Intraocular hemorrhage
    D. Secondary glaucoma
    E. Prolonged or permanent hazing of vitreous and posterior lens surface
    F. Extension to anterior uvea

Retinal Detachments

Definition

I. Separation of the neurosensory retina from the underlying retinal pigmented epithelium (RPE).
II. Types of detachments
    A. Rhegmatogenous detachments occur when holes or tears in the retina allow fluid from vitreous body to flow under the retina and cause it to separate from the retinal pigment epithelium layer.
    B. Nonrhegmatogenous detachments may be transudative, exudative, or hemorrhagic.

Causes

I. Rhegmatogenous
    A. Lenticular diseases
    B. Glaucoma
    C. Intraocular inflammation
    D. Developmental aphakic (rare)
    E. Idiopathic retinal disinsertion (dialysis)
    F. Trauma, intraocular surgery
II. Nonrhegmatogenous
    A. Lenticular diseases: hypermature cataracts, luxation
    B. Panuveitis: infectious, immune-mediated
    C. Neoplasia: lymphosarcoma, metastatic tumors
    D. Vitreoretinal fibroplasia: postinflammatory fibrous strands placing traction on the retina
    E. Secondary to systemic disorders: viral, bacterial, or mycotic infections, hypertension, bleeding disorders, uremia, toxins
    F. Trauma: nonsurgical, surgical (lens extraction)
    G. Idiopathic: Shih Tzu
    H. Congenital: retinal dysplasia, collie eye anomaly, multiple ocular anomalies, colobomas
    I. Associated with vitreous displacement or degeneration
    J. Secondary to retrobulbar abscess or mass

Pathophysiology

I. The retina is only firmly attached at the ora ciliaris and the optic disk.
II. Separation occurs as the result of several factors.
    A. Accumulation of inflammatory exudates or transudates, or tumor cells between the retina and RPE
    B. Contraction of cyclitic membranes
    C. Leakage of liquefied vitreous humor through retinal tears, most commonly at the vitreous base
    D. Coalescence of edema within the retina cell layers that cleaves the inner and outer retinal layers (retinoschisis)
III. Once detached, the retina may remain attached at the ora ciliaris and the optic disk, creating a ''morning glory–like'' appearance, or it may tear away from the ora ciliaris, falling into the ventral vitreal space. The optic disk is often obscured from view with the latter.

Clinical Signs

I. Breeds with primary, spontaneous detachments and age at onset are listed below.
    A. Basenji: 2 years
    B. Dachshund: 8 months
    C. English springer spaniel: 1–2 years
    D. Poodle, miniature, standard, and toy: 8 months
    E. Rottweiler: 2–3 years
    F. Shih Tzu: 2–4 years
    G. Akita, Boston terrier, collie, German shepherd dog, Labrador retriever, Old English sheep dog, Shetland sheep dog, Siberian husky: age variable
II. Vision varies from normal, if unilateral, to total blindness, if bilateral.
III. Signs of systemic disease may or may not be apparent.

Diagnosis

I. Pupillary light reflex
    A. Normal in focal or acute detachments
    B. Abnormal in total or chronic detachments
II. Diagnosis of actual detachment
    A. Direct ophthalmic examination with penlight or transilluminator: gray vascular veil of tissue visible behind the pupil or lens
    B. Indirect funduscopy
        1. Focal to diffuse sheet-like elevations obscuring underlying choroid/tapetum
        2. Focal hemorrhages within the detached retina
        3. Holes, tears, or folds in the retina
        4. Associated vitreous degeneration
    C. Scleral depression to detect small tears along vitreous base
III. Ultrasonography, computed tomography, magnetic resonance imaging
    These imaging techniques help delineate the detached retina when the interior of the eye cannot be seen through an opaque cornea or cloudy ocular media.
IV. Aspiration and examination of subretinal fluid or exudates: may help isolate cause

Treatment

I. Treatment of underlying cause (if possible)
II. Medical therapy for detachment
    A. Consider prednisone 0.5–2 mg/kg PO BID.

B. Mannitol 1–2 g/kg IV may be useful in transudative detachments.

III. Surgical therapy for detachment
   A. Complete retinal detachments: vitrectomy, aspiration of subretinal fluid, and the use of expandable gases to push the neurosensory retina back to the surface of the retinal pigment epithelium layer followed by laser therapy or cryotherapy, or the placement of retinal tacks to secure the retina have had limited success in dogs (Vainisi et al., 1990).
   B. Retinal tears: remove the subretinal fluid, then follow with laser therapy, cryotherapy, or some tacking procedure.
   C. Scleral buckling procedures in which a prosthetic ''belt'' is used to bring the choroid into apposition with the detached retina are difficult to perform in animals.
   D. Prophylactic treatment with cryotherapy or laser therapy to create firm adhesions of retina to the choroid/sclera along the edge of partial detachments may be performed (Hendrix et al., 1993).
   E. Cryotherapy or laser therapy may also be applied prophylactically prior to cataract surgery in cases at risk.

Patient Monitoring

I. Many detachments seen in animals are incidental findings, unless there are obvious visual deficits, and are too chronic to recommend surgical correction.

II. When the retina separates, degeneration of the photoreceptor cell outer segments is complete within 2 weeks; however, the photoreceptor inner segments and cell bodies may remain unaffected for months after the separation.

III. Prognosis with treatment is uncertain.
   A. In cases caused by trauma, inflammation, or infection, retinal reattachment and return of vision are variable.
   B. If reattachment occurs early, vision may return in dogs but does so only rarely in cats.
   C. If the detachment has been present for a month or more, the prognosis for return of vision is guarded.
   D. Those associated with metabolic or immune-mediated diseases may recur.

IDIOPATHIC DISORDERS

Sudden Acquired Retinal Degeneration

Definition

I. Sudden total and permanent blindness in otherwise healthy animals

II. Also known as silent retina syndrome, toxic metabolic retinopathy

Causes

I. The cause of sudden acquired retinal degeneration (SARD) is unknown.

II. Proposed theories include neurotoxicity from excitotoxins present in food additives or from elevations of melanocyte-stimulating hormone (Riis, 1990; van der Woerdt et al., 1991).

Pathophysiology

I. An acute loss of the photoreceptor outer segments is seen histologically.

II. All parts of the retina are affected equally and acutely.

III. Transient increases in blood levels of neurotoxins or excitotoxins such as found in food additives and by-products (e.g., glutamate, biotenic acid, aspartame, cysteine sulfonic acid) have been proposed as responsible for destroying these neurons.

Clinical Signs

I. Acute onset of vision loss

II. Predilection for middle-aged (6–14 years), overweight, neutered female dogs

III. Brittany spaniel, dachshund, and miniature schnauzer possibly at higher risk

Diagnosis

I. A history of acute onset of blindness (within weeks) in an adult, obese dog creates suspicion of SARD.

II. Ocular examination is often nondiagnostic.
   A. Pupils are often fixed, dilated, and unresponsive to light.
   B. Early in the disease the fundus often appears normal or may have subtle beading of the primary arterioles.
   C. Later there is complete retinal degeneration with vessel attenuation and increased tapetal reflectivity.

III. Nonspecific laboratory abnormalities may be present.
   A. Elevated serum alkaline phosphatase, aspartate aminotransferase, cholesterol
   B. Increased adrenocorticotropic hormone (ACTH) response test compatible with hyperadrenocorticism; variable dexamethasone suppression test results

IV. ERG is mandatory for diagnosis. It is completely extinguished in SARD.

Differential Diagnosis

I. Retrobulbar optic neuritis
   A. The ERG is normal, but the VER is abnormal or absent.
   B. It may respond to anti-inflammatory therapy.

II. Cortical blindness
   A. Pupillary light reflexes are usually normal.
   B. ERG findings are normal, but VER is absent.
   C. Cerebrospinal fluid analysis may indicate inflammatory disease.

III. PRA
  A. Funduscopic appearance is indistinguishable from long-standing SARD.
  B. ERG is attenuated but present in early phases, whereas in SARD the ERG is extinguished early; later ERG recordings are indistinguishable.

Treatment and Monitoring

  I. No treatment is available.
  II. Animal is irreversibly blind.

NUTRITIONAL DISORDERS

Taurine Deficiency Retinal Degeneration

Definition

  I. It is a retinopathy unique to felines caused by their limited ability to produce endogenous taurine from cysteine.
  II. It has also been called feline central retinal degeneration (FCRD).

Cause and Pathophysiology

  I. The disease occurs in animals fed diets deficient in taurine or its precursors, e.g., casein.
  II. Similar lesions have been reproduced following hypoxia.
  III. Disruption of the normal cone outer segment develops, followed by rapid degeneration, with the area centralis affected first.
  IV. Similar changes occur in the rods, but at a slower rate.

Clinical Signs

  I. Early in the disease, cats have normal vision and behavior, and lesions are found incidentally on physical examination.
  II. Later in the disease, vision diminishes to total blindness.

Diagnosis

  I. Funduscopic findings are highly suggestive.
    A. Lesions are bilateral and symmetrical.
    B. Lesions demonstrate a uniform progression.
      1. Sharply delineated, highly reflective oval lesion is first seen in the area centralis temporal to the optic disk.
      2. A second lesion then develops nasal to the disk.
      3. Eventually the two lesions join dorsal to the disk to form a horizontal streak.
      4. Late in the disease, the entire retina degenerates and appears similar to chronic PRA.
  II. ERG shows abnormal cone response.
  III. Also look for evidence of dilatative cardiomyopathy (see Chap. 10).

Treatment and Monitoring

  I. Lesions can be minimized by taurine supplementation early in the disease.
  II. Give taurine 250 mg/kg PO SID-BID in capsule or powder form.
  III. In later stages, supplementation with taurine stops further progression but does not reverse lesions.
  IV. In 1989, commercial food manufacturers in the United States increased the levels of taurine found in cat foods, and this has resulted in a significant reduction in the incidence of FCRD (Riis, 1990).

NEOPLASIA

Definition and Causes

  I. Primary
    A. Malignant teratoid medulloepithelioma
    B. Choroidal melanoma (rare)
    C. Neurosensory tumors: glioma, astrocytoma, etc.
  II. Secondary
    A. Meningioma
    B. Hemangiosarcoma
    C. Rhabdomyosarcoma
    D. Post-traumatic ocular sarcomas of cats: fibrosarcoma, anaplastic sarcoma, osteosarcoma
  III. Metastatic
    A. Lymphosarcoma (most common)
    B. Adenocarcinomas: mammary gland, thyroid, kidney, pancreas
    C. Others: transmissible venereal tumor, seminoma

Pathophysiology

  I. Primary tumors originate from cells within the retina or choroid or the optic nerve.
  II. Secondary and metastatic tumors develop from hematogenous localization or by direct extension from adjacent structures. The vascular nature of the choroid makes it a likely site for tumor metastasis.
  III. Intraocular sarcoma in the cat appears to be a delayed effect of penetrating trauma and lens rupture.

Clinical Signs

  I. Some animals present with obvious ocular signs.
    A. Mass protruding through the pupil from the posterior chamber, or inability to see the fundus
    B. Uveitis, scleral injection
    C. Anisocoria, retinal detachment, blindness
    D. Glaucoma with corneal edema
    E. Hemorrhage in the vitreous chamber
  II. Occasionally there is a history of prior ocular trauma or cancer elsewhere in the body.
  III. Other animals are presented with evidence of systemic disease.

Diagnosis

  I. Ocular findings may be suspicious.
  II. Ultrasonography is useful when the posterior segment cannot be seen.

III. In cases where the fundus cannot be seen, vitreal aspirate may demonstrate neoplastic cells, but intraocular hemorrhage can result.
IV. Perform a complete systemic work-up, including thoracic radiography to look for both primary or metastatic lesions.
V. Histopathology of the enucleated globe allows a definitive diagnosis.

Treatment

I. Enucleation is the treatment of choice when diagnosis is in doubt or if the eye is painful (see technique in Chap. 103).
II. Adjunct chemotherapy may be indicated for lymphosarcoma and other tumors.
III. Cryosurgery and laser surgery have been applied to successfully treat some focal neoplasms of the retina.

Patient Monitoring

I. The prognosis for primary tumors varies.
  A. Choroidal melanomas are rare in the dog and cat, and the probability of metastasis is uncertain; enucleation is advised (Wilcock, 1985).
  B. Metastasis has not been reported for medulloepitheliomas.
II. Prognosis for secondary and metastatic tumors is guarded.
  A. Ocular lymphosarcoma is usually accompanied or preceded by systemic lymphosarcoma.
  B. Post-traumatic ocular sarcomas in cats commonly extend to the brain or metastasize.
  C. Optic nerve meningiomas are slow growing but may extend posteriorly into the brain.

Bibliography

Acland GM: Diagnosis and differentiation of retinal diseases in small animals by electroretinography. Semin Vet Med Surg 3(1):15, 1988

Acland GM, Aguirre GD: Retinal degenerations in the dog: IV. Early retinal degeneration (erd) in Norwegian elkhounds. Exp Eye Res 44:491, 1987

Acland GM, Aguirre GD: Retinal dysplasia in the Samoyed dog is the heterozygous phenotype of the gene (drds) for short-limbed dwarfism and ocular defects. Proc Am Coll Vet Ophthalmol 22:44, 1991

Acland GM, Blanton SH, Hershfield B et al: XLPRA: an X-linked form of progressive retinal atrophy in Siberian husky dogs. Proc Am Coll Vet Ophthalmol 24:37, 1993

Aguirre GD: Pathogenesis of progressive rod-cone degeneration in miniature poodles. Invest Ophthalmol Vis Sci 23:610, 1982

Aguirre GD, Acland GM: Variation in retinal degeneration phenotype inherited at the prcd locus. Exp Eye Res 46:663, 1988

Aguirre GD, Rubin LF: Rod-cone dysplasia (progressive retinal atrophy) in Irish setters. J Am Vet Med Assoc 166:157, 1975

Aguirre G, Parshall C, Acland GM: Progressive retinal atrophy in the miniature schnauzer. Proc Am Coll Vet Ophthalmol 17:226, 1986

Barnett KC: The diagnosis of central progressive retinal atrophy in the Labrador retriever. J Small Anim Pract 8:631, 1967

Barnett KC, Knight GC: Persistent pupillary membrane and associated defects in the Basenji. Vet Rec 85:242, 1969

Bedford PGC: Collie eye anomaly in the border collie. Vet Rec 111:34, 1982

Bedford PGC: Retinal pigment epithelial dystrophy (CPRA): study of the disease in the briard. J Small Anim Pract 25:129, 1984

Brown GC, Shields JA, Patty BE: Congenital pits of the optic nerve head. I. Experimental studies in collie dogs. Arch Ophthalmol 97:1341, 1979

Burger IH, Barnett KC: The taurine requirement of the adult cat. J Small Anim Pract 24:533, 1983

Carrig CB, MacMillan AD, Brundage S et al: Retinal dysplasia associated with skeletal abnormalities in Labrador retrievers. J Am Vet Med Assoc 170:49, 1974

Carrig CB, Sponenberg UP, Schmidt GM et al: Inheritance of associated ocular and skeletal dysplasia in Labrador retrievers. J Am Vet Med Assoc 193:1269, 1988

Curtis R, Barnett KC, Leon A: An early-onset retinal dystrophy with dominant inheritance in the Abyssinian cat. Invest Ophthalmol Vis Sci 28:131, 1987

Dubielzig RR, Everitt J, Shadduck JA, Albert DM: Clinical and morphologic features of post-traumatic ocular sarcomas in cats. Vet Pathol 27:62, 1990

Hendrix DV, Nasisse MP, Cowen P, Davidson MG: Clinical signs, concurrent diseases and risk factors associated with retinal detachment in dogs. Prog Vet Comp Ophthalmol 3:87, 1993

Jacobson JB, Kemp CM, Borraut FX et al: Rhodopsin topography and rod-mediated function in cats with the retinal degeneration of taurine deficiency. Exp Eye Res 45:481, 1987

Kern TJ, Riis RC: Optic nerve hypoplasia in three miniature poodles. J Am Vet Med Assoc 178:49, 1981

Lavach JD, Murphy JM, Severin GA: Retinal dysplasia in the English springer spaniel. J Am Anim Hosp Assoc 14:192, 1978

Lindley DM, Pickett P, Boosinger TR, Toivio-Kinnucan M: Stationary night blindness in a collie. Proc Am Coll Vet Ophthalmol 21:149, 1990

MacMillan AD, Lipton DE: Hereditability of multifocal retinal dysplasia in the American cocker spaniel. J Am Vet Med Assoc 172:568, 1978

Millichamp NJ, Curtis R, Barnett KC: Progressive retinal atrophy in the Tibetan terrier. J Am Vet Med Assoc 192:769, 1988

Narfstrom K: Hereditary PRA in the Abyssinian cat. J Hered 74:273, 1983

Riis R: Electron microscopic observation of a SARD case. Proc Am Coll Vet Ophthalmol 21:112, 1990

Riis R, Aguirre G: The briard problem. Proc Am Coll Vet Ophthalmol 14:62, 1983

Rubin LF, Bourne TKR, Lord LH: Hemeralopia in dogs: heredity of hemeralopia in Alaskan malamutes. Am J Vet Res 28:355, 1967

Saunders LZ: Congenital optic nerve hypoplasia in collie dogs. Cornell Vet 42:67, 1952

Schmidt GM, Ellersieck MR, Wheeler CA et al: Inheritance of retinal dysplasia in the English springer spaniel. J Am Vet Med Assoc 174:1089, 1979

Vainisi S, Schmidt GM, West CS et al: Metabolic toxic retinopathy—a preliminary report. Proc Am Coll Vet Ophthalmol 14:76, 1983

Vainisi S, Packo K, Schmidt G: Retinal detachment in the Shih tzu. Proc Am Coll Vet Ophthalmol 21:115, 1990

van der Woerdt A, Nasisse MP, Davidson MG: Sudden acquired retinal degeneration in the dog: clinical and laboratory findings in 36 cases. Prog Vet Comp Ophthalmol 1:11, 1991

West-Hyde L, Buyukmihci N: PRC degeneration in a family of cats. J Am Vet Med Assoc 181:243, 1982

Wilcock BP: The eye and ear. p. 339. In Jubb RUF, Kennedy PC, Palmer N (eds): Pathology of Domestic Animals. Academic Press, San Diego, California, 1985

101

Ocular Manifestations of Systemic Disease

James F. Swanson

Ocular examination may provide important clues aiding in the diagnosis of systemic disorders. This chapter provides a series of tables, which is by no means all inclusive, of systemic diseases that have associated ocular findings.

Table 101–1. **Inborn Errors of Metabolism**

Disorder	Enzyme Deficiency	Species/Breed	Clinical Signs
Chediak-Higashi syndrome	Undetermined	Cats, mink, mice, cattle	Partial oculocutaneous albinism Photophobia, pale irides, hypopigmented fundus
Gyrate atrophy	Ornithine-δ-aminotransferase	Domestic shorthair cat	Generalized retinal atrophy
Tyrosinemia	Tyrosine aminotransferase	Dog	Persistent corneal erosions and vascularization Conjunctivitis, cataracts
α-Mannosidosis	α-Mannosidase	Persian cat	Corneal opacity Posterior subcapsular cataract Gray, granular discoloration of area centralis
Mucopolysaccharidosis I	α-L-Iduronidase	Plott hound, cat	Granular corneal opacity Facial dysmorphism
Mucopolysaccharidosis VI	Arylsulfatase B	Siamese cat	Corneal opacities Facial dysmorphism
Mucopolysaccharidosis VII	β-Glucuronidase	Dog	Corneal opacities Facial dysmorphism
GM$_1$ gangliosidosis	β-Galactosidase	Cats, dogs	Fine granular opacification of posterior cornea (cats) Multifocal intraretinal white to gray spots
GM$_2$ gangliosidosis	α- and β-Hexosaminidase	Cats, dogs	Corneal opacities Diffusely scattered gray-white retinal foci
Fucosidosis	α-L-Fucosidase	English springer spaniel	Facial dysmorphism Decreased pupil responses

Table 101–2. **Ocular Manifestations of Infectious Diseases**

Infectious Agent	Route of Infection	Ocular Findings
Systemic Mycoses		
Blastomyces dermatitidis	Inhalation	Rarely subclinical Severe keratitis, corneal edema Anterior uveitis, panuveitis, chorioretinitis Glaucoma, orbital cellulitis Endophthalmitis, panophthalmitis Episcleritis, episcleral granulomas
Histoplasma capsulatum	Inhalation, possibly ingestion	Conjunctivitis, eyelid granuloma Granulomatous chorioretinitis Retinal detachment, optic neuritis Endophthalmitis, panophthalmitis
Coccidioides immitis	Inhalation, skin inoculation	Conjunctivitis, keratitis Iritis, hyphema, hyalitis Chorioretinitis, retinal detachment Secondary glaucoma, orbital cellulitis
Cryptococcus neoformans	Uncertain, possibly inhalation	Blindness, retinal detachment Iritis (rare), optic neuritis Granulomatous chorioretinitis
Bacterial Infections		
Brucella canis	Oral, vaginal, conjunctival exposure	Corneal opacity Nongranulomatous anterior uveitis
Leptospira pomona, L. icterohaemorrhagiae	Mucous membranes, abraded skin	Conjunctivitis, scleral icterus Intraocular hemorrhage, uveitis
Clostridium tetani	Skin wounds	Enophthalmos, decreased palpebral fissure size Protrusion of third eyelid, inconsistent miosis Risus sardonicus
Mycobacterium tuberculosis, M. bovis	Inhalation	Ocular granulomas
Septicemias	Disseminated from various organs	Conjunctival congestion Uveitis, iridal and retinal hemorrhages
Borrelia burgdorferi	Ticks (*Ixodes*)	Conjunctivitis, anterior uveitis Chorioretinitis, retinal hemorrhages and detachment
Viral Infections		
Canine distemper	Respiratory, urine, other secretions	Purulent conjunctivitis, mild anterior uveitis Multifocal to diffuse chorioretinitis, especially in nontapetal fundus Optic neuritis and blindness Keratoconjunctivitis sicca (KCS)
Infectious canine hepatitis	Urine and other body secretions, fomites	Corneal endothelial inflammation with "blue-eye" corneal edema Severe anterior uveitis, secondary glaucoma
Rabies	Bite wounds	Anisocoria, mydriasis, areflexic pupils Chorioretinitis, optic neuritis
Canine herpesvirus	Oronasal exposure	Neonates: keratitis, panuveitis, cataracts, retinal necrosis, atrophy and dysplasia; optic neuritis Adults: mild conjunctivitis
Feline herpesvirus	Oronasal, conjunctival exposure	Kittens: severe, often ulcerative keratoconjunctivitis, symblepharon formation Young adults: chronic conjunctivitis, KCS, dendritic corneal ulcers, corneal stromal vascularization, proliferative/eosinophilic keratitis, corneal sequestrum formation, optic neuritis

Table 101–2. **Ocular Manifestations of Infectious Diseases** (Continued)

Infectious Agent	Route of Infection	Ocular Findings
Viral Infections Continued		
Feline leukemia	Saliva and other secretions	Chronic anterior uveitis
		Secondary cataracts, lens luxation
		Glaucoma, dyscoria, anisocoria
		Retinal dysplasia (kittens)
		Ocular and orbital lymphoma
Feline immunodeficiency virus	Bite wounds probably	Chronic anterior uveitis
		Secondary glaucoma, pars planitis
		Cataracts, lens luxation
Feline panleukopenia	In utero exposure	Focal to multifocal retinal dysplasia
Feline infectious peritonitis	Ingestion or inhalation probably	Conjunctivitis early
		Chronic anterior uveitis with keratic precipitates
		Chorioretinitis with perivascular sheathing
		Retinal hemorrhages and detachments
Rickettsial Infections		
Rickettsia rickettsii	Ticks (Dermacentor)	Nystagmus, conjunctival, and iridal hemorrhages
		Anterior uveitis, retinitis
		Retinal hemorrhages and vasculitis
Ehrlichia canis	Ticks (Rhipicephalus)	Acute phase: conjunctivitis, conjunctival hemorrhages, anterior uveitis, hyalitis, chorioretinitis, retinal hemorrhages, optic neuritis
		Subacute and chronic phase: multifocal perivascular retinal lesions
Ehrlichia platys	Ticks (Rhipicephalus)	Uveitis
Hemobartonella felis	Blood-sucking arthropods, bite wounds	Scleral icterus
		Focal retinal hemorrhages
Protozoal Infections		
Toxoplasma gondii	In utero, ingestion	Cats: chronic anterior uveitis, acute chorioretinitis
		Dogs: anterior uveitis, focal retinitis, optic neuritis, extraocular muscle myositis
Neospora caninum	Transplacental	Puppies: mild iridocyclitis and choroiditis, focal retinitis, infestation of extraocular muscles
Leishmania spp.	Sandflies	Conjunctivitis, keratitis, hyalitis
		Panuveitis, chorioretinitis
Encephalitozoon cuniculi	Unknown	Multifocal superficial corneal opacities
Miscellaneous Infections		
Chlamydia psittaci	Ocular, nasal secretions	Recurrent conjunctivitis with chemosis and vesicle formation
Prototheca zopfii, P. wickerhami	Exposure to contaminated food, water, soil (dog)	Panuveitis, blindness
		Leukocoria from vitreal exudates and/or retinal detachment
Parasitic Infestations		
Dirofilaria immitis	Ocular larva migrans	Stage 5 larvae within anterior or posterior chamber
		Uveitis
Toxocara canis or Ancylostoma spp.	Ocular larva migrans	Intraretinal hemorrhage, larval tracks
		Retinal necrosis, atrophy, and detachment
		Chorioretinal granulomas, panuveitis, blindness
Cuterebra spp.	Ophthalmomyiasis interna/externa	Uveitis, meandering retinal scars
		Larvae visible in anterior chamber, vitreous, subretinal space, or choroid
		Retinal atrophy

Table 101–3. Ocular Manifestations of Metabolic and Endocrine Disorders

Disorder	Species Affected	Ocular Findings
Diabetes mellitus	Dog	Cataracts, retinal microangiopathy
Inherited hyperchylomicronemia	Cat	Lipemia retinalis Horner's syndrome, facial nerve paralysis
Hyperlipidemia	Dog	Corneal arcus lipoides, lipemia retinalis Lactescent aqueous with uveitis
Hypothyroidism	Dog	Facial nerve palsy Blepharitis, keratoconjunctivitis sicca Corneal arcus lipoides, other lipid keratopathies Lipemia retinalis
Hyperadrenocorticism	Dog	Persistent corneal erosions Calcium ("band") keratopathies
Hypocalcemia	Dog	Multifocal punctate to linear cortical lens opacities

Table 101–4. Ocular Changes Associated with Certain Drugs and Toxins

Drug	Species Affected	Ocular Findings
Corticosteroids	Dog, cat	Lipid keratopathy, cataracts Recrudescence of latent infections
Dinitrophenol	Dog	Cataracts
Dithizone and diethylthiocarbamate	Dog	Retinal edema and detachment
Estradiol cypionate	Dog	Retinal hemorrhages from pancytopenia
Ethambutol	Dog	Transient discoloration of tapetum
Ethylene glycol	Dog	Uveitis, retinal edema and detachment
Ketamine with methylnitrosourea	Cat	Blindness, retinal degeneration
Rafoxanide	Dog	Optic disk edema
Strychnine	Dog	Facial spasm
Sulfonamides	Dog	Keratoconjunctivitis sicca, subretinal bullae
Vasodilators	Dog	Linear discoloration of tapetum dorsal to disk

Table 101–5. Ocular Manifestations of Immune-Mediated Disorders

Disorder	Species Affected	Ocular Findings
Uveitis/poliosis/vitiligo syndrome (Vogt-Koyanagi-Harada–like syndrome)	Dog	Corneal edema, eyelid and skin depigmentation Anterior and panuveitis, secondary glaucoma Uveal and retinal depigmentation Retinal edema and detachment, blindness
Autoimmune hemolytic anemia	Dog, cat	Scleral icterus, conjunctival pallor Periocular crusting, focal retinal hemorrhages Blanching of retinal vasculature
Immune thrombocytopenia	Dog, cat	Conjunctival and iridal petechiation Hyphema; pre-, intra-, or subretinal hemorrhages Retinal edema and detachment, blindness
Systemic lupus erythematosus	Dog, cat	Crusting and ulceration of face and eyelids Possible keratoconjunctivitis sicca, uveitis
Pemphigus complex	Dog, cat	Early: papular, pustular lesions of eyelid margins Late: ulceration, crusting of affected areas
Sjögren's syndrome	Dog	Keratoconjunctivitis sicca
Allergic reactions	Dog, cat	Urticaria, blepharoedema, chemosis Eyelid self-trauma from pruritus
Juvenile cellulitis	Dog	Eyelid inflammation with crusting, alopecia, erythema, and microabscessation, and purulent discharge

Table 101–6. **Vasculopathies and Coagulopathies Causing Ocular Signs**

Disorder	Types	Ocular Findings
Coagulopathies	Inherited clotting factor deficiencies Disseminated intravascular coagulopathy Platelet abnormalities Vitamin K–related disorders	Orbital, conjunctival, intraocular hemorrhages Anterior uveitis Serous or hemorrhagic retinal detachments
Hypertension	Primary Secondary Idiopathic	Hyphema, anterior uveitis Retinal and vitreal hemorrhages Retinal detachments, blindness Secondary glaucoma
Hyperviscosity syndrome	Monoclonal gammopathies Polyclonal gammopathies	Retinal vasculature congestion and tortuosity Retinal hemorrhages, edema, and detachment Optic disk edema, blindness
Polycythemia	Absolute Relative	Conjunctival erythema Retinal vasculature engorgement, tortuosity, hemorrhage Retinal detachment, blindness Folds in nontapetal retina
Anemia	Pre- and post-transfusion retinopathy	Multifocal retinal hemorrhages

Table 101–7. **Ocular Signs Associated with Nutritional Disorders**

Disorder	Species Affected	Ocular Findings
Taurine deficiency	Cat	Early: granular appearance to area centralis, retinal degeneration in area centralis Late: retinal degeneration progressing to affect entire retina
Vitamin A deficiency	Dog, cat	Xerophthalmia (KCS), keratomalacia Nyctalopia
Riboflavin deficiency	Dog	Corneal vascularization, punctate keratitis Purulent ocular discharge
Riboflavin deficiency (with high-fat diet)	Cat	Cortical and nuclear cataracts
Vitamin E deficiency (experimental)	Dog	Retinal degeneration

Bibliography

Angell JA, Merideth RE, Shively JN, Sigler RL: Ocular lesions associated with coccidioidomycosis in dogs: 35 cases (1980–1985). J Am Vet Med Assoc 190:1319, 1987

Armstrong PJ, Ford RB: Hyperlipidemia. p. 1046. In Kirk RW (ed): Current Veterinary Therapy X: Small Animal Practice. WB Saunders, Philadelphia, 1989

Blouin P, Cello RM: Experimental ocular cryptococcosis, preliminary studies in cats and mice. Invest Ophthalmol Vis Sci 19:21, 1980

Bovee KC, Littman MP, Crabtree BJ et al: Essential hypertension in a dog. J Am Vet Med Assoc 195:81, 1989

Braund KG, Everett RM, Albert RA: Neurologic manifestations of monoclonal IgM gammopathy associated with lymphocytic leukemia in a dog. J Am Vet Med Assoc 172:1407, 1978

Brooks DE, Wolf ED, Merideth RE: Ophthalmomyiasis interna in two cats. J Am Anim Hosp Assoc 20:157, 1984

Buyukmihci N: Ocular lesions of blastomycosis in the dog. J Am Vet Med Assoc 180:426, 1982

Buyukmihci N, Rubin LF, Depaoli A: Prototvecosis with ocular involvement in a dog. J Am Vet Med Assoc 167:158, 1975

Campbell L, Reed C: Ocular signs associated with feline infectious peritonitis in two cats. Feline Pract 5:32, 1975

Center SA, Smith JF: Ocular lesions in a dog with serum hyperviscosity secondary to an IgA myeloma. J Am Vet Med Assoc 181:811, 1982

Cowgill LD, Kallett AJ: Systemic hypertension. p. 360. In Kirk RW (ed): Current Veterinary Therapy IX. WB Saunders, Philadelphia, 1986

Davidson MG, Breitschwerdt EB, Nasisse MP et al: Ocular manifestations of Rocky Mountain spotted fever in dogs. J Am Vet Med Assoc 194:777, 1989

Dubey JP: Toxoplasmosis in dogs. Canine Pract 12:7, 1985

English RV, Davidson MG, Nasisse MP et al: Intraocular disease associated with feline immunodeficiency virus infection in cats. J Am Vet Med Assoc 196:1116, 1990

Feldman BF, Thomason KJ, Jain NC: Quantitative platelet disorders. Vet Clin North Am [Small Anim Pract] 18:38, 1988a

Feldman BF, Thomason KJ, Jain NC: Autoimmune hemolytic anemia. Vet Clin North Am [Small Anim Pract] 18:308, 1988b

Fischer CA: Retinal and retinochoroidal lesions in early neuropathic canine distemper. J Am Vet Med Assoc 158:740, 1971

Garmer NL, Naeser P, Bergman AJ: Reticulosis of the eyes and the central nervous system in a dog. J Small Anim Pract 22:39, 1981

Glaze MB, Gaunt SD: Uveitis associated with *Ehrlichia platys* infection in a dog. J Am Vet Med Assoc 188:916, 1986

Greene CE, Dreesen DW: Rabies. p. 365. In Greene CE (ed): Infectious Diseases of the Dog and Cat. WB Saunders, Philadelphia, 1990

Greene CE, Shotts EB: Leptospirosis, p. 498. In Greene CE (ed): Infectious Diseases of the Dog and Cat. WB Saunders, Philadelphia, 1990

Gwin RM, Yakley TA, Wyman M, Werling K: Multifocal ocular histoplasmosis in a dog and cat. J Am Vet Med Assoc 176:638, 1980

Halliwell REW, Gorman NT: Autoimmune and other immune-mediated skin diseases. p. 285. In: Veterinary Clinical Immunology. WB Saunders, Philadelphia, 1989a

Halliwell REW, Gorman NT: Autoimmune blood diseases. p. 308. In: Veterinary Clinical Immunology. WB Saunders, Philadelphia, 1989b

Hass JA, Shell L, Sounders G: Neurological manifestations of toxoplasmosis: a literature review and case summary. J Am Anim Hosp Assoc 25:253, 1989

Jezyk PF, Haskins ME, Newman LR: Alpha-mannosidosis in a Persian cat. J Am Vet Med Assoc 189:1483, 1986

Johnson BW, Helper LC, Szajerdki MF: Intraocular *Cuterebra* in a cat. J Am Vet Med Assoc 193:829, 1988

Jones BR, Johnstone AC, Hancock WS et al: Inherited hyperchylomicronemia in the cat. Feline Pract 16:7, 1986

Kern TJ, Riis RC: Ocular manifestations of secondary hyperlipidemia associated with hypothyroidism and uveitis in a dog. J Am Anim Hosp Assoc 16:907, 1980

Kern TJ, Walton DK, Riis RC et al: Uveitis associated with poliosis and vitiligo in six dogs. J Am Vet Med Assoc 187:408, 1985

Luttgen PJ: Inflammatory disease of the central nervous system. Vet Clin North Am [Small Anim Pract] 18:623, 1988

Meyers SM, Vasil ML, Yammamoto L: Pathologic mechanisms of multifocal choroiditis with retinal detachment after carotid injection of *Streptococcus mutans* and other bacteria in dogs. Invest Ophthalmol Vis Sci 22:165, 1982

Morgan RV: Systemic hypertension in four cats: ocular and medical findings. J Am Anim Hosp Assoc 22:615, 1986

Nasisse MP, Guy J, Davidson MG et al: Experimental ocular herpesvirus infection in the cat. Invest Ophthalmol Vis Sci 30:1758, 1989

Olin DD, Rogers WA, MacMillan AD: Lipid-laden aqueous humor associated with anterior uveitis and concurrent hyperlipemia in two dogs. J Am Vet Med Assoc 168:861, 1976

Paulsen ME, Allen TA, Jaenke RS et al: Arterial hypertension in two canine siblings: ocular and systemic manifestations. J Am Anim Hosp Assoc 25:287, 1989

Romatowski J: A uveodermatological syndrome in an akita dog. J Am Anim Hosp Assoc 21:777, 1985

Rutgers C, Kowalske J, Cole CR: Severe Rocky Mountain spotted fever in five dogs. J Am Anim Hosp Assoc 21:361, 1985

Sarfaty D, Carrillo JM, Greenlee PG: Differential diagnosis of granulomatous meningoencephalomyelitis, distemper, and suppurative meningoencephalitis in the dog. J Am Vet Med Assoc 188:387, 1986

Sparger EE, Yamamoto JK: Feline immunodeficiency virus infection. p. 530. In Kirk RW (ed): Current Veterinary Therapy X: Small Animal Practice. WB Saunders, Philadelphia, 1989

Swanson JF: Uveitis associated with *Ehrlichiá canis* infection. Proc Am Coll Vet Ophthalmol 13:102, 1982

Wilkinson GT: Feline cryptococcosis: a review and seven case reports. J Small Anim Pract 20:749, 1979

Yamamoto JK, Sparger E, Ho EW et al: Pathogenesis of experimentally induced feline immunodeficiency virus infection in cats. Am J Vet Res 49:1246, 1988

102

Neuro-ophthalmology

Steven M. Roberts

DISORDERS OF THE PUPIL

Mydriasis: Afferent Anisocoria

Definition

I. It is a neurologic lesion of the retina, cranial nerve (CN) II, optic chiasm, or optic tract resulting in near-maximal mydriasis under darkened room conditions.
II. Pupillary light reflexes (PLRs) and menace response vary depending on the site of the lesion. A vision deficit is present in one or both eyes.

Causes

I. Prechiasmal (most common)
  A. Retinal degeneration (see Chap. 100)
    1. Primary: progressive retinal atrophy, feline generalized retinal degeneration
    2. Secondary: post–inflammatory disease, glaucoma, retinal detachment
  B. Optic nerve disease: congenital, inflammatory, neoplastic, or traumatic (see Chap. 100)
II. Chiasmal and optic tract
  A. Infectious disease: canine distemper
  B. Inflammatory: granulomatous meningoencephalitis (GME)
  C. Vascular
  D. Neoplastic: meningioma or neoplasia involving the hypophyseal fossa
  E. Traumatic

Pathophysiology

I. Neural pathway involved in this disorder includes the retina, optic nerve, chiasm (the nasal fibers cross over at the chiasm), optic tract, and pretectal area (most fibers that cross at the chiasm cross over again in the pretectal area).
II. Lesions may be complete or incomplete and cause bilateral or unilateral signs.

Clinical Signs

I. Prechiasmal lesion
  A. Unilateral lesions may produce partial mydriasis

in normal room light, and bilateral lesions cause maximal mydriasis.
    1. Ophthalmoscopic abnormalities (if the fundus is involved) such as retinal thinning, retinal vascular attenuation, and optic nerve atrophy
    2. Afferent PLR deficit: loss of direct PLR in affected eye and of indirect PLR in unaffected eye
    3. Normal direct PLR in unaffected eye and normal indirect PLR in affected eye
    4. Unilateral visual deficit with no menace response in affected eye
  B. Bilateral lesions result in mydriasis and blindness.
II. Chiasmal disorders
  A. Partial or complete visual deficit
  B. Bilateral dilated, unresponsive pupils if lesion is complete
  C. Partial direct PLR function if lesion is incomplete
  D. Normal fundus
III. Optic tract disorders
  A. Unilateral lesions
    1. Hemianopia (deficit in half of the visual field of both eyes)
    2. Normal PLR, possibly slight slowing of PLR in contralateral eye
    3. Possible mydriasis contralateral
    4. Miosis ipsilateral that persists irrespective of the eye illuminated
  B. Bilateral lesions
    1. Partial to complete visual deficit
    2. Dilated unresponsive pupils
  C. Normal fundus

Diagnosis

I. Perform an ophthalmoscopic examination to detect retinal thinning, optic neuritis, or optic nerve atrophy. If there is no retinal or optic disk involvement, then the ophthalmoscopic examination is normal.
II. Perform PLR testing (Table 102–1). In the case of prechiasmal lesions, the swinging flashlight test

Table 102–1. Neuro-ophthalmic Examinations and Reflexes

Test	Afferent Innervation	Efferent Innervation	Testing Procedure	Normal Response	Interpretation of Abnormal Response[a]
Blink reflex	Ophthalmic division of trigeminal nerve: cornea and medial canthus Maxillary division of trigeminal nerve: lateral canthus	Motor portion of facial nerve: eyelids Trigeminal nerve: muscles of mastication	Apply a light tactile stimulus to cornea, medial canthus, and lateral canthus. Do not elicit a pain response.	Rapid closure of eyelids with possible movement of the mouth	Dysfunction of trigeminal or facial nerve motor innervation
Dazzle reflex	Retina, optic nerve, and central visual pathways	Facial nerve: orbicularis oculi muscle	Direct a bright light at first one eye and then the other.	Partial closure of eyelids (squinting)	Dysfunction of retina, optic nerve, or facial nerve
Maze response	Retina, optic nerve, and central visual pathways	Various motor pathways	Allow animal to move freely among randomly placed objects under normal, reduced, and darkened room light conditions.	Avoidance of all objects under normal, reduced, and darkened room light conditions. Allow several minutes for dark adaptation before performing the test.	Partial to total vision loss (peripheral or central) or ataxia
Menace response	Retina, optic nerve, and central visual pathways	Facial nerve: orbicularis oculi muscle Abducens nerve: retractor bulbi muscles	Rapidly present a threatening or sudden visual stimulus without causing a trigeminal sensory response.	Partial to complete blinking of the eyelids with possible retraction of the globe and momentary protrusion of the nictitating membrane	Vision loss, facial or abducens nerve dysfunction
Motion detection	Retina, optic nerve, and central visual pathways	Motor to the eye, head, and neck	Quietly roll a ball or tape roll across the visual field.	Movement of the eyes, head, ears, and neck to track the object	Partial to total vision loss or motor innervation dysfunction

Test	Structures (afferent)	Structures (efferent/motor)	Method	Normal response	Abnormal response[a]
Optokinetic nystagmus reflex	Retina, optic nerve, and central visual pathways (including vestibular system and medial longitudinal fasciculus)	Motor to extraocular muscles (cranial nerves III, IV, VI)	A tape, drum, or cathode ray tube with vertical dark and light bars is viewed by the animal. The bars are caused to move horizontally, and the resulting eye movement is noted.	Nystagmus with slow phase in the direction of bar movement and fast phase opposite the direction of bar movement	Partial or total vision loss or dysfunction of cranial nerves III, IV, VI
Pupillary light reflex (PLR)	Retina, optic nerve, optic tracts, pretectal nucleus, and oculomotor nucleus	Oculomotor nerve (cranial nerve III), ciliary ganglion, and short ciliary nerves	Shine a light into one pupil while observing the contralateral pupil with dim illumination, or swing a light quickly between the eyes after 2–4 seconds of illumination.	Bilateral miosis (direct: miosis of stimulated eye; indirect: miosis of contralateral eye)	Loss of direct reflex: dysfunction of ipsilateral retina, optic nerve, or oculomotor nerve. Loss of indirect reflex: dysfunction of contralateral retina, optic nerve, ipsilateral oculomotor nerve
Trigemino-abducens reflex	Ophthalmic division of trigeminal nerve: cornea and medial canthus. Maxillary division of trigeminal nerve: lateral canthus	Abducens nerve: retractor bulbi muscles and lateral rectus muscle	Apply light tactile stimulus to cornea, medial canthus, or lateral canthus. Do not elicit a pain response.	Retraction of the globe and protrusion of the nictitating membrane	Dysfunction of trigeminal nerve, abducens nerve, or orbital mass preventing retraction
Vestibulo-ocular reflex	Labyrinthine semicircular canals, medial longitudinal fasciculus	Motor to extraocular muscles (cranial nerves III, IV, VI)	Move the head (usually horizontally) while observing the direction of eye motion.	Nystagmus with fast phase in the direction of head movement	Dysfunction of vestibular system, extraocular muscle innervation, or orbital disease
Visual placing response	Retina, optic nerve, central visual pathways	Various motor pathways	Holding the animal off the floor, bring it toward the edge of a table surface.	Elevation and placement of the forepaws on the table surface.	Dysfunction of visual pathways or motor innervation to forelimbs

[a]Abnormal responses may result from problems other than neuro-ophthalmic conditions.

shows a loss of the direct PLR but a normal indirect PLR on the affected side.

III. Loss of dazzle reflex, menace response, motion detection, optokinetic nystagmus reflex, and visual placing response in the affected eye occur (see Table 102–1).

IV. Consider pharmacologic testing (Table 102–2) with 0.5% physostigmine or 0.1% pilocarpine to confirm functional status of the pupil.

V. Computed axial tomography scans or magnetic resonance imaging may be indicated if an orbital or intracranial mass is suspected.

VI. An electroretinogram (ERG) confirms dysfunction or degeneration of retinal photoreceptors.

Differential Diagnosis

I. Efferent mydriasis: see later

II. Central blindness: lesions of the optic radiation or visual cortex do not result in an abnormal PLR and often are associated with other neurologic abnormalities

III. Intraocular diseases that may cause mydriasis as a result of pupil dysfunction
   A. Iris atrophy
   B. Glaucoma
   C. Posterior synechia

Treatment

I. Treat the underlying cause.
   A. Antineoplastic treatment if warranted (see Chap. 23)
   B. Anti-inflammatory agents for inflammatory cause (see Chaps. 23 and 100)
   C. Antimicrobials for infectious cause (see Section XV, Infections Diseases)

II. No treatment may be available if degenerative changes predominate.

Patient Monitoring

I. Monitor for progression of neuro-ophthalmic signs, development of other neurologic signs, and involvement of other body systems.

II. Pupil and visual deficit changes may be permanent.

Efferent Mydriasis

Definition

I. Internal ophthalmoplegia is paralysis of intraocular muscles of the iris sphincter and ciliary body.
   A. Pupillotonia (Gerding et al., 1986)
   B. Tonic pupil (Goldfarb and Swann, 1984)
   C. CN III dysfunction

II. Afferent pathways are normal.

III. Persistent ipsilateral mydriasis with a normal menace response occurs.

Causes

I. Use of topical parasympatholytic agents (e.g., atropine) or ingestion of belladonna, alkaloid-containing plants

II. Orbital disease causing loss of CN III function

III. Cavernous sinus syndrome (see Chap. 23)

IV. Midbrain lesions involving the CN III nucleus and proximal nerve: infectious, neoplastic, traumatic, or vascular processes

V. Idiopathic lesions

Pathophysiology

I. The neural pathway involved includes the following.
   A. CN III nucleus and nerve
      1. Parasympathetic fibers are superficial and medial in the nerve.
      2. Compression affects the parasympathetic fibers first.
   B. Ciliary ganglion
      The CN III motor component does not enter the ciliary ganglion, so motor involvement indicates a lesion proximal to the ganglion.
   C. Short ciliary nerves
      1. Dogs have five to eight short ciliary nerves.
      2. Cats have two short ciliary nerves (nasal and malar).

II. Lesions anywhere along the pathway can cause mydriasis.

III. Midbrain swelling may compress the CN III nucleus and/or nerve.

Clinical Signs

I. Persistent ipsilateral mydriasis with a normal menace response is found (see Table 102–1).

II. There is no response to direct or indirect PLR in the affected eye.

III. The unaffected eye has a normal pupil response.

IV. Anisocoria is accentuated in lighted room conditions.

V. Concurrent ptosis and extraocular muscle abnormalities are possible with proximal CN III lesions affecting the levator palpebrae, superior rectus, inferior rectus, medial rectus, and inferior oblique muscles.

Diagnosis

I. Preganglionic lesion (see Table 102–2)
   A. 0.5% Physostigmine test: miosis of affected eye within 20 minutes
   B. 0.1% Pilocarpine test: no miosis

II. Postganglionic lesion
   A. Dog
      1. Short ciliary nerves carry both parasympathetic and sympathetic innervation, so concurrent loss of sympathetic innervation is possible.
         a) If unilateral, ipsilateral miosis may occur during dark room examination.
         b) There may be concurrent loss of pupillary dilator function.
      2. With the 0.5% physostigmine test, the affected eye remains dilated.
      3. Challenge with 0.1% pilocarpine produces miosis within 20 minutes because of denervation hypersensitivity.

Table 102–2. Pharmacologic Testing of the Pupil[a,b]

Pharmacologic Agent	Indication	Testing Procedure	Mode of Action	Interpretation of Responses
Indirect Acting				
1% Hydroxyamphetamine (Paredrine)[c]	Horner's syndrome Dysautonomia	Instill 1 drop to test eye several times over 30–60 min	Endogenous norepinephrine release from postganglionic presynaptic junction to stimulate the iris dilator muscle	Normal: mydriasis Preganglionic or central lesion: mydriasis
4% Cocaine HCl	Horner's syndrome Dysautonomia	Instill 1 drop to test eye and repeat in 5 min (evaluate at 30 and 60 min)	Prevents uptake of endogenous norepinephrine at postganglionic postsynaptic junction to stimulate the iris dilator muscle	Normal: mydriasis Horner's syndrome: no mydriasis (central lesion may show mydriasis)
Eserine (0.25% physostigmine)[d]	Internal ophthalmoplegia	Instill 1 drop to test eye and repeat in 5 min (evaluate at 20, 40, and 60 min)	Reversible anticholinesterase that prevents breakdown of acetylcholine at the postganglionic postsynaptic junction thus causing stimulation of the iris sphincter muscle	Normal: miosis Preganglionic or central oculomotor lesion: rapid miosis in 20 min Postganglionic oculomotor lesion: no miosis
Direct Acting				
1% Phenylephrine (Neo-Synephrine) or 0.1% epinephrine (1 : 1000)[e]	Horner's syndrome Dysautonomia	Instill 1 drop to test eye and evaluate at 20, 40, and 60 min	Stimulation on postsynaptic junction of iris dilator muscle	Normal: minimal mydriasis Postganglionic lesion: mydriasis in 20 min Preganglionic lesion: mydriasis in 40–60 min Dysautonomia: retraction of nictitating membrane
0.1% Pilocarpine	Dysautonomia Internal ophthalmoplegia	Instill 1 drop to test eye and evaluate at 20, 40, and 60 min	Stimulation of postsynaptic junction of oculomotor nerve	Normal: no miosis Postganglionic lesion: miosis in 20 min Preganglionic lesion: miosis in 40–60 min

[a]Before testing, determine which pupil is abnormal. Perform all tests under identical lighting conditions. If both eyes are evaluated, use identical dosage and instillation methods. Indirect agents should be used first, followed at least 24 hours later by direct-acting agents.
[b]Rule out pharmacologic or structural pupil blockades if both indirect- and direct-acting agents fail to elicit a response.
[c]This test is considered unreliable by many veterinarians. Available from Pharmics, Inc., Salt Lake City, UT, (800) 456-4138.
[d]Irreversible anticholinesterase agents such as echothiophate iodide (Phospholine Iodide) and demecarium bromide (Humorsol) are not recommended because of their prolonged duration of action.
[e]For dysautonomia testing, 0.01% epinephrine (1 : 10,000) is recommended.

B. Cat
   1. Parasympathetic innervation separate from sympathetic
   2. Two short ciliary nerves
      a) Nasal short ciliary nerve innervates the medial half of the iris.
         (1) "D-shaped" pupil if right eye involved
         (2) "Reverse-D" pupil if left eye involved
      b) Malar short ciliary nerve innervates the lateral half of the iris.
         (1) "D-shaped" pupil if left eye involved
         (2) "Reverse-D" pupil if right eye involved
   3. Pharmacologic testing as for the dog

Differential Diagnosis

I. Afferent mydriasis
II. Intraocular disease
   A. Developmental abnormalities of the iris sphincter
   B. Glaucoma
   C. Iris atrophy with sphincter involvement
   D. Lens luxation
   E. Posterior synechia
III. Dysautonomia

Treatment

I. If possible, institute specific therapy for any underlying neurologic condition.
II. For symptomatic therapy, instill indirect long-acting miotic agents such as echiothiophate iodide or demecarium bromide once daily to mask the mydriasis.

Patient Monitoring

I. Mydriasis from parasympatholytic agents such as topical atropine wears off in 1–2 weeks.
II. Watch for other ocular signs or neurologic dysfunction indicating more diffuse disease.
III. Bilateral midbrain lesions warrant a grave prognosis, whereas unilateral lesions warrant a guarded prognosis.
IV. Caudal brain stem lesions causing partially dilated, fixed pupils are life-threatening problems and warrant a grave prognosis.

Horner's Syndrome

Definition

I. Loss of cervical sympathetic innervation to the eye and periorbita results in the following.
   A. Enophthalmos
   B. Ptosis
   C. Nictitans protrusion
   D. Miosis
II. Location of nerve involvement may be central, preganglionic, or postganglionic.

Causes

I. Brain stem, cervical cord, and cranial thoracic cord lesions
   A. Trauma
   B. Ischemia: vascular, embolic
   C. Neoplasia
   D. Infectious or inflammatory diseases
II. Preganglionic lesions
   A. Mediastinal and thoracic masses
      1. Neoplasia: lymphosarcoma, hemangiosarcoma, etc.
      2. Abscess, foreign body
      3. Hematoma formation
      4. Cranial lung lobe disease
   B. Trauma
      1. Brachial plexus avulsion
      2. Bite wounds to the neck
      3. Carotid sheath manipulations: venipuncture and catheterization
      4. Surgical manipulations in the ventral neck region
   C. Neoplasia: thyroid adenocarcinoma
III. Postganglionic lesions
   A. Otitis media, ear cleaning, or bulla osteotomy
   B. Retrobulbar disease: injury, neoplasia, and abscess
   C. Cavernous sinus vascular or neoplastic abnormalities
   D. Peripheral neuropathy associated with hypothyroidism
IV. Idiopathic
   A. Most common in dogs
   B. Increased prevalence in golden retrievers

Pathophysiology

I. Sympathetic neurons originate in the hypothalamus and descend via the tectotegmentospinal system of the cord.
II. Preganglionic cell bodies are characterized as follows.
   A. These are located in the intermediate gray column of the first three or four thoracic segments.
   B. Axons leave the cord via the ventral gray horn, pass through the ventral roots, thoracic sympathetic trunk, and synapse in the cranial cervical ganglion.
III. Postganglionic axons travel as follows.
   A. They travel in a plexus around the internal carotid artery with the pupillomotor fibers, joining the tympanic branch of the glossopharyngeal nerve in the middle ear.
   B. Axons exit the middle ear and join the ophthalmic branch of CN V in the cavernous sinus.
   C. Axons enter the orbit through the orbital fissure.
IV. Loss of sympathetic tone from a lesion anywhere along the pathway results in clinical signs. Lower motor neuron lesions involving the thoracic and cervical sympathetic trunk and postganglionic lesions are most common in companion animals.

Clinical Signs

I. Miosis and anisocoria: the most consistent signs
II. Enophthalmos from loss of tone to the orbital smooth muscle
III. Ptosis from loss of tone to Müller's muscle in the upper lid or enophthalmos-related narrowing of the palpebral fissure
  A. Drooping of the upper lid: there is some question as to the significance of this Müller's muscle in dogs and cats.
  B. Narrowed palpebral fissure: posterior displacement of the globe allows upper and lower eyelids to approach each other.
IV. Protrusion of the nictitating membrane due to failure to passively retract it and loss of orbital smooth muscle tone
V. Enophthalmos, ptosis, and nictitating membrane protrusion often subtle

Diagnosis

I. History often reveals an acute onset but may not delineate a cause.
II. Diagnosis requires the presence of at least three of the four cardinal signs.
III. Anisocoria that becomes greater in the dark as the normal pupil dilates fully is a classic finding.
IV. Physical findings of nonocular clinical signs can be used to localize the sympathetic lesion.
V. Consider ancillary diagnostic tests.
  A. Pharmacologic localization of the lesion is helpful in some cases and has limited prognostic value (see Table 102–2).
    1. 4% Cocaine: usually only the normal pupil dilates
    2. 1% Hydroxyamphetamine: postganglionic lesions do not dilate
    3. 1% Phenylephrine or 0.1% epinephrine
      a) Postganglionic lesions dilate rapidly within 20 minutes.
      b) Preganglionic lesions may show some dilation in 40–60 minutes.
  B. Suspected preganglionic lesions may warrant further work-up.
    1. Radiography and computed tomography of the chest, neck, and skull
    2. Hematology and serum chemistries to rule out systemic disease
    3. Thyroid function testing (see Chap. 2)
    4. Complete neurologic examination to rule out brain and spinal cord lesions
    5. Cerebrospinal fluid (CSF) tap and analysis if central disease is suspected
  C. For suspected postganglionic lesions, consider skull radiographs and myringotomy for detection of otitis media.

Differential Diagnosis

I. Enophthalmos
  A. Reduction in orbital contents from dehydration and debilitation with loss of retrobulbar fat pad
  B. Atrophy and postinflammatory fibrosis of the muscles of mastication
II. Protrusion of nictitating membrane
  A. Enophthalmos
  B. Idiopathic protrusion in cats (see Chap. 94)
  C. Tetanus
  D. Dysautonomia
III. Miosis
  A. Corneal ulcers
  B. Anterior uveitis
  C. Spastic pupil syndrome in cats
  D. Drug-induced: topical parasympathomimetic agents and systemic organophosphate toxicity
  E. Central neurologic lesions

Treatment

I. Treat any specific underlying problem.
II. Symptomatic treatment of postganglionic lesions with topical sympathomimetics may be considered if the nictitating membrane protrusion causes obscured vision.

Patient Monitoring

I. Central lesions have less favorable prognosis than peripheral lesions.
II. Many lower motor neuron cases resolve spontaneously in 6–8 weeks.

Feline Spastic Pupil Syndrome

Definition

I. It is a static anisocoria in cats that is seen in some FeLV-positive animals (Brightman et al., 1991).
II. Autonomic nerve, and thus pupillary, dysfunction is possible in any domestic species.

Causes

I. Short ciliary nerves and ciliary ganglia in some cats contain a C-type RNA virus on electron microscopy and immunofluorescence.
II. Lymphosarcoma infiltration of ciliary ganglia can occur (Brightman et al., 1977).

Pathophysiology

I. Pupillary changes may precede systemic disease by several months.
II. It is most often seen in cats with lymphoreticular lymphosarcoma.

Clinical Signs and Diagnosis

I. There is often a history of abnormal pupillary movements.
II. Pupils may be miotic to partially mydriatic.
III. Anisocoria persists in darkness, i.e., the lack of light stimulus does not result in significant mydriasis.
IV. Vision is normal.

V. Many cats test FeLV positive or have lymphosarcoma.

Differential Diagnosis

I. Afferent mydriasis
II. Other causes of efferent mydriasis
III. Intraocular disease producing odd-shaped pupils or affecting pupil mobility
   A. Congenital pupil abnormalities, traumatic iris lesions, sphincter muscle atrophy
   B. Anterior uveitis, posterior synechia

Treatment

I. There is no specific treatment for the mydriasis.
II. Antineoplastic treatment may be considered for lymphosarcoma.

Patient Monitoring

I. If initially there is no evidence of systemic neoplastic involvement, monitor for its development at a later date.
II. Some cats may show dysfunction of other autonomic ganglia, such as urinary incontinence.

Dysautonomia

Definition

I. Dysautonomia is a dysfunction of the autonomic nervous system, both sympathetic and parasympathetic, characterized by mydriasis, dry mucous membranes, megaesophagus, and constipation.
II. Feline dysautonomia has also been called the Key-Gaskell syndrome, dilated pupil syndrome, and autonomic polyganglionopathy.
III. Canine dysautonomia is a rare disorder.

Causes

I. Feline dysautonomia
   A. Unknown cause
   B. Acute onset and sporadic
      1. Multiple cases were reported from 1982 to 1986 in and originating from the United Kingdom, Scandinavia, and the United States.
      2. Prevalence and severity of cases have declined since 1987.
      3. It usually occurs in young cats, <3 years of age.
II. Canine dysautonomia: unknown cause

Pathophysiology

I. An abnormal protein synthetic pathway in certain autonomic and nonautonomic neurons, especially CN III, V, VII, and XII, may exist.
II. Pre- and postganglionic sympathetic and parasympathetic neuronal degeneration occurs.

A. Chromatolytic changes develop in neurons of autonomic ganglia, intermediate gray columns of the spinal cord, certain cranial nerve nuclei, and sympathetic chain axons. These changes may be evident only within the first few weeks of the disorder.
   B. Early, characteristic neuronal electron microscopic changes consist of large cisternae and complex membranous stacks (Griffiths et al., 1985).
   C. Postganglionic receptors remain intact.
III. Chronic cases show neuronal depletion and increases in non-neuronal cells in autonomic ganglia.
IV. Most signs are caused by parasympathetic denervation.
V. Protrusion of the nictitating membrane and bradycardia are caused by sympathetic denervation.
VI. Lesions are similar to grass sickness in horses.

Clinical Signs

I. Acute or chronic onset
II. Dogs often young (median age, 15 months) and large breeds (Longshore et al., 1995)
III. Nonspecific signs
   A. Lethargy and depression
   B. Anorexia
   C. Dry nose
   D. Bradycardia and hypotension
IV. Gastrointestinal signs
   A. Dry mouth
   B. Megaesophagus or reduced esophageal motility
   C. Retching, regurgitation, vomiting
   D. Delayed gastric emptying
   E. Fecal incontinence
   F. Anal areflexia
V. Ocular signs
   A. Reduced lacrimation with associated signs of keratoconjunctivitis sicca
   B. Mydriasis (possible anisocoria) and photophobia
   C. Reduced or absent PLRs
   D. Protruding nictitating membrane
   E. Normal vision
VI. Other possible abnormalities
   A. Proprioceptive deficits
   B. Dysuria and urinary incontinence with bladder distention
   C. Transient syncopal episodes due to hypotension
   D. Aspiration pneumonia

Diagnosis

I. Clinical signs are usually suggestive.
II. Radiographic studies may reveal reduced esophageal motility, megaesophagus, slow gastric emptying, or aspiration pneumonia.
III. Pharmacologic testing may be helpful (see Table 102–2).
   A. Sympathetic system
      1. 1% Hydroxyamphetamine: no mydriasis
      2. 1% Phenylephrine or 0.1% epinephrine: rapid mydriasis
   B. Parasympathetic system

1. 0.5% Physostigmine: no miosis
2. 0.1% Pilocarpine: rapid miosis
C. Systemic testing
1. Systemic pharmacologic testing of the cardiovascular system with intravenous ephedrine, epinephrine, edrophonium, and methacholine should be done with care, as signs may be exacerbated. Topical epinephrine can induce fatal arrhythmias.
2. Atropine (0.04 mg/kg SQ) can be used to determine whether the sympathetic system is functional. With a normal sympathetic nervous system, the heart rate increases following atropinization.
3. Failure to demonstrate a wheal and flare reaction to intradermal histamine (1:1000) indicates a defect in sympathetic innervation of cutaneous blood vessels.
IV. Plasma and urine catecholamine levels in sympathetic insufficiency are low.
V. Necropsy with typical histopathology findings confirms the diagnosis.

Differential Diagnosis

I. Afferent mydriasis
II. Efferent mydriasis
III. Spastic pupil syndrome

Treatment

I. No curative treatment is available.
II. Supportive treatment includes the following.

A. Correct hypovolemia, hypothermia, hypoglycemia, and electrolyte abnormalities.
B. Consider nasogastric or gastrostomy intubation for alimentation.
C. Manually express the bladder as needed.
D. Administer laxatives and enemas for constipation.
III. Topical and oral parasympathomimetic agents have had mixed results.
A. Topical
1. 1% Pilocarpine solution OU QID
2. 0.25% Physostigmine ointment OU TID
B. Oral
1. Bethanechol 2.5–7.5 mg PO BID-TID
2. Metoclopramide 0.3 mg/kg PO TID to reduce vomiting

Patient Monitoring

I. Recovery period in cats is prolonged.
A. Complete recovery is possible but uncommon.
B. Recovery failures and complications occur despite best efforts.
C. Overall prognosis is guarded to poor.
II. Some cats, on recovery, have a "D-shaped" pupil in the left eye and a "reverse-D" pupil in the right eye.
III. All affected dogs have either died or been euthanized (Longshore et al., 1995)

Miscellaneous Causes of Anisocoria

See Table 102–3.

*Table 102–3. **Miscellaneous Causes of Anisocoria***

Cause	Pathophysiology	Clinical Signs
Cerebral or thalamic disease	Decreased higher control center inhibition of oculomotor nucleus	Miosis Miosis progressing to mydriasis: a grave prognosis
Cerebellar disease	Asymmetrical lesions may cause anisocoria from altered input to oculomotor nucleus	Mydriasis of the eye contralateral to the lesion Normal PLR and vision Concurrent cerebellar signs
Drugs: topical, ingested, inhalant, or parenteral		
Gaseous anesthetics, sedatives, and morphine	Decreased higher control center parasympathetic inhibition or alteration in sympathetic tone	Miosis: sedatives and deep anesthesia Mydriasis: ketamine, excitement during general anesthesia, and near-terminal depth of anesthesia
Parasympatholytic agents	Blockade of the postganglionic oculomotor neuron	Mydriasis
Parasympathomimetic agents	Stimulation of the postganglionic oculomotor neuron	Miosis
Ocular disease		
Corneal disease	Trigeminal nerve stimulation through corneal or adnexal irritation	Miosis
Iridocyclitis	Local production of inflammatory mediators including prostaglandins	Miosis
Glaucoma	Afferent optic nerve lesion caused by compression of ganglion cells and nerve fiber layer axons, and pressure-induced paralysis of iris sphincter muscle	Mydriasis

VISION ABNORMALITIES

Definition

I. Partial or complete loss of vision
II. Result from lesions of visual pathway
   A. Retina
   B. Optic nerve
   C. Optic tract
   D. Lateral geniculate body (LGB)
   E. Optic radiation
   F. Visual cortex

Causes

Note: Before assuming that a neuro-ophthalmic problem exists, rule out vision loss from problems of opaque ocular media such as a large corneal opacity, cataract, and inflammation of anterior segment or vitreous.

I. Retinal disease: progressive retinal atrophy, retinal detachment, retinal dysplasia, sudden acquired retinal degeneration, ganglion cell hypoplasia, congenital stationary night blindness, inflammatory disease (see Chap. 100)
II. Optic nerve disease: CN II atrophy, aplasia, or hypoplasia, glaucomatous cupping, optic neuritis, neoplasia, trauma (see Chap. 100)
III. Intracranial disease (see Chap. 23)
   A. Optic tract lesions
      1. Inflammatory disease: canine distemper, granulomatous meningoencephalitis (GME), etc.
      2. Neoplasia
      3. Trauma
   B. LGB, optic radiation, and visual cortex
      1. Feline cerebral vascular disease
      2. Hydrocephalus
      3. Inflammatory disease: canine distemper, GME, toxoplasmosis, abscess
      4. Ischemic cerebral hypoxia: apnea, cardiac arrest
      5. Metabolic storage diseases
      6. Neoplasia
      7. Tentorial herniation
      8. Trauma

Pathophysiology

I. The normal visual pathway has several components.
   A. Retina to LGB
      1. First-order neuron: photoreceptor
      2. Second-order neuron: bipolar cell
      3. Third-order neuron: ganglion cell with axons projecting to the LGB
      4. Point-to-point retinogeniculate projection
         a) Each ganglion cell projects an axon to a specific point of synapse in the LGB (Howard, 1973).
         b) If this organization is lost or disorganized, vision is impaired or lost.
   B. LGB to visual cortex
      1. LGB neuron cell bodies project axons to the visual cortex.
      2. Point-to-point geniculocortical projection also exists.
         a) LGB neurons project their axons to specific visual cortex synaptic connections.
         b) Loss of this orderly arrangement causes loss of vision.
II. Lesion location determines the clinical signs.
III. Final common tissue response of the nervous system to any insult is cellular necrosis and degeneration, a process that is usually permanent.

Clinical Signs

I. Generalized lesions of the retina involving photoreceptors and bipolar cells
   A. Partial to complete vision loss
   B. Afferent PLR deficit in involved eye
   C. Reduced or absent menace response in involved eye
   D. Probable ophthalmoscopic abnormalities in involved eye
   E. Electroretinogram abnormalities in involved eye
II. Ganglion cell and CN II lesions
   A. Partial to complete vision loss
   B. Afferent PLR deficits on involved side
   C. Reduced or absent menace response on involved side
   D. Possible optic disk changes visible on ophthalmoscopy of the involved side
   E. Normal ERG
   F. Abnormal visual evoked response (VER)
III. Optic tract, LGB, and visual cortex lesions
   A. Bilateral lesions
      1. Partial to total vision loss
      2. Dilated unresponsive pupils if optic tract involved
      3. Normal PLR if LGB or visual cortex involved
      4. Normal on ophthalmoscopy
      5. Normal ERG
      6. Abnormal VER
      7. Possible tetraparesis and other neurologic deficits
   B. Unilateral lesions
      1. Afferent PLR deficit if optic tract involved
      2. Normal PLR if LGB or visual cortex involved
      3. Normal ocular fundus
      4. Hemianopia detectable with careful examination
      5. Normal ERG
      6. Abnormal VER
      7. Possible contralateral hemiparesis
IV. Lesions causing congenital blindness (severe retinal dysplasia, ganglion cell and optic nerve hypoplasia, and cataract)
   A. These are usually associated with a searching or wandering nystagmus.
   B. Do not confuse this nystagmus with that commonly noted in Siamese and Himalayan cats.

Diagnosis and Differential Diagnosis

I. Clinical examination (see Table 102–1)
   A. Ocular examination to detect cloudy ocular media, retinal disease, and optic disk disease
   B. Neuro-ophthalmologic examination to detect afferent or efferent mydriasis
   C. Dazzle reflex, maze response, menace response, motion detection, and optokinetic nystagmus reflex testing to determine extent of vision loss
   D. ERG to differentiate photoreceptor dysfunction from optic nerve or vision cortex dysfunction
   E. Visual evoked potentials to identify ganglion cell to visual cortex dysfunction
II. Radiographic examination: computed tomography and magnetic resonance imaging to detect orbital and intracranial lesions

Treatment

I. No specific treatment is available for the vision loss.
II. Treatment is directed at the underlying disease.
   A. Antimicrobial drugs for infectious causes
   B. Anti-inflammatory medications for inflammation
   C. Antineoplastic treatment when indicated
III. Conditions that are degenerative in nature are not treatable.

Patient Monitoring

I. There is always a guarded to poor prognosis for vision return if vision loss is total; caused by dysfunction of the retina, optic nerve, or central vision pathways; and of a duration exceeding several weeks.
II. Monitor for progressive loss of vision or the occurrence of neurologic signs indicating disease progression.
III. Visually impaired companion animals make acceptable pets.

Bibliography

Bichsel P, Jacobs G, Oliver JE Jr: Neurologic manifestations associated with hypothyroidism in four dogs. J Am Vet Med Assoc 192:1745, 1988

Bistner S, Rubin L, Cox TA, Condon WE: Pharmacologic diagnosis of Horner's syndrome in the dog. J Am Vet Med Assoc 157:1220, 1970

Boydell P: Idiopathic Horner's syndrome in the golden retriever. J Small Anim Pract 36:328, 1995

Braund KG: Neoplasia of the nervous system. Compend Contin Educ Pract Vet 6:717, 1984

Brightman AH, Macy DW, Gosselin Y: Pupillary abnormalities associated with feline leukemia complex. Feline Pract 11:24, 1977

Brightman AH II, Ogilvie GK, Tompkins M: Ocular disease in FeLV-positive cats: 11 cases (1981–1986). J Am Vet Med Assoc 198:1049, 1991

Bullmore CC, Sevedge JP: Canine meningoencephalitis. J Am Anim Hosp Assoc 14:387, 1978

Canton DD, Sharp NJH, Aguirre GD: Dysautonomia in a cat. J Am Vet Med Assoc 192:1293, 1988

Carpenter JL, King NW Jr, Abrams KL: Bilateral trigeminal nerve paralysis and Horner's syndrome associated with myelomonocytic neoplasia in a dog. J Am Vet Med Assoc 191:1594, 1987

Collins BK, O'Brien D: Autonomic dysfunction of the eye. Semin Vet Med Surg 5:24, 1990

Cuddon PA, Smith-Maxie L: Reticulosis of the central nervous system in the dog. Compend Contin Educ Pract Vet 6:23, 1984

Gerding PA, Brightman AH, Brogdon JD: Pupillotonia in a dog. J Am Vet Med Assoc 189:1477, 1986

Glauberg A, Beaumont PR: Sudden blindness as the presenting sign of eosinophilic myositis: a case report. J Am Anim Hosp Assoc 15:509, 1979

Goldfarb S, Swann PG: Case report—idiopathic tonic pupil or Adie's syndrome in the dog. Aust Vet Pract 14:20, 1984

Griffiths IR, Sharp NJH, McCullouch MC: Feline dysautonomia (the Key-Gaskell syndrome): an ultrastructural study of autonomic ganglia and nerves. Neuropathol Appl Neurobiol 11:17, 1985

Howard DR, Breazile JE: Optic fiber projections to dorsal lateral geniculate nucleus in the dog. Am J Vet Res 34:419, 1973

Hutchison CP, Buxton DF, Garrett PD: Anatomic basis for the examination of olfactory and visual cranial nerve function in dogs. Compend Contin Educ Pract Vet 6:751, 1984

Kornegay JN: Small animal neuro-ophthalmology. Compend Contin Educ Pract Vet 2:923, 1980

Lewis GT, Blanchard GL, Trapp AL, DeCamp CE: Ophthalmoplegia caused by thyroid adenocarcinoma invasion of the cavernous sinuses in the dog. J Am Anim Hosp Assoc 20:805, 1984

Longshore RC, O'Brien DP, Johnson GC et al: Canine dysautonomia: a retrospective study of ten cases. J Vet Intern Med 10:207, 1995

Morgan RV, Zanotti SW: Horner's syndrome in dogs and cats: 49 cases (1980–1986). J Am Vet Med Assoc 194:1096, 1989

Neer TM: Horner's syndrome: anatomy, diagnosis, and causes. Compend Contin Educ Pract Vet 6:740, 1984

Neer TM, Carter JD: Anisocoria in dogs and cats: ocular and neurologic causes. Compend Contin Educ Pract Vet 9:817, 1987

Rochlitz I: Feline dysautonomia (the Key-Gaskell or dilated pupil syndrome): a preliminary review. J Small Anim Pract 25:587, 1984

Scagliotti RH: Neuro-ophthalmology. Prog Vet Neurol 1:157, 1990

Sharp NJH: Feline dysautonomia. Semin Vet Med Surg (Small Anim) 5:67, 1990

Sharp NJH, Nash AS, Griffiths IR: Feline dysautonomia (the Key-Gaskell syndrome): a clinical and pathological study of forty cases. J Small Anim Pract 25:599, 1984

Shell L: Cranial nerve disorders in dogs and cats. Compend Contin Educ Pract Vet 4:458, 1982

Shell LG: The cranial nerves of the brain stem. Prog Vet Neurol 1:233, 1990

Sorjonen DC: Clinical and histopathological features of granulomatous meningoencephalitis in dogs. J Am Anim Hosp Assoc 26:141, 1990

Twitchell MJ: Amaurosis due to nonsuppurative meningoencephalitis. J Am Anim Hosp Assoc 13:500, 1977

van den Broek AHM: Horner's syndrome in cats and dogs: a review. J Small Anim Pract 28:929, 1987

Wise LA, Lappin MR: Canine dysautonomia. Semin Vet Med Surg (Small Anim) 5:72, 1990

103) Diseases of the Orbit

Cynthia S. Cook

CONGENITAL DISORDERS

Microphthalmia

Definition

A congenitally small globe, often accompanied by multiple ocular defects, including anterior segment dysgenesis, cataract, retinal dysplasia

Causes

I. Sporadic in all breeds, cause unknown
II. Inherited in some breeds
    A. Australian shepherd: associated with merle coat color and defect in retinal pigmented epithelium (RPE) differentiation during embryogenesis
    B. Cavalier King Charles spaniel
    C. Doberman pinscher: associated with persistent hyperplastic tunica vasculosa lentis and persistent hyperplastic primary vitreous
    D. Miniature schnauzer: associated with congenital cataracts

Pathophysiology

I. Most cases are genetic in origin.
II. Microphthalmia can be induced by teratogenic insult during the first month of gestation that results in cell death and subsequent growth deficiency of the neural plate and optic vesicle.
III. Persistence of the optic fissure can result in failure to establish intraocular pressure necessary for optic cup expansion later in embryogenesis.

Clinical Signs

I. Globe appears small and is often noticeably abnormal in appearance.
II. Third eyelid is prominent.
III. Secondary entropion may be present and may result in keratitis and corneal ulceration.
IV. Vision is often impaired, although if the microphthalmia is unilateral, it may not be apparent.

V. Accumulation of discharge occurs because of increased depth of conjunctival sac and inadequate tear film circulation and drainage. As a result, affected eyes are more susceptible to surface ocular infections.

Diagnosis

I. History of congenital origin
II. Predisposed breeds
III. Ocular examination: look for presence of other ocular anomalies

Differential Diagnosis

I. Enophthalmos (globe size is normal)
    A. Conformational
        1. Large, dolichocephalic breeds
        2. Bilateral and symmetrical
    B. Pain-induced
        1. Pain from eyelid irritation, foreign body, uveitis, etc. results in retraction of the globe with secondary enophthalmos.
        2. If pain is corneal in origin, partial or complete resolution occurs following application of topical anesthesia.
    C. Loss of retrobulbar fat
        1. Previous retrobulbar disease
        2. Senile
            a) Cats affected more often than dogs
            b) Bilateral
            c) Often associated with weight loss
    D. Neurogenic: Horner's syndrome (see Chap. 102)
        1. Protrusion of third eyelid and ptosis may appear similar.
        2. Miosis is a cardinal sign.
II. Phthisis bulbi
    A. History of prior injury, inflammation
    B. Acquired, not congenital
    C. Clinical examination
        1. Corneal edema, scarring, and pigmentation
        2. Evidence of chronic inflammation
III. Anophthalmos (congenital absence of globe)
    A. Extreme of microphthalmos spectrum, same causes

B. Rare; usually some globe tissue can be found
C. Management same as for microphthalmos

Treatment and Monitoring

I. Treatment is usually not required.
II. Discharge that accumulates in the conjunctival sac may be periodically removed by lavage.
III. If the cosmetic appearance is objectionable or if chronic secondary entropion results in ocular irritation and/or corneal ulceration, enucleation may be performed.

DEGENERATIVE DISORDERS

Phthisis Bulbi

Definition

Irreversible ocular damage results in shrinkage of the globe.

Causes

I. Trauma
II. Inflammation
III. Acquired, not congenital (although can occur in puppies)

Pathophysiology

Damage to the ciliary body results in the inability to secrete adequate aqueous humor to maintain intraocular pressure.

Clinical Signs and Diagnosis

I. Shrinkage of globe
II. Accumulation of ocular discharge
III. Prolapse of third eyelid
IV. Possible secondary entropion
V. Corneal edema, scarring, pigmentation
VI. Collapse of anterior chamber
VII. Low intraocular pressure (often not recordable)
VIII. Blind in affected eye

Differential Diagnosis

I. Microphthalmia: congenital, not acquired
II. Extreme enophthalmos

Treatment and Monitoring

I. Often none required unless ocular inflammation persists
II. Enucleation
  A. Indications are as follows.
    1. Objectional appearance
    2. Irreparable ocular trauma
    3. Ocular or orbital neoplasia
    4. Persistent, uncontrollable ocular inflammation and/or pain associated with irreversible vision loss

Table 103–1. *Surgical Technique for Enucleation*

1. A lateral canthotomy is performed to maximize exposure.
2. A 360° bulbar conjunctival incision is made just posterior to the limbus.
3. Blunt dissection is used to separate the globe from the bulbar conjunctiva and Tenon's capsule from the limbus to the posterior pole.
4. The extraocular muscles are transected at their insertions on the globe.
5. The optic nerve and ophthalmic arteries and veins may be isolated and ligated with 4-0 absorbable suture or small hemoclips to minimize hemorrhage.
6. Hemostasis can also be accomplished by packing the orbit with gauze and applying digital pressure for a few moments if necessary.
7. Insertion of a methylmethacrylate sphere (16–22 mm) may help avoid a sunken appearance to the orbit (Nasisse et al., 1988; Hamor et al., 1993).
   a. The sphere is inserted within the sac created by the retained orbital septum, which is a reflection of the orbit periosteum.
   b. The conjunctiva is closed over the sphere with a continuous or interrupted layer of 4-0 absorbable suture.
   c. Rarely, the sphere may be extruded during the first 3–4 weeks postoperatively, necessitating a second surgical procedure to debride and close the orbit.
      (1) This appears to be a more common complication in cats than dogs.
      (2) Implantation of an orbital sphere is contraindicated if there is suspicion of an infectious or neoplastic process with extraocular extension.
8. The third eyelid is transected at its base.
9. The eyelid margins are excised to include all hair follicles and meibomian glands.
10. The subcutis is closed in a continuous pattern using 4-0 absorbable suture.
11. The skin is sutured in an interrupted pattern with 4-0 nonabsorbable suture.

    5. May include eyes that are painful and blind as a result of chronic glaucoma; however, alternative procedures may be suitable for such cases (see Chap. 98)
  B. Surgical technique is described in Table 103–1.
  C. Postoperative considerations include the following.
    1. Although an injection of a long-acting antibiotic may be administered postoperatively, oral antibiotics are usually required only if an infectious process exists.
    2. Postoperative swelling is to be expected and may resolve more rapidly if the owner is able to apply warm compresses to the surgical site several times daily for the first week.
    3. Orbital emphysema may rarely occur (Martin, 1971; Bedford, 1979).

INFLAMMATORY CONDITIONS

Orbital Cellulitis/Abscess

Definition

I. Orbital inflammation may be suppurative or nonsuppurative.

II. Cellulitis indicates diffuse inflammation; an abscess is a localized pocket of purulent material and may develop as a sequela to an initial cellulitis.

Causes and Pathophysiology

I. Migrating foreign body
    A. Foxtail and other plant awns
    B. Wood debris such as sticks
    C. Long blades of grass
    D. Porcupine quills
    E. Sewing needles
II. Secondary to dental disease
    A. Upper carnassial (fourth premolar) and molar root disease
    B. More common in brachycephalic dogs and cats
III. Extension of maxillary or frontal sinusitis
    A. Uncommon association with *Pneumonyssus caninum* frontal sinusitis (Roberts and Thompson, 1969)
    B. Nasal or sinus aspergillosis, penicilliosis
IV. Migrating parasite larvae (uncommon)
    A. *Dirofilaria immitis*
    B. *Ancylostoma* spp.
V. Eosinophilic infiltrate: uncommon, possibly immune-mediated condition described in a cat (Dziezyc et al., 1992)
VI. Etiology often undiagnosed

Clinical Signs

I. Exophthalmos
    A. Nearly always unilateral
    B. Typically acute, rarely chronic
    C. If severe, lagophthalmos and secondary exposure keratitis
    D. Globe deviation less common than with orbital neoplasia
    E. Resistance to retropulsion of the globe
    F. Pain with attempt to retropulse globe
II. Pupillary dilation ± blindness
    A. Indicates involvement of afferent (optic nerve) or efferent (pupillary branches of the oculomotor nerve) pupillary pathways
        1. Evaluation of menace response and consensual pupillary light responses necessary to differentiate

            a) Optic nerve involvement results in absent response of either pupil to light directed into the affected eye. Menace reflex is also absent.
            b) Oculomotor nerve involvement (rare) results in a positive consensual response in the contralateral eye even though the affected pupil fails to respond to direct light stimulus.
        2. Poor prognostic indicator if optic nerve involved
    B. Relatively uncommon in acute cases
III. Chemosis
IV. Protrusion of the third eyelid caused by passive pressure from orbital contents
V. Pain on opening jaw
    A. Caused by pressure of the ramus of the mandible on the orbital contents
    B. Often severe and may result in resistance to eating, particularly hard food
VI. Oral changes
    A. Swelling and possible draining tract in oral mucosa behind last molar on affected side
    B. Evidence of dental disease
VII. Variable pyrexia, leukocytosis
VIII. Normal intraocular pressure

Diagnosis

I. Clinical signs and history of acute onset are suggestive.
II. Identify any draining oral fistula or swelling behind the last upper molar.
III. Skull radiographs can be helpful to help rule out foreign bodies and neoplasia, but ultrasonography and biopsy may be ultimately required because most causes are not radiopaque.
IV. If surgical drainage is performed, material is obtained for cytology as well as culture and sensitivity.

Differential Diagnosis

I. Orbital neoplasia (Table 103–2)
    A. Usually older animals (>7 years old)
    B. More gradual onset (weeks to months)
    C. Absence of pyrexia, pain, leukocytosis
        1. However, necrosis and secondary infection

Table 103–2. **Differential Diagnosis of Exophthalmos**

Condition	Onset	Symmetry	Pain	Other Findings
Orbital cellulitis/abscess	Usually acute	Unilateral	Yes	Swelling behind last molar, fever
Zygomatic salivary gland adenitis	Gradual	Unilateral	Yes	± Purulent exudate from zygomatic papilla in mouth
Mucocele/dacryops	Gradual	Unilateral	No	Fluctuant periorbital swelling on retropulsion
Masticatory myositis	Gradual	Bilateral	Yes	Pain and localized warmth associated with masticatory muscles
Orbital neoplasia	Gradual	Unilateral	No	± Bony involvement, systemic signs of metastasis
Proptosis	Acute, traumatic	Unilateral	Yes	Evidence of trauma, marked lagophthalmos, xerophthalmia

may occur in an orbital neoplasm, making differentiation difficult.

2. Surgical exploration and biopsy may be necessary to rule out neoplasia.
   D. Deviation of globe more common
II. Traumatic proptosis
   A. History of possible or probable trauma
   B. Other evidence of trauma: hyphema, periocular contusions and fractures, systemic injuries
III. Orbital cyst/mucocele
   A. Nonpainful, nonfebrile, noninflammatory
   B. Usually gradual onset
   C. Retropulsion possible with simultaneous bulging of periorbital structures
IV. Masticatory myositis (see Chap. 80)
   A. Usually bilateral
   B. Breed predisposition: larger breeds
      1. German shepherd dog: most common
      2. Weimaraner
V. Zygomatic salivary adenitis (see Chap. 28)
   A. Divergent strabismus may rarely be seen.
   B. Purulent exudate may be present from zygomatic duct opening in the oral mucosa.
VI. Glaucoma with megophthalmos
   A. Increase in intraocular pressure is diagnostic.
   B. Presence of pain, ± pupillary dilation, and scleral injection may appear similar to exophthalmos associated with cellulitis.
   C. Severe chemosis as is seen in orbital cellulitis is not typical.
   D. Other differentiating signs of glaucoma include corneal edema, no pain on opening mouth, absence of pyrexia and leukocytosis, and no resistance to retropulsion.

Treatment

I. Administer broad-spectrum systemic antibiotics.
   A. Ampicillin 5–10 mg/kg PO TID for 10–14 days
   B. Specific antibiotic therapy based on culture and sensitivity if available
II. Apply topical ocular lubricants/antibiotic ointment liberally 3–4 times daily if lagophthalmos exists.
III. Surgical incision and drainage are indicated to relieve pressure if exophthalmos is severe and/or there is suspicion of a foreign body.
   A. A 5- to 10-mm incision is made in the oral mucosa behind last upper molar on affected side.
   B. Blunt dissection with hemostats is used to establish ventral drainage from the orbit.
   C. A temporary tarsorrhaphy may be indicated to protect the cornea.
IV. Treat other primary diseases if present.
   A. Dental disease requires extraction of affected tooth.
   B. Sinusitis may require surgical exploration.

Patient Monitoring

I. If no response to medical therapy alone occurs within 48 hours or if exophthalmos becomes severe, surgical intervention (drainage and possible biopsy) should be performed.

II. Skull radiographs and ultrasonography are indicated for recurrences that do not respond to medical and surgical therapy.

Orbital Cyst/Mucocele

Definition

I. Relatively uncommon causes of exophthalmos
II. Sialocele: rupture of the duct of the zygomatic salivary gland with leakage of saliva into the orbit (see Chap. 28)
III. Dacryops: accumulation of lacrimal secretion from ruptured lacrimal gland ducts and/or from ectopic lacrimal tissue (Martin et al., 1987)

Causes

I. Trauma
II. Congenital
III. Often unknown

Clinical Signs

I. Slowly progressive exophthalmos, usually unilateral
II. Nonpainful, noninflammatory swelling
III. Afebrile
IV. Fluctuant orbital swelling with minimal resistance to retropulsion of globe; simultaneous bulging of periorbital structures
V. Protrusion of third eyelid
VI. Bulge behind last molar (rare)

Diagnosis

I. Clinical examination findings of a fluctuant, nonpainful orbital swelling are suggestive.
II. Aspiration of the periorbital swelling often yields a thick, golden or blood-tinged fluid.
III. Cytology helps confirm the presence of a mucinous, noninflammatory fluid but does not differentiate the source.
IV. Orbital ultrasonography may reveal a hypoechoic, cystic structure behind or ventral to the globe.
V. Sialography and/or magnetic resonance imaging (MRI) may be used to confirm the involved salivary gland.

Differential Diagnosis

I. Abscess, cellulitis: acute, painful, febrile, inflammatory
II. Orbital neoplasia
   A. Most are nonfluctuant.
   B. Most difficult to rule out is myxoma/myxosarcoma, which may produce sialomucin resulting in a fluctuant swelling.
   C. Radiography of the skull, computed tomography (CT), or MRI may be needed to rule out mucin-producing tumors.

Treatment

I. Exploration of orbit with extirpation of cyst is the definitive treatment.

Table 103–3. **Orbital Neoplasms**

Tumor Origin	Reference(s)
Primary	
Osteosarcoma: most frequent	Magrane, 1965; Knecht and Greene, 1977; Kern, 1985; Cottrill et al., 1987; McCalla et al., 1989
Mast cell tumor	Kern, 1985
Reticulum cell sarcoma	Kern, 1985
Fibrosarcoma	Blodi and Ramsey, 1967; Kern, 1985
Chondrosarcoma	Magrane, 1965
Chondroma rodens (parosteal osteoma)	Pletcher et al., 1979
Meningioma of optic nerve	Barron et al., 1963; Geib, 1966; Langham et al., 1971; Andrews, 1973; Frith, 1975; Buyukmihci, 1977
Neurofibrosarcoma	Barron et al., 1963; Kern, 1985
Rhabdosarcoma (skeletal extraocular muscles)	Magrane, 1965; Siebold, 1974
Glioma of optic nerve	Williams et al., 1961; Magrane, 1965; Barnett and Grimes, 1972
Hemangiosarcoma	Gwin et al., 1982; LeCouteur et al., 1982
Secondary by Extension	
Regional adenocarcinoma	
Nasal	Gelatt et al., 1970; Peiffer et al., 1978; Kern, 1985
Salivary (usually zygomatic)	Magrane, 1965; Buyukmihci et al., 1975
Lacrimal	Magrane, 1965; Hayden, 1976; Rebhun and Edwards, 1977
Squamous cell carcinoma (from sinuses, eyelids, mouth; more common in cats)	Rebhun and Edwards, 1977; Kern, 1985; Gilger et al., 1992
Melanoma (extension from globe, lids)	Gwin et al., 1982
Myxoma/myxosarcoma	
Metastatic	
Multicentric lymphosarcoma	Saunders and Barron, 1964; Gwin et al., 1982; Lavach, 1984; Kern, 1985; Gilger et al., 1992
Adenocarcinoma	
Uterus	Bellhorn, 1972
Mammary gland	Bellhorn, 1972
Kidney	Barron et al., 1963; Bellhorn, 1972
Thyroid	Barron et al., 1963
Sweat gland	Jabara and Finnie, 1978; Berryman et al., 1981; Moise et al., 1982
Hemangiosarcoma	Gilger et al., 1992
Squamous cell carcinoma	Cook et al., 1984; Hamilton et al., 1984
Melanoma	Barron et al., 1963
Transitional cell carcinoma	Szymanski et al., 1984
Fibrosarcoma	Lavach, 1984; Gilger et al., 1992

II. Removal of involved salivary gland is indicated for zygomatic sialocele (see Chap. 28).

NEOPLASIA

Definition and Causes (Table 103–3)

  I. Primary orbital neoplasia may arise from any of the tissues present in the orbit.
  II. Secondary neoplasia occurs by extension of tumors from a primary site in adjacent tissues.
  III. Metastatic tumors invade the orbit from distant sites.

Clinical Signs

  I. Slowly progressive, unilateral exophthalmos
  II. Globe deviation: direction depends on location of tumor mass
  III. Protrusion of third eyelid, chemosis
  IV. Rarely enophthalmos from neoplastic destruction of periorbital fascia (Pentlarge et al., 1989)

  V. Resistance to retropulsion: often not painful, although this is inconsistent
  VI. Blindness, ± pupillary dilation
    A. May be caused by secondary retinal detachment and/or retinal degeneration (Barnett and Grimes, 1972; Frith, 1975)
    B. May indicate involvement of afferent (optic nerve) or efferent (pupillary branches of the oculomotor nerve) pupillary pathways
    C. Evaluation of menace response and consensual pupillary light responses necessary to differentiate
    D. Poor prognostic indicator
  VII. Extraocular findings: presence of palpable masses associated with orbital rim, sinuses, oral cavity
  VIII. Evidence of systemic disease in cases of metastatic neoplasia

Diagnosis

  I. History and clinical signs of slowly progressive, nonpainful exophthalmos
  II. Plain skull radiographs

A. Differentiate soft tissue density from fluid accumulation
B. Identify bone alterations
III. Ultrasonography: increased echogenicity of retrobulbar tissues with indentation and deformation of globe
IV. CT scan, MRI: define extent of neoplastic invasion (Calia et al., 1994; Ramsey et al., 1994; Morgan et al., 1996)
V. Biopsy and histopathology
Approach depends on localization of mass and requires general anesthesia.
A. Lateral percutaneous
B. Subconjunctival
C. Via oral cavity
D. Following exenteration
VI. Systemic work-up to detect metastatic disease
A. Physical examination, palpation of lymph nodes and abdomen
B. Thoracic radiography
C. Serum biochemistries

Differential Diagnosis

I. Orbital cellulitis
II. Masticatory myositis
III. Orbital cyst or mucocele
IV. Megophthalmos vs. exophthalmos

Treatment

I. Surgical therapy
A. Lateral orbitotomy ± zygomatic arch resection (Slatter and Abdelbaki, 1979; Gilger et al., 1994)
1. Indications
a) Procedure for excision of orbital mass while potentially preserving the globe intact; can be converted to exenteration intraoperatively if necessary
b) For laterally located (e.g., lacrimal gland) tumors
c) If globe is visual and not directly involved with the neoplasm
2. Can be used for partial tumor excision, palliative therapy if tumor is extensive
B. Orbital exenteration
1. May be required for tumor excision even if globe is visual, because adequate exposure of medial orbit is not possible without globe removal
2. Indications
a) Orbital tumor or ocular tumor with extraocular extension
b) Procedure the same as for enucleation except that orbital contents (extraocular muscles, orbital fat, and all conjunctivae) are also removed
II. Adjunct therapy (depending on tumor type)
A. Chemotherapy is the primary mode of treatment for lymphosarcoma and mast cell tumors.
B. Doxorubicin has been used for orbital sarcoma (Schoster and Wyman, 1978).

C. Radiation therapy may be tried (Adams et al., 1987; Roberts et al., 1987; Evans et al., 1989).
1. In general, carcinomas are more responsive than sarcomas.
2. Both teletherapy and brachytherapy have been used in this area with limited success.
III. Indications for euthanasia
A. Extension of orbital tumor has exceeded surgical options.
B. Systemic disease due to metastasis is unresponsive to adjunct therapy.

Patient Monitoring

I. Prognosis for orbital tumors, primary or secondary, is guarded. In one survey, 91.3% of orbital tumors were malignant, with only 3 of 23 dogs surviving beyond 3 years (Kern, 1985).
II. Following palliative partial tumor excision, regrowth can be expected within 3–12 months unless there is a response to adjunct therapy.

TRAUMATIC PROPTOSIS

Definition

Forward displacement or prolapse of the globe beyond the eyelid margins

Causes and Pathophysiology

I. Most common in brachycephalic breeds
A. Large palpebral fissures
B. Shallow orbit
II. Caused by blunt trauma, dog fight, overzealous restraint, progressive retrobulbar disease

Clinical Signs and Diagnosis

I. Acute exophthalmos
II. Lagophthalmos with secondary corneal exposure, drying, ulceration
III. Subconjunctival hemorrhage, severe chemosis from secondary occlusion of vortex veins
IV. Deviation of the globe if one or more extraocular muscles have ruptured (rupture of the medial rectus most common, results in exotropia)
V. Pupillary dilation and blindness
A. Indicates damage to optic nerve
B. May be temporary or permanent but justifies a guarded prognosis for return of vision
VI. Other evidence of ocular trauma
A. Hyphema
B. Periocular contusions, fractures

Differential Diagnosis

I. Exophthalmos due to orbital space-occupying lesion
A. Absence of history or other evidence of trauma
B. Lids usually able to partially cover globe
II. Anatomic macropalpebral fissure (see Chap. 93)

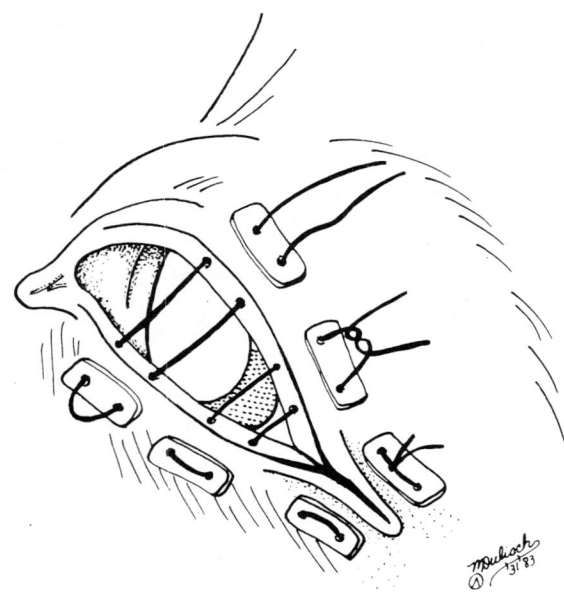

Figure 103–1. Technique for temporary tarsorrhaphy. Sutures are passed through the lid margins at the opening of the meibomian glands and anchored with elastic stents, effectively closing the eyelids. (From Morgan, 1985, with permission.)

Treatment

I. Surgical therapy: goals
   A. Reestablish venous return and relieve chemosis
   B. Relieve lagophthalmos and exposure keratitis
   C. Relieve tension on optic nerve and maximize opportunity for return of vision
II. Surgical technique (Fig. 103–1)
   A. A lateral canthotomy is often needed.
   B. A peritomy has been recommended when chemosis is severe but is rarely necessary.
   C. The upper and lower eyelid margins are apposed, and a temporary tarsorrhaphy is performed using stents and 4-0 suture.
      1. A small opening is left nasally to facilitate application of topical medication.
      2. Care is taken not to invert or evert the lid margins.
III. Postoperative care
   A. Broad-spectrum systemic antibiotics
   B. Topical antibiotic ointment
   C. Application of warm compresses TID to facilitate resolution of orbital swelling
   D. Elizabethan collar to prevent rubbing at sutures

Patient Monitoring

I. Tarsorrhaphy sutures are removed after 10–14 days.
II. Possible postoperative sequelae include the following.
   A. Blindness
      1. Not uncommon; a guarded visual prognosis should always be given (Gilger et al., 1995).
      2. Persistent pupillary dilation indicates damage to optic nerve and a poor prognosis.
      3. Loss of menace response confirms blindness.
      4. Blindness may occur despite a normal-appearing optic disk on fundic exam.
   B. Permanent deviation of globe
      1. Usually lateral deviation occurs as a result of rupture of medial rectus and/or inferior oblique muscles.
      2. Globe may be repositioned using nylon anchoring suture nasally.
      3. A permanent medial canthoplasty conceals exposed sclera, results in improved cosmetic appearance, and provides better protection of the cornea.
   C. Persistent anterior displacement of globe with lagophthalmos
      1. Temporary tarsorrhaphy may be repeated for an additional 10–14 days.
      2. Semipermanent tarsorrhaphy may be left in place for 3–6 months.
   D. Corneal dryness
      1. Deficient tear function due to damage to lacrimal gland or ducts
      2. Secondary to lagophthalmos and poor distribution of tear film
      3. Detected by Schirmer's tear tests and corneal staining with rose bengal
   E. Abnormal fundus examination
      1. Optic nerve damage may result in secondary retinal degeneration.
      2. This is a long-term sequela; initially the optic nerve may appear normal even if irreversibly damaged.

Bibliography

Adams WM, Withrow SJ, Walshaw R et al: Radiotherapy of malignant nasal tumors in 67 dogs. J Am Vet Med Assoc 191:311, 1987

Andrews EJ: Clinicopathologic characteristics of meningiomas in dogs. J Am Vet Med Assoc 163:151, 1973

Barnett KC, Grimes TD: Retrobulbar tumour and retinal detachment in a dog. J Small Anim Pract 13:315, 1972

Barron CN, Saunders LZ, Jubb KV: Intraocular tumors in animals. III. Secondary intraocular tumors. Am J Vet Res 24:835, 1963

Bedford PGC: Orbital pneumatosis as an unusual complication to enucleation. J Small Anim Pract 20:551, 1979

Bellhorn RW: Secondary ocular adenocarcinoma in three dogs and a cat. J Am Vet Med Assoc 160:302, 1972

Bergsjo T, Arnesen K, Heim P, Nes N: Congenital blindness with ocular developmental anomalies, including retinal dysplasia, in Doberman pinscher dogs. J Am Vet Med Assoc 184:1383, 1984

Berryman FC, de Lahunta A, Summers BA, Rendano VT: Metastatic intracranial carcinoma in a cat. J Am Anim Hosp Assoc 17:387, 1981

Bertram T, Coignoul F, Cheville N: Ocular dysgenesis in Australian shepherd dogs. J Am Anim Hosp Assoc 20:177, 1984

Blodi FC, Ramsey FK: Ocular tumors in domestic animals. Am J Ophthalmol 64:627, 1967

Buyukmihci N: Orbital meningioma with intraocular invasion in a dog. Vet Pathol 14:521, 1977

Buyukmihci N, Rubin LF, Harvey CE: Exophthalmos secondary to zygomatic adenocarcinoma in a dog. J Am Vet Med Assoc 167:162, 1975

Calia C, Kirschner S, Baer K, Stefanacci J: The use of computed tomography scan for the evaluation of orbital disease in cats and dogs. Prog Vet Comp Ophthalmol 4:24, 1994

Cook CS, Peiffer RL, Stine PE: Metastatic ocular squamous cell carcinoma in a cat. J Am Vet Med Assoc 185:1547, 1984

Cottrill N, Carter J, Pechman R et al: Bilateral orbital parosteal osteoma in a cat. J Am Anim Hosp Assoc 23:405, 1987

Dziezyc J, Apolonio Santo J, Barton C: Exophthalmia in a cat caused by an eosinophilic infiltrate. Prog Vet Comp Ophthalmol 2:91, 1992

Evans SM, Goldschmidt M, McKee LJ, Harvey CE: Prognostic factors and survival after radiotherapy for intranasal neoplasms in dogs: 70 cases (1974–1985). J Am Vet Med Assoc 194:1460, 1989

Frith CH: Meningioma in a young dog resulting in blindness and retinal degeneration. Vet Med Small Anim Clin 70:307, 1975

Geib LW: Ossifying meningioma with extracranial metastasis in a dog. Pathol Vet 3:247, 1966

Gelatt KN, McGill LD: Clinical characteristics of microphthalmia with colobomas of the Australian shepherd dog. J Am Vet Med Assoc 162:393, 1973

Gelatt KN, Ladds PW, Guffy MM: Nasal adenocarcinoma with orbital extension and ocular metastasis in a dog. J Am Anim Hosp Assoc 6:132, 1970

Gelatt KN, Samuelson DA, Barrie KP et al: Biometry and clinical characteristics of congenital cataracts and microphthalmia in the miniature schnauzer. J Am Vet Med Assoc 183:99, 1983

Gilger BC, McLaughlin SA, Whitley RD, Wright JC: Orbital neoplasms in cats: 21 cases (1974–1990). J Am Vet Med Assoc 201:1083, 1992

Gilger BC, Whitley RD, McLaughlin SA: Modified lateral orbitotomy for removal of orbital neoplasms in two dogs. Vet Surg 23:53, 1994

Gilger BC, Hamilton HL, Wilkie DA et al: Traumatic ocular proptoses in dogs and cats: 84 cases (1980–1993). J Am Vet Med Assoc 206:1186, 1995

Gilmour MA, Morgan RV, Moore FM: Masticatory myopathy in the dog: a retrospective study of 18 cases. J Am Anim Hosp Assoc, 1992

Gwin RM, Gelatt KN, Williams LW: Ophthalmic neoplasms in the dog. J Am Anim Hosp Assoc 18:853, 1982

Hamilton HB, Severin GA, Nold J: Pulmonary squamous cell carcinoma with intraocular metastasis in a cat. J Am Vet Med Assoc 185:307, 1984

Hamor RE, Roberts SM, Severin GA: Use of orbital implants after enucleation in dogs, horses, and cats: 161 cases (1980–1990). J Am Vet Med Assoc 203:701, 1993

Hayden DW: Squamous cell carcinoma in a cat with intraocular and orbital metastases. Vet Pathol 13:332, 1976

Jabara AG, Finnie JW: Four cases of clear-cell hidradenocarcinomas in the dog. J Comp Pathol 88:525, 1978

Kern TJ: Orbital neoplasia in 23 dogs. J Am Vet Med Assoc 186:489, 1985

Knecht CD, Greene JA: Osteoma of the zygomatic arch in a cat. J Am Vet Med Assoc 171:1087, 1977

Knecht CD, Slusher R, Guibor EG: Zygomatic salivary cyst in a dog. J Am Vet Med Assoc 155:625, 1969

Langham RF, Bennett RR, Zydeck FA: Primary retrobulbar meningioma of the optic nerve of a dog. J Am Vet Med Assoc 159:175, 1971

Lavach JD: Disseminated neoplasia presenting with ocular signs: a report of two cases. J Am Anim Hosp Assoc 20:459, 1984

LeCouteur RA, Fike JR, Scagliotti RH: Computed tomography of orbital tumors in the dog. J Am Vet Med Assoc 180:910, 1982

Magrane WG: Tumors of the eye and orbit in the dog. J Small Anim Pract 6:165, 1965

Martin CL: Orbital emphysema: a complication of ocular enucleation in the dog. Vet Med Small Anim Clin 66:86, 1971

Martin CL, Kaswan RL, Doran CC: Cystic lesions of the periorbital region. Compend Contin Educ Pract Vet 9:1022, 1987

McCalla TL, Moore CP, Turk J et al: Multilobular osteosarcoma of the mandible and orbit in a dog. Vet Pathol 29:92, 1989

Moise NS, Riis RC, Allison NM: Ocular manifestations of metastatic sweat gland adenocarcinoma in a cat. J Am Vet Med Assoc 180:1100, 1982

Morgan RV: Manual of Small Animal Emergencies. Churchill Livingstone, New York, 1985

Morgan RV: Ultrasonography of retrobulbar diseases of the dog and cat. J Am Anim Hosp Assoc 25:393, 1989

Morgan RV, Ring RD, Ward DA, Adams WH: Magnetic resonance imaging of ocular and orbital disease in 5 dogs and a cat. Vet Radiol Ultrasound 37:185, 1996

Narfstrom K, Dubielzig R: Posterior lenticonus, cataracts and microphthalmia; congenital ocular defects in the Cavalier King Charles spaniel. J Small Anim Pract 25:669, 1984

Nasisse MP, van Ee RT, Munger RJ, Davidson MG: Use of methylmethacrylate orbital prostheses in dogs and cats: 78 cases (1980–1986). J Am Vet Med Assoc 192:539, 1988

Neuman NB: Chronic ocular discharge associated with a carnassial tooth abscess. Can Vet J 15:128, 1974

Peiffer RL, Fischer CA: Microphthalmia, retinal dysplasia, and anterior segment dysgenesis in a litter of Doberman pinschers. J Am Vet Med Assoc 183:875, 1983

Peiffer RL Jr, Spencer C, Popp JA: Nasal squamous cell carcinoma with periocular extension and metastasis in a cat. Feline Pract 8:43, 1978

Pentlarge VW, Powell-Johnson G, Martin CL et al: Orbital neoplasia with enophthalmos in a cat. J Am Vet Med Assoc 195:1249, 1989

Pletcher JM, Koch S, Stedham MA: Orbital chondroma rodens in a dog. J Am Vet Med Assoc 175:187, 1979

Ramsey D, Gerding P, Losonsky J et al: Comparative value of diagnostic imaging techniques in a cat with exophthalmos. Prog Vet Comp Ophthalmol 4:198, 1994

Rebhun WC, Edwards NJ: Two cases of orbital adenocarcinoma of probable lacrimal gland origin. J Am Anim Hosp Assoc 13:691, 1977

Roberts SR, Thompson TJ: *Pneumonyssus caninum* and orbital cellulitis in the dog. J Am Vet Med Assoc 155:731, 1969

Roberts SM, Lavach JD, Severin GA et al: Ophthalmic complications following megavoltage irradiation of the nasal and paranasal cavities in dogs. J Am Vet Med Assoc 190:43, 1987

Saunders LZ, Barron CN: Intraocular tumours in animals. IV. Lymphosarcoma. Br Vet J 120:25, 1964

Schmidt GM, Betts CW: Zygomatic salivary mucoceles in the dog. J Am Vet Med Assoc 172:940, 1978

Schoster J, Wyman M: Remission of orbital sarcoma in a dog, using doxorubicin therapy. J Am Vet Med Assoc 172:101, 1978

Siebold HR: Juvenile alveolar rhabdomyosarcoma in a dog. Vet Pathol 11:558, 1974

Slatter DH, Abdelbaki Y: Lateral orbitotomy by zygomatic arch resection in the dog. J Am Vet Med Assoc 175:1179, 1979

Stades FC: Persistent hyperplastic tunica vasculosa lentis and persistent hyperplastic primary vitreous (PHTVL/PHPV) in 90 closely related Doberman pinschers: clinical aspects. J Am Anim Hosp Assoc 16:739, 1980

Stades FC: Persistent hyperplastic tunica vasculosa lentis and persistent hyperplastic primary vitreous in Doberman pinschers: techniques and results of surgery. J Am Anim Hosp Assoc 19:393, 1983a

Stades FC: Persistent hyperplastic tunica vasculosa lentis and persistent hyperplastic primary vitreous in 90 Doberman pinschers: pathological aspects. J Am Anim Hosp Assoc 19:791, 1983b

Stades FC: Persistent hyperplastic tunica vasculosa lentis and persistent hyperplastic primary vitreous in Doberman pinschers: genetic aspects. J Am Anim Hosp Assoc 19:957, 1983c

Szymanski C, Boyce R, Wyman M: Transitional cell carcinoma of the urethra metastatic to the eyes in a dog. J Am Vet Med Assoc 185:1003, 1984

Wilkinson GT, Sutton RH, Grono LR: *Aspergillus* spp. infection associated with orbital cellulitis and sinusitis in a cat. J Small Anim Pract 23:127, 1982

Williams J, Garlick E, Beard D: Glioma of the optic nerve of a dog. J Am Vet Med Assoc 138:377, 1961

Williams LW, Gelatt KN, Gwin RM: Ophthalmic neoplasms in the cat. J Am Anim Hosp Assoc 17:999, 1981

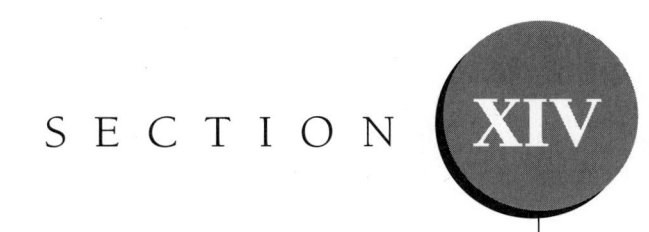

Diseases of the Ear

104

Introduction

Sandra R. Merchant

GENERAL INFORMATION

I. Diseases of the ear are common, and chronic cases are often referred to a veterinary specialist.
II. Diseases of the external ear may be a reflection of, or intimately associated with, an underlying dermatologic condition and are best evaluated with a complete dermatologic/otic examination.
III. Chronic disease with compromise of the external ear canal or involvement of the middle ear may require surgical intervention for resolution of clinical signs.
IV. Diseases of the inner ear most often present with neurologic signs, including head tilt, nystagmus, and asymmetrical limb ataxia. A complete neurologic evaluation is indicated if such signs are present.
V. Deafness requires a complete clinical examination including behavioral and electrophysiologic assessments.

DEFINITIONS

I. Otitis externa is acute or chronic inflammation of the epithelium of the external auditory meatus, which may also involve the pinna.
II. Otitis media is acute or chronic inflammation of the structures of the middle ear, including the tympanic membrane, the tympanic cavity, the tympanic nerve, the auditory tube, and the three auditory ossicles.
III. Otitis interna is inflammation of the inner ear structures, including the cochlea, the vestibule, and the semicircular canals.
IV. The definitions here are extended to incorporate neoplastic processes that do not necessarily cause inflammation.
V. Deafness is the lack or loss of the sense of hearing and may be either conductive or sensorineural in origin.
   A. Conductive deafness occurs when the transmission and/or transduction of sound is compromised in the external or middle ear.
   B. Sensorineural deafness occurs when the physics or hydrodynamics of the inner ear are altered or when there is abnormality in the receptor cell of the cochlea or any part of the auditory pathway from the acoustic nerve to the auditory cortex.

ANATOMY OF THE EAR

I. Pinna
   A. The shape of the pinna is breed-specific in the dog, but there is little breed variation in the cat.
   B. The function of the pinna is to funnel and transmit sound from the external environment to the tympanic membrane.
   C. The movement of the pinna is controlled by 19 muscles, all innervated by branches of the facial nerve (cranial nerve VII). The mobility supplied by these muscles contributes to the well-developed directional hearing.
   D. The pinna and the vertical canal are supported by the cone-shaped auricular cartilage, which provides both the shape and stability. The portion that gives the pinna its shape is the helix.
II. External auditory meatus (external ear canal)
   A. The external ear canal is 5–10 cm in length and 4–5 mm in width.
   B. The vertical canal is essentially a continuation of the pinna. The anatomic marker that divides the pinna from the vertical canal is the large tubercle (prominence) of the antihelix, which is located on the medial aspect of the ear canal as the cartilage begins to form a complete tube.
   C. The longer vertical canal runs ventrally and slightly rostrally before bending into the shorter horizontal canal.
   D. The annular cartilage gives shape to the horizontal canal and is attached to the auricular cartilage by an annular ligament.
   E. The vertical and horizontal canal is lined by skin that is similar to the rest of the body.
      1. The epithelium is relatively flat and does not form rete ridges.
      2. The dermis constitutes the major thickness of the skin.
      3. The most superficial glands are the sebaceous

glands that become larger and more numerous deeper down the ear canal.

4. The ceruminous glands are modified apocrine glands and are in the deep dermis.
5. The combination of these two glandular secretions and desquamating stratum corneum cells make up normal earwax.
6. Hair follicles are fewer in number and smaller than those in normal skin.
7. Hair follicle density and apocrine gland density vary between dog breeds. The cocker spaniel, English springer spaniel, and Labrador retriever have more hair follicles and apocrine glands when compared with greyhound and mongrel dogs (Stout-Graham et al., 1990).
8. In the cat, sebaceous and apocrine glands are more numerous in the proximal one third of the horizontal canal, although the glands are present throughout the external meatus.
9. Studies in humans and the guinea pig have proved that there is a self-cleaning function achieved by a process called epithelial migration. Epithelial cells move off the tympanic membrane distally along the canal wall and transport debris passively toward the canal opening (Logas, 1994).

F. The tympanic membrane separates the external ear from the middle ear.
1. It is thin in the center, becoming thicker near its periphery.
2. It has a small upper portion, the pars flaccida, and a large lower part, the pars tensa.
3. The pars flaccida appears opaque pink or white with small branching blood vessels.
4. The pars tensa is thick, tough, and usually pearl gray and translucent to transparent. It occasionally contains opaque radiating strands.
5. The outline of the manubrium of the malleus may sometimes be seen through the pars tensa.

III. Middle ear
A. The middle ear is composed of the tympanic cavity located in the petrous temporal bone and the eustachian tube.
B. The air-filled tympanic bulla forms the ventral part of the cavity. The dorsal portion of the cavity contains the ear ossicles.

C. The three ear ossicles—the malleus, incus, and stapes—form a bony chain from the tympanic membrane to the inner ear, where the base of the stapes attaches to the vestibular or oval window. The function of the ossicles is to amplify sound waves striking the tympanic membrane and transmit them to the vestibular window.
D. The opening of the eustachian tube is on the anteromedial surface of the cavity.
E. The cochlear or round window is located in the tympanic cavity ventral to the ossicle, serving as a potential route of communication between the middle and inner ear.

IV. Inner ear
A. The inner ear is located in the petrous temporal bone. Within its osseous labyrinth is a membranous labyrinth filled with fluid.
B. The inner ear consists of the cochlea and the vestibular apparatus.
C. The vestibular apparatus contains the communicating compartments of the saccule and the utricle, which connect the vestibule and the semicircular canals. This portion of the inner ear allows the animal to alter eye, trunk, and limb posture in relation to head position.
D. The purpose of the cochlear portion of the inner ear is to transmit motion from the oval window (caused by sound wave vibrations on the ossicles) through the perilymph to eventually produce vibration of the basilar membrane and the organ of Corti. This stimulation is then sent for interpretation by the brain.

DISEASES OF THE EAR

I. Chap. 105 covers diseases of the external ear and pinna.
II. Chap. 106 discusses diseases of the middle and inner ear.
III. Chap. 107 examines deafness and its various causes.

Bibliography

Logas DB: Diseases of the ear canal. Vet Clin North Am [Small Anim Pract] 24:905, 1994

Stout-Graham M, Kainer RA, Whalen LR, Macy DW: Morphologic measurements of the external horizontal ear canal of dogs. Am J Vet Res 51:990, 1990

105

Diseases of the External Ear and Pinna

Sandra R. Merchant
Paul E. McCarthy

OTITIS EXTERNA

Definition

I. Otitis externa is an acute or chronic inflammation of the epithelium of the external auditory meatus (external ear canal).

II. There may be concurrent pinnal disease and/or otitis media.

III. Etiology of chronic otitis externa is usually multifactorial.

Causes

I. Causes of otitis externa can be categorized as primary factors, predisposing factors, and perpetuating factors.

II. Primary factors are those that directly cause otitis externa.

   A. Parasites

      1. *Otodectes cynotis* is the most common otic parasite.

         a) It is responsible for 50% of the otitis externa in the cat and 5–10% in the dog.

         b) Many cats acquire an immune response that prevents further infestation.

      2. *Demodex* infestation can be localized to the ear, but usually other areas of the skin are also involved. It causes a ceruminous otitis externa when infesting the ear of a cat.

      3. *Sarcoptes* spp., *Notoedres* spp., fleas, flies, and lice usually affect the pinna and rarely cause external canal disease.

      4. Hard ticks and the chigger *Eutrombicula alfreddugesi* can affect the pinna and the external ear canal.

      5. The spinous ear tick, *Otobius megnini*, causes disease in the external ear canal.

   B. Foreign bodies

      1. Plant material: grass awns, foxtails

      2. Dirt, debris

      3. Dried medication

      4. Displaced hair

   C. Atopy

      1. Of atopic dogs, >50% have allergic otitis externa.

      2. Otitis externa may be the only clinical complaint.

   D. Food allergy

      1. Of food allergic dogs, 80% have allergic otitis externa.

      2. Otitis externa may be the only clinical complaint.

   E. Contact allergy

      Contact allergy is suspected in any case in which the ear disease worsens significantly while undergoing treatment.

   F. Disorders of keratinization

      1. Seborrheic disease is the most common problem seen (see Chap. 88).

      2. Fatty acids can be irritating to the ear canal epithelium.

      3. Other causes of keratinization disorders include hypothyroidism, male feminizing syndrome, Sertoli or interstitial cell tumors, and ovarian imbalance.

   G. Immune-mediated skin diseases

      1. These include pemphigus foliaceus, pemphigus erythematosus, cutaneous lupus erythematosus, systemic lupus erythematosus, pemphigus vulgaris, bullous pemphigoid, and drug eruptions.

      2. Pinnal involvement is usually more pronounced than vertical or horizontal canal involvement.

   H. Neoplasia

      1. Inflammatory polyps in cats may present as recurrent unilateral otitis externa.

2. Other neoplasms include sebaceous gland tumor, basal cell tumor, mast cell tumor, ceruminous gland tumor, fibroma, fibrosarcoma, chondroma, chondrosarcoma, squamous cell carcinoma, and trichoepithelioma (Scott et al., 1995).

  I. Miscellaneous diseases
  1. Juvenile cellulitis (puppy strangles)
  2. Zinc-responsive dermatosis
  3. Lethal acrodermatitis of bull terriers
III. Predisposing factors increase the likelihood that an animal will develop otitis externa.
  A. Conformation abnormalities
    1. Narrow ear canals, hair in the ear canal, and floppy, heavy ears decrease aeration and increase heat and moisture.
    2. The Labrador retriever, the American cocker spaniel, and the English springer spaniel have greater numbers of hair follicles and apocrine glands when compared with greyhound and mongrel dogs.
  B. Ear canal epithelial compromise
    1. It may be secondary to chronically wet ears or improper drying after cleaning.
    2. Maceration of the epidermis with loss of the stratum corneum barrier function is seen.
  C. Obstruction of the ear canal
    1. Epithelial swelling from an acute inflammatory process can compromise the ear canal diameter.
    2. Tumors may also occlude the ear canal.
  D. Systemic diseases
    1. Diseases that cause impairment of cell-mediated immunity may predispose to otitis externa. These diseases include feline leukemia virus, feline immunodeficiency virus, canine parvovirus, and canine distemper virus.
    2. Other systemic diseases that are infrequently associated with otitis externa include hyperadrenocorticism and diabetes mellitus.
IV. Perpetuating factors do not usually cause clinical disease alone but prevent resolution or actually worsen an existing otitis externa.
  A. Bacteria
    1. Bacteria colonize the external ear canal given the appropriate environment or ear canal alterations.
    2. Low numbers of bacteria are found in normal ears.
    3. The most common bacteria associated with otitis externa are *Staphylococcus intermedius, Staphylococcus epidermidis, Streptococcus* spp., *Pseudomonas* spp., *Proteus* spp., and *Escherichia coli.*
  B. Fungi
    1. *Malassezia* spp. are the most common fungi to affect the ears.
     a) Low numbers of *Malassezia* are found in normal ears.
     b) It colonizes the external ear canal given the opportunity.
     c) Overgrowth is often associated with ceruminous otitis.
     d) Recurrent infection is often associated with allergic otitis externa.
    2. Other fungi and yeast that can cause ear disease include *Candida, Aspergillus, Trichophyton*, and *Microsporum* spp.
  C. Otitis media
    1. Although otitis media can cause recurrent otitis externa, more often recurrent otitis externa is the cause of otitis media.
    2. Otitis media is usually bacterial in origin (see Chap. 106).
  D. Progressive pathologic changes
    1. They occlude the canal and cause increased wax formation, decreased natural cleaning (epithelial migration), and decreased ability to manually clean the ear or apply topical medication.
    2. They include tissue hyperplasia and glandular dilation and hyperactivity.

Pathophysiology

  I. Although there are many causes for otitis externa, a common pathway exists for the development of otitis externa (Logas, 1994).
  II. In the acute stage, the canal becomes erythematous and swollen. As the disease continues, thickening of the epidermis occurs with hyperkeratosis and acanthosis, dermal vasodilation and edema, and an increase in migration of inflammatory cells into the dermis and epidermis.
  III. Natural epithelial migration is inhibited.
  IV. The sebaceous and apocrine glandular activity is increased. The composition of the cerumen that is produced is also altered.
  V. The combination of increased epidermal thickness, increased glandular activity, and decreased epithelial migration leads to excessive wax production and entrapment in the canal, and this further leads to increased bacterial and yeast infections.
  VI. Persistent inflammation and infection can lead to permanent changes such as calcification/ossification of the auricular cartilages, dermal fibrosis, and permanent stenosis of the ear canal lumen.

Clinical Signs

  I. Pruritus is a common clinical sign and is manifested as head shaking, periauricular self-trauma with excoriations and alopecia, and rubbing the side of the head.
  II. A painful ear may cause the animal to tilt the head with the affected side down.
  III. A discharge or foul odor may be noted.
  IV. Erythema of the pinna and vertical canal with little to no erythema of the horizontal canal is most commonly associated with allergic otitis externa.
  V. Erosions and ulceration of the ear are most commonly seen with gram-negative bacterial infections or contact dermatitis.

VI. Chronic infection/inflammation may lead to ear canal stenosis, palpable ossification of the external ear canal, and possibly decreased hearing.

Diagnosis

I. A complete dermatologic history and examination are imperative because the ear is an extension of the skin.
II. An otoscopic examination is required.
  A. The unaffected or least affected ear is examined first.
  B. If a culture is indicated, this is performed first with a sterile Culturette.
  C. Cytology of the ear canal exudate is advised every time the animal is examined.
    1. Cytologic stains used include Gram's stain, Wright-Giemsa stain, modified Wright-Giemsa stain (Diff-Quik), and new methylene blue.
    2. The smear is evaluated for number and morphology of bacteria, number of yeast, and presence of fungal hyphae, parasites, white blood cells, cerumen, or neoplastic cells.
    3. A few yeast and a few gram-positive cocci can be seen in normal ears. Evaluation of the significance of numbers of bacteria and yeast also needs to take into account the amount of exudate and reaction of the ear canal.
    4. Evidence of white blood cells may indicate systemic response to the inflammation/infection and the need for systemic therapy.
  D. Note the severity or presence of erythema, erosion/ulceration, tissue hyperplasia, exudate (color and odor), or masses.
  E. Assess the state of the tympanic membrane.
    1. Lack of a membrane or abnormalities such as discoloration, thickening, or abnormal tension (bulging outward or caving inward) may indicate active or previous middle ear disease.
    2. A normal tympanic membrane does not rule out middle ear disease.
III. A definitive diagnosis may require further diagnostic tests or therapeutic trials.
  A. Bacterial or fungal culture and sensitivity
  B. Skin scraping and trial scabicidal therapy
  C. Hypoallergenic diet trial
  D. Intradermal skin testing or in vitro blood testing for allergies
  E. Discontinuation of any topical or systemic drugs if drug reaction is suspected
  F. Biopsy if neoplasia or immune-mediated disease are considerations
  G. Evaluation of estrogen/testosterone levels or surgical intervention (spaying, castration) for sex hormonal diseases
  H. Thyroid evaluation
  I. Evaluation for any systemic disease that may manifest with ear involvement

Differential Diagnosis

I. A diagnosis of otitis externa is a clinical description and does not imply any specific underlying cause. A differential diagnosis list is based on the history, as well as physical, dermatologic, and otoscopic examinations.
II. All primary, predisposing, and perpetuating factors must be identified.
III. Rule out a concurrent otitis media/interna if the ear disease has been chronic and/or recurrent.

Treatment

I. Ear cleaning
  A. Ear cleaning both in hospital and at home is a vital part of successful treatment.
  B. Excessive wax and purulent debris may prevent interaction of the topical drug with the infectious agent or decrease its efficacy.
  C. Aggressive cleaning and flushing may remove foreign bodies, degenerating cellular debris, and bacterial toxins that can exacerbate the otic inflammation.
  D. Hair is plucked and clipped away from the canal and pinna.
  E. Ceruminolytic agents may be necessary to micelialize the wax and aid in its removal.
    1. They may be irritating and must be thoroughly flushed from the canal.
    2. These agents and some topical medications may be contraindicated in animals with ruptured tympanic membranes.
  F. Cleaning solutions can be instilled in the ear with a bulb syringe, squeezed directly from the bottle (if packaged appropriately), or delivered through a tom cat catheter or rubber feeding tube.
    1. Water pulsating devices can be used.
    2. Sedation or general anesthesia may be needed.
  G. Ear loops or ear curettes are helpful for removing wax, crust, debris, and foreign bodies that remain after flushing.
  H. Drying the ear removes any residual material suspended in the flushing solution.
    1. Drying may be performed with low-powered suction devices (syringes attached to tom cat catheters or rubber feeding tubes and then attached to surgical vacuum suction).
    2. Cotton balls and use of drying agents and solution can be used both in hospital and at home.
    3. Use of cotton swabs is avoided because of potential damage to the ear canal epithelium and potential for pushing the exudate farther down the canal.
II. Topical therapy
  A. Most cases of otitis externa require daily topical medication.
  B. The majority of otic preparations are various combinations of antibacterial, antifungal, antiinflammatory, and antiparasiticidal agents.
  C. In using combination medications, match the potency of each drug to the severity of each etiologic component.
  D. Antibacterial agents are chosen based on cytologic evaluation or culture and sensitivity.

E. Antifungal agents are needed when significant yeast is seen cytologically.

F. Anti-inflammatory medication is needed to decrease erythema, tissue edema, and cerumen production and for management of allergic otitis. Low-potency glucocorticoids are used if long-term management is required.

III. Systemic therapy

A. Systemic therapy is warranted if otitis externa is complicated by otitis media.

B. Antibiotic therapy is based on bacterial culture and sensitivity.

C. Short-term oral glucocorticoid therapy (prednisone or prednisolone at 0.25–0.5 mg/lb PO SID) is often helpful in decreasing tissue inflammation and edema.

D. Antifungal agents such as ketoconazole (5–10 mg/kg PO SID) may be needed for *Malassezia* infections that will not resolve.

IV. Lateral ear canal resection

A. Indications

1. It is indicated for animals with persistent otitis externa confined to the vertical ear canal.

2. Surgery facilitates topical treatment of the ear canal, allows drainage, and changes the microenvironment by altering the temperature and humidity of the horizontal ear canal.

3. It does not cure otitis externa.

B. Technique (McCarthy and McCarthy, 1994)

1. Two parallel skin incisions are made along the vertical ear canal from the dorsal opening of the canal to below the level of the horizontal ear canal ventrally.

2. The length of the skin incisions is 1.5 times the actual length of the vertical ear canal.

3. The skin incisions are connected ventrally to form a U-shaped incision.

4. The cartilage of the vertical ear canal is resected using scissors, making sure the incisions in the cartilage do not converge at the level of the horizontal canal. The distance between the two parallel incisions is kept maximal.

5. The cartilaginous incision extends down to the ventral limit of the horizontal ear canal in order to allow the free flap of cartilage to hinge ventrally.

6. One third to one half of the cartilaginous flap is excised, and the remainder of the hinged flap is pulled ventrally.

7. If the flap partially occludes the opening to the horizontal ear canal, the cartilage incisions are extended more ventrally.

8. The mucosa of the ear canal is apposed to the skin margin using a 4-0 nonabsorbable or absorbable monofilament suture material.

9. Sutures do not engage the cartilage unless the mucosa is judged to have suboptimal holding potential.

10. The ear(s) are bandaged over the head until suture removal in 10–14 days.

V. Vertical ear canal resection

A. Indications

1. Similar to lateral ear canal resection

2. End-stage otitis externa when the horizontal ear canal is determined to be patent

a) It is used when the client is not willing to accept the risks of total ear canal ablation.

b) The horizontal ear canal must be relatively disease free.

c) It may need to be combined with a ventral bulla osteotomy.

3. Traumatic separation of the external ear canal at the annular ligament

B. Technique (McCarthy and McCarthy, 1994)

1. A skin incision encircles the external opening of the ear canal and is extended ventrally along the vertical ear canal to a level 1 cm below the junction with the horizontal ear canal.

2. Dissection continues as close to the perichondrium as possible using a combination of sharp and blunt dissection.

3. The facial nerve courses horizontally just ventral to the horizontal ear canal and care must be taken during dissection in this area.

4. The vertical ear canal is dissected free to the level of the annular cartilage, where it is transected.

5. Samples are obtained for cytology, culture, and sensitivity, and the entire canal is submitted for histopathology.

6. The mucosa of the horizontal ear canal is sutured circumferentially to the surrounding skin. The remainder of the skin dorsal to the canal is sutured in the form of a "T" using a simple interrupted pattern.

VI. Total ear canal ablation and lateral bulla osteotomy

A. Indications

1. End-stage otitis externa and concurrent otitis media

2. Failed lateral or vertical ear canal resection

3. Neoplasia of the external ear canal

4. Traumatic separation of the external ear canal at either the annular ligament or the external acoustic meatus

B. Goals of surgery

1. Remove the epithelial source of infection

2. Enlarge the opening of the external acoustic meatus and allow granulation tissue to fill the tympanic bulla

3. Establish temporary drainage of the tympanic bulla and periauricular tissues

C. Technique (McCarthy and McCarthy, 1994)

1. An incision is made encircling the external opening of the ear canal.

2. The skin incision is extended ventrally along the vertical ear canal to a point 1 cm below the level of the horizontal ear canal.

3. Dissection is continued as close to the perichondrium as possible, using a combination of sharp and blunt dissection.

4. The entire ear canal is dissected free to the

level of its connection with the petrous temporal bone at the external acoustic meatus.

5. The facial nerve is identified and protected.
6. Retraction of soft tissues ventral and cranial to the external acoustic meatus is done with extreme care. Hemorrhage from the retroglenoid recess cranially or the maxillary artery ventrally may result in uncontrollable blood loss.
7. The ear canal is separated from the petrous temporal bone.
8. The opening to the tympanic bulla is enlarged with rongeurs or a pneumatic drill and bur.
9. All epithelium around the external acoustic meatus and within the tympanic bulla is removed. Care is taken not to damage structures located dorsomedially in the bulla.
10. Culture and sensitivity testing of the bulla contents and histopathology of the canal are performed.
11. Either a Penrose drain or a closed suction drain is placed within the bulla. The Penrose drain exits ventral to the surgical site.
12. The surgical incision is closed in two layers with the resulting suture line forming a "T" shape.

Patient Monitoring

I. Postoperative monitoring is as follows.
   A. Patient monitoring and complications following lateral ear resection
      1. Sedating the animal facilitates suture removal and cleansing of the ear canal.
      2. Small areas of dehiscence not associated with the horizontal canal opening can be allowed to heal by second intention.
      3. Larger areas of dehiscence or areas involving the opening of the horizontal ear canal are managed by débriding and resuturing to avoid stenosis of the horizontal ear canal.
      4. Stenosis of the horizontal ear canal is usually the result of an inadequate ventral reflection of the vertical ear canal cartilaginous flap and can be treated by revision of the canal or by total ear canal ablation.
      5. Failure of the surgery is often due to misapplication of the procedure rather than poor surgical technique.
   B. Patient monitoring and complications following vertical ear canal resection
      1. The ear can be bandaged or an Elizabethan collar placed until suture removal in 10 days.
      2. Sedation may be needed for suture removal and to allow assessment of the ear canal opening.
      3. Areas of dehiscence around the canal opening are resutured to avoid stenosis.
      4. Other complications include facial nerve palsy and failure of the pinna to stand erect.
   C. Patient monitoring and complications following ear canal ablation
      1. The head is bandaged, taking precautions not to interfere with respiratory function.
      2. If a Penrose drain is used, the bandage is changed daily to monitor the drainage.
      3. If a closed suction system is used, the collection tubes are changed frequently to maintain suction.
      4. Drains can usually be removed on the third day postoperatively. At the same time, the bandage is removed and an Elizabethan collar is placed until suture removal.
      5. Dehiscence of the suture line may be allowed to heal by second intention or can be resutured.
      6. Facial nerve palsy occurs in about 50% of the cases, but 80% of these regain function within a few weeks.
      7. Inner ear damage may result from overly aggressive curettage of the tympanic bulla.
      8. Periauricular abscessation and fistulation may occur anytime postoperatively, usually as the result of infected epithelial tissue remaining in or near the tympanic bulla. Such an event warrants re-exploration of the lateral bulla osteotomy.
      9. Animals undergoing a total ear canal ablation with lateral bulla osteotomy may be partially deaf.
         a) Transmission of sound via bone conduction may still allow for some auditory function.
         b) Subjectively, most dogs postoperatively appear to hear about the same as prior to surgery.
II. Regardless of the type or severity of otitis externa/media, client education and follow-up evaluation are extremely important.
   A. Clients must be instructed on the appropriate method to clean and dry the ear canal or how to examine a suture line.
   B. Continued re-evaluation of the ear canal every 1–2 weeks is performed until the cytologic evaluation and otoscopic examination are normal.
   C. Long-term, indefinite, maintenance therapy may be needed in animals with unresolvable underlying diseases or non-correctable predisposing factors or in animals with significant ear canal stenosis, especially if surgery is not a viable option.

DERMATOSES OF THE PINNA

See Table 105–1 and Chap. 83.

Aural Hematoma

Definition and Causes

I. An aural hematoma is an accumulation of serosanguineous fluid or blood in the pinna.
II. Scratching and/or shaking of the head is the primary cause and is often due to underlying otitis externa.

Table 105–1. Diseases of the Pinna

Disease	Areas Affected	Clinical Lesions	Diagnosis	Treatment
Demodicosis	#	A, B, C, D	Skin scrape	Local—no Tx; systemic—amitraz, ivermectin, milbemycin
Dermatophytosis	#	A, B, C, D	Culture	Topical antifungal agent, griseofulvin or itraconazole PO
Alopecia areata	#	B	Biopsy	No Tx
Pinnal alopecia	*	B	Rule out Dx	No Tx
Periodic alopecia	*	B	Rule out Dx	No Tx
Congenital alopecia	#	B	Rule out Dx	No Tx
Hypothyroidism	¶	B, D	Thyroid testing	T_4 supplementation
Atopy	#	A	Skin test, blood test	Desensitization vaccine, topical steroids
Food allergy	#	A	Food trial	Avoidance, topical steroids
Actinic (solar) dermatitis	*	A, B, D, E	Biopsy	Limit sun exposure, sunscreens
Contact dermatitis	*	A, B, C, D, E	Provocative exposure	Avoidance
Dermatomyositis	#	A, B, D, E	Muscle, skin Bx, EMG	None; pentoxifylline?
T-cell lymphoma	¶	A, E, F	Biopsy	Chemotherapy
Juvenile cellulitis	¶	A, B, D, E	Biopsy	Steroids ± antibiotics
Ear margin dermatosis	*	A, B, D, E	Rule out Dx	Topical antiseborrheic therapy
Fly strike	*	A, C, D	Clinical signs	Fly control; topical steroids
Sarcoptiform mange	#	A, B, D	Skin scrape, response to Tx	Lime sulfur, ivermectin
Keratinization disorders	#	B, D	Rule out Dx	Topical antiseborrheic Tx
Lichenoid-psoriasiform dermatosis of springer spaniels	*	A, C, D	Biopsy	None, antibiotics?
Zinc responsive dermatosis	¶	A, D	Biopsy	Zinc supplementation
Pemphigus foliaceus, erythematosus	¶	C, D	Biopsy	Immunosuppressive drug therapy
Staphylococcal folliculitis	¶	C, D	Biopsy, response to therapy	Antibiotics
Subcorneal pustular dermatosis	¶	C, D	Biopsy	Avlosulfon
Sterile eosinophilic pinnal folliculitis	*	C, D	Biopsy	Topical and systemic steroids
Systemic lupus erythematosus	¶	B, D, E	Biopsy, work-up systemic disease	Immunosuppressive drug therapy
Cutaneous lupus erythematosus	¶	B, D, E	Biopsy	Topical, systemic steroids, tetracycline niacinamide
Bullous pemphigoid/pemphigus vulgaris	¶	E	Biopsy	Immunosuppressive drug therapy
Vasculitis	#	D, E	Biopsy, work-up underlying disease	Immune modulating drugs
Cold agglutinin disease	#	D, E	Biopsy, positive 4°C Coombs	Systemic steroids
Frostbite	#	D, E	Clinical signs	Warm area
Proliferative thrombovascular necrosis	*	E	Biopsy	Surgery
Squamous cell carcinoma	*	A, B, D, E	Biopsy	Surgery
Insect-induced granuloma	¶	A, B, D, F	Biopsy	Avoidance
Neoplasia	#	F	Biopsy	Surgery; chemotherapy
Linear granuloma	¶	F	Biopsy	Systemic steroids
Deep/subcutaneous mycotic disease	¶	E, F	Biopsy, culture	Systemic antifungal therapy
Aural hematoma	*	F	See text	

* = pinna affected only; # = pinna and sometimes other body areas affected; ¶ = pinna and other body areas affected; A = erythema; B = alopecia; C = pustule/papule; D = scale/crust; E = ulcer/scar; F = nodule; Tx = treatment; Dx = diagnosis; Bx = biopsy; EMG = electromyogram.

III. An autoimmune component may play a primary or secondary role in its development (Kuwahara, 1986).
IV. Trauma to the vasculature of the pinna results in a hematoma developing within the auricular cartilage.

Clinical Signs

I. Fluctuant to firm swelling usually involving the concave surface of the pinna
II. Concurrent otitis externa/media

Diagnosis

I. Aspiration may reveal a serosanguineous fluid.
II. Aspiration for fluid may be negative with organized blood clots.

Differential Diagnosis

Clinical signs and physical exam findings are usually diagnostic.

Treatment

I. Aspiration can be tried for temporary relief of pain or if owners do not allow surgical drainage.
II. Surgical drainage is indicated to reduce the likelihood of recurrence and to reduce disfiguring contracture of the pinna.
III. Methods of surgical drainage include the following.
   A. Teat cannula placement (McCarthy and McCarthy, 1994)
      1. Placement can usually be done under heavy sedation or with a short-acting anesthetic.
      2. After surgical preparation, a stab incision is made in the concave surface at the most dependent aspect of the hematoma (with the ear in its normal position).
      3. The screw cap of a teat cannula is removed, and two holes are made in the collar of the cannula using a 19-gauge needle.
      4. The cannula is introduced into the hematoma through the stab incision and secured with a suture placed through the skin and collar.
      5. A second suture may be placed through the skin around the end of the tube.
      6. An Elizabethan collar may be needed.
   B. Incisional drainage (McCarthy and McCarthy, 1994)
      1. It is indicated for more chronic, organized hematomas and requires general anesthesia.
      2. A straight or "S"-shaped curvilinear incision is made over the hematoma on the concave surface of the pinna.
      3. Fluid and clots are removed.
      4. Full-thickness mattress sutures are placed parallel to the long axis of the pinna to avoid compromising the vasculature.
      5. A bandage or Elizabethan collar is applied.

Patient Monitoring

I. Cannula technique
   A. Owners are instructed to keep the opening of the cannula free of debris and milk out any fluid that accumulates.
   B. The cannula is removed after 3 weeks, and the stab incision is left to heal by second intention.
II. Incisional technique
   A. Sutures are removed in 10 days.
   B. Some disfigurement of the pinna may be seen.

Bibliography

Boothe HW, Hobson HP: Traumatic separation of auricular and annular cartilages in three dogs. Proc Am Coll Vet Surg (Miami, Florida) 3, 1992

Dubielzig RR, Wilson JW, Seireg AA: Pathogenesis of canine aural hematomas. J Am Vet Med Assoc 185:873, 1984

Gregory CR, Vasseur PB: Clinical results of lateral ear resection in dogs. J Am Vet Med Assoc 182:1087, 1983

Griffin C: Pinnal disease. Vet Clin North Am [Small Anim Pract] 24:897, 1994

Henderson JT, Radasch RM: Total ear canal ablation with lateral bulla osteotomy for the management of end-stage otitis in dogs. Compend Contin Educ Pract Vet 17:157, 1995

Joyce JA, Day MJ: Investigation into the immunopathogenesis of canine aural hematoma. Proc Euro Coll Vet Surg (Utrecht, The Netherlands) 262, 1996

Krahwinkel DJ, Pardo AD, Sims MH et al: Effect of total ablation of the external acoustic meatus and bulla osteotomy on auditory function in dogs. J Am Vet Med Assoc 202:949, 1993

Kuwahara J: Canine and feline aural hematoma: clinical, experimental and clinicopathologic observations. Am J Vet Res 47:2300, 1986

Logas DB: Diseases of the ear canal. Vet Clin North Am [Small Anim Pract] 24:905, 1994

Marino DJ, MacDonald JM, Mattiesen DT et al: Results of surgery and long-term follow-up in dogs with ceruminous gland adenocarcinoma. J Am Anim Hosp Assoc 29:560, 1993

Marino DJ, MacDonald JM, Mattiesen DT et al: Results of surgery in cats with ceruminous gland adenocarcinoma. J Am Anim Hosp Assoc 30:54, 1994

McAnulty JF, Hattel A, Harvey CE: Wound healing and brain stem auditory evoked potentials after experimental total ear canal ablation with lateral tympanic bulla osteotomy in dogs. Vet Surg 24:1, 1995

McCarthy PE, McCarthy RJ: Surgery of the ear. Vet Clin North Am [Small Anim Pract] 24:953, 1994

McCarthy PE, Hosgood G, Pechman RD: Traumatic ear canal separation and para-aural abscessation in three dogs. J Am Anim Hosp Assoc 31:419, 1995

McCarthy RJ, Caywood DD: Vertical ear canal resection for end-stage otitis externa in dogs. J Am Anim Hosp Assoc 28:545, 1992

Scott DW, Miller WH, Griffin CE: Small Animal Dermatology. WB Saunders, Philadelphia, 1995

Wilson JW: Treatment of auricular hematoma using a teat tube. J Am Vet Med Assoc 182:1081, 1983

106

Diseases of the Middle and Inner Ear

Kim Knowles

OTITIS MEDIA

Definition

I. Otitis media is defined as inflammation of the middle ear regardless of cause or duration of the disease.

II. Middle ear effusions can either be infected (suppurative otitis media) or noninfected (serous otitis media).

Causes

I. Infectious agents
   A. Bacterial otitis media is the most common type of middle ear infection.
      1. Most common bacterium is *Staphylococcus intermedius*.
      2. Other frequent pathogens include other *Staphylococcus* spp., *Pseudomonas aeruginosa*, *Proteus*, and *Streptococcus*.
   B. Fungi such as *Malassezia (Pityrosporon)* and *Candida* may occasionally be isolated, but infections with *Paecilomyces* and *Aspergillus* are extremely rare.
   C. Upper respiratory viral disease in cats has been suggested as a cause.

II. Noninfectious agents
   A. Mechanical obstruction of the eustachian tube may result in noninfectious or serous otitis media. Chronic inflammation of the pharynx or tonsils can compromise the lumen of the eustachian tube or act as a focus for spread of infection to the middle ear.
   B. Allergic disease (atopy) is a common cause of persistent bilateral otitis externa in the dog, and perforation of the tympanic membrane, in chronic cases, results in spread of inflammation to the middle ear.
   C. Inflammatory polyps in cats commonly originate in the tympanic cavity or eustachian tube and can produce a serous or suppurative inflammatory response.
   D. Tumors of the nasopharynx and tonsils may metastasize to the middle ear or result in eustachian tube obstruction, usually resulting in unilateral otitis media.
   E. Middle ear effusions can occur after radiation therapy owing to osteoradionecrosis of the bulla or disturbed lymphatic drainage of the nasopharynx.
   F. Serous middle ear effusions may become secondarily infected and evolve into suppurative otitis media.

III. Cases of chronic or recurrent unilateral otitis media indicate the need to rule out the following causes.
   A. Foreign bodies (plant awns, insects)
   B. Trauma
   C. Neoplasia (London et al., 1996)
      1. Benign tumors of external ear canal, middle ear
         a) Dogs: polyps, papilloma, sebaceous gland adenoma, basal cell tumor, ceruminous gland adenoma, histiocytoma
         b) Cats: polyps, ceruminous gland adenoma, papilloma
      2. Malignant tumors of external ear canal, middle ear
         a) Dogs: ceruminous gland adenocarcinoma, squamous cell carcinoma, round cell tumor, sarcoma, malignant melanoma
         b) Cats: ceruminous gland adenocarcinoma, squamous cell carcinoma, sebaceous gland adenocarcinoma

Pathophysiology

I. Inflammation of the middle ear can occur through three basic pathways.
   A. Direct spread across a diseased or ruptured tympanic membrane (most common)
   B. Retrograde extension through the eustachian tube from the pharynx

C. Hematogenous dissemination: suspected with septicemia

II. Multiple factors are involved in the pathogenesis of otitis media.

A. The mucous membrane lining of the middle ear and eustachian tube is an extension and modification of the ciliated respiratory epithelium.

1. Ciliated cells in the middle ear actively function in evacuating foreign material from the middle ear through the eustachian tube to the nasopharynx.

2. Pathologic changes in the epithelium from inflammation can reduce clearance of foreign material and secretions from the middle ear.

B. Mechanical or functional eustachian tube obstruction causes a decrease in intratympanic pressure as a result of oxygen resorption from the middle ear space.

1. Because the walls of the middle ear cannot collapse, negative intratympanic pressure is maintained and transudation of fluid from the vasculature into the tympanum may result.

2. This results in an environment with lowered oxygen that permits long-term, low-grade infections with microorganisms.

C. Cellular defense mechanisms are important in removing material from the tympanic bulla.

1. Ciliated epithelial cells secrete lysosomes, which aid in defense.

2. In bacterial otitis media, polymorphonuclear leukocytes predominate at first.

3. In chronic cases, macrophages increase in number.

4. Phagocytes aid in clearing foreign material from the middle ear.

D. Inflammatory mediators, including histamine, prostaglandins, and leukotrienes, have been identified in middle ear effusions in humans; they may play a role in animals.

E. Microorganisms are capable of eroding or ulcerating the epithelial tissue and tympanic membrane and can cause severe pathologic changes in the tympanic cavity, such as erosion of the mucosal lining, metaplasia of the epithelium, degeneration or proliferative changes of the osseous bulla, and accumulation of inflammatory debris in the tympanic cavity.

III. There are predisposing factors that place an animal at risk for developing otitis media.

A. Dog breeds with pendulous ears have a higher incidence of chronic otitis externa.

1. Chronic otitis externa provides a focus of infection for middle ear infections.

2. American cocker spaniels, springer spaniels, and Labrador retrievers are predisposed, possibly because of more ceruminous glands in their external ear canal (Stout-Graham et al., 1990).

B. In a recent study, cocker spaniels represented the largest population of dogs with benign and malignant aural tumors (London et al., 1996).

C. Inadequate antibiotic therapy, in cases of purulent otitis media, is implicated in causing a lingering, low-grade infection of the middle ear.

Clinical Signs

I. Head shaking

II. Pawing or rubbing the involved ear

III. Pain when ear is touched

IV. Affected ear tilted downward

V. Signs of otitis externa; foul smelling aural discharge

VI. Ipsilateral complete or partial Horner's syndrome: miosis, ptosis, enophthalmos, protrusion of third eyelid

VII. Ipsilateral hemifacial spasms (rare)

VIII. Impaired hearing

IX. Pain when chewing hard food or opening the jaw

A. The pain is secondary to involvement of the temporomandibular joint with fibrous connective tissue or bony proliferation.

B. Mild trismus (limitation of jaw opening) may be caused by pain or mechanical factors.

X. Ipsilateral facial nerve paresis/paralysis; asymmetry of the face, drooping of the lip, eyelid, ear, drooling on affected side, widened palpebral fissure, inability to close the palpebral fissure

A. Ipsilateral keratoconjunctivitis sicca (KCS) with or without exposure keratitis may occur with facial nerve paralysis.

B. *Note*: Clinically apparent involvement of the facial nerve occurs only if the inflammatory process extends to the inner ear.

Diagnosis

I. A careful history is important.

A. Onset of problem: sudden, gradual, recurrent

B. History of upper respiratory signs or a cough

C. Precipitating factors such as swimming, ear cleaning, generalized skin disease

D. Review of all previous treatments (topical, systemic)

II. A thorough physical, dermatologic, and neurologic exam is performed.

A. Dermatologic exam can rule out generalized skin or systemic diseases such as immune-mediated conditions, generalized seborrhea, atopy, and hypothyroidism

B. The neurologic exam is conducted with emphasis on signs suggestive of vestibular disease, Horner's syndrome, facial palsy, and KCS.

C. Regional lymph nodes, the oral cavity, and the pharynx are examined.

D. The ear canal, salivary and thyroid glands, mastoid region, and temporomandibular joints are palpated for pain or swelling.

E. Examine the ear canal for ectoparasites, foreign bodies, and tumors.

1. Assess inflammation and the nature and amount of exudate, and if indicated, obtain specimens for culture, cytology, and histology.

2. Good lighting, magnification, and cleaning

wax and debris from the external ear canal are important; this usually requires general anesthesia.
3. If the tympanum is obscured, a small curette can be used to remove wax and debris.
4. The ear canal may need to be gently flushed with warm saline and dried or suctioned to visualize the tympanum.
5. If a perforation or rupture of the tympanum is suspected, extreme caution is used when flushing because material may be pushed into the middle ear.
F. Assess the tympanic membrane.
1. The normal tympanic membrane is slightly concave, translucent, and pearly-gray. The malleus and fine radially distributed vessels should be apparent.
2. Discoloration of the tympanic membrane is a sign of disease.
a) Reddish color usually indicates acute otitis media.
b) Opaque white color associated with small white plaques may occur with healed perforations.
c) Opaque amber or yellow color is common in purulent otitis media.
d) Blue to purple is seen with intratympanic hemorrhage.
3. Perforations are usually associated with chronic otitis media. Polyps, granulation tissue, and tumors may protrude through a tympanic membrane perforation.
4. Bulging is usually seen when pus, blood, or serum accumulates behind the eardrum.
5. Isolated or generalized retraction of the tympanic membrane into the bulla is seen with chronic disease and suggests a partially filled tympanic cavity or an obstructed eustachian tube.
III. Laboratory tests are usually helpful.
A. Cytologic preparations of exudates can be made with Diff-Quik or new methylene blue.
B. Obtain samples for culture (aerobic, fungal, anaerobic) near the tympanum or from the middle ear if the tympanic membrane is ruptured.
1. In the presence of a rupture, a small volume of saline may be flushed into the middle ear and then aspirated for cytology and culture.
2. If the tympanum is intact, paracentesis through the ventral half of the tympanum using a spinal needle attached to a syringe may be used to obtain a sample for culture and cytology.
C. Biopsies are indicated when raised, ulcerated, or pedunculated soft tissue masses are noted on otoscopic exam.
IV. Radiologic studies include ventrodorsal, lateral, oblique, and open-mouth views. Open-mouth views are the most useful for evaluating the bulla.
A. Clouding or increased density within the normally air-filled bulla, sclerosis, or evidence of

osteomyelitis of the bulla or adjacent temporomandibular joint may be seen in chronic cases.
B. Unfortunately, normal radiographs do not rule out middle ear disease. In one report, 25% of surgically confirmed cases of otitis media had no radiographic evidence of disease (Remedios et al., 1991).
C. Computed tomography (CT) appears to be more sensitive than plain radiography in detecting changes in the bulla and surrounding soft tissues.
D. Lytic bone changes on CT images or plain radiographs strongly suggest neoplasia.
V. Evaluation for allergies may be essential in dogs with recurring middle ear infections. Hyposensitization has been very beneficial when definite allergies are demonstrated by skin testing.
VI. Audiologic examination may also be indicated (see Chap. 107).
A. Although rarely a complaint, conductive hearing loss would be expected to occur in most cases of otitis media.
B. Brain stem auditory evoked response testing usually shows an elevated threshold.
C. Impedance audiometry, an objective method of assessing the integrity of the middle ear conducting system, is one of the best ways to document a conductive hearing loss from otitis media.
VII. Surgical exploration may be required for definitive diagnosis (see later).

Differential Diagnosis

I. Avoid missing subclinical cases of otitis media, especially if concurrent otitis externa is present. Because otitis interna may occur concurrently, differentials should include causes of infectious and noninfectious labyrinthitis (see causes of otitis interna below).
II. Lesions in several parts of the nervous system may cause Horner's syndrome.
A. A combination of the animal's history and associated physical and neurologic signs usually establishes location of the lesion.
B. See Table 106–1 for examples of lesion locations and causes of Horner's syndrome.

Treatment

I. The goals of treatment are to remove any infected material or debris from the middle ear to provide an avenue for ventilation and drainage, to eliminate and control any predisposing causes, and to minimize recurrence, complications, and sequelae.
II. Deep ear cleaning requires general anesthesia.
A. Small pieces of wax can be easily removed with a curette.
1. Alligator forceps may be used to remove larger particulate material and hair.
2. Care is taken to avoid traumatizing the ear canal and producing abrasions and bleeding.
B. Discharge from the external ear canal is easily removed with gentle suction (small metal suction

*Table 106–1. **Lesion Location and Causes of Horner's Syndrome***

Location	Lesion
Preganglionic	
Hypothalamus, midbrain	Trauma, neoplasia, inflammatory diseases
Cervical and T1-T3 spinal cord	Trauma, neoplasia, embolic myelopathy
T1-T3 ventral roots or proximal peripheral nerves	Trauma (brachial plexus avulsion), neoplasia
Cranial thoracic sympathetic trunk	Neoplasia, cranial lung or mediastinal disease, trauma
Cervical sympathetic trunk	Surgical trauma, neoplasia, drug injections, bite wounds, jugular IV catheters
Postganglionic	
Middle ear	Otitis media, neoplasia, trauma (hemorrhage), iatrogenic (bulla osteotomy, ear cleaning)
Retrobulbar	Neoplasia, infections, trauma
Cavernous sinus	Neoplasia, infections, trauma

tip or open-ended tom cat catheter attached to a 12-ml syringe).

C. In severe cases, where the external ear canal is narrowed, repeated deep cleansing is usually necessary at weekly intervals until infection is controlled.

D. If the tympanic membrane is intact and concurrent otitis externa is present, an acidifying and drying agent such as Burow's solution can be used to flush the external ear canal.
   1. In cases of a perforation or when the integrity of the eardrum is unknown, irrigation with warm saline is the safest solution.
   2. If a perforation is present, flushing the middle ear may be repeated until the fluid recovered is clear of debris and blood.

III. Antibiotics are usually indicated.
   A. Systemic antibiotics
      1. Selection is based on cytologic, culture, and sensitivity results from the middle ear effusion.
      2. Commonly used antibiotics are amoxicillin with clavulanic acid, first-generation cephalosporins, enrofloxacin, and chloramphenicol.
      3. Long-term (3–6 weeks) therapy is usually required.
   B. Topical antibiotics
      1. Commercially available ear drops, with an acid pH and containing a combination of antibiotics effective against *Staphylococcus* and gram-negative organisms, with a steroid may be used.
      2. Be alert to the potential hypersensitivity and ototoxic properties of neomycin. The hypersensitivity reaction may be masked by the accompanying steroid.
      3. In the presence of an open middle ear, avoid lipid-based and ototoxic preparations.
      4. If *Malassezia* organisms are present in large numbers, acidify the external ear canal with either Burow's solution or 1 part acetic acid to 2–3 parts water (Rosychuk, 1994), and consider ketoconazole or itraconazole.

IV. Surgical management includes the following.
   A. Indications
      1. Recurrent otitis media that fails to respond to proper medical management
      2. Middle ear polyps, neoplasia, foreign bodies, or osteomyelitis of the tympanic bulla
      3. Intractable polypoid mucosal changes of the external ear canal associated with otitis media
   B. Surgical techniques (see Chap. 105)
      1. Lateral or ventral bulla osteotomy and curettage can be performed as a separate procedure or in combination with vertical ear canal resection in cases of uncomplicated otitis externa.
      2. Total ear canal ablation with an osteotomy is used in animals with end-stage ear canal disease and concurrent otitis media. A success rate of 90–95% is reported (Seim, 1993).
      3. Ventral bulla osteotomy provides excellent exposure of the tympanic cavity, allowing careful examination of its contents and adequate ventral drainage (Seim, 1993).

Patient Monitoring

I. Otoscopic exam
   A. Follow-up otoscopic examinations are the most important factor in the successful management of otitis media. Recheck every 1–2 weeks until adequate response is seen.
   B. In cases of severe concurrent otitis externa, repeated débridement and cleaning of the external ear canal under general anesthesia may be necessary until infection is controlled.
   C. Owner compliance is imperative; any predisposing factors such as swimming should be minimized.
II. Repeat culture and cytology
   A. Repeat culture and cytology of the external or middle ear are indicated with any failure to respond to therapy.
   B. If the culture remains positive and cytology indicates continued inflammation/infection, continue

systemic/topical antibiotic therapy for an additional 3–6 weeks.

C. Surgical intervention, with excision of all regional infected or inflammatory foci, coupled with bulla culture and curettage is strongly considered at this point.

III. Neurologic signs

A. Horner's syndrome and facial palsy are often permanent even when the inflammatory or infectious disorder has resolved.

1. Some cases regain incomplete recovery of various components of the facial nerve over time.

2. In those with permanent facial paralysis, contracture of facial muscles usually occurs over several months.

B. The labyrinthine segment of the facial nerve that carries the parasympathetic secretory fibers to the lacrimal gland is affected when otitis media spreads to the petrous temporal bone.

1. Exposure keratitis and KCS may occur.

2. Keep the globe moist with lubricants and artificial tears, try topical cyclosporine, and consider surgical blepharoplasties (see Chaps. 93 and 95).

IV. Complications and sequelae

A. Chronic otitis media usually occurs when antibiotic treatment has not extinguished but merely diminished a smoldering infection. Common signs include persistent aural discharge, continued pain on palpation of the bullae, and occasional fever.

B. A cholesterol granuloma (cholesteatoma) is a type of epidermoid cyst lined by keratinized squamous epithelium (Braund, 1994).

1. It is formed from pockets of the tympanic membrane and can invade the middle ear and temporal bone, producing a foreign body reaction.

2. Cholesteatoma may cause recurrent infection and extensive erosion and remodeling of adjacent bone.

3. Surgical débridement and drainage of the middle ear is required.

C. Conductive hearing loss can result from effusion into the middle ear or disruption of the ossicular chain, but it is usually reversible with antibiotics.

D. Osteomyelitis of the petrous temporal bone may occur as the result of direct spread of infection from the middle ear with inadequately treated otitis media.

1. Signs of peripheral vestibular disease develop, and surgical drainage of the middle ear coupled with intensive long-term antibiotic therapy is indicated.

2. Sensorineural hearing loss is common and not usually reversible.

E. Meningitis and intracranial abscess can occur in chronic cases of purulent otitis media and labyrinthitis.

1. Infection spreads to the central nervous system through pre-formed pathways such as the round window or by direct bony erosion.

2. Hematogenous dissemination may also play a role.

3. It has a high mortality rate.

4. Clinical signs include fever, neck pain, ipsilateral cranial nerve V–VII deficits, ipsilateral hemiparesis/hemiplegia, and cerebellar signs.

5. Examination of cerebrospinal fluid reveals inflammatory cells and a high protein content.

6. Treatment is usually a combination of surgery (eradication of infection in middle ear) and intense long-term antibiotic therapy.

OTITIS INTERNA (LABYRINTHITIS)

Definition

I. Otitis interna, or labyrinthitis, applies to a group of inflammatory conditions of the inner ear.

II. These conditions can be grouped into two categories: infectious and noninfectious.

Causes

I. Infectious causes

A. Usually arise when bacteria associated with otitis media invade the inner ear

1. *Staphylococcus* spp.

2. *Streptococcus* spp.

3. *Proteus mirabilis*

4. *Pseudomonas* spp.

5. *Escherichia coli*

B. Fungal

1. *Malassezia*

2. *Candida*

3. *Paecilomyces* spp.

4. *Aspergillus*

II. Noninfectious causes

A. Congenital peripheral vestibular syndrome (usually seen in young purebred animals)

1. English cocker spaniels

2. German shepherd dogs

3. Beagles

4. Doberman pinschers

5. Akita

6. Burmese and Siamese cats

B. Idiopathic vestibular syndromes

1. Old dogs

2. Cats (usually adults)

C. Trauma

D. Polyneuropathy

E. Hypothyroidism (Jaggy et al., 1994)

F. Aminoglycoside antibiotics

G. Neoplasia

1. Tumors originating in the temporal bone or bulla

2. Neurofibromas, neurofibrosarcomas of the cranial nerve VIII

3. Metastatic tumors: tonsillar, thyroid adenocarcinoma
4. Meningiomas

Pathophysiology

I. Infectious disease
   A. Extension of infection from otitis media is the most common.
      1. Bacteria invade the round window membrane or annular ligament of the oval window.
      2. Extension of infection may also occur by direct bony erosion.
   B. Hematogenous spread from distant or systemic infections is rare but may occur with systemic fungal infections.
II. Noninfectious disease
   A. Degeneration of vestibular and auditory receptors with aminoglycoside antibiotics
   B. Direct invasion or encroachment of bony labyrinth by tumors
   C. Severe head trauma resulting in temporal bone fractures

Clinical Signs

I. In most unilateral labyrinthitic conditions, the clinical signs consist of asymmetrical loss of balance with preservation of strength.
II. Common signs with acute peripheral vestibular lesions are as follows.
   A. Head tilt toward side of lesion
   B. Falling, rolling toward side of lesion
   C. Spontaneous or positional jerk-type nystagmus (horizontal or rotary) with the fast phase away from lesion and direction not altered with changes in head position
   D. Circling with short radii toward side of lesion
   E. Decrease in extensor tone on affected side, increase in extensor tone on contralateral side
   F. Positional, nonparalytic ventral or ventrolateral strabismus on affected side
   G. Nausea or vomiting common in dogs, especially in the acute phase
III. Animals with mild or insidious lesions may have subtle clinical signs due to compensation. Blindfolding the animal usually makes a head tilt and vestibular ataxia more obvious.
IV. Examining the vestibular animal requires detection of subtle vestibular signs in a compensated animal and distinguishing peripheral (labyrinth) from central (brain stem) disease.
   A. Evaluate mental status, cranial nerves, and motor and sensory systems.
   B. Vestibular function tests are used to detect which side the lesion is on in an animal that no longer has spontaneous nystagmus or other apparent signs.
      1. Normal vestibular nystagmus (doll's eye test, oculocephalic response)
         a) Reflex eye movements are induced by passively moving the head from side to side and up and down. Normally the eyes slowly deviate in the direction opposite to head movement and then quickly flick back in the direction of head movement.
         b) Absent normal vestibular nystagmus in an ambulatory, alert animal may indicate bilateral peripheral vestibular disease.
         c) Absent or disconjugate eye movements could also indicate a lesion involving the medial longitudinal fasciculus; CNs III, IV, VI, or their nuclei; or the extraocular muscles.
      2. Rotational tests (difficult to perform in large dogs)
         a) Rapidly rotating an animal several times elicits a horizontal nystagmus in the direction of the turn.
         b) The turning is suddenly stopped and horizontal nystagmus is evoked to the opposite side; postrotatory nystagmus is elicited by the opposite labyrinth.
         c) Absence of postrotatory nystagmus or a gross difference in nystagmus duration between the two sides indicates a past or present vestibular problem.
      3. Positional nystagmus testing
         a) Head position is rapidly changed by dorsiflexion of the head or hanging the head over a table.
         b) The character of the positional nystagmus is noted.
         c) Animals with chronic vestibular disease may have diminishing nystagmus with repeated maneuvers.
      4. Examination of hearing via the brain stem auditory evoked response (BAER)
         a) Pathologic processes in the vestibular labyrinth may also affect the cochlea, resulting in deafness.
         b) Animals with severe labyrinth disease may have no waveforms on BAER testing, indicating an irreversible sensorineural deafness.

Diagnosis

I. Infectious labyrinthitis
   A. A history of chronic recurrent otitis media/externa increases the likelihood of extension of infection into the inner ear.
   B. The rate of onset of vestibular signs is variable, with signs appearing acutely or subacutely over a 2–3-week period.
      1. Clinical signs are consistent with a unilateral peripheral vestibular lesion.
      2. Ipsilateral facial palsy, Horner's syndrome, and KCS are common.
      3. Head shaking, pawing, or rubbing of the ear and an inflammatory aural discharge may be seen.
   C. Diagnostic procedures are similar to those for middle ear disease.

1. Otoscopic examination
2. Cytology, culture, and sensitivity of external ear/middle ear discharge
3. Radiography of the bulla and petrous temporal bones
4. Computed tomography in chronic cases if radiographs normal
5. Surgical exploration of the middle ear
6. Fundic exam if systemic fungal disease suspected
7. Schirmer tear test if facial nerve palsy present
8. BAER test if unilateral hearing loss suspected

II. Noninfectious labyrinthitis
   A. History
      1. Onset of signs, sequence of events, and progression of signs vary depending on cause.
      2. History of aminoglycosides may be suggestive.
      3. Neoplasia often has a slowly progressive course.
      4. Age and breed are helpful in idiopathic and congenital vestibular syndromes.
   B. Clinical signs
      1. Signs are consistent with peripheral vestibular disease.
      2. Facial palsy, KCS, and Horner's syndrome may accompany tumors originating in the temporal bone.
      3. Facial palsy, KCS, and Horner's syndrome are not seen with aminoglycoside intoxication

or congenital or idiopathic vestibular syndromes.
   C. Diagnostic procedures
      1. The same diagnostic procedures listed for infectious labyrinthitis are often indicated.
      2. Perform serial neurologic exams in cases of idiopathic syndromes.
      3. Assess thyroid profiles if hypothyroidism is suspected.

Differential Diagnosis

I. The findings on physical and neurologic exam help distinguish peripheral from central disease (Table 106–2). Special attention is focused on detecting deficits in neural structures in close proximity to the peripheral vs. the central vestibular systems.
   A. Neuroanatomic structures near the peripheral vestibular system
      1. Facial nerve (facial palsy)
      2. Postganglionic sympathetic fibers of the middle ear (Horner's syndrome)
      3. Parasympathetic fibers to the lacrimal gland (dry eye)
      4. Cochlear nerve (deafness)
   B. Neuroanatomic structures near the central (brain stem) vestibular system
      1. Trigeminal nucleus (atrophy of masticatory muscles, reduced facial sensation)
      2. Facial nucleus (facial palsy)

Table 106–2. **Clinical Findings of the Common Causes of Vestibular Disease**

Cause	Findings on Ear Exam	Type of Nystagmus	Other Cranial Nerve (CN) Deficits	Other Neurologic Findings
Peripheral (labyrinth)				
Bacterial labyrinthitis	Often exudate in ear canal or abnormal tympanum	Horizontal or rotary to side opposite of lesion	Horner's syndrome (if middle ear involved), CN VIII	Mentation normal
Idiopathic vestibular syndrome	Negative	Horizontal or rotary to side opposite of lesion	None	Mentation normal
Trauma to petrous temporal bone	Often hemorrhage in ear canal or behind tympanum	Horizontal/rotary to side opposite of lesion	Often CN VII, Horner's syndrome (if middle ear involved)	Mentation normal
Neoplasia of petrous temporal bone	Negative	Horizontal/rotary to side opposite of lesion	Often CN VII, ± Horner's syndrome (if middle ear involved)	Mentation normal
Polyneuropathy	Negative	Horizontal/rotary to side opposite of lesion	Often CN V, VII	Mentation normal
Central (brain stem)				
Brain stem/cerebellar tumors or trauma	Negative	Horizontal, rotary vertical or direction-changing	Often CN V, VI, VII, IX, X, or XII	Mentation variable (depression to coma) Ipsilateral hemiparesis, cerebellar signs
Inflammatory/infectious diseases (feline infectious peritonitis, toxoplasmosis systemic fungal infections, distemper, Rickettsial diseases)	Negative	Horizontal, rotary vertical or direction-changing	Often CN V, VI, VII Other CNs may be involved	Mentation variable (depression to coma) Ipsilateral (hemiparesis) Cerebellar signs Cervical pain Fever

3. Abducens nucleus (lack of retractor oculi reflex, medial strabismus)
4. Cerebellum (head tremor, truncal ataxia, drunken gait)
5. Upper motor neuron paresis and general proprioceptive deficits
6. Altered mentation

II. Unilateral deafness is consistent with labyrinthitic lesions, as cochlear and vestibular fibers diverge upon entering the brain stem and are thus anatomically separated. Impaired hearing or deafness from lesions of the central auditory pathway, without other neurologic signs, is rare (DeLahunta, 1983).

III. Lesions in the cerebellopontine angle and ascending central vestibular pathways are primarily caused by neoplasia, infectious disease, granulomatous meningoencephalomyelitis, head trauma, thiamine deficiency, or lysosomal storage disease (see Chap. 23).

Treatment

I. Infectious otitis interna
   A. Refer to section on treatment of otitis media.
   B. Selection of antibiotics for bacterial brain abscesses and meningitis secondary to labyrinthitis depends on results of culture and sensitivity on samples of cerebrospinal fluid (CSF) or middle ear effusions (see Chap. 23).
   C. Systemic fungal infections with labyrinth involvement are often treated with amphotericin B and oral antifungal agents, but treatment is difficult and relapses are common.

II. Noninfectious otitis interna
   A. No specific treatment alters the course of congenital or idiopathic syndromes.
   B. Corticosteroids and supportive care are indicated in cases of trauma.
   C. Surgical management of labyrinth or caudal fossa tumors is usually not attempted because of the advanced stage of disease at the time of diagnosis and difficulty in the surgical approach.
      1. Radiation therapy may prolong survival in many cases (Heidner et al., 1991).
      2. Adjunct chemotherapy has been tried with mixed success (Fulton and Steinberg, 1990).

Patient Monitoring

I. Follow-up examination is the same as for otitis media. Consider an underlying disease such as diabetes or hyperadrenocorticism in animals for whom therapy is ineffective.

II. Deafness, facial palsy, and KCS are usually permanent.

III. With proper treatment, the head tilt usually becomes less pronounced over time as a result of compensation; it may occasionally become more apparent during periods of stress.

IV. Acute vestibular signs usually improve within a few weeks. Enduring or waxing and waning signs require reevaluation of the original diagnosis.

V. Prognosis is variable.
   A. Chronic bacterial labyrinthitis is difficult to treat but can usually be managed with long-term antibiotic therapy.
   B. Intracranial complications of bacterial labyrinthitis can be fatal; however, if diagnosed and treated early, some cases resolve.
   C. Long-term prognosis of fungal labyrinthitis is poor, but local control of disease may sometimes be achieved.
   D. The prognosis for malignant tumors of the petrous temporal bone is poor; however, benign polyps (if completely resected) warrant a favorable prognosis.
   E. Trauma of the petrous temporal bone usually carries a favorable prognosis if it is not accompanied by massive intraparenchymal hemorrhage within the brain stem.

Bibliography

Birken EA, Brookler KH: Surface tension lowering substance of the canine eustachian tube. Ann Otol Rhinol Laryngol 81:268, 1972

Braund KG: Neurological diseases. p. 284. In Braund KG (ed): Clinical Syndromes in Veterinary Neurology. 2nd Ed. Mosby, St. Louis, 1994

DeLahunta A: Auditory system—special somatic afferent system. p. 307. In DeLahunta A (ed): Veterinary Neuroanatomy and Clinical Neurology. 2nd Ed. WB Saunders, Philadelphia, 1983

Fulton LM, Steinberg HS: Preliminary study of lomustine in the treatment of intracranial masses in dogs following localization by imaging techniques, p. 241. In Fenner WR (ed): Neuro-oncology. Semin Vet Med Surg (Small Anim) 5:241, 1990

Heidner GL, Kornegay JN, Page RL et al: Analysis of survival in a retrospective study of 86 dogs with brain tumors. J Vet Intern Med 5:219, 1991

Jaggy A, Oliver JE, Duncan FC et al: Neurological manifestations of hypothyroidism: a retrospective study of 29 dogs. J Vet Intern Med 8:328, 1994

Kornegay JN, Anson LW: Musculoskeletal infections. p. 91. In Greene CE (ed): Infectious Diseases of the Dog and Cat. WB Saunders, Philadelphia, 1990

London CA, Dubilzeig RR, Vail DM et al: Evaluation of dogs and cats with tumors of the ear canal: 145 cases (1978–1992). J Am Vet Med Assoc 208:1413, 1996

Neer TM, Howard PE: Otitis media. Compend Contin Educ Pract Vet 4:410, 1982

Paparella MM, Jung TTK, Goycoolea MV: Otitis media with effusion. p. 1322. In Paparella MM, Shumrick DA, Gluckman JL, Meyerhoff WL (eds): Otolaryngology. 3rd Ed. WB Saunders, Philadelphia, 1991

Remedios AM, Fowler JD, Pharr JW: A comparison of radiographic versus surgical diagnosis of otitis media. J Am Anim Hosp Assoc 27:183, 1991

Rosychuk RAW: Management of otitis externa. Vet Clin North Am [Small Anim Pract] 24:921, 1994

Sade J: Middle ear mucosa. Arch Otolaryngol 84:132, 1966

Seim HB: Middle ear. p. 1568. In Slatter D (ed): Textbook of Small Animal Surgery. 2nd Ed. WB Saunders, Philadelphia, 1993

Stout-Graham M, Kainer RA, Whalen LR et al: Morphologic measurements of the external horizontal ear canal of dogs. Am J Vet Res 51:990, 1990

107

Deafness

Kim Knowles

Definition and Classification

I. Deafness is defined as the lack of or deficiency of hearing.

II. Deafness or impaired hearing may be bilateral or unilateral and be partial or complete.

III. Hearing disorders are classified as conductive or sensorineural, based on the site of pathology.

IV. The external ear canal, tympanic membrane, and ossicles form the conductive component of hearing, and the hair cells of the organ of Corti and their neural connections form the sensory component of hearing.

   A. Conductive hearing loss results from lesions involving the external or middle ear.

   B. Sensorineural hearing loss results from lesions of the hair cells or the organ of Corti and/or auditory division of cranial nerve (CN) VIII.

Causes

I. Conductive hearing loss

   A. Lesions of the external ear canal

      1. Impacted cerumen

      2. Foreign body

      3. Otitis externa with stenosis of the ear canal

      4. Trauma resulting in hemorrhage in the external ear canal

      5. Neoplasia

   B. Lesions of the middle ear

      1. Otitis media

      2. Thickening or perforation of the tympanic membrane

      3. Neoplasia of the middle ear (primary or metastatic)

      4. Trauma resulting in hemorrhage in the middle ear

      5. Obstruction of the eustachian tube causing a fluid-filled middle ear space

      6. Irradiation of the head and neck region resulting in a serous otitis media (see Chap. 106)

II. Sensorineural hearing loss

   A. Congenital and hereditary deafness in dogs

      1. It invariably produces a total hearing loss in the affected ear and is the most common cause in young animals.

      2. Numerous breeds are affected with congenital deafness (Strain, 1991). See Table 107–1 for reported breeds.

   B. Inherited deafness: seen in some white cats with blue irises

   C. Infectious labyrinthitis

   D. Trauma

      1. Fractures of the petrous temporal bone

      2. Acoustic trauma

      3. Surgical trauma or high-pressure flushing of the bulla

   E. Primary or metastatic neoplasia of the petrous temporal bone or CN VIII

   F. Hypothyroidism

Table 107–1. Breeds with Congenital Deafness

Akita	Ibizan hound
American cocker spaniel	Jack Russell terrier
American Staffordshire terrier	Kuvasz
Australian cattle dog	Maltese
Australian shepherd	Miniature pinscher
Beagle	Miniature poodle
Border collie	Mongrel
Boston terrier	Norwegian dunkerhound
Boxer	Old English sheepdog
Bulldog	Papillon
Bull terrier	Pit bull terrier
Catahoula leopard dog	Pointer
Collie	Rhodesian ridgeback
Dalmatian	Rottweiler
Dappled dachshund	Saint Bernard
Doberman pinscher	Schnauzer
Dogo Argentino	Scottish terrier
English setter	Sealyham terrier
English springer spaniel	Shetland sheepdog
Foxhound	Shropshire terrier
Fox terrier	Siberian husky
German shepherd dog	Toy poodle
Great Dane	Walker American foxhound
Great Pyrenees	West Highland white terrier

G. Ototoxins (Merchant, 1994)
   1. Systemic and topical aminoglycosides
   2. Some topical otic agents: polymyxin B, chlorhexidine
   3. Diuretics: furosemide, bumetanide
   4. Salicylates
   5. Cisplatin
H. Degenerative changes of the organ of Corti associated with aging (presbycusis)
I. Neuropathy following radiation to the head (Thomas and Holdorff, 1993)
J. Severe hydrocephalus causing damage to the auditory cortex

Pathophysiology

I. Conduction deafness
   A. Normally the tympanic membrane and ossicles act as a transformer by amplifying airborne sound and efficiently transferring it to the inner ear fluids for receptor stimulation.
   B. If the normal pathway is obstructed, there is a loss of transmission of auditory stimuli to the hair cells of the organ of Corti.
   C. Transmission of auditory stimuli may still occur across the skin and through bones of the skull (bone conduction), but it is much less efficient.
   D. Diseases causing external ear canal occlusion, rigidity or rupture of the tympanum, damage to the ossicular chain, or effusion into the middle ear result in conduction hearing loss or deafness.
   E. Most causes of conductive deafness are acquired.
II. Sensorineural deafness
   A. Under normal conditions, acoustic vibrations from the middle ear ossicles are transmitted to inner ear fluids.
      1. These vibrations result in fluid waves that cause an upward displacement of the basilar membrane, which lifts the hair cells of the organ of Corti.
      2. Hair cells of the organ of Corti then undergo a shearing effect with the tectorial membrane, ultimately generating nerve impulses in the cochlear nerve.
      3. Sensory hair cells of the organ of Corti mechanically analyze the frequency content of sound.
      4. Sensory cells in the basal turn are activated by high-frequency tones, whereas for low-frequency tones, maximal stimulation occurs at the apex of the cochlea.
   B. Conditions that cause degeneration of the sensory cells of the cochlea or cochlear nerve (see earlier) result in sensorineural hearing loss due to loss of receptor function.
      1. The majority of conditions cause hair cell loss in the basal region, resulting in a high-frequency hearing loss.
      2. Histologic features and development and pathogenesis of the inner ear degeneration in the white cat with blue irises have been extensively studied.
         a) It is a cochleosaccular degeneration with a dominant mode of inheritance.
         b) The bony labyrinth, membranous utricle, and semicircular canals are fully formed.
         c) Deafness results from initial degeneration of the vascular supply to the cochlea (stria vascularis) followed by degeneration of the hair cells of the organ of Corti.
         d) Strial atrophy and progressive degeneration of the organ of Corti occur from base to apex of the cochlea and are at an advanced stage by 3 weeks of age.
      3. Congenital deafness in the dalmatian is linked to the extreme piebald gene.
         a) Mode of inheritance is unclear and probably is multifactorial.
         b) Histologic features of the degeneration are consistent with a cochleosaccular degeneration like that seen in the white cat.
         c) Degeneration of the hair cells of the organ of Corti is essentially complete by 4–5 weeks of age.
      4. Infectious labyrinthitis, trauma, and neoplasia result in deafness and often peripheral vestibular dysfunction due to destruction of the membranous structures within the inner ear.
      5. Hearing loss and deafness in old dogs and cats (presbycusis) are degenerative and associated with atrophy and loss of spiral ganglion cells.
         a) Loss of ganglion cells is present in all areas of the cochlea but is consistently found in the basal region of the cochlea.
         b) Loss of ganglion cells is probably secondary to loss of hair cells and supporting cells in the organ of Corti (Knowles et al., 1989).
      6. Ototoxicity from systemic and topical aminoglycosides results in severe cochlear hair cell degeneration initially in the basal turn of the cochlea.
         a) The main reason aminoglycosides are toxic is their ability to concentrate in the perilymph and endolymph of the membranous labyrinth.
         b) The degeneration can spread to the remainder of the cochlea if therapy is prolonged.

Clinical Signs

I. Generalizations regarding signs of deafness
   A. Complete bilateral deafness is usually peripheral (labyrinth) in origin and is generally caused by dysfunction or degeneration of the organ of Corti.
   B. Central sensorineural deafness, unaccompanied by severe neurologic deficits, is rare because of the large percentage of afferent fiber decussation in the central auditory pathway.
      1. The complexity of this pathway accounts for the fact that a small isolated central lesion

would be unlikely to produce bilateral deafness.

2. Diagnosis of central deafness requires cognitive testing and is therefore difficult to document in animals.

C. Deafness is difficult to objectively diagnose when there is incomplete bilateral or complete unilateral hearing loss.

D. Cochlear and vestibular receptors as well as the facial nerve are closely related anatomically, so signs often involve all three of these nerves with peripheral lesions.

II. Signs of cochlear deafness

A. Animal sleeps more soundly, even in noisy environments, and cannot be aroused with loud noises.

B. When awake and alert, animal fails to respond to squeak toys or spoken commands of different intensities (whisper, conversation, shouting).

C. Animals startle easily and may bite if approached without visual cues.

D. In cases of congenital deafness, animals are difficult to train (without hand signals) and resist being restrained.

E. Animals with unilateral deafness behave almost normally but have difficulty in localizing sounds.

III. Signs of cochlear deafness associated with vestibular signs

A. See cochlear signs listed previously.

B. Aural pain or discharge, head tilt, nystagmus, Horner's syndrome, facial palsy, and keratoconjunctivitis sicca (KCS) cause suspicion of infectious, traumatic, or neoplastic disorders of the petrous temporal bone.

Diagnosis

I. Sensorineural deafness

A. Congenital/hereditary deafness

1. History indicates the age of onset to be <5 weeks, and the course is nonprogressive.

2. Check for breed predisposition as well as familial history of congenital deafness.

3. There is usually no history of previous ear disease, and otoscopic exam is normal.

4. Brain stem auditory evoked response (BAER) testing is usually necessary for definitive diagnosis.

B. Acquired sensorineural deafness

1. Infectious labyrinthitis and neoplasia (see Chap. 106)

a) Adult to older animals are more frequently affected.

b) Onset of signs is usually gradual, and course of problem is progressive.

c) History of chronic, recurrent otitis is common.

2. History of ototoxic agents or trauma

3. Signs suggestive of hypothyroidism

4. Age-related hearing loss

a) Usually occurs in older animals

b) Is often bilaterally symmetrical with a gradual onset

c) May occur concurrently with conductive hearing loss

II. Conductive deafness

A. As this type of deafness may improve with treatment, the diagnostic work-up is designed to rule out all possible causes of external and middle ear disease.

B. Note any history of recurrent ear infections.

C. See diagnostic procedures for otitis media/interna in Chap. 106.

III. Auditory testing

A. Behavioral evaluation

1. Observation

a) Examiner stands behind animal to avoid visual and tactile cues and observes animal's behavioral response to sounds of different intensities.

b) Interpretation of an animal's response is subjective, and the response may be influenced by the animal's level of interest, its temperament, and the presence or absence of distracting environmental factors.

2. Conditioned audiometry (Anderson et al., 1968)

a) This involves training an animal to show a behavioral response to a pure tone at selected frequencies that is terminated in conjunction with a mild electrical shock. Eventually the animal learns to respond to the test tone and the shock is omitted.

b) An audiogram is constructed based on the animal's reaction to sound of varying intensities and frequencies.

c) It is time consuming, unsuitable for young animals, and does not detect unilaterally deaf animals.

B. Electrodiagnostic tests

1. These tests do not require conscious cooperation on the part of the animal and provide a more objective assessment of auditory function.

2. They are particularly useful in testing young animals, in which behavioral responses are difficult to assess.

3. They can be used to evaluate both conductive and sensorineural deafness.

4. Electroencephalographic (EEG) audiometry is based on an arousal phenomenon (Redding, 1987).

a) Record an EEG with the animal in a relaxed state, then present auditory stimuli to the animal and note changes in the EEG tracing.

b) A normal response consists of an increase in frequency and decrease in voltage in the EEG at the time of auditory stimulus application.

5. Brain stem auditory evoked response (BAER) consists of a series of 4–7 waves at approximately 1 msec intervals after presentation of

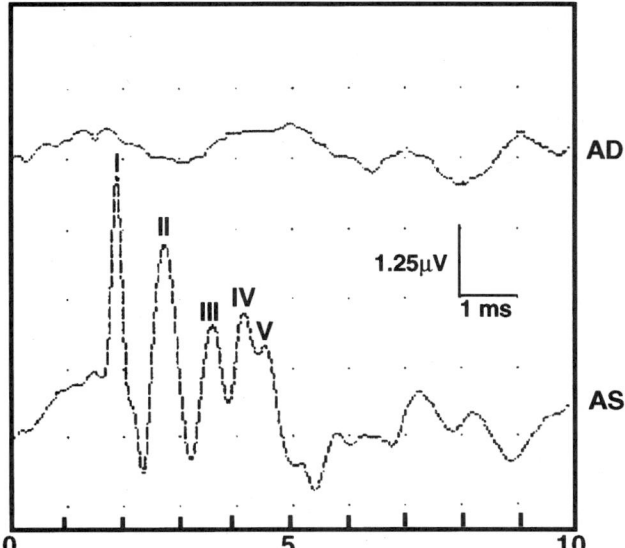

Figure 107–1. Brain stem auditory evoked response (BAER) from a 6 week old dalmatian with unilateral deafness of the right ear. Each trace is an average of 1000 click stimuli presented at an intensity of 87 dB hearing level. The peaks from the left ear are labeled with roman numerals and are produced by neural generators in the cranial nerve (CN) VIII and brain stem. No response is elicited from the right ear, indicating lack of cochlear/ CN VIII function. AD = right ear; AS = left ear.

sound stimuli; waves reflect electrical activity in the cochlear nerve and brain stem.

   a) Short-duration auditory stimuli in the form of clicks are delivered to the external auditory canal, and signal-averaged responses are recorded from scalp electrodes.

   b) The organ of Corti and cochlear nerve are the neural structures responsible for initiation of the BAER.

   c) Complete deafness resulting from labyrinthitis, presbycusis, or congenital/hereditary causes results in a flat-line recording.

   d) As each ear is tested independently, unilateral deafness can be diagnosed (Fig. 107–1).

   e) When different intensities of auditory stimuli are used, an elevated threshold may be seen with a conductive loss.

6. Impedance audiometry is an objective method of assessing the integrity of the middle ear, cochlea, CN VII and VIII, and brain stem auditory pathways (Penrod and Coulter, 1980).

   a) Tympanometry, acoustic (stapedial) reflex, and the physical volume test are examples of tests that use impedance audiometry.

   b) It is very useful when combined with a complete battery of impedance testing coupled with diagnostic judgments.

   c) The technique is still in varying stages of development and is of limited availability.

Treatment

  I. Congenital/hereditary deafness is not reversible, and there is no treatment.

  II. Many cases of conductive hearing loss from otitis media benefit from antibiotic therapy (see Chap. 106).

  III. Recovery of auditory function is usually minimal following treatment of bacterial labyrinthitis.

  IV. Age-related hearing loss is not reversible.

    A. However, some older dogs may suffer a combination of sensorineural and conductive changes.

    B. Emphasis of diagnostic testing is to exclude all possible causes of external and middle ear disease.

  V. A hearing aid may be tried in animals with conductive hearing loss that is not amendable to medical or surgical management.

    A. Hearing aids may also be useful in acquired sensorineural hearing loss.

    B. Most animals do not appear to tolerate the model currently available (Marshall, 1990).

Patient Monitoring

  I. Although the prognosis for most animals with congenital/hereditary or acquired sensorineural deafness is poor, dogs or cats with unilateral congenital/hereditary deafness still make excellent pets.

  II. Sire, dam, and littermate screening using the BAER test is employed for breeds at high risk for congenital deafness.

  III. Owners of animals with congenital deafness should be strongly discouraged from breeding them.

  IV. Conductive deafness secondary to otitis media has a more favorable prognosis with aggressive long-term therapy.

Bibliography

Anderson H, Henricson B, Lundquist PG et al: Genetic hearing impairment in the Dalmation dog. Acta Otolaryngol [Suppl] 232:5, 1968

Bohne BA, Rabbitt KD: Holes in the reticular lamina after noise exposure: implication for continuing damage in the organ of Corti. Hearing Res 11:41, 1983

Delack JB: Hereditary deafness in the white cat. Compend Contin Educ Pract Vet 6:609, 1984

Hayes HM, Wilson GPJ, Fenner WR et al: Canine congenital deafness: epidemiologic study of 272 cases. J Am Anim Hosp Assoc 17:473, 1981

Huizing EH, deGroot JCM: Human cochlear pathology in aminoglycoside ototoxicity. Acta Otolaryngol 436:117, 1987

Jaggy A, Oliver JE, Ferguson DC et al: Neurological manifestations of hypothyroidism: a retrospective study of 29 dogs. J Vet Intern Med 8:328, 1994

Knowles K, Blauch B, Leipold H et al: Reduction of spiral

ganglion neurons in the aging canine with hearing loss. J Vet Med (Series A) 36:188, 1989

Liberman MC, Kiang NYS: Acoustic trauma in cats. Cochlear pathology and auditory-nerve activity. Acta Otolaryngol [Suppl] 358:6, 1978

Marshall AE: Hearing loss in aged dogs. Adv Small Animal Med Surg 2(12):6, 1990

Merchant SR: Ototoxicity. Vet Clin North Am [Small Anim Pract] 24:971, 1994

Penrod JP, Coulter DB: The diagnostic uses of impedance audiometry in the dog. J Am Anim Hosp Assoc 16:941, 1980

Redding RW: Electrophysiologic diagnosis. p. 111. In Oliver JE, Hoerlein BF, Mayhew IG (eds): Veterinary Neurology. WB Saunders, Philadelphia, 1987

Sims MH, Moore RE: Auditory-evoked response in the clinically normal dog: early latency components. Am J Vet Res 45:2019, 1984

Strain GM: Congenital deafness in dogs and cats. Compend Contin Educ Pract Vet 13:245, 1991

Thomas PK, Holdorff B: Neuropathy due to physical agents. p. 990. In Dyck PJ, Thomas PK (eds): Peripheral Neuropathy. 3rd Ed. WB Saunders, Philadelphia, 1993

Wurster CF, Krespi PI, Curtis AW: Osteoradionecrosis of the temporal bone. Otolaryngol Head Neck Surg 90:126, 1982

SECTION **XV**

Infectious Diseases

108

Introduction

Johnny D. Hoskins

IMPORTANCE OF INFECTIOUS DISEASES

I. Infectious diseases continue to be an important daily management concern in practice.

II. The relative importance of individual diseases and our clinical understanding of each are undergoing change.

   A. Since the mid-1970s, canine parvovirus type 2 has undergone genetic alterations, and development of new viral strains has occurred, which means clinical presentations are different and vaccination programs need to be changed.

   B. The importance of zoonotic diseases has become more apparent because of the spread of human immunodeficiency virus and increased prevalence of various immunocompromised conditions in the human population.

   C. Feline and wildlife rabies is still a major zoonotic problem in many local communities.

   D. Other increasingly important zoonotic concerns include bartonellosis (cat-scratch disease), *Helicobacter* spp. infections, cryptosporidiosis, campylobacteriosis, bite wound–associated infections, and microsporidiosis.

   E. Anaerobic bacteria are now being recognized as significant pathogens in animals, and anaerobic bacteria are also being found that do not cause clinical infections.

   F. In the 1990s the importance of tick-transmitted diseases such as ehrlichiosis, Lyme borreliosis, and other newly emerging, yet unnamed, diseases continues to be addressed.

NEW DEVELOPMENTS

I. Enzyme-linked immunosorbent assay (ELISA) techniques

   A. ELISA technology is currently the state of the art in diagnostic procedures.

   B. ELISA testing procedures may be either antigen-based or antibody-based, depending on which infectious agent or disease is of concern.

   C. The real challenge in practice is in the interpretation of the ELISA test results as they relate to the clinical animal—i.e., is the result a true positive, false positive, true negative, or false negative.

II. Polymerase chain reaction (PCR) techniques

   A. PCR is the newest technology that allows for amplification of a gene product a billionfold in just hours and has clinical application for increasing the sensitivity for detecting infectious agents.

     1. With PCR technology, probes (primers) of short sequences of DNA seek complementary regions of the target viral, bacterial, or fungal gene sequence. When the probes find and bind the target gene, the PCR occurs.

     2. An enzyme, taq polymerase, shuttles back and forth between the complementary probe sequences. It uses them as a double-stranded starting template to create DNA copies of the viral, bacterial, or fungal gene.

     3. The DNA sequence is then copied as many as one billion times. The result is a product that is easily visualized on an agarose gel as a specific band, constituting a positive PCR test.

   B. Commercial DNA/PCR materials that include primers and positive controls are available for screening or confirming for *Ehrlichia canis, Rickettsia rickettsii, Chlamydia psittaci, Borrelia burgdorferi, Bartonella henselae, Yersinia pestis, Mycobacterium tuberculosis, M. avium, M. bovis,* feline leukemia virus, feline infectious peritonitis virus, rabies, feline immunodeficiency virus, feline herpesvirus-1, and *Coccidioides immitis.*

   C. Other PCR primers and positive controls for infectious agents will continue to be developed, and the PCR technology will be refined with advancing laboratory techniques.

III. Therapeutic advances

   A. New vaccines have been developed for canine parvovirus type 2, Lyme borreliosis, *Micro-*

sporum canis, rabies, and *Bordetella bronchiseptica*.

  B. New antibiotics such as aminoglycosides, fluoroquinolones, penicillins, carbapenems, and combined beta-lactamase inhibitors with beta-lactam antimicrobials have been used with increasing frequency.

  C. Oral azole derivatives (fluconazole or itraconazole) with an improved spectrum of activity and safety are now commonly used for systemic mycoses.

IV. Disadvantages

  A. Even with the newer antibiotics and antifungal agents, indiscriminate use will increase the levels of resistant bacteria and fungi, with subsequent development of very resistant nosocomial infections.

  B. The overall costs for using these newer antibiotics and antifungal agents or performing the emerging PCR technology will be, or will remain, frustrating to the dog or cat owners with limited income but a real love for their animal.

FUTURE PROSPECTS

I. Despite great strides, our understanding of many or emerging diseases remains baffling and provides us the opportunity to develop better means of diagnosis, treatment, and potential vaccination for these diseases.

II. The following chapters in this section address the major infections encountered in small animals.

109

Systemic Mycoses

Joseph Taboada

BLASTOMYCOSIS

Definition

I. Blastomycosis is a systemic fungal infection that usually originates in the lungs and then disseminates to the lymphatics, skin, eyes, bones, and other organs.
II. A variety of mammalian species are affected, including dogs, cats, ferrets, horses, and humans.
III. Young, male, large-breed dogs (especially sporting breeds and hounds) living near water are at increased risk; most animals live within one-quarter mile of water.
IV. Dogs have been used as a sentinel animal for human disease, as the incidence in dogs is about 10 times higher.

Causes

I. It is caused by the dimorphic fungus *Blastomyces dermatitidis.*
II. *B. dermatitidis* characteristics are as follows.
   A. In tissue or when cultured at 37°C, the organism is a thick-walled yeast that usually has a single bud attached to the mother cell by a broad base.
   B. When cultured at 25°C, the organism grows as a white cottony mold that may become tan as it ages.
   C. Colonies grow slowly and contain branching septate (1–2 μm) mycelia that form round to pyriform-shaped (2–10 μm) conidia, resembling the microconidia of *Histoplasma capsulatum.*
III. *B. dermatitidis* is probably a soil saprophyte, but the natural reservoir remains unidentified.
   A. When found, it is grown from wet, acidic, or sandy soil containing decaying wood, animal feces, or other organic enrichment.
   B. Moisture is important for growth and transmission; therefore, the organism is primarily endemic along the Mississippi, Ohio, Missouri, Tennessee, and St. Lawrence Rivers; in the southern Great Lakes; and in the southern Mid-Atlantic states.

Pathophysiology

I. Infection is most commonly via inhalation of infective conidia from the environment, but direct inoculation may result in localized cutaneous disease.
II. Blastomycosis is not a contagious disease; however, it is an occupational hazard to laboratory workers and veterinary personnel when handling infective materials or cultures. Activities that disrupt the soil such as digging or construction may also play a role in the aerosolization of spores.
III. After inhalation, conidia are phagocytized by alveolar macrophages and transformed from the mycelial phase to the yeast phase, which induces a marked suppurative to pyogranulomatous response.
   A. Phagocytized yeast are then transported into the pulmonary interstitium, where access is gained to the lymphatic and vascular systems.
   B. Hematogenous and lymphatic dissemination results in multisystemic disease.
   C. Although dissemination may affect any organ system, the lymph nodes, eyes, skin, bones, subcutaneous tissue, and prostate gland are commonly affected in dogs, and the skin, subcutaneous tissue, eyes, central nervous system (CNS), and lymph nodes are affected in cats.
IV. Incubation period varies in dogs from 5–12 weeks.
V. Immune response determines the severity of clinical disease.
   A. Antibody production occurs in most cases, with higher serologic titers found in severe disseminated disease.
   B. Recovery is probably dependent on cell-mediated immune response.
      1. Adequate immune response may result in mild respiratory disease that resolves spontaneously or may result in disease in other organ systems without apparent pulmonary involvement.
      2. A poor or weak immune response results in severe pulmonary and disseminated disease.

Clinical Signs

I. High-risk breeds include bluetick coonhounds, treeing-walker coonhounds, pointers, and Weimaraners (Rudmann et al., 1992).

1113

A. Male dogs are affected more than females; any age dog can be affected, but 2–4 year olds have the highest incidence.

B. Exposure to possible environmental sources, close proximity to water, and likelihood of being housed in outdoor kennels probably explain the breed association.

II. Clinical findings are variable.

A. Nonspecific signs such as anorexia, depression, weight loss, cachexia, and fever (about 40%) are common.

B. The lungs are the portal of entry for organisms; thus, pulmonary signs are seen in 65–85% of dogs (Legendre et al., 1981; Wolf and Troy, 1995; Arceneaux and Taboada, 1996).

1. Signs range from mild respiratory distress to severe dyspnea.

2. Hypoxemia results in cyanosis in the most severely affected cases.

C. A dry, hacking cough is common from enlargement of perihilar lymph nodes with compression of primary bronchi and from bronchointerstitial and alveolar disease.

D. Rapid shallow respiratory efforts are occasionally caused by pleural effusion and pleuritic pain.

E. Chylothorax and solid pulmonary masses are uncommon.

III. Diffuse lymphadenopathy occurs in about 40–60% of dogs (Arceneaux and Taboada, 1996).

IV. Cutaneous signs occur in about 30–50% of dogs and are commonly noted in cats (Arceneaux and Taboada, 1996).

A. Skin lesions are usually single or multiple papules, nodules, or plaques that may ulcerate and drain a serosanguineous to purulent exudate.

B. Large abscesses occasionally occur.

C. Paronychia is common in dogs, so the feet and nailbeds should be closely examined.

V. Ocular involvement is noted in 20–50% of the cases, with approximately 50% having bilateral involvement (Brooks et al., 1991; Arceneaux and Taboada, 1996).

A. Posterior segment disease usually occurs first and may progress to endophthalmitis, panophthalmitis, and/or secondary glaucoma.

B. Posterior segment disease includes chorioretinitis, retinal detachment, subretinal granulomas, or vitreitis.

C. Optic neuritis is occasionally noted.

D. Anterior segment disease is usually secondary to posterior segment disease.

1. It includes conjunctivitis, keratitis, episcleritis, or anterior uveitis.

2. Secondary glaucoma is common in dogs with anterior segment disease.

E. Long-term effects on vision.

1. Dogs that have vision and only focal chorioretinitis have a better prognosis for vision than those with anterior segment disease or endophthalmitis (Brooks et al., 1991).

2. It is unlikely that dogs with severe visual impairment will regain vision even with appropriate therapy.

VI. Lameness is noted in about 25% of dogs (Arceneaux and Taboada, 1996).

A. Osteomyelitis is noted in about 10–15% of dogs, usually involving the epiphyseal regions below the elbow or stifle (as a single lesion).

B. Paronychia may cause pain and lameness.

C. Mono- or polyarthritis is a rare cause of lameness.

VII. Reproductive system is affected in approximately 10% of dogs (Arceneaux and Taboada, 1996).

A. Orchitis was seen in 16% of 61 intact male dogs with blastomycosis at Louisiana State University (Arceneaux and Taboada, 1996).

B. Prostatitis or mastitis is seen in <5% of dogs.

VIII. The CNS is affected in <5% of dogs; a higher percentage of cats have CNS involvement.

IX. Other potential sites of infection include liver, spleen, kidney, and nasal cavity.

X. Feline blastomycosis is not common.

A. Most clinical signs seen in dogs also occur in cats.

B. Large abscesses are more common.

C. Neurologic signs are more common.

Diagnosis

I. Hematologic and serum chemistry findings

A. They are often normal, but mild nonregenerative anemia and mature neutrophilia or neutrophilia with mild left shift may be seen.

B. Hypoalbuminemia is the most consistent abnormality seen on serum chemistries.

C. Hypercalcemia is noted in <5% of cases.

II. Radiographic findings (Walker, 1981; Arceneaux and Taboada, 1996)

A. Interstitial patterns are observed in about 70% of dogs (nodular interstitial [41%], diffuse interstitial [24%], and bronchointerstitial [5%]).

B. Alveolar or mixed interstitial/alveolar patterns are observed in about 20%.

C. Tracheobronchial lymphadenopathy is noted in about 30%.

D. Mediastinal mass (8%) or solitary pulmonary mass (8%) is uncommon.

E. Pleural effusion (7%) may obscure the pulmonary parenchyma.

F. Pneumothorax (1%) is rare.

G. Most bony lesions (66%) are solitary osteomyelitis lesions.

1. Most lesions (75%) occur in the extremities.

a) Lesions are osteolytic and typically at the ends of the long bones.

b) The forelimbs are affected more than the rear limbs.

c) Most extremity lesions are below the elbow or the stifle.

2. Periosteal proliferation and soft tissue swelling is noted in about 50% of lesions.

III. Organism identification

A. Cytologic findings from tissue are as follows.

1. Suppurative or pyogranulomatous inflammation is present, often with thick-walled yeast (8–12 μm in diameter with a 0.5–0.75 μm thick wall) that bud to form daughter cells from a broad base.
2. The yeast cells lack a capsule, helping to differentiate them from *Cryptococcus*.
3. Infected skin yields organisms in about 80% of impression smears, skin scrapings, or fine-needle aspirates of nodular lesions.
4. Vitreal aspirates yield organisms from most affected eyes.
5. Lymph node aspirates yield organisms approximately 60% of the time.
6. Bone and lung aspirates, transtracheal wash, and bronchoalveolar lavage each yield organisms <50% of the time.
7. Urine sediment or prostatic wash rarely shows organisms.
   B. Histopathologic findings are as follows.
1. Purulent to pyogranulomatous lesions with broad-based organisms are usually apparent.
2. Special stains (periodic acid–Schiff [PAS], Gridley's fungal, and Gomori methenamine silver) demonstrate the organisms best in tissue.
   C. Fungal culture and identification are as follows.
1. They are not needed for definitive identification in clinical cases.
2. Mycelial growth on Sabouraud's dextrose agar may require 1–4 weeks at 37°C, whereas yeast will grow on blood or brain-heart infusion agar in 1–2 weeks at 25°C.
3. Culturing the organisms from the environment is rarely achieved.
   IV. Serology
   A. It is used primarily when a high degree of suspicion exists or repeated attempts fail to demonstrate the organisms.
   B. Agar-gel immunodiffusion (AGID) test is most commonly used; it detects antibodies directed against the fungal organism (sensitivity and specificity of approximately 90%).
   C. It may be negative in early disease.
   D. It is not useful in following response to therapy.

Differential Diagnosis

I. Other multisystemic granulomatous, neoplastic, and immune-mediated diseases
II. Skin involvement
   A. Bacterial diseases include actinomycosis, mycobacteriosis, botryomycosis, brucellosis, or *Rhodococcus equi* infection.
   B. Mycotic and other infectious diseases include cryptococcosis, coccidioidomycosis, sporotrichosis, basidiobolomycosis, conidiobolomycosis, phaeohyphomycosis, hyalohyphomycosis, eumycotic mycetoma, dermatophytic mycetoma, prototothecosis, pythiosis, and nodular leishmaniasis.
   C. Non-infectious pyogranulomatous diseases include foreign body reaction, idiopathic nodular

panniculitis, sebaceous nodular adenitis, and canine cutaneous sterile pyogranuloma/granuloma syndrome.
   D. Neoplasia includes squamous cell carcinoma, cutaneous lymphoma, mycosis fungoides (cutaneous T-cell lymphoma), and cutaneous histiocytosis.
   E. Miscellaneous diseases include systemic lupus erythematosus, systemic vasculitis, and cutaneous embolic disease.
III. Ocular involvement
   A. Fungal disease, including cryptococcosis, coccidioidomycosis, geotrichosis, histoplasmosis, and aspergillosis
   B. Neoplastic disease, including lymphosarcoma and metastatic neoplasia
   C. Other diseases, including prototothecosis, brucellosis, toxoplasmosis, neosporosis, or leishmaniasis
IV. Lymph node involvement
   A. Lymphosarcoma
   B. Other fungal infections, rickettsial diseases, or brucellosis
   C. Mycobacteriosis, prototothecosis, or leishmaniasis
V. Bone involvement
   A. Primary or metastatic neoplasia
   B. Other fungal or bacterial osteomyelitis

Treatment

I. Spontaneous recovery from symptomatic blastomycosis has been reported in humans but rarely occurs in dogs; symptomatic disease in dogs and cats is always treated.
II. Itraconazole is the preferred treatment.
   A. Give dogs 5 mg/kg PO SID for 2–3 months or until active disease is inapparent. Cats may require 5 mg/kg PO BID.
   B. It requires an acidic gastric pH for maximal oral bioavailability and is always given with food. Antacids such as H_2-receptor blockers or proton-pump inhibitors should not be used concurrently.
   C. Response is minimal in the initial 1–2 weeks of treatment; a loading dose of 10 mg/kg PO SID for the first 3 days of treatment may minimize this lag time.
   D. Drug-induced side effects include the following.
1. Liver enzymes are monitored monthly while itraconazole is administered.
   a) Mild to moderate increases in serum alanine transaminase (ALT), aspartate transaminase (AST), and alkaline phosphatase (AP) activities occur in about 50% of dogs and cats treated.
   b) Therapy is discontinued if liver enzyme elevations are marked or if they are accompanied by anorexia, vomiting, or abdominal pain.
   c) Therapy can be reinstituted at a lower dose following return of liver enzyme activities to normal ranges.
2. Anorexia is the most common side effect; it is dose-related and more common in cats.

Cyproheptadine (2 mg/cat PO SID-BID) or oxazepam (2–3 mg/cat PO SID-BID) may be used as an appetite stimulant.

3. Cutaneous-induced vasculitis (ulcerative skin lesions that look like recurrence of blastomycosis) is rarely seen.
4. Behavioral changes such as fearful behaviors (hiding, submission) are rare complications in dogs.

E. It does not cross the blood-brain, blood-ocular, or blood-prostatic barriers well but is still effective in some CNS, ocular, and prostatic infections.

F. It concentrates well in the skin, making it highly effective in treating cutaneous infections.

G. Severely ill or hypoxemic dogs may have a better outcome if they are treated initially with itraconazole and amphotericin B in combination or with intravenous fluconazole.

III. Ketoconazole is another choice.

A. Give dogs or cats 5–15 mg/kg PO BID for a minimum of 3 months (with food and not concurrently with antacids).

B. The response rate is much lower and relapses are higher when compared with itraconazole treatment, and dogs generally have to be treated for a longer time period.

C. Anorexia, vomiting, hepatic toxicity, and adrenal insufficiency are more likely with ketoconazole.

IV. Fluconazole may also be used.

A. Give dogs or cats 2.5–5 mg/kg PO or IV SID.

B. It does not require a low gastric pH for maximal bioavailability and is not affected by the presence or absence of food.

C. Fluconazole is excreted in the urine; crosses the blood-brain, blood-ocular, and blood-prostatic barriers well; and may be the preferred treatment for urinary tract, prostatic, and CNS infection.

D. The availability of an IV form is useful in severely affected or hypoxemic animals.

E. Side effects are similar to those of itraconazole.

V. Amphotericin B is still used in selected cases.

A. It has good efficacy against *Blastomyces* organisms, but nephrotoxicity is the primary limiting side effect.

1. Fever is another major side effect that is usually ameliorated by pretreatment with nonsteroidal anti-inflammatory drugs.
2. Other side effects include thrombophlebitis, hypokalemia, distal renal tubular acidosis, hypomagnesemia, cardiac arrhythmias, and nonregenerative anemia.

B. It is recommended in combination with itraconazole or ketoconazole for severely affected or hypoxemic cases.

1. Reconstitute with 5% dextrose in water (D5W) and infuse as a rapid infusion over 10–15 minutes or continuous infusion over 1–6 hours. The longer infusion rate or pretreatment saline diuresis is less likely to cause nephrotoxicity.
2. Dosage is 0.5 mg/kg (dog), 0.25 mg/kg (cat) IV QOD to a total dose of 4 mg/kg (total dose of 8 mg/kg if amphotericin B is the sole treatment).
3. Renal function is monitored before each treatment; therapy is discontinued if the animal becomes azotemic (BUN >50 mg/dl, creatinine >3 mg/dl).

C. Amphotericin B lipid complex (Abelcet; The Liposome Co., Princeton, NJ) allows higher total doses to be used and may reduce nephrotoxicity. Recommended dose is 1 mg/kg IV QOD to a total dose of 12 mg/kg for dogs.

D. Efficacy of amphotericin B when combined with ketoconazole or itraconazole is equal to that of itraconazole alone.

Patient Monitoring

I. Initial in-hospital monitoring includes daily vital signs, body weight, and physical/ocular examinations.

II. Monthly recheck examinations on therapy also include a serum chemistry profile.

III. After 2 months of itraconazole therapy, consider whether to discontinue the drug.

A. Discontinue therapy if the animal is normal at home, there is no evidence of active ocular disease, and thoracic radiographs have improved substantially.

B. Thoracic radiographs often continue to improve after discontinuing therapy.

C. If doubt exists about the presence or absence of active disease, the animal is treated for the additional month.

IV. If ketoconazole is used, treatment is continued at least 1 month beyond complete clinical remission.

A. It usually requires at least 3 months.

B. Thereafter, animals are reevaluated 3 and 6 months after discontinuing therapy.

V. Prognosis is as follows.

A. Approximately 70–75% of dogs treated with either itraconazole or ketoconazole/amphotericin B combination respond completely to therapy (Legendre et al., 1984; Arceneaux and Taboada, 1996).

B. Dogs most often die of severe respiratory disease and hypoxemia; however, dogs that live through the first 10 days of therapy do well.

C. Hypoxemia and involvement of three or more body systems warrant a poor prognosis.

D. Relapse occurs in 15–20% of treated dogs, usually in the first 6 months.

E. Relapses are treated similar to any new infection.

HISTOPLASMOSIS

Definition

I. Histoplasmosis is a systemic fungal infection that usually originates in the lungs or gastrointestinal (GI) tract and then disseminates to the lymphatics, liver, spleen, bone marrow, eyes, and other organs.

II. It occurs in a wide variety of mammals, with cats being more susceptible than dogs.

III. Dogs <4 years old and young cats are at an increased risk, but any age can be affected; no apparent sex predilection exists.

IV. Pointers, Brittany spaniels, and Weimaraners are the most commonly affected breeds.

Causes

I. It is caused by the dimorphic fungus *Histoplasma capsulatum*.

II. *H. capsulatum* characteristics are as follows.
  A. In tissue or when cultured at 30–37°C, the organism is a yeast and is usually found intracellularly.
  B. When cultured at 25°C, the organism grows as a white cottony or buff-brown mold that requires 7–10 days for colony growth.

III. *H. capsulatum* is a soil saprophyte that survives in a wide range of moistures and temperatures. Nitrogen-rich soil (those containing bird or bat guano) appears ideal for its growth.

IV. *H. capsulatum* is endemic to most temperate and subtropical regions of the world and mostly occurs in the central United States along the Mississippi, Ohio, and Missouri Rivers.

Pathophysiology

I. Infection is most commonly via inhalation or ingestion of infective conidia from the environment.
  A. Inhalation is probably the primary route of infection for cats, dogs, and humans.
  B. Ingestion of conidia may occur in dogs.

II. After inhalation or ingestion, conidia transform from the mycelial phase to yeast phase and are phagocytized by cells of the macrophage-monocyte system, where they grow as facultative intracellular organisms.
  A. Hematogenous and lymphatic dissemination results in multisystemic disease.
  B. Although dissemination may affect any organ system, the lungs, GI tract, lymph nodes, liver, spleen, bone marrow, eyes, and adrenal glands are commonly affected in dogs, whereas lungs, liver, lymph nodes, eyes, and bone marrow are most commonly affected in cats.

III. Incubation period is 12–16 days in dogs.

IV. Like blastomycosis, the immune response determines the severity of clinical disease.

V. Subclinical infection is probably common.

VI. Point-source outbreaks of disease are usually associated with exposure to areas heavily contaminated with *Histoplasma* organisms (chicken coops, bat habitats, or starling roosts).

Clinical Signs

I. Feline histoplasmosis
  A. Signs are usually insidious in onset and nonspecific, such as depression, anorexia, fever, pale mucous membranes, or weight loss.
  B. Pulmonary signs, including dyspnea, tachypnea, or abnormal lung sounds, are seen in about 50% of animals.
  C. Hepatomegaly, splenomegaly, or lymphadenopathy is noted in about one third of animals.
  D. Ocular signs include eyelid granulomas, retinal pigment proliferation, retinal edema, granulomatous chorioretinitis, anterior uveitis, panophthalmitis, and optic neuritis. Retinal detachment and secondary glaucoma are uncommon.
  E. Lameness in one or more limbs may occur from lytic bone lesions and soft tissue swelling.
  F. Cutaneous lesions consisting of multiple, small nodules that either ulcerate and drain or crust over are uncommon.
  G. GI signs other than anorexia are uncommon. Oral and lingual ulceration has been reported as an atypical manifestation; icterus is occasionally seen with hepatic involvement.

II. Canine histoplasmosis
  A. Subclinical infection is probably common following inhalation of organisms.
  B. GI signs occur most commonly.
    1. Large intestinal diarrhea with tenesmus and passage of mucus and fresh blood is most common in early disease.
    2. Small intestinal diarrhea (possibly voluminous and associated with malabsorption and/or protein-losing enteropathy) may be apparent with progressive disease.
  C. Elaboration of inflammatory mediators (tumor necrosis factor, interleukin-1) may cause nonspecific signs of fever, anorexia, depression, and severe weight loss.
  D. Abnormal lung sounds with or without coughing, tachypnea, or dyspnea are seen in <50% of dogs.
  E. Splenomegaly, hepatomegaly, and lymphadenopathy occur occasionally.
  F. Oral ulceration, lameness from bony involvement, neurologic signs, nodular skin disease, ocular involvement, and adrenal insufficiency are less common.

Diagnosis

I. Hematologic and serum chemistry findings
  A. Normocytic, normochromic nonregenerative anemia is the most commonly seen hematologic abnormality and results from chronic inflammation, GI blood loss, or bone marrow infection.
  B. Neutrophilia and monocytosis are often seen, but total leukocyte counts are variable.
    1. Neutropenia and/or pancytopenia are unusual occurrences, especially in cats.
    2. Organisms are rarely seen within monocytes, neutrophils, or eosinophils.
  C. Thrombocytopenia from increased platelet utilization or destruction is common.
  D. Hypoalbuminemia is the most consistent abnormality seen in serum chemistries.
  E. Increased serum ALT, AST, AP, and total bilirubin levels indicate hepatic involvement.

F. Hypercalcemia may occur, especially in cats.
II. Radiographic findings
  A. Thoracic radiography often shows a diffuse interstitial or linear interstitial pattern that may coalesce into a nodular interstitial pattern. Alveolar infiltrates are rare.
  B. Hilar lymphadenopathy is common in dogs but unusual in cats.
  C. Calcified pulmonary infiltrates or hilar lymph nodes usually indicate inactive disease.
  D. Bony lesions of the distal appendicular skeleton (especially carpal and tarsal bones) are rarely seen.
III. Organism identification
  A. Cytologic examination may show *Histoplasma* organisms in phagocytic cells of the mononuclear-phagocyte system.
    1. Some organisms are released from infected cells during slide preparation and seen as free organisms on slides stained with a Wright-Giemsa stain.
    2. Evidence of pyogranulomatous inflammation may exist with numerous intracellular small round to oval yeast cells (2–4 μm in diameter, basophilic center, and light halo caused by shrinkage of its cell wall during fixation).
    3. In cats, aspirates from the bone marrow or lymph nodes, or cells from a tracheal wash or bronchoalveolar lavage, are most likely to yield organisms.
    4. In dogs, cells from rectal scrapings or biopsies; aspirates from bone marrow, liver, lymph nodes, or spleen; or cells from a tracheal wash or bronchoalveolar lavage are most likely to yield organisms.
    5. Buffy coat smears, aspirates of lytic bone lesions, or aspirates or impression smears of nodular skin lesions may also yield organisms.
  B. Histopathologic findings are as follows.
    1. Pyogranulomatous lesions with multiple intracellular organisms are usually apparent.
    2. Special stains (PAS, Gridley's fungal, and Gomori methenamine silver) best demonstrate organisms in tissue.
  C. Fungal culture and identification are as follows.
    1. It is not needed for definitive identification.
    2. Buff-brown mycelial growth on Sabouraud's dextrose agar usually takes 7–10 days at room temperature, whereas yeast produces white moist colonies on blood agar at 30–37°C.
    3. Attempts at culture in a clinical practice are not warranted because of the potential public health risk.
IV. Other tests
  A. Serology is presently an ineffective method of diagnosis; both false-positive and false-negative results occur commonly.
  B. Cats with histoplasmosis are typically negative for feline leukemia virus (FeLV) and feline immunodeficiency virus (FIV).

Differential Diagnosis

I. Blastomycosis or other systemic fungal diseases
II. Other GI diseases
  A. Large intestinal disease: see Chap. 33
  B. Small intestinal disease: see Chap. 32

Treatment

I. Treatment is similar to that described for blastomycosis, although azole antifungal usage is not as well studied.
II. Longer treatment times are probably needed with the azole antifungals but are variable depending on the severity of the infection and the response of the animal.
III. Pulmonary disease may be self-limited, but antifungal treatment is still recommended because of the potential for chronic dissemination.
IV. Feline histoplasmosis is treated as follows.
  A. Itraconazole (5 mg/kg PO BID) for at least 2–4 months is the treatment of choice (Hodges et al., 1994).
  B. Ketoconazole is effective in about one third of cats.
  C. Fluconazole may be effective, but it has not been well researched.
  D. Amphotericin B may be added to the treatment protocol in severely affected cats.
V. Canine histoplasmosis requires the following.
  A. Ketoconazole has been described as the preferred treatment, but amphotericin B is added in fulminant cases.
  B. Itraconazole or fluconazole is safer and may have better efficacy.

Patient Monitoring

I. Resolution of clinical signs is the best means of monitoring therapy.
II. Initially, in-hospital monitoring includes daily vital signs, body weight, and physical/ocular examinations.
III. Monthly recheck examinations also include a serum chemistry profile.
IV. Treatment is continued for 1 month beyond complete resolution of clinical signs.
V. Animals are reevaluated 3 and 6 months after discontinuing therapy to assess for relapse.
VI. Serology is not useful in monitoring response to therapy or evaluating for relapse.
VII. Prognosis is variable.
  A. Prognosis is good for dogs with only pulmonary signs.
  B. Dogs with GI or severe disseminated signs have a guarded prognosis.
  C. The prognosis is fair to good for cats treated with itraconazole, although long-term therapy may be required.
  D. Severely debilitated cats have a guarded prognosis.

COCCIDIOIDOMYCOSIS

Definition

I. Coccidioidomycosis (valley fever, San Joaquin Valley fever) is a systemic fungal infection that typically originates in the lungs and may disseminate to the lymphatics, bones, and other organs.

II. It can occur in most mammals and in some cold-blooded vertebrates; dogs are affected more often than cats.

III. Young large and medium-sized male dogs housed outside are most commonly affected, with the likelihood of infection decreasing with advancing age.

IV. Boxers, pointers, Australian shepherd dogs, beagles, Scottish terriers, Doberman pinschers, and cocker spaniels may be at an increased risk (Davidson, 1995; Wolf and Troy, 1995).

V. No breed or sex predilection occurs in domestic cats.

VI. Epizootics occur in endemic areas when drought conditions are followed by periods of rain, dust storms, earthquakes, or other conditions that spread soil-derived arthrospores into the air.

Causes

I. It is caused by the geophilic dimorphic fungus *Coccidioides immitis.*

II. *C. immitis* characteristics are as follows.
   A. In tissue or when cultured at 37°C, the organism grows as large spherules that gradually enlarge to 20–200 μm. Endospores are produced by cleavage from the wall of the spherule.
   B. In the environment or when cultured at 25°C, the organism grows as a mycelium that forms square to rectangular (2–4 μm by 3–10 μm) multinucleate arthrospores.

III. *C. immitis* is a soil saprophyte that is restricted to the lower Sonoran life zone.
   A. It grows only in areas with sandy alkaline soils, semi-arid conditions, high summer and moderate winter temperatures, and low geographic elevations (sea level to a few hundred feet).
   B. It is endemic to the desert southwest (California, Arizona, Texas, New Mexico, Nevada, Utah) and to Mexico, Central America, and parts of South America.

Pathophysiology

I. Infection is usually via inhalation of infective arthrospores from the environment or direct inoculation of arthrospores into the skin.
   A. During periods of high temperature and low rainfall, the mycelia lie dormant below the soil surface.
   B. Following periods of rain, the organism then returns to the surface, sporulates, and releases large numbers of arthrospores that are disseminated by the wind.
   C. After drought periods, large numbers of arthrospores may be released, resulting in disease epidemics in endemic areas.
   D. Coccidioidomycosis is not a contagious disease.

II. Inhalation of <10 arthrospores produces clinical disease.
   A. Following inhalation, arthrospores move from the peribronchial tissue to the subpleural area, and spherules form to produce endospores, which become more spherules.
   B. Respiratory signs result from the endospore formation and subsequent inflammatory responses.
   C. Hematogenous and lymphatic dissemination occurs uncommonly and results in multisystemic disease.
   D. While dissemination may occur to any organ system, bones and joints, spleen, liver, kidney, heart, reproductive organs, eyes, brain, and spinal cord are affected most commonly. The skin is often affected in cats.

III. The incubation period varies from 1–3 weeks in dogs.

IV. The immune response determines the severity of clinical disease.
   A. Recovery is dependent on cell-mediated immunity, but a humoral response is present in most dogs living in endemic areas.
      1. An adequate immune response results in subclinical or mild respiratory disease that resolves spontaneously; most cases in dogs and cats are probably subclinical.
      2. A poor immune response results in severe pulmonary and disseminated disease.
   B. Recovered humans are usually immune, but it is unknown whether the same immunity occurs in dogs and cats.

Clinical Signs

I. Most affected dogs and cats probably show no or only mild respiratory signs before mounting an effective immune response.

II. Disseminated feline coccidioidomycosis is uncommon.
   A. Cats are more resistant to infection when compared with dogs.
   B. No age, sex, or breed predisposition exists.
   C. Clinical findings are variable because of the multisystemic nature of the disease. Typically, signs of disease are present for <1 month prior to diagnosis.
   D. Nonspecific signs of depression, anorexia, fever, and weight loss are common.
   E. Pulmonary involvement (dyspnea, tachypnea, or abnormal lung sounds) is seen in about 25% of cats.
   F. Skin lesions (draining lesions, subcutaneous masses, abscesses) are seen in >50% of cats. Localized lymphadenopathy is noted in a third of the cats with skin lesions.
   G. Lameness develops in approximately 20% of cats.
   H. Ocular involvement (granulomatous chorioretini-

tis with retinal detachment, uveitis, or panophthalmitis) is noted in approximately 10% of cats.
  I. CNS involvement is uncommon.
III. Disseminated canine coccidioidomycosis often occurs in dogs <4 years of age.
  A. Males are affected twice as often as females.
  B. The clinical findings are related to the severity of pulmonary involvement and the extent of systemic dissemination.
    1. Clinically inapparent infection is common following inhalation of organisms.
    2. When clinical signs develop, they are often present for 1–6 months before the initial diagnosis.
  C. The most common presenting complaint is usually a chronic cough.
  D. Prolonged intermittent fever, anorexia, depression, and weight loss are common.
  E. Lameness associated with osteomyelitis and painful periarticular swelling is common.
    1. Multiple osseous lesions may be seen in as many as 65% of dogs.
    2. The distal portion of long bones is affected most commonly.
  F. Approximately 20% of dogs have cutaneous lesions characterized by nodules, abscesses, ulcers, and draining tracts.
    1. Skin lesions usually occur as an extension from an infected osseous lesion.
    2. Primary skin and subcutaneous infections following direct cutaneous inoculation in dogs are rare.
    3. Regional lymphadenopathy associated with cutaneous or osseous lesions is common, but generalized peripheral lymphadenopathy is unusual.
  G. Visceral organ involvement may result in icterus, renal failure with renomegaly, or GI signs.
  H. Cardiac involvement may result in right- or left-sided heart failure, pericardial effusion, arrhythmias, and syncope.
  I. Seizures, ataxia, behavioral changes, and coma have been associated with CNS involvement.
  J. Ocular lesions often involve both the posterior and anterior segments, but they are not as common as with other systemic fungal infections.
    1. Anterior segment disease (iritis, granulomatous uveitis) is usually an extension of posterior segment disease.
    2. Glaucoma occurs in almost half of affected eyes (Angell et al., 1987).
    3. Granulomatous chorioretinitis with or without retinal detachment is common but may not be apparent because of the severity of the anterior segment disease.
    4. Lesions are usually unilateral, but bilateral disease may develop.

Diagnosis

  I. Hematologic and serum chemistry findings
    A. A mild normocytic, normochromic nonregenerative anemia is common.
    B. Moderate neutrophilia, usually with a left shift, and monocytosis are often seen.
    C. Hypoalbuminemia and hyperglobulinemia are consistent abnormalities.
    D. Increased serum ALT, AST, AP, and total bilirubin levels indicate hepatic involvement.
    E. Azotemia and hyperphosphatemia may indicate renal involvement.
    F. Hypercalcemia may occur.
  II. Radiographic findings
    A. Numerous abnormalities may be found on thoracic radiographs.
      1. Hilar and central lung regions (peripheral lung regions are less commonly affected) often reveal an ill-defined diffuse interstitial or peribronchiolar pattern, with alveolar infiltrates being uncommon.
      2. Hilar lymphadenopathy is seen in approximately 80% of dogs.
      3. Mediastinal widening due to mediastinal lymph node enlargement is less common.
      4. Pleural involvement as evidenced by pleural thickening or effusion is seen in almost 65% of dogs (Millman et al., 1979).
    B. Osseous lesions consisting of periosteal and endosteal new bone formation and osteolysis are noted in approximately 20% of dogs.
      1. Bones of the distal appendicular skeleton are affected about three times more frequently than bones of the axial skeleton.
      2. The distal diaphysis, metaphysis, and epiphysis are affected most often.
      3. Multiple osseous lesions are usually evident.
      4. Hypertrophic osteopathy may occur secondary to pulmonary or hilar lymph node involvement.
  III. Cytologic findings
    A. Fewer numbers of spherules make cytologic demonstration more difficult than demonstration of the yeast forms in other systemic fungal infections.
    B. Exudate from draining skin lesions and pleural fluid are most likely to yield organisms.
    C. Tracheal wash or bronchoalveolar lavage samples, lymph node aspirates, or aspirates from affected tissue may also yield organisms.
    D. Bone aspirates do not usually yield organisms.
    E. Spherules appear as large (20–200 μm), round, double-walled structures with endospores.
      1. The walls are refractile appearing on wet preps or potassium hydroxide (KOH) preps.
      2. They stain blue when hematoxylin and eosin (H&E) type stains are used.
      3. They stain deep red to purple with PAS, whereas the endospores stain bright red.
      4. They stain purple-black with Papanicolaou's (Pap) stain, whereas the cytoplasm stains yellow and the endospores stain red-brown.
  IV. Histopathologic findings
    A. Biopsy is more likely to demonstrate organisms than cytology.
    B. Multiple biopsy samples are taken when biop-

sying bone to increase the likelihood of finding organisms.

    C. Special stains (PAS, Gridley's fungal, or Gomori methenamine silver) best demonstrate the organisms.

V. Fungal culture and identification

    A. *C. immitis* grows readily on a wide variety of agars at room temperature as a white cotton-like mold that changes to tan or brown with age.

    B. Arthrospores from cultures are highly infectious.

VI. Serology

    A. It is used in dogs and cats from endemic areas to make a presumptive diagnosis when clinical signs are suggestive but organisms cannot be demonstrated.

    B. Precipitin antibodies are thought to represent IgM and are detectable 2–4 weeks after initial infection.

        1. The precipitin test may become negative after 4–5 weeks and then positive again in those animals in which dissemination has occurred.

        2. False-negative results may occur in early infections, fulminant disease, chronic infections, and immunosuppressed animals.

    C. Complement-fixing (CF) antibodies are thought to represent IgG and are detectable shortly after precipitin antibodies.

        1. An agar gel immunodiffusion test (AGID) is used as a screening test for CF antibodies.

        2. The CF titer generally increases with the severity of disease.

        3. Low titers (<1:16) may indicate early, very chronic, localized or past infection.

        4. Titers >1:32 are suggestive of active, disseminated disease.

        5. Higher titers are generally seen in more severe disease.

Differential Diagnosis

Rule out blastomycosis or other systemic fungal diseases.

Treatment

I. Ketoconazole (5–15 mg/kg PO BID) or itraconazole (5–10 mg/kg PO SID) is the preferred treatment.

    A. Ketoconazole is generally used because it is less expensive, but side effects are more likely.

    B. Ketoconazole treatment is continued for at least 2 months beyond clinical remission; treatment is often needed for at least 6–12 months.

    C. Itraconazole treatment may allow for a shorter course of treatment, but limited studies exist in dogs.

    D. Chronic low-dose therapy beyond the initial treatment period may be necessary to keep some animals in remission.

II. Coccidioidomycosis is less responsive to amphotericin B than the other systemic fungal infections.

Patient Monitoring

I. Resolution of clinical signs is the best means of monitoring response to therapy.

II. Initial in-hospital monitoring includes daily vital signs, body weight, and physical/ocular examinations.

III. Monthly recheck examinations also include a serum chemistry profile to evaluate liver enzyme activities for animals receiving azole antifungals.

IV. Cataracts may occur in dogs on long-term (>12 months) ketoconazole.

V. Animals are reevaluated 3 and 6 months after discontinuing therapy to assess for relapse.

VI. Serology has been used to monitor response to therapy or evaluate for relapse.

    A. CF titers may stay elevated for a year or more following therapy.

    B. CF titers should be <1:16 when therapy is discontinued.

    C. CF titers often increase with relapse of clinical disease.

VII. Prognosis is variable.

    A. The prognosis is good for dogs and cats with only pulmonary signs.

    B. The prognosis is guarded for dogs and cats with disseminated disease. Most animals respond well initially but relapse when treatment is discontinued.

    C. If untreated, disseminated disease is usually fatal.

CRYPTOCOCCOSIS

Definition

I. Cryptococcosis is an opportunistic systemic fungal infection of worldwide significance that usually originates in the nasal cavity, paranasal tissue, or lungs and is then disseminated to the skin, eyes, or CNS.

II. It occurs in a wide variety of mammalian species, but cats are most commonly affected.

III. Unlike the other systemic mycoses, it does not follow any specific geographic boundaries.

Causes

I. Cryptococcosis is caused by *Cryptococcus neoformans,* a saprophytic, round, yeast-like organism with a restricted ecologic niche that is related to the rust and smut fungal organisms of higher plants.

II. *C. neoformans* var. *neoformans* is the subspecies that most commonly causes clinical disease in cats and is usually associated with pigeon droppings in the environment or other avian habitats.

    A. *C. neoformans* var. *gattii* is a second subspecies that is capable of causing clinical disease and is associated with bark and leaf litter of certain *Eucalyptus* trees.

    B. In tissue and often when cultured, the organism is a variably sized yeast (3.5–7 μm) with a large heteropolysaccharide capsule (1–30 μm thick).

    C. The organism primarily reproduces by budding from a narrow base.

    D. Under controlled laboratory conditions the organism undergoes sexual reproduction, but most infections are thought to be caused by environmental exposure to the yeast-like phase.

III. Pigeons are thought to be the most important vector of *C. neoformans.*
   A. The organism can be found in high numbers in pigeon roosts, barn lofts, hay mows, and along cupolas and cornices where pigeons often sit.
   B. In the desiccated state, the organism may be no larger than 1 μm and survive up to 2 years.
   C. Direct exposure to sunlight or soil quickly kills the organisms.

Pathophysiology

I. Infection is most commonly via inhalation of yeast organisms from the environment.
   A. Most yeast are probably too large to be inhaled directly into the lungs but tend to settle in the nasal passages.
   B. Small desiccated forms of the yeast are infective and can be inhaled directly into the small airways and alveoli.
II. After inhalation, nasal, paranasal sinus, or pulmonary granulomas form.
   A. Dissemination may occur by direct extension or by hematogenous spread.
      1. Direct extension through the cribriform plate to the CNS or to the paranasal soft tissue or skin is common.
      2. Although dissemination can occur to any organ, the skin, eyes, and CNS are most commonly affected.
   B. Lesions often exist as either granulomatous inflammation with few organisms or gelatinous masses of organisms with little inflammation.
   C. The capsule surrounding the cryptococcal organism contributes its pathogenicity by inhibiting phagocytosis, plasma cell function, and leukocyte migration.
III. The immune response determines the severity of clinical disease.
   A. Antibodies are not protective.
   B. Recovery is dependent on cell-mediated immunity.
      1. Immunosuppression has not been as apparent in infected cats and dogs.
      2. An association with FeLV and FIV infections in cats may exist.
      3. Prolonged glucocorticoid use may be a predisposing factor.
IV. Cryptococcosis is not a contagious disease.

Clinical Signs

I. Feline cryptococcosis
   A. No apparent breed or sex predilection exists.
   B. Clinical findings are usually related to upper respiratory, cutaneous, ocular, or CNS involvement.
   C. Depression and anorexia are common in chronic cases, but fever is uncommon.
   D. Upper respiratory signs related to nasal cavity involvement are seen in 50–80% of cats.
      1. Sneezing and unilateral or bilateral mucopuru-

lent nasal discharge, with or without blood, are typically seen.
      2. Proliferative soft tissue masses or ulcerative lesions within the nasal passage or on the bridge of the nose are seen in approximately 70% of cases with upper respiratory involvement (Malik et al., 1992).
   E. The lungs are affected less often than by the other systemic mycoses.
   F. Oral ulcerations are occasionally noted.
   G. The skin or subcutaneous tissue is affected in approximately 30–50% of cats (Malik et al., 1992; Wolf and Troy, 1995).
      1. Papules or nodules are the primary lesions; multiple lesions are typical, and larger lesions are usually ulcerated.
      2. Regional lymphadenopathy is common.
   H. The eyes are affected in 20–25% of cats, especially those with CNS involvement.
      1. Granulomatous chorioretinitis with or without exudative retinal detachment is the most common lesion and may lead to a panophthalmitis.
      2. Optic neuritis may cause acute blindness.
      3. Anterior uveitis is present in some cats.
   I. CNS involvement is reported in approximately 25% of cats (Wolf and Troy, 1995).
      1. Behavior changes, seizures, circling, and ataxia occur.
      2. Head pressing, cranial nerve deficits, and paresis also occur.
   J. Hematogenous spread from the respiratory tract may result in lameness secondary to osteomyelitis, renal failure with kidney involvement, and generalized lymphadenopathy.
II. Canine cryptococcosis
   A. Dogs <4 years of age are most commonly affected, with over-representation of American cocker spaniels, Labrador retrievers, Great Danes, and Doberman pinschers.
   B. Clinical findings are most often related to CNS, upper respiratory, ocular, or cutaneous involvement.
   C. Depression and anorexia are common, but fever is uncommon.
   D. CNS involvement occurs in approximately 50–80% of dogs (Berthelin et al., 1994a, 1994b).
      1. The brain is most often affected, but involvement of the spinal cord may also occur.
      2. Neurologic signs include mental depression, vestibular syndrome, ataxia, cranial nerve (CN) deficits (especially CN V, VII, VIII), seizures, paresis, blindness, hypermetria, and cervical pain.
      3. Most dogs with CNS involvement have other organ systems affected.
   E. Upper respiratory tract or perinasal tissues are affected in approximately 50% of dogs (Malik et al., 1995).
      1. Caudal nasal passages and frontal sinuses are affected more commonly than are the rostral nasal passages.

2. Respiratory signs include upper airway stridor, nasal discharge and sneezing, epistaxis, and firm swellings on the bridge of the nose or periorbitally.

F. Eyes and/or periorbital tissue are affected in approximately 20–40% of dogs.
   1. Granulomatous chorioretinitis with or without exudative retinal detachment is the most common lesion and can lead to panophthalmitis.
   2. Retinal hemorrhage or retinal scarring may be seen.
   3. Optic neuritis may cause acute blindness.
   4. Anterior uveitis is less common than posterior segment disease.

G. The skin is affected in approximately 10–20% of dogs.
   1. Subcutaneous nodules with ulcerative draining lesions are typical.
   2. The head, footpads, nail beds, and oral mucous membranes are common sites.

H. Proliferative lesions in the external ear canals may result from cryptococcal otitis, and direct extension from the ear canals to the CNS may also occur.

I. Multiorgan dissemination is common and may either be subclinical or result in clinical signs.

Diagnosis

I. Hematologic and serum chemistry findings
   A. They are often normal, but mild nonregenerative anemia and mature neutrophilia or neutrophilia with mild left shift may be seen.
   B. Serum chemistry findings are usually normal.

II. Cerebrospinal fluid (CSF) analysis
   A. Pressure and protein levels are often increased, and a mixed mononuclear and neutrophilic pleocytosis is common.
   B. Organisms are visualized in approximately 90% of dogs with CNS involvement.

III. Radiographic findings
   A. Thoracic radiographs are usually normal, but a nodular to interstitial lung pattern, pleural effusion, and tracheobronchial lymphadenopathy do occur.
   B. Nasal radiographs may demonstrate increased soft tissue density and bone destruction in the nasal passages and frontal sinuses.

IV. Organism identification
   A. Cytology is the quickest and easiest means of identifying cryptococcal organisms.
      1. Nasal swabs, exudate from cutaneous lesions, or aspirates from soft tissue masses, subretinal sites, or vitreal areas often reveal organisms.
      2. Organisms may not be apparent in approximately 25% of animals (Medleau and Barsanti, 1990).
      3. The organism's thin wall and large capsule help differentiate it from *Blastomyces* as well as its budding with a narrow base.
   B. Histopathologic findings are as follows.
      1. Nodular to diffuse granulomatous lesions or

areas of degeneration with limited inflammation are seen in infected tissue, and yeast-like organisms are usually numerous.
      2. Special stains (PAS, Gridley's fungal, and Gomori methenamine silver) best demonstrate the organisms.
      3. Mucicarmine stains demonstrate the organism's capsule.
   C. Fungal culture can also be used for identification.
      1. The organism can be cultured from infected tissue, exudate, CSF, urine, joint fluid, and blood if sufficient samples are submitted.
      2. Yeast-like growth occurs in 2–42 days on Sabouraud's dextrose agar.
      3. Hyphae rarely grow, even at 37°C.

V. Serology
   A. It is very useful when cytology fails to demonstrate organisms.
   B. Latex agglutination (LA) detects cryptococcal capsular antigen and is the preferred test.
   C. The commercially available LA tests can be used on serum, urine, or CSF.
      1. CSF is the preferred sample in animals with neurologic signs.
      2. Serum is the preferred sample in animals with other signs.
   D. False-negative LA antigen titers may occur with localized disease.
   E. False-positive LA antigen titers are uncommon and are usually related to technique or interfering substances such as rheumatoid factor.
   F. The LA antigen titer tends to correlate well with the extent of disease and may be used to evaluate the effectiveness of treatment.
   G. Detection of serum or CSF antibodies is not a useful diagnostic tool.

Differential Diagnosis

I. Other upper respiratory diseases: primary nasal neoplasia, nasal aspergillosis, other nasal fungal infection, nasal foreign body, chronic viral sinusitis in cats, oronasal or oroantral fistula, tooth root abscess

II. CNS disease: toxoplasmosis (primary differential in cats)

III. Cutaneous disease: see Blastomycosis section earlier

IV. Ocular disease: see Blastomycosis section earlier

Treatment

I. Amphotericin B is the most effective drug (in vitro) against the various cryptococcal isolates.
   A. Amphotericin B is synergistic with flucytosine (25–50 mg/kg PO QID), and the combination is especially useful in CNS infections.
      1. CSF concentrations of flucytosine approach those of serum.
      2. Cryptococcal organisms may rapidly develop resistance to flucytosine, so it has limited efficacy as a single treatment agent.
      3. Toxicity to flucytosine includes ulcerative drug eruptions of the skin (especially of the

face and mucocutaneous junctions), enterocolitis, leukopenia, and thrombocytopenia.
4. The dose of flucytosine is decreased in animals with advancing renal failure.
B. Amphotericin B in combination with azole antifungals or flucytosine has been used to successfully treat feline and canine cryptococcosis.
   1. Amphotericin B (0.5–0.8 mg/kg) is diluted in 0.45% saline/2.5% dextrose solution (400 ml for cats, 500 ml for dogs <20 kg; 1000 ml for dogs >20 kg) and administered SQ 2–3 times per week.
   2. This protocol may allow for larger cumulative doses of amphotericin B with reduced toxicity.
   3. Concentrations >20 mg/L of amphotericin B result in local irritation.
II. Fluconazole (50 mg/cat PO BID) is very effective and may be the preferred treatment in cats because there are fewer side effects when compared with amphotericin B.
III. Itraconazole (10 mg/kg PO SID) is also effective in cats and dogs, whereas ketoconazole (10–30 mg/kg PO BID) is slightly less effective.

Patient Monitoring

I. Resolution of clinical signs is the best means of monitoring response to therapy.
II. In-hospital monitoring includes daily vital signs, body weight, and physical/ocular examinations.
III. Monthly recheck examinations also include a serum chemistry profile to evaluate liver enzyme activities for animals receiving azole antifungals.
IV. Treatment is continued for 2 months beyond complete resolution of clinical signs.
V. Animals are reevaluated 3 and 6 months after discontinuing therapy to assess for relapse.
VI. Cryptococcal LA antigen titers are useful in monitoring treatment progress when interpreted together with clinical remission.
   A. Negative LA antigen titers are occasionally seen in animals with localized disease, so negative titers do not always indicate a clinical cure.
   B. Clinical "cures" have also been seen in animals that maintain a positive LA antigen titer.
VII. The prognosis is good for cats with extraneural disease.
VIII. The prognosis is guarded for dogs with any form of the disease and for cats with CNS involvement.

PYTHIOSIS

Definition

I. Pythiosis is an uncommon infectious disease of dogs, cats, horses, cattle, and humans.
II. Horses and dogs are the most common species infected; cats are very rarely infected.
III. It occurs primarily in tropical and subtropical areas of the world. In the United States it occurs primarily along the Gulf of Mexico, mostly in southern Louisiana, Texas, Alabama, and Florida.

Causes

I. Pythiosis is caused by a protistan member of the Oomycetes class, *Pythium insidiosum,* which is evolutionarily more closely related to algae than to true fungi.
II. *P. insidiosum* grows in tissue and in the environment as thick-walled septated hyphae; in aquatic environment, it produces motile zoospores.

Pathophysiology

I. The infective stage is thought to be the motile zoospore.
   A. Zoospores are released into a warm water environment, where they are able to chemotactically orient themselves toward certain aquatic plants and animal hair.
   B. They enter the host through damaged skin or mucous membranes.
II. *P. insidiosum* is considered to be a true pathogen rather than an opportunist because immune suppression is not an apparent prerequisite for infection.
III. Three forms of pythiosis occur: cutaneous disease (most common in horses and cats), GI disease (predominantly in dogs), and the rare multisystemic metastatic disease.
IV. In the GI form of the disease, any part of the GI tract may be affected, but the stomach and proximal small intestine are affected most commonly.
   A. Occasionally only the mesenteric lymph nodes are affected.
   B. Diffuse to irregular transmural thickening of a 5–25 cm segment of the GI tract with variable irregular mucosal ulceration is noted.
V. Arterial thrombosis and arterial disruption from the growing *Pythium* and the inflammatory processes may occur and probably account for those rare cases of multisystemic involvement.

Clinical Signs

I. Canine GI pythiosis
   A. Male, large-breed (especially hunting breeds) dogs <3 years old are most likely to be infected.
   B. Vomiting, pronounced weight loss, and a palpable abdominal mass are typical clinical findings.
   C. Other signs may include regurgitation if the esophagus is involved, diarrhea if the distal small intestine is affected, or hematochezia if the colon is involved.
   D. Presentation is often late in the disease, because affected dogs usually remain bright and alert.
   E. Signs of systemic illness occur when intestinal obstruction, infarction, or perforation occurs.
II. Canine cutaneous pythiosis
   A. Cutaneous disease is less common than the GI disease in dogs. The German shepherd dog may be predisposed.

B. Cutaneous lesions may occur anywhere.
1. Slightly pruritic, poorly defined nodules that soon become ulcerated are typical.
2. Multiple tracts may drain a serosanguineous or purulent exudate.
3. Rarely, complicated by GI involvement.
III. Feline pythiosis
A. Cats are very rarely infected.
B. Most cases involve the cutaneous form of disease.
C. Nasal and retrobulbar disease has been seen in one case (Bissonnette et al., 1991).

Diagnosis

I. Hematologic and serum chemistry findings are usually normal.
II. Radiographic and sonographic findings are variable.
A. An abdominal mass with or without an obstructive pattern may be seen on abdominal radiographs.
B. *Pythium*-induced esophagitis may result in megaesophagus.
C. Ultrasonography may reveal markedly thickened intestinal or gastric walls with loss of the normal layered pattern.
III. Organism identification involves the following.
A. Histopathologic findings are as follows.
1. Presumptive diagnosis can be made based on the morphology of the hyphal organisms and the inflammatory response pattern.
2. A pronounced granulomatous or eosinophilic inflammatory response is seen.
3. *Pythium* organisms do not stain well on H&E stain.
4. Gridley-stained or Gomori methenamine silver–stained sections are best used to identify hyphae.
5. An indirect immunoperoxidase technique is also useful in identifying hyphal organisms such as *Pythium*.
B. Fungal culture and identification are as follows.
1. *Pythium* is relatively easy to culture on a variety of fungal culture media.
2. Failure to grow the organism is usually related to sample handling.
3. *Pythium* is sensitive to temperature stress and dehydration; therefore, chilling or freezing samples results rapidly in organism death.

Differential Diagnosis

I. With the GI form of disease, rule out neoplasia such as lymphosarcoma or adenocarcinoma.
II. True zygomycetes such as *Mucor, Absidia,* or *Rhizopus* infections as well as *Basidiobolus* and *Conidiobolus* infections must be differentiated from pythiosis.
III. Differential considerations for cutaneous form of disease are the same as for blastomycosis.

Treatment

I. Wide surgical excision is the preferred treatment.
II. Amphotericin B and ketoconazole have been unsuccessful in resolving the disease.
III. Itraconazole (10 mg/kg PO SID-BID) is efficacious in approximately 20% of dogs (Taboada, 1996b).
IV. The prognosis is generally poor.

Patient Monitoring

I. Resolution of clinical signs and weight gain are the primary monitoring tools.
II. It may take a month or more before improvement occurs with itraconazole therapy.
III. Abdominal palpation or ultrasonography can be used to assess the size of the abdominal mass.

Bibliography

Angell JA, Merideth RE, Shively JN et al: Ocular lesions associated with coccidioidomycosis in dogs: 35 cases (1980–1985). J Am Vet Med Assoc 190:1319, 1987

Arceneaux KA, Taboada J: Unpublished data, 1996

Baumgardner DJ, Paretsky DP, Yopp AC: The epidemiology of blastomycosis in dogs: north central Wisconsin, USA. J Med Vet Mycol 33:171, 1995

Berthelin CF, Bailey CS, Kass PH et al: Cryptococcosis of the nervous system in dogs, part 1: epidemiologic, clinical, and neurologic features. Prog Vet Neurol 5:88, 1994a

Berthelin CF, Legendre AM, Bailey CS et al: Cryptococcosis of the nervous system in dogs, part 2: diagnosis, treatment, monitoring, and prognosis. Prog Vet Neurol 5:136, 1994b

Bissonnette KW, Sharp NJH, Dykstra MH et al: Nasal and retrobulbar mass in a cat caused by *Pythium insidiosum*. J Med Vet Mycol 29:39, 1991

Brooks DE, Legendre AM, Gum GG et al: The treatment of canine ocular blastomycosis with systemically administered itraconazole. Prog Vet Comp Ophthal 1:263, 1991

Clinkenbeard KD, Wolf AM, Cowell RL et al: Feline disseminated histoplasmosis. Compend Contin Educ Pract Vet 11:1223, 1989a

Clinkenbeard KD, Wolf AM, Cowell RL et al: Canine disseminated histoplasmosis. Compend Contin Educ Pract Vet 11:1347, 1989b

Davidson AP: Canine coccidioidomycosis update. Proc Am Coll Vet Intern Med 13:808, 1995

Davies C, Troy GC: Deep mycotic infections in cats. J Am Anim Hosp Assoc 32:380, 1996

Flatland B, Greene RT, Lappin MR: Clinical and serologic evaluation of cats with cryptococcosis. J Am Vet Med Assoc 209:1110, 1996

Foil CSO: A report of subcutaneous pythiosis in five dogs and a review of the etiologic agent *Pythium* spp. J Am Anim Hosp Assoc 20:959, 1984

Garma-Aviña A: Cytologic findings in 43 cases of blastomycosis diagnosed ante-mortem in naturally-infected dogs. Mycopathologia 131:87, 1995

Greene RT, Troy GC: Coccidioidomycosis in 48 cats: a retrospective study (1984–1993). J Vet Intern Med 9:86, 1995

Hodges RD, Legendre AM, Adams LG et al: Itraconazole for the treatment of histoplasmosis in cats. J Vet Intern Med 8:409, 1994

Legendre AM, Walker M, Buyukmihci N et al: Canine blastomycosis: a review of 47 clinical cases. J Am Vet Med Assoc 178:1163, 1981

Legendre AM, Selcer BA, Edwards DF et al: Treatment of canine blastomycosis with amphotericin B and ketoconazole. J Am Vet Med Assoc 184:1249, 1984

Malik R, Wigney DI, Muir DB et al: Cryptococcosis in cats: clinical and mycological assessment of 29 cases and evaluation of treatment using orally administered fluconazole. J Med Vet Mycol 30:133, 1992

Malik R, Dill-Macky E, Martin P et al: Cryptococcosis in dogs: a retrospective study of 20 consecutive cases. J Med Vet Mycol 33:291, 1995

Malik R, Craig AJ, Wigney DI et al: Combination chemotherapy of canine and feline cryptococcosis using subcutaneously administered amphotericin B. Aust Vet J 73:124, 1996

Medleau L, Barsanti JA: Cryptococcosis. p. 687. In Greene CE (ed): Infectious Diseases of the Dog and Cat. WB Saunders, Philadelphia, 1990

Medleau L, Greene CE, Rakich PM: Evaluation of ketoconazole and itraconazole for treatment of disseminated cryptococcosis in cats. Am J Vet Res 51:1454, 1990

Miller RI: Gastrointestinal phycomycosis in 63 dogs. J Am Vet Med Assoc 186:473, 1985

Millman TM, O'Brien TR, Suter PF et al: Coccidioidomycosis in the dog: its radiographic diagnosis. Vet Radiol 20:50, 1979

Patton CS, Hake R, Newton J et al: Esophagitis due to *Pythium insidiosum* infection in two dogs. J Vet Intern Med 10:139, 1996

Richter KP: Feline cryptococcosis. Proc Am Coll Vet Intern Med 13:804, 1995

Rudmann DG, Coolman BR, Perez CM et al: Evaluation of risk factors for blastomycosis in dogs: 857 cases (1980–1990). J Am Vet Med Assoc 201:1754, 1992

Taboada J: Oomycosis (pythiosis): biology, clinical disease, and therapeutic implications. Proc Am Coll Vet Intern Med 10:715, 1992

Taboada J: Blastomycosis. Proc Am Coll Vet Intern Med 14:605, 1996a

Taboada J: Unpublished data, 1996b

Taboada J, Merchant SR: Treatment of fungal diseases: antifungal agents used in the treatment of systemic diseases. Proc Am Coll Vet Intern Med 13:800, 1995

Taboada J, Werner BE, Legendre AM: Successful management of gastrointestinal pythiosis with itraconazole in two dogs. J Vet Intern Med 8:176, 1994

Walker MA: Thoracic blastomycosis: a review of its radiographic manifestations in 40 dogs. Vet Radiol 22:22, 1981

Wolf AM, Troy GC: Deep mycotic diseases. p. 439. In Ettinger SJ, Feldman EC (eds): Textbook of Veterinary Internal Medicine, 4th Ed. WB Saunders, Philadelphia, 1995

110

Viral Infections

Johnny D. Hoskins

CANINE DISTEMPER

Definition

Canine distemper virus (CDV) causes a highly contagious disease of dogs and all animals in the Canidae family (dingo, fox, coyote, wolf, jackal), the Mustelidae (ferret, mink, skunk, badger, marten, weasel, otter), and the Procyonidae family (raccoon, panda, kinkajou, coati).

Cause

I. Virus characteristics
  A. CDV is caused by a morbillivirus, a large RNA virus that is closely related to measles and rinderpest viruses.
  B. CDV is environmentally labile and inactivated by heat, sunlight, most detergents, soaps, and various chemicals (0.75% phenol, 0.3% quaternary ammonium compounds, 0.1% formalin).
II. Epidemiology
  A. CDV is shed via all body excretions, especially respiratory exudates.
  B. Recovering dogs may shed CDV for several weeks but not after full recovery.
  C. CDV induces prolonged but not lifelong immunity.
  D. Young puppies (3–6 months old) are most susceptible; and the natural incidence of disease decreases with age.
  E. A susceptible puppy can be safely introduced into a household 1 month after removal of a puppy that died of CDV infection.

Pathophysiology

I. Systemic infection
  A. CDV spreads by aerosol droplets and replicates in macrophages of the lower respiratory tract and associated lymphoid tissue.
  B. Degree and duration of viremia parallel serum antibody titer.
  C. CDV spreads rapidly to most epithelial tissues and the central nervous system (CNS).

II. CNS infection
  A. Young or immunodeficient puppies have direct viral injury to the CNS and develop acute encephalomyelitis.
  B. Slightly older or immunocompetent puppies develop nonsuppurative encephalomyelitis.
  C. Older and immunocompetent dogs develop an immune-mediated demyelinating or chronic progressive encephalomyelitis.

Clinical Signs

I. Inapparent or mild disease
  A. Mild disease is associated with fever (40–41.1°C; 104–106°F), transient anorexia, depression, and mild serous conjunctivitis.
  B. Localizing signs are not evident.
II. Severe multisystemic disease
  A. Fever is usually present but may sometimes be unnoticed.
  B. Ocular and nasal discharges are initially serous but later become mucopurulent.
  C. Depression, anorexia, diarrhea, vomiting, dehydration, and/or intestinal intussusception may occur.
  D. Initially a dry cough occurs, but it rapidly becomes moist and productive.
III. Neurologic signs
  A. They are usually evident 1–3 weeks after recovery from systemic disease and are progressive and variable.
  B. Focal neurologic signs suggesting a local brain or cord lesion may occur, but more often neurologic signs are multifocal.
    1. Signs may include seizures, hyperesthesia, pacing, circling, and behavioral changes.
    2. Disturbances in gait and posture include ataxia, asynergy, paraparesis, and tetraparesis.
    3. Rhythmic motor movements (referred to as chorea, tic, or myoclonus) are sometimes noted.
IV. Ancillary signs
  A. Multifocal chorioretinitis (usually in peripheral

and midperipheral nontapetal fundus) and optic neuritis may be present.
B. Keratoconjunctivitis and rarely a transient keratitis are evident.
C. Nasal and digital hyperkeratosis (hardpad disease) is a chronic manifestation.

V. Transplacental infection
A. Abortion, stillbirths, or birth of weak puppies occurs in the absence of multisystemic signs in the dam.
B. Neurologic signs are variable in puppies within the first 4–6 weeks of life.
C. Puppies only a few weeks old usually die quicker than older puppies.

Diagnosis

I. History: unvaccinated puppies or stressed, exposed older animals
II. Compatible clinical signs
III. Hematologic and cytologic findings
A. Lymphopenia and mild neutrophilia are usually present.
B. Inclusions are rare in peripheral blood cells during viremia. Buffy coat and bone marrow examination may improve the chances of finding inclusions.
C. Occasionally inclusions are found in imprint preparations of conjunctiva or vagina during viremia.
IV. Biochemical findings
A. Serum results are nonspecific.
1. Decreased albumin and/or increased globulin levels during initial and advanced stages of disease
2. Hypoglobulinemia in prenatally and neonatally infected animals
B. Cerebrospinal fluid (CSF) may reveal the following.
1. Increased protein (>25 mg/dl, primarily IgG) and cells (>10/µl, predominantly lymphocytes)
2. Specific CDV neutralizing antibody found with distemper encephalitis
a) Absent in vaccinated dogs or dogs recovered from mild CDV infection
b) Absent in dogs that have died from acute CDV infection
V. Pulmonary radiography
A. Interstitial pattern is noted in early or uncomplicated disease.
B. Mixed interstitial/alveolar pattern occurs with secondary bacterial infection and severe bronchopneumonia.
VI. Immunocytology
A. Cellular material is stained with fluorescein-conjugated anti-CDV antibody.
B. Antigen can be detected in the following at appropriate times.
1. Buffy coat smears: 2–5 days after infection
2. Cytologic smears of conjunctival and vaginal epithelium: 5–21 days after infection

3. Footpad biopsy: up to 60 days
C. Immunoperoxidase technique detects CDV antigen in formalin-fixed, paraffin-embedded tissue.
VII. Immunologic testing
A. Virus neutralization results in the following.
1. A high serum titer may indicate relative immune protection.
2. Paired serum samples taken 10–14 days apart with a fourfold rise in titer confirm active infection.
3. Increased CSF titer indicates chronic distemper encephalitis if blood contamination is excluded, and the CSF titer is high in comparison with serum titer.
B. Enzyme-linked immunosorbent assay (ELISA) is more sensitive than virus neutralization but is less widely used.
VIII. Viral isolation
A. Isolation of CDV is difficult in most tissue culture systems.
B. Primary cultivation of canine lymphocytes and macrophages provides the most successful viral replication.
C. CDV can be isolated from nasal or conjunctival swabs and from CSF of dogs with acute distemper encephalitis.

Differential Diagnosis

I. Respiratory diseases: infectious tracheobronchitis, bacterial pneumonia
II. Gastroenteritis: canine parvovirus-2 infection, bacterial infection
III. CNS diseases
A. Other causes of seizures
B. Other causes of encephalomyelitis: toxoplasmosis, neosporosis, rickettsial diseases, herpesvirus infection

Treatment

I. Supportive care
A. Keep animal in a clean, warm, draft-free environment; keep eyes and nose free of discharges.
B. Give broad-spectrum antibiotics for secondary infections; initial choices may include ampicillin, amoxicillin, and trimethoprim/sulfadiazine.
C. Discontinue food and water if vomiting and diarrhea are present.
D. Give polyionic isotonic fluids as needed for vomiting, diarrhea, and maintenance of hydration.
E. Inhalation therapy, bronchodilators, and mucolytics aid removal of exudate in respiratory passages.
F. If intestinal parasitism exists, specific treatment is indicated.
II. Management of CNS disturbances
A. Anticonvulsant drugs may help partially control seizures and are recommended at the start of systemic disease (prior to development of seizures).
B. Myoclonus is untreatable and irreversible.

C. Glucocorticoid therapy may help in cases of blindness caused by optic neuritis.

D. Despite ineffective therapy, dogs should not be euthanized unless the neurologic disturbances are progressive or incompatible with good quality of life.

Patient Monitoring and Prevention

I. Maternal immunity
   A. Vaccinate dam before breeding to increase level of maternal antibody. Do not administer attenuated live CDV vaccine to pregnant animals.
   B. Duration of maternal antibodies is 9–12 weeks in most puppies that received colostrum and only 1–2 weeks in colostrum-deprived puppies.

II. Immunization
   A. Vaccination may be effective in preventing systemic distemper if it is performed using attenuated products within 4 days of exposure.
   B. Active immunization is ineffective until there is a decrease in maternal antibodies.
      1. At least two vaccinations 3–4 weeks apart are required, with annual boosters recommended.
      2. Combined CDV and measles virus vaccine is sometimes used as the first vaccination for puppies in order to break through maternal antibodies against CDV.
         a) It should be followed by at least two CDV vaccines later in the series.
         b) It should be used in puppies 6–12 weeks of age because passive transfer of antibodies to measles virus can occur to offspring if the dog is bred on the first heat cycle (Brown, 1975).
   C. Postvaccinal complications and vaccine interference may occur.
      1. Encephalitis has been associated with the use of commercial, attenuated CDV vaccines.
      2. Attenuated CDV vaccines should not be given to animals with fever (>40°C; 104°F) or those debilitated or immunodeficient.
      3. Inactivated CDV vaccine can be used during pregnancy or immunosuppression, but duration of active immunity is uncertain.

INFECTIOUS CANINE HEPATITIS

Definition

Infectious canine hepatitis (ICH) is a multisystemic viral disease that primarily affects the liver of dogs and foxes.

Cause

I. Virus characteristics
   A. ICH is caused by canine adenovirus type 1 (CAV-1), a DNA virus. CAV-1 is closely related to canine adenovirus type 2 (CAV-2).
   B. CAV-1 is rapidly destroyed by heat (in 10 minutes at 56°C) and inactivated by ultraviolet light, most disinfectants, or organic iodides.

II. Epidemiology
   A. CAV-1 has been isolated from all body tissues and excretions.
   B. Dogs and foxes serve as reservoirs for CAV-1, which can be shed in urine for 6–9 months.
   C. CAV-1 is highly contagious and transmitted by contact with infected animals, contaminated fomites, and ectoparasites.

Pathophysiology

I. After oronasal exposure, CAV-1 localizes in the tonsils with subsequent viremia.

II. Cytologic injury primarily occurs to the liver, kidney, and eyes.

III. Antibody titer determines the outcome of CAV-1 infection.
   A. High titer clears CAV-1 from tissues.
   B. Low titer results in disseminated disease.
   C. Intermediate titer is associated with immune-complex disease.

IV. Ocular lesions are seen in 20% of naturally occurring cases and in <1% of dogs after attenuated CAV-1 vaccination (even more rarely after attenuated CAV-2 vaccination) (Mansfield, 1996).

Clinical Signs

Signs of naturally occurring ICH are seen exclusively in unvaccinated dogs <1 year of age.

I. Peracute disease
   A. Fever of 39.4–41.1°C (103–106°F) is usually present.
   B. Abdominal pain may be noted.
   C. Petechiae are seen in the mucous membranes.
   D. Progressive nervous system signs may develop, including seizures and coma.
   E. Dogs may be moribund or dead within hours after onset of signs.

II. Severe, nonfatal disease
   A. Depression, weakness, and disorientation are noted.
   B. Anorexia, some vomiting (hematemesis), and diarrhea may be present.
   C. A fever of 41.1°C (106°F) that is transient or biphasic may occur.
   D. Icterus may be noted.
   E. Lymphadenopathy occurs.

III. Mild clinical disease
   A. Signs are like those listed previously but milder.
   B. "Blue eye" from anterior uveitis occurs days to weeks later.

IV. Inapparent or subclinical disease
   A. Most naturally occurring cases have only pharyngitis or tonsillitis.
   B. Up to 40–50% of unvaccinated dogs are resistant to CAV-1 infection.

V. Chronic disease
   A. Cirrhosis and chronic inflammation of the liver

develop with ascites, hepatic encephalopathy, and weight loss.
   B. CAV-1 persists asymptomatically in the kidney for long periods.
VI. Complications
   A. Glaucoma may occur.
   B. Immune-complex glomerulonephritis is generally present.
   C. Disseminated intravascular coagulation (DIC) may develop (see Chap. 66).

Diagnosis

I. History: unvaccinated dogs <1 year of age
II. Compatible clinical signs
III. Hematologic findings
   A. Leukopenia and lymphopenia occur.
   B. Neutropenia occurs early in the disease; neutrophilia and lymphocytosis occur in recovering animals.
IV. Biochemical findings
   A. Increased serum alanine transaminase (ALT) and aspartate transaminase (AST) and alkaline phosphatase levels are noted.
   B. Bilirubinuria and proteinuria are detected.
   C. Increased bile acids occur.
   D. Hypoglycemia may be detected.
   E. Coagulation abnormalities suggestive of DIC occur.
V. Serology
   A. Serologic tests are available but are seldom performed.
   B. A fourfold rising titer is required to determine active infection.
VI. Viral isolation
   A. Cytopathologic effects and intranuclear inclusion bodies are noted in tissue cultures.
   B. Antemortem samples include oropharyngeal swabs, urine, and feces.
   C. Postmortem samples include liver, kidney, and tonsils.

Differential Diagnosis

I. Canine distemper
II. Leptospirosis
III. Certain poisons, especially anticoagulant rodenticides

Treatment

I. Supportive therapy may include broad-spectrum antibiotics and fluid therapy with polyionic isotonic fluids.
II. Treatment includes management of DIC and hepatic encephalopathic signs.
III. Corticosteroid therapy is indicated for immune-mediated ocular manifestations.

Patient Monitoring and Prevention

I. Maternal immunity
   A. Vaccinate dam before breeding to increase level of maternal antibody.

   B. Puppies acquire maternal antibodies via colostrum, but these antibodies decrease by 5–7 weeks of age.
II. Immunization
   A. Recovery from ICH, regardless of severity of illness, results in long-lasting immunity. The actual duration of immunity has not been established.
   B. Available vaccines for ICH protect dogs against both types of canine adenoviruses. CAV-2 vaccine protects dogs against itself and against ICH.
   C. Active immunization is ineffective until there is a decrease in maternal antibodies.
      1. At least two vaccinations 3–4 weeks apart are required, with annual boosters recommended.
      2. Attenuated CAV-2 vaccine is now preferred to attenuated CAV-1 vaccine, because it does not usually produce the ocular or renal disease associated with CAV-1 vaccines.

CANINE HERPESVIRUS INFECTION

Definition

Canine herpesvirus (CHV) primarily causes severe illness and death in puppies <3 weeks of age.

Cause

I. Virus characteristics
   A. CHV is an enveloped DNA virus that is species-specific.
   B. CHV is very labile and is rapidly inactivated by most disinfectants.
II. Epidemiology
   A. CHV has worldwide distribution and may be isolated from clinically normal adult dogs.
   B. CHV is transmitted by transplacental infection, during passage through the birth canal, or by direct contact with infected dogs or littermates.

Pathophysiology

I. Transplacental infection: abortion of stillborn or delivery of weak puppies
II. Systemic infection
   A. After oronasal exposure, CHV replicates in nasal and pharyngeal epithelium and tonsils.
   B. CHV dissemination to many tissues in hypothermic puppies causes multifocal hemorrhages and necrosis.
III. Adult genital infection
   A. It can occur in the presence of circulating antibody titers.
   B. It is usually asymptomatic but is an important means of venereal transmission.
IV. Resistance factors
   A. Older animals (>3 weeks of age) and normother-

mic neonates (99–100°F; 37.2–37.7°C) are relatively protected from systemic spread of CHV.
B. Maternal antibody may have a role in protection against systemic infection.

Clinical Signs

I. Pregnant dam aborts in last one third of gestation or gives birth to stillborn or weak puppies.
II. Signs noted in puppies from birth to 3 weeks of age include the following.
  A. Listlessness, weakness, and unwillingness to nurse
  B. Passage of bright yellow, fluid stools
  C. Persistent crying until exhausted, and evidence of abdominal pain on palpation
  D. Serous to mucopurulent or hemorrhagic nasal discharge, petechial hemorrhages on mucous membranes, and erythematous rash and subcutaneous edema of the ventral abdomen and inguinal region
  E. May lose consciousness, show opisthotonos or seizure, with subnormal rectal temperatures just before death
  F. Death within 24–48 hours after onset of clinical signs
  G. Persistent neurologic deficits of ataxia, blindness, cerebellar signs in recovered puppies
III. Older puppies (3–5 weeks of age) show mild respiratory signs with subsequent recovery.
IV. Adult dogs often exhibit the following signs.
  A. Mild, serous nasal discharge
  B. Genital infections
    1. Female dogs develop small areas of mucosal vesicles in the vagina and a slight serous discharge.
    2. Male dogs develop similar lesions over the base of the penis and preputial reflection and have a preputial discharge.
  C. Transient conjunctivitis of 4–6 days duration

Diagnosis

I. History: unvaccinated dogs <1 year of age
II. Compatible clinical signs
III. Hematologic findings
  A. Leukopenia and lymphopenia may be noted.
  B. Neutropenia occurs early in the disease; neutrophilia and lymphocytosis occur in recovering animals.
IV. Biochemical findings
  A. Increased serum ALT and AST and alkaline phosphatase levels
  B. Bilirubinuria and proteinuria
  C. Increased bile acids
  D. ± Hypoglycemia
  E. Coagulation abnormalities suggestive of DIC
V. Serology
  A. Serologic tests are available using routine methods.
  B. A fourfold rising titer is required to determine active infection.

VI. Viral isolation
  A. Cytopathologic effects and intranuclear inclusion bodies are noted in tissue cultures.
  B. Antemortem samples include oropharyngeal swabs, urine, and feces.
  C. Postmortem samples include liver, kidney, and tonsils.

Differential Diagnosis

I. Neonatal bacterial septicemia
II. Canine parvovirus type 1 infection
III. Canine brucellosis
IV. Malnutrition

Treatment

I. Institute supportive therapy with broad-spectrum antibiotics and polyionic isotonic fluids supplemented with 5% dextrose.
II. Maintain body temperature at 99–100°F (37.2–37.7°C).
III. One injection of 1–2 ml of hyperimmune serum may reduce the mortality in neonates.
IV. Provide adequate nutritional support by feeding appropriate amounts of milk replacers.

Patient Monitoring and Prevention

I. Vaccines are not currently available.
II. Keeping puppies warm and providing adequate nutrition for steady weight gain are especially important during the first 3 weeks of life.

CANINE PARVOVIRUS INFECTION

Definition

I. Canine parvovirus type 2 (CPV-2) is a virus of domestic dogs, bush dogs, coyotes, crab-eating foxes, maned wolves, and raccoons that causes a severe gastroenteritis in susceptible animals.
II. Canine parvovirus type 1 (CPV-1), previously called minute virus of canines or MVC, is widespread in dogs and is restricted to causing clinical disease in puppies <3 weeks of age (Harrison et al., 1992) (see Table 110–1).
III. The following discussion pertains to CPV-2 infection.

Cause

I. Virus characteristics
  A. CPVs, members of the family Parvoviridae, are small non-enveloped DNA viruses (Parrish et al., 1991).
    1. CPV-2 has an affinity for rapidly dividing cells.
    2. CPV-1 is serologically distinct from CPV-2 (Macartney et al., 1988).

B. Parvoviruses persist in the environment for long periods but can be inactivated by formalin, sodium hypochlorite (household bleach), and glutaraldehyde.

II. Epidemiology

A. CPV-2 is shed in the feces and may also be shed in the saliva and vomitus.

B. Contaminated fomites and mechanical vectors (insects and humans) are the primary sources.

C. CPV-2 persistence in the environment is more important in perpetuating the virus than are chronic carriers.

D. Dogs and other members of the Canidae family are primary reservoirs of CPV-2. Domestic cats are susceptible but show no clinical signs.

E. Most adults are immune from vaccination or previous infection, so the disease is now almost exclusively observed in puppies 6 weeks to 6 months of age.

F. Risk factors include type of breed, overcrowding, stress, and concurrent disease (Houston et al., 1996).

Pathophysiology

I. Intestinal disease

A. After oronasal exposure, CPV-2 replicates in lymphoid tissues of the oropharynx, mesenteric lymph nodes, and thymus, producing a viremia 2–4 days later.

B. CPV-2 then replicates in tissue with rapidly dividing cells, such as bone marrow, lymphopoietic tissue, and intestinal crypt epithelium.

C. The course and severity of infection depend on the strain of CPV-2 and type of breed affected.

II. Myocardial disease

A. Found in puppies <2 weeks of age because myocyte mitosis is rapid enough to support CPV-2 replication

B. Less prevalent now that maternal immunity is often passed to neonates

Clinical Signs

I. Intestinal disease

A. Depression, anorexia, vomiting, and lethargy

B. Fever of 40–41°C (104–106°F)

C. Gray or yellow-gray to blood-streaked or grossly bloody diarrhea and hematochezia

D. Dehydration and weight loss 24–48 hours after gastrointestinal signs begin

E. Death within 24–48 hours if the animal deteriorates rapidly

F. Recovery within 5–7 days of clinical presentation in uncomplicated cases

II. Myocardial disease

A. It occurs in dogs 3 weeks to 27 months old.

B. The dog is found dead with signs of congestive heart failure.

C. Although it is uncommon, mortality can be >50% of the litter.

Diagnosis

I. History: puppies 6 weeks to 6 months of age

II. Compatible clinical signs

III. Hematologic findings

A. Leukopenia is inconsistent but, when present, may be proportional to the severity of the disease.

B. Lymphopenia is more characteristic than neutropenia.

C. Leukocytosis may develop if the animal survives.

D. Abnormalities may not occur in dogs with myocardial disease.

IV. Biochemical and radiographic findings: nonspecific

V. Electrocardiographic findings

A. Abnormalities are sometimes detected in acute and chronic myocarditis.

B. However, death occurs so suddenly in acutely ill puppies that changes can be missed.

VI. Virus detection

A. It is the most specific means of confirming CPV-2 infection.

B. It is limited to a period of 3–12 days during clinical illness.

C. Methods include electron microscopy, fecal hemagglutination, virus isolation, or fecal ELISA assay.

VII. Serologic testing

A. It is used to make a diagnosis and to evaluate the animal's immune status after vaccination.

B. A single high IgM titer or a fourfold elevation in IgG titer is required to diagnose active infection.

C. Methods include hemagglutination-inhibition, virus neutralization, and ELISA assays.

Differential Diagnosis

I. Salmonellosis

II. Campylobacteriosis

III. Canine coronavirus infection

IV. Canine distemper

V. Other enteric viruses (Table 110–1)

Treatment

I. Discontinue ingestion of foods and liquids if vomiting is present.

II. Provide supportive therapy with broad-spectrum antibiotics and IV polyionic isotonic fluids supplemented with potassium chloride (with or without 5% dextrose).

III. Hyperimmune serum or plasma transfusion may reduce the mortality and can be helpful for dogs with hypoalbuminemia.

IV. Antiemetic drugs (e.g., chlorpromazine 0.5 mg/kg IM TID or 0.05 mg/kg IV TID; metoclopramide 0.2–0.4 mg/kg SQ TID or 0.01–0.02 mg/kg/h continuous IV infusion; or prochlorperazine 0.1 mg/kg IM TID-QID) are used if vomiting is persistent and uncontrollable.

V. Adjunctive therapy may also include administration of recombinant human granulocyte colony-stimulat-

Table 110–1. Other Enteric Viruses of Dogs and Cats

Affected Species	Virus	Significance	Clinical Signs	Diagnosis
Dog	Canine parvovirus type 1 (CPV-1) (Harrison et al., 1992)	Isolated in clinically healthy dogs; clinical disease in puppies birth to 21 days old; fecal spread similar to CPV-2	Mild diarrhea in adults; puppies usually present with diarrhea, vomiting, dyspnea, and constant crying; sudden death may be only sign	Virus isolation, virus neutralization, hemagglutination-inhibition
Dog	Rotaviruses (England and Poston, 1980; Johnson et al., 1983)	Adults dogs infected; problem in young (<12 week old) puppies	Mucoid to watery diarrhea	Virus isolation, ELISA, electron microscopy
Dog	Herpesvirus (Evermann et al., 1982)	Related to feline rhinotracheitis virus	Diarrhea, vomiting	Not available or impractical
Dog	Calicivirus (Evermann et al., 1985; Schaffer et al., 1985)	Isolated from feces of dogs with enteritis, sometimes alone and sometimes with other enteric pathogens	Bloody diarrhea, vomiting, anorexia	Not available or impractical
Dog	Astrovirus	Isolated from stools of clinically healthy and diarrheic dogs	Diarrhea	Not available or impractical
Cat	Feline enteric coronavirus	Severity is age-related	Mild and transient diarrhea; leukopenia in severe cases	Not available or impractical
Cat	Feline astrovirus	Transmission probably by direct contact	Persistent, green watery diarrhea; vomiting and dehydration; fever; gas-distended loops of small intestines	Electron microscopy

ing factor (G-CSF) (Rewerts et al., 1996) and antiendotoxin hyperimmune plasma (Dimmitt, 1991).

VI. If intestinal parasitism coexists, specific treatment is indicated.

VII. Provide adequate nutritional and water support 24–48 hours after cessation of the vomiting and reduction of diarrhea.

Patient Monitoring

I. Animals with septic shock and hemorrhagic diarrhea have a much poorer prognosis.

II. Animals surviving intestinal disease are fed small portions of highly digestible, low-fiber, moderately low-fat diet (cooked rice or cereal supplemented in a 4:1 ratio with low-fat cottage cheese, boiled lean ground beef, chicken, or commercial baby food) 3–6 times daily.
   A. Commercial diets specifically formulated for acute gastrointestinal disease may also be prescribed.
   B. Over several days, the amount of homemade or commercial food fed is gradually increased to meet the animal's needs.

III. Because the myocardial disease is progressive, prognosis is poor. Although therapy for heart failure may help, it is usually frustrating to manage.

IV. Recovery time is usually 3–10 days or longer depending on severity of the illness. Some animals have persistent or intermittent diarrhea for weeks thereafter.

Prevention

I. Maternal immunity
   A. Maternal antibodies may be too low to protect against infection but may still be able to suppress the puppy's response to vaccination.
   B. Puppies become susceptible to virulent CPV-2 as early as 6–12 weeks but in some cases may not respond to vaccination for up to 16 weeks of age.

II. Passive immunity
   A. Immediate plasma administration to colostrum-deprived puppies may provide antibody protection until they are 5–6 weeks of age, at which time they can be vaccinated.
   B. Puppies are then vaccinated at 3–4 week intervals until they are 16 weeks of age.

III. Immunization
   A. Inactivated CPV-2 products may be used.
      1. Can be used safely in pregnant animals
      2. Vaccine virus not shed in the feces
      3. Do not prevent shedding of virulent virus
      4. Produce short-lived immunity
   B. Attenuated CPV-2 products are available.
      1. Not to be used in pregnant animals
      2. Prevent shedding of virulent virus
      3. Transient lymphopenia 4–6 days after administration
      4. Replicate in intestinal tract and briefly shed in feces

C. Attenuated CPV-2 vaccine from a highly immunogenic strain produced at high titer is now preferred to attenuated CPV-2 vaccine produced at low titer or to the inactivated CPV-2 products (Schultz et al., 1995).
      1. It actively immunizes puppies with low to moderate levels of maternal or passive immunity (Greenwood et al., 1995).
      2. Vaccinate with a high-titer attenuated CPV-2 vaccine at 6, 9, 12, and possibly 15 weeks of age, and then revaccinate annually, especially high-risk breeds such as the rottweiler.
      3. Checking serologic titers for CPV-2 after vaccination at 15–20 weeks of age is recommended.

IV. Environmental control
   A. Isolate acutely ill animals.
   B. Disinfect contaminated areas and utensils, and properly dispose of infected feces.

CANINE CORONAVIRUS INFECTION

Definition

Canine coronavirus (CCV) is a cause of gastroenteritis in most Canidae.

Cause

I. Virus characteristics
   A. CCV, an enveloped RNA virus, is a member of Coronaviridae.
   B. CCV is fairly resistant and remains infectious for long periods during winter months. CCV is inactivated by most commercial detergents and disinfectants.

II. Epidemiology
   A. CCV is host-specific and is shed in the feces.
   B. CCV is highly contagious and spreads rapidly through groups of susceptible dogs.
   C. Neonates are more severely affected than puppies of weaning age or adults.
   D. Immunity to CCV is short-lived.
   E. Risk factors include overcrowding, stress, and concurrent disease (Tennant et al., 1993).

Pathophysiology

I. Following its ingestion, CCV infects the mature epithelial cells of the villi of the small intestine (Tennant et al., 1991).

II. After uptake by the epithelial cell, it rapidly replicates in the cell within cytoplasmic vacuoles.

III. CCV is shed in the feces of infected dogs for 3–14 days after initial infection.

IV. Other enteric microflora such as *Clostridium perfringens*, *Campylobacter* spp., and *Salmonella* spp. may increase the severity of a CCV infection.

Clinical Signs

I. Signs vary from inapparent to rapidly fatal gastroenteritis.

II. It is difficult to distinguish from other causes of gastroenteritis.

III. Depression, anorexia, vomiting, and lethargy are common. Fever is not constant.

IV. Yellow-green to orange and malodorous diarrhea begins simultaneously with vomiting and persists or is intermittent for up to 3–4 weeks. There may be variable amounts of mucus or blood.

V. Recovery is noted within 8–10 days.

Diagnosis

I. History: any age affected, but puppies 6 weeks to 6 months of age more severely affected

II. Compatible clinical signs

III. No specific hematologic or biochemical findings

IV. Rarely leukopenia

V. Serologic testing

A. A single high IgG titer indicates exposure only.

B. A fourfold rising IgG titer confirms infection.

VI. Virus identification includes detection via electron microscopy, growth in tissue culture, or detection via immunofluorescence assay.

Differential Diagnosis

I. Salmonellosis

II. Campylobacteriosis

III. Canine parvovirus infection

IV. Canine distemper

V. Giardiasis or other endoparasitism

Treatment

See Canine Parvovirus Infection, earlier.

Patient Monitoring and Prevention

I. CCV vaccines (inactivated and attenuated live virus cell line origin) are presently available. Two doses 3–4 weeks apart and annual revaccination are recommended (Pardo and Mackowiak, 1995).

II. It is difficult to assess the role of CCV vaccines in protection against disease because CCV infections are usually inapparent.

III. Strict isolation of affected animals and sanitation within the kennel are needed.

FELINE PANLEUKOPENIA

Definition

Feline panleukopenia, also called feline infectious enteritis and feline distemper, is a disease of domestic cats that causes a severe gastroenteritis in susceptible animals.

Cause

I. Virus characteristics

A. Feline panleukopenia virus (FPV) is a parvovirus.

B. Parvoviruses persist in the environment for long periods but can be inactivated by formalin, sodium hypochlorite (household bleach), and glutaraldehyde.

II. Epidemiology

A. FPV causes disease in members of the family Felidae and in other animals such as the raccoon, ferret, coati, ringtail cat, and mink.

B. FPV is transmitted directly from infected animals and their secretions, especially feces.

C. Fomites are important because of the environmental persistence of FPV.

D. The highest incidence of feline panleukopenia occurs in kittens 3–5 months of age.

Pathophysiology

I. Requires rapidly multiplying cells

A. Lymphoid tissue, bone marrow, and intestinal mucosal crypts are most affected.

B. Neonatal or prenatal infections can result in ocular and CNS lesions.

II. Transplacental infection: early fetal death, resorption, or abortion

III. Systemic infection: severity of lesions increased by intestinal bacteria

IV. CNS infection: damage to the cerebellum, optic nerve, and retina during prenatal or early neonatal development

Clinical Signs

I. Fever of 40–41°C (104–106°F) is common.

II. Depression and anorexia may be seen.

III. Bile-tinged vomiting, unrelated to eating, and dehydration are noted.

IV. Diarrhea, when present, occurs later in the course of the disease.

V. Small intestines have a "rope-like" consistency and may be painful on palpation.

VI. Mesenteric lymphadenopathy can occur.

VII. Death can follow if signs are severe and complicated by secondary infections.

VIII. Pregnant queens may show infertility, abortion, or birth of dead or mummified fetuses.

IX. Kittens may show signs of cerebellar ataxia.

X. Prenatally infected kittens may have retinal dysplasia, folding, or streaking.

Diagnosis

I. History: kittens 3–5 months of age

II. Compatible clinical signs

III. Hematologic and biochemical findings

A. Initially, leukopenia develops, but white blood cell (WBC) numbers rebound within 24–48 hours.

B. Neutropenia is more common than lymphopenia.

C. Marked anemia is uncommon unless there is severe intestinal blood loss.

D. Mild to moderate increases in serum ALT and AST or bilirubin levels reflect hepatic involvement.

E. Azotemia may be present from prerenal or nonrenal causes.

IV. Serologic testing: available but rarely used in practice

V. Virus detection

A. Samples most commonly examined include feces, intestine, mesenteric lymph nodes, lung, and pharyngeal swabs.

B. Canine fecal ELISA assays for CPV-2 antigen can be used, but infected cats infrequently shed virus and only in small amounts.

C. Positive canine fecal ELISA assay is helpful.

Differential Diagnosis

I. Salmonellosis

II. Campylobacteriosis

III. Feline coronavirus infection

IV. Feline leukemia virus infection

Treatment

I. Withhold food and water when vomiting is present.

II. Provide supportive therapy with broad-spectrum antibiotics and IV polyionic isotonic fluids supplemented with potassium chloride.

III. Whole blood transfusion may be needed to correct the anemia.

IV. Antiemetic drugs (e.g., metoclopramide 0.3 mg/kg SQ TID or 0.01 mg/kg/h continuous IV infusion) are used if vomiting is persistent.

V. If intestinal parasitism coexists, specific treatment is indicated.

VI. Institute adequate nutritional and water support 24–48 hours after cessation of the vomiting and reduction of diarrhea.

Patient Monitoring

I. Recheck hemogram for a resurgence of leukopoiesis within 24–48 hours.

II. Resume feeding small portions of highly digestible, low-fiber, moderately low-fat diet (cooked rice or cereal supplemented in a 4:1 ratio with low-fat cottage cheese, boiled lean ground beef, chicken, or commercial baby food) 3–6 times daily.

A. Commercial diets specifically formulated for acute gastrointestinal disease may also be prescribed.

B. Over several days, the amount of homemade or commercial food fed is gradually increased to meet the animal's needs.

III. Recovery usually occurs within 3–5 days, but some animals have persistent or intermittent diarrhea for weeks thereafter.

Prevention

I. Maternal immunity

A. Maternal antibodies are received via colostrum and last 8–14 weeks.

B. Successful vaccination can be achieved in 12 week old kittens.

II. Passive immunity

A. Immediate plasma administration to colostrum-deprived kittens may provide antibody protection for 2–4 weeks, at which time they can be vaccinated.

B. Kittens are then vaccinated at 3-week intervals until they are 12 weeks of age.

III. Immunization

A. Inactivated FPV products

1. They can be used safely in pregnant animals, in kittens ≤4 weeks of age, or in debilitated cats.

2. Minimum of two doses is needed to achieve the same protection as one dose of attenuated FPV vaccine.

B. Attenuated FPV products

1. They are not to be used in pregnant cats or kittens ≤4 weeks of age.

2. They prevent shedding of virulent virus.

3. Because of the breakthrough of maternal antibody, it is recommended that at least one or more doses be given 3 weeks apart.

4. One attenuated or two inactivated doses probably confer lifelong immunity; however, annual vaccination is recommended to produce an anamnestic response.

FELINE CORONAVIRUS INFECTION

Definition

Feline coronavirus infection, also called feline infectious peritonitis (FIP), is a highly fatal viral disease of cats that has two primary forms: effusive and noneffusive.

Cause

I. Virus characteristics

A. Feline coronavirus, the preferred term, is often referred to as FIP virus.

B. Feline coronavirus is an enveloped RNA virus related to feline enteric coronavirus (FECV); it has numerous strains that vary in virulence.

C. Feline coronaviruses are labile and readily inactivated by disinfectants.

II. Epidemiology

A. The highest prevalence of disease occurs in cats <2 years of age.

B. Feline coronavirus is spread by contaminated feces; fomites may also play a role.

C. Feline leukemia virus (FeLV) and feline immunodeficiency virus (FIV) act as potentiators of feline coronavirus infection.

III. Forms of the disease
   A. The effusive (wet) form is characterized by peritoneal and/or pleural effusion.
   B. The noneffusive (dry) form is characterized by localized pyogranulomatous lesions with no or limited peritoneal and/or pleural effusion.

Pathophysiology

I. General features
   A. Ingestion and inhalation are the most common routes of infection, but in utero infection is possible.
   B. Unlike FECV, feline coronavirus enters the systemic circulation after intestinal replication; macrophages are the primary target cells.
   C. Deposits of immune complexes (virus-antibody-complement) localize in the walls of small blood vessels and produce vasculitis, with escape of fibrin-rich serum into intercellular spaces.
   D. Cats with strong cell-mediated immunity eliminate the infection and recover, or show no clinical illness.
II. Effusive lesions
   A. Lesions develop as a result of a disseminated vasculitis.
   B. Cell-mediated immunity is ineffective, and increased humoral antibody response is unable to eliminate the virus.
   C. Humoral antibody response may be harmful in that it reacts with virus and complement, producing an Arthus-like reaction.
III. Noneffusive lesions
   A. Lesions develop in cats with partial cell-mediated immunity.
   B. Pyogranulomatous reactions occur at isolated foci of persistent virus.

Clinical Signs

I. General signs
   A. Onset of signs may be sudden or slow over weeks to months.
   B. Early signs are nonspecific of anorexia, weight loss, depression, and dehydration.
   C. Fevers of 39.5–40.6°C (103.1–105.1°F) are antibiotic-resistant and wax and wane.
II. Effusive form
   A. Fever may be present.
   B. Ascites typically is present.
   C. Tachypnea or dyspnea, muffled heart sounds, and/or pale mucous membrane may be additional observations.
III. Noneffusive form
   A. Onset of signs is insidious.
   B. Fever and weight loss are common.
   C. Signs reflect the specific organ that is involved.
      1. Abdominal organs (kidneys, lymph nodes, peritoneum and omentum, liver) are the most common sites affected.
      2. CNS signs can be of any type, depending on the sites affected.
      3. Ocular lesions include pyogranulomatous uveitis, hyphema, retinal hemorrhages, perivasculitis, or focal chorioretinitis.

Diagnosis

I. History: cats younger than 2 years of age
II. Compatible clinical signs
III. Hematologic and biochemical findings
   A. Leukocyte count may be variable, but usually there is neutrophilia, eosinophilia, and lymphopenia.
   B. Anemia (mild to moderate normocytic, normochromic) may occur from hematopoietic suppression associated with chronic illness and/or other concurrent infections.
   C. Serum protein is often increased (>7.8 g/dl).
   D. Levels of liver enzymes and total bilirubin may also be increased.
   E. Azotemia may be present when kidney involvement occurs.
   F. Hyperfibrinogenemia and DIC may result.
IV. Evaluation of effusive fluid
   A. Typically, the fluid is light to dark yellow with sticky honey-like consistency.
   B. Protein content is usually ≥5–12 g/dl.
   C. The fluid often clots on standing and with exposure to room air.
   D. It is highly cellular, with 1600–25,000 WBCs/μl (primarily neutrophils) expected.
V. CSF findings
   A. CSF is normal if lesions are focal or localized to subependymal areas.
   B. CSF may show increased protein (≥90–2000 mg/dl) and cells, especially with extensive meningeal involvement.
VI. Serologic testing
   A. Because currently available antibody tests lack specificity, they are unable to distinguish antibody titers from effusive or noneffusive disease from those of feline enteric coronavirus infections.
   B. The indirect fluorescent antibody test and ELISA assays are the most popular.
   C. Titers vary among laboratories.
      1. A single positive titer (>1:1600) or a fourfold rise in antibody titer over at least a 2-week period along with a careful review of clinical and clinicopathologic information can be helpful in making a diagnosis.
      2. A single negative titer does not rule out coronavirus-related disease.
VII. Polymerase chain reaction (PCR) findings
   A. PCR techniques can detect extremely low levels of viral RNA in tissue and various body fluids.
   B. Specificity of PCRs for feline coronavirus diagnosis is based on the following assumptions.
      1. That feline infectious peritonitis (FIPV) is found within tissue, whereas FECV is found only in feces
      2. That it is possible to differentiate feline coronavirus strains from FECV based on the ge-

nomic maps of known strains of FECV (FECV-79-1683) and the feline coronaviruses
C. Feline coronavirus genome is detected by PCR in the blood of many healthy cats in endemic households.

Differential Diagnosis

I. Toxoplasmosis
II. FeLV infection
III. FIV infection
IV. Other causes of abdominal/pleural effusion
V. Other causes of ocular lesions

Treatment and Monitoring

I. There is no curative therapy once clinical signs of effusion or organ involvement are evident.
II. Treatment is supportive.
   A. It is most successful when used on cats that are still eating and have not lost much weight.
   B. Treatment provides short-term remissions.
   C. Administer prednisolone (4 mg/kg PO SID) alone or in combination with cyclophosphamide (2 mg/kg PO SID). Monitor for bone marrow suppression, kidney dysfunction, and serum potassium abnormalities.
   D. Manage ocular and neurologic signs, when present.
III. Prognosis is guarded.
   A. Survival time is variable but is usually 5–7 weeks from onset of clinical signs.
   B. The noneffusive form has a more protracted clinical course than the effusive form.
   C. Ocular signs alone carry the best long-term prognosis.

Prevention

I. A safe intranasal vaccine is presently available.
   A. It increases secretory and cell-mediated immune responses, thereby reducing the ability of the virus to enter the body and persistently infect cells.
   B. At least two vaccinations are needed and are given 3–4 weeks apart with yearly boosters thereafter.
   C. Protection afforded is not 100% but may reduce the risk of infection after exposure.
   D. The vaccine is recommended primarily for use in catteries, shelters, and multi-cat households, where the disease is more likely to exist.
II. Proper litter and fecal management helps reduce contaminated fecal exposure.
III. Testing and elimination of carrier animals can be difficult because of ambiguity of serologic and PCR results.

FELINE LEUKEMIA VIRUS (FeLV) INFECTION

Definition

FeLV causes spontaneous neoplasia and suppresses the bone marrow and immune systems of primarily domestic cats.

Cause

I. Virus characteristics
   A. FeLV is a retrovirus that replicates in cells of the bone marrow, salivary glands, and respiratory epithelium.
   B. FeLV is not cytopathic and buds from the cell membrane of infected cells.
   C. There are three viral subgroups: A, B, and C.
   D. Feline oncornavirus cell membrane antigen (FOCMA) antibody is involved in immunity to tumor development.
II. Epidemiology
   A. FeLV is transmitted directly, primarily by ingesting virus in saliva.
   B. Close, prolonged direct contact is required for the spread of FeLV.
   C. FeLV is susceptible to most disinfectants, soaps, heating, and drying.

Pathophysiology

I. Sequential findings
   A. Most cats are exposed to FeLV early in life.
   B. After ingestion, FeLV initially infects lymphoid tissue of the nasopharynx.
   C. With inadequate immune response, FeLV spreads to the bone marrow, infecting hematopoietic precursor cells.
   D. Some cats that do not completely eliminate FeLV may harbor it in a latent form in bone marrow cells and possibly in mammary gland and CNS cells.
   E. With stress or immunosuppression, latent FeLV may reactivate.
   F. A partial immune response (before FeLV suppresses the bone marrow) allows some cats to become immune carriers and a source of infection for other cats.
II. Environmental influences
   A. Crowding and stress increase the risk of infection in exposed, uninfected kittens.
   B. Persistent FeLV-infected cats have a much higher risk of death associated with lymphosarcoma development or non-neoplastic immunosuppressive disorders.
   C. Cats in multi-cat households have a higher prevalence of FOCMA antibody titer, indicating FeLV-induced cell transformation.
   D. Certain strains of FeLV may be defective and require a helper virus, such as feline sarcoma virus, to replicate.

Clinical Signs

I. Neoplastic diseases
   A. Lymphosarcoma occurs most often.
   B. Leukemias and myeloproliferative disease may also occur.
   C. Fibrosarcoma (combination FeLV and feline sarcoma virus infection) rarely occurs.
II. Bone marrow suppression
   A. Secondary nonregenerative anemia may be present.
   B. Leukocyte count is usually normal, but granulocytopenia and lymphopenia may be present, especially in recently infected cats.
   C. Bone marrow is usually normocellular but may be hypocellular.
III. Other disorders
   A. Glomerulonephritis with nephrotic syndrome
   B. Reproductive disorders: infertility and abortion with bacterial endometritis
   C. Lymphadenopathy, especially of submandibular lymph nodes
   D. Osteochondromas and osteopetrosis
   E. Urinary incontinence
   F. Immunosuppression with secondary bacterial, viral, protozoal, fungal, or rickettsial infections

Diagnosis

I. History: usually young cats
II. ± Compatible clinical signs
III. Serologic testing
   A. Indirect fluorescent antibody (IFA) is a definitive test.
      1. It measures presence of viral core antigen.
      2. It is not diagnostic of leukemia, lymphosarcoma, or any disease, but it shows that the cat is viremic.
   B. ELISA is a screening test.
      1. It measures presence of viral core antigen.
      2. It is not diagnostic of leukemia, lymphosarcoma, or any disease, but it shows that the cat is viremic.
      3. It is more sensitive than IFA and detects lower levels of antigen than IFA.
IV. Detection of lymphosarcoma

Differential Diagnosis

I. Other causes of anemia such as hemobartonellosis, immune-mediated hemolytic anemia
II. Panleukopenia and panleukopenia-like syndromes
III. Feline immunodeficiency virus infection

Treatment

I. Myelosuppressive diseases
   A. Blood transfusions may be given for nonregenerative anemias.
   B. Oxymetholone (1–5 mg/kg PO SID) or other testosterone derivatives may be tried, but their efficacy is unproven.
   C. Glucocorticoids increase the life span and production of red blood cells and are useful if thrombocytopenia is present.
   D. Therapy with oral low-dose human recombinant interferon (1 U/day) improves the quality of life of some cats.
II. Lymphosarcoma: see Chap. 67
III. Lymphocytic leukemia: see Chap. 64
IV. Myeloproliferative diseases: see Chap. 65
V. Management of the FeLV-infected cat
   A. Keep indoors to protect it from contact with other sources of infections such as respiratory viruses and bite wounds.
   B. Keep other vaccinations current.
      1. Attenuated panleukopenia, upper respiratory, and feline infectious peritonitis vaccines can be used safely.
      2. Use inactivated rabies vaccine because of risk of vaccine-induced disease in the immunosuppressed cat.
   C. Monitor closely for onset of systemic illnesses.

Patient Monitoring and Prevention

I. Test and elimination program
II. Immunization
   A. Inactivated and recombinant FeLV vaccines are available.
   B. At least two vaccinations are needed, given 3 weeks apart, with yearly boosters thereafter.
   C. Protection afforded is not 100% but may reduce the risk of infection after exposure.
   D. Cats do not test positive for viral core antigen from the vaccine with IFA or ELISA tests.
   E. Because vaccination has little benefit in FeLV-infected cats, they should be tested at 1–3 months and vaccinated only if they are not infected.

FELINE IMMUNODEFICIENCY VIRUS (FIV) INFECTION

Definition

FIV is associated with acquired immunodeficiency states primarily in domestic cats.

Cause

I. Virus characteristics
   A. FIV is a lentivirus that is isolated from peripheral blood leukocytes.
   B. FIV causes clinical disease in cats that is similar to acquired immunodeficiency syndrome (AIDS) in people.
II. Epidemiology
   A. Primary mode of transmission is via a bite wound. Free-roaming male cats are approximately three times more likely to be infected with FIV as female cats.
   B. FIV can be isolated from serum, plasma, saliva,

and CSF. The ease of recovery of FIV from cells and fluids correlates with the stage of infection.

  C. Placental or colostral transmission of FIV from a queen to her offspring occurs infrequently.

  D. FIV is not directly associated with FeLV infection; combination FeLV and FIV infections are uncommon.

Pathophysiology

  I. Following the initial exposure, FIV appears in regional lymph nodes, where it replicates in T lymphocytes. Generalized lymphadenopathy then occurs in 3–7 weeks.

  II. An asymptomatic stage, which develops within 7 months, is dependent on environmental, nutritional, immunologic, and genetic factors.

  III. Secondary pathogens may play a facilitative role in the development of FIV infection and clinical disease.

Clinical Signs

  I. Acute stage
    A. Lymphadenopathy, fever, and malaise are typically present.
    B. Diarrhea or signs of anemia may develop.

  II. Latent stage
    A. It follows resolution of the acute stage.
    B. Mild lymphadenopathy is usually present.
    C. Duration of the latent period is unknown.

  III. Chronic stage
    A. Stomatitis, gingivitis, and periodontitis: hallmark signs
    B. Chronic nonresponsive diarrhea
    C. Persistent upper respiratory infections
    D. Wasting and fevers of unknown origin
    E. Neurologic signs such as behavioral changes, psychotic behavior, dementia, facial twitching movements, and/or seizures
    F. Increased susceptibility to opportunistic infections

Diagnosis

  I. History: cats usually 5 years of age or older
  II. Compatible clinical signs
  III. Hematologic findings: neutropenia, often with severe leukopenia and anemia
  IV. Serologic testing
    A. Antibody detection using IFA, ELISA, or Western blot techniques can be performed at diagnostic laboratory facilities.
    B. ELISA can be performed using in-hospital test kits.
  V. Virus isolation and PCR techniques
    A. FIV isolated from leukocytes of a suspect cat can be co-cultivated in cell culture.
    B. PCR techniques are used as a research tool but are not available yet as a clinical diagnostic test.

Differential Diagnosis

  I. Other causes of anemia, leukopenia, or immunosuppression
  II. FeLV infection and associated diseases

Treatment and Prevention

  I. There is no curative therapy for FIV.
  II. Treatment is usually directed at control of secondary bacterial infections.
  III. Therapy with azidothymidine (AZT) (5 mg/kg PO, SQ BID) reduces virus replication and often improves the quality of life of FIV-infected cats (Hartmann et al., 1995).
  IV. There is no vaccine currently available.

FELINE SYNCYTIUM-FORMING VIRUS (FeSFV) INFECTION

Definition

FeSFV causes a progressive polyarthritis in infected cats.

Cause

  I. Virus characteristics: retrovirus that produces a multinucleated syncytium in rapidly growing cell cultures
  II. Epidemiology
    A. FeSFV spreads primarily by bite wounds.
    B. Free-roaming and outdoor cats are at greater risk than indoor cats.
    C. Transplacental transmission can occur.

Pathophysiology

  I. Most cats infected with FeSFV do not exhibit clinical disease.
  II. Most infected cats also have FeLV or FIV infections.
  III. Arthritis probably results from chronic antigenic stimulation and immune-complex deposition.
  IV. Cats are infected for life and develop persistent nonprotective antibody titers to FeSFV.

Clinical Signs

  I. Asymptomatic
  II. Chronic progressive polyarthritis, especially in male cats 1.5–5 years of age
    A. Swollen joints and stiff gait
    B. Peripheral lymphadenopathy

Diagnosis

  I. Joint fluid abnormalities include increased numbers of neutrophils and large mononuclear cells.
  II. Serologic testing for antibody involves agar gel immunodiffusion and IFA techniques.
  III. Culture of buffy coat cells from peripheral blood of kittens may be done for detection of FeSFV.

Differential Diagnosis

Rule out other forms of arthritis (see Chap. 78).

Treatment and Prevention

I. There is no known cure for FeSFV infection, but infections may be temporarily responsive to immunosuppressive therapy.

II. Infected cats should be identified and eliminated, especially in a cattery.

RABIES

Definition

Rabies is an acute viral encephalitis characterized by altered behavior, aggressiveness, progressive paralysis, and death in all warm-blooded animals.

Cause

I. Virus characteristics
   A. Rabies virus is an enveloped, bullet-shaped rhabdovirus that has worldwide distribution.
   B. Diagnostic antigenic differences occur in the various isolates from wildlife hosts.
   C. Rabies virus is labile and readily inactivated by sunlight, heat, and most disinfectants but remains viable in a carcass at room or refrigerated temperatures for 24–48 hours.

II. Epidemiology
   A. Transmission usually occurs via the bite of an infected animal or less commonly via other body excreta.
   B. A few animals have survived clinical rabies, and serologic evidence of infection without clinical disease has been found in bats, foxes, raccoons, cats, and dogs.
   C. Rabies has become an increasing problem in wildlife reservoirs (fox, skunk, raccoon, bobcat, coyote, bat, mongoose, and other small carnivorous mammals).
      1. Transport of infected wildlife into new areas has been initially responsible for this increase.
      2. Urbanization of rural areas has also increased the risk of exposure to rabid animals.
   D. Rabies occurs in cats more frequently than in dogs.

Pathophysiology

I. Incubation is variable, depending on the site of the bite, amount of virus introduced, strain of virus, and the species and age of animal bitten, but it is believed to range from 3 weeks to ≥6 months.

II. After muscle penetration, the virus enters terminal axons, ascends the peripheral nerve, and spreads in the CNS.

III. After replication in the CNS, the virus moves into other body tissues via peripheral sensory and motor nerves.

Clinical Signs

I. Prodromal stage
   A. It usually lasts 2–3 days and sometimes only a few hours.
   B. Changes in behavior and temperament occur, such as restlessness, snapping at imaginary objects, or vocalization at the slightest provocation.
   C. Mydriasis and/or sluggish palpebral or corneal reflexes may be noted.
   D. Slight rise in body temperature is recorded.

II. Furious stage
   A. It usually lasts 1–7 days.
   B. There is an increased response to auditory and visual stimulation including restlessness, photophobia, hyperesthesia, eating unusual objects, aggression, and/or attacking any live or inanimate objects.
   C. Self-mutilation may be present.
   D. Muscular incoordination and seizures occur.

III. Paralytic (dumb) stage
   A. It develops 2–10 days after clinical signs and usually last 2–4 days.
   B. It may begin at the bite area and progress until the entire CNS is involved.
   C. Change in tone of vocalization, dysphagia, protrusion of third eyelids, pupil dilation, or pupil constriction may occur.
   D. "Jaw drop" and excessive salivation may be noted.
   E. Following paralysis of the head and neck, the entire body becomes paralyzed.
   F. Coma and/or respiratory paralysis resulting in death follows within 2–4 days.

Diagnosis

I. History
II. Compatible clinical signs
III. Hematologic and biochemical findings: minimal or no specific changes in hemogram, serum, or CSF biochemistries
IV. Direct immunofluorescence
   A. It detects rabies virus antigen in fresh (preferred) or paraffin-embedded tissue.
   B. Nervous tissue is preferred, but skin at the nape of the neck or sensory vibrissae from the maxillary areas have also been used.
   C. It becomes positive rapidly and before clinical signs appear.
   D. It is widely available in diagnostic laboratory facilities and is currently the diagnostic test of choice.
V. Direct immunoperoxidase method: available in some laboratories
VI. Intracellular inclusions (Negri bodies)
   A. When present, they are found in the CNS, but they are usually not detected until neurologic signs are apparent.
   B. They are not commonly found in cats and resemble inclusions of other viral diseases.

VII. Monoclonal antibody
  A. It helps to distinguish the actual source of rabies virus (originating animal).
  B. It can differentiate between vaccine and virulent strains of rabies virus.

Differential Diagnosis

  I. Dogs: canine distemper, polyradiculoneuritis, certain toxicoses, and pseudorabies
  II. Cats: feline coronavirus infection, FIV and FeLV infection, toxoplasmosis, certain toxicoses, and pseudorabies

Treatment

Because of the threat to the public, rabies-infected animals should be euthanized.

Prevention

  I. Vaccination is the best way to control rabies in the pet animal population. Inactivated products are the only type available.
  II. Annual recommendations concerning current acceptable vaccine products are made by the National Association of State and Public Health Veterinarians.
  III. Postexposure advice is as follows.
    A. Any cat or dog that is bitten or scratched by a bat or carnivorous (wild or domestic) animal that is not available for testing should be regarded as having been exposed to rabies.
    B. When bitten by a rabid animal, unvaccinated dogs and cats should undergo one of the following options.
      1. It is destroyed immediately.
      2. It is quarantined in strict isolation for 6 months at the owner's risk and vaccinated 1 month before its release.
    C. Vaccinated dogs and cats (when bitten) are revaccinated immediately and closely observed for 90 days.

PSEUDORABIES

Definition

Pseudorabies, primarily a disease of swine, affects the CNS of dogs and cats.

Cause

  I. Virus characteristics
    A. Pseudorabies virus (PRV) is an enveloped DNA virus that belongs to the herpesvirus group.
    B. PRV is stable in the environment.
  II. Epidemiology
    A. Pigs, the primary reservoir of PRV, usually have subclinical infection.
    B. PRV in dogs and cats occurs worldwide, especially in areas where the disease is endemic in pigs.

Pathophysiology

  I. After ingestion, PRV enters nerve endings and travels through the nerves to the brain.
  II. Nervous tissue injury is caused by inflammatory changes and direct neuronal injury associated with viral replication.

Clinical Signs

  I. Sudden change in behavior
  II. Dyspnea, diarrhea, vomiting, and/or hypersalivation
  III. Intense pruritus that usually occurs on the head, limbs, and sometimes neck and shoulders
  IV. Self-mutilation resulting in erythema and ulcerative skin lesions
  V. Cranial nerve deficits including anisocoria, mydriasis, trismus, paresis and paralysis, and vocal changes
  VI. Seizures and subsequently death

Diagnosis

  I. History often reveals a CNS disease after contact with pigs.
  II. Compatible clinical signs are highly suggestive.
  III. Laboratory findings are nonspecific.
    A. No hematologic and biochemical changes are found.
    B. CSF may have a slightly increased protein content, which is nonspecific and can be associated with any viral encephalitis.
  IV. Fluorescent antibody tests detect PRV in smears or frozen sections of the brain and tonsils.
  V. Serologic testing can be performed using virus neutralization, immunodiffusion, or ELISA techniques.
  VI. PCR techniques in dogs and cats are primarily a research tool at the present.

Differential Diagnosis

  I. Rabies
  II. Canine distemper
  III. Bilateral trigeminal nerve paralysis
  IV. Other causes of seizures

Treatment

  I. Treatment is usually futile.
  II. Death is the expected outcome.

Prevention

  I. Prevent contact with infected pigs; especially avoid feeding raw pork products to dogs and cats.
  II. Vaccination is usually not performed except in endemic areas.

Bibliography

Brown AL: Canine distemper-measles vaccination: studies on three practical aspects. Canine Pract 2:47, 1975
Dimmitt R: Clinical experience with cross-protective antiendo-

toxin antiserum in dogs with parvoviral enteritis. Canine Pract 16:23, 1991

England JJ, Poston RP: Electron microscopic identification and subsequent isolation of a rotavirus from a dog with fatal neonatal diarrhea. Am J Vet Res 41:782, 1980

Evermann JF, McKeirman AJ, Ott RL et al: Diarrheal condition in dogs associated with viruses antigenically related to feline herpesvirus. Cornell Vet 72:285, 1982

Evermann JF, McKeirman AJ, Smith AW et al: Isolation and identification of caliciviruses from dogs with enteric infections. Am J Vet Res 46:218, 1985

Greenwood NM, Chalmers WSK, Baxendale W et al: Comparison of isolates of canine parvovirus by restriction enzyme analysis, and vaccine efficacy against field strains. Vet Rec 136:63, 1995

Harrison LR, Styer EL, Pursell AR et al: Fatal disease in nursing puppies associated with minute virus of canines. J Vet Diagn Invest 4:19, 1992

Hartmann K, Donath A, Kraft W: AZT in the treatment of feline immunodeficiency virus infection, part 1. Feline Pract 23:16, 1995

Houston DM, Ribble CS, Head LL: Risk factors associated with parvovirus enteritis in dogs: 283 cases (1982–1991). J Am Vet Med Assoc 208:542, 1996

Johnson CA, Snider TG, Fulton RW et al: Gross and light microscopic lesions in neonatal gnotobiotic dogs inoculated with a canine rotavirus. Am J Vet Res 44:1687, 1983

Macartney L, Parrish CR, Binn LN et al: Characterization of minute virus of canines (MVC) and its pathogenicity for pups. Cornell Vet 78:131, 1988

Mansfield PD: Vaccination of dogs and cats in veterinary teaching hospitals in North America. J Am Vet Med Assoc 208:1242, 1996

Pardo C, Mackowiak M: Efficacy of a new canine origin, modified live virus vaccine against canine coronavirus. Rhone Merieux, Inc, Athens, GA, 1995

Parrish CR, Aquadro CF, Strassheim ML et al: Rapid antigenic-type replacement and DNA sequence evolution of canine parvovirus. J Virol 65:6544, 1991

Rewerts JM, Harrington DP, McCaw D et al: Effect of rhG-CSF administration on the clinical outcome of neutropenic parvovirus-infected puppies. J Vet Intern Med 10:178, 1996

Schaffer FL, Soergel ME, Black JW et al: Characterization of a new calicivirus isolated from feces of a dog. Arch Virol 84:181, 1985

Schultz RD, Larson LJ, McCoy KP et al: An evaluation of canine vaccines for their ability to provide protective immunity against challenge with canine parvovirus. Proc North Vet Conf Symp 9:19, 1995

Tennant BJ, Gaskell RM, Kelly DF et al: Canine coronavirus infection in the dog following oronasal inoculation. Res Vet Sci 51:11, 1991

Tennant BJ, Gaskell RM, Jones RC et al: Studies on the epizootiology of canine coronavirus. Vet Rec 132:7, 1993

111

Bacterial Infections

Johnny D. Hoskins

CANINE BRUCELLOSIS

Definition

Canine brucellosis is a contagious bacterial disease of dogs that causes primarily reproductive abnormalities.

Causes

I. Canine brucellosis is caused by several species of the genus *Brucella,* the most common of which is *Brucella canis* (previously referred to as *B. suis* biotype 5).

II. Canine brucellosis has also been attributed to *B. abortus, B. suis,* and *B. melitensis.*

III. *Brucella* species are small gram-negative, aerobic, non-spore-forming coccobacilli.

IV. Cats infected with *B. canis* have only a low degree of bacteremia and serum antibody response. The disease does not appear to be important in cats.

Pathophysiology

I. Organisms penetrate mucous membranes and proliferate in tissue macrophages in the lymph nodes, spleen, uterus, placenta, bone, and prostate gland.

  A. Male infertility is caused by proliferation of *B. canis* in the epididymis, phagocytosis of sperm, and extratubular leakage of phagocytized sperm, which results in antisperm antibodies.

  B. The mechanism of infertility and abortion in the bitch is unknown, although necrosis of the chorionic villi occurs.

    1. Abortions usually occur after day 30.

    2. Affected puppies may be stillborn or die perinatally.

    3. Necrosis and hemorrhage of multiple organs and perivascular infiltration of the liver with lymphocytes are prominent features.

II. Other tissue such as the uveal tract, vertebrae, and kidneys may also be infected.

III. Bacteremia may persist for as long as 2 years.

IV. Transmission occurs at the time of mating or after exposure to infected aborted tissue, vaginal discharge, or milk.

Clinical Signs

I. Most infected dogs are asymptomatic.

II. Most infected dogs are not seriously ill, and mortality does not occur in infected adults.

III. Physical examination findings are nonspecific and include fever, peripheral lymphadenopathy, lethargy, weight loss, and mild splenomegaly.

IV. Reproductive abnormalities are the most common clinical problem.

  A. Female dogs

    1. Abortion often occurs between days 45 and 55 of gestation, followed by brown or greenish gray vaginal discharge.

    2. Reduced fertility exists.

      a) Apparent conception failures or early fetal death (10–20 days after breeding) may occur.

      b) Reduced litter size may also occur.

      c) Increased neonatal mortality occurs.

  B. Male dogs

    1. In the first 3 months of infection, orchitis, epididymitis, scrotal enlargement, or dermatitis is usually evident.

    2. Chronic infection is associated with unilateral or bilateral testicular atrophy.

    3. Abnormal semen, such as azoospermia, head-to-head agglutination and clumping of sperm, and/or increased neutrophils and monocytes, occurs.

V. Diskospondylitis may be present, with back pain and variable neurologic findings.

VI. Recurrent uveitis and immune-complex glomerulonephritis may be seen.

Diagnosis

I. Definitive diagnosis requires the isolation of *B. canis* from blood, semen, or tissue (fetus, placenta, spleen, lymph nodes, bone marrow, prostate gland, epididymides, intervertebral disk space).

A. Successful isolation of *B. canis* is difficult because of low levels of bacteremia.

B. Blood can be inoculated into tryptose broth or brain-heart infusion broth or inoculated directly onto blood agar plates.

II. Hematologic and serum biochemical findings are nonspecific.

III. Serologic tests are the most widely used means of diagnosing canine brucellosis (Johnson and Walker, 1992).

A. Rapid slide agglutination test (RSAT) is a screening procedure.

  1. It measures the presence of antibodies to *B. canis*.

  2. False-negatives may occur with early infections (<8 weeks); however, 99% of negative RSATs are also culture-negative.

  3. False-positives are common (up to 50%).

  4. RSAT becomes positive 2 weeks after infection.

  5. Interpretation is difficult in dogs treated with antibiotics within 4 weeks of the testing.

B. Tube agglutination (TAT) and 2-mercaptoethanol modification (2ME-TAT) are more definitive tests.

  1. They are used to confirm a positive RSAT.

  2. Absolute titers obtained in different laboratories cannot be accurately compared because of lack of standards; however, the following guidelines are useful.

   a) TAT titer >1:200 or 2ME-TAT titer >1:100 indicates active infection.

   b) Titer of 1:50–1:100 indicates suspicion of active infection; repeat titer 4–6 weeks later.

   c) Titer >1:50 indicates early or recovering infection.

  3. They become positive 3–4 weeks after infection.

  4. With titers indicative of active infection, attempt to isolate *B. canis* from blood, semen, or appropriate tissue.

C. Agar-gel immunodiffusion (AGID) is a confirmational test.

  1. This test is the preferred serologic test for the diagnosis of active infection.

  2. It uses either somatic (cell wall) or cytoplasmic antigens.

   a) Somatic antigen AGID may be negative in male dogs with only reproductive tract disease.

   b) Cytoplasmic antigen AGID becomes positive earlier (<1 week) and persists longer (>12 months).

D. Enzyme-linked immunosorbent assay (ELISA) is available but not generally recommended.

Differential Diagnosis

I. Canine herpesvirus infection

II. Canine parvovirus-1 infection

III. Lymphosarcoma

IV. Testicular inflammation or tumor

V. Intervertebral disk disease

VI. Other causes of recurrent uveitis

Treatment

I. *B. canis* is often resistant to antibiotic therapy because of its intracellular location.

A. Successful treatment is not currently available.

B. Because organisms can persist in sequestered sites such as the prostate gland and bones, cures are difficult to achieve.

II. Antibiotic therapy is recommended.

A. Minocycline is given at 12.5 mg/kg PO BID for 14–21 days and then off 3 weeks.

B. Tetracycline HCl is given at 10–20 mg/kg PO TID for 3 weeks and then off 3 weeks.

C. Enrofloxacin is given at 10–15 mg/kg PO BID for 3 weeks and then off 3 weeks.

D. Enrofloxacin is probably the best initial choice and may be repeated 1–3 times.

E. Antibiotic therapy is repeated 2 months later if cultures and titers fail to improve.

III. Control of the disease involves the following.

A. Eliminate all infected animals from the breeding program and, if possible, from the kennel.

B. Neuter all infected dogs if kept as pets.

C. Warn owners of the uncertain outcome of treatment, of the consequences of keeping infected animals with sequestered organisms, and of their zoonotic potential.

Patient Monitoring and Prevention

I. Spontaneous recovery may occur 1–3 years after infection.

A. Bacteremia may be continuous or intermittent during this time.

B. When bacteremia ceases, the serologic titer decreases within 2–6 months, although a nidus of infection may persist.

II. Cultures and serologic tests are repeated 2 months after treatment.

III. Prevention of the disease involves the following.

A. Because an acceptable vaccine is not currently available, prevention of disease relies on preventing exposure to the organism.

B. Breeders mate their dogs only to ones that have been tested and are *Brucella*-negative.

C. Once infection has been confirmed within a kennel, euthanize all animals with positive blood or tissue cultures.

D. Before being introduced into a kennel, all new dogs are placed in isolation until they have two negative serologic tests 1 month apart.

E. The carrier state of infected dogs is a more important reservoir for the organism than environmental contamination, as survival of *B. canis* outside the host appears to be short-lived.

F. *B. canis* is killed by quaternary ammonium compounds and iodophors.

CAMPYLOBACTERIOSIS

Definition

Campylobacteriosis is a potential cause of infectious gastroenteritis in dogs, cats, humans, and other animals.

Causes

I. Campylobacteriosis is caused by *Campylobacter jejuni.*
  A. It apparently induces diarrhea in some animals, whereas other animals shed the organism in their feces while remaining clinically asymptomatic.
  B. It may affect the clinical manifestations of other infectious gastrointestinal infections such as canine parvovirus-2 infection.
  C. Although infected dogs and cats represent a zoonotic risk, the disease is most often associated with poor sanitation.
II. *C. jejuni* are gram-negative, curved-shaped rods with single polar flagella. The bacterium is motile, requires a microaerophilic environment for growth, and grows only at 42–43°C.
III. *Campylobacter* survives poorly outside the host, but viable organisms can persist in feces for as long as 4 weeks and can be found in fresh and salt water.
IV. The organism is difficult to culture but grows best on selective media especially enriched for the *Campylobacter* spp.

Pathophysiology

I. The status of *C. jejuni* and other *Campylobacter* species as primary pathogens is unknown. *Campylobacter,* like *Salmonella,* is probably a pathogen of opportunistic nature.
II. A higher incidence of isolation is found in kenneled or stray animals, in animals with access to poultry, and in those stressed by transport or other disease.
III. Transmission occurs through the feces.
  A. It is shed in feces for 1–4 months or more.
  B. It contaminates food and water via feces.
IV. Incubation period is 1–7 days.
V. Gastrointestinal lesions involve the jejunum, ileum, and colon.
  A. Colonization occurs with epithelial invasion.
  B. Thickening and congestion occur and are worse distally.
  C. Fluid sequestration occurs within the lumen, and associated lymph nodes are enlarged and congested.
  D. Clinical signs may occur from elaboration of an enterotoxin.

Clinical Signs

I. Most animals are asymptomatic carriers.
II. Clinical signs are most severe in young animals.
  A. Vomiting is generally present.
  B. Hemorrhagic or watery mucoid diarrhea occurs for 1–2 weeks.

C. Fever occurs with an associated bacteremia.
III. Clinical signs are generally self-limited (5–15 days).

Diagnosis

I. Isolation procedures
  A. Feces are the preferred sample, but blood cultures can be performed.
  B. Inoculate onto selective plate media (Blaser's Camy-BAP medium).
  C. Alternatively, rectal swabs can be stored in Cary-Blair medium at 4°C.
  D. Culture plates are incubated in evacuatable anaerobic jars.
  E. Isolation of *C. jejuni* from feces of a diarrheic animal does not establish a definitive diagnosis.
II. Direct examination
  A. Diluted fecal smears examined by darkfield or phase-contrast microscopy show large numbers of darting, motile, corkscrew-shaped organisms.
  B. The presence of these descriptive organisms in feces of a diarrheic animal does not establish a definitive diagnosis.
  C. The presence of blood and leukocytes is variable.
III. Serology
  A. A passive hemagglutination serotyping technique for somatic (O) antigen has been developed.
  B. The significance of antibody titers as a marker of disease or infection in dogs and cats has not been defined.

Differential Diagnosis

I. Coronavirus or parvovirus diarrhea
II. Dietary-related diarrhea
III. *Salmonella* enteritis

Treatment

I. Antibiotic therapy is indicated if the following signs are present.
  A. Bloody diarrhea is present for 3–4 days.
  B. High fever and neutrophilic leukocytosis exist.
II. Antibiotic therapy may also be indicated when diarrheic animals are found shedding *Campylobacter* in their feces.
III. The organism is susceptible to many antibiotics (except those strains that produce beta-lactamase, which accounts for their resistance to penicillin), but antibiotic efficacy is unknown in dogs and cats.
  A. Erythromycin is given to dogs at 20 mg/kg PO BID and to cats at 10 mg/kg PO TID.
  B. Chloramphenicol is given at 25–50 mg/kg PO BID-TID for 5 days.
  C. Most strains are also susceptible to aminoglycosides, tetracyclines, furazolidone, and clindamycin.
  D. Less effective antibiotics include penicillin, polymyxin B, cephalosporins, trimethoprim-sulfonamide, and vancomycin.
IV. The effectiveness of treatment is confirmed by fecal cultures performed 1 and 4 weeks following therapy.

V. Antibiotic therapy does not appear to increase the convalescent carrier state, as it does with salmonellosis.

Patient Monitoring and Prevention

I. *Campylobacter* organisms are destroyed by common disinfectants such as household bleach, iodophors, and quaternary ammonium compounds.
II. Reduce moist areas in the environment where *Campylobacter* can survive.
III. As far as zoonosis is concerned, current medical opinion advocates simple hygienic measures such as handwashing and isolation of diarrheic animals from people.

SALMONELLOSIS

Definition

Salmonellosis is an important cause of infectious gastroenteritis in dogs, cats, humans, and other animals.

Causes

I. *Salmonella* spp. are gram-negative organisms of the family Enterobacteriacae that can be isolated on selective media from infected tissue, surgical wounds, feces, and oral or conjunctival membranes.
II. Primary animal pathogens include *S. typhimurium, S. enteritidis, S. arizonae,* and *S. choleraesuis.*
   A. Certain serotypes have affinity for particular animals.
   B. The species most commonly isolated from infected dogs and cats is *S. typhimurium.*

Pathophysiology

I. Epizootiology
   A. The most common sources of *Salmonella* organisms are contaminated water, food, and fomites.
   B. *Salmonella* can survive for prolonged periods in the environment.
   C. Unprocessed or improperly cooked food from infected swine, cattle, or poultry is a potential source.
   D. Processed pet foods may be contaminated by rodents, insects, and birds during storage.
   E. Nosocomial infection has been associated with fomites such as water bowls, food dishes, animal cages, bathing facilities, and endoscopic equipment, as well as exposure to infected hospital personnel.
II. Pathogenesis
   A. After ingestion of the organism, invasion of the lymphoid tissue of the pharynx and possibly the small intestine and colon occurs.
   B. Organisms may also reside in lymph nodes, liver, or spleen.
   C. Shedding in the feces occurs for 3–6 weeks, depending on the amount of exposure, the strain of *Salmonella,* and host immune response.
      1. Shedding is continual for the first week and then intermittent.
      2. Stress, concurrent infection with an enteropathogen, or immunosuppression can cause a recrudescence of clinical disease or shedding.
   D. Any changes that cause alteration in endogenous microflora increase the susceptibility to *Salmonella* infection when exposed.
   E. Gastrointestinal signs are caused by the invasion of epithelial cells and the subsequent inflammatory response.
   F. Necropsy abnormalities are rare, even in animals with severe clinical disease.

Clinical Signs

I. Several clinical syndromes are possible (Dow et al., 1989).
   A. Gastroenteritis
   B. Bacteremia and endotoxemia
   C. Asymptomatic carrier state
II. Gastroenteritis syndrome is common.
   A. Severity is variable and influenced by factors such as age, number of infecting organisms, infecting *Salmonella* strain, host immune status, and concurrent stress and infection.
   B. Signs develop 3–5 days after oral exposure and include fever, lethargy, anorexia, vomiting, diarrhea, and abdominal pain.
   C. The diarrhea may be watery or mucoid and contain fresh blood and inflammatory cells.
III. Bacteremia and endotoxemia syndrome may also occur.
   A. This syndrome may be subclinical and transient in some animals.
   B. Depression, weakness, and collapse can occur with or without diarrhea.
   C. Fever and lethargy may be the only manifestations.
   D. It occurs most often in very young or immunocompromised animals.
IV. Most infected animals recover in 3–4 weeks. After that, the carrier state may be established.
V. Other problems may rarely be associated with *Salmonella* infection.
   A. In utero transmission may result in death and abortion of the fetuses or the birth of weak or ill puppies or kittens.
   B. Vaginal discharge, placental tissue and fluid, and meconium may contain *Salmonella* organisms.
   C. Central nervous system (CNS) signs may include hyperexcitability, incoordination, posterior paresis, blindness, and convulsions.

Diagnosis

I. Salmonellosis is suspected whenever acute or chronic gastrointestinal signs are present.
II. Definitive diagnosis is made by bacterial isolation of *Salmonella* organisms.
   A. A negative culture does not eliminate the possibility of clinical salmonellosis, as it can be diffi-

cult to isolate *Salmonella* spp. in the presence of other organisms and after the use of antibiotics.
  B. Samples obtained from the pharynx or intestinal tract are cultured in selective enrichment broths such as selenite or tetrathionate to increase yield, and then plated on selective media such as deoxycholate after 24 hours incubation.
  C. Demonstration of the organism in urine, blood, or tracheal/bronchial lavage suggests bacteremia.
III. The presence of leukocytes in diarrheic feces suggests invasion of the intestinal mucosa by *Salmonella* organisms.
IV. Hematologic abnormalities include nonregenerative anemia (chronic disease) and leukopenia (sepsis).

Differential Diagnosis

  I. Coronavirus or parvovirus diarrhea
 II. Dietary-related diarrhea
III. *Campylobacter* enteritis
IV. Clostridial diarrhea

Treatment

  I. Antibiotic therapy for salmonellosis is controversial.
  A. Gastroenteric signs are probably unaltered by antibiotic treatment, and the shedding of organisms and development of a chronic carrier state may actually be enhanced.
  B. Antibiotics are indicated if signs of *Salmonella* septicemia are present.
    1. Enrofloxacin, chloramphenicol, gentamicin, or trimethoprim-sulfonamide can be used initially.
    2. Definitive therapy is based on sensitivity testing because of an increasing resistance to antibiotics.
 II. Supportive therapy is indicated for gastrointestinal signs.
  A. Withhold food and water, and replace fluid losses with polyionic isotonic fluids parenterally.
  B. Blood or plasma transfusions may be given to replace blood loss and manage a hypoproteinemic state (see Chap. 69).
  C. If intestinal parasitism exists, specific treatment is indicated.
  D. Provide adequate nutritional and water support after 24–48 hours of cessation of vomiting and reduction of diarrhea.

Patient Monitoring and Prevention

  I. *Salmonella* organisms are destroyed by common disinfectants such as household bleach, iodophors, and quaternary ammonium compounds.
 II. As far as zoonosis is concerned, current medical advice includes simple hygienic measures such as handwashing and isolation of diarrheic animals from people.

LEPTOSPIROSIS

Definition

Leptospirosis, a bacterial disease of dogs, cats, humans, and other animals, is important as both a clinical and a zoonotic disease.

Causes

  I. The genus *Leptospira* is divided into saprophytic and pathogenic groups. Pathogenic leptospires are maintained in nature by particular animal reservoirs.
 II. All pathogenic leptospires are classified under one species, *Leptospira interrogans.*
III. Most clinical cases of leptospirosis in dogs are caused by several serovars of the genus *Leptospira interrogans,* including *L. canicola, L. icterohaemorrhagiae, L. grippotyphosa,* and *L. pomona* (Rentko and Ross, 1992).

Pathophysiology

  I. Organisms enter through mucous membranes or abraded skin. After 4–10 days, the host becomes bacteremic, and invasion of internal organs occurs.
 II. Kidneys may become infected.
  A. Renal tubular epithelial cells are infected, with subsequent shedding in urine (possible in seronegative carriers).
  B. Complete recovery is possible, although progressive renal failure may be a sequela to acute leptospiral infections.
III. Liver may become involved.
  A. Icterus, even without pronounced histopathology, may occur with *L. icterohaemorrhagiae.*
  B. Severe, acute hepatitis may occur.
  C. *L. grippotyphosa* may cause chronic active hepatitis.
IV. Anterior uveitis results from immunologic mechanisms.
 V. Coagulopathies may also develop.

Clinical Signs

  I. Clinical signs vary from subclinical to chronic.
 II. Peracute infections can be rapidly fatal.
  A. Initial signs include fever (103–104°F; 39.5–40°C), lethargy, vomiting, and dehydration.
  B. Subsequently, signs of shock and bleeding diatheses develop.
III. Acute to subacute infections may occur.
  A. Fever, anorexia, polydipsia, vomiting, dehydration, petechial and ecchymotic hemorrhages, injected mucous membranes, oliguria or anuria, sublumbar pain and reluctance to move, icterus, and anterior uveitis may be present.
  B. With acute *L. pomona* and *L. grippotyphosa* infections, signs of acute renal failure usually dominate.
IV. Dogs with severe irreversible renal damage or

chronic active hepatitis often develop signs of advancing organ failure.

V. Cats show minimal to no clinical signs, although there may be histopathologic evidence of hepatic and renal involvement.

Diagnosis

I. Hematologic findings show the following.
  A. Leukopenia occurs during the initial leptospiremia, but leukocytosis develops later.
  B. Thrombocytopenia may or may not be present.
II. Biochemical findings are as follows.
  A. Increased serum blood urea nitrogen (BUN), creatinine, and phosphorus are seen with renal injury.
  B. Increased serum alanine transaminase (ALT), aspartate transaminase (AST), and bilirubin levels occur with liver involvement.
  C. Electrolyte abnormalities usually reflect the severity of signs associated with renal and gastrointestinal involvement.
III. Urinalysis findings include bilirubinuria, proteinuria, pyuria, and/or hematuria.
IV. Severely affected dogs often develop coagulation abnormalities such as thrombocytopenia and increased fibrin degradation products (FDPs).
V. Serology usually aids in the diagnosis.
  A. The microscopic agglutination test (MAT) has been widely used but is relatively nonspecific.
    1. Antibodies to multivalent bacterins can produce false-positive reactions.
    2. Demonstration of a fourfold rise in titer on samples taken 2–4 weeks apart confirms the diagnosis.
    3. MAT titers parallel IgM rather than IgG activity.
  B. An ELISA test is currently being used in many laboratories.
    1. It is more sensitive than MAT, so that ''shedding'' animals can be detected.
    2. Increased IgM-ELISA titers occur 1 week after exposure; IgG-ELISA titers develop in 2–3 weeks.
    3. Vaccinated dogs show a high IgG-ELISA titer with a low or negative IgM-ELISA titer.
  C. A microscopic microcapsular agglutination test also exists.
    1. Serum titers increase soon after initial infection.
    2. Titers parallel IgM activity, thereby detecting recent infections.
VI. Successful isolation of leptospires is difficult because of their fastidious growth requirements and susceptibility to environmental factors.
  A. Urine or blood is submitted for culture.
    1. Special media are required for their growth. Stuart's and Fletcher's are available and are supplemented with hemoglobin or serum.
    2. Leptospires are long, slender, spiral-shaped organisms with a hook at one or both ends.
  B. Rapid identification of leptospires in urine samples and cultures can sometimes be accomplished with darkfield microscopy.

Differential Diagnosis

I. Other causes of acute renal failure
II. Other causes of anterior uveitis
III. Other causes of liver disease

Treatment

I. Procaine penicillin (40,000 U/kg IM, SQ SID or divided BID for 2 weeks or longer) is most effective in arresting the leptospiremia, although it does not prevent the carrier state.
II. Chloramphenicol (50 mg/kg PO TID), tetracycline (5–10 mg/kg PO BID-TID), and doxycycline (5 mg/kg PO loading dose, then 2.5 mg/kg PO BID-SID for 2 weeks or longer) have all been effective in treating infected dogs.
III. Enrofloxacin (5 mg/kg PO BID) and ciprofloxacin (10–15 mg/kg PO BID) are also effective.
IV. Supportive therapy is usually needed.
  A. Type of therapy depends on the presence and severity of renal and hepatic dysfunction and related problems such as dehydration, electrolyte abnormalities, bleeding problems, and shock.
  B. See Chap. 47 for treatment of renal failure.
  C. See Chap. 66 for therapy of bleeding diatheses.

Patient Monitoring and Prevention

I. It is best prevented and controlled through immunization.
  A. Inadequately vaccinated dogs may become asymptomatic shedders and possibly infect other animals as well as humans.
  B. Some of the currently available vaccines may produce a hypersensitivity reaction and subsequently anaphylactic shock.
II. Bacterins for serovars *L. canicola* and *L. icterohaemorrhagiae* provide immunity that persists for 6 months to 1 year after immunization.
III. Vaccinated dogs may become infected and develop clinical disease when exposed to the nontraditional serovars of *L. pomona* and *L. grippotyphosa.*
IV. Leptospires are easily killed by heat and common disinfectants.

LYME BORRELIOSIS

Definition

Lyme borreliosis is a spirochete infection in humans and animals that may result in skin lesions, limb-joint dysfunction, and other associated organ dysfunctions.

Causes

I. Lyme borreliosis is caused by *Borrelia burgdorferi,* a member of the family Spirochaetacae.

II. Multiple strains of *Borrelia* exist; some may be non-pathogenic in the dog and cat.

III. *B. burgdorferi* is transmitted primarily but not exclusively through the bite of an infected ixodid tick. In the United States, two ixodid ticks are commonly involved.

    A. East Coast, Southeast, and Midwest: *Ixodes scapularis*

    B. West coast: *Ixodes pacificus*

Pathophysiology

I. Epidemiology

    A. *Borrelia* spp. infect humans, dogs, cats, horses, and cattle (Angulo, 1986).

    B. The dog is more susceptible than the cat to infection and disease.

    C. Young outdoor dogs (<5 years old) have a greater chance of exposure to tick vectors and are most often affected.

    D. Most cases occur from May through November, corresponding to the feeding times of infective ticks.

    E. *B. burgdorferi* have been recovered from the urine of feral white-footed mice (*Peromyscus leucopus*), humans, and dogs. Contact transmission has occurred between white-footed mice and dogs.

II. Pathogenesis

    A. Bites from infected ticks may produce no clinical signs, or clinical signs may appear 2–5 months later.

    B. Direct or indirect mechanisms may account for the clinical signs.

        1. Direct mechanisms include pyrogen-producing lipopolysaccharide, endotoxin, or cell wall peptidoglycan.

        2. Indirect mechanisms may be mediated through immune-complex formation deposited primarily in joints.

Clinical Signs

I. *B. burgdorferi* infection is often asymptomatic in the dog and cat.

II. Only a small percentage of infected dogs and cats develop clinical signs. Signs occur approximately 2–5 months after exposure (Burgess, 1992; Appel et al., 1993).

    A. Fever of 103–106°F (40–41°C) may occur.

    B. Anorexia and lethargy may be noted.

    C. Painful muscles or joints make the animal reluctant to move.

    D. Weight-bearing lameness is noted, usually with no history of trauma.

        1. Lameness involves a single joint or multiple joints, predominantly carpus, elbow, tarsus, and stifle.

        2. There is usually minimal joint swelling.

        3. Lameness may be intermittent.

    E. Mild peripheral lymphadenopathy may occur.

F. Skin, renal, cardiac, and neurologic lesions and/or signs are rarely seen.

Diagnosis

I. Clinical diagnosis is based on a combination of history, clinical signs, serologic tests, and response to therapy.

II. There may be a history of recent exposure or finding ticks on the animal.

III. Immunofluorescent antibodies (IFA), ELISA, and immunoblot serology are available; there is variation in IFA and ELISA titer results among individual laboratories.

    A. There is considerable overlap of titers in symptomatic and asymptomatic dogs and cats.

    B. It is not known whether asymptomatic animals with titers develop disease and whether continued monitoring is important.

    C. A fourfold increase in titer over 2–4 weeks is considered diagnostic.

IV. Isolation and detection by polymerase chain reaction (PCR) techniques may be done.

    A. *Borrelia* spp. are difficult to culture; specific culture media such as Barbour-Stoener-Kelly are required for isolation from skin biopsy, joint fluid, or blood samples.

    B. Detection by PCR techniques is most successful from skin biopsy samples at the site of the tick bite.

V. Rapid response of clinical signs to antibiotic therapy is also supportive of a diagnosis of Lyme borreliosis.

Differential Diagnosis

I. Ehrlichiosis

II. Rocky Mountain spotted fever

III. Other causes of lameness

Treatment

I. Antibiotics are indicated.

    A. Tetracycline HCl is given at 25 mg/kg PO TID for 14–28 days. Other anthracyclines, including doxycycline and minocycline, are similarly effective.

    B. Other effective antibiotics include penicillin, ampicillin, amoxicillin, ceftriaxone, and cefotaxime.

II. Supportive care such as nonsteroidal anti-inflammatory drugs and restricted activity may be used to alleviate joint pain.

Patient Monitoring and Prevention

I. Limit exposure of the dog or cat to tick vectors in endemic areas.

II. Use insect repellents such as 0.5% permethrin or 20–30% DEET, or apply topical insecticidal products for ticks.

III. Vaccination is still controversial.

    A. Canine *B. burgdorferi* vaccine, available as killed bacteria and recombinant products, provides protection against Lyme borreliosis (Levy et al., 1993).

B. According to manufacturers currently marketing canine *B. burgdorferi* vaccines, puppies 9–12 weeks of age or older should receive 2 doses administered at 2- to 3-week intervals, with annual revaccination with a single dose recommended.

C. The manufacturers have shown protection for up to 6 months against one or more strains of organism after parenteral challenges.

D. Questions exist whether the vaccines protect against the other strains of pathogenic *B. burgdorferi* or *Borrelia* spp. or against challenges with infected ticks.

PLAGUE

Definition

Plague is a bacterial zoonotic disease that infects cats and dogs in the western United States.

Cause

I. Feline plague is caused by the coccobacillus *Yersinia pestis,* which is a member of the family Enterobacteriaceae (Chomel et al., 1994).

II. Sylvatic plague is established in the United States in wild animal populations in all the states west of the Great Plains.

A. The primary hosts for plague in the Upper Sonoran Life Zone Habitat of New Mexico, Arizona, and southern Colorado are rock squirrels *(Spermophilus variegatus)* and their fleas *(Diamanus montanus).*

B. The Upper Sonoran Life Zone Habitat is characterized by juniper and piñon vegetation.

Pathophysiology

I. Transmission is as follows.

A. The organisms cannot penetrate unbroken skin but can invade mucous membranes.

B. Naturally infected cats acquire the disease by eating infected rodents.

II. The incubation period is usually 2–6 days.

III. Infection can occur in three forms.

A. The bubonic form is the most common and occurs after the bite of an infected flea or introduction of *Y. pestis* through a break in the skin.

1. Lymphadenopathy develops in the regional lymph nodes.

2. The suppurative lymph node is called a bubo.

B. Septicemic plague can develop without evidence of lymphadenopathy.

1. Septicemia may also develop in the bubonic form if the animal is not treated.

2. It may be more common in immunocompromised hosts.

C. Pneumonic plague occurs from primary infection of the respiratory tract or secondary to the bubonic or septicemic forms.

IV. Modes of animal-to-human transmission are as follows.

A. Mechanical transport of *Y. pestis*–infected rodent fleas by cats and dogs to humans is most common.

B. Veterinarians or animal health technicians may become infected by contact with tissue of infected animals or by bites or scratches from infected animals.

C. Direct tissue contact with infected rabbits, hares, prairie dogs, bobcats, and coyotes may occur.

Clinical Signs

I. Cats are more susceptible than dogs, and plague in cats has a high mortality rate (50%).

II. Cats may exhibit the following signs (Eidson et al., 1991).

A. Fever, anorexia, lethargy, and lymphadenopathy may be seen.

B. Buboes on the head or neck may rupture and form fistulous tracts with a creamy, purulent discharge.

C. Drooling or sneezing associated with oral or upper respiratory tract involvement may be seen.

D. Primary pneumonic plague has not been seen in the cat, but bacteremia may cause splenic, hepatic, or pulmonary lesions.

E. Death may occur within 7 days, or chronic emaciation occurs, with death within 2–4 weeks.

III. Dogs often exhibit more nonspecific signs.

A. *Y. pestis* infection is uncommon and not well documented.

B. Infected dogs may become septicemic and develop high fever and lymphadenopathy.

Diagnosis

I. It is based on microscopic and bacteriologic examination of lymph node aspirates and blood.

A. Aspirate fluid from a bubo, air-dry, fix in absolute methanol for 5 minutes, and apply either Gram's or Giemsa's stain.

1. *Y. pestis* is a small, gram-negative, bipolar coccobacillus.

2. If it is not aspirated on the first attempt, inject sterile saline solution and re-aspirate the area.

3. If smears are suspicious, send to a reference laboratory.

B. Direct fluorescent antibody test can also be performed on exudate.

C. Detection by PCR techniques can also be performed on exudate and lymph node aspirates.

II. Obtain blood for hemogram, bacterial culture, and acute-phase passive hemagglutination titers.

A. Infected cats have neutrophilia with a left shift.

B. Blood is directly inoculated into a liquid blood culture medium such as trypticase soy broth.

C. Convalescent-phase titers develop within 10–14 days of exposure.

III. Thoracic radiography is recommended to assess the potential of aerosol transmission to humans.

Differential Diagnosis

I. Cat fight abscess
II. Other causes of sepsis
III. Other causes of splenic, hepatic, or pulmonary inflammatory disease

Treatment

I. *Y. pestis* is susceptible to a variety of antibiotics.
   A. Aminoglycosides such as gentamicin or streptomycin are the drugs of choice.
   B. Tetracycline and chloramphenicol are acceptable alternatives.
II. Regardless of whether fleas are present, the cat or dog is treated with an appropriate flea control product.
III. During treatment of plague or suspected plague, precautions should be taken to reduce the risk of human exposure.
   A. Limit the number of individuals involved in treatment to an absolute minimum.
   B. It is best to house the suspected animal in an isolation room.
   C. Wear gloves, gowns, and single-use high-filtration surgical masks.
   D. It is best to use parenteral rather than oral antibiotics.

Patient Monitoring and Prevention

I. *Y. pestis* survives for only several days in the environment unless the organism is protected by organic material such as exudate; therefore, disinfection of directly contaminated surfaces and equipment with phenolic or quaternary ammonium compounds is effective.
II. After recovery, the animal presents no risk of plague transmission.

TETANUS

Definition

Tetanus is a bacterial disease of warm-blooded animals characterized by localized or generalized muscle spasms that can rapidly progress to death.

Causes

I. Tetanus is caused by the effect of an exotoxin of *Clostridium tetani* on the dog's or cat's CNS.
II. *C. tetani* is a motile, gram-positive, anaerobic, spore-forming bacillus that is commonly found in the feces of many domestic animals, including dogs and cats.

Pathophysiology

I. Infection is established at the site of contaminated puncture wounds under anaerobic conditions and can also occur in surgical wounds or during eruption of teeth.
II. *C. tetani* produces three toxins: a tetanospasmin, a hemolysin, and a peripherally active nonspasmogenic toxin.
   A. The tetanospasmin is responsible for the characteristic clinical features of tetanus. It enters the axons of motor nerves and travels retrograde to the neuronal cell body within the spinal cord.
      1. It inhibits the inhibitory interneurons in the gray matter of the spinal cord and brain stem.
      2. The net result is a release of inhibition on motor neurons and an extensor rigidity of muscles all over the head and body.
   B. The hemolysin causes local tissue necrosis and creates more favorable conditions for multiplication of *C. tetani*. The toxin is hemolytic for erythrocytes.
   C. The action of the nonspasmogenic toxin is poorly defined but may play a role in the peripheral paralytic action of tetanus toxin.
III. The incidence of tetanus in dogs and cats is much lower than in horses and humans and may be related to the relative susceptibility of these species to tetanospasmin.

Clinical Signs

I. Although clinical signs can be seen within 5–8 days after the organism has entered body tissue, as long as 3 weeks may elapse before enough toxin is produced to cause signs.
   A. It may be difficult to locate the site where the organism entered the animal's body by the time clinical signs appear (Dieringer and Wolf, 1991).
   B. Generalized muscle spasms usually begin in the temporal muscles and progress until the animal assumes opisthotonos.
   C. The temporal muscle spasms result in prolapse of the third eyelids, elevation of the upper eyelids, retraction of the lips, and dorsal retraction of the earflaps.
   D. The muscle spasms then progress further, causing dysphagia, difficulty opening the mouth (''lockjaw''), and difficulty breathing.
   E. Hypersensitivity to external stimuli results from a lowered neural threshold that is apparent early in the disease.
   F. Pyrexia occasionally occurs owing to increased muscle activity.
   G. The heart and pulse rates usually remain normal.
II. Secondary complications such as nutritional deficiencies, electrolyte and water imbalances, airway obstruction, and pneumonia are usually the result of dysphagia, muscle paralysis, and prolonged recumbency.
III. When tetanus is fatal, death usually occurs within 5 days of the onset of clinical signs.

Diagnosis

I. Diagnosis is based on clinical findings and history of a prior wound.

II. Although isolation of the organism enables a positive diagnosis, the site of infection cannot always be identified.

Differential Diagnosis

I. Antifreeze poisoning
II. Organophosphate poisoning
III. Polymyositis

Treatment

I. Treatment involves an attempt to destroy the toxin-producing bacteria and to neutralize the free toxin.
  A. Surgical débridement of necrotic areas is indicated.
    1. Drain abscesses and remove any foreign bodies.
    2. The wound is then instilled with intralesional 1,000,000 U aqueous penicillin G, and 10,000 U tetanus antitoxin is administered.
    3. The wound is not closed, as this would provide the anaerobic environment needed by the organism.
  B. Antitoxin is administered to neutralize free toxin.
    1. Give a test dose of 0.1–0.2 ml SQ and observe for 30 minutes for anaphylaxis.
    2. Dose is 1000 U/kg/day IV divided into 3 doses for the first 2–3 days only.
  C. Antibiotics are used.
    1. Give potassium penicillin G 40,000 U/kg IV, followed by 20,000 U/kg IM BID.
    2. Other antibiotics effective against anaerobic organisms can be used.
II. Supportive and symptomatic care is helpful.
  A. A dark, quiet environment is provided, with minimal handling.
  B. Use sedation to control muscle spasms, extensor rigidity, and anxiety.
    1. Give acepromazine 0.5–2 mg/kg IM, SQ BID.
    2. Another choice is phenobarbital IM or pentobarbital IV, given to effect.
  C. Fluid therapy and nutritional support are given as needed.
  D. Recumbent animals need special nursing care to prevent or treat decubital ulcers.
  E. Tracheal intubation and administration of oxygen with a respirator are necessary when respiratory paralysis is imminent.

Patient Monitoring and Prevention

I. Dogs and cats that recover exhibit signs for 30 days or longer before the muscle rigidity completely resolves. Once recovered, there are no permanent neurologic deficits.
II. A guarded prognosis is indicated when generalized signs are present; it is more favorable when the condition is localized.
III. Active immunoprophylaxis or postexposure prophylaxis with tetanus toxoid is not usually recommended in the dog and cat.

IV. In high-risk environments, postexposure prophylaxis with tetanus antitoxin can be administered before wound débridement as outlined earlier.

NOCARDIOSIS

Definition

Nocardiosis is a bacterial disease that infrequently causes exudative skin lesions, pyothorax, and/or widely disseminated infection in dogs and cats.

Causes

I. *Nocardia asteroides, N. brasiliensis,* and *N. caviae* are gram-positive bacteria that form branching rods and filaments (hyphae) (Hardie, 1990).
II. These organisms are aerobic saprophytes that originate from soil and are members of the order Actinomycetales.

Pathophysiology

I. *Nocardia* organisms enter through injured skin or may be inhaled or ingested.
II. Once infection is established, the organism may be disseminated in widely scattered sites, including the thorax, skin, lymph nodes, or CNS.

Clinical Signs

I. Skin infections
    There is typically a history of a wound and a resultant nonhealing ulcerated lesion or draining fistulous tract (Marino and Jaggy, 1993)
II. Pyothorax
  A. Respiratory distress and weight loss are usually present.
  B. Evidence of a penetrating thoracic wall injury may not be apparent.
III. Disseminated nocardiosis
  A. Signs may mimic those of canine distemper or systemic fungal infection.
  B. Signs include cough, respiratory distress, fever, anorexia, neurologic signs, cachexia, and ocular and nasal discharges.

Diagnosis

I. The *Nocardia* organisms can usually be demonstrated in exudates.
  A. They are gram-positive, branching, and beaded filaments.
  B. They stain acid-fast or partially acid-fast.
II. Pleural effusion has a typical "cream of tomato soup" appearance. Sulfur granules (clumps of organisms) may or may not be present; when present, they are not pathognomonic for nocardiosis.
III. Hematologic and serum chemistry findings are nonspecific and often reflect the degree of inflammation or organ dysfunction present.

IV. Isolation of the organism may be performed from exudate or sulfur granules on blood agar or plain Sabouraud's dextrose agar plates.

V. *Nocardia* may not be seen with routine hematoxylin and eosin (H&E) stain; modified acid-fast stain of tissue may be necessary to demonstrate the organism.

Differential Diagnosis

I. Other causes of draining skin or lymph node lesions
II. Other causes of pyothorax
III. Canine distemper
IV. Systemic fungal diseases
V. Actinomycosis

Treatment

I. Drainage and lavage of the infected site
  A. Chest tube insertion and lavage are used for pyothorax (see Chap. 19).
  B. Surgical exploration and drainage of closed body cavity infections may be necessary to address walled-off areas of infection. Thoroughly search for any foreign bodies.
II. Long-term antibiotic therapy
  A. Antibiotics are administered for at least 1 month beyond detectable evidence of *Nocardia* lesions.
  B. The antibiotic susceptibility patterns of *Nocardia* spp. vary.
  C. Drugs of choice are sulfadiazine 220 mg/kg initial dose, then 110 mg/kg PO BID, and trimethoprim/sulfadiazine 15–30 mg/kg PO, SQ BID.
III. Fluid therapy and nutritional support

Patient Monitoring

I. Cytology, radiology, and repeated cultures can be used to determine the duration of therapy; however, months of continuous therapy may be required.
II. The prognosis for complete, uncomplicated recovery from pyothorax or disseminated disease is guarded.

ACTINOMYCOSIS

Definition

I. Actinomycosis is a bacterial disease that infrequently causes subcutaneous abscesses, pyothorax, and/or other localized infections in dogs and cats.
II. Clinical features of actinomycosis are similar to those of nocardiosis, as discussed earlier.

Causes

I. *Actinomyces* spp. are gram-positive filaments that branch and break into coccobacilli; they are non-acid-fast and anaerobic or microaerophilic (Hardie, 1990).
II. These organisms are members of the order Actinomycetales.

III. *Actinomyces* spp. are often constituents of the normal oral microflora of dogs and cats.
IV. *A. viscosus* and *A. hordeovulneris* are the species isolated from dogs.

Pathophysiology

I. *Actinomyces* organisms enter through injured skin or may be inhaled or ingested.
II. Examples of clinical disease include pleuritis, pyothorax, septic arthritis, peritonitis, vertebral osteomyelitis, and cutaneous draining tracts or subcutaneous abscesses.

Clinical Signs

I. Signs vary, depending on the site of involvement.
II. With subcutaneous or skin infections, there is typically a history of a wound and a resultant nonhealing ulcerated lesion, draining fistulous tract, or subcutaneous abscess.
III. With pyothorax, respiratory distress and weight loss are usually present. Evidence of a penetrating thoracic wall injury may not be apparent.
IV. The disseminated form of actinomycosis is uncommon.

Diagnosis

I. The *Actinomyces* organisms can usually be demonstrated in exudates as gram-positive, non-acid-fast, branching filaments (Edwards et al., 1988).
II. Pleural effusion has a typical "cream of tomato soup" appearance. Sulfur granules (clumps of organisms) may or may not be present; when present, they are not diagnostic for actinomycosis.
III. Hematologic and serum chemistry findings are nonspecific and often reflect the degree of inflammation or organ dysfunction present.
IV. Isolation of the organism may be performed from exudate or sulfur granules on blood agar or plain Sabouraud's dextrose agar plates. Samples for culture are obtained and maintained under anaerobic conditions.

Differential Diagnosis

I. Other causes of draining skin lesions
II. Other causes of pyothorax, such as nocardiosis
III. Systemic fungal diseases

Treatment

I. Drainage and lavage of the infected site (see Nocardiosis, earlier)
II. Long-term antibiotic therapy for at least 1 month beyond detectable evidence of *Actinomyces* lesions
  A. The antibiotic susceptibility patterns of *Actinomyces* spp. vary.
  B. Typically, penicillins are considered first-choice drugs.
  C. Favorable clinical responses may be seen with

Table 111–1. *Other Bacterial Infections*

Disease	Organism	Species Affected	Clinical Significance	Treatment
Tuberculosis (Carpenter et al., 1988)	*Mycobacterium tuberculosis, M. bovis*	Dog, cat	*M. bovis* usually enters through the GI tract and most frequently results in subclinical infection. Clinical disease in *M. tuberculosis* results in respiratory signs.	Isoniazid, rifampin
Tyzzer's disease (Boschert et al., 1988; Myerslough, 1988)	*Bacillus piliformis*	Dog, cat	Dogs and cats are relatively resistant to infection. Young animals are infected most often. Infection may result in watery diarrhea and dehydration.	Tetracycline, penicillins, erythromycin

Streptococcal infection	Streptococcal groups A, B, C, G, L, M, D, E
	
	Groups B, G
		Dog
		
		Cat
			Group A: tonsils
			        B: urogenital
			        C: skin, genitourinary
			        G: tonsils, genital
			        L: genital
			        M: asymptomatic
			        D: asymptomatic
			        E: asymptomatic
				Penicillins, erythromycin, chloramphenicol, cephalexin

Atypical mycobacterial infection (Walsh and Losco, 1984; Monroe et al., 1988)	*Mycobacterium fortuitum, M. chelonei*	Cat, dog	Draining, poor-healing abscesses at wound penetration site and associated bacteremia. Occasionally associated with pneumonia (Turnwald et al., 1988).	Enrofloxacin, gentamicin, trimethoprim/sulfonamide; management of abscesses by surgical removal and drainage (Studdert and Hughes, 1992)
Botulism (VanNes, 1986)	*Clostridium botulinum*	Dog, cat	Ingestion of contaminated food or water that contains the exotoxin results in ascending flaccid paralysis beginning with hindlimbs.	Penicillins, amoxicillin/clavulanate, clindamycin
Bartonellosis (Groves et al., 1993; Koehler et al., 1994)	*Bartonella henselae*	Cat, dog	Cats are infected but asymptomatic. Humans have slow-healing wounds from bites or scratches, fever, lymphadenopathy, malaise, or headaches. Dogs develop bacteremia and endocarditis.	Antibiotic therapy in humans includes doxycycline, erythromycin, rifampin, penicillin, gentamicin, ceftriaxone, ciprofloxacin, and azithromycin (Maurin and Raoult, 1993)
Listeriosis	*Listeria monocytogenes*	Dog, cat	Infection after ingestion of contaminated foodstuffs results in fever, diarrhea, vomiting, and occasionally abortion and neurologic disease.	Penicillins, erythromycin, ampicillin, chloramphenicol, aminoglycosides, trimethoprim/sulfonamide
Anthrax	*Bacillus anthracis*	Dog, cat	Infection after ingestion of contaminated meat results in upper GI inflammation progressing to septicemia.	Penicillins; care in handling infected tissue is advised
Bite wound infection (Greene et al., 1990)	*Bacteroides* spp., *Fusobacterium* spp., *Pasteurella* spp.	Cat, dog	Bite wounds or contamination by oral fluids results in abscessation at bite wound site and/or bacteremia.	Penicillins, cephalosporins; management of wound sites and bacteremia
Helicobacter infection (Fox et al., 1995)	*Helicobacter pylori*	Cat, dog	Organisms have been isolated from the stomach of cats and dogs; probably results in gastric ulcers.	Combination therapy: clarithromycin/metronidazole, roxithromycin/amoxicillin, amoxicillin/metronidazole, tetracycline/metronidazole, amoxicillin/clarithromycin
Eugonic fermenter type 4 (EF-4) infection	Gram-negative bacterium	Dog, cat	Bite wounds or contamination by oral fluids results in abscessation at bite wound site and/or bacteremia.	Penicillins, cephalosporins; management of wound sites and bacteremia
Tularemia	*Francisella tularensis*	Dog, cat	Animals become infected by tick bites or by ingestion of infected rabbits or contaminated water. Infection results in fever, anorexia, lymphadenopathy, splenomegaly, icterus, abscesses, and hepatomegaly.	Gentamicin, tetracycline, chloramphenicol
Shigellosis	*Shigella* spp.	Dog	Becomes infected after consuming food or water contaminated by infected human/primate feces. Enterotoxins result in severe diarrhea and endotoxins in systemic manifestations.	Ampicillin, sulfonamides, tetracycline
L-form bacterial disease (Caro et al., 1989)	Cell wall deficit bacteria similar to mycoplasma	Dog, cat	L-form bacteria have been found in cats with fever, persistent draining tracts, spreading cellulitis of the extremities, and arthritis.	Tetracyclines, erythromycin, chloramphenicol

ampicillin, chloramphenicol, clindamycin, doxycycline, tetracycline, and erythromycin.

III. Fluid therapy and nutritional support are given as needed.

Patient Monitoring

I. Cytology, radiology, and repeated cultures can be used to determine the duration of therapy; however, months of continuous therapy may be required.

II. The prognosis for complete, uncomplicated recovery from pyothorax or systemic infections is poor.

OTHER BACTERIAL INFECTIONS

See Table 111–1.

Bibliography

Angulo AB: Lyme disease in cats. Southwest Vet 37:108, 1986

Appel MJG, Allan S, Jacobson RH et al: Experimental Lyme disease in dogs produces arthritis and persistent infection. J Infect Dis 167:651, 1993

Boschert KR, Allison N, Clair Allen TL et al: *Bacillus piliformis* in an adult dog. J Am Vet Med Assoc 192:791, 1988

Burgess EC: Experimentally induced infection of cats with *Borrelia burgdorferi.* Am J Vet Res 53:1507, 1992

Carpenter JL, Myers AM, Conner MW et al: Tuberculosis in five basset hounds. J Am Vet Med Assoc 192:1563, 1988

Caro T, Pedersen NC, Beaman BL et al: Subcutaneous abscesses and arthritis caused by a probable bacterial L-form in cats. J Am Vet Med Assoc 194:1583, 1989

Chomel BB, Jay MT, Smith CR et al: Serological surveillance of plague in dogs and cats, California, 1979–1991. Comp Immunol Microbiol Infect Dis 17:111, 1994

Dieringer TM, Wolf AM: Esophageal hiatal hernia and megaesophagus complicating tetanus in two dogs. J Am Vet Med Assoc 199:87, 1991

Dow SW, Jones RL, Henik RA et al: Clinical features of salmonellosis in cats: six cases (1981–1986). J Am Vet Med Assoc 194:1464, 1989

Edwards DF, Nyland TG, Weigel JP: Thoracic, abdominal, and vertebral actinomycosis: diagnosis and long-term therapy in three dogs. J Vet Intern Med 2:184, 1988

Eidson M, Thilsted JP, Rollag OJ: Clinical, clinicopathologic and pathological features of plague in cats: 119 cases (1977–1988). J Am Vet Med Assoc 200:1191, 1991

Fox JG, Batchelder M, Marini R et al: *Helicobacter pylori*–induced gastritis in the domestic cat. Infect Immun 63:2674, 1995

Greene CE, Lockwood R, Goldstein EJC: Bite and scratch infections. p. 614. In Greene CE (ed): Infectious Diseases of the Dog and Cat. WB Saunders, Philadelphia, 1990

Groves MG, Hoskins JD, Harrington KS: Cat scratch disease: an update. Compend Contin Educ Pract Vet 15:441, 1993

Hardie EM: Actinomycosis and nocardiosis. p. 585. In Greene CE (ed): Infectious Diseases of the Dog and Cat. WB Saunders, Philadelphia, 1990

Johnson CA, Walker RD: Clinical signs and diagnosis of *Brucella canis* infection. Compend Contin Educ Pract Vet 14:763, 1992

Koehler JE, Glaser CA, Tappero JW: *Rochalimaea henselae* infection: a new zoonosis with the domestic cat as a reservoir. JAMA 271:531, 1994

Levy SA, Dombach DM, Barthold SW et al: Canine Lyme borreliosis. Compend Contin Educ Pract Vet 15:833, 1993

Marino DJ, Jaggy A: Nocardiosis: a literature review with selected case reports in two dogs. J Vet Intern Med 7:4, 1993

Maurin M, Raoult D: Antimicrobial susceptibility of *Rochalimaea quintana, Rochalimaea vinsonii,* and the newly recognized *Rochalimaea henselae.* J Antimicrob Chemother 32:587, 1993

Monroe WE, August JR, Chickering WR et al: Atypical mycobacterial infections in cats. Compend Contin Educ Pract Vet 10:1044, 1988

Myerslough N: Tyzzer's disease in puppies. Vet Rec 122:238, 1988

Rentko VT, Ross LA: Canine leptospirosis. p. 260. In Kirk RW, Bonagura JD (eds): Current Veterinary Therapy XI: Small Animal Practice. WB Saunders, Philadelphia, 1992

Studdert VP, Hughes KL: Treatment of opportunistic mycobacterial infections with enrofloxacin in cats. J Am Vet Med Assoc 201:1388, 1992

Turnwald GH, Pechman RD, Turk JR et al: Survival of a dog with pneumonia caused by *Mycobacterium fortuitum.* J Am Vet Med Assoc 192:64, 1988

VanNes JJ: Electrophysiological evidence of peripheral nerve dysfunction in 6 dogs with botulism type C. Res Vet Sci 40:372, 1986

Walsh KM, Losco PE: Canine mycobacteriosis: a case report. J Am Anim Hosp Assoc 20:295, 1984

112

Mixed Infections

Johnny D. Hoskins

CANINE UPPER RESPIRATORY INFECTION COMPLEX

Definition

Any contagious respiratory disease of dogs that is manifested by coughing and is not caused by canine distemper is referred to as infectious tracheobronchitis or kennel cough.

Causes

I. Incriminated viruses include canine adenovirus-2 (CAV-2), parainfluenza (CPI), adenovirus-1 (CAV-1), canine reovirus-1, canine reovirus-2, canine reovirus-3, and canine herpesvirus. CAV-2 and CPI may damage the respiratory epithelium to such an extent that invasion by various bacteria and/or mycoplasmas results in severe airway disease.

II. Many different bacteria contribute to the clinical signs. *Bordetella bronchiseptica* (even in the absence of other pathogens) produces signs that are indistinguishable from other bacterial causes (Bemis, 1992).

III. *Pseudomonas, Escherichia coli, Klebsiella, Pasteurella, Streptococcus, Mycoplasma,* and other bacterial species are equally capable of causing signs of tracheobronchitis, but they may be opportunists.

Pathophysiology

I. The pathogenesis usually involves an initiating injury and/or viral infection of respiratory epithelium, followed by invasion of damaged tissue by bacterial organisms that results in further damage and clinical signs.

II. The most common bacterial isolate is *B. bronchiseptica* (Bemis, 1992).
   A. It may occur in dogs of all ages and often develops in the presence of preexisting subclinical airway disease such as congenital anomalies, chronic bronchitis, or bronchiectasis.
   B. It attaches to the cilia of the bronchial epithelium and produces stasis of the cilia.

C. It infects a number of animal species, but there is no evidence of cross-species transmission.

III. CPI is an important causative agent.
   A. The virus alone does not produce typical clinical signs, but it does cause subclinical bronchitis and bronchiolitis.
   B. If there is a concurrent infection with other agents, clinical signs are more pronounced.
   C. It is spread rapidly by aerosol exposure.

IV. CAV-2 may also be involved.
   A. CAV-2 produces mild pharyngitis, tonsillitis, and tracheobronchitis.
   B. Active viral shedding and rapid aerosol spread are limited to the first 8 days after exposure.

V. Several other viruses have also been incriminated.
   A. Canine herpesvirus has been associated with respiratory disease in older puppies and adults.
      1. Dogs >3 weeks of age develop mild respiratory signs when infected.
      2. The virus is activated by stress and is difficult to transmit between dogs.
   B. Canine reoviruses have been sporadically isolated, but their importance in this complex is questionable.

VI. The role of *Mycoplasma* is uncertain.
   A. *Mycoplasma* may be part of the normal microflora of the upper respiratory tract of dogs (Bemis, 1992).
   B. Although its role is not scientifically understood, *Mycoplasma* seems to contribute to the clinical signs.

Clinical Signs

I. Signs are related to the degree of respiratory tract damage and the age of the affected dog. They may range from an uncomplicated cough to severe, life-threatening pneumonia (Ford and Vaden, 1990).

II. Typically, there is a history of possible exposure at a pet shop, animal shelter, research or veterinary facility, or boarding or training kennel.

III. Uncomplicated tracheobronchitis is usually a mild, self-limiting infection, with a duration of 5–14 days.

A. A dry and hacking, soft and dry, moist and hacking, or paroxysmal cough is prominent, followed by gagging or expectoration of mucus.
B. If untreated, dry coughs may become moist during the course of the disease.
C. Excitement, exercise, changes in temperature or humidity of the inspired air, or gentle pressure on the trachea induce a paroxysm of coughing.
D. Serous nasal or ocular discharges are unusual.
E. Except for coughing, the dog usually appears to be healthy.
IV. Severe tracheobronchitis presents as an entirely different disease.
A. Constant low-grade or fluctuating fever and anorexia may be present.
B. Coughing is often less apparent and, if present, is moist and productive.
C. Within 24–48 hours, a serous nasal discharge is present, and the discharge rapidly becomes mucoid or mucopurulent.
D. Other clinical signs may include lethargy, dyspnea, and exercise intolerance.
E. Lung sounds may be normal, but an increased intensity of normal lung sounds, crackles, or, less frequently, wheezes may be detected.
F. Severe, life-threatening pneumonia is usually seen in puppies that are 6 weeks to 6 months old.
G. *B. bronchiseptica* infection or canine distemper virus may be associated with these more serious cases.

Diagnosis

I. Diagnosis is based on a typical history of exposure to infected dogs 5–10 days before acute development of clinical signs and supportive physical examination findings.
II. Hematologic findings are variable.
A. Although an early mild leukopenia may be present that coincides with the onset of coughing, it does not occur often, nor does it persist for more than 2–3 days.
B. A neutrophilic leukocytosis with a left shift is frequently found with severe pneumonia.
III. Serum chemistry profile and urinalysis are usually normal.
IV. In most cases of uncomplicated disease, thoracic radiography is unremarkable and of value primarily for ruling out noninfectious causes of a cough.
A. Thoracic radiographs may show an interstitial and alveolar lung pattern with a cranioventral distribution (typical of bacterial pneumonia), a diffuse interstitial lung pattern (typical of viral pneumonia), or a mixed lung pattern (typical of secondary bacterial pneumonia).
B. In *B. bronchiseptica* infection, the radiographic changes tend to be characteristic of bacterial pneumonia.
V. If severe infectious tracheobronchitis is suspected, transtracheal washing or tracheobronchial lavage via bronchoscopy is done. The antibiotic sensitivity pattern of cultured bacteria aids in providing effective treatment.

Differential Diagnosis

The diagnosis is established provisionally by eliminating noninfectious causes of coughing.

Treatment

I. Outpatient therapy is recommended for uncomplicated disease. All treatments are given at home after the initial examination is completed.
A. Enforced rest for at least 14–21 days or until radiographic evidence of pneumonia has subsided
B. Suppression of dry, nonproductive cough with butorphanol 0.05–0.1 mg/kg PO BID–TID or hydrocodone bitartrate 0.22 mg/kg PO BID-QID
II. Inpatient therapy is recommended for dogs with complicated tracheobronchitis and/or pneumonia (Padrid, 1992).
A. Antibiotic therapy is recommended if pneumonia or systemic signs are present.
1. Amoxicillin/clavulanate (11–22 mg/kg PO TID) or trimethoprim/sulfonamide (15–30 mg/kg PO, SQ, IV BID) is appropriate for initial therapy.
2. In severe cases, gentamicin (2–4 mg/kg IV, IM, SQ BID-TID) or amikacin (5–7.5 mg/kg IV, IM, SQ BID-TID) and a first-generation cephalosporin (cefazolin 15–30 mg/kg IV, IM TID) or enrofloxacin (5–10 mg/kg PO, IV, SQ BID) are effective if used in combination (Hoskins and Taboada, 1994).
3. Ideally, the choice of antibiotic is based on culture and sensitivity results from a transtracheal washing or tracheobronchial lavage via bronchoscopy.
B. Adequate hydration is maintained.
1. Steam or cold mist vaporizers may provide supportive care.
2. Airway hydration can be maximized if nebulization is done for 15–30 minutes TID with normal saline solution.
C. Bronchodilators may be indicated.
D. Rest is enforced for at least the duration of radiographic evidence of pneumonia.
E. Nutritional support is provided by forced feeding or other feeding means, depending on the general health of the animal.

Patient Monitoring and Prevention

I. Isolate the affected dog from other animals. Infected dogs can transmit the agent(s) before the onset of clinical signs and until immunity is established.
II. Affected dogs with uncomplicated disease usually respond within 10–14 days.
A. In severe cases, thoracic radiography is repeated weekly until at least 7 days beyond complete resolution of lung lesions.

B. The typical course of severe disease is 2–6 weeks.
III. Once the disease spreads in a kennel, it can be controlled by evacuation of the kennel for 1–2 weeks and disinfection with sodium hypochlorite (1:30 dilution), chlorhexidine, or benzalkonium.
IV. Immunoprophylaxis involves the following.
   A. Both intranasal and parenteral vaccines are marketed for control of the primary agents.
      1. Inactivated whole cell *B. bronchiseptica* vaccine can cause pain at the injection site but not systemic signs.
      2. Avirulent live strains of *B. bronchiseptica* for intranasal vaccination are available alone or in combination with attenuated parainfluenza virus.
   B. Vaccination is performed with parenteral vaccines at least 10 days before anticipated exposure; with intranasal vaccines, at least 72 hours before exposure.
   C. Puppies 2–4 weeks of age or older are vaccinated intranasally without interference from maternal antibody, followed by annual revaccination. Mature dogs can receive a one-dose intranasal vaccination at the same time as their puppies or at the time they receive their annual vaccinations.
   D. Duration of immunity varies for different agents.
      1. *B. bronchiseptica* immunity lasts for >6 but <14 months.
      2. CPI immunity lasts for at least 2 years.
      3. CAV-2/CAV-1 vaccination probably induce a lifetime immunity.
   E. Vaccination protects against clinical disease but not infection, and it will not stop the spread of infection between dogs.
V. Minimizing transmission is difficult.
   A. Whenever feasible, unvaccinated dogs should be quarantined before entering a breeding establishment.
   B. Adequate ventilation (12–15 air changes per hour) must be maintained in all areas housing multiple dogs.
   C. Avoid excessive moisture, and disinfect with sodium hypochlorite (1:30 dilution), chlorhexidine, or benzalkonium.

FELINE UPPER RESPIRATORY INFECTION COMPLEX

Definition

Any contagious upper respiratory disease of cats that is manifested by oculonasal discharge and sneezing is considered to be part of the feline upper respiratory infection complex.

Causes

I. There are several causative agents.
   A. Feline rhinotracheitis virus (herpesvirus)
   B. Feline calicivirus
   C. *Chlamydia psittaci* (Wills et al., 1988)
   D. *Bordetella bronchiseptica* (McArdle et al., 1994)
   E. *Mycoplasma* spp. and reoviruses
II. Feline rhinotracheitis virus and feline calicivirus account for approximately 85–90% of the feline upper respiratory infection complex.

Pathophysiology

I. Mode of transmission is by direct contact between susceptible cats and infected cats or contact with contaminated fomites.
   A. Transmission may occur via upper respiratory secretions produced by sneezing cats (can travel a maximum distance of 4 feet).
   B. The most common method of spread appears to be by fomites such as hands, feeding/water bowls, litter pans, clothing, and cages.
II. Most cats develop a carrier state after acute natural infection with feline rhinotracheitis virus, feline calicivirus, and *C. psittaci.*
   A. Clinical signs in carrier cats may be inapparent or extremely subtle, e.g., persistent sneezing and/or oculonasal discharge in an otherwise healthy cat.
   B. Calicivirus is shed continuously from the oropharynx of carrier cats.
   C. Rhinotracheitis virus and *C. psittaci* are shed intermittently from the oropharynx and conjunctiva, respectively, particularly after stressful events.
   D. Several days of close contact appear to be necessary for a carrier cat to infect a susceptible cat.
III. Natural immunity exists.
   A. Immunity after natural infection is of short duration (approximately 3–4 months).
   B. The duration of maternal immunity to rhinotracheitis virus is 2–10 weeks of age; for calicivirus, it is 10–14 weeks of age; and for *C. psittaci,* it is 6–8 weeks of age.
IV. *B. bronchiseptica* infection appears to be more common in multicat households with a history of respiratory disease (Jacobs et al., 1993).
V. The role of mycoplasmas or reoviruses in feline respiratory disease is not clear.

Clinical Signs

I. Typical clinical signs include the following.
   A. Fever and depression may be present.
   B. Sneezing and coughing rarely occur.
   C. Serous to mucopurulent oculonasal discharge is usually present.
   D. Reluctance to eat, oropharyngeal vesicles/ulcers, and hypersalivation are often present in severe cases.
   E. Dehydration and weight loss occur.
II. Upper respiratory signs are more severe in kittens and immunosuppressed cats.
III. Feline rhinotracheitis virus, calicivirus, and chlamydial infection can cause ocular disease with or without accompanying respiratory signs.

IV. Cats with histories of prolonged or intermittent sneezing, mucopurulent nasal discharge, and gingivitis may be chronic carriers.
V. Typical clinical signs of *B. bronchiseptica* infection include fever, sneezing, nasal discharge, mandibular lymphadenopathy, spontaneous or induced cough, and increased lung sounds on auscultation.

Diagnosis

I. Diagnosis is usually based on history and clinical signs.
II. Identification of the specific causative agent is difficult.
  A. Causative agents cannot be differentiated based solely on clinical signs.
  B. Identification is indicated for a recurrent problem in a cattery or multicat household or in an individual cat with recurrent signs.
III. Isolation procedures via cell culture are available for feline rhinotracheitis virus, calicivirus, and the chlamydial agent.
  A. Virus isolation and identification from nasal, ocular, or oropharyngeal swabs may be tried from samples collected within 1 week of the onset of signs.
  B. *Chlamydia* isolation and identification from a firmly taken conjunctival swab may be tried from samples collected within 1 week of the onset of signs.
    1. Giemsa-stained conjunctival smears may show basophilic cytoplasmic inclusions that are most numerous in the first 4–7 days of clinical disease.
    2. Either immunofluorescence or histochemical stains can be used to confirm or identify cytoplasmic inclusions in cell cultures or conjunctival scrapings.
IV. Paired serum samples may be submitted for titers 2 weeks apart; a fourfold rise in titer is considered diagnostic.
V. Bacterial culture can be done.
  A. Bacterial cultures of nasal or ocular discharge are rarely of diagnostic value, as it is difficult to differentiate pathogens from normal microflora.
  B. Bacterial culture for *B. bronchiseptica* is best done from a pharyngeal swab and/or tracheobronchial lavage via bronchoscopy (Willoughby et al., 1991).

Differential Diagnosis

The diagnosis is established provisionally by eliminating noninfectious causes of sneezing and other upper respiratory signs.

Treatment

I. Supportive care is the most important aspect (Hawkins, 1988).
  A. Cats capable of eating and maintaining normal hydration are best treated on an outpatient basis.
    1. Keep the eyes and nares free of discharge.
    2. Humidify the upper airway with a steam or cold-mist vaporizer or confinement to a bathroom with the shower running.
    3. Provide a warm, well-ventilated, well-lighted environment and good nutritional support.
  B. Cats with hypersalivation caused by oropharyngeal vesicles or ulcers usually require hospitalization for fluid therapy and assisted feeding.
    1. Administer polyionic isotonic fluids supplemented with potassium chloride (dosage is based on serum potassium concentration) IV, SQ, or PO.
    2. Feed a liquid diet by means of intermittent nasogastric or gastric tube, or via a continuous indwelling nasogastric tube.
II. Antibiotics are recommended for the secondary bacterial infections that cause complications.
  A. Give ampicillin or amoxicillin 10–22 mg/kg PO BID-TID as the initial choice.
  B. Give doxycycline 2.5–5 mg/kg PO BID as a second choice.
  C. Give chloramphenicol 25 mg/kg PO BID-TID only if cats are still eating.
III. Pregnant queens with *C. psittaci* infections may be treated with erythromycin 10–15 mg/kg PO TID or tylosin 25 mg PO TID.
IV. If ocular involvement is present, topical ophthalmic preparations are indicated (see Chap. 94).
V. If *B. bronchiseptica* infection is present, doxycycline is the drug of choice.

Patient Monitoring and Prevention

I. Immunoprophylaxis
  A. Although vaccination does not provide complete protection from the clinical disease or prevention of the carrier state, timely spaced vaccinations are recommended with attenuated or inactivated rhinotracheitis virus and calcivirus vaccine.
    1. Parenteral and intranasal products are available.
    2. Vaccination is recommended at 8–12 and 14–16 weeks of age, followed by annual revaccination.
    3. Protection with parenteral vaccine usually takes 3–4 weeks, whereas the intranasal vaccine may show protection within 4 days.
  B. Vaccination against *C. psittaci* is not recommended for individual cats because of the low incidence of this agent in single-cat households. The use of *C. psittaci* vaccine in catteries and research facilities is advisable.
  C. Vaccination against *B. bronchiseptica* using the current canine products is not recommended for individual cats.
II. Prevention
  A. Control of spread within a veterinary hospital or cattery requires management practices that reduce transmission via direct contamination or fomites.

B. House all cats in separate cages with solid partitions at least 4 feet apart.

C. Clean cages thoroughly with a virucidal agent and leave vacant for 2 days, if possible. An excellent virucidal product is sodium hypochlorite (household bleach diluted 1:32), and it is applied to the contaminated surface for at least 10 minutes.

D. Ventilation providing at least 12 air changes per hour is recommended.

E. Disposable food and water bowls and litter pans are used, or appropriate disinfection procedures are followed (e.g., cleaned in dishwasher or autoclaved).

F. Change clothing after handling infected cats, and wash hands thoroughly.

Bibliography

Bemis DA: *Bordetella* and *Mycoplasma* respiratory infection in dogs. Vet Clin North Am [Small Anim Pract] 22:1173, 1992

Ford RB, Vaden SL: Canine infectious tracheobronchitis. p. 259. In Greene CE (ed): Infectious Diseases of the Dog and Cat. WB Saunders, Philadelphia, 1990

Hawkins EC: Chronic viral upper respiratory disease in cats: differential diagnosis and management. Compend Contin Educ Pract Vet 10:1003, 1988

Hoskins JD, Taboada J: Specific treatment of infectious causes of respiratory disease in dogs and cats. Vet Med May:443, 1994

Jacobs AAC, Chalmers WSK, Pasman J et al: Feline bordetellosis: challenge and vaccine studies. Vet Rec 133:260, 1993

McArdle HC, Dawson S, Coutts AJ et al: Seroprevalence and isolation rate of *Bordetella bronchiseptica* in cats in the UK. Vet Rec 135:506, 1994

Padrid P: Chronic lower airway disease in the dog and cat. Prob Vet Med 4:320, 1992

Willoughby K, Dawson S, Jones MRC et al: Isolation of *B. bronchiseptica* from kittens with pneumonia in a breeding cattery. Vet Rec 129:407, 1991

Wills JM, Howard PE, Gruffydd-Jones TJ et al: Prevalence of *Chlamydia psittaci* in different cat populations in Britain. J Small Anim Pract 29:327, 1988

113

Rickettsial Infections

Thomas N. Hribernik
Johnny D. Hoskins

EHRLICHIOSIS

Definition

I. Canine ehrlichiosis is a worldwide tick-borne infectious disease.
II. Although several *Ehrlichia* species may infect the dog, ehrlichiosis is generally attributed to *E. canis* infection.

Causes

I. The causative organism is the obligate intracellular parasite *E. canis.*
II. Transmission occurs primarily via the brown dog tick *(Rhipicephalus sanguineus)* or rarely vis-à-vis transfusion of infected blood.
III. Other *Ehrlichia* species may also cause disease.
   A. *E. platys* causes an infectious cyclic thrombocytopenia (see later).
   B. *E. equi* may infrequently cause naturally occurring disease.
   C. *E. risticii* may infrequently cause naturally occurring disease.
   D. *E. ewingii* is frequently associated with lameness in dogs.
   E. *E. chaffeensis,* an ehrlichial species of humans, may also infrequently cause naturally occurring disease in dogs.

Pathophysiology

I. Three phases have been recognized experimentally.
   A. Acute phase lasts 2–4 weeks.
      1. Replication in infected mononuclear cells
      2. Hematogenous spread to multiple organs
      3. Vasculitis from dissemination, particularly in microvasculature
      4. Nonregenerative anemia, leukopenia, and/or thrombocytopenia
      5. Mildly elevated liver enzymes
      6. Mildly decreased serum albumin
   B. Subclinical phase may last for an extended period (occasionally years).
      1. Associated with organism persistence and antibody production
      2. Variety of laboratory abnormalities, including those seen in acute phase
   C. Chronic phase represents an ineffective immune response by the host.
      1. Severity of the disease appears to be related to breed susceptibility, age, concomitant disease, and host immunocompetence.
      2. Mild chronic disease may have the same abnormalities as described for the acute phase.
      3. Severe chronic disease, seen particularly in the German shepherd dog, may have profound bone marrow hypoplasia and organ system failure, with or without sepsis.
II. It is difficult to distinguish the various phases on a clinical basis.
III. Pathologic findings are variable.
   A. Petechiae and ecchymoses
   B. Lymphadenopathy, splenomegaly, and hepatomegaly
   C. Bone marrow hyperplastic to hypoplastic
   D. Lymphoplasmacytic infiltrate of some organs
   E. Evidence of sepsis in severe chronic disease

Clinical Signs

I. Clinical and subclinical infections may occur.
II. The most common clinical findings are as follows.
   A. Depression, lethargy, and anorexia
   B. Weight loss
   C. Fever
   D. Pale mucous membranes
   E. Lymphadenopathy and splenomegaly
   F. Bleeding tendencies: petechiae, ecchymoses, epistaxis
   G. Vomiting
   H. Anterior and/or posterior uveitis

I. Neurologic abnormalities such as ataxia, seizures, vestibular dysfunction, generalized or localized hyperesthesia
J. Lameness associated with joint pain
K. Peripheral edema
L. Signs of specific organ failure (e.g., kidney and liver)

Diagnosis

I. Definitive diagnosis is made in several ways.
   A. Positive indirect immunofluorescence test (most commonly used)
   B. Western immunoblotting assay
   C. Polymerase chain reaction (PCR) assay
   D. Demonstration of organisms within mononuclear cells (seldom possible)
II. Evidence of the following clinical and/or laboratory abnormalities in endemic areas raises suspicion for the disease.
   A. Thrombocytopenia, nonregenerative anemia, and/or leukopenia
   B. Hyperproteinemia, hyperglobulinemia, hypoalbuminemia
   C. Polyclonal gammopathy; monoclonal gammopathy on occasion
   D. Mildly to moderately elevated alanine aminotransferase (ALT) and serum alkaline phosphatase (SAP), hyperbilirubinemia occasionally
   E. Azotemia, proteinuria occasionally
   F. Altered coagulation tests (e.g., prolonged activated clotting time [aCT], prolonged one-stage prothrombin time [OSPT], prolonged activated partial thromboplastin time [aPTT], and elevated fibrin-fibrinogen degradation products [FDPs])
   G. Hyperplastic to hypoplastic bone marrow
   H. Elevated protein and mononuclear pleocytosis in cerebrospinal fluid
   I. Positive blood cultures in severe chronic disease

Differential Diagnosis

I. Rocky Mountain spotted fever
II. Other causes of fever of undetermined origin, thrombocytopenia, nonregenerative anemia, leukopenia, lymphadenopathy, and splenomegaly

Treatment

I. Medical therapy
   A. Tetracycline 22 mg/kg PO TID for 14–21 days
      1. Occasionally longer (months) in small number of animals that show disease recrudescence
      2. IV therapy if vomiting present
   B. Doxycycline 5–10 mg/kg PO BID for 10–21 days
      1. IV therapy if vomiting present
      2. May result in lower incidence of relapse
   C. Chloramphenicol 15–25 mg/kg PO TID for 14–21 days
      1. IV therapy if vomiting present
      2. Used in puppies <5 months of age

3. May be more effective than tetracycline in eliminating infection
   D. Imidocarb dipropionate 5 mg/kg IM, single injection (not licensed in the United States)
      1. Highly efficacious
      2. Possible lower relapse rate than with tetracycline
II. Supportive therapy
   A. Fluid therapy for dehydrated animals and those in renal failure
   B. Blood transfusion in severely anemic animals
   C. Broad-spectrum bactericidal antibiotics for septic animals
   D. Tick control (e.g., dipping of animals and premise spraying with approved pesticides)

Patient Monitoring

I. Animals afflicted with less than severe chronic disease usually show a positive response within 48–72 hours.
II. Severe, chronically infected animals tend to have a poor response to therapy and a poor prognosis.
III. Recovered animals are apparently susceptible to reinfection.
IV. Tetracycline may be administered at 6.6 mg/kg PO SID prophylactically for at least 6 months in endemic areas.

INFECTIOUS CYCLIC THROMBOCYTOPENIA

Definition and Causes

I. This is an infectious disease of dogs with low morbidity and insignificant mortality.
II. The etiologic agent is the obligate intracellular parasite *E. platys.*
III. Natural mode of transmission probably involves ticks.
IV. Co-infection with *E. canis* may be seen.

Pathophysiology

I. Experimentally, organisms parasitize platelets, resulting in intermittent thrombocytopenia, at 1- to 2-week intervals.
II. Thrombocytopenia may be the result of direct injury of platelets and/or immune-mediated mechanisms.
III. Generalized lymphadenopathy is the only gross morphologic finding.
IV. Histologic lesions are generally confined to lymphoid hyperplasia, plasmacytosis, and Kupffer's cell hyperplasia in the liver.

Clinical Signs

I. Clinical signs are often lacking.
II. Co-infection with *E. canis* or other *Ehrlichia* species gives rise to signs attributable to ehrlichiosis.

III. There is occasional evidence of bleeding (e.g., epistaxis, petechiation).
IV. Anterior uveitis has been observed.

Diagnosis

I. Demonstration of organisms within platelets on stained blood smears
II. Serology, using indirect fluorescent antibody techniques

Differential Diagnosis

I. *E. canis* infection
II. Other causes of thrombocytopenia (see Chaps. 66 and 67) and uveitis (see Chap. 97)

Treatment

I. Tetracycline 22 mg/kg PO TID for 14 days
II. Chloramphenicol 15–25 mg/kg PO TID for 14 days
III. Treatment for uveitis as outlined in Chap. 97
IV. Tick control with dipping of animals and spraying of premises with approved pesticides

Patient Monitoring

Most animals have a dramatic response to specific and supportive care.

ROCKY MOUNTAIN SPOTTED FEVER

Definition

I. Rocky Mountain spotted fever (RMSF) is a tick-borne, infectious disease of the dog found throughout the United States, with the highest prevalence occuring in the eastern regions.
II. It has also been observed in portions of Canada, Mexico, and several Central and South American countries.

Causes

I. The etiologic agent is the obligate intracellular parasite *Rickettsia rickettsii.*
II. Transmission occurs via the bite of an infected tick *(Dermacentor variabilis* or *Dermacentor andersoni).*

Pathophysiology

I. Entry into the circulatory system results in invasion and replication of the organism in endothelial cells of small vessels.
II. Resultant vasculitis can cause alterations in the coagulation system, edema formation, and various organ system dysfunctions or failures.
III. Common pathologic findings include evidence of hemorrhage (petechiae, ecchymoses), lymphadenopathy, splenomegaly, and necrotizing vasculitis.
IV. *R. rickettsii* is not detected by routine histologic staining methods.
V. The infective dose of rickettsiae, and perhaps breed predisposition, may play a role in determining the severity of illness.

Clinical Signs

I. Clinical and subclinical infections may occur.
II. Purebred dogs, particularly the German shepherd dog and Siberian husky, appear to be more prone to clinical illness.
III. It is most commonly observed from March to October.
IV. The course of illness is generally short (<2 weeks) in symptomatic animals.
V. Signs may reflect widespread organ involvement.
   A. Fever: early and consistent finding in acute cases
   B. Anorexia, depression, weight loss, and dehydration
   C. Lameness from joint and/or muscle pain
   D. Vomiting and/or diarrhea
   E. Ocular and/or nasal discharges
   F. Dyspnea, cough
VI. The following are often detected on physical examination.
   A. Fever
   B. Petechiae and/or ecchymotic hemorrhages of the skin and/or mucous membranes
   C. Peripheral edema
   D. Retinal hemorrhages
   E. Lymphadenopathy, splenomegaly, hepatomegaly
   F. Neurologic signs, including paresthesia, ataxia, vestibular signs, stupor, seizures, and coma
   G. Dyspnea, cough
   H. Evidence of dermal necrosis

Diagnosis

I. Clinical signs alone do not allow differentiation from other rickettsial and nonrickettsial diseases.
II. Seasonal occurrence, particularly March to October, is suggestive.
III. Hematologic findings may include thrombocytopenia, leukopenia to leukocytosis, and anemia.
IV. Potential biochemical abnormalities are hypoalbuminemia, elevated SAP, ALT, and aspartate aminotransferase (AST), hypocalcemia, hypercholesterolemia, hyponatremia, hypochloremia, metabolic acidosis, hyperbilirubinemia, and elevated serum urea nitrogen and creatinine.
V. Cerebrospinal fluid analysis may reveal mildly elevated protein and increased numbers of neutrophils or mononuclear cells.
VI. Synovial fluid analysis often shows a neutrophilic inflammatory response.
VII. Prolonged aCT, aPPT, and OSPT and elevated FDPs are occasionally observed.
VIII. The diagnosis may be confirmed by direct immunofluorescence (DIF) testing for *R. rickettsii* in skin

biopsies or serologic testing using microscopic immunofluorescence (Micro-If) methodology.
  A. DIF testing is not readily available, and prior treatment for 48–72 hours may result in false-negatives.
  B. Micro-IF measuring IgG usually requires a four-fold or greater increase in titers over 2–3 weeks to document infection. Markedly increased single titers ($\geq$1:1024 in East; $\geq$1:256 in West) may indicate active infection.
  C. Micro-IF measuring IgM permits more specific diagnosis of recent infection with a single convalescent titer (Greene and Breitschwerdt, 1990).

Differential Diagnosis

  I. Ehrlichiosis
  II. Other causes of thrombocytopenia, fever of unknown origin, splenomegaly, lymphadenopathy, and any of the other signs seen with RMSF

Treatment

  I. Tetracycline 22 mg/kg PO TID for 7–14 days, IV therapy when vomiting or coma is present
  II. Chloramphenicol 15–25 mg/kg PO TID for 7–14 days, IV therapy when vomiting or coma is present
  III. Doxycycline 5–10 mg/kg PO BID for 7 days, IV therapy when vomiting or coma is present
  IV. Enrofloxacin 5–10 mg/kg PO BID for 7–14 days, IV therapy when vomiting or coma is present
  V. Antibiotics most successful if given before advanced pathologic changes
  VI. Supportive care (e.g., judicious use of balanced electrolyte fluid therapy for shock, dehydration, or renal failure, or blood transfusion in severely anemic animals)
  VII. Tick control (e.g., dipping of animals and spraying of premises with approved pesticides, safe removal of attached ticks manually)

Patient Monitoring

  I. A rapid response to therapy (24–48 hours) is noted in most animals.
  II. Antibiotics are most successful if given before advanced pathologic changes.
  III. RMSF may be fatal if left untreated.
  IV. Recovered dogs are immune to reinfection for at least 6–12 months.

SALMON POISONING DISEASE

Definition and Causes

  I. It is a frequently fatal helminth-transmitted disease of wild and domestic Canidae seen most commonly on the western slopes of the Cascade Mountains from northern California to central Washington State.
  II. The etiologic agent is *Neorickettsia helminthoeca*.

  III. The vector is *Nanophyetus salminocola,* a trematode that can infest salmonid fish and certain nonsalmonids.

Pathophysiology

  I. Ingestion of raw, metacercariae-infected fish leads to adult fluke development in the small intestine.
  II. Adult flukes attach to the intestinal mucosa and release the rickettsiae by unknown mechanisms.
  III. Rickettsial replication initially occurs in the intestine, with subsequent spread to the lymph nodes, tonsils, thymus, spleen, liver, lungs, and brain.
  IV. Lymphadenopathy with lymphoid hyperplasia and foci of necrosis, splenomegaly, and hemorrhagic enteritis often occur.

Clinical Signs

  I. Signs usually develop 5–7 days after ingestion of infected fish.
  II. Fever is noted initially, with the temperature gradually decreasing to normal or subnormal levels over the following 4–10 days.
  III. Anorexia, depression, vomiting, dehydration
  IV. Diarrhea, particularly with blood
  V. Nasal and ocular discharges
  VI. Generalized lymphadenopathy

Diagnosis

  I. Demonstration of operculated trematode eggs on fecal examination increases the index of suspicion for salmon poisoning disease.
  II. Fine-needle aspiration biopsies of enlarged lymph nodes may reveal the presence of intracytoplasmic rickettsial bodies.
  III. Hematologic and biochemical findings are generally nonspecific in nature.

Differential Diagnosis

  I. Canine distemper
  II. Canine parvovirus-2 infection
  III. Ehrlichiosis
  IV. Other causes of lymphadenopathy, splenomegaly, hemorrhagic enteritis, and fever of undetermined origin

Treatment

  I. Treatment initiated early in the course of disease markedly improves the chances for survival.
  II. Medical therapy includes the following.
    A. Tetracycline 22 mg/kg PO TID for 3–5 days, IV route preferable in vomiting animals
    B. Praziquantel 10–30 mg/kg PO, SQ once is highly effective against fluke infestation; given when tetracycline treatment has been completed
  III. Provide supportive care (e.g., IV balanced electrolyte solutions when dehydration exists, and exogenous heat sources for hypothermic animals).

Patient Monitoring

I. If treated early, most animals survive, but if left untreated, the disease is often fatal.
II. It can be prevented by prohibiting dogs from eating raw fish in endemic areas.
III. Freezing or thorough cooking of fish kills both the metacercariae and the rickettsiae.

HAEMOBARTONELLOSIS

Definition and Causes

I. Haemobartonellosis is a rickettsial disease of cats and, to a lesser extent, dogs that results in an anemia.
II. *Haemobartonella felis* and *Haemobartonella canis* are the epicellular rickettsial parasites of erythrocytes that infect the cat and dog, respectively.
III. Transmission in the cat is by several ways.
  A. Most commonly via blood-sucking arthropods
  B. Queen to offspring: exact mechanism unknown
  C. Transfusion of infected blood
IV. Transmission in the dog is thought to be primarily by the brown dog tick *(Rhipicephalus sanguineus).*

Pathophysiology

I. Feline haemobartonellosis
  A. Regenerative anemia develops after extravascular erythrophagocytosis by macrophages in the spleen, liver, lungs, and bone marrow.
  B. Immune-mediated mechanisms against erythrocytes may also play a role in anemia development.
  C. Parasitemias can be cyclic and of short duration.
  D. Icterus may develop because of hemolysis.
  E. Death results in one third of untreated cases.
  F. Recovered animals are probably infected for life.
  G. Stress, debilitating conditions, or immunosuppression may reactivate acute episodes of the disease.
  H. Parasites may be observed occasionally in normal animals.
II. Canine haembartonellosis
  A. The disease seldom occurs in nonsplenectomized or immunocompetent animals.
  B. Hemolytic anemia caused by extravascular hemolysis may occur in splenectomized or immunosuppressed animals.

Clinical Signs

I. Dogs are usually asymptomatic unless splenectomized or immunosuppressed.
II. Signs in cats are related to hemolysis.
  A. Anorexia, depression, weakness, pyrexia, weight loss
  B. Pale mucous membranes, splenomegaly, icterus
  C. Acute collapse, dyspnea, potentially death

Diagnosis

I. Detection of the parasite in blood smears is necessary to confirm the diagnosis.
II. Absence of the organism does not rule out the disease, particularly in cats.
III. Clinicopathologic findings include the following.
  A. Regenerative anemia
  B. Neutrophilic leukocytosis, hyperbilirubinemia, bilirubinuria
  C. Hypoglycemia in moribund animals
  D. ± Direct Coombs' test
  E. ± Positive for feline leukemia virus and feline immunodeficiency virus

Differential Diagnosis

Consider all potential causes of regenerative anemia, as described in Chap. 63.

Treatment

I. Doxycycline 5–10 mg/kg PO BID for 10–14 days
II. Oxytetracycline
  A. Cats 20 mg/kg PO TID for 3 weeks
  B. Dogs 22–40 mg/kg PO TID for 3 weeks
III. Chloramphenicol in dogs: 15–25 mg/kg PO TID for 2–3 weeks
IV. Enrofloxacin 5 mg/kg PO BID for 10–14 days
V. Prednisolone to severely anemic animals at 2.2 mg/kg PO, tapered gradually; possible helpful in some animals being treated concurrently with the preceding antibiotics (Harvey, 1990b).
VI. Supportive care, particularly blood transfusions for severely anemic animals
VII. Control of blood-sucking arthropods

Patient Monitoring

I. Hemogram is checked periodically for response.
II. Monitor for drug-induced fever in cats receiving tetracyclines and switch to enrofloxacin or chloramphenicol if its occurs.
III. Educate the owner that once infected, parasitemia and clinical signs may occur throughout life with stress or other illnesses.

Bibliography

Comer KM: Rockey Mountain spotted fever. Vet Clin North Am [Small Anim Pract] 21:27, 1991
Gorham JR, Foreyt WJ: Salmon poisoning disease. p. 397. In Greene CE (ed): Infectious Diseases of the Dog and Cat. WB Saunders, Philadelphia, 1990
Greene CE, Breitschwerdt EB: Rocky Mountain spotted fever and Q fever. p. 419. In Greene CE (ed): Infectious Diseases of the Dog and Cat. WB Saunders, Philadelphia, 1990
Harvey JW: Ehrlichia platys infection (infectious cyclic thrombocytopenia of dogs). p. 415. In Greene CE (ed): Infectious Diseases of the Dog and Cat. WB Saunders, Philadelphia, 1990a
Harvey JW: Haemobartonellosis. p. 434. In Greene CE (ed): Infectious Diseases of the Dog and Cat. WB Saunders, Philadelphia, 1990b

Hoskins JW: Canine haemobartonellosis, canine hepatozoonosis, and feline cytauxzoonosis. Vet Clin North Am [Small Anim Pract] 21:129, 1991

Iqbal Z, Chaichanasiriwithaya W, Rikihisa Y: Comparison of PCR with other tests for early diagnosis of canine ehrlichiosis. J Clin Microbiol 32:1658, 1994

Iqbal Z, Rikihisa Y: Reisolation of *Ehrlichia canis* from blood and tissues of dogs after doxycycline treatment. J Clin Microbiol 32:1644, 1994

Troy GC, Forrester SD: Canine ehrlichiosis. p. 404. In Greene CE (ed): Infectious Diseases of the Dog and Cat. WB Saunders, Philadelphia, 1990

Woody BJ, Hoskins JD: Ehrlichial diseases of dogs. Vet Clin North Am [Small Anim Pract] 21:75, 1991

114

Protozoal Infections

Michael R. Lappin

ENTERIC PROTOZOAL INFECTIONS

Giardiasis

Definition and Causes

I. Giardiasis is a gastrointestinal syndrome caused by a protozoan parasite that infects many vertebrates, including dogs, cats, and people.
II. The genus *Giardia* contains multiple species of flagellated protozoans that are indistinguishable morphologically.
III. Host specificity is minimal for *Giardia* spp.

Pathophysiology

I. Epidemiology
   A. Distribution is worldwide, with a wide host range.
   B. The organism exists in the gastrointestinal tract as a motile trophozoite or a nonmotile cyst.
      1. Trophozoites live in the upper small intestine of dogs and the lower small intestine of cats.
      2. Trophozoites are more common in diarrheic stools and are not environmentally resistant.
      3. Cysts form in the cecum of dogs, are common in both normal and diarrheic stools, and can survive in the environment for days to weeks. They are considered immediately infective.
II. Transmission
   A. Primarily from exposure to cysts from fecal–oral contact or exposure to cysts on fomites or in contaminated water
   B. Ingestion of trophozoites in diarrheic stools or paratenic hosts
   C. Prepatent period
      1. Dog: 5–12 days, mean = 8 days
      2. Cat: 5–16 days, mean = 10 days
III. Pathogenesis
   A. After oral exposure to cysts, gastric and duodenal secretions trigger release of trophozoites.
   B. Parasites inhibit host enzymatic actions and cause rapid sloughing of microvillus cells, resulting in malabsorption.
   C. Virulence differences among strains of *Giardia* may determine the development of clinical disease, and immunologic responses to the organism may potentiate clinical signs.
   D. Host immune status may help determine the development of clinical disease.
   E. Animals housed in groups are more likely to have *Giardia* infections.

Clinical Signs

I. Subclinical infections are common; infection may also be self-limited in 27–35 days.
II. Acute small bowel diarrhea that is occasionally watery and accompanied by borborygmus is common.
III. Chronic small bowel diarrhea may also occur.
   A. Greasy, semiformed diarrhea
   B. Evidence of weight loss or poor weight gain
   C. Continuous or intermittent clinical signs
IV. Large bowel diarrhea is uncommon, but mixed bowel diarrhea can occur.
V. Vomiting or fever is uncommon.

Diagnosis

I. Direct smear of feces may demonstrate trophozoites.
II. Direct saline preparations may demonstrate trophozoites.
   A. Phase-contrast or darkfield microscopy is superior to bright-field microscopy.
   B. Trophozoite motion is erratic.
   C. Addition of 1 drop of iodine to the specimen immobilizes the trophozoites and stains them for easier identification.
III. Fecal flotation with zinc sulfate centrifugal flotation technique (specific gravity of 1.18–1.20) is the optimal technique for the demonstration of cysts. Sugar and other salt solutions lead to distortion of cysts.
IV. Formalin–ethyl acetate sedimentation is the best technique for demonstration of cysts in steatorrheic stools.
V. Endoscopic or peroral string sampling of duodenal

secretions for trophozoites can be performed but is not applicable in the cat because of the mid to distal small bowel location of the parasite.

VI. Cysts are shed intermittently, and their presence does not correlate to clinical signs of disease. At least three stool specimens are examined every other day.

VII. Enzyme-linked immunosorbent assay (ELISA) for detection of *Giardia* antigens in stool may have false-positive and false-negative reactions.

Differential Diagnosis

I. Other causes of acute small bowel diarrhea, intermittent chronic small bowel diarrhea, steatorrhea, protein-losing enteropathies, weight loss, and failure to grow, including pancreatic exocrine insufficiency, gastrointestinal helminth infections, and inflammatory bowel diseases

II. Rarely, causes of large bowel diarrhea or mixed bowel diarrhea

III. Other enteric protozoal infections (Table 114–1)

A. Differentiation of *Giardia* trophozoites from *Pentatrichomonas hominis* trophozoites

B. Differentiation of *Giardia* cysts from coccidian oocysts

Treatment

I. Dog treatment options include the following.
   A. Metronidazole 15–25 mg/kg PO BID for 8 days
   B. Fenbendazole 50 mg/kg PO SID for 3–7 days
   C. Albendazole 25 mg/kg PO BID for 2–7 days
   D. Quinacrine 9 mg/kg PO SID for 6 days; gastrointestinal irritation common
   E. Tinidazole 44 mg/kg PO SID for 3 days
   F. Ipronidazole 126 mg/L of water PO ad libitum for 7 days

II. Cat treatment options include the following.
   A. Metronidazole 10–25 mg/kg PO SID-BID for 5–7 days; treatment of choice
   B. Furazolidone 4 mg/kg PO BID for 7–10 days; not to be used in pregnancy

Table 114–1. Enteric Protozoal Infections

Disorder	Organism[a]	Species Affected	Transmission	Clinical Signs	Diagnosis	Therapy
Giardiasis	*Giardia* spp.	Dog, cat	Fecal–oral cysts and trophozoites Ingestion of paratenic hosts	Small, large, or mixed bowel diarrhea	See text	See text
Trichomoniasis	*Pentatrichomonas hominis*	Dog, cat	Fecal–oral trophozoite only	Subclinical Rarely, large bowel diarrhea	Direct smear of feces Direct saline preparation of feces	Metronidazole Dog: 15–30 mg/kg PO SID-BID for 5–7 days Cat: 10–25 mg/kg PO SID-BID for 5–7 days
Amebiasis	*Entamoeba histolytica*	Dog, cat	Fecal–oral trophozoite only	Rare in the dog and cat Large bowel diarrhea Extraintestinal disease is rare	Direct smear of feces Staining of fecal smears Biopsy demonstration of organism Fecal flotation fails because of lack of cysts	As for trichomoniasis
Balantidiasis	*Balantidium coli*	Dog	Fecal–oral cysts or trophozoites Cysts are directly infectious	Large bowel diarrhea Extraintestinal infection is rare	Direct saline preparation of feces Acidic methyl green staining of fecal smear Zinc sulfate centrifugal flotation	As for trichomoniasis
Enteric coccidiosis	*Cystoisospora* spp. *Besnoitia* spp. *Hammondia* spp. *Sarcocystis* spp. Only *Cystoisospora* spp. pathogenic for dogs and cats	Dog, cat See Table 114–2	Fecal–oral contact with sporulated oocysts Ingestion of paratenic hosts See text	Small, large, or mixed bowel diarrhea See text	Fecal flotation and identification of oocysts	See text
Cryptosporidiosis	*Cryptosporidium parvum*	Dog, cat	Fecal–oral contact with oocysts	Small bowel diarrhea predominant sign Occasional large bowel diarrhea and vomiting	See text	See text
Toxoplasmosis	*Toxoplasma gondii*	Cat	See text	No clinical signs with enteroepithelial cycle	See text	See text

[a]See Table 114–2 for description of the identifying features of enteric protozoal infections.

C. Quinacrine 11 mg/kg PO SID for 12 days
D. Fenbendazole 50 mg/kg PO SID for 3–7 days; efficacy unknown
E. Albendazole 25 mg/kg PO BID for 2–7 days; efficacy unknown

III. Treatment failures may be common.

IV. Combination metronidazole and quinacrine therapy may resolve some resistant infections.

V. Because clinical signs induced by *Giardia* spp. can be intermittent and because giardiasis may be zoonotic, subclinically infected animals should be treated.

VI. Metronidazole also kills *Pentatrichomonas, Balantidium,* and *Entamoeba.*

Patient Monitoring

I. Resolution of clinical signs usually occurs within 7 days.

II. Because cyst shedding can be intermittent, it is difficult to use fecal flotation results to predict a cure.

III. Prevention involves boiling or filtering water collected from the environment before drinking and disinfecting premises contaminated with infected feces with quaternary ammonium compounds.

IV. In resistant or recurrent cases, evaluate for other underlying disorders such as inflammatory bowel diseases, exocrine pancreatic insufficiency, bacterial overgrowth, and immunodeficiency.

Enteric Coccidiosis

Definition

I. Coccidiosis is a common parasitism of dogs and cats.

II. Clinical signs of disease are rare but may include small, large, or mixed bowel diarrhea.

Causes

I. Coccidian parasites with an enteric life cycle include *Cystoisospora, Besnoitia, Hammondia, Sarcocystis, Cryptosporidium,* and *Toxoplasma* (Tables 114–1 and 114–2).

II. Dogs and cats are the definitive hosts for these genera and as such shed oocysts in feces.

III. Only *Cystoisospora, Toxoplasma,* and *Cryptosporidium* are known pathogens in dogs and cats.

IV. Clinical disease associated with a *Sarcocystis*-like organism has been described in a dog (Dubey et al., 1991).

V. Although dogs and cats are the definitive hosts for *Besnoitia, Hammondia,* and *Sarcocystis,* clinical disease generally develops only in the intermediate hosts.

Pathophysiology

I. Epidemiology
 A. *Cystoisospora* spp. have a worldwide distribution.
 B. Oocysts are passed unsporulated. Sporulation occurs within 8 hours.

C. Once ingested, sporozoites are released and penetrate the intestinal mucosa.

D. Some sporozoites initiate the production of schizonts and meronts (asexual reproduction), culminating in the production of gamonts, sexual reproduction, and oocyst production.

II. Transmission
 A. Sporulated oocysts
 B. Ingestion of infected paratenic hosts
  1. Primarily mammals; the mouse for *Cystoisospora felis*
  2. Monozoic cyst formation in extraintestinal tissues, primarily lymphoid tissues
  3. Monozoic cyst development in the definitive host: possible source of repeat gastrointestinal tract infection
 C. Variable prepatent periods (5–11 days) for different species of *Cystoisospora*

III. Pathogenesis
 A. Asexual and sexual reproduction in the gastrointestinal tract generally is a subclinical infection.
 B. Clinical disease in immunocompetent animals may result because of co-infection with other infectious agents.
 C. Clinical disease is more common in puppies and kittens younger than 6 months of age.
 D. Coccidial infections are seen most commonly in group situations.
 E. Exacerbation of disease may occur during stressful periods.

Clinical Signs

I. Small, large, or mixed bowel diarrhea

II. Occasional vomiting, dehydration, depression, anorexia, and weight loss

III. Most animals subclinically infected

Diagnosis

I. Oocyst identification can occur with any fecal flotation procedure.

II. The size of the oocyst can help identify the species of *Cystoisospora* (see Table 114–2).

Differential Diagnosis

I. All causes of small, large, or mixed bowel diarrhea, including infectious diseases such as parvoviruses and coronaviruses, inflammatory bowel diseases, obstructive enteropathies, and gastrointestinal helminth infections, must be considered.

II. *Eimeria* spp. oocysts can pass through the gastrointestinal tract of dogs and cats after the ingestion of feces or intestinal content of rodents and herbivores.

Treatment

I. Treatment of clinically ill animals is indicated.

II. Supportive care is administered as needed.

III. Dog treatment options include the following.

Table 114–2. **Identifying Features of Enteric Protozoal Infections**

Organism	Class	Fecal Form	Size (μm)
Giardia	Flagellate	Trophozoite	$15 \times 10 \times 3$
		Cyst	10×8
Pentatrichomonas hominis	Flagellate	Trophozoite	$5–20 \times 3–14$
Entamoeba histolytica	Amoeba	Trophozoite	10–30
		Cyst	5–20
Balantidium coli	Ciliate	Trophozoite	60×35
		Cyst	50
Cystoisospora spp.	Coccidian		
Cat			
C. felis		Oocyst	30×40
C. rivolta		Oocyst	20×25
Dog			
C. canis		Oocyst	30×38
C. ohioensis		Oocyst	19×23
C. neorivolta		Oocyst	11×13
C. burrowsi		Oocyst	17×20
Sarcocystis spp.	Coccidian		
Cat			
S. hirsuta		Oocyst	12×8
S. tenella		Oocyst	12×8
S. porcifelis		Oocyst	13×8
S. muris		Oocyst	10×8
S. leporum		Oocyst	13×10
Dog			
S. cruzi		Oocyst	16×11
S. capracams		Oocyst	—
S. ovicanis		Oocyst	15×10
S. miescheriana		Oocyst	13×10
S. bertrami		Oocyst	15×10
S. fryeri		Oocyst	12×8
S. hemionilatrantis		Oocyst	14×9
S. idiciukeicabus		Oocyst	11×15
Hammondia spp.	Coccidian		
Cat			
H. hammondi		Oocyst	12×11
Dog			
H. heydorni		Oocyst	11×12
Besnoitia spp.	Coccidian		
Cat			
B. besnoiti		Oocyst	15×13
B. wallacei		Oocyst	17×12
B. darlingi		Oocyst	12×12
Cryptosporidium spp.	Coccidian	Oocyst	3–6
Toxoplasma gondii	Coccidian	Oocyst	10×12

A. Trimethoprim-sulfonamide 15 mg/kg PO SID-BID for 5 days
B. Sulfadimethoxine/ormetroprim (55 mg/kg sulfadimethoxine and 11 mg/kg ormetroprim) PO SID for up to 23 days
C. Sulfadimethoxine 50–60 mg/kg PO once, then 25 mg/kg PO SID for 5–20 days
D. Furazolidone 4–10 mg/kg PO SID-BID for 5 days
E. Amprolium 200 mg total dose PO SID for 5 days
F. Quinacrine, spiramycin, toltrazuril, and roxithromycin used on a limited basis
IV. Cat treatment options include the following.
  A. Trimethoprim-sulfonamide 15 mg/kg PO SID-BID for 5 days

B. Sulfadimethoxine 50–60 mg/kg PO once, then 25 mg/kg PO SID for 5–20 days
C. Furazolidone 4–10 mg/kg PO SID-BID for 5 days
D. Amprolium 60–100 mg total dose PO SID for 5 days

Patient Monitoring

I. Clinical signs usually resolve within several days after initiation of drug therapy.
II. Most infections are self-limiting.
III. Clinical disease is not associated with the extraintestinal phase.
IV. Sanitation is the most important form of prevention.

A. Avoid fecal contamination of food and water dishes.
B. Incinerate feces.
C. Steam clean runs, cages, and dishes.
D. Alternatively, clean with 5% ammonium solutions.
V. Avoid contact with intermediate hosts.
VI. Control mechanical vectors, such as flies.
VII. Anticoccidial drugs can be administered to infected bitches after whelping.
VIII. Sulfonamides can cause macrocytic anemia, keratoconjunctivitis sicca, type III hypersensitivity reactions (primarily Doberman pinschers), and acute hepatic necrosis.
IX. Amprolium can cause anorexia, diarrhea, depression, and central nervous system (CNS) signs caused by induction of thiamine deficiency.

Cryptosporidiosis

Definition and Causes

I. Cryptosporidiosis is an acute or chronic gastrointestinal syndrome usually caused by *Cryptosporidium parvum.*
II. Cross-infection between mammals occurs, but reptile and avian species do not infect mammals.

Pathophysiology

I. Epidemiology
A. There is a high seroprevalence, suggesting that the organism infects animals commonly.
B. Infection occurs primarily in the ileum.
C. Life cycle is as follows.
1. After exposure to oocysts, parasitophorous vacuoles form on the microvillus surface, and asexual and sexual reproduction occurs, resulting in the production of oocysts by days 3–8 after infection.
2. Thick-walled oocysts are excreted in feces, whereas thin-walled oocysts excyst in the intestinal tract, infecting other cells (autogenous reinfection).
II. Fecal–oral transmission
A. Fecal contamination of food or drinking water is common.
B. Very few oocysts are required to induce infection.
III. Pathogenesis
A. It is unknown whether pathogenesis is related to parasite-derived effects or immune responses against the parasite.
B. Microvillus enzyme systems are attenuated.
C. Malabsorption may occur secondary to blunting of microvillus.
D. Clinical disease is less severe in immunocompetent individuals than in immunosuppressed individuals.
E. Concurrent infections with other gastrointestinal pathogens can accentuate clinical illness.

Clinical Signs

I. Cats
A. Small, large, or mixed bowel diarrhea
B. Anorexia, weight loss, and dehydration
II. Dogs
A. Clinical disease described infrequently
B. Persistent diarrhea
C. Dyspnea, lymphocytic-plasmacytic enteritis, and malabsorption syndromes, rarely

Diagnosis

I. Fecal examination
A. Oocysts are approximately 5 μm in diameter and thus are very difficult to identify. Phase-contrast microscopy is superior for evaluation of unstained samples.
B. Mix one part 100% formaline with nine parts liquefied feces to inactivate the oocysts.
C. Sheather's sugar centrifugation is the optimal flotation procedure for the demonstration of oocysts.
D. Direct smears of feces followed by staining procedures may aid in the identification of oocysts.
1. Kinyoun's modified carbolfuchsin
2. Crystal violet
3. Acid-fast staining using dimethyl sulfoxide (DMSO)
4. Fluorescein-labeled monoclonal antibody
II. Alternative procedures for the detection of infection include ELISA for fecal antigens, laboratory animal inoculation of feces, and intestinal biopsy.
III. Evaluation for *Cryptosporidium* is performed on all animals with chronic diarrhea, in particular, those that are immunocompromised.

Differential Diagnosis

I. Rule out other causes of acute or chronic small, large, or mixed bowel diarrhea and malabsorption syndromes, including inflammatory bowel diseases, gastrointestinal helminth infections, obstructive enteropathies, and infectious diseases, including parvoviruses and coronaviruses.
II. Oocysts must be differentiated from yeast and fat droplets.

Treatment

I. Infection of immunocompetent animals is usually self-limited, and only supportive care is needed.
II. Paromomycin 125–165 mg/kg PO BID for 5 days is effective in dogs and cats, but repeated treatments may be necessary.
III. Tylosin 11 mg/kg PO BID for 28 days has blocked oocyst shedding in some cats.

Patient Monitoring

I. Monitor for resolution of clinical signs of disease and cessation of oocyst shedding.

II. Cryptosporidiosis is a common zoonosis. People are infected primarily from calves with diarrhea, but infection has also been documented after exposure to infected cats and dogs.

III. The following protocols have been shown to inactivate oocysts.

A. 10% formalin for 18 hours

B. 5% ammonia solution for 18 hours

C. 50% ammonia solution for 30 minutes

D. Steam cleaning

E. Freezing

F. Thorough drying

EXTRAINTESTINAL PROTOZOAL DISEASES

Babesiosis

Definition

Babesiosis of dogs and cats is caused by protozoans that parasitize red blood cells, leading to progressive anemia.

Causes

I. Dogs

A. *Babesia gibsoni*: single, annular bodies, 1×3.2 μm

B. *B. canis*: paired, piriform bodies, 2.4×5.0 μm; 3 subspecies

1. *B. canis vogeli*

2. *B. canis canis*

3. *B. canis rossi*

II. Cats

A. *B. cati*: 1×2.5 μm

B. *B. felis*: single or paired annular bodies, 1×2.3 μm

C. *B. herpailuri*: single or paired piriform bodies, 1.3×3.4 μm

D. *B. pantherae*: 1.2×2.2 μm

Pathophysiology

I. Epidemiology and distribution

A. Dogs

1. *B. canis*: worldwide, including Africa, Asia, Australia, Europe, Central America, South America, Japan, and the United States; *B. canis vogeli* is the primary subspecies in the United States

2. *B. gibsoni*: United States, Japan, India, Sri Lanka, Korea, Malaysia, and Egypt

3. *B. vogeli*: Africa and Asia

B. Cats

1. *B. cati*: India

2. *B. felis*: South Africa and Sudan

3. *B. herpailuri*: South America and Africa

4. *B. pantherae*: Kenya

C. Most canine cases in the United States: Gulf coast states, south-central and southwestern states, except for individual epizootics in Massachusetts, Pennsylvania, and New Jersey

II. Transmission

A. The primary vectors in dogs are ticks.

1. *B. canis: Rhipicephalus sanguineus, Dermacentor* spp., *Haemaphysalis leachi,* and *Hyalomma plumbeum*

2. *B. gibsoni: Haemaphysalis bispinosa* and *R. sanguineus*

3. *B. vogeli: R. sanguineus*

B. The vector(s) of the species infecting cats is unknown.

C. Ticks transmit *Babesia* while taking a blood meal.

D. Ticks transmit *B. canis* and *B. gibsoni* transstadially and transovarially.

E. Transmission can occur transplacentally and by blood transfusion.

III. Pathogenesis

A. The tick must feed 2–3 days for transmission to occur.

B. The incubation period varies from 10 days to 3 weeks.

C. Organisms replicate by binary fission in erythrocytes, leading to hemolytic anemia.

D. Acute disease is primarily an intravascular hemolysis with resultant hemoglobinemia, hyperbilirubinemia, hemoglobinuria, and bilirubinuria.

E. Infected animals are commonly Coombs-positive, but it is unknown to what extent red blood cell breakdown is caused by immune-mediated events.

F. Hypoxia induced by severe anemia can induce disseminated intravascular coagulation.

G. The *Babesia* spp. infecting cats produce similar clinical signs of disease, but there appears to be strain differences in virulence.

H. Severity of clinical disease appears to be dependent on the immune status of the host.

I. Chronic infections occur with the organism maintained in the body in a quiescent state by host immune reactions (premunition).

Clinical Signs

I. Dogs

A. Subclinical, hyperacute, acute, chronic, and atypical infections occur (Taboada, 1995).

B. History may reveal the following.

1. Depression, anorexia, and weakness; acute death in hyperacutely infected puppies

2. Variable history of stress, immunosuppressant drug administration, or splenectomy

3. History of tick exposure frequently unknown

C. Physical examination findings are frequently nonspecific.

1. Elevated body temperature

2. Pale mucous membranes

3. Occasional petechiation, icterus, hepatosplenomegaly

D. Chronically infected dogs commonly have intermittent fever, weight loss, and anorexia.

E. Atypical cases can present with ascites, gastrointestinal or neurologic signs, peripheral edema,

and clinical evidence of cardiopulmonary disease.
II. Cats
   A. Usually young
   B. History of anorexia, weakness, depression, increased respiratory rate, diarrhea, and rough haircoats
   C. Pale mucous membranes, tachycardia, and tachypnea (common)
   D. Fever and icterus (unusual)

Diagnosis

I. Hematologic findings
   A. Regenerative hemolytic anemia in dogs, macrocytic hypochromic anemia in cats
   B. Occasional thrombocytopenia, particularly with *B. gibsoni*
   C. Occasional demonstration of the organism with Wright's or Giemsa's stain; blood from ear vein or toenail increases odds of organism identification
II. Chemistry abnormalities
   A. Metabolic acidosis and azotemia
   B. Polyclonal gammopathy and renal casts
   C. Bilirubinemia, bilirubinuria
   D. Hemoglobinuria
   E. Increased activities of alanine transaminase (ALT), aspartate transaminase (AST), and creatine kinase (CK)
III. Serology with immunofluorescent antibody (IFA) assay
   A. There is cross-reactivity between *B. canis* and *B. gibsoni,* but some IFA tests may differentiate (Yamane et al., 1993).
   B. Titers ≥1:80 are generally considered positive.
   C. False-negative results can occur in peracute cases, immature dogs, and immunosuppressed dogs.
IV. Inoculation of suspect blood into a splenectomized dog
V. Identification of species important for therapeutic selection (see later)
VI. Diagnosis usually based on a combination of clinical findings, history, clinical laboratory findings, and positive serology

Differential Diagnosis

I. Other causes of hemolytic anemia (in particular, immune-mediated hemolytic anemia), thrombocytopenia, and disseminated intravascular coagulopathy
II. *Haemobartonella canis*
III. *Haemobartonella felis* and *Cytauxzoon felis* (Table 114-3)

Treatment

I. Dogs
   A. Diminazene aceturate
      1. Effective for *B. canis* and *B. gibsoni*
      2. 10% solution: 3.5 mg/kg IM once

3. Pain at injection site, weakness, tremors, polyneuritis, and paralysis possible; encephalomalacia and CNS hemorrhage with overdose
      4. Clinical response usually within 2–3 days, with resolution of anemia in 2–3 weeks
      5. Unavailable in the United States
      6. Relapses possible
   B. Phenamidine isethionate
      1. Effective for *B. canis* and *B. gibsoni*
      2. 5% solution: 15 mg/kg SQ SID for 2 days
      3. Nausea, vomiting, abscess formation at injection site, CNS hemorrhage, and relapses possible
      4. Available in the United States
   C. Imidocarb dipropionate
      1. Effective for *B. canis*
      2. Dose: 2–6 mg/kg SQ or IM once
      3. Transient salivation, diarrhea, dyspnea, lacrimation, and depression possible (usually responsive to atropine)
      4. Variable responses (0–90%)
      5. Unavailable in the United States
   D. Clindamycin
      1. Possibly effective
      2. Used if other drugs not available
      3. Dose: 25 mg/kg PO divided BID for 2–3 weeks
   E. Glucocorticoids contraindicated
   F. Potentially effective drugs
      1. Tetracyclines
      2. Metronidazole 25–65 mg/kg PO daily for 2–3 weeks for *B. gibsoni*
II. Cats: primaquine phosphate
   A. Effective for *B. felis*
   B. Dose: 0.5 mg/kg PO or IM once
   C. Vomiting common; death with dosages ≥1 mg/kg
   D. Unavailable in the United States
III. Supportive care: blood transfusion, sodium bicarbonate therapy for acidosis, and fluid therapy

Patient Monitoring

I. Because of the variable effect of drug therapy, some animals need repeated treatments.
II. Failure to respond to drug therapy may indicate other underlying disease, in particular, *E. canis* infection.
III. Tick control in the environment is indicated.
IV. There is no current evidence to suggest that *Babesia* spp. infecting dogs and cats can cause human disease.

Leishmaniasis
Definition

Leishmaniasis is a group of cutaneous, mucocutaneous, and visceral diseases of dogs, people, and other mammals.

Causes

I. *Leishmania* spp. are flagellates that have a life cycle involving both a vertebrate and an invertebrate host.

Table 114–3. Extraintestinal Protozoal Infections

Disorder	Organism	Class	Species Affected	Transmission	Clinical Signs	Diagnosis	Therapy
Acanthamebiasis	Acanthamoeba castellani A. culbertsoni	Amoeba	Dog	Unknown	Similar to canine distemper virus Fever, oculonasal discharge, cough, anorexia, ataxia, seizures	Culture Histopathology Laboratory data nonspecific	Unknown in dogs Sulfonamides effective in mice
Babesiosis	Babesia spp. See text	Piroplasmia	Dog, cat	Tick vector Transplacentally Blood transfusion See text	See text	See text	See text
Cytauxzoonosis	Cytauxzoon felis	Piroplasmia	Cat	Unknown, but likely tick-borne—Dermacentor variabilis	Fever, anorexia, dyspnea, depression, icterus, pale mucous membranes, death	Regenerative anemia Leukocytosis and thrombocytopenia Parasitized red blood cells Definitive diagnosis based on demonstration of the organism in red blood cells or in macrophages in the bone marrow, spleen, liver, or lymph nodes	Parvaquone 15–30 mg/kg IM, SQ SID for 2–3 days Buparvaquone 10 mg/kg IM, SQ Thiacetarsamide 0.1 mg/kg IV BID for 2 days Variable response; generally fatal
Leishmaniasis	Leishmania spp. See text	Flagellate	Dog, cat	Sandflies	Multiple See text	Primarily on organism demonstration See text	See text
American trypanosomiasis	Trypanosoma cruzi	Flagellate	Dog, cat	Reduviid bugs (kissing bugs) Blood transfusions Ingestion of infected tissues Congenital Infected milk	Reported only in the dog Acute: lymphadenopathy, myocarditis Chronic: dilatative cardiomyopathy	Thoracic radiographs Electrocardiography, echocardiography Laboratory abnormalities nonspecific Definitive diagnosis based on organism demonstration, culture, laboratory animal inoculation, and serology	Nitrofurtimox 2–7 mg/kg PO QID for 3–5 mo Benzimidazole 5 mg/kg PO SID for 2 mo Treat heart failure and arrhythmias as needed

Disease	Organism	Type	Host	Transmission	Clinical Signs	Diagnosis	Treatment
Hepatozoonosis	*Hepatozoon canis*	Coccidian	Dog, cat	Ingestion of *Rhipicephalus sanguineous*; Ingestion of infected tissues	Dog: subclinical, fever, weight loss, anorexia, hyperesthesia, diarrhea; Cat: depression, cholangiohepatitis; See text	See text	See text
Encephalitozoonosis	*Encephalitozoon cuniculi*	Microspora	Dog, cat	Oronasal contact with urine infected with spores	Dogs: stunted growth, signs of renal failure, depression, seizures, blindness; Cats: depression, paralysis, superficial corneal infection, generalized muscle spasms	Laboratory abnormalities are nonspecific. Immunochemical identification of spores in urine is definitive. Serologic tests can document exposure.	No known effective therapy. Fumagillin, an antibiotic, has been tried but is toxic to dogs and cats.
Pneumocystosis	*Pneumocystis carinii*	Unknown	Dog, cat	Direct transfer from animal to animal	Primarily subclinical. Weight loss and dry cough common. See text	Organism demonstration. See text	See text
Neosporosis	*Neospora caninum*	Coccidian	Dog, cat	Oral ingestion of tachyzoites and cysts; Transplacental	Ascending paralysis and extensor rigidity. See text	Organism demonstration. Serology. See text	See text
Toxoplasmosis	*Toxoplasma gondii*	Coccidian	Dog, cat	Sporulated oocyst ingestion; Ingestion of tachyzoites or tissue cysts	Enteroepithelial cycle is subclinical. Multiple syndromes seen with extraintestinal cycle. See text	See text	See text

II. Diseases in humans induced by *Leishmania* spp. have been divided by geographic location into New World leishmaniasis and Old World leishmaniasis, as well as by clinical manifestation of disease into cutaneous, mucocutaneous, and visceral forms.

III. Human leishmaniasis has several causes.
  A. Old World leishmaniasis
    1. Cutaneous: *L. tropica* complex
    2. Mucocutaneous: rare disease
    3. Visceral: *L. donovani* complex
  B. New World leishmaniasis
    1. Cutaneous: *L. mexicana* complex and *L. braziliensis* complex
    2. Mucocutaneous: *L. braziliensis* complex
    3. Visceral: *L. donovani* complex

IV. Dogs are major reservoir hosts for many Old World and New World *Leishmania* spp.
  A. Old World leishmaniasis
    1. Cutaneous: *L. tropica* complex
    2. Visceral: *L. donovani* complex and *L. tropica* complex
  B. New World leishmaniasis
    1. Cutaneous: *L. donovani* complex and *L. braziliensis* complex
    2. Mucocutaneous: *L. braziliensis* complex
    3. Visceral: *L. donovani* complex

V. Clinically affected cats in Texas were infected by *L. mexicana* (Craig et al., 1986; Barnes et al., 1993).

Pathophysiology

I. Epidemiology and transmission
  A. Sand flies (*Phlebotomus* spp. and *Lutzomyia* spp.) are the vectors.
  B. Rodents and dogs are primary reservoirs; people and cats are probably incidental hosts.
  C. Amastigotes (nonflagellated, 2.5–5 μm × 1.5–2 μm) form in macrophages in the vertebrate host and are available to the sand fly via cutaneous lesions.
  D. Promastigotes (flagellated) form in the sand fly and are injected into the vertebrate host when the sand fly feeds.
  E. Some cases of canine leishmaniasis in the United States have been in animals transported from other endemic areas.

II. Pathogenesis
  A. After initiation of infection by sand fly bites, promastigotes are engulfed by macrophages, and disseminated infection occurs.
  B. The incubation period is 1 month to 7 years.
  C. Because the organism is intracellular, the humoral and cell-mediated immune responses are extreme, leading to polyclonal gammopathy, proliferation of macrophages, histiocytes, and lymphocytes in lymphoreticular organs, and immune complex formation and deposition, especially in the glomerulus, uvea, and synovium.
  D. Protective immunity is cell-mediated; if T-lymphocyte function is poor, disseminated disease occurs.

Clinical Signs

I. Dogs
  A. Primarily visceral involvement, with approximately 90% having nonpruritic cutaneous manifestations
  B. Dermal signs
    1. Hyperkeratosis, scaling, thickening of the skin, mucocutaneous ulcers, and occasional intradermal nodules are the most prominent lesions.
    2. The muzzle, pinna of the ears, and footpads are the most common locations (see Chap. 84).
  C. Visceral clinical signs and findings
    1. Weight loss in the face of a normal to increased appetite
    2. Polyuria, polydipsia
    3. Muscle wasting, depression
    4. Vomiting, diarrhea, melena
    5. Cough, epistaxis, sneezing
    6. Splenomegaly, lymphadenopathy
    7. Fever, icterus, hepatomegaly
    8. Uveitis, keratitis, conjunctivitis
    9. Polyarthritis
II. Cats
  A. Usually subclinically infected
  B. Cutaneous nodules on the ear pinna and muzzle

Diagnosis

I. Laboratory abnormalities
  A. Hyperglobulinemia, hypoalbuminemia, proteinuria
  B. Increased liver enzymes, azotemia
  C. Thrombocytopenia, lymphopenia, and leukocytosis with left shift
  D. Anemia; occasional positive direct Coombs' test or antinuclear antibody test
  E. Increased numbers of lymphocytes and neutrophils in synovial fluid
II. Definitive diagnosis
  A. Organism identification
    1. Wright- or Giemsa-stained lymph node aspirate, bone marrow aspirate, or skin imprints
    2. Histopathologic, immunoperoxidase, or polymerase chain reaction (Ashford et al., 1995) evaluation of skin or organ biospy
  B. Culture of the organism from skin lesions or tissue aspirates
  C. Inoculation of hamsters with material from skin biopsy
  D. Serologic testing
    1. Multiple types of tests are available.
    2. A true-positive test indicates infection, because dogs are unlikely to eliminate infection.
    3. IgG titers develop 14–28 days after infection and decline 45–80 days after treatment.

Differential Diagnosis

Rule out other causes of focal dermatitis, splenomegaly, immune-complex disease, polyclonal gammopathy, weight loss, and muscle wasting, including immune-mediated diseases such as systemic lupus erythematosus, neoplasia, and infectious diseases such as *E. canis*.

Treatment

I. Administer meglumine antimonate 100 mg/kg IV or SQ SID for 3–4 weeks.
II. Alternatively, give sodium stibogluconate 30–50 mg/kg IV or SQ SID for 3–4 weeks.
III. Administer liposomal amphotericin B 3–3.3 mg/kg IV QOD for 3–5 treatments (Oliva et al., 1995).
IV. Administer ketoconazole 10 mg/kg PO TID for 3 weeks.
V. Administer allopurinol 20 mg/kg PO BID for up to 9 months (Ferrer et al., 1995).
VI. Prognosis varies; most cases are recurrent.
VII. Surgically excised cutaneous nodules usually recur.

Patient Monitoring

I. The presence of renal insufficiency usually denotes a poor prognosis.
II. In endemic areas, confine animals to the indoors during nighttime hours and control breeding places of sand flies with insecticides and moisture control.
III. A zoonotic potential exists both from the dog being a reservoir host and from direct contact with lesions (rare).

Hepatozoonosis

Definition and Causes

I. Hepatozoonosis is a polysystemic protozoal disease of dogs and cats that results in clinical signs including fever and hyperesthesia (see Table 114–3).
II. It is caused by *Hepatozoon canis* in dogs and *H. canis* or *Hepatozoon* spp. in cats.

Pathophysiology

I. Epidemiology and life cycle
   A. The disease occurs in Africa, southern Europe, Asia, and the United States, especially along the Texas Gulf coast and in Louisiana and Oklahoma.
   B. The vector is the brown dog tick, *R. sanguineus*.
   C. After ingestion of an infected tick or infected tissues, sporozoites are released that infect mononuclear phagocytes and endothelial cells of the spleen, liver, muscle, lungs, and bone marrow, leading to merogony.
   D. Cysts develop containing macromeronts and micromeronts. Micromeronts develop into micromerozoites, which develop into gamonts in leukocytes and are capable of infecting the invertebrate vector.
   E. Vertical transmission can occur (Murata et al., 1993)
II. Pathogenesis
   A. Susceptibility may be age dependent; it is more common in young animals.

B. Concurrent infections or immunosuppression worsens clinical disease.
C. Clinical disease is likely related to the pyogranulomatous response of the body to the tissue stages and to immune-complex formation and deposition.
D. The pyogranulomatous changes in muscles commonly lead to periosteal bone reactions.
E. Amyloidosis may occur secondary to chronic inflammation and immune-complex disease.

Clinical Signs

I. Most infected dogs are subclinically infected.
II. Most clinically affected dogs develop fever and weight loss.
III. Anorexia, anemia, depression, hyperesthesia over the paraspinal regions, oculonasal discharge, and bloody diarrhea are common.
IV. Fever and hyperesthesia are intermittent and recurrent.
V. Cholangiohepatitis caused by a parasite resembling *H. canis* was reported in a cat from Hawaii (Ewing, 1977).
VI. Fever (cat), weakness, and gametocytes in neutrophils were reported in two cats from Israel (Baneth et al., 1995).

Diagnosis

I. Laboratory abnormalities (nonspecific)
   A. Neutrophilic leukocytosis (20,000–200,000 cells/μl) with a left shift
   B. Eosinophilia, regenerative anemia
   C. Hypoalbuminemia, hypoglycemia, increased serum alkaline phosphatase
II. Radiographic changes
   A. Periosteal bone reaction may be found on most bones except the skull.
   B. Periosteal reactions are most common in young dogs, do not occur in every case, and are not pathognomonic.
III. Definitive diagnosis
   A. Identification of gamonts in neutrophils or monocytes in Giemsa- or Leishman-stained blood smears
   B. Identification of the organism in muscle biopsy sections
   C. Most dogs with gamonts in blood cells seropositive by IFA assay (Thkap et al., 1994).

Differential Diagnosis

Rule out other causes of fever, neutrophilic leukocytosis, muscle hyperesthesia, and periosteal bone reaction, including immune-mediated polyarthritis, immune-mediated myositis, neoplasia, and other infectious disease syndromes such as diskospondylitis.

Treatment

I. The following drugs are potentially useful for the treatment of dogs.

A. Diminazene aceturate 3.5 mg/kg IM once
B. Imidocarb dipropionate 5 mg/kg SQ once
C. Imidocarb dipropionate 5 mg/kg SQ once every 14 days combined with tetracycline 22 mg/kg PO TID for 14 days
D. Primaquine phosphate 0.5 mg/kg SQ once
E. Toltrazuril 5–10 mg/kg SQ, PO SID for 3–5 days
F. Clarithromycin 5–10 mg/kg PO BID for 14–21 days

II. The following drugs are potentially useful for the treatment of cats.
A. Primaquine phosphate 2 mg/kg PO once with oxytetracycline 50 mg/kg PO BID for 7 days
B. Toltrazuril 5–10 mg/kg SQ, PO SID for 3–5 days
C. Doxycycline 5 mg/kg PO SID for 10 days

III. Because of the limited number of cases treated with the preceding medications, it is not possible to make definitive recommendations concerning therapy.

IV. Each of these drugs is potentially toxic (see treatment of babesiosis, earlier).

V. Symptomatic therapy with nonsteroidal anti-inflammatory agents such as buffered aspirin 10–25 mg/kg PO BID may control discomfort in most cases.

VI. Glucocorticoid administration may exacerbate clinical disease.

Patient Monitoring

I. Monitor clinical signs of disease and blood smears for the presence of the organism.
A. Time to clinical response is variable.
B. Anti-*Hepatozoon* drugs are commonly ineffective.

II. Tick control is the best form of prevention.

III. Zoonotic potential is minimal.

IV. Radiographic changes may never resolve.

Pneumocystosis

Definition and Causes

I. Pneumocystosis has been associated with respiratory tract disease in a number of mammalian hosts.

II. It is caused by *Pneumocystis carinii*, which is classified by some as a protozoan in the subphylum Sarcodina but also has characteristics of fungi.

Pathophysiology

I. Epidemiology
A. Worldwide distribution
B. Normally a saphrophytic organism of the mammalian respiratory tract
C. Life cycle completed in alveolar spaces
D. Extrapulmonary infection rare

II. Transmission: direct transfer

III. Pathogenesis
A. Immunodeficiency or concurrent pulmonary disease results in growth of large numbers of the organism.
B. Overpopulation interferes with gaseous exchange in the alveoli.

C. Infiltrates of lymphocytes, plasma cells, and macrophages worsen clinical disease and can lead to fibrosis.

Clinical Signs

I. It is a rare disease, with most dogs and all cats subclinically infected.

II. Progressive weight loss and dry cough are the most common clinical signs.

III. Vomiting, diarrhea, and exercise intolerance occur.

IV. Physical examination may reveal dry respiratory sounds, dyspnea, cachexia, and potential cyanosis.

Diagnosis

I. Laboratory abnormalities are nonspecific.

II. Thoracic radiographic abnormalities include a mixed alveolar and interstitial lung pattern.

III. Cor pulmonale can arise from chronic respiratory disease.

IV. Serologic tests are not commercially available for use with animal serum.

V. Organisms may be demonstrated in sputum, transthoracic aspirates, transtracheal wash specimens, or lung biopsies.

VI. *Pneumocystis* antigens can be detected in sputum or airway washings using ELISA, fluorescent antibody, and polymerase chain reaction (Furuta et al., 1994).

Differential Diagnosis

I. Infectious tracheobronchitis

II. Bacterial and mycotic pneumonitis

III. Heart failure

Treatment

I. Trimethoprim-sulfonamide 15 mg/kg PO BID for 2 weeks

II. Phenamidine isethionate 4 mg/kg IM SID for 2 weeks

III. Supportive care such as bronchodilators and airway humidification for respiratory signs

Patient Monitoring

I. If pneumocystosis is documented, evaluate the animal for immunodeficiency.

II. Monitor for resolution of cough and dyspnea after initiation of treatment (clinical course and outcome variable).

III. There is little to no zoonotic potential.

Neosporosis

Definition and Causes

I. Neosporosis is a protozoal disease caused by *Neospora caninum,* a protozoan in the phylum Apicomplexa.

II. The organism is morphologically similar to *Toxoplasma gondii* but antigenically distinct.

Pathophysiology

I. Epidemiology
    A. Cases have been reported in North America, Europe, Scandinavia, United Kingdom, Australia, New Zealand, South Africa, and Japan.
    B. The host range appears to be extensive.
        1. Natural infections: dogs, calves, lambs, and horses
        2. Experimental infections: sheep, goats, fox, macaques, cats, dogs, mice, and rats
    C. The life cycle stages recognized to date include tachyzoites and cysts, which are found in many tissues.
    D. The sexual stages have not been determined.
II. Transmission
    A. Tachyzoites and cysts are infective orally.
    B. Transplacental infection has been proved.
    C. The definitive host and source of the organism have not been discovered.
III. Pathogenesis
    A. Destruction of host cells occurs by intracellular replication.
    B. Mononuclear cell infiltrates are found in spinal nerves, muscle, and CNS tissues and progress to fibrosis.
    C. Immune-mediated events directed against the parasite may increase tissue damage.

Clinical Signs

I. Young dogs tend to develop ascending paralysis.
    A. Hyperextension of the affected limbs is common.
    B. Progressive ascending weakness starts in the rear limbs, advances cranially, and ultimately results in death.
    C. Not all puppies born to an infected bitch are clinically affected.
II. Adult clinical syndromes are as follows.
    A. Multifocal CNS disease
    B. Myocarditis
    C. Chorioretinitis, iridocyclitis
    D. Ulcerative or nodular dermatitis
    E. Pneumonia
    F. Hepatitis
III. Clinical disease can be exacerbated by glucocorticoids.

Diagnosis

I. Nonspecific laboratory abnormalities include lymphocytosis and increased serum liver and muscle enzymes.
II. Cerebrospinal fluid (CSF) abnormalities include increased protein concentrations and a mixed cellular pleocytosis (mononuclear cells predominate).
III. Organism demonstration allows a definitive diagnosis.
    A. Occasionally, tachyzoites are found in CSF.
    B. Tissue biopsy may be submitted for specialized tests.
        1. Electron microscopic differentiation or immu-

nohistochemical differentiation from *T. gondii* is undertaken.
        2. Intracellular *N. caninum* are located in cell cytoplasm, whereas *T. gondii* are found in a parasitophorous vacuole.
    C. Serology using an IFA technique is available, but positive results do not correlate to clinical disease.
    D. Presumptive diagnosis can be made based on appropriate clinical signs, positive *Neospora* serology, and negative *T. gondii* serology.

Differential Diagnosis

I. *T. gondii* as a cause of ascending paralysis, intraocular inflammation, and tissue cysts
II. Other causes of chorioretinitis, such as neoplasia, systemic fungal infection, and canine distemper virus infection (see Chap. 100)

Treatment

I. Several dogs have survived infection after being treated (Ruehlmann et al., 1995).
    A. Trimethoprim-sulfadiazine 15 mg/kg PO BID for 4 weeks and pyrimethamine 1 mg/kg PO SID for 4 weeks
    B. Trimethoprim-sulfadiazine 15 mg/kg PO BID for 4 weeks and clindamycin 10 mg/kg PO TID for 4 weeks
    C. Clindamycin 7.5 mg/kg PO BID for 6–7 weeks (Dubey, 1995)
II. Early diagnosis and treatment may lessen severity of clinical signs.
III. Pelvic limb rigidity may not resolve.

Patient Monitoring

I. So few dogs have been treated that survival and drug efficacy are yet to be determined.
II. Zoonotic potential is unknown.
III. Repeated transplacental transmission occurs, so bitches whelping an infected litter should not be rebred.

Toxoplasmosis

Definition and Causes

I. Toxoplasmosis is a polysystemic protozoal disease infecting most vertebrates, including dogs, cats, and people.
II. It is caused by *T. gondii,* a tissue protozoan in the phylum Apicomplexa.

Pathophysiology

I. Epidemiology
    A. It is one of the most ubiquitous parasites in the world.
    B. Toxoplasmosis is found everywhere there are cats.

C. Seroprevalence of infection is approximately 40% in cats and humans in the United States, but it varies by region.

II. Life cycle
  A. Enteroepithelial cycle (cat only)
    1. Asexual and sexual reproduction in the intestinal tract results in the production and passage of oocysts in feces.
    2. Oocysts are passed unsporulated and are not infectious until sporulated.
    3. Sporulation occurs after 1–5 days when exposed to oxygen and appropriate humidity and temperature.
  B. Extraintestinal phase
    1. After exposure to sporulated oocysts or tissue cysts, sporozoites (oocysts) or bradyzoites (tissue cysts) penetrate the intestinal tract and disseminate in blood and lymph as tachyzoites (rapidly dividing stage).
    2. Tachyzoites penetrate almost all cells of the body and divide asexually until the host cell is destroyed or immune responses attenuate replication.
    3. If immune responses are appropriate, replication is slowed, leading to the development of tissue cysts containing bradyzoites (slowly dividing stage).
    4. Bradyzoites form in multiple tissues, especially the CNS, skeletal muscles, and visceral organs.
    5. It is likely that bradyzoites live in the body for the life of the host in a state of premunition with the immune system.

III. Transmission
  A. Sporulated oocyst ingestion
  B. Ingestion of tissue cysts during carnivorous feeding
  C. Transplacental transmission possible in people, dogs, cats, goats, and sheep when the primary exposure is during pregnancy

IV. Pathogenesis
  A. Clinical disease is determined by the immune status and age of the host, number and stage of organisms ingested, strain of *T. gondii*, and presence of concurrent infections.
  B. Clinical disease may be induced by organism replication or breakdown of tissue cysts (rare) or may be induced by immune-mediated reactions against the parasite.
  C. Glucocorticoid administration can exacerbate clinical disease and may reinduce oocyst shedding.

Clinical Signs

I. Cats
  A. Stillbirths and abortion can occur.
  B. Neonates have the most severe disease.
    1. CNS and pulmonary signs are most common.
    2. Fever, cough, dyspnea, depression, ascites, hepatomegaly, seizures, and death may occur.
  C. Adults display a variety of clinical signs, which are listed in decreasing frequency.
    1. Intraocular inflammation: anterior and posterior uveitis (see Chaps. 97 and 100)
    2. Fever
    3. Muscle hyperesthesia
    4. Depression, anorexia, weight loss
    5. Respiratory signs: cough, dyspnea
    6. CNS signs: seizures, vestibular syndromes
    7. Icterus
  D. Clinical signs are often recurrent or chronic, particularly when the CNS or eyes are involved.
  E. Many cats are older when initially clinically affected and have stable antibody titers.
  F. Feline immunodeficiency virus (FIV) and feline leukemia virus (FeLV) co-infected cats have similar clinical signs to virus-naive cats but seem to be more resistant to therapy.

II. Dogs
  A. Respiratory signs: cough, dyspnea
  B. Gastrointestinal abnormalities: vomiting, diarrhea
  C. Generalized signs
    1. Usually in dogs <1 year old
    2. Fever, dyspnea, vomiting, diarrhea, icterus, and myocardial disease
  D. Neuromuscular signs
    1. Dependent on location
    2. Myositis with weakness, abnormal gait, and stiffness
    3. Ataxia, seizures, and cranial nerve deficits
    4. Possible paraparesis and tetraparesis
  E. Ocular disease: less common than in cats

Diagnosis

I. Variable leukogram abnormalities
  A. Leukopenia is more common in acute disease, and leukocytosis is more common in chronic disease.
  B. Normocytic, normochromic, nonregenerative anemia is seen in some cats.

II. Chemistry abnormalities
  A. Dependent on organ system involvement
  B. Increased serum liver and muscle enzymes
  C. Hyperbilirubinemia, bilirubinuria
  D. Both hyper- and hypoproteinemia; polyclonal gammopathies with chronic recurrent disease in cats

III. Fecal examination
  A. Oocysts are generally shed only 1–6 weeks after primary exposure.
  B. Sheather's sugar centrifugation is the best method for demonstration of oocysts (10 × 12 μm).
  C. Other coccidians have similar-sized oocysts (see Table 114–2), but only *T. gondii* is pathogenic for cats, dogs, or people.
  D. Any oocyst 10 × 12 μm should be considered to be *T. gondii*, and the case should be handled appropriately (see later).

E. Six years after primary exposure, gut immunity is incomplete.
F. Extremely high doses of glucocorticoids can induce repeat oocyst shedding, but clinical doses appear to be safe (Lappin et al., 1991).
G. Concurrent infection by FeLV or FIV does not appear to increase oocyst numbers, increase the length of time oocysts are shed, or reinduce oocyst shedding in chronically infected cats.

IV. Serology
A. IgG antibody testing
1. IgG antibodies develop within 3–4 weeks after inoculation and may persist for the life of the cat.
2. IgG antibodies develop in approximately 100% of experimentally infected cats.
3. High IgG antibody titers do not necessarily correlate with recent or active infection.
4. Increasing IgG antibody titers can indicate recent or active infection but do not correlate with clinical disease.
5. Some clinically ill animals do not have increasing IgG antibody titers.
B. IgM antibody testing
1. IgM antibodies generally develop within 2 weeks after infection and are nondetectable by 16 weeks.
2. Approximately 90% of experimentally infected cats develop positive IgM titers.
3. The presence of an IgM titer ≥1:256 generally indicates recent or active infection.
4. IgM antibody titers can persist >16 weeks in some chronically ill cats, especially those coinfected with FIV.
5. IgM titers can be induced transiently after repeat infection or glucocorticoid administration.
6. Many cats with clinical toxoplasmosis have positive IgM titers.
7. Some chronically infected cats, especially those with FIV, have IgM antibodies in serum (without IgG antibodies) for months after infection.
8. Latex agglutination and indirect hemagglutination kits detect all antibody classes against *T. gondii* in human serum but fail to consistently detect IgM in cat serum (Lappin and Powell, 1991).
9. Modified agglutination tests can aid in the diagnosis of recent or active infection but are not commercially available (Dubey et al., 1990).
C. Antigen testing
1. Circulating *T. gondii* antigens can be detected in serum, CSF, and aqueous humor of cats by ELISA.
2. Antigenemia can be intermittent or recurrent and occurs in both sick and healthy cats.
3. It also occurs in the face of antibodies and thus is not beneficial in determining oocyst shedding periods, recent or active infection, or clinical disease.

4. The presence of antigen without antibody suggests peracute infection or severe immunosuppression.
5. Some cats with clinical toxoplasmosis have had detectable antigen without antibody in serum.
V. Aqueous humor and CSF
A. IgG and IgA antibodies are produced in the eyes and CNS of experimental cats.
B. IgM has been detected in eyes of only naturally exposed cats with uveitis.
C. *T. gondii* has been detected in aqueous humor of naturally exposed and experimentally inoculated cats with or without uveitis.
VI. Protozoal identification
A. Histopathology
B. Immunohistochemical staining: helps differentiate from *N. caninum*
C. Animal inoculation: fecal material, tissue homogenates
D. Polymerase chain reaction: aqueous humor
VII. Antemortem diagnosis: requires combination of the following
A. Serologic evidence of active or recent infection
1. IgM titer >1:256
2. Increasing IgG titer
3. Antigen without antibody
B. Clinical signs of disease referable to toxoplasmosis
C. Exclusion of other etiologies inducing similar clinical signs
D. Response to an anti-*Toxoplasma* drug or demonstration of the organism
VIII. Other tests
A. CSF analysis reveals increased protein and mixed inflammatory cell infiltrates; tachyzoites are occasionally seen cytologically during acute disease.
B. Tachyzoites are occasionally seen in pleural effusions, peritoneal effusions, and blood and on transtracheal wash cytology during acute infection.
C. Interstitial infiltrates, alveolar densities, and pleural effusion may be detected on thoracic radiography.
D. Enlarged mesenteric lymph nodes and peritoneal effusion may be detected radiographically or on palpation.
E. Prediction of oocyst shedding is not possible via serology; cat owners are given detailed preventive measures as discussed later.

Differential Diagnosis

I. Cats
A. Ocular disease: feline infectious peritonitis (FIP), FeLV, FIV, and systemic mycoses (e.g., cryptococcosis)
B. Other polysystemic diseases
1. FIP, FIV, FeLV
2. Haemobartonellosis
3. Immune-mediated diseases

4. Neoplasia
II. Dogs
  A. *N. caninum* in dogs with neuromuscular disease
  B. Acute viral gastrointestinal diseases
  C. Ocular inflammation: see earlier under Neosporosis
  D. Combined inflammatory CNS and ocular diseases (e.g., canine distemper virus, systemic mycoses, protothecosis)

Treatment

I. Cats
  A. Polysystemic disease (extraintestinal cycle)
    1. Clindamycin 12.5 mg/kg PO, IM BID for 3–6 weeks
      a) Causes occasional vomiting and diarrhea
      b) Can be used parenterally in anorectic animals
      c) May be effective for the treatment of CNS toxoplasmosis
    2. Trimethoprim-sulfonamide 15 mg/kg PO, SQ BID for 3–6 weeks
      a) The author has successfully treated several CNS cases with this combination.
      b) It can potentially induce folic acid deficiency with long-term use.
    3. Sulfonamides 30 mg/kg PO BID for 2 weeks combined with pyrimethamine 0.25–0.5 mg/kg PO BID for 2 weeks
      a) Severe anorexia and depression are commonly induced by this combination.
      b) Bone marrow suppression is common but can be prevented with the concurrent administration of folinic acid 5 mg/day PO or brewer's yeast 100 mg/kg PO SID.
  B. Oocyst shedding (enteroepithelial cycle)
    1. Clindamycin 12.5 mg/kg PO, IM BID for 1–2 weeks
    2. Sulfonamides 100 mg/kg PO SID for 1–2 weeks combined with pyrimethamine 0.5 mg/kg PO BID for 1–2 weeks
    3. Monensin administered as a 0.02% concentration in dry weight of food, PO daily for 1–2 weeks
    4. Toltrazuril 5–10 mg/kg PO SID for 2 weeks
  C. Ocular toxoplasmosis (see Chap. 101)
II. Dogs
  A. Clindamycin 10–20 mg/kg PO, IM BID for 3–6 weeks
  B. Sulfonamides 30 mg/kg PO BID for 2 weeks combined with pyrimethamine 0.25–0.5 mg/kg PO BID for 2 weeks

Patient Monitoring

I. Zoonotic potential
  A. Because oocysts have to sporulate and cats are fastidious, direct contact with cats is unlikely to result in infection.
  B. Transmission to people can be prevented.

    1. Do not feed raw meat to cats or allow them to hunt.
    2. Remove feces from litter box daily, flush or incinerate feces, rinse litter box periodically with scalding water, or use litter box liners.
    3. Cover children's sandboxes.
    4. Wear gloves when gardening.
    5. Wear gloves when handling meats or wash hands thoroughly.
    6. Cook meat to at least medium-well.
    7. Boil water collected from the environment before drinking.
    8. Control mechanical vectors such as earthworms and cockroaches.
II. Clinically affected animals generally have an antibiotic response within 48 hours.
  A. Resolution of fever and hyperesthesia
  B. Improved appetite
III. Laboratory abnormalities generally resolve within weeks.
IV. The organism is probably not cleared from the body, so recurrence of clinical signs is common.
V. Cats undergoing oocyst shedding are monitored with repeat fecal examinations and are kept isolated; feces are disposed of daily.

PROTOTHECOSIS

Definition and Causes

I. Protothecosis is a disseminated disease in the dog and a cutaneous disease in the cat.
II. *Prototheca zopfii* and *P. wickerhamii* are the two species in this genus of green algae incriminated as pathogens.

Pathophysiology

I. The organisms are found in sewage and animal wastes.
II. Transmission is by ingestion of contaminated food, water, or soil.
III. Individuals with decreased cell-mediated immune responses are more likely to develop clinical disease.
IV. There may be strain differences in virulence.

Clinical Signs

I. Dogs
  A. Common in collies
  B. Disseminated disease
    1. Large bowel diarrhea
    2. Weight loss
    3. CNS disease: depression, ataxia, paresis
    4. Ocular disease: exudative retinal detachment, blindness, intraocular inflammation
  C. Cutaneous disease
    1. Crusty exudates of the trunk, extremities, and mucous membranes
    2. Draining ulcers

II. Cats
   A. Only cutaneous protothecosis reported
   B. Firm nodules on the limbs, feet, and head

Diagnosis

I. Laboratory findings are nonspecific.
II. CSF changes include pleocytosis with either lymphocytes or granulocytes as the predominant cell type and increased total protein.
III. Organism isolation or identification is easiest from CSF, rectal scrapings or biopsies, or vitreal aspirates.

Differential Diagnosis

I. Other inflammatory ocular and CNS diseases in the dog, such as canine distemper virus, systemic mycoses, and granulomatous meningoencephalitis
II. Other causes of large bowel diarrhea, including histoplasmosis, trichuriasis, inflammatory bowel disease, and neoplasia

Treatment

I. Excision of cutaneous lesions
II. Drugs used in the treatment of canine protothecosis
   A. Amphotericin B 0.25–0.5 mg/kg IV three times weekly to a cumulative dosage of 8 mg/kg with tetracycline 22 mg/kg PO TID
   B. Ketoconazole 10–15 mg/kg PO BID for 28–42 days; only effective against *P. wickerhamii*
   C. Itraconazole 5 mg/kg PO SID-BID

Patient Monitoring

I. Systemic protothecosis appears to be resistant to therapy. Although progression of the disease may be slowed, it is usually fatal.
II. Multifocal cutaneous abscesses may respond to ketoconazole, but long-term therapy is usually needed (months).
III. There is no zoonotic risk.

Bibliography

Ashford DA, Bozza M, Freire M et al: Comparison of the polymerase chain reaction and serology for the detection of canine visceral leishmaniasis. Am J Trop Med Hyg 53:251, 1995

Baer S, Baker D, Markovits J: Trypanosomiasis and laryngeal paralysis in a dog. J Am Vet Med Assoc 188:1307, 1986

Baker DG, Strombeck DR, Gershwin LJ: Laboratory diagnosis of *Giardia duodenalis* infection in dogs. J Am Vet Med Assoc 190:53, 1987

Baneth G, Levy E, Presentey B et al: *Hepatozoon* sp. parasitemia in a domestic cat. Feline Pract 23:10, 1995

Barnes JC, Stanley O, Craig TM: Diffuse cutaneous leishmaniasis in a cat. J Am Vet Med Assoc 202:416, 1993

Barr SC, Bowman DD, Heller RL: Efficacy of fenbendazole against giardiasis in dogs. Am J Vet Res 55:988, 1994

Barr SC, Bowman DD, Heller RL et al: Efficacy of albendazole against giardiasis in dogs. Am J Vet Res 54:926, 1993

Barton CL, Russo EA, Craig TM, Green RW: Canine hepatozoonosis: a retrospective study of 15 naturally occurring cases. J Am Anim Hosp Assoc 21:125, 1985

Bennett M, Baxby D, Blundell N et al: Cryptosporidiosis in the domestic cat. Vet Rec 117:73, 1985

Blogg JR, Sykes JE: Sudden blindness associated with protothecosis in a dog. Aust Vet J 72:147, 1995

Botha WS, VanRensburg IBJ: Pneumocytosis: a chronic respiratory distress syndrome in the dog. J S Afr Vet Assoc 50:173, 1979

Bravo L, Frank LA, Brenneman KA: Canine leishmaniasis in the United States. Compend Contin Educ Pract Vet 15:699, 1993

Buckner RG, Ewing SA: Trichomoniasis. p. 772. In Kirk RW (ed): Current Veterinary Therapy V. WB Saunders, Philadelphia, 1974

Cole JR, Sangster LT, Sulzer CR et al: Infections with *Encephalitozoon cuniculi* and *Leptospira interrogans,* serovars, grippotyphosa, and ballum in a kennel of foxhounds. J Am Vet Med Assoc 180:435, 1982

Conrad P, Thomford J, Yamane I et al: Hemolytic anemia caused by *Babesia gibsoni* infection in dogs. J Am Vet Med Assoc 199:601, 1991

Craig TM, Barton CL, Mercer SH et al: Dermal leishmaniasis in a Texas cat. Am J Trop Med Hyg 35:1100, 1986

Dubey JP: A review of *Sarcocystis* of domestic animals and of other coccidia of cats and dogs. J Am Vet Med Assoc 169:1061, 1976

Dubey JP: Toxoplasmosis in dogs. Canine Pract 12:7, 1985

Dubey JP: Toxoplasmosis in cats. Feline Pract 16:12, 1986

Dubey JP: Duration of immunity to shedding of *Toxoplasma gondii* oocysts by cats. J Parasitol 81:410, 1995

Dubey JP, Carpenter JL: Histologically confirmed clinical toxoplasmosis in cats: 100 cases (1952–1990). J Am Vet Med Assoc 203:1556, 1993

Dubey JP, Cosenza SF, Lipscomb TP et al: Acute sarcocystosis-like disease in a dog. J Am Vet Med Assoc 198:439, 1991

Dubey JP, Hattel AL, Lindsay DS, Topper MJ: Neonatal *Neospora caninum* infection in dogs: isolation of the causative agent and experimental transmission. J Am Vet Med Assoc 193:1259, 1988

Dubey JP, Koestner A, Piper RC: Repeated transplacental transmission of *Neospora caninum* in dogs. J Am Vet Assoc 197:857, 1990

Dubey JP, Metzger FL, Hattel AL et al: Canine cutaneous neosporosis: clinical improvement with clindamycin. Vet Dermatol 6:37, 1995

Dubey JP, Thulliez PH: Serologic diagnosis of toxoplasmosis in cats fed *Toxoplasma gondii* tissue cysts. J Am Vet Med Assoc 194:1297, 1989

Ewing GO: Granulomatous cholangiohepatitis in a cat due to a protozoan resembling *Hepatozoon canis*. Feline Pract 7:37, 1977

Farwell GE, LeGrand EK, Cobb CC: Clinical observations on *Babesia gibsoni* and *Babesia canis* infections in dogs. J Am Vet Med Assoc 180:507, 1982

Ferrer L, Aisa MJ, Roura X et al: Serological diagnosis and treatment of canine leishmaniasis. Vet Rec 136:514, 1995

Finnie JW, Coloe PJ: Cutaneous protothecosis in a cat. Aust Vet J 57:307, 1981

Fox JC, Ewing SA, Buckner RG et al: *Trypanosoma cruzi* infection in a dog from Oklahoma. J Am Vet Med Assoc 189:1583, 1986

Furuta T, Nagami S, Kojima J et al: Spontaneous *Pneumocystis carinii* in the dog with generalized demodicosis. Vet Rec 134:423, 1994

Gaunt SD, McGrath RK, Cox HU: Disseminated protothecosis in a dog. J Am Vet Med Assoc 185:906, 1984

Geulfi JF: Use of imidocarb dipropionate to treat babesiosis in dogs: chemoprophylaxis trial. Rev Med Vet 133:617, 1982

Glenn BL, Stair EL: Cytauxzoonosis in domestic cats: report of two cases in Oklahoma, with a review and discussion of the disease. J Am Vet Med Assoc 184:822, 1984

Gossett KA, Gaunt SD, Aja DS: Hepatozoonosis and ehrlichiosis in a dog. J Am Anim Hosp Assoc 21:265, 1985

Greene CE, Cook JR, Mahaffey EA: Clindamycin for treatment of *Toxoplasma* polymyositis in a dog. J Am Vet Med Assoc 187:631, 1985

Greene CE, Jacobs GJ, Prickett D: Intestinal malabsorption and cryptosporidiosis in an adult dog. J Am Vet Med Assoc 197:365, 1990

Haberkorn A: Chemotherapy of human and animal coccidioses: state and perspectives. Parasitol Res 82:193, 1996

Hagler DN, Kim CK, Walzer PD: Feline leukemia virus and *Pneumocystis carinii* infection. J Parasitol 73:1284, 1987

Hay WH, Shell LG, Lindsay DS, Dubey JP: Diagnosis and treatment of *Neospora caninum* infection in a dog. J Am Vet Med Assoc 197:87, 1990

Kier AB, Wagner JE, Morehouse LG: Experimental transmission of *Cytauxzoon felis* from bobcats (*Lynx rufu*) to domestic cats (*Felis domesticus*). Am J Vet Res 43:97, 1982

Kirkpatrick CE: Giardiasis. Vet Clin North Am [Small Anim Pract] 17:1377, 1987

Kirkpatrick CE, Dubey JP: Enteric coccidial infections. *Isospora, Sarcocystis, Cryptosporidium, Besnoitia,* and *Hammondia.* Vet Clin North Am [Small Anim Pract] 17:1405, 1987

Kirkpatrick CE, Farrell JP, Goldschmidt MH: *Leishmania chagasi* and *L. donovani*: experimental infections in domestic cats. Exp Parasitol 58:125, 1984

Kontos UJ, Koutinas AF: Old World canine leishmaniasis. Compend Contin Educ Pract Vet 15:949, 1993

Lappin MR, Burney DP, Dow SW et al: Polymerase chain reaction for the detection of *Toxoplasma gondii* in aqueous humor of cats. Am J Vet Res 57:1589, 1996

Lappin MR, Dawe DL, Lindl PA et al: The effect of glucocorticoid administration on oocyst shedding, serology, and cell-mediated immune responses of cats with acute or chronic toxoplasmosis. J Am Anim Hosp Assoc 27:625, 1991

Lappin MR, George JW, Pedersen NC et al: Primary and secondary *Toxoplasma gondii* infection in normal and feline immunodeficiency virus infected cats. J Parasitol (in press)

Lappin MR, Greene CE, Winston S et al: Clinical feline toxoplasmosis: serologic diagnosis and therapeutic management of 15 cases. J Vet Intern Med 3:139, 1989

Lappin MR, Powell CC: Comparison of latex agglutination, indirect hemagglutination, and ELISA techniques for the detection of *Toxoplasma gondii*–specific antibodies in the serum of cats. J Vet Intern Med 5:299, 1991

Lappin MR, Roberts SM, Davidson MG et al: Enzyme-linked immunosorbent assays for the detection of *Toxoplasma gondii*–specific antibodies and antigens in the aqueous humor of cats. J Am Vet Med Assoc 201:1010, 1992

Lindsay DS, Blagburn BL: Practical treatment and control of infections caused by canine gastrointestinal parasites. Vet Med 5:441, 1995

McCully RM, Lloyd J, Kuys D, Schneider DJ: Canine *Pneumocystis* pneumonia. J S Afr Vet Assoc 50:207, 1979

Moon HW, Woodmansee DB: Cryptosporidiosis. J Am Vet Med Assoc 189:643, 1986

Moore FM, Schmidt GM, Chandler FW: Unsuccessful treatment of disseminated prototothecosis in a dog. J Am Vet Med Assoc 186:705, 1984

Moore JA, Blagburn BL, Lindsay DS: Cryptosporidiosis in animals including humans. Compend Contin Educ Pract Vet 10:275, 1988

Mtambo MMA, Nash AS, Blewett DA et al: Comparison of staining and concentration techniques for detection of *Cryptosporidium* oocysts in cat faecal specimens. Vet Parasitol 45:49, 1992

Murata T, Inoue M, Tateyama S et al: Vertical transmission of *Hepatozoon canis* in dogs. J Vet Med Sci 55:867, 1993

Oliva G, Gradoni L, Ciaramella P et al: Activity of liposomal amphotericin B (AmBisome) in dogs naturally infected with *Leishmania infantum*. J Antimicrob Chemother 36:1013, 1995

Patton S, Legendre AM, McGavin MD, Pelletier D: Concurrent infection with *Toxoplasma gondii* and feline leukemia virus. J Vet Intern Med 5:199, 1991

Pearce JR, Powell HS, Chandler FW, Visvesvara GS: Amebic meningoencephalitis caused by *Acanthamoeba castellani* in a dog. J Am Vet Med Assoc 187:951, 1985

Rakich PM, Latimer KS: Altered immune function in a dog with disseminated prototothecosis. J Am Vet Med Assoc 185:681, 1984

Ruehlmann D, Podell M, Oglesbee M et al: Canine neosporosis: a case report and literature review. J Am Anim Hosp Assoc 31:174, 1995

Sisk DB, Gosser HS, Styer EL: Intestinal cryptosporidiosis in two pups. J Am Vet Med Assoc 184:835, 1984

Snider TG: Myocarditis caused by *Trypanosoma cruzi* in a native Louisiana dog. J Am Vet Med Assoc 177:247, 1980

Taboada J: Canine babesiosis. p. 315. In Bonagura JD (ed): Kirk's Current Veterinary Therapy XII. WB Saunders, Philadelphia, 1995

Thkap V, Baneth G, Pipano E: Circulating antibodies to *Hepatozoon canis* demonstrated by immunofluorescence. J Vet Diagn Invest 6:121, 1994

Turrel JM, Pool RR: Bone lesions in four dogs with visceral leishmaniasis. Vet Radiol 23:243, 1982

Yamane I, Thomford JW, Gardner IA et al: Evaluation of the indirect fluorescent antibody test for diagnosis of *Babesia gibsoni* infections in dogs. Am J Vet Res 54:1579, 1993

Behavioral Disorders

115

Introduction

Karen L. Overall

GENERAL COMMENTS

I. Behavioral medicine is the newest specialty to be board certified in the United States by the American Veterinary Medical Association.
   A. It is estimated that more animals are euthanized for behavioral complaints than for complaints associated with any other specialty.
   B. The American Animal Hospital Association estimates that the average practice loses almost $20,000 per annum in services that are not delivered because clients get rid of pets because of behavioral complaints.
   C. Veterinarians have increasingly become aware of the importance of preventive and therapeutic behavioral medicine.
II. Behavior is complex, and structured thought processes are useful in distinguishing nonspecific signs or symptoms from behavioral diagnoses.
   A. Behavioral medicine uses terminology that may require specific interpretation and definition of terms.
   B. A behavioral diagnosis should be considered a hypothesis to be tested, so that the clinician can postulate a specific mechanism for that diagnosis and then formulate specific responses to treatment as tests of the hypothesis. For example, assessing responses to behavior modification designed to desensitize a dog to the approach of a stranger may help distinguish a diagnosis of dominance aggression from one of fearful aggression.
   C. Tests of these hypotheses may include therapeutic trials using drugs. For pharmacologic intervention to be used rationally, it is essential to have a specific working diagnosis, because medications have defined mechanisms of action.

BEHAVIOR VS. BEHAVIORAL PROBLEMS

I. Behavior (whether appropriate or not) results from the integration of all organ system responses to perceived and actual environmental stimuli.
   A. Inherent in this definition is integration of all external and internal stimuli and the interactions of the physical, physiologic, social, demographic, and resource environments.
   B. Behavior can be both an event and a process. When one discusses "a behavior," one is discussing the physical manifestations of both the event and the process. This complexity becomes important when discussing the issue of the context in which the behavior occurs.
II. Behaviors can be normal, in-context, or they can be abnormal, out-of-context.
   A. Some behaviors are appropriate when considered within the framework or context of a species-specific or species-typical behavior but may be inappropriate if they are exhibited to another species.
   B. Many behaviors are "normal" behaviors that clients find undesirable.
   C. For the purposes of these chapters, most contextual distinctions focus on whether the behavior is warranted given the circumstances and whether the behavior is contextual given the scope, intensity, and range of behaviors exhibited.
   D. The extent to which a behavior is inappropriate may not reflect the extent to which it is potentially dangerous or poses a risk.
III. Most behavioral diagnoses are phenomenologic or phenotypic ones (Table 115–1).
   A. Table 115–1 displays a hierarchical ranking for

Table 115–1. Levels of Causality or Mechanism to Consider in Any Behavioral Diagnosis

1. Phenotype
   - Role of underlying broad genotype × environment interactions
   - Role of phenomenologic diagnoses
2. Neuroanatomy
   - Role of localization of activity
   - Role of neuroanatomic diagnoses
3. Neurophysiology/neurochemistry
   - Role of chemical/substrate interaction
   - Role of most mechanistic pathophysiologic diagnoses
4. Molecular
   - Role of gene regulation and interaction with substrate
   - Role of most etiologic diagnostic refinements
5. Genotype
   - Role of heritability

different levels of mechanism or causality that operate for all behavioral diagnoses.

B. The first level, the phenotypic, is the one on which most behavioral diagnoses are based.
  1. Such diagnoses are based on the recognition of a constellation of related signs that are correlates of the necessary and sufficient elements defining the condition.
  2. The phenotypic level is the one that is the least specific and the most sensitive to client and clinician interpretation.
  3. It is the level at which behavior modification is aimed and is also the relevant level for assessment of changes in signs attendant with treatment or progression of the condition.
C. The neuroanatomic level is associated with structural pathology that contributes to behavioral problems (e.g., circling caused by a space-occupying lesion).
  1. This level becomes elucidated as imaging techniques become more specific.
  2. This is the level at which pharmacologic intervention is aimed.
D. The molecular level focuses on the activity of gene product interactions and neurochemical receptor activity and is poorly understood for most behavioral issues.
E. The genotypic level is defined by the mode of heritability and issues related to gene and base-pair sequences and stereochemistry.
  1. In behavioral medicine, the disorder is usually understood at the phenotypic level and at the level of simple mendelian inheritance, with little mechanistic understanding at any other level.
  2. Understanding the mode of inheritance of behavioral disorders helps prevent them through cautious breeding and facilitates understanding of the regulation of neurochemical-substrate interactions.

GENERAL APPROACHES TO TREATMENT

I. The behavioral, social, physical, and pharmacologic (both endogenous and exogenous) environments can be modified.
  A. Modifying the physical and social environments can be as simple as excluding an animal from one area or creating a time- and space-sharing environment.
  B. Pharmacologic intervention can be accomplished by altering the endogenous environment, generally through ovariohysterectomy or castration, or through the use of behavioral pharmacology.
II. Behavior modification uses six main tactics: habituation, extinction, desensitization, counterconditioning, flooding, and avoidance/aversive conditioning. Other techniques such as shaping are often associated with these.
  A. Habituation
    1. Habituation is an elementary form of learning that involves no rewards.
    2. It is merely the cessation of or decrease in a response to a stimulus that is the result of repeated or prolonged exposure to that stimulus. The stimulus can be positive, neutral, or negative.
    3. Stimuli associated with potentially adverse consequences (negative stimuli) might be more difficult to extinguish with habituation than other stimuli.
    4. If responses are even occasionally rewarded, the habituation response will be inhibited.
  B. Spontaneous recovery
    1. Spontaneous recovery is a phenomenon that is associated with habituation.
    2. If there is an extended period between the animal's last experience of a stimulus (to which it had previously been habituated) and its re-exposure to the stimulus, the animal may react. This is spontaneous recovery.
    3. Rehabituation is quick and simple if no overt fearful associations are involved.
  C. Dishabituation
    1. Dishabituation is the reinstatement of a habituated response as a result of exposure to a stimulus that provokes a response similar to the original.
    2. The classic examples of this involve mildly fearful responses. If habituation has just occurred to a certain hand gesture and another movement occurs that is also worrisome for the animal, the animal could dishabituate to the hand gesture.
    3. Rehabituation is the rule unless the event is compounded and made more fearful or unless the animal's reaction is extreme (suggesting something innate about the animal's response).

D. Conditioning
   1. Conditioning refers to associations between stimuli and responses.
   2. Classic conditioning does not involve a reward structure to make these associations.
   3. Operant or instrumental conditioning uses a reward structure.
   4. With operant conditioning, learning is fastest if the positive reinforcer occurs immediately (within 0.5 seconds).
   5. Delayed and intermittent reinforcements slow the acquisition of the response but work well to reinforce its maintenance (they enhance resistance to extinction).
   6. In addition to timing (quantity), value (quality) is important.
      a) The more an animal values a reinforcer, the more quickly and reliably it will acquire the response.
      b) Hence, a food treat that dogs do not usually get (e.g., cheese) is more effective than their standard dog kibble in teaching them new behavior.
   7. Designing behavior modification programs that have a high probability of success requires understanding what the animal values and incorporating that into the program.
E. Reinforcement
   1. Reinforcement is a process that involves a stimulus or an event that increases the probability that a certain behavior or class of behaviors will be performed in the future.
   2. A positive reinforcer is a stimulus or an event that occurs after a response that leads to an increase in that response in the future.
   3. A negative reinforcer is an aversive event or stimulus that increases the frequency of a behavior but does so through escape or avoidance.
   4. Negative reinforcement is *not* to be confused with punishment.
F. Punishment
   1. Punishment is the application of an aversive or negative stimulus as a response is occurring or immediately after it has occurred.
   2. It is done in an attempt to decrease the frequency of the response.
G. Second-order reinforcers
   1. Second-order reinforcers are signals that can be used at a distance and convey that the reward or the valuable stimulus is coming.
   2. Commonly used second-order reinforcers are words (''good girl''), hand signals, and clicks or whistles.
   3. By carefully pairing these with the reward, second-order reinforcers can elicit the same response as the reward would (at least temporarily).
H. Stimulus and response generalization
   1. Stimulus and response generalization is what occurs when an operantly or classically conditioned response is provoked not only by the object or event that originally provoked it but also by objects or events that are similar to the original stimulus.
   2. The most common example of stimulus response generalization in dogs is to people in uniforms. If a delivery man or meter reader initially scared the dog or provoked a protective response, this response may then be generalized to others in uniform, although the circumstances might not be the same.
   3. The more similar the original and subsequent stimuli, the more similar and intense the response.
I. Extinction
   1. Extinction is the cessation of a response that occurs when reinforcement is stopped.
   2. The classic example of extinction of a response is a dog that jumps on people for attention. If people pet the dog, the behavior continues; if they stop the petting at once and forever, the dog will eventually extinguish its response because the reward is no longer there.
   3. The same example is also classic for resistance to extinction. Any form of intermittent reinforcement (even occasional petting of the dog in response to the jumping) enhances continuation of the response.
J. Overlearning
   1. Overlearning is a phenomenon that is frequently employed in training for specific events but may be underused in preventing fearful responses in dogs.
   2. Overlearning is the repeated evocation and expression of an already learned response.
   3. This accomplishes three things.
      a) It delays forgetting.
      b) It increases the resistance to extinction.
      c) It increases the probability that the response will become a knee-jerk one, or the response of first choice, when the circumstances are similar.
      d) This last aspect can be extremely useful in teaching an animal to overcome a fear or anxiety.
K. Shaping
   1. Shaping is a learning technique that works well for animals that do not know what a perfect response would be.
   2. It works through gradual approximations and allows the animal to be rewarded initially for any behavior that resembles the one desired as the final outcome.
   3. For instance, when teaching a puppy to sit, rewarding a slight squat with food enhances the probability that squatting will be repeated. This squatting behavior is then rewarded only when it becomes more exaggerated, and finally, when it becomes a true sit.
L. Flooding

1. Flooding involves prolonged exposure at a level that *provokes* the response so that the animal eventually gives up.
2. This is exactly the opposite of the approach taken in desensitization.
3. Flooding is far more stressful than any of the other therapeutic strategies and, when used inappropriately, could damage the animal.
4. One of the risks is the potential worsening and intensification of the fear.
5. In most cases, flooding is a last resort and should always be executed as humanely as possible.

Bibliography

Blanchard RJ, Blanchard DC: The organization and modeling of animal aggression. p. 529. In Brain PF, Benton D (eds): The Biology of Aggression. Sitjhoff and Noordhoff, Rockville, 1981

Moyer KE: Kinds of aggression and their physiological basis. Comm Behav Biol A 2:62, 1968

Overall KL: Animal models for human psychiatric illness: obsessive-compulsive disorders (abstract). American Veterinary Medical Association, Pittsburgh, 1995

Overall KL: Clinical Behavioral Medicine for Small Animals. Mosby, St. Louis, 1997

Voith VL: Principles of learning. Vet Clin North Am [Equine Pract] 2:485, 1986

116

Canine Behavioral Disorders

Karen L. Overall

CANINE AGGRESSION

Dominance Aggression

Definition

I. Dominance aggression is the abnormal, inappropriate, or out-of-context aggression (threat, challenge, or attack) consistently exhibited by dogs toward people under any circumstance involving passive or active control of the dog's behavior or the dog's access to the behavior.

II. This is a discrete definition of dominance aggression and has the advantage of not including the challenge to food (food-related aggression), toys (possessive aggression), or space (territorial aggression).
   A. These aggressions can all be correlates of dominance aggression and may be indicative of a more severe situation.
   B. Most of the problems with diagnosing the condition arise from a misunderstanding of canine social systems, canine signaling, and anxieties associated with endogenous uncertainty about contextually appropriate responses.

III. This form of aggression is among the most common behavioral diagnoses for dogs and is the main diagnosis that results in euthanasia.

IV. Males that are socially mature (≥18–24 months) are overrepresented.

V. There is another population of young (<1 year), unspayed females that exhibits a profound form of dominance aggression. In these females, ovariohysterectomy may enhance the development of dominance aggression.

Clinical Signs

I. Signs include staring at people; resisting having the feet manipulated, muzzle and head handled, or pressure put on the neck, dorsum, or rump; leaning forcefully against people and moving to press on them every time they move; and resisting having a leash, collar, or harness put on when doing so requires the person to move his or her hand over the dog's head.

II. These dogs also lean over people, particularly children in play, or put their paws on a person's shoulders and attempt to press their heads over the person's head.

III. Dogs may also lick a person's face (which owners refer to as kissing), but they do not do so in the deferential manner associated with small licks at the corner of the mouth. These dogs direct their licking to the entire head and face area and do not exhibit body postures otherwise associated with deferential behaviors.

IV. Disturbing dogs while they are sleeping, or stepping over them in a passageway, can provoke the aggression, and dogs choose to lie in areas where people have to go around or over them.

V. When requested to move or change their behavior, the dogs often grumble, snort, sneeze, stamp their feet, "talk back," or "bill pop" (a behavior that involves turning the head away from and then back to the person and popping the jaws; the teeth do not have to snap).

VI. These dogs intensify their aggression if they are verbally or physically corrected or disciplined (such corrections include a stare).

VII. The behavior, once it begins, becomes more visible and consistent, but data on early signs, patterns of change with experience, and changes in intensity are lacking.

Diagnosis

I. Training behaviors, including dominance downs and alpha rolls, that are touted to prevent and treat these aggressive behaviors usually provoke or worsen them in dogs manifesting signs of dominance aggression and should be avoided.

II. Dominance aggression is generally associated with anxiety about the social situation.

A. Not all people who interact with the dog are equally the target of its aggression.

B. Because anxiety is worsened by decreased behavioral and environmental predictability, there may be aggression-free periods (consistent environment). This may lead the owner to believe that the outbursts of aggression are sporadic and unpredictable, but they are usually not so.

Treatment

I. Avoid all circumstances known to be associated with an inappropriate response from the dog.
   A. Avoidance keeps the people involved safe and does not reinforce the inappropriate behavior.
   B. Every time the dog successfully threatens a person, the dog's inappropriate behavior is reinforced.

II. Behavior modification is both active and passive.
   A. Passive behavior modification is designed to enforce deferential behaviors in the dog.
      1. The dog must sit quietly and wait for every form of interaction that occurs with people (e.g., getting food, going for walks, going through a door, getting into the car, playing, loving).
      2. Do not proceed with the activity if the dog is vocalizing, moving, or not lying down or sitting.
      3. If the dog resists, the owner does not become forceful but walks away.
      4. Eventually the dog will want something badly enough that it will exhibit the canine deferential behavior of lowering its posture by sitting or lying down.
      5. This passive behavior modification is lifelong.
   B. Active behavior modification is designed to teach the dog to sit or lie down (some dogs are more comfortable and less reactive if they are lying down), to stay, and to take all the cues as to the appropriateness of its behavior from the owner.
      1. Such behavior modification involves a programmed approach to desensitization and counterconditioning.
      2. First, this is practiced involving benign, non-provocative circumstances; gradually, more provocative behaviors are addressed.
      3. These programs are best executed with the help of someone familiar with them and who can, at first, monitor the dog's responses.
      4. Everyone who regularly interacts with the dog must either practice these programs or stop interacting with the dog, because people who choose to ignore this advice make good victims.

III. If the dog is male and intact, castrate him.
   A. The loss of testosterone decreases the overall reactivity of the dog, which can facilitate behavior modification.
   B. Earlier castration is better, because learning factors into any behavioral problem.

IV. Young females (≤6 months at the onset of the aggression) who are already showing signs of dominance aggression (rare) may get worse if subjected to early ovariohysterectomy.
   A. They are not spayed until they have had at least one heat cycle.
   B. All other bitches can be spayed immediately.

V. Many forms of dominance aggression appear heritable, and most appear to follow a pattern of simple mendelian inheritance for dominant traits, so it is inappropriate to breed such dogs.

VI. Head collars (Gentle Leader, Promise) that put humane pressure on the back of the dog's neck if the dog lunges can greatly aid in treatment.
   A. Owners can interrupt the behavior before it becomes full-blown and can lead the dog from a confrontational situation.
   B. Head collars can also be used to prevent bites by pulling forward on the end of the leash and closing the dog's mouth.
   C. Prong collars, choke collars, and electronic shock collars can worsen the behaviors and render the dog more dangerous.

VII. Physical punishment intensifies the aggression.
   A. Caution owners not to direct their anger toward the dog.
   B. Owners need to understand that these dogs are abnormal, not simply misbehaving and ignoring them.

VIII. Environmental modification may involve the use of baby gates, doors, and crates to control access to areas over which a conflict may erupt.
   A. These can also be effective devices to minimize contact with young children who cannot be controlled.
   B. If visitors are unwilling to comply with the passive behavior modification, the dog can be placed in a safe area (or even boarded) so that its inappropriate behaviors are not reinforced, behavior modification programs are not sabotaged, and visitors are protected.

IX. Medications can be extremely helpful in an integrated treatment program.
   A. They are used both to decrease the anxiety-related responses associated with dominance aggression and to facilitate the implementation of behavioral and environmental modification.
   B. They are preceded by a thorough physical examination, including cardiac auscultation, a complete blood count, and a serum biochemistry profile.
      1. Because many of the medications used are tricyclic antidepressants, which may be arrhythmogenic (primarily tachycardic), an electrocardiogram is warranted.
      2. Long-term treatment requires repeated monitoring every 6–12 months or as warranted by clinical signs.
   C. Obtain a signed informed consent statement that details possible side effects (tachycardia, gastrointestinal distress, transient sedation).
   D. Drugs that can be tried include the following.
      1. Amitriptyline 1–2 mg/kg PO BID (i.e., q 12 h) for 30 days
         a) Steady-state levels appear to be attained

within about 3–5 days, and the half-life is approximately 8–12 hours.

b) Start at 1 mg/kg PO BID for the first 10 days and increase the dose if there is no change.

2. Fluoxetine 1 mg/kg PO SID (i.e., q 24 h) for 60 days
   a) Attainment of steady-state levels is slow and the compound is protein bound, so owners are warned not to expect any effect for up to 3–5 weeks.
   b) A 6- to 8-week trial is instituted to assess efficacy.

3. Clomipramine 2 mg/kg PO BID for 60 days or 1 mg/kg PO BID for 14 days, then 2 mg/kg PO BID for 14 days, then 3 mg/kg PO BID for 28 days
   a) Attainment of steady-state levels is slow and the compound is protein bound, so owners may not see any effect for 3–5 weeks.
   b) A 6- to 8-week trial is instituted to assess efficacy.

4. Sertraline (not widely used)
   a) It is very potent.
   b) It may reach steady-state levels more quickly than fluoxetine and clomipramine.

Patient Monitoring

I. Animals are monitored for changes in behavior.
II. Once the behavior is improved and relatively constant, treatment is continued for at least a month (to assess reliability) and then gradually decreased.
III. If the dog experiences a relapse or a worsening of signs, the minimum effective dose has been defined.
IV. If owners are reluctant to decrease their pets' medication for fear of a relapse, they must comply with strict monitoring procedures.

Territorial Aggression

Definition

I. It is defined as aggression that is consistently demonstrated in the vicinity of a circumscribed mobile (e.g., car) or stationary (e.g., yard) area when that area is approached by another individual in the absence of an actual contextual threat from that individual and that intensifies with decreasing distance, despite attempts at intervention, correction, or the desire to interact on the part of the approaching individual.
II. This aggression is included in the class of aggressions associated with aberrant social contextual perception, and it may be an anxiety disorder.

Clinical Signs and Diagnosis

I. Intact males may patrol more than other groups of dogs, but intact females or those with pups may also exhibit large amounts of territorial marking.
II. Crates, doghouses, fences (invisible and not), chaining, tying, and runs can all worsen the intensity of the behavior and render the dog more confident in the execution of the aggression.
III. The territorial response can be directed toward humans or other animals.
IV. The response may intensify at social maturity.
   A. Fearful aggression can occur concurrently with territorial aggression, and both problems worsen at social maturity.
   B. In dogs exhibiting signs associated with uncertainty about their territorial behavior (e.g., piloerection over the shoulder and pelvic girdles, ears retracted, pattern of approach-retreat behaviors), both the fearful and the territorial aspects of their behavior are addressed.
V. This aggression may occur with dominance aggression but is not a sign of it.

Treatment and Monitoring

I. Unless the behavior is associated with patrol and marking behaviors, castration or ovariohysterectomy only modulates the reactivity response; it does not suppress the territorial one.
II. Do not sequester these dogs in fenced areas, runs, or pens, because this removes any degree of uncertainty for them and augments their response.
III. Implement passive and active behavior modification programs (see treatment of dominance aggression, earlier).
   A. Counterconditioning and desensitization are aimed at teaching the dog not to react to the trigger stimulus and at aborting the behavior early.
   B. In the absence of the owner and the reinforcement, relapse is likely, so treatment is aimed at control.
IV. Head collars (Gentle Leader, Promise) help correct and interrupt the response as the sequence of behaviors preceding it is developing. These dogs are leash-walked to enforce this.
V. Bark collars that spray the dog with citronella (ABS System, Aboistop) may be a useful treatment adjuvant if the dog's first response to an "intruder" is to bark.
VI. Breeds selected for guarding, protecting, and herding behaviors appear to be overrepresented in this diagnosis and may exhibit the breed-characteristic behaviors of their selected response in territorial situations (e.g., herding dogs may nip at intruders' ankles).
VII. Medication can be extremely helpful as part of an integrated treatment program.
   A. It can be used both to decrease the anxiety-related responses associated with the aggression and to facilitate the implementation of behavioral and environmental modification.
   B. Medications such as amitriptyline and clomipramine are used for the aggressor.
   C. It may also be necessary to treat the animal victim with amitriptyline, or another tricyclic antidepressant may be tried (see also Fears and Anxieties, later).

Protective Aggression

Definition

I. It includes aggression that is consistently demonstrated when an individual or class of individuals is approached by a third party, in the absence of an actual contextual threat from that third party.

II. The aggression intensifies with decreasing distance or with vocal or physical cues that could indicate excitement or threat, despite attempts at intervention, correction, or the desire to interact on the part of the individual being "protected."

III. Protective and territorial aggression are often lumped under one diagnosis.

Clinical Signs and Diagnosis

I. It is important to acknowledge that some degree of in-context, innate "protectiveness" is desired in most pet dogs. Diagnosis of protective aggression must be made only after the relevance of the context in which it occurs has been evaluated.

II. Dogs that are exhibiting protective behaviors may be subtle and may only place themselves between any "intruder" and the object of their protection.

A. The extent to which they assess the situation and make a reasonable response may clarify when the behavior is normal and when it becomes abnormal.

B. The actual behaviors are similar to those seen in territorial aggression.

Treatment and Monitoring

I. Implement passive and active behavior modification programs.

A. Counterconditioning and desensitization are aimed at teaching the dog not to react to the trigger stimulus and at aborting the behavior early.

B. In the absence of the owner, the behaviors may not occur.

C. Treatment is aimed at control and encouraging the dog to take its cue as to the appropriateness of its behavior from the owner.

II. Head collars can help owners correct and interrupt the response as the sequence of behaviors preceding it is developing.

A. Leash-walk these dogs to enforce this.

B. The head collar can also be used indoors, so that the owner can teach the dog that visitors are not threats.

III. Bark collars that spray the dog with citronella may be a useful treatment adjuvant if the dog's first response to an "intruder" is to bark.

IV. Breeds selected for guarding, protecting, and herding behaviors appear to be overrepresented.

V. Medication can be extremely helpful as part of an integrated treatment program.

A. It is used to decrease the anxiety-related responses associated with the aggression and to facilitate the implementation of behavioral and environmental modification.

B. The medications used are the same as for territorial aggression.

Interdog Aggression

Definition

I. Interdog aggression is a consistent, volitional, proactive aggression that is not contextual given the social signals, threat circumstances, or response received.

II. There is usually no threatening signal or interaction from the animal that is attacked.

III. At some level, the behaviors involved with aggression are normal behaviors.

A. This diagnostic category does not depend on either hierarchy or social maturity; it depends on the contextual response.

B. This is an important distinction that supports the contention that social shifts and occasional threats can be normal.

Clinical Signs and Diagnosis

I. Involved dogs can include those within the household and social network, as well as those outside of it (e.g., unknown dogs on the street).

II. When only dogs outside of the household are involved, there may be a response to dogs of only one sex (usually the same sex), one size, or one morphology (e.g., shaggy).

III. When only dogs within the household are involved, there may be a response to a dog that is actually passively or actively challenging or posturing toward the aggressor, or the aggressor may perceive a challenge where there might not be one.

A. In the former case, the problem is with the interaction between the dogs as the relative roles in the social hierarchy shift with alteration in physical condition or impending social maturity of one of the participants.

B. In the latter case, the problem is with how the aggressor perceives the social structure of the group.

1. In this instance, the aggressor persists in its aggression even if the challenged dog actively defers to it.

2. The victim is potentially at profound risk.

Treatment and Monitoring

I. It is imperative to separate all involved dogs and to avoid aggressive interactions that cannot be aborted.

A. This may involve feeding the dogs in different rooms and behind closed doors.

B. Subtle threats must be avoided.

II. Emphasis is placed on treating the entire social environment and on enforcement of a structure that the dogs can maintain.

A. If one dog is actively challenging another, the dog most able to hold the status is enforced by feeding, walking, and paying attention to it first.

B. There is no hard rule about enforcement of younger over older or vice versa.

C. Ability to hold status depends on physical capabilities, sensory capabilities, and discretion in, or control over, social interactions.

D. If one dog is primarily the aggressor, the victim must be given status so that the aggressor understands that this dog has a right to be there. Reinforcement of the aggressor in this circumstance is inappropriate.

III. In some situations, the safest choice may be to place the victim in another home or to incarcerate the aggressor.

A. It is generally a mistake to incarcerate the victim, even transiently.

B. Because this disorder involves control over social hierarchies and the anxieties associated with those, behaviors designed to protect the victim by removing it can make the behavior worse.

IV. Also institute passive and active behavior modification programs (see Dominance Aggression, earlier).

A. In the absence of the owner, relapse can occur, so separation when unsupervised may be desirable.

B. For some profoundly aggressive dogs, treatment is aimed at control, not diminution or elimination, of the behaviors.

V. Head collars can help owners correct and interrupt the response as the sequence of behaviors unfolds.

A. Head collars can be used in the house and to control all interactions between dogs.

B. Sometimes placing only the aggressor in a head collar can passively lower its status while raising that of the dog being attacked. This works only if the victim does not run and hide.

VI. Medication can be extremely helpful as part of an integrated treatment program.

A. It is used both to decrease the anxiety-related responses associated with the aggression and to facilitate the implementation of behavioral and environmental modification.

B. Drugs to be tried include amitriptyline, fluoxetine, clomipramine, and possibly sertraline.

Predatory Aggression

Definition

I. Predatory aggression includes quiet aggression, or behaviors congruent with subsequent predatory behavior (e.g., staring, salivating, stalking, body lowering and tail twitching), consistently exhibited in circumstances associated with predation or toward victims that usually include infants, or young or ill animals.

II. Instances include quiet, unheralded attacks, generally involving at least one fierce bite and shake, consistently exhibited toward species-contextual prey items (e.g., cats and birds) or toward individuals that exhibit uncoordinated movements and sudden sleep and wake cycles (human infants, young or ill animals, geriatric humans).

Clinical Signs and Diagnosis

I. When sufficient conditions are met, this diagnosis is unassailable; however, there is some leeway in interpretation, and one seldom knows whether an actual attack will occur.

II. Discrete analyses of the behaviors involved elucidate different forms of this behavior and the role that the victim's behavior plays in determining the form the aggression will take.

A. This is important, because predatory aggression can also be used to describe aggression toward joggers and bicyclists.

B. In the latter case, territorial concerns must be ruled out, but when predatory aggression involves sentient adult humans, it is likely to be categorically different from ''true'' predatory aggression.

III. The entire range of predatory behaviors can be exhibited toward human infants or any small animal, although young animals may be more at risk.

IV. Stalking, staring, and drooling may be the only signs noticed.

V. Attacks can be prompted by sudden movement; high-pitched, unpredictable sounds; and correlates of the sudden sleep-wake cycles that characterize infant sleep.

VI. The infant eventually grows out of looking like a prey item to the dog, so the dog and child can have a normal relationship later. (But for this to happen, owners have to be realistic and responsible.)

Treatment and Monitoring

I. Dogs that stalk and kill small animals are considered at risk to exhibit the same behavior in the presence of a human infant.

II. Most dogs must not have unrestrained access to infants.

III. Dogs with predatory aggression are not punished for their behavior, nor are they removed whenever the infant is present.

A. Instead, locked gates, crates, and restraint systems can allow the dog to see the child and participate in some level of interaction that can be favorable for the dog without putting the child at risk.

B. The infant at risk must always have an adult supervising it and another adult supervising and/or restraining the dog when they are in the same environment.

IV. Unsupervised, sleeping infants must be kept behind a secured door in a room with a baby monitor.

V. Desensitization and counterconditioning are not implemented, because any doubt about their reliability makes them too risky.

VI. These dogs can sometimes be safely placed in other homes with older children.

VII. If the owner wishes to keep the dog, the dog is introduced to the baby in the manner recommended earlier and then graduates to introductions using head collars and harnesses, using positive reinforcement

Table 116–1. **Miscellaneous Aggressions**

Definition	Clinical Signs	Treatment
Redirected aggression: Aggression that is consistently directed toward a third party when the animal is thwarted or interrupted from exhibiting aggressive behavior to its primary target. The aggression is not accidental, and the animal actively pursues the third party.	A. This is seldom a solitary diagnosis and may act as a flag for other problem behaviors. B. Redirected aggression may co-exist with dominance aggression but is not a sign of it. C. It is important to distinguish redirected aggression from a truly accidental bite that is inflicted on a person who is, for example, trying to separate fighting dogs.	A. Treatment involves anticipation and avoidance. B. An accurate diagnosis of the primary problem, the interruption from which the redirected aggression is a response, is necessary. The primary aggressive diagnosis is then pursued.
Food-related aggression: Consistent aggression that is exhibited only in the presence of pet food, bones, rawhides, biscuits, blood, or human food (in the absence of torture or starvation).	A. This diagnosis serves to highlight that food is *not* a possession, but rather something very different from a possession. B. Although food-related aggression may be associated with dominance aggression, it is absolutely, categorically different, based on the necessary and sufficient criteria listed for each. C. When food-related aggression and dominance aggression co-occur, the development of food-related aggression usually precedes the development of dominance aggression.	A. The easiest and safest treatment, if the aggression focuses on rawhide, real bones, or treats, is to delete them from the dog's diet. B. If the dog is aggressive only for scraps or treats that are hand-fed, they can be offered only in the dog's dish. C. If the dog is aggressive when its food dish is approached, passive and active behavior modification programs should be implemented. D. In profound cases involving feeding meals, it may be easiest and safest to feed the dog behind a locked door and leave it undisturbed until the meal is finished. E. Head collars (Gentle Leader, Promise) can help correct and interrupt the response.
Possessive aggression: Aggression that is consistently directed toward other individuals when they approach or attempt to obtain a non-food object or toy that the aggressor possesses or to which the aggressor controls access.	A. This diagnostic category includes *only* non-food, non-gustatory items. B. Although this aggression may be correlated with the occurrence of dominance aggression, the latter is about control of activity or access—it is *not* about control of objects. C. The objects protected by the dog may not seem rational to the owner.	A. Avoidance of the object or class of objects can be an easy and effective treatment. B. If avoidance is not possible, passive and active behavior modification programs are implemented. Counterconditioning and desensitization are aimed at teaching the dog to relinquish toys or other objects on command and to not otherwise react in their presence. C. Any other problem aggressions must be addressed.
Pain aggression: Consistent aggressive behavior, in excess of that required to indicate concern and to effect restraint, demonstrated only in a context known or potentially associated with pain but that may not be painful itself.	A. This is a diagnosis of degree and correlation: conditions that are known to cause pain (e.g., fractured legs) could render the animal resistant to manipulation. B. In order for this diagnosis to be made, fear must not be primary (although anticipation of pain and the attendant anxiety may be involved), and the behaviors must be in excess of those required to indicate the animal's concern.	A. Treatment of the primary painful condition is mandatory. B. Medications designed to relieve or control pain are used and may minimize the frequency with which pain aggression develops. C. Avoidance of the approaches known to correlate with the response helps. D. Punishment has no role here. E. If avoidance is not possible, passive and active behavior modification programs are implemented.

techniques. The dog will probably cease to react to the child when the child can sit up and begins to appear human to the dog.

VIII. Young children can be taught to ask dogs to sit for food treats, but dogs are not encouraged to clean children's faces or to steal their food.

Miscellaneous Aggressions

See Table 116–1.

CANINE ELIMINATION DISORDERS

Incomplete Housebreaking

Definition and Clinical Signs

I. This disorder involves consistent and age-inappropriate elimination in undesirable locations or at undesir-

Table 116–1. **Miscellaneous Aggressions** (*Continued*)

Definition	Clinical Signs	Treatment
Maternal aggression: Consistent aggression (threat, challenge, or contest) directed toward puppies, or an individual approaching those puppies, in the absence of pain, challenges, or threats to the mother or the puppies.	A. When this is profound, it is extremely easy to recognize. B. The more common manifestation of this diagnosis is when the bitch is experiencing a false pregnancy or a pseudocyetic event. In this case, toys or nests are protected. C. Approach distances may be huge and if the aggression is directed toward individuals other than the puppies, the main aggressive signs might be prolonged growling without intensification of aggressive behaviors.	A. If the bitch is attacking the puppies, the puppies are removed and hand-reared. The bitch is not rebred. B. If the bitch is aggressive only when approached by other animals or humans, approaches are avoided. C. Passive and active behavior modification programs are implemented. Counterconditioning and desensitization are aimed at teaching the dog to relax when gradually approached. D. If the aggression is associated with a pseudocyetic event, recidivistic events can be prevented by spaying the dog after the cessation of the false pregnancy. E. The use of progestins and androgens is not encouraged, because of the risks they pose for future breeding. The better choice is to spay the dog.
Play aggression: Out-of-context, consistent aggression in circumstances in which play is relevant or that occurs in instances consistent with the solicitation of play, but involves actions that would discourage play (biting, pain).	A. The difficulty here is to distinguish rough play that the animals have learned in their interactions with other animals or people from truly abnormal behavior. B. Dogs will use their mouths and paws to play rambunctiously. These behaviors can be normal but must be channeled to more appropriate activities.	A. Avoidance of all situations that elicit the behavior is paramount. B. From the outset, rough play with dogs is not tolerated. Physical roughhousing with dogs involves only toys. C. Mouthing is not tolerated. Anyone who experiences mouthing says ''no'' and freezes. D. Aerobic play (e.g., agility training, Frisbee, fly ball) is encouraged.

Fear aggression: Aggression that consistently occurs concomitantly with behavioral and physiologic signs of fear as identified by withdrawal, passive, and avoidance behaviors associated with the sympathetic branch of the autonomic nervous system.	A. The actual behaviors associated with fear, fear aggression, and any other aggression that is driven primarily by anxiety are poorly qualified.
	B. Note that this aggression does not have to occur consistently, although identification of the fearful stimuli permits assessment of the extent to which the behaviors are consistent and pose a predictable risk.
		A. Identification of the stimuli that initiate the response is critical.
		B. Counterconditioning and desensitization are aimed at teaching the dog to relax in the presence of the fear-eliciting stimulus.
		C. Head collars (Gentle Leader, Promise) can help correct and interrupt the response.
		D. Bark collars that spray the dog with citronella (ABS System, Aboistop) may be useful.
		E. This is one of the few diagnoses for which flooding may be an option.
		F. Medication can be extremely helpful as part of an integrated treatment program.
		  1. Amitriptyline
		  2. Fluoxetine
		  3. Clomipramine
		  4. ± Sertraline
		  5. Propranolol (limited success).

Idiopathic aggression: Aggression that occurs in an unpredictable, toggle-switch manner in contexts not associated with stimuli noted for any other behavioral aggressive diagnosis and in the absence of any underlying causal physical or physiologic condition.	A. This aggression must be distinguished from that associated with any neurologic condition. B. It is necessary to rule out undiagnosed or subtle dominance aggression. C. This condition has been labeled ''rage,'' a term that should not be used.	A. If this condition exists, it is almost impossible to avoid because of its unpredictability, and it may be difficult to treat. B. Preliminary treatment with lithium and carbamazepine (Tegretol) has been investigated.

able times and is not associated with any lack of access or opportunity, other behavioral conditions, or any physical or physiologic condition.

II. This diagnosis is applied to animals for which this has always been true and for which the complaint does not involve a change in behavior.

Diagnosis

I. The only way to make this diagnosis is through an exhaustive history and examination of actual behaviors.

II. Diagnosis is confirmed by a positive response following institution of a rigorous housebreaking paradigm.

Differential Diagnosis

I. Insufficient access
  A. It includes the denial of access to an appropriate substrate, at an appropriate time, in a manner consistent with the individual dog's needs.
  B. Inherent in this diagnosis are changes that might occur with age (e.g., arthritis) and ambient environmental conditions (e.g., ice) that could cause dogs to be denied access to an area where they would otherwise eliminate.
  C. This diagnosis also includes temporal situations that exceed an individual dog's particular physiologic limits.
  D. This is a management-related problem that involves identification of the factors involved in lack of access and correcting them.

II. Substrate preference
  A. It is the consistent elimination in an area or areas that are linked by some common sensory aspect, and avoidance or rejection of alternative materials or conditions.
  B. This is the normal condition for well-housebroken dogs; however, in those situations, the substrate they prefer is also one that is acceptable to the owners.
  C. This becomes a diagnosis only when there is an owner-pet preference mismatch.
  D. Kenneled, crated, or pet store dogs may have either no preference (and no inhibition) or a preference for a substrate that the owner considers undesirable.
  E. Stray dogs, even if adults, are not automatically housebroken; they often have little inhibition and no preference for substrate, although they may have well-developed marking behaviors.
  F. Treatment focuses on positively reinforcing preferred substrates.

Treatment and Monitoring

I. It is difficult to teach a puppy to go outside to urinate and defecate after it has learned to use newspaper.
  A. It is preferable to teach the dog to go outside from the outset, but this may not fit into the owner's schedule.
  B. If the puppy is to be trained to paper or a litter box, place it in one location, preferably close to a door.

II. Housebreaking is done as follows.
  A. The puppy is taken outside every 1–2 hours when awake.
  B. The puppy is taken to the desired area upon awakening; 15–30 minutes after eating, after having a treat, and after playing; and when the puppy slows down during play.
  C. The puppy is permitted to sniff but not to play until it has eliminated.
  D. The pup is praised for using the right substrate every time it squats.
  E. After elimination, the pup is permitted to play and explore.
  F. Crate training can facilitate housebreaking, because it decreases elimination in inappropriate places.
    1. Crates are not used for punishment and are not a substitute for attention.
    2. They need to be large enough for the dog to be able to fully extend and turn around.
  G. Punishment has almost no role in housebreaking a dog.
    1. Startling the dog at the onset of the inappropriate behavior (e.g., sniffing, circling, beginning to squat) can be useful.
    2. Reprimanding the dog after the act can teach the dog to fear the owner.
  H. If the pup has a bell placed on its collar, it can be monitored as it moves through the house. When the bell becomes silent, the client should run to check on the dog.

Miscellaneous Elimination Disorders

See Table 116–2.

FEARS AND ANXIETIES

Fear

Definition and Clinical Signs

I. These behaviors occur concomitantly with behavioral and physiologic signs of fear, as identified by withdrawal, passive, and avoidance behaviors associated with the sympathetic branch of the autonomic nervous system, and in the absence of any aggressive behavior.

II. Fear and anxiety have signs that overlap.
  A. Some nonspecific signs such as avoidance, shaking, and trembling can be characteristic of both.
  B. The physiologic signs probably differ at some very refined level, and the neurochemistry of each is probably very different.

Treatment and Monitoring

I. Treatment addresses the identified provocative stimuli.

Table 116–2. **Miscellaneous Elimination Disorders**

Definition	Clinical Signs	Treatment
Anxiety, primarily separation anxiety: Physical or behavioral signs of distress exhibited by the animal only in the absence of or lack of access to the owner.	A. The elimination is exhibited only in the virtual or actual absence of the owner. B. The behaviors are most severe within the first 15–20 min of separation. C. Any anxiety-provoking stimulus can induce an elimination response.	A. Identification of the provocative stimulus is necessary. B. Treatment based on desensitization and counterconditioning to address the anxiety-provoking stimulus is necessary. C. Antianxiety drugs can help with the treatment of the anxiety (see Separation Anxiety).
Marking behavior: Urination or defecation that occurs in frequencies and/or locations inconsistent solely with evacuation of bladder and bowel, but consistent with social and olfactory stimuli and with species-typical postures distinct from those used in simple elimination.	A. Postures and associated behaviors are sufficiently well described in a circumscribed manner that is not consistent with anxiety, excitement, incomplete housebreaking, or aversions and perferences. B. Marking functions can also be part of normal elimination that does not involve behavior that is distasteful to the owner.	A. Castration (if prepubertal) can prevent or decrease marking behaviors in about ⅔ of all dogs that are castrated. B. Ovariohysterectomy decreases seasonal marking in females in heat and removes a source of stimulation for reciprocal marking behaviors. C. Odor eliminators may be useful in helping to alter perception for repeated marking.
Submissive behavior: Urination that occurs in an otherwise housebroken animal only when the animal is exhibiting species-specific postures associated with deferential behavior.	A. Any confusion about whether this diagnosis is the appropriate one can be eliminated by evaluation of the history and concomitant behaviors. B. Discrete description of the posture in which this behavior occurs is diagnostic.	A. Treatment is aimed at decreasing the extent to which deferential and submissive behaviors are exhibited. B. Dogs are not rewarded for any submissive behaviors. C. Using desensitization and counterconditioning, owners teach dogs that they are ignored if they exhibit the behaviors attendant with submissive urination.
Excitement urination: Urination that occurs only when the dog is actively engaged in active behavior and is concomitantly demonstrating physical and physiologic signs of excitement.	A. The urination occurs when the animal is not sitting or lying down, or approaching sitting or lying down, and the animal may exhibit no signs of awareness. B. This diagnosis can be difficult to distinguish from submissive urination, incomplete housebreaking, or intense need for micturition.	A. Treatment is aimed at not rewarding the behavior associated with excitement. B. These dogs receive attention only after they have emptied their bladders. C. Punishment makes this worse. D. Young pups may exhibit this behavior more often than older dogs. Most pups grow out of this as they strengthen urinary sphincter tone. E. Dogs that have decreased urinary sphincter tone can benefit from ancillary use of phenylpropanolamine 1–2 mg/kg PO PRN.
Attention-seeking behavior: The presence of vocal or physical behaviors that result in obtaining passive or active attention from people when the people are engaged in passive or active activities not directly involving the animal.	A. This may be an undesirable behavior, but it is common and may be a variant of normal; it is certainly a behavior that people unconsciously reinforce in their pets. B. In extreme cases, the animal may exhibit postures associated with elimination (or actually eliminate) because people then get up and take them out.	A. The dog must be taught to sit and stay for all attention. Once it does this, it must get attention. It is neither sufficient nor acceptable to recommend ignoring the dog. B. The dog is taken out and exercised on a regular schedule. Most dogs that exhibit elimination associated with attention-seeking behavior otherwise get little attention or affection.

II. In situations involving developing fear, mild fear, or anxiety, counterconditioning and desensitization can be efficacious; early intervention is desirable.

III. Prevention can be useful.
   A. Dogs are most sensitive to learning about new stimuli at 5–14 weeks of age.
   B. They should be broadly exposed to all stimuli and allowed to explore at their own pace, provided they demonstrate no overt signs of profound fear or panic.

IV. It is never acceptable to terrorize a dog to ''treat'' its fear. This is very different from flooding.

V. If the fearful stimulus is solitary, nongeneralized, and identifiable, flooding can work if counterconditioning and desensitization fail. The risk is that the fear will be worsened.

VI. Medications can be extremely useful as part of an integrated treatment program.
  A. See the general drug discussion under Dominance Aggression, earlier.
  B. Drugs that may be efficacious include amitriptyline, fluoxetine, clomipramine, propranolol, and possibly sertraline.

Non–Noise-Related Phobias

Definition

I. A phobia is a consistent, sustained, and extreme nongraded response, manifested as intense and active avoidance, escape, or anxiety behaviors associated with the activities of the sympathetic branch of the autonomic nervous system.
II. If the consistent, sustained, sudden, profound, nongraded response is to unfamiliar objects and circumstances, the condition is termed neophobia. Dogs kept in restrictive and isolated circumstances through 14 weeks of age are at increased risk for the development of neophobia.

Clinical Signs and Diagnosis

I. Behaviors associated with a phobic response can include catatonia or mania concomitant with decreased sensitivity to pain or social stimuli; repeated exposure results in an invariant pattern of response.
II. The stage at which a fear becomes a phobia is unknown but is epistemologically important.
III. Patterns related to the development of fears and phobias involve evaluation of the frequency, intensity, and qualification of actual behaviors.
IV. Risks associated with the development of related behaviors are unknown for animals already exhibiting fear or anxiety.
V. There seems to be a strong genetic component to the development of a phobic response.

Treatment and Monitoring

I. Early prevention aimed at encouraging normal responses to a variety of stimuli is encouraged.
II. Early treatment using counterconditioning and desensitization is strongly recommended.
III. Medication may be an essential part of the treatment paradigm.
  A. Amitriptyline 1–2 mg PO BID (i.e., q 12 h) for 30 days
  B. Fluoxetine 1 mg/kg PO SID (i.e., q 24 h) for 60 days
  C. Clomipramine 2 mg/kg PO BID for 60 days or 1 mg/kg PO BID for 14 days, then 2 mg/kg PO BID for 14 days, then 3 mg/kg PO BID for 28 days
  D. Propranolol 5–10 mg/dog PO BID-TID
  E. Sertraline (dose not well defined)
  F. Alprazolam (Xanax) 0.01–1 mg/kg PO PRN 1 hour before provocation, not to exceed 4 mg/day
    1. Use very low dosages (1–2 mg/dog)
    2. Sedation and incoordination can be profound, but if panic is associated with the phobic

response, this can be an excellent medication to use alone or in combination with one of the preceding.

Noise- and Thunderstorm-Related Phobias

Definition

Noise phobia is a sudden, profound, nongraded, extreme response to noise manifested as intense and active avoidance, escape, or anxiety behaviors.

Clinical Signs and Diagnosis

I. Behaviors can include catatonia or mania concomitant with decreased sensitivity to pain or social stimuli; repeated exposure results in an invariant pattern of response.
II. Patterns related to the development of fears and phobias involve evaluation of the frequency, intensity, and qualification of actual behaviors. Risks associated with the development of related behaviors are unknown for animals already exhibiting fear or anxiety.
III. If the response is associated only with thunderstorms, it is termed a thunderstorm phobia.
  A. The response can be to any aspect of thunderstorms (noise, dark, changes in barometric pressure, changes in ozone levels).
  B. Many animals with thunderstorm phobias may have generalized phobias, but this specific diagnosis relies on other related cues that are associated with other sensory systems (olfaction, vision), not just the auditory one.
  C. It is likely that all animals with noise phobias have a thunderstorm phobia, but the converse might not be true.

Treatment and Monitoring

I. Treatment is aimed at protecting the dog during the phobic event and at diminishing the dog's response.
II. Counterconditioning and desensitization can be useful for very early noise phobias. Tape recordings that also convey the vibrations and atmospheric effects are commercially available and should be played at increasingly loud levels while the dog relaxes.
III. Almost without exception, medication is essential in treatment.
  A. Medication must be administered before the onset of the stimulus and before the dog begins to display any signs of distress.
  B. Short-term treatment involves the following.
    1. Diazepam 0.55–2.2 mg/kg PO PRN
      a) This short-acting medication can help relieve anxiety and render the dog less sensitive to the environmental stimuli.
      b) Sedation and incoordination are common side effects.
    2. Clorazepate (Tranxene) 0.55–2.2 mg/kg PO PRN

This is a longer-acting drug than diazepam and may be a better choice if the dog is to be left alone for more than a few hours.

3. Alprazolam (see Non–Noise-Related Phobias, earlier)

C. Long-term or chronic treatment may take 3–5 weeks to take effect.
   1. Clomipramine (see Dominance Aggression, earlier)
   2. Buspirone (BuSpar): relatively free of side effects, a nonspecific partial serotonin agonist that relieves situational anxiety
   3. Fluoxetine (see Dominance Aggression, earlier)

Separation Anxiety

Definition

It includes physical or behavioral signs of distress (consistent or intensive destruction, elimination, vocalization, or salivation) exhibited by the animal only in the absence of or lack of access to the owner.

Clinical Signs and Diagnosis

I. Behaviors are most severe within the first 15–20 minutes of separation, and many anxiety-related behaviors (autonomic hyper-reactivity, increased motor activity, and increased vigilance and scanning) may become apparent as the owner displays behaviors consistent with the intention to leave.

II. The extent to which animals exhibiting separation anxiety have other anxious behaviors or experience self-mutilation, phobias, or fears is unknown.

III. No study has demonstrated that it is more common in animals with very attentive owners.

IV. It is important to rule out other situations that could be associated with the common signs of separation anxiety: incomplete housebreaking, teething, play, and a response to a truly scary, unique event (e.g., a robbery).

Treatment and Monitoring

I. Protecting the dog from itself and protecting the environment from the dog are important.
   A. Barriers (gates, crates) may help.
   B. Caution is urged, because confinement makes some of these dogs worse.

II. While treatment is ongoing, dogs are accompanied by a human when possible.

III. Obtaining another pet has not traditionally ameliorated the condition, but the loss of an animal companion can worsen it.

IV. Counterconditioning and desensitization can be used to change the dog's response to cues associated with the onset of the owner's departure (e.g., briefcases, keys, hair dryers) and to accustom the dog to increasingly longer separations.

V. If vocalization is caused by separation anxiety, bark collars neither treat the symptoms (the dog overrides them) nor help the condition (the barking is the symptom, not the problem).

VI. Medication is an integral part of treatment for this condition.
   A. Unless the complaint has just developed, effective treatment is unlikely without pharmacologic intervention.
   B. Medications to try include amitriptyline, clomipramine, fluoxetine, sertraline, and alprazolam.
   C. If panic is involved, combination drug treatment using alprazolam and one of the other medications may be advantageous.

Generalized Anxiety

Definition

I. Generalized anxiety is the consistent exhibition of increased autonomic hyper-reactivity, increased motor activity, and increased vigilance and scanning that interferes with a normal range of social interaction in the absence of any provocative stimuli.

II. This condition can easily be misdiagnosed in the absence of critical thought or an incomplete history. It is a diagnosis of last resort, and all the signs must be present concomitantly under conditions in which any of these signs would have subsided in a normal or nonsymptomatic animal.

Clinical Signs

I. Hyperactivity may be associated with generalized anxiety.
   A. Hyperactivity is defined as motor activity that occurs in a consistent manner in excess of that warranted by the animal's age and stimulation level.
      1. It does not respond to correction, redirection, or restraint.
      2. It is concomitant with sympathetic signs (increased heart rate, increased respiratory rate, vasodilatation), even when at rest.
      3. It occurs in the absence of other signs or significant laboratory data associated with thyroid disease.
      4. The dog responds to treatment with amphetamine or methylphenidate with a paradoxic decrease in motor activity.
   B. Most dogs that owners call hyperactive (a diagnosis that does *not* depend on the dog's exercise level compared with its needs) are actually overactive.

II. Hyperactivity is a specific diagnosis for which specific behavioral signs have been poorly elucidated.

Treatment and Monitoring

I. Early recognition of deviations from normal and excessive behavior is important.

II. Counterconditioning and desensitization to stimuli that appear to be correlated with the behavior can be useful.

III. Medications may be useful as ancillary treatment that raises the threshold for the trigger of the anxious response and renders the behavior modification more efficacious.

IV. Therapy can be instituted with amitriptyline, clomipramine, fluoxetine, or sertraline.

Obsessive-Compulsive Disorder (OCD)

Definition and Clinical Signs

I. OCD is repetitive, stereotypic motor, locomotor, grooming, ingestive, or hallucinogenic behaviors that occur out of context to their normal occurrence or in a frequency or duration that is in excess of that required to accomplish the ostensible goal.

II. These behaviors occur in a manner that interferes with the animal's ability to otherwise normally function in its social environment.

III. It is debatable whether animals can obsess.

IV. Separate from the obsession issue is the one of relative intensity.
   A. Whether a behavior is excessive or a manifestation of OCD may be a determination of degree.
   B. Careful description and recording of behaviors and their durations provide data that permit evaluation of the extent to which such behaviors develop as a continuum.

Diagnosis

I. Good histories and observation are important, because in some peculiar forms, OCD can resemble seizure-like activity.

II. By definition, some epileptic or seizure-like activity is stereotypic, which is one reason that a diagnosis of OCD is preferable to that of stereotypy.

Treatment and Monitoring

I. Treatment is aimed at teaching the dog to relax in circumstances under which the OCD would become pronounced.

II. Counterconditioning and desensitization can help as part of an integrated treatment program.

III. Unless the behavior has just started, the key to treatment is pharmacologic.

IV. Maintenance drug therapy with amitriptyline, clomipramine, fluoxetine, or sertraline may be necessary (see Dominance Aggression, earlier).

Cognitive Dysfunction

Definition and Clinical Signs

I. It is a change in interactive, elimination, or navigational behaviors attendant with aging that are not caused by primary failure of any organ system.

II. This is a potential animal model for the age-dependent cognitive changes that occur in people. The affiliated behaviors may be associated with Alzheimer's-like lesions (senile dementia of the Alzheimer type).

III. It is unclear whether this is associated with age-dependent changes in dopaminergic function or with microembolic events or is a form of old-age–onset separation anxiety.

Diagnosis

I. The main method for evaluating cognitive dysfunction in people is not applicable to domestic pet animals.

II. Refinements of cognitive tests based on learning and navigational skills should provide future enhancements.

Treatment and Monitoring

I. Treatment is currently directed at the signs that may be related to adult-onset separation anxiety (see earlier).

II. Medications to try include the following.
   A. Amitriptyline 1–2 mg PO BID for 30 days
   B. Selegiline (deprenyl) 1 mg/kg PO SID indefinitely

Bibliography

Archer J: The Behavioral Biology of Aggression. Cambridge University Press, New York, 1988

Baerends GP: The functional organization of behaviour. Anim Behav 24:726, 1976

Bateson P: How do sensitive periods arise and what are they for? Anim Behav 27:470, 1979

Baum M: Veterinary use of exposure techniques in the treatment of phobic domestic animals. Behav Res Ther 9:249, 1971

Borchelt PL: Aggressive behavior of dogs kept as companion animals: classification and influence of sex, reproductive status and breed. Appl Anim Ethology 10:45, 1983

Borchelt PL, Voith VL: Diagnosis and treatment of separation-related behavior problems in dogs. Vet Clin North Am [Small Anim Pract] 12:625, 1982

Borchelt PL, Voith VL: Dominance aggression in dogs. Compend Contin Educ Pract Vet 8:36, 1986

Boulenger JP, Squilace K, Simon P et al: Buspirone and diazepam: comparison of subjective, psychomotor, and biological effects. Neuropsychobiology 22:83, 1989

Chapman BL, Voith VL: Behavioral problems in old dogs. J Am Vet Med Assoc 196:944, 1990

Cummings BJ, Su JH, Cotman CW et al: Beta-amyloid accumulation in aged canine brain: a model of early plaque formation in Alzheimer's disease. Neurobiol Aging 14:547, 1993

deLuca RV, Holborn SW: A comparison of relaxation training and competing response training to eliminate hair pulling and nail biting. J Behav Ther Exp Psychiatry 15:67, 1984

Domjan M, Burkhard B: The Principles of Learning and Behavior. 2nd Ed. Brooks/Cole, Pacific Grove, 1985

Elliot O, Scott JP: The development of emotional distress reactions to separation in puppies. J Genet Psychol 99:3, 1961

Fält L: Inheritance of behavior in the dog. p. 183. In Anderson RS (ed): Nutrition and Behavior in Dogs and Cats. Pergamon Press, New York, 1984

Floody OR: Hormones and aggression in female mammals. p. 39. In Svare BB (ed): Hormones and Aggressive Behavior. Plenum, New York, 1983

Free NK, Winget CN, Whitman RM: Separation anxiety in panic disorder. Am J Psychiatry 150:595, 1993

Freedman DG, King JA, Elliot O: Critical periods in the social development of dogs. Science 133:1016, 1961

Gasperini M, Gatti F, Bellini L et al: Perspective in clinical psychopharmacology of amitriptyline and fluoxetine. Neuropsychobiology 26:186, 1992

Gosling LM: A reassessment of the function of scent-marking in territories. Z Tierpsych 60:89, 1982

Hopkins SG, Schubert TA, Hart BL: Castration of adult male dogs: effects on roaming, aggression, urine spraying, and mounting. J Am Vet Med Assoc 168:1108, 1976

Jenkins SC, Maruta T: Therapeutic use of propranolol for intermittent explosive disorders (review). Mayo Clin Proc 62:204, 1987

Kalin NH: The neurobiology of fear. Sci Am 268:94, 1993

Line S, Voith VL: Dominance aggression of dogs towards people: behavior profile and response to treatment. Appl Anim Behav Sci 16:77, 1986

Marder AR: Psychotropic drugs and behavior therapy. Vet Clin North Am [Small Anim Pract] 21:329, 1991

Mason GJ: Stereotypies: a critical review. Anim Behav 41:1015, 1991

McCrave EA: Diagnostic criteria for separation anxiety in the dog. Vet Clin North Am [Small Anim Pract] 21:247, 1991

Milgram NW, Head E, Weiner E, Thomas E: Cognitive functions and aging in the dog: acquisition of non-spatial visual tasks. Behav Neurosci 108:57, 1994

Milgram NW, Ivy GO, Head E et al: The effect of L-deprenyl on behavior, cognitive function, and biogenic amines in the dog (review). Neurochem Res 18:1211, 1993

Montgomery SA, Bullock T, Fineberg B: Serotonin selectivity for obsessive-compulsive and panic disorders. J Psychiatry Neurosci 16:30, 1991

O'Farrell V, Peachey E: Behavioral effects of ovariohysterectomy on bitches. J Small Anim Pract 31:595, 1990

Overall KL: Practical pharmacological approaches to behavior problems. Purina Specialty Review—Behavioral Problems in Small Animals 36, 1992a

Overall KL: Recognition, diagnosis, and management of obsessive-compulsive disorders. Part I. Canine Pract 17:40, 1992b

Overall KL: Use of clomipramine to treat ritualistic stereotypic motor behavior in three dogs. J Am Vet Med Assoc 205:1733, 1994

Overall KL: Clinical Behavioral Medicine for Small Animals. CV Mosby, St. Louis, 1997

Serpell J, Jagoe JA: Early experience and the development of behaviour. p. 80. In Serpell J (ed): The Domestic Dog: Its Evolution, Behaviour, and Interactions with People. Cambridge University Press, Cambridge, 1995

Spreat S, Spreat SR: Learning principles. Vet Clin North Am [Small Anim Pract] 12:593, 1982

Voith VL, Wright JC, Danneman PJ: Is there a relationship between canine behavior problems and spoiling activity, anthropomorphism, and obedience training? Appl Anim Behav Sci 34:262, 1992

Vom Saal FS: Sexual differentiation in litter-bearing mammals: influence of sex of adjacent fetuses in utero. J Anim Sci 67:1824, 1989

Young MS: Treatment of fear-induced aggression in dogs. Vet Clin North Am [Small Anim Pract] 12:645, 1982

117

Feline Behavioral Disorders

Ann D. Beebe
Karen L. Overall

FELINE ELIMINATION DISORDERS

Definition

I. The most common feline behavioral complaint involves inappropriate or undesirable elimination.
   A. By 3 weeks of age, kittens no longer rely on the urogenital reflex and can voluntarily eliminate.
   B. Kittens are not trained to litter boxes but have a natural attraction to explore and eliminate in loose particle material.
II. Elimination patterns are affected by observation of the queen and by olfactory stimulation.
   A. Elimination patterns for voiding urine or feces usually involve a squatting posture with the pelvic limbs abducted and the tail rigid and pointed caudally.
   B. Many cats dig a small hole in the litter material before urinating or defecating.
   C. Some cats cover their urine and/or feces, but lack of digging and covering can also be part of the normal range of feline elimination behaviors.

Causes and Clinical Signs

I. Role of medical problems
   A. Medical problems that influence the frequency, urgency, volume, and pain of urination and defecation may contribute to inappropriate elimination patterns. These can include components of feline lower urinary tract disease, renal disease, metabolic disorders, anatomic abnormalities, or orthopedic conditions.
   B. Recent data indicate that most medical problems are not manifested as behavioral elimination disorders, and most behavioral elimination disorders are not caused by an underlying physical problem (Beebe et al., in preparation)

II. Environmentally related inappropriate elimination
   A. Substrate preferences and aversions
      1. Substrates are materials chosen for elimination and are associated with tactile sensations that occur during an elimination sequence.
      2. Cats may preferentially choose a material for urination and/or defecation that is offered as a litter.
      3. Aversions to litter types may be associated with negative experiences, punishment, or a frightening encounter while in the litter box. They can occur with a new litter type or a dirty litter box.
   B. Location preferences and aversions
      1. Busy traffic areas or locations that present maneuvering difficulties can lead the cat to seek alternative areas for elimination.
      2. This can encourage a cat to develop a location preference.
      3. Cats that experience an aversive event in the area of the litter box may avoid the present litter box location.
III. Socially related inappropriate elimination
   A. Cats are social animals and are affected by a variety of daily stressors that influence patterns of elimination.
      1. Intact animals use marking behaviors more frequently than do neutered animals. These include spraying, nonspraying urine marking, and marking with feces.
      2. Marking behaviors occur more often in the complex social environment of multicat households.
   B. Nonspraying urine marking consists of urine found on a horizontal surface.
      1. The behavior is usually associated with social interactions with other cats or people and is a normal form of feline communication.

2. The urine puddle may be of various sizes and is often found by doorways, windows, beds, and owner clothing.

C. Marking with feces is another form of feline social communication, especially at entry/exit areas or areas of social contact.

IV. Urine spraying

   A. Males and females can urine spray.

     1. The cat usually sniffs an object, turns so the hind end is pointed at the object, and directs a small amount of urine at a vertical target.

     2. One characteristic of urine spraying is the classic upright tail quiver at the time of the urine spray.

   B. This form of feline communication is closely associated with both reproductive status and conflict or anxiety in social encounters.

   C. Cats that urine spray normally use their litter box for urination and defecation.

Diagnosis

I. Obtain medical and behavioral histories related to elimination.

   A. Determine patterns of elimination complaints and behaviors such as postures, frequencies, surfaces, and locations of inappropriate elimination.

   B. Determine the number, location, and style of litter boxes; the type of litter material used; and the maintenance and care of litter boxes.

   C. Establish the number of people and pets and their interactions in the household.

II. Perform a urinalysis and fecal analysis, and consider other tests to rule out organic disease of the urinary or gastrointestinal tract.

III. The cat is given a physical exam, complete blood count, and serum biochemistry profile to establish baseline values to detect underlying renal or hepatic conditions that would affect the symptoms or drug therapy.

Treatment

I. Treat medical problems as indicated.

II. Institute treatment for the behavioral disorder.

   A. Environmental treatment

     1. Clean soiled areas with enzymatic products; heavily soiled rugs or furniture may have to be removed.

     2. Offer multiple boxes, a variety of substrates (clumpable, fine, or silicate litters are more universally preferred), different locations, and alternative style boxes, and vary the litter depth.

     3. Remove urine and feces soon after deposited.

     4. Dump litter and clean boxes 1–2 times per week.

     5. Avoid scented litters and cleaning products, liners, and hooded boxes (unless the cat prefers a hooded box).

     6. Use deterrents such as heavy plastic, food/ water, plants, and blockades in elimination areas.

     7. Use positive reinforcement such as food treats and praise for appropriate litter box use.

     8. Interrupt inappropriate elimination by startling the cat (foghorns, whistles, squirt gun) in the first 30 seconds.

     9. Confinement of the cat when it is not actively supervised may be necessary.

    10. Give the cat set play and attention times—at least 5–10 minutes twice a day.

    11. If necessary, slowly change litter preferences or box locations over a period of weeks.

    12. Address social influences of the elimination disorder; practice behavior modification, desensitization, and counterconditioning techniques such as positive reintroduction to the cat or person causing anxiety.

    13. Neuter intact animals, provide more vertical space per cat, and decrease the number of cats in the household.

   B. Pharmacologic treatment

     1. Elimination disorders are complex, and multiple diagnoses are common. Many elimination disorders are the result of underlying anxiety about environmental or social aspects of elimination.

     2. Medications that address the anxiety component of inappropriate elimination are used in conjunction with environmental modifications to control the problem.

     3. Antianxiety medications have also begun to play a role in the treatment of feline lower urinary tract disease when neurogenic inflammation and stress or anxiety are components of its etiology.

     4. Elimination disorders that include marking behaviors are reflections of anxiety about social encounters.

      a) Medication may be needed to control marking.

      b) The environmental changes of cleaning, deterrents, and behavior modification to change the anxiety components of social encounters are necessary to manage the elimination disorder.

     5. Owners must sign an informed consent if the use of antianxiety medications is extra-label (most), and this statement must list potential side effects.

     6. Medications that have been used with success include amitriptyline (Elavil), diazepam (Valium), buspirone (BuSpar), clomipramine (Anafranil), and megestrol acetate (Ovaban) (Table 117–1).

     7. Side effects of all the preceding medications can include lethargy, vomiting, diarrhea, appetite change, and cardiac arrhythmias, particularly for the tricyclic antidepressants. The possible side effects of progestins are diabetes, gynecomastia, and bone marrow suppression.

Table 117–1. Commonly Used Medications for the Treatment of Feline Elimination Disorders, Aggression, and Obsessive-Compulsive Disorders

Drug	Dose
Amitriptyline (tricyclic antidepressant)	0.5–1 mg/kg PO q 12–24 h (general range: 2.5–5 mg/cat PO q 12–24 h)
Buspirone (nonspecific anxiolytic)	0.5–1 mg/kg PO q 12–24 h (general range: 5–10 mg/cat PO q 12–24 h)
Diazepam (benzodiazepine)	0.2–0.4 mg/kg PO q 12–24 h (general range: 1–2 mg/cat PO q 12–24 h)
Clomipramine (tricyclic antidepressant)	0.5 mg/kg PO q 24 h
Hydrocodone (narcotic agonist)	0.25–0.5 mg/kg PO q 12–24 h (general range: 1.25–2.5 mg/cat PO q 12–24 h)
Fluoxetine (serotonin-specific reuptake inhibitor)	0.5 mg/kg PO q 24 h
Megestrol acetate (progestin)	1–2 mg/kg PO q 24 h × 7 days, then taper (general range: 5–10 mg/cat PO q 24 h × 7 days, then taper)

Patient Monitoring

I. Schedule a re-examination appointment or phone update within 2 weeks of the initial exam to evaluate environmental and pharmacologic changes.

II. Prognosis is generally good for management of the problem.

III. Prognosis may depend on duration of the problem, frequency of the behavior, and owner compliance.

IV. Cats on medication have blood work every 8–12 months (every 6 months for older animals) or if the cat becomes ill.

V. After successful treatment, some cats can be weaned from medications over a 1- to 2-week period.

FELINE AGGRESSION

Definition

I. The second most common feline behavioral problem is aggression.

II. Aggressive interactions can be subtle, with stares or body postures, or they can be active encounters involving hissing, growling, swatting, chasing, and biting.

III. Aggression is affected by feline social hierarchies. These can be complex and are often poorly defined.

IV. Many aggressions develop during social maturity between 2 and 4 years of age, when issues related to social status become important.

Causes and Clinical Signs

I. Aggression caused by lack of socialization
   A. The sensitive period for cats is between 2 and 12 weeks of age, when many appropriate interactions with other cats and people are learned.
   B. The most important time to expose a cat to people is 2–7 weeks of age.
   C. Cats that have missed aspects of social exposure are at risk for abnormal social responses.
   D. Aggressive actions quickly escalate when these cats are restrained, confined, or corrected.

II. Play aggression
   A. Kittens that have been bottle raised and have not been corrected by their mother or other littermates for rough play may not inhibit their bites or scratches during play bouts.
   B. People may become targets of inappropriate play if they use their hands as play objects and if they encourage rough play.

III. Fearful aggression
   A. These cats display escalating aggression when frightened. The cat takes a defensive posture but will attack if provoked.
   B. The cat usually exhibits ears flattened against the back of the head, teeth bared, nose wrinkled, back arched, and piloerection.

IV. Pain aggression
   A. A cat that has a current or previous medical condition or experiences a painful procedure may react aggressively when approached or manipulated.
   B. The cat may try to escape or avoid situations that it associates with pain.

V. Intercat aggression
   A. Intercat aggression is common between intact males competing for mates.
   B. In a household, intercat aggression may develop in relation to social maturity issues and environmental changes that are separate from any sexual or mating behaviors.
   C. One cat is usually the aggressor, and the other is the victim.
   D. The aggressor visually and physically monitors one or many areas of the environment, whereas the victim usually hides and actively avoids social encounters.

VI. Maternal aggression
   A. A queen may solidly defend her kittens and nest area from intruders, especially during the periparturient period.
   B. A threatening display as the other cat or intruder approaches usually aborts the encounter.
   C. The queen may attack if the confrontation escalates.

VII. Predatory aggression
   A. Cats may naturally stalk small animals.
   B. The postures associated with aggression include lowered head; tense body; silent, slow movements or no movement; and tail twitch.
   C. Cats can also direct predatory aggression toward children or adults (feet, hands) as an out-of-context event.

VIII. Territorial aggression
   A. Cats may defend an area from other animals or people.

B. The area usually has distinct boundaries where the cat may patrol and mark with urine or feces or other scent marking.

IX. Redirected aggression

A. Redirected aggression most often occurs when a cat is in a highly aroused state.

B. The target that provokes the arousal is unavailable or unattainable, and the response is shifted to another individual by interruption of the event.

C. The cat may be agitated for an extended period following redirected aggression.

D. This aggression may be directed toward other cats (common) or to other species, including humans.

X. Assertion or status-related aggression

A. Cats' social hierarchies can include interactions with humans.

B. Some cats are controlling and pushy and display aggression toward people when petted or held.

C. The cat may block the owner's path and exhibit attention-seeking behaviors, such as rubbing, or challenge behaviors, such as staring.

D. Rubbing and bunting behaviors are marking behaviors in this context.

XI. Idiopathic aggression

A. Unlike with status-related aggression or redirected aggression, targets are not identifiable, and neither the target nor the context may be consistent.

B. It is often seen as an unprovoked, rapidly escalating aggression.

Diagnosis

I. Obtain a behavioral history that includes the following.

A. The age at which the pet was obtained, and from what source
B. Medical history
C. Number of people and pets in the household
D. Description of events
E. Chronology, frequency, and intensity of behavior
F. Number of bites and identification of victim
G. How the cat interacts with people and pets in the house
H. Amount of play and attention given
I. Concurrent marking/elimination problems

II. Rule out medical conditions such as metabolic, endocrine (hyperthyroidism), neurologic, and vascular (ischemic event) disorders.

III. Perform a physical exam, complete blood count, and serum biochemistry profile.

Treatment

I. Environmental treatment

A. Learn to recognize postures associated with aggressive events.

1. Intervene within the first few seconds of the event or 30–60 seconds after the onset of the process.

2. Use startles such as foghorns, whistles, or water pistols to interrupt the event.

B. Gently correct young kittens, do not use hands to play with the cat, and stop play if the cat is highly aroused.

C. Set daily play and attention times and increase the time spent in active play.

D. Do not approach reactive cats; wait until grooming or eating behaviors are observed.

E. Place light jingle bells on the aggressor to give warning to victims.

F. Reward the cat for nonreactive postures.

G. Separate cats in different rooms.

1. Provide neutral areas for both cats, or a more valued area or free range for the victim.
2. Cats should also be separated when not strictly supervised.

H. Gradually reintroduce cats (to cats or people) using positive reinforcement techniques such as food treats or by using cat carriers, leashes, and harnesses to control the situation.

I. Trim nails short or use nail caps.

II. Pharmacologic treatment

A. Cats that are anxious or abnormal during social encounters may benefit from medication that addresses underlying physiologic causes of the behavior.

B. Medications that have been used with success include amitriptyline (Elavil), buspirone (BuSpar), diazepam (Valium), clomipramine (Anafranil), and fluoxetine (Prozac) (see Table 117–1).

1. Obtain an informed consent from the owners.
2. Side effects of these drugs include lethargy, vomiting, diarrhea, and cardiac arrhythmias.

Patient Monitoring

I. Schedule a re-examination appointment or phone update within 2 weeks of the initial visit to evaluate environmental and pharmacologic therapy.

II. Prognosis is generally good for management of aggression.

III. Prognosis may depend on severity and frequency of the aggression, as well as owner compliance.

IV. Repeat blood work every 8–12 months (every 6 months for older animals) or if the cat is ill.

V. After successful treatment, some cats can be weaned from medications over a 1- to 2-week period.

OBSESSIVE-COMPULSIVE DISORDERS

Definition

I. Obsessive-compulsive disorders are usually defined as repetitive, ritualistic behaviors performed in excess of those required for normal function, the execution of which interferes with normal daily activities.

II. Many of the behaviors are species typical, but they are performed in exaggerated motions and durations.

III. These behaviors are complex, and medical causes of

or contributions to these activities must be investigated.
    IV. The abnormal behaviors usually increase if the cat is anxious.
    V. Multiple etiologies for obsessive-compulsive disorders have been postulated, and the most commonly cited mechanism is aberrant neuropharmacologic activity in the brain.

Causes and Clinical Signs

    I. Grooming
        A. Cats may overgroom by barbering and licking, and they may traumatize or mutilate their skin.
        B. The areas most often affected include the flank, ventral abdomen, and tail.
        C. The animals may vocalize, hide, or locomote to escape from the activity.
    II. Consumptive
        A. Cats may ingest, chew, or suck on items such as wool, cloth, leather, plastic, and a variety of other objects.
        B. Many cats actively seek out these objects and spend a large part of the day performing the behavior.
    III. Hallucinatory
        A. Some cats stare at or follow imaginary objects.
        B. This may be associated with predator-like motions.
        C. Other cats shriek and run after seeming to visualize an unknown stimulus.

Diagnosis

    I. Cats are evaluated for dermatologic and neurologic conditions.
    II. Obtain a behavioral history that includes the following items.
        A. Signalment
        B. Age at onset of behavior
        C. Duration and frequency of behavior
        D. Description of typical events, including the average duration and intensity of each episode
        E. Any changes in the pattern of behavior
        F. Events that occur before or after the behavior
        G. Methods that stop the behavior
        H. Attitude while performing the behavior
        I. A 24-hour schedule that includes pet-owner interactions and daily activities
        J. Any animal relative with similar behavior
    III. The history elucidates the extent to which the behaviors are performed in a stylized manner, excessively, or out of context.
    IV. Evaluate a complete blood count and serum biochemistry profile for renal and hepatic dysfunction that may be associated with signs or preclude the use of medication.

Treatment

    I. Treat any underlying medical conditions.
    II. Reward the cat with praise, food treats, or long gentle strokes for normal activities.

    III. Anticipate and interrupt behavior.
    IV. Give the cat set play and attention times.
    V. Identify any stimulus that elicits the behavior, and avoid or decrease exposure to that stimulus.
    VI. Pharmacologic therapy is often beneficial (see Table 117–1).
        A. Medications to consider include amitriptyline (Elavil), buspirone (BuSpar), clomipramine (Anafranil), hydrocodone (Tussigon), and fluoxetine (Prozac).
        B. Side effects can include lethargy, vomiting, diarrhea, and cardiac arrhythmias.

Patient Monitoring

    I. Most cats need medication for the duration of their life.
    II. Prognosis is good for greatly decreasing the frequency of the behavior.
    III. Blood work is monitored every 8–12 months (every 6 months for older cats) or if the cat is ill.

MISCELLANEOUS FELINE BEHAVIORAL COMPLAINTS

Attention Seeking

    I. Cats may solicit the owner for affection, play, and food.
    II. Attention seeking can be decreased by having fixed schedules for feeding and attention and by ignoring the cat (walking away, not petting or talking to the cat) in that circumstance.
    III. A variety of interactive toys and environmental stimuli can help engage the cat in activities other than attention seeking.
    IV. The addition of another cat may decrease attention-seeking behaviors, because the cat can interact with the other cat instead of the owner.

Scratching

    I. Scratching is a normal behavior for cats that serves to sharpen and unsheath claws, as well as provide visual and olfactory marking functions.
    II. Many cats respond to cloth, wood, or cardboard scratching posts that mimic the attractive household material.
    III. Undesirable scratching areas can be covered, and the cat can be interrupted as it approaches the location.
    IV. Nails can be trimmed, covered with caps, or surgically removed as a last resort.
    V. Cats can learn appropriate scratching locations and substrates if reinforced early and consistently.

Destruction

    I. This behavior can occur in a play, attention, or anxiety context.

II. The behavior can be controlled by adhering to set activity schedules, providing a variety of stimulating toys, and identifying or changing anxiety patterns.

III. If there is another cat in the household, many of the destructive behaviors can be redirected to that individual.

Vocalization

I. Excessive vocalization can be part of attention-seeking or anxiety behaviors.

II. Many cats decrease vocalizations if they are ignored and then rewarded for other more desirable activities.

Overactivity

I. Many cats exhibit bursts of activity that are usually associated with play.

II. Young energetic cats can benefit from channeled bouts of aerobic play.

III. This type of cat may benefit from an age- and size-matched play partner.

Bibliography

Beaver B: Feline Behavior: A Guide for Veterinarians. WB Saunders, Philadelphia, 1992

Beebe AD, Overall KL, Dunham AC: The influence of medical problems on feline elimination disorders (in preparation)

Bradshaw JW: The Behavior of the Domestic Cat. CAB International, Oxford, 1992

Buffington CA, Chew DJ: Lower urinary tract disease in cats: new directions. Vet Clin Nutr 1:53, 1991

Buffington CA, Chew DJ: Lower urinary tract disease in cats: new problems, new parodigms. J Nutr 124(12 Suppl), 1994

Hart BL, Hart LA: Canine and Feline Behavioral Therapy. Lea & Febiger, Philadelphia, 1985

Marder AR, Voith VL (eds): Advances in companion animal behavior. Vet Clin North Am [Small Anim Pract] 21:401, 1991

Overall KL: Clinical Behavioral Medicine for Small Animals. CV Mosby, St. Louis, 1997

Perse T: Obsessive-compulsive disorder: a treatment review. J Clin Psychiatry 49:48, 1988

Turner DC, Bateson P: The Domestic Cat: The Biology of Its Behavior. Cambridge University Press, New York, 1988

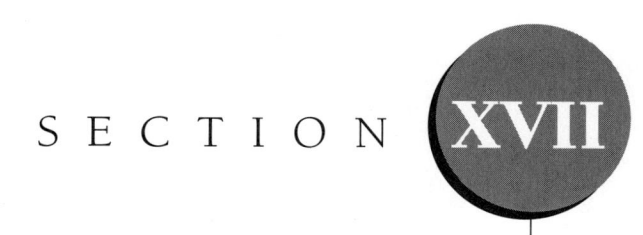

SECTION **XVII**

Nutritional Disorders

118

Introduction

David A. Dzanis

DEFINITIONS

Nutritional Adequacy

I. This is the condition wherein all required dietary nutrients are supplied in sufficient but safe quantities and qualities to allow for proper health and function for a given life stage, i.e., "complete and balanced."

II. Dogs and cats require nutrients, not ingredients.
   A. The quality of a diet cannot be judged on the presence or absence of a specific ingredient.
   B. The overall balance of nutrients as supplied by the ingredient formulation is used as the basis for determining the adequacy of a diet.

Nutritional Deficiency

I. One or more required nutrients are lacking in the diet or are present but not able to be sufficiently used.

II. Types of deficiencies include the following.
   A. Absolute lack in the diet relative to physiologic need
   B. Present in adequate quantities in a poorly bioavailable form
   C. Present in sufficient amount and form but compromised in utility by the presence of an interfering dietary substance

Nutritional Excess

I. One or more nutrients are present in excess in the diet.

II. The excess can exert direct toxic effects or cause a secondary deficiency in another nutrient by interfering with absorption or metabolism.

This chapter was written by Dr. Dzanis in his private capacity. No official support or endorsement by the Food and Drug Administration is intended or should be inferred.

ESTABLISHING NUTRITIONAL ADEQUACY

Association of American Feed Control Officials (AAFCO)

I. AAFCO is an advisory body composed of state feed control officials. It has no direct regulatory function.

II. AAFCO publishes models for state feed bills and associated feed regulations, which state governments are free to adopt.

III. Approximately 30 states have adopted the AAFCO models.

IV. Included in the AAFCO model pet food regulations are two methods to substantiate the nutritional adequacy of all "complete and balanced" dog and cat foods sold in the United States (AAFCO, 1996).
   A. The product is formulated so that essential nutrient levels fall within the ranges set in the AAFCO Dog or Cat Food Nutrient Profiles.
   B. The product successfully passes a feeding trial following AAFCO protocols.
   C. Other programs or methods (e.g., National Research Council [NRC], Nutritional Assurance Program [NAP], Canadian Veterinary Medical Association [CVMA]) are not recognized by AAFCO at this time.

AAFCO Dog and Cat Food Nutrient Profiles

I. The AAFCO Dog and Cat Food Nutrient Profiles are one means by which nutritional adequacy can be substantiated.

II. Dog or cat foods meeting all the minimum and maximum nutrient levels and ratios may state "(Product name) is formulated to meet the AAFCO Dog (Cat) Food Nutrient Profiles for (life stage)."

III. The profiles replace the label statement "(Product name) meets or exceeds the National Research Council (NRC) recommendations" (Dzanis, 1994).

A. Historically, AAFCO recognized the NRC recommendations as the basis for "complete and balanced" claims for dog and cat foods.
B. Because the best available scientific information on nutrient requirements was based on studies with purified diets, nutrient recommendations for dogs and cats in the NRC's latest revisions (NRC, 1985, 1986) were based on the assumption of 100% bioavailability of nutrients. Thus, they did not account for differences in the bioavailability of commonly used ingredients in practical formulations of commercial pet foods.
C. Because the recommendations in the latest revisions did not reflect the needs of the pet food industry or AAFCO, pet food adequacy remained based on the recommendations from the previous revisions (NRC, 1974, 1978). However, these proved inadequate in that they no longer reflected up-to-date knowledge of dog and cat nutrition.
IV. The AAFCO Dog and Cat Food Nutrient Profiles set minimums and maximums for nutrient levels and ratios in pet foods.
A. Minimum nutrient levels are the presumed lowest levels that will supply nutritionally adequate amounts (see Table 120–1).
1. Minimum nutrient levels are expressed as a proportion of dry matter at a set caloric density (3.5 kcal metabolizable energy [ME] per kg for dogs, 4 kcal ME/kg for cats).
2. Separate minimums are set for adult maintenance and growth/reproduction. Foods that meet the minimums for growth/reproduction meet the adult maintenance requirements by default and hence qualify as adequate for "all life stages."
3. The bioavailability of nutrients from ingredients commonly used in dog and cat food formulations is considered. For example, the minimum calcium level for growth and reproduction in dogs is 1%, based on the available calcium requirement of 0.59% (NRC, 1985) and the presumption of no more than 40% loss owing to poor bioavailability.
B. Maximum nutrient levels are the presumed highest amounts that will not cause nutritional toxicity in any life stage of the dog or cat (see Table 121–2).
1. Maximums are established for calcium, phosphorus, most trace minerals, and fat-soluble vitamins for dogs, and methionine, zinc, and vitamins A and D for cats.
2. Lack of an established maximum does not imply safety at any level but reflects the lack of studies performed to define a safe upper level.
C. Minimum and maximum nutrient ratios are established for calcium and phosphorus for dogs, where the relative as well as the absolute amounts of the two may be nutritionally significant.

V. Substantiation of nutritional adequacy by meeting the profiles (vs. passage of a feeding trial) has advantages and disadvantages.
A. Advantages include the following.
1. State feed control officials can easily verify the truthfulness of the claim by laboratory analysis of a sample.
2. It does not rely on industry testing, where a potential conflict of interest may exist.
3. A problem with the formulation can be easily detected and corrected.
B. Disadvantages include the following.
1. Because products are not tested on animals, acceptability, palatability, and other factors are not assessed.
2. Formulations may be at least partially based on "book" values for the nutrient content of ingredients, which may or may not reflect actual content.
   a) Macronutrient levels may vary widely for the same ingredient, depending on the source of the ingredient and other factors, so the final product may not contain the nutrient levels estimated from the formulation.
   b) For many micronutrients, estimates of content in the diet from calculations may be better than analysis of the final product, because methods for determining amounts of nutrients in vitamin/mineral premixes are more reliable than those performed on the final product.
3. Although the bioavailability of nutrients in commonly used ingredients is taken into account, these considerations have their practical limits (Morris and Rogers, 1994).
   a) A pet food that "looks good on paper" may not offer nutritionally adequate amounts of all nutrients.
   b) Of particular concern is the availability of some micronutrients, such as copper and iron.

AAFCO Feeding Trial Protocols

I. Successful passage of a feeding trial following AAFCO minimum protocols is recognized as an alternative means of substantiating nutritional adequacy.
II. Foods that pass a feeding trial are exempt from the requirement to meet the profiles and may make the label statement "Animal feeding tests following AAFCO procedures substantiate that (product name) is complete and balanced for (life stage)."
A. Although few, if any, products bear both profile and feeding trial statements, most products bearing the "animal feeding tests" claim also meet the AAFCO nutrient profile standards.
B. Exceptions include some therapeutic diets and adult maintenance foods that are lower in nutrients such as protein and phosphorus.

III. Adult maintenance protocols are performed on a minimum of eight healthy adult dogs or cats of optimal body weight.
- A. The test diet is offered as the sole source of nutrition (except water) for a minimum of 6 months.
- B. Requirements for passage of the test include the following.
    1. Maintenance of body weight to within 10% of initial average weight, or same degree weight change as a concurrent control group offered a product that previously passed the feeding trial
    2. Maintenance of normal blood hemoglobin, packed cell volume, serum albumin, serum alkaline phosphatase, and taurine (cats only)
    3. Lack of clinical signs indicative of nutritional deficiency or toxicity
- C. Alternatively, passage of either the growth or the gestation/lactation protocols presumes that the criteria for the adult maintenance protocols have been met.

IV. Growth protocols are carried out using a minimum of eight weaned healthy puppies ≤8 weeks of age or kittens ≤9 weeks of age.
- A. The test diet is offered as the sole source of nutrition (except water) for a minimum of 10 weeks.
- B. Requirements for passage of the test include the following.
    1. Normal gain in body weight, based on statistical comparison with a historic or concurrent control group offered a product that previously passed the feeding trial
    2. Normal blood hemoglobin, packed cell volume, serum albumin, and taurine (kittens only)
    3. Lack of clinical signs indicative of nutritional deficiency or toxicity

V. Gestation/lactation protocols are performed on a minimum of eight healthy dams or queens.
- A. The test diet is offered as the sole source of nutrition (except water) from breeding until puppies are 4 weeks of age and until kittens are 6 weeks of age.
- B. Requirements for passage of the test include the following.
    1. Maintenance of body weight in the adults, based on statistical comparison with a historic or concurrent control group offered a product that previously passed the feeding trial, or, in cats, maintenance within 10% of starting weight
    2. Normal blood hemoglobin, packed cell volume, serum albumin, and taurine (queens only) in the adults
    3. Normal litter performance, based on a minimum 80% survivability, and normal litter size and weight
    4. Lack of clinical signs indicative of nutritional deficiency or toxicity in the adults or offspring

VI. "All life stages" protocols are achieved by the following.
- A. Sequential passage of the gestation/lactation and growth protocols, using the offspring obtained from the former for the latter trial
- B. Adult maintenance met by default

VII. Feeding trials have advantages and disadvantages compared with the nutrient profiles.
- A. Feeding trials are advantageous in that they assess bioavailability, palatability, and other factors not assessed by the profiles (Morris and Rogers, 1994).
- B. Disadvantages include the following.
    1. AAFCO does not conduct the feeding trials itself, so a conflict of interest is possible.
    2. The manufacturer or a private testing facility performs the studies and attests to a product's successful passage.
    3. Although AAFCO and state feed control officials have the ability to review the data, they must still rely on the integrity and competence of the persons conducting and reporting on the studies.
- C. The feeding trial protocols may not be sensitive enough to disclose all instances of nutritional inadequacy.
    1. Particularly for adult maintenance trials, signs of subtle chronic deficiencies and toxicities may be missed.
    2. Depending on the nutritional status of the animal going into the trial, abundant body reserves of some nutrients (e.g., vitamin A, calcium) may compensate for a deficient diet over the course of the trial.
- D. Not all products bearing an "animal feeding tests" statement are actually tested.
    1. "Family members" deemed "nutritionally similar" to the tested product may also bear the same statement.
        - a) Under its original intent, this provision justifiably allows virtually identical products (i.e., minor flavor variations) to be marketed without the need for redundant testing.
        - b) The concept has been liberally applied by some pet food manufacturers, making the relationship among "family members" less clear.
    2. At worst, products deemed family members on the basis of similar profiles assume all the disadvantages of reliance on a nutrient profile.

Bibliography

Association of American Feed Control Officials: Official Publication. AAFCO, Atlanta, 1996

Dzanis DA: The Association of American Feed Control Officials Dog and Cat Food Nutrient Profiles: substantiation of nutritional adequacy of complete and balanced pet foods in the United States. J Nutr 124:2535S, 1994

Morris JG, Rogers QR: Assessment of the nutritional adequacy of pet foods through the life cycle. J Nutr 124:2520S, 1994

National Research Council: Nutrient Requirements of Dogs. National Academy of Sciences, Washington, DC, 1974

National Research Council: Nutrient Requirements of Cats. National Academy of Sciences, Washington, DC, 1978

National Research Council: Nutrient Requirements of Dogs. National Academy Press, Washington, DC, 1985

National Research Council: Nutrient Requirements of Cats. National Academy Press, Washington, DC, 1986

119

Nutrition Through the Life Cycle

David A. Dzanis

BIRTH TO ADULTHOOD

Neonate

Definition

Life stage between birth and weaning

Requirements

I. Energy/fat
   A. Energy needs are proportional to increased metabolic size and rapid growth rate.
      1. At peak growth, needs may approach 300 kcal metabolizable energy (ME) per kg body weight (BW).
      2. To meet these needs, milk or milk replacer must be very energy dense. The density of dam's milk is 100–130 kcal ME/100 ml, which is over 5000 kcal ME/kg on a dry-matter (DM) basis (Lewis et al., 1987).
   B. To achieve this degree of caloric density, fat levels must be high. Estimates of fat content of milks are as follows (Lewis et al., 1987).
      1. Bitch's milk: 9.8% fat (43% DM)
      2. Queen's milk: 5.1% fat (27.6% DM)
      3. Cow's milk (for comparison): 3.8% fat (30.6% DM)
II. Protein/amino acids
   A. Protein levels are also high and are proportional to the high caloric density (Lewis et al., 1987).
      1. Amounts in dam's milk presumed adequate
      2. Bitch's milk: 8.1% protein (35.5% DM)
      3. Queen's milk: 8.1% protein (43.8% DM)
      4. Cow's milk (for comparison): 3.3% protein (26.6% DM)
   B. Amino acid deficiencies in some commercial products have been linked to cataract formation (Glaze and Blanchard, 1983).
III. Minerals
   A. Calcium (Ca) and phosphorus (P) are critical in neonatal dogs.
      1. Estimates of bitch's milk Ca content (Lewis et al., 1987)
         a) 0.28% Ca (1.23% DM)
         b) Ca:P ratio = 1.3:1
      2. Reports (to the Food and Drug Administration) exist of Ca deficiency observed at the time of weight-bearing when animals were fed a commercial product that supposedly met National Research Council (NRC) recommendations for growth.
   B. Ca needs are apparently less critical in the neonatal cat. Estimates of Ca content of queen's milk are as follows (Lewis et al., 1987).
      1. 0.035% Ca (0.19% DM)
      2. Ca:P ratio = 0.5:1
   C. Requirements for other minerals are unknown. Those levels required for growth (adjusted to caloric density) are probably adequate for neonates.
IV. Vitamins and other nutrients
   A. Little is known of true vitamin needs of neonates.
   B. Requirements for growth, adjusted for increased caloric density, are probably adequate.
   C. Neonates are likely to have obligate needs for other nutrients (e.g., carnitine), but such needs are unproven to date.

Feeding Management

I. Type
   A. Access to a lactating dam is preferred in all cases.
   B. Supplement large litters and runts with suitable milk replacer.
   C. Orphaned puppies and kittens are totally reliant on milk replacers.

This chapter was written by Dr. Dzanis in his private capacity. No official support or endorsement by the Food and Drug Administration is intended or should be inferred.

1219

1. The Association of American Feed Control Officials (AAFCO) Dog and Cat Food Nutrient Profiles and AAFCO feeding trial protocols do not address neonatal formula needs (AAFCO, 1996). Thus, there is no unbiased authority upon which to judge the nutritional adequacy of commercial products (see Chap. 118).
2. Many home formulations have been recommended, but the nutritional adequacy of most is unknown.
3. Regardless of whether a commercial or homemade formula is used, careful scrutiny of performance is critical. Animals that do poorly are switched to another formula.
   D. As neonates become weight-bearing and mobile (after the third week), offer a gruel of milk replacer and growth diet, gradually replacing milk replacer with water. Neonates raised on the dam may be weaned onto a gruel of growth food and water.
   E. As neonates become accustomed to a separate water source, decrease the amount of water in the gruel until the food is at normal feeding consistency.
II. Amount
   A. Assuming the energy density of replacer is similar to that of dam's milk (100–130 kcal/100 ml), offer the following (Hoskins, 1992; Case et al., 1995).
      1. First week: 13 ml/100 g BW
      2. Second week: 17 ml/100 g BW
      3. Third week: 20 ml/100 g BW
      4. Thereafter: same as third week; taper off as weaned
   B. For the first few feedings, offer replacer at slightly lower amounts and slightly diluted, until the animal can accommodate full volume and strength.
   C. Suspect that the daily amount of milk replacer may be inadequate with these signs.
      1. Constant crying
      2. Depression, inactivity
      3. Failure to gain weight every day (not just weight loss)
   D. Offer free access to as much gruel/growth formula as can be consumed within 15 minutes. Supervise group feedings.
III. Frequency
   A. More frequent feedings are better.
      1. For neonates in their first week, every 2 hours is not too frequent.
      2. By the time of weaning, 4 times a day is usually adequate.
   B. Total estimated daily intake is divided equally.
   C. Attempts to feed larger volumes at night usually fail to achieve the desired effect of extending the time between feedings.

Growth
Definition
I. Life stage between weaning and completion of skeletal growth

II. Most of the experimental studies on the nutritional requirements of dogs and cats performed with growing animals

Requirements
I. Energy/fat
   A. Energy
      1. Caloric requirements per kg BW are greater than those for adult maintenance (see Maintenance, later). These higher levels taper off as the animal approaches adulthood.
      2. Dog requirements are as follows (NRC, 1985).
         a) Weaning: 2 times maintenance
         b) 40% of adult weight: 1.6 times maintenance
         c) 80% of adult weight: 1.2 times maintenance
      3. Cat requirements are as follows (NRC, 1986).
         a) 10 weeks: 250 kcal ME/kg BW
         b) 20 weeks: 130 kcal ME/kg BW
         c) 40 weeks: 80 kcal ME/kg BW
   B. Fat
      1. Dogs and cats do not have a nutritional requirement for fat per se. However, it is needed in the diet.
         a) Source of essential fatty acids
         b) Carrier and aid to absorption of fat-soluble vitamins
         c) Provider of adequate caloric density (as recognized by the higher level of fat for growth and reproduction in the AAFCO Dog Food Nutrient Profile)
         d) Palatability enhancer
      2. Essential fatty acids
         a) In the dog, linoleic acid is the only essential fatty acid required in the diet. The other fatty acids can be synthesized in the body if the linoleic acid supply is adequate.
         b) Cats also have a need for a dietary source of arachidonic acid.
II. Protein/amino acids
   A. Protein
      1. Dogs and cats do not have a nutritional requirement for protein per se, but it is needed as a source of essential amino acids.
      2. Dietary protein must be of sufficient quantity and quality to supply adequate amounts of all essential amino acids. Higher-quality proteins can be given in a lower quantity.
   B. Essential amino acids
      1. Dogs and cats have an absolute requirement for 10 essential (indispensable) amino acids.
      2. The remaining 12 nonessential (dispensable) amino acids found in protein can be synthesized by the body.
III. Minerals
   A. Macrominerals: calcium (Ca), phosphorus (P), potassium (K), sodium (Na), chloride (Cl), magnesium (Mg), iron (Fe)

1. Adequate Ca and P are critical to optimal growth, but excessive amounts are contraindicated.
2. The source of Fe is important; Fe from oxide or carbonate sources are poorly available (Chausow and Czarnecki-Maulden, 1987).
   B. Microminerals: copper (Cu), manganese (Mn), zinc (Zn), iodine (I), selenium (Se)
   1. Balanced commercial diets offer adequate quantities.
   2. Supplementation does not improve performance and is potentially harmful.
   3. Cu oxide is poorly available (Czarnecki-Maulden et al., 1993).
IV. Vitamins and other nutrients
   A. Vitamin A
   1. Cats lack the enterocytic dimerase to utilize beta carotene from plants, so they require preformed vitamin A (NRC, 1986).
   2. Most commercial dog and cat foods are supplemented with preformed vitamin A, so additional amounts are usually unnecessary and potentially harmful.
   B. Vitamin D
   1. Dogs and cats have a relative lack of 7-dehydrocholesterol in their skin, a precursor of vitamin D that is transformed upon exposure to ultraviolet light (Wheatley and Sher, 1961; Morris, 1996).
   2. Exposure to sunlight as an adequate source cannot be presumed, so a dietary source is needed.
   3. Vitamin D_2 (ergocalciferol) is the plant form of vitamin D.
      a) The animal-source form is vitamin D_3 (cholecalciferol).
      b) Both are used effectively by dogs and cats, although cholecalciferol is typically used in commercial food formulation (NRC 1985, 1986).
   C. Other nutrients
   1. Intestinal microbial production of vitamin K and biotin is probably adequate, but these vitamins are often added as "insurance."
   2. Vitamin E requirements increase with diets high in polyunsaturated fat, especially fish oil–based foods.
   3. Taurine needs in cats fed canned foods are greater than in those fed extruded foods (Douglass et al., 1991). Processing and the type of protein sources affect the metabolic disposition of taurine, resulting in increased losses with canned food.

Feeding Management

I. Type
   A. Form (e.g., canned, dry) may be dictated by owner preference. Most dogs and cats do well on dry foods, and these should be the first choice in most instances.
   B. Many cat owners feed combinations of forms.

Dry may be offered as the mainstay, with very small meals of canned or semi-moist food offered as treats.
   C. Foods adequate for growth or "all life stages" are generally sufficient, regardless of breed.
   1. Smaller dogs and cats may be able to accommodate more nutrient-dense diets, but they may be economically wasteful.
   2. Larger breeds of dogs and/or breeds predisposed to obesity should be offered foods more closely meeting the minimum requirements (e.g., 22% DM protein, 8% DM fat).
II. Amount
   A. Amount is based on an estimation of energy requirements and the energy density of food.
   B. If the caloric density is not stated on the label, it can be estimated from the label "guaranteed analysis" values using the formula in Table 119–1.
   1. The formula may underestimate the caloric density of highly digestible food by up to 20%.
   2. The formula may overestimate the caloric density of poor-quality, less digestible food.
   C. Feeding directions on the label are a good starting point but typically overestimate true needs.
   D. Time-controlled feedings (i.e., free access to food, but with a 15-minute time limit for each

Table 119–1. *Estimating Calorie Content of a Pet Food from the Label "Guaranteed Analysis" Values*

Step 1:	Multiply the percentage of crude protein by 3.5.
Step 2:	Multiply the percentage of crude fat by 8.5.
Step 3:	Add the percentages of crude protein, crude fat, crude fiber, moisture, and ash, and subtract the total from 100. This provides the percentage of nitrogen-free extract (NFE), which is the carbohydrate portion.
Step 4:	Multiply the percentage of NFE from Step 3 by 3.5.
Step 5:	Add the results from Steps 1, 2, and 4, and multiply the total by 10. The result is the calorie content in kcal metabolizable energy (ME) per kg "as fed" (AF).
Step 6:	To determine calories on a dry-matter (DM) basis, divide the result from Step 5 by the proportion of DM in the product [(100 − % moisture)/100].

Example:	Crude protein	24% × 3.5 = 84
	Crude fat	10% × 8.5 = 85
	Crude fiber	3%
	Moisture	10%
	Ash	5%
		52%
	NFE (100 − 52 = 48)	48% × 3.5 = 168
		Total 337

$$337 \times 10 = 3370 \text{ kcal ME/kg AF}$$

$$\frac{3370}{(100 - 90)/100} = 3744 \text{ kcal ME/kg DM}$$

feeding) work well in most puppies. Supervise group feedings.

E. Adjustments are made to maintain ideal body condition score (BCS) as needed, regardless of previous estimates or feeding directions.

F. Several methods to judge body condition have been suggested, but a nine-point system (vs. a five-point system) allows for more precise assessments (Table 119–2).

G. It is especially important for large- or giant-breed dogs to maintain ideal, if not slightly low, BCS (4 to 5).

III. Frequency

A. Multiple feedings (3–4 times per day) important in younger dogs and cats

B. May decrease number of feedings as animals approach maturity (9–12 months)

ADULTHOOD

Maintenance

Definition

Life stage characterized by the absence of nutritional stressors (i.e., non-growing, non-reproducing, non-working)

Requirements

I. Energy/fat

A. Energy

1. Energy needs are proportional to metabolic body size.

2. Smaller animals need more calories per kg BW than larger animals. This takes on greater

Table 119–2. Body Condition Score (BCS)

Score	Body Condition	Clinical Signs: Dog	Clinical Signs: Cat
1	Emaciated	Ribs, lumbar vertebrae, pelvic bones, and all bony prominences are evident from a distance. There is no discernible body fat, and there is obvious loss of muscle mass.	Ribs are visible on shorthaired cats. There is no palpable fat. Severe abdominal tuck is evident. Lumbar vertebrae and wing of ilia are easily palpated.
2	Very thin	Ribs, lumbar vertebrae, and pelvic bones are easily visible. There is no palpable fat, some evidence of other bony prominences, and minimal loss of muscle mass.	Signs include shared characteristics of BCS 1 and 3.
3	Thin	Ribs are easily palpated and may be visible with no palpable fat. Tops of lumbar vertebrae are visible. Pelvic bones are becoming prominent. There are an obvious waist and abdominal tuck.	Ribs are easily palpable with minimal fat covering. Lumbar vertebrae are obvious. There is an obvious waist behind ribs, and minimal abdominal fat.
4	Underweight	Ribs are easily palpable, with minimal fat covering. Waist is easily noted, viewed from above. Abdominal tuck is evident.	Signs include shared characteristics of BCS 3 and 5.
5	Ideal	Ribs are palpable without excess fat covering. Waist is observed behind ribs when viewed from above. Abdomen is tucked up when viewed from side.	Animal is well proportioned. Waist is observed behind ribs. Ribs are palpable with slight fat covering. Abdominal fat pad is minimal.
6	Overweight	Ribs are palpable with slight excess fat covering. Waist is discernible viewed from above but is not prominent. Abdominal tuck is apparent.	Signs include shared characteristics of BCS 5 and 7.
7	Heavy	Ribs are palpable with difficulty, with heavy fat cover. There are noticeable fat deposits over lumbar area and base of tail. Waist is absent or barely visible. Abdominal tuck may be absent.	Ribs are not easily palpated, with moderate fat covering. Waist is poorly discernible. There is an obvious rounding of abdomen, with a moderate abdominal fat pad.
8	Obese	Ribs are not palpable under very heavy fat cover, or palpable only with significant pressure. There are heavy fat deposits over lumbar area and base of tail. Waist is absent. There is no abdominal tuck. Obvious abdominal distention may be present.	Signs include shared characteristics of BCS 7 and 9.
9	Grossly obese	There are massive fat deposits over thorax, spine, and base of tail. Waist and abdominal tuck are absent. There are fat deposits on neck and limbs, and obvious abdominal distention.	Ribs are not palpable under heavy fat cover. There are heavy fat deposits over lumbar area, face, and limbs. There is distention of the abdomen, with no waist. Extensive abdominal fat deposits are evident.

Adapted with permission, Ralston Purina Company, St. Louis. (Laflamme DP: Body condition scoring and weight maintenance. Proc North Am Vet Conf, Jan 16–21, 1993, Orlando, FL, pp 290–291; Laflamme DP, Kealy RD, Schmidt DA: Estimation of body fat by body condition score. J Vet Intern Med 8:154, 1994; Laflamme DP, Kuhlman G, Lawler DF et al: Obesity management in dogs. J Vet Clin Nutr 1:59, 1994.)

significance in dogs, where differences in mature body sizes are extreme.

3. Estimation of the metabolizable energy (ME) requirement uses the following formulas.
   a) Dogs
      (1) ME (kcal) = 132 BW(kg)$^{0.75}$, or
      (2) ME (kcal) = 144.4 + 62.2 BW(kg) (NRC, 1985)
   b) Cats
      ME (kcal) = 60–80 BW(kg) (NRC, 1986)

B. Fat
   1. A decline in the need for calorie-dense diets reduces the need for fat.
   2. Adequate amounts are still required to supply sufficient essential fatty acids, fat-soluble vitamins, and so forth.

II. Protein/amino acids
   A. Protein needs decline upon completion of growth.
   B. Amino acid needs are unknown for adult dogs, but it is presumed that needs decrease in proportion to the decrease in protein needs (approximately 15% lower than growth needs) in the AAFCO Dog Food Nutrient Profiles (AAFCO, 1996).
   C. In cats, the need for some amino acid levels cannot be presumed to be lower than growth needs, so there is no difference in the AAFCO Cat Food Nutrient Profiles for some amino acids.

III. Minerals
   A. Requirements for Ca and P decline with completion of skeletal growth.
   B. NaCl requirements are probably the same as those for growth. They are lower in the AAFCO Dog Food Nutrient Profiles because of the artificially high level in the "growth and reproduction" profile to accommodate heavy lactation needs.
   C. The requirements for other minerals for maintenance are unknown, but those established for growth are presumed to be adequate by default.

IV. Vitamins and other nutrients
   A. The requirements for vitamins A and D are probably lower with completion of skeletal growth.
   B. Requirements for the other vitamins for maintenance are not known, and growth requirements are presumed to be adequate.

Feeding Management

I. Type
   A. Most animals do well on dry foods. However, other forms of food (as dictated by owner preference) may be used.
   B. Regardless of form, nutrient density should be adequate but not excessive.
   C. Although there is no evidence that an "all life stage" diet is necessarily harmful, its higher nutrient level is usually unnecessary and more expensive and may lead to excess calorie consumption.

II. Amount
   A. Amount is based on an estimation of energy requirements and the energy density of food.
   B. Feeding directions on the label are a good starting point but typically overestimate true needs.
   C. Adjust amounts as needed to maintain the animal's ideal BCS, regardless of previous estimates or feeding directions.

III. Frequency
   A. Many dogs do well on a once-a-day feeding schedule.
   B. Multiple daily feedings may alleviate boredom and prevent gorging, begging, and destructive behaviors. They may also lower risk factors for acute canine gastric dilatation-volvulus (Bataller, 1995).
   C. Cats can be offered free access to dry food if intake is regulated sufficiently.

Reproduction

Definition

I. This discussion pertains to the gestating or lactating bitch or queen.
II. Although adequate nutrition is critical to satisfactory reproductive performance, there is little evidence that nutritional needs of the non-gestating, non-lactating female or the reproducing male are significantly above maintenance.

Requirements

I. Energy/fat
   A. Energy needs in early gestation are not significantly different from maintenance.
   B. In late gestation, energy needs may increase 25–50% (Case et al., 1995).
   C. Lactation energy needs are directly proportional to litter size.
      1. Needs may approach 3–4 times maintenance (Case et al., 1995).
      2. Peak demands occur at approximately 4 weeks for dogs, 6 weeks for cats.

II. Protein/amino acids
   A. Protein needs increase with late gestation/lactation to accommodate fetal growth and milk production.
   B. Although true requirements are not well known, levels needed for growth appear to be adequate.

III. Minerals
   A. Sufficient NaCl is needed for adequate milk production. Balanced "all life stage" food should have adequate amounts of salt.
   B. Demand for Ca and P may be higher with heavy lactation, but the animal should be able to accommodate with body stores. Requirements are presumed to be the same as for growth.
   C. Little is known regarding other minerals, but growth requirements are presumed to be adequate.

IV. Vitamins and other nutrients
  A. Controlled data on true needs are lacking.
  B. Requirements for growth are presumed to be adequate.

Feeding Management

I. Type
  A. Prebreeding, first half of gestation: feed same as maintenance
  B. Second half of gestation: begin higher-energy diet (>4000 kcal ME/kg DM)
  C. Lactation: maintain on higher-energy diet until weaning
II. Amount
  A. Prebreeding
    1. Adjust amounts so the animal enters breeding season at ideal BCS.
    2. If weight loss is needed, it should be done much earlier, so the animal can enter the breeding period on an increased plane of nutrition.
  B. First half of gestation: same as prebreeding
  C. Second half of gestation
    1. Switch to higher-density food.
    2. Offer approximately the same amount of maintenance food as offered in prebreeding and early gestation.
  D. Intake adjusted as needed to accommodate increasing need, and tapered off as puppies or kittens become used to solid food
III. Frequency
  A. Prebreeding, gestation: retain normal schedule
  B. Lactation
    1. More frequent feedings may be needed to accommodate increased demand.
    2. Free access to a source of dry food may be necessary during peak needs.

Work

Definition

I. Life stage of growing and adult animals that is characterized by increased physical exertion above "normal" activities (e.g., hunting, racing, herding).
II. Although environmental stress (such as outdoor housing in cold temperatures) may increase energy needs, there is no evidence that "mental stress" (e.g., confinement, showing) significantly increases requirements over maintenance needs.
III. For obvious reasons, "work" rarely (if ever) pertains to cats.

Requirements

I. Energy/fat
  A. Depending on the amount of work and the environmental conditions, energy expenditures may be as little as 20% over maintenance or as high as 4 times maintenance (NRC, 1986).
  B. Because of its high caloric value, fat is the preferred source of additional energy.

    1. A high-fat diet (vs. a high-carbohydrate diet) improves muscle glycogen stores and endurance in trained animals (Reynolds et al., 1996).
    2. Increasing the fat level is done at the expense of fiber and complex carbohydrates.
      a) Protein and other nutrients are increased proportionally with fat.
      b) Simply adding fat to a maintenance diet may inadvertently result in deficiencies in other nutrients.
  C. Simple carbohydrate supplementation may be helpful.
    1. Administration of readily utilized carbohydrates (e.g., glucose-based fluids, sports drinks) immediately after exertion improves recovery and repletion of muscle glycogen (Reynolds et al., 1996).
    2. The same simple carbohydrate source may be used to supplement animals prone to "hunting dog hypoglycemia" during work.
II. Protein/amino acids
  A. Protein needs are poorly understood but are likely higher than maintenance.
    1. Muscle growth
    2. Muscle and other tissue repair
  B. Increases in protein density should be proportional to increases in fat and calorie increase (optimum protein-to-fat ratio is 3:2).
III. Minerals
  A. Little known
  B. Probably not significantly different from maintenance
IV. Vitamins and other nutrients
  A. Requirements for B vitamins are likely to be increased with increased work.
  B. Increased needs are met by increased consumption of an appropriately balanced diet.
  C. Requirements for other vitamins are probably not significantly different from maintenance.

Feeding Management

I. Type
  A. If work is relatively light or during off-season, offer the same food as required for maintenance.
  B. With increased demand by work or environmental stress, the need for higher energy density (>4500 kcal ME/kg DM) is more likely. High-fat (>20% DM), high-protein (>30% DM), low-fiber diets are most effective.
II. Amount
  A. Dogs should enter working season well-fleshed but not heavy (i.e., BCS score of 5–6).
  B. As energy expenditures increase, adjust the amount, striving toward maintenance of ideal BCS.
III. Frequency
  A. With profound caloric demand, multiple feedings may be needed to accommodate daily needs.
  B. Feeding after performance improves recovery.

C. Do not feed dogs for 4 hours before performance of work.

Senior

Definition

I. Senior describes an older dog or cat, characterized by a slowly progressive decline in physical activity, metabolic rate, and normal body functions.

II. Many have attempted to define ranges of years for the senior life stage of dogs and cats.
   A. In general, giant- and large-breed dogs have proportionally shorter life spans than small dogs and cats.
   B. Great individual variation makes it impossible to assign a specific chronologic age as "senior."

Requirements

I. Energy
   A. A decline in lean body mass and metabolic rate generally lowers energy requirements compared with maintenance of a younger adult.
   B. Most senior pet foods are lower in caloric density based on this generalization.
   C. However, a decreased ability to consume, digest, and absorb nutrients may actually increase, rather than decrease, the need for calorie-dense food.
   D. High fiber may further interfere with the ability to absorb nutrients and receive adequate energy.

II. Protein/amino acids
   A. Because of a decline in gastrointestinal function and efficiency, true protein/amino acid requirements are probably higher with age.
   B. Many commercial senior foods are lower in protein, based on the premise that it will retard the progression of yet-undetected chronic renal disease.
      1. No evidence exists in dogs or cats that low-protein diets prevent or significantly retard renal aging (Brown, 1996).
      2. A low-protein diet likely exacerbates loss of lean body mass, further depressing physical activity and ability to function.
      3. Because of potential adverse effects, low-protein diets are reserved for animals displaying clinical evidence of renal disease.

III. Minerals
   A. Commercial diets formulated for seniors are often lower in P, for the same reason as protein.
      1. There is no clear demonstration of benefit in nonclinical animals (Finco et al., 1996).
      2. Ca is also usually lower, to maintain the Ca:P balance, but the need for Ca may be increased in older animals.
   B. NaCl needs are the same as for maintenance.
      1. Restricted salt content may adversely affect palatability, especially if the animal is accustomed to a higher level and taste acuities are declining.

      2. Salt restriction is limited to animals with demonstrated clinical need (e.g., cardiovascular insufficiency).
   C. True requirements for other minerals are unknown, but maintenance requirements are presumed to be adequate.

IV. Vitamins and other nutrients
   A. Little is known about the requirements for vitamins or other nutrients.
   B. Requirements for maintenance are presumed to be adequate.
   C. Some propose the use of antioxidants and other nutrients to retard the effects of aging (Machlin, 1996).
      1. There is a paucity of controlled studies in dogs and cats to conclude that these substances do as claimed.
      2. There are no data on the proper dosages or metabolic fates of many of these substances.
         a) The doses recommended most likely have absolutely no effect. At best, they do no harm.
         b) Characterization of these substances as "food" or "natural" cannot be the basis for a presumption of safety.

Feeding Management

I. Type
   A. The type of food is individually tailored to the animal's needs, not its age.
      1. Maintaining body weight and reasonable health
         A change to a commercial senior diet is often unnecessary and potentially contraindicated.
      2. Propensity to gain weight
         a) A slightly lower energy-dense food may be offered.
         b) If the animal is obese, institute a weight-reduction program (see Chap. 121). Aggressive weight loss aggravates loss of lean body mass.
      3. Propensity to lose weight/lean body mass
         a) A higher-calorie, lower-fiber food may be indicated.
         b) Nutritional need, rather than labeled intended use, should be the primary factor. In some cases, a puppy or kitten food is required.
      4. Chronic disease
         a) Restricted protein, P, and Na may be necessary to help ameliorate signs of chronic renal, cardiovascular, or other degenerative disease.
         b) Use appropriately restricted diets to ameliorate clinical signs.
   B. If dental or other problems compromise the ability to eat sufficient dry food, the food should be moistened and/or the animal switched to a canned product.

II. Amount
   A. As with type, the amount of food is dependent on many individualized factors.
   B. If the animal has maintained weight well through its adulthood, adjust the amount to anticipate a 20% decrease in caloric need in old age.
   C. The amount offered is adjusted, with the goal being to maintain ideal BCS.
III. Frequency
   A. The animal is retained on its normal feeding schedule unless a change in condition dictates otherwise.
   B. Adherence to a routine is especially important in the senior animal. Skipped meals must be avoided.
   C. More frequent feedings may be needed if the animal's capacity to ingest larger volumes becomes compromised.

Bibliography

Association of American Feed Control Officials: Official Publication. AAFCO, Atlanta, 1996

Bataller N: Risk factors and debate of diet in canine gastric dilatation volvulus. Vet Clin Nutr 2:87, 1995

Brown S: The protein debate. p. 12. In: Proceedings, Focus on Geriatric Nutrition, Chicago, 1996

Case LP, Carey DP, Hirakawa DA: Canine and Feline Nutrition—A Resource for Companion Animal Professionals. CV Mosby, St. Louis, 1995

Chausow DG, Czarnecki-Maulden GL: Estimation of the dietary iron requirement for the weanling puppy and kitten. J Nutr 117:928, 1987

Czarnecki-Maulden GL, Rudnick RC, Chausow DG: Copper bio-availability and requirement in the dog: comparison of copper oxide and copper sulfate (abstract). FASEB J 7:A306, 1993

Douglass GM, Fern EB, Brown RC: Feline plasma and whole blood taurine levels as influenced by commercial dry and canned diets. J Nutr 121:S91, 1991

Finco DR, Brown SA, Crowell WA: Effects of dietary protein and phosphorus on the kidneys of dogs. p. 123. In Carey DP, Norton SA, Bolser SM (eds): Recent Advances in Canine and Feline Nutritional Research: Proceedings of the 1996 Iams International Nutrition Symposium. Orange Frazer Press, Wilmington, OH, 1996

Glaze MB, Blanchard GL: Nutritional cataracts in a Samoyed litter. J Am Anim Hosp Assoc 19:951, 1983

Hoskins JD: Nutritional disorders of the neonate. p. 1273. In Morgan RV (ed): Handbook of Small Animal Practice. 2nd Ed. Churchill Livingston, New York, 1992

Lewis LD, Morris ML, Hand MS: Small Animal Clinical Nutrition III. Mark Morris Associates, Topeka, KS, 1987

Machlin LJ: Are antioxidants anti-aging? p. 28. In: Proceedings, Focus on Geriatric Nutrition, Chicago, 1996

Morris JG: Vitamin D synthesis by kittens. In: Proceedings, Purina Nutrition Forum, St. Louis, 1996

National Research Council: Nutrient Requirements of Dogs. National Academy Press, Washington, DC, 1985

National Research Council: Nutrient Requirements of Cats. National Academy Press, Washington, DC, 1986

Reynolds AJ, Taylor CR, Hoppeler H et al: The effect of diet on sled dog performance, oxidative capacity, skeletal muscle microstructure, and muscle glycogen metabolism. p. 181. In Carey DP, Norton SA, Bolser SM (eds): Recent Advances in Canine and Feline Nutritional Research: Proceedings of the 1996 Iams International Nutrition Symposium. Orange Frazer Press, Wilmington, OH, 1996

Wheatley VR, Sher DW: Studies of the lipid of dog skin. J Invest Dermatol 36:169, 1961

120

Disorders of Nutritional Deficiency

David A. Dzanis

PROTEIN AND FAT

Protein/Calorie Malnutrition (PCM)

Definition

I. PCM is an inadequate caloric intake relative to the animal's physiologic needs.
II. Although a protein deficiency can exist with adequate calorie consumption, the converse is not possible, because protein is metabolized for its energy value in the face of calorie deficiency.

Causes

I. Insufficient amount of food offered to meet needs
  A. High physiologic needs (e.g., lactation, work)
  B. Competition with other individual animals
II. Bulk-limited diet (insufficient caloric density to meet needs when offered ad lib)
III. Extremely poor palatability of food

Pathophysiology

I. With short-term deprivation, glycogen stores are mobilized to supply glucose for glucose-obligate tissues.
II. As glycogen supplies are exhausted, proteins are catabolized into amino acids for use in gluconeogenesis. New protein synthesis for normal tissue repair, serum proteins, and so forth is hindered.
III. As calorie deficiency continues, there are metabolic adaptations to promote survival.
  A. The body becomes more dependent on hepatic ketogenesis, provided from catabolized fats.
  B. Activity and energy expenditure are reduced, with a decrease in metabolic rate.
  C. Protein catabolism is minimized but persistent.

IV. With depletion of fat stores, protein catabolism is resumed at higher rates.

Clinical Signs

I. Body condition score (BCS) <3 (see Table 119–2)
II. Lack of body fat
III. Muscle wasting
IV. Hypoglycemia, hypoproteinemia, hypoalbuminemia
V. Low serum urea nitrogen
VI. Weakness, inactivity

Diagnosis

I. Clinical signs are suggestive.
II. It may be difficult to obtain an accurate diet history because of the owner's guilt regarding the animal's level of care.
III. Nonjudgmental, open-ended questioning may be most revealing.

Differential Diagnosis

I. Anorexia as a result of some pathologic condition, e.g., chronic renal failure
II. Increased energy expenditure owing to parasitic infestation, burns, trauma, or other pathologic conditions characterized by a hypermetabolic instead of a hypometabolic state

Treatment

I. Severely weakened animals may require intensive support until they can eat and tolerate regular food.
II. Feeding management is critical to recovery.
  A. Type
    1. A balanced, highly digestible and palatable food is offered initially.
    2. The food contains moderate protein (25–30% dry matter [DM]) and fat (8–12% DM) levels.

This chapter was written by Dr. Dzanis in his private capacity. No official support or endorsement by the Food and Drug Administration is intended or should be inferred.

3. Many premium foods intended for adult maintenance are suitable.
    B. Amount
        1. Initial amounts offered provide no more than 50–75% of normal energy requirements, as the animal is still hypometabolic and may not be able to tolerate abrupt changes (Donoghue, 1989).
        2. As a return to normal metabolic state is achieved, a gradual increase in caloric intake is indicated to accommodate maintenance needs as well as a moderate rate of weight gain.
    C. Frequency
        Frequent small meals are offered initially until the animal can accommodate a more normal feeding pattern.

Patient Monitoring

I. Animals are monitored for progressive weight gain and restoration to ideal body condition, with intake adjusted accordingly.
II. As the animal's condition permits, exercise is encouraged. This increases lean body mass and prevents a rebound of fat deposition.

Protein/Amino Acid Deficiency

Definition

I. This deficiency is an inadequate protein or essential amino acid intake relative to physiologic needs (Table 120–1).
II. Lack of a single essential amino acid can cause deficiency, despite adequate or even overabundant amounts of protein.

Causes

I. Product intended for adult maintenance offered to growing or reproducing animals
II. Low-protein diets
III. Improperly balanced diets, especially vegetarian

Pathophysiology

I. Protein is required for myriad biologic processes, including growth, tissue turnover and repair, serum protein synthesis, and immune function.
II. Obligate needs not met by diet are met through catabolism of protein stores, primarily muscle.
III. Lack of a single essential amino acid is compensated for by catabolism.
IV. Excess amino acids that are not required for new protein synthesis are deaminated and used for energy.

Clinical Signs

I. Muscle wasting
II. Poor growth
III. Edema, ascites
IV. Rough, dull hair coat
V. Hypoproteinemia, hypoalbuminemia
VI. Compromised immune function, resistance to disease
VII. Lethargy, weakness
VIII. Depressed milk production

Diagnosis

I. Clinical signs
II. Dietary history

Differential Diagnosis

I. Excessive protein loss from a pathologic condition
    A. Burns
    B. Infection
    C. Parasitic infestation
    D. Protein-losing enteropathy or nephropathy
II. Cardiac or cancer cachexia

Treatment

I. The animal is offered a balanced diet appropriate for its life stage.
II. Attempts to correct a deficient diet through protein supplementation are less successful than switching to a proven balanced food, and excessive protein does not replete protein stores more rapidly.
III. Amounts of food offered are appropriate for the animal's life stage; attempts at rapid correction are ill-advised.

Patient Monitoring

I. The animal is monitored for adequate return of body condition and function.
II. Serum protein and albumin concentrations can be used to assess general protein status.

Essential Fatty Acid Deficiency

Definition

This deficiency is an inadequate intake of essential fatty acids relative to physiologic needs (linoleic acid in dogs, and linoleic and arachidonic acids in cats).

Causes

I. Low-fat diets in adults
II. Young or reproducing animals offered an adult maintenance food
III. Inadequately preserved or rancid diets

Pathophysiology

I. Essential fatty acids are required for normal cell membrane function and fluidity and for the production of prostaglandins, leukotrienes, and other compounds.
II. Dogs can synthesize sufficient fatty acids as long as dietary linoleic acid is adequate.

Table 120–1. AAFCO Dog and Cat Food Nutrient Profile Minimum Requirements

Nutrient	Units DM Basis	Dog Food Minimum[a]	Cat Food Minimum[a]
Protein	%	22.0 (18.0)	30.0 (26.0)
Arginine	%	0.62 (0.51)	1.25 (1.04)
Histidine	%	0.22 (0.45)	0.31
Isoleucine	%	0.45 (0.37)	0.52
Leucine	%	0.72 (0.59)	1.25
Lysine	%	0.77 (0.63)	1.10 (0.83)
Methionine-cystine	%	0.53 (0.43)	1.10
Methionine	%	ND	0.62
Phenylalanine-tyrosine	%	0.89 (0.73)	0.88
Phenylalanine	%	ND	0.42
Threonine	%	0.58 (0.48)	0.73
Tryptophan	%	0.20 (0.16)	0.25 (0.16)
Valine	%	0.48 (0.39)	0.62
Fat	%	8.0 (5.0)	9.0
Linoleic acid	%	1.0	0.5
Arachidonic acid	%	ND	0.02
Minerals			
Calcium	%	1.0 (0.6)	1.0 (0.6)
Phosphorus	%	0.8 (0.5)	0.8 (0.5)
Ca:P	—	1:1	ND
Potassium	%	0.6	0.6
Sodium	%	0.3 (0.06)	0.2
Chloride	%	0.45 (0.09)	0.3
Magnesium	%	0.04	0.08 (0.04)
Iron	mg/kg	80	80
Copper	mg/kg	7.3	15 (5)
Manganese	mg/kg	5.0	5
Zinc	mg/kg	120	7.5
Iodine	mg/kg	1.5	75
Selenium	mg/kg	0.11	0.35 0.1
Vitamins and others			
Vitamin A	IU/kg	5000	9000 (5000)
Vitamin D	IU/kg	500	750 (500)
Vitamin E	IU/kg	50	30
Vitamin K	mg/kg	ND	0.1
Thiamine	mg/kg	1.0	5.0
Riboflavin	mg/kg	2.2	4.0
Pantothenic acid	mg/kg	10	5.0
Niacin	mg/kg	11.4	60
Pyridoxine	mg/kg	1.0	4.0
Folic acid	mg/kg	0.18	0.8
Biotin	mg/kg	ND	0.07
Vitamin B$_{12}$	mg/kg	0.022	0.02
Choline	mg/kg	1200	2400
Taurine (extruded)	%	ND	0.10
Taurine (canned)	%	ND	0.20

DM = dry matter; ND = not determined.
[a]Values in parentheses are for foods intended for adult maintenance only.
Adapted with permission. Association of American Feed Control Officials: Official Publication. AAFCO, Atlanta, 1996. (Copies may be obtained from Charles P. Frank, AAFCO Treasurer, Georgia Department of Agriculture, Capitol Square, Atlanta, GA 30334, 404-656-3637.)

III. Lack of a desaturating enzyme in cats requires an obligate source of arachidonic acid.
IV. Essential fatty acids in the food are prone to oxidation and degradation.
   A. Outdated, poorly preserved, or poorly stored foods may be deficient.
   B. The trend away from the use of synthetic antioxidant preservatives (e.g., ethoxyquin) in commercial foods may increase the risk.
V. A lack of fatty acids affects epidermal cell fluidity and results in a decrease in water retention in the stratum corneum.
VI. This pathophysiology is distinct from the conditions treated with omega-3 fatty acid supplementation.

A. In the latter case, the goal is to pharmacologically overwhelm the metabolism of fatty acids away from inflammatory prostaglandin synthesis.
B. There is no true dietary deficiency in omega-3 fatty acids (Campbell, 1992).

Clinical Signs

I. Predominant sign is seborrheic skin disease (Miller, 1989).
II. Rough, dry coat may be the initial finding.

Diagnosis

I. Clinical signs of characteristic skin lesions
II. History of prolonged use of low-fat diet in adults, or feeding of inappropriate or outdated food to young or reproducing animals

Differential Diagnosis

I. Zinc deficiency
II. Energy deficiency, protein deficiency
III. Other causes of seborrhea (see Chap. 88)

Treatment

I. Offering fresh food appropriate for life stage
II. Short-term use of fatty acid supplements
A. A variety of commercial fatty acid supplements are available, with or without other nutrients (see Chap. 90).
B. Corn oil is a less expensive alternative for use in dogs (Kallfelz and Dzanis, 1989).
C. Cats require an animal-source fat supplement to supply arachidonic acid, such as chicken or bacon fat.

Patient Monitoring

I. Discontinue supplementation with resolution of signs and change to an appropriately balanced food. Overuse may increase the risk for vitamin E deficiency and supply excess calories.
II. Failure of signs to resolve within 2 months suggests another diagnosis and/or some multiple-component disease (Miller, 1989).

MINERALS

Calcium Deficiency

Definition

An absolute, relative, or functional deficiency of dietary calcium (Ca) resulting in one of a number of disorders collectively referred to as metabolic bone disease (see Table 120–1).

Causes

I. Absolute dietary Ca deficiency, e.g., all-meat homemade diet without adequate calcium supplementation

II. Vitamin D deficiency
III. Phosphorus (P) deficiency (rare in dogs and cats)
IV. P excess, or low Ca:P ratio (Fowler, 1978; Kallfelz, 1987)

Pathophysiology

I. Low Ca intake
A. Low intake results in a transient drop in serum ionized Ca, stimulating the parathyroid glands.
B. Elevated serum parathormone (PTH) stimulates bone resorption, 1,25-dihydroxyvitamin D production, and renal Ca resorption.
C. Normocalcemia is restored, but at the expense of higher circulating PTH.
D. Osteopenia from excessive bone resorption and lack of calcification of organic matrix occurs.
E. High circulating PTH may also have direct toxic effects.
II. Inadequate vitamin D
A. Inhibits intestinal absorption of Ca, renal Ca resorption
B. Results in functional Ca deficiency
III. Excess dietary P, inverse Ca:P ratio (<1:1)
A. This causes a transient hyperphosphatemia, which results in a drop in serum ionized Ca.
B. High dietary P may inhibit intestinal Ca absorption.
C. This results in functional Ca deficiency.
D. Cats are more tolerant of inverse ratio than dogs (Kealy et al., 1995).

Clinical Signs

I. Lameness, inability to stand or walk, bone pain
II. Pathologic fractures, bowing deformities
III. Radiographic evidence of poorly mineralized bone, thin cortices, loss of lamina dura dentes early in course
IV. Serum Ca likely within normal range
V. Alkaline phosphatase activity increased (reliable indication only in mature, nonreproducing animals)
VI. High circulating PTH (see Chap. 42)

Diagnosis

I. Clinical signs are more likely in growing animals, because they are more sensitive to the effects of Ca deficiency.
II. Because of large body reserves, an adult can go many months on a deficient diet before signs are evident.
III. Diet history of an all-meat homemade diet is typical.
IV. Low serum 25-hydroxyvitamin D is diagnostic of vitamin D deficiency (<10 ng/ml).

Differential Diagnosis

I. Chronic renal disease (renal secondary hyperparathyroidism)
II. Primary hyperparathyroidism, pseudohyperparathyroidism

III. Vitamin D toxicity: similar gross and radiographic bone lesions

Treatment

I. Institute balanced diet appropriate for life stage.
II. Supplemental Ca and vitamin D are not recommended. Abrupt influx of Ca could result in aberrant calcification of damaged tissues (Kallfelz, 1987).
III. Institute appropriate medical or surgical repair of fractures or deformities, with confinement until improvement.

Patient Monitoring

I. Monitor improvement with radiographs every 2–4 weeks.
II. Allow closely supervised exercise as the animal's condition permits, to prevent disuse osteoporosis and further aggravation of bone demineralization.

Potassium Deficiency

Definition

I. An inadequate dietary potassium (K) deficiency relative to physiologic needs (see Table 120–1)
II. Seen primarily in cats with renal dysfunction offered presumed adequate diets (kaliopenic polymyopathy/nephropathy)

Causes

I. Preexisting hyperkaluria, increasing physiologic need
II. Renal dysfunction, hyperadrenocorticism, metabolic acidosis
III. Use of diets promoting diuresis or urine acidification (Buffington et al., 1991)
IV. Use of potassium-wasting diuretics

Pathophysiology

I. Adequate intracellular K is fundamental to a large number of biochemical processes.
II. Excessive urinary loss may not be accommodated by presumed normal dietary levels.
III. Neuromuscular, cardiovascular, and renal functions are compromised.

Clinical Signs

I. Acute onset of weakness, abnormal gait, reluctance to walk
II. Characteristic ventroflexion of neck
III. Serum K concentrations unreliable; severe depletion of intracellular K levels before extracellular levels affected
IV. Azotemia, hyperkaluria

Diagnosis

I. Characteristic clinical signs
II. History of renal dysfunction, use of diuretics, acidifying diets

Differential Diagnosis

I. Ventroflexion of neck may be confused with thiamine deficiency.
II. Plantigrade stance may also occur with other polyneuropathies.

Treatment

I. Severe cases may require intensive support with parenteral fluids with intravenous K (see Chap. 80).
II. Oral K supplementation is instituted.
   A. K gluconate is generally more palatable than other salts such as chloride.
   B. Administer 2–6 mEq per day, depending on estimation of depletion and size of cat (Dow and Fettman, 1992).
III. Discontinue use of offending diuretics and acidifying diets.
IV. Feed cat food containing ≥0.6% K DM.

Patient Monitoring

I. Significant response is usually seen in several days.
II. Continue oral K supplementation as a preventative, using caution with cats in advanced renal failure.
III. Reassess serum K and renal function every 2 months.

Zinc Deficiency

Definition

A primary or secondary deficiency in dietary zinc (Zn) relative to physiologic needs (see Table 120–1)

Causes

I. Secondary deficiency is caused by competing factors in poor-quality diets (high Ca, phytates), i.e., "generic dog food syndrome" (Sanecki et al., 1982; Sousa et al., 1988).
II. Oversupplementation with Ca can cause a secondary deficiency.
III. There is a familial tendency in Siberian huskies, malamutes, and other breeds (Miller, 1989).

Pathophysiology

I. Poor-quality diets may contain large concentrations of phytates from plant sources or Ca from high-ash meat and bone meal. A high-Ca product is indicative of poorer-quality ingredients.
II. Competing factors inhibit adequate absorption.
III. A genetic abnormality in some breeds affects Zn absorption or metabolism. Zn levels in normally balanced, good-quality foods may be insufficient.
IV. Zn deficiency disrupts normal epidermal integrity.

Clinical Signs

I. Alopecia, crusting, erythema
II. May affect footpads, mucocutaneous junctions initially
III. Parakeratotic hyperkeratosis on skin biopsy

Diagnosis

I. Typical clinical signs, with positive response to Zn supplementation
II. Diet history of poor-quality food
III. Breed predisposition

Differential Diagnosis

I. Essential fatty acid deficiency
II. Pyoderma
III. Autoimmune skin diseases

Treatment

I. Animals on poor-quality diets are switched to a higher-quality food appropriate for the life stage.
II. Discontinue use of Ca supplements.
III. Institute Zn supplementation (see Chap. 90).

Patient Monitoring

I. Response to therapy is seen within 3 weeks.
II. Zn supplementation in breeds previously on poor-quality diets (i.e., non–genetically affected) may be discontinued with resolution of signs.
III. Supplementation for dogs of affected breeds is permanent.

Other Mineral Deficiencies

See Table 120–2.

VITAMINS AND OTHER NUTRIENTS

Vitamin E Deficiency

Definition

I. It is an inadequacy of dietary vitamin E relative to physiologic needs (see Table 120–1).
II. On a clinical basis, it is observed mainly in cats (pansteatitis).

Causes

I. Diets containing high levels of polyunsaturated fatty acids (PUFAs), such as those containing large portions of tuna or other fish, are the usual cause.
II. Unbalanced diets not containing supplemental vitamin E may also be a cause.
III. The trend away from reliance on synthetic antioxidants (e.g., ethoxyquin) and toward the use of "natural preservatives," such as mixed tocopherols, in commercial foods may increase the risk, especially with high-fat dry foods.

Pathophysiology

I. High dietary PUFA content increases the requirement for vitamin E (NRC, 1986).

II. Vitamin E requirement is raised 10 IU per gram of fish oil per kg of diet (AAFCO, 1996).
III. PUFAs are prone to oxidative damage, both in the food and in the body.
IV. Vitamin E (mixed tocopherols) prevents oxidation of PUFAs but is sacrificed in the effort.
V. High PUFA/low vitamin E results in peroxidation of fatty deposits and fat necrosis.

Clinical Signs

I. Firm, granular subcutaneous fat
II. Generalized pain upon palpation
III. Fever
IV. Anorexia, lethargy
V. Neutrophilia with left shift
VI. Fat necrosis and inflammation upon biopsy

Diagnosis

I. Clinical signs characteristic
II. History of high fish intake, especially tuna or other fish intended for human consumption that is not supplemented with vitamin E

Differential Diagnosis

I. Generalized trauma
II. Bite wounds, infections

Treatment

I. Discontinue fish and fish-based cat foods.
II. Begin oral vitamin E supplementation at 10–20 IU/kg PO BID (Hoskins, 1992).
III. Short-term use of corticosteroids may reduce inflammation and alleviate pain.

Patient Monitoring

I. Improvement is usually observed within a few weeks.
II. Supplementation may be discontinued with resolution of signs and continued feeding of a balanced diet.

Vitamin K Deficiency

Definition

I. It implies a functional inadequacy of vitamin K relative to physiologic needs.
II. A simple vitamin K deficiency is rare in dogs and cats.

Causes

I. Antibiotic therapy, especially in young animals
II. Excess of dietary vitamin E (Nichols et al., 1989)
III. Commercial fish-based cat foods (Strieker et al., 1996)

Table 120–2. **Other Nutritional Deficiencies**

Nutrient	Causative Factors/Incidence	Clinical Signs
Phosphorus	Rare in dogs and cats	See Calcium Deficiency
Sodium chloride	Rare with commercial foods owing to wide availability of NaCl in ingredients	Aberrant water balance, fatigue, decreased milk production in heavily lactating animals
Magnesium	Feeding of Mg-restricted adult maintenance diets to kittens	Poor growth, anorexia, hyperextension of front legs
Iron	Feeding unsupplemented diets, diets containing poorly bioavailable sources (Fe oxide, carbonate)	Decreased hemoglobin synthesis, leading to a macrocytic, hypochromic anemia
Copper	Feeding diets containing poorly bioavailable source (Cu oxide)	Anemia, lightening of coat color
Manganese	Deficiency not reported in dogs or cats	Impaired growth, skeletal abnormalities, impaired reproduction in males and females of other species
Iodine	Naturally occurring deficiency uncommon	Goiter, alopecia, cretinism in young animals
Selenium	Naturally occurring deficiency rare	Myocardial and skeletal muscle degeneration experimentally; may exacerbate signs of vitamin E deficiency
Vitamin A	Feeding vegetarian diets to cats without source of preformed vitamin A or liver	Xerophthalmia, corneal lesions, reproductive failure, abnormal bone growth, neurologic defects
Vitamin D	Rare as single factor	Exacerbates signs of metabolic bone disease (see Calcium Deficiency)
Riboflavin	Rare owing to utilization of intestinal microbial synthesis	Anorexia, poor growth, weakness, skin lesions
Pantothenic acid	Rare	Depressed growth, anorexia, other nonspecific signs; emaciation, convulsions, death with severe deficiency
Niacin	Rare; readily available in animal tissues (cat has higher obligate need, but not of practical concern)	Anorexia, weight loss, ulcerations of the mouth
Pyridoxine	Rare	Anorexia, poor growth, microcytic hypochromic anemia, convulsions
Folic acid	Rare owing to intestinal microbial synthesis; difficult to reproduce without purified diet and administration of sulfa drugs	Anorexia, weight loss, anemia, leukopenia
Biotin	Rare owing to intestinal microbial synthesis and wide distribution among foodstuffs (raw egg whites contain avidin, which can bind biotin, but it is easily destroyed by cooking)	Poorly described in dogs and cats, but characterized by hyperkeratosis or other skin lesions
Vitamin B_{12}	Rare except when fed an unsupplemented vegetarian diet	Hypoplasia of the erythropoietic system (pernicious anemia in humans)
Choline	Uncommon, as dietary methionine partially replaces the need for choline (but only if methionine needs are met)	Fatty infiltration of the liver, liver dysfunction

Pathophysiology

I. Vitamin K is essential to the normal clotting cascade.
II. Adequate production of vitamin K usually occurs from gut bacterial synthesis.
III. Antibiotics or other substances may disrupt normal synthesis.
IV. The pathogenesis involved in clinical vitamin K deficiency from fish-based cat foods has not been determined or reproduced experimentally.

Clinical Signs

I. Mild to severe hemorrhage, bruising
II. Prolonged activated clotting time, prothrombin time
III. Hypoprothrombinemia

Diagnosis

I. Clinical signs of bleeding disorder
II. History of antibiotic or other medical treatment

III. Laboratory findings compatible with vitamin K deficiency (see Chap. 66)

Differential Diagnosis

I. Ingestion of coumarin-containing rodenticides or rodents dead or dying from such consumption
II. Other coagulopathies

Treatment

I. Parenteral vitamin K (see Chap. 66)
II. Supportive care, parenteral fluids, transfusions (see Chap. 69)

Patient Monitoring

I. Response to vitamin K treatment is rapid, but recovery from blood loss may be slow.
II. The animal can return to normal activity and diet as its condition permits.

Thiamine Deficiency

Definition

I. An inadequate dietary thiamine intake relative to physiologic needs (see Table 120–1)
II. More common in cats
III. Chastek's paralysis

Causes

I. Feeding of raw fish
II. Feeding of "complementary" pet food (i.e., not "complete and balanced") (Davidson, 1992)
III. Overprocessed food
IV. Sulfites in diet

Pathophysiology

I. Many species of fish contain a thiaminase that is easily destroyed by normal cooking (Smith and Proutt, 1944; Loew et al., 1970).
II. Thiamine is also very heat-labile.
   A. Normal processing of pet foods can destroy up to 90% of the added thiamine (AAFCO, 1996). For that reason, thiamine is generally added at far higher levels than needed to account for losses.
   B. Rare instances of overprocessing may destroy excessive amounts, however.
III. Sulfites in foods may interfere with thiamine absorption. The use of sulfites such as sodium metabisulfite is not allowed in products intended to serve as a source of thiamine.
IV. Thiamine deficiency compromises the metabolism of pyruvate to coenzyme A in the Krebs' cycle, disrupting normal production of energy.

Clinical Signs

I. Ventroflexion of neck
II. Muscle weakness, ataxia, convulsions

III. Elevated serum pyruvate and lactate
IV. Mydriasis, usually with normal vision

Diagnosis

I. Clinical signs
II. History of feeding raw fish

Differential Diagnosis

I. Potassium deficiency (especially with neck ventroflexion)
II. Other causes of weakness, mydriasis

Treatment

I. Administer parenteral thiamine (25–50 mg IM, SQ SID) for several days or until recovery (Hoskins, 1992).
II. Discontinue feeding of raw fish or suspect deficient food.

Patient Monitoring

I. Response to therapy confirms diagnosis.
II. Severe neural damage may not fully resolve.

Taurine Deficiency

Definition

I. Taurine deficiency is an inadequate dietary taurine intake relative to physiologic needs (see Table 120–1).
II. Manifestations of deficiency in cats include central retinal degeneration and dilated cardiomyopathy.
III. Dogs appear to synthesize adequate quantities for normal function, although taurine-sensitive cardiomyopathy may occur in some breeds.

Causes

I. Homemade diets with inadequate supplementation, especially vegetarian diets, are often low in taurine.
II. Dog foods are not typically adequate in taurine for cats.
III. Feeding of canned foods increases the excretion of taurine via the enterohepatic circulation (Douglass et al., 1991). Increased levels are required in canned food to accommodate the loss.

Pathophysiology

I. Taurine is required for normal retinal neurotransmission and cardiac function.
II. It is present in highest concentrations in animal tissues and is lowest in plant foodstuffs.
III. Although most animals are able to synthesize adequate quantities from dietary methionine and/or cysteine, cats lack sufficient enzyme capacity to produce adequate levels (NRC, 1986).

IV. Cats are also less capable of recirculating taurine via the enterohepatic circulation, which results in a continual loss from the gut.

Clinical Signs

I. There is permanent degeneration of neurosensory retina, with slowly progressive loss of photoreceptor cells (see Chap. 100).

II. Kittens from taurine-deficient queens may also show signs of poor growth and neural damage. Reproductive performance of the queen is compromised.

III. Dilated cardiomyopathy occurs in adults, with subsequent signs of cardiac insufficiency (Pion et al., 1987) (see Chap. 10).

Diagnosis

I. Clinical signs are strongly suggestive.

II. Diet history of feeding a homemade diet or dog food is common.

III. Low plasma (<60 nmol/ml) or whole blood (<200 nmol/ml) taurine levels are diagnostic.

Differential Diagnosis

I. Inherited progressive retinal degeneration (atrophy)

II. Other cardiomyopathies

Treatment

I. Taurine supplements at 250–500 mg PO BID

II. Feeding a balanced commercial diet

Patient Monitoring

I. Further retinal damage may be minimized, but existing damage is permanent.

II. Signs of taurine-responsive cardiomyopathies are reversible with supplementation.

III. Supplementation can be discontinued with resolution of signs, provided normal blood taurine levels are restored and the cat remains on balanced food.

Other Vitamin Deficiencies

See Table 120–2.

Bibliography

Association of American Feed Control Officials: Official Publication. AAFCO, Atlanta, 1996

Buffington CAT, DiBartola SP, Chew DJ: Effect of low potassium commercial nonpurified diet on renal function of adult cats. J Nutr 121:S91, 1991

Campbell KL: Therapeutic indications for dietary lipids. p. 36. In Kirk RW, Bonagura JD (eds): Current Veterinary Therapy XI: Small Animal Practice. WB Saunders, Philadelphia, 1992

Davidson MG: Thiamine deficiency in a colony of cats. Vet Rec 130:94, 1992

Donoghue S: Nutritional support of hospitalized patients. Vet Clin North Am [Small Anim Pract] 19:475, 1989

Douglass GM, Fern EB, Brown RC: Feline plasma and whole blood taurine levels as influenced by commercial dry and canned diets. J Nutr 121:S91, 1991

Dow SW, Fettman MJ: Renal disease in cats: the potassium connection. p. 820. In Kirk RW, Bonagura JD (eds): Current Veterinary Therapy XI: Small Animal Practice. WB Saunders, Philadelphia, 1992

Fowler ME: Metabolic bone disease. p. 55. In Fowler ME (ed): Zoo and Wild Animal Medicine. WB Saunders, Philadelphia, 1978

Hoskins JD: Juvenile nutritional disorders. p. 1277. In Morgan RV (ed): Handbook of Small Animal Practice. 2nd Ed. Churchill Livingstone, New York, 1992

Kallfelz FA: Skeletal and neuromuscular diseases. p. 12–1. In Lewis LD, Morris ML, Hand MS (eds): Small Animal Clinical Nutrition III. Mark Morris Associates, Topeka, 1987

Kallfelz FA, Dzanis DA: Overnutrition: an epidemic problem in pet animal practice? Vet Clin North Am [Small Anim Pract] 19:433, 1989

Kealy RD, Lawler DF, Ballam JM: Dietary calcium:phosphorus ratio for adult cats. Proceedings, Purina Nutrition Forum, 1995

Loew FM, Martin CL, Dunlop RH et al: Naturally-occurring and experimental thiamine deficiency in cats receiving commercial cat food. Can Vet J 11:109, 1970

Miller WH: Nutritional considerations in small animal dermatology. Vet Clin North Am [Small Anim Pract] 19:497, 1989

National Research Council: Nutrient Requirements of Dogs. National Academy Press, Washington, DC, 1985

National Research Council: Nutrient Requirements of Cats. National Academy Press, Washington, DC, 1986

Nichols DK, Wolff MJ, Phillips LG et al: Coagulopathy in pink-backed pelicans (*Pelecanus rufenscens*) associated with hypervitaminosis E. J Zoo Wildl Med 20:57, 1989

Pion PD, Kittleson MD, Rogers QR et al: Myocardial failure in cats associated with low plasma taurine: a reversible cardiomyopathy. Science 237:764, 1987

Sanecki RK, Corbin JE, Forbes RM: Tissue changes in dogs fed a zinc-deficient ration. Am J Vet Res 43:1642, 1982

Smith DC, Proutt LM: Development of thiamine deficiency in the cat on a diet of raw fish. Proc Soc Exp Biol Med 56:1, 1944

Sousa CA, Stannard AA, Ihrke PJ: Dermatosis associated with feeding generic dog food: 13 cases (1981–1982). J Am Vet Med Assoc 192:676, 1988

Strieker MJ, Morris JG, Feldman BF et al: Vitamin K deficiency in cats fed commercial fish-based diets. J Small Anim Pract 37:322, 1996

121

Disorders of Nutritional Excess

David A. Dzanis

ENERGY

Obesity

Definition

I. Obesity is the excess accumulation of fat in the adipose tissues.
   A. An animal is overweight at any level over its ideal body weight.
   B. An animal is considered obese if its accumulation of fat reaches a point where it may compromise the normal functions or activities of the animal.
II. Many definitions of obesity attempt to ascribe a specified percentage over ideal body weight (generally between 15 and 25%). However, because the ideal body weight of an individual animal is difficult to ascertain, such attempts are of limited usefulness, especially for dogs.
III. A better criterion is the body condition score, or BCS (see Table 119–2) (Laflamme et al., 1994). Dogs or cats with BCS >7 are considered obese.

Causes

I. Increased calorie consumption
   A. Feeding management
      1. Unrestricted access to food
      2. Offering highly palatable, high–energy density food (>4000 kcal metabolizable energy [ME]/kg dry matter [DM]
      3. Excessive offering of table scraps or treats
      4. Unsupervised group feeding
   B. Pet factors
      1. Boredom, emotional stress
      2. Competition with other animals
      3. Finicky behavior by the animal, inducing the owner to offer more palatable, energy-dense foods
II. Decreased energy expenditure
   A. Sedentary lifestyle
   B. Limited opportunities for exercise
   C. Decreased metabolic activity associated with age
   D. Decreased activity associated with neutering
   E. Loss of lean body mass and metabolic activity from previous weight loss
III. Genetic predispositions
   A. Certain breeds of dogs (beagles, Labrador retrievers) and cats (Persians) may be prone to excess weight gain.
   B. More sedentary temperaments and greater efficiency in using energy may be predisposing factors.

Pathophysiology

I. In its initial phase, calorie consumption exceeds expenditure. Excess energy is stored as fat.
II. Fat stores require less energy expenditure to maintain than does lean tissue.
   A. As the animal enters the static phase of obesity, calorie consumption may be less than that required to maintain the same animal at its ideal body weight.
   B. A finicky animal may actually consume very small portions of food.
III. Excess weight can hinder locomotor abilities, cardiovascular function, and heat/exercise tolerance.
   A. Intra-abdominal fat can put pressure on the diaphragm, compromising pulmonary capacity.
   B. These factors can result in a further decrease in activity, lowering metabolic rate, and loss of lean body mass.
   C. The conditions leading to obesity are thus exacerbated.

This chapter was written by Dr. Dzanis in his private capacity. No official support or endorsement by the Food and Drug Administration is intended or should be inferred.

Clinical Signs

I. Excess accumulation of subcutaneous fat
  A. Accumulation of fat distorts palpation of ribs and other bony prominences (ilia, dorsal processes of vertebrae), progressing to overt palpable or visible accumulations along trunk, ventral abdomen, brisket, and tail head.
  B. In cats, accumulation along the ventral abdomen may be the most evident initial site.
II. Excess accumulation of intra-abdominal fat
  A. Loss of abdominal tuck when viewed from the side, progressing to distention of abdomen below ventral level of thorax
  B. Loss of waist when viewed from above
III. Loss of functional capacity
  A. Decreased physical activity
  B. Heat or exercise intolerance
  C. Decreased locomotor ability, waddling gait

Diagnosis

I. Clinical signs are readily evident in pronounced cases.
  A. BCS of every animal should be assessed by visible exam and palpation.
  B. Corrective measures are more successful and easier to implement in the initial stages of weight gain, before the animal becomes obese.
II. Diet history may reveal problems in feeding management.

Differential Diagnosis

I. Endocrine imbalances affecting metabolic rate or satiety
  A. Hypothyroidism
  B. Diabetes mellitus
  C. Hyperadrenocorticism
  D. Pituitary or hypothalamic abnormality
II. Drug-induced polyphagia (megestrol, anticonvulsants)
III. Edema or ascites
  A. Cardiovascular disease
  B. Liver failure
  C. Hypoproteinemia from parasite infestation, protein deficiency

Treatment

I. Decrease calorie intake.
  A. Amount
    1. Many recommend reducing the calorie intake to 60–70% of the amount needed to maintain ideal body weight.
    2. However, because ideal weight is at best an arbitrary judgment, and the true energy expenditure may be less than that required to maintain the nonobese animal, such formulas may not work in all cases.
    3. A decrease in energy consumption to 50% of that required to maintain the weight of the

*Table 121–1. **Maximum Calorie Content (kcal ME/kg AF)***

Category (% Moisture)	Dog Food	Cat Food
Dry (<20%)	3100	3250
Semi-moist (≥20%, <65%)	2500	2650
Canned (≥65%)	900	950

obese animal may be a reasonable starting point.
    4. Adjustments in amount offered are made to achieve a weight loss rate of approximately 0.5–2% of initial body weight per week (Burkholder, 1996).
  B. Type
    1. A comparable amount of a less calorie-dense product than that normally fed may increase the chances for success.
    2. Reduced amounts of the same food may not sate the animal, leading to the pet's begging, and breakdown of owner compliance.
    3. Care must be taken to compare the calorie densities of available products. Depending on the brand, many commercial "lite" products may have more calories per weight than another brand's regular maintenance food.
    4. Recommendations for maximum "as fed" (AF) calorie densities of products to be used for the treatment of obesity are given in Table 121–1.
  C. Frequency
    1. More frequent feedings may help maintain satiety and prevent animal boredom.
    2. The prescribed daily amount is offered as three small meals rather than one large meal.
II. Increase energy expenditure.
  A. The chance for long-term success in a weight-loss program is minimal unless activity is increased.
  B. Exercise helps ameliorate the decrease in lean body mass and metabolic rate associated with calorie deprivation.
  C. Unless contraindicated by cardiovascular, pulmonary, or musculoskeletal impairment, a progressive daily exercise program is instituted.
    1. Owner-supervised activities (e.g., walking, fetching) are better at assuring increased activity than owner-passive encouragements such as increased access to outdoors.
    2. Although more difficult in indoor-confined cats, exercise can be induced through the use of toys, catnip, or play with other animals.

Patient Monitoring

I. Frequent veterinarian-owner-animal interaction is critical to long-term compliance. Initial biweekly visits (to assess progress and recommend adjustments

to the amount fed and degree of exercise) can be gradually extended to bimonthly.
II. Body weight and BCS are measured at each visit.
   A. Emphasis is placed on a thorough reassessment of BCS.
   B. Progress in loss of subcutaneous fat, tuck of abdomen, and so forth, is noted and pointed out to the pet owner.
III. Especially for finicky cats, care is taken to ensure that the animal continues to eat reasonable quantities of a new food. Obese cats that refuse to eat for protracted periods (1–2 months) are at a greatly increased risk for hepatic lipidosis.
IV. As the animal approaches its ideal BCS, a gradual relaxation in the amount or type of food can be made.
   A. Return to the pre-obese intake level is unlikely.
   B. The exercise program is retained.

Overnutrition of Large- and Giant-Breed Dogs

Definition

I. Numerous joint or skeletal problems are associated with the "excessive" growth of juvenile large- or giant-breed dogs.
II. Such problems include osteochondrosis dissecans, hip dysplasia, valgus deformities, and wobbler syndrome.

Causes

I. Unrestricted or poorly restricted access to highly energy- and nutrient-dense foods in the growing animal (Hedhammer et al., 1974; Kealy et al., 1992)
II. High dietary intake of specific nutrients, particularly calcium (Hazewinkel, 1989) (Table 121–2)
III. Large- and giant-breed dogs (e.g., Great Dane, German shepherd dog) predisposed
IV. No evidence of vitamin C deficiency as cause (Teare et al., 1979)

Pathophysiology

I. Excessive gain in body weight (fat or lean) may place undue strain on the still-developing bone and joint structures.
II. Skeletal growth of dogs cannot "exceed" predetermined genetic factors. However, genetic selection that allows for growth or growth rates above that of the prototypical dog (i.e., above 20 kg adult weight) may not provide for optimum skeletal development.
III. High dietary calcium, with or without a concurrently high dietary phosphorus level, adversely affects endochondral ossification and bone remodeling.

Clinical Signs

I. Lameness, reluctance to move
II. Joint or bone pain upon palpation
III. Radiographic signs of skeletal deformity or joint defect

IV. Well-fleshed appearance (BCS ≥6), with or without excess fat deposits

Diagnosis

I. Clinical signs
II. Diet history

Differential Diagnosis

I. Other causes of lameness or musculoskeletal pain (see Section XI)
II. Other causes of bone deformity

Treatment

I. Many skeletal defects are irreversible or can be ameliorated only by surgical intervention. Prevention and early detection are paramount.
II. Medical and/or surgical intervention is instituted as needed to alleviate clinical signs (see Section XI).
III. Feeding management is important.
   A. Restrict calorie intake to ≤75% of usual intake.
   B. If a very nutrient-dense product is offered, switch to a less-dense product that still provides adequate nutrition for normal growth.
      1. Many of the premium dog foods intended for adults are suitable for all life stages.
      2. The nutritional adequacy statement on the back panel should be consulted rather than relying on the front-panel life-stage designation.
   C. If the animal is greater than its ideal BCS, adjust intake to allow it to "grow into" a more suitable condition.
   D. Vitamin C supplementation has no benefit and may be contraindicated (Teare et al., 1979).

Patient Monitoring

I. Monitor growth rate. Feed with the goal of achieving an ideal (if not slightly low) BCS of 4–5.
II. As the animal's condition permits, allow moderate exercise to promote proper growth of skeleton and adequate musculature.

MINERALS

See Table 121–3.

VITAMINS AND OTHER NUTRIENTS

Vitamin A Toxicity

Definition

I. Hypervitaminosis A occurs with chronic intake of dietary vitamin A 50–100 times the dietary requirement.

Table 121–2. **AAFCO Dog and Cat Food Nutrient Profile Maximum Permitted Levels**

Nutrient	Units DM Basis	Dog Food Maximum	Cat Food Maximum
Protein	%	ND	ND
Arginine	%	ND	ND
Histidine	%	ND	ND
Isoleucine	%	ND	ND
Leucine	%	ND	ND
Lysine	%	ND	ND
Methionine-cystine	%	ND	ND
Methionine	%	ND	1.5
Phenylalanine-tyrosine	%	ND	ND
Phenylalanine	%	ND	ND
Threonine	%	ND	ND
Tryptophan	%	ND	ND
Valine	%	ND	ND
Fat	%	ND	ND
Linoleic acid	%	ND	ND
Arachidonic acid	%	ND	ND
Minerals			
Calcium	%	2.5	ND
Phosphorus	%	1.6	ND
Ca: P	—	2:1	ND
Potassium	%	ND	ND
Sodium	%	ND	ND
Chloride	%	ND	ND
Magnesium	%	0.3	ND
Iron	mg/kg	3000	ND
Copper	mg/kg	250	ND
Manganese	mg/kg	ND	ND
Zinc	mg/kg	1000	2000
Iodine	mg/kg	50	ND
Selenium	mg/kg	2	ND
Vitamins and others			
Vitamin A	IU/kg	250,000	750,000
Vitamin D	IU/kg	5000	10,000
Vitamin E	IU/kg	1000	ND
Vitamin K	mg/kg	ND	ND
Thiamine	mg/kg	ND	ND
Riboflavin	mg/kg	ND	ND
Pantothenic acid	mg/kg	ND	ND
Niacin	mg/kg	ND	ND
Pyridoxine	mg/kg	ND	ND
Folic acid	mg/kg	ND	ND
Biotin	mg/kg	ND	ND
Vitamin B_{12}	mg/kg	ND	ND
Choline	mg/kg	ND	ND
Taurine	%	ND	ND

DM = dry matter; ND = not determined.

Adapted with permission. Association of American Feed Control Officials: Official Publication. AAFCO, Atlanta, 1996. (Copies may be obtained from Charles P. Frank, AAFCO Treasurer, Georgia Department of Agriculture, Capitol Square, Atlanta, GA 30334, 404-656-3637.)

II. Dogs and cats appear to be more tolerant than most other species (the presumed safe level is 10 times the requirement for others) (Cline et al., 1995; Goldy et al., 1996).

Causes

I. Excessive feeding of diets containing large amounts of liver
II. Injudicious use of vitamin A–containing supplements, especially fish liver oils
III. Most clinical cases in cats

Pathophysiology

I. Vitamin A toxicity adversely affects bone ossification, resulting in dystrophic calcification and aberrant bone remodeling (Seawright et al., 1967).
II. Clinical manifestation is most often characterized as deforming cervical spondylosis in an adult cat. The predilection for this effect on the cervical vertebrae is not well understood.
III. The skeletal changes limit movement of the region and may impinge on nerves in the area of the lesions.

Clinical Signs

I. Postural changes: marsupial position—sitting with front feet raised
II. Lameness, neck or joint pain
III. Cutaneous hyperesthesia
IV. Lethargy, anorexia
V. Radiographic evidence of new bone formation, especially around the cervical vertebrae; periosteal bone formation and bony arthrodesis (see Chap. 79)

Diagnosis

I. Clinical signs, radiographic evidence
II. History of feeding large amounts of liver or oversupplementation with fish liver oil

Differential Diagnosis

I. Trauma to cervical region
II. Intervertebral disk disease

Treatment

I. Discontinue all dietary sources of vitamin A.
II. Provide supportive care.

Patient Monitoring

I. Although clinical signs may diminish with time, skeletal changes are unlikely to resolve.
II. It may take months to years for the accumulated vitamin A in the liver to be metabolized.

Vitamin D Toxicity

Definition

Hypervitaminosis D occurs with chronic intake of dietary vitamin D exceeding 10–20 times the requirement, or acute intake exceeding 100 times the requirement.

Causes

I. Rodenticides containing cholecalciferol as the active ingredient (Dzanis and Kallfelz, 1988; Dougherty et al., 1990)
II. Injudicious use of vitamin D–containing supplements, especially fish liver oils
III. Possibly some fish-based canned cat foods (Morris, 1996)
IV. *Cestrum diurnum* (day-blooming jessamine), an ornamental houseplant containing a 1,25-dihydroxycholecalciferol (1,25-diOH D3) analogue (Dzanis and Kallfelz, 1988)

Pathophysiology

I. Metabolism of vitamin D to 25-hydroxycholecalciferol (25-OH D3) is poorly regulated. High circulating levels of 25-OH D3 compete for 1,25-diOH D3 receptors in intestine and bone.
II. Increased influx of calcium (Ca) and phosphorus (P) occurs from the intestine, and increased bone mineral is released by enhanced osteoclasia and osteonecrosis.
III. Hypercalcemia is directly or indirectly responsible for most clinical signs and lesions in acute cases.

Clinical Signs

I. Acute stage
   A. Hypercalcemia: most distinguishing characteristic
   B. Acute renal failure
   C. Anorexia, weight loss, emesis, lethargy, diarrhea, polyuria/polydipsia
II. Chronic disease
   A. Bone lesions
      1. Thin, poorly mineralized bone
      2. Pathologic fractures
      3. Osteoblastic and osteocytic atrophy, osteonecrosis, enhanced osteoclasia
   B. Soft tissue necrosis, calcification
      1. Predominant sites: kidneys, heart, aorta, lungs, stomach, vocal cords
      2. Secondary sites: joints, periarticular tissues, tendons, ligaments
   C. Bone pain, lameness

Diagnosis

I. Clinical signs consistent with acute or chronic intoxication
II. History of rodenticide ingestion or oversupplementation

Table 121–3. **Other Nutritional Excesses**

Nutrient	Causative Factors/Incidence	Clinical Signs
Calcium	"Generic dog food syndrome," oversupplementation	May adversely affect absorption of other minerals, such as zinc (see Chap. 120, under Zinc Deficiency); associated with overnutrition of juvenile large-breed dogs (see text)
Phosphorus	All-meat homemade diet	May cause nutritional secondary hyperparathyroidism (see Chap. 120, under Calcium Deficiency)
Potassium	Injudicious use of urine-alkalinizing agents (e.g., potassium citrate) for the prevention of calcium oxalate urolithiasis	May interfere with magnesium absorption and increase the risk of struvite urolithiasis by increasing urine pH
Sodium chloride	Unlikely in a dog or cat with normal cardiac and renal function and continuous access to fresh, potable water	High levels (>3%) adversely affect palatability of dog and cat foods; food refusal is more likely to occur before clinical signs are manifested
Magnesium	Poor-quality foods containing high-ash meat and bone meal or poultry meal	Direct toxic effects rare in dogs and cats; may be a risk factor in development of lower urinary tract disease in cats when urine pH >6.4 (AAFCO, 1996); not all individual cats offered an "acidifying" commercial diet will maintain an acidic urine; when the urine pH of individual cats at potential risk is unknown or not monitored occasionally, magnesium content of the food should not exceed 0.12% DM (250 mg/ 1000 kcal ME)
Iron (Fe)	Highly dependent on chemical form (Fe sulfate [in human supplements] more toxic than Fe oxide [approved color additive for pet foods up to 0.25%])	May cause vomiting, diarrhea, anorexia, gastrointestinal damage; Fe sulfate induces gastrointestinal lesions at approximately eight times the dietary requirement; Fe oxide does not cause signs at levels up to 1% of the diet (NRC, 1980)
Copper (Cu)	Rare except in predisposed breeds	Cu storage disease (autosomal recessive disorder) in dogs arises from impaired excretion of Cu from liver in bile and results in excess accumulation, even at levels typically found in most foods; it causes a chronic progressive liver disease with hepatolenticular degeneration (see Chap. 34)
Manganese	No documented reports in dogs and cats	Metabolic alterations, growth retardation, and other signs seen in other species
Zinc (Zn)	Consumption of zinc-containing objects (hardware, pennies, toys) or zinc oxide ointments	Most Zn salts are readily absorbed from the gastrointestinal tract; signs include vomiting, diarrhea, anorexia, icterus, hemolytic anemia
Iodine	Injudicious use of kelp or other iodine supplements	Signs of toxicity mimic deficiency (goiter, hypothyroidism, reduced reproductive performance)

Table 121–3. **Other Nutritional Excesses** *(Continued)*

Nutrient	Causative Factors/Incidence	Clinical Signs
Selenium	Unlikely; cats may be more tolerant than dogs	Clinical signs of toxicity include depression, anorexia, emaciation, loss of hair; cats fed fish-based cat foods containing up to 10 mg/kg DM apparently do not suffer adverse effects; inhibition of absorption by competing trace minerals may be a factor
Vitamin E	Injudicious use of antioxidant supplements	High dietary levels may interfere with absorption of vitamins D and K; vitamin K–responsive coagulopathy observed in piscivorous birds fed large amounts of vitamin E (Nichols et al., 1989)
Vitamin K	Parenteral administration of synthetic form (menadione), but nontoxic orally	Parenteral administration may cause hemolytic anemia, which is potentially lethal; acute renal failure observed in horses given amounts within therapeutic dosage range; LD_{50} of dogs = 75–200 mg/kg BW (NRC, 1987)
Thiamine	Parenteral administration, but essentially nontoxic orally	Parenteral administration may cause respiratory paralysis, cardiac failure, and death; LD_{50} in dogs = 50–125 mg/kg BW (NRC, 1987)
Riboflavin	Nontoxic orally	Dogs given 250 times the dietary requirement for 5 mo showed no adverse effects; no studies reported in cats
Pantothenic acid	Nontoxic orally	No adverse effects reported at levels up to 10 g/kg of food
Niacin	Essentially nontoxic	Eighty times the dietary requirement caused slight proteinuria in dogs after 2 mo; higher levels (300 times) produced bloody feces and convulsions in a few animals; no studies reported in cats
Pyridoxine	Essentially nontoxic	At several thousand times the requirement, dogs show signs of neuromuscular impairment; no studies in cats reported
Folic acid	Essentially nontoxic	No adverse effects documented
Biotin	Essentially nontoxic	No studies in dogs or cats on toxic effects reported
Vitamin B_{12}	Essentially nontoxic	Essentially nontoxic orally; presumed safe at several hundred times the dietary requirement
Choline	Oversupplementation	Dogs appear intolerant of excess choline; as little as three times the dietary requirement may result in reduction of erythrocyte counts; no reports of adverse effects in cats from excess choline
Taurine	Nontoxic	No reports of toxicity in either dogs or cats
Methionine	Oversupplementation for purposes of urinary acidification in cats; supplemental methionine added to that already present in commercial diet, causing total diet to exceed AAFCO maximum	Hemolytic anemia, methemoglobinemia, and Heinz body formation observed in cats fed high levels (Fau et al., 1987); may cause metabolic acidosis when used with acidifying diet
Vitamin C	Megadose supplementation	No adverse effects reported in short-term studies in dogs offered 3 g/day and cats offered 0.5 g/day (NRC, 1987); no long-term studies on effects in dogs or cats reported; megadoses of vitamin C can result in oxaluria and reduced urine pH, both risk factors for calcium oxalate urolithiasis; megadoses may cause diarrhea, excessive iron absorption

III. Elevated serum or plasma 25-OH D3 diagnostic (>60 ng/ml), except for *C. diurnum* ingestion
IV. Depressed serum alkaline phosphatase activity (not as reliable in young or reproducing animals)

Differential Diagnosis

I. Hypercalcemia
   A. Cancer: lymphosarcoma, adenocarcinoma, bone tumors
   B. Infection: fungal or bacterial osteomyelitis, granulomatous diseases
   C. Primary hyperparathyroidism
II. Bone lesions
   A. Metabolic bone disease (see Chaps. 79 and 120)
   B. Chronic renal failure

Treatment

I. Control hypercalcemia, renal failure (see Chaps. 47, 71, and 123).
II. Feeding management is as follows.
   A. Discontinue use of all supplements and foods (if possible) containing vitamin D.
   B. Although Ca is not needed in the diet in cases of acute toxicity, a dietary source is provided in chronic cases, because Ca will continue to be drawn from bone resorption owing to high circulating 25-OH D3.

Patient Monitoring

I. Monitor renal status and serum calcium, and modify therapy as needed (see Chaps. 47 and 123).
II. A gradual return to normal food (containing appropriate levels of vitamin D) is not instituted until serum or plasma 25-OH D3 approaches the normal range.
III. The approximate serum half-life of 25-OH D3 is 12–30 days, although higher levels may induce more rapid metabolic disposition (Dzanis and Kallfelz, 1988; Dougherty et al., 1990).

Other Vitamin Excesses

See Table 121–3.

Bibliography

Association of American Feed Control Officials: Official Publication. AAFCO, Atlanta, 1996
Burkholder W: Fighting obesity. p. 90. In: Proceedings, Focus on Geriatric Nutrition, Chicago, 1996
Cline JL, Czarnecki-Maulden GL, Lonosky JM et al: Effect of vitamin A on bone density and mucosal epithelium in dogs (abstract). J Anim Sci 73(Suppl 1):192, 1995
Dougherty SA, Center SA, Dzanis DA: Salmon calcitonin as adjunct treatment for vitamin D toxicosis in a dog. J Am Vet Med Assoc 196:1269, 1990
Dzanis DA, Kallfelz FA: Recent knowledge of vitamin D toxicity in dogs. Proc Am Coll Vet Intern Med 6:289, 1988
Fau D, Smalley KA, Rogers QR et al: Effect of excess dietary methionine on weight gain and plasma amino acids in kittens. J Nutr 117:1838, 1987
Goldy GG, Burr JR, Longardner CN et al: Effects of measured doses of vitamin A fed to healthy beagle dogs for 26 weeks. Vet Clin Nutr 3:42, 1996
Hazewinkel HAW: Calcium metabolism and skeletal development in dogs. p. 293. In Burger IH, Rivers JPW (eds): Nutrition of the Dog and Cat. Cambridge University Press, Cambridge, 1989
Hedhammer AF, Wu F, Krook L et al: Overnutrition and skeletal disease: an experimental study in growing Great Dane dogs. Cornell Vet 64(Suppl 5):1, 1974
Kealy RD, Olsson SE, Monti KL et al: Effects of limited food consumption on the incidence of hip dysplasia in growing dogs. J Am Vet Med Assoc 201:857, 1992
Laflamme DP, Kuhlman G, Lawler DF et al: Obesity management in dogs. Vet Clin Nutr 1:59, 1994
Morris JG: Vitamin D synthesis by kittens. In: Proceedings, Purina Nutrition Forum, St. Louis, 1996
National Research Council: Mineral Tolerance of Domestic Animals. National Academy of Sciences, Washington, DC, 1980
National Research Council: Vitamin Tolerance of Animals. National Academy Press, Washington, DC, 1987
Nichols DK, Wolff MJ, Phillips LG et al: Coagulopathy in pink-backed pelicans *(Pelecanus rufenscens)* associated with hypervitaminosis E. J Zoo Wildl Med 20:57, 1989
Seawright AA, English PB, Gartner RJW: Hypervitaminosis A and deforming cervical spondylosis of the cat. J Comp Pathol 77:29, 1967
Teare JA, Hintz H, Krook L et al: Ascorbic acid deficiency and hypertrophic osteodystrophy in the dog: a rebuttal. Cornell Vet 69:384, 1979

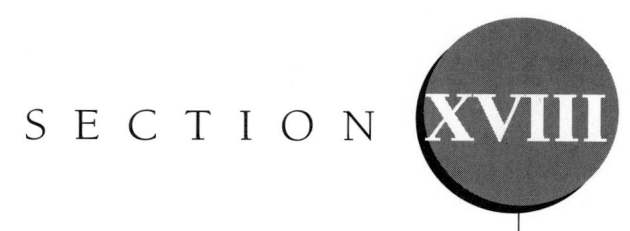

SECTION XVIII

Toxicology

122

Introduction

Gary D. Osweiler
Thomas L. Carson

POISONINGS

I. The symptoms of intoxication in small animals are often severe and have a rapid onset.
   A. These circumstances can be extremely distressing to the owner of the animal.
   B. A preplanned course of action and ready availability of equipment and drugs are essential.
II. This section discusses the source, action, clinical signs, diagnosis, and treatment of the more frequently encountered intoxications in small animal medicine.
   A. Clinical signs and treatment objectives are listed in chronologic order.
   B. A general protocol for emergency treatment of poisonings as well as a list of equipment and drugs for an ''antidote crash cart'' are outlined.

EMERGENCY PROTOCOL

I. Preliminary instructions to owners to prevent further exposure to a toxicant are as follows.
   A. Bathe with large volumes of water when skin or eyes are exposed. Instruct owners to protect themselves from exposure with gloves and aprons.
   B. Get the animal into fresh air after exposure to inhaled toxicants.
   C. Induce emesis—best if within 2 hours of ingestion.
      1. Contraindications: central nervous system (CNS) depression; ingestion of petroleum distillates, acids, alkalis, tranquilizers, other emetics
      2. Household remedies: syrup of ipecac (1–2 ml/kg PO), hydrogen peroxide (1–5 ml/kg PO), maximum 50 ml, liquid dishwashing detergent (mix 1:8 in water and give 10 ml/kg PO)

         Do not use laundry detergents or automatic dishwasher detergents, which are very irritating. Syrup of ipecac is an effective emetic, but the other methods are only about 50% effective.
   D. Allow the animal to drink water.
   E. Keep the animal calm.
   F. Owners are instructed to bring vomitus and/or suspected material with the animal for possible analysis.
II. Prevent further absorption of toxicant.
   A. Induction of emesis
      1. Induction of emesis and gastric lavage, if accomplished immediately after ingestion, remove at best only 60–70% of the gastric contents.
      2. Emesis is most effective when the stomach contains food or liquids.
      3. Apomorphine is an effective emetic; however, it may aggravate CNS and respiratory depression.
         a) Dose is 0.04 mg/kg IV or 0.08 mg/kg SQ.
         b) A tablet placed in the conjunctival sac induces vomiting but can result in moderate to severe conjunctivitis, so thoroughly flush conjunctival sac with sterile saline when vomiting starts.
         c) Apomorphine is of questionable safety in cats; therefore, syrup of ipecac is used.
         d) Naloxone (0.04 mg/kg IV) is an effective antagonist to apomorphine.
      4. Xylazine 1.1 mg/kg IM induces emesis in a high proportion of cats. Any secondary CNS or respiratory depression can be reversed with yohimbine (0.1 mg/kg IV).
   B. Gastric lavage: best if performed within 2 hours of ingestion
      1. Institute anesthesia with cuffed endotracheal tube in place. Tube should extend at least 2 in. beyond teeth to prevent aspiration.
      2. Use large-bore stomach tube.
      3. Premeasure tube from nose to last rib.
      4. Lower head slightly below body.
      5. Do not force stomach tube.
      6. Use 5–10 ml lavage solution/kg body weight for each washing; use low pressure.
      7. Aspirate with large bulb or 60-ml syringe.
      8. Repeat 10 times.

C. Gastrointestinal adsorbents
1. Activated charcoal is best; tablets are easiest to administer.
2. Slurry of 1–2 g activated charcoal/5 ml water may be used.
3. Dosage is 10 ml slurry/kg body weight.
4. Allow last lavage to sit 30 minutes and then give a cathartic.
D. Cathartics
1. Sodium sulfate is readily available; dosage is 1 g/kg PO.
2. Sorbitol (70%) 3 ml/kg PO is an effective alternative cathartic.
E. Enemas
1. Use warm soapy water.
2. Avoid hexachlorophene soaps.

III. Apply specific antidotes as outlined in the following chapters.

IV. Hasten elimination of absorbed toxicant.
A. Maintain renal function and urine output.
1. Fluid therapy
2. Diuretics
a) Be sure that the animal is well hydrated first.
b) Give mannitol 1–2 g/kg IV; if diuresis does not develop within 30 minutes, mannitol is not repeated.
c) Give furosemide (Lasix) 2–4 mg/kg IV; it may be repeated TID.
B. Attempt ion trapping.
1. Ionized compounds traverse cell membranes less readily than do nonionized compounds; hence ionized compounds are poorly reabsorbed by renal tubules.
2. Alkaline urine facilitates ionization of acid compounds (e.g., aspirin, barbiturates). To alkalinize the urine, give sodium bicarbonate 50 mg/kg PO BID-TID.
3. Acidic urine ionizes basic compounds (e.g., amphetamines, strychnine). To acidify the urine, give ammonium chloride 100–200 mg/kg/day PO in 3–4 divided doses.
4. Ion trapping may also be used in conjunction with gastric lavage (e.g., use of a 1–2% tannic acid solution for lavage in animals with strychnine poisoning).
C. Peritoneal dialysis may be tried for dialyzable toxins (e.g., ethylene glycol).

V. Give supportive therapy.
A. Respiratory support
1. Maintain airway.
2. Provide oxygen and artificial respiration if necessary.
B. Cardiovascular support
1. Treat shock.
2. Correct cardiac arrhythmias.
3. Correct electrolyte abnormalities.
4. Correct acid–base imbalances.
5. Maintain normal hydration.
C. Body temperature control
1. Hypothermia: blankets, heat lamps (use cautiously), circulating water pads

2. Hyperthermia: fluid therapy, fans, cold water baths
D. CNS
1. Depression: oxygen and respiratory support
2. Hyperactivity and/or seizures
a) Diazepam 0.5 mg/kg IV as needed
b) Phenobarbital 2–10 mg/kg IV, IM
c) Pentobarbital IV to effect
Note: Seizures may cause cerebral edema, and therapy with mannitol and/or dexamethasone may be appropriate.
E. Control of pain: meperidine (Demerol)
1. Dogs: 5–10 mg/kg IM PRN
2. Cats: 1–4 mg/kg IM PRN

VI. Equipment and drugs to stock in an emergency toxicity treatment cart are as follows.
A. Equipment
1. Endotracheal tubes, several sizes
2. Laryngoscope, with light
3. Oxygen source
4. Mechanical respirator or respirator (Ambu) bag
5. Gauze and tape
6. Intravenous catheters
7. Needles
8. Syringes
9. Fluid administration sets and IV extension tubing
10. Thermometer
11. Large funnel or pump for stomach tube
12. Stomach tubes, several sizes
13. Aspirator bulb
14. Enema bag and hose
15. Urinary catheters, several sizes
16. Small sterile surgery kit for venostomy or tracheostomy
17. Mild soap or detergent
18. Pen light
19. Blanket, heat lamps, circulating water heating pad
20. Clean specimen vials
B. Drugs
1. Acepromazine 0.05 mg/kg IV, IM, or SQ for amphetamine toxicosis
2. Acetylcysteine (Mucomyst) 140 mg/kg PO initially, and then 70 mg/kg PO QID for 3–5 treatments for acetaminophen toxicosis
3. Activated charcoal 1 g/5 ml water as a gastrointestinal adsorbent per 1–2 g/kg body weight
4. Ammonium chloride 100–200 mg/kg/day PO divided QID for urine acidification
5. Amphetamine sulfate (Benzedrine) 4.4 mg/kg SQ for CNS stimulation
6. Apomorphine (dogs) 0.04 mg/kg IV or 0.08 mg/kg SQ for induction of emesis
7. Ascorbic acid (vitamin C) 30 mg/kg PO or parenterally QID for seven treatments for reduction of methemoglobin
8. Atropine sulfate 0.2–0.5 mg/kg for cholinergic signs; one fourth of the dosage IV, the rest SQ or IM
9. Barbiturates, phenobarbital, pentobarbital IV slowly to effect for CNS hyperactivity
10. Calcitonin (salmon) 4–6 IU/kg SQ every 2–3

hours for hypercalcemia in cholecalciferol toxicosis

11. Calcium EDTA (Versenate) 100 mg/kg/day as 10 mg/ml in 5% dextrose/water (D/W) SQ divided QID for 5 days for lead poisoning

12. Calcium gluconate 10% for hypocalcemia: dogs, 10–30 ml IV slowly; cats, 5–15 ml IV slowly while monitoring electrocardiogram

13. 5% D/W

14. Diazepam (Valium) 2.5–20 mg IV as needed for CNS hyperactivity

15. Dimercaprol (BAL) 4 mg/kg IM QID for no more than 4 days for arsenic toxicosis

16. Diphenhydramine (Benadryl) 1–4 mg/kg PO TID for nicotinic receptor overload

17. Diphenylthiocarbazone (Dithizone) 50–70 mg/kg PO TID for thallium toxicosis

18. 20% ethanol for ethylene glycol toxicosis: dogs, 5.5 ml/kg IV every 4 hours for five treatments and then QID for four more treatments; cats, 5 ml/kg IV QID for five treatments and then TID for four more treatments

19. Ferric cyanoferrate (Prussian blue) 100 mg/kg PO TID for thallium toxicosis

20. Furosemide (Lasix) 2–4 mg/kg IV for diuresis

21. Glyceryl guaiacolate (Geocolate) 110 mg/kg IV as needed for muscle relaxation

22. Glyceryl monoacetate 0.55 mg/kg IM hourly to total dose of 2–4 mg/kg for sodium fluoroacetate toxicosis

23. Kaolin (Kaopectate) 1–2 ml/kg PO QID as a gastrointestinal protectant

24. Lactated Ringer's solution

25. Lidocaine (without epinephrine) (Xylocaine) for ventricular arrhythmias: dogs, 1–2 mg/kg IV bolus followed by IV drip of 0.1% solution at 30–50 µg/kg/minute

26. Lime water 5 ml/kg PO for alkaline gastric lavage

27. 20% mannitol 1–2 g/kg IV for diuresis or cerebral edema

28. Meperidine HCl (Demerol) for sedation and pain: dogs, 5–10 mg/kg IM; cats, 1–4 mg/kg IM

29. 10% methocarbamol (Robaxin) 150 mg/kg IV for muscle relaxation

30. 4-Methylpyrazole 5% solution for ethylene glycol toxicosis: dogs, 20 mg/kg IV, then 15 mg/kg IV at 12 and 24 hours, then 5 mg/kg IV at 36 hours

31. Naloxone HCl (Narcan) 0.04 mg/kg IV for narcotic antagonism

32. Nicotinamide (nicotinic acid, niacin) 50–100 mg IM for 2 weeks for Vacor poisoning

33. Normal saline

34. D-penicillamine (Cuprimine) 50 mg/kg PO divided QID for 7–14 days for lead poisoning

35. Phenylephrine (Neo-Synephrine) 0.15 mg/kg IV for CNS stimulation

36. Phenytoin (Dilantin): dogs, 8–15 mg/kg PO TID or 50–100 mg IV over 5 minutes (maximum dose 24 mg/kg) for arrhythmias

37. Potassium chloride (Kay Ciel) PO and IV for hypokalemia and thallium toxicosis

38. Potassium permanganate (1:2000) 5 ml/kg for gastric lavage for strychnine toxicosis

39. Pralidoxime chloride (2-PAM, Protopam) 20 mg/kg IV BID for organophosphate toxicity

40. Propranolol (Inderal): dogs, 0.2–1 mg/kg PO TID for arrhythmias

41. Sodium bicarbonate, PO and IV to effect for metabolic acidosis and for alkalinization of urine

42. Sodium sulfate (GoLYTELY) 1 g/kg PO for catharsis

43. Sodium thiosulfate 20% solution: 40–50 mg/kg IV TID for arsenic toxicosis

44. Syrup of ipecac 1–2 ml/kg PO for induction of emesis

45. 1–2% tannic acid for gastric lavage in strychnine toxicosis

46. Thiamine (vitamin B$_1$) 10–100 mg/day PO for ethylene glycol toxicosis

47. Vitamin K$_1$ (AquaMEPHYTON) 2–5 mg/kg SQ divided BID, 2–3 mg/kg PO divided TID for warfarin and other anticoagulant toxicosis

48. Whole fresh blood (<2 weeks old) 10–20 ml/kg IV slowly for anemia and blood clotting disorders

49. Xylazine (Rompun) 1.1 mg/kg IV for sedation and muscle relaxation

Bibliography

Atkins CE, Johnson RR: Clinical toxicities of cats. Vet Clin North Am 5:623, 1975

Baily EM: Emergency and general treatment of poisonings. p. 116. In Kirk RW (ed): Current Veterinary Therapy X: Small Animal Practice. WB Saunders, Philadelphia, 1989

Beasley VR (ed): Toxicology of selected pesticides, drugs and chemicals. Vet Clin North Am [Small Anim Pract] 20:283, 1990

Clarke EGC, Clarke ML: Veterinary Toxicology. Williams & Wilkins, Baltimore, 1975

Dormann DC: Emergency treatment of toxicoses. p. 211. In Bonagura JD (ed): Current Veterinary Therapy XII: Small Animal Practice. WB Saunders, Philadelphia, 1995

Fenner WR: Intoxications. p. 565. In Fenner WR (ed): Quick Reference to Veterinary Medicine. JB Lippincott, Philadelphia, 1982

Goodman LS, Gilman A: The Pharmacologic Basis of Therapeutics. 7th Ed. Macmillan, New York, 1985

Harris WF: Clinical toxicities of dogs. Vet Clin North Am 5:605, 1975

Meester WD: Emesis and lavage. Vet Hum Toxicol 22:225, 1980

Oehme FW: Emergency kit for treatment of small animal poisoning (antidotes, drugs, equipment). p. 92. In Kirk RW (ed): Current Veterinary Therapy VIII. WB Saunders, Philadelphia, 1983a

Oehme FW: Toxicologic problems. p. 175. In Ettinger SJ (ed): Textbook of Veterinary Internal Medicine. 2nd Ed. WB Saunders, Philadelphia, 1983b

Osweiler GD: Toxicology. Williams & Wilkins, Philadelphia, 1996

Osweiler GD, Carson TL, Buck WB, Van Gelder GA: Clinical and Diagnostic Veterinary Toxicology. 3rd Ed. Kendall-Hunt Publishing, Dubuque, 1985

123

Rodenticides

Thomas L. Carson
Gary D. Osweiler

STRYCHNINE

Source

I. Alkaloid used as rat, mole, gopher, and coyote poison; most approvals for subsoil use
II. Sweet-tasting pellets or coating on rodent food, usually dyed purple, red, or green
III. Usually formulated as ≤0.3% baits (a 0.3% bait contains 3 mg/g)
IV. Weak organic base, ionized in stomach
V. Lethal dosage
  A. Dogs: 0.75 mg/kg
  B. Cats: 2 mg/kg
VI. Narrow margin between toxic and lethal dosage

Action

I. Interferes with postsynaptic neuronal inhibition in spinal cord and medulla
II. Antagonizes glycine in spinal cord and medulla, where glycine is an inhibitory transmitter
III. Allows spinal reflex activity to proceed unchecked

Clinical Signs

I. They appear within 10 minutes to 2 hours after ingestion.
II. Early signs are apprehension, nervousness, stiffness.
III. Rigid abdominal and cervical musculature may be evident.
IV. Violent tetanic seizures appear spontaneously or secondary to stimuli (e.g., bright light, sound, touch).
V. All striated muscles are affected, but more powerful extensors predominate, giving rigid, symmetrical "sawhorse" stance
VI. Tetanic spasms become more frequent and powerful.
  A. Legs and body are stiff.
  B. Ears are erect.
  C. Lips are pulled back over teeth (risus sardonicus).
  D. Mydriasis is present.
  E. Breathing stops.
  F. No paddling, chomping, or salivation is noted.
VII. Death is caused by hypoxia secondary to respiratory distress.
VIII. Postmortem examination shows the following.
  A. No gross or microscopic lesions
  B. Stomach usually full of undigested food or bait

Diagnosis/Differential Diagnosis

I. It is based on a history of ingestion or exposure, characteristic clinical signs, and absence of lesions; it often occurs in large-breed male dogs.
II. Hyperesthetic response to a sharp handclap can be a diagnostic aid.
III. Chemical analysis of stomach contents may be helpful.
IV. Differential diagnosis includes hypocalcemia, chlorinated hydrocarbons, lead, zinc phosphide, metaldehyde, compound 1080, tetanus, 4-aminopyridine, nicotine, caffeine.

Treatment

I. Prevent absorption.
  A. Induce vomiting if the animal is not hyperesthetic or convulsive.
  B. Gastric or enterogastric lavage with 1–2% tannic acid or 1:2000 potassium permanganate, followed by activated charcoal and sodium sulfate, may be helpful.
II. Maintain relaxation and prevent hypoxia.
  A. Pentobarbital IV to effect
  B. Endotracheal tube, oxygen, and artificial respiration for respiratory failure
  C. Inhalation anesthesia
  D. Diazepam 2.5–20 mg IV as needed
  E. Glyceryl guaiacolate 110 mg/kg IV as needed
  F. Methocarbamol 150 mg/kg IV—average initial dose
  G. *Caution:* morphine contraindicated because of its

spinal cord stimulant and respiratory depressant properties

III. Hasten elimination of absorbed toxicant.
  A. Establish diuresis.
  B. Acidify urine with NH_4Cl 100–200 mg/kg/day PO divided QID. Do not administer NH_4Cl until diuresis is established.
  C. Elimination is usually complete by 24–48 hours.

COUMARINS AND RELATED COMPOUNDS

Source

I. First-generation anticoagulants are moderately toxic but have a relatively short residence time in the body.
  A. Coumarin type: warfarin and related compounds
    1. Concentration of active ingredients varies from 0.025% in baits and throw packs to 1% in tracking powders.
    2. Commercial products include Coumafene, D-Con, Banarat, Rosex, Ratox, and Prolin.
  B. Indanedione type
    1. Concentration of active ingredients is similar to coumarins.
    2. Chemical names contain the suffix ''1,3 indanedione.''
    3. Generic products include pindone, diphacinone, and chlorophacinone.
    4. Commercial products include Chemrat, Drat, Rozol, Ramik, and Diphacin.
II. Second-generation anticoagulants have been developed within the past 15 years.
  A. They are more potent and are designed to control rodents resistant to first-generation agents.
  B. Many are available in pellets or weather-resistant blocks and are colored green or blue.
  C. Generic products include brodifacoum, bromadiolone, and difethiolone.
  D. Commercial products include Talon, De-mize, Rodend, Havoc, Bolt, Ropax, D-Con Mouse Prufe II, Maki, D-Cease, and Contrac.
III. Certain factors enhance toxicosis.
  A. Oral antibiotics that reduce intestinal vitamin K synthesis
  B. Displacement from binding with plasma proteins by other drugs such as sulfonamides, phenylbutazone, corticosteroids
  C. Biliary obstruction
  D. Liver disease
IV. The acute oral LD_{50} dose varies among products.
  A. Warfarin: 5–50 mg/kg for the dog and cat
  B. Pindone: 5–75 mg/kg for the dog
  C. Diphacinone: 0.9–8 mg/kg for the dog, 15 mg/kg for the cat
  D. Brodifacoum: 0.2–4 mg/kg for the dog, 25 mg/kg for the cat
  E. Bromadiolone: 11–15 mg/kg for the dog, >25 mg/kg for the cat
V. The cumulative toxic dosage is as follows.

  A. Warfarin: 1–5 mg/kg for 5–15 days for dogs, 1 mg/kg for 5 days for cats
  B. Cumulative toxicity of diphacinone and bromadiolone enhanced by long half-life

Action

I. Coumarins inhibit vitamin K epoxide reductase.
II. Decreased vitamin K epoxide reductase inhibits the activation of vitamin K.
III. Active vitamin K is necessary for the synthesis of coagulation factors II, VII, IX, and X in the liver.

Clinical Signs

I. Clinical signs depend on amount and source of hemorrhage.
II. There is a latent period of 2–7 days before coagulation defects occur.
III. With acute poisoning, animals may be found dead, especially with brain, pericardial, or intrathoracic hemorrhage.
IV. Subacute poisoning may produce these signs.
  A. Anemia, weakness
  B. External hemorrhage: epistaxis, hematemesis, hematuria, melena, hematochezia
  C. Internal hemorrhage
    1. Dyspnea with thoracic and/or abdominal hemorrhage
    2. Neurologic signs with brain and/or spinal cord hemorrhage
    3. Lameness with hemarthrosis
    4. Subcutaneous hematomas and ecchymoses secondary to minor trauma or handling
    5. Hyphema

Diagnosis/Differential Diagnosis

I. Coagulation profile
  A. Prolonged one-stage prothrombin time occurs first, inasmuch as factor VII has the shortest half-life (6.2 hours) of affected factors.
  B. Activated partial thromboplastin time is prolonged (early, it may be normal).
  C. Activated coagulation time is prolonged (early, it may be normal).
  D. Platelet count, fibrinogen, and fibrin split products (FSPs) are usually normal in early stages of intoxication. Later, the platelet count and fibrinogen may be decreased and FSPs may increase.
  E. *Caution:* Use a peripheral vein, not the jugular vein, for venipuncture, as it is easier to control cephalic and saphenous bleeding than jugular bleeding.
II. Plasma or liver anticoagulant levels
III. Response to vitamin K_1
  High vitamin K epoxide levels and high vitamin K epoxide:vitamin K_1 ratios occur in dogs exposed to anticoagulant rodenticides after treatment with vitamin K_1.
IV. Differential diagnosis for vitamin K–responsive co-

agulopathies: chronic cholestasis, malabsorption syndromes, gut sterilization with antibiotics

Treatment

I. Prevent absorption; induce vomiting if early after ingestion.
II. Acute cases are treated as follows.
    A. Handle the animal gently to prevent bruising; avoid IM injections.
    B. Give fresh, whole blood transfusion 10–20 ml/kg IV; give first half rapidly and second half at 20 drops/minute.
    C. Give oxygen if hypoxic or severely anemic.
    D. If dyspneic, consider radiography and thoracentesis for intrathoracic hemorrhage.
    E. Give vitamin K_1 (see later).
III. Subacute cases are treated as follows.
    A. Give vitamin K_1 (phytonadione) 2–5 mg/kg/day PO, followed by a fatty meal (e.g., moist dog food) to promote absorption. Oral administration is more effective than parenteral dosing and avoids the potential hemorrhage of an injection.
    B. If vitamin K_1 must be administered parenterally (3–5 mg/kg), the smallest-bore needle possible should be used. *Caution:* Anaphylactic reactions have been reported following IV vitamin K.
    C. Follow with daily vitamin K_1 2–5 mg/kg PO for 7–14 days, keeping in mind that the longer-acting rodenticides (diphacinone, brodifacoum) may require vitamin K_1 therapy for as long as 30 days.
    D. *Caution:* Vitamin K_3 is much less effective than vitamin K_1.
    E. Repeat coagulation profile when therapy is discontinued.
IV. Hasten elimination of absorbed toxicant.
    A. Sedation or light anesthesia with barbiturates may aid with gentle handling of animals and may also increase hepatic biotransformation of those compounds with longer half-lives.
    B. Elimination of warfarin is usually complete within 48–96 hours; however, diphacinone and brodifacoum may have half-lives of 15–20 days.
V. Oral vitamin K_1 is given to animals that have been exposed to coumarins even if ingestion is questionable.

ZINC PHOSPHIDE

Source

I. Gray-black powder; water-insoluble; used as grain fumigant; incorporated into bread, sugar, and grain baits at 2–5%
II. Often used by pest control operators
III. Has a faint acetylene or rotten fish odor
IV. Toxic dosage for most animals: 20–50 mg/kg
V. Toxicity enhanced by recent ingestion of food, from increased gastric acidity

Action

I. Phosphine gas is released from zinc phosphide in the presence of acidic pH; phosphine gas causes respiratory distress and asphyxia.
II. Intact phosphide may also cause liver and kidney damage and gastrointestinal hemorrhage.

Clinical Signs

I. Onset of signs is usually within 15 minutes to 4 hours.
II. Anorexia and lethargy are followed by dyspnea and tachypnea.
III. Vomitus often contains dark blood, and abdominal pain is common.
IV. Ataxia and running and yelping fits have been observed.
V. Animals are often acidotic and hyperthermic.
VI. Terminal gasping and struggling, as well as hyperesthesia and convulsions, may occur.
VII. Death is caused by hypoxia.

Diagnosis/Differential Diagnosis

I. Phosphine or acetylene odor to breath or vomitus
II. Analysis of stomach contents
III. Differential diagnosis: strychnine, compound 1080

Treatment

I. Prevention of absorption
    A. Gastric lavage with 5% sodium bicarbonate if early after ingestion
    B. Oral 5% sodium bicarbonate to increase gastric pH and decrease the release of phosphine gas
    C. Withholding of food for 24 hours to decrease gastric acid production
II. No specific antidotes
III. Supportive care
IV. Correction of acidosis

CHOLECALCIFEROL

Source

I. Grain-like baits containing 0.075% active ingredient
II. Brand-name products: Quintox, Rampage, Ortho Mouse-B-Gone and Rat-B-Gone
III. Commonly available in 25- to 30-g packets
IV. LD_{50} dose reported to be 88 mg/kg; minimum toxic dose estimated to be 2–3 mg/kg
    A. Smaller animals are more susceptible.
    B. Ingestion of one packet has been fatal in dogs <20 lb.

Action

I. Cholecalciferol is vitamin D_3.
II. It is converted in the liver to 25-hydroxycholecalciferol.

III. It causes hypercalcemia with dystrophic calcification in the kidneys, liver, and gastrointestinal tract.
IV. Although recently introduced as a safer, alternative rodenticide to the coumarins, reports of toxicity in dogs and cats are increasing.

Clinical Signs

I. Usually occur 18–36 hours after ingestion
II. Vomiting
III. Anorexia, lethargy
IV. Polydipsia, polyuria
V. ±Hyperthermia

Diagnosis/Differential Diagnosis

I. Known ingestion
II. Evidence of acute hypercalcemia (calcium >12 mg/dl) in an otherwise healthy animal, especially if young
III. Clinical laboratory findings
  A. Hypercalcemia, hyperphosphatemia
  B. Azotemia, hyposthenuria, proteinuria, glycosuria
  C. Elevated serum or tissue cholecalciferol metabolites (normal serum 25-hydroxyvitamin D_3 is 10–40 ng/ml)
IV. Postmortem findings
  A. Pitted and mottled kidneys
  B. Pale, enlarged thyroid glands
  C. Aortic calcification
  D. Soft tissue mineralization
V. Differential diagnosis: other causes of hypercalcemia (see Chap. 71), ingestion of other grain-like bait rodenticides

Treatment

I. Prevent absorption.
  A. Induce vomiting if soon after ingestion.
  B. Administer activated charcoal 1 g/5 ml water.
  C. Consider sodium sulfate for catharsis.
II. Measure serum calcium levels on entry and at 24, 48, and 96 hours.
III. Therapy for hypercalcemia includes the following.
  A. Diuresis with normal saline 60–80 ml/kg/day IV
  B. Furosemide 2–4 mg/kg SQ, IV TID
  C. Corticosteroids
    1. Prednisone 1–2 mg/kg PO BID-TID
    2. Dexamethasone 1 mg/kg SQ divided QID
  D. Calcitonin (salmon)
    1. Begin with 4–6 IU/kg SQ q 2–3 h.
    2. Moderate therapy when the calcium levels stabilize.
    3. Maintain serum calcium <12 mg/dl.
  E. Enteric phosphate binders
    1. Reduces phosphorus absorption in the intestinal tract
    2. Aluminum hydroxide 10–30 mg/kg PO BID-TID
VI. Prophylactic therapy with IV normal saline may be

instituted when small animals have ingested moderate amounts (½ packet) of the toxin.
V. Low-calcium diets and avoidance of sunlight may be helpful in the first week after exposure to the toxin.

BROMETHALIN

Source

I. It is a new rodenticide developed for use against warfarin-resistant rats and mice.
II. It is available in green or tan pellets containing 0.01% bromethalin.
III. Packs contain 16–42.5 g of bait.
IV. Commercial products include Assault, Vengeance, and Trounce.
V. LD_{50} of technical material is reported to be 4.7 mg/kg for dogs and 0.54 mg/kg for cats.
  A. Estimated minimal toxic dose of a 0.01% bait is 16.7 g/kg in the dog and 3 g/kg in the cat.
  B. Estimated minimal lethal dose of a 0.01% bait is 25 g/kg in the dog and 4.5 g/kg in the cat.

Action

I. It is a neurotoxin that probably uncouples oxidative phosphorylation, resulting in alterations of the Na/K ATPase pump and causing cerebral edema.
II. It is rapidly absorbed from the intestinal tract, has a plasma half-life of 5.6 days, and is metabolized in the liver.

Clinical Signs

I. The central nervous system (CNS) is affected, with signs being dose dependent.
II. Acute signs following high doses include muscle tremors, hyperexcitability, paddling, ataxia, hyperesthesia, pyrexia, and seizures precipitated by sound or light.
III. Lower dosages similar to that seen with bait ingestion cause a delayed syndrome that develops 1–2 days after ingestion, manifested by posterior paresis, ascending ataxia, hyporeflexia, muscle tremors, depression, anisocoria, and vomiting.
IV. Recovery from mild toxicosis occurs within 1–2 weeks.

Diagnosis/Differential Diagnosis

I. History of exposure with characteristic clinical signs
II. Electroencephalographic changes: spike-and-wave activity, marked voltage depression, abnormal high-voltage slow-wave activities
III. Diffuse vacuolization of the white matter of the CNS on histopathology
IV. Chemical confirmation of residues in tissues (not readily available)
V. Differential diagnosis: strychnine, organophosphates, chlorinated hydrocarbons, DEET, rabies

Table 123–1. Miscellaneous Uncommon Rodenticides

Rodenticide	Source	Action	Clinical Signs	Treatment
Alpha-chlorohydrin (3-chloro-1,2-propanediol)	Available only to exterminators; not widely used in the United States	Exerts a strong antifertility effect in males, characterized by reduced spermatozoa	Large doses cause depression, anorexia, renal failure, and possible bone marrow suppression	Infertility in dogs is apparently reversible, although no treatment is described
ANTU (alpha naphthyl-thio-urea)	Rarely used today	Increases capillary permeability of pulmonary vessels; cyanosis leads to death	Vomiting, salivation, gastric pain, lacrimation, urination, severe dyspnea, and air hunger; lesions are massive pulmonary edema and hydrothorax	Treatment is ineffective, although silicone aerosols have been recommended
Alpha-chloralose	Has been used as an anesthetic; rarely used as a rodenticide; old product	Depressed neurons of the ascending reticular formation	Early excitement followed by depression; severe depression to deep anesthesia develops and may progress to apnea and death; glucuronide is excreted in urine	Restraint of excited animals; diazepam to control seizures; analeptics to correct depression or anesthesia
Crimidine (2-chloro-4-dimethylamino-6-methylpyrimidine)	Old rodenticide; used mainly in Europe	Antagonist of vitamin B$_6$	Acute convulsive seizures 0.5–1 h after consumption	Animals may recover quickly; pyridoxine HCl (20 mg/kg IV); diazepam or barbiturates for seizures
Norbormide	Developed as a "safe" rodenticide against rats; never widely used	Peripheral vasoconstriction in rats	Rats are ataxic, restless, dyspneic, and weak	Not applicable
Pyriminil (Vacor)	Used in the 1970s, withdrawn from registration	Nicotinamide antagonist	Hyperglycemia, nausea, vomiting, depression, miosis, lethargy, possible muscle tremors; dogs may develop night blindness and other visual deficits	Nicotinamide (50–100 mg IM) is effective if given early or before signs develop; therapy is continued for 7–10 days
Red squill (*Urginea maritima*)	Rarely used in the United States	Cardioactive glycoside; unpalatable, strong emetic	Vomiting and nausea early; bradycardia and cardiac arrest at toxic dosages	Treat hyperkalemia with insulin, glucose, and sodium bicarbonate; atropine or lidocaine for cardiac effects
Sodium fluoroacetate (compound 1080), fluoroacetamide	Restricted to licensed exterminators	Blocks intermediary metabolism by replacing acetyl coenzyme A	Hyperirritability, defecation, urination, wild running, hysteria, tonoclonic seizures	Emetics, gastric lavage, barbiturates, glycerol monacetate; prognosis guarded
Thallium	Use stopped in 1965, old products	Blocks sulfhydryl enzymes	Acute: gastroenteritis, diarrhea, abdominal pain; Subacute: gastrointestinal signs, dermal erythema and necrosis; Chronic: anorexia, skin necrosis, alopecia	Early decontamination, prussian blue, forced diuresis, supportive care

Treatment

I. Decrease absorption.
  A. Best results occur if it is performed within 2 hours of ingestion.
  B. Feed the animal a small meal, and then administer an emetic.
  C. Follow with repeated doses of activated charcoal and a cathartic every 4–8 hours for at least 2–3 days.
II. Minimize cerebral edema.
  A. Mannitol and dexamethasone are recommended in the early stages.
  B. Therapy does not appear to be effective as the clinical course progresses.
III. Control seizures and tremors with diazepam or phenobarbital.
IV. Provide supportive care, especially supplemental feeding.

MISCELLANEOUS UNCOMMON RODENTICIDES

See Table 123–1.

Bibliography

Beasley VR, Buck WB: Warfarin and other anticoagulant poisonings. p. 101. In Kirk RW (ed): Current Veterinary Therapy VIII. WB Saunders, Philadelphia, 1983

Blakely BR: Epidemiologic and diagnostic considerations of strychnine poisoning in the dog. J Am Vet Med Assoc 184:46, 1984

Carothers M, Chew DJ: Management of cholecalciferol rodenticide toxicity. Compend Contin Educ Pract Vet 13:1058, 1991

Dorman DC: Bromethalin rodenticide toxicosis. p. 175. In Kirk RW, Bonagura J (eds): Current Veterinary Therapy XI: Small Animal Practice. WB Saunders, Philadelphia, 1992

Dorman DC, Beasley VR: Diagnosis of and therapy for cholecalciferol toxicosis. p. 148. In Kirk RW (ed): Current Veternary Therapy X: Small Animal Practice. WB Saunders, Philadelphia, 1989

Dorman DC, Harlin KS, Simon J, Buck WB: Diagnosis of bromethalin poisoning in the dog. J Vet Diagn Invest 2:123, 1990

Dorman DC, Parker AJ, Dye JA, Buck WB: Electroencephalographic changes associated with bromethalin toxicosis in the dog. Vet Hum Toxicol 33:9, 1991

Mount ME, Feldman BF: Mechanism of diphacinone rodenticide toxicosis in the dog and its therapeutic implications. Am J Vet Res 44:2009, 1983

Murphy MS, Gerken DF: The anticoagulant rodenticides. p. 143. In Kirk RW (ed): Current Veterinary Therapy X: Small Animal Practice. WB Saunders, Philadelphia, 1989

Osweiler GD: Strychnine poisoning. p. 98. In Kirk RW (ed): Current Veterinary Therapy VIII. WB Saunders, Philadelphia, 1983

Stowe CM, Metz AL, Arendt TD et al: Apparent brodifacoum poisoning in a dog. J Am Vet Med Assoc 182:817, 1983

124

Insecticides and Molluscacides

Thomas L. Carson
Gary D. Osweiler

METALDEHYDE

Source

I. Metaldehyde is a snail, slug, and rat poison that is used especially in the southern lowlands and Pacific coastal areas of the continental United States and in the Hawaiian Islands.
II. It is a palatable liquid, powder, or pelleted bait used around vegetable and ornamental gardens, usually formulated as <4% baits.
III. Preparations used in Europe may contain 50% metaldehyde.
IV. Older preparations also contained arsenic compounds.
V. Toxic dosage for dogs is 100–1000 mg/kg.

Action

I. Mechanism of action is largely unknown.
II. It was thought to be primarily the result of acetaldehyde released during metaldehyde hydrolysis, but that now appears unlikely.
III. Effects may be caused by metaldehyde itself.
IV. Levels of gamma-aminobutyric acid and 5-hydroxy-tryptamine decrease, and monoamine oxidase activity in the brain increases, causing central nervous system (CNS) dysfunction.
V. Severe metabolic acidosis secondary to acetaldehyde oxidation may also play a role.

Clinical Signs

I. Appear within 1–4 hours
II. Anxiety, hyperesthesia, ataxia
III. Tachycardia, tachypnea, hypersalivation
IV. Muscle fasciculations and tremors, not affected by external stimuli
V. ± Vomiting and diarrhea (not characteristic of early stages)
VI. Nystagmus in cats
VII. Severe hyperthermia—as high as 108°F (42.5°C)
VIII. Severe metabolic acidosis
IX. Loss of consciousness, decreased respiration, cyanosis
X. Death caused by respiratory failure

Diagnosis/Differential Diagnosis

I. Geographic region and compatible clinical signs
II. Bait found in vomitus or lavage material
III. Acetaldehyde odor on breath or from stomach contents
IV. Laboratory analysis of stomach contents
V. Differential diagnosis: strychnine, compound 1080, chlorinated hydrocarbons, organophosphates, bromethalin

Treatment

I. Prevent absorption.
   A. Induce vomiting if the animal is conscious.
   B. Begin gastric lavage with milk, lime water, or sodium bicarbonate solutions, followed by activated charcoal.
II. Maintain relaxation, and prevent hypoxia.
   A. Diazepam 2.5–20 mg IV as needed
   B. Muscle relaxants
      1. Methocarbamol 150 mg/kg IV
      2. Xylazine 1.1 mg/kg IV
   C. Barbiturates used cautiously, because they compete with enzymes that degrade acetaldehyde
   D. Endotracheal tube, oxygen, and artificial respiration for respiratory failure
III. Supportive care to combat dehydration and acidosis

ORGANOPHOSPHATES

Source

I. Veterinary products are common sources: dips, sprays, powders, flea collars, and oral products, as well as numerous agricultural insecticides and home and garden products.
  A. Dichlorvos (Vapona)
  B. Tyrichlorfon (Dipterex, Neguvon)
  C. Dimethoate (Cygon)
  D. Crufomate (Ruelene)
  E. Malathion (Cythion)
  F. Parathion (Bladan)
  G. Ronnel (Korlan)
  H. Diazinon (Spectracide)
  I. Chlorpyrifos (Dursban)
  J. Fonofos (Dyfonate)
  K. Phosmet (Imidan)
  L. Disulfoton (Di-Syston)
  M. Coumaphos (Co-ral)
  N. Famphur (Warbex)
  O. Phorate (Thimet)
  P. Fenthion (Spotton)
II. Toxic dose is variable, depending on the product. Some organophosphates are highly toxic (e.g., 1–3 mg/kg), and exposure may constitute an acute medical emergency.

Action

I. Organophosphates inhibit acetylcholinesterase enzymes at the muscarinic, nicotinic, and neuromuscular synapse. Consequently, symptoms of muscarinic and nicotinic stimulation are observed.
II. Inhibition of cholinesterase enzymes by many organophosphates can become irreversible over time.
III. Some organophosphates are well absorbed after dermal exposure.

Clinical Signs

I. Signs may appear within minutes to several hours after exposure.
II. Not all signs are seen in every instance. In advanced cases, muscarinic signs may be minimal.
  A. Muscarinic effects
    1. Salivation
    2. Lacrimation
    3. Defecation; watery diarrhea
    4. Gastrointestinal hypermotility; abdominal pain
    5. Miosis, occasionally mydriasis
    6. Pallor
    7. Cyanosis
    8. Dyspnea
    9. Emesis
  B. Nicotinic effects: twitching of facial and tongue muscles progressing to all musculature, followed by paralysis
  C. CNS effects
    1. Extreme depression
    2. Tonoclonic seizures (rare)
III. Cats with chlorpyrifos intoxication often have a delayed onset of signs (1–5 days after dermal exposure).
  A. Predominantly neurologic signs
  B. Tremors, ataxia, depression, seizures that persist for 2–4 weeks
IV. Death is caused by hypoxia: respiratory muscle paralysis, bronchoconstriction, excessive pulmonary secretions, pulmonary edema, and bradycardia.

Diagnosis/Differential Diagnosis

I. History of exposure and characteristic clinical signs
II. Analysis of stomach contents or hair
III. Evaluation of acetylcholinesterase activity in whole blood. Severe clinical signs associated with inhibition of 75–80%
IV. Response to atropine
V. Differential diagnosis: strychnine, chlorinated hydrocarbons, metaldehyde, bromethalin

Treatment

I. Prevent further exposure and absorption.
  A. Remove flea collar.
  B. Bathe skin with soapy water if exposure is topical.
  C. Induce emesis if ingestion is witnessed.
  D. Lavage stomach with activated charcoal slurry.
  E. Protect the people involved with therapy from exposure by having them wear gloves and aprons.
II. Give specific antidotes.
  A. Atropine sulfate does not affect the extent of cholinesterase inhibition but, rather, blocks muscarinic receptors.
    1. Dosage is 0.2 mg/kg to effect (mydriasis and reduced salivation).
    2. Usually one fourth of the dose is given IV and three fourths SQ or IM; may need to be repeated at 3–6 hours for 1–2 days, depending on the response.
  B. The oxime agent pralidoxime HCl (2-PAM) acts on the organophosphate–enzyme complex, binding the phosphate and thereby releasing the cholinesterase.
    1. Early treatment before the complex has stabilized or "aged" (within 12 hours of exposure) is required for 2-PAM to be effective.
    2. Treatment with 2-PAM beyond 12 hours of exposure is usually not indicated.
    3. Repeated use of 2-PAM may help correct nicotinic signs.
    4. Dosage is 20 mg/kg IV BID.
  C. Diphenhydramine (Benadryl) may be useful in animals showing predominantly nicotinic signs.
    1. This drug acts to decrease the nicotinic receptor overload.
    2. Dosage is 1–4 mg/kg PO TID.
III. Give supportive care.
  A. Ventilation and oxygen for respiratory failure

B. Contraindicated drugs: morphine, succinylcholine, phenothiazine tranquilizers

CARBAMATES

Source

I. Numerous insecticide products are potential sources.
   A. Carbaryl (Sevin)
   B. Methomyl (Lannate)
   C. Propoxur (Baygon)
   D. Bendiocarb (Ficam)
   E. Aldicarb (Temik)
   F. Carbofuran (Furadan)
II. Toxic dose is variable, depending on the product.

Action

I. There is inhibition of acetylcholinesterase enzymes at the muscarinic, nicotinic, and neuromuscular synapses similar to the organophosphates.
II. Inhibition of acetylcholinesterase by carbamates is reversible, and no acetylcholinesterase aging occurs.
III. With the exception of aldicarb, the carbamates have lower dermal toxicity than the organophosphates.

Clinical Signs and Diagnosis

I. Similar signs to those seen with organophosphate intoxication, but of shorter duration
II. Similar diagnostic results to organophosphate intoxication, except that serum cholinesterase activity must be measured early after exposure

Treatment

I. Similar to organophosphate intoxication, except that 2-PAM is not considered effective for carbamate toxicoses because hydrolysis of the acetylcholinesterase–carbamate bond occurs fairly rapidly (i.e., within 2–24 hours).
II. As with organophosphate intoxication, protect the people involved in therapy from exposure.

CHLORINATED HYDROCARBONS

Source

I. Most of the products listed are no longer approved for use or have very limited approval. Few commercial preparations are still available.
   A. Veterinary products: powders, sprays, dips
      1. Methoxychlor
      2. Toxaphene
      3. Lindane
      4. Chlordane
   B. Agricultural products: insecticides
      1. DDT
      2. TDE

   3. Dieldrin
   4. Aldrin
   5. Endrin
   6. Chlordecone (Kepone)
   7. Endosulfan (Thiodan)
II. Toxic dose is variable, depending on the product; cats are particularly susceptible.
III. Dermal absorption is low for DDT and methoxychlor but is high for lindane, aldrin, dieldrin, and endrin.

Action

I. Lipid-soluble products are absorbed through skin or ingested.
II. These agents behave as diffuse CNS stimulants or depressants; exact mechanism is unknown (except DDT).
III. DDT decreases the nerve membrane action potential threshold.

Clinical Signs

I. Onset can be observed within minutes to days of exposure, although it is usually noted within several hours.
II. Apprehension, hypersensitivity, hypersalivation, exaggerated response to stimuli, and vomiting are present (if insecticide was ingested).
III. Muscle twitching of face and neck progresses posteriorly to severe fasciculations and tremors.
IV. Intermittent clonic-tonic seizures are seen, with paddling and foaming around the mouth.
V. Hyperthermia is common.
VI. These compounds distribute to fat, and the clinical course may be protracted. Many of the compounds have long half-lives.

Diagnosis/Differential Diagnosis

I. History of exposure and characteristic clinical signs
II. Analysis of brain, liver, or perhaps stomach contents, (samples submitted in glass containers only)
III. Poor correlation of tissue concentrations with clinical signs
IV. Differential diagnosis: strychnine, compound 1080, metaldehyde, 4-aminopyridine, caffeine, garbage intoxication, lead, organophosphates, degenerative cerebellar disease

Treatment

I. Prevent further exposure and absorption.
   A. Wash with copious amounts of warm, soapy water in cases of dermal exposure.
   B. Induction of emesis may initiate seizures.
   C. Perform gastric lavage with saline and activated charcoal, after seizures are controlled.
   D. Protect people involved with therapy from exposure by having them wear rubber gloves and plastic aprons.
II. Control seizures.
   A. Specific antidotes do not exist.

B. Give diazepam 2.5–20 mg IV as needed.

C. Give pentobarbital IV to effect.

III. Give sedatives for excitability if seizures are not present.

A. Give diazepam 2.5–20 mg IV as needed.

B. Do not use phenothiazines, as they lower the seizure threshold.

IV. Maintain hydration and urine output, as the chlorinated hydrocarbons are eliminated primarily in the urine.

V. Chlorinated hydrocarbons persist in the environment, so sources should be disposed of by the proper authorities.

AMITRAZ

Source

I. Amitraz is a formamidine insecticide with broad acaricidal activity that is used topically for controlling ticks, keds, lice, and mites on animals.

II. Amitraz is available as a 19.9% liquid concentrate (Mitaban, Upjohn) for topical use on dogs for the treatment of generalized demodicosis, and as a 12.5% liquid concentrate (Taktic, Hoechst-Roussel) for controlling mites, lice, and ticks on livestock.

III. Amitraz-impregnated collars for dog tick control have also been ingested.

IV. Amitraz products should not be used on cats.

Action

The mechanism of amitraz is not well established, but it appears to act like a local anesthetic at the membrane level.

Clinical Signs

I. Clinical signs are dose related.

II. With therapeutic doses, transient sedation of 2–6 hours duration and mild gastrointestinal signs of anorexia, vomiting, and diarrhea may be seen.

III. With higher doses, CNS depression, mydriasis, ataxia, hypothermia, bradycardia, hypotension, muscular weakness, emesis, uncontrolled vocal spasm, and micturition have been noted.

Diagnosis

Diagnosis is based on a history of exposure to amitraz-containing products and recognition of compatible clinical findings.

Treatment

I. With adverse signs following therapeutic doses, no treatment is needed.

II. In overdose situations, decontamination by bathing is used for topical exposure, and induction of emesis, gastric lavage, or activated charcoal is instituted for ingestion.

III. In dogs, yohimbine 0.1–0.2 mg/kg IV (start with the lower level) can be used to reverse the bradycardia and depression and prevent hypotension. Treatment may have to be repeated, as the half-life of yohimbine is only 1.5–2 hours.

IV. Supportive care with IV fluids, antiemetics, and body warming may also be indicated.

PYRETHRINS AND PIPERONYL BUTOXIDE

Source

I. Naturally occurring (pyrethrum flower extract) and synthetic (allethrin) insecticides that are used for their ''knock-down'' properties are sources.

II. Piperonyl butoxide is a cytochrome P-450 inhibitor that is often used in combination with other insecticides (e.g., organophosphates, carbamates, and pyrethrins).

III. Many veterinary insecticide products contain these substances.

IV. Household insecticide products are sources as single or combination products.

V. Toxicity of pyrethrins is thought to be low; however, they are often used in combination with other insecticides that may be more toxic or prolong the half-life of the pyrethrins.

A. Oral toxicity is usually quite low.

B. Products with LD_{50} values <100 mg/kg include resmethrin, fenpropanthrin, decamethrin, and flucythrinate.

C. Respiratory exposure is considered hazardous.

Action

I. Pyrethrins cause slight depolarization of the nerve membrane, increase the negative afterpotential, induce repetitive afterdischarges, and eventually block the action potential by affecting sodium and potassium channels.

II. Piperonyl butoxide inhibits pyrethrin metabolism.

Clinical Signs

I. Usually observed only with very high dosages

II. Contact dermatitis

III. Vomiting, diarrhea, hypersalivation

IV. Ataxia, CNS excitation, seizures

V. Hypothermia, hyperthermia, dyspnea

VI. Paralysis and death caused by respiratory failure

Diagnosis/Differential Diagnosis

I. Known exposure

II. Characteristic clinical signs

III. Difficult or impossible to confirm by clinical analysis

IV. Differential diagnosis: metaldehyde, lead poisoning, organophosphates, carbamates, chlorinated hydrocarbons, nicotine

Treatment

    I. Prevent further absorption and exposure.
    II. Control CNS excitability and/or seizures as outlined for chlorinated hydrocarbons.
       A. Methocarbamol 150 mg/kg IV
       B. Phenothiazines contraindicated
    III. Maintain hydration and urine output, as pyrethrins are excreted in urine.
    IV. Use vitamin E ointment for dermatitis.

NAPHTHALENE

Source

    I. Naphthalene is a coal tar derivative and is found in various compounds.
       A. Mothballs, moth repellents
       B. Some insect repellents
    II. Hemolytic anemia occurs with exposures >411 mg/kg in dogs.

Action

    I. Gastrointestinal irritation is common.
    II. Oxidative stress and hemolytic anemia may result.
    III. Renal damage can occur secondary to hemoglobinuria.
    IV. Retinal damage and cataract formation have been observed in rabbits.

Clinical Signs

    I. Vomiting and diarrhea
    II. Hemolytic anemia, hemoglobinuria
    III. ± Liver and kidney damage
    IV. Seizures and/or severe CNS depression (rare)

Diagnosis/Differential Diagnosis

    I. Known exposure or finding mothballs in vomitus or gastric lavage material
    II. Hemolytic anemia with Heinz bodies; methemoglobinemia in cats
    III. Differential diagnosis: organophosphates, carbamates, chlorinated hydrocarbons, and other causes of hemolytic anemia (e.g., onions and acetaminophen)

Treatment

    I. Prevent further exposure and absorption by inducing emesis and administering activated charcoal, followed by a saline cathartic.
    II. Blood transfusions may be indicated for severe hemolytic anemia.
    III. Steroids may reduce the amount of hemolysis.
    IV. Give ascorbic acid 30 mg/kg PO QID for seven treatments for methemoglobinemia.
    V. Alkalinize urine with sodium bicarbonate 50 mg/kg PO BID–TID to facilitate excretion.

BORATE

Source

    I. Borate and its sodium salts (borates) are often used for roach control.
    II. Borates may also be incorporated in antiseptic agents (e.g., toilet bowl cleaners and sanitizers, diaper rinses, and ointments).
    III. Rat LD_{50} is approximately 5 g/kg PO.

Action

    I. Exact mechanism of toxicity is unknown.
    II. Borates are absorbed through denuded or inflamed skin and the gastrointestinal tract.
    III. Local irritation results.
    IV. Renal damage often occurs owing to the high concentration of borate in the kidneys during excretion.

Clinical Signs

    I. Local dermatitis
    II. Vomiting and diarrhea, often with blood and mucus
    III. Muscle weakness and tremors
    IV. Seizures
    V. Evidence of renal damage: oliguria, azotemia, proteinuria, hematuria, casts in urine sediment
    VI. Metabolic acidosis

Diagnosis/Differential Diagnosis

    I. Known exposure
    II. Characteristic clinical signs
    III. Evidence of renal damage in urinalysis: proteinuria, casts, red blood cells
    IV. Boric acid analysis in urine
    V. Differential diagnosis: arsenic, metaldehyde, lead poisoning, garbage intoxication, nonspecific gastroenteritis

Treatment

    I. Flush with large amounts of warm, soapy water in cases of dermal exposure.
    II. Perform gastric lavage with activated charcoal followed by a cathartic.
    III. No specific antidotes exist; give supportive care.
       A. Maintain hydration.
       B. Correct acidosis.
       C. Induce diuresis.
       D. Consider peritoneal dialysis.

ROTENONE

Source

    I. Extract from the *Derris* and *Lonchocarpus* plants
    II. Used as a topical insecticide for lice and mites: not absorbed through intact skin

III. Not common in veterinary products, but active ingredient in Sebumsol
IV. Oral LD$_{50}$ dose: 10–30 mg/kg
  A. Cats more susceptible than dogs
  B. Most toxic to birds and fish

Action

Inhibits mitochondrial electron transport

Clinical Signs

  I. Local effects are dermatitis, conjunctivitis, pharyngitis, and rhinitis.
 II. If swallowed, rotenone preparations produce gastrointestinal irritation, nausea, and vomiting.
III. Liver damage has been reported in cats that have licked rotenone preparations off their fur.
IV. Inhalation is extremely hazardous and may be followed by depression and seizures.

Diagnosis

  I. Known exposure
 II. Hypoglycemia (reported to occur frequently)

Treatment

  I. Decrease absorption with emesis or gastric lavage and cathartics.
 II. Bathe with a detergent.

DEET

Source

  I. DEET (*N,N*-diethyltoluamide) is a common ingredient in over-the-counter insect repellents.
  A. Human products: Off, Deep Woods Off, Cutter's Jungle Formula, Muskol
  B. Veterinary products: DMT-50 (50% DEET)
  C. May be combined (9% DEET) with fenvalerate (0.09%)
 II. Approximately 50% of applied dose is rapidly absorbed through the skin within 6 hours.
III. It is metabolized by the liver and excreted in the urine.
IV. Recent studies have established toxic dosages in dogs and cats.
  A. Approximately 1.8 g/kg is lethal dermally for cats. This represents 10% of a 7-oz can applied per kilogram body weight.
  B. Small dogs may be mildly intoxicated by 40% of a 7-oz can applied per kilogram body weight.
  C. Accidental spraying into the mouth or self-grooming by cats may increase the probability of toxicosis 50-fold.

Action

  I. The agent is a neurotoxin, but the exact mechanism of action is not defined.

 II. It is lipophilic and crosses the blood-brain barrier.
III. DEET may enhance the dermal absorption of other drugs.

Clinical Signs

  I. Signs are similar in the dog and cat, but cats are more likely to die from acute toxicosis.
 II. Severe, acute clinical signs occur within 5–10 minutes after oral exposure.
  A. Restlessness, aimless gazing, defecation, chewing and tongue thrusting motions, hypersalivation, trembling, hypermetria, intention tremors
  B. Recumbency by 30 minutes after exposure
  C. ± Seizures
  D. Also paddling, opisthotonos, vocalization, depression, and dyspnea in cats
III. Restlessness, hypersalivation, and tremors are signs of mild poisoning.
IV. Intoxicated animals are generally aware of their surroundings; the syndrome appears to affect primarily the cerebellum.
 V. Mild cases may be normal within 4 hours. More severe cases may recover within 48–72 hours.

Diagnosis/Differential Diagnosis

  I. History of excessive use of agent, especially if a combination product
 II. Clinical signs compatible with cerebellar dysfunction
III. Chemical analysis for DEET and/or fenvalerate
  A. DEET appears in the serum (>20 ppm) and urine (>1 ppm) of intoxicated dogs and cats.
  B. Collect blood, urine, brain, liver, skin, and stomach contents if death occurs.
IV. Differential diagnosis: organophosphate insecticides, metaldehyde, nicotine, inflammatory cerebellar disease, neoplasia, trauma

Treatment

  I. Remove and inactivate the pesticide from skin or gastrointestinal tract.
  A. Emesis, gastric lavage, activated charcoal, cathartics
  B. Bathing of skin with soap and water
 II. Control seizures and administer supportive care for respiratory distress.

Bibliography

Booze TF, Oehme FW: Metaldehyde toxicity: a review. Vet Hum Toxicol 27:11, 1985
Dorman DC, Beasley VR: Neurotoxicity of pyrethrin and the pyrethroid insecticides. Vet Hum Toxicol 33:238, 1991
Dorman DC, Buck WB, Trammel HL et al: Fenvalerate/*N,N*-diethyl-*m*-toluamide (DEET) toxicosis in two cats. J Am Vet Med Assoc 196:100, 1990
Fikes JD: Organophosphorus and combamode insecticides. In Beasley VR (ed): Toxicology of selected pesticides, drugs, and

chemicals. Vet Clin North Am [Small Anim Pract] 20:353, 1990

Fikes JD: Feline chloropyrifos toxicosis. p. 188. In Kirk RW, Bonagura JD (eds): Current Veterinary Therapy XI: Small Animal Practice. WB Saunders, Philadelphia, 1992

Maddy KT, Peoples SA: Poisoning of dogs in California with pesticides. Calif Vet May:9, 1977

Mount ME, Moller G, Cook J et al: Clinical illness associated with a commercial tick and flea product in dogs and cats. Vet Hum Toxicol 33:19, 1991

Mull RL: Metaldehyde poisoning. p. 106. In Kirk RW (ed): Current Veterinary Therapy VIII. WB Saunders, Philadelphia, 1983

Van Gelder GA: Chlorinated hydrocarbon insecticide toxicosis. p. 141. In Kirk RW (ed): Current Veterinary Therapy VI. WB Saunders, Philadelphia, 1977

125

Herbicides

Gary D. Osweiler
Thomas L. Carson

GENERAL CONSIDERATIONS

I. Inorganic forms include arsenicals and chlorates, which are generally banned from use or used very little.
II. The commonly used modern herbicides are organic synthetic herbicides.
III. Properly applied herbicides generally do not persist in soil beyond the normal growing season.
   A. Most applications result in concentrations in lawn grasses of 5–300 parts per million (ppm).
   B. For most dogs and cats, a body weight dosage of 1 mg/kg is equivalent to a dietary concentration (e.g., if grass is consumed) of 40 ppm.
   C. Greatest exposure and risk are immediately after application, before the herbicide is dried.
IV. Commercial granular herbicides may be applied in combinations that include fertilizers (urea, nitrates) and insecticides (see Chap. 124).
V. Urban use is increasing in recent years with increasing emphasis on high-maintenance lawn care.

CHLORINATED PHENOXY DERIVATIVES

Source

I. Chlorinated phenoxy esters of fatty acids are used in commercial products such as 2,4-D, MCPP, MCPA, and Silvex.
II. Occasional anecdotal reports of toxicosis exist in dogs with access to freshly sprayed lawns.
III. These esters are absorbed readily from the stomach and intestinal tract, but dermal absorption is slower and less complete.
IV. They are rapidly distributed to liver, kidney, and brain.
V. They are metabolized to less toxic products.
   A. Half-life of 2,4-D is approximately 18 hours.
   B. As organic acids, their excretion is markedly enhanced by ion trapping using alkaline diuresis.
   C. Dogs have relatively slow excretion of phenoxy herbicides.

Action

I. Biochemical pathways affected include ribonuclease synthesis and uncoupling of oxidative phosphorylation.
II. Alteration of the clinical electromyogram occurs in dogs.
III. Major organ systems affected include gastrointestinal tract, kidneys, and skeletal muscle.
IV. Toxicosis is not expected under recommended conditions of use.
   A. Oral LD_{50} of 2,4-D in dogs is approximately 100 mg/kg, and the multiple lethal dosage in dogs is 6 days at 25 mg/kg.
   B. Dogs may tolerate 500 ppm of 2,4-D in their diet for 2 years with no adverse effects.
   C. Table 125–1 lists the toxicity of other common chlorophenoxy herbicides.

Clinical Signs

I. Vomiting, diarrhea, bloody feces at high acute dosage
II. Myotonia, ataxia, and posterior weakness
III. Periodic clonic spasms or seizures (only at high dosages)
IV. Altered electromyogram with increased insertional activity

Diagnosis

I. History of known exposure
II. Slightly increased serum alkaline phosphatase, lactate dehydrogenase, and creatine phosphokinase consistent with liver, kidney, and muscle damage
III. Chemical analysis of grass, sprays, urine, or kidney to confirm exposure
IV. Pathologic lesions of swollen liver, renal congestion, enlarged kidneys, and tubular degeneration

Table 125–1. Toxicity of Selected Common Lawn Herbicides in Dogs

Common Name	Usual Concentration on Treated Lawn[a]	Estimated Toxic Exposure Rate (Dosage in Dietary ppm)	Effects
Atrazine	150 ppm	>150 ppm	No effect at 150 ppm
Bensulide	1000 ppm	8000 ppm is lethal	Dose-related decrease in cholinesterase; signs typical of cholinesterase inhibition
2,4-D and other chlorophenoxys	150 ppm	4000 ppm lethal	See text for details
Dicamba	5–7 ppm	250 ppm	Mild jaundice, no other health effects; poisoning not likely
Glyphosate	150 ppm	>2000 ppm (nontoxic)	Wide safety margin; toxic dose not reported in dogs; see text
MCPP	300 ppm	640 ppm chronic toxicity 2560 ppm acute toxicity	Reduced weight gain; anemia
Paraquat	75–150 ppm	300 ppm	Long-term exposure leads to chronic pulmonary fibrosis; narrow margin of safety for chronic effects
Pendimethalin	80–120 ppm	>500 ppm	Dose-related increase in serum alkaline phosphatase; no permanent effects
Triclopyr	5–30 ppm	1200 ppm	Wide safety margin; anorexia, reduced weight gain, enlarged liver and kidneys, nephrosis

[a]Estimated at 150 ppm for each pound applied per acre. Data supplied by TrueGreen-Chemlawn.

Treatment

I. Administer activated charcoal for recent (<2 days) oral exposure.
II. For dermal exposure, wash skin and hair with soap and water.
III. Institute IV fluids to promote diuresis, and administer sodium bicarbonate 50 mg/kg PO BID–TID to promote urinary excretion.
IV. Feed a bland, high-quality diet in convalescing animals.
V. Monitor renal function in all animals.
VI. Prognosis for recovery is good if exposure is moderate and decontamination is used early.

TRIAZINES

Source

I. Synthetic herbicides used with many crops, especially corn
   A. Atrazine
   B. Prometone
II. Also used as algacides in ponds (Simazine)

Action

I. Exact mechanism of toxicity is unknown.
II. LD_{50} values are in the range of 200–1000 mg/kg for most triazines.

Clinical Signs

I. Anorexia, depression, weakness
II. Salivation, dyspnea, muscular spasms, ataxia
III. Recumbency and death

Diagnosis

I. There may be a history of a known exposure.
II. Most symptoms are not specific, making diagnosis difficult.

Treatment

I. Decrease exposure and absorption.
II. Give supportive care and establish diuresis.

DIPYRIDYL COMPOUNDS

Source

I. These are synthetic, contact herbicides.
   A. Paraquat
   B. Diquat
II. LD_{50} values for these compounds in dogs are 25–50 mg/kg.
III. Dietary concentrations of >150 ppm for 2 months may cause anorexia, dyspnea, lung fibrosis, and death.
IV. Spray-can products are available for home use in the spot treatment of weeds.
V. In some agricultural areas, paraquat has been used as a malicious poison against dogs.

Action

I. Paraquat is poorly absorbed orally but is absorbed dermally; diquat is absorbed poorly both orally and dermally.
II. Herbicidal action and mechanism of toxicity in mammals are thought to be mediated by the production

of free radicals during cyclic oxidation-reduction of the dipyridyl compounds.

III. Paraquat oxidation-reduction produces superoxide radicals that cause lipid membrane damage.

IV. Both compounds have short half-lives, with most of the absorbed substance being excreted unchanged via the kidneys.

V. Paraquat is concentrated in the lungs by transport into alveolar cells by an energy-dependent process; therefore, alveolar cells may have significant concentrations after most of the dose has been cleared by the kidneys.

Clinical Signs

I. Paraquat
  A. Mucosal irritation, vomiting, hyperexcitability, and ataxia are common.
  B. Seizures are possible.
  C. Proximal tubular necrosis and renal failure occur more readily in the dog than in other species.
  D. After a delay of 3 days or more, significant pulmonary complications begin.
    1. Pulmonary edema and congestion with tachypnea and dyspnea are seen.
    2. Thoracic radiographs reveal pulmonary infiltrates.
    3. Necrosis of alveolar cells occurs, causing decreased production of surfactant and eventual scarring and fibrosis.
    4. Respiratory signs may be delayed 2–7 days.
  E. Death is caused by respiratory failure.
II. Diquat
  A. Hyperexcitability and seizures are common.
  B. Gastroenteritis is usually present. Large volumes of fluid and electrolytes are lost, and dehydration may be severe.
  C. Renal failure ensues, similar to that seen with paraquat toxicity.
  D. Death is caused by acute fluid loss and electrolyte imbalance.

Diagnosis/Differential Diagnosis

I. History of exposure and characteristic clinical signs
II. Differential diagnosis: organophosphates, carbamates, chlorinated hydrocarbons, ANTU (pulmonary effects are not delayed as with paraquat), allergic reactions, ethylene glycol, garbage intoxication, viral gastroenteritis
III. Analysis of urine or suspect baits if done within 2–3 days after exposure stops

Treatment

I. Prevent further exposure and absorption.
  A. Bentonite and/or Fuller's earth (activated clays) are more effective than charcoal against paraquat.
  B. Ground, clay-based cat litter has been suggested as an emergency alternative to Fuller's earth, but its effectiveness is not documented.

C. Protect people involved with therapy from exposure.
II. Control hyperexcitability or seizures.
  A. Diazepam 2.5–20 mg IV as needed
  B. Barbiturates IV to effect
III. Superoxide dismutase (Pallosein) and acetylcysteine (Mucomyst) are theoretically beneficial, but data on effectiveness are lacking.
IV. Give supportive care.
  A. Maintain fluid and electrolyte balance.
  B. Diuresis should aid in excretion and may lessen kidney damage.
  C. Use of oxygen is contraindicated.
V. Prognosis for clinically affected dogs is grave.

GLYPHOSATE

Source

I. Roundup: agricultural herbicide
II. Kleenup: spray for home use, commonly available in dilute formulations

Action

I. Irritant
II. Low order of toxicity when applied properly

Clinical Signs

I. Dermal irritation with contact
II. Gastroenteritis, with possible vomiting and diarrhea
III. Possible central nervous system (CNS) depression, coma

Diagnosis

I. Known exposure
II. No characteristic clinical signs

Treatment

I. Gastrointestinal cleansing
  A. Emesis
  B. Gastric lavage with activated charcoal
  C. Sodium sulfate cathartic
II. Supportive and symptomatic therapy

ALGACIDES

Source

I. Products for home aquariums often containing triazines or diquat
II. Monuron (Telvar)
III. Dichlone (Phygon), a fungicide-algacide
IV. Toxicity: LD_{50} for monuron and dichlone in rats approximately 1.5 g/kg

Action

I. See Triazines and Dipyridyl Compounds, earlier.
II. Dichlone is a CNS depressant and reacts with thiol enzymes.

Clinical Signs

I. Dermatitis with skin contact
II. Depression, lethargy, gastroenteritis
III. Ataxia and hyporeflexia
IV. With large doses, death caused by cardiac or respiratory arrest
V. Liver and kidney damage: common in animals that ingest nonlethal doses

Diagnosis

History of exposure and clinical signs

Treatment

I. Prevent absorption with emesis or gastric lavage and catharsis.
II. Give supportive care.

Bibliography

Gee BR, Farrow CS, White RJ et al: Paraquat toxicity resulting in respiratory distress syndrome in a dog. J Am Anim Hosp Assoc 14:256, 1978

Longstaffe JA, Humphreys DJ, Hayward AHS et al: Paraquat poisoning in dogs and cats—differences between accidental and malicious poisoning. J Small Anim Pract 22:153, 1981

Yeary RA: Oral intubation of dogs with combinations of fertilizer, herbicide, and insecticide chemicals commonly used on lawns. Am J Vet Res 45:288, 1984

Yeary RA: Herbicides. p. 153. In Kirk RW (ed): Current Veterinary Therapy IX. WB Saunders, Philadelphia, 1986

126

Bacterial and Mold Toxins

Gary D. Osweiler
Thomas L. Carson

ENTEROTOXEMIAS AND ENDOTOXEMIAS ASSOCIATED WITH GARBAGE- AND FOOD-BORNE INTOXICATION

Source

I. Ingestion of food or garbage that contains preformed toxins (e.g., *Staphylococcus, Streptococcus, Bacillus*)
II. Sporulation of enteric *Clostridium perfringens* with production of enterotoxin
III. Ingestion of food that is grossly contaminated with bacteria (e.g., *Escherichia coli, Salmonella*)
IV. More common in warmer climates and during summer months with ingestion of food contaminated with bacteria or preformed toxins
V. Animal products (e.g., milk, infected by-products) or spoiled foods of animal origin: high-risk sources of *Staphylococcus aureus* enterotoxin

Action

I. Most enterotoxins activate intestinal epithelial secretory mechanisms, causing loss of fluid and electrolytes. Absorptive mechanisms may be intact.
II. Some enterotoxins cause morphologic changes in the mucosa. Epithelium may be eroded, resulting in hemorrhage.
III. Some enterotoxins disrupt the gut's absorptive capabilities.
IV. Endotoxins affect the thermoregulatory center and the reticuloendothelial system and can cause margination of white blood cells, thrombocytopenia, blood clotting abnormalities, and circulatory disturbances.

Clinical Signs

I. Signs usually appear within 15 minutes to 6 hours of ingestion.
II. Vomiting and cranial abdominal pain may be present.
III. Diarrhea may be hemorrhagic.
IV. Abdomen may be distended with gas.
V. Restlessness, weakness, and ataxia may be seen.
VI. Shock can result from hypovolemia or toxemia and may be accompanied by hypoglycemia and leukopenia.
VII. Chronic diarrhea may be observed in dogs with clostridial enteritis.

Diagnosis/Differential Diagnosis

I. History of ingestion of garbage or carrion
II. Abdominal radiographs revealing stasis and dilatation of the gut, or bones or garbage material in the gastrointestinal tract
III. Bacterial culture or serologic identification of staphylococcal toxins or clostridial enterotoxins
IV. Endotoxin assays (e.g., limulus assay) or other methods to detect endotoxin not routinely available
V. Differential diagnosis: viral gastroenteritis; lead, arsenic, salmon poisoning; hemorrhagic gastroenteritis

Treatment

I. Cleansing of the gastrointestinal tract
   A. Emetics
   B. Gastric lavage
   C. Enemas
   D. Enteral antibiotics
      1. See Chaps. 32 and 33.
      2. Avoid aminoglycosides if endotoxemia is suspected, to reduce possible interaction in depressing the myocardium.
II. Supportive therapy
   A. Treatment of shock (see Chap. 131)
   B. Gastrointestinal protectants such as Kaopectate 1–2 ml/kg PO QID

BOTULISM

Source

I. *Clostridium botulinum* is a saprophytic, anaerobic, gram-positive, spore-forming rod bacterium that is ubiquitous in the environment.
II. It is a normal enteric inhabitant in many species and is frequently found in feces.
III. Food, garbage, or carrion that contains preformed *C. botulinum* neurotoxin is ingested. The toxin can also be elaborated in the gastrointestinal tract after ingestion of the organism, but it is thought to be a minor source.
IV. Type C and D botulinum toxins are most common in dogs.

Action

I. *C. botulinum* neurotoxin causes a generalized neuromuscular blockade from inhibition of the presynaptic release of acetylcholine.
II. The syndrome is rare in dogs and cats, owing to relatively high resistance to the toxins.

Clinical Signs

I. Onset is usually within 6 days of ingestion.
II. Progressive, symmetrical, generalized, lower motor neuron dysfunction (flaccid paralysis) of spinal and cranial nerves is present (see Chap. 25).
III. There is no loss of mental alertness.
IV. Pain perception is intact and normal.

Diagnosis/Differential Diagnosis

I. History of exposure to carrion
II. Suggestive clinical signs
III. Electromyography: decreased amplitude of muscle action potentials
IV. Identification of toxin from serum or carrion: neutralization with type-specific antitoxin
V. Differential diagnosis: tick paralysis, polyradiculoneuritis, myasthenic disease, aminoglycoside neuromuscular blockade, hypocalcemia

Treatment

I. Empty the stomach via lavage or induction of emesis.
II. Give supportive nursing care, especially providing assisted ventilation; if respiratory failure occurs, prognosis is grave.
III. Antitoxin is of no proven value, although it is most likely effective if given early in the course of the disease.
IV. Enteric antibiotics are of questionable value.
V. Guanidine hydrochloride has been shown to increase the release of acetylcholine in some people with botulism.
VI. Prevent toxicity by avoiding access to spoiled foods or by boiling questionable foods for 5 minutes.

TETANUS

Source

I. *Clostridium tetani* is a gram-positive spore-forming anaerobic bacterium.
II. These bacteria are found in soil and feces of various animals.
III. Germination occurs in necrotic or infected wounds.
IV. Dogs and cats are relatively resistant to the disease.

Action

I. The bacterium produces a neurotoxin that reaches the central nervous system (CNS) via peripheral nerves and the circulation.
II. The toxin inhibits the activity of inhibitory interneurons (Renshaw cells) in the CNS that function to limit the duration, intensity, and distribution of motor neuron discharges.
III. Persistent increased motor reflex excitability results.

Clinical Signs

I. Incubation period of usually 5–8 days
II. Localized spasms of facial and cervical musculature
   A. Elevation of upper eyelids
   B. Wrinkling of forehead skin
   C. Retraction of lipfolds (risus sardonicus)
   D. Erect ear carriage
   E. Prolapse of third eyelids
   F. Masticatory and pharyngeal muscle spasms, resulting in trismus (lockjaw)
III. Exaggerated response to external stimuli
IV. Generalized muscle spasticity
   A. Exaggerated clonus in response to tendon motor reflexes
   B. Rigid extension of limbs and tail (sawhorse stance)
V. Death caused by respiratory paralysis

Diagnosis/Differential Diagnosis

I. History of laceration or puncture wound, prior surgery, recent parturition, or teething
II. Characteristic clinical signs: continuous spasticity, in contrast to the alternating periods of spasticity seen with strychnine
III. Anaerobic and aerobic bacterial cultures
IV. Differential diagnosis: strychnine, canine distemper, rabies, meningitis, chlorinated hydrocarbons, metaldehyde, hypocalcemia

Treatment

I. Maintain relaxation and respiration similar to therapy for strychnine poisoning.
   A. Pentobarbital IV to effect
   B. Endotracheal tube, oxygen, and mechanical respiration for respiratory muscle paralysis
   C. Inhalation anesthesia

D. Diazepam 2.5–20 mg IV as needed
E. Glyceryl guaiacolate 110 mg/kg IV as needed
F. Methocarbamol 150 mg/kg IV (the average initial dose)

II. *Caution:* Morphine is contraindicated because of its spinal cord stimulant and respiratory depressant properties.

III. Specific therapy involves the following (see also Chap. 111).
A. Systemic penicillin G is the treatment of choice.
1. Dose: 20,000 U/kg IV initially
2. Followed by aqueous penicillin at 20,000 U/kg IV QID or procaine penicillin G 22,000 U/kg IM BID
B. Tetanus antitoxin neutralizes free or unbound toxin before it reaches the CNS.
1. It is ineffective against toxin already in nerve cells.
2. Dose is 30,000–100,000 U IV after a test dose of 0.1–0.2 ml SQ and 30 minutes observation for anaphylactic reaction.

IV. Surgical debridement of wound and local installation of 10,000 U of tetanus antitoxin and 1,000,000 U of aqueous penicillin G may be tried.

V. Supportive care is essential.
A. Quiet, darkened kennel
B. Fluid therapy
C. Assisted alimentation
D. Ventilation with oxygen for respiratory failure and secondary pneumonia

AFLATOXIN

Source

I. Aflatoxins are produced by *Aspergillus flavus* and/or *A. parasiticus* in molded corn or other feed grains (cottonseed, milo).
II. High humidity, drought stress, and insect damage favor aflatoxin production.
III. Dogs or pet birds fed low-quality foods produced from moldy grains are at risk.

Action

I. Aflatoxins affect nucleic acid–directed protein synthesis and secondarily interfere with enzyme synthesis and fat mobilization.
II. High dosages (dietary concentrations >200 ppb) result in hepatic dysfunction, icterus, hepatic lipidosis, and bile duct hyperplasia.
III. Aflatoxins may be immunosuppressive, affecting both humoral and cell-mediated immunity.

Clinical Signs

I. Acute signs are anorexia, vomiting, hematemesis, icterus, and hemorrhages.
II. Subacute to chronic signs are weight loss, rough hair coat, mild icterus, anemia, and moderately elevated serum liver enzymes.

Diagnosis

I. History of exposure to moldy grain is highly suggestive, especially if analysis reveals more than 200 ppb aflatoxin.
II. Elevated serum bile acids, bilirubinemia and bilirubinuria, increased serum levels of liver-specific enzymes, hypoalbuminemia, and increased prothrombin time are characteristic of aflatoxicosis.
III. Liver biopsy or postmortem histopathology reveals hepatic lipidosis, fibrosis, and bile duct hyperplasia.

Treatment

I. Remove contaminated foods from the diet.
II. For acute cases, give activated charcoal PO to bind aflatoxin in the gastrointestinal tract.
III. Provide supportive therapy for potential liver failure and anemia or hypoprothrombinemia.
IV. Supplement diet with vitamin E and selenium and provide high-quality, easily digestible protein sources.

TREMORGENIC MYCOTOXINS

Source

I. Fungi of the genus *Penicillium* (*P. crustosum, P. cyclopium, P. puberulum*) produce fungal tremorgens with an indole structure similar to that of lysergic acid.
II. Common substrates for growth and toxin production are cream cheese, moldy walnuts, and other spoiled foods.
III. Moldy walnuts may serve as a source of tremorgens even before harvest and are a significant problem in California.

Action

I. Tremorgens decrease the function of inhibitory neurotransmitters glycine and gamma-aminobutyric acid (GABA), allowing excitatory influences to predominate.
II. Cerebral vasoconstriction may contribute to CNS signs as well.

Clinical Signs

I. Acute onset of excitement, ataxia, tremors, hypermetria, opisthotonos and seizures is typical.
II. Signs subside or are less prominent when animals are at rest but exacerbate when they are handled or stressed.
III. Morbidity may be high, but mortality is low if animals are handled carefully and removed from contaminated food sources.

Diagnosis

I. History of consumption of moldy foods with high potential for tremorgens
II. Characteristic clinical signs
III. Isolation and identification of tremorgens, especially penitrem A, from suspect food sources or stomach contents
IV. Analysis of toxin in tissue not usually available

Treatment

I. Remove animals from suspected food source.
II. Provide protection from weather, and administer parenteral fluids to reduce probability of dehydration.
III. Keep affected animals in a quiet, protected environment.
IV. Detoxify the gastrointestinal tract with activated charcoal and saline cathartics.

Bibliography

Barsanti JA, Walser M, Hatheway CL et al: Type C botulism in American foxhounds. J Am Vet Med Assoc 172:809, 1978
Coppock RW: Garbage-, food-, and water-borne intoxication. p. 163. In Kirk RW (ed): Current Veterinary Therapy VIII. WB Saunders, Philadelphia, 1983
Coppock RW, Mostrom MS: Intoxication due to contaminated garbage, food, and water. p. 221. In Kirk RW (ed): Current Veterinary Therapy IX. WB Saunders, Philadelphia, 1986
Eberhart GW: Garbage- and food-borne intoxications (enterotoxemias). p. 176. In Kirk RW (ed): Current Veterinary Therapy VI. WB Saunders, Philadelphia, 1977
Franco DA: Botulism. p. 361. In Beran GW (ed): Handbook of Zoonoses. 2nd Ed. CRC Press, Boca Raton, FL, 1994
Lambe DW Jr, Kloos WE, Lachica RV: Staphylococcal food poisoning. p. 369. In Beran GW (ed): Handbook of Zoonoses. 2nd Ed. CRC Press, Boca Raton, FL, 1994
Nicholson SS: Mycotoxicosis. p. 225. In Kirk RW (ed): Current Veterinary Therapy IX: Small Animal Practice. WB Saunders, Philadelphia, 1986

127

Household and Metal Toxicants

Gary D. Osweiler
Thomas L. Carson

LEAD

Source

  I. Household items
    A. Linoleum
    B. Rug padding
    C. Lead toys
    D. Drapery weights
    E. Lead-base paints (lead content <0.06% since 1977)
    F. Decorative glazes
  II. Construction items
    A. Putty and caulking material
    B. Plumbing materials
    C. Solder
    D. Roofing materials
    E. Lead-base paint
  III. Automotive items
    A. Batteries
    B. Wheel weights
    C. Uncommon: antiknock gasoline additives, crankcase oil, grease
  IV. Sporting goods
    A. Fishing sinkers
    B. Pellets and lead shot

Action

  I. Lead interferes with thiol-containing enzymes.
  II. Anemia may occur but is usually mild.
    A. Increased red blood cell (RBC) fragility and premature destruction
    B. Inhibition of hemoglobin synthesis in bone marrow
  III. Central nervous system (CNS) is affected by edema caused by damaged capillaries.
  IV. Peripheral nerves undergo segmental demyelination, causing slowed nerve conduction.

Clinical Signs

  I. Usually appear within 3–15 days after ingestion
  II. Gastrointestinal signs
    A. Anorexia
    B. Abdominal pain or "lead colic," especially in younger animals
    C. Vomiting and diarrhea
    D. Megaesophagus (uncommon)
  III. Neurologic signs
    A. Hysteria, aggression, nervousness, barking
    B. Ataxia, tremors
    C. Clonic-tonic seizures
    D. Blindness, deafness, dementia
  IV. Polyuria, polydipsia, especially in older animals

Diagnosis/Differential Diagnosis

  I. History
    A. Usually a younger animal, <1.5 years old, except in high-lead environments
    B. Males more commonly affected than females
    C. Often from inner-city environment, where buildings and furnishings are old and poverty rates are high
    D. Recent home remodeling, including scraping or sanding of lead-based paint
  II. Suspicious clinical signs: gastrointestinal and nervous system involvement
  III. Laboratory tests
    A. Nucleated RBCs on peripheral smears are the most common hematologic abnormality found (up to 54% of cases).
    B. Basophilic stippling occurs less often (25%). Examine fresh blood smears, as anticoagulants can make visualization of stippling difficult.
    C. Leukocytosis (25%), elevated liver enzymes (15%), and anemia (8%) may also be found (Morgan et al., 1991a).

D. Acceptable blood levels of lead for animals are poorly defined.
 1. Although blood lead concentrations ≥35 μg/dl (0.35 ppm) are considered diagnostic, clinical signs have been observed in dogs with blood lead concentrations as low as 12 μg/dl (Morgan, 1994).
 2. Diagnostic levels are >10 ppm in liver and kidney.
E. Aminolevulinic acid levels in urine are increased.
F. Free RBC zinc protoporphyrin is increased.
IV. Radiography
 A. Diffuse radiopaque material (lead or metallic foreign bodies) may be seen in the gastrointestinal tract.
 B. Lead lines may develop in the metaphyses of long bones in chronically exposed immature dogs.
V. Differential diagnosis: canine distemper, epilepsy, thallium, strychnine, zinc, and chlorinated hydrocarbons

Treatment and Monitoring

I. Prevention of further absorption from gastrointestinal tract
 A. Gastric lavage
 B. Enemas
 C. Surgery: to remove large lead objects from the stomach or intestinal tract
II. Specific antidotes
 A. Ca EDTA (Versenate) chelates lead and hastens excretion. Be sure there is no lead in the gastrointestinal tract before using Ca EDTA.
 1. Dosage: 100 mg/kg SQ divided into four daily doses in 5% dextrose/water (D/W) for 5 days. Some dogs require an additional 5 days of treatment after ending the first treatment, especially if initial blood levels are ≥100 μg/dl (0.10 ppm).
 2. Daily dose cannot exceed 2 g and cannot be continued for more than 5 consecutive days, because Ca EDTA may cause renal or gastrointestinal damage.
 3. It is highly effective, with signs abating within a few days.
 B. Penicillamine is an effective oral chelating agent that may be used as an alternate or adjunct to Ca EDTA.
 1. Dosage is 35–50 mg/kg/day divided QID for 7 days; this regimen can be repeated after 7 days off therapy.
 2. If vomiting occurs, dramamine 2–4 mg/kg PO 0.5 hour before the pencillamine is often helpful.
 3. Give at least 30 minutes before daily meals to reduce chelation of essential minerals.
 4. It may affect animals with penicillin allergies.
 C. Succimer is a new oral heavy metal chelator that has been used successfully in dogs.
 1. Dosage: 10 mg/kg PO TID for 10 days

 2. Does not require that the gastrointestinal tract be free of lead prior to treatment
 3. Effective, but expensive
III. Supportive care
 A. Fluid, electrolyte, and acid–base therapy
 B. Control of seizures
IV. Blood lead assay repeated 10–14 days after treatment; chelation therapy repeated if lead is ≥40 μg/dl
V. Prevention of re-exposure and promotion of owner education
 A. The source of the lead is identified if possible.
 B. Owners of lead-poisoned animals with young children should be advised to consult with their pediatricians and local health officials.

ARSENIC

Source

I. Current sources are limited but may include trivalent organic forms such as monosodium methanearsonate (MSMA) and disodium methanearsonate (DMSA) that are used as herbicides.
II. Thiacetarsamide is a trivalent arsenical used for heartworm disease in dogs.
III. Sodium or potassium arsenate baits are available to control ants and may be ingested by cats.

Action

I. Arsenic compounds bind to sulfhydryl groups (lipoic acid) and prevent entry to the tricarboxylic acid cycle, with inhibition of cellular respiration.
II. Tissues with high oxidative energy requirements (intestinal epithelium, kidney, liver, skin) are most affected.
III. Effects on capillary integrity result in edema and loss of fluids.
IV. Inorganic trivalent arsenic is toxic at 1–25 mg/kg for most species.
V. Among domestic animals, cats are most susceptible.

Clinical Signs

I. Vomiting, gastritis, and colic
II. Severe, watery diarrhea within 24 hours
III. Weakness, ataxia, tremors, and recumbency
IV. Weak, rapid pulses with circulatory shock, dehydration, and hypothermia
V. Subacute poisoning: watery diarrhea with shedding of necrotic intestinal mucosa (rice-water stools) within 3–5 days
VI. Survivors of gastrointestinal damage: oliguria, proteinuria that progresses to polyuria with dilute urine from renal damage

Diagnosis

I. Dehydration, increased hematocrit, elevated blood urea nitrogen, proteinuria, and urinary casts are characteristic.

II. Test the arsenic concentration in urine, vomitus, or feces from live affected animals and in the liver and kidney of dead animals.

Treatment

I. Institute gastrointestinal detoxification and supportive therapy.
II. Treat shock, acidosis, and dehydration with appropriate fluid therapy (see Chap. 131).
III. Specific antidotes contain sulfhydryl groups to complex with arsenic.
  A. British antilewisite (BAL or dimercaprol) is the classic treatment.
    1. It is not effective unless given very early.
    2. Give 3–5 mg/kg IM QID for 5 days, then evaluate renal function to avoid BAL nephrotoxicity.
  B. Succimer or mesodimercaptosuccinic acid is a new therapy.
    1. Experimentally effective but not widely used for arsenic intoxication
    2. Dosage: 10 mg/kg PO TID for 5 days, then BID for 5 days
IV. Give convalescent animals bland diets with high-quality protein and supplemental vitamins.

COPPER

See Chap. 34.

IRON

Source

I. Excessive accidental or intentional consumption of oral iron supplements containing ferrous or ferric salts
II. Overdosage of parenteral iron solutions used as hematinics

Action

I. Excessive oral or parenteral iron exceeds the iron binding capacity of transferrin.
II. Free plasma iron triggers several adverse actions.
  A. Free radical damage to cell membranes of liver, heart, and brain
  B. Increased capillary permeability and vascular dilatation, leading to venous pooling, shock, and metabolic acidosis
III. Exposure to >20 mg/kg may be toxic, dosages >60 mg/kg are severely toxic, and dosages >200 mg/kg are potentially lethal.
IV. Phosphate absorption may be impaired by dietary iron concentrations above 0.5%.

Clinical Signs

I. Depression, vomiting, and hemorrhagic diarrhea appear within several hours after toxic oral ingestion.

II. Serious toxicosis causes continued vomiting and diarrhea, dehydration, hepatic necrosis, circulatory shock, and acidosis within 24 hours.

Diagnosis

I. Total serum iron >300 μg/dl indicates excessive exposure.
II. Clinical signs and laboratory evidence of shock, acidosis, and liver damage strongly suggest iron toxicosis.
III. Icterus, hemoglobinuria, and hepatic necrosis are prominent lesions.

Treatment

I. Early emptying of the gastrointestinal tract followed by milk of magnesia to precipitate iron in the intestinal tract is the treatment of choice.
II. Control shock, dehydration, and acidosis with appropriate fluid therapy (see Chap. 131).
III. Deferoxamine 15 mg/kg/h IV has been recommended to chelate iron.
  A. Treatment must be monitored carefully to prevent arrhythmias and hypotension.
  B. Deferoxamine 40 mg/kg IM QID has also been used.
IV. Iron excretion is enhanced by oral ascorbic acid.
V. Serum iron levels are checked 2–3 days later to determine whether iron concentrations have returned to normal.

ZINC

Source

I. Zinc-containing objects: nuts, bolts, galvanized metal utensils or cages, batteries
II. Pennies minted after 1983
III. Unintentional ingestion of zinc-containing ointments

Action

I. Zinc salts are directly irritating and damaging to the gastrointestinal mucosa.
II. Zinc antagonizes the role of copper and iron in hematopoiesis, leading to anemia and mild hemolysis.
III. Toxic dosage may be 50–100 mg/kg PO, or ≥1–3 pennies.

Clinical Signs

I. Early in the course, depression, vomiting, diarrhea, and anorexia occur.
II. Advanced signs include icterus, hemoglobinuria, hematuria, and mild to moderate anemia.
III. Zinc toxicosis may be lethal if the source is not removed and supportive or chelation therapy is not provided.

Diagnosis

I. Nucleated erythrocytes and basophilic stippling
II. Elevated serum liver enzymes
III. Elevated serum zinc concentration (>0.7 μg/ml); collected in trace element–free tube
IV. Radiography to demonstrate intact metallic objects in the gastrointestinal tract

Treatment

I. Remove any zinc objects from the gastrointestinal tract.
II. Monitor and treat anemia, thrombocytopenia, and disseminated intravascular coagulation as needed (see Chap. 66).
III. Chelation therapy with Ca EDTA at 100 mg/kg SQ divided QID for 3–5 days may be instituted.
IV. Oral penicillamine may be used for long-term chelation at 35 mg/kg PO divided QID for 7–14 days.

ETHYLENE GLYCOL

Source

I. Automobile antifreeze-antiboil radiator solutions are 95% ethylene glycol. They may be used as a malicious poison.
II. Color film processing solutions in home darkrooms may contain ethylene glycol.
III. Toxicity, or minimum lethal dosage, is as follows.
  A. Dogs: 6.6 ml/kg
  B. Cats: 1.5 ml/kg

Action

I. Ethylene glycol is oxidized by the liver and kidney to toxic metabolites.
II. Glycoaldehyde is toxic to the CNS.
III. Glycolate and glyoxylate contribute to metabolic acidosis.
IV. Pulmonary edema can occur, but the mechanism is unknown.
V. Glycolate and oxalate cause severe renal tubular epithelial necrosis.

Clinical Signs

I. Signs vary with stage of intoxication and dosage.
II. Stage one occurs 30 minutes to 12 hours after ingestion; it is similar to alcohol intoxication. CNS signs predominate. Massive doses cause death in less than 12 hours.
  A. Polydipsia, polyuria
  B. Nausea and vomiting
  C. Ataxia
  D. Metabolic acidosis
  E. Coma and death with ingestion of large doses
III. Stage two occurs 12–24 hours after ingestion. Signs in animals are nondescript, and animals often appear to be recovering.

IV. Stage three occurs 24–72 hours after ingestion. Renal signs predominate.
  A. Severe depression
  B. Oliguria
  C. Anorexia and vomiting, oral ulcers (common)
  D. Death caused by acute, anuric renal failure and acidosis

Diagnosis/Differential Diagnosis

I. History of ingestion or exposure
II. Usually a young animal
III. Severe metabolic acidosis
IV. High serum osmolality and large anion and osmolal gap
V. Calcium oxalate crystalluria 6 hours after ingestion
VI. Serum or urine ethylene glycol levels
VII. Acute, anuric renal failure
  A. Early in the course, there is marked polyuria.
  B. Azotemia does not occur until 36–72 hours after ingestion in dogs and 12–24 hours after ingestion in cats.
VIII. Examination of renal biopsy under polarized light for presence of calcium oxalate crystals
IX. Diffuse hyperechoic pattern in kidneys on ultrasonography, from dystrophic calcification
X. Differential diagnosis: other causes of acute renal failure, ketoacidotic diabetes mellitus, pancreatitis, gastroenteritis, garbage intoxication, primary CNS disorders

Treatment and Monitoring

I. Prevent gastrointestinal absorption if <4 hours after ingestion.
  A. Emesis
  B. Gastric lavage and activated charcoal
II. Specific antidotes block metabolism of ethylene glycol by inhibiting liver alcohol dehydrogenase and allowing the intact ethylene glycol to be excreted by the kidneys.
  A. Prognosis varies inversely with time between ingestion and initiation of therapy.
  B. Therapy to block metabolism beyond 24 hours after ingestion is of questionable value.
  C. Give 20% ethanol.
    1. Dosage for dogs: 5.5 ml/kg IV q 4 h for five treatments and then QID for four more treatments
    2. Dosage for cats: 5 ml/kg IV QID for five treatments, then TID for four more treatments
  D. 4-Methylpyrazole 5% is a potent alcohol dehydrogenase inhibitor that has been used in dogs with success. It does not depress the CNS, as does ethanol.
    1. Dosage used in dogs is 20 mg/kg IV, then 15 mg/kg IV at 12 and 24 hours, then 5 mg/kg IV at 36 hours.
      a) 4-Methylpyrazole has been approved for dogs and is available as Antizol-Vet (Orphan Medical, Minnetonka, MN).
    2. 4-Methylpyrazole is not effective in cats.

E. Thiamine (10–100 mg/day PO) and pyridoxine do not inhibit alcohol dehydrogenase but facilitate conversion of glyoxylate to nontoxic metabolites.

III. Provide supportive care.
 A. Fluid and electrolyte therapy is given to maintain urine output.
 B. Sodium bicarbonate is given to combat metabolic acidosis.
  1. Dosage is based on plasma bicarbonate levels.
  2. If blood gases are unavailable, give 6 mEq/kg in IV fluids slowly q 4–6 h.
 C. Diuretics may be used to maintain urine output if the animal is well hydrated.
 D. Peritoneal dialysis is the best therapy if the animal presents in renal failure. The nephrosis may be reversible with time, but the prognosis is guarded.

AROMATIC HYDROCARBONS

Source

 I. Wood preservatives: creosote, creosol, pine tar
 II. Solvents: toluene, xylene
 III. Disinfectants, sanitizers: phenol, cresol, hexachlorophene
 IV. Herbicides, fungicides, insecticides (dinitroorthocresol)
 V. Mothballs (naphthalene)
 VI. Toxicity: cats and young dogs especially susceptible, owing to a deficiency of metabolizing enzymes

Action

 I. Phenolic compounds are rapidly absorbed from the gastrointestinal tract or through intact skin.
 II. Phenolic compounds cause necrosis of mucous membranes, cerebral edema, hepatopathy, and nephropathy.
 III. Many phenolic metabolites inhibit mitochondrial respiration and result in methemoglobin formation.
 IV. It is also hypothesized that phenol causes accumulation of acetylcholine at the myoneural junction.

Clinical Signs

 I. With ingestion of concentrated solutions: corrosion of oral mucous membranes
 II. Depression, vomiting
 III. Incoordination, ataxia
 IV. Muscle fasciculations, seizures
 V. Coma, respiratory failure
 VI. With slower absorption from chronic skin exposure: increased RBC fragility, hemolysis, icterus

Diagnosis/Differential Diagnosis

 I. History and clinical signs
 II. Urine test for phenols
   Add 1 ml of 20% ferric chloride to 10 ml urine; a blue-purple color is positive.

III. Differential diagnosis: chlorinated hydrocarbons, hypocalcemia, garbage intoxication, metaldehyde, Vacor

Treatment

 I. Prevent further absorption
 A. Wash with soap and water if skin is exposed.
 B. If there is evidence of corrosion of the mouth, induction of vomiting is contraindicated. Milk or egg whites are given immediately to decrease the corrosive action.
 C. Institute gastric lavage with activated charcoal.
 II. Supportive therapy
 A. Fluids, electrolytes, acid–base therapy
 B. Gastrointestinal protectants
 C. Control of seizures

GLUES AND ADHESIVES

Source

Numerous household products contain one of the following.
 I. Cyanoacrylate
 II. Epoxy resins
 III. Toluene
 IV. Plastic resins
 V. Methylethyl ketones

Action

Local irritants

Clinical Signs

 I. Dermatitis
 II. Irritation and/or ulceration of mucous membranes
 III. Possible hyperesthesia or listlessness
 IV. Possible gastroenteritis

Diagnosis

Known exposure and clinical signs

Treatment

 I. Try to remove from the skin with warm, soapy water. Be careful with the use of other solvents, as they may also cause toxicity.
 II. Give supportive and symptomatic therapy.

DETERGENTS AND SOAPS

Source

 I. Anionic detergents: sodium, potassium, or ammonium salts of sulfated higher alcohols and sodium sulfonates of long-chain alkyl derivatives of benzene
 A. Dishwashing soaps

B. Shampoos
C. Laundry soaps
II. Cationic detergents: usually alkyl or aryl quaternary ammonium compounds; used to destroy bacteria on skin, surgical instruments, cooking equipment, sickroom supplies, and diapers
   A. Diaparene
   B. Zephiran
   C. Phemerol
   D. Ceepryn
III. Nonionic detergents containing alkyl and aryl polyether sulfates, alcohols or sulfonates, alkyl phenol, polyglycol, polyethylene glycol, and aryl ethers
   A. These compounds are only slightly irritating to skin; however, glycolic acid and oxalate are potential toxic metabolites.
   B. Cats and young dogs have decreased ability to metabolize phenolic compounds.
IV. Hexachlorophene soaps: pHisoHex

Action

I. Mechanism of damage is not known.
II. They are dermal irritants that remove natural skin oils.
III. They produce corrosive damage to mucous membranes.
IV. Some cationic detergents are broken down to compounds that can cause methemoglobinemia.
V. Hexachlorophene has caused marked vacuolation of the white matter of the brain and spinal cord in puppies.

Clinical Signs

I. Erythematous dermatitis or mucous membrane damage is common.
II. Stomatitis and pharyngitis are possible with ingestion and may result in hypersalivation, gagging, and respiratory distress.
III. Vomiting, diarrhea, and gastrointestinal distention are often seen.
IV. Collapse, ataxia, severe depression, and seizures are possible.
V. Hexachlorophene produces vomiting, hypersalivation, tachypnea, depression, and generalized tremors.

Diagnosis/Differential Diagnosis

I. History of exposure
II. Characteristic clinical signs
III. Differential diagnosis: phenolic compounds, corrosives and caustics, paint thinners and turpentine

Treatment

I. Maintain a patent airway if laryngeal swelling exists.
II. Flush skin with copious amounts of warm water.
III. Cationic detergents can be neutralized or inactivated before absorption with ordinary soaps.
IV. Consider gastric lavage with milk or activated char-

coal or induction of emesis after administration of milk or activated charcoal.
V. Follow lavage or emesis with a sodium sulfate cathartic.
VI. Give supportive care.

CORROSIVES AND CAUSTICS

Source

I. Corrosives and caustics are substances that cause destruction of tissue by chemical action.
   A. Acids (e.g., battery acid, acetic acid, cleaning and etching compounds) are often referred to as corrosives.
   B. Alkalis (e.g., lye, cleaning preparations, refrigerants, grease solvents) are often referred to as caustics.
II. Toxicity is variable, depending on the strength of the acid or base and the route of exposure.

Action

I. Corrosives and caustics cause necrosis of skin and mucous membranes on contact.
II. Severe corrosion of skin and mucous membranes may result in systemic intoxication.

Clinical Signs

I. Stomatitis and pharyngitis occur with ingestion. Mucous membranes appear grayish-white or inflamed, and with time, the tissue may turn black and become wrinkled.
II. Vomiting and thirst usually occur when these compounds are ingested.
III. Dyspnea and asphyxia may occur secondary to swelling and edema of the larynx and glottis.
IV. Skin exposure can vary from mild dermatitis to severe necrosis.

Diagnosis/Differential Diagnosis

I. History of exposure
II. Characteristic clinical signs
III. Differential diagnosis: detergents and soaps, paint thinners and turpentine, phenolic compounds

Treatment

I. Maintain a patent airway with an endotracheal tube or tracheostomy if necessary.
II. Copiously flush the dermally exposed areas with warm, soapy water; 5% sodium bicarbonate may be used to neutralize dermal exposure to acids.
III. Do not induce emesis until the acid or base has been neutralized.
   A. Four egg whites in a quart of warm water, 1–5 g of magnesium oxide 1:25 in warm water, or 1–15 ml of milk of magnesia is given orally after ingestion of acids.

B. Vinegar (diluted 1:4), 1–5% acetic acid, or lemon juice is given orally with four egg whites in a quart of warm water after ingestion of an alkali.

IV. After the acid or base has been neutralized, emesis is induced, followed by a sodium sulfate cathartic.

V. Damaged skin or gastrointestinal mucosa is protected as much as possible.

   A. Gastrointestinal protectants (e.g., kaolin or pectin)

   B. Bandages and topical antibiotics for dermal lesions

FERTILIZERS AND PLANT FOOD

Source and Action

I. Numerous household products that contain nitrogen, phosphorus, potassium, and, in some cases, ammonia, metal salts, potash, and sulfur

II. Local irritants with possible systemic effects secondary to absorption of nitrogen, phosphorus, potassium, and metals

Clinical Signs

I. Hypersalivation, stomatitis, gastroenteritis, abdominal pain

II. Fever, tachypnea

III. Weakness, muscle tremors, possible seizures

IV. Cyanosis caused by methemoglobin formation with some nitrate-based fertilizers

Diagnosis/Differential Diagnosis

I. Known exposure or ingestion

II. Clinical signs

III. Possible methemoglobinemia, hyperkalemia, hyperphosphatemia, hyperosmolality, increased blood ammonia concentrations

IV. Differential diagnosis: phenolic compounds, acetaminophen, naphthalene, onions, soaps and detergents

Treatment

I. Perform gastric lavage with milk or activated charcoal and water or induce emesis after the animal has ingested milk or water.

II. Give supportive care; monitor serum electrolytes.

PAINTS AND VARNISHES

Source

I. Many household products, including lead-base, oil-base, latex, and acrylic paints

II. Many products containing petroleum distillates, xylene, toluene

III. Wood stains, polyurethane, varnishes

IV. Paint chips from peeling walls and furniture

Action

I. Many paints act as local irritants in the gastrointestinal tract.

II. Petroleum distillates are fat solvents that can alter CNS function and cause pulmonary edema as well as liver and kidney damage.

III. Ingestion of lead-base paints can result in lead poisoning.

Clinical Signs

I. Anorexia, depression, hypersalivation, vomiting, diarrhea

II. Tachypnea/dyspnea; sometimes CNS hyperactivity or depression with coma or seizures secondary to ingestion of petroleum distillates

Diagnosis

Witnessed ingestion or the presence of paint or varnish on hair coat

Treatment

I. Perform gastric lavage with activated charcoal followed by a sodium sulfate cathartic.

II. Bathe skin with warm water and mild soap.

III. Give supportive and symptomatic therapy.

IV. See also Lead, earlier.

PAINT THINNERS AND TURPENTINE

Source

I. Numerous paint thinners and paint stripping compounds contain methyl chloride, mineral spirits, phenols, cresols, or alkalis.

II. Turpentine is a common household solvent that is also known as gum turpentine, oil of turpentine, and spirits of turpentine.

Action

I. They are local irritants that cause dermatitis with dermal exposure and stomatitis, pharyngitis, and gastroenteritis with ingestion.

II. Absorption of these compounds can result in hyperesthesia, ataxia, CNS depression, seizures, hepatic damage, and hemoglobinemia (see Aromatic Hydrocarbons, earlier).

III. Turpentine may cause renal damage.

IV. Inhalation of toxic fumes may cause respiratory damage.

Clinical Signs

I. Local irritation of skin and mucous membranes

II. Anorexia, vomiting, abdominal pain

III. Hyperesthesia, CNS depression, ataxia

IV. Ingestion of phenols and/or alkalis: seizures, hepatic damage, hemoglobinemia/hemoglobinuria
V. Ingestion of turpentine: proteinuria, hematuria, glycosuria
VI. Polypnea, dyspnea

Diagnosis/Differential Diagnosis

I. History of exposure
II. Characteristic clinical signs
III. Differential diagnosis: phenolic compounds, corrosives and caustics, detergents and soaps, petroleum distillates

Treatment

I. Flush with copious amounts of warm, soapy water in cases of contact exposure.
II. Gastric lavage with activated charcoal followed by a sodium sulfate cathartic is indicated if these compounds are ingested.
III. Give supportive therapy; maintain hydration and urine output. (See also Chap. 133.)

Bibliography

Bratton GR, Kowalczyk DF: Lead poisoning. p. 152. In Kirk RW (ed): Current Veterinary Therapy X: Small Animal Practice. WB Saunders, Philadelphia, 1989

Center SA: Suspected calcium EDTA intoxication in a dog. J Am Vet Med Assoc 183:884, 1983

Coppock RW, Mostrom MS, Smetzer DL: Volatile hydrocarbons (solvents, fuels) and petrochemicals. p. 197. In Kirk RW (ed): Current Veterinary Therapy IX: Small Animal Practice. WB Saunders, Philadelphia, 1986

Dial SM, Thrall MA, Hamar DW: Efficacy of 4-methlypyrazole for treatment of ethylene glycol intoxication in dogs. Am J Vet Res 55:1762, 1994

Grauer GF, Thrall MA: Ethylene glycol (antifreeze) poisoning. p. 206. In Kirk RW (ed): Current Veterinary Therapy IX: Small Animal Practice. WB Saunders, Philadelphia, 1986

Grauer GF, Thrall MA, Henre BA et al: Early clinicopathologic findings in dogs ingesting ethylene glycol. Am J Vet Res 45:2299, 1984

Grauer GF, Thrall MA, Henre BA, Hjelle JJ: Comparison of the effects of ethanol and 4-methylpyrazole on the pharmacokinetics and toxicity of ethylene glycol in the dog. Toxicol Lett 35:307, 1987

Greentree WF, Hall JO: Iron toxicosis. p. 240. In Bonagura JD (ed): Kirk's Current Veterinary Therapy XII: Small Animal Practice. WB Saunders, Philadelphia, 1995

Meurs KM, Breitschwerdt EB: Zinc toxicity. p. 238. In Bonagura JD (ed): Kirk's Current Veterinary Therapy XII. WB Saunders, Philadelphia, 1995

Morgan RV: Lead poisoning in small companion animals: an update (1987–1992). Vet Hum Toxicol 36:18, 1994

Morgan RV, Moore FM, Pearce LK, Rossi T: Clinical and laboratory findings in small companion animals with lead poisoning: 347 cases (1977–1986). J Am Vet Med Assoc 199:93, 1991a

Morgan RV, Pearce LK, Moore FM, Rossi T: Demographic data and treatment of small companion animals with lead poisoning: 347 cases (1977–1986). J Am Vet Med Assoc 199:98, 1991b

Ramsey DT, Casteel SW, Faggella AM et al: Use of orally administered succimer (meso-2,3-dimercaptosuccinic acid) for treatment of lead poisoning in dogs. J Am Vet Med Assoc 208:371, 1996

Scott DW, Bolton GR, Lorenz MD: Hexachlorophene toxicosis in dogs. J Am Vet Med Assoc 162:947, 1973

Thrall MA, Grauer GF, Mero KN: Clinicopathologic findings in dogs and cats with ethylene glycol intoxication. J Am Vet Med Assoc 184:377, 1984

128

Household Drugs

Gary D. Osweiler
Thomas L. Carson

ACETAMINOPHEN AND OTHER OXIDANT DRUGS

Source

I. Acetaminophen analgesic, antipyretic drugs, in regular strength (325 mg) and extra strength (500 mg) oral dosage forms
  A. Tylenol
  B. Excedrin
  C. Anacin-3
  D. Datril
  E. Tempra
  F. Phenacetin alone or in aspirin-phenacetin-caffeine tablets: rapidly metabolized to acetaminophen
II. Phenazopyridine (urinary analgesic)
III. Methylene blue (urinary antiseptic)
IV. Allylpropyl disulfide (onions, raw and cooked)
V. Naphthalene (mothballs)
VI. Toxic dosage
  A. Cats: acetaminophen 50–100 mg/kg (½ to 1 tablet per cat) one time and phenazopyridine 65 mg/kg/day for 3 days
  B. Dogs: acetaminophen 200 mg/kg one time

Action

I. Acetaminophen is rapidly absorbed (within 1 hour) from the gastrointestinal tract.
  A. It is detoxified by conjugation with glucuronide, sulfate, or glutathione.
  B. Cats lack the ability to conjugate glucuronides, so are particularly susceptible.
  C. Both dogs and cats have a low ability to conjugate by sulfation.
II. The toxic metabolite of acetaminophen (*N*-acetyl-*p*-benzoquinone) causes severe oxidative stress to red blood cells (RBCs) and hepatocytes.
III. Ferrous iron (Fe^{2+}) is oxidized to ferric iron (Fe^{3+}), converting hemoglobin to methemoglobin, which does not carry oxygen.
IV. Oxidation of hemoglobin also forms disulfide bonds, resulting in hemoglobin precipitation and Heinz body (erythrocyte refractile body) formation.
V. Heinz bodies are removed by macrophages in the spleen and liver, causing the RBC to lose surface area, thereby decreasing its life span.
VI. Some of these drugs also cause liver damage, particularly toxic doses of acetaminophen in dogs.

Clinical Signs

I. Hypersalivation and facial edema in cats (acetaminophen)
II. Depression, weakness, anorexia, vomiting
III. Tachypnea, tachycardia
IV. Methemoglobinemia, cyanosis, brown mucous membranes in cats within 6–12 hours after ingestion
V. Hematuria, hemoglobinemia
VI. With naphthalene, seizures or central nervous system (CNS) depression
VII. Acute anemia (see Chap. 63)
VIII. Acute hepatic necrosis with associated signs in dogs
IX. Lacrimation and pruritus (cats)

Diagnosis/Differential Diagnosis

I. History of administration of the drugs or feeding table scraps containing onions
II. Heinz bodies
III. Elevated methemoglobin levels (normal 0–1%)
IV. Icterus (increased total and direct bilirubin serum levels); elevated serum glutamic-pyruvic transaminase (alanine aminotransferase) and alkaline phosphatase
V. Differential diagnosis: phenolic compounds, detergents and soaps, chlorates and nitrites

Treatment

I. Induce emesis if early after ingestion, followed by activated charcoal and cathartic.
  A. Emetics are contraindicated if animal is hypoxic.

B. Detoxification early with activated charcoal and osmotic cathartics is recommended.
II. Give specific antidotes.
   A. Acetylcysteine (Mucomyst)
      1. It supplements available glutathione by replenishment or substitution.
      2. Dosage is initially 140–280 mg/kg PO or 140 mg/kg IV in 5% dextrose/water, followed by 70 mg/kg PO QID for 2–3 days.
      3. Activated charcoal may inactivate acetylcysteine given PO.
   B. Ascorbic acid
      1. It reduces methemoglobin to hemoglobin.
      2. Dosage is 30 mg/kg PO or SQ QID for seven treatments.
   C. Methylene blue may be used for methemoglobinemia in cats at a dosage not to exceed 1.5 mg/kg.
III. Hasten elimination.
   A. Alkaline urine increases excretion of naphthalene.
   B. Give sodium bicarbonate 50 mg/kg PO BID–TID.
IV. Give supportive care.
   A. Transfusions
   B. Fluid, electrolyte, acid–base therapy
   C. Corticosteroids and antihistamines not indicated

ASPIRIN/SALICYLATES

Source

I. Accidental ingestion or administration of improper dose may be responsible.
II. Cats and young dogs are more susceptible, owing to a deficiency in metabolizing enzymes, particularly those responsible for glucuronide formation.
III. Potentially toxic single dose in cats and dogs is >60 mg/kg.
IV. For cats, >25 mg/kg PO TID may be toxic if given for more than 5–7 days.

Action

I. Prostaglandin inhibitors
   A. High doses uncouple oxidative phosphorylation.
   B. Hyperglycemia may result.
II. Initial stimulation and then depression of respiration
III. Metabolic acidosis
IV. Gastric ulceration
V. Decreased platelet aggregation
VI. Bone marrow hypoplasia

Clinical Signs

I. Tachypnea early, then respiratory depression
II. Hyperthermia
III. Anorexia, vomiting, ulcerative gastritis
IV. Metabolic acidosis, which can lead to coma
V. Renal damage

VI. Hemorrhage
VII. Nonregenerative anemia with long-term administration
VIII. Occasionally seizures

Diagnosis/Differential Diagnosis

I. History is usually helpful.
II. Metabolic acidosis, aciduria, and increased anion gap may be seen.
III. Serum or urine salicylate levels may be diagnostic.
   Add 3 drops of 10% ferric chloride to 1 ml acidified urine; red color indicates salicylates are present.
IV. Differential diagnosis includes other causes of gastritis and severe metabolic acidosis, ethylene glycol exposure, and other nonsteroidal anti-inflammatory drugs such as ibuprofen.

Treatment

I. Prevent absorption if early after ingestion with induction of emesis, gastric lavage, activated charcoal, and cathartics.
II. Hasten elimination with alkalinization of urine for 36–48 hours.
   A. Give sodium bicarbonate 50 mg/kg PO BID-TID.
   B. It also combats metabolic acidosis, which is common.
III. Supportive care
   A. Fluid, electrolyte, acid–base therapy
   B. Gastrointestinal protectants and histamine receptor antagonists (e.g., cimetidine, ranitidine)
   C. Alkaline peritoneal dialysis for severe cases

IBUPROFEN

Source

I. Common nonsteroidal anti-inflammatory drug (NSAID)
II. Commercial products: Advil, Medipren, Midol 200, Motrin, Nuprin
III. Other potentially toxic NSAIDs: naproxen, piroxicam, indomethacin, phenylbutazone
IV. Narrow range of safety
   A. Therapeutic dosage: 5 mg/kg
   B. Gastrointestinal irritation and hemorrhage: dogs, 8 mg/kg/day; single dosages of 50 mg/kg in cats or 100 mg/kg in dogs
   C. Renal failure and death: dosages ≥300 mg/kg in either dogs or cats

Action

I. Reduced prostaglandin synthesis via inhibition of prostaglandin synthetase
II. May decrease cytoprotective effects of prostaglandins, especially in the stomach
III. May be cellular antioxidants
IV. Bound to plasma albumin, so may displace other drugs or toxicants that are also protein bound

Clinical Signs

I. Early signs, at lower dosages
    A. Nausea, vomiting, colic, diarrhea
    B. Depression, drowsiness
    C. Evidence of metabolic acidosis
II. Severe signs, at higher dosages
    A. Continued vomiting and dark, tarry stools
    B. Ataxia, weakness
    C. Oliguria from interstitial nephritis, acute renal failure

Diagnosis

I. History of exposure
II. Suspicious gastrointestinal and renal signs
III. Laboratory findings
    A. Uremia and hyperkalemia in acute toxicosis
    B. Hematuria, proteinuria, possibly pyuria
IV. Histopathologic lesions
    A. Gastrointestinal irritation, ulceration, hemorrhage
    B. Renal tubular or papillary necrosis, interstitial nephritis

Treatment and Monitoring

I. Prevent absorption with emesis, gastric lavage, activated charcoal, and saline cathartic, if ≤4 hours after ingestion.
II. Treat gastrointestinal ulcers symptomatically.
    A. Cimetidine 4–8 mg/kg IV (dog) or 5 mg/kg IV (cat) TID–QID
    B. Ranitidine 2 mg/kg PO (dog) or 0.5 mg/kg PO (cat) BID
    C. Sucralfate 1 g PO TID (dog) or 40 mg/kg PO TID (cat)
    D. Metoclopramide 0.2–0.4 mg/kg PO, SQ QID (dog)
III. Misoprostol (Cytotec), a synthetic prostaglandin E analogue, may help prevent gastric mucosal damage from NSAIDs. Dosage in dogs is 3–5 μg/kg PO TID-QID.
IV. Treat acute renal failure as outlined in Chap. 47.

METHYLXANTHINES

Source

I. Caffeine
    A. Over-the-counter and prescription preparations
        1. Diet pills
        2. Mood elevators
        3. Fatigue reduction drugs: 200 mg/tablet
    B. Tea leaves, coffee products, cola soft drinks
II. Theobromine
    A. Milk chocolate: 40–60 mg theobromine/oz
    B. Semisweet chocolate: 140 mg/oz
    C. Baking chocolate: 390–450 mg/oz
III. Toxic dosage for dogs: 100–150 mg/kg

Action

I. Caffeine is a powerful CNS stimulant that can cause hyperesthesia and spinal cord reflex excitability.
II. Xanthines antagonize adenosine receptors and inhibit phosphodiesterase, which increases cyclic adenosine monophosphate (cyclic AMP) concentrations.
    A. Xanthines stimulate the myocardium directly, causing increased rate and force of contraction.
    B. Xanthines strengthen skeletal muscle contraction, probably through increased release of acetylcholine at the neuromuscular junction.
    C. Xanthines increase gastric secretion and may cause mucosal ulceration.
III. Diuresis occurs because of increased cardiac output and increased urinary sodium and chloride excretion.

Clinical Signs

I. Restlessness, hyperesthesia, hyperirritability
II. Tachycardia, extrasystoles
III. Vomiting
IV. Polyuria
V. Tense skeletal musculature
VI. Convulsions (may be epileptiform or tetanic)
VII. Death caused by cardiac and respiratory arrest

Diagnosis/Differential Diagnosis

I. History of ingestion or exposure and characteristic clinical signs
II. Analysis of vomitus, plasma, and urine for caffeine, theobromine
III. Differential diagnosis: strychnine, zinc phosphide, nicotine, amphetamines, metaldehyde

Treatment and Monitoring

I. Prevention of absorption, if it is early after ingestion, with induced emesis, gastric lavage, or cathartics
II. Supportive therapy
    A. Oxygen and artificial respiration for respiratory arrest
    B. Control of seizures
        1. Diazepam 2.5–20 mg IV as needed
        2. Barbiturates IV if diazepam ineffective
    C. Control of tachyarrhythmias with lidocaine (dogs), propranolol, or metoprolol (see Chap. 7)
    D. Fluid, electrolyte, acid–base therapy
    E. Gastrointestinal protectants

NICOTINE

Source

I. Nicotine-containing darts used by dog wardens
II. Ingestion of cigarettes and/or cigars (0.5–2 mg/cigarette)
III. Some insecticides (Black Leaf 40)
IV. Toxicity: minimum lethal dose for dogs and cats, 20–100 mg

V. Nicotine solutions (Black Leaf 40) absorbed quickly through skin and oral mucosa

Action

I. Small doses stimulate all autonomic ganglia.
II. Large doses block the autonomic ganglia and myoneural junction.

Clinical Signs

I. Salivation, excitement, tachypnea, tachycardia
II. Vomiting, diarrhea
III. Muscle tremors, ataxia, seizures
IV. Slow and shallow respiration, flaccid paralysis
V. Death caused by respiratory arrest

Diagnosis/Differential Diagnosis

I. History and characteristic clinical signs
II. Parts of cigarettes and/or cigars in vomitus or stomach contents
III. Differential diagnosis: strychnine, xanthines, organophosphates, carbamates

Treatment

I. Prevention of absorption
   A. Emesis
   B. Gastric lavage with 1:2000 potassium permanganate solution or with activated charcoal
   C. Dermal exposure: wash with soap and water
II. Supportive care
   A. Oxygen and artificial respiration for respiratory arrest
   B. Sedation early: diazepam 2.5–20 mg IV as needed
   C. Stimulants later
      1. Phenylephrine 0.15 mg/kg IV (slowly)
      2. Amphetamine sulfate 4.4 mg/kg SQ
   D. Fluid, electrolyte, acid–base therapy

MARIJUANA, HASHISH

Source and Action

I. *Cannabis sativa* (hemp plant) is the source.
II. Active ingredient tetrahydrocannabinol causes CNS depression, visual hallucinations, and changes in sensory perception in people.

Clinical Signs

Note: Signs can rapidly change in nature.
I. Drowsiness, depression, hypothermia
II. Ataxia, poor vision
III. Salivation, vomiting
IV. Mydriasis (common)
V. Bradycardia

Diagnosis/Differential Diagnosis

I. History from owner
II. Suspect materials; vomitus and urine analyzed to confirm exposure
III. Differential diagnosis: ethanol or early ethylene glycol, ingestion of tranquilizers, depressants, muscle relaxants

Treatment

I. Prevent absorption. Remove gastrointestinal contents via emesis or lavage, followed by activated charcoal and a cathartic.
II. Give supportive care.
   A. Allow time in a quiet, darkened environment.
   B. Maintain normal body temperature.
   C. Bradycardia may respond to atropine.

AMPHETAMINES

Source

I. Amphetamine sulfate, dextroamphetamine, methamphetamine
II. Diet pills, mood elevators, fatigue reducers
III. Toxicity: minimum lethal dose 10–23 mg/kg

Action

I. They are potent stimulants of the CNS and cardiovascular system.
II. Amphetamines increase the amount of catecholamine at nerve endings by increasing release and inhibiting reuptake and metabolism.
III. They stimulate the respiratory center and reticular activating system.

Clinical Signs

I. Hyperexcitability, hyperesthesia
II. Tachycardia, hypertension
III. Hyperthermia, panting
IV. Mydriasis
V. Vomiting, diarrhea
VI. Trembling, seizures

Diagnosis/Differential Diagnosis

I. History and clinical signs
II. Laboratory analysis of urine or stomach contents
III. Lactic acidosis and hypoglycemia suggestive
IV. Differential diagnosis: strychnine, zinc phosphide, metaldehyde, nicotine, xanthines

Treatment

I. Prevent absorption by emesis, gastric lavage, activated charcoal, cathartics.
II. Provide sedation.
   A. Acetylpromazine maleate has been recom-

mended, although it may lower the seizure threshold

B. Give diazepam 2.5–20 mg IV as needed.

C. Give barbiturates IV to effect. *Caution:* They may worsen poststimulant CNS depression.

III. Hasten elimination of amphetamine by acidifying urine with 100–200 mg NH$_4$Cl/kg/day PO divided QID.

IV. Give supportive care. Cold-water baths may be necessary for severe hyperthermia, but they must be used with caution, as hypothermia may follow.

ETHANOL (ETHYL ALCOHOL)

Source

I. Wine, beer, mixed drinks, and other ethanol-containing beverages

II. Commercial products containing ethanol

Action

I. Ethanol is rapidly absorbed and distributed throughout the body, where it acts as an anesthetic agent by reversibly blocking action potentials of neurons.

II. In dogs, the LD$_{50}$ of 95% ethanol is 5.5–6.6 ml/kg.

III. Doses as low as one-half the LD$_{50}$ can be life-threatening.

Clinical Signs

I. Behavioral changes, including excitability, vocalizing, and incontinence

II. Emesis

III. Ataxia and incoordination

IV. Drowsiness or depression

V. Unconsciousness

VI. Loss of reflexes

VII. Respiratory depression

VIII. Respiratory and cardiac arrest

IX. Death

Treatment

I. Early decontamination
   A. Emetics

B. Gastric lavage with isothermic water

C. Activated charcoal

II. Supportive care

A. Maintain ventilation with respiratory stimulants, oxygen, and mechanical support as needed.

B. Monitor blood acid–base, electrolyte, and fluid balance; lactic acid–containing fluids are contraindicated.

C. Maintain body temperature.

Bibliography

Davis LE: Clinical pharmacology of salicylates. J Am Vet Med Assoc 176:65, 1980

Farkas MC, Farkas JN: Hemolytic anemia due to ingestion of onions in a dog. J Am Anim Hosp Assoc 10:65, 1974

Foor J, Stowe CM: Acute fatal caffeine toxicosis in a dog. J Am Vet Med Assoc 167:379, 1975

Gaunt SD, Baker DC, Green RA: Clinicopathologic evaluation of N-acetylcysteine therapy in acetaminophen toxicosis in the cat. Am J Vet Res 42:1982, 1981

Glauberg A, Blumenthal HP: Chocolate poisoning in the dog. J Am Anim Hosp Assoc 19:246, 1983

Godbold JC, Hawkins BJ, Woodward MG: Acute oral marijuana poisoning in the dog. J Am Vet Med Assoc 175:1101, 1979

Harvey JW, Kornick HP: Phenazopyridine toxicosis in the cat. J Am Vet Med Assoc 169:327, 1976

Hjelle JJ, Grauer GF: Acetaminophen induced toxicity in dogs and cats. J Am Vet Med Assoc 188:742, 1986

Hooser SB, Beasley VR: Methylxanthine poisoning (chocolate and caffeine toxicosis). p. 191. In Kirk RW (ed): Current Veterinary Therapy IX: Small Animal Practice. WB Saunders, Philadelphia, 1986

Kore AM: Toxicology of nonsteroidal antiinflammatory drugs. Vet Clin North Am [Small Anim Pract] 20:419, 1990

Kore AM: Ibuprofen. p. 191. In Kirk RW, Bonagura J (eds): Current Veterinary Therapy XI: Small Animal Practice. WB Saunders, Philadelphia, 1992

Kore AM, Kiesche-Nesselrodt A: Toxicology of household cleaning products and disinfectants. Vet Clin North Am [Small Anim Pract] 20:525, 1990

Lees GE, Polzin DJ, Perman V et al: Idiopathic Heinz body hemolytic anemia in three dogs. J Am Anim Hosp Assoc 15:143, 1979

Oehme FW: Aspirin and acetaminophen. p. 188. In Kirk RW (ed): Current Veterinary Therapy IX: Small Animal Practice. WB Saunders, Philadelphia, 1986

Papich MG: Toxicoses from over-the-counter human drugs. Vet Clin North Am [Small Anim Pract] 20:431, 1990

Stowe CM, Werdin RE, Barnes DM et al: Amphetamine poisoning in dogs. J Am Vet Med Assoc 168:504, 1976

129

Toxic Plants and Zootoxins

Gary D. Osweiler
Thomas L. Carson

GENERAL CONSIDERATIONS

I. Ingestion of plants by cats and dogs occurs fairly frequently.
   A. The incidence appears to increase during winter months, when both plants and pets are likely to be indoors.
   B. Predisposing factors include age (young animals), boredom, change in the environment, behavioral problems, and offering of plants by owners.
II. In some cases, animals do not exhibit clinical signs after ingestion of toxic plants, although vomiting and diarrhea are frequent symptoms.
III. Diagnosis is often difficult unless ingestion is witnessed or plant material is found in the vomitus or gastric contents.
IV. Therapy is usually symptomatic and supportive after cleansing the gastrointestinal (GI) tract to prevent further absorption.
V. Although there is always the potential for serious poisoning, lethal plant toxicoses are seldom reported in small animals.

INSOLUBLE OXALATE-CONTAINING PLANTS

Source

I. *Philodendron* spp.
II. *Dieffenbachia* (dumbcane)
III. *Caladium* spp.
IV. Jack-in-the-pulpit (*Arisaema* spp.)
V. Elephant ears (*Colocasia* spp.)

Action

I. Severe oral and pharyngeal irritation is caused by needle-like crystals of calcium oxalate and proteolytic enzymes.

II. Destruction of small blood vessels often results in hemorrhage.

Clinical Signs

I. Hypersalivation, swelling of tongue and throat, scratching or pawing at lips and face, local necrosis, possible dyspnea
II. Anorexia, vomiting
III. Tongue paralysis (possible)
IV. Renal failure (rarely)

Treatment

I. Induce emesis (unless oral swelling is severe).
II. Perform gastric lavage with activated charcoal.
III. Rinse mouth; cold-pack the lips.
IV. Tracheostomy may be necessary in cases of severe pharyngeal swelling.
V. Steroids and antihistamines may be beneficial.
VI. GI demulcents such as kaolin and activated charcoal may be useful.
VII. Fluid therapy is given to prevent renal failure.

GASTROINTESTINAL IRRITANTS

Source

I. Poinsettia (*Euphorbia* spp.)
II. Mistletoe (*Phoradendron* spp.); may also result in cardiovascular collapse caused by the amines phenylethylamine and tyramine
III. Aloe vera
IV. Crown of thorns (*Euphorbia* spp.)
V. Snow-on-the-mountain (*Euphorbia* spp.)
VI. Azalea (*Rhododendron* spp.)
VII. Bulbs of tulip, daffodil, iris, amaryllis

1284

VIII. Castor bean (*Ricinus communis*)
IX. Rosary pea (*Abrus precatorius*)
X. English ivy (*Hedera helix*)
XI. Daphne (*Daphne mezereum*)
XII. Christmas rose (*Helleborus niger*)
XIII. Holly (*Ilex* spp.)
XIV. Privet (*Ligustrum vulgare*)

Action and Clinical Signs

I. Mainly GI
II. Secondary effects in other organs by some plants
III. Irritation, vesiculation of mucous membranes
IV. Gastroenteritis, abdominal pain
V. Slowed pulse with mistletoe, similar to digitalis intoxication; cardiac arrhythmias

Treatment and Monitoring

I. Begin gastric lavage or emesis to prevent further absorption, followed by activated charcoal and a cathartic.
II. Most GI plant toxicoses respond to oral decontamination (emesis, activated charcoal) accompanied by supportive therapy to compensate for vomiting and diarrhea.
III. Monitoring the electrocardiogram (ECG) may be important in the case of plants that cause cardiovascular toxicosis along with GI signs (see Cardiac Glycosides, Andromedotoxin).
   A. Evaluate serum potassium, as hypokalemia and hyperkalemia can contribute to arrhythmias.
   B. Phenytoin, propranolol, or lidocaine may be useful in controlling ventricular arrhythmias.
IV. Monitor for secondary liver and kidney abnormalities.
V. Administer GI demulcents, such as kaolin.

TAXINE ALKALOID

Source

I. Evergreen shrubs with alternate "two-ranked" (blades of a feather) leaves
   A. English yew (*Taxus baccata*)
   B. Japanese yew (*Taxus cuspidata*)
II. Toxic at 0.1% of body weight
III. Entire plant, except ripe fruit, toxic

Action

I. It depresses cardiac conduction by inhibition of depolarization in cardiac muscle.
II. Heart stops in diastole.

Clinical Signs

I. Trembling, weakness, collapse
II. Dyspnea
III. Bradycardia, asystole

IV. Coma, convulsions, sudden death (leaves or twigs may still be in the animal's mouth)
V. Gastroenteritis with survival for more than 6–8 hours

Treatment

I. Perform gastric lavage or emesis followed by activated charcoal and cathartics. However, because of the rapid absorption of these toxins, removal of GI contents may be ineffective.
II. Give symptomatic and supportive therapy.
III. Atropine, given early, may counteract cardiac depression.

CARDIAC GLYCOSIDES

Source

I. Oleander (*Nerium oleander*)
II. Lily of the valley (*Convallaria majalis*)
III. Foxglove (*Digitalis purpurea*)

Action

Similar to digitalis intoxication, with conduction blockade, arrhythmias, and asystole

Clinical Signs

I. Depression, dizziness, mydriasis, blurred vision
II. Gastroenteritis (common)
   A. Often the first or most obvious sign
   B. Abdominal pain, nausea, vomiting
III. Cardiac arrhythmias
IV. Coma, convulsions
V. Respiratory and cardiac arrest

Treatment and Monitoring

I. Gastric lavage or emesis to prevent further absorption, followed by activated charcoal and sodium sulfate
II. Monitoring of ECG
   A. Evaluate serum potassium, as hypokalemia and hyperkalemia can contribute to arrhythmias.
   B. Phenytoin, propranolol, or lidocaine may be useful in controlling ventricular arrhythmias.
   C. Antidigitalis antibody fragment (FAB) may be needed for severe digitalis glycoside toxicosis. Consult a local pharmacist for sources.
   D. Avoid calcium-containing solutions.
III. Symptomatic and supportive care

NEPHROTOXIC PLANTS

Source

I. Lilies (*Lilium* spp.): Easter lily, tiger lily, Asiatic hybrids
II. Daylily (*Hemerocallis* spp.)

Action

Unknown toxins in the leaves and blooms produce renal tubular necrosis in cats.

Clinical Signs

I. Vomiting within 1–24 hours after ingestion
II. Progressive depression, apprehension, and anorexia over next 12 hours
III. At 12–36 hours after ingestion, polyuria and dehydration, with urine containing tubular epithelial casts, protein, and glucosuria, indicating severe renal damage
IV. Renal failure at 48–96 hours after ingestion

Treatment

I. If recognized <6 hours after ingestion, administration of an emetic, activated charcoal, saline cathartic, and fluid diuresis usually results in a good recovery.
II. If recognized >18 hours after exposure, prognosis is poor, with renal failure and death usually occurring.

SOLUBLE OXALATES

Source

I. Rhubarb (*Rheum* spp.)
II. Beet tops (*Beta vulgaris*)
III. Sorrel (*Oxalis* spp.)
IV. Dock (*Rumex* spp.)

Action

I. Oxalate is absorbed into the bloodstream and chelates calcium.
II. Once filtered by the glomerulus, the calcium oxalate crystals may precipitate and cause renal tubular blockage and necrosis.

Clinical Signs

I. Vomiting and diarrhea
II. Hypocalcemic tetany
III. Calcium oxalate crystalluria
IV. Acute renal failure

Treatment

I. Remove GI contents.
  A. Induce emesis.
  B. Lavage with activated charcoal.
  C. Give calcium hydroxide or calcium gluconate solution PO to precipitate soluble oxalate as calcium salts.
  D. Give sodium sulfate cathartic.
II. Protect the GI tract with demulcents (e.g., kaolin).
III. Give supportive care.
  A. Fluid therapy, especially for renal failure
  B. Diuresis
  C. Calcium solutions IV for hypocalcemia

TOXALBUMINS OR PHYTOTOXINS

Source

I. Castor bean (*Ricinus communis*)
II. Black locust (*Robinia pseudoacacia*)
III. Rosary pea (*Abrus precatorius*)

Action

I. Toxalbumins or phytotoxins are proteolytic enzymes that break down natural proteins.
II. These toxins also act as antigens and can cause agglutination of red blood cells.
III. A dosage of these toxins as small as 0.0001 mg/kg is the minimum lethal dosage for most mammals when injected; however, the oral toxic dosage is much higher, owing to poor GI absorption.
IV. Toxicity is from ingestion of seeds.
V. Toxicity is much greater if the seed coat is broken or seeds are chewed.

Clinical Signs

I. Stomatitis, glossitis
II. GI irritation: vomiting and diarrhea
III. Muscle trembling, ataxia
IV. Kidney damage: hematuria, azotemia, casts in urine sediment

Treatment

I. Remove GI contents with emesis or lavage, followed by activated charcoal and catharsis.
II. Give supportive and symptomatic care.

SOLANACEOUS ALKALOIDS

Source

I. Nightshade (*Solanum nigrum*)
II. Jerusalem cherry (*Solanum pseudocapsicum*)
III. European bittersweet (*Solanum dulcamara*)

Action

I. Solanaceous alkaloids contain a toxic glycoalkaloid that is a poorly absorbed irritant and a central nervous system (CNS) depressant.
II. GI and CNS signs predominate.
III. Some *Solanum* spp. plants also inhibit cholinesterase, leading to signs similar to organophosphate toxicosis.

Clinical Signs

I. Anorexia, salivation
II. Vomiting and diarrhea, sometimes bloody from ulceration
III. Abdominal pain
IV. Listlessness, weakness, muscle trembling, paralysis

Treatment

    I. Remove GI contents with emesis or lavage, followed by activated charcoal and a cathartic.

    II. Give supportive and symptomatic care.

ANDROMEDOTOXIN (GRAYANTOXIN)

Source

    I. Azalea (*Rhododendron* spp.)

    II. Numerous toxin derivatives in various plant parts

      A. Some components are toxic at <1 mg/kg.

      B. Leaves contain approximately 0.025% toxin.

Action

    I. Hypotension

    II. Depression of respiration and CNS

Clinical Signs

    I. Anorexia, depression, weakness

    II. Vomiting, diarrhea

    III. Ataxia

    IV. Bradycardia, hypotension, respiratory depression

    V. CNS depression

Treatment

    I. Remove GI contents with emesis or lavage, followed by activated charcoal and cathartics.

    II. Give supportive care.

      A. Ephedrine sulfate has been used in people with severe depression caused by andromedotoxin.

      B. Atropine may be effective for bradycardia.

CONTACT IRRITANTS

Source

    I. Asparagus fern (*Asparagus* spp.)

    II. Poison ivy, oak, and sumac (*Toxicodendron* spp.)

    III. Nettles: spurge, stinging, and wood (*Urtica* spp.)

    IV. Trumpet creeper or cow itch (*Campsis* spp.)

    V. Giant hogweed (*Heracleum* spp.)

Clinical Signs

    I. Dermatitis

    II. Stomatitis, glossitis

    III. Vomiting

Treatment

    I. Wash skin with copious amounts of warm, soapy water. Protect people involved with therapy from dermal exposure.

    II. Remove GI contents with emesis or lavage, followed by activated charcoal and cathartics.

    III. Apply topical therapy for blisters or ulcerations.

COMMON PLANTS WITH HIGH POTENTIAL FOR TOXICOSIS

See Table 129–1.

MUSHROOMS

Source and Action

    I. *Amanita phalloides*: cholinergic effects with GI and nervous system signs

Table 129–1. *Common Toxic Plants with High Potential for Toxicosis*[a]

Plants Causing Primarily GI Signs

Autumn crocus (*Colchicum autumnale*)
Castor bean (*Ricinus communis*)
Chinaberry tree (*Melia azedarach*)
Christmas rose (*Helleborus niger*)
Daphne (*Daphne mezereum*)
English holly (*Ilex* spp.)
English ivy (*Hedera helix*)
Iris or flag (*Iris* spp.)
Jack-in-the-pulpit (*Arisaema triphyllum*)
Mistletoe (*Phoradendron* spp.)
Narcissus, daffodil, jonquil (*Narcissus* spp.)
Philodendron (*Monstera* and *Philodendron* spp.)
Poinsettia (*Euphorbia pulcherrima*)
Rosary pea or precatory bean (*Abrus precatorius*)
Wisteria (*Wisteria* spp.)

Plants Causing Primarily CNS Signs (Seizures or Abnormal Behaviors)

Angel's trumpet (*Datura* spp.)
Bleeding heart (*Dicentra* spp.)
Moonseed (*Menispermum canadense*)
Morning glory (*Ipomoea purpurea* and *I. tricolor*)

Plants Causing Cardiovascular Signs (Often Preceded or Accompanied by GI Signs)

Azalea (*Rhododendron* spp.)
Lily of the valley (*Convallaria majalis*)
Oleander (*Nerium oleander*)
Yew (*Taxus cuspidata* and *T. baccata*)

Plants Causing Renal Damage

Daylily (*Hemerocallis* spp.)
Lily, including Easter lily, tiger lily (*Lilium* spp.)
Rhubarb (leaves) (*Rheum rhaponticum*)

Plants Causing Nonspecific Signs Involving GI, CNS, and Cardiovascular Systems

Golden chain (*Laburnum anagyroides*)
Yellow jessamine (*Gelsemium semper-virens*)

[a]Toxic potential is based on a combination of toxicity of plant parts and availability and palatability of plants in typical small-animal environments.

II. *Gyromitra* spp.: hemolysis; liver, kidney, and CNS damage
III. *Coprinus atramentarius*: arrhythmias and hypotension
IV. *Inocybe* and *Clitocybe* spp.: cholinergic effects

Clinical Signs

I. Muscarinic signs
   A. Hypersalivation
   B. Vomiting and diarrhea, often with mucus and blood 6–24 hours after digestion
II. Ataxia, paralysis, coma
III. Liver and kidney damage (*Amanita phalloides* toxicosis)
   A. Icterus, azotemia 8–12 hours after acute hemorrhagic gastroenteritis
   B. May be delayed; usually very serious or lethal
IV. Psychotic effects
   Ibotenic acid, muscimol, and psilocybin can cause euphoria, hallucinations, and other CNS effects in people.

Treatment and Monitoring

I. Perform emesis and gastric lavage with 1:2000 potassium permanganate or activated charcoal, followed by cathartics.
II. Physostigmine has been recommended for muscarinic mushrooms, but efficacy is questionable. If used, dosage is 0.02 mg/kg IM BID.
III. Propranolol has been used to treat cardiac arrhythmias.
IV. Penicillin may reduce toxin uptake by the liver.
V. Give symptomatic and supportive therapy, and monitor liver function.

BLUE-GREEN ALGAE

Source

I. *Microcystis aeruginosa, Anabaena flos-aquae,* and *Aphanizomenon flos-aquae* are the most common sources.
II. Algae blooms on lakes or ponds in the upper midwestern United States and Canada during hot, dry, summer weather.
III. Pets ingest the endotoxin when they drink pond water.

Action

I. Anatoxin-a is a fast-acting depolarizing neurotoxin.
II. Anatoxin-s is an anticholinesterase agent.
III. Microcystin is a cyclic peptide toxin that is hepatotoxic.
IV. Lipopolysaccharides (endotoxin) in cell walls may contribute to signs.

Clinical Signs

I. Rapid onset within 15–45 minutes of ingestion (anatoxin-a)

   A. Rigidity, muscle tremors
   B. Paralysis, cyanosis
   C. Occasional seizures
II. Nausea, vomiting, diarrhea, abdominal pain (microcystin)
III. Death, frequently within 1–2 hours of ingestion, caused by the "fast death factor," which is a cyclic polypeptide

Treatment

I. Remove GI contents with emesis or lavage, followed by activated charcoal and cathartics.
II. Give symptomatic and supportive care only.
III. Surviving animals may have liver damage.

TOAD POISONING

Source

I. Colorado River toad (*Bufo alvarius*) is a potential source.
II. Marine toad (*Bufor marinus*) is the most toxic and dangerous.
III. Most toxic varieties are located in the desert in the southwestern and southeastern United States and Hawaii.
IV. Evening, night, and early morning are the most frequent times for exposure, and dogs are most commonly exposed when they attack and mouth toads.

Action

I. Toxins secreted by the parotid glands contain catecholamines, indole alkyl amines, and cardiac glycosides.
II. Toxins affect the parasympathetic nervous system and heart.

Clinical Signs

I. Profuse hypersalivation and oral pain with pawing at the mouth are immediate signs.
II. Excitement and vocalization are common.
III. Buccal mucous membranes may be brick red, and dyspnea can be prominent.
IV. Marked cardiac ventricular arrhythmia can be followed by seizures and/or collapse.
V. Hyperthermia may occur and predispose dogs to secondary heatstroke.
VI. Serum potassium may be elevated.

Treatment

I. Decontaminate the oral cavity by flushing the mouth with large amounts of water.
II. Control hyperthermia with cool-water baths.
III. Some toad intoxications can be fatal, and rapid evaluation of cardiovascular function is important to survival.
IV. Begin therapy for secondary heatstroke (see Chap. 134).

V. Atropine 0.05 mg/kg IM, SQ controls salivation and helps prevent aspiration. It is also useful for bradycardia, heart block, or other digitalis-like effects.

VI. Administration of propranolol 2.5 mg/kg IV, PO may be used for cardiac arrhythmias.

PIT VIPERS

Source

I. Pit vipers include the following species.
  A. *Crotalus* spp.: rattlesnakes
  B. *Sistrurus* spp.: pygmy rattlesnakes, massasaugas
  C. *Agkistrodon* spp.: copperheads, cottonmouth water moccasins

II. A triangular head with a ''pit'' between the eye and nostril, as well as elliptical pupils, are characteristics of pit vipers.

III. In addition, rattlesnakes have dry rings at the tail, which provide an audible ''rattle'' when the snake is in an attack or defensive posture.

IV. Rattlesnake venoms are generally more toxic than those of water moccasins or copperheads.

Action

I. A variety of proteolytic enzymes, coagulation factors, phospholipases, and neurotoxins are present in pit viper venoms.

II. Tissue destruction, impaired blood coagulation, cardiovascular collapse, edema, shock, weakness, and respiratory depression result from the combination of toxins in the venom.

Clinical Signs

I. Nearly immediate pain at the site of the bite is the first clinical response.

II. Examination reveals puncture wounds, local tissue swelling, and hemorrhage.

III. Petechial and ecchymotic hemorrhages develop in tissues and mucous membranes.

IV. Shock, hypotension, tachycardia, and shallow respiration develop quickly.

V. Nausea and excessive salivation are typical secondary responses.

Diagnosis

I. Laboratory findings include hemoconcentration, thrombocytopenia, hypokalemia, and elevated serum creatine kinase.

II. Prolonged activated clotting, prothrombin, and partial thromboplastin times occur, and fibrin split products develop.

III. Urinalysis may reveal elevated hemoglobin and myoglobin owing to hemolysis and rhabdomyolysis.

IV. The ECG may show ventricular arrhythmias.

Treatment

I. Treat as a true emergency: first aid is limited to calming the animal and providing rapid transport to a veterinarian.

II. Administer antivenin (Crotalidae Polyvalent, equine origin, Ft. Dodge, or Wyeth) by slow IV infusion, with careful monitoring for possible allergic reactions. Diphenhydramine can be used to counteract allergic reactions.

III. Cautions in the treatment of pit viper bites include the following.
  A. Incision and suction are not usually recommended.
  B. Corticosteroids are not recommended.
  C. Heparin may be indicated for disseminated intravascular coagulation.

Bibliography

Clay BR: Poisoning and injury by plants. p. 179. In Kirk RW (ed): Current Veterinary Therapy VI. WB Saunders, Philadelphia, 1977

Ellenhorn MJ, Barceloux DG: Plants—mycotoxins—mushrooms. p. 1209. In: Medical Toxicology: Diagnosis and Treatment of Human Poisoning. Elsevier, New York, 1988

Fowler ME: Plant Poisoning in Small Companion Animals. Ralston Purina, St. Louis, 1981

Garland T, Bailey EM: Toxic ornamental and garden plants. p. 217. In Bonagura JD (ed): Kirk's Current Veterinary Therapy XII. WB Saunders, Philadelphia, 1995

Meerdink G, Peterson ME: Venomous bites and stings. p. 175. In Kirk RW (ed): Current Veterinary Therapy X: Small Animal Practice. WB Saunders, Philadelphia, 1989

Ruhr LP: Ornamental toxic plants. p. 216. In Kirk RW (ed): Current Veterinary Therapy IX: Small Animal Practice. WB Saunders, Philadelphia, 1986

Spoerke D, Evans B, Linaburg B: The Hidden Hazards in House and Garden Plants. Pictorial Histories Publishing Co., Missoula, MT, 1991

Stephans HA: Poisonous Plants of the Central United States. Regents Press of Kansas, Lawrence, 1980

Stowe CM, Fangmann G: Schefflera toxicosis in a dog. J Am Vet Med Assoc 167:74, 1975

130

Adverse Drug Reactions

Gary D. Osweiler
Thomas L. Carson

Definition

I. Adverse drug reactions are defined as noxious reactions to normal doses of common therapeutic drugs.
II. These reactions may also result from excessive drug use or failure to establish a specific therapeutic dosage range or end point.
III. Idiosyncrasies in the metabolism of individual animals may also be involved.
IV. Drug interactions and incompatibilities may also occur.
V. Concurrent diseases (e.g., abnormal liver or kidney function) can be a factor.
VI. For a more complete list of certain adverse drug reactions, see Aronson and Riviere, 1983, 1986; Madewell and Simonson, 1989.

Causes in Dogs

I. Analgesics
   A. Acetaminophen: methemoglobinemia, liver necrosis
   B. Aspirin: bleeding disorders, gastric irritation and/or ulceration
   C. Phenylbutazone: anemia, leukopenia, thrombocytopenia, emesis, bleeding disorders, enteritis, elevated liver enzymes, gastric irritation
II. Central nervous system (CNS) depressants
   A. Acetylpromazine: atypical behavior, aggression, prolonged action, injection site pain, cardiac effects, urination, defecation, hypotension, hypothermia, potentiation of seizures, interference with ovulation
   B. Fentanyl-droperidol: atypical behavior, aggression, hyperthermia, seizures, cardiac effects, respiratory effects
   C. Halothane: cardiac effects, hyperthermia, nystagmus, torticollis, emesis, hepatitis
   D. Ketamine: seizures, cardiac arrest, ineffective anesthesia, death
   E. Lidocaine: facial and laryngeal edema, seizures, tremors, ataxia

F. Methoxyflurane: cardiac arrest, delayed hepatic damage, renal damage
   G. Oxymorphone: bradycardia, tachypnea, vomiting, diarrhea
   H. Thiamylal: cardiac and respiratory arrest, prolonged action, ventricular arrhythmias, sinus bradycardia
   I. Thiopental: cardiac arrest, perivascular damage, prolonged recovery, pulmonary edema
   J. Tiletamine and zolazepam: vocalization, seizures, hyperactivity, hypersalivation, cyanosis, prolonged recovery, ataxia, death
   K. Xylazine: aggression, bradycardia, cardiac arrest, vomiting
III. Anticonvulsants
   A. Phenytoin: hepatic damage, emesis, leukopenia, ataxia, gingival hyperplasia, death
   B. Primidone: hepatic damage, polydipsia, polyuria, alopecia, emesis, death
IV. Antiparasitics
   A. Amitraz: lethargy, depression, recumbency, paddling, ataxia, seizures, death
   B. Arecoline: mydriasis, ataxia, diarrhea, abdominal pain, inability to walk
   C. Bunamidine: dyspnea, ataxia, gastroenteritis, seizures, death
   D. Butamisole: dyspnea, tremors, ataxia, collapse, injection site pain
   E. Dichlorophene-toluene: ataxia, seizures, mydriasis, death
   F. Dichlorvos: gastroenteritis, ataxia, tremors, organophosphate toxicity, death
   G. Diethylcarbamazine (DEC): anaphylactoid reactions, gastroenteritis, death
   H. DEC-oxibendazole: hepatotoxicity, vomiting, diarrhea, anorexia, lethargy, death
   I. DEC-styrylpyridinium: gastroenteritis, sterilization, teratogenesis, thrombocytopenia, death
   J. Disophenol (DNP): hyperthermia, respiratory effects, injection site reaction, staining of hair coat, collapse, death
   K. Dithiazanine iodide: gastroenteritis, depression,

apprehension, fever, diarrhea, discoloration of feces that stains carpet
  L. Fenbendazole: depression, vomiting, icterus, hepatoxicity
  M. Ivermectin: anorexia, vomiting, diarrhea, depression, ataxia, seizures
  N. Levamisole: emesis, dyspnea, pulmonary edema, neurologic disorders, skin eruptions
  O. Mebendazole: emesis, hepatic damage
  P. Metronidazole: lethargy, weakness, peripheral neuropathy
  Q. Piperazine: paralysis, death
  R. Pyrantel pamoate: emesis
  S. Thiacetarsamide: emesis, liver and kidney damage, perivascular damage, bleeding disorders, death
  T. Trichlorfon: weakness, lethargy
V. Hormones
  A. Dexamethasone: polydipsia, polyuria, hemorrhagic gastroenteritis, tachypnea, osteoporosis, infertility, hepatopathy, adrenal suppression
  B. Estradiol cypionate: bone marrow suppression, pyometra, injection site pain, cystic endometrial hyperplasia
  C. Megestrol acetate: polyphagia, uterine disorders, depression, diabetes mellitus, death
  D. Mibolerone: abnormal behavior, vaginal discharge, liver damage, urinary incontinence, clitoral hypertrophy
  E. Prednisolone: polydipsia, polyuria, polyphagia, hepatopathy, anemia, iatrogenic hypercortisolism, adrenal suppression
  F. Triamcinolone: hypercortisolism, depression, emesis, muscle wasting, alopecia, adrenal suppression
VI. Antibiotics/antibacterials
  A. Amoxicillin: skin rash, emesis
  B. Amphotericin B: renal damage, perivascular irritation, hypokalemia, gastrointestinal irritation
  C. Ampicillin: skin wheals, gastroenteritis
  D. Cephalexin: salivation, tachypnea, excitability
  E. Cephaloridine: proximal tubular nephrotoxicity
  F. Cephalothin: injection irritation
  G. Chloramphenicol: depression, gastroenteritis, ataxia, bone marrow depression, depression of microsomal enzymes, death
  H. Clindamycin: vomiting, hematemesis and other evidence of bleeding, elevated serum alkaline phosphatase
  I. Erythromycin: emesis
  J. Gentamicin: facial edema, injection site inflammation, renal tubular damage (especially when used in conjunction with furosemide), ototoxicity, neuromuscular blockade
  K. Hetacillin: emesis
  L. Lincomycin: gastroenteritis, shock after IM injection
  M. Potassium penicillin G: tachypnea, tachycardia
  N. Procaine penicillin G: ataxia, dyspnea, edema
  O. Sulfasalazine: keratoconjunctivitis sicca, allergic dermatitis, emesis, cholestatic jaundice, decreased sperm counts

  P. Tetracycline: emesis, hepatotoxicity, dental staining in immature animals
  Q. Trimethoprim-sulfadiazine: keratoconjunctivitis sicca, gastroenteritis, polyarthritis, pustular dermatitis, erythema multiforme, blood dyscrasias, hepatic necrosis
VII. Miscellaneous
  A. Aminophylline: excitability, emesis, polyphagia, polydipsia, polyuria
  B. Atropine: paradoxic bradycardia, heart block
  C. Digoxin: emesis, anorexia, arrhythmias, diarrhea
  D. Theophylline: diarrhea

Causes in Cats

I. Analgesics
  A. Acetaminophen: prolonged half-life; depression, methemoglobinemia, anemia, hematuria, death
  B. Aspirin: prolonged half-life; depression, excitability, tachypnea, bone marrow suppression, anemia, gastritis, death
  C. Phenylbutazone: anorexia, weight loss, severe depression, emesis, death
II. CNS depressants
  A. Acetylpromazine: prolonged half-life; cardiac arrest, hyperactivity, seizures, death
  B. Halothane: cardiac arrest, apnea
  C. Ketamine: prolonged half-life/ineffective recovery; behavioral changes, seizures, tremors, liver and kidney damage, pulmonary edema, apnea, cardiac arrest, death
  D. Methoxyflurane: ataxia, death
  E. Thiamylal: prolonged half-life; cardiac and respiratory arrest, ataxia, arrhythmias, death
  F. Xylazine: prolonged half-life; apnea, seizures
III. Antiparasitic agents
  A. Bunamidine: seizures, hypersalivation, pulmonary edema, sudden death
  B. Dichlorophene-toluene: ataxia, tremors, seizures, tachycardia, hypersalivation, death
  C. Dichlorvos: organophosphate toxicity, death
  D. Levamisole: salivation, gastroenteritis, excitement, mydriasis
  E. N-butylchloride: hyperactivity, vocalization, vomiting
  F. Niclosamide: depression, ataxia, hypothermia
  G. Piperazine: emesis, dementia, ataxia, salivation
IV. Hormones
  A. Medroxyprogesterone acetate: hair color change over injection site
  B. Megestrol acetate: adrenal suppression, polyphagia, uterine and mammary disorders, diabetes mellitus
  C. Triamcinolone: nervousness, disorientation, salivation, syncope, hypercortisolism, adrenal suppression
V. Antibacterials/antifungals
  A. Amoxicillin: emesis, injection site pain, ataxia, nystagmus, urticaria
  B. Amphotericin B: renal damage after a single dose
  C. Ampicillin: diarrhea
  D. Cephalexin: emesis, fever

E. Chloramphenicol: prolonged half-life; anaphylactoid-like reactions, anorexia, gastroenteritis, ataxia, neutropenia, bone marrow suppression, death

F. Gentamicin: pruritus, alopecia, erythema, renal damage, ototoxicity

G. Griseofulvin: bone marrow suppression

H. Lincomycin: gastroenteritis, shock after IM injection

I. Miconazole: erythema, alopecia

J. Procaine penicillin–dihydrostreptomycin: ataxia

K. Tetracycline: fever, malignant hyperthermia, emesis

L. Trimethoprim-sulfadiazine: salivation, emesis, mydriasis, ataxia, seizures

VI. Miscellaneous

A. Bethanechol: emesis, tenesmus

B. Digoxin: anorexia, emesis, diarrhea

C. Morphine: excitement

D. Phosphate-containing urinary acidifiers: hyperphosphatemia, azotemia, acidosis

Bibliography

Aronson AL, Riviere JE: Adverse drug reactions. p. 122. In Kirk RW (ed): Current Veterinary Therapy VIII. WB Saunders, Philadelphia, 1983

Aronson AL, Riviere JE: Adverse drug reactions. p. 169. In Kirk RW (ed): Current Veterinary Therapy IX: Small Animal Practice. WB Saunders, Philadelphia, 1986

CVM Annual Report of Adverse Drug Reactions—1989. FDA Veterinarian. Vol V, p. I-1 and Vol VI, p. I-13. Center for Veterinary Medicine, Food and Drug Administration, Rockville, MD, 1990

Davis LE: Clinical management of adverse drug reactions. p. 176. In Kirk RW (ed): Current Veterinary Therapy IX: Small Animal Practice. WB Saunders, Philadelphia, 1986

Dodds WJ: Sulfonamides and blood dyscrasias. J Am Vet Med Assoc 196:681, 1990

Madewell BR, Simonson ER: Special considerations in drug preparation and administration. p. 475. In Kirk RW (ed): Current Veterinary Therapy X: Small Animal Practice. WB Saunders, Philadelphia, 1989

Talbot RB (ed): Veterinary Pharmaceuticals and Biologicals 1991/92. Veterinary Medicine Publishing, Lenexa, KS, 1990

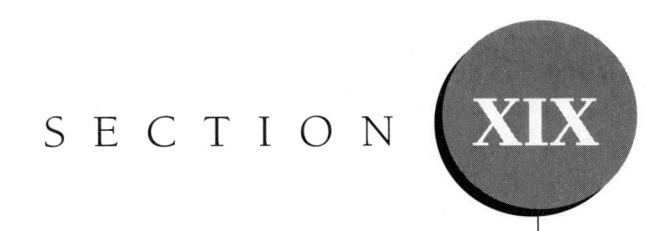

Environmental Injuries

131

Introduction to Critical Care

Alicia M. Faggella

TRIAGE AND PRIMARY SURVEY

Definition

I. Triage is a system of examination and rapid classification of emergency cases by the urgency with which treatment is required.
II. Classifications include stable, potentially unstable, and unstable.
III. Primary survey is the initial assessment of an animal for life-threatening conditions.

Priorities

I. Airway, respiratory system
   A. Keep airway clear, extend head, pull tongue forward if necessary.
   B. Assess respiratory rate, depth, rhythm, and effort.
   C. Auscultate, percuss thorax, inspect thoracic wall for trauma.
   D. Check mucous membrane color: absence of cyanosis does not assure normal lung function.
   E. Check pulse oximetry for oxygen saturation.
II. Cardiovascular system
   A. Evaluate heart rate and rhythm.
   B. Assess pulse rate, rhythm, and quality simultaneously with cardiac auscultation.
   C. Control major hemorrhage.
III. Other systems
   A. All life-threatening emergencies of the respiratory or cardiovascular system are treated before completion of the physical examination.
   B. Then a complete systematic physical examination is performed (see Chap. 1).

GOALS OF RESUSCITATION

Ventilation

I. If the animal cannot adequately ventilate, establish an airway via endotracheal tube or tracheostomy as needed.
II. Provide supplemental oxygen.
   Goal is Pa_{O_2} >70 mmHg and Pa_{CO_2} of 35–45 mmHg.
III. Correct underlying problem if possible.

Cardiovascular and Circulatory Support

I. Maintain effective circulating blood volume.
   Establish IV access through a central line to allow rapid fluid administration and measurement of central venous pressure.
II. Correct life-threatening cardiac dysrhythmias (see Chap. 7).
III. Prevent or reverse shock.
IV. Prevent or attenuate the systemic inflammatory response syndrome (SIRS), which may lead to multiple organ dysfunction syndrome (MODS).

SHOCK, SIRS, MODS

Definition

I. Shock is a multifactorial syndrome that results in failure of the microcirculation caused by maldistribution and inadequate blood flow.
   A. Microcirculatory failure resulting in decreased oxygen delivery ($\dot{D}_{O_2}$) to the tissues
   B. Also decreased tissue oxygen consumption ($\dot{V}_{O_2}$), causing tissue hypoxia, increased oxygen debt, cellular injury, and death (Shoemaker, 1995)

II. SIRS
  A. SIRS is the widespread inflammatory response of the body to a variety of inciting causes, including trauma, ischemia, sepsis, infection, and immune-mediated disease (Bone et al., 1992).
  B. In animals, two or more of the following must be present (Kirby, 1995).
    1. Temperature <100°F or >103.5°F
    2. Heart rate >160 beats/min (dog); >250 beats/min (cat)
    3. Respiratory rate >20 breaths/minute or Pa_{CO_2} <32 mmHg
    4. White blood cell count >12,000, <4000, or >10% bands
III. MODS
  A. MODS is altered function in more than one organ, such that homeostasis cannot be maintained without therapeutic intervention (Kirby, 1995).
  B. The organ insult may be primary or secondary.

Classification of Shock

  I. Hypovolemic
    A. Exogenous fluid loss: blood loss, vomiting and diarrhea, massive burns
    B. Endogenous: anaphylaxis
  II. Obstructive
    A. Aortic embolism
    B. Caval syndrome of heartworm disease
    C. Pericardial tamponade
  III. Cardiogenic
    A. Congestive heart failure, cardiomyopathy
    B. Dysrhythmias
  IV. Distributive
    A. Low resistance: arterial-venous shunting or failure to exchange oxygen in capillaries
      1. Peritonitis
      2. Pneumonia
      3. Sepsis
    B. High resistance: sequestering of blood in veins caused by increased capacity of the venous intravascular space, systemic resistance normal to increased
      1. Endotoxemia, early sepsis
      2. Anesthetic overdose
      3. Surgical trauma
  V. Classification schemes possibly misleading, as more than one process may be present

Pathophysiology

  I. Circulatory insult causes compensatory responses in cardiopulmonary function, which are mediated via neurohormonal pathways.
  II. End result is a maldistribution of cardiac output (which may be normal, decreased, or increased) between and within organs and at the microcirculatory level.
  III. Oxygen delivery and consumption are inadequate.
  IV. Cellular hypoxia, increased oxygen debt, anaerobic metabolism, and buildup of lactic acid and other toxic metabolites cause continued cell injury and death.
  V. Death occurs after activation of the complement and the arachidonic acid cascade systems; release of histamine, bradykinins, and serotonin; and production of free radicals with decreased integrity of the reticuloendothelial system and continued intravascular fluid loss.

Treatment

  I. Fluid therapy (Table 131–1).
    A. Administer restricted volumes in shock caused by cardiac failure.
    B. Aggressive fluid therapy is required for other kinds of shock.
    C. Numerous choices of fluids are available.
      1. Crystalloids: ionized substances capable of passing through a semipermeable membrane
      2. Colloids: solutions that contain particles not capable of crossing membranes; exert an oncotic effect
      3. Blood products (see Chap. 69)
    D. Realize that there is a distinction between total body water, plasma volume, extracellular fluid volume, and the intracellular fluid volume.
      1. The goal is to increase the plasma volume.
      2. An animal with pulmonary or peripheral edema may still have a contracted vascular volume and require aggressive fluid therapy.
  II. Inotropic support, after volume loading
    A. Dobutamine: dog, 2–10 μg/kg/min IV infusion to effect; cat, 0.5–3 μg/kg/min IV infusion to effect
    B. Dopamine 2–5 μg/kg/min IV infusion
  III. Vasopressors
    A. Administered for persistently low peripheral vascular resistance and low blood pressure
    B. Dopamine 10–20 μg/kg/min IV infusion (predominantly α-adrenergic vasoconstriction at this dosage)
    C. Methoxamine 0.1–0.2 mg/kg IV
    D. Phenylephrine 0.13 mg/kg IV
  IV. Oxygen supplementation: nasal oxygen catheter, oxygen cage, face mask, oxygen hood, oxygen blanket
  V. Antibiotics for septic shock
  VI. Corticosteroids for early septic, hypovolemic shock
    A. Dexamethasone sodium phosphate 3–4 mg/kg IV once
    B. Prednisolone sodium succinate 11 mg/kg IV once
    C. Methylprednisolone sodium succinate 30 mg/kg IV once
  VII. Nonsteroidal anti-inflammatory drugs (Hardie, 1992)
    A. Possibly beneficial when given in first 2 hours of septic shock
    B. Flunixin meglumine: dog, 1 mg/kg IV once; cat, 0.5 mg/kg IV once
  VIII. Gastrointestinal protectants
    A. Decreases risk of ulceration
    B. Sucralfate (Carafate)
      1. Dog: 1 g/25 kg PO TID-QID
      2. Cat: 250–500 mg PO TID
  IX. Sodium bicarbonate

Table 131–1. **Comparison of Fluid Therapies in Shock**

Fluid Type	IV Dosage	Indications for Use	Benefits	Potential Complications	Miscellaneous Data
Isotonic crystalloids Lactated Ringer's (LRS) Normal saline solution	Initial dog: 40–90 ml/kg Initial cat: 20–60 ml/kg	Intravascular volume expansion	Readily available Inexpensive Easy to use Help correct electrolyte imbalances	Dilutional anemia Hypoproteinemia Pulmonary/peripheral edema Stay in intravascular space only a short time	Lactate in LRS does not potentiate lactic acidemia
Hypertonic crystalloids Hypertonic saline (3%, 7%)	3%: 5–20 ml/kg 7%: 4–8 ml/kg Infusion: 1 ml/kg/min	Intravascular volume expansion	Small volume required Rapid improvement of cardiovascular function Positive inotropic effect	Reflex bradycardia, hypotension Potential hypokalemia, hypernatremia	Contraindicated in hyperosmolar or hypernatremic states, heart failure, dehydration
Colloids Dextrans 40, 70	10–20 ml/kg/day Infusion: 2 ml/kg/h	Intravascular volume expansion Promotion of peripheral blood flow	Small volume required Osmotically active Holds fluid in vascular space Remains in vascular space longer than crystalloids Volume expansion may persist for 4–8 h Protentiates microcirculatory blood flow—coats endothelial surfaces Reduces incidence of thromboembolism	May decrease platelet function Renal failure possible if animal is oliguric and hypovolemia not corrected, owing to renal tubular obstruction Anaphylaxis (rare) Osmotic diuresis May interfere with cross-matching of blood May temporarily decrease immune competence Relatively expensive	Contraindicated in thrombocytopenia, oliguric or anuric renal failure, heart failure
Dextran 70 + hypertonic saline (3%, 7%)	4 ml/kg over 5–10 min	Intravascular volume expansion in hypovolemic and septic shock	Longer dwell time in intravascular space than hypertonic saline alone Other benefits as listed above	As above for hypertonic saline, dextrans	As above for hypertonic saline, dextrans
Hydroxyethyl starch (Hetastarch)	20 ml/kg/day	Intravascular volume expansion	Small volume needed Remains in intravascular space longer than crystalloids Osmotically active	Expensive Rarely: anaphylaxis Rarely: coagulopathy at high doses (>20 ml/kg/day) Pulmonary edema if volume overload occurs	Increases serum amylase but does not alter pancreatic function
VetaPlasma (Marshalton Veterinary Group)	5 ml/kg every 4–6 h PRN Infusion: 2–4 ml/min	Intravascular volume expansion Hypoproteinemia	Remains in vascular space longer than crystalloids Less coating of platelets than dextrans Can be repeated frequently	Relatively expensive Do not use in dehydrated animal.	Approved for use in dog and cat
Blood products (see Chap. 69)				Osmotic diuresis	

A. Administration is based on blood gas analysis. Calculate need: mEq needed = 0.3 × body weight (kg) × base deficit.

B. Replace one-fourth to one-third calculated deficit over 15–20 minutes, and an equal volume over 6–8 hours.

C. Use with caution when metabolic acidosis is accompanied by respiratory acidosis.

X. Energy substrates (Crowe et al., 1996)

A. Controversial but may be helpful in septic shock or prolonged shock of other etiologies

B. Glucose 0.3 g/kg/h IV followed by regular insulin 0.3 U/kg/h and KCl 0.2 mEq/kg/h IV

C. Experimental: secondary or intermediate energy substrates (e.g., fructose 1,6 diphosphate)

XI. Glucose: keep serum glucose between 100 and 180 mg/dl

XII. Nutrition

A. Start within 12–24 hours.

B. Use enteral route whenever possible.

XIII. Analgesics: for trauma or painful metabolic conditions

Patient Monitoring

I. Parameters such as heart rate and rhythm, respiratory rate, blood pressure, temperature, and urine output are not sensitive indicators of circulatory function (see Appendix I).
   A. Changes in their values do not occur early enough in shock to provide good warning of circulatory failure.
   B. In striving to return these variables to "normal," complete decompensation of the animal may occur.

II. The best parameters to monitor are those related to oxygen delivery and consumption.
   A. Hematocrit/hemoglobin (reflects oxygen binding capacity)
   B. Arterial and venous blood gases
   C. Arterial oxygen saturation
   D. Central venous pressure
   E. Blood lactate

III. Monitor return of perfusion.
   A. Kidneys: urine output
   B. Nervous system: mentation
   C. Liver: bilirubin
   D. Peripheral circulation: capillary refill time, warmth of extremities

IV. Best predictors of survival are the oxygen transport variables, especially $\dot{D}O_2$ and $\dot{V}O_2$ (Shoemaker, 1995).

Bibliography

Bone RD, Sprung CL, Sibbald WJ: Definitions for sepsis and organ failure. Crit Care Med 20:724, 1992

Crowe DT, Devey J, Reinhart GA et al: Metabolic demands and their management in the severe septic peritonitis patient. Proc ACVECC Postgraduate Course 1:9, 1996

Hardie EM: Sepsis vs. septic shock. p. 176. In Murtaugh RJ, Kaplan PM (eds): Veterinary Emergency and Critical Care Medicine. Mosby Yearbook, St. Louis, 1992

Kirby R: Septic shock. p. 139. In Bonagura JD (ed): Kirk's Current Veterinary Therapy XII: Small Animal Practice. WB Saunders, Philadelphia, 1995

Shoemaker WC: Diagnosis and treatment of the shock syndromes. p. 85. In Shoemaker WC, Ayres SM, Grenvik A et al (eds): Textbook of Critical Care. 3rd Ed. WB Saunders, Philadelphia, 1995

132

Electric Cord and Smoke Inhalation Injuries

Alicia M. Faggella

ELECTRIC CORD INJURY

Definition and Causes

I. Electric cord injury usually results from chewing on a live wire of a household appliance (usually 120 V).
II. It is most often seen in puppies and kittens.

Pathophysiology

I. Electrical current causes thermal injury as it passes through the tissues from the generation of heat.
   A. Coagulation necrosis happens at the points of highest thermal intensity (point of entry).
   B. As the current travels over a wider surface area, the intensity dissipates.
II. Electrical current alters the electrophysical patterns of organ systems, resulting in seizures, dysrhythmias, ventricular fibrillation, or cardiopulmonary arrest.
III. Neurogenic changes result in pulmonary edema.
IV. Bowel infarction or ileus causes signs of acute abdomen.

Clinical Signs

I. Vary according to current intensity, duration of exposure, and pathway of current through the body
II. Oral and cutaneous burns
   A. Often at commissures of the lips
   B. Pale yellow, tan, or gray, well-circumscribed lesions
   C. ± Copper deposits at site
III. Respiratory distress
   A. Tachypnea
   B. Orthopnea
   C. ± Cyanosis
   D. May progress to apnea
IV. Muscle spasms
V. Generalized seizures
VI. Vomiting, abdominal pain
VII. Cardiac arrest

Diagnosis

I. History
   A. The injury is not often witnessed.
   B. Respiratory distress with or without collapse in a young animal raises the index of suspicion.
II. Physical examination
   A. Burns or erosions to mouth, tongue, and lips, especially the commissures
   B. Cutaneous burns
   C. Pulmonary rales, crackles
III. Radiography
   A. May be normal
   B. Usually pulmonary edema with interstitial or alveolar pattern
   C. Air bronchograms most commonly seen in diaphragmatic lobes first
   D. May progress to other lung fields
IV. ± Ventricular dysrhythmias
V. Biochemistry, hemogram: generally unremarkable

Differential Diagnosis

I. Other causes of oral burns or erosions
   A. Chemical
   B. Metabolic
II. Other causes of alveolar lung pattern on radiographs
   A. Heart failure
   B. Hemorrhage
   C. Infection

Treatment

I. First aid at site
   A. Shut off electricity.
   B. Unplug cord and remove animal.
   C. If it is not breathing, administer mouth-to-nose resuscitation.
II. Clearance of airway
   A. Suction any mucus or vomitus.
   B. Check for airway obstruction from oropharyngeal or laryngeal edema.
   C. Intubate if the animal is unconscious or the airway is compromised.
III. Ventilation
   A. If the animal is not breathing well or is unconscious, provide mechanical ventilatory support.
   B. Administer 100% oxygen initially.
   C. Wean to lowest supplementation possible to support oxygenation.
IV. Intravenous fluids
   A. Use with caution to avoid further pulmonary edema.
   B. Base fluid therapy on degree of existing shock.
   C. Consider colloids for volume expansion to maintain oncotic pressure and decrease chance of aggravating edema.
V. Diuretics for pulmonary edema
   A. Dog: furosemide 2–4 mg/kg IV TID-QID
   B. Cat: furosemide 0.5–2 mg/kg IV TID
VI. Bronchodilators
   A. Give terbutaline 0.01 mg/kg SQ TID-QID.
   B. Give aminophylline as follows.
      1. Dog: 6–11 mg/kg IV TID
      2. Cat: 4 mg/kg IM BID
   C. Do not use both together.
VII. Corticosteroids
   Steroids increase the risk of infection and are not indicated.
VIII. Treatment of oral and cutaneous burns (see Chap. 133)

Patient Monitoring

I. Watch for delayed onset of respiratory signs (up to 48 hours).
II. Monitor vital signs, and auscultate lung fields.
III. Consider using pulse oximetry to assess oxygen saturation and the need for mechanical ventilation. Maintain oxygen saturation at $\geq$90%.
IV. Measure arterial blood gases every 1–4 hours.
   A. Use for severe respiratory involvement to monitor need for ventilation.
   B. Titrate oxygen therapy to maintain Pa_{O_2} >70 mmHg.
V. Continuously monitor the electrocardiogram for the initial 48 hours to watch for ventricular dysrhythmias.
VI. Radiograph the lungs every 24–48 hours until all changes resolve.

SMOKE INHALATION

Definition and Causes

I. Smoke inhalation injury is an insult to the airways or lung parenchyma caused by exposure to smoke and by-products of combustion.
II. Smoke inhalation injuries may be the result of the following.
   A. Thermal injury
   B. Simple asphyxia
      Oxygen is consumed in fires, decreasing the available oxygen (FI_{O_2} <21%) content for breathing.
   C. Chemical injury
      1. Carbon monoxide
      2. Hydrogen cyanide
      3. Acrolein
   D. Inhalation of particulate matter
III. Tissue damage and decreased pulmonary defense mechanisms are caused primarily by the chemical injury, not the heat.

Pathophysiology

I. Thermal injury
   A. Usually restricted to upper airway
      1. Air exchange mechanism cools air prior to reaching the lungs.
      2. Dry air has low heat-carrying capacity.
      3. Steam heat has 4000 times the heat-carrying capacity, and may damage the entire pulmonary tree.
   B. May cause edema and sloughing of mucosa
   C. $\pm$ Secondary upper airway obstruction
II. Chemical injury
   A. A variety of chemical by-products are contained in smoke.
   B. Carbon monoxide (CO) is a by-product of combustion of carbon-containing compounds (e.g., wood).
      1. Interferes with oxygen uptake and delivery rather than causing direct lung injury
      2. Binds preferentially to hemoglobin (250 times greater affinity than oxygen)
      3. Decreases the delivery of oxygen to tissues by shifting oxyhemoglobin curve to the left
      4. Acts at cellular level to impair oxidative phosphorylation
      5. Direct myocardial depressant, causing low cardiac output (Ruddy, 1994)
      6. Net result: profound hypoxemia and tissue hypoxia
   C. Hydrogen cyanide (HCN) is a by-product of partial combustion of plastics and acrylics.
      1. Acts at the cellular level, binding to cytochrome oxidase, preventing oxygen use by mitochondria
      2. Interferes with aerobic metabolism, causing increased lactate levels
      3. Net result: tissue hypoxia, metabolic acidosis

D. Acrolein is a by-product of combustion of wood, cotton, polypropylene, and polyethylene (Weiss and Lakshminarayan, 1994).
   1. Impairs ciliary function
   2. Denatures mucosal proteins, causing edema and sloughing
   3. Causes pulmonary edema
   4. Interferes with chemotactic and alveolar macrophage function
   5. Net result: airway compromise, increased risk of pneumonia
III. Respiratory injury
   A. Early injury (1–12 hours): acute respiratory distress
      1. Upper airway damage/obstruction
         a) Thermal injury
         b) Particulate matter: edema, obstruction
      2. Bronchoconstriction, bronchospasm
         a) Toxic gases, irritants
         b) Release of inflammatory mediators, activation of neutrophils, macrophage injury
      3. Pulmonary consolidation
         a) Surfactant inhibition and loss
         b) Atelectasis
      4. Tissue hypoxia (end-organ damage)
         a) Low inspired oxygen
         b) CO, HCN
         c) Abnormal pulmonary gas exchange, intrapulmonary shunting
         d) Poor perfusion
      5. Damage to mucociliary clearance function
   B. 6–72 hours after injury
      1. Pulmonary edema occurs as a result of increased pulmonary capillary permeability from chemical injury (Nieman et al., 1994).
         a) Pulmonary vascular injury
         b) Inflammatory mediators, oxygen free radicals
         c) Fluid therapy may exacerbate
         d) May progress to adult respiratory distress syndrome (ARDS)
      2. If accompanying a burn injury, the lung may have an exaggerated or accelerated response to the injury (Clark, 1992).
   C. 2–3 days after injury
      1. Pneumonia
         a) Decreased pulmonary defense mechanism from damaged mucociliary clearance and decreased alveolar macrophage clearance of bacteria
         b) Poor lung compliance, pulmonary atelectasis
      2. Systemic effect of burns increases susceptibility to sepsis

Clinical Signs

I. Variable, may be normal on presentation
II. Odor of smoke on fur, soot on fur
III. ± Burns, singed hair and whiskers
IV. Cough, upper airway stridor
V. Tachypnea, dyspnea, respiratory distress
VI. Cherry red or brick red mucous membranes
VII. Conjunctival and/or corneal edema, excoriation of eyelids
VIII. Nasal and ocular discharge
IX. Weakness, collapse
X. Respiratory, cardiac arrest

Diagnosis

I. History
   A. Determine type and length of exposure
   B. Discern preexisting diseases
   C. Identify any current medications
II. Suggestive clinical signs
III. Physical examination
   A. Diagnosis may be obvious or may be reached from indirect information.
   B. Respiratory signs are variable and progressive. Initially, there may be no evidence of respiratory compromise.
   C. Respiratory signs may include the following.
      1. Dry, unproductive cough
      2. Wheezing, upper airway stridor
      3. Upper airway obstruction
      4. Tachypnea, increased respiratory effort
      5. Cyanosis: not reliable, may be absent if CO a major component
      6. Pulmonary rales, crackles
   D. Other signs that support the diagnosis are as follows.
      1. Conjunctival irritation/edema
      2. Corneal ulcers
      3. Burns to any part of the body
      4. Soot in oropharynx
IV. Clinicopathologic data
   A. Arterial blood gas analysis may reveal a normal PaO_2 until alveolar collapse occurs (Clark, 1992).
      1. Calculated oxygen saturation may be normal.
      2. Calculated oxygen content (vol %) is decreased.
   B. A venous blood gas analysis showing persistently elevated PvO_2 with metabolic acidosis may indicate cyanide toxicity.
   C. Plasma lactate is a good indicator of cyanide toxicity independent of hypoxemia (Ruddy, 1994).
   D. Biochemistries and complete blood counts are variable.
V. Pulse oximetry
   A. It is unreliable if CO is present.
   B. It will be normal or falsely elevated with CO present in the blood.
VI. Carboxyhemoglobin level
   A. A normal value does not rule out CO toxicity.
   B. Levels are affected by time since exposure and any supplemental oxygen.
   C. Signs of CO toxicity start at levels of 20%.
VII. Hydrogen cyanide level
   Toxic in humans: >1.0 mg/L
VIII. Radiography
   A. Chest films are often normal for the first 12–36 hours.

B. Initial radiographic changes may be patchy interstitial patterns with peribronchial changes.

C. Progression to an alveolar pattern with air bronchograms may be seen with pneumonia.

D. Radiographic changes consistent with ARDS may be seen in severe smoke-inhalation injuries.

IX. Cytologic exam of respiratory secretions

A. It is not usually needed for diagnosis.

B. Bronchoscopy may help determine the severity of airway lesions but does not correlate with mortality, and anesthetic risk may outweigh benefits (Clark, 1992).

C. Saliva from oropharyngeal region may contain soot.

D. Cytology from transtracheal aspirate or bronchoscopy may show absence of cilia on ciliated cells, soot, or other particulate material.

Differential Diagnosis

I. Other causes of respiratory distress, pulmonary edema, or pneumonia

II. Other causes of facial burns

Treatment

I. Airway maintenance

A. Manually clear or suction the oropharynx.

B. If there is a decreased level of consciousness or upper airway obstruction, consider the following.
1. Intubation
2. Tracheostomy

C. Use high-volume, low-pressure cuffs. Do not overinflate, as tracheal mucosa is already compromised.

II. Oxygen therapy

A. Initially 100% provided
1. It decreases the half-life of CO to 30–60 minutes.
2. Removal of CO is more dependent on alveolar Po_2 than alveolar ventilation.
3. Wean to lowest oxygen supplementation to maintain Pao_2 after initial treatment to avoid oxygen toxicity.

B. Oxygen delivery
1. Oxygen hood
2. Oxygen blanket
3. Oxygen cage
4. Nasal oxygen: avoid with severe facial burns
5. Ventilator

III. Ventilation

A. Positive pressure ventilation may be indicated.
1. Marked decrease in the level of consciousness
2. Impending respiratory insufficiency or failure

B. Mode of ventilation is controversial.
1. Positive pressure ventilation with positive end-expiratory pressure (PEEP) may increase interstitial fluid when surfactant is deficient.
2. High-frequency ventilation is the administration of small tidal volumes at very rapid rates and requires a specialized ventilator.

C. Humidify all gases.

IV. Fluid therapy

A. Requirements vary, depending on the degree of burns on the body.

B. Aggressive fluid therapy is needed if burns are severe, but the risk of pulmonary complications increases.

C. If possible, avoid rapid bolus administration, which may increase pulmonary microvascular pressure and increase extravascular water (Clark et al., 1988).

D. Balanced replacement crystalloid solutions are indicated when large volumes not required.

E. Consider colloids if volume expansion is needed.

V. Bronchodilators

A. Beta-adrenergic agonists are preferred.
1. Terbutaline (Brethine) 0.01 mg/kg SQ TID-QID or 0.03 mg/kg PO TID
2. Albuterol 0.02–0.04 mg/kg PO BID-TID
3. Not to be used in conjunction with aminophylline or theophylline

B. If beta-adrenergic agonists are not available, consider the following.
1. Aminophylline 6–11 mg/kg IV TID in the dog and 4 mg/kg IM BID in the cat
2. Theophylline 1–2 mg/kg IV TID-QID in the dog and 1–2 mg/kg IV TID in the cat

VI. Corticosteroids

A. Not usually indicated
1. Do not modify the pathophysiologic response (Clark, 1992)
2. Increase morbidity and mortality

B. May be indicated
1. If upper airway edema is a major component of injury
2. If airway constriction is nonresponsive to beta-adrenergic drugs (Weiss and Lakshminarayan, 1994)

VII. Diuretics

A. Indicated for pulmonary edema

B. May not be effective, because pulmonary edema is noncardiogenic in origin

C. May contribute to fluid and electrolyte imbalances

D. Mechanical ventilation considered better option for treating severe pulmonary edema

VIII. Exercise

A. Induce frequent position changes.

B. Encourage the animal to stand and walk when stable.

C. Perform chest wall coupage every 4–6 hours.

IX. Analgesics

A. May improve ventilation by decreasing pain-associated tachypnea

B. Butorphanol tartrate
1. Dog: 0.2–0.4 mg/kg IV, IM, SQ q 4–6 h
2. Cat: 0.2–0.8 mg/kg IV, IM, SQ q 4–6 h

C. Buprenorphine
1. Dog: 0.005–0.015 mg/kg IV, IM, SQ BID-TID
2. Cat: 0.01 mg/kg IV, IM, SQ BID-TID

D. Morphine sulfate
1. Dog: 0.2–1 mg/kg IV, SQ, IM BID-QID

2. Cat: 0.05–0.1 mg/kg SQ, IM BID
  E. Meperidine
    1. Dog: 3–5 mg/kg IM, SQ as needed; 2–4 mg/kg IV q 2 h
    2. Cat: 2–4 mg/kg IM, SQ as needed
Note: All the preceding analgesics may be given as continuous-rate infusions. All listed dosages are starting points; dosages can be increased and intervals shortened.
X. Antibiotics
  A. Do not use prophylactically, because suprainfections and resistant infections may occur.
  B. Bacterial pneumonia is common 2–3 days after a burn injury.
  C. If pneumonia occurs, obtain a culture and sensitivity, and start broad-spectrum antibiotics. Once the culture is completed, use the most narrow-spectrum antibiotic appropriate.

Patient Monitoring

I. Trends are as important as absolute numbers.
  A. Vital signs, lung sounds
  B. Arterial blood pressure
  C. Central venous pressure
  D. Level of consciousness
  E. Arterial blood gases (see Diagnosis, earlier)
  F. Hemograms
  G. Radiography
II. Monitor for adequate perfusion.
  A. Urine output
  B. Packed cell volume, total solids
  C. Mentation

  D. Bilirubin level (levels rise with poor hepatic perfusion)
  E. Capillary refill time
  F. Limb warmness
III. Factors that affect prognosis include the following.
  A. Mortality increases when body burns are present.
    1. Burns and burn therapy make the lungs more susceptible to further damage and dysfunction (Clark, 1992).
    2. There is a greater chance for sepsis, systemic inflammatory response syndrome (SIRS), and multiple organ dysfunction syndrome (MODS).
  B. The need for prolonged mechanical ventilation worsens prognosis.
  C. Early, fulminant pulmonary edema warrants a poor prognosis.
  D. Secondary complications (e.g., sepsis, SIRS, disseminated intravascular coagulation, ARDS, MODS) warrant a poor prognosis.

Bibliography

Clark WR: Smoke inhalation: diagnosis and management. World J Surg 16:24, 1992
Clark WR, Nieman GF, Goyette D et al: Effects of crystalloid on lung fluid balance after smoke inhalation. Ann Surg 208:56, 1988
Nieman GF, Cigada M, Paskanik AM et al: Comparison of high-frequency jet to conventional mechanical ventilation in the treatment of severe smoke inhalation injury. Burns 20:157, 1994
Ruddy RM: Smoke inhalation injury. Pediatr Clin North Am 41:31, 1994
Weiss SM, Lakshminarayan S: Acute inhalation injury. Clin Chest Med 15:103, 1994

133

Burns

Nishi Dhupa
Michael M. Pavletic

Definition

I. There are three main types of burn injuries: thermal, chemical, and electrical.
  A. Thermal injury is caused when skin comes into contact with a source of sufficient temperature to cause cell injury and death via protein coagulation.
  B. Chemical injuries result from thermal energy produced, coagulation necrosis, vascular thrombosis, and collagen denaturation and precipitation when strong acids or alkalis contact skin.
  C. Electrical injury occurs when electric current damages tissue by the conversion of electric energy into heat.
II. In small animals, electric heating pads, hot-air dryers, and scalding water are common causes of thermal burns.
  A. Thermal burns associated with flame trauma are less common.
  B. Flame trauma and contact with heated surfaces or scalding water result in immediate thermal wounds, whereas lesions resulting from electric heating pads and hot-air dryers may not be apparent for several days.

Causes

I. Thermal injuries
  A. Direct heat (dry)
    1. Electric heating pads
    2. Heat lamps
    3. Radiators
    4. Stoves
    5. Heat packs, hot water bottles
  B. Direct heat (wet)
    1. Scalding
    2. Hot tar
  C. Flame trauma
    1. Household fires
    2. Outdoor (forest and camp) fires
    3. Malicious dousing with flammable liquids
II. Chemical injuries
  A. Strong acids
  B. Strong alkalis
  C. Household agents
    1. Corrosives
    2. Dehydrating agents
  D. Solvents, petroleum distillates
    1. Phenols
    2. Turpentine
    3. Gasoline
    4. Kerosene
  E. Concentrated flea dip solutions
III. Electrical injuries
  A. High voltage (>2000 V)
    1. Lightning
    2. High-tension power transmission lines
  B. Low voltage (<1000 V): electric cord exposure (AC, DC)

Classification

I. Burn severity
  A. The severity of burn injury is determined by evaluating both the degree or depth of injury as well as a percentage of total body surface area (TBSA) involved.
  B. Thermal burns are additionally classified into three concentric zones of tissue injury, with the central zone of coagulative necrosis being the most severely damaged, the middle zone of vascular stasis and compromised tissue perfusion being moderately damaged, and the outermost zone of hyperemia being the least damaged.
II. Depth of injury
  A. Superficial burns (first degree)
    1. They involve injury to the outermost layer of the epidermis only.
    2. The skin is erythematous, dry to the touch, without blister formation, and hyperesthetic. Desquamation of the epidermis occurs, and healing may be complete within 5 days.
    3. Systemic reaction is absent or mild.

B. Partial-thickness burns (second degree burns)
 1. Superficial partial-thickness burns
  a) These involve injury to the epidermis and a limited portion of the dermis.
  b) Damage to dermal blood vessels results in congestion and leakage of plasma.
  c) Blister formation occurs, and the skin is exquisitely painful to touch.
  d) Hair follicles remain intact.
  e) Healing occurs in 10–21 days with minimal scarring.
  f) Systemic effects are present.
 2. Deep dermal partial-thickness burns
  a) These involve destruction of the epidermis and dermis with only the hair follicles remaining intact.
  b) Injured tissue is dark or yellow-white, contains ruptured bullae, and has decreased skin sensation to a pinprick but intact sensation for deep pressure.
  c) The healing process is prolonged and often results in extensive scarring and marked contracture of tissues without surgical intervention.
  d) Significant systemic effects are present.
C. Full-thickness burns (third degree)
 1. Involves destruction of all layers of skin and may include subcutaneous tissue, fat, fascia, muscle, and bone.
 2. Injured tissue appears charred, dry, and leathery. Increased permeability of intact deep vessels results in marked edema of the subcutis.
 3. The site is insensitive.
 4. Skin grafts and skin flaps are required for closure of larger skin wounds.
 5. Significant, often life-threatening systemic effects may occur when large surface areas are involved.
III. TBSA involved
 A. The percentage of TBSA involved can be roughly estimated in small animals by allotment of specific percentages to various body areas. The loose elastic skin of animals obscures accurate estimation.
  1. The head and neck account for 9%.
  2. Each forelimb accounts for 9%.
  3. Each rear limb accounts for 18%.
  4. The thorax and abdomen each account for 18%.
 B. Burns affecting more than 20% TBSA may impair cardiac, respiratory, and immune function.
 C. If partial- or full-thickness burns involve >50% of TBSA, chances of recovery are poor.

Pathophysiology

I. Burn wound pathology in extensive thermal wounds
 A. Direct thermal injury results in coagulative necrosis of tissue.
 B. The local release of vasoactive mediators results in a peripheral zone of dermal capillary occlusion.

C. Loss of capillary endothelial integrity results in tissue edema due to leakage of fluid, electrolytes, and proteins from the intravascular space.
D. The most dramatic fluid loss occurs within the first 12 hours.
E. Degree of local damage is related to the depth of the burn injury.
II. Systemic effects of burn shock in extensive thermal wounds
 A. Cardiovascular effects
  1. Loss of fluid into burn tissue and via evaporation may result in significant hypovolemia if >20% of TBSA is involved.
  2. Fluid losses may be estimated as 1 ml/kg body weight × % TBSA affected.
  3. The combination of hypovolemia and the release of myocardial depressant factors from burned tissue results in decreased cardiac output.
  4. The initial catecholamine surge results in an increase in heart rate, peripheral vasoconstriction, and an increase in arterial blood pressure.
  5. As further fluid loss occurs, compensatory mechanisms are overwhelmed and hypovolemic shock occurs.
  6. Low-voltage electric cord injuries may result in fatal ventricular arrhythmias and death. Life-threatening pulmonary edema may be noted.
  7. The ultimate consequence of cardiovascular failure is tissue hypoxemia.
 B. Hematologic effects
  1. Fluid loss results in initial hemoconcentration.
  2. Red cell hemolysis may occur as a result of direct thermal injury, passage through damaged microcirculation, and disseminated intravascular coagulation (DIC).
  3. The development of anemia is exacerbated by depressed hematopoiesis.
  4. A stress leukogram may persist for days.
 C. Respiratory effects
  1. Hot air inhalation to the upper airway results in mucosal damage and tissue edema, as well as inactivation of cilia and surfactant.
  2. Inhalation of soot and toxic byproducts of combustion can cause additional pulmonary injury.
  3. Alveolar injury results in atelectasis and pulmonary edema causing abnormal gas exchange.
  4. Chest wall burns may decrease compliance and result in hyperventilation.
  5. Untreated muscle catabolism causes respiratory muscle weakness.
  6. High-voltage electrical injuries may cause neurogenic pulmonary edema, with a typical distribution in the caudodorsal lung lobes.
 D. Renal effects
  1. Hypovolemia may result in reduced renal tissue perfusion and oliguria.

2. Hemoglobinuria and myoglobinuria contribute to the development of acute renal failure.
E. Gastrointestinal effects
   1. Increased mucosal permeability and disruption of the intestinal barrier result in increased bacterial translocation and endotoxin absorption.
   2. Hepatic dysfunction due to congestion and necrosis as well as reticuloendothelial cell dysfunction predisposes to immunosuppression and septicemia.
   3. Gastrointestinal ulceration may result in bleeding (Curling's ulcers).
F. Immunologic effects
   1. These may occur if >20% of TBSA is affected.
   2. Both humoral and cell-mediated immunity are affected.
   3. Loss of immunoglobulins and fibronectin occurs into the burn wound.
   4. Reduced albumin, acute phase protein and glutamine levels, and increased cortisol levels affect both humoral and cell-mediated immunity.
G. Miscellaneous
   1. The production of cytokines, such as interleukin-6, results in a hypermetabolic state and eventual negative nitrogen balance.
   2. Daily protein loss may exceed 2 g/kg/day.
   3. Inflammatory mediators contribute to a systemic inflammatory response and lead to multiorgan dysfunction.
   4. Increased susceptibility to infection results from gastrointestinal and hepatic dysfunction, protein catabolism cytokine release, and the impairment of humoral and cell-mediated immunity.
   5. Thermoregulation may be impaired from evaporative heat loss from the surface areas of large thermal wounds.

Clinical Signs

I. Thermal burns
   A. Local damage
      1. Superficial burns
         a) Hyperemia, no blister formation, pain
         b) Desquamation of epidermis prior to healing
      2. Superficial partial-thickness burns
         a) Marked pain, blister formation
         b) Hair follicles intact
      3. Deep dermal partial-thickness burns
         a) Yellow-white tissue, decreased sensation, ruptured blisters (rare)
         b) Marked scarring upon healing
      4. Full-thickness burns
         a) Charred, dry, leathery tissue, no pain sensation
         b) Hair loss
   B. Systemic effects
      1. These may occur with deep dermal partial-thickness burns and full-thickness burns over large surface areas, in part depending on the medical management instituted.
      2. The systemic clinical course changes with time.
         a) Effects immediately after burn injury include cardiovascular compromise, increased vascular permeability, immunocompromise, red blood cell hemolysis, DIC, upper airway edema, and reduced urine output.
         b) From days 2–6, clinical signs may include anemia, DIC, immune dysfunction, small airway obstruction, and early burn wound infection.
         c) From day 7 to wound closure, clinical signs may include hyperthermia, hyperventilation, pneumonia, sepsis, and wound demarcation and healing.
         d) Electrolyte and acid–base disturbances may include hypernatremia, hyponatremia, hyper- or hypokalemia, and acidosis (metabolic and/or respiratory).
II. Electrical burns
   A. Oral cavity injuries may be pale yellow, tan, or gray.
   B. Oronasal fistulas may occur.
   C. High-voltage skin injury may cause charred, leathery indented skin at the entry point.
   D. If arcing of the current occurs, a copper deposit may be present.
   E. Seizures, pulmonary edema, respiratory arrest, or ventricular fibrillation may occur.
   F. There is no pain at the site.
III. Chemical burns
   A. Pain is a feature.
   B. Superficial damage results in erythema.
   C. Deeper tissue damage results in coagulative necrosis and alopecia.

Diagnosis

I. History
   A. Determine events surrounding occurrence.
   B. Determine duration and type of exposure.
II. Physical examination
   A. Primary survey of animal in order to assess airway patency, breathing, and circulation
   B. Secondary survey
      1. Full physical exam
      2. Assessment of severity and extent of burn injury (depth of tissue damage and % TBSA affected)
      3. Assessment of systemic effects
   C. Supplemental tests
      1. Thoracic radiography
      2. Hemogram, serum electrolytes
      3. Assessment of acid–base status and oxygenation via blood gas analysis

Treatment of Thermal Burns

I. Principal objectives
   A. Removal of animal from source of injury

B. Acute airway management and oxygen supplementation

C. Acute treatment of cardiovascular and metabolic alterations

D. Prevention of wound sepsis

E. Monitoring for immunosuppression and multiorgan dysfunction

F. Pain relief

G. Wound closure

II. Airway and oxygenation

A. If upper airway stridor indicates foreign material obstruction, clean out pharyngeal area with fingers or suction.

B. Persistent inspiratory stridor or cyanosis may indicate laryngeal edema, necessitating immediate intubation.

C. Emergency tracheostomy is performed if extensive airway damage precludes intubation.

D. Supplemental oxygen (preferably humidified) is mandatory.

E. Positive pressure ventilation may be indicated.

F. Bronchodilator therapy may help maintain patency of small airways.

G. In the presence of bacterial pneumonia, cultures of respiratory tract are obtained followed by antibiotic therapy.

III. Shock resuscitation

A. Anticipate possible hypovolemic shock if >20% of the body surface is affected by partial- or full-thickness burn injury.

B. The ideal resuscitation fluid should remain in the vascular compartment in order to avoid complications such as pulmonary edema and burn tissue edema.

C. Balanced electrolyte crystalloid solutions are recommended within the first 24 hours.

D. Initial shock dose is 80–90 ml/kg IV during the first hour.

E. As microvascular permeability stabilizes by 18–24 hours, subsequent IV fluid therapy can include a colloid solution, such as plasma, hetastarch, or dextrans. It is desirable to maintain serum protein between 3.5 and 6.5 g/dl.

1. Plasma dose is 0.5 ml × body weight (kg) × % burn.

2. Hetastarch/dextran dose is 20 ml/kg/day.

F. The total fluid delivery rate within the first 24 hours is 1–4 ml/kg × % TBSA burned.

G. Consider blood transfusion if hematocrit and total protein levels decrease significantly, but only after the first 12 hours have passed. Maintain hematocrit above 25%.

H. After 48 hours, mobilization of retained fluids in the burn wounds occurs. Longer term fluid therapy requires lower total fluid rates and a greater use of colloidal solutions.

IV. Nutritional support

A. Hypermetabolic energy requirements for wound healing necessitate a high-calorie, high-protein diet (approximately 2–2.5 times standard maintenance requirements).

B. Daily caloric requirements are (25 × kg body weight) × (50 × % TBSA burned).

C. Vitamin and mineral supplementation (especially vitamins A and C and zinc) is recommended.

D. A combination of enteral (pharyngostomy, nasogastric tube, forced feeding) and parenteral (partial or total parenteral) nutrition may be used.

V. Wound management

A. The primary goal in burn management is promoting the earliest possible wound closure. Medical management is directed at stabilizing the animal, controlling pain, preventing infection, and providing those elements necessary to support optimal wound healing.

B. Chilled fluids, applied to small burns within 2 hours after the insult, can reduce heat retention and the depth of injury.

1. Chilled water or preferably sterile saline, at a temperature of 3–17°C, can be applied to local burns for 30 minutes.

2. The area can be immersed in the chilled fluids, or they can be applied as cold compresses.

3. Avoid their use over large surface areas to reduce the serious risk of hypothermia.

C. Systemic antibiotics are reserved for use with life-threatening infection. Topical antimicrobial agents are the primary means of preventing infection in burns.

1. Minor burns may be treated with a variety of topical ointments. Water-miscible ointments may be preferable because they are easier to rinse from the wound surface for periodic visual inspection of the injury.

2. Major burns are best treated with topical silver sulfadiazine because it has excellent penetration of the burn eschar and has a broad spectrum of activity.

3. Topical management is indicated for several days as the depth and extent of the wound is determined.

D. Débridement, the removal of devitalized tissue, is a key component to the management of deep partial- and full-thickness burns, once the delineation between viable and nonviable tissue is determined.

1. Removal of dead tissues helps prevent and control infection.

a) Its removal, in turn, helps promote a viable vascular wound bed suitable for closure more quickly than retention of this dead skin.

b) It may take up to 7–10 days before the full extent and depth of a thermal wound is known.

2. There are several options to promote the removal of necrotic tissue.

3. Topical enzymatic débriding agents can be useful in the removal of necrotic tissue. Their use is best restricted to smaller areas of necrotic skin when surgical débridement is unnecessary or inadvisable.

a) Sutilains (Travase ointment)
b) Bromelains (Ananase)
c) Collagenase (Santyl ointment)
d) Papain (Panafil ointment)
e) Trypsin–balsam Peru–castor oil (Granulex-V)
f) Dakin's solution 0.125–0.25% (sodium hypochlorite buffered with sodium bicarbonate in water)

4. Hydrotherapy, or the application of warm fluids to the wound surface, can be used to hydrate and soften necrotic tissue and promote its manual removal with surgical scissors and forceps.

a) Hydrotherapy is preferred to remove well-demarcated necrotic skin that is adhered to the body.
b) Softening the dry necrotic skin facilitates its surgical removal.
c) Normally hydrotherapy techniques are required for no more than 3–5 days to facilitate débridement.
d) Small animals can be immersed or bathed in warm isotonic solutions for 20–30 minutes by placing them in sterilized buckets. For larger animals, tubs or large containers can be lined with sterilized plastic liners.
e) In some cases, wet dressings can be applied to areas as a practical alternative to immersion of large patients.
f) Softened necrotic tissues are grasped with forceps and gently pulled or trimmed from the body.

5. Surgical débridement can be used for the removal of definite deep partial- to full-thickness skin necrosis.

a) This aggressive form of débridement is essentially wound excision.
b) It is easiest to perform when there is a delineation between the dead tissue and underlying viable tissues and the dead skin is not firmly adhered to underlying structures.
c) Otherwise, hydration of the dead tissue may be considered to facilitate its removal.
d) After excision, topical management may be instituted for a variable period of time, followed by wound closure.

E. Wound closure can be accomplished by several means, depending on the depth and surface area of the burn.

1. Superficial and most partial-thickness burns can heal by epithelialization from surviving dermal adnexa and any surviving germinal epithelium. Topical wound management is used to promote this process of healing.
2. Small full-thickness burns may heal by second intention with supportive care, presuming the wound is not located in an important body region.

3. Larger full-thickness burns can be closed with several surgical techniques, depending on the surface area and location of the burn.
a) Skin grafts
b) Skin flaps, including axial pattern flaps
c) Myocutaneous flaps
d) Skin stretching techniques

VI. Pain management
A. Pain control is paramount for the animal's comfort.
B. Uncontrolled pain contributes to hypermetabolism, a catabolic state, and immune dysfunction.
C. Good systemic analgesics include the following.
1. Oxymorphone 0.02–0.06 mg/kg IV q 4 h (dogs)
2. Butorphanol 0.05–0.2 mg/kg IV BID-QID (dogs, cats)
3. Morphine sulfate 0.2–0.5 mg/kg SQ, IM q 4 h (dogs)
D. Treatment of surface pain involves these measures.
1. Application of cold water to injured tissue within the first 2 hours
2. Prevention of decubital sores on pressure points
3. Motion exercises to reduce edema formation and maintain preburn mobility and function

VII. Adjunctive therapy
A. Antibiotics
1. Systemic antibiotic therapy is avoided except in systemic sepsis.
2. Topical antibiotic therapy is indicated.
B. Tetanus toxoid
1. Although tetanus is rare, consider toxoid administration in partial- or full-thickness burn injuries involving >20% of TBSA.
2. Recommended dose is 30,000–100,000 U IV or IM, following a test dose of 0.2 ml SQ (watch for anaphylaxis).
C. Heparin
1. In cases of severe burn injury and suspected DIC, heparin may be used to decrease thrombosis and vascular occlusion.
2. Dose is 50–150 U/kg SQ QID.
D. Environmental temperature control
1. Maintain ambient temperature at 75–80°F.
2. This modifies hypermetabolic and stress responses.

Treatment of Electrical Burns

I. Initial therapy
A. Remove animal from electric source.
B. With high-voltage injuries, treat pulmonary edema with oxygen supplementation and diuretics.

II. Fluid therapy
A. Fluid requirements for initial resuscitation may be two or three times that of an equivalent surface burn. Reduce fluid rates in case of pulmonary edema.
B. Fluid therapy is important in preventing renal

tubular damage associated with hemoglobinuria and myoglobinuria.

III. Wound management
   A. Circumferential burns on the extremities may require escharotomy and fasciotomy to maintain circulation in the face of massive edema formation.
   B. Aggressive removal of devitalized tissue is important.
   C. Topical antimicrobial therapy is recommended.
   D. Minor lesions may heal by second intention.

Treatment of Chemical Burns

I. Initial therapy
   A. Remove animal from source.
   B. Lavage affected area with large volumes of water.
   C. Lavage eyes copiously with sterile saline.
II. Specific therapy to be considered following copious lavage
   A. Acids, alkalis, household chemicals
      1. Neutralize acid burns with magnesium hydroxide or sodium bicarbonate solution, applied in the form of soaked gauze sponges held in place for 20 minutes.
      2. Neutralize alkali burns with weak (0.5–5%) acetic acid or lemon juice, applied in the form of soaked gauze sponges held in place for 20 minutes.
      3. Deep chemical burns may eventually require deep surgical excision.
   B. Hot tar
      1. Clip matted hair.
      2. Liberally apply an emulsifying agent such as Neosporin ointment.
      3. Wash mixture away with soap and water.
III. Adjunctive therapy
   A. Analgesic administration
   B. Sedation or general anesthesia during painful dressing changes or surgical débridement
   C. Prevention of self-trauma by using Elizabethan collar or sedation

Patient Monitoring

I. Monitor vital systems throughout the clinical course.
   A. Respiratory rate and pattern
   B. Assessment of oxygenation via pulse oximetry or blood gas analysis
   C. Heart rate and rhythm
   D. Femoral pulse strength or blood pressure
   E. Body temperature
   F. Mentation
   G. Urine output and presence of pigmenturia (output may be as high as 3–4 ml/kg/h in first 24 hours)
   H. ±Central venous pressure monitoring during acute phase of fluid administration
II. Assess the following for the first 12–24 hours.
   A. Monitor vital systems.
   B. Assess hemogram, chemistry profile, and urinalysis prior to fluid therapy.
      1. A high hematocrit level indicates hemoconcentration from excessive fluid loss.
   2. Monitor hematocrit every 4–6 hours, using fluid therapy to maintain it above 25% (ideally in a range of 40–45%).
   3. Ketolysis and hemoglobinuria are associated with severe brain injury.
   4. Hyperkalemia may occur secondary to metabolic acidosis, hemolysis, and tissue damage. (See treatment in Chap. 47.) Hypokalemia may occur as a result of accelerated renal excretion.
   5. Hypernatremia or hyponatremia may occur early in the clinical course. Either is corrected with appropriate balanced electrolyte solutions.
   C. Calculate serum osmolality using the following formula.
      1. $2[Na + K (mEq/L)] + \dfrac{glucose (mg/dl)}{20} + \dfrac{BUN (mg/dl)}{3}$
      2. If calculated osmolality is in excess of 340 mOsm/kg (normal = 300 mOsm/kg), increase fluid therapy using a hypotonic solution such as 0.45% NaCl.
   D. Monitor serum albumin levels or total solids. If total solids fall to <4 g/dl or serum albumin <1.5 g/dl, consider supplemental colloid therapy (hetastarch or dextrans at 1 ml/kg/h IV to a total daily dose of 20 ml/kg) after the first 8 hours have passed.
III. Assess the following for the second 24 hours.
   A. Monitor vital signs.
   B. Monitor hematocrit and total solids BID.
      1. If total solids fall below 25%, consider packed red cell or whole blood transfusion.
      2. If total solids fall below 4 g/dl, consider synthetic colloid or plasma transfusion (10 ml/kg IV).
   C. Monitor serum electrolytes once daily.
   D. Monitor hemogram.
      1. Expect a neutrophilic leukocytosis (≥30,000/μl) within 24 hours and persisting for 5–10 days.
      2. Mild anemia may develop and persist for 50–60 days.
   E. Monitor blood urea nitrogen (BUN) and creatinine.
      1. If azotemia develops, assess and treat any hypovolemia.
      2. Monitor urine output; become concerned if oliguria (normal output ≥ 0.5 ml/kg/h) develops.
      3. Look for casts in urine as an early indicator of renal tubular damage.
IV. From day 3 onward, assess the following.
   A. Monitor vital signs.
   B. Monitor hematocrit and total solids daily.
   C. Monitor serum electrolytes QOD.

Bibliography

Achauer BM, Martinez SE: Burn wound pathophysiology and care. Crit Care Clin 1:47, 1985

Aikawa N, Yamamoto S: Clinical analysis of multiple organ failure in burned patients. Burns 13:103, 1987

Baxter CR, Waecherie JF: Emergency treatment of burn injury. Am Emerg Med 17:1305, 1988

Demling RH: Fluid replacement in burn patients. Surg Clin North Am 67:15, 1987

Demling RH, Buerstatte RPH, Perea A: Management of hot tar burns. J Trauma 20:242, 1980

Lee-Parritz DE, Pavletic MM: Burns. p. 199. In Murtaugh RJ, Kaplan PM (eds): Veterinary Emergency and Critical Care Medicine. CV Mosby, St. Louis, 1992

Mozingo DW, Smith AA, McManus WF et al: Chemical burns. J Trauma 28:642, 1988

Warden ED: Immunologic response to burn injury. p. 113. In Boswick JA (ed): The Art and Science of Burn Care. Aspen, Rockville, MD, 1987

134

Heat Prostration

Ann Marie Manning
Robert J. Murtaugh

Definition

Heat prostration (heatstroke, hyperthermia) is a medical emergency defined as an elevation in body temperature that exceeds the animal's compensatory mechanisms for dissipating heat and results in direct thermal damage to tissues and potentially life-threatening multiple organ dysfunction.

Causes

I. Factors contributing to decreased heat dissipation
  A. Lack of acclimatization
  B. Humidity: high ambient temperature
  C. Confinement/poor ventilation
  D. Water deprivation
  E. Brachycephalic breeds
  F. Obesity
  G. Extremes of age
  H. Drugs
    1. Anticholinergics
    2. Phenothiazines
II. Factors contributing to increased heat production
  A. Exercise
  B. Drugs
    1. Aspirin
    2. Thyroid supplements
    3. Amphetamines
  C. Fever
III. Preexisting medical problems that predispose to heatstroke
  A. Cardiovascular disease
  B. Central nervous system disease: status epilepticus, disorders of the hypothalamic region
  C. Laryngeal paralysis
  D. Hypokalemia
  E. Endocrine disorders
    1. Hyperthyroidism
    2. Diabetes mellitus
    3. Pheochromocytoma
    4. Addisonian crisis
  F. Prior heatstroke (mechanism unknown)

Pathophysiology

I. Causes of organ system dysfunction are multifactorial and include thermal destruction of cellular membrane lipids and chemical bonds, denaturation and inactivation of enzymes, and development of tissue hypoxia, with resultant acidosis. All these factors contribute to cell necrosis.
II. Cardiovascular changes include the following.
  A. Increased metabolic rate and oxygen consumption
  B. Inadequate cardiac output, leading to insufficient perfusion of vital organs, acidosis, and muscle degeneration
  C. Myocardial necrosis and pulmonary hypertension
  D. Arrhythmias secondary to myocardial necrosis and ischemia, systemic acidosis, hyper- or hypokalemia, and hypoxia
  E. Hypovolemic shock
III. Hyperthermia may result in permanent neurologic damage; however, most changes resolve with correction of underlying disorders and resolution of hyperthermia.
  A. Cerebral edema
  B. Neuronal degeneration, necrosis, and diffuse petechial hemorrhages (occurring mostly in the cerebellum)
  C. Febrile seizures
IV. Direct thermal injury to gastrointestinal mucosa and hypoperfusion result in breakdown of the mucosal barrier and leakage of bacteria and bacterial endotoxins into the circulation. Gastrointestinal bleeding is a common sequela.
V. Renal changes may occur early in the course.
  A. Acute tubular necrosis develops from direct thermal injury, intravascular thrombosis, hypoperfusion, hypoxia, and myoglobinuria.
  B. Myoglobin and uric acid may crystallize in renal tubules, causing an obstructive uropathy.
VI. Hepatic changes may also arise.
  A. Hepatocellular necrosis
  B. Cholestasis

C. Reticuloendothelial system damage, leading to compromise of the immune system
VII. Musculoskeletal changes include rhabdomyolysis secondary to direct thermal injury to muscle, hypoperfusion, and increased muscular activity.
  A. Myoglobinuria
  B. Precipitation of calcium in damaged muscle: hypocalcemia
VIII. Adult respiratory distress syndrome (ARDS) can occur in association with disseminated intravascular coagulation (DIC) in severe heatstroke.
IX. Coagulogram findings are consistent with DIC and can result from any of the following.
  A. Direct thermal injury to the vascular endothelium, with increased capillary permeability
  B. Thermal inactivation of clotting factors and destruction of platelets
  C. Impaired synthesis of clotting factors owing to hepatic necrosis
  D. Release of thromboplastic substances
  E. Initiation of fibrinolysis
X. Acid–base changes are variable.
  A. Early stages: respiratory alkalosis (decreased PCO_2) caused by panting
  B. Later stages
    1. Metabolic acidosis develops in association with dehydration.
    2. Dehydration causes hypotension and insufficient perfusion of tissues, with resultant lactic acidosis.
    3. Mixed respiratory alkalosis and metabolic acidosis are also possible.
XI. Electrolyte abnormalities are common.
  A. Hypokalemia occurs early as a result of vomiting and respiratory alkalosis.
  B. Hyperkalemia develops later and results from metabolic/lactic acidosis, tissue destruction, and impaired renal function.
  C. Hypernatremia and hyperchloridemia occur secondary to dehydration. A free water deficit develops from panting and lack of available water for compensatory oral intake.
  D. Hypophosphatemia and hypomagnesemia occur, although the mechanism is unknown.

Clinical Signs

I. Early stages
  A. Tachypnea, hyperventilation, panting
  B. Tachycardia, hyperdynamic femoral pulse
  C. Hyperemic, dry mucous membranes
  D. Hypersalivation
  E. Altered mentation (depression, stupor, coma), seizures
  F. Hypotension
  G. Weakness, collapse
  H. Vomiting, diarrhea
  I. Bleeding
II. Severe or protracted heatstroke
  A. Weak femoral pulses
  B. Pale, gray mucous membranes

C. Shallow respirations progressing to apnea
D. Seizures, coma
E. Vomiting and diarrhea (often bloody)
III. Delayed signs
  Whereas organ failure and coagulation abnormalities can occur within hours of the development of heatstroke, these clinical signs may occur as late as 3–5 days after apparent recovery.
  A. Oliguria
  B. Icterus
  C. Cardiac arrhythmias
  D. Sepsis
  E. Seizures
  F. DIC
  G. ARDS

Diagnosis

I. History of exercise or confinement in a hot or humid environment
II. Physical findings of heatstroke concomitant with an elevated body temperature
III. Hemogram
  A. Hematocrit (packed cell volume) often elevated
  B. Anemia possible later from red blood cell injury, shortened red blood cell life span, bleeding, and hemolysis
  C. Thrombocytopenia common
  D. Leukocytosis possible
IV. Biochemistry profile
  A. Elevated blood urea nitrogen and creatinine
  B. Elevated liver and muscle enzymes
    1. Increased aspartate aminotransferase, alanine aminotransferase, and bilirubin
    2. Increased creatine phosphokinase
  C. Hypoglycemia
  D. Hypocalcemia
  E. Hypokalemia (early), hyperkalemia (late)
  F. Hypernatremia and hyperchloridemia
  G. Hypomagnesemia and hypophosphatemia
V. Urinalysis
  A. Proteinuria
  B. Hematuria
  C. Myoglobinuria
  D. Renal tubular casts
VI. Coagulogram
  A. Increased prothrombin time, partial thromboplastin time, fibrin degradation products, and activated clotting time
  B. Hypofibrinogenemia and thrombocytopenia

Differential Diagnosis

I. Inflammatory or infectious diseases
  A. Encephalitis, meningitis
  B. Septic shock
  C. Rickettsial diseases
II. Status epilepticus
III. Salicylate intoxication
IV. Space-occupying lesion of the hypothalamic region

Treatment

I. Successful treatment of hyperthermia requires early recognition and aggressive support. The main goals of therapy are as follows.
   A. Cool the animal.
   B. Provide cardiovascular support.
   C. Control seizures.
   D. Diagnose and treat any underlying disorder.
   E. Monitor for and treat developing complications such as DIC, ARDS, renal or hepatic failure.
II. Maintain patent airway.
   A. Intubate if poor gag reflex is present.
   B. Supplement with 100% oxygen until temperature is controlled.
   C. Provide mechanical ventilation with positive end-expiratory pressure (PEEP) if ARDS develops.
III. Attempt to correct hyperthermia quickly with the following methods.
   A. Remove the animal from hot environment.
   B. Bathe with cool water and blow air over the animal with a fan to promote evaporation.
   C. Apply ice packs to axillary, groin, and neck regions.
   D. Begin IV fluids (room temperature).
      1. Initial dosage is 90 ml/kg of lactated Ringer's solution over 1 hour.
      2. Follow with maintenance fluids and additional amounts to correct dehydration and ongoing losses.
   E. Gastric lavage with cool water, cool-water enemas, and peritoneal dialysis with cool dialysate promote cooling without causing peripheral vasoconstriction.
      1. Cool-water enemas may interfere with rectal temperature monitoring.
      2. These procedures are usually reserved for refractory cases.
   F. Massage feet to promote circulation.
   G. Cool to a body temperature of 103°F, then stop cooling procedures and monitor temperature to avoid hypothermia.
IV. Initiate cardiovascular support.
   A. Treat for shock if present.
      1. Give initial dosage of IV fluids (balanced electrolyte solution), then reassess.
         a) Dogs: 90 ml/kg over 1 hour
         b) Cats: 70 ml/kg over 1 hour
      2. Steroids are not indicated for treatment of shock.
   B. If hypotension persists, consider the following.
      1. Additional crystalloids
      2. Colloidal support
         a) Hetastarch or dextrans 20 ml/kg/24 hours IV
         b) Can be administered as a bolus if necessary
      3. Vasopressors
         a) Dopamine: 5–20 μg/kg/min continuous IV infusion
         b) Dobutamine: 2.5 μg/kg/min continuous IV infusion
         c) Norepinephrine contraindicated, as it causes vasoconstriction and impairs heat dissipation
         d) Vasopressors delayed until adequate volume expansion attained
V. Control seizures and increased muscle activity
   A. Diazepam 0.5 mg/kg IV
   B. Pentobarbital constant rate infusion at 0.2–1 mg/kg/h IV
      1. Intubate.
      2. Continuously monitor electrocardiogram (ECG).
   C. Paralyzing agents and mechanical ventilation if muscle activity uncontrollable with the preceding drugs
      1. Atracurium 0.3–0.5 mg/kg IV loading dose, followed by 4–9 μg/kg/min IV
      2. Pancuronium 0.04–0.1 mg/kg IV initial bolus, followed by 0.06–0.1 mg/kg/h IV
   D. To treat cerebral edema
      1. Dexamethasone 2 mg/kg IV
      2. 20% mannitol 0.5–2 g/kg slowly IV over 30–45 minutes

Patient Monitoring

I. Monitor cardiovascular function.
   A. Continuous ECG monitoring for arrhythmias
   B. Blood pressure and central venous pressure measurements
      1. Desired blood pressure is 120/80.
      2. If possible, use central venous pressure (target is 8–10 cm H_2O) to assess adequacy of fluid support.
II. Monitor renal function.
   A. Creatinine and electrolytes are measured daily.
   B. Measure urine output with an indwelling urinary catheter.
   C. If creatinine rises or urine output decreases, attempt diuresis with the following.
      1. Fluid challenge with 50 ml/kg as IV bolus followed by furosemide or dopamine, as necessary.
      2. Furosemide 2 mg/kg IV bolus, repeated in 20 minutes if no results, or constant rate infusion at 0.1–1 mg/kg/hour IV
      3. Dopamine 1–5 μg/kg/minute IV
      4. Peritoneal dialysis
   D. Note presence of myoglobinuria.
III. Monitor for signs of DIC.
   A. Serial measurements of clotting parameters are made throughout the clinical course.
   B. Evidence of DIC includes, but is not limited to, the following.
      1. Ecchymoses, petechiae
      2. Bleeding from venipuncture sites
      3. Epistaxis, hematemesis, melena
      4. Abnormal coagulogram
   C. If evidence of DIC is present, treat aggressively.
      1. Fresh frozen plasma (FFP) 10 ml/kg IV incubated with 75 U/kg heparin

    2. Heparin 150–200 U/kg SQ QID, following administration of FFP

IV. Monitor acid–base status.
    A. Administer sodium bicarbonate for metabolic acidosis.
    B. Sodium bicarbonate requirement is 0.3 × body weight (kg) × bicarbonate deficit.

V. Monitor for seizures.

VI. Monitor for development of sepsis.
    A. Consider prophylactic use of broad-spectrum antibiotics if significant gastrointestinal disruption is present.
    B. Monitor for signs of sepsis and initiate antibiotics after obtaining blood for culture.

VII. Avoid use of the following drugs.
    A. Nonsteroidal anti-inflammatory drugs (NSAIDs) can contribute to gastrointestinal bleeding.
    B. Glucocorticoid administration has not been proved to be beneficial in heatstroke and is reserved for specific indications, such as cerebral edema.
    C. Phenothiazines are not used to prevent shivering, as they interfere with thermoregulation.

VIII. Prevention involves the following.
    A. Avoid confinement in hot or humid environments.
    B. Avoid exercise under hot or humid conditions.
    C. Provide free access to water at all times.
    D. Provide adequate shade.

Bibliography

Clowes GH, O'Donnell TF: Heatstroke. N Engl J Med 291:564, 1974

Dhupa N, Shaffran N: Continuous rate infusion formulas. p. 2130. In Ettinger SJ, Feldman EC (eds): Textbook of Veterinary Internal Medicine. 4th Ed. WB Saunders, Philadelphia, 1995

El-Kassim FA, Al-Mashhadani S, Abdullah AK et al: Adult respiratory distress syndrome and disseminated intravascular coagulation complicating heatstroke. Chest 90:571, 1986

Graham BS, Lichtenstein MJ, Hinson JM: Nonexertional heatstroke: physiologic management and cooling in 14 patients. Arch Intern Med 146:87, 1986

Holloway SA: Heatstroke in dogs. Compend Contin Educ Pract Vet 14:1598, 1992

Johnson KE: Pathophysiology of heatstroke. Compend Contin Educ Pract Vet 4:141, 1982

Krum SH, Osborne CA: Heatstroke in dogs: a polysystemic disorder. J Am Vet Med Assoc 170:531, 1977

Mustafa MY, Khogali M, Gumaa KA: Central nervous system, blood clotting and respiratory functions associated with heatstroke. p. 277. In Hales JR, Richards DB (eds): Heat Stress: Physical Exertion and Environment. Elsevier Science Publishers BV, Sydney, 1987

Mustafa MY, Omer O, Khogali M et al: Blood coagulation and fibrinolysis in heat stroke. Br J Haematol 61:517, 1985

Olson KR, Benowitz NL: Environmental and drug-induced hyperthermia: pathophysiology, recognition, and management. Emerg Clin North Am 2:459, 1984

Schall WD: Heatstroke (heat stress, hyperpyrexia). p. 195. In Kirk RW (ed): Current Veterinary Therapy VII: Small Animal Practice. WB Saunders, Philadelphia, 1980

Simon HB: Hyperthermia. N Engl J Med 329:483, 1993

Vicario SJ, Okabajue R, Haltom T: Rapid cooling in classic heatstroke: effect on mortality rates. Am J Emerg Med 4:394, 1986

135

Hypothermia and Frostbite

Nishi Dhupa

Definition

I. Hypothermia is a state of body temperature that is below normal in a homeothermic organism.
II. Frostbite is a state of actual freezing of body tissue.
III. Mild hypothermia is a core body temperature of 90–99°F, moderate hypothermia is in the range of 82–90°F, and severe hypothermia is any body temperature below 82°F.
IV. Hypothermia results from prolonged exposure to cold from an inability to maintain thermal homeostasis.

Causes

I. Hypothermia
   A. Decreased heat production
      1. Neonates: reduced muscle, fat, and glycogen reserves
      2. Cachexia: reduced energy stores
      3. Impaired thermoregulation
         a) Endocrine disorders: hypothyroidism, adrenal insufficiency
         b) Anesthetics and sedatives
      4. Immobility
         a) Unconsciousness
         b) Leg-hold traps
         c) Trauma or debility
   B. Increased heat loss
      1. Increased surface area to body mass
         a) Small dogs, cats
         b) Neonates
      2. Inadequate behavioral responses
         a) Geriatric animals
         b) Neonates
         c) Debility, e.g., trauma, unconsciousness
      3. Large evaporative and conductive heat loss
         a) Cold water immersion
         b) Burns
         c) Trauma
         d) Surgery
II. Frostbite
   A. Exposure to high winds on chilly days
   B. Prolonged contact with snow or ice
   C. Contact with cold metals or volatile liquids

Pathophysiology

I. Hypothermia
   A. During mild hypothermia, compensatory mechanisms such as increased metabolic rate, shivering, peripheral vasoconstriction, increased cardiac output, piloerection, and heat seeking go into effect.
   B. During moderate hypothermia, thermoregulation begins to fail. Metabolic processes, heart rate, and respiratory rate slow; blood pressure and cardiac output drop; central nervous system depression becomes evident.
   C. Atrial and ventricular cardiac muscle irritability results in dysrhythmias. Ventricular fibrillation is common during severe hypothermia.
   D. Despite decreased oxygen consumption, metabolic demands of vital tissues may be met for some time through decreased cellular metabolism.
   E. Decreased tissue perfusion results in metabolic acidosis.
   F. Effects on coagulation include reversible platelet dysfunction and reversible coagulation factor dysfunction.
II. Frostbite
   A. Hypothermic animals are prone to frostbite of ears, tail, digits, and external genitalia.
   B. Frostbite occurs from a combination of tissue ischemia secondary to peripheral vasoconstriction, intracellular and extracellular ice formation, and thrombosis related to vascular wall injury.
   C. Damaged tissue may slough several days after exposure.

Clinical Signs

I. Hypothermia
   A. Obtundation, stupor

B. Bradycardia, cardiac dysrhythmias
C. Hypotension: weak peripheral pulses
D. Shallow, slow respirations
E. Shivering (or muscle rigidity below 90°F)
F. Dilated pupils
G. Lethargy, impaired gait, or recumbency
H. Coma

II. Frostbite
A. Pale, bluish appearance of frozen tissue
B. Anesthesia of affected tissue

Diagnosis

I. History
A. Exposure to cold
B. Underlying illness or trauma
II. Suspicious clinical signs
III. Verification of hypothermia
A. Standard rectal thermometers measure temperatures as low as 94°F.
B. Rectal or esophageal probes, specialized low-temp thermometers, or indirect tympanic thermometers record temperatures to 75°F.

Treatment

I. Aims
A. Support vital organ systems
B. Prevent further heat loss
C. Rewarm animal and thaw frozen tissue
D. Prevent complications such as life-threatening dysrhythmias

II. Protocol
A. Airway management
1. Establish patency, or intubate and ventilate.
2. Provide oxygen supplementation (warmed, humidified).
B. Intravenous access
1. Institute volume expansion via rapid infusion with a warmed isotonic balanced electrolyte solution at 30–90 ml/h.
2. Warm IV fluids to 104–109°F in an incubator, water bath, or microwave oven.
3. Supplement fluids with 2.5% dextrose to provide an energy substrate.
C. Rewarming methods
1. Passive rewarming for mild hypothermia (90–99°F)
a) Remove the animal from the cold environment.
b) Provide insulation with blankets, tin foil, or bubble wrap.
c) The animal must activate its own heat-production mechanisms.
2. Active external rewarming for moderate hypothermia (82–90°F)
a) Expose the animal to an exogenous heat source such as hot water bottles, recirculating water blankets, heating pads, or radiant heat.
b) Do not place external heat sources in direct contact with the animal's skin, as thermal injury can result.
c) Radiant heat sources are placed at least 75 cm from the animal.
d) Direct heat is applied to the thorax preferentially, keeping the extremities cool and allowing selective warming of the heart. This also guards against peripheral vasodilation and shunting of blood away from the core.
3. Core rewarming for severe hypothermia (<82°F)
a) Infusion of warmed IV fluids
b) Airway rewarming (warm, humidified air)
c) Gastric or colonic lavage with warm saline
d) Peritoneal dialysis
(1) Use a warm (109°F) balanced electrolyte solution.
(2) Infuse 50 ml/kg body weight via a peritoneal dialysis or Foley catheter.
(3) Remove immediately.
(4) Repeat procedure until core body temperature is >96°F; may require 6–8 exchanges.
D. Thawing frozen tissue
1. Remove from source of cold.
2. Immerse affected tissue in warm water (104–108°F) for 20 minutes.
3. Do not rub or massage frozen tissue.
4. After thawing, apply dry protective bandages to protect affected tissue.
5. Necrotic tissue may require careful debridement and application of topical antiseptics.
6. Consider administration of analgesics.

III. Adjunctive therapy
A. Cardiac dysrhythmias
1. At temperatures <82°F, excessive handling of the animal may precipitate a lethal ventricular dysrhythmia.
2. At temperatures <82°F, the heart is refractory to atropine, antiarrhythmic agents, and electroconversion therapy.
3. Rewarming the animal is very important.
4. If cardiopulmonary resuscitation is necessary, external cardiac massage and mechanical ventilation may be performed at half the normal rate.
B. Metabolic acidosis
1. Treat with IV fluids to improve tissue perfusion and oxygenation.
2. It does not usually require bicarbonate supplementation.
C. Pulmonary complications
1. Anticipate pulmonary edema and/or pneumonia after rewarming.
2. Consider antibiotic therapy with broad-spectrum antibiotics such as ampicillin or cephalexin.
D. Cerebral edema
1. Increasing unresponsiveness following re-

warming may be related to cerebral edema and increased intracranial pressure.

2. Treatment involves the use of dexamethasone sodium phosphate at a dose of 0.25 mg/kg and mannitol at 0.5 g/kg IV over 20 minutes.

E. Analgesics for pain associated with thawing tissue (in a normothermic animal)
   1. Morphine sulfate 0.2–0.5 mg/kg IM
   2. Meperidine HCl 3–5 mg/kg IM
   3. Oxymorphone 0.05–0.10 mg/kg IM or IV

Patient Monitoring

I. Body temperature
  A. Once body temperature reaches 97°F, active rewarming techniques are moderated to avoid hyperthermia.
  B. Constant monitoring and adjustments in exogenous heat may be required to maintain body temperature in the normal range until thermoregulation normalizes.

II. Cardiovascular monitoring
  A. Monitor the electrocardiogram closely for the first 24–48 hours. Dysrhythmias (e.g., ventricular tachycardia) resulting in hemodynamic compromise require treatment (see Chap. 7).
  B. Monitor blood pressure or pulse strength. Weak peripheral pulses or a mean arterial pressure <65 mmHg indicates the need for IV fluid infusion or antiarrhythmic drug therapy.

III. Respiratory monitoring
  A. Monitor oxygenation by pulse oximetry or arterial blood gas measurement.
  B. Thoracic radiography may be used to evaluate for possible pneumonia.

IV. Urine output
  A. The development of oliguria or anuria may indicate hypotension, hypovolemia, or acute renal insufficiency.
  B. Urine output should exceed 0.5 ml/kg/h.

V. Central nervous system monitoring
  A. Monitor mentation, muscle strength, and pupillary light reflexes.
  B. Any deterioration in function may indicate developing cerebral edema.

VI. Laboratory evaluation
  A. Monitor hematocrit and total solids to maintain normal hydration.
  B. Monitor urea nitrogen, creatinine, and serum electrolytes daily until the animal is stable.

VII. Nutritional status
  A. Monitor body weight closely.
  B. Institute a high-protein, high-calorie diet.
  C. Feed via nasogastric tube or parenteral nutrition if necessary.

VIII. Frostbitten tissues
  A. Monitor for return of blood flow, warmth, and sensation.
  B. Persistence of avascular, anesthetic skin warrants a guarded prognosis for affected tissue.
  C. Monitor for demarcation of nonviable tissue. Once this occurs (may take 4–15 days), surgical debridement or amputation of affected tissue can be performed.

Bibliography

Ahn AH: Hypothermia. p. 157. In Bonagura JD (ed): Kirk's Current Veterinary Therapy XII. WB Saunders, Philadelphia, 1995

Dhupa N: Hypothermia in the dog and cat. Compend Contin Educ Pract Vet 17:61, 1995

Hansen BD, Morgan RV: Hypothermia and frostbite. p. 1373. In Morgan RV (ed): Handbook of Small Animal Practice. 2nd Ed. WB Saunders, Philadelphia, 1992

Lee-Parritz DE, Pavletic MM: Accidental hypothermia. p. 196. In Murtaugh RJ, Kaplan PM (eds): Veterinary Emergency and Critical Care Medicine. Mosby–Year Book, St. Louis, 1992

Otto RJ, Metzler MH: Rewarming from experimental hypothermia: comparison of heated aerosol inhalation, peritoneal lavage, and pleural lavage. Crit Care Med 16:869, 1988

Reuler JB: Hypothermia: pathophysiology, clinical setting, and management. Ann Intern Med 89:519, 1978

Normal Physiologic Values

Normal Hematologic Values

Parameter	Dog	Cat
PCV (%)	37–55	27–45
Hemoglobin (g/dl)	12–18	9–15
Erythrocytes ($10^6/\mu l$)	5.5–8.5	6–10
MCV (fl)	60–77	37–50
MCHC (g/dl)	32–36	30–36
RBC life span (days)	120	70
Reticulocyte count (%)	0–1.5	0–0.4
Leukocytes (/μl)	6000–17,000	5000–19,500
Segmented neutrophils (/μl)	3000–11,500	2500–12,500
Band neutrophils (/μl)	0–300	0–300
Lymphocytes (/μl)	1000–4800	1500–7000
Monocytes (/μl)	150–1350	0–850
Eosinophils (/μl)	100–750	0–750
Basophils (/μl)	Rare	Rare
Total solids (g/dl)	6–8	6–8

Corrections for Reticulocyte Counts

(1) Corrected reticulocyte count (%) = observed reticulocyte count (%) $\times$ actual PCV/normal PCV

(2) Reticulocyte index = reticulocyte count (%) $\times \dfrac{\text{actual PCV}}{\text{normal PCV}} \times \dfrac{1}{\text{reticulocyte maturation time (days)}}$

Reticulocyte Maturation Time for Various PCVs

PCV (%)	Maturation Time (days)
45	1.0
35	1.5
25	2.0
15	2.5

Insert corresponding maturation time into Equation 2.

Bone Marrow Evaluation

Cell Types	Dog	Cat
M:E ratio (range)	0.75–2.50:1.00	0.6–3.9:1.0
M:E ratio (average)	1.15:1.00	2.47:1.00
Erythrocytic series (%)		
Rubriblasts	0.2	1.71
Prorubricytes	3.9	12.50
Rubricytes	27.0	—
Metarubricytes	15.3	11.68
Total	46.4	25.89
Granulocytic series (%)		
Myeloblasts	0	1.74
Progranulocytes	1.3	0.88
Neutrophilic myelocytes	9.0	9.76
Eosinophilic myelocytes	0	1.47
Neutrophilic metamyelocytes	7.5	7.32
Eosinophilic metamyelocytes	2.4	1.52
Band neutrophils	13.6	25.80
Band eosinophils	0.9	—
Neutrophils	18.4	9.24
Eosinophils	0.3	0.81
Basophils	0	0.002
Total	53.4	58.542
Others (%)		
Lymphocytes	0.2	7.63
Plasma cells	0	1.61
Reticulum cells	0	0.13
Mitotic cells	0	0.61

From Bentinck-Smith J, 1983, with permission.

Normal Chemistry Values[a]

Chemistry	Common Units			Système International d'Unités		
	Dog	*Cat*	*Unit*	*Dog*	*Cat*	*SI Unit*
Glucose	60–110	70–150	mg/dl	3.9–6.1	3.9–8.0	mmol/L
BUN	10–25	17–30	mg/dl	3.5–7.1	5.9–10.5	mmol/L
Creatinine	0.6–2.0	0.6–2.0	mg/dl	50–180	50–180	μmol/L
Calcium	8.8–11.2	8.8–10.4	mg/dl	2.2–2.7	2.2–2.5	mmol/L
Phosphorus	2.5–5.9	1.8–7.0	mg/dl	0.8–1.6	0.58–2.2	mmol/L
Sodium	140–155	146–158	mEq/L	140–155	146–158	mmol/L
Potassium	3.5–5.0	3.5–5.2	mEq/L	3.5–5.0	3.5–5.2	mmol/L
Chloride	105–125	114–126	mEq/L	105–125	114–126	mmol/L
Magnesium	1.8–3.0	1.90–2.28	mg/dl	0.8–1.2	0.8–0.9	mmol/L
Iron	80–122	70–215	μg/dl	14–32	12–38.5	μmol/L
Total iron binding	280–340	170–400	μg/dl	63–81	30–71	μmol/L
Triglyceride	10–42	6–58	mg/dl	0.56	0.56	mmol/L
Cholesterol	100–265	87–171	mg/dl	2.5–5.9	2.1–4.3	mmol/L
Bilirubin						
Total	0.1–0.6	0.1–0.6	mg/dl	2–17	2–17	μmol/L
Direct	0–0.14	0–0.15	mg/dl	0–2	0–2	μmol/L
Indirect	0.07–0.60	0.09–0.20	mg/dl	0–15	0–15	μmol/L
Total protein	5.0–7.1	5–8	g/dl	50–71	50–80	g/L
Albumin	2.8–4.0	2.3–3.5	g/dl	28–40	23–35	g/L
Globulin	3.0–4.7	2.6–5.0	g/dl	30–47	26–50	g/L
SAP	20–150	10–100	U/L	20–150	10–100	U/L
SALT (SGPT)	15–70	10–50	U/L	15–70	10–50	U/L
SAST (SGOT)	10–50	10–40	U/L	10–50	10–40	U/L
LDH	50–495	75–495	U/L	50–495	75–495	U/L
GGT	1–11.5	1–10	U/L	1–11.5	1–10	U/L
Bile acids, fasting	<10	<5	μmol/L	<10	<5	μmol/L
Bile acids, postprandial	<25	<15	μmol/L	<25	<15	μmol/L
Amylase	300–2000	500–1800	IU/L	300–2000	500–1800	U/L
Lipase	25–750	25–375	IU/dl	25–750	25–375	U/L
CK	30–200	26–450	U/L	30–200	26–450	U/L
CO$_2$	22–27	20–23	mEq/L	22–28	20–25	mmol/L
HCO$_3$	25	25	mEq/L	25	25	mmol/L
NH$_3$	<120–150		μg/dl	69–87		μmol/L
Lactate	5–20		mg/dl	0.5–2.0		mmol/L
Pyruvate	0.1–0.2		mEq/L			
pH	7.31–7.42	7.24–7.40				
Osmolality	280–305	280–305	mOsm/kg	280–305	280–305	mmol/kg
Blood lead	<25	<25	μg/dl	<1.21	<1.21	μmol/L

[a]It is important to realize that normal values vary among individual laboratories.

BUN = blood urea nitrogen; SAP = serum alkaline phosphatase; SALT = serum alanine transaminase; SGPT = serum glutamate pyruvate transaminase; SAST = serum aspartate transaminase; SGOT = serum glutamic-oxaloacetic transaminase; LDH = lactate dehydrogenase; GGT = γ-glutamyltransferase; CK = creatine kinase; CO$_2$ = carbon dioxide; HCO$_3$ = bicarbonate; NH$_3$ = ammonia.

Modified from Lumsden JH, 1982, with permission.

Normal Urinalysis Values

Parameter	Dog	Cat
Color	Light yellow	Yellow
Turbidity	Clear	Clear
Specific gravity	1.015–1.045	1.015–1.060
Osmolality (mOsm/kg)	500–2400	1200–3200
Volume (ml/kg/day)	24–40	22–30
Semiquantitative tests		
Protein	0–1	0–1
Ketones, glucose	0	0
Urobilinogen	0–1	0–1
Bilirubin	1$^+$	0–1
pH	5.0–7.0	5.0–7.0
Quantitative tests		
Creatinine (mg/dl)	100–300	110–280
Urea (g/dl)	1.0–2.5	1.0–3.0
Protein (mg/dl)	0–30	0–20
Sodium (mEq/L)	20–165	
Potassium (mEq/L)	20–120	
Calcium (mEq/L)	2–10	
Phosphorus (mEq/L)	50–180	
Amylase (SU)	50–150	3–120

Modified from Bentinck-Smith J, 1983, with permission.

Normal Coagulation Values

Test	Dog	Cat
Platelet count (/μl)	175,000–500,000	175,000–500,000
Clot retraction at 37°C (h)	1–2	1–2
Bleeding time (min)	2–4	1–5
Cuticle bleeding time (min)	1–5	1–5
Partial thromboplastin time (aPTT) (sec)	14–25	14–28
Activated clotting time (ACT) (sec)	60–120	70–120
Prothrombin time (PT) (sec)	7–10	5–9
Russell's viper venom time (RVVT) (sec)	8–14	8–14
Thrombin time (TT) (sec)	6–9	6–9
Fibrinogen (mg/dl)	150–200	150–200
Fibrin split products (FSP) (μg/ml)	<10	<10

NORMAL SERUM PROTEIN ELECTROPHORESIS

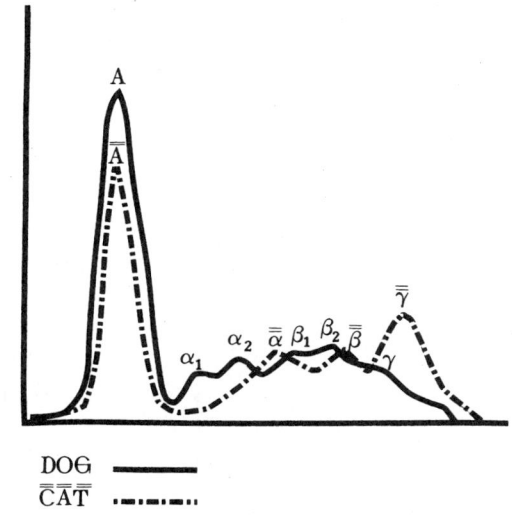

DOG ———
$\overline{\overline{\text{CAT}}}$ ·—·—·—·

Figure A–1. Normal serum protein electrophoretic patterns in the dog and cat.

Protein Component	Common Units (g/dl)		SI Units (g/L)	
	Dog	Cat	Dog	Cat
Albumin	2.3–3.4	2.3–3.5	23–34	23–35
Globulins	3.0–4.7	2.6–5.0	30–47	26–50
Alpha 1	0.3–0.8	0.3–0.5	3–8	3–5
Alpha 2	0.5–1.3	0.4–1.0	5–13	4–10
Beta	0.7–1.8	0.6–1.9	7–18	6–19
Gamma	0.4–1.0	0.5–1.5	4–10	5–15
Total protein	5.5–8.0	6–8	55–80	60–80

Modified from Tvedten HW, 1981, and Bentinck-Smith J, 1983, with permission.

Normal Cerebrospinal Fluid Values

Parameter	Dog	Cat
Color	Clear, colorless	Clear, colorless
Pressure (mm H_2O)	<170	<100
Cell count/μl		
Mononuclear WBCs	<5–8	<5–8
RBCs	None	None
Cell types	Small lymphocytes, few monocytes	
Protein (mg/dl)	<25	<20
Glucose (mg/dl)	61–116	85

Modified from Bentinck-Smith J, 1983, with permission.

Normal Parameters for Patient Monitoring

Parameter	Normal Value
Body temperature	101.5°F (37°C)
Heart rate (beats/min)	
Dog	70–160
Cat	140–210
Respiratory rate (breaths/min)	
Dog	16–20
Cat	20–24
Capillary refill time (CRT) (sec)	<2
Blood pressure (mmHg) (Weiser et al., 1977; Morgan, 1986)	
Systolic	130–180
Diastolic	60–100
Urine output (ml/kg/h)	1–2
Central venous pressure (CVP) (cm H_2O)	
Normal	0–10
Shock	0
Overhydration	8–12
Heart failure	20
Cardiac tamponade	22–25
Arterial blood gases (room air)	
pH	7.35–7.45
PCO_2 (mmHg)	29–36
PO_2 (mmHg)	85–95
HCO_3 (mEq/L)	17–25
Venous blood gases	
pH	7.35–7.45
PCO_2 (mmHg)	29–42
PO_2 (mmHg)	40–60
Lactic acid (mmol/L)	<1.0

Modified from Morgan RV, 1985, with permission.

Commonly Used Equations

Serum Osmolality

$$2 \, (Na + K \, mEq/L) + \frac{glucose \, (mg/dl)}{20} + \frac{BUN \, (mg/dl)}{3}$$

Normal = 305 mOsm/kg

Adjusted Calcium Values (Dogs)

Adjusted calcium = calcium (mg/dl) − albumin (g/dl) + 3.5
= calcium (mg/dl) − 0.4 × total protein + 3.3

Hypocalcemia < 6.5 mg/dl
Hypercalcemia > 12.0 mg/dl

Amended Insulin: Glucose Ratio

$$\frac{Serum \, insulin \, (\mu U/ml) \times 100}{Glucose \, (mg/dl) - 30} \quad Normal < 30$$

Base Deficit

Bicarbonate need (mEq/L) = base deficit × 0.3 × body weight (kg)

Fluid Therapy

I. Replacement needs: Need (L) = % dehydration × body weight (kg) × 1 L + losses from vomiting, diarrhea

II. Maintenance requirements: Maintenance = 10 − 15 ml × body weight (kg) QID

Bibliography

Bentinck-Smith J: A roster of normal values for dogs and cats. p. 1206. In Kirk RW (ed): Current Veterinary Therapy VIII. WB Saunders, Philadelphia, 1983

Feldman BF, Thomason KJ: Useful indexes, formulas, and ratios in veterinary laboratory diagnostics. Compend Contin Educ Pract Vet 11:169, 1989

Lumsden JH: SI units in veterinary medicine. Can J Comp Med 4:103, 1982

Meuter DJ, Chew DJ, Capen CC, Kociba GJ: Relationship of serum total calcium to albumin and total protein in dogs. J Am Vet Med Assoc 180:63, 1982

Meyer DJ, Coles EH, Rich LJ: Veterinary Laboratory Medicine. WB Saunders, Philadelphia, 1992

Morgan RV: Manual of Small Animal Emergencies. Churchill Livingstone, New York, 1985

Morgan RV: Chronic hypertension in four cats: ocular and medical findings. J Am Anim Hosp Assoc 22:615, 1986

Tvedten HW: Hematology of the normal dog and cat. Vet Clin North Am 11:209, 1981

Weiser MG, Spangler WL, Gribble DH: Blood pressure measurement in the dog. J Am Vet Med Assoc 171:364, 1977

Units, Abbreviations, Equivalents

Units

Weights

oz	ounce
lb	pound
kg	kilograms (10^3 g)
g	gram (1 g)
mg	milligram (10^{-3} g)
µg	microgram (10^{-6} g)
ng	nanogram (10^{-9} g)
pg	picogram (10^{-12} g)
gr	grain (1 gr = 65 mg)

Fluids

L	liter (10^3 ml)
dl	deciliter (10^2 ml)
ml	milliliter (1 ml or 10^{-3} L)
µl	microliter (10^{-6} L)
tsp	teaspoon
tbsp	tablespoon

Pressure

mmHg	millimeters of mercury
cm H_2O	centimeters of water

Distance

mm	millimeters
cm	centimeters
in.	inches
m^2	square meter

Time

sec	second
min	minute
h	hour
q	every
d	day
mo	month
yr	year
wk	week

Concentration of Solutions

mEq/L	milliequivalents per liter
g/dl	grams per deciliter
mg/dl	milligrams per deciliter
pg/dl	picograms per deciliter
mOsm/kg	milliosmoles per kilogram
µU/ml	microunits per milliliter
µg/dl	micrograms per deciliter
µmol/L	micromoles per liter
mmol/L	millimoles per liter
pmol/L	picomoles per liter
mmol/kg	millimoles per kilogram
g/L	grams per liter
U/L	units per liter
IU/L	international units per liter
ppm	parts per million

Modified from Morgan RV: Manual of Small Animal Emergencies. Churchill Livingstone, New York, 1985, with permission.

Abbreviations

Routes of Administration

PO	per os, oral
IC	intracardiac
IM	intramuscular
IV	intravenous
SQ	subcutaneous
IT	intrathecal

Dosage Schedules

QID	four times daily; every 6 hours
TID	three times daily; every 8 hours
BID	twice daily; every 12 hours
SID	once daily; every 24 hours
QOD	once every other day; every 48 hours
q	every

Equivalents of Centigrade (Celsius) and Fahrenheit Temperatures

°C	°F
23	73.4
24	75.2
25	77.0
26	78.8
27	80.6
28	82.4
29	84.2
30	86.0
31	87.8
32	89.6
33	91.4
34	93.2
35	95.0
36	96.8
37	98.6
38	100.4
39	102.2
40	104.0
41	105.8
42	107.6
43	109.4
44	111.2
45	113.0
46	114.8

Calibration Tables for the Schiøtz Tonometer

Tables have been devised for both the dog and the cat that convert the numbers read from the Schiøtz instrument to values that represent mmHg for each species.

Calibration Table for Schiøtz Tonometry in Dogs

Schiøtz Scale Reading	IOP (mmHg) 5.5 g wt	IOP (mmHg) 7.5 g wt	IOP (mmHg) 10.0 g wt
0.5	46	61	75
1.0	44	59	73
1.5	43	56	70
2.0	40	53	66
2.5	33	47	61
3.0	26	40	55
3.5	23	35	49
4.0	21	32	44
4.5	20	29	41
5.0	19	27	38
5.5	18	26	36
6.0	17	24	33
6.5	16	23	31
7.0	15	22	30
7.5	—	20	28
8.0	14	19	27
8.5	13	—	25
9.0	—	18	24
9.5	12	17	23
10.0	—	16	22
10.5	11	15	21
11.0	—	—	20
11.5	10	14	19
12.0	—	13	18
12.5	—	—	17
13.0	—	12	16
13.5	8	11	15
14.0	—	—	—
14.5	—	10	14
15.0	7	—	13
15.5	—	9	12
16.0	—	—	—
16.5	6	8	11
17.0	—	—	10
17.5	—	7	—
18.0	5	—	9
18.5	—	6	—
19.0	—	—	8
19.5	—	—	7
20.0	—	5	—

From Pickett JP, Miller PE, Majors LJ: Calibration of the Schiøtz tonometer for the canine and feline eyes. Proc Am Coll Vet Ophthalmol 19:47, 1988, with permission.

Calibration Table for Schiøtz Tonometry in Cats

Schiøtz Scale Reading	IOP (mmHg) 5.5 g wt	IOP (mmHg) 7.5 g wt	IOP (mmHg) 10.0 g wt
0.5	44	73	—
1.0	42	71	—
1.5	40	68	—
2.0	37	65	80
2.5	33	61	76
3.0	30	56	71
3.5	27	48	66
4.0	25	42	61
4.5	24	37	56
5.0	22	34	51
5.5	21	31	47
6.0	20	29	44
6.5	18	27	40
7.0	—	25	37
7.5	17	24	35
8.0	16	22	33
8.5	15	21	31
9.0	14	20	29
9.5	13	19	27
10.0	—	18	25
10.5	—	17	23
11.0	12	16	22
11.5	11	15	20
12.0	—	14	19
12.5	10	13	18
13.0	—	12	17
13.5	9	—	15
14.0	—	11	14
14.5	8	10	13
15.0	—	—	12
15.5	—	9	11
16.0	7	8	10
16.5	—	—	9
17.0	6	7	8
17.5	—	6	7
18.0	—	—	6
18.5	5	5	5
19.0	—	—	—
20.0	—	—	—

From Pickett JP, Miller PE, Majors LJ: Calibration of the Schiøtz tonometer for the canine and feline eyes. Proc Am Coll Vet Ophthalmol 19:47, 1988, with permission.

APPENDIX **IV**

Recommended Drug Dosages

Every effort has been made to provide precise dosages for specific clinical situations; however, individual needs or circumstances may necessitate alterations in both the dosage and the frequency of administration of any of the medications listed on the following pages. Dosages are designated for either "Dog" or "Cat." If neither word appears, the dosage is applicable to both the dog and cat. Note: Multiple uses for drug are listed under original drug entry. A key to the abbreviations can be found on the last page of the table.

Drug (Brand Name or Abbreviation)	Purpose or Use	Chapters Where Cited	Dosage
Acetazolamide (Diamox)	Hydrocephalus Glaucoma	23 98	0.1 mg/kg PO TID Dog: 5–10 mg/kg IV × 1–2 doses
Acetohydroxamic acid (Lithostat)	Struvite urolithiasis	49	Dog: 12.5 mg/kg PO BID
Acetylcysteine (Mucomyst)	Degenerative myelopathy Acetaminophen toxicosis	24 63, 122, 128	70 mg/kg PO TID × 2 wk, then TID QOD Cat: 140–240 mg/kg PO, then 70 mg/kg PO QID × 7 Rx or 140 mg/kg IV
Acetylpromazine (Acepromazine)	Restraint, sedation	37, 79, 111	Dog: 0.025–0.2 mg/kg IV; max 2.5 mg or 0.1–0.25 mg/kg IM, PO Cat: 0.05–0.1 mg/kg IV; max 1 mg
	Arterial thromboembolism	10	0.1–0.2 mg/kg SQ TID
	Scotty cramps	23	Dog: 0.1–0.75 mg/kg PO BID
	Preanesthetic		Dog: 0.1–0.2 mg/kg IV, IM; max 2.5 mg
	Amphetamine toxicosis	128	0.05–1 mg/kg IV, IM, SQ
Acetylsalicylic acid (aspirin)	Glomerulonephritis	47	Dog: 0.5–5 mg/kg PO SID-BID
	Antithrombic, antiprostaglandin effects	18	Dog: 10 mg/kg PO BID
			Cat: 6 mg/kg PO q 48–72 h
	Musculoskeletal pain, inflammation	24, 78, 79	Dog: 10–25 mg/kg PO BID-TID
	Antipyretic, ocular effects	71, 84, 97, 99, 100	Dog: 5–10 mg/kg PO SID-BID Cat: 3–6 mg/kg PO q 48–72 h
Actinomycin D (Cosmegen)	Chemotherapy	70	Dog: 0.5–0.9 mg/m² IV slowly q 3 wk
Activated charcoal (Actidose-Aqua, Requa)	Gastrointestinal adsorbent	122–130	1 g/5 ml water: give 10 ml of slurry/kg PO
Albendazole	*Paragonimus*, capillariasis, giardiasis	18, 47, 114	25–50 mg/kg PO BID × 7–10 days
Albuterol (Ventolin, Proventil)	Bronchodilator	16, 17, 132	Dog: 0.02–0.045 mg/kg PO SID-TID
Allopurinol (Zyloprim)	Urate urolithiasis	47, 49	Dog: 10–15 mg/kg PO BID × 30 days, then 10 mg/kg PO SID
	Leishmaniasis	114	Dog: 20 mg/kg PO BID
Alprazolam (Xanax)	FUS	49	Cat: 0.1–0.2 mg PO SID-BID
	Certain behavioral disorders	116	Dog: 1–2 mg PO PRN; max = 4 mg/day
Aluminum hydroxide (ALternaGEL, Amphojel, Maalox)	Phosphate binder	123	30–90 mg/kg PO SID-TID with meals
Amikacin (Amikin, Amiglyde-V)	Serious infections, endocarditis	9, 18, 79, 112	Dog: 10 mg/kg IM, IV, SQ BID-TID Cat: 10 mg/kg IM, SQ, IV TID

Table continued on following page

1339

Drug (Brand Name or Abbreviation)	Purpose or Use	Chapters Where Cited	Dosage
Aminocaproic acid (Amicar)	Degenerative myelopathy	24	Dog: 500 mg PO TID
Aminophylline (Aminophyllin, Somophyllin)	Bronchodilator	9, 18, 132	Dog: 6–11 mg/kg IM, SQ, PO TID Cat: 4–6 mg/kg PO, IM BID
Amitraz (Mitaban)	Demodicosis	87	Dog: 5.3 ml/gal water; dip wet dog and air-dry q 7–14 days × 3–6 Rx
	Ear mites	87	Mix 1 ml amitraz in 10–20 ml mineral oil, apply topically QOD × 3 wk
Amitriptyline HCl (Elavil, Amitriptyline)	Certain behavioral disorders, FUS	49, 116, 117	Dog: 1–2 mg/kg PO BID Cat: 2.5–5 mg PO SID-BID
	Acral lick granuloma, allergic dermatitis	86, 89	Dog: 0.5–1 mg/kg PO BID
Amlodipine (Norvasc)	Hypertension	47	Dog: 0.5–1 mg/kg PO SID Cat: 0.625 mg PO SID
Ammonium chloride (NH₄Cl)	Urinary acidifier	122, 123, 128	Dog: 100–200 mg/kg/day PO dd TID-QID Cat: 20 mg/kg PO BID
Amoxicillin (Amoxi-Drops, Amoxi-Tabs)	Routine infections	14, 17, 27, 30, 34	10 mg/kg PO, SQ, IV BID-TID
	Serious infections	36, 51, 84, 112	20 mg/kg PO, SQ, IV, IM BID-TID
Amoxicillin/clavulanic acid (Clavamox)	Resistant, serious infections	17, 18, 27, 79, 85	12–22 mg/kg (amoxicillin) PO BID-TID
Amphetamine SO₄ (Adderall)	CNS stimulation during certain toxicoses, chlorpromazine overdose	128	Dog: 1–4 mg/kg SQ PRN Cat: 5 mg PO SID × 4 days
Amphotericin B (Fungizone)	Systemic mycoses, prototothecosis	32, 109, 114	a) 0.25–0.5 mg/kg in 0.5–1 L 5% D/W IV over 6–8 h; QOD to total dose of 8–10 mg/kg or BUN and creatinine levels rise b) 0.5–0.8 mg/kg diluted in saline and dextrose SQ 2–3 times weekly (cryptococcosis)
Amphotericin, liposomal (Abelcet)	Leishmaniasis, systemic mycoses	109, 114	Dog: 1–3 mg/kg IV QOD to total dose of 12 mg/kg
Ampicillin (Omnipen, Polycillin, Polyflex)	Various infections	24, 31–33, 59, 100, 103	22 mg/kg PO TID or 11–22 mg/kg IV, SQ, IM TID-QID
Amprolium (Corid)	Coccidiosis	114	Dog: 200 mg in food or water PO SID × 7–10 days Cat: 60–100 mg in food or water PO SID × 5 days

Drug	Indication	Reference	Dosage
Amrinone (Inocor)	Low-output heart failure		Dog: 0.75 mg/kg IV over 2–3 min, then 5–10 µg/kg/min IV
Antazoline 0.5% (Naphcon)	Allergic conjunctivitis	94	Apply topically SID
Antidiuretic hormone	See *Desmopressin acetate*		
Apomorphine	Induction of vomiting	122	Dog: 0.04 mg/kg IV or 0.08 mg/kg IM, SQ or crush small amount into conjunctival sac
Ascorbic acid (vitamin C)	Reduction of methemoglobin (acetaminophen, naphthalene toxicity)	124, 127, 128	30 mg/kg PO, SQ QID × 7 Rx
	Urinary acidifier		Dog: 100–500 mg PO SID-TID; Cat: 100 mg PO SID-TID
Asparaginase (Elspar)	Lymphosarcoma, lymphocytic leukemia, mastocythemia	64, 67, 70	Dog: a) 10,000 IU/m² IM weekly in a protocol b) 400 IU/kg IP, IM in a protocol
	Sterile pyogranulomas, sebaceous adenitis	85	Dog: 10,000 U IM once weekly × 1–3 Rx
Atenolol (Tenormin)	Supraventricular tachycardia	7, 9, 10	Dog: 0.2–1 mg/kg PO SID-BID or 6.25–12.5 mg/dog PO BID; Cat: 6.25–12.5 mg PO SID-BID
	Hypertension	47	2 mg/kg PO SID-BID
Atracurium besylate (Tracrium)	Paralytic agent	134	Dog: 0.1–0.5 mg/kg IV
Atropine SO₄	Sinus bradycardia, SA block, AV block	7, 8	0.01–0.04 mg/kg IM, SQ, IV PRN
	Atropine response test	7	0.044 mg/kg IM
	Preanesthetic		0.02–0.04 mg/kg SQ, IM
	Hypersialism	28	0.02 mg/kg SQ PRN
	Cholinergic toxins	124, 125, 129	0.2–0.5 mg/kg; give one fourth of dose IV, the rest SQ, IM
Auranofin (Ridaura)	Autoimmune skin diseases	89	Dog: 0.1–0.2 mg/kg PO BID
Aurothioglucose (Solganal)	Pemphigus complex, plasmacytic stomatitis and pododermatitis, immune-mediated arthritis	27, 78, 89	Test dose of 1–5 mg IM, then 1 mg/kg IM weekly until remission, then biweekly or monthly
Azathioprine (Imuran)	Refractory acquired myasthenia gravis	25	Dog: 2 mg/kg PO SID-QOD
	Lymphocytic/plasmacytic, eosinophilic stomatitis, gastritis or enteritis	27, 30, 32	Dog: 1–2.5 mg/kg PO SID-QOD; Cat: 0.2–0.3 mg/kg PO SID-QOD
	Chronic active hepatitis, glomerulonephritis	47	Dog: 2–2.5 mg/kg PO SID
	Immune hemolytic anemia	63	Dog: 2 mg/kg PO SID-QOD

Table continued on following page

Drug (Brand Name or Abbreviation)	Purpose or Use	Chapters Where Cited	Dosage
Azathioprine (Imuran) (*Continued*)	Immune thrombocytopenia (dog)	66	a) 2 mg/kg PO SID, taper to 0.5–1 mg/kg PO QOD
			b) 50 mg/m² PO SID, taper to 25 mg/m² PO QOD
	Immune skin diseases, SLE, sterile pyogranulomas	74, 85, 89	Dog: 2.2 mg/kg or 50 mg/m² PO SID-QOD
	Rheumatoid and immune-mediated arthritis	78	Dog: 2 mg/kg PO SID × 14–21 days, then QOD
	Blepharitis, episcleritis	93, 96, 97	Dog: 2 mg/kg PO SID
	Immune polymyositis, masticatory myositis	80	Dog: 2 mg/kg PO SID
AZT	FIV	110	Cat: 5 mg/kg PO, SQ BID
Baclofen (Lioresal)	Functional urethral obstruction	50	Dog: 1–2 mg/kg PO TID
BAL	*See Dimercaprol*		
Benazepril (Lotensin)	Hypertension	9, 47	Dog: 0.25–0.5 mg/kg PO SID-BID
Benzimidazole	Trypanosomiasis	114	5 mg/kg PO SID × 2 mo
Betamethasone (Celestone)	Pannus, episcleritis, uveitis	96, 100	Dog: 1–2 mg subconjunctivally
Betaxolol 0.5% (Betoptic)	Selective beta-blocker for glaucoma		Apply 1 drop to affected eye twice daily
Bethanechol (Urecholine)	Bladder atony, dysautonomia	50, 102	Dog: 2.5–10 mg SQ TID or 5–25 mg PO TID
			Cat: 1.25–5 mg PO BID-TID
Bisacodyl (Dulcolax)	Stool softener		Dog: 10 mg PO SID PRN
			Cat: 5 mg PO SID PRN
Bismuth (Pepto-Bismol)	GI tract protectant, *Helicobacter*	30, 32, 33	Dog: 0.25–2 ml/kg PO TID-QID
Bleomycin (Blenoxane)	Chemotherapy		Dog: 10 mg/m² IV, SQ SID × 4 days, then 10 mg/m² weekly to max dose 200 mg/m²
Bretylium (Bretylium)	Ventricular fibrillation	8	Dog: 4 mg/kg IV; repeat in 5 min
Brewer's yeast	Source of B vitamins		0.2 g/kg PO q 24–96 h
Buprenorphine (Buprenex)	Analgesia	70, 132	Dog: <11 kg: 15 μg/kg IM, IV BID
			11–23 kg: 10 μg/kg IM, IV BID
			>23 kg: 5 μg/kg IM, IV BID
			Cat: 5–10 μg/kg IM, IV, SQ BID-TID or 3–5 μg/kg IV in normal saline BID

Drug	Indication	References	Dosage
Buspirone (BuSpar)	Anxiolytic drug	117	Dog: 2.5–10 mg PO BID-TID Cat: 5–10 mg PO SID-BID
Busulfan (Myleran)	Chronic myelocytic leukemia		Dog: 4 mg/m² or 0.1 mg/kg PO SID
Butorphanol tartrate (Torbutrol, Torbugesic)	Cough suppressant Preanesthetic Analgesia, sedation	15–17, 112 4, 24, 35, 37, 70, 132, 133	Dog: 0.5–1 mg/kg PO, SQ BID-TID 0.05 mg/kg IV or 0.4 mg/kg SQ, IM Dog: 0.1–0.2 mg/kg IV or 0.2–0.4 mg/kg SQ, IM 2–6 h Cat: 0.1–0.8 mg/kg IM, SQ 4–6 h
Calcitonin (Calcimar)	Hypercalcemia, cholecalciferol toxicosis	42, 71, 123	Dog: 4–6 IU/kg SQ, IM q 2–12 h
Calcitriol (Rocaltrol)	Hypocalcemia Chronic renal failure	42 47, 49	0.03–0.06 µg/kg/day PO 0.025–0.05 µg/kg/day PO
Calcium carbonate (Caltrate, Tums, Calcet)	Hypocalcemia, eclampsia	42, 60	100–150 mg/kg PO dd BID-TID
Calcium chloride	Ventricular asystole	8	10% soln: 0.2 ml/kg IV
Calcium EDTA (Versenate)	Lead and zinc poisoning	127	100 mg/kg/day × 5 days = total dose; make soln of 1 g Versenate/100 ml 5% D/W, divide total quantity of milliliters into 20 aliquots, give 1 dose SQ QID × 5 days
Calcium gluconate (Calcet, Ca gluconate injection)	Ventricular asystole Hypocalcemia, hyperkalemia	8 42, 44, 47, 60, 61	10% soln: 0.4–0.6 ml/kg IV PRN 10% soln: a) 0.5–1 ml/kg IV up to 10 ml in 5% D/W over 20–30 min; may repeat at 6–8 h intervals b) 20 mg/kg IV infusion in 5% D/W at 22 ml/kg/8 h Tab: 150–250 mg/kg PO BID-TID 30–100 mg/kg/day PO
Calcium lactate (Calcet, Calphosan)	Eclampsia Hypocalcemia	60 42, 60	130–200 mg/kg PO TID
Captan powder 50% (Orthocide)	Dermatomycoses	84	Mix 2 tbsp/gal water, use topically twice weekly; do not rinse after applying
Captopril (Capoten)	Vasodilator, congestive heart failure	9	Dog: 0.5–2 mg/kg PO BID-TID Cat: 0.25–0.5 mg/kg PO BID
Carbamazepine (Tegretol)	Aggressive behavior		Cat: 25 mg PO SID-BID
Carbenicillin (Geocillin, Geopen)	Serious infections		15 mg/kg PO, IV TID

Table continued on following page

Drug (Brand Name or Abbreviation)	Purpose or Use	Chapters Where Cited	Dosage
Carbimazole (not available in the United States)	Feline hyperthyroidism	41	Cat: 5 mg PO BID-TID
Carboplatin (Paraplatin)	Chemotherapy, in a protocol	27, 70, 79	Dog: 300 mg/m² IV q 3 wk Cat: 210 mg/m² IV q 3 wk
Carprofen (Rimadyl)	Hip dysplasia, DJD	78	Dog: 2.2 mg/kg PO BID
L-Carnitine (Tyson)	Nutritional supplement, cardiomyopathy		Dog: 100 mg/kg PO BID or 220 mg/kg/day IV Cat: 50–100 mg/kg/day PO
Carteolol 1% (Ocupress)	Nonselective topical beta-blocker for glaucoma		Apply 1 drop to affected eye BID
Cefaclor (Ceclor)	Serious infections		4–20 mg/kg PO TID
Cefadroxil (Cefa-Tabs, Duricef)	Serious infections	85	20 mg/kg PO BID
Cefazolin sodium (Ancef, Kefzol)	Serious infections, endocarditis Acute abdomen syndrome, osteomyelitis	9, 112 37, 79	15–30 mg/kg IV, IM QID 20 mg/kg IV, IM, SQ TID-QID
Cefotaxime (Claforan)	Acute pancreatitis, osteomyelitis, meningitis	24	Dog: 20–40 mg/kg IV, IM, SQ TID-QID
Cefoxitin sodium (Mefoxin)	Resistant or serious infections	36	Dog: 15–30 mg/kg SQ, IM, IV TID
Ceftiofur (Naxcel)	Resistant or serious infections		Dog: 2 mg/kg SQ SID
Cephalexin (Keflex)	*Staphylococcus* diskospondylitis; stomatitis Mastitis Borreliosis Serious infections	24, 27 59 78 31, 36, 79, 84, 85	Dog: 20 mg/kg PO, IM, SQ TID 30 mg/kg PO BID × 21 days Dog: 22 mg/kg PO TID 20–30 mg/kg PO, SQ, IM, IV BID-TID
Cephalothin (Keflin)	Serious infections	35, 51	20–35 mg/kg IM, SQ, IV TID-QID
Cephamandole (Mandol)	Resistant infections		6–40 mg/kg IM, IV TID-QID
Cephapirin (Cefadyl)	Resistant infections		10 mg/kg IM, IV TID-QID
Cephradine (Anspor, Velosef)	Liver disease		20 mg/kg PO TID
Charcoal, activated (Requa, Actidose-Aqua)	Adsorbent during poisonings	122–130	Mix 1 g charcoal in 5 ml water, give 10 ml slurry/kg PO

Drug	Indication	Ref.	Dosage
Chlorambucil (Leukeran)	Lymphoplasmacytic stomatitis	27	Dog: 1–2 mg/kg PO SID-QOD Cat: 0.25–0.33 mg/kg PO q 3 days
	Chronic lymphocytic leukemia	64	a) Dog: 2–8 mg/m² PO SID × 3 wk beyond remission, then 1.5 mg/m² PO SID × 15 days, then q 3rd day Cat: 1.5 mg/m² PO SID as above b) Dog: 15 mg/m² PO SID × 5 days, then q 3 wk
	Macroglobulinemia, mast cell tumor	70	Dog: 0.2 mg/kg PO SID × 10 days, then 0.1 mg/kg PO SID, with prednisone 0.1–0.2 mg/kg PO QOD, with prednisone
Chloramphenicol (Chloromycetin)	Bacterial, rickettsial infections	16, 17, 52, 84, 100, 111–113	Dog: 25–50 mg/kg IV, PO TID Cat: 25 mg/kg PO BID
Chlordiazepoxide-clidinium (Librax)	Irritable colon syndrome	33	Dog: 1–2 tab PO BID
Chlorothiazide (Diuril)	Partial ADH deficiency, diuretic	40	20–40 mg/kg PO BID
Chlorpheniramine (Chlor-Trimeton, Novahistine)	Urticaria, antihistamine, allergic skin disease	74, 89	Dog: 0.5–1 mg/kg PO BID-TID Cat: 1–2 mg PO BID-TID
	Excessive grooming, self-trauma	85	Cat: 2–4 mg PO BID
Chlorpromazine (Thorazine)	Tranquilization Antiemetic	30, 32, 35, 37, 110	Dog: 0.8–2.2 mg/kg PO BID-TID Dog: 0.05–0.1 mg/kg IV TID-QID or 0.25–0.5 mg/kg SQ, IM SID-QID Cat: 0.01–0.025 mg/kg IV
	Muscle relaxation during tetanus	126	Dog: 2 mg/kg IM BID
Chlorpropamide (Diabinese)	Partial ADH deficiency	40	Dog: 10–40 mg/kg/day PO
Cholestyramine (Questran)	Short bowel syndrome	32	Dog: 200–300 mg/kg PO BID
Chorionic gonadotropin, human (HCG, Follutein, Profasi)	Luteinize a follicular cyst Induce descent of inguinal testis Male hypogonadism	54 55 60	Dog: 500–1000 IU IM; repeat in 48 h 100–1000 IU IM q 5 days for 4 Rx 500 IU SQ twice weekly × 4 wk, then start pregnant mare serum (PMS)
	Induce ovulation	57, 60, 61	Dog: 500–1000 IU SQ SID × 2 days, after FSH Cat: 250 IU IM on days 1 and 2 of estrus
Cimetidine (Tagamet)	Esophagitis, gastric ulceration Chronic gastritis, GI tract ulceration, EPI	29, 37 30–32, 35	Dog: 1–4 mg/kg PO, IV, IM TID-QID Dog: 5–10 mg/kg PO, IV, IM TID-QID Cat: 5 mg/kg PO, IV TID-QID
	Chronic renal failure	47	Dog: 4 mg/kg PO, IV, SQ BID-TID
	Effects of mast cell tumors	71	Dog: 4–6 mg/kg PO, IV, SQ BID-QID
	Protectant, with use of NSAIDs	78, 84, 129	Dog: 5–10 mg/kg PO TID

Table continued on following page

Drug (Brand Name or Abbreviation)	Purpose or Use	Chapters Where Cited	Dosage
Ciprofloxacin (Cipro)	Resistant infections, mycoplasmosis	79, 111	Dog: 10–15 mg/kg PO BID
Cisapride (Propulsid)	Gastric motility disorders, megacolon	29–31, 33	Dog: 0.1 mg/kg PO BID-TID or 2.5–5 mg PO TID Cat: 0.3–0.5 mg/kg PO BID-TID or 2.5 mg PO BID-TID
Cisplatin (Platinol)	Chemotherapy, in a protocol	27, 41, 59, 70, 79	Dog: 40–70 mg/m² IV q 3 wk with saline infusion
Clarithromycin (Biaxin)	Hepatozoonosis	114	Dog: 5–10 mg/kg PO BID × 14–21 days
Clemastine (Tavist)	Antihistamine, allergic skin disease	89	Dog: 0.05–0.1 mg/kg PO BID Cat: 0.67 mg PO BID
Clindamycin (Cleocin, Antirobe)	Rhinitis Protozoal polymyositis/neuritis Stomatitis, acute pancreatitis Toxoplasmosis, prostatitis Anaerobic infections Bacterial folliculitis, cellulitis	14 25, 80 27 52, 114 79 84	12.5 mg/kg PO BID 10 mg/kg PO TID-QID 10 mg/kg IV, IM TID 10–20 mg/kg PO, IM BID × 3–6 wk 11 mg/kg PO, IM, IV BID-TID 5 mg/kg PO BID
Clofazimine (Lamprene)	Feline leprosy	84	Cat: 8 mg/kg/day PO × 6 wk
Clomiphene citrate (Clomid, Serophene)	Antiestrogen agent, male infertility	60	Dog: 25 mg/kg PO SID
Clomipramine (Anafranil)	Certain behavioral disorders	116, 117	Dog: 1–3 mg/kg PO SID-BID, in a protocol Cat: 0.5 mg/kg PO SID
Clonazepam (Klonopin)	Anticonvulsant		Dog: 0.1–0.5 mg/kg PO TID, with phenobarbital
Clorazepate dipotassium (Tranxene-SD)	Seizures Anxiolytic drug	22 116	Dog: 2 mg/kg PO BID Cat: 3.75 mg PO BID Dog: 0.55–2.2 mg/kg PO PRN
Clotrimazole (Lotrimin, Mycelex)	Dermatophytosis, fungal rhinitis	14, 84	Apply topically as directed
Cloxacillin (Tegopen)	*Staphylococcus* diskospondylitis	24	10 mg/kg PO QID
Cobalamin	*See Vitamin B₁₂*		

Drug	Indication	Ref.	Dosage
Colchicine (Colchicine, ColBenemid)	Chronic hepatic fibrosis	34	Dog: 0.03 mg/kg PO SID
Cortisone acetate (Cortone Acetate)	Hypoadrenocorticism	44	1 mg/kg/day PO, IM
Coumarin (non-anticoagulant form)	Lymphedema	68	Dog: 400 mg/day PO
Cromolyn sodium 4%	Allergic conjunctivitis	94	Apply topically 4–6 times daily
Cyclophosphamide (Cytoxan)	Glomerulonephritis, granulomatous urethritis	47, 51	Dog: 2.2 mg/kg PO SID × 4 days/wk
	Feline mammary cancer	59	Cat: 100 mg/m² PO q 3 wk, with doxorubicin
	Immune thrombocytopenia (use with caution)	66	Dog: 50 mg/m² PO SID × 4 days/wk × 3–4 wk
	Immune hemolytic anemia	63	2 mg/kg PO, IV SID × 4 days/wk
	Lymphosarcoma, myeloproliferative disorders, multiple myeloma, as part of a protocol	64, 67, 68, 70, 75	a) 50 mg/m² PO QOD-SID b) 250–300 mg/m² PO, IV q 3 wk
	Rheumatoid, immune-mediated arthritis	78	Dog: 1.5–2.5 mg/kg PO SID × 4 days/wk
	Autoimmune skin diseases, SLE	74, 89	Dog: 50 mg/m² PO SID × 4 days/wk or QOD
	Polymyositis	80	1 mg/kg PO SID × 4 days/wk
	Feline infectious peritonitis	110	Cat: 2 mg/kg PO SID × 4 days/wk, with prednisone
Cyclosporine (Sandimmune)	Glomerulonephritis	47	Dog: 15 mg/kg PO SID
	Immune hemolytic anemia or thrombocytopenia, SLE, sebaceous adenitis	63, 74, 85	Dog: 5–10 mg/kg PO SID × 5 days, off 2 days, then 2.5–5 mg/kg PO SID × 5 days, then taper
Cyclosporine (Optimmune)	KCS, pigmentary keratitis, plasmoma of third eyelid, immune conjunctivitis	94–96	Dog: Apply to affected eye BID
Cyproheptadine (Periactin)	Appetite stimulant	34, 70, 71, 109	Dog: 3 mg/kg PO BID-TID Cat: 1–2 mg/kg PO SID-BID
	Antihistamine, urticaria	74	1.1 mg/kg PO BID-TID
Cytarabine (Cytosar)	Lymphosarcoma, myeloproliferative disorders, as part of a protocol	67, 70	100 mg/m² IV SID × 4 days or 300 mg/m² SQ BID × 2 days
Dacarbazine (DTIC)	Chemotherapy	70	Dog: 200 mg/m² IV SID × 5 days; repeat cycle q 3 wk
Danazol (Danocrine)	Thrombocytopenia	63, 66	Dog: 2–5 mg/kg PO BID-TID
Dantrolene (Dantrium)	Functional urethral obstruction	50	Dog: 1–5 mg/kg PO BID-TID Cat: 0.5–2 mg/kg PO TID or 1 mg/kg IV

Table continued on following page

Drug (Brand Name or Abbreviation)	Purpose or Use	Chapters Where Cited	Dosage
Dapsone (Avlosulfon)	Feline mycobacteriosis Cutaneous vasculitis	84 87	Cat: 1 mg/kg PO BID × 4–6 wk Dog: 1 mg/kg PO TID × 14 days, then taper
Deferoxamine (Desferal)	Iron toxicity	127	40 mg/kg IM QID or 15 mg/kg/h IV (with caution) × 1–2 days
Dehydrocholic acid (Decholin)	Cholangitis, cholelithiasis		Dog: 15 mg/kg PO TID until urine negative for bilirubin
Demeclocycline (Declomycin)	Inappropriate ADH secretion	71	Dog: 3–6 mg/kg PO SID-BID
L-Deprenyl	*See Selegiline*		
Desmopressin acetate (DDAVP)	Central diabetes insipidus	40	Dog: 2–4 drops BID-TID intranasally, conjunctivally
	von Willebrand's disease	66	Dog: 1 μg/kg SQ, IV 90 min prior to surgery
Desoxycorticosterone acetate (DOCA, Percorten)	Hypoadrenocorticism	44	0.2–0.4 mg/kg IM, SQ SID; max = 5 mg
Desoxycorticosterone pivalate (DOCP, Percorten Pivalate)	Hypoadrenocorticism	44	a) 25 mg IM = 1 mg/day DOCA released × 25 days b) 125 mg pellet SQ = 0.5 mg/day DOCA released × 6 mo c) Dose = 1–1.5 mg/kg IM, SQ q 25–28 days
Dexamethasone NaPO₄ (Azium-SP, Dexate)	Anti-inflammatory	14	0.2–2.2 mg/kg IV
	Brain trauma	23	2–4 mg/kg IV; repeat in 6–8 h, then taper
	Spinal cord trauma or inflammation, disk disease	24	1–2 mg/kg IV, then 1 mg/kg SQ, IV BID-TID × 24 h, then taper
	Shock, anaphylaxis, CPR	8, 31, 44, 74, 131	1–4 mg/kg IV slowly
	Immune-mediated skin diseases	89	Cat: 0.2–0.4 mg/kg PO SID, then taper
	Cerebral edema	134, 135	0.25–2 mg/kg IV, then 0.25–1 mg/kg SQ TID-QID in tapering doses
Dextran 40 (Rheomacrodex)	Shock	37, 131	10–20 ml/kg/day IV or 2 ml/kg/h IV infusion
	Anaphylaxis	74	5 ml/kg IV bolus, not to exceed 20 ml/kg/day
	Frostbite, heat prostration	134	20 ml/kg/day IV in 5% D/W
Dextroamphetamine (Dexedrine)	Hyperkinesis		Dog: 0.2–1.3 mg/kg PO PRN
Dextrose, 50%	Hypoglycemia, insulin overdosage	43, 45	2 ml/kg PO or 0.25–1 ml/kg IV

Drug	Indication	References	Dosage
Diazepam (Valium)	Restraint, pain relief	3, 4, 8	0.2–0.6 mg/kg IV
	Seizures	22	a) Cat: 2.5 mg PO TID, max = 7.5 mg PO TID b) Rectal administration: Dog: 1–3 mg/kg Cat: 0.5 mg/kg
	Status epilepticus, certain toxicoses	22, 122–130	0.5–1 mg/kg IV in increments of 5–20 mg, to effect
	Acquired tremors, Scotty cramps	23	Dog: 0.25–0.5 mg/kg PO TID-QID
	Preanesthetic		Dog: 0.1–0.2 mg/kg IV slowly
	Sedation	37, 134	Dog: 0.5–2.2 mg/kg PO PRN
	Functional urethral obstruction	49, 50	Dog: 2–10 mg PO TID
			Cat: 1–2.5 mg PO TID or 0.5 mg/kg IV
	Appetite stimulant	71	Cat: 0.05–0.15 mg/kg IV SID-QOD or 1 mg PO SID
	Urine marking, anxiety, psychogenic alopecia	86, 117	Cat: 1–2 mg PO SID-BID
	Certain behavioral disorders	116	Dog: 0.5–2.2 mg/kg PO PRN
Diazoxide (Proglycem)	Hypoglycemia	45, 71	Dog: 5–13 mg/kg PO BID-TID; max = 40 mg/kg/day
Dichlorphenamide (Daranide)	Glaucoma	98	Dog: 2–4 mg/kg PO BID-TID Cat: 1 mg/kg PO BID-TID
Diclofenac 0.1% (Voltaren)	Conjunctivitis	94	Apply 1 drop to affected eye BID-TID
Dicloxacillin (Pathocil)	Resistant *Staphylococcus* infections	10–20 mg/kg	PO TID-QID
Dicyclomine (Bentyl)	Decrease bladder contractility	50	Dog: 10 mg PO TID
	Acute colitis, irritable colon		Dog: 0.15 mg/kg PO TID
Diethylcarbamazine (Carbam)	Heartworm prophylaxis	12	Dog: 6.6 mg/kg PO SID
Diethylstilbestrol (DES, Stilphostrol)	Hormone-responsive incontinence	50	Dog: 0.1–1 mg PO SID × 5 days, then q 5–14 days
		83	Cat: 0.625 mg IM, with testosterone 5–14 days
	Feline symmetrical alopecia	88	Dog: 0.02 mg/kg PO SID × 14 days, then QOD × 3 mo; max = 1 mg/day
	Estrogen responsive dermatosis		
Digoxin (Lanoxin)	Congestive heart failure, supraventricular tachyarrhythmias	7, 9, 10	Dog: 0.005–0.01 mg/kg PO BID or 0.22 mg/m² PO BID
			Cat: 0.005–0.008 mg/kg PO QOD-SID or 0.0312 mg PO QOD-SID
Digoxin immune Fab (Digibind)	Digoxin toxicity	7	Dog: 40 mg IV (over 30 min) per mg digoxin ingested
Dihydrotachysterol (Hytakerol, DHT)	Hypocalcemia	42	0.03 mg/kg/day PO × 2 days, then 0.01–0.02 mg/kg/day PO

Table continued on following page

1349

Drug (Brand Name or Abbreviation)	Purpose or Use	Chapters Where Cited	Dosage
1,25-Dihydroxyvitamin D₃	See Calcitriol		
Diltiazem (Cardizem)	Hypertrophic cardiomyopathy, supraventricular tachyarrhythmias	7, 9, 10	Dog: 0.5–1.5 mg/kg PO TID Cat: 1.5–2.4 mg/kg PO BID-TID
Dimenhydrinate (Dramamine)	Motion sickness, urticaria	74	Dog: 25–50 mg PO SID-TID Cat: 12.5 mg PO SID-TID
Dimercaprol (BAL)	Arsenic toxicosis	127	3–5 mg/kg IM QID × 5 days
Dimethyl sulfoxide, 40% (DMSO)	Spinal cord trauma		Dog: 1 g/kg IV in 5% D/W SID × 3–4 days
Diminazene aceturate (Berenil) (not available in the United States)	Babesiosis, trypanosomiasis	63, 114	Dog: 3.5 mg/kg IM once
Dioctyl sulfosuccinate (Colace, Surfak, docusate)	Stool softener	33, 36	Small dog, cat: 25 mg PO SID-BID Medium/large dog: 50–100 mg PO SID-BID
Diosmin	Lymphedema	68	Dog: 3 g/day PO
Diphenhydramine HCl (Benadryl)	Rhinitis Counteract effects of mast cell tumors Anaphylaxis, urticaria, angioneurotic edema Antipruritic, allergic skin disease	14 71 74 74, 89	Dog: 2–4 mg/kg PO TID 1 mg/kg IM BID 2–4 mg/kg IM, IV slowly Dog: 2–4 mg/kg PO, IM BID-QID
Diphenoxylate HCl (Lomotil)	Acute colitis, irritable colon syndrome Antidiarrheal	33	Dog: 0.05–0.1 mg/kg PO TID-QID Cat: 0.063 mg/kg PO TID Dog: 2.5 mg PO BID-QID Cat: 0.6–1.2 mg PO BID-TID
Diphenylthiocarbazone (Dithizone)	Thallium toxicosis	122	50–70 mg/kg PO TID
Disodium EDTA	Calcium keratopathy	96	a) 0.37% soln: lavage cornea × 15–20 min b) 1% soln: 1–2 drops topically BID × several wk
Disopyramide PO₄ (Norpace)	Ventricular dysrhythmias		Dog >18 kg: 100 mg PO TID-QID
Dobutamine HCl (Dobutrex)	Inotropic agent	8, 31, 131, 134	Dog: 2–25 µg/kg/min IV infusion Cat: 0.5–3 µg/kg/min IV
Dopamine HCl (Dopamine)	Inotropic agent Renal vasodilator: acute renal failure	8, 31, 131, 134 47	2–25 µg/kg/min IV infusion 1–3 µg/kg/min IV infusion in 5% D/W
Doxapram (Dopram)	Respiratory stimulant		5–10 mg/kg IV

Drug	Indication	References	Dosage
Doxorubicin (Adriamycin)	Chemotherapy	41, 59, 64, 67, 68, 70, 79, 103	Dog: 30 mg/m² IV in 150 ml 5% D/W q 2–9 wk; max cumulative dose = 250 mg/m² Cat: 25 mg/m² IV q 3 wk; max cumulative dose = 150 mg/m²
Doxycycline (Vibramycin, Doryx)	Rickettsial infections, leptospirosis, tuberculosis, borreliosis	16, 18, 27, 47, 66, 78, 84, 111–114	Dog: Acute disease: 5–10 mg/kg PO, IV BID × 10–14 days Chronic disease: 10 mg/kg PO SID × 7–21 days Cat: 2.5–5 mg/kg PO BID
	Mycoplasmal infection	60	Dog: 5 mg/kg PO once, then 2.5 mg/kg PO SID × 10 days; repeat in 10 days
Edrophonium Cl (Tensilon, Enlon)	Tensilon test	25	Dog: 0.1–0.2 mg/kg IV; max = 5 mg Puppies: 0.1–0.5 mg IV
Eicosapentaenoic acid	See Essential fatty acids		
Enalapril (Enacard, Vasotec)	Hypertension, heart failure, valvular insufficiency	9, 10, 47	Dog: 0.5 mg/kg PO SID-BID Cat: 0.25–0.5 mg/kg PO SID-QOD
Enflurane (Ethrane)	Anesthesia		Induction: 2–3% Maintenance: 1.5–3%
Enilconazole (not available in the United States)	Nasal aspergillosis		Administer 5% solution topically BID × 7–10 days
Enrofloxacin (Baytril)	Resistant infections, mycoplasmal infections	16, 17, 24, 31, 32, 60, 84, 112	Dog: 2.5–5 mg/kg PO, SQ IV BID Cat: 1–2 mg/kg PO, SQ BID
	Diskospondylitis, osteomyelitis	24, 79	Dog: 11–15 mg/kg PO BID
	Brucellosis	111	Dog: 10–15 mg/kg PO BID
	Rickettsial infections	113	Dog: 5–10 mg/kg PO BID × 7–14 days
Ephedrine (Mudrane GG, Quadrinal)	Bronchodilator		Dog: 5–15 mg PO BID-TID Cat: 2–5 mg PO BID-TID
	Urethral sphincter incompetence	50	Dog: 1.2 mg/kg PO TID Cat: 2–4 mg PO TID
Epinephrine (Adrenalin)	Cardiac arrest	8	1:10,000 soln: 0.1 ml/kg IV, intraosseously or 0.2–0.4 ml/kg IT
	Anaphylaxis	74	1:10,000 soln: At site: 0.2–0.5 ml SQ, IM IV: 0.5–1 ml; repeat in 30 min
	Urticaria	74	1:10,000 soln: 0.5–2 ml SQ
Epsiprantel (Cestex)	Dipylidium, Taenia		Dog: 5 mg/kg PO Cat: 2.5 mg/kg PO

Table continued on following page

Drug (Brand Name or Abbreviation)	Purpose or Use	Chapters Where Cited	Dosage
Ergocalciferol	*See Vitamin D₂*		
Erythromycin (E-Mycin, Ilotycin)	*Campylobacter*, actinomycosis, URI in cats, mastitis, prostatitis Bacterial folliculitis	32, 52, 59, 111, 112 84	Dog: 10–40 mg/kg PO BID-TID Cat: 10–15 mg/kg PO TID 10–15 mg/kg PO TID
Erythropoietin (Epogen)	Anemia from renal failure	47, 63	50–100 U/kg SQ 2–3 ×/wk PRN
Esmolol (Brevibloc)	Supraventricular tachycardia	7	250–500 µg/kg slowly IV or 50–200 µg/kg/min IV
Essential fatty acids	Atopy, fatty acid deficiency	89, 90, 120	Dog: DermCaps: 1 cap/10–20 kg or 1 ml/10 kg PO SID EFA-2 plus: 2.5 ml/5 kg PO SID PET-Tabs/FA granules: 1 tsp/5 kg PO SID
Ethacrynate sodium (Edecrin)	Diuretic: pulmonary edema	71	0.2–0.4 mg/kg IV, IM q 4–12 h
Ethambutol (Myambutol)	Tuberculosis	18	Dog: 15 mg/kg PO SID
Ethanol 20%	Ethylene glycol toxicosis	127	Dog: 5.5 ml/kg IV q 4 h × 5 Rx, then q 6 h × 4 Rx Cat: 5 ml/kg IV q 6 h × 5 Rx, then q 8 h × 4 Rx
Etidronate disodium (Didronel)	Hypercalcemia	71	Dog: 10–30 mg/kg PO, IV × 1–2 Rx
Etretinate (Tegison)	Squamous cell carcinoma Primary seborrhea	70 88	Dog: 2–3 mg/kg PO TID Dog: 1 mg/kg PO SID
Famotidine (Pepcid)	Gastric ulcers, esophagitis	29, 30, 34	0.5–1 mg/kg PO, SQ SID-BID
Felbamate (Felbatol)	Seizures	22	Dog: <10 kg: 200 mg PO TID initially >10 kg: 400 mg PO TID initially
Fenbendazole (Panacur)	*Oslerus, Capillaria* Hookworms, whipworms, round-worms, *Taenia* *Paragonimus*, pancreatic flukes *Crenosoma vulpis, Giardia canis*	16, 47 32, 33 35 114	Dog: 50 mg/kg/day PO × 6–30 days Dog: 50 mg/kg (1 ml/2 kg) PO SID × 3 days; repeat in 3 wk Dog: 50 mg/kg PO SID × 3–6 days Cat: 30 mg/kg PO SID × 3–6 days Dog: 50 mg/kg PO SID × 3–7 days
Fentanyl transdermal patch (Dur-agesic)	Analgesic	70	Dog: 3–5 µg/kg as needed
Fentanyl/droperidol (Innovar-Vet)	Tranquilization Preanesthetic		Dog: 0.3–0.5 ml/55 kg IV Dog: 1 ml/20 kg IM

Drug	Indication	Reference	Dosage
Ferric cyanoferrate (Prussian blue)	Thallium toxicosis	122	100 mg/kg PO TID
Ferrous sulfate (Feosol, Iberet)	Dietary iron supplement, iron deficiency anemia	63	Dog: 100–300 mg PO SID; Cat: 50–100 mg PO SID
Flavoxate (Urispas)	Detrusor hyperspasticity, urge incontinence		Dog: 100–200 mg PO TID-QID
Fluconazole (Diflucan)	Fungal rhinitis and stomatitis, systemic mycoses	14, 27, 109	Dog: 1.25–2.5 mg/kg PO, IV BID; Cat: 50 mg PO BID or 2.5–5 mg/kg PO, IV SID
Flucytosine (Ancobon)	*Cryptococcus*	109	25–50 mg/kg PO QID
Fludrocortisone (Florinef)	Hypoadrenocorticism	44	0.02 mg/kg/day PO
Flumethasone (Flucort)	Anti-inflammatory		Dog: 0.06–0.25 mg PO SID; Cat: 0.03–0.125 mg PO SID
Flunixin meglumine (Banamine)	Acral lick dermatitis	86	Dog: mix 3 ml in one bottle Synotic, apply topically BID-TID
	Antiprostaglandin effects for ocular disease	94, 100	Dog: 0.5 mg/kg IV SID-BID × 1–2 Rx
	Shock	131	Dog: 1 mg/kg IV once
5-Fluorouracil (Efudex)	Colonic adenocarcinoma, in a protocol		Dog: 150 mg/m^2 IV once weekly
Fluoxetine (Prozac)	Certain behavioral disorders	58, 116, 117	Dog: 1 mg/kg PO SID; Cat: 0.5 mg/kg PO SID
Fluoxymesterone (Android F, Halotestin)	Testosterone responsive dermatosis	88	Dog: 0.5 mg/kg PO QOD × 12 wk; max = 30 mg/day
Flurazepam (Dalmane)	Appetite stimulant		0.2–0.4 mg/kg PO q 4–7 days
Flurbiprofen 0.03% (Ocufen)	Allergic conjunctivitis, anterior uveitis	94, 97	Apply topically BID-TID to affected eye
Folic acid (Feosol Plus)	Dietary supplement	32, 63	Dog: 1–5 mg/day PO or 4–10 µg/kg/day PO; Cat: 2.5 mg/day PO
	Supplement to pyrimethamine	114	1 mg/day PO
Follicle-stimulating hormone (FSH-P; pregnant mare serum, PMS)	Male hypogonadism	60	Dog: 25 mg SQ once weekly or 1 mg/kg IM QOD
	Induction of estrus	61	Dog: 20 IU/kg SQ SID × 10 days, then 500 IU HCG SID × 2 days; Cat: FSH-P = 2 mg IM SID × 5 days
Furazolidone (Furoxone)	*Giardia*, coccidiosis	114	4–10 mg/kg PO SID-BID × 5 days

Table continued on following page

Drug (Brand Name or Abbreviation)	Purpose or Use	Chapters Where Cited	Dosage
Furosemide (Lasix)	Diuresis: heart failure	8–10	Dog: 2–4 mg/kg IV, IM, SQ BID-QID, then taper to 1–2 mg/kg PO SID-BID Cat: 1–3 mg/kg IV, IM, SQ BID-TID, then taper
	Diuresis: pulmonary edema	18, 132	Dog: 2–4 mg/kg IV, IM, PO q 4–12 h Cat: 0.5–2 mg/kg IV TID
	Hydrocephalus, brain edema	23	Dog: 1–2 mg/kg PO BID
	Diuresis: ascites from hepatic failure	34	0.25–0.5 mg/kg PO, SQ SID-BID
	Diuresis: hypercalcemia	42, 71, 123	1–2 mg/kg IV, IM, SQ, PO BID-TID
	Hypertension	47	1 mg/kg PO SID-BID
	Institute diuresis in acute renal failure, certain toxicoses	47, 122	2–5 mg/kg IV TID or PRN
Gallium nitrate	Hypercalcemia	71	Dog: 2.5 μg/kg IV SID × 5 days
Gamma globulin, human (Iveegam)	Immune hemolytic anemia	63	Dog: 0.5–1.5 g/kg IV over 12 h
Gentamicin (Gentocin)	Serious infections Osteomyelitis	9, 31, 32, 112 79	2–4 mg/kg IV, SQ, IM TID 6 mg/kg IV, IM, SQ SID
Glipizide (Glucotrol)	Feline diabetes mellitus	43	Cat: 5 mg PO SID-BID
Glucagon (Glucagon)	Transient improvement in hypoglycemia	43, 71	Dog: 0.03 mg/kg IV, IM, SQ
	Induce gastric hypomotility	4	0.1–0.35 mg IV
Glucose 40% o.o.	Corneal edema, nonhealing erosions	96	Apply ⅛ in. topically 2–6 times daily
Glycerin	Acute glaucoma	98	Dog: 1–2 ml/kg PO × 1–2 Rx
Glyceryl guaiacolate (Geocolate)	Muscle relaxation during certain toxicoses	122–129	110 mg/kg IV PRN
Glyceryl monoacetate	Sodium fluoroacetate toxicosis	122	0.55 mg/kg IM hourly to 2–4 mg/kg
Glycopyrrolate (Robinul)	Sinus bradycardia, heart block	7	0.005–0.01 mg/kg IV, IM or 0.01–0.02 mg/kg SQ PRN
	Hypersialism Preanesthetic	28	0.01 mg/kg SQ PRN 0.01–0.02 mg/kg SQ, IM
Gonadotropin-releasing hormone (Lutrepulse)	Luteinize an ovarian follicular cyst	54	50–100 μg IM/day × 1–3 Rx
	Stimulate descent of inguinal testis Stimulate ovulation	55 57, 61	Dog: 50–100 μg IV, SQ weekly for 2 Rx Dog: 50 μg IV Cat: 25 μg IM after mating, or on day 2 of estrus

Drug	Indication	Reference	Dosage
Granulocyte colony-stimulating factor (Neupogen)	Neutropenia	64	5 µg/kg/day SQ
Griseofulvin (Fulvicin)	Dermatomycoses	84	Microsized: 10–30 mg/kg PO BID × 4–6 wk Ultramicrosized: 2.5–3 mg/kg PO SID-BID × 4–6 wk
Growth hormone (Protropin; Bovine GH)	Pituitary dwarfism Adult hyposomatotropism	40, 73 88	Dog: 0.1 IU/kg SQ SID 3 days/wk × 4–6 wk Dog: 0.1 IU/kg SQ QOD × 30 days
Halothane (Fluothane)	Anesthesia		Induction: 3% Maintenance: 0.5–1.5%
Heparin	Arterial thromboembolism, thrombophlebitis DIC	10, 18 37, 133, 134	Cat: 100 IU/kg SQ TID 75–100 U/kg IV QID or 150–200 U/kg SQ QID
Hetastarch (Hespan)	Shock, hypoproteinemia, CPR	8, 37, 131, 133, 134	Dog: 20 ml/kg/day IV Cat: 10–15 ml/kg IV
Hydralazine (Apresoline)	Vasodilator: heart failure Hypertension	9	Dog: 0.5–2 mg/kg PO BID Cat: 2–5 mg PO BID Dog: 0.5–2 mg/kg PO BID-TID Cat: 2.5 mg PO BID
	Acute arterial thromboembolism	18	Dog: 0.5–2 mg/kg PO, IM BID Cat: 2.5 mg PO BID
Hydrochlorothiazide (HydroDIURIL)	Diuretic: pulmonary edema Nephrogenic diabetes insipidus Hypoglycemia Hypertension	9 40 45, 71 47	2–4 mg/kg PO SID-BID 2.5–5 mg/kg PO BID Dog: 2–4 mg/kg PO BID, with diazoxide Dog: 0.5–5 mg/kg PO SID-BID Cat: 1–2 mg/kg PO BID
Hydrochlorothiazide/spironolactone	See Spironolactone/hydrochlorothiazide		
Hydrocodone bitartrate (Hycodan)	Cough suppressant Feline compulsive disorders	15–17, 112 117	Dog: 0.22 mg/kg PO BID-QID Cat: 1.25–2.5 mg PO SID-BID
Hydrocortisone sodium succinate (Solu-Cortef)	Shock Feline asthma		10 mg/kg IV Cat: 1–3 mg/kg IV
Hydrogen peroxide 3%	Emetic	122	1.5 ml/kg PO × 1–2 Rx

Table continued on following page

Drug (Brand Name or Abbreviation)	Purpose or Use	Chapters Where Cited	Dosage
Hydroxyurea (Hydrea)	Primary polycythemia, thrombocytosis	63, 65, 70	Dog: a) 15–25 mg/kg PO SID-BID or 0.5 g/m² PO BID × 5–7 days, then 15 mg/kg PO SID b) 80 mg/kg PO q 3 days
	Feline hypereosinophilic syndrome	64	Cat: 25 mg/kg PO 3 times weekly
	Chronic granulocytic leukemia	65	Cat: 15 mg/kg/day PO Dog: 20–25 mg/kg or 0.5 g/m² PO BID × 4–6 wk, then 50 mg/kg PO twice weekly
Hydroxyzine (Atarax)	Antihistamine, allergic skin disease, urticaria	74, 89	Dog: 2.2 mg/kg PO BID-TID
Hyoscyamine (Levsin)	Irritable bowel syndrome	33	Dog: 0.003–0.006 mg/kg PO BID-TID
Hypertonic saline (3–7%)	Shock, CPR	8, 31, 131	4–5 ml/kg IV slowly
Idoxuridine (Herplex)	Ocular herpesvirus infection	94, 96	Apply topically 3–6 times daily
Ifosfamide (Ifex)	Lymphosarcoma	70	Dog: 350–375 mg/m² IV, with mesna, q 2–3 wk
Imidacloprid (Advantage)	Flea adulticide	87	Apply topically once monthly, as directed
Imidocarb dipropionate (Imizol) (not available in the United States)	Babesiosis, ehrlichiosis	63, 113, 114	Dog: 5 mg/kg IM, SQ; repeat in 14 days
Imipramine (Tofranil)	Narcolepsy Urethral sphincter incompetence	22 50	Dog: 0.5–1 mg/kg PO TID Dog: 5–15 mg PO BID Cat: 2.5–5 mg PO BID-TID
Insulin, NPH	Diabetes mellitus	43	Dog: <15 kg: 1 U/kg SQ SID-BID >25 kg: 0.25–0.5 U/kg SQ SID-BID Cat: 1–3 U SQ SID-BID
Insulin, regular	Diabetic ketoacidosis	43	Dog: 0.2 U/kg IM, IV, then 0.1 U/kg IM, IV hourly until glucose <250 mg/dl or 2.2 U/kg IV per 24 h
	Uncomplicated diabetes mellitus	43	Dog: 0.5 U/kg SQ q 3–8 h Cat: 0.25 U/kg SQ q 3–8 h
Insulin, Ultralente	Diabetes mellitus	43	Dog: 0.5 U/kg SQ SID Cat: 1–3 U SQ SID
Interferon, human recombinant (Alferon, Intron)	FeLV	110	Cat: 1 U/day PO

Drug	Indication	Reference	Dosage
Iohexol (Omnipaque)	Myelography	4	0.25 ml/kg
Iopamidol (Isovue-200)	Myelography	4	0.25 ml/kg
Ipecac syrup	Induce vomiting	122	1–2 ml/kg PO
Ipronidazole	Giardiasis	114	Dog: 126 mg/L water PO ad libitum × 7 days
Isoflurane (Forane, AErrane)	Anesthesia		Induction: 4–5% Maintenance: 1.5–2.5%
Isoniazid (Rifamate, Rifater)	Tuberculosis	18	10–20 mg/kg PO SID
Isopropamide/prochlorperazine (Darbazine)	Antiemetic, antidiarrheal		Dog: 0.14–0.22 mg/kg SQ BID
Isoproterenol (Isuprel)	Bradycardia, heart block	7	0.01 µg/kg/min IV infusion as 0.2–0.5 mg in 250 ml 5% D/W
	Feline asthma		Cat: 0.2 mg in 100 ml 5% D/W IV TID to effect or 0.004–0.006 mg IM q 30 min PRN
Isosorbide dinitrate (Isordil)	Vasodilator		Dog: 1–2 mg/kg PO TID
Isotretinoin (Accutane)	Sebaceous adenitis, schnauzer comedo syndrome	85, 88	Dog: 1 mg/kg PO SID-BID Cat: 5 mg PO SID
Itraconazole (Sporanox)	Systemic mycoses, dermatophytosis, protothecosis, fungal stomatitis	14, 27, 32, 84, 88, 109, 114	5 mg/kg PO SID-BID × 2–3 mo
Ivermectin (Heartgard)	Heartworm prophylaxis	12	Dog: 6–12 µg/kg PO once monthly Cat: 24 µg/kg PO once monthly
	Microfilaricide	12	Dog: 50 µg/kg PO; repeat in 10 days Cat: 24 µg/kg PO
	Pneumonyssus, Capillaria, Oslerus	14, 16, 18, 47	Dog: 0.2–0.3 mg/kg PO, SQ; repeat in 3 wk (Do not use this dosage in collies or shelties.)
	Intracranial *Cuterebra*	23	0.3 mg/kg SQ QOD × 3 Rx (Not to be used in collies or shelties.)
	Spirocercosis		Dog: 0.2 mg/kg PO once (Not to be used in collies or shelties.)
	Cheyletiellosis, notoedric and sarcoptic mange	87	Dog: 0.2–0.3 mg/kg PO, SQ; repeat in 2 wk (Not to be used in collies or shelties.)
	Demodicosis	87	Dog: 0.4–0.6 mg/kg PO SID × 30 days (Do not use in collie-type, English, or Australian sheepdogs.)
Kanamycin (Kantrim)	Routine infections GI tract bacterial overgrowth	18	5 mg/kg SQ BID 5 mg/kg PO BID-TID

Table continued on following page

Drug (Brand Name or Abbreviation)	Purpose or Use	Chapters Where Cited	Dosage
Kaolin/pectin (Kaopectate)	GI tract protectant	122, 126	1–2 ml/kg PO BID-QID
Ketamine HCl (Ketaject, Ketamine)	Restraint	3, 4	Cat: 0.2–0.6 mg/kg IV, with diazepam or acetylpromazine
	Anesthesia, sedation	4	Dog: 6–10 mg/kg IV Cat: 22–33 mg/kg IM or 2.2–4.4 mg/kg IV
Ketoconazole (Nizoral)	Systemic, oral, and cutaneous mycoses; prototheecosis	14, 27, 32, 84, 88, 93, 109, 114	Dog: 5–15 mg/kg PO BID Cat: 10–15 mg/kg PO SID-BID
	Hyperadrenocorticism	44	Dog: 5–15 mg/kg PO BID
	Malassezia otitis	105	Dog: 5–10 mg/kg PO SID
	Leishmaniasis	114	10 mg/kg PO TID × 3 wk
Ketorolac 0.5% (Acular)	Conjunctivitis	94	Apply 1 drop to affected eye BID-TID
Lactulose (Enulose, Cholac)	Hepatic encephalopathy, stool softener	23, 33, 34	0.25–0.5 mg/kg (2–10 ml) PO TID-QID until feces are soft
Leucovorin (Leucovorin)	Counteract toxicity of methotrexate		Dog: 3 mg/m² IM within 3 h of methotrexate
Levamisole (Ripercol, Tramisol)	*Aleurostrongylus, Oslerus*	16, 18	Dog: 7.5 mg/kg PO SID × 10–30 days
Levobunolol 0.25%, 0.5% (Betagan)	Nonselective beta-blocker for glaucoma	98	Apply 1 drop to affected eye SID-BID
Lidocaine	Ventricular arrhythmias	7, 8, 10, 31	Dog: a) 1–2 mg/kg IV bolus up to a total dose of 8 mg/kg in 10 min b) 25–80 µg/kg/min IV infusion Cat: a) 0.25–0.75 mg/kg IV bolus b) 10–40 µg/kg/min IV infusion
Lime sulfur suspension	Sarcoptic mange	84	Dog: 1:20 dilution Cat: 1:40 dilution Dip, air-dry; repeat weekly × 6 wk
Lime water	Alkaline gastric lavage	122–129	5 ml/kg PO
Lincomycin (Lincocin)	Mastitis	59	15 mg/kg PO TID × 21 days
	Bacterial folliculitis	84	20 mg/kg PO BID
Liothyronine, T₃	*See Triiodothyronine*		
Lisinopril (Prinivil)	Heart failure	9	Dog: 0.5 mg/kg PO SID

Drug	Indication	References	Dosage
Lithium carbonate (Lithonate, Litho-tabs)	Cyclic neutropenia, pancytopenia	64, 66, 73	Dog: 11 mg/kg PO SID
	Inappropriate secretion of ADH	71	Dog: 25 mg PO SID
Lomotil (diphenoxylate HCl with atropine)	Antidiarrheal		Dog: 2.5 mg PO BID-TID
Lomustine (CeeNU)	Brain tumors	70	Dog: 90 mg/m² PO q 3-4 wk
Loperamide (Imodium)	Antidiarrheal, acute colitis	32, 33	Dog: 0.08-0.2 mg/kg PO TID-QID Cat: 0.04 mg/kg PO SID-BID; use with caution
Lufenuron (Program)	Flea growth inhibitor	87	Dog: 10 mg/kg PO once monthly Cat: 30 mg/kg PO once monthly
8-L-Lysine vasopressin (Diapid)	Central diabetes insipidus		1-2 sprays in each nostril SID-TID
Magnesium hydroxide (Milk of Magnesia)	Antacid		Dog: 5-30 ml PO SID-BID Cat: 5-10 ml PO SID-BID
	Cathartic		3-5 × the antacid dosage
Mannitol 20%	Cerebral edema, spinal cord trauma, acute glaucoma	8, 23, 98, 122, 134	1-2 g/kg IV slowly
	Acute renal failure	47	0.5-1 g/kg IV slowly
Meclizine (Bonine)	Motion sickness, urticaria	23, 74	Dog: 4 mg/kg PO SID Cat: 2 mg/kg PO SID
Meclofenamic acid (Arquel)	Degenerative joint disease	78	Dog: 1.1 mg/kg PO SID × 4-7 days, then 0.5 mg/kg
Medium-chain triglyceride (MCT Oil, Portagen)	Chylothorax	19	1-2 ml/kg/day PO
	Primary lymphangiectasis, EPI	32, 35	0.5-1 oz/10 kg PO dd TID-QID; max = 1 tbsp per meal or 1-2.2 ml/kg/day PO with food
Medroxyprogesterone acetate (Depo-Provera, Provera)	Aggressive masculine behavior Urine marking, anxiety, intraspecies aggression		Dog: 10 mg/kg IM, SQ PRN Cat: 10-20 mg/kg SQ, IM
Megestrol acetate (Ovaban, Megace)	Lymphoplasmacytic stomatitis	27	Cat: 2.5 mg PO SID-QOD × 10 days, then 1-2 ×/wk
	Urethritis, FUS, prostatic hyperplasia	52	Dog: 0.55 mg/kg PO SID × 4 wk Cat: 2.5-5 mg PO SID-QOD
	Prevent estrus	60	Dog: Proestrus: 2.2 mg/kg/day PO × 8 days; Anestrus: 0.55 mg/kg/day PO × 32 days
	Endocrine alopecia	88	Cat: 2.5-5 mg PO SID × 10 days, then QOD
	Eosinophilic keratitis, hypereosinophilic syndrome	64, 96	Cat: 0.5 mg/kg/day PO × 7-14 days

Table continued on following page

Drug (Brand Name or Abbreviation)	Purpose or Use	Chapters Where Cited	Dosage
Megestrol acetate (Ovaban, Megace) (*Continued*)	Unacceptable masculine behavior, urine marking, anxiety, intraspecies aggression	117	Dog: 1.1–2.2 mg/kg PO SID PRN Cat: 2.5–10 mg PO SID × 7 days, then taper
Meglumine antimonate	Leishmaniasis	114	Dog: 100 mg/kg IV, SQ SID × 3–4 wk
Melarsomine (Immiticide)	Heartworm adulticide	12	Dog: 2.5 mg/kg IM BID × 2 days or 2.5 mg/kg IM, wait 30 days, then give 2 more doses 24 h apart
Melatonin	Primary acanthosis nigricans	82	Dog: 1–2 mg SQ SID × 3–5 days
Melphalan (Alkeran)	Multiple myeloma	70, 75	Dog: a) 0.1 mg/kg PO SID × 10 days, then 0.05 mg/kg PO SID × 2 wk, then 0.05 mg/kg PO QOD b) 7 mg/m² PO SID × 5 days q 3 wk c) 1.5 mg/m² PO SID × 7–10 days; repeat every 3 wk
Meperidine HCl (Demerol)	Preanesthetic Analgesia Sedation	31 35, 132, 135 122	Dog: 0.5 mg/kg IV Dog: 3–5 mg/kg IM PRN or 2–4 mg/kg IV q 2 h Cat: 2–4 mg/kg IM, SQ PRN Dog: 5–10 mg/kg IM Cat: 1–4 mg/kg IM
2-Mercaptopropionyl glycine, Tiopronin (Thiola)	Cystinuria	49	Dog: 15–25 mg/kg PO BID
6-Mercaptopurine (Purinethol)	Chronic myelocytic leukemia, lymphoma	67	Dog: 50 mg/m² PO SID or 2 mg/kg PO SID, in a protocol
Metaraminol (Aramine)	Vascular support during shock		0.01–0.1 mg/kg IV slowly or 10 mg in 250 ml 5% D/W IV to effect
Methazolamide (Neptazane)	Glaucoma	98	Dog: 1–2 mg/kg PO TID Cat: 1–2 mg/kg PO BID
Methimazole (Tapazole)	Hyperthyroidism	41	Cat: 5 mg PO SID-TID to effect
Methocarbamol (Robaxin)	Muscle relaxation: intervertebral disk disease Muscle relaxation for certain toxicoses	122–129	Dog: 15–20 mg/kg PO TID Dog: 10% soln: 150 mg/kg IV
Methohexital (Brevital)	Anesthesia induction		2.5% soln: 11 mg/kg IV

Drug	Indication	References	Dosage
Methotrexate Na (Methotrexate)	Chemotherapy	67, 70	Dog: 2.5 mg/m² PO SID-BID or 0.3–0.8 mg/kg IV weekly, in a protocol Cat: 0.8 mg/kg IV, PO q 4 wk
Methoxamine HCl (Vasoxyl)	Vasopressor: cardiac arrest, shock	131	Dog: 0.1–0.8 mg/kg IV slowly
Methylphenidate (Ritalin)	Narcolepsy Hyperkinesis	22	Dog: 0.25 mg/kg PO SID-BID Dog: 2–4 mg/kg PO PRN
Methylprednisolone (Medrol)	Chorioretinitis	100	0.2 mg/kg PO BID
Methylprednisolone acetate (Depo-Medrol)	Eosinophilic ulcers and linear granulomas, lymphoplasmacytic stomatitis Pannus, episcleritis, anterior uveitis	27, 85 96, 97	Cat: 20–40 mg SQ, IM q 2–6 wk × 2–6 Rx Dog: 4–12 mg subconjunctivally
Methylprednisolone sodium succinate (Solu-Medrol)	Brain or spinal trauma Shock	23, 24 131	30 mg/kg IV, then 15 mg/kg IV 2 h later, then 15 mg/kg IV QID × 2 days 30 mg/kg IV once
4-Methylpyrazole (Antizol-Vet)	Ethylene glycol toxicosis	127	Dog: 20 mg/kg IV, then 15 mg/kg IV at 12 and 24 h, then 5 mg/kg IV at 36 h
Methyltestosterone (Metandren, Android-25)	Galactorrhea Anabolic drug Testosterone-responsive dermatosis	59 83, 88	Dog: 1–2 mg/kg PO SID × 5–7 days; max = 25 mg/day 1–2 mg/kg PO SID; max = 30 mg/day Dog: 0.5–1 mg/kg PO QOD; max = 30 mg/day
Metipranolol 0.3% (OptiPranolol)	Nonselective beta-blocker for glaucoma		Apply 1 drop to affected eye BID
Metoclopramide (Reglan)	Gastric motility disorders, antiemetic Gastric reflux Dysautonomia	29–35, 37, 110 29, 128 102	Dog: 0.2–0.5 mg/kg PO, SQ TID-QID or 0.01–0.05 mg/kg/h IV infusion Cat: 0.1–0.2 mg/kg PO TID or 0.01 mg/kg/h IV infusion Dog: 0.2–0.4 mg/kg PO TID-QID Cat: 0.3 mg/kg PO TID
Metoprolol (Lopressor)	Atrial fibrillation, hypertrophic cardiomyopathy		Dog: 0.5–1 mg/kg PO TID Cat: 12.5–25 mg PO BID
Metronidazole (Flagyl)	Hepatic encephalopathy, GI bacterial overgrowth, acute colitis Meningitis Stomatitis Osteomyelitis, cellulitis Giardia, Entamoeba, Trichomonas, Balantidium	23, 30, 32–35, 37 24 27 79, 84 114	Dog: 7.5–15 mg/kg PO TID or 7–10 mg/kg IV slowly over 30 min TID Cat: 10 mg/kg/day PO or 25–100 mg PO BID Dog: 10–20 mg/kg PO TID 15 mg/kg PO BID-TID 15–25 mg/kg PO, IV BID Dog: 10–25 mg/kg PO BID × 8 days Cat: 10–25 mg/kg PO SID-BID × 5–7 days

Table continued on following page

1361

Drug (Brand Name or Abbreviation)	Purpose or Use	Chapters Where Cited	Dosage
Mexiletine (Mexitil)	Ventricular arrhythmias	7, 31	Dog: 5–8 mg/kg PO BID-TID
Mibolerone (Cheque)	Galactorrhea	59	Dog: 16 mg/kg PO SID × 5 days
	Prevent estrus (dogs only)	60	Dog: 1–11 kg: 30 µg/day PO 12–22 kg: 60 µg/day PO 23–45 kg: 120 µg/day PO >45 kg, GSD, GSDx: 180 µg/day PO (GSD = German shepherd dog; GSDx = German shepherd dog cross)
	Pseudocyesis	60	Dog: 10 times above dosage × 5 days PO
Miconazole (Conofite)	Dermatophytosis	84	Apply topically as directed
	Ocular fungal infections (Monistat i.v.)	94, 96	Apply topically 4–12 times daily
Midazolam (Versed)	Preanesthetic, sedation	3	Dog: 0.1–0.2 mg/kg IM, SQ, IV
Milbemycin oxime (Interceptor)	Heartworm, hookworm, and whip-worm prophylaxis, microfilaricide	12, 33	Dog: 0.5 mg/kg PO monthly
	Demodicosis in adult dogs	87	Dog: 2 mg/kg PO SID × 60–90 days PRN
	Sarcoptic mange	87	Dog: 0.75 mg/kg PO SID × 30 days
Milrinone (Primacor)	Low-output heart failure		Dog: 0.5–1 mg/kg PO BID
Minocycline (Minocin)	Brucellosis, diskospondylitis	18, 24, 55, 111	Dog: 12.5 mg/kg PO BID with gentamicin 2.2 mg/kg IM TID
Misoprostol (Cytotec)	Gastric protectant	128	Dog: 1–5 µg/kg PO TID-QID
Mithramycin (Mithracin)	Hypercalcemia	42, 71	0.1–0.5 µg/kg IV SID × 2 Rx
Mitotane (Lysodren)	Pituitary-dependent hyperadrenocorti-cism	44, 88	Dog: 25–50 mg/kg/day PO SID × 5–10 days, then q 4–7 days or PRN
	Functional adrenocortical tumors	44, 70	Dog: 50–75 mg/kg PO dd BID initially, then 75–100 mg/kg/wk PO
Mitoxantrone (Novantrone)	Chemotherapy, in a protocol	41, 70	Dog: 2.5–6 mg/m² IV q 3 wk Cat: 6.5 mg/m² IV q 3 wk
Morphine SO₄	Supraventricular premature beats	8, 9	Dog: 0.1–0.2 mg/kg IM, IV, SQ PRN
	Analgesia	24, 79, 132, 133, 135	Dog: 0.2–0.5 mg/kg SQ, IM every 4–6 h or 0.1 mg/kg IV BID-QID Cat: 0.05–0.1 mg/kg SQ, IM BID
Nafcillin (Unipen)	Resistant *Staphylococcus* infections		10 mg/kg PO, IM QID
Nalmefene (not licensed in the United States)	Stereotypic behavior		Dog: 1–4 mg/kg SQ

Drug	Indication	Ref.	Dosage
Nalorphine HCl (Nalline)	Narcotic antagonist		0.1 mg/kg IV: dog, max = 5 mg; cat, max = 1 mg
Naloxone HCl (Narcan)	Stereotypic behavior Narcotic antagonist	122	Dog: 20 mg SQ 0.02–0.04 mg/kg IV
Naltrexone (Trexan)	Acral lick granuloma	90	Dog: 1 mg/kg SQ or 2.2 mg/kg PO SID
Nandrolone decanoate (Deca-Durabolin)	Anabolic effects	71	Dog: 1–5 mg/kg/wk IM; max = 200 mg Cat: 10–20 mg/wk IM
Natamycin (Pimaricin)	Ocular fungal infections	94, 96	Apply topically 3–8 times daily
Neostigmine (Prostigmin)	Myasthenia gravis	25	Dog: 0.05 mg/kg IM TID-QID
Niacinamide (Glutofac)	Pemphigus, discoid lupus	89	Dog: 2.5–5 mg/kg PO TID, with tetracycline
Nicotinamide (niacin, nicotinic acid)	Vacor toxicosis	122, 123	50–100 mg IM
Nifurtimox (Lampit)	Trypanosomiasis	114	Dog: 2 mg/kg PO QID × 3 mo
Nitroglycerin 2% ointment (Nitro-Bid, Nitrol)	Dilatative cardiomyopathy, heart failure	9	Dog: 0.25–1 in. cutaneously q 4–6 h Cat: ⅛–¼ in. cutaneously QID
Nitroprusside (Nipride, Nitropress)	Vasodilator for acute congestive heart failure	9	Dog: 1–10 μg/kg/min IV infusion
Nizatidine (Axid)	Gastric ulcers		Dog: 5 mg/kg PO SID
Norfloxacin (Noroxin)	Resistant infections Salmonellosis		Dog: 11–22 mg/kg PO BID Dog: 22 mg/kg PO BID
Nystatin (Mycolog, Nystatin)	Candidiasis	84	Apply topically BID-TID × 1–2 wk
Octreotide acetate (Sandostatin)	Insulinoma	45	10–20 μg PO, SQ BID-TID
Omeprazole (Prilosec)	Reflux esophagitis, GI ulceration	29, 30	Dog: 0.7–2 mg/kg PO SID
o,p'-DDD	See Mitotane		
Ormetroprim/sulfa (Primor)	See Sulfadimethoxine/ormetroprim		
Oxacillin (Oxacillin)	Staphylococcus infections	79, 84, 93	10–22 mg/kg PO, IV, IM TID-QID
Oxazepam (Serax)	Appetite stimulant	109	Cat: 2–3 mg PO SID-BID
Oxybutynin (Ditropan)	Detrusor hyperspasticity	50	Dog: 1.25–5 mg PO BID-TID Cat: 0.5–1.25 mg PO BID-TID

Table continued on following page

Drug (Brand Name or Abbreviation)	Purpose or Use	Chapters Where Cited	Dosage
Oxymetholone (Anadrol-50)	Anabolic agent	63, 110	1 mg/kg PO SID-BID
Oxymorphone (Numorphan)	Sedation	3	Dog: 0.05–0.1 mg/kg IV or 0.1–0.2 mg/kg IM, SQ Cat: 0.02 mg/kg IV
	Analgesia	8, 24, 37, 79, 133, 135	Dog: 0.025–0.2 mg/kg IV, IM, SQ q 4–6 h Cat: 0.025–0.05 mg/kg IV, SQ q 4–6 h
	Preanesthetic, during gastric dilatation	31	Dog: 0.1–0.2 mg/kg IV; max = 3 mg
Oxytetracycline (Medamycin, Terramy-cin)	Haemobartonellosis, EPI	35, 113	Dog: 20–40 mg/kg PO TID × 3 wk Cat: 15–30 mg/kg PO BID-TID × 3 wk
Oxytocin (Pitocin, Syntocinon)	Uterine prolapse	56	Dog: 5–20 U IM once Cat: 5 U IM once
	Stimulate milk letdown		Spray intranasally in the bitch 5–10 min before nursing
	Uterine inertia	60, 61	Dog: a) 5–20 U IM or IV infusion; may repeat in 30–60 min b) 10 U in 5% D/W IV over 30 min Cat: 2–5 U IM, SQ; may repeat in 45 min
Pancreatic enzymes (Viokase)	Pancreatic exocrine insufficiency	35	Dog: 1–2 tsp/20 kg with each meal until nor-mal, then taper Cat: 0.5 tsp/5 kg with food until normal, then taper
Pancuronium bromide (Pavulon)	Paralytic agent	134	Dog: 0.1 mg/kg IV or 0.06 mg/kg/h IV
Paregoric	Antidiarrheal		0.06 mg/kg PO BID-TID
Paromomycin (Humatin)	Cryptosporidiosis	114	125–165 mg/kg PO BID × 5 days
D-Penicillamine (Cuprimine)	Copper hepatopathy	34	Dog: 125–250 mg/day PO
	Cystine urolithiasis	49	Dog: 15 mg/kg PO BID with food
	Lead, arsenic, zinc poisoning	127	Dog: 35–50 mg/kg/day PO dd QID × 7 days; wait 7 days, then repeat
Penicillin, aqueous (K or Na)	Meningitis, bacterial endocarditis	9, 24	20,000–40,000 U/kg IV q 4–6 h
	Actinomycosis, tetanus	111, 126	22,000 U/kg IV QID or 1,000,000 U intrale-sionally
Penicillin, procaine (Wycillin)	Leptospirosis, actinomycosis	47, 111, 126	20,000–40,000 U/kg IM, SQ BID
Penicillin V (Pen-Vee K)	Routine infections		10 mg/kg PO TID
Pentamidine (phenamidine) isethionate (Pentam)	Babesiosis	114	Dog: 15 mg/kg SQ SID × 2 days
	Pneumocystis carinii	114	Dog: 4 mg/kg IM, SQ SID × 2 wk

Drug	Indication	Reference	Dosage
Pentobarbital (Nembutal)	Status epilepticus, strychnine and other toxicities	22, 122, 123, 126	2–15 mg/kg IV to effect
	Sedation	134	2–4 mg/kg IV or 1 mg/kg/h IV
	Anesthesia		10–30 mg/kg IV to effect
Pentoxifylline (Trental)	Ear margin seborrhea	88	Dog: 200–400 mg PO SID
Phenobarbital	Antitussive	15	Dog: 2 mg/kg PO at bedtime
	Seizures	22, 23	Dog: 1–2.5 mg/kg PO BID initially; some require up to 20 mg/kg/day
			Cat: 2.5 mg/kg PO SID
	Status epilepticus	22, 122	2–4 mg/kg IV repeated to effect; max = 20 mg/kg, or ≤100 mg/min IV until serum level = 25 μg/ml
	Sedation		Dog: 1–2 mg/kg PO BID-TID
			Cat: 1 mg/kg PO BID
	Psychogenic alopecia	86	Cat: 4–8 mg PO BID
Phenoxybenzamine HCl (Dibenzyline)	Acute hypertension from pheochromocytoma	44	Dog: 0.2–1.5 mg/kg PO BID
	Functional urethral obstruction	50	Dog: 0.25 mg/kg PO BID
			Cat: 1.25–7.5 mg PO SID-BID
Phentolamine (Regitine)	Hypertension from pheochromocytoma		Dog: 0.02–0.1 mg/kg IV
Phenylbutazone (Butazolidin)	Analgesia		Dog: 8–10 mg/kg PO TID; max = 800 mg/day
	Anti-inflammatory: arthritis	78	Dog: 13 mg/kg PO TID × 48 h, then taper dose to lowest effective dose; max = 800 mg/day
Phenylephrine (Neo-Synephrine)	Vasopressor	128, 131	Dog: 0.13 mg/kg IV
Phenylpropanolamine HCl (Dexatrim, Ornade, Triaminic)	Urethral sphincter incompetence	50	Dog: 12.5–50 mg PO TID or 1.5 mg/kg PO TID
			Cat: 1.5–2.2 mg/kg PO BID-TID
Phenytoin (Dilantin)	Ventricular arrhythmias		Dog: 2–4 mg/kg IV in increments; max = 10 mg/kg
Physostigmine (Antilirium)	Muscarinic mushroom intoxication	129	Dog: 0.5–3 mg IM
			Cat: 0.25–0.5 mg IM
Physostigmine 0.25% o.o. (Eserine)	Dysautonomia	102	Cat: Apply ⅛ in. topically TID

Table continued on following page

Drug (Brand Name or Abbreviation)	Purpose or Use	Chapters Where Cited	Dosage
Phytomenadione	*See Vitamin K₁*		
Pilocarpine 1% ophthalmic soln	Dysautonomia	102	Cat: Apply 1 drop topically QID
	To induce miosis	99	Apply 1 drop to affected eye BID-TID
Piroxicam (Feldene)	Transitional cell carcinoma	49, 51, 52, 70	Dog: 0.3 mg/kg PO SID
Plasma, fresh frozen	DIC	134	10 ml/kg IV
Plicamycin	*See Mithramycin*		
Polymyxin (Aerosporin)	Mycobacterial infections	84	Dog: 2 mg/kg IM BID
Polysulfated glycosaminoglycans (Adequan)	Degenerative joint disease	78	Dog: 5 mg/kg IM once weekly × 6–8 wk
Potassium bromide	Seizures	22	Dog: 20–40 mg/kg PO SID with food
			Cat: 30 mg/kg PO SID
Potassium chloride (Kaon-Cl, Kolyum)	Potassium supplementation	47	0.1–0.25 ml/kg PO TID; dilute 1:1 with water
Potassium chloride, injectable	Hypokalemic polymyopathy	80	0.5–1 mEq/kg/h as 40–80 mEq KCl per liter IV fluids
	Serum potassium deficit	43	2–10 mEq/kg/day added to IV fluids
Potassium citrate (Citrolith)	Chronic renal failure	47	30 mg/kg PO BID
	Urine alkalization	49	40–75 mg/kg PO BID
Potassium gluconate (Kolyum, Tumil-K)	Hypokalemic polymyopathy	47, 80, 120	Cat: 2–6 mEq PO SID-BID
Potassium iodide (SSKI Solution)	Sporotrichosis, pythiosis	84	Dog: 0.4 ml/kg/day PO
Potassium permanganate (1:2,000)	Strychnine and nicotine toxicosis	123, 128	5 ml/kg in gastric lavage
Pralidoxime Cl (2PAM, Protopam)	Organophosphate toxicosis	124	20 mg/kg IV BID
Praziquantel (Droncit, Drontal Plus)	*Paragonimus* infection	18	5 mg/kg PO TID × 3 days
	Tapeworms: *Taenia, Dipylidium*		Dog: 0.5 tab/2.5 kg PO; max = 5 tab
			Cat: 1.8 kg: 0.5 tab PO
			2.3–5 kg: 1 tab PO
			>5 kg: 1.5 tab PO
	Pancreatic flukes	35	Cat: 40 mg/kg PO SID × 3 days
	Nanophyetus salmincola	113	Dog: 10–30 mg/kg PO, SQ once

Drug	Indication	Ref.	Dosage
Prazosin (Minipress)	Vasodilator: heart failure	47	Dog: 1 mg/15 kg PO TID
	Systemic hypertension	50	Dog: 1 mg/10–15 kg PO BID-TID
	Decrease urethral resistance		Dog: 1 mg/15 kg PO TID Cat: 0.5 mg PO TID or 0.03 mg/kg IV
Prednisolone, prednisone (Deltasone)	Allergic bronchitis and rhinitis, asthma, heartworm disease	12, 14, 17	0.5–2 mg/kg IM, PO BID
	Chronic bronchitis, tracheitis	15–17	Dog: 0.1–0.5 mg/kg PO BID
	Lymphosarcoma, myeloproliferative disorders, eosinophilic leukemia, in a protocol	15, 64, 65, 67, 70	a) 1 mg/kg PO SID × 4 wk, then QOD b) 30–40 mg/m² PO SID × 4 wk, then QOD
	Pulmonary eosinophilic infiltrates	18	0.5–1 mg/kg/day PO
	Acquired tremors	23	Dog: 1–2 mg/kg PO BID
	Cerebral edema from brain or spinal tumors	23, 24	Dog: 0.5–1 mg/kg PO SID-QOD
	Idiopathic, eosinophilic meningitis, granulomatous meningoencephalitis	23	Dog: 1–2 mg/kg IM, PO BID, then taper
	Brain trauma	23	0.5–1 mg/kg PO BID × several days
	Meningitis-arteritis	24	Dog: 4 mg/kg/day PO × 7–14 days, then taper to 0.5 mg/kg PO QOD × 6 mo
	Intervertebral disk disease, spondylopathy, cauda equina syndrome	24	Dog: 0.5 mg/kg PO SID
	Acquired myasthenia gravis	25	Dog: 0.25 mg/kg PO SID initially; slowly increase to 2 mg/kg/day PO until remission, then taper to QOD
	Relapsing neuropathy	25	Cat: 2 mg/kg PO BID
	Eosinophilic ulcers, lymphoplasmacytic gingivitis	27, 85	Dog: 1–2.2 mg/kg PO SID × 7 days, then taper dose to QOD Cat: 1–2 mg/kg PO BID
	Plasmacytic/lymphocytic gastritis, enteritis	30, 32	Dog: 1–2 mg/kg PO BID, taper dose weekly
	Eosinophilic gastritis, enteritis, colitis	32, 33	Cat: 2–4 mg/kg/day PO, then taper
	Lymphocytic cholangitis, chronic active hepatitis, copper hepatopathy	34	1–3 mg/kg PO SID, taper to QOD 1 mg/kg PO BID, then taper
	Hypercalcemia	42, 71, 123	a) 2–3 mg/kg PO, SQ SID-BID b) 40 mg/m² PO BID
	Hypoadrenocorticism	44	0.2–0.4 mg/kg PO SID-QOD
	Hypoglycemia	45	0.25–2 mg/kg PO BID
	Urethritis, persistent hematuria	49, 51	1.1 mg/kg PO BID × 14 days, then taper
	Immune hemolytic anemia	63	1–2 mg/kg/day PO BID
	Mast cell tumors, mastocytosis	64, 68, 70, 71	Dog: 30–40 mg/m² PO SID × 4 wk, then QOD, or 1–2 mg/kg PO SID-BID Cat: 40 mg/m² PO SID × 1 wk, then 20 mg/m² PO QOD
	Immune thrombocytopenia	66	2–3 mg/kg/day PO, IM dd BID, taper to 0.5–1 mg/kg PO q 2–3 days
	Angioneurotic edema, urticaria	74	2 mg/kg PO, IM BID
	Immune skin diseases, SLE	74, 89	1.1–2.2 mg/kg PO BID until remission, then taper

Table continued on following page

Drug (Brand Name or Abbreviation)	Purpose or Use	Chapters Where Cited	Dosage
Prednisolone, prednisone (Deltasone) (Continued)	Multiple myeloma, macroglobulinemia	75	0.5 mg/kg PO SID, in a protocol
	SLE or rheumatoid arthritis	78	1–2 mg/kg PO SID-BID, taper to ≦1 mg/kg PO QOD
	Panosteitis, hypertrophic osteopathy	79	Dog: 0.25–0.5 mg/kg PO SID
	Immune polymyositis, masticatory myositis	80	1–2 mg/kg PO, IM SID-BID × 3–4 wk, then taper
	Canine atopy, contact allergy, flea allergy, acanthosis nigricans	82, 84, 89	Dog: 0.5 mg/kg PO BID × 5–10 days, then taper
	Sterile pyogranulomas	85	Dog: 2–4 mg/kg/day PO
	Juvenile cellulitis	85	Dog: 2.2 mg/kg PO SID
	Food allergy, parasite hypersensitivity	89	0.5 mg/kg PO SID-BID, taper weekly
	Blepharitis, episcleritis, uveitis, chorio-retinitis	93, 96, 97, 99, 100	0.5–2 mg/kg PO BID
	Feline infectious peritonitis	110	Cat: 4 mg/kg PO SID, with cyclophosphamide
Prednisolone acetate 1% (Econopred)	Anterior uveitis	97, 99	Apply 1 drop to affected eye 2–12 × daily
Prednisolone sodium succinate (Solu-Delta-Cortef)	Shock, CPR	8, 31, 131	11–30 mg/kg IV
	Allergic bronchitis, asthma	17	0.5–1 mg/kg IV, IM
	Brain trauma	23	10–30 mg/kg IV
	Hypoglycemia	45	1–2 mg/kg IV
Primaquine PO₄ (Primaquine) (not available in the United States)	Babesiosis	114	Cat: 0.5 mg/kg PO, IM, SQ once
Procainamide (Procainamide, Procan SR)	Ventricular arrhythmias	7, 8, 10, 31	Dog: a) 10–20 mg/kg IM, PO TID-QID b) 6–24 mg/kg IV over 5 min c) 500–1000 mg in 500 ml 5% D/W, slow IV infusion at 25–50 μg/kg/min or to effect Cat: a) 3–8 mg/kg PO TID-QID b) 1–2 mg/kg IV bolus c) 10–20 μg/kg/min IV in 5% D/W
Prochlorperazine (Compazine)	Antiemetic	110	Dog: 0.1 mg/kg IM TID-QID
Prochlorperazine/isopropamide	See Isopropamide/prochlorperazine		
Promethazine (Phenergan)	Antihistamine, urticaria	74	0.2–0.4 mg/kg PO TID-QID
Propantheline (Pro-Banthine)	Sinus bradycardia	7	0.5–1 mg/kg PO TID or 3.75–7.5 mg PO BID-TID
	Irritable colon syndrome	33	Dog: 0.25 mg/kg PO BID
	Decrease bladder contractility	50	Dog: 7.5–15 mg PO SID-TID Cat: 5–7.5 mg PO SID-TID

Drug	Indication	References	Dosage
Propofol (Rapinovet, Diprivan)	Status epilepticus Anesthesia	22	Dog: 4–8 mg/kg IV to effect or 8–12 µg/kg/h IV Cat: Induction: 7 mg/kg IV Maintenance: 0.51 mg/kg/min IV Dog: Induction: 2.5–3 mg/kg IV, with premedication
Propranolol (Inderal)	Ventricular arrhythmias	7, 9	Dog: 0.02–0.06 mg/kg IV over 5–10 min or 0.2–1 mg/kg PO TID; max = 1 mg/kg/day PO
	Tachyarrhythmias from endocrinopathies, certain toxicoses	7, 41, 44, 129	Dog: 0.15–0.5 mg/kg PO TID or 0.03–0.1 mg/kg IV Cat: 2.5–5 mg PO BID-TID
	Acquired tremors	23	Dog: 1 mg/kg PO TID
	Hypertrophic cardiomyopathy, valvular insufficiency	41	Dog: 0.3–1 mg/kg PO TID; max = 120 mg/day Cat: ≤4.5 kg: 2.5 mg PO BID-TID ≥5 kg: 5 mg PO BID-TID
	Hypertension	44, 47	Dog: 2.5–80 mg PO BID-TID Cat: 2.5–10 mg PO BID-TID
	Certain behavioral disorders	116	Dog: 5–10 mg PO BID-TID
Prostaglandin $F_{2\alpha}$ (Lutalyse)	Pyometritis, open	56, 60	Dog: 0.1–0.25 mg/kg SQ SID-BID × 5–7 days Cat: 0.1 mg/kg SQ SID × 5 days
	Abortifacient	60	Dog: 0.1–0.25 mg/kg SQ BID × 4 days
Pseudoephedrine (Actifed, Sudafed)	Rhinitis	14	Dog: 15–50 mg PO BID-TID; max = 4 mg/kg Cat: 2–4 mg/kg PO BID-TID
Psyllium (Metamucil, Alarmucil)	Bulk laxative		Dog: 2–4 tsp PO PRN in food Cat: 1–2 tsp PO SID-BID in food
Pyrantel pamoate (Nemex, Strongid-T)	Roundworms, hookworms	32	5–10 mg/kg (1 ml/10 kg) PO; repeat in 3 wk
Pyridostigmine bromide (Mestinon)	Myasthenia gravis	25	Dog: 0.2–2 mg/kg PO BID-TID
Pyridoxine HCl	Crimidine toxicosis	123	Dog: 20 mg/kg IV
Pyrimethamine (Daraprim)	Toxoplasmosis	25, 80, 114	0.25–1 mg/kg PO BID × 2 wk, with sulfonamides
Quinacrine (Atabrine)	Giardia	114	9–11 mg/kg PO SID × 6–12 days
Quinidine Q. gluconate (Quinaglute) Q. polygalacturonate (Cardioquin) Q. sulfate (Quinidex)	Ventricular arrhythmias	7	6–20 mg/kg IM, PO TID-QID

Table continued on following page

Drug (Brand Name or Abbreviation)	Purpose or Use	Chapters Where Cited	Dosage
Ranitidine HCl (Zantac)	Esophagitis, gastric reflux Chronic gastritis, GI tract ulceration, EPI Hypergastrinemia from chronic renal failure	29 30–32, 35, 71, 128 47	Dog: 2 mg/kg PO BID-TID Dog: 0.5–2 mg/kg IV, SQ BID-TID Cat: 0.5 mg/kg IV BID Dog: 1–2 mg/kg PO BID or 0.5 mg/kg IV, SQ BID
Rifampin (Rifamate, Rifadin)	Tuberculosis	18	10–20 mg/kg PO BID-TID
Rutin	Lymphedema	19, 68	Dog: 3 g/day PO or 50 mg/kg PO TID
Selegiline (Eldepryl, Anipryl)	Hyperadrenocorticism Cognitive disorders	44 116	Dog: 1–2 mg/kg PO SID Dog: 1 mg/kg PO SID
Sodium bicarbonate	CPR Hyperkalemia Renal failure Urine alkalization Certain toxicoses	8 47 47 49 122–129	0.5–1 mEq/kg IV q 10 min 0.5–2 mEq/kg IV over 20–30 min 15 mg/kg PO TID 10–90 gr/day PO 50 mg/kg PO BID-TID
Sodium chloride (salt tablets)	Hypoadrenocorticism	44	1–5 g/day PO
Sodium chloride 5% o.o. (Muro 128)	Corneal edema, nonhealing erosions	96	Apply ⅛ in. topically 2–6 times daily
Sodium chloride, 3–7% soln	See Hypertonic saline		
Sodium iodide, 20% soln	Sporotrichosis	84	Cat: 0.5 ml/5 kg/day PO
Sodium phosphate (K-Phos)	Hypercalcemia		Dilute 1–3 g with water (1:1); give 10–20 ml PO SID-TID until stools are soft
Sodium stibogluconate; antimony (Pentostam)	Leishmaniasis	114	Dog: 30–50 mg/kg IV, SQ SID × 3–4 wk
Sodium sulfate (GoLYTELY)	Cathartic	122	1 g/kg PO
Sodium thiopental (Pentothal)	Anesthesia		3–15 mg/kg IV to effect
Sorbitol 70% (Actidose with Sorbitol)	Cathartic	122	3 ml/kg PO
Spironolactone (Aldactone)	Diuretic: heart failure, hypertension Primary hyperaldosteronism, hepatic insufficiency	9, 47 34	Dog: 1–2 mg/kg PO SID-BID Dog: 1–2 mg/kg PO BID Cat: 12.5 mg PO SID
Spironolactone/hydrochlorothiazide (Aldactazide)	Diuretic, antihypertensive agent		2 mg/kg PO SID-BID

Drug	Indication	Reference	Dosage
Stanozolol (Winstrol)	Anabolic agent	71	Dog: 1–4 mg PO BID Cat: 1–2 mg PO BID
Streptomycin (Streptomycin)	Leptospirosis, endocarditis, tuberculosis *Yersinia pestis*	18, 47 111	Dog: 10 mg/kg IM BID-QID Cat: 10 mg/kg IM QID
Succimer (Chemet)	Lead and arsenic poisoning	127	Dog: 10 mg/kg PO TID × 10 days
Succinylcholine (Anectine)	Paralytic: controlled anesthesia		Dog: 0.07 mg/kg IV Cat: 0.06 mg/kg IV
Sucralfate (Carafate)	GI tract ulceration	29, 30, 32, 37, 78, 128, 131	Dog: 0.5–1 g/25 kg PO TID-QID or 1 g crushed and mixed with 10 ml water, give 5–10 ml slurry PO TID-QID Cat: 250–500 mg PO BID-TID
Sulfadiazine (Sulfadiazine)	Toxoplasmosis	25	30–50 mg/kg PO BID × 14 days, with pyrimethamine
	Nocardiosis	111	220 mg/kg PO × 1 Rx, then 110 mg/kg PO BID
Sulfadimethoxine (Bactrovet, Albon)	Coccidiosis	114	50 mg/kg PO SID once, then 25 mg/kg PO SID × 5–20 days
Sulfadimethoxine/ormetroprim (Primor)	Bacterial infections Coccidiosis	84 114	Dog: 27 mg/kg/day PO × 14 days 55 mg/kg PO SID × 10–23 days
Sulfasalazine (Azulfidine)	Chronic colitis Cutaneous vasculitis	33 89	Dog: 10–20 mg/kg PO TID; max = 3 g/day Cat: 10 mg/kg PO SID-BID; use with caution Dog: 10 mg/kg PO TID until remission, then taper
Suprofen 1% (Profenal)	Allergic conjunctivitis, anterior uveitis	94, 97	Apply 1 drop to affected eye BID-TID
Tamoxifen (Nolvadex)	Mammary neoplasia	59	Dog: 0.42 mg/kg/day PO
Taurine	Dilatative cardiomyopathy Central retinal degeneration	10, 120 100, 120	Dog: 500 mg PO BID Cat: 250–500 mg PO BID Cat: 250–500 mg PO SID-BID
Terbutaline (Brethine)	Bronchodilator	16, 17, 132	Dog: a) 1.25–2.5 mg PO BID-TID b) 0.03 mg/kg PO TID c) 0.01 mg/kg IM, SQ Cat: 0.625 mg PO BID
Terfenadine (Seldane)	Antihistamine, allergic skin disease	74, 89	Dog: 2.5–5 mg/kg PO BID

Table continued on following page

Drug (Brand Name or Abbreviation)	Purpose or Use	Chapters Where Cited	Dosage
Testosterone cypionate (Depo-Testosterone)	Hormone-responsive incontinence	50	Dog: 200 mg IM monthly
Testosterone, methyl	See Methyltestosterone		
Testosterone propionate (in oil)	Hormone-responsive incontinence	50	Dog: 2 mg/kg SQ, IM 3 times/wk Cat: 5–10 mg IM PRN Cat: 12.5 mg IM, with estrogen
	Feline symmetrical alopecia	83, 88	
Tetanus toxoid	Tetanus treatment	111, 133	Dog: Give 0.2 ml SQ as a test dose, watch for anaphylaxis × 30 min; then give 30,000–100,000 U IM, IV or 1000 U kg/day divided TID × 2–3 days
Tetracycline HCl (Achromycin V, Panmycin)	Acute bronchitis	17	Cat: 10 mg/kg PO TID
	GI bacterial overgrowth, acute colitis, stomatitis	27, 32	Dog: 10–22 mg/kg PO BID-TID
	Brucellosis, chronic leptospirosis, borreliosis	47, 55, 60, 78, 111	Dog: 10–20 mg/kg PO TID × 28 days
	Rickettsial diseases	63, 66, 113	Dog: 20–22 mg/kg PO TID × 14–21 days Cat: 15 mg/kg PO TID × 21 days
	Mycobacterial infections	84	22 mg/kg PO TID
Tetramisole	Oslerus infestation	18	Dog: 2 mg/kg SQ × 2–4 Rx
Theophylline (Quibron, Quadrinal)	Bronchodilator	12, 17, 132	Dog: 1–2 mg/kg IV or 5 mg/kg PO TID-QID Cat: 1–2 mg/kg IV or 4 mg/kg PO TID Theo-Dur: Dog: 10–20 mg/kg PO BID Cat: 25 mg/kg PO SID at night Slo-bid: Dog: 25 mg/kg PO BID
Thiabendazole (Mintezol)	Oslerus infestation	16, 18	Dog: 70 mg/kg PO BID × 2 days, then 35 mg/kg PO BID × 20 days
Thiacetarsamide (Caparsolate)	Heartworm adulticide	12	2.2 mg/kg IV BID × 2 days
Thiamine (vitamin B₁)	Seizures	22	25–50 mg IM
	Thiamine deficiency, malabsorption	32, 120	Cat: 25–50 mg/kg IM, SQ SID until signs abate, then 10 mg/kg PO SID × 21 days
	Ethylene glycol toxicosis	127	10–100 mg/kg PO SID
Thiamylal sodium (Surital, BioTal)	Anesthesia		8–20 mg/kg IV to effect
Thioridazine (Mellaril)	Stereotypic and aggressive behavior		Dog: 1.1 mg/kg PO
L-Thyroxine, T₄ (Soloxine, Synthroid)	Hypothyroidism, feline symmetrical alopecia	40, 41, 83, 88	Dog: 22 µg/kg or 0.5 mg/m² PO BID Cat: 20–30 µg/kg/day PO SID or dd BID

Drug	Indication	Reference	Dosage
Tiletamine/zolazepam (Telazol)	Short-duration anesthesia		Dog: 6–13 mg/kg IM Cat: 9–12 mg/kg IM
Timolol maleate 0.25%, 0.5% (Timoptic)	Nonselective beta-blocker for glaucoma	98	Apply 1 drop to affected eye BID
Tinidazole	Giardiasis	114	Dog: 44 mg/kg PO SID × 3 days
Tissue plasminogen activator, alteplase (Activase)	Anterior chamber fibrinolytic	97	0.1 ml of 250 µg/ml solution intracamerally
Tobramycin (Nebcin)	Resistant *Pseudomonas* infections		Dog: 1 mg/kg SQ, IM, IV TID
Tocainide (Tonocard)	Ventricular arrhythmias	7, 31	Dog: 10–20 mg/kg PO TID
Tocopherol	*See Vitamin A*		
Toltrazuril	Hepatozoonosis, toxoplasmosis	114	5–10 mg/kg SQ, PO SID × 10–14 days
Tretinoin (Retin-A)	Canine and feline acne, nasal hyperkeratosis	88	Apply topically SID
Triamcinolone (Vetalog)	Feline plasmacytic pharyngitis, podo-dermatitis Anti-inflammatory effects	89	Cat: 2–4 mg PO SID-QOD or 0.4–0.8 mg/kg PO SID, then taper Dog: 0.05 mg/kg PO BID-TID
Triamcinolone ophthalmic soln (Kenalog)	Pannus, eosinophilic keratitis, episcleritis	96, 97	Dog: 4–8 mg subconjunctivally Cat: 4 mg subconjunctivally
Trientine (Syprine)	Copper hepatopathy	34	Dog: 10–15 mg/kg PO SID-BID
Trifluridine ophthalmic soln (Viroptic)	Ocular herpesvirus infection	94, 96	Apply topically 3–8 times daily
Triiodothyronine, T3 (Cytobin)	Hypothyroidism, feline symmetrical alopecia	41, 83	Dog: 4–6 µg/kg PO TID Cat: 4.4 µg/kg PO BID-TID
Trimeprazine (Temaril)	Antihistamine, allergic skin disease, urticaria	74, 89	Dog: 0.5–2 mg/kg PO BID
Trimethobenzamide (Tigan)	Antiemetic		Dog: 3 mg/kg IM BID-TID
Trimethoprim/sulfadiazine (Tribrissen)	Routine infections Meningitis Mastitis, prostatitis, urethritis, URI Toxoplasmosis, coccidiosis, nocardiosis Bacterial folliculitis *Pneumocystis carinii* infection	18, 32, 100, 114 24 51, 52, 59, 112 80, 111, 114 84, 85 114	15 mg/kg PO, SQ BID 15–20 mg/kg PO, IM BID 15–30 mg/kg PO BID × 21 days 15–30 mg/kg PO, SQ BID 30 mg/kg PO BID Dog: 15 mg/kg PO BID-TID × 14 days

Table continued on following page

Drug (Brand Name or Abbreviation)	Purpose or Use	Chapters Where Cited	Dosage
Tripelennamine (PBZ)	Antihistamine, urticaria	74	1 mg/kg PO BID
Tylosin (Tylan)	GI bacterial overgrowth, chronic colitis	32, 33	Dog: 10–40 mg/kg PO BID Cat: 5–10 mg/kg PO BID
	Feline URI	112	Cat: 25 mg PO TID
	Cryptosporidiosis	114	11 mg/kg PO BID × 28 days
Ursodeoxycholate (Actigall)	Chronic hepatitis	34	10–15 mg/kg PO SID
Vancomycin (Vancocin)	GI bacterial overgrowth		Dog: 3 mg/kg PO BID-TID
Vecuronium bromide (Norcuron)	Paralytic agent for controlled anesthesia		Dog: 10–20 µg/kg IV Cat: 20–40 µg/kg IV
Verapamil HCl (Calan, Isoptin)	Supraventricular arrhythmias	7	Dog: 0.05–0.15 mg/kg IV bolus over 5 min; repeat q 10–30 min to max dose of 0.2 mg/kg
Vidarabine o.o. (Vira-A)	Ocular herpesvirus infection	94, 96	Apply ⅛ in. topically 3–6 times daily
Vinblastine (Velban)	Mast cell tumor, lymphosarcoma	70	1–2 mg/m² IV once weekly, in a protocol
Vincristine (Oncovin)	Transmissible venereal tumor	58, 70	Dog: 0.025 mg/kg or 0.5 mg/m² IV once weekly × 4–6 wk
	Lymphosarcoma, mastocythemia	64, 67, 68, 70	0.5–0.75 mg/m² IV once weekly, in a protocol
	Immune thrombocytopenia	66	Dog: 0.02 mg/kg IV or 0.25–0.3 mg/m² IV
Vitamin A (Aquasol A)	Dietary supplement	32, 35	100–500 IU/kg PO, IM SID × 10–30 days
	Vitamin A–responsive dermatosis	90	Dog: 10,000 IU PO SID indefinitely
Vitamin B₁	See Thiamine		
Vitamin B₁₂ (Cyanocobalamin)	Dietary supplement	32, 63	Dog: 100–200 µg/day PO, SQ Cat: 50–100 µg/day PO, SQ
	Inherited vitamin B₁₂ malabsorption	32, 35, 64	Dog: 0.25–1 mg SQ, IM weekly for 1 mo, then q 3 mo
Vitamin C	See Ascorbic acid		
Vitamin D₂, ergocalciferol (Calciferol)	Hypocalcemia	42	4000–6000 U/kg/day PO initially; 1000–2000 U/kg/day PO maintenance

Drug	Indication	Ref	Dosage
Vitamin E (E-Gems, Pure-E)	Scotty cramps	23	Dog: 125 IU/kg/day PO
	Degenerative myelopathy	24	Dog: 2000 IU/day PO
	Vitamin E–deficient myositis, dermatomyositis	80, 82, 86	Dog: 100–200 IU PO SID-BID
	Acanthosis nigricans	82	Dog: 200 IU PO BID indefinitely
	Discoid lupus, panniculitis	85, 89	Dog: 200–800 IU PO, topically BID
	Steatitis	120	Cat: 10–20 IU/kg PO BID
Vitamin K₁ (AquaMEPHYTON, Mephyton)	Cirrhosis	35, 66, 120, 123	1–2 mg/kg SQ BID or 0.5–1 mg/kg PO TID
	Warfarin toxicosis, vitamin K deficiency		Dog: 0.5–1.5 mg/kg SQ, PO BID-TID × 7–14 days, then 1 mg/kg/day PO × 4–6 wk Cat: a) 5 mg PO SID or 10 mg PO twice weekly b) 5–20 mg SQ BID
Warfarin (Coumadin)	Prevent thromboembolism	10, 18	Dog: 0.1 mg/kg PO SID Cat: 0.1–0.2 mg/kg PO SID Maintain prothrombin time 2–2.5 times normal
Xylazine (Rompun)	Sedation, muscle relaxant for certain toxicoses	124	1.1 mg/kg IM, IV
	Emetic	122	Cat: 1.1 mg/kg IM
Yohimbine (Yobine)	Narcolepsy	22	Dog: 50–100 μg/kg SQ BID-TID
	Reverse effects of xylazine and certain toxicoses	122, 124	0.1–0.2 mg/kg IV
Zinc acetate	Copper hepatotoxicosis, chronic hepatitis	34	Dog: 50–200 mg PO SID
Zinc methionine (Virbac)	Zinc deficiency	90, 120	Dog: 1.7 mg/kg PO SID
Zinc sulfate (Zinc-220, Vi-Zac)	Zinc deficiency	90, 120	Dog: 10 mg/kg PO SID; crushed and mixed with food

Rx = treatment(s); max = maximum; dd = divided; PRN = as needed; soln = solution; D/W = dextrose in water; tab = tablet; o.o. = ophthalmic ointment. ADH = antidiuretic hormone; AV = atrioventricular; CNS = central nervous system; CPR = cardiopulmonary resuscitation; DIC = disseminated intravascular coagulation; DJD = degenerative joint disease; EPI = exocrine pancreatic insufficiency; FeLV = feline leukemia virus; FIV = feline immunodeficiency virus; FSH = follicle-stimulating hormone; FUS = feline urologic syndrome; GI = gastrointestinal; KCS = keratoconjunctivitis sicca; NSAID = nonsteroidal anti-inflammatory drug; SA = sinoatrial; SLE = systemic lupus erythematosus; URI = upper respiratory infection.

Index

Note: Page numbers in *italics* refer to illustrations. Page numbers followed by t indicate tables.

K

Kanamycin (Kantrim), dosage of, 1357t
  for mycobacterial infection, of lung, 178
Kaofeed II feeding tube, 18t
Kaolin, in poisoning management, 1249
  with pectin (Kaopectate), dosage of, 1358t
    for food-borne toxins, 1267
    in poisoning management, 1249
Karo syrup, for hypoglycemia, insulin-induced, in diabetes mellitus, 467
Kaswan-Martin technique, for third eyelid gland prolapse, 987t, 988
Keflex (cephalexin). See *Cephalexin.*
Keflin. See *Cephalothin.*
Kefzol. See *Cefazolin.*
Kenalog. See *Triamcinolone.*
Kennel cough, 1158–1160
  and laryngitis, 149–150
Kepone, toxicity of, 1258
Kerat-. See also *Cornea.*
Keratectomy, for dermoid, 991
Keratinization, disorders of, and otitis externa, 1089
  in hyperkeratosis, 870, 934t
    nasal, tretinoin for, 1373t
    of footpad, congenital, 873t
  in protein deficiency, 955–956
  in seborrhea, 928–932, 929t, 930t, 933t, 934t
  in vitamin A–responsive dermatosis, 958
  pinnal, 1094t
Keratitis, and corneal calcium infiltration, 1009
  eosinophilic, 1016–1017
    drugs for, 1359t, 1373t
  in distemper, 1128
  pigmentary, 1015
  tear film lipid abnormalities and, 1002
  ulcerative, 1011–1013, 1013t
  with eyelid agenesis, 973, 974
Keratoacanthoma, 963t
Keratoconjunctivitis, in distemper, 1128
  in ectropion, 976
  in symblepharon, 991
  in third eyelid gland prolapse, 986–988
Keratoconjunctivitis sicca, 1000–1002
  mucin deficiency in, 1003
  sulfonamides and, in colitis management, 379
Keratoplasty, for persistent pupillary membranes, 1020
Kerion, fungal infection and, 894
  vs. granulomatous dermatitis, 906t
Ketamine, dosage of, 1358t
  in anesthesia, in gastric dilatation, with volvulus, 348
  in sedation, for angiography, 35
    for intubation, in bronchial asthma, 171
    for nasal feeding tube placement, 25
    for pneumocolonography, 43
    for thoracentesis, 19
    for transtracheal aspiration, 22
    for upper gastrointestinal tract imaging, 41
    of blood donors, 742
  toxicity of, 1290, 1291
    ocular signs of, 1062t
Ketoacidosis, diabetic, 467–470, 469t
Ketoconazole, dosage of, 1358t
  for blastomycosis, 1116
  for candidiasis, of skin, 897
  for coccidioidomycosis, 1121
  for fungal infection, in blepharitis, 981
    in otitis externa, 1092
    in rhinitis, 142–143
    of skin, 895–896

Ketoconazole *(Continued)*
  of small intestine, 359
    subcutaneous, 897t
    with seborrhea, 931, 934t
  for hyperadrenocorticism, pituitary-dependent, 477, 478
  for leishmaniasis, 1179
  for *Malassezia* infection, of skin, 899
  for oral inflammation, 302
  for prototothecosis, 1185
  with trimethoprim, toxicity of, to liver, 397t
Ketones, methylethyl, toxicity of, 1275
Ketorolac, for conjunctivitis, 1358t
Kidney(s), amyloidosis of, 507–508
  calculi in, 519–520
  contrast imaging of, 44–45
  disorders of, 497–523
    and coagulation factor deficiencies, 713, 714
    and corneal calcium deposition, 1009
    and drug excretion, in hypothyroidism, 450
    and gastric ulcers, 339
    and hypercholesterolemia, 482
    and polycythemia, 671
    as contraindication to intravenous urography, 44
    burns and, 1305–1306, 1308–1309
    familial, 498t
    heartworm and, 124
    immune-mediated, 792t
    perirenal cysts and, 497
    potassium deficiency in, 1231
    ureteral obstruction and, 528, 529
    ureterocele and, 527
    with ectopic ureters, 525, 526
    with vesicoureteral reflux, 528
  erythropoietin synthesis in, abnormalities of, 484–485
  failure of, acute, 508–512, 510t–512t
    in glomerulonephritis, 506
    mannitol for, 1359t
    toxicity and, 503, 504
    and erythropoietin abnormalities, 484, 485
    and platelet disorders, 707
    bicarbonate for, 1370t
    chronic, 512–516
      anemia with, 668
      hypergastrinemia in, ranitidine for, 1370t
      potassium citrate for, 1366t
      vs. acute, 510, 510t
    contrast media and, 35
    hemodialysis for, 518–519
    in amyloidosis, 507
    in ibuprofen toxicity, 1280, 1281
    peritoneal dialysis for, 516–518
    transplantation for, 519
  function of, after cardiopulmonary resuscitation, 90
    assessment of, blood urea nitrogen in, 493
      glomerular filtration rate in, 493–494
      laboratory tests in, 13t
      proteinuria in, 494
      serum creatinine in, 493
      urine concentration in, 494–496, *495*
  hormones produced by, 437
  in diabetes insipidus, 443–445
  in diabetic ketoacidosis, 468
  in heat prostration, 1311, 1313
  in hyperparathyroidism, 459–461
  in hyperthyroidism, 451
  in hyperviscosity syndrome, paraneoplastic, 769

Kidney(s) *(Continued)*
  in hypoadrenocorticism, 471, 472
  in leptospirosis, 1149–1150
  in multiple myeloma, 801
  in systemic lupus erythematosus, 793
  inflammation of, in glomerulonephritis, 504–507, 505t
    drugs for, 1339t, 1341t, 1347t
    heartworm and, 124
    in systemic lupus erythematosus, 793
  in pyelonephritis, 500–502
  leptospirosis of, 498–500
  neoplasia of, 520–522
  palpation of, in physical examination, 7
  parasitosis of, 502–503
  toxicity to, 503–504
    chemotherapy and, 503, 751t, 754
    ethylene glycol and, 1274, 1275
    herbicides and, 1263, 1265
    plants and, 1285–1286
  transplantation of, 519
  trauma to, 522–523
Killer cells, 776
Kirschner wires, in fracture fixation, 842
Klebsiella infection, in pyelonephritis, 500, 501
  in pyothorax, 200t
Kleenup herbicide, toxicity of, 1264t, 1265
Klonopin, for seizures, 1346t
Korlan, toxicity of, 1257
K-Phos, for hypercalcemia, 1370t

L

L-form bacterial disease, 1156t
Labor, dystocia in, canine, 637–639
  feline, 649–650
Labrador retriever, axonopathy in, 257t
Labyrinthitis, 1100–1103, 1102t
Lacrimal system, dacryops of, 999–1000
  disorders of, signs of, 972t
  imperforate punctum in, 998–999
  in keratoconjunctivitis sicca, 1000–1002
  inflammation of, 1004–1005
  neoplasia of, 1005–1006
Lactate, normal blood level of, 1323t
Lactate dehydrogenase, normal blood level of, 1323t
Lactation, arrest of, 617
  excessive, 617
  in galactostasis, 616–617
  in mastitis, 615–616
  in neonatal nutrition, 1219–1220
  in pseudocyesis, 630–631
  nutrition in, 1223–1224
    feeding trials in, 1217
Lactic acid, normal laboratory value for, 1326t
Lactulose, for hepatic encephalopathy, 246–247, 385, 1358t
  for megacolon, 372, 1358t
Lagophthalmos, 979–980
  in keratitis, pigmentary, 1015
    ulcerative, 1011
Lameness, biceps brachii injury and, 858t
  blastomycosis and, 1114
  bone cysts and, 836, 837
  coccidioidomycosis and, 1119, 1120
  collateral ligament rupture and, 827
  cruciate ligament rupture and, 825, 826
  evaluation of, 811–812
  examination for, 5, 8
  fractures and, 842
  hip dysplasia and, 816
  histoplasmosis and, 1117
  hypertrophic osteopathy and, 837